D1034092

Pediatric Gastrointestinal and Liver Disease

Commissioning Editor: **Karen Bowler**
Project Development Manager: **Joanne Scott**
Editorial Assistant: **Amy Head**
Project Manager: **Alan Nicholson**
Designer: **Andy Chapman**
Marketing Manager(s) (UK/USA): **Amy Hey / Kathleen Neely**

Pediatric Gastrointestinal and Liver Disease

Pathophysiology / Diagnosis / Management

THIRD EDITION

Editors

Robert Wyllie MD
Chairman
Department of Pediatric Gastroenterology, Hepatology and Nutrition
The Children's Hospital
Cleveland Clinic
Cleveland OH
USA

Jeffrey S Hyams MD
Head, Division of Digestive Diseases and Nutrition
Connecticut Children's Medical Center, Hartford CT
and Professor, Department of Pediatrics
University of Connecticut School of Medicine
Farmington CT
USA

Associate Editor

Marsha Kay MD
Staff Physician
Department of Pediatric Gastroenterology
The Cleveland Clinic Foundation
Cleveland OH
USA

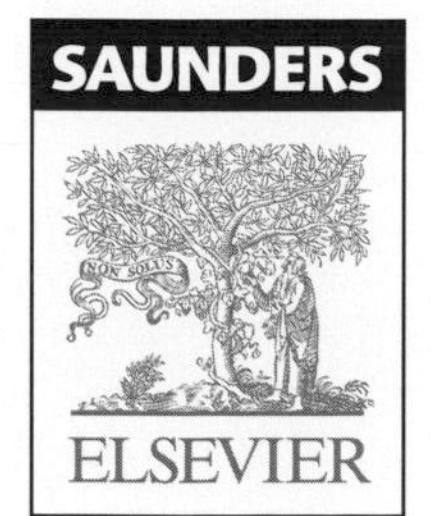

SAUNDERS
ELSEVIER
Saunders is an affiliate of Elsevier Inc.

First edition 1993
Second edition 1999
Third edition 2006

ISBN 10: 0-7216-3924-0
ISBN 13: 978-0-7216-3924-6

British Library Cataloguing in Publication Data
A catalogue record for this book is available from the British Library

Library of Congress Cataloging in Publication Data
A catalog record for this book is available from the Library of Congress

Notice
Medical knowledge is constantly changing. Standard safety precautions must be followed, but as new research and clinical experience broaden our knowledge, changes in treatment and drug therapy may become necessary or appropriate. Readers are advised to check the most current product information provided by the manufacturer of each drug to be administered to verify the recommended dose, the method and duration of administration, and contraindications. It is the responsibility of the practitioner, relying on experience and knowledge of the patient, to determine dosages and the best treatment for each individual patient. Neither the Publisher nor the author assume any liability for any injury and/or damage to persons or property arising from this publication.

The Publisher

Printed in the Netherlands

Last digit is the print number: 9 8 7 6 5 4 3 2 1

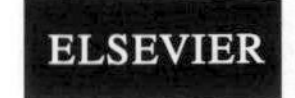

Contents

List of Contributors

H Hesham A-Kader MD MSc
Associate Professor of Pediatrics
Chief, Division of Gastroenterology, Hepatology and Nutrition
Department of Pediatrics
University of Arizona
Tucson AZ
USA

Frederick Alexander MD FACS FAAP
Chairman
Department of Pediatric Surgery
The Cleveland Clinic Foundation
Cleveland OH
USA

Estella M Alonso MD
Professor of Pediatrics
Medical Director
Liver Transplant Program
Children's Memorial Hospital
Chicago IL
USA

Dean L Antonson MD
Associate Professor of Pediatrics and Internal Medicine
Section of Pediatric Gastroenterology
Nebraska Medical Center
Omaha NE
USA

Marjorie J Arca MD
Assistant Professor of Surgery
Division of Pediatric Surgery
Children's Hospital of Wisconsin
Medical College of Wisconsin
Milwaukee WI
USA

Sundeep Arora MBBS MD
Fellow, Pediatric Gastroenterology, Hepatology and Nutrition
Rainbow Babies and Children's Hospital
Case Western Reserve University
Cleveland OH
USA

Arthur B Atlas MD
Director, Respiratory Center for Children
Atlantic Health System
Assistant Professor of Pediatrics
University of Medicine and Dentistry of New Jersey
Morristown NJ
USA

Salvatore Auricchio MD
Professor of Pediatrics
Department of Pediatrics
Faculty of Medicine and Surgery
Universita Degli Studi Di Napoli Federico II
Naples
ITALY

Susan S Baker MD PhD
Professor of Pediatrics
Co-Director, Digestive Diseases and Nutrition Center
Children's Hospital
SUNY
Buffalo NY
USA

Robert D Baker MD PhD
Professor of Pediatrics
University at Buffalo, SUNY
Co-Chief, Digestive Disease and Nutrition Center
Womens and Children's Hospital of Buffalo
Buffalo NY
USA

Dorsey M Bass MD
Associate Professor
Department of Pediatrics
Stanford University School of Medicine
Stanford CA
USA

Phyllis R Bishop MD
Professor of Pediatrics
Division of Pediatric Gastroenterology
University of Mississippi Medical Center
Jackson MS
USA

Samra S Blanchard MD
Assistant Professor
Case Western Reserve University
Rainbow Babies and Children's Hospital
Cleveland OH
USA

Athos Bousvaros MD MPH
Associate Director Inflammatory Bowel Disease Program
Division of Gastroenterology and Nutrition
Boston Children's Hospital
Boston MA
USA

John T Boyle MD
Chief, Division of Pediatric Gastroenterology and Nutrition
Children's Hospital of Alabama
Professor of Pediatrics
University of Alabama, Birmingham School of Medicine
Birmingham AL
USA

Steven W Bruch MD FACS
Clinical Associate Professor of Surgery
University of Michigan Medical School
CS Mott Children's Hospital
Ann Arbor MI
USA

Linda Casey MD FRCPC MSc
Assistant Professor of Pediatrics
Stollery Children's Hospital
Edmonton AB
CANADA

Michael G Caty MD FACS FAAP
Chief of Surgery, Associate Professor
Division of Pediatric Surgery
Women and Children's Hospital of Buffalo
Buffalo NY
USA

Dennis L Christie MD
Professor of Pediatrics, University of Washington
Head, Division of Pediatric Gastroenterology
Children's Regional Hospital and Medical Center
Seattle WA
USA

Mitchell B Cohen MD
Professor and Director
Pediatric Gastroenterology, Hepatology and Nutrition
Cincinnati Children's Hospital Medical Center
Cincinnati OH
USA

Stanley A Cohen MD FAAP
Pediatric Gastroenterologist
Children's Center for Digestive Health Care
Children's Healthcare of Atlanta
and Adjunct Clinical Professor of Pediatrics
Emory University School of Medicine
Atlanta GA
USA

Frances L Connor MBBS FRACP
Paediatric Gastroenterologist
Queensland Paediatric Gastroenterology, Hepatology and Nutrition Service
Royal Children's Hospital
Brisbane
Queensland
AUSTRALIA

Claudia A Conkin MS RD LD
Director, Department of Food and Nutrition Services
Texas Children's Hospital
Houston TX
USA

Donald R Cooney MD
Professor of Surgery and Pediatrics
Texas A&M University College of Medicine
Texas A&M Health Science Center
Division of Pediatric Surgery
Scott & White Memorial Hospital
Temple TX
USA

Arnold G Coran MD
Professor of Surgery and Head, Pediatric Surgery
University of Michigan Medical School
Surgeon-in-Chief, CS Mott Children's Hospital
University of Michigan Medical School
Ann Arbor MI
USA

Steven J Czinn MD
Professor and Chairman
Department of Pediatrics
University of Maryland School of Medicine
Chief of Pediatrics
University of Maryland Medical Center
Baltimore MD
USA

David Devadason MB BS MRCP(UK)
Specialist Registrar
Paediatric Gastroenterology
Bristol Children's Hospital
Bristol
UK

Carlo Di Lorenzo MD
Professor of Clinical Pediatrics
The Ohio State University and
Chief, Division of Pediatric Gastroenterology
Children's Hospital of Columbus
Columbus OH
USA

Ranjan Dohil MBBch MRCP(UK) MRCPCH
DCH(UK)
Associate Professor of Pediatrics
University of California
and Children's Hospital and Health Center
San Diego CA
USA

Maryanne L Dokler MD
Pediatric Surgeon
Nemours Children's Clinic
Jackonsville FL
USA

Lisa Feinberg MD
Clinical Associate
Department of Pediatric Gastroenterology
Cleveland Clinic Foundation
Cleveland OH
USA

Laura S Finn MD
Associate Professor
Department of Pathology
University of Washington
Children's Hospital and Regional Medical Center
Seattle WA
USA

Joseph F Fitzgerald MD FAAP MACG
Professor of Pediatrics
Division of Pediatric Gastroenterology, Hepatology and Nutrition
Indiana University School of Medicine
Indianapolis IN
USA

Dean R Focht III MD MAJ MC
Pediatric Gastroenterology
Department of Pediatrics
Tripler Army Medical Center
Honolulu HI
USA

Jacqueline L Fridge MD
Associate Gastroenterologist
Pediatric Gastroenterology, Hepatology and Nutrition
Children's Hospital and Research Center
Oakland CA
and Adjunct Clinical Assistant Professor
LPCH Stanford University School of Medicine
Palo Alto CA
USA

Reinaldo Garcia-Naveiro MD
Assistant Professor
University Hospitals Health System
Division of Pediatric, Hepatology, Gastroenterology and Nutrition
Cleveland OH
USA

Michael WL Gauderer MD FACS FAAP
Professor of Surgery and Pediatrics
University of South Carolina School of Medicine
Chief, Division of Pediatric Surgery
Children's Hospital Greenville Hospital System
Greenville SC
USA

Donald E George MD
Co-Clinical Associate Professor of Pediatrics
University of Florida
Chief, Division of Gastroenterology and Nutrition
Nemours' Children's Clinic
Jacksonville FL
USA

Fayez K Ghishan MD
Horace W Steele Endowed Chair in Pediatric Research
Professor and Head, Department of Pediatrics
Director, Steele Memorial Children's Research Center
University of Arizona Health Sciences Center
Tucson AZ
USA

Mark A Gilger MD
Professor of Pediatrics
Head, Section of Pediatric Gastroenterology, Hepatology and Nutrition
Baylor College of Medicine
Chief of Service
Department of Gastroenterology, Hepatology and Nutrition
Texas Children's Hospital
Houston TX
USA

Elizabeth Gleghorn MD
Director, Department of Gastroenterology, Hepatology and Nutrition
Children's Hospital and Research Center, Oakland
Oakland CA
USA

Glenn R Gourley MD
Professor of Pediatrics
and Chief, Division of Pediatric Gastroenterology
Oregon Health and Science University
Portland OR
USA

Terry L Gramlich MD
Director of Hepatopathology
AmeriPath Institute of Gastrointestinal Pathology and Digestive Disease
Oakwood Village OH
USA

Richard J Grand MD
Director, Center for Inflammatory Bowel Disease
Professor of Pediatrics
Children's Hospital Boston
Boston MA
USA

Moises B Guelrud MD
Gastroenterologist
Tufts New England Medical Center
Tufts University School of Medicine
Boston MA
USA

Sandeep K Gupta MD
Associate Professor of Clinical Pediatrics
Division of Pediatric Gastroenterology, Hepatology and Nutrition
James Whitcomb Riley Hospital for Children
Indiana University School of Medicine
Indianapolis IN
USA

Nedim Hadžić MD MSc FRCPCH
Consultant and Senior Lecturer in Paediatric Hepatology
Paediatric Liver Services
Institute of Liver Studies
King's College Hospital
London
UK

Eric Hassall MBChB FRCPC
Professor of Pediatrics
Division of Gastroenterology
BC Children's Hospital
University of British Columbia
Vancouver BC
CANADA

James E Heubi MD
Professor of Pediatrics
University of Cincinnati College of Medicine
Division of Pediatric Gastroenterology, Hepatology and Nutrition
Cincinnati Children's Hospital Medical Center
Cincinnati OH
USA

Vera F Hupertz MD
Staff Physician
Department of Pediatric Gastroenterology, Hepatology and Nutrition
and Division of Transplant Surgery
Cleveland Clinic Foundation
Cleveland OH
USA

Jeffrey S Hyams MD
Head, Division of Digestive Diseases and Nutrition
Connecticut Children's Medical Center Hartford
and Professor of Pediatrics
University of Connecticut School of Medicine
Farmington CT
USA

Paul E Hyman MD
Professor of Pediatrics
Chief, Pediatric Gastroenterology
Kansas University Medical Center
Kansas City KS
USA

Maureen M Jonas MD
Associate Professor of Pediatrics
Harvard Medical School
Division of Gastroenterology
Children's Hospital
Boston MA
USA

Adrian Jones MD FRCPC
Pediatric Gastroenterologist
Division of Pediatric Gastroenterology and Nutrition
University of Alberta
Edmonton AB
CANADA

Nicola L Jones MD FRCPC PhD
Staff Gastroenterologist
Division of Gastroenterology, Hepatology
and Nutrition
Hospital for Sick Children
and Associate Professor of Paediatrics
and Physiology
University of Toronto
Toronto ON
CANADA

Binita M Kamath MD
Postdoctoral Fellow
Abramson Research Center
The Children's Hospital of Philadelphia
Philadelphia PA
USA

Barbara Kaplan MD
Staff Pediatric Gastroenterologist
Department of Pediatric Gastroenterology
Cleveland Clinic Foundation
Cleveland OH
USA

Stuart S Kaufman MD
Medical Director, Intestinal Rehabilitation
and Transplantation Program
Georgetown University Transplant Institute and
Children's National Medical Center
Washington DC
USA

Marsha Kay MD
Staff Physician
Department of Pediatric Gastroenterology
The Cleveland Clinic Foundation
Cleveland OH
USA

Deirdre Kelly MD FRCP FRCPI FRCPH
Professor of Paediatric Hepatology
The Liver Unit
Birmingham Children's Hospital
University of Birmingham
Birmingham
UK

Marilyn Kennedy-Jones BHEc RD
Clinical Dietitian
Pediatric Home Nutrition Support
Stollery Children's Hospital
Edmonton
CANADA

Samantha Kim RD CNSD CDE LDN
Clinical Dietician
The Children's Hospital of Philadelphia
Philadelphia PA
USA

Robert M Kliegman MD
Professor and Chair
Department of Pediatrics
Executive Vice President, Childrens Research
Institute
Medical College of Wisconsin
Milwaukee WI
USA

Samuel Kocoshis MD
Professor of Pediatrics
Director, Nutrition and Intestinal Transplantation
Cincinnati Children's Hospital Medical Center
Cincinnati OH
USA

Tzuyung Doug Kou MPH MA
Doctoral Student
Department of Epidemiology and Biostatistcs
Case Western Reserve University
Cleveland OH
USA

ST Lau MD
Fellow in Pediatric Surgery
Department of Pediatric Surgery
Women and Children's Hospital of Buffalo
Buffalo NY
USA

Marc A Levitt MD
Associate Director
Colorectal Center for Children
Cincinnati Children's Hospital
Cincinnati OH
USA

BU K Li MD
Director of Gastroenterology
Division of Gastroenterology, Hepatology
and Nutrition
and Professor of Pediatrics
Feinberg School of Medicine
Northwestern University
Chicago IL
USA

Chris A Liacouras MD
Professor of Pediatric Gastroenterology
Division of Gastroenterology and Nutrition
University of Pennsylvania School of Medicine
and Medical Director, Clinical Trials Office
Division of Gastroenterology and Nutrition
The Children's Hospital of Philadelphia
Philadelphia PA
USA

Danny C Little MD
Texas A&M University College of Medicine
Temple TX
USA

Vera Loening-Baucke MD
Professor of Pediatrics
Department of Pediatrics
University of Iowa Hospitals and Clinics
Iowa City IA
USA

James K Madison PhD
Assistant Professor and Director of Psychology
Department of Psychiatry
Creighton University
Omaha NE
USA

David K Magnuson MD FACS FAAP
Chief, Division of Pediatric Surgery
Rainbow Babies and Children's Hospital
Case Western Reserve University
Cleveland OH
USA

Lori A Mahajan MD
Pediatric Gastroenterologist
Department of Pediatric Gastroenterology
Cleveland Clinic Foundation
Cleveland OH
USA

Jonathan E Markowitz MD MSCE
Assistant Professor of Pediatrics
Division of Gastroenterology and Nutrition
The Children's Hospital of Philadelphia
Philadelphia PA
USA

James F Markowitz MD
Professor of Pediatrics
NYU School of Medicine
Division of Pediatric Gastroenterology
Schneider Children's Hospital
New Hyde Park NY
USA

Maria R Mascarenhas MBBS
Associate Professor of Pediatrics
and Section Chief, Nutrition
School of Medicine, Division of GI and Nutrition
Children's Hospital of Philadelphia
Philadelphia PA
USA

Valerie A McLin MD
Assistant Professor of Pediatrics
Baylor College of Medicine
Texas Children's Liver Center
Houston TX
USA

Adam G Mezoff MD CPE
Professor of Pediatrics
Department of Pediatric Gastroenterology
Children's Medical Center
Wright State University
Dayton OH
USA

Giorgina Mieli-Vergani MD PhD FRCP FRCPCH
Alex Mowat Professor of Paediatric Hepatology
and Director, Paediatric Liver Service
Department of Liver Studies and Transplantation
King's College Hospital
London
UK

Tracie L Miller MD
Professor of Pediatrics
Department of Pediatrics
University of Miami School of Medicine
Miami FL
USA

Robert K Montgomery MD PhD
Instructor
Division of Gastroenterology and Nutrition
Children's Hospital Boston
Boston MA
USA

Kathleen J Motil MD PhD
Associate Professor Pediatrics
Baylor College of Medicine
Houston TX
USA

Simon H Murch BSc PhD FRCP FRCPCH
Professor of Paediatrics and Child Health
Warwick Medical School
University of Warwick
Coventry
UK

Karen F Murray MD
Director, Hepatobiliary Program
Children's Hospital and Regional Medical Center
Seattle WA
USA

Hillel Naon MD
Clinical Assistant Professor of Pediatrics
Keck School of Medicine
University of Southern California
and Pediatric Gastroenterology
Children's Hospital Los Angeles
Los Angeles CA
USA

Aruna Navathe MA RD LD CSP
Nutrition Co-ordinator
Children's Healthcare of Atlanta at
Scottish Rite
Atlanta GA
USA

Vicky Lee Ng MD FRCPC
Assistant Professor of Pediatrics
University of Toronto
Division of Gastroenterology and Nutrition
Hospital for Sick Children
Toronto ON
CANADA

Richard J Noel MD PhD
Assistant Professor of Pediatrics
Pediatric Gastroenterology and Nutrition
Medical College of Wisconsin
Milwaukee WI
USA

Michael J Nowicki MD
Associate Professor of Pediatrics
Division of Pediatric Gastroenterology
and Nutrition
Blair E Batson Children's Hospital,
University of Mississippi Medical Center
Jackson MS
USA

Keith T Oldham MD
Professor and Chief
Division of Pediatrics
Medical College of Wisconsin
Surgeon-in-Chief and Marie Z Uihlein Chair
Children's Hospital of Wisconsin
Milwaukee WI
USA

Bankole Osuntokun MD
Clinical Fellow
Division of Pediatrics, Gastroenterology and Nutrition
Cincinnati Children's Hospital Medical Center
Cincinnati OH
USA

Harpreet Pall MD
Attending in Gastroenterology
Gastroenterology/Nutrition Medicine
Children's Hospital Boston
Boston MA
USA

Alberto Peña MD
Director, Colorectal Center for Children
Division of Surgery
Cincinnati Children's Hospital Medical Center
Cincinnati OH
USA

Robert E Petras MD FCAP FACG
Associate Professor of Pathology
Northeastern Ohio Universities College of Medicine
and National Director, Gastrointestinal Pathology Services
AmeriPath, Inc.
Oakwood Village OH
USA

Marian D Pfefferkorn MD FAAP
Associate Professsor of Clinical Pediatrics
Department of Pediatrics
Indiana University School of Medicine
Indianapolis IN
USA

Sara M Phillips MS RD/LD
Manager Nutrition Support
Instructor of Pediatrics
Department of Gastroenterology, Hepatology and Nutrition
Clinical Care Center
Baylor College of Medicine
Houston TX
USA

Cathleen A Piazza MD PhD
Director, Feeding Disorders Program
Marcus Institute
Atlanta GA
USA

Daniel L Preud'Homme MD CNS
Associate Professor of Pediatrics
Pediatric Gastroenterology
Children's Medical Center
Wright State University
Dayton OH
USA

Kadakkal Radhakrishnan MD MBBS MD(Ped)
DCH MRCP (UK) MRCPCH FAAP
Fellow in Pediatric Gastroenterology
Cleveland Clinic Foundation
Cleveland OH
USA

Elyanne Ratcliffe MD FRCPC
Assistant Professor of Pediatrics
Pediatric Gastroenterology, Hepatology and Nutrition
Morgan Stanley Children's Hospital of New York-Presbyterian
Columbia University Medical Center
New York NY
USA

Douglas G Rogers MD
Department of Pediatric Endocrinology
The Childrens Hospital
Cleveland Clinic
Cleveland OH
USA

Joel R Rosh MD
Director, Pediatric Gastroenterology
Atlantic Health System
Associate Professor of Pediatrics
University of Medicine and Dentistry New Jersey
Medical School
New Jersey NJ
USA

Colin D Rudolph MD PhD
Professor and Chief
Division of Pediatric Gatroenterology and Nutrition
Medical College of Wisconsin
Milwaukee WI
USA

Shehzad A Saeed MD FFAP
Assistant Professor of Pediatrics and
Nutrition Sciences
Division of Gastroenterology and Nutrition
Department of Pediatrics
University of Alabama at Birmingham
and The Children's Hospital of Alabama
Birmingham AL
USA

Bhupinder Sandhu MD MBBS FRCP FRCPCM
Consultant Paediatric Gastroenterologist
and Professor of Paediatric Gastroenterology and Nutrition
Royal Hospital for Children
Bristol
UK

Thomas T Sato MD
Associate Professor of Surgery
Division of Paediatric Surgery
Medical College of Wisconsin
Milwaukee WI
USA

Marshall Z Schwartz MD
Professor of Surgery and Pediatrics
Drexel University School of Medicine
and Thomas Jefferson University
Director, Pediatric Surgery Research Laboratory
St Christopher's Hospital for Children
Philadelphia PA
USA

Lesley Smith MD MBA FRCP(C)
Professor of Clinical Pediatrics
Division of Pediatric Gastroenterology, Hepatology and Nutrition
Morgan-Stanley Children's Hospital of New York–Presbyterian
Columbia University Medical Center
New York NY
USA

Manu R Sood FRCPCH MD
Associate Professor of Pediatrics
Department of Pediatrics
Division of Pediatric Gastroenterology and Nutrition
Medical College of Wisconsin
Milwaukee WI
USA

Maya Srivastava MD PhD
Division of Allergy and Immunology
Cleveland Clinic Foundation
Cleveland OH
USA

Anthony Stallion MD
Associate Professor of Surgery
Case Western Reserve University
Department of Pediatric Surgery
Cleveland Clinic Foundation
Cleveland OH
USA

Rita Steffen MD
Staff Physican, Pediatric Gastroenterology
Department of Pediatric Gastroenterology
The Children's Hospital Cleveland Clinic Foundation
Cleveland OH
USA

Shikha S Sundaram MD MSCI
Assistant Professor of Pediatrics
Gastroenterology and Hepatology
Children's Memorial Hospital
Northwestern University
Chicago IL
USA

Bhanu K Sunku MD
Fellow in Pediatric Gastroenterology
Division of Gastroenterology, Hepatology and Nutrition
Children's Memorial Hospital
Chicago IL
USA

James L Sutphen MD PhD
Department of Pediatrics
Division of Gastroenterology
University of Virginia Medical Center
Charlottesville VA
USA

Francisco A Sylvester MD
Associate Professor of Pediatrics
Department of Pediatrics
Connecticut Children's Hospital
Hartford CT
USA

Jan Taminiau MD PhD
Director, Pediatric Gastroenterology, Hepatology and Nutrition
Academic Medical Center
and Emma Children's Hospital
Amsterdam
THE NETHERLANDS

Jonathan E Teitelbaum MD
Assistant Professor
Drexel University School of Medicine
and Chief, Pediatric Gastroenterology and Nutrition
Monmouth Medical Center
Long Branch NJ
USA

Daniel W Thomas MD
Associate Professor of Pediatrics,
Keck School of Medicine at the University of Southern California
and Head of Liver and Intestinal Transplantation
Children's Hospital Los Angeles
Los Angeles CA
USA

Mike A Thomson MB ChB DCH MRCP FRCPCH FRCP MD
Consultant Paediatric Gastroenterologist
and Director of Paediatric Endoscopy Training Centre
Centre for Paediatric Gastroenterology
Sheffield Children's Hospital
Sheffield
UK

Shaheen J Timmapuri MD
General Surgery Resident
and Research Fellow
Department of Surgery
Thomas Jefferson University
Philadelphia PA
USA

Vasundhara Tolia MD
Professor of Pediatrics
Wayne State University
Detroit MI
USA

William R Treem MD
Professor of Pediatrics
Vice-Chair, Department of Pediatrics for Clinical Development
Director, Division of Pediatric Gastroenterology, Hepatology, and Nutrition
SUNY Downstate Medical Center
Brooklyn NY
USA

Riccardo Troncone MD
Professor of Paediatrics
Department of Pediatrics
and European Laboratory for the Investigation of Food Induced Diseases
University Federico II
Naples
ITALY

Aaron Turkish MD FAAP
Pediatric Gastroenterology, Hepatology and Nutrition
Morgan Stanley Children's Hospital of New York-Presbyterian
Columbia University Medical Center
New York NY
USA

John N Udall Jr MD PhD
Professor and Chairman
Department of Pediatrics
Robert C. Byrd Health Sciences Center
West Virginia University
Charleston WV
USA

Yvan Vandenplas MD PhD
Professor of Pediatrics
Department of Pediatrics
Academic Children's Hospital
Free University Brussels
Brussels
BELGIUM

Gigi Veereman-Wauters MD PhD
Pediatric Gastroenterologist
Department of Pediatric Gastroenterology, Hepatology and Nutrition
Queen Paolo Children's Hospital and University Hospital
Antwerp
BELGIUM

Ghassan Wahbeh MD
Assistant Professor of Pediatric Gastroenterology
Children's Hospital and Regional Medical Center
University of Washington
Seattle WA
USA

Thomas D Walters MBBS FRACP
Research Fellow
Division of Gastroenterology and Nutrition
Hospital for Sick Children
Toronto ON
CANADA

Charles Winans MD
Staff Surgeon
Department of General Surgery
Transplant Centre
Cleveland Clinic Foundation
Cleveland OH
USA

Robert Wyllie MD
Chairman, Department of Pediatric Gastroenterology, Hepatology and Nutrition
The Children's Hospital
Cleveland Clinic
Cleveland OH
USA

Nada Yazigi MD
Assistant Professor of Clinical Pediatrics
Division of Gastroenterology and Nutrition
Cincinnati Children's Hospital Medical Center
Cincinnati OH
USA

Qian Yuan MD PhD
Instructor in Pediatrics
Department of Pediatrics
Harvard Medical School
Division of Pediatric Gastroenterology and Nutrition
Massachusetts General Hospital
Boston MA
USA

Preface

More than a century ago pediatrics emerged as a specialty in response to the recognition that health problems in children differ from those of adults and the response to illness varies with age. The goal of the Third Edition of *Pediatric Gastrointestinal Disease: Pathophysiology, Diagnosis and Management* is to incorporate the rapid changes in medical knowledge into a framework that is useful to those providing care to children.

All chapters have been updated and many written by new authors who bring their own expertise. Readers will note a markedly increased international roster of authors who we hope will bring new perspectives. The book is organized into distinct sections starting with basic aspects of gastrointestinal function, followed by common clinical problems and organ specific diseases. The last section focuses on nutritional issues. The scope of the Third Edition has been expanded and includes a new section on diseases of the liver and bile ducts.

We would like to express our appreciation to the editorial staff at Elsevier for their support and encouragement. Special thanks to Karen Bowler and Joanne Scott who have fielded our many inquires and nudged the book to completion. We also thank Alan Nicholson, Amy Head, Sven Pinczewski, Sue Hodgson and Rolla Couchman for their assistance along the way.

The greatest reward in the editing of the previous editions is from the kind reports of students, residents and staff who found it useful in caring for children with gastrointestinal and liver disease. Producing the book is always a team effort and would not be possible without the dedication of the chapter authors who took time from their busy schedules to contribute to the book. These are the people who by their effort again demonstrate their commitment to the care of children with gastrointestinal disorders.

Robert Wyllie MD
Jeffrey S Hyams MD
2006

Dedicated to

our families

and colleagues

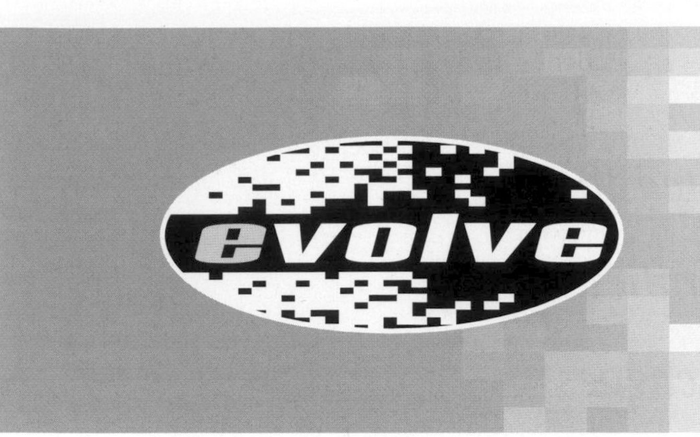

The latest evolution in learning

Evolve provides online access to free learning resources and activities designed specifically for the textbook you are using in your class. The resources will provide you with information that enhances the material covered in the book and much more.

Visit the Web address listed below to start your learning evolution today!

LOGIN: http://evolve.elsevier.com/wyllie/pediatricGI/

Wyllie and Hyams
Pediatric Gastrointestinal and Liver Disease: Pathophysiology/ Diagnosis / Management THIRD EDITION

Evolve Learning Resources

- **500 case-study, self-assessment questions – with answers – along with color clinical images, helps you test your knowledge**

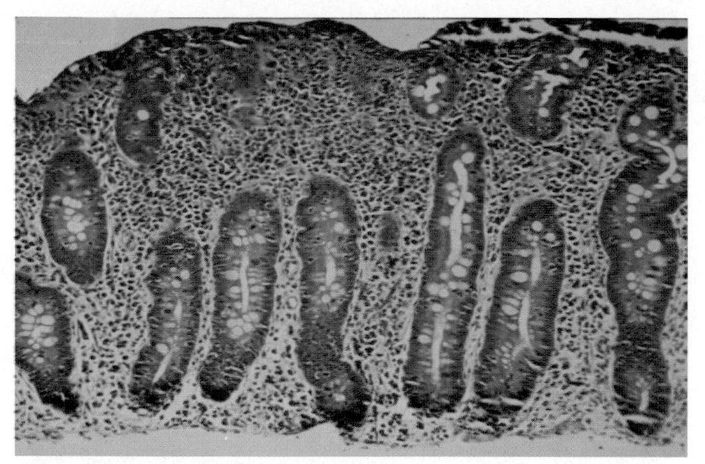

Figure 9.1: Small bowel biopsy from patient with celiac disease demonstrating villous atrophy and increased number of intraepithelial lymphocytes.

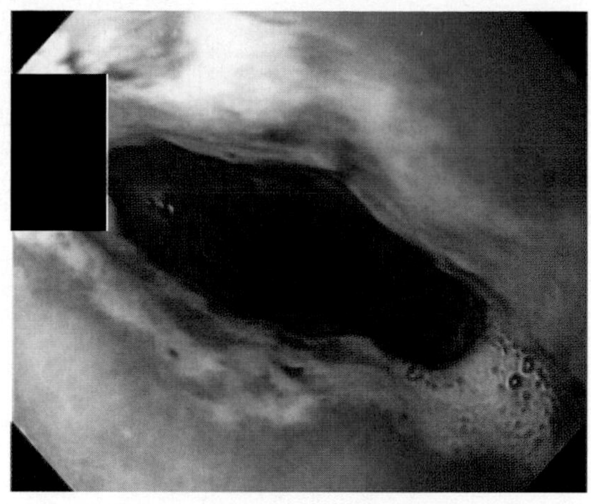

Figure 17.1: 'Pill esophagitis' in a teenage girl on doxycycline.

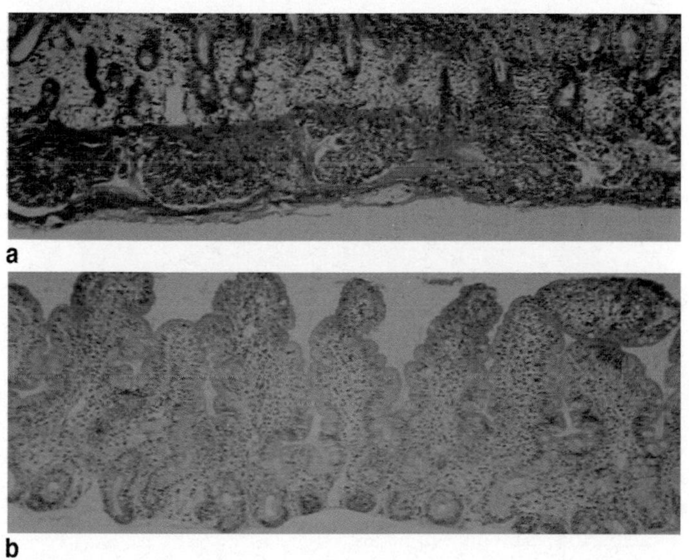

Figure 9.2: Small bowel biopsy (**a**) prior to and (**b**) after soy challenge in child with soy allergy. After the challenge the epithelium is damaged: villi are destroyed and the mucosa is invaded by a dens cellular infiltrate.

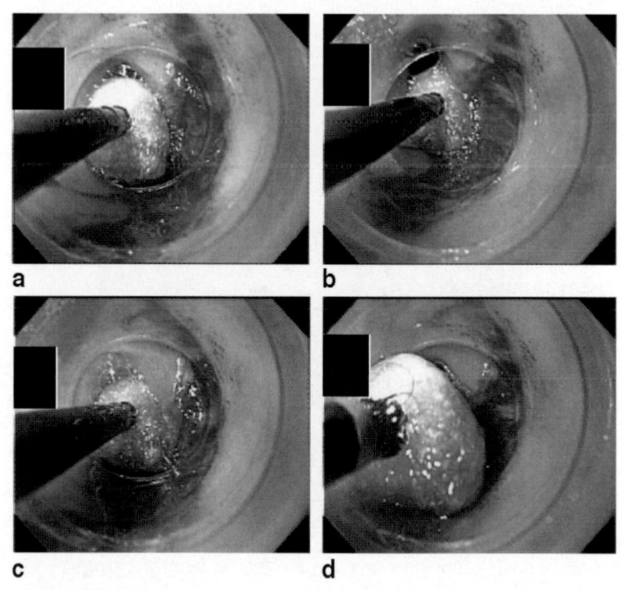

Figure 17.6: Application of mitomycin C to dilated stenotic area in esophagus. (**a**) Dry pledget is advanced from clear plastic hood on scope. (**b**) Mitomycin C is injected down forceps sheath onto pledget. (**c**) Pledget is held on mucosa at site of dilation. (**d**) Pledget is withdrawn into hood for safe removal.

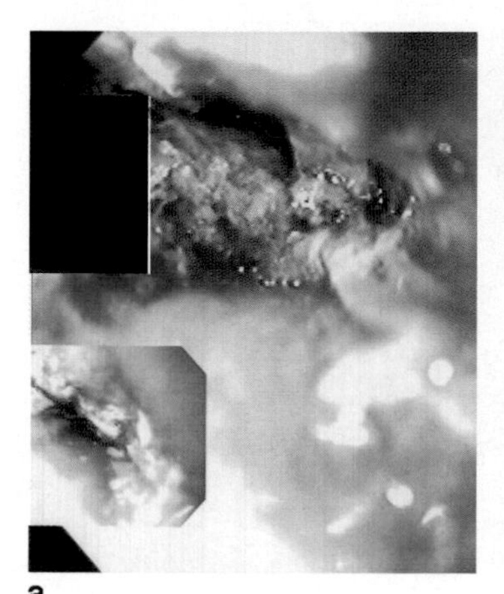

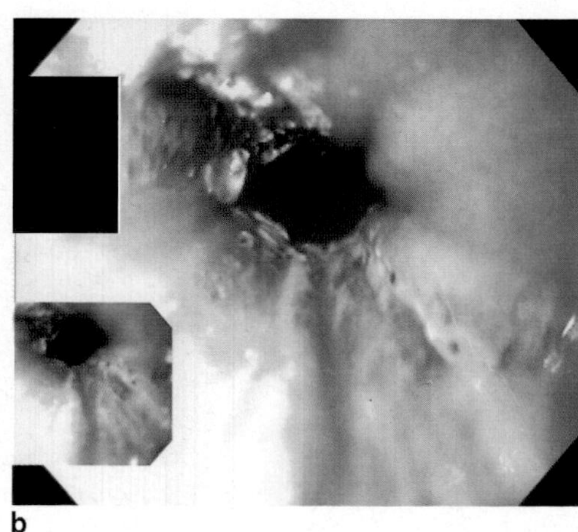

Figure 17.8: (**a**) Disk battery in esophagus with necrotic debris at burn site. (**b**) Typical bilateral esophageal burn after removal of disk battery.

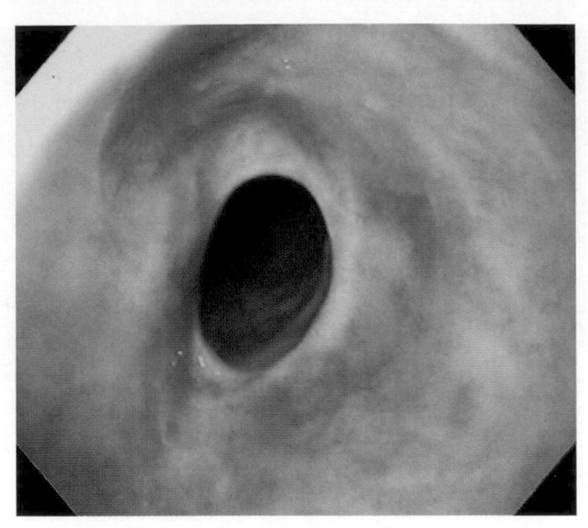

Figure 17.9: Esophageal stenosis in a toddler resulting from ingestion of oven cleaner.

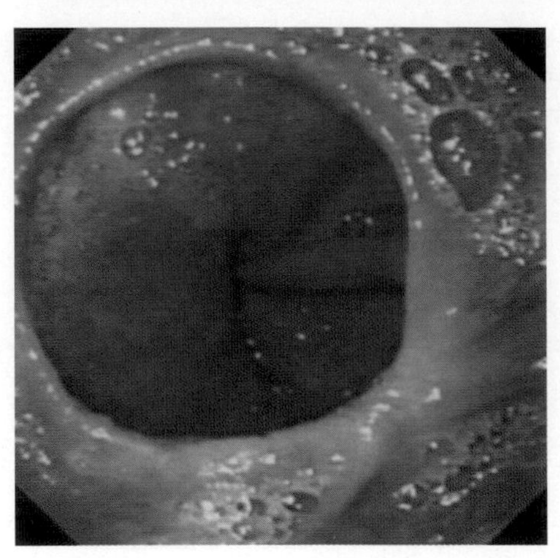

Figure 18.14: Endoscopic view of the distal esophagus revealing a Schatzki ring.

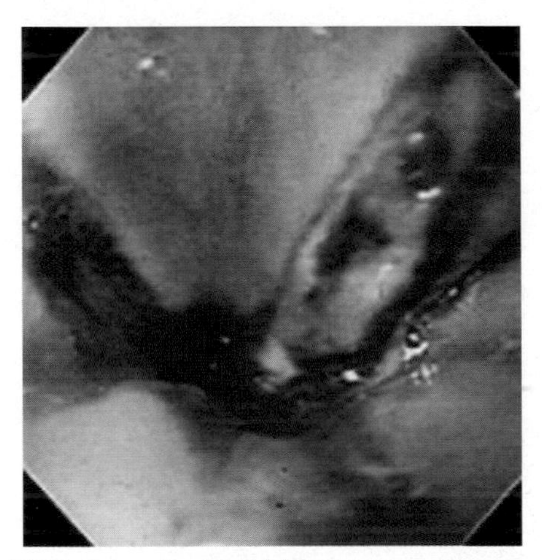

Figure 18.11: Endoscopic view of the distal esophagus revealing thickened folds resulting from edema, often a sign of chronic esophagitis.

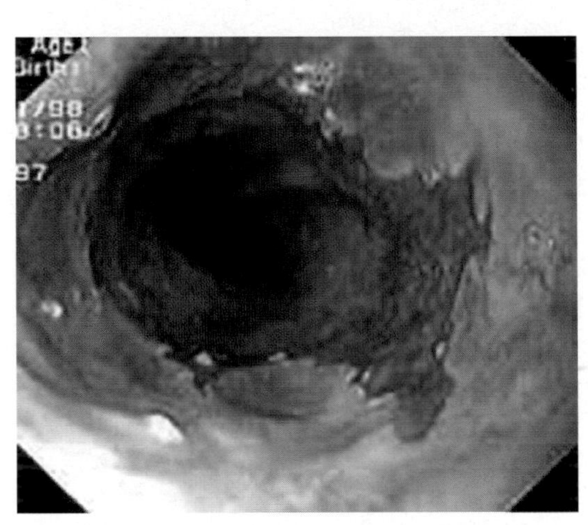

Figure 20.4: Barrett's esophagus.

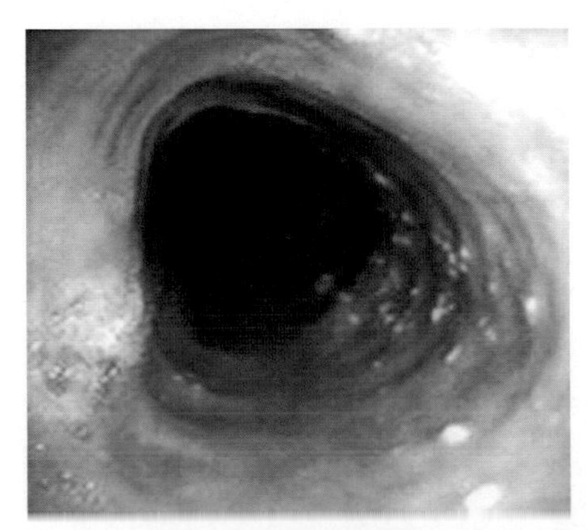

Figure 18.12: Endoscopic view of the distal esophagus revealing circumferential furrows, a sign of eosinophilic esophagitis.

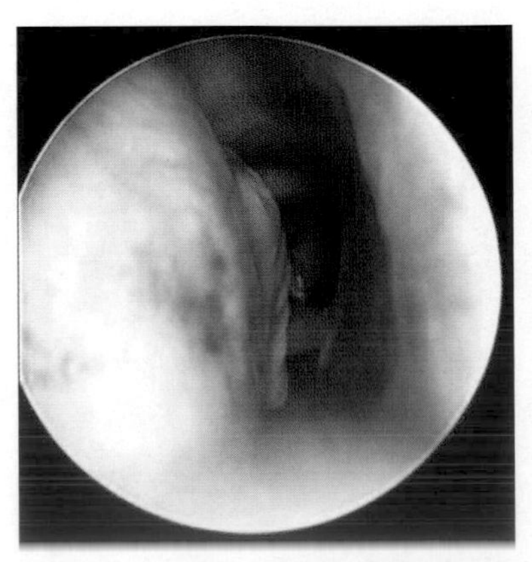

Figure 19.7: Tracheomalacia after repair of esophageal atresia and tracheo-esophageal fistula.

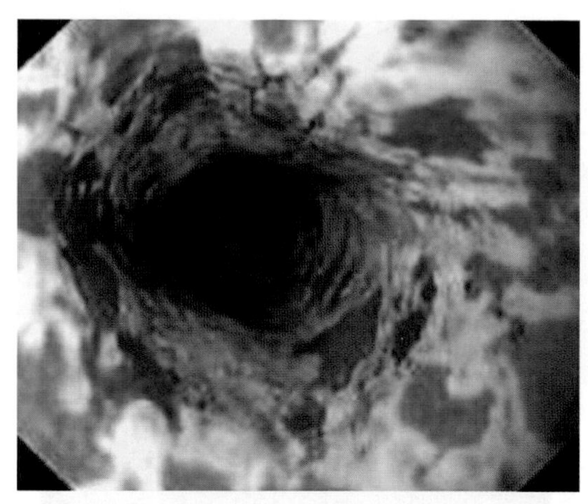

Figure 20.5: Endoscopic view of severe (reflux) esophagitis.

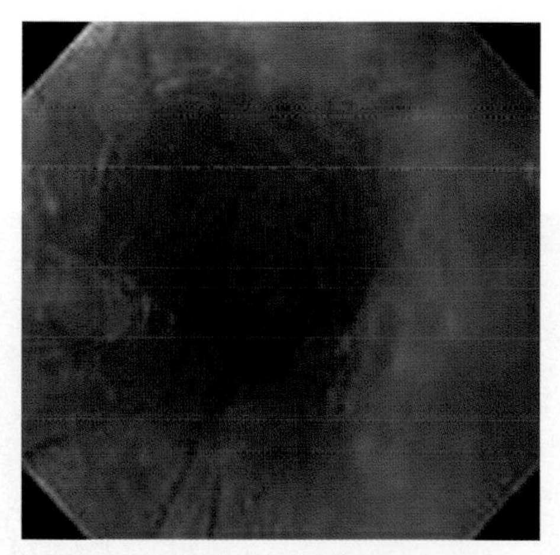

Figure 20.6: Normal esophagus. The distal redness is normal, due to an increased number of small blood vessels at the cardiac region.

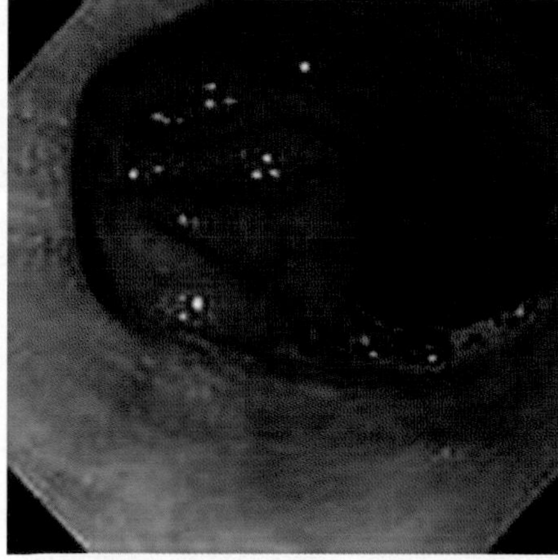

Figure 20.7: Endoscopic view of sliding hernia. The stomach is protruding into the esophagus through the cardia.

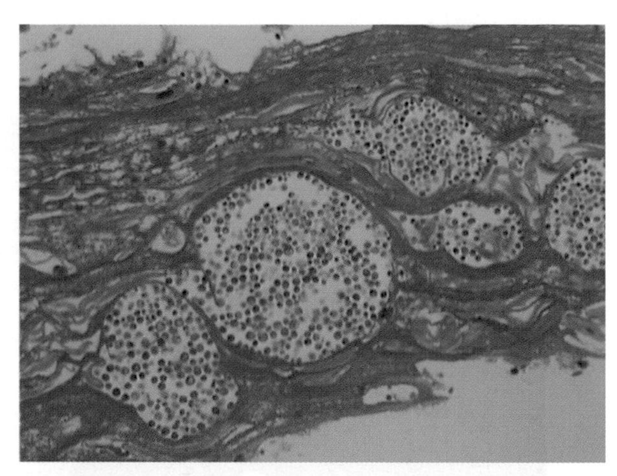

Figure 22.1: Invasive candida esophagitis. The mucosa is necrotic and the yeasts are within the mucosa (H&E, ×132). (Courtesy David R. Kelly, MD, Children's Hospital of Alabama and University of Alabama).

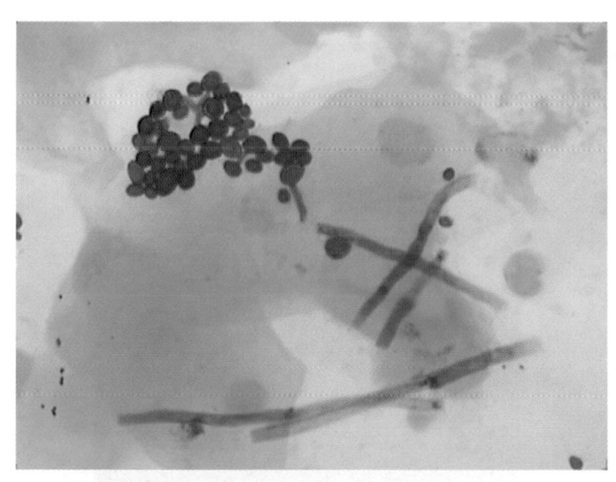

Figure 22.2: Yeasts, germ tubes (chlamydospores) and pseudohyphae of candida in esophageal brushing specimen (GMS, ×330) (Courtesy David R. Kelly, MD, Children's Hospital of Alabama and University of Alabama).

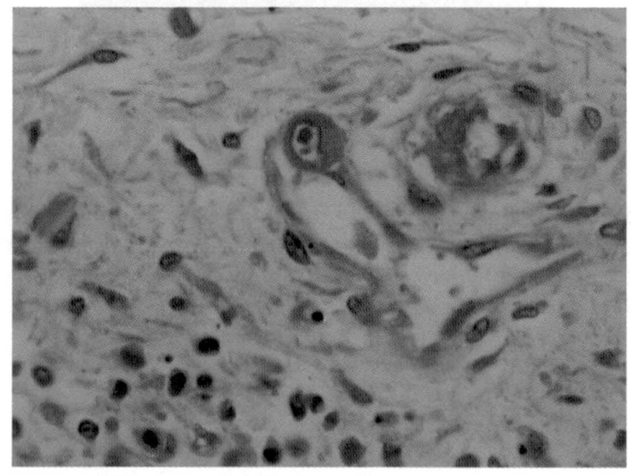

Figure 22.3: CMV esophagitis. This virus typically is characterized by a prominent eosinophilic intranuclear inclusion and displays vascular tropism (H&E, ×330). (Courtesy David R. Kelly, MD, Children's Hospital of Alabama and University of Alabama).

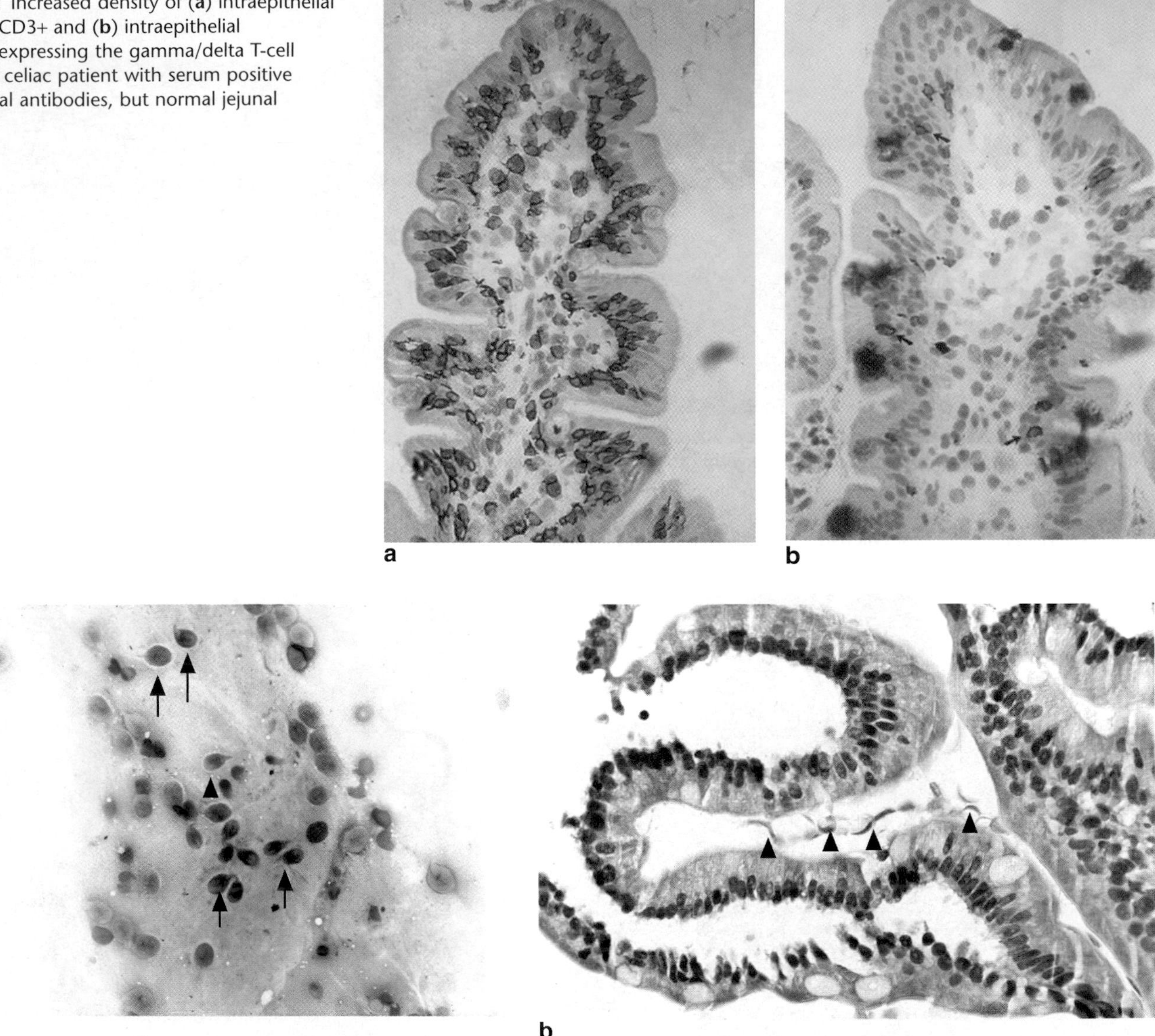

Figure 33.3: Increased density of (**a**) intraepithelial lymphocytes CD3+ and (**b**) intraepithelial lymphocytes expressing the gamma/delta T-cell receptor, in a celiac patient with serum positive antiendomysial antibodies, but normal jejunal architecture.

Figure 37.1: Trophozoites (arrows) of *Giardia lamblia* from small bowel biopsy. (**a**) Giemsa stain of touch prep. (**b**) Routine section (H&E). (Courtesy of Drs Gerald Berry and Terry Longacre).

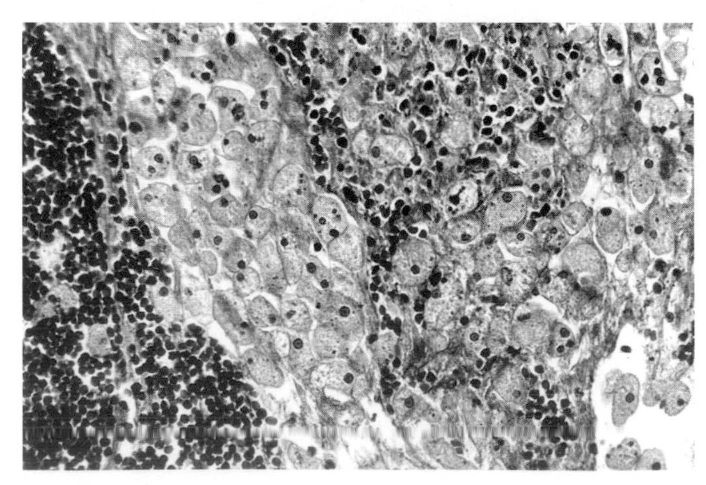

Figure 37.2: *Entamoeba histolytica* trophozoites in a colonic biopsy. (Courtesy of Drs Gerald Berry and Terry Longacre).

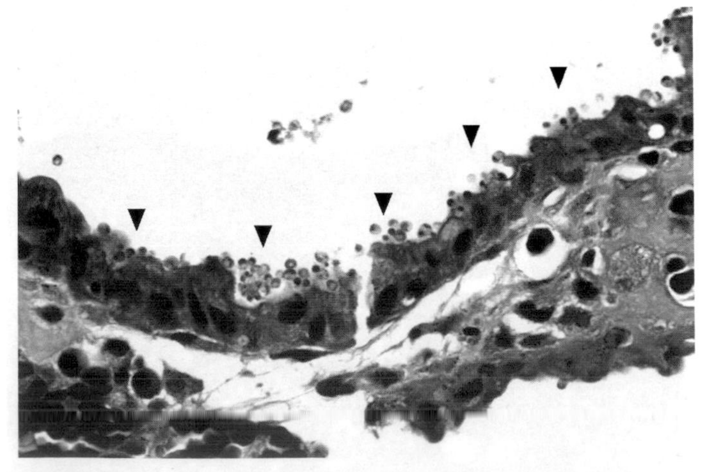

Figure 37.3: Cryptosporidia on the surface of a small intestinal biopsy. (Courtesy of Drs Gerald Berry and Terry Longacre).

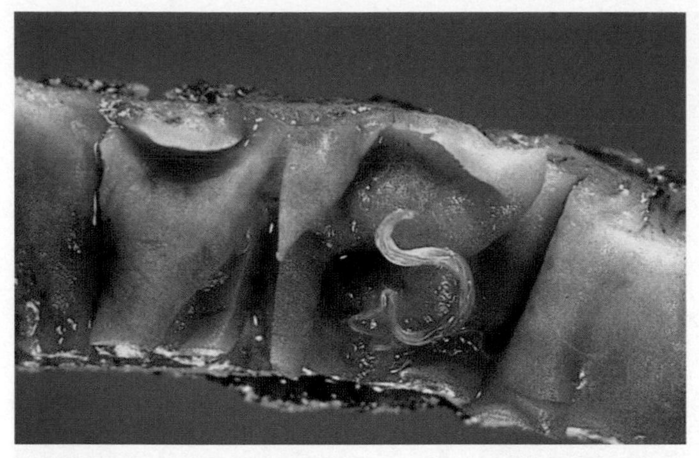

Figure 37.4: *Trichuris trichiura* in a resected colon. (Courtesy of Drs Gerald Berry and Terry Longacre).

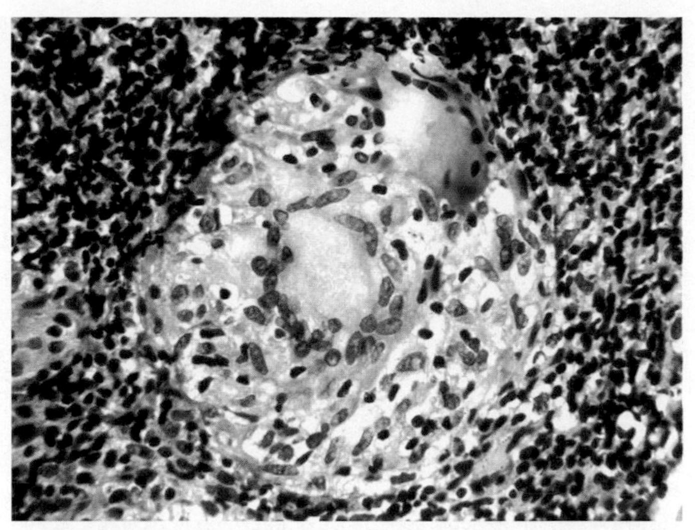

Figure 40.9: Epitheliod granuloma with multinucleated giant cells.

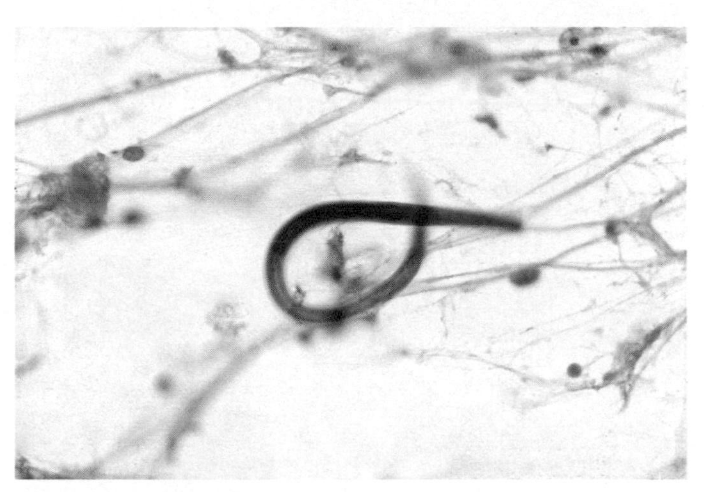

Figure 37.5: Strongyloides stercoralis (adult form). (Courtesy of Drs Gerald Berry and Terry Longacre).

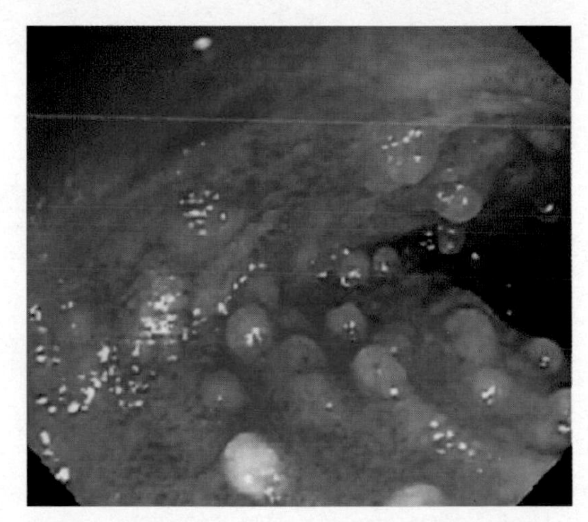

Figure 40.14: Marked lymphoid hyperplasia in Crohn's disease.

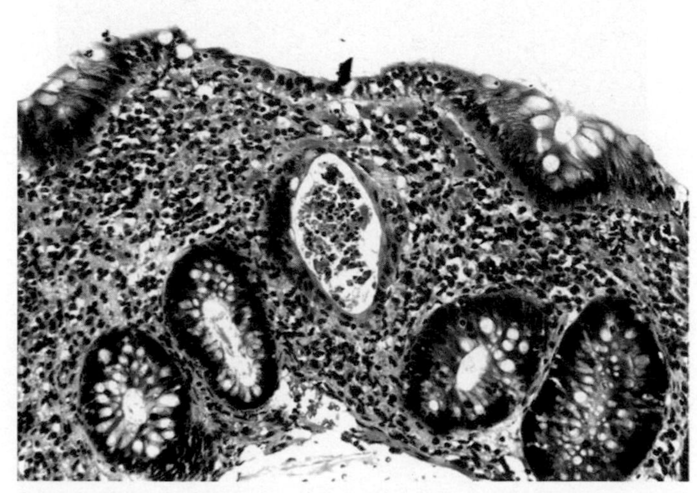

Figure 40.8: Neutrophilic crypt abscess and crypt architectural distortion.

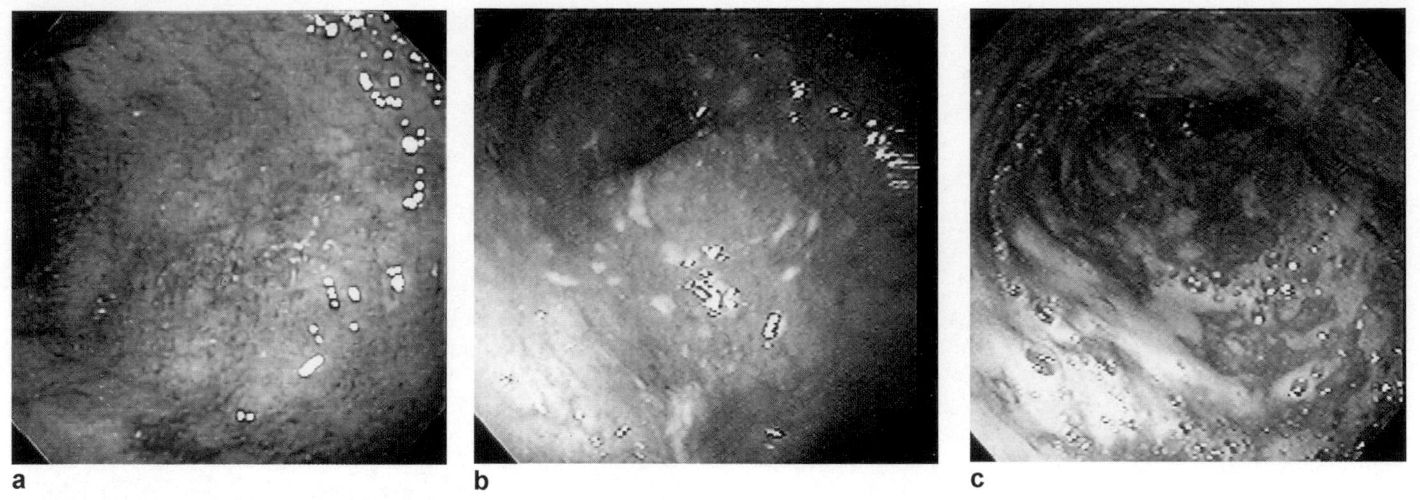

Figure 41.1: Endoscopic appearance of the colon in ulcerative colitis. (**a**) Mild inflammation. (**b**) Moderate inflammation. (**c**) Severe inflammation.

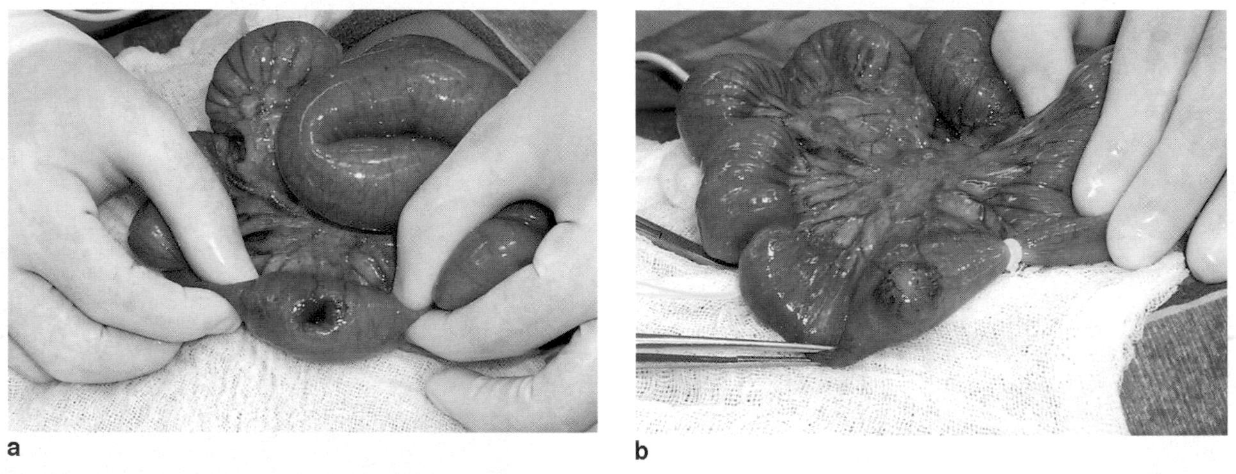

Figure 45.1: Surgically reduced ileocolic intussusception secondary to Meckel's diverticulum as lead point. (**a**) Inverted diverticulum as lead point. (**b**) Everted diverticulum in normal orientation.

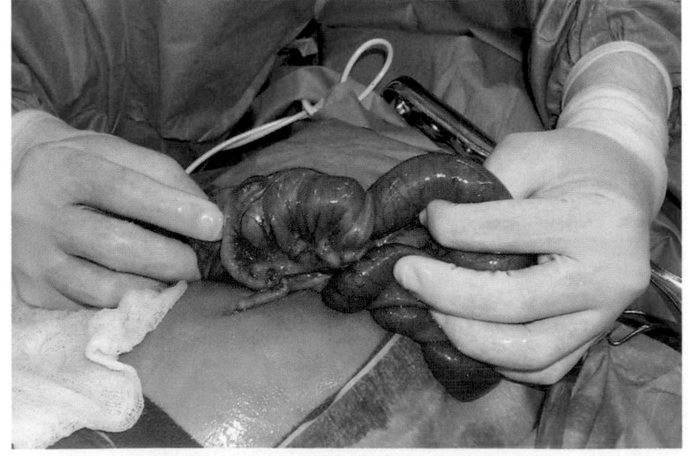

Figure 45.8: Intraoperative photograph of an ileocolic intussusception through the ileocecal valve. The absence of ischemic changes predicts successful manual reduction.

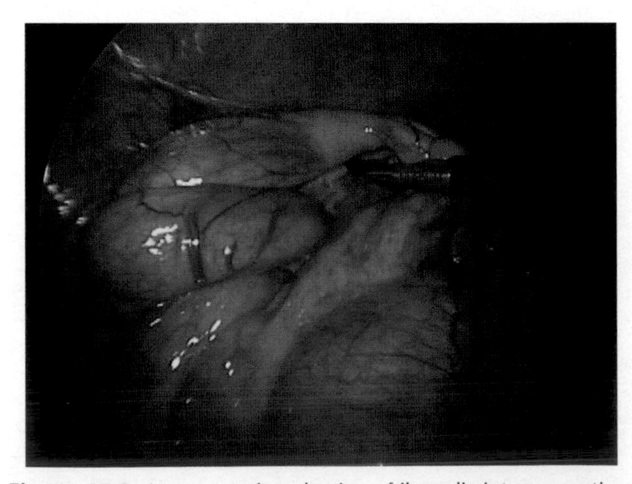

Figure 45.9: Laparoscopic reduction of ileocolic intussusception.

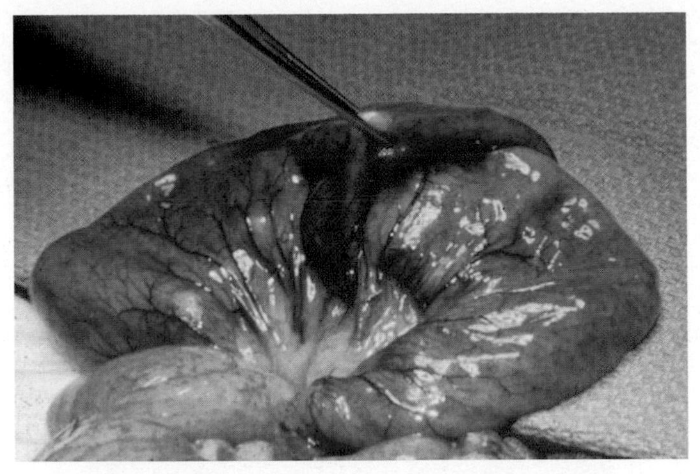

Figure 45.10: Small intestinal (enteroenteric) intussusception.

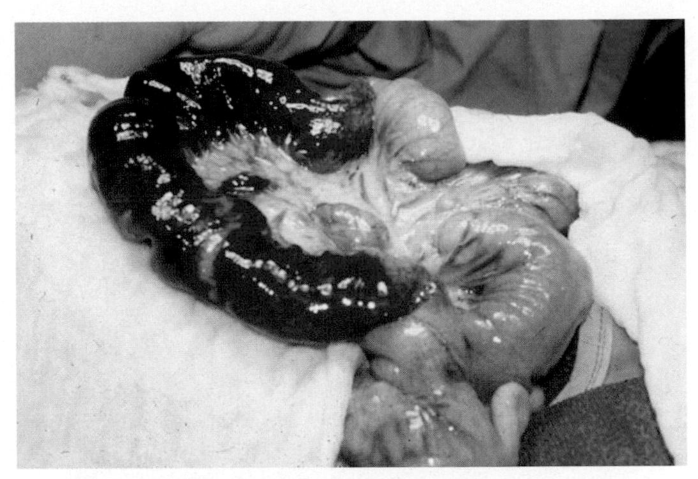

Figure 45.11: Intramural hemorrhage in small intestine secondary to Henoch–Schönlein purpura.

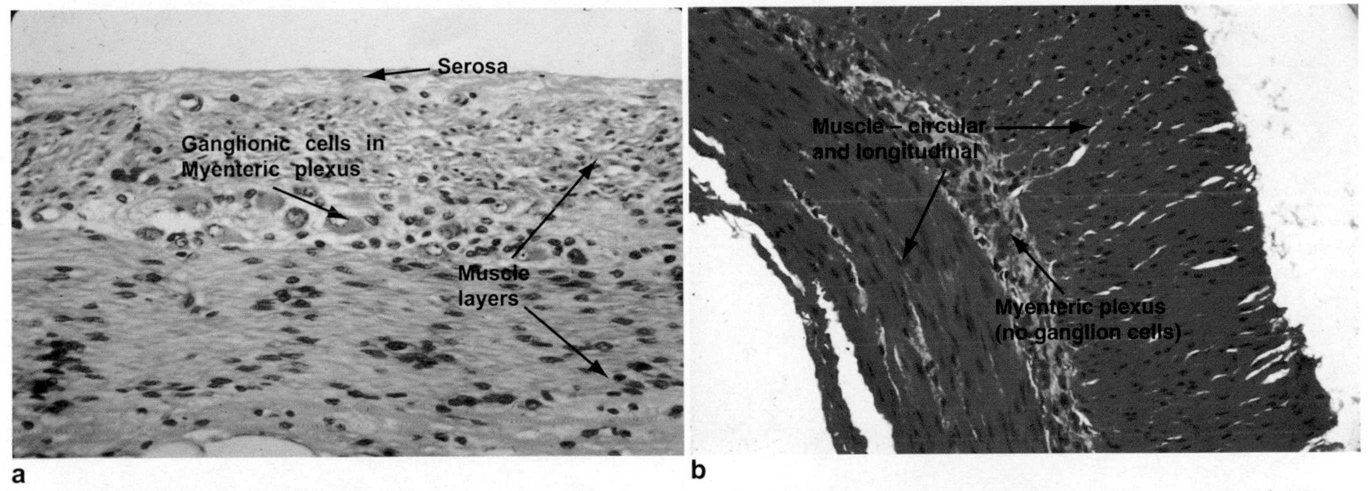

Figure 48.2: Hematoxylin and eosin stain of colonic biopsy showing myenteric plexus from (**a**) a normal subject and (**b**) a patient with HD.

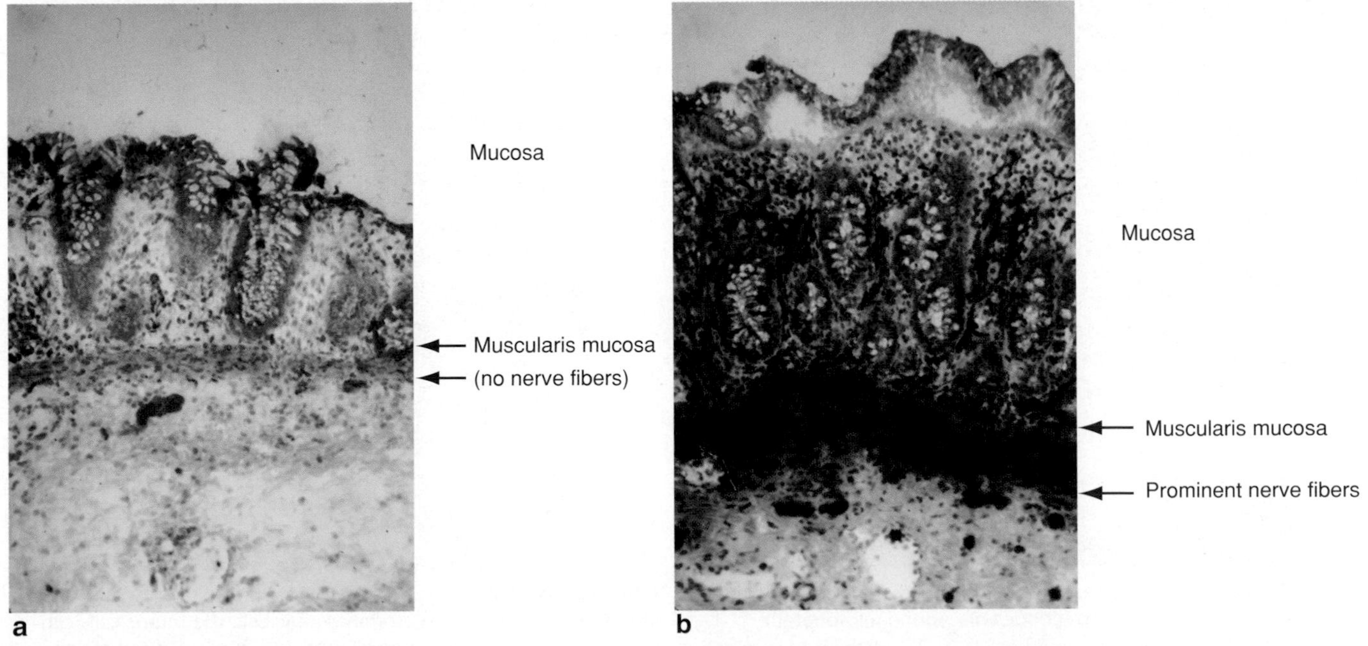

Figure 48.3: Acetylcholinesterase staining of colonic biopsy from (**a**) a normal subject and (**b**) a patient with HD.

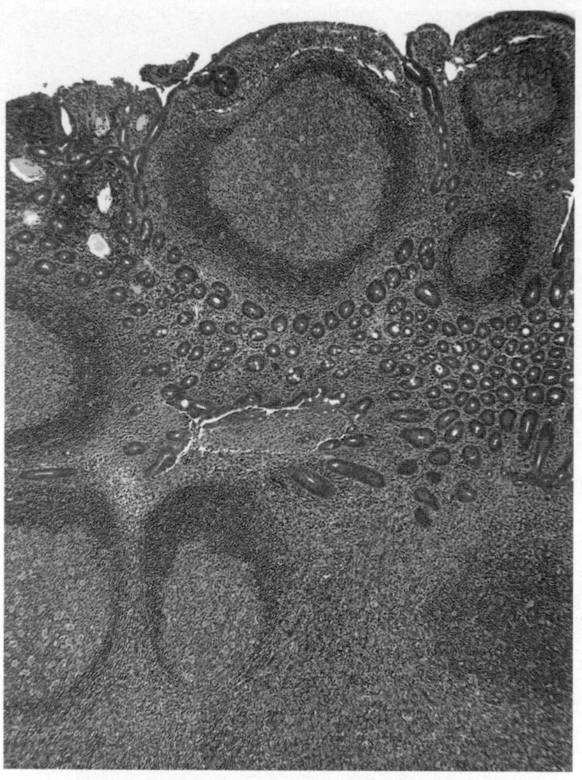

Figure 55.1: Lymphonodular hyperplasia. Numerous reactive germinal centers distort the normal villous architecture of the small bowel.

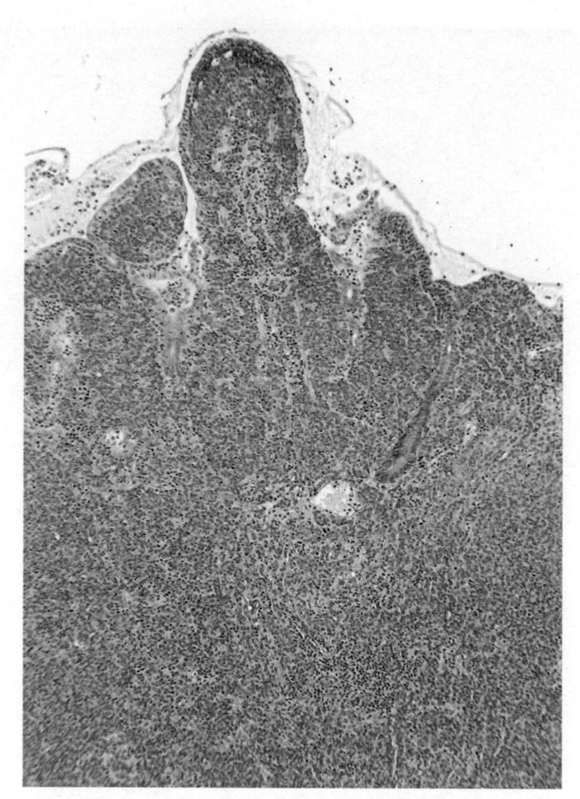

Figure 55.3: Burkitt lymphoma. The neoplastic lymphoid cells diffusely infiltrate the mucosa, overrunning the epithelium. Contrast with the benign lymphoid reaction in Figure 55.1.

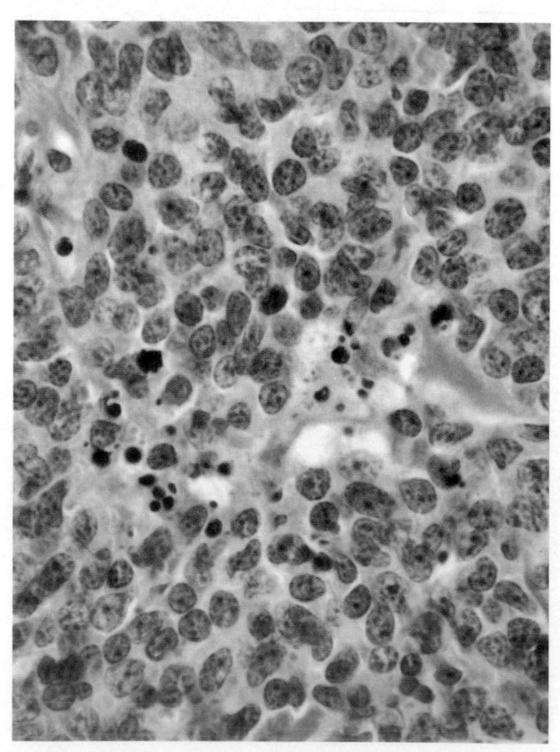

Figure 55.2: Burkitt lymphoma. Sheets of monotonous intermediate sized lymphoid cells have indiscreet nucleoli. Abundant apoptotic nuclear debris is present centrally.

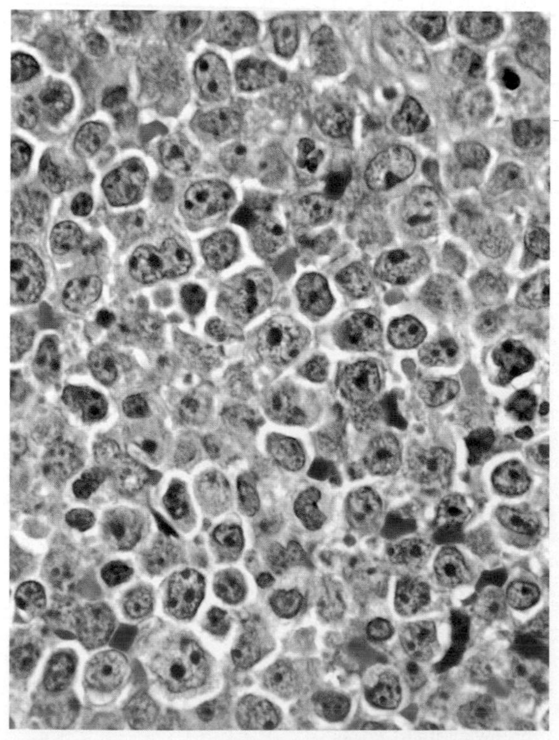

Figure 55.4: Diffuse large cell lymphoma. Sheets of large, immunoblastic cells have prominent nucleoli; the tumor cells can diffusely infiltrate the bowel wall similar to Burkitt lymphoma.

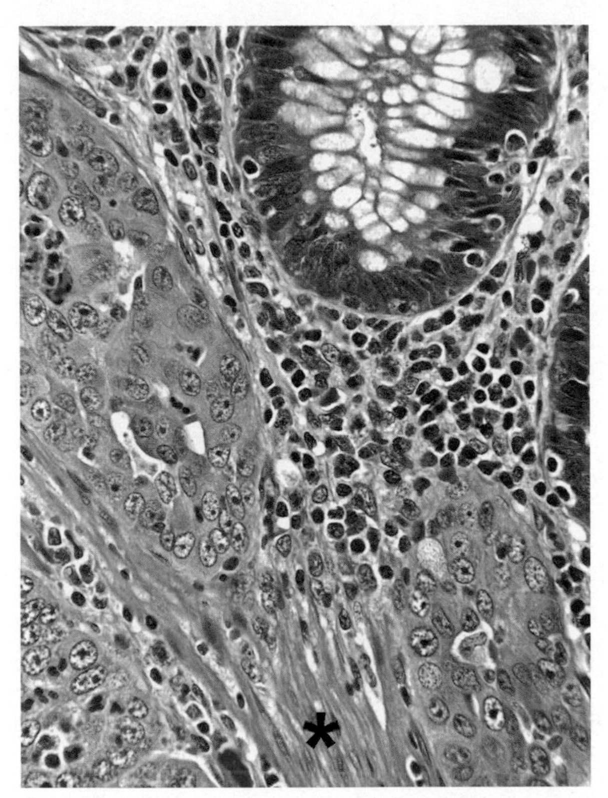

Figure 55.5: Adenocarcinoma, well differentiated. Malignant glands with complex architecture invade the muscularis (*) and are comprised of crowded large epithelial cells with prominent nucleoli. By contrast, the overlying normal glands have a regimented nuclear polarization and obvious goblet cells.

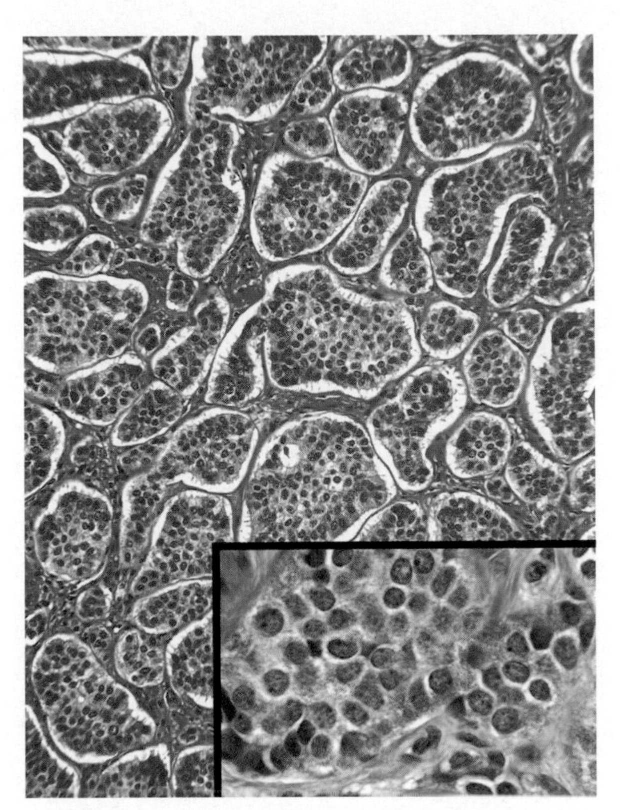

Figure 55.7: Carcinoid tumor. Fibrous stroma surrounds numerous well-demarcated islands of tumor cells. Uniform cells with faintly granular cytoplasm and round, bland nuclei that contain finely stippled chromatin are characteristic features of endocrine cell neoplasms (inset).

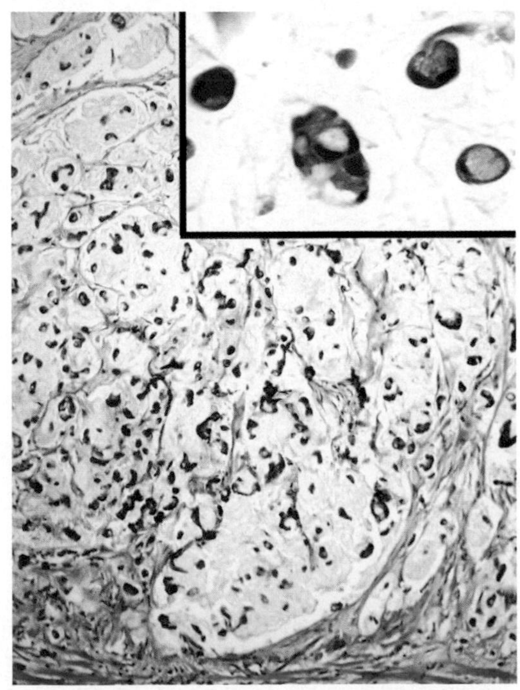

Figure 55.6: Adenocarcinoma, poorly differentiated (signet-ring cell carcinoma). Malignant epithelial cells float in pools of mucin. A 'signet-ring' cell is created by a large mucin vacuole that fills the cytoplasm and displaces the nucleus (inset).

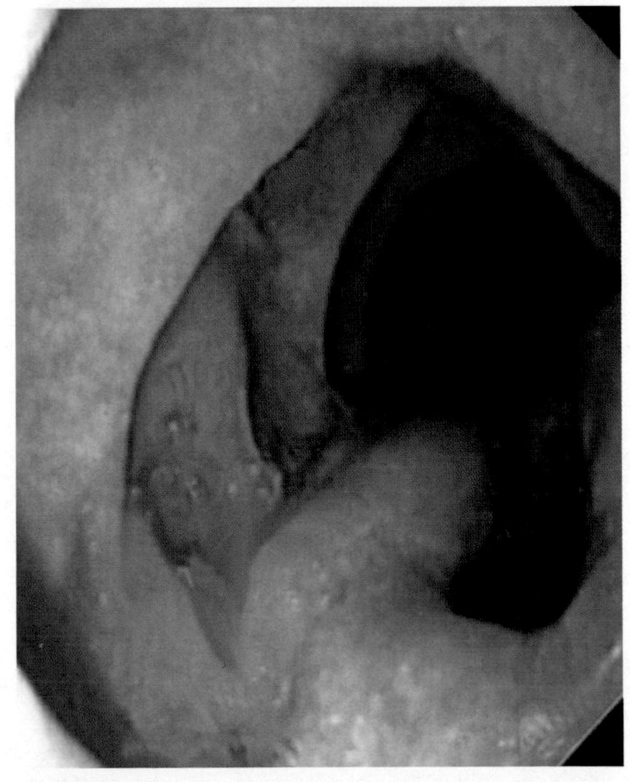

Figure 55.8: Primitive neuroectodermal tumor of the duodenum, endoscopic view.

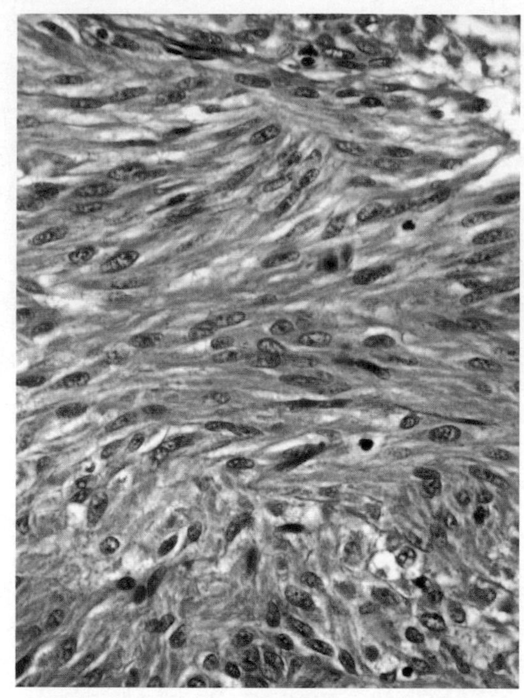

Figure 55.9: Gastrointestinal stromal cell tumor (GIST). Interlacing fascicles of plump cigar-shaped cells with tapered ends, comprise the spindle cell GIST.

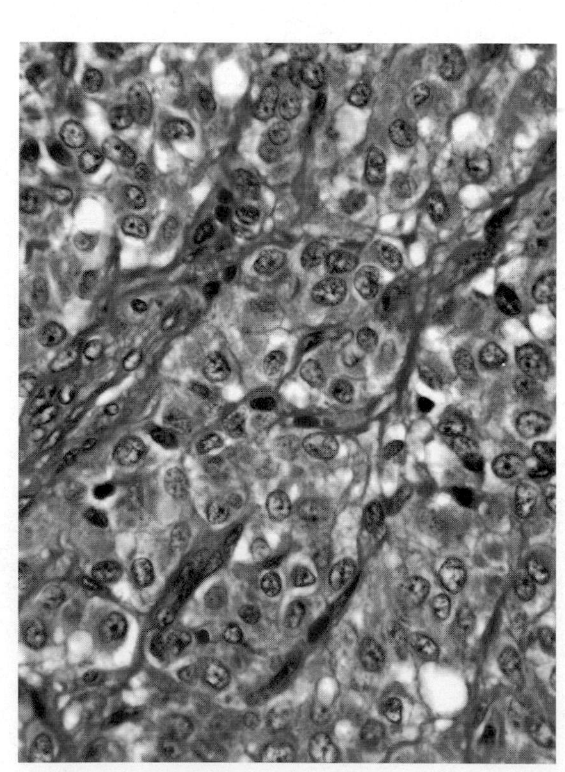

Figure 55.10: Gastrointestinal stromal cell tumor (GIST). Nests of medium-sized epithelioid cells with a moderate amount of eosinophilic cytoplasm comprise the epithelioid GIST.

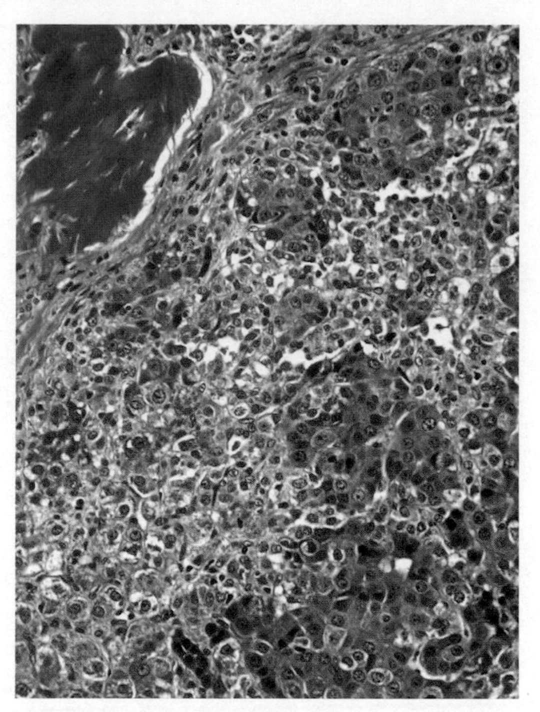

Figure 55.11: Hepatoblastoma. Trabeculae of hepatocyte-like cells resembling the fetal liver (lower right) mingle with the smaller 'embryonal' cells (center); this bi-phasic pattern helps distinguish a primary liver tumor as hepatoblastoma. Homogenous eosinophilic osteoid-like material is a common mesenchymal element (top left).

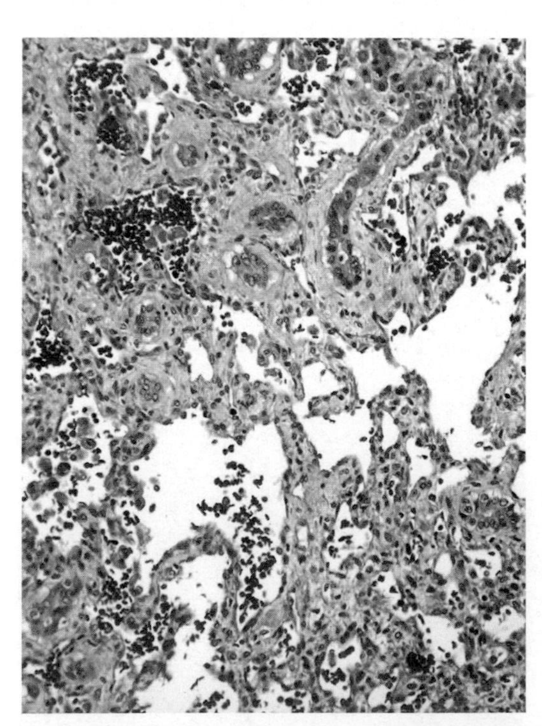

Figure 55.12: Infantile hemangioendothelioma. Slightly ectatic vascular spaces are lined by plump endothelial cells and contain erythrocytes. Scattered hepatocytes and bile ducts may be entrapped (top).

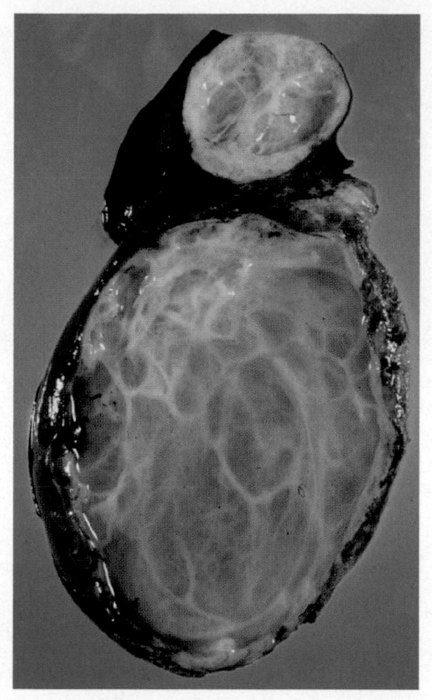

Figure 55.13: Mesenchymal hamartoma. The bisected multiloculated mass has fibrous septa dividing the lesion into cysts that contain viscous clear fluid. A thin rim of liver parenchyma is noted (upper left).

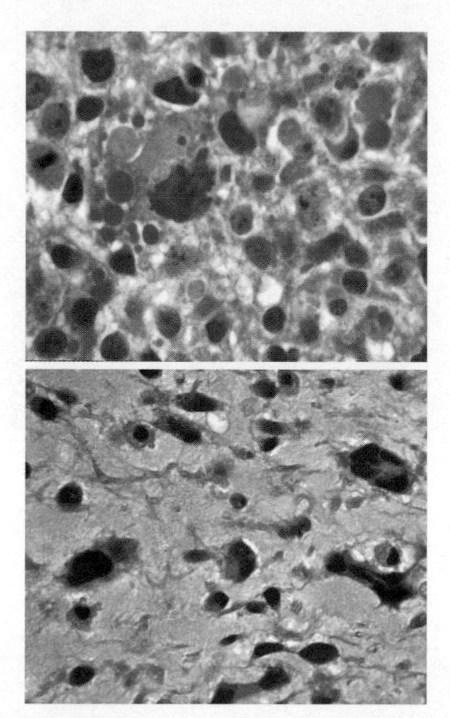

Figure 55.14 Undifferentiated embryonal sarcoma. Marked pleomorphism is characteristic and cellular density is variable. Scattered atypical hyperchromatic multinucleated cells are sporadically distributed within abundant myxoid stroma (bottom). Another more cellular tumor has abundant eosinophilic hyaline globules (top).

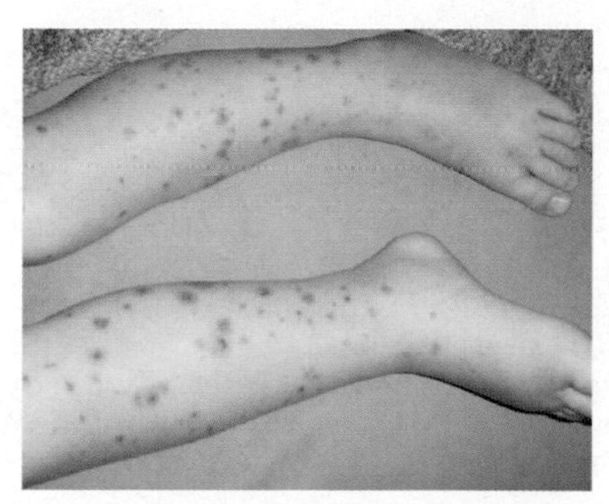

Figure 56.1: Palpable purpura on the back and legs of a four year old with abdominal pain from Henoch–Schönlein purpura.

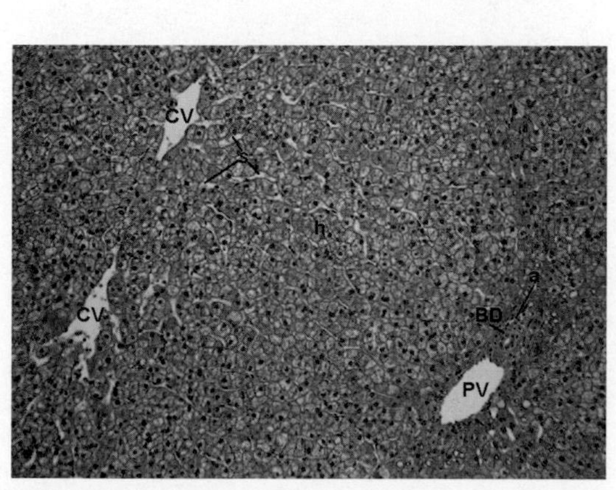

Figure 57.8: Microscopic functional unit of the liver: the liver lobule, from a mature child. a, Arteriole; BD, bile duct; CV, central vein; h, hepatocytes; PV, portal vein; s, sinusoids.

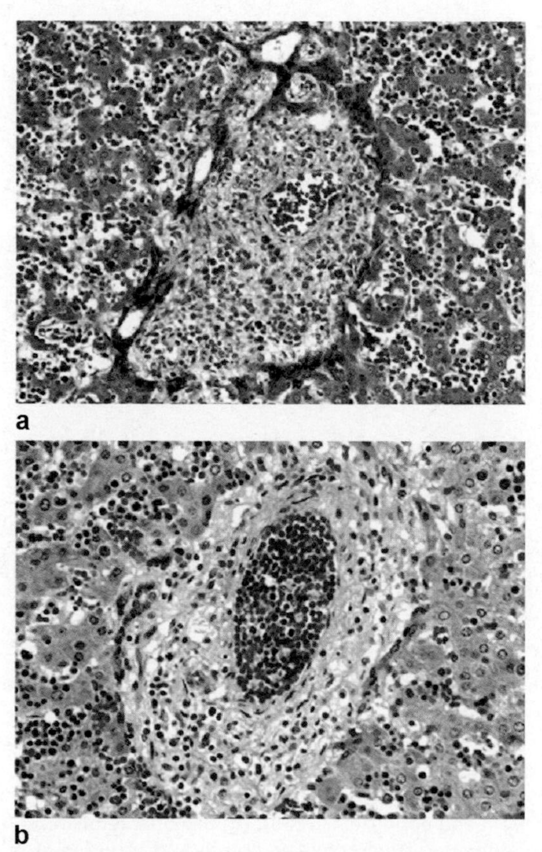

Figure 57.4: Human fetal liver tissue at weeks 16 (**a**) and 20 (**b**). (**a**) Remodeling of the ductal plate. (From Lemaigre, 2003, with permission).[11]

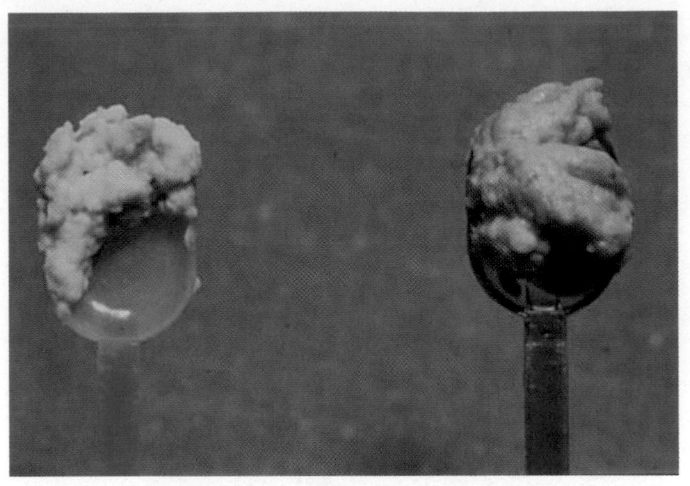

Figure 59.1: Acholic stool (left) strongly suggestive of a surgical problem during neonatal period. Children with biliary atresia can, however, have initially pigmented stools (right). (With permission from The Medicine Publishing Company.)

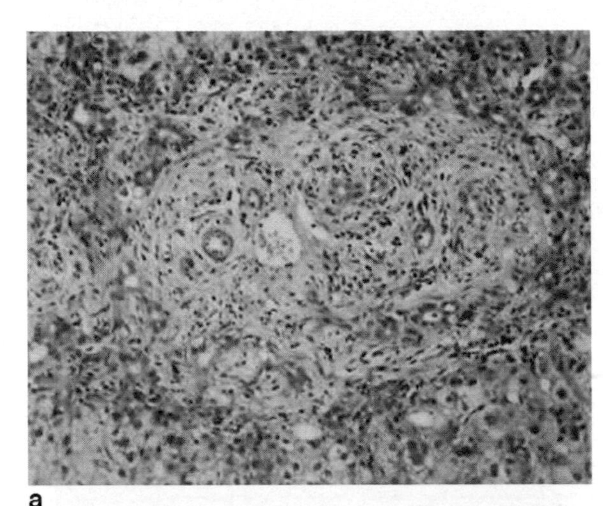

a

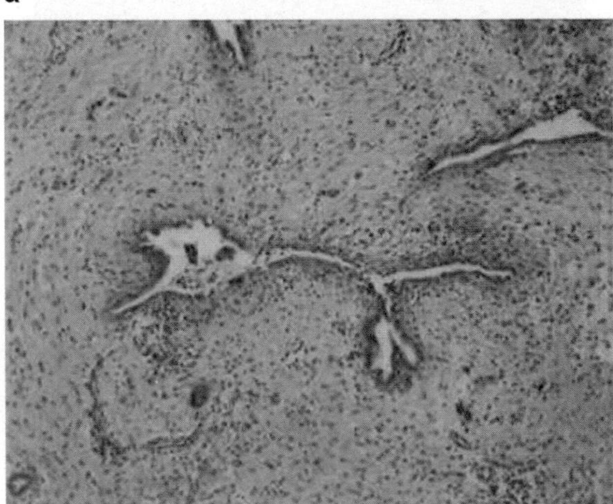

b

Figure 59.2: Histological appearance of biliary atresia. (**a**) Liver biopsy showing typical changes – edematous portal tract with increased fibrosis, duplicating bile ducts and cholestatic plugs (hematoxylin and eosin stain, ×250). (**b**) Bile duct remnant obtained at Kasai portoenterostomy showing fibrosis and occlusion of extrahepatic bile ducts (hematoxylin and eosin stain, ×125). (With permission from The Medicine Publishing Company.)

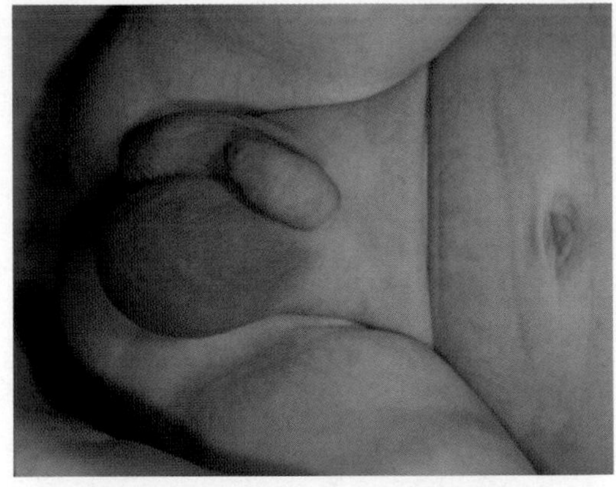

Figure 59.6: Green-yellow discoloration of scrotum and umbilicus due to intra-abdominal presence of bile following spontaneous perforation of the bile duct.

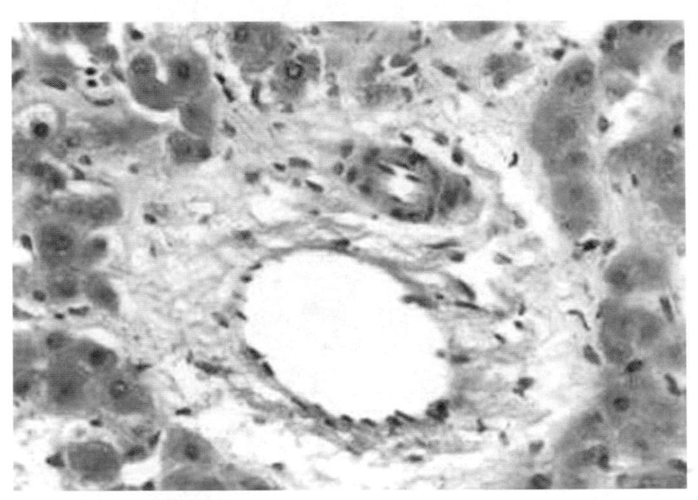

Figure 59.8: Alagille syndrome. (**a**) Liver biopsy showing absence of bile duct in the portal tract (hematoxylin and eosin stain, ×320). (**b**) Classic facial appearance – triangular face, deep-set eyes, mild hypertelorism, prominent forehead, small pointed chin, low set ears. (**c**) Typical appearance of a 'butterfly' vertebra (arrow) on spinal radiography. (**d**) Disfiguring xanthomas on the hands. (With permission from The Medicine Publishing Company.)

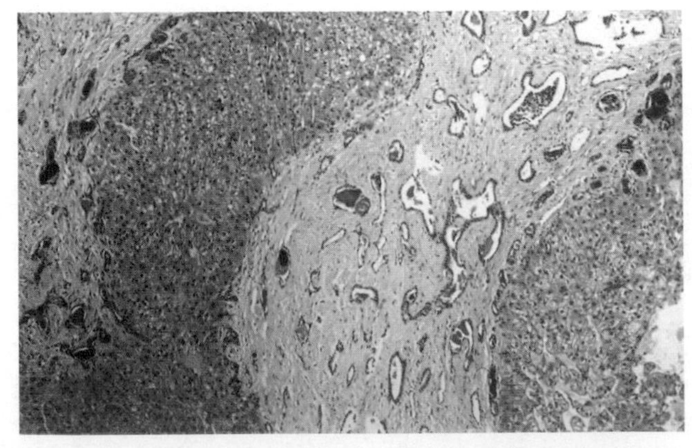

Figure 59.10: Liver biopsy in the ductal plate malformation; loose fibrous tissue containing small irregular bile ducts, some of them dilated and containing bile (hematoxylin and eosin stain, ×125).

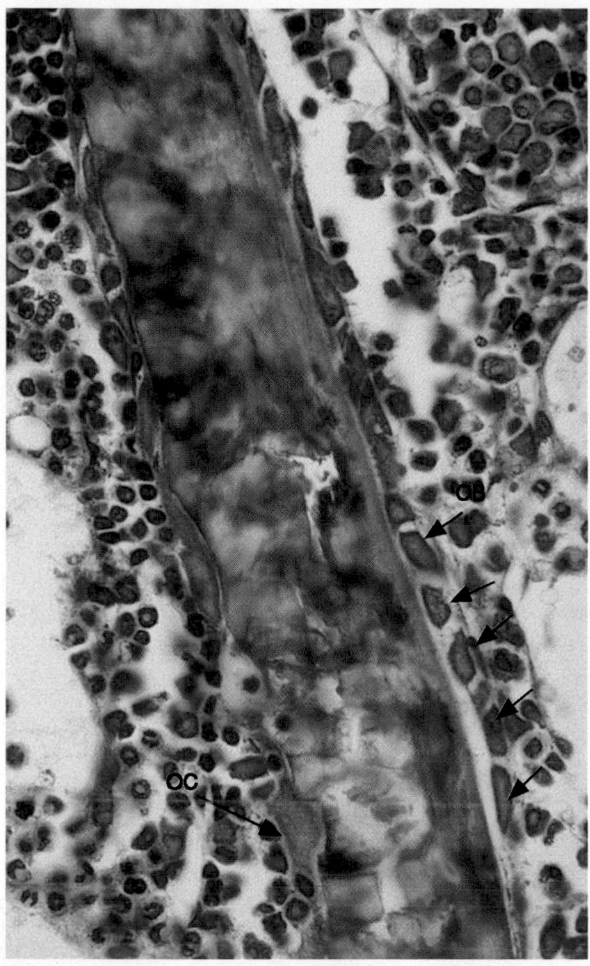

Figure 77.2: Bone mass is regulated by the balance between osteoblast and osteoclast activities. Photomicrograph from a bone trabecula of mouse femur (×400) lined by osteoblasts (OB, short arrows) and osteoclasts (OC, long arrow).

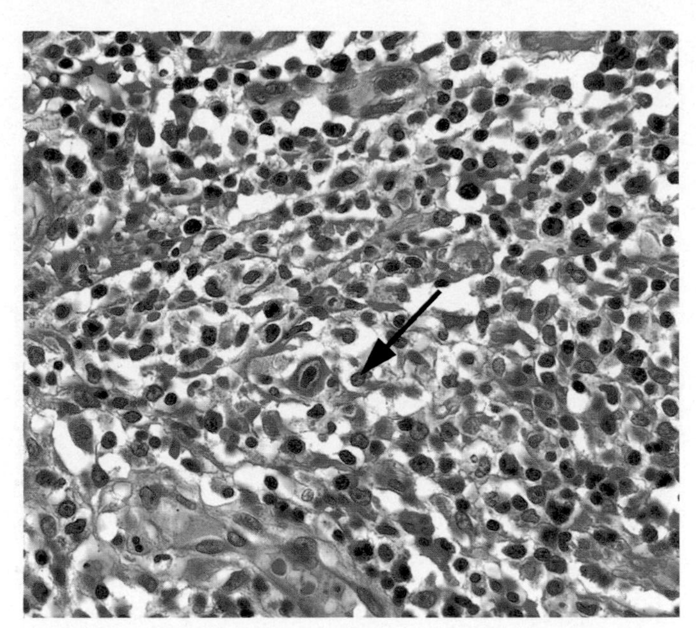

Figure 79.2: Cytomegalovirus inclusion found in ulcer base (arrow). The infected mesenchymal cell shows cellular enlargement. The nucleus contains a large basophilic inclusion body with surrounding halo and preservation of the nucleolus.

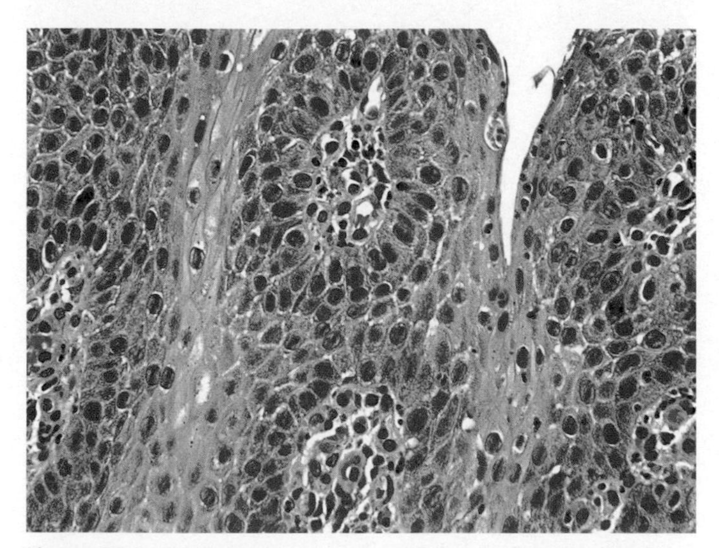

Figure 79.1: Esophageal squamous epithelial changes of reflux. In addition to papillomatosis, an increase in the squamous basal cell layer and increased intraepithelial lymphocytes and eosinophils, surface neutrophils are also present.

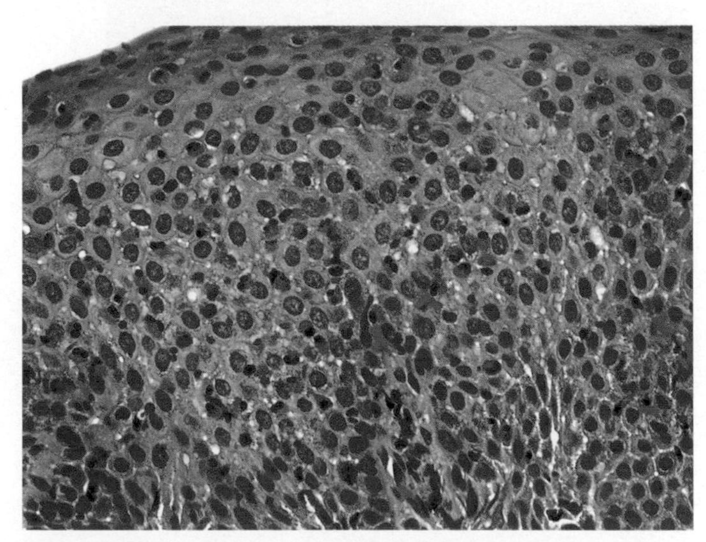

Figure 79.3: Eosinophilic esophagitis. Sections show squamous papillomatosis, a marked increase in the squamous epithelial basal cell layer and numerous intraepithelial eosinophils leukocytes.

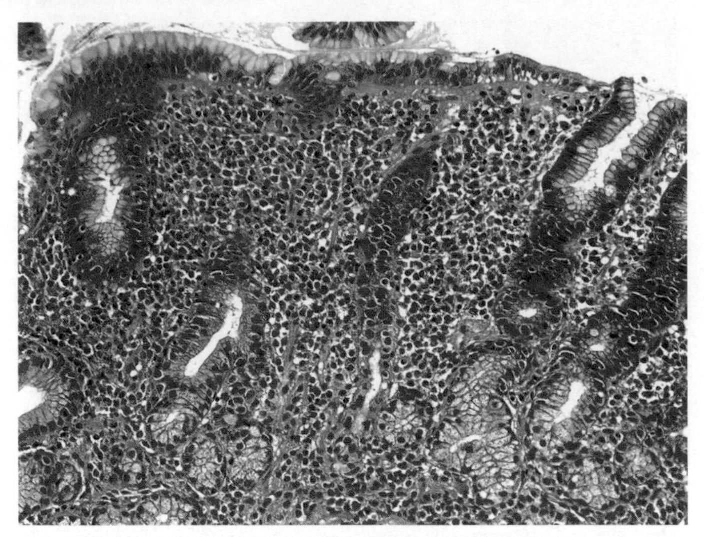

Figure 79.4: *Helicobacter pylori*-associated gastritis. Sections show a dense chronic inflammatory cell infiltrate of the lamina propria associated with some acute inflammation.

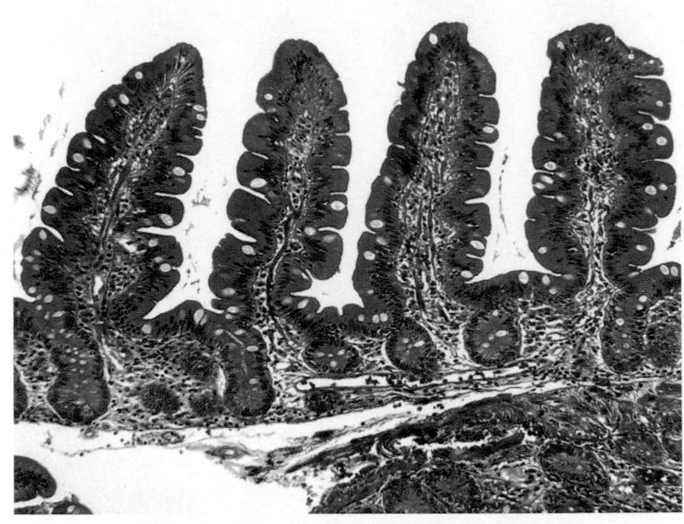

Figure 79.6: Normal small-bowel mucosa. The villi are long and slender. The ratio of villus : crypt length is approximately 4 : 1. Enterocyte nuclei are basilar in location and evenly aligned. Occasional intraepithelial lymphocytes are present.

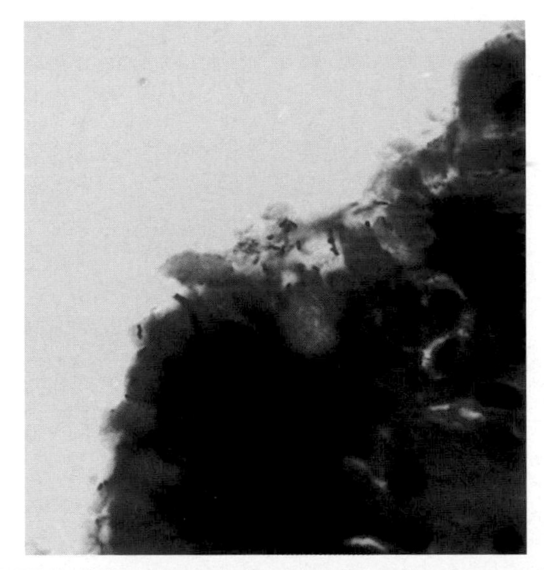

Figure 79.5: *Helicobacter pylori*-associated gastritis, giemsa stain. Note the curved bacilli within the mucous layer.

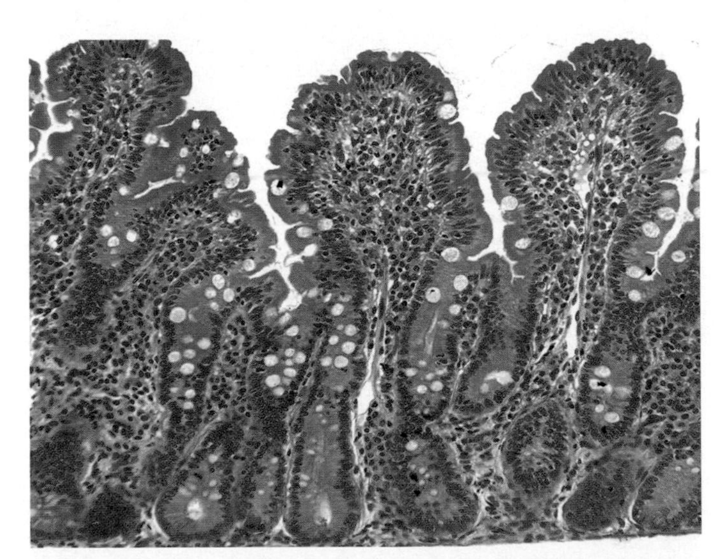

Figure 79.7: Severe villous abnormality typical of celiac sprue. The villus : crypt length is less than 1 : 1. Inflammatory cells are increased within the lamina propria. Numerous intraepithelial lymphocytes are also present.

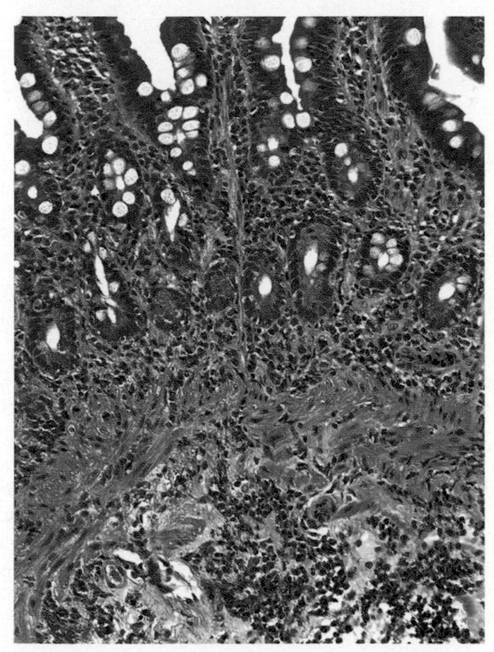

Figure 79.8: Small bowel with eosinophilic gastroenteritis. Note the large collection of eosinophils within the submucosa with lesser numbers infiltrating the muscularis mucosae and lamina propria.

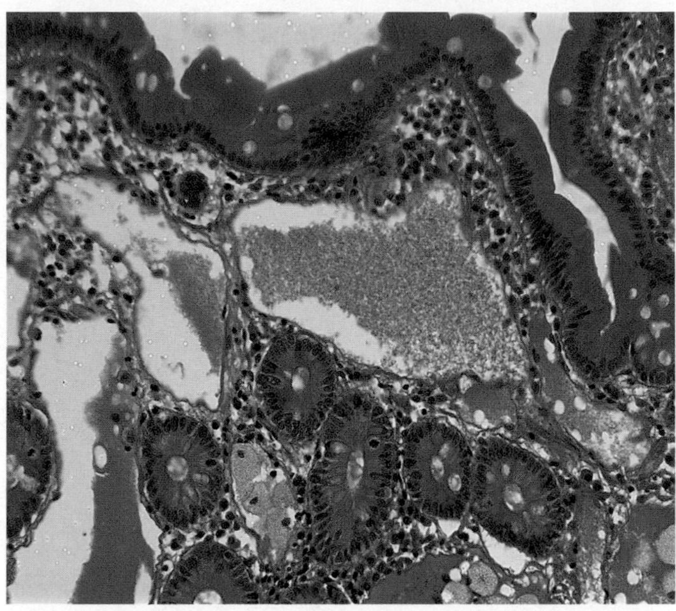

Figure 79.10: Intestinal lymphangiectasia. The primary and secondary forms appear identical in histologic sections, demonstrating dilated lymphatic located in otherwise normal mucosa.

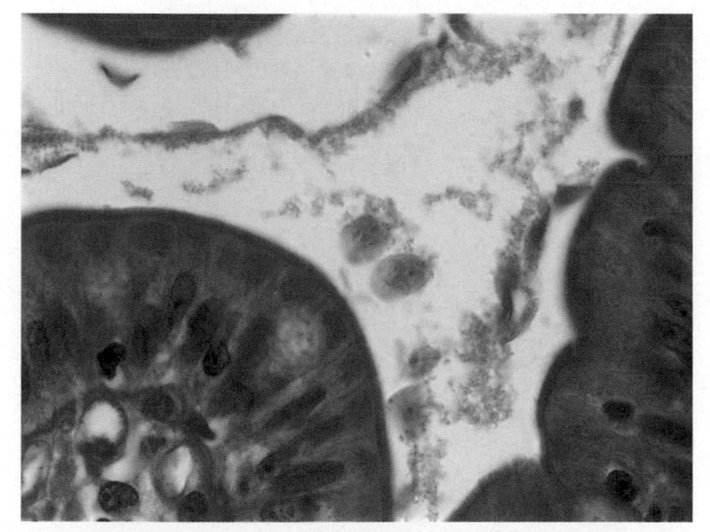

Figure 79.9: Giardiasis. In this small bowel specimen, the diagnosis rests on demonstration of the trophozoite in tissue section. Seen *en face*, *Giardia lamblia* is pear-shaped and demonstrates prominent paired nuclei.

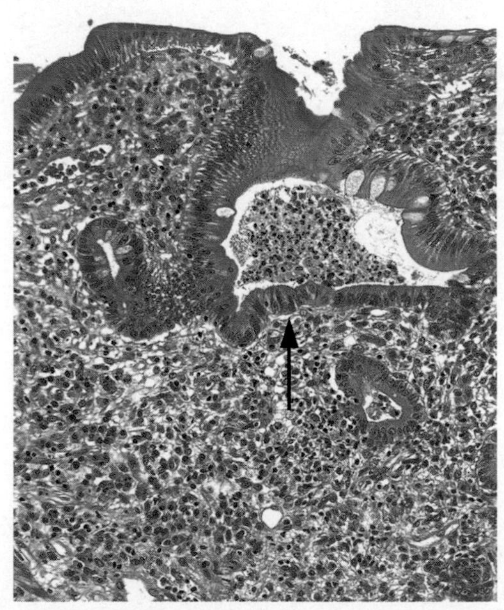

Figure 79.11: Ulcerative colitis in an active phase. Sections show diffuse architectural change, prominent lamina proprial plasmacytosis and crypt abscess formation (arrow).

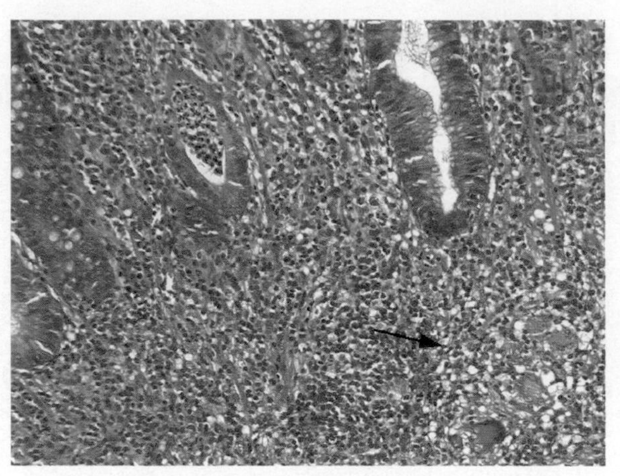

Figure 79.12: Colonic Crohn's disease showing focal active colitis with an intramucosal non-necrotizing granuloma (arrow).

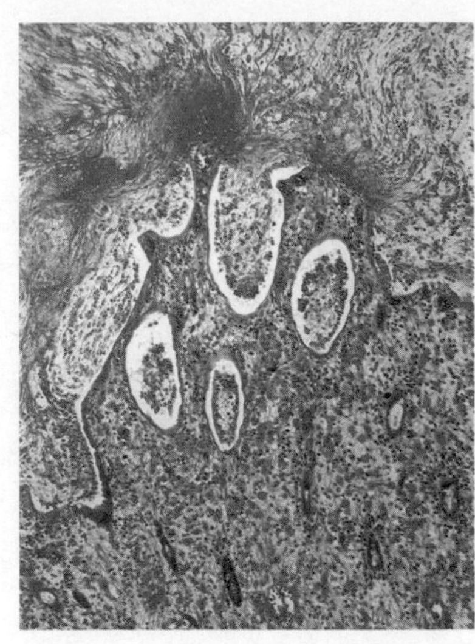

Figure 79.15: *Clostridium difficile*-associated pseudomembranous colitis. An inflammatory pseudomembrane exudes from dilated degenerating crypts in an erosive fashion. The karyorrhectic debris and neutrophils within the pseudomembrane tend to align in a linear configuration within the mucus.

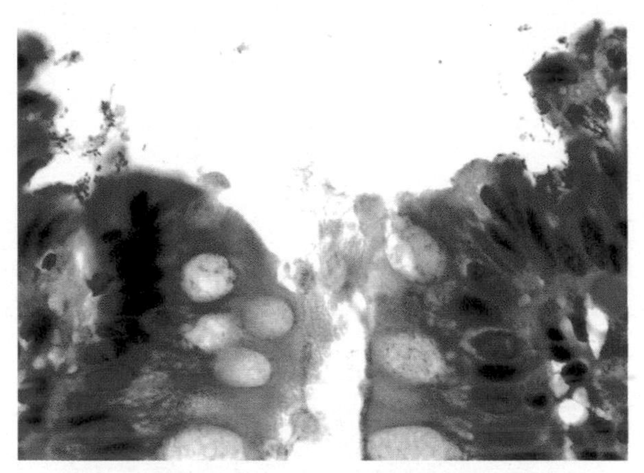

Figure 79.13: Enteroadherent *Escherichia coli*. Note the surface epithelial changes with adherent rod-shaped bacteria.

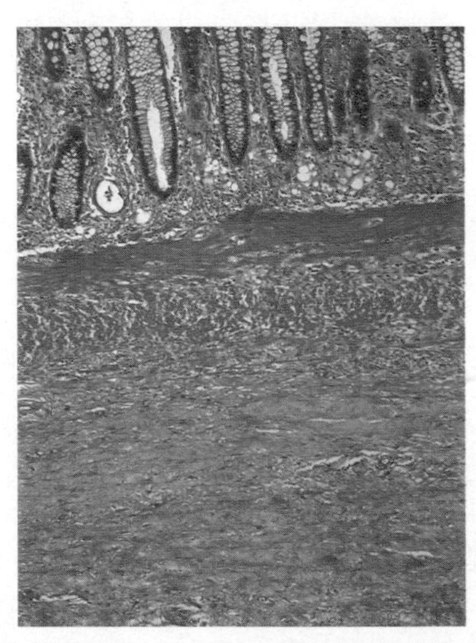

Figure 79.16: Biopsy specimen from patient with Hirschsprung's disease illustrating an absence of ganglion cells associated with marked hypertrophy of the muscularis mucosae.

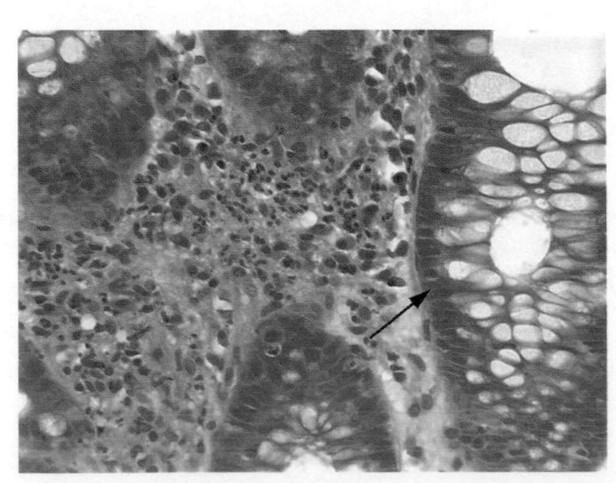

Figure 79.14: Infectious-type focal active colitis pattern of injury from patient with culture-proved *E. coli* O157:H7 infection. Sections show a collection of lamina proprial neutrophils adjacent to a relatively normal colonic crypt (arrow)

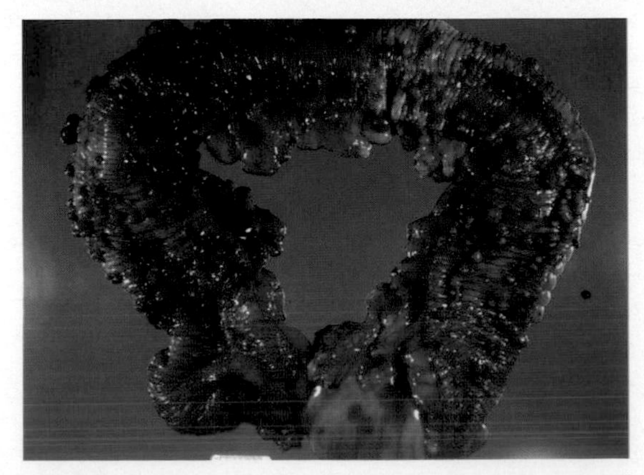

Figure 79.17: Resected colonic resection specimen from familial adenomatous polyposis.

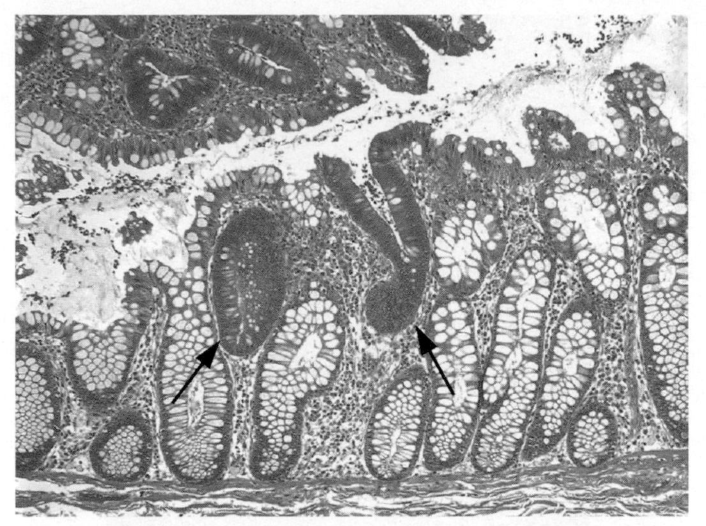

Figure 79.18: Familial adenomatous polyposis. Sections show tubular adenomas including one gland adenomas (arrow) typical for the syndrome.

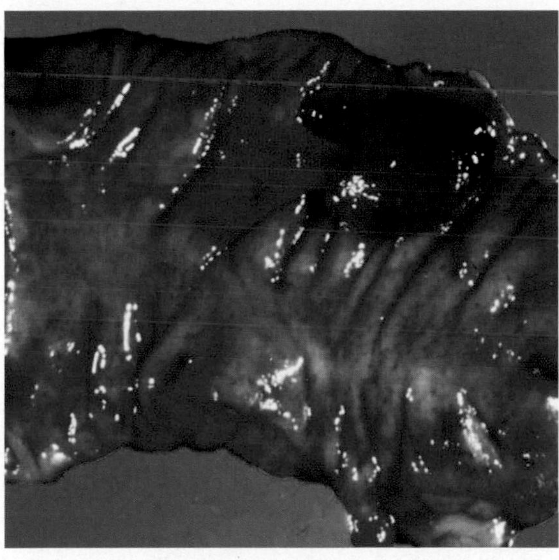

Figure 79.19: Resected colonic juvenile polyp. Note the spherical red polyp attached by an elongate pedicle.

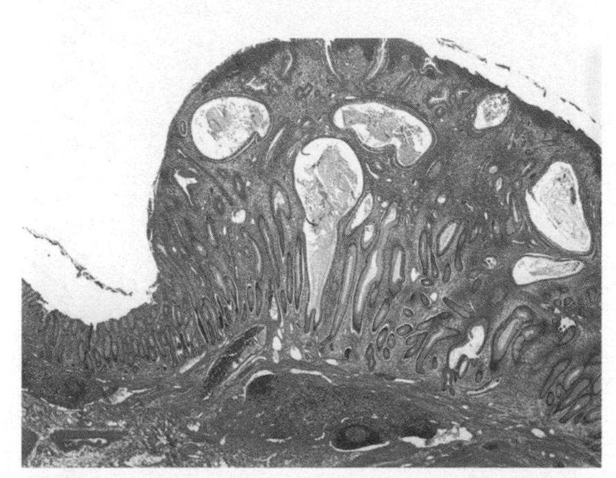

Figure 79.20: Juvenile polyp demonstrating edematous and inflammatory expansion of the lamina propria with colonic mucosal epithelial microcyst formation.

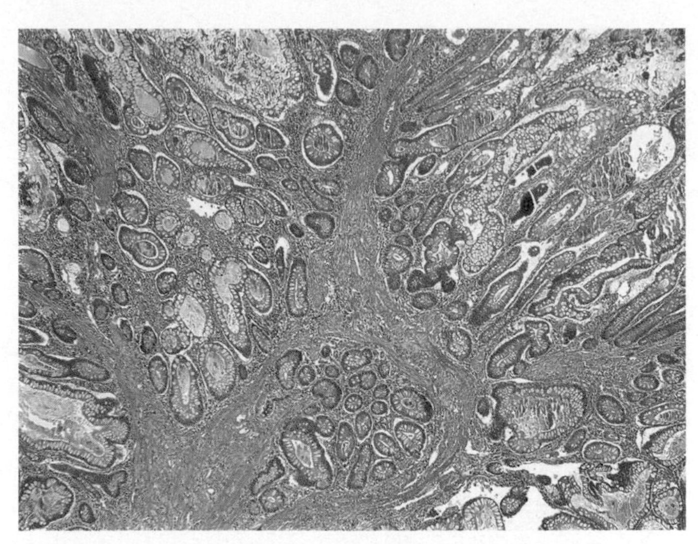

Figure 79.21: Peutz–Jeghers polyp composed of fairly normal epithelium and lamina propria lining an abnormal arborizing overgrowth of the smooth muscle of the muscularis mucosae.

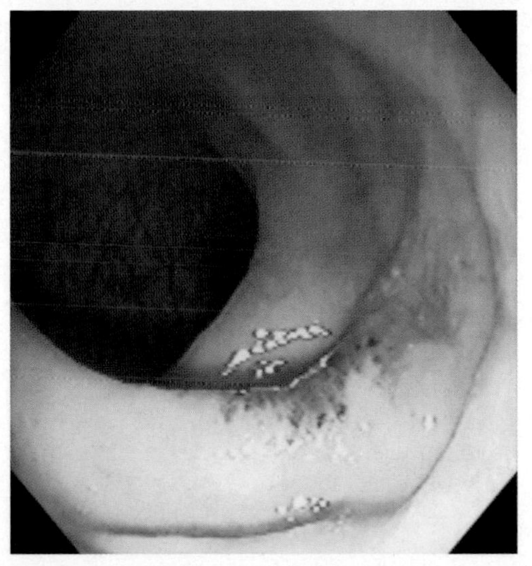

Figure 81.1: Endoscopic appearance of the rectum in a patient with mucosal prolapse. Note localized friability due to repetitive prolapse with an otherwise normal mucosal appearance.

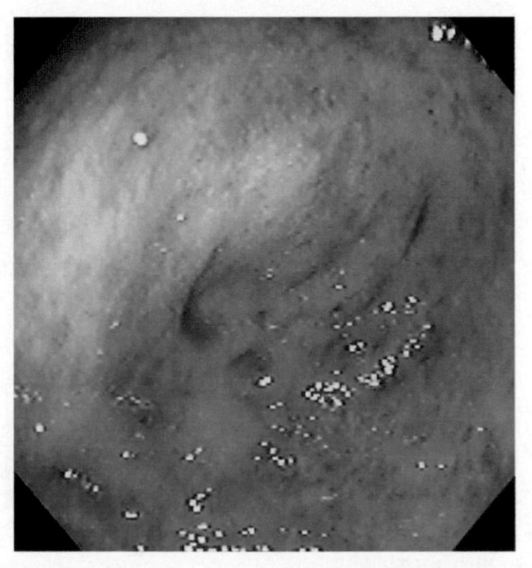

Figure 81.4: Typical appearance of the appendiceal orifice at colonoscopy.

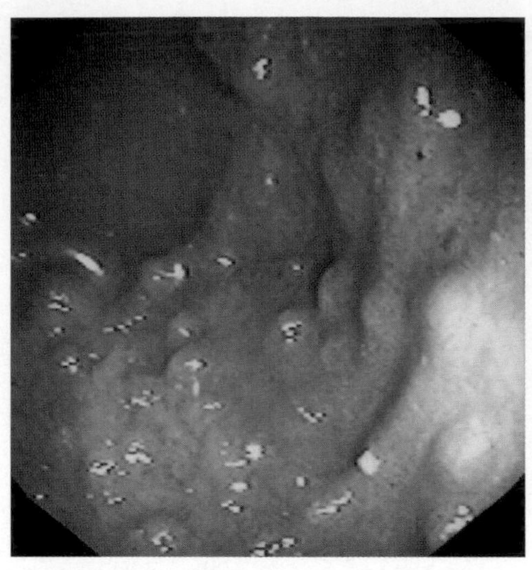

Figure 81.5: Lymphonodular hyperplasia of the terminal ileum. Note glistening mucosa and nodularity without erosions, which is characteristic.

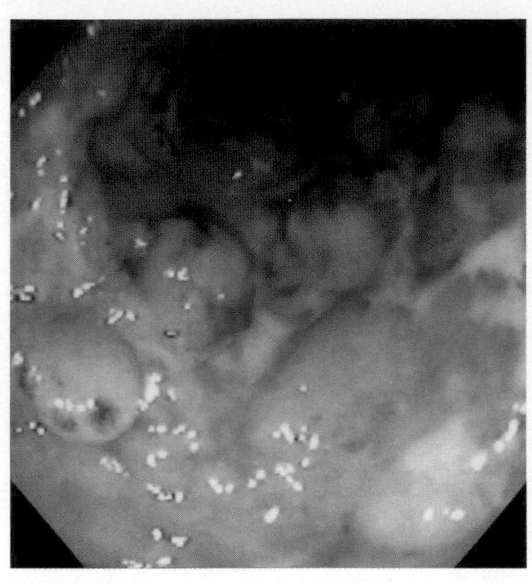

Figure 81.19: Endoscopic appearance of Crohn's colitis involving the transverse colon. Note marked nodularity, mucosal erosions and overlying exudate in contrast to the appearance in Figure 81.16.

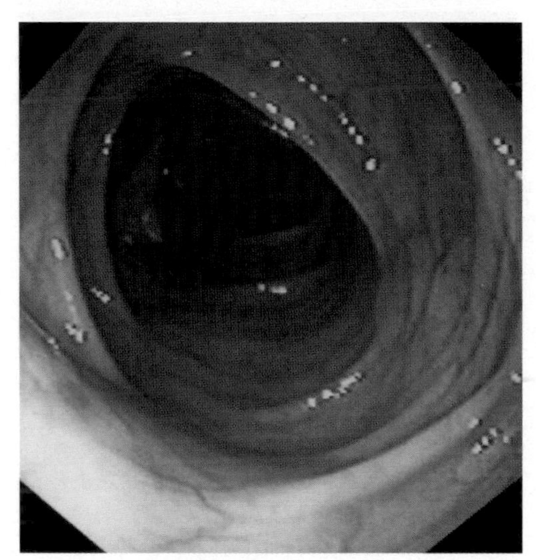

Figure 81.16: Normal colonic mucosal appearance of the transverse colon. Triangular shape of the folds is typical of this area.

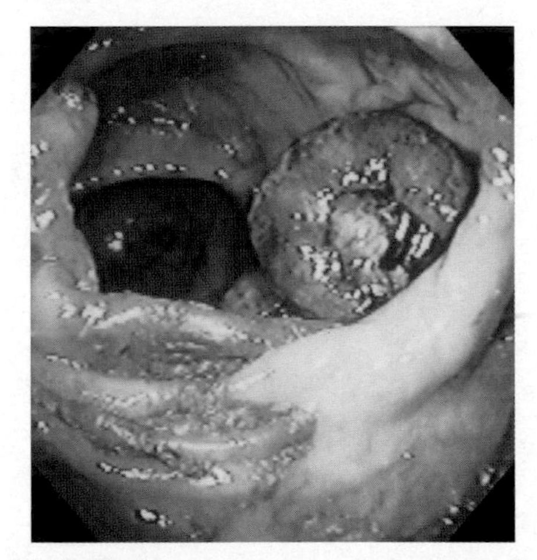

Figure 81.25: Head of a resected and coagulated juvenile polyp. Note the whitish area in the center of the polyp representing the area of coagulation.

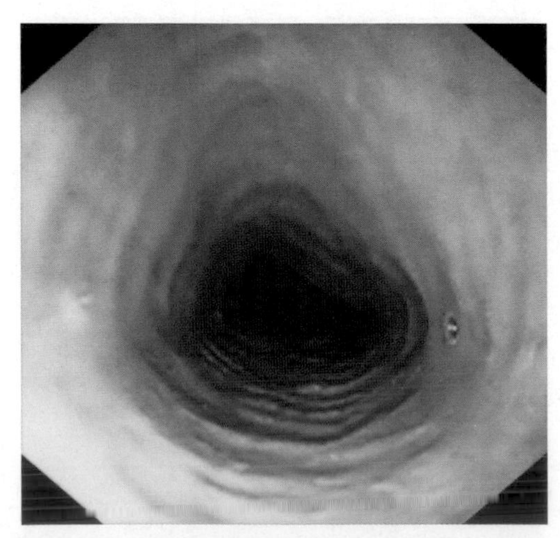

Figure 81.18: Rings of the proximal and mid-esophagus in a patient with eosinophilic esophagitis.

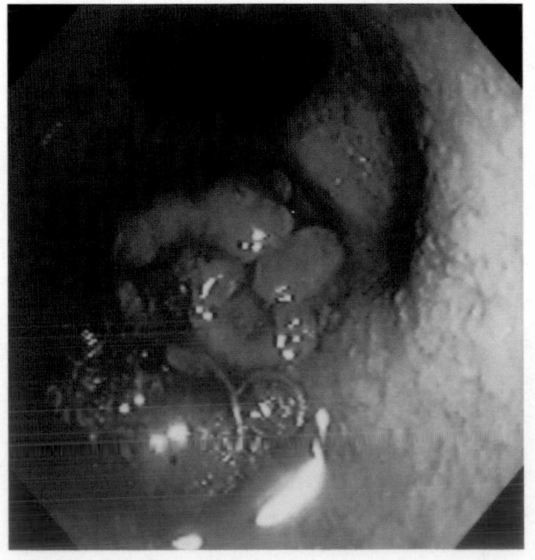

Figure 81.2[illegible]: Large right sided sessile polyp in a patient with long-standing Crohn's disease.

SECTION ONE
BIOLOGIC ASPECTS OF GASTROINTESTINAL FUNCTION

Chapter 1
Development of the gastrointestinal tract

Robert K. Montgomery and Richard J. Grand

Organogenesis of the human gastrointestinal tract and liver is essentially complete by 12 weeks of gestation. At 4 weeks, the gastrointestinal tract is a straight tube, with identifiable organ primordia. Subsequently, the intestine elongates and begins to form a loop, which protrudes into the umbilical cord. By a process of growth and rotation during the following weeks, the intestine increases in length and turns through 270°, then retracts into the abdominal cavity. The crypt–villus structure is established during this process, as well as the patterns of expression of digestive enzymes and transporters. The intestine elongates approximately 1000-fold from the 5th to the 40th week of gestation, so that at birth the small intestine is approximately three times the crown–heel length of the infant. A number of the critical genetic regulators of morphogenesis of the gastrointestinal tract have been identified and their mechanisms of action are being elucidated.

MORPHOGENESIS

Proliferation of cells from the fertilized egg gives rise to the blastocyst. The embryo will develop from a compact mass of cells on one side of the blastocyst, called the inner cell mass. It splits into two layers, the epiblast and hypoblast, which form a bilaminar germ disk from which the embryo develops. At the beginning of the third week of gestation, the primitive streak appears as a midline depression in the epiblast near the caudal end of the disk. During gastrulation, epiblast cells detach along the primitive streak and migrate down into the space between the two germ layers.

The process of gastrulation generates the endoderm cells that will form the epithelia lining the gastrointestinal tract. Some of the cells migrating inward through the primitive streak displace the lower germ layer (hypoblast) and form the definitive endoderm. Gastrulation establishes the bilateral symmetry and the dorsal–ventral and craniocaudal axes of the embryo. Formation of the three germ layers brings into proximity groups of cells that then initiate inductive interactions and give rise to the organs of the embryo. As described below, the molecular mechanisms of many of these processes are now being elucidated.

The gut tube is formed by growth and folding of the embryo. The tissue layers formed during the third week differentiate to form primordia of the major organ systems. A complex process of folding, driven by differential growth of different parts of the embryo, converts the flat germ disk into a three-dimensional structure. As a result, the cephalic, lateral and caudal edges of the germ disk are brought together along the ventral midline, where the endoderm, mesoderm and ectoderm layers fuse to the corresponding layer on the opposite side. Thus, the flat endodermal layer is converted into the gut tube (Fig. 1.1).

Folding of the embryo forms a closed gut tube at both cranial and caudal ends. The anterior and posterior ends of the developing gut tube where the infolding occurs are designated the anterior and posterior (or caudal) intestinal portals. Initially, the gut consists of blind-ending cranial and caudal tubes – the foregut and hindgut – separated by the future midgut, which remains open to the yolk sac. As the lateral edges continue to fuse along the ventral midline, the midgut is progressively converted into a tube, while the yolk sac neck is reduced to the vitelline duct (Fig. 1.2).

Three pairs of major arteries develop caudal to the diaphragm to supply regions of the developing abdominal gut. The regions of vascularization from these three arteries provide the anatomic basis for dividing the abdominal gastrointestinal tract into foregut, midgut and hindgut. The celiac artery is the most superior of the three. It develops branches that vascularize the foregut from the abdominal esophagus to the descending segment of the duodenum, as well as the liver, gallbladder and pancreas, which are derived from the foregut. The superior mesenteric artery supplies the developing midgut, the intestine from the descending segment of the duodenum to the transverse colon. The inferior mesenteric artery vascularizes the hindgut – the distal portion of the transverse colon, the descending and sigmoid colon, and the rectum. The sepa-

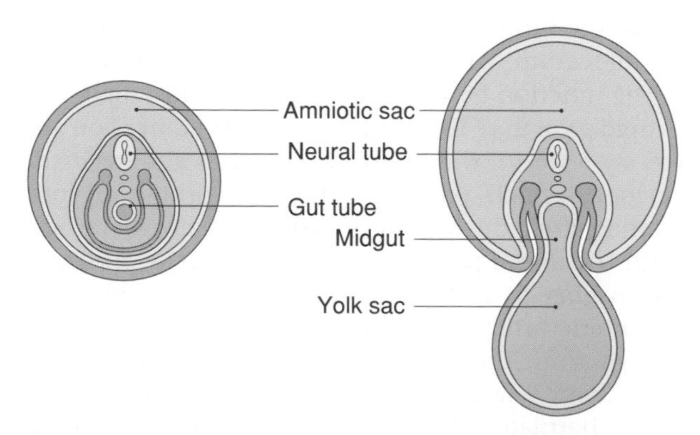

Figure 1.1: Folding forms a closed gut tube at both cranial and caudal ends of the growing embryo. The midgut remains open, but is progressively reduced to the vitelline duct, which remains connected to the yolk sac. (Reproduced from Unit 35, Undergraduate Teaching Project of the American Gastroenterological Association, by permission of Milner-Fenwick, Inc.)

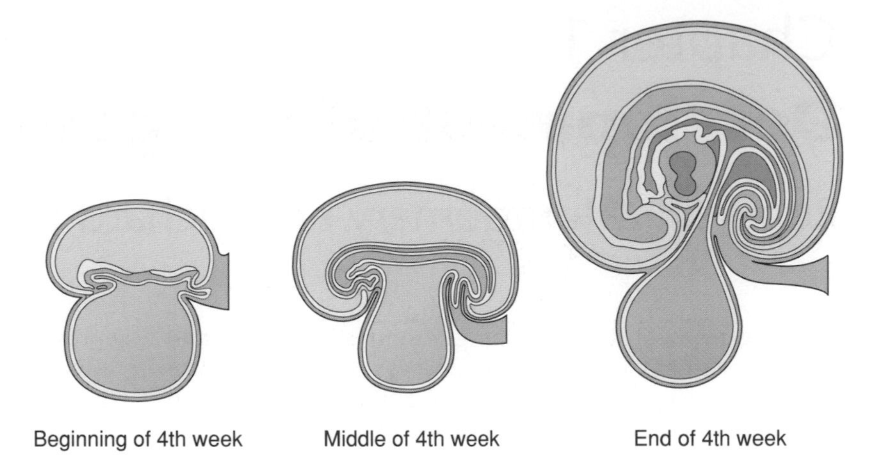

Figure 1.2: Growth and folding of the embryo form the gut tube – sagittal sections through embryos. (Reproduced from Unit 35, Undergraduate Teaching Project of the American Gastroenterological Association, by permission of Milner-Fenwick, Inc.)

rately derived inferior end of the anorectal canal is supplied by branches of the iliac arteries.

During the early part of the fourth week, the caudal foregut just posterior to the septum transversum expands slightly to initiate formation of the stomach. Continued expansion gives rise to a spindle-shaped or fusiform region. The dorsal wall of this fusiform expansion of the foregut grows more rapidly than the ventral wall, producing the greater curvature of the stomach during the fifth week. The fundus of the stomach is formed by continued differential expansion of the superior portion of the greater curvature. A rotation of 90° around a craniocaudal axis during the seventh and eighth weeks makes the original left side the ventral surface and the original right side the dorsal surface of the fetal stomach. Thus, the left vagus nerve supplies the ventral wall of the adult stomach and the right vagus innervates the dorsal wall. Additional rotation about a dorsal–ventral axis results in the greater curvature facing slightly caudal and the lesser curvature slightly cranial.

By about the third week of gestation, the gut is a relatively straight tube demarcated into three regions: the foregut, which will give rise to the pharynx, esophagus, stomach and proximal duodenum; the midgut, which is open ventrally into the yolk sac and will produce the remainder of the duodenum, small intestine and proximal colon; and the hindgut, which will develop into the distal colon and rectum. The hepatic and pancreatic anlagen arise at the junction between the foregut and midgut.

The rapid growth of the midgut causes its elongation and rotation. By 5 weeks, the intestine elongates and begins to form a loop, which protrudes into the umbilical cord. Shortly thereafter, the ventral pancreatic bud rotates and fuses with the dorsal pancreatic bud. At 7 weeks, the small intestine begins to rotate around the axis of the superior mesenteric artery, moving counterclockwise (viewing the embryo from the ventral surface) approximately 90° (Fig. 1.3). From 9 weeks onward, growth of the intestine forces it to herniate into the umbilical cord. The midgut continues to rotate as it grows, then returns to the abdominal cavity. By about 10 weeks, rotation has completed approximately 180°. By about 11 weeks, rotation has continued an additional 90° to complete 270°, and then the intestine retracts into the abdominal cavity, which has gained in capacity not only by growth, but by regression of the mesonephros and reduced hepatic growth (Fig. 1.4). The control of re-entry has not been elucidated, but it occurs rapidly, with the jejunum returning first and filling the left half of the abdominal cavity, and the ileum filling the right half. The colon enters last, with fixation of the cecum close to the iliac crest and the upward slanting of the ascending and transverse colon across the abdomen to the splenic flexure. Later growth of the colon leads to elongation and establishment of the hepatic flexure and transverse colon. The position of the abdominal organs is completed as the ascending colon attaches to the posterior abdominal wall. By 12 weeks of gestation, this process is completed (Fig. 1.5).

Small intestinal villus and crypt formation occurs through a process of epithelial and mesenchymal reorganization, in a proximal to distal progression. Morphologic

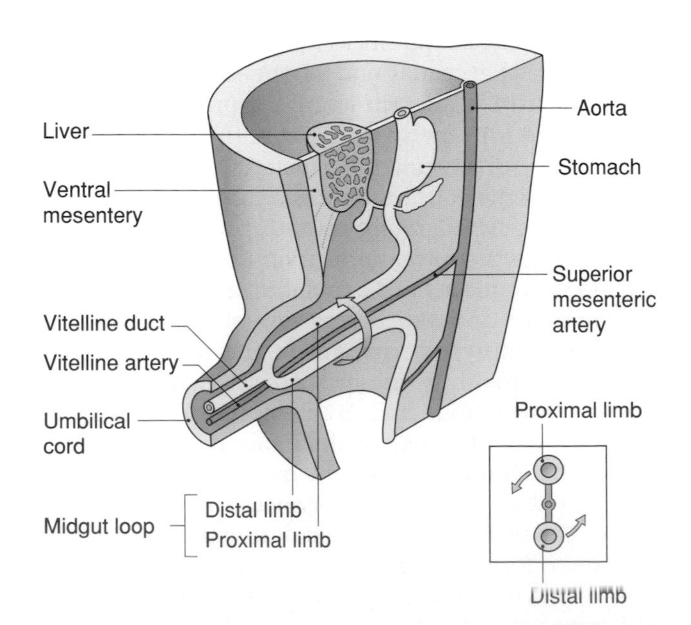

Figure 1.3: Rapid growth of the midgut causes its elongation and rotation. (Reproduced from Unit 35, Undergraduate Teaching Project of the American Gastroenterological Association, by permission of Milner-Fenwick, Inc.)

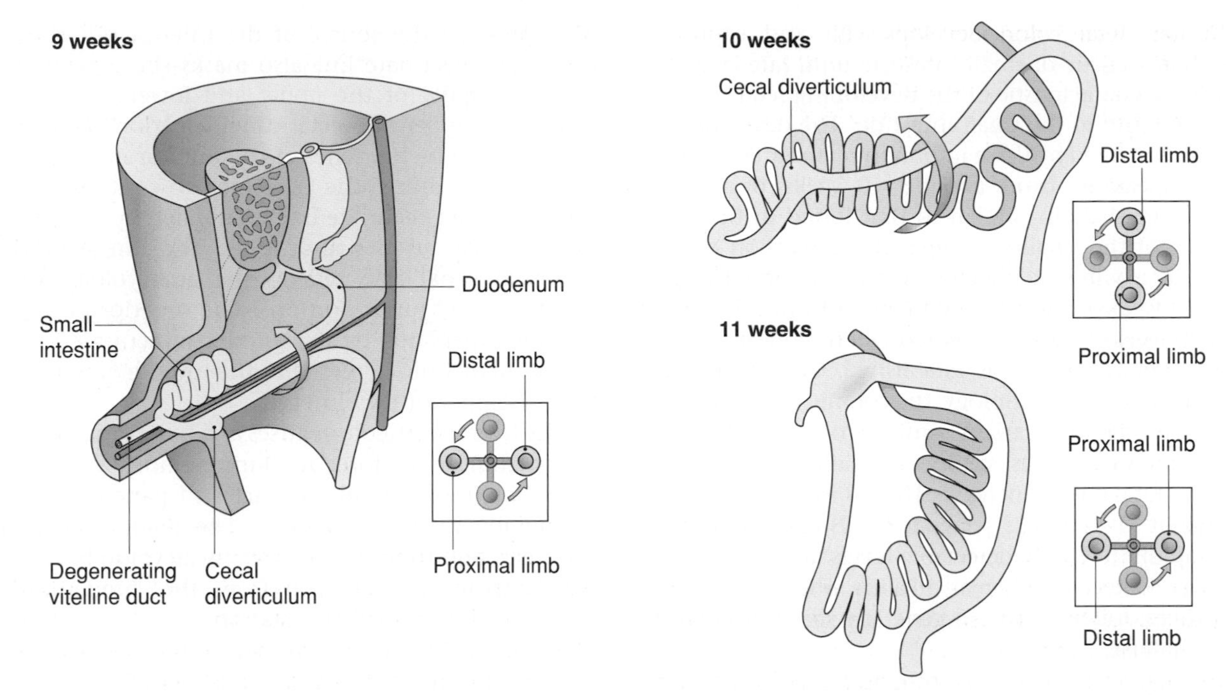

Figure 1.4: The growing midgut continues to rotate and returns to the abdominal cavity. (Reproduced from Unit 35, Undergraduate Teaching Project of the American Gastroenterological Association, by permission of Milner-Fenwick, Inc.)

analysis of human fetal small intestine by scanning electron microscopy demonstrates the first appearance of villi as rounded projections during the eighth week. The stratified epithelium is converted to a single layer of columnar epithelium through a process of secondary lumina formation and mesenchymal upgrowth. By 12 weeks, crypts with a narrow lumen lined with simple columnar cells are present. Between the 10th and 14th weeks the villi increase in height and develop a more finger-like appearance. The microvilli become more regular and more dense on the apical surface of the enterocytes over this same period. Between 17 and 20 weeks, the first indications of muscularis mucosa develop near the base of the crypts.

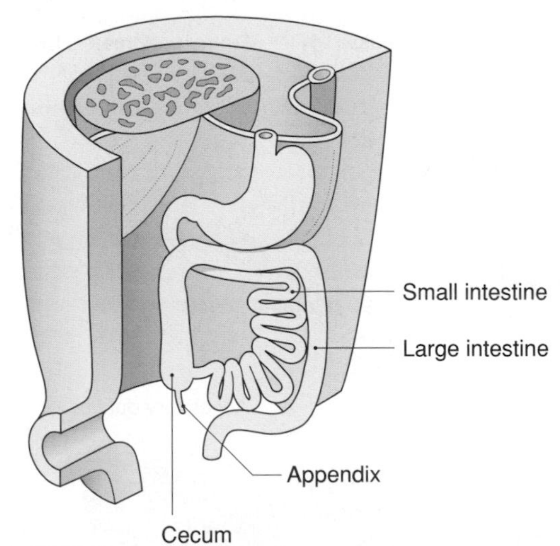

Figure 1.5: The position of the abdominal organs is completed as the ascending colon attaches to the posterior abdominal wall. (Reproduced from Unit 35, Undergraduate Teaching Project of the American Gastroenterological Association, by permission of Milner-Fenwick, Inc.)

Most small intestinal microvillus enzymes begin to appear at 8 weeks. Enzyme analysis of fetal human intestine has detected activities of sucrase, maltase, alkaline phosphatase and aminopeptidase at 8 weeks of gestation, essentially simultaneous with villus morphogenesis. By 14 weeks, activity levels were comparable with those of adult intestine. These observations contrast with those in the well studied rodent models, where enzyme activities are detectable following villus morphogenesis late in gestation, but major changes in levels of activity occur postnatally during weaning. In particular, sucrase in rodents is present only at very low levels until an abrupt upsurge at weaning. In contrast to other hydrolases examined, human lactase activity remains low until nearly the end of gestation, when it rises abruptly. This has been suggested to be a potential problem for premature infants, but the ability of premature infants to digest milk lactose is potentiated by bacterial fermentation in the colon of unabsorbed lactose and absorption of resultant short-chain fatty acids. Microvillus membrane enzymes demonstrate proximal to distal gradients as early as 17 weeks' gestation. The topographic distribution of lactase activity is known to be regulated genetically. In all mammals studied, maximal activity is in the mid-jejunum, with activity levels declining proximally and distally. Even at 17 weeks, lactase activity demonstrates this pattern, which is maintained throughout life.

The human fetal colon develops villi and expresses enzymes characteristic of small intestine until late in gestation. A striking characteristic of the developing fetal colon is its initial similarity to the small intestine. The development of the colon is marked by three important cytodifferentiative stages: the appearance (from about 8–10 weeks) of a primitive stratified epithelium, similar to that found in the early development of the small intestine; the conversion of this epithelium to a villus architecture with developing crypts (about 12–14 weeks); and the remodeling of the epithelium at around 30 weeks of gestation when villi disappear and the adult-type crypt epithelium is established. Consistent with the presence of villus morphology, the colonic epithelial cells express differentiation markers similar to those in small intestinal enterocytes. Thus, sucrase–isomaltase is detectable at 8 weeks in fetal colon, increases 10-fold as villus architecture emerges at 11–12 weeks, peaks at 20–28 weeks, and then decreases rapidly to barely detectable levels at term. Lactase has not been detected, whereas alkaline phosphatase and aminopeptidase follow a pattern generally similar to that of sucrase–isomaltase.

The cloaca gives rise to the rectum and urogenital sinus. Early in embryogenesis, the distal hindgut expands to form the cloaca. Between the fourth and sixth weeks, the cloaca is divided into a posterior rectum and anterior primitive urogenital sinus by the growth of the urorectal septum. Thus, the upper and lower parts of the anorectal canal have distinct embryologic origins. The original cloacal membrane is divided by the urorectal septum into an anterior urogenital membrane and a posterior anal membrane. The anal membrane separates the endodermal and ectodermal portions of the anorectal canal. The former location of the anal membrane, which breaks down during the eighth week, is marked by the pectinate line in the adult. The distal hindgut gives rise to the upper two-thirds of the anorectal canal, while the ectodermal invagination called the anal pit represents the source of the inferior one-third of the canal. The pectinate line also marks the separation of the vascular supply of the upper and lower segments of the canal. The upper anorectal canal superior to the pectinate line is served by branches of the inferior mesenteric artery, and veins draining the hindgut. By contrast, the region inferior to the pectinate line is supplied by branches of the internal iliac arteries and veins. The innervation of the anorectal canal also reflects the embryologic origins of the upper and lower portions. The superior portion of the canal is innervated by the inferior mesenteric ganglia and pelvic splanchnic nerves, and the inferior canal is supplied from the inferior rectal nerve.

The liver diverticulum arises as a bud from the most caudal portion of the foregut. During embryogenesis, specification of the liver, biliary tract and pancreas occurs in a temporally regulated pattern. The liver, gallbladder and pancreas, and their ductal systems, develop from endodermal diverticulae that bud from the duodenum in the fourth to sixth weeks of gestation.

At about 30 days of embryogenesis, the pancreas consists of dorsal and ventral buds, which originate from endoderm on opposite sides of the duodenum. The dorsal bud grows more rapidly, whereas the ventral bud grows away from the duodenum on the elongating common bile duct (Fig. 1.6). As the duodenum grows unequally, torsion occurs and the ventral pancreas is brought dorsal so that it lies adjacent to the dorsal pancreas in the dorsal mesentery of the duodenum; the two primordia thus fuse at about the seventh week. The head and uncinate process of the mature pancreas stem from the ventral primordium, whereas the remainder of the body and tail is derived from the dorsal primordium. Subsequently, the ducts originally serving each bud join to form the duct of Wirsung, although the proximal original duct of the dorsal bud often remains as the accessory duct of Santorini.

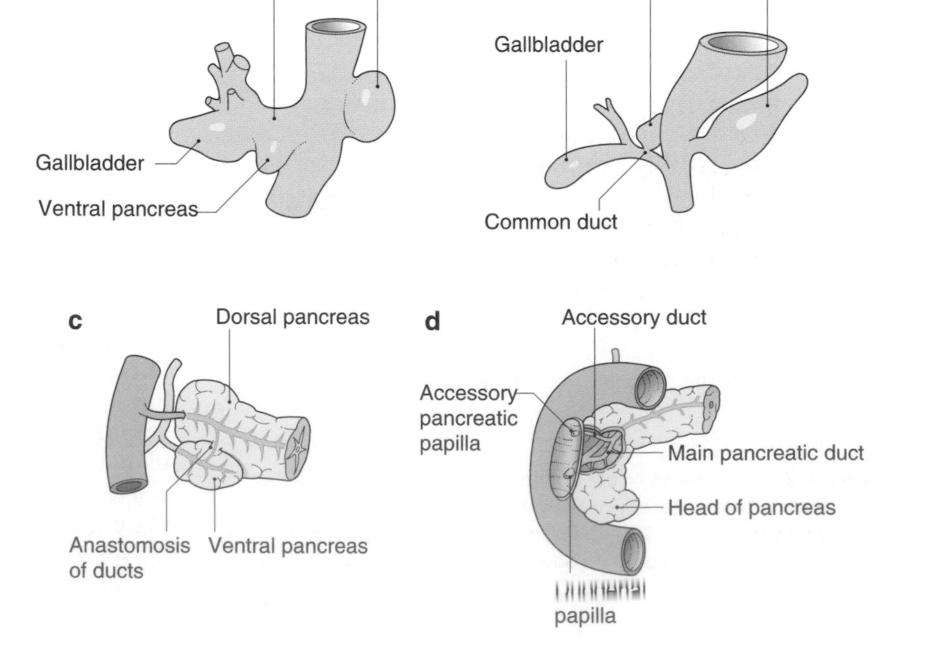

Figure 1.6: Development of the pancreas. (**a**) At 4 weeks, dorsal and ventral buds are formed. (**b**) At 6 weeks, the ventral pancreas extends toward the dorsal pancreas. (**c**) At 7 weeks, fusion of the dorsal and ventral pancreas occurs. (**d**) At 40 weeks, the pancreas is a single organ and ductular anastomosis is complete. (From Sleisenger & Fordtran, 1989, with permission).[29]

The prevertebral sympathetic ganglia develop next to the major branches of the descending aorta. The postganglionic sympathetic axons from these ganglia grow out along the arteries and come to innervate the same tissues that the arteries supply with blood. The postganglionic fibers from the celiac ganglia innervate the distal foregut region from the abdominal esophagus to the entrance of the bile duct into the duodenum. Fibers from the superior mesenteric ganglia innervate the midgut, the remaining duodenum, jejunum, ileum, ascending colon and two-thirds of the transverse colon. The inferior mesenteric ganglia innervate the hindgut, the distal third of the transverse colon, the descending and sigmoid colon, and the upper two-thirds of the anorectal canal.

The vagus nerve and the pelvic splanchnic nerves provide preganglionic parasympathetic innervation to ganglia embedded in the walls of visceral organs. Unlike the sympathetic ganglia, parasympathetic ganglia form close to the organs they innervate and produce only short postganglionic fibers. The central neurons of the parasympathetic pathways reside in either the brain or the spinal cord. Preganglionic parasympathetic fibers associated with cranial nerve X form the vagus nerve, which extends into the abdomen where these fibers synapse with the parasympathetic ganglia in target organs including the liver and the gastrointestinal tract proximal to the colon. Parasympathetic preganglionic fibers arising from the spinal cord form the pelvic splanchnic nerves, which innervate ganglia in the walls of the descending and sigmoid colon and rectum. Neural crest cells that migrate into the developing intestinal tract form a critical component of the enteric nervous system.

Under normal conditions, the human gastrointestinal tract at term exhibits essential structural and functional maturity, although some functions, such as bile salt conjugation, mature postnatally.

MOLECULAR MECHANISMS

Gastrulation, during which the axes of the embryo are determined and formation of the gastrointestinal tract is initiated, is an essential early step in development of all multicellular organisms. Regionalization and development of specialized organs along the gut tube appear early in evolution, suggesting that the mechanisms regulating gut formation are likely to be very early evolutionary developments, and similar in most organisms. Current research suggests that the mechanisms governing these processes are indeed highly conserved throughout evolution. Therefore data from model organisms are directly relevant to human development.

There are three major developmental milestones in the formation of the gastrointestinal tract. First is the initial specification of the endoderm. Second is formation and patterning of the gut tube that establishes the anterior–posterior axis and the boundaries between different organs. Third is the initiation of formation of organs that are outgrowths of the gut tube, such as liver and pancreas. Experiments in model organisms have identified families of genes involved in endoderm specification that are highly conserved in evolution, whereas other genes may be specific to vertebrate gut development. This overview focuses on current understanding of the molecular basis of these major milestones in gastrointestinal development and the roles of the best understood genes.

Specification of the endoderm

Specification of the endoderm can be traced to the earliest stages of embryo formation. Classic experiments demonstrated that explants of chick embryos prior to gastrulation were capable of gastrointestinal development, indicating that their fate had already been specified. Evidence is accumulating in support of the hypothesis that the original patterning of the endoderm is cell autonomous, but that full development of the organs requires a reciprocal interaction between the endoderm and mesoderm. Six gene families that act to specify endoderm have now been identified in a number of model organisms. One class of genes encodes transcription factors that directly activate target genes. A second class encodes signaling molecules that mediate cellular interactions. At least some of the transcription factors involved in specification of the endoderm continue to be expressed in the gastrointestinal tract throughout development, such as the forkhead-related factors (*FOX* genes) and GATA factors. Signaling pathways, such as those mediated by members of the transforming growth factor β (TGF-β) superfamily of growth factors, including TGF-β and the bone morphogenetic proteins (BMPs), and the hedgehog pathways, act at different times and in different locations to regulate gastrointestinal development.

From its earliest stages, the endoderm is in close apposition to mesoderm throughout the gastrointestinal tract. Tissue recombination experiments have shown that patterning of the endoderm and its differentiation into separate organs results from signaling between the mesoderm and the endoderm. The earliest identified step in anterior–posterior patterning in mouse endoderm requires signaling from mesoderm to endoderm by fibroblast growth factor 4 (FGF-4).[1] Other members of the FGF family and their receptors are critical in liver development. Three other important gene families mediating mesoderm–endoderm signaling are sonic hedgehog, the BMPs, and the *hox* genes.

It remains unclear whether a single 'master gene' initiates the formation of the endoderm, setting in motion the process of gastrointestinal development. In some of the model systems, genes have been identified that appear to be both necessary and sufficient to specify endoderm, for example the *mixer* gene in *Xenopus*.[2] In other model organisms, genes have been identified that are necessary, but may not be sufficient.

Two GATA transcription factor genes are essential in specification of the cells that give rise to the intestinal epithelium of *Caenorhabditis elegans*, whereas a *Drosophila* GATA factor is encoded by the gene *serpent*, previously demonstrated to be required for differentiation of gut endoderm. Three members of the GATA family are expressed in vertebrate intestine. Distinct functions for GATA-4, -5 and -6 in intestinal epithelial cell proliferation and differentiation have been suggested, but their role in early development of the mammalian intestine remains unresolved. In addition to the GATA factors, members of the forkhead-related (Fox) family and members of the wnt/Tcf signaling pathway are critical regulators of endoderm formation. Members of the TGF-β superfamily critical in the initiation of endoderm formation have been identified in vertebrates. One of the effector molecules in this pathway, Smad2, has also been shown to be critical for early endoderm formation. A scaffolding molecule important in the TGF pathway, ELF-3, is also required, as null mice lack intestinal endoderm.[3]

Many transcription factors initially identified as liver specific have key roles in the intestine. When analyzed in mouse development, several of these transcription factors have been found to be expressed in patterns, suggesting that they may also regulate intestinal development. For example, hepatic nuclear factor 3β (HNF-3β; now Fox-A2) has been shown to be critical for the earliest differentiation of the gastrointestinal tract and continues to be expressed in the adult progeny of the endoderm.[4] Homozygous null mutants of HNF-3β do not form a normal primitive streak that gives rise to the gut tube and other structures. HNF-3β is critical to formation of the foregut and midgut, but not the hindgut.[5] Multiple members of this family have been identified, some of which display intestine-enriched or intestine-specific expression. One of the family members, normally expressed in the intestinal mesoderm, is a critical mediator of epithelial–mesenchymal interactions. Its elimination led to abnormal epithelial cell proliferation and aberrant intestinal development.[6] Thus, it appears likely that during intestinal development multiple members of the Fox family interact in a complex mechanism, which remains to be elucidated.

Several mouse homeobox genes related to *Drosophila caudal* are expressed specifically in the intestine. One, *Cdx-1*, is restricted to the adult intestine, but is expressed widely in the developing embryo. Another, *Cdx-2*, is expressed in visceral endoderm of the early embryo, but restricted to the intestine at later stages. Forced expression of *Cdx-2* induces differentiation in an intestinal cell line that does not normally differentiate.[7] *Cdx-2* is clearly a critical intestine-specific differentiation factor, but its role in early development of the intestine remains unclear.

Formation of the gut tube

The gut tube is formed from a layer of endoderm by a process of folding that begins at the anterior and posterior ends of the embryo. Reciprocal signaling between endoderm and mesoderm continues to be critical to the developmental process.

A key mechanism that has emerged as a mediator of endoderm–mesoderm interactions in the organization of the gastrointestinal tract involves the sonic (Shh) and Indian hedgehog (Ihh) signaling proteins. Both Shh and Ihh play critical roles in anterior–posterior patterning and concentric patterning of the developing gastrointestinal tract, at least in part through their role in development of muscle from the mesoderm.[8] One target of this signaling pathway is a second family of signaling molecules, the BMPs, members of the TGF-β superfamily.[9,10]

Shh is first detectable in the primitive endoderm of the embryo, later in the endoderm of the anterior and posterior intestinal portals, and subsequently throughout the gut endoderm and in the adult crypt region. *Bmp4* is expressed in the mesoderm adjacent to the intestinal portals and can be induced ectopically in the visceral mesoderm by Shh protein. The endoderm of the intestinal portals is the source of Shh; the portal regions can act as polarizing centers if transplanted. Shh also induces the expression of *hox* genes. Producing abnormal epithelial cell proliferation later in development, Shh likely has its effect through reduced expression of *Bmp2* and *Bmp4*. Shh is a critical regulator of both foregut and hindgut development, as null mice display foregut anomalies such as esophageal atresia and tracheo-esophageal fistula, and hindgut anomalies such as persistent cloaca.[11]

Organ development

Patterning

In *Drosophila*, the large family of homeotic genes is expressed in the body in a precise anterior to posterior order. The homeotic genes encode transcription factors, incorporating a conserved homeobox sequence, which regulate segmentation and pattern formation. Vertebrates have homologous *hox* genes, which play important roles in the formation of distinctly delineated regions of the brain and skeleton. There are four copies of the set of vertebrate genes, *hoxa–d*, which form groups of paralogs, e.g. *hoxa-1*, *hoxb-1* and *hoxd-1*. Within each group, the genes are expressed in the embryo in an anterior to posterior sequence of regions with overlapping boundaries, for example *hoxa-1* in the occipital vertebrae to *hoxa-11* in the caudal vertebrae.

A detailed study of the developing chick hindgut demonstrated a correlation between the boundaries of expression of *hoxa-9*, *-10*, *-11* and *-13* in the mesoderm and the location of morphologic boundaries. Regional differences in expression of homeobox genes in the developing mouse intestine have also been demonstrated.[12] Interference with the expression of specific *hox* genes produces organ-specific gastrointestinal defects. Disruption of *hoxc-4* gave rise to esophageal obstruction due to abnormal epithelial cell proliferation and abnormal muscle development. Alteration of the expression pattern of *hox3.1* (now *hoxc-8*) to a more anterior location caused distorted development of the gastric epithelium. Loss of mesenchymal *hoxa-5* alters gastric epithelial cell phenotype.[13] Mice with disrupted *hoxd-12* and *hoxd-13* genes display defects in formation of the anal musculature. Expression of the human homologs of a number of homeobox genes has also been shown to be region specific.[14] These data indicate that the *hox* genes are critical early regulators of proximal to distal organ specific patterning. Ectopic expression of hox genes in chicken has suggested that the morphology of the intestine may be altered.[9,10] The *caudal* genes are members of a divergent homeobox gene family and regulate the anterior margins of *hox* gene expression as well as having gastrointestinal-specific roles. Almost all of the *hox* genes analyzed are expressed in mesodermal tissue, likely affecting endodermal development via epithelial–mesenchymal interactions.[15]

Regional specification

Organs such as the stomach are first identifiable by thickening in the mesodermal layer. Early in the process of patterning, *Bmp4* is expressed throughout the mesoderm. Sonic hedgehog is expressed in the endoderm and is an upstream regulator of *Bmp4*. The patterning of *Bmp4* expression in the mesoderm regulates growth of the stomach mesoderm and determines the sidedness of the stomach. Location of the pyloric sphincter is dependent upon the interaction of *Bmp4* expression and inhibitors of that expression.[16] Patterning of the concentric muscle layer structure is dependent upon Shh signaling that induces formation of lamina propria and submucosa, while inhibiting smooth muscle and enteric neuron development near the endoderm.[8,17]

Indirect analysis indicates that the small intestinal crypts contain the stem cells of the small intestine. Despite many years of effort, the exact location and specific markers for the stem cell remain unknown. Studies of mouse development suggest that expression of the gene *Musashi-1* may mark the stem cell or a larger progenitor cell compartment.[18,19] Knockout of Tcf-4, a component of the wnt signaling pathway, results in a loss of proliferating cells, suggesting that wnt signaling is critical to the maintenance of the stem cell compartment, in addition to regulating cell proliferation.[20,21] Recent evidence suggests that the location of crypts, likely reflecting the location of the stem cells, is determined by a gradient of BMP.[17]

Development of organs from outgrowths

Liver The liver diverticulum emerges from the most caudal portion of the foregut just distal to the stomach. It is first detectable as a thickening in the endoderm of the ventral duodenum. Hepatogenesis is initiated through an instructive induction of ventral foregut endoderm by cardiac mesoderm. A series of elegant experiments have identified a number of signaling pathways involved in the complex process of development of the liver. The immediate signal is provided by fibroblast growth factors from the cardiac mesoderm that bind to specific receptors in the endoderm.[22] The appearance of messenger RNA for the liver-specific protein albumin in endodermal cells of the liver diverticulum is one of the earliest indications of hepatocyte induction. Endothelial precursor cells provide another critical factor for hepatogenesis, indicating the importance of interaction between blood vessels and the endoderm.[23] After formation of the liver bud, hepatocyte growth factor (HGF) is required for continued hepatocyte proliferation. The hepatic diverticulum grows into the septum transversum and gives rise to the liver cords, which become the hepatocytes. During this process, a combination of signals from the cells of the septum transversum, including BMP, is necessary for liver development.[24]

Pancreas Development of the pancreas has provided one of the classic examples of epithelial–mesenchymal interactions. Previous investigations showed that growth and differentiation of the pancreas required the presence of mesenchyme, although both endocrine and exocrine cells develop from the foregut endoderm. Analysis of the development of separated endoderm and mesenchyme under different conditions indicated that the 'default pathway' of pancreatic differentiation leads to endocrine cells, whereas a combination of extracellular matrix and mesenchymal factors is required for complete organogenesis.[25]

The dorsal pancreatic bud arises in an area where *Shh* expression is repressed by factors from the notochord. Expression of the *pdx-1* gene in cells of the pancreatic bud is one of the earliest signs of pancreas development. The protein was found to be expressed in the epithelium of the duodenum immediately surrounding the pancreatic buds, as well as in the epithelium of the buds themselves. Examination of an initial *pdx-1* knockout mouse indicated that, although development of the rest of the gastrointestinal tract and the rest of the animal was normal, the pancreas did not develop. A second group, which independently made a *pdx-1* null mouse, found that the dorsal pancreas bud did form, but its development was arrested.[26] The defect due to the *pdx* knockout was restricted to the epithelium, as the mesenchymal cells maintained normal developmental potential. In addition, the most proximal part of the duodenum in the null mice was abnormal, forming a vesicle-like structure lined with cuboidal epithelium, rather than villi lined by columnar cells, indicating that *pdx-1* influences the differentiation of cells in an area larger than that which gives rise to the pancreas, consistent with the earlier delineated domain of expression. A case of human congenital pancreatic agenesis has been demonstrated to result from a single nucleotide deletion in the human *pdx-1* gene.[27]

Key regulators of gastrointestinal development have been identified. Some of the genes critical in epithelial–mesenchymal interaction, long known to be a fundamental developmental process, are now known. Analysis of the expression pattern of the *hox* genes suggests that they act to pattern the gastrointestinal tract. The hedgehog proteins mediate several aspects of early development, but inhibition experiments suggest that after organ formation their role is largely complete. Targeted disruption of several genes that regulate intestinal growth indicate that BMP secretion has a key developmental role in cell proliferation, villus morphology and crypt location. Most of the signaling pathways identified are short range. With the exception of epidermal growth factor (EGF), there is little compelling evidence for a critical developmental role for any circulating or luminal growth factor in the development of the intestine.

Microarray analysis of gene expression profiles indicates that the organs of the adult gastrointestinal tract display distinct patterns.[28] Furthermore, the analysis identified some common regulatory elements, including those for HNF-1 and GATA factors, in the 5′ flanking sequences of groups of genes expressed in specific regions, suggesting organ-specific regulation. A combination of work on critical individual genes with examination of cell- and organ-specific developmental gene expression profiles should provide a deeper understanding of the regulation of gastrointestinal development.

Acknowledgment

Supported by grant R37 DK32658 from the National Institutes of Health.

References

1. Wells J, Melton D. Early mouse endoderm is patterned by soluble factors from adjacent germ layers. Development 2000; 127:1563–1572.
2. Henry GL, Melton DA. *Mixer*, a homeobox gene required for endoderm development. Science 1998; 281:91–96.
3. Ng AY, Waring P, Ristevski S, et al. Inactivation of the transcription factor Elf3 in mice results in dysmorphogenesis and altered differentiation of intestinal epithelium. Gastroenterology 2002; 122:1455–1466.
4. Ang SI, Wierda A, Wong D, et al. The formation and maintenance of the definitive endoderm lineage in the mouse: involvement of HNF3/forkhead proteins. Development 1993; 119:1301–1315.
5. Dufort D, Schwartz L, Kendraprasad H, et al. The transcription factor HNF3beta is required in visceral endoderm for normal primitive streak morphogenesis. Development 1998; 125:3015–3025.
6. Kaestner KH, Silberg DG, Traber PG, et al. The mesenchymal winged helix transcription factor Fkh6 is required for the control of gastrointestinal proliferation and differentiation. Genes Dev 1997; 11:1583–1595.
7. Suh E, Traber PG, An intestine-specific homeobox gene regulates proliferation and differentiation. Mol Cell Biol 1996; 16:619–625.
8. Ramalho-Santos M, Melton DA, McMahon AP. Hedgehog signals regulate multiple aspects of gastrointestinal development. Development 2000; 127:2763–2772.
9. Roberts DJ, Johnson Rl, Burke AC, et al. Sonic hedgehog is an endodermal signal inducing *Bmp-4* and *Hox* genes during induction and regionalization of the chick hindgut. Development 1995; 121:3163–3174.
10. Roberts DJ, Smith DM, Goff DJ, et al. Epithelial–mesenchymal signaling during the regionalization of the chick gut. Development 1998; 125:2791–2801.
11. Motoyama J, Liu J, Mo R, et al. Essential function of Gli2 and Gli3 in the formation of lung, trachea and oesophagus. Nat Genet 1998; 20:54–57.
12. Pitera JE, Smith VV, Thorogood P, et al. Coordinated expression of 3′ *hox* genes during murine embryonal gut development: an enteric Hox code. Gastroenterology 1999; 117:1339–1351.
13. Aubin J, Dery U, Lemieux M, et al. Stomach regional specification requires Hoxa5-driven mesenchymal–epithelial signaling. Development 2002; 129: 4075–4087.
14. Walters JR, Howard A, Rumble HE, et al. Differences in expression of homeobox transcription factors in proximal and distal human small intestine. Gastroenterology 1997; 113:472–477.
15. Kawazoe Y, Sekimoto T, Araki M, et al. Region-specific gastrointestinal Hox code during murine embryonal gut development. Dev Growth Differ 2002; 44:77–84.
16. Smith DM, Tabin CJ. BMP signalling specifies the pyloric sphincter. Nature 1999; 402:748–749.
17. Haramis A-PG, Begthel H, van den Born M, et al. *De novo* crypt formation and juvenile polyposis on BMP inhibition in mouse intestine. Science 2004; 303:1684–1686.
18. Potten CS, Booth C, Tudor GL, et al. Identification of a putative intestinal stem cell and early lineage marker; musashi-1. Differentiation 2003; 71:28–41.
19. Kayahara T, Sawada M, Takaishi S, et al. Candidate markers for stem and early progenitor cells, Musashi-1 and Hes1, are expressed in crypt base columnar cells of mouse small intestine. FEBS Lett 2003; 535:131–135.
20. Korinek V, Barker N, Moerer P, et al. Depletion of epithelial stem-cell compartments in the small intestine of mice lacking *Tcf-4*. Nat Genet 1998; 19:379–383.
21. Pinto D, Gregorieff A, Begthel H, et al. Canonical Wnt signals are essential for homeostasis of the intestinal epithelium. Genes Dev 2003; 17:1709–1713.
22. Jung J, Zheng M, Goldfarb M, et al. Initiation of mammalian liver development from endoderm by fibroblast growth factors. Science 1999; 284:1998–2003.
23. Matsumoto K, Yoshitomi H, Rossant J, et al. Liver organogenesis promoted by endothelial cells prior to vascular function. Science 2001; 294:559–563.
24. Zaret KS. Regulatory phases of early liver development: paradigms of organogenesis. Nat Rev Genet 2002; 3:499–512.
25. Gittes GK, Galante PE, Hanahan D, et al. Lineage-specific morphogenesis in the developing pancreas: role of mesenchymal factors. Development 1996; 122:439–447.
26. Offield MF, Jetton Tl, Laboskyl PA, et al. PDX-1 is required for pancreatic outgrowth and differentiation of the rostral duodenum. Development 1996; 122:983–995.
27. Stoffers DA, Zinkin NT, Stanojevic V, et al. Pancreatic agenesis attributable to a single nucleotide deletion in the human *IPF1* gene coding sequence. Nat Genet 1997; 15:106–110.
28. Bates MD, Erwin CR, Sanford LP, et al. Novel genes and functional relationships in the adult mouse gastrointestinal tract identified by microarray analysis. Gastroenterology 2002; 122:1467–1482.
29. Sleisenger MH, Fordtran JS. Gastrointestinal Disease, 4th edn. Philadelphia, PA: WB Saunders, 1989.

Further reading

Grapin-Botton A, Melton DA. Endoderm development: from patterning to organogenesis. Trends Genet 2000; 16:124–130.

Kim SK, Hebrok M. Intercellular signals regulating pancreas development and function. Genes Dev 2001; 15:111–127.

Montgomery RK, Mulberg AE, Grand RJ. Development of the human gastrointestinal tract: twenty years of progress. Gastroenterology 1999; 116:702–731.

Roberts DJ. Molecular mechanisms of development of the gastrointestinal tract. Dev Dyn 2000; 219:109–120.

Shivdasani RA. Molecular regulation of vertebrate early endoderm development. Dev Biol 2002; 249:191–203.

Zaret KS. Molecular genetics of early liver development. Annu Rev Physiol 1996; 58:231–251.

Chapter 2
Basic aspects of digestion and absorption

Ghassan T. Wahbeh and Dennis L. Christie

INTRODUCTION

Through a highly coordinated process, the gastrointestinal tract carries the task of receiving nutrients, processing, digesting and absorbing the breakdown products. In addition to the enteral intake, an even larger cumulative volume of intestinal and secreted fluids, electrolytes, proteins, and bile acids is recycled daily. The efficiency of this system is such that only a minimal fraction of all nutrients is wasted in feces. A complex network of neural and hormonal factors regulates the function of specialized gastrointestinal cells (epithelial, muscular and glandular). An ample surface area is provided for digestion and absorption by virtue of intestinal folding, villi and microvilli. The neonatal gut has distinct physiologic features that evolve to accommodate to a wider array of nutrients as the infant grows. A significant degree of intestinal adaptation to dietary environmental and anatomic changes exists. Nevertheless, an alteration in the physiology of the gastrointestinal system can result in significant morbidity and mortality. Understanding different aspects of digestion and absorption provides a solid base to appreciate how disease states happen and can be managed. Utilizing some of the known concepts of electrolyte absorption, mortality from acute diarrhea has fallen from 5 million to 1.3 million deaths annually with the use of Oral Rehydration Salts.[1] This chapter provides an overview of the basic aspects of digestion and absorption of the major constituents of our diet, which – besides water – include carbohydrates, proteins, fats, nucleic acids, vitamins and minerals.

Carbohydrates

Dietary forms

Carbohydrates account for around 50% of calories in the Western adult diet. The dominant forms of consumed carbohydrates are age variable and include disaccharides, starch (main form of plant carbohydrate storage) and glycogen from animal sources. Some carbohydrates are ingested but poorly digested or absorbed (see Non-digestible carbohydrates, below).

The predominant carbohydrate (CHO) in breast milk and cow milk-based infant formulas is lactose, a disaccharide of glucose and galactose. For many children, lactose consumption in milk continues into adolescence and adulthood. Soy-based formulas as well as hypoallergenic formulas are lactose free and contain corn syrup, starch or sucrose (glucose and fructose). With the introduction of solid food, the amount of consumed starch as amylose and amylopectin increases comprising around 50% of the total adult CHO intake. Amylose (molecular weight 10^6) is a linear polymer of glucose molecules linked by α1,4 bonds, while amylopectin (molecular weight 10^9) contains additional α1,6 bonds that allow for a branched chain form. Most starches contain more amylopectin than amylose. Starch granules vary in size (potato>wheat>rice) and shape. Wheat is a unique form of starch since the carbohydrate component is encased in a protein shell. Such differences account for the variable degrees of digestion and absorption among different types of starch.[2] Food processing and preparation may alter the susceptibility of the molecular bonds in starch to enzymatic digestion.[3,4] Fructose is present in fruits and vegetables as well as soft drinks and processed foods along with corn syrup, oligo- and polysaccharides. Table sugar is sucrose derived from cane or beet. Glycogen contains α1,4 linked glucose molecules. It accounts for a small fraction of total carbohydrate intake. Poorly digestible monosaccharides like lactulose, sorbitol and sucrulose are frequently consumed, the latter two commonly as sweeteners in sugar-free foods. Other 'unavailable' carbohydrates are discussed below.

Luminal digestion

Digestion of starch CHO begins in the oral cavity upon exposure to saliva mainly from the parotid gland, although limited due to the brief exposure time prior to swallowing. Salivary α-amylase is produced in the neonatal period. Although inactivated by gastric acid, some α-amylase activity may be present within the food bolus. Amylase is present in breast milk and plays a more significant role in neonates – especially premature – where pancreatic amylase production is low (Fig. 2.1).[5]

The majority of starch digestion occurs in the duodenum through the effect of pancreatic amylase. This activity is not restricted to the lumen since amylase may adsorb to the enterocyte luminal surface. α-Amylase is an endoenzyme that cleaves the α1,4 internal links in amylose leaving oligosaccharides: maltose (two glucose molecules) and maltriose (three glucose molecules). Since α-amylase does not cleave α1,6 or adjacent α1,4 bonds, digestion of amylopectin also leaves branched oligosaccharides termed α-limit dextrins. Amylase activity produces a small amount of free glucose molecules. Only severe pancreatic insufficiency that leaves less than 10% normal amylase levels affects starch breakdown.[6]

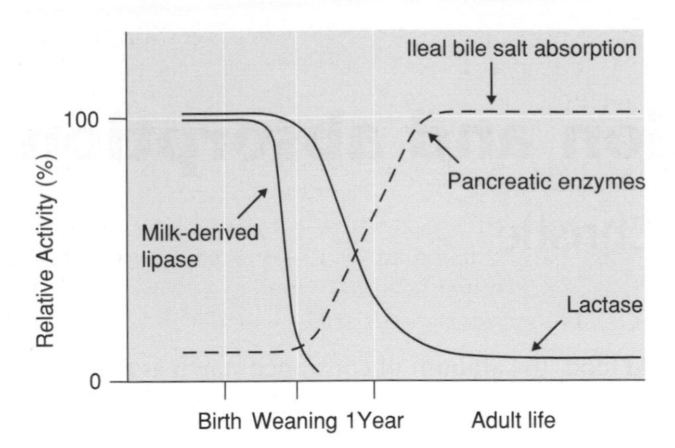

Figure 2.1: Major changes in digestive function in neonates. (From Marsh and Riley, 1998, with permission).[15]

Enzyme	Carbohydrate substrate	Product
Lactase	Lactose	Glucose, galactose
Maltase (Glucoamylase)	Oligosaccharides with α1,4 bonds, 5–9 units long	Glucose
Sucrase	Sucrose	Glucose, fructose
Isomaltase	Branches oligosaccharides with α1,6 links (α limit dextrins)	Glucose
Trehalase	Trehalose	Glucose

Table 2.1 Brush border membrane enzymes in carbohydrate digestion

Brush border digestion

Only monosaccharides can be absorbed across the enterocyte membrane. Therefore, further digestion of the luminal products of starch and ingested disaccharides takes place at the brush border by different membrane hydrolases (Table 2.1). Maltase (glucoamylase) acts on the α1,4 links in oligosaccharides 5–9 glucose molecules long. Isomaltase (aka α-dextrinase) possesses the ability to break α1,6 bonds, acting as a debranching enzyme. It functions in conjunction with sucrase (Fig. 2.2), both having their genetic coding on chromosome 3.[7] Sucrase hydrolyzes a sucrose molecule leaving glucose and fructose. Sucrase-isomaltase complex cleaves its substrate by a ping-pong bibi mechanism (two substrates, two products with only one substrate bound to the catalytic site at one time).[2,8]

Lactase breaks down lactose into glucose and galactose. The human lactase gene is located on the long arm of chromosome 2.[9] Lactose digestion in the premature neonate may be incomplete in the small intestine but partially salvaged through colonic fermentation. Lactase level declines from a peak at birth to less than 10% of the pre-weaning infantile level in childhood as dietary lactose consumption falls (Fig. 2.1).[10] The decline in lactase in other mammals occurs even if weaning is prolonged.[11] In certain human populations where dairy products are consumed into adulthood (e.g. North Europe), lactase activity may persist.[12] This phenotype is inherited as an autosomal recessive trait, with intermediate activity levels in heterozygotes. Thus the aberrant allele in the human population is considered to be the one that leads to persistence of the enzyme, not the deficiency.[13] Trehalase breaks down the disaccharide trehalose present in mushrooms. The significance of having a dedicated enzyme to a sugar that may not be frequently consumed is unclear.

With the exception of lactase, where enzyme activity is the rate-limiting step for digestion, brush border hydrolases are inducible by presence of the substrate. Thus the rate of uptake of carbohydrate monomers is the limiting step for their absorption. Disaccharidases are synthesized in the endoplasmic reticulum of the enterocyte, modified

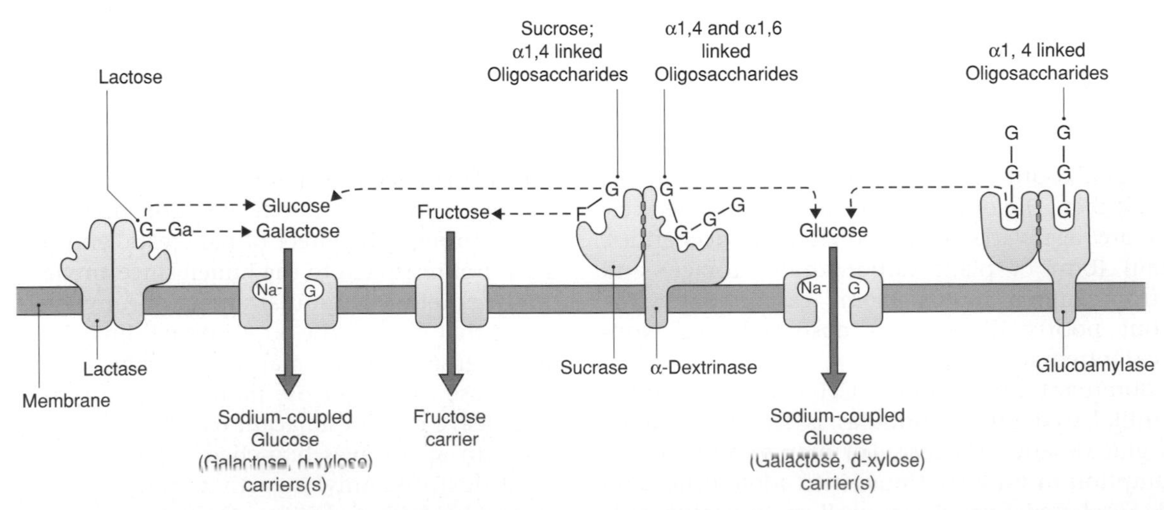

Figure 2.2: Overview of brush border digestion and absorption of carbohydrate. The α1,4 and α1,6 linked oligosaccharides are products of intraluminal amylase digestion of starch. Sucrase-dextrinase and sucrase-isomaltase represent the same enzyme complex. G, glucose; Ga, galactose; F, fructose. (Modified from Van Dyke RW. Mechanisms of digestion and absorption of food. In: Wyllie R and Hyams JS, eds. Paediatric Gastrointestinal Disease, 1st edn. 1999:18, with permission)

in the Golgi apparatus and integrate into the brush border membrane, anchored by a hydrophobic portion in their structure. Pancreatic enzymes play a role in carbohydrases' modification and turnover.[14] The half life of sucrase-isomaltase drops from 20 h during fasting to 4.5 h after meals.[15] Activity of mucosal carbohydrases is maximal in the duodenum and jejunum, decreasing distally along the small intestine.[16] Most carbohydrate digestion is complete by mid-jejunum.

Transport after digestion

Monosaccharides cross the enterocyte apical membrane via carrier mediated transport since their size is too large to allow for significant passive diffusion (Fig. 2.2). For glucose and galactose, co-transport with sodium down a sodium gradient takes place. A gradient is generated when a Na^+, K^+ ATPase pump located in the basolateral membrane exchanges $3Na^+$ out of the enterocyte for 2 K^+ (Fig. 2.3). Activation of the Na^+, glucose transport protein allows water, electrolytes and possibly smaller digested molecules (including glucose and oligopeptides) to pass into the intercellular space through relaxation of the tight junctions.[17,18] Fructose is transported through facilitated diffusion, which allows a faster rate than simple diffusion down its concentration gradient.[19] All monosaccharides exit the enterocyte by facilitated diffusion across the basolateral membrane in to the portal circulation. A small amount of hexoses may be utilized within the cell for metabolism.

Non-digestible carbohydrates

Approximately 10% of ingested starch is not digested in the small intestine. Digestion-resistant starch includes complex molecules that resist amylase activity or are physically inaccessible as in intact grains.[20] Some lactose and fructose may escape complete digestion and pass to the large intestine along with poorly digestible monosaccharides like lactulose, sorbitol and sucrulose. Cellulose and hemicellulose are present in fruit and vegetable structure. Cellulose is a polymer of glucose molecules linked by β1,4 bonds that, unlike α1,4 bonds, resist digestion by α-amylase. Hemicellulose is a polymer of pentose and hexose molecules in straight and chained form. Resistant starches constitute dietary 'fiber' together with non-digestible non-carbohydrate components present in plant cell wall (e.g. phytates, lignins). Non-digestible carbohydrates are fermented by colonic bacteria leaving short chain fatty acids that are readily absorbed and may account for a minute caloric source in healthy state, in addition to possibly having cellular trophic properties.[21] By-products of this process are lactic, acetic, propionic and butyric acids, with methane and hydrogen accounting for flatus. While excessive consumption of non-digestible carbohydrates can result in undesirable gastrointestinal symptoms, dietary fiber offers multiple health benefits.[22]

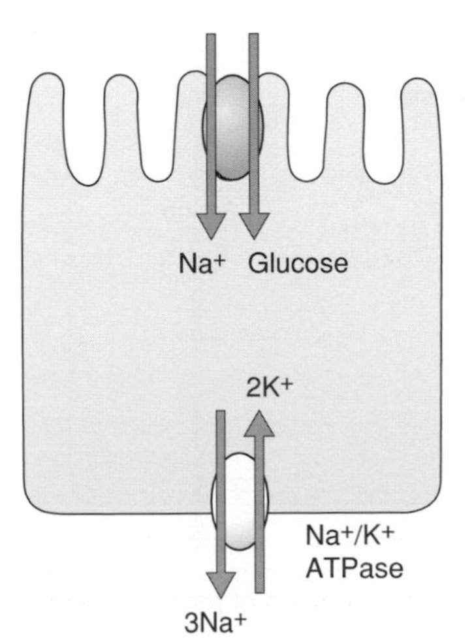

Figure 2.3: Sodium, glucose co-transport.

PROTEINS

Protein sources

Intake of proteins must be accompanied by other calorie sources to prevent the use of amino acids for energy production. In addition to dietary protein, the gastrointestinal tract recycles endogenous proteins in digestive juices and shed epithelial cells amounting up to 65 g daily in adults.[23] The quality of dietary protein relates to its content of essential amino acids (valine, leucine, isoleucine, phenylalanine, lysine, tyrosine, methionine, tryptophan and histidine) that cannot be synthesized in humans. An egg has a high-protein biologic value since it is rich in essential amino acids. Plant proteins are less digestible than animal proteins and contain fewer essential amino acids. Processing of protein (e.g. heat) and co-ingestion with reducing sugars like fructose can alter its molecular structure and affect digestibility.[24,25] Proteins with high proline content (e.g. casein, gluten, collagen and keratin) are incompletely digested by pancreatic proteases.[2,26] Other proteins that escape digestion include secretory IgA and intrinsic factor.[27] In the neonatal period, uptake of whole polypeptide macromolecules occurs possibly by pinocytosis or receptor mediated endocytosis, allowing for passage of such molecules as immunoglobulins in the first 3 months of life.[28]

Luminal digestion

Gastric phase

Digestion of proteins begins in the stomach with exposure to pepsin and hydrochloric acid. In addition to its role in pepsinogen activation, gastric acid denatures protein. Pepsin is secreted by chief cells as pepsinogen. It acts as an endopeptidase, breaking peptide bonds within the polypeptide and leaves shorter polypeptides and a small number of amino acids. Three pepsin isoenzymes have been identified, all optimally active at a pH range of 1–3. The duodenal alkaline medium irreversibly inactivates pepsin. Both pepsin and gastric acid production and secretion are stimulated by gastrin, acetylcholine and histamine.[29] The gastric phase does not seem critical in protein breakdown since patients with decrease acid output and/or gastrectomy do not necessarily lose protein.[30]

Intestinal phase

The main protein digestion site is the proximal small intestine upon exposure to the pancreatic fluid. Unlike amylase, pancreatic proteases are secreted as proenzymes. The presence of food in the duodenum stimulates the influx of bile with contractions of the gallbladder and secretion of pancreatic fluid. Although mediators of pancreatic stimulation are incompletely understood, the cholinergic intestinal system appears to have greater influence than cholecystokinin for pancreozymes, while secretin mainly promotes bicarbonate flow. In response to the presence of bile acids and trypsinogen, enterokinase (enteropeptidase) is released from the brush border cells.[31,32] Enterokinase's only substrate, trypsinogen, is the most abundant proenzyme in pancreatic juices. The subsequent removal of a hexapeptide from the N-terminus of trypsinogen yields the active form, trypsin, which activates the other zymogens as well as its own precursor (Fig. 2.4). Pancreatic proteases are either endo- or exopeptidases depending on the site of the peptide bonds each acts upon (Table 2.2). Endopeptidases cleave peptide bonds within the polypeptide chain while exopeptidases remove a single amino acid from the carboxyl terminal. About 30–40% of the products of this process are amino acids, and 60–70% are oligopeptides up to six peptides long.[33] Endogenous proteins are digested and processed in a similar manner to exogenous proteins.

Pancreatic enzymes also release cobalamine (vitamin B_{12}) from the R protein allowing the former to bind to intrinsic factor. The enzymes may also play a role in gut immunity against microbials[26] and interact in the modification – regulation of different brush border enzymes like disaccharidases. Exposure to trypsin changes pro-colipase to colipase, a key player in the assimilation of fat. Bicarbonate secreted from the pancreas assures an alkaline pH above 5 required for its enzymes optimal function. An over-acidic environment, as seen in Zollinger-Ellison syndrome, deactivates pancreatic enzymes.

Enzyme	Protein substrate
Endopeptidases	
Trypsin	Basic amino acids (lysine, arginine)
	Pancreatic proenzymes
Chymotrypsin	Aromatic amino acids (glutamine, leucine, methionine)
Elastase	Aliphatic (nonpolar) amino acids
Exopeptidases	
Carboxypeptidase A	Aromatic, alipathic amino acids
Carboxypeptidase B	Basic amino acids

Table 2.2. Pancreatic proteases

Brush border and intracellular digestion

Brush border

In contrast to carbohydrates where only monosaccharide units are transported across the enterocyte membrane, small polypeptides are absorbed as such from the lumen (Fig. 2.5), possibly through a more efficient mechanism than that for amino acids (Fig. 2.6).[34–36] Since almost all protein that enters the portal vein is in the form of amino acids, further digestion of the oligopeptides must take place at the brush border level and within the enterocytic cytoplasm. It has been shown in animals with pancreatic insufficiency secondary to pancreatic duct ligation, that nearly 40% of ingested proteins were absorbed.[37]

The brush border peptidases include an array of aminopeptidases, carboxypeptidases, endopeptidases and dipeptidases that are active at neutral pH. They possess a combined ability to digest hexapeptides or smaller chains into amino acids, di- and tripeptides that are actively transported across the luminal enterocyte membrane. Oligopeptidases are predominantly aminopeptidases; removing

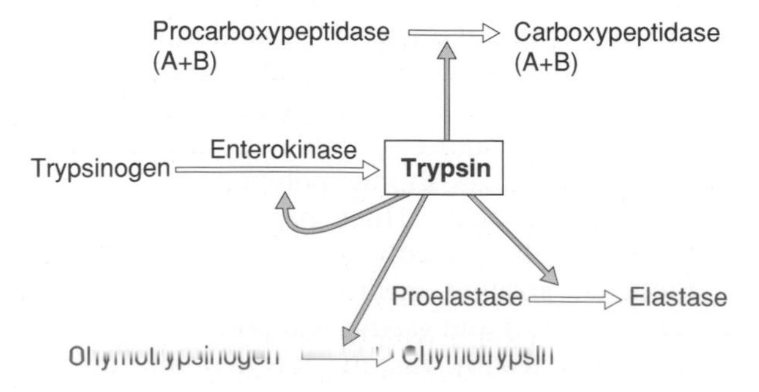

Figure 2.4: Pancreatic enzyme activation.

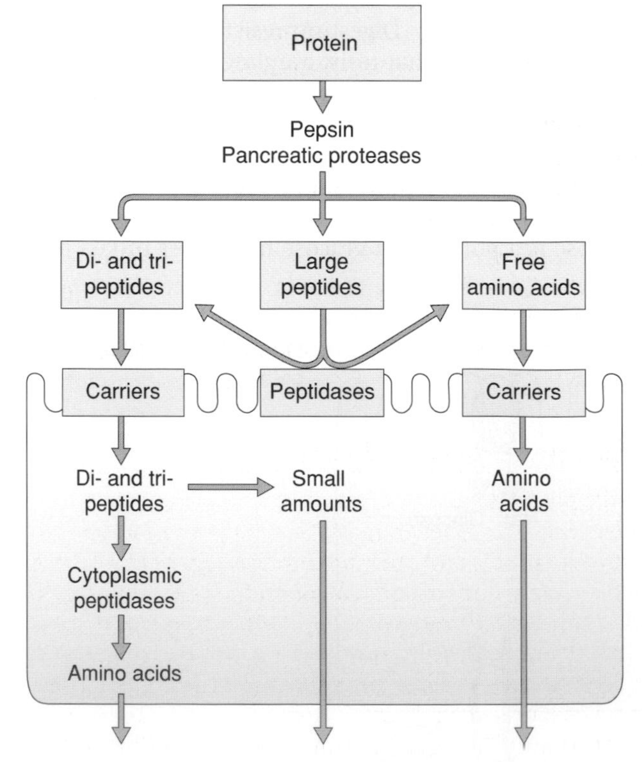

Figure 2.5: Overview of digestion and absorption of protein. (From Johnson, 1997, with permission).

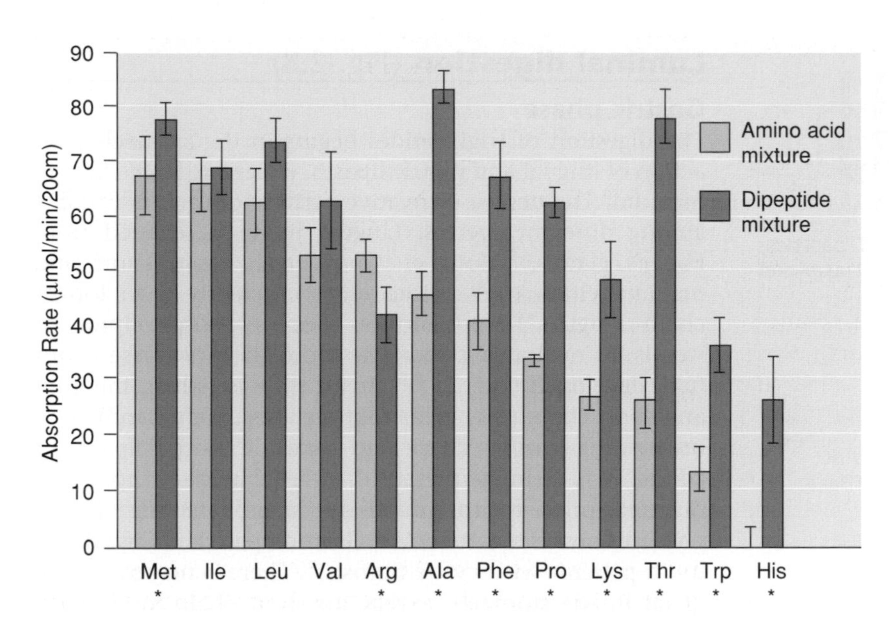

Figure 2.6: Rate of absorption of amino acids from amino acid *vs* dipeptide mixture. An asterisk signifies a statistically significant difference. (Reproduced from Steinhardt HJ, Adibi SA. Kinetics and characteristics of absorption from an equimolar mixture of 12 glycyl-dipeptides in human jejunum. Gastroenterology 1986; 90:579, with permission from the American Gastroenterological Association.)

amino acids from the amino terminus of the peptide. A polypeptide's length determines the rate and the site (brush border versus intracellular) of its assimilation. Synthesis of the brush border peptidases occurs in the rough endoplasmic reticulum with little post-translational enzyme modification within the cell or by pancreatic enzymes at the brush border, in contrast to disaccharidases.[38,39] Mucosal enzymes also include folate conjugase needed to hydrolyze ingested folate, and angiotensin converting enzyme.

Cytoplasm

Cytosol peptide hydrolases differ in structure and electrophoretic mobility from those in the brush borders, and are predominantly di- and tri-peptidases. Further assimilation of small polypeptides into free amino acids takes place in the cytoplasm, however the capacity to digest peptides more than three amino acids long is lacking. Imino-dipeptidase (aka prolidase) is an intracellular hydrolase with specificity to proline containing dipeptides, which resist luminal digestion but pass into the cytoplasm. In contrast to the brush border enzymes, cytosol peptidases are not exclusive to the intestine and are present in other body tissues.

Transport after digestion

Amino acids

Given the rich heterogeneity of amino acid structures, the complex process of transmembrane movement remains incompletely understood. Oligopeptides and amino acids do not compete for transport (Fig. 2.5). Amino acid transport proteins are numerous and group specific for neutral, basic and acidic amino acids with some overlap. A few transport proteins have been extensively studied and characterized.[40,41] Absorption is maximal in the proximal intestine and occurs by active diffusion, Na^+-co-transport and to a lesser extent, simple and facilitated diffusion.[42] The rate of absorption varies for different amino acid groups, being highest for branched chain amino acids.[43] Vasointestinal polypeptide and somatostatin slow these processes down. As noted in glucose transport, activating the cotransport protein may allow paracellular movement of intestinal contents.

Polypeptides

In contrast to amino acids, oligopeptides are carried by a single membrane transporter with a broad substrate specificity. This transporter utilizes an H^+ gradient and is uniform along the small intestines.[44] The human peptide transporter has been cloned.[45] A brush border Na^+, H^+ exchange pump, along with Na^+,K^+ ATPase in the basolateral membrane maintain this confined acidic milieu (Fig. 2.7). Oligopeptide transport into the enterocyte contributes to the lack of specific amino acid deficiency in hereditary disorders of amino acid transport, as seen in Hartnup disease and cystinuria.[46] Both substrates of these carriers are absorbed normally in disease states if presented in the form of small peptides.

Exit from the enterocyte

The movement of amino acids across the basolateral membrane occurs by facilitated and active transport.[47] This is handled by transport proteins different from those in the brush border membrane. In addition to exporting amino acids into the portal circulation, such a transport mechanism takes up amino acids into the enterocyte for use in fasting periods. The basolateral membrane also possesses a peptide transport system similar to the one in the brush border membrane, allowing a small amount of intact peptides to enter the blood stream.[38]

About 10% of the amino acids absorbed into the mucosa are used for enterocyte protein synthesis *in vitro*.[48] Luminal protein sources are more readily used than systemic protein, especially in apical villous cells.[49] It has been shown in animals that exclusive parenteral nutrition can lead to mucosal atrophy.[50]

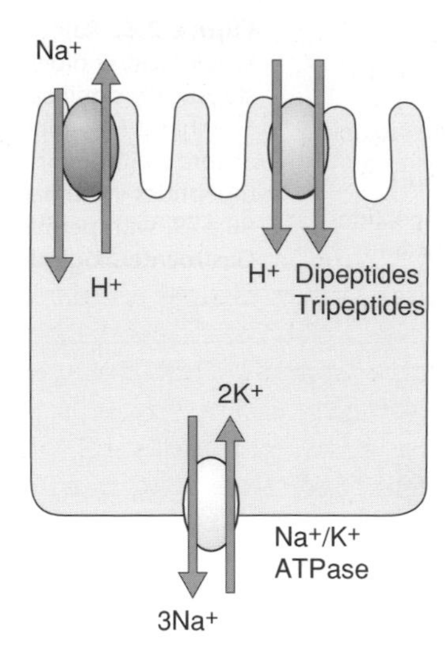

Figure 2.7: Polypeptide-proton cotransport into the enterocyte.

LIPIDS

Dietary forms

Up to 90% of the consumed fat in the average human diet is in the form of trigylcerides, along with phospholipids, plant and animal sterols. In a triglyceride, a backbone of glycerol carries three fatty acids of variable structures. Animal derived triglycerides generally have long chain-saturated fatty acids (more than C14 units), the majority being oleate and palmitate. Plant fatty acids are polyunsaturated and include linoleic and linolenic acids that cannot be synthesized *de novo* in humans and are therefore essential. Medium chain triglycerides have fatty acids with 8–12 carbons. Processing of vegetable fat involves hydrogenation, which increases the melting point, saturates the covalent bonds within the fatty acid and changes double bonds from *cis* to *trans* isomers.[51] A phospholipid is composed of a backbone of lysophosphatidylcholine and one fatty acid. The average adult diet contains 1–2 g of phospholipids, while 10–20 g are secreted daily in bile.[52,53] Phospholipids are also recycled from cell membranes of shed enterocytes. The main dietary phospholipid is phosphatidylcholine (lecithin) and the predominant fatty acids in phospholipids are linoleate and arachidonate. Cholesterol, in animal fat, is the main dietary sterol in the Western diet. Fat-soluble vitamins are discussed later in this chapter.

Lipids are divided into polar and non-polar, depending on the nature of their interactions with water. Triglycerides are insoluble in water and form an unstable layer while the polar phospholipids can shape into a more stable form. This is key to understanding the dynamics of lipid digestion and absorption across the water phase in the intestinal lumen, epithelial membrane lipid phase and later lymphatic and blood water phase. To provide a better exposed, more stable enzyme substrate, ingested lipids are mechanically and enzymatically broken down to smaller units, then appropriately coated with such hydrophilic molecules as phospholipids and bile salts to cross through different aqueous phases.

Luminal digestion (Fig. 2.8)

Gastric phase

The digestion of triglycerides begins in the stomach with action of lingual and gastric lipases, which are stable in acid medium. The degree of relative activity of each is variable among different species. Lingual lipase is secreted from Ebner's glands.[54] Both enzymes break down short and medium chain triglycerides more efficiently than longer chain lengths,[55] and cannot process phospholipids or sterols. In neonates, pancreatic production of lipase is not fully developed (Fig. 2.1).[56] Breast milk is rich in medium and short chain fatty acids that are adequately handled by breast milk-derived lipase and infantile gastric lipase. In adults, it is estimated that 10–30% of ingested lipids are digested prior to the duodenal stage, yielding diacylglycerols and free fatty acids. Gastric lipase has high activity in patients with cystic fibrosis.[57] There is no absorption of fat in the stomach, except for short chain fatty acids. Nevertheless, the stomach is the major site of fat emulsification. This is achieved in part by the mechanical fragmenting of larger lipid masses. Breast milk fat emulsion droplets are relatively small.[58] In addition, gastric lipase releases some fatty acids together with dietary phospholipids that 'coat' intact triglycerides to provide a suspension of emulsified fat droplets. The coordinated gastric propulsion – retropulsion contractions leave lipid droplets smaller than 0.5 μm that are squirted through the pylorus.

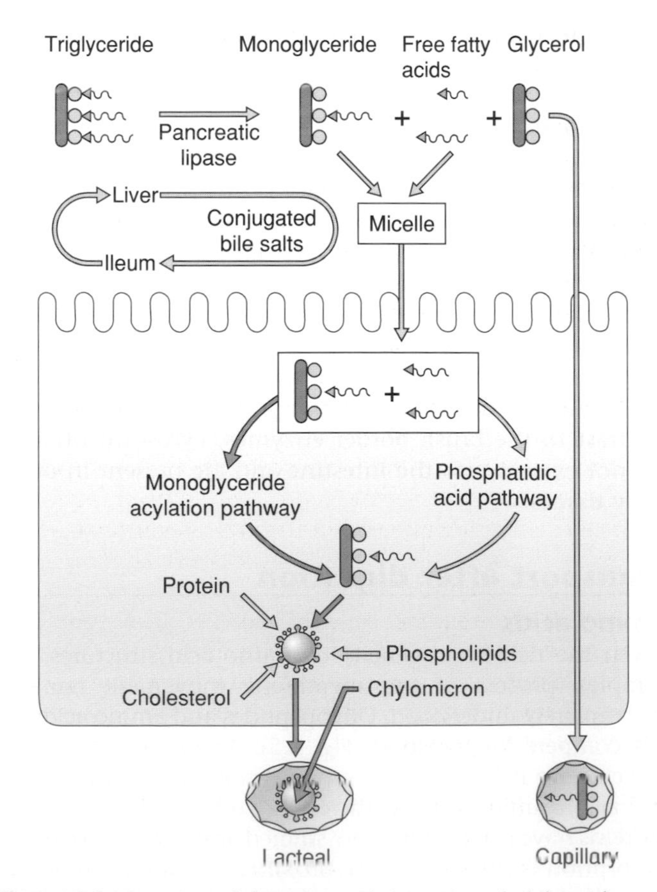

Figure 2.8: Overview of digestion and absorption of triglyceride. (From Johnson, 1997, with permission).

Small intestinal phase

Bile acids and biliary phospholipids further stabilize the lipids presented to pancreatic lipase in the duodenum. As such, the hydrophobic portion of the lipid where lipase acts is contained deep within the emulsion droplet. To allow exposure to lipase, pancreatic phospholipase A_2 is activated by bile acids and calcium to digest the phospholipid coat leaving fatty acids and lysophosphatidylcholine. The optimal action of phospholipase A_2 requires a bile salt to phosphatidylcholine ratio of 2:1 moles.[59] It has been shown that the presence of bile acids inactivates lipase, which led to the discovery of its cofactor, colipase in 1963.[60] Colipase is secreted form the pancreas as pro-colipase at 1:1 ratio to lipase, which it carries to close proximity to the triglyceride. A by-product of pro-colipase's activation by trypsin is a pentapeptide, enterostatin, thought to play a role in satiety after fat ingestion.[61,62] The products of lipase's activity are 2-monoacylglycerols and free fatty acids. Most ingested cholesterol is in the free sterol form and a small amount is in cholesterol-ester form that requires digestion by cholesterol esterase, also called non-specific lipase. The luminal end products of lipid digestion are fatty acids, 2-monoglycerides, glycerol, lysophosphatidylcholine and free cholesterol; all insoluble in water except short/medium chain fatty acids and glycerol which are soluble enough to pass through the unstirred water layer that lines the intestinal epithelium.

Bile acids

After meal ingestion, vagal stimulation and cholecystokinin release stimulate gallbladder contractions and relaxation of the sphincter of Oddi allowing bile flow into the duodenum. In addition to bile acids, bile is a rich source of phospholipids. The three main bile acids are cholic, deoxycholic and chenodeoxycholic acids. Bile acids are amphipathic compounds since they have both hydrophilic and lipophilic molecules. The concentration of bile acids is usually well above a critical level where micelles (water soluble aggregates) are formed upon mixing with digested lipids. Micelles are 100–500 times smaller in diameter than emulsion particles, which makes for a water-clear micellar solution in the proximal small intestine. The orientation within a micellar structure is such that the hydrophobic bile acid parts cover the insoluble molecules within, while the hydrophilic portion lines the outer layer, allowing movement through the luminal aqueous phase. Bile acids are secreted almost exclusively in conjugated form, predominantly to glycine and less so taurine.[63] Such modification enhances the water solubility of bile acids, even in slightly acidic medium, by lowering the critical micellar concentration.[64] Conjugation also confers some resistance to pancreatic digestion and prevents calcium-bile salt precipitation.[65]

Enterohepatic bile circulation

Liver cells synthesize and conjugate bile acids from cholesterol and conjugate bile acids reabsorbed through the enterohepatic circulation. Both processes are in balance to keep an adequate bile acid pool. Since conjugated bile acids are in ionized form in the alkaline intestinal milieu, they cannot be absorbed passively across the enterocyte membrane. It has been shown that active transport of these bile acids takes place in the distal ileum.[66] Ileal bile acid absorption involves Na^+ cotransport down a gradient secured by the basolateral membrane Na^+, K^+ ATPase (Fig. 2.9). Within the enterocyte, bile acids are carried by binding proteins that protect against cellular injury induced by free cellular acids.[67,68] Bacterial enzymatic action in the distal small and large intestine leads to deconjugation of bile acids that escape ileal absorption, and removal of the 7-hydroxy group leaving deoxy bile acid forms. A fraction of the unconjugated bile acids are readily absorbed into the gut epithelium, given their lipophylic properties. The acidic environment in the colon results in the change of bile acids to solid form.[64] Only a small amount of bile acids is lost in feces.

Transport of fat digestion products

The next step is the transport of the hydrophobic digestion products, carried in water-stable micelles from the small intestinal lumen, into the brush border membrane. In addition to the micellar form, digested lipids may be shuttled into the enterocyte through other mechanisms. With the lipid emulsion droplets shrinking in size as lipolysis continues, liquid crystalline structures are formed at the surface.[69,70] These vesicular uni- and multi-lamellar bodies bud off the lipid droplets and carry their hydrophobic contents into the cell. The presence of non-micellar transport structures may explain how, in the absence of bile salts, 50% or more of dietary triglycerides may be absorbed.[15] The adequacy of bile acids usually obviates the need for such soluble forms.[53]

Monoglycerides, fatty acids, cholesterol and lyophospholipids can pass through the enterocyte membrane by passive diffusion. Since passive diffusion is dependent on the concentration gradient across the membrane, bile acid micellar forms elegantly allow for a high concentration of hydrophobic lipolysis products to be carried into the unstirred aqueous layer (40 μm deep) adjacent to the brush border (Fig. 2.10).[71] Once approximated to the brush

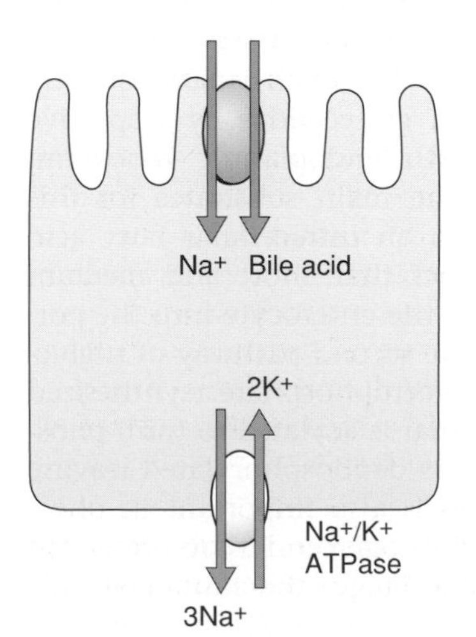

Figure 2.9: Sodium, bile acid cotransport

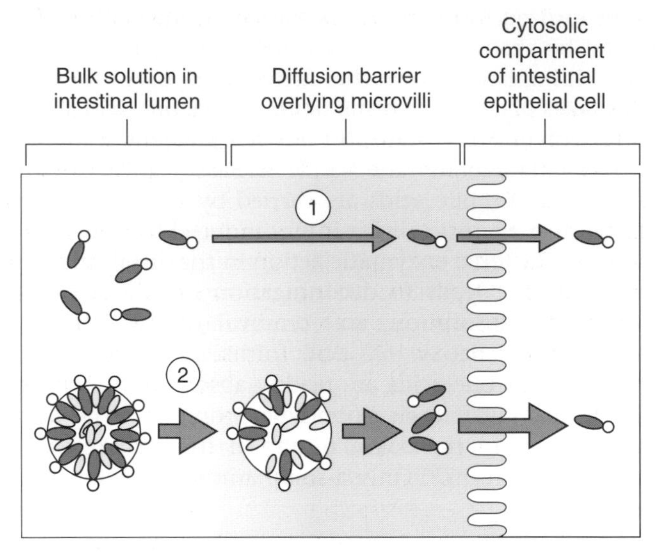

Figure 2.10: Role of bile acid micelles in optimizing diffusion of lipids into intestinal cells. In the absence of bile acids (arrow 1), individual lipid molecules must diffuse across the unstirred aqueous layer. Therefore their uptake is diffusion limited. In the presence of bile acids (arrow 2), large amounts of the lipid molecules are delivered directly to the aqueous-membrane interface so that the rate of uptake is greatly enhanced. (From Westergaard and Dietschy, 1976).[72]

border membrane, the digested lipids are released from their micellar form in the slightly acid medium maintained at the unstirred water layer on the surface of the epithelium.[72] The presence of a Na^+, H^+ exchange pump keeps a pH of 5–6 in the enterocyte's luminal vicinity (Fig. 2.7). Because of their adequate solubility in the unstirred water layer, glycerol, short and medium chain fatty acids diffuse through, independent of micellar formation. There is recent evidence that other carrier mediated transport exists for cholesterol and other lipids.[73,74]

Intracellular phase of fat assimilation

Once in the enterocyte, triglycerides are re-synthesized from 2-monoacylglycrerol and fatty acids as a result of two processes: monoglyceride acylation and phosphatidic acid pathways (Fig. 2.8). In the first, Acyl-CoA synthetase adds an acyl group to a free fatty acid, which is subsequently incorporated into mono- and diglycerides by respective acyltransferases in the smooth endoplasmic reticulum. Long chain fatty acids are the main substrates for this process because of binding to an intracellular fatty acid binding protein[75] and the fact that short and medium chain fatty acids pass through the enterocyte into the portal circulation in free form. The second pathway of triglyceride resynthesis utilizes α-glycerophosphate (synthesized from glucose) as a backbone that is acylated to form phosphatidic acid which, in turn, is dephosphorylated leaving diglyceride. Phosphatidic acid is also important in phospholipid synthesis. When 2-monoglycerides are present in abundance, as in postprandial stage, the monoglyceride acylation pathway predominates. In the fasting state, the phosphatidic acid part provides triglycerides. Lysophosphatidylcholine is either re-acylated to form phosphatidylcholine or hydrolyzed to release a fatty acid and glycerol-3-phosphoylcholine. Endogenous and absorbed cholesterol is re-esterified. Triglycerides, phospholipids and cholesterol esters are packaged into chylomicrons and very low-density lipoproteins (VLDL).

Exit from the enterocyte

Chylomicrons are made only in intestinal cells, while VLDLs are also synthesized in the liver. To form a chylomicron, triglycerides, fat-soluble vitamins and cholesterol are coated with a layer of apolipoprotein (apo A and B types),[76] cholesterol ester and phospholipids. Chylomicrons are made in the endoplasmic reticulum and later processed in the Golgi complex where glycosylation of the apoprotein takes place. It has been suggested that apo B is involved in the movement of chylomicrons from the endoplasmic reticulum to the Golgi apparatus, as lipids accumulate in the former in patients with abetalipoproteinemia.[77] VLDLs are smaller in size than chylomicrons. They are synthesized through a different pathway and seem to be predominant in fasting states. Chylomicrons exit the enterocyte by exocytosis. Although they are too large to pass through capillary pores, chylomicrons and VLDL easily cross into the lacteal endothelial gaps that are present in the postprandial phase.[78] Medium chain triglycerides move directly into the portal circulation.

DIGESTION AND ABSORPTION IN INFANTS

The progressive development of the neonatal gut, to take on new digestive tasks as the nutrient repertoire expands, is a complex process that remains to be further elucidated.

Carbohydrates

Lactose digestion in the premature neonate may be incomplete in the small intestine but partially salvaged from the colon. Lactase level declines from a peak at birth to less than 10% of the pre-weaning infantile level in childhood (Fig. 2.1). The decline in lactase in other mammals occurs even if weaning is prolonged.[11] Lactase activity may persist in some populations where dairy products are consumed into adulthood.[12] Although non-lactose disaccharides are not abundant in breast milk or standard cow milk-based formulas, other disaccharidases besides lactase are present in the young infant intestinal brush border. The presence of these glucosidases reflects a genetically determined sequence, apparently independent from substrate availability.[79] However, the appearance of pancreatic amylase later in the first year of life as starches are introduced (Fig. 2.1) suggests that substrate exposure may play a role in genetic expression of some gastrointestinal enzymes. Amylase is also present in saliva and breast milk.

Proteins

In neonates, pepsin and gastric acid production is lower than that in adults. Acid secretion shows less response to pentagastrin stimulation[80,81] While this fact belittles the gastric acid role in proteolysis it may allow longer lingual amylase and lipase activity and leave some breast milk antibodies intact.

Pancreatic production of trypsin in the neonate is close to adult level, while other pancreatic proteases are low. Pancreatic acinar cells are not as responsive to hormonal stimulation.[82] Enterokinase is present at birth, and mucosal peptidases seem well developed. The role of breast milk proteases remains to be further clarified.

It has been shown that in the neonatal period, uptake of whole polypeptide macromolecules occurs, allowing for passage of such molecules as immunoglobulins.[28]

Lipids

Several factors facilitate the digestion and absorption of triglycerides in the first few months of life. Aside from pancreatic lipase, production of which is low at birth, some triglyceride assimilation is achieved by breast milk, lingual and gastric lipases (see above). Breast milk lipase requires bile acids to be activated.[83] Triglycerides are uniquely packaged in breast milk, such that they are present in small emulsion droplets. Breast milk is rich in medium and short chain fatty acids, which pose less of a digestive challenge. In neonates and young infants, the bile salt pool is smaller than that in adults, possibly because of immature ileal reabsorption.

VITAMINS AND MINERALS

Vitamins are crucial for normal human metabolism; they are classified as either fat or water soluble. (Table 2.3).

Water soluble vitamins

Water soluble vitamins are absorbed generally by passive diffusion, but some, such as ascorbic acid, thiamine, vitamin B_2 and folate are absorbed by carrier mediated processes.

Vitamin	Water soluble	Fat soluble
A		+
Ascorbic acid	+	
Biotin	+	
Cobalamine (B_{12})	+	
D		+
E		+
Folic acid	+	
K		+
Niacin	+	
Pantothenic acid	+	
Pyridoxine (B_6)	+	
Riboflavin (B_2)	+	
Thiamine (B_1)	+	

Table 2.3 Solubility of vitamins

Vitamin B_{12}

Vitamin B_{12} (cobalamine) is available predominantly from animal sources. Gastric acid releases cobalamine from any associated dietary proteins. At acidic pH, cyanocobalamine has a high affinity to R protein produced by salivary glands, gastric parietal cells and the pancreas. Digestion by trypsin in the duodenum frees cobalamine from R protein, allowing it to bind to intrinsic factor, produced by parietal cells.[80,84] Intrinsic factor protects cobalamine from digestion by pancreatic enzymes. It has been shown that receptors for the cobalamine-intrinsic factor complexes exist in the distal ileum.[81,85] Gastric pathology may decrease intrinsic factor production and therefore allow for loss of ingested vitamin B_{12}. Moreover, pancreatic insufficiency leaves vitamin B_{12}-R protein forms that are unabsorbable. Diseases involving the terminal ileum or distal bowel resection can compromise the absorption of cobalamine. Further processing of bound cobalamine within the enterocyte is incompletely understood; vitamin B_{12}-intrinsic factor complex is cleaved and the free form leaves the cell into plasma, where it binds transcobalamine 2.[38]

Vitamin C, folate

Vitamin C (ascorbic acid) intake in adequate doses prevents scurvy. Fresh fruits and juices are abundant sources of ascorbic acid. Vitamin C is taken up by the enterocyte by active and Na^+ dependent processes.[79,86] Folic acid is absorbed after hydrolysis of dietary polyglutamates at the brush border membrane by folate conjugase. Malabsorption of folic acid occurs with severe mucosal disease of the proximal small intestine. Patients with inflammatory bowel disease who take sulfasalazine are at risk of folate deficiency because the drug is a competitive inhibitor of several folate dependent systems.

Other water soluble vitamins

For biotin, pantothenic acid, riboflavin and thiamin, a vitamin specific active transport process has been demonstrated.[87] Pyridoxine is absorbed by simple diffusion.

Fat soluble vitamins

Fat-soluble vitamins include vitamins A, D, E and K. Being water insoluble; they require bile acid micelle formation for absorption, thus mirroring the absorption of dietary fat.

Vitamin A

Vitamin A (retinol) is present in dairy products, eggs and fish oils. β-carotene is the most abundant of carotenoids; the plant derived precursors of vitamin A. Cellular uptake of carotenoids occurs by passive diffusion. Cleavage of carotenoids yields apocarotenoids and retinol, subsequently converted to retinol and retinoic acid, respectively. Animal retinol precursors are mostly available as retinyl esters. Retinyl esters are hydrolyzed to free retinol by pancreatic enzymes and brush border retinyl ester hydrolase.[88] Retinol passes into the enterocyte in micellar form by carrier mediated passive diffusion. Within the enterocyte, retinol is re-esterified and packaged together with free carotenoids and apocarotenoids, into chylomicrons. Hepatocytes as well as hepatic stellate cells (Ito cells) store vitamin A as retinyl esters.[89]

Vitamin D

The two main dietary forms of vitamin D are vitamin D_2 (ergocalciferol) and D_3 (cholecalciferol). The assimilation of vitamin D is highly dependent on bile salts.[90] Synthetic forms of vitamin D (25(OH)-vitamin D_3 and 1,25$(OH)_2$-vitamin D_3) are less bile-salt dependent given some water solubility. Absorption of vitamin D occurs mainly in the proximal and mid small intestine[91] and occurs by passive diffusion. Little intracellular metabolism of vitamin D seems to take place once in the enterocyte, where it is carried in chylomicrons to the lymphatics. Transfer of vitamin D between lymph chylomicrons and plasma Vitamin D binding proteins takes place. It has been suggested that an alternate transport pathway exists, where Vitamin D directly passes into the portal circulation.[92]

Vitamin K, Vitamin E

Vitamin K is available in two forms: K_1 (phytomenadione) derived from plants and K_2 (multiprenyl menaquinones) from intestinal bacteria. Dietary vitamin K requires micelle formation and is absorbed by an active carrier mediated transport process. Vitamin K_2's absorption is passive.[38] Absorption of vitamin E also occurs by passive diffusion.

MINERALS AND TRACE ELEMENTS

The sites and absorption mechanisms of different minerals and trace elements are displayed in Table 2.4.

Calcium

About one-third of total ingested calcium is absorbed. As calcium binds strongly to oxalate, phytate and dietary fiber, its absorption is decreased when co-ingested. The duodenum is the major site of calcium active uptake probably through a specific calcium channel. Passive paracellular transport (across tight junctions) also occurs throughout the small intestine.[93] Both pathways are enhanced by vitamin D.[94] In the cytoplasm, calcium is carried by a specific binding protein, calbindin D_{28K}.[95,96] Exit to the portal circulation occurs against concentration gradient via Ca^{2+} ATPase. Some calcium absorption may take place in the colon.[97]

Compound	Proposed site of absorption	Probable mechanism
Calcium	Duodenum	Active
	Remainder small intestine	Passive
Magnesium	Distal small intestine	Active, Passive
Iron	Duodenum	Active
Zinc	Small intestine, colon	Active
Copper	Stomach, small intestine	Active

Table 2.4 Absorption of minerals and trace elements

Iron

Iron is more abundant and bioavailable in animal dietary sources than plant. Lactoferrin in breast milk is an iron binding protein with a specific brush border receptor securing high absorption.[98] Iron is absorbed in the proximal small intestine. Factors enhancing absorption are Fe^{2+} form, gastric acid, ascorbic acid and co-ingestion with amino acids and sugars. Heme is absorbed as such. The enterocyte not only handles iron uptake from the intestinal lumen but also exclusively regulates iron balance. Specific iron binding proteins are thought to exist within the brush border membrane. Once in the cytoplasm, iron is processed and routed to the circulation as ferritin. Some iron may bind to non-ferritin proteins, which 'trap' excess iron and are discarded with shedding of the intestinal epithelium.

Magnesium, phosphorus, zinc, copper

Magnesium is mainly absorbed in the distal small intestines, both by carrier mediated and paracellular routes. Phosphorus is taken up more efficiently proximally in the duodenum and ileum. Zinc is absorbed through passive and carrier mediated transport in the distal small bowel. It undergoes an enterohepatic circulation, similar to bile acids.[99] Copper is absorbed by active transport and at high concentrations competes with zinc.

References

1. World Health Organization. Press Release 35. World Health Organization; 2002:8 May.
2. Alpers D. Digestion and absorption of carbohydrates and proteins. In: Johnson L, ed. Physiology of the Gastrointestinal Tract. New York, NY: Raven Press; 1994:1723–1749.
3. Snow P, O'Dea K. Factors affecting the rate of hydrolysis of starch in food. Am J Clin Nutr 1981; 34:2721–2727.
4. Anderson H, Levine AS, Levitt MD. Incomplete absorption of the carbohydrate in all purpose wheat flour. N Eng J Med 1981; 304:890–892.
5. Zoppi G, Andreotti G, Pajno-Ferrara F, et al. Exocrine pancreas function in premature and full term neonates. Pediatr Res 1972; 6:880.
6. Layer P, Zinsmeister AR, DiMagno EP. Effects of decreasing intraluminal amylase activity on starch digestion and postprandial gastrointestinal function in humans. Gastroenterology 1986; 91:41.
7. Wu GD, Wang W, Traber PG. Isolation and characterization of the human sucrase-isomaltase gene and demonstration of intestine-specific transcriptional elements. J Biol Chem 1992; 267:7863.
8. Hunziker W, Spiess M, Semenza G, et al. The sucrase-isomaltase complex: primary structure, membrane orientation and evolution of a stalked intrinsic brush border protein. Cell 1986; 46:227–234.

9. Kruse TA, Bolund L, Byskov A. Mapping of the human lactase-phlorizin hydrolase gene to chromosome 2. Cytogenet Cell Genet 1989; 51:1026.
10. Koldovsky O. Developmental dietary and hormonal control of intestinal disaccharidases in mammals (including man). In: Randle JP, Steiner DF, Whelan WJ, Whelan WP, eds. Carbohydrate Metabolism and its Disorders. London: Academic Press; 1981:418–522.
11. Henning SJ. Postnatal development: coordination of feeding, digestion, and metabolism. Am J Physiol Gastrointest Liver Physiol 1981; 241:G199–G214.
12. Semenza G, Auricchio S. Small intestinal disaccharidases. In: Scriver CR, Beaudet AL, Sey WS, Valle D, eds. The Metabolic Basis of Inherited Disease, 4th edn. New York, NY: McGraw-Hill; 1989:2975.
13. Traber P. Carbohydrate assimilation. In: Yamada T, ed. Textbook of Gastroenterology, 4th edn. Philadelphia, PA: Lippincott Williams & Wilkins; 2003:400.
14. Das BC, Gray CM. Intestinal sucrase: in vivo synthesis and degradation. Clin Res 1970; 18:378.
15. Marsh MN, Riley SA. Digestion and absorption of nutrients and vitamins. In: Feldman M, Scharschmidt BF, Sleisenger MH, eds. Sleisenger & Fordtran's Gastrointestinal and Liver Disease: Pathophysiology, Diagnosis, Management, 6th edn. Philadelphia, PA: WB Saunders; 1998:1471–1500.
16. Newcomer AD, McGill DB. Distribution of disaccharidase activity in the small bowel of normal and lactase deficient subjects. Gastroenterology 1966; 51:481–488.
17. Madara JL. Loosening tight junctions: Lessons from the intestine. J Clin Invest 1989; 83:1089–1094.
18. Atisook K, Madara JL. An oligopeptide permeates intestinal tight junctions at glucose-elicited dilatations. Gastroenterology 1991; 100:719–724.
19. Guy MJ, Deren JJ. Selective permeability of the small intestine for fructose. Am J Physiol 1971; 221:1051–1056.
20. Englyst HN, Kingman SM. Dietary fiber and resistant starch. A nutritional classification of plant polysaccharides. In: Kritchevsky D, Bonfield C, Anderson JW, eds. Dietary Fiber. New York, NY: Plenum Press; 1990:49–65.
21. Livesey G. The energy values of dietary fiber and sugar alcohols for man. Nutr Res Rev 1992; 5:61–84.
22. Aggett PJ, Agostoni C, Axelsson I, et al. Nondigestible carbohydrates in the diets of infants and young children: a commentary by the ESPGHAN committee on nutrition. J Pediatr Gastroenterol Nutr 2003; 36(3):329–337.
23. Erickson RH, Kim YS. Digestion and absorption of dietary proteins. Annu Rev Med 1990; 41:133–139.
24. Ford JE. Some effects of overheating of protein on the digestion and absorption. In: Mathews DM, Payne JW, eds. Peptide Transport in Protein Nutrition. Amsterdam: North-Holland Press; 1975:183–203.
25. Friedman M. Dietary impact of food processing. Annu Rev Nutr 1992; 12:119–137.
26. Mellander O, Folsch G. Enzyme resistance and metal binding of phosphorylated peptides. In: Bigwood EJ, ed. International Encyclopedia of food and nutrition. Oxford: Pergamon Press; 1972:569–579.
27. Seetharam B, Alpers DH. Cellular uptake of cobalamine. Nutr Rev 1985; 43:97–102.
28. Udall JN, Walker WA. The physiologic and pathologic basis for the transport of macromolecules across the intestinal tract. J Pediatr Gastroenterol Nutr 1982; 1:295.
29. Samloff IN. Pepsins, peptic activity, and peptic inhibitors. J Clin Gastroenterol 1981; 3:91.
30. Freeman HG, Sleisenger MH, Kim YS. Human protein digestion and absorption. Clin Gastroenterol 1983; 12:357–378.
31. Nordstrom C. Release of enteropeptidase and other brush border enzymes from the small intestine wall in the rat. Biochim Biophys Acta 1972; 289:376–377.
32. Hermon-Taylor J, Perrin J, Grant DAW. Immunofluorescent localization of enterokinase in human small intestine. Gut 1987; 28:259–265.
33. Nixon SE, Mawer GE. The digestion and absorption of protein in man. 2. The form in which digested protein is absorbed. Br J Nutr 1970; 24:241–258.
34. Adibi S. Glycyl-dipeptides: New substrates for protein nutrition. J Lab Clin Med 1989; 113:665.
35. Adibi S. Evidence for two different modes of tripeptide disappearance in human intestine. Uptake by peptide carrier systems and hydrolysis by peptide hydrolases. J Clin Invent 1975; 56:1355–1363.
36. Steinhardt HJ, Adibi SA. Kinetics and characteristics of absorption from an equimolar mixture of 12 glycyl-dipeptides in human jejunum. Gastroenterology 1986; 90:579.
37. Curtis KJ, Gaines HD, Kim YS. Protein digestion and absorption in rats with pancreatic duct occlusion. Gastroenterology 1978; 74:1271–1276.
38. Farrel J. Digestion and absorption of nutrients and vitamins. In: Feldman M, Friedman LS, Sleisenger MH, eds. Sleisenger and Fordtran's Gastrointestinal and Liver Disease: Pathophysiology, Diagnosis, Management, 7th edn. Philadelphia, PA: Saunders; 2002:1731.
39. Ahnen D, Mircheff A, Santiago N. Intestinal surface amino-oligopeptidase. Distinct molecular forms during assembly in intra-cellular membranes in vivo. J Biol Chem 1983; 258:5960.
40. Kekuda R, Torres-Zamorano V, Fei YJ, et al. Molecular and functional characterization of intestinal Na^+-dependent neutral amino acid transporter. Am J Physiol 1997; 272:G1463.
41. Hoshide R, Ikeda Y, Karashima S, et al. Molecular cloning, tissue distribution and chromosomal localization of human cationic amino acid transporter 2. Genomics 1996; 38:174–178.
42. Hopfer U. Membrane transport mechanisms for hexoses and amino acids in the small intestine. In: Johnson LR, ed. Physiology of the Gastrointestinal Tract, 2nd edn. New York, NY: Raven Press; 1987:1499–1526.
43. Adibi SA, Gray SJ, Menden E. The kinetics of amino acid absorption and alteration of plasma composition of free amino acids after intestinal perfusion of amino acid mixtures. Am J Clin Nutr 1967; 20:24–33.
44. Leibach FH, Ganapathy V. Peptide transporters in the intestine and the kidney. Annu Rev Nutr 1996; 16:99.
45. Liang R, Fei YJ, Prasad PD, et al. Human intestinal H^+ peptide cotransporter. Cloning, functional expression and chromosomal localization. J Biol Chem 1995; 270:6456.
46. Silk DBA. Disorders of nitrogen absorption. Clin Gastroenterol 1982; 11:47–72.
47. Ganapathy V, Brandsch M, Lelbach F. Intestinal transport of amino acids and peptides. In Johnson LR, ed. Physiology of the Gastrointestinal Tract. New York, NY: Raven Press; 1994:1782.
48. Garlick PJ. Protein turnover in the whole animal and specific tissue. In: Florkin M, Neuberger A, Deenen LLM Van, eds. Comprehensive Biochemistry: Protein Metabolism. Amsterdam: Elsevier Science; 1980:77–152.
49. Alpers DH. Protein synthesis in intestinal mucosa: the effect of route of administration of precursor amino acids. J Clin Invest 1972; 51:167–173.

50. Levine GM, Deren JJ, Steiger S, Zunio R. Role of oral intake in maintenance of gut mass and disaccharidase activity. Gastroenterology 1974; 67:975–982.
51. British Nutrition Foundation. Report of the Task Force on Trans Fatty Acids. London: British Nutrition Foundation; 1987.
52. Borgstrom B. Phospholipid absorption. In: Rommel K, Goebell H, Bohmer R, eds. Lipid absorption: biochemical and clinical aspects. London: MTP Press; 1976:65–72.
53. Carey MC, Small DM, Bliss CM. Lipid digestion and absorption. Annu Rev Physiol 1983; 45:651–677.
54. Hamosh M, Burns WA. Lipolytic activity of human lingual glands (von Ebner). Lab invest 1977; 37:603–608.
55. Liao TH, Hamosh M. Fat digestion by lingual lipase: mechanism of lipolysis in the stomach and upper small intestine. Pediatr Res 1984; 18:402–409.
56. Grand RJ, Watkins JB, Torti FM. Development of the human gastrointestinal tract: a review. Gastroenterology 1976; 70:790–810.
57. Armand M, Hamosh M, Philpott JR, et al. Gastric function in children with cystic fibrosis: effect of diet on gastric lipase levels and fat digestion. Pediatr Res 2004; 55(3):457–465.
58. Hernell O, Blackberg L, Bernback S. Digestion of human milk fat in early infancy. Acta Pediatr Scand 1989; 351:57.
59. Nalbone G, Larion D, Charbonnier-Augeire M, et al. Pancreatic phospholipase A2 hydrolysis of phosphatidyl cholines in various physicochemical states. Biochim Biophys Acta 1980; 620:612–625.
60. Baskys B, Klein E, Lever WF. Lipases of blood and tissues. III. Purification and properties of pancreatic lipase. Arch Biochem Biophys 1963; 102:201–209.
61. Erlanson-Albertsson C, Larsson A. The activation peptide of pancreatic procolipase decreases food intake in rats. Regul Peptides 1988; 22:325–331.
62. Okada S, York DA, Bray GA. Erlanson-Albertsson C. Enterostatin (Val-Pro-Asp-Pro-Arg), the activation peptide of procolipase, selectively reduces fat intake. Physiol Behav 1991; 49:1185–1189.
63. Haslewood GAD. The Biological Importance of Bile Salts. Amsterdam: North-Holland; 1978.
64. Hoffman AF. Intestinal absorption of bile acids and biliary constituents. In: Johnson LR, ed. Physiology of the Gastrointestinal Tract. New York, NY: Raven Press; 1994:1845–1865.
65. Hoffman AF, Mysels KJ. Bile acid solubility and precipitation in vitro and in vivo: the role of conjugation, pH and Ca2+. J Lipid Res 1992; 33:617–626.
66. Weiner IM, Lack L. Bile salt absorption: enterohepatic circulation. In: Code CF, ed. Handbook of Physiology. Alimentary Canal. Washington, DC: American Physiological Society; 1968:1439–1455.
67. Weinberg SL, Bruckhardt G, Wilson FA. Taurocholate transport by rat intestinal basolateral membrane vesicles. Evidence for the presence of an anion exchange transport system. J Clin Invest 1986; 78:44–50.
68. Kraehenbuehl S, Talos C, Reichen J. Mitochondrial toxicity of hydrophobic bile acids and partial reversal by ursodeoxycholate. Hepatology 1992; 16:156A.
69. Hernell O, Staggers JE, Carey MC. Physical-chemical behavior of dietary and biliary lipids during intestinal digestion and absorption. 2. Phase analysis and aggregation states of luminal lipids during duodenal fat ingestion in healthy adult human beings. Biochemistry 1990; 29:2041.
70. Holt PR, Fairchild BM, Weiss JA. Liquid crystalline phase in human intestinal contents during fat digestion. Lipids 1986; 21:444.
71. Strocchi A, Levitt MD. A reappraisal of the magnitude and implications of the intestinal unstirred layer. Gastroenterology 1991; 101:843.
72. Westergaard H, Dietschy JM. The mechanism whereby bile acid micelles increase the rate of fatty acid and cholesterol uptake into the mucosal cell. J Clin Invest 1976; 58:97–108.
73. Stremmel W. Uptake of fatty acids by jejunal mucosal cells is mediated by a fatty acid binding membrane protein. J Clin Invest 1988; 82:2001–2010.
74. Bhat SG, Brockman HL. The role of cholesteryl ester hydrolysis and synthesis in cholesterol transport across rat intestinal mucosal membrane: a new concept. Biochem Biophys Res Commun 1982; 109:486–492.
75. Ockner RK, Manning JA. Fatty acid binding protein in small intestine. Identification, isolation and evidence for its role in cellular fatty acid transport. J Clin Invest 1974; 54:326–338.
76. Davidson NO, Magun AM, Brasitus TA, et al. Intestinal apolipoprotein A-I and B-48 metabolism: effects of sustained alterations in dietary triglyceride and mucosal cholesterol flux. J Lipid Res 1987; 28:388–402.
77. Dobbins WO. An ultrastructural study of the intestinal mucosa in congenital β-lipoprotein deficiency with particular emphasis on intestinal absorptive cells. Gastroenterology 1970; 50:195–210.
78. Sabesin SM, Frase S. Electron microscopic studies of the assembly, intracellular transport and secretion of chylomicrons by rat intestine. J Lipid Res 1977; 18:496.
79. Lebenthal E. Impact of digestion and absorption in the weaning period on infant feeding practices. Pediatrics 1985; 75(1):207–213.
80. Deren JS. Development of structure and function in the fetal and newborn stomach. Am J Clin Nutr 1971; 24:144.
81. Christie DL. Development of gastric function during the first month of life. In: Lebenthal E, ed. Textbook of Gastroenterology and Nutrition in Infancy. New York, NY: Raven Press; 1981:109–120.
82. Lebenthal E, Lee PC. Development of functional response in human exocrine pancreas. Pediatrics 1980; 66:556.
83. Hernell O. Specificity of human milk bile salt stimulated lipase. J Pediatr Gastroenterol Nutr 1985; 4:517–519.
84. Allen RH, Seetheram B, Podell E, et al. Effect of proteolytic enzymes on the binding of cobalamine to R protein and intrinsic factor. In vitro evidence that a failure to partially degrade R protein is responsible for cobalamine malabsorption in pancreatic insufficiency. J Clin Invest 1978; 61:47.
85. Hagedorn C, Alpers D. Distribution of intrinsic factor vitamin B12 receptors in human intestine. Gastroenterology 1977; 73:1010.
86. Siliprandi L, Vanni P, Kessler M, et al. Na+-dependent, electroneural L-ascorbate transport across brush border membrane vesicles from guinea pig small intestine. Biochim Biophys Acta 1979; 552:129.
87. Rose RC. Intestinal absorption of water soluble vitamins. In: Johnson LR, ed. Physiology of the Gastrointestinal Tract, 2nd edn. New York, NY: Raven Press; 1987:1581.
88. Rigtrup KM, Ong DE. A retinyl ester hydrolase activity intrinsic to the brush border membrane of rat small intestine. Biochemistry 1992; 31:2920–2926.
89. Levin MS. Intestinal absorption and metabolism of vitamin A. In: Johnson L, ed. Physiology of the Gastrointestinal Tract. New York, NY: Raven Press; 1994:1957–1978.
90. Brasitus TA, Sitrin MD. Absorption and cellular actions of vitamin D. In: Johnson L, ed. Physiology of the Gastrointestinal Tract. New York, NY; Raven Press; 1994:1935–1955.

91. Hollander D. Mechanism and site of small intestinal uptake of vitamin D3 in pharmacological concentrations. Am J Clin Nutr 1976; 29:970–975.

92. Sitrin MD, Pollack KL, Bolt MJG, Rosernberg IH. Comparison of vitamin hydroxyvitamin D absorption in the rat. Am J Physiol 1982; 242:G326–G332.

93. Bronner F. Intestinal calcium transport: The cellular pathway. Miner Electrolyte Metab 1990; 16:94.

94. Krejs GJ, Nicar MJ, Zerwekh JE, et al. Effect of 1,25-dihydro yvitamin D3 on calcium and magnesium absorption in the healthy human jejunum and ileum. Am J Med 1983; 75:973.

95. Civitelli R, Avioli LV. Calcium, phosphate and magnesium absorption. In: Johnson L, ed. Physiology of the Gastrointestinal Tract. New York, NY: Raven Press; 1994:2173–2181.

96. Nemere I, Norman AW. Transcaltachia, vesicular calcium transport and microtubule-associated calbindin-D28K: Energizing views of 1,25-dihydroxyvitamin D3-mediated intestinal calcium absorption. Miner Electrolyte Metab 1990; 16:109–114.

97. Favus MJ, Kathpalia SC, Coe FL. Kinetic characteristics of calcium absorption and secretion by rat colon. Am J Physiol 1981; 240:G350.

98. Cox T, Mazurier G, Spik G. Iron binding proteins and influx across the duodenal brush border. Evidence for specific lactotransferrin receptors in the human intestine. Biochim Biophys Acta 1969; 588:120.

99. Taylor CM, Bacon JR, Aggett PJ, Bremner I. Homeostatic regulation of zinc absorption and endogenous losses in zinc-deprived men. Am J Clin Nutr 1991; 53:755–763.

Further Reading

Johnson L, ed. Physiology of the Gastrointestinal Tract. New York, NY: Raven Press; 1994.

Feldman M, Friedman LS, Sleisenger MH, eds. Gastrointestinal and Liver Disease Pathology, Diagnosis, Management, 3rd edn. Amsterdam: Elsevier Science; 2002.

Johnson LR. Gastrointestinal Physiology – Year Book Inc. St. Louis, MO: Mosby; 1997.

Chapter 3
Bile acid physiology and alterations in the enterohepatic circulation

James E. Heubi and Dean R. Focht

INTRODUCTION

Bile acids are important in the processing of dietary lipids and serve three major functions. Bile acids aggregate and form micelles in the upper small intestine, which help solubilize lipolytic products, cholesterol and fat soluble vitamins, thus facilitating absorption across the intestinal epithelium. They also stimulate bile flow during their secretion across the biliary canaliculus. Finally, bile acids are major regulators of sterol metabolism and serve as a major excretory pathway for cholesterol from the body.

Bile acids undergo an enterohepatic circulation within the liver, biliary tract, intestinal tract, and the portal and peripheral circulations. This carefully regulated enterohepatic circulation allows for conservation of bile acids. Any alteration in this circulatory pathway can lead to a loss of bile acids from the body and associated clinical manifestations. This chapter will first review the normal physiology of bile acids and will be followed by a discussion of the clinical manifestations of defects of bile acid biosynthesis and clinical conditions associated with alterations in bile acid transport in the liver and gastrointestinal tract.

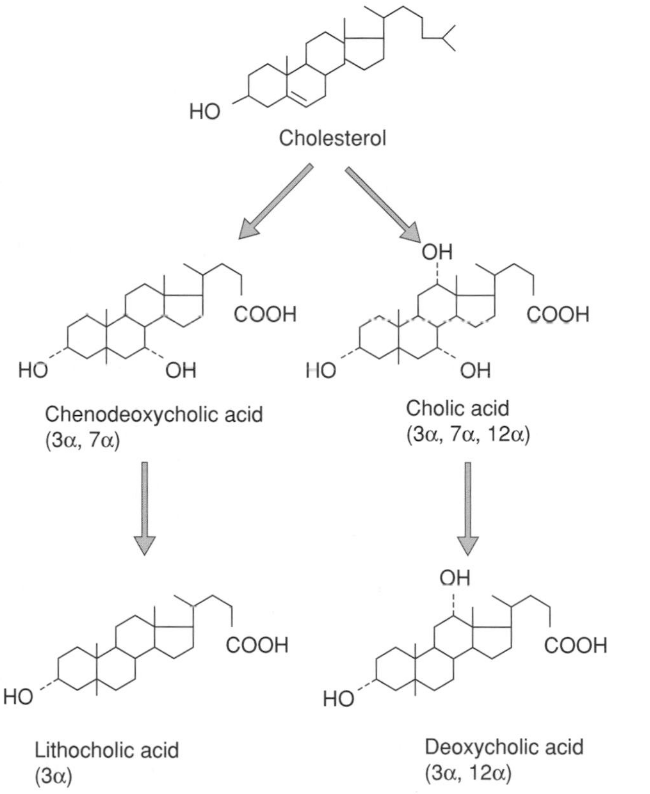

HO
Cholesterol
OH
COOH
COOH
HO
OH
HO
OH
Chenodeoxycholic acid
(3α, 7α)
Cholic acid
(3α, 7α, 12α)
OH
COOH
COOH
HO
HO
Lithocholic acid
(3α)
Deoxycholic acid
(3α, 12α)

Figure 3.1: Primary bile acids synthesized in liver from cholesterol, and the secondary bile acids produced by bacterial 7α-dehydroxylation.

BIOSYNTHESIS

The two primary bile acids, cholic acid (3a, 7a, 12a-trihydroxy-5β-cholanoic acid) and chenodeoxycholic acid, (3a, 7a-dihydroxy-5β-cholanoic acid) are synthesized in the liver from cholesterol (Fig. 3.1). The synthesis of these acids occurs through a tightly regulated enzymatic cascade within hepatocytes involving at least 14 different enzymes.[1] Modifications to the cholesterol nucleus occur via two different biosynthetic pathways: the classic, or neutral, pathway and the alternative, or acidic, pathway. Both pathways work to convert a hydrophobic cholesterol molecule into hydrophilic primary bile acids.

The neutral pathway of bile acid biosynthesis involves the formation of a cholic acid (CA) to chenodeoxycholic acid (CDCA) ratio of approximately 1:1.[2] The initial step of cholesterol synthesis in the neutral pathway involves the 7a-hydroxylation of cholesterol by the rate-limiting enzyme, cholesterol 7a-hydroxylase. Compared with the neutral pathway, the alternative pathway of bile acid biosynthesis predominately yields CDCA with smaller amounts of CA. While the neutral pathway is felt to be the quantitatively more important pathway of bile acid synthesis, the alternative pathway is likely more functional early in life, and alterations in this pathway may have devastating consequences.[3,4]

Virtually all primary bile acids are conjugated with either glycine or taurine after being synthesized by hepatocytes. This conjugation effectively decreases the permeability of bile acids to cholangiocyte cellular membranes, thereby delivering higher concentrations to the intestines.[5] Conjugation also inhibits digestion of bile acids by pancreatic carboxypeptidases.[6]

ENTEROHEPATIC CIRCULATION

The bile acid pool in man is typically made up of the primary bile acids, cholic and chenodeoxycholic acid, and the secondary bile acids, deoxycholic and lithocholic acid. Ursodeoxycholic acid accounts for an additional small percentage of the bile acid pool size. This pool of bile acids circulates through the liver, biliary tract, intestine, portal circulation and peripheral serum in response to meal stimuli. Maintenance of a pool of bile acids is essential to normal fat absorption and bile secretion.

For most individuals, newly synthesized bile acids only account for approximately 2–5% of the total bile acid pool.[7] This percentage can be greatly increased in patients with impaired bile acid reabsorption such as in patients who have undergone ileal resection commonly encountered in Crohn's Disease. Once synthesized by hepatocytes, bile acids are excreted into the canalicular lumen. In addition to bile acids, a sodium ion is excreted which creates a gradient to passively draw water into the biliary canalicula. This flow of bile acids and water serves as the major stimulus for bile flow. While bile acids make up the major solute of bile, other components include phospholipids, organic anions, inorganic anions (especially chloride) and cholesterol.[8]

Most of the bile acids secreted from the liver are stored in the gallbladder as mixed micelles accompanied by phospholipid and cholesterol. Upon consumption of a meal, the gallbladder contracts and the bile acid micelles are delivered to the small intestine (Fig. 3.2). In the proximal small bowel, bile acids form mixed micelles with dietary lipolytic products, fatty acids and monoglycerides. Cholesterol, phospholipids, and fat-soluble vitamins are also solubilized in a similar manner. The lipolytic products are initially absorbed by the small intestine and this is followed by reabsorption of the bile acids. Bile acids may be reabsorbed by either passive non-ionic diffusion along the length of the gastrointestinal tract or by a sodium-dependent mechanism in the ileum. Reabsorption is limited in the upper small bowel because the pKa of bile acids tends to be too low to be absorbed by non-ionic diffusion although there is some absorption of unconjugated and glycine-conjugated bile acids.

Upon initial entry into the small intestines, bile acids have a net negative charge. As the bile acids pass through the more distal small intestine, the colonized bacteria deconjugate the bile acids. This deconjugation confers a neutral charge to the bile acids and thus permits rapid uptake by intestinal endothelial cells via passive diffusion.[7] The combination of both passive and active reuptake of bile acids provides a very efficient method of recycling bile acids in humans. With each of the 8–12 enterohepatic cycles every day, there is loss of approximately 3–5% of the pool of bile acids largely due to an efficient absorption by the combination of passive and active transport systems in the intestine.

A small percentage of bile acids escape reabsorption in the small intestine and are delivered to the large intestine where bacterial transformation of the bile acids occurs. After conjugated bile acids are deconjugated, bacterial 7a-dehydroxylation of CA and CDCA may occur, causing formation of the secondary bile acids deoxycholic acid (3a,12a-dihydroxy-5β cholanoic acid) and lithocholic acid (3a-hydroxy-5β cholanoic acid) (Fig. 3.1).

A small amount of bile acids are lost in the stool each day. While the amount varies by diet and individual, up to 30 g of bile acids are reabsorbed by the intestines, with 0.2 to 0.6 g being eliminated in the stool daily.[9] The bile acids which are lost in the stool are replaced by newly synthesized bile acids in the liver through a tightly controlled negative feedback system. The rate limiting enzyme for bile acid synthesis in the neutral pathway, cholesterol 7a-hydroxylase, is tightly regulated by feedback inhibition from the bile acids returning to the liver. This feedback inhibition mechanism insures that the bile acid pool remains constant in healthy humans, thereby ensuring adequate bile acids to promote bile flow, micelle formation and cholesterol excretion.

Bile acids enter the portal venous system upon absorption by intestinal endothelial cells. These bile acids are bound to albumin and other proteins as they are transported in the portal vein to the liver. Up to 90% of these bile acids are removed by the liver during their first pass.[7]

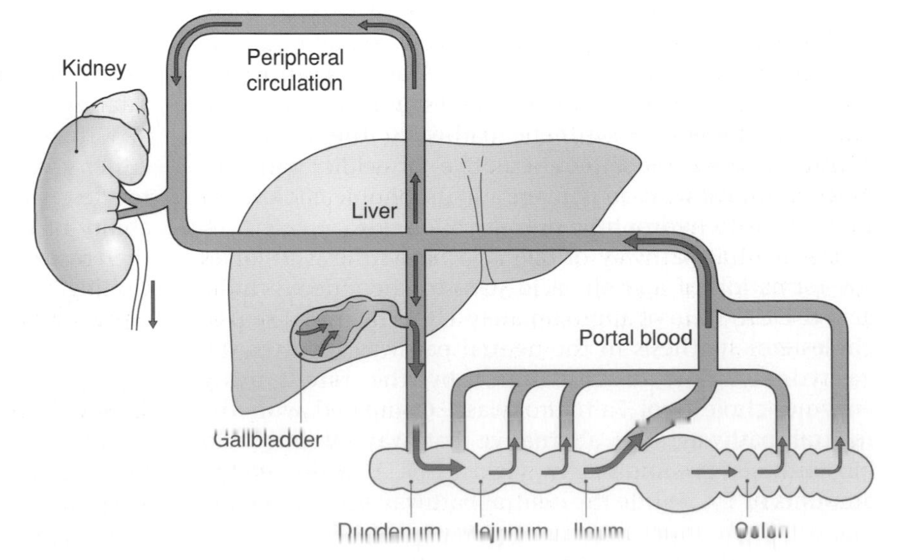

Figure 3.2: The enterohepatic circulation of bile acids. Upon contraction of the gallbladder, bile acids are expelled into the duodenum. Small arrows indicate passive intestinal absorption, while the large arrow in the ileum represents the active uptake of bile acids. The bile acids return to the liver via the portal system. A small fraction of the bile acids spill over into the systemic circulation and are excreted by the kidneys. (Adapted from Heubi JE. In: Banks RO, Sperelakis N, eds. Essentials of Basic Science: Physiology. Boston: Little, Brown and Company; 1993, with permission.)

Most of the reuptake is performed by periportal hepatocytes which then secrete the bile acids into the canalicular space, the rate-limiting step of bile acid transport. A small fraction of the circulating bile acids in the portal blood escape removal by the hepatocytes and spill over into the systemic circulation. Therefore, with each cycling of bile acids, there is a characteristic small spillover of bile acids in the serum that can be measured. The postprandial rise of bile acids may be a reasonable indicator that the enterohepatic circulation is intact. The serum bile acids undergo filtration by the kidney and can either be excreted in the urine or reabsorbed in the renal tubules for transport back to the liver.

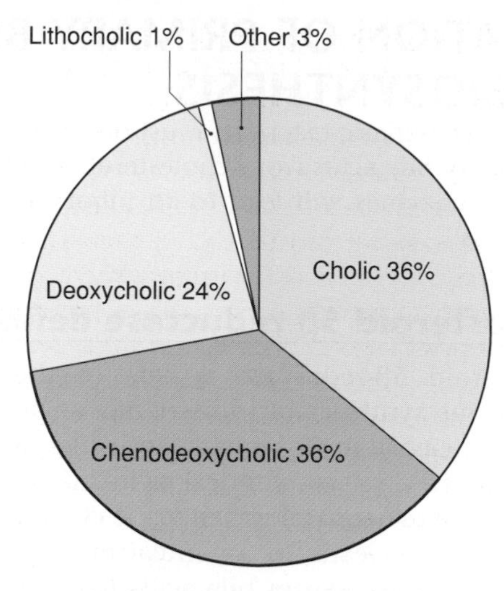

Figure 3.3: Normal concentration of biliary bile acids.

MATURATION OF THE ENTEROHEPATIC CIRCULATION

Neonates are born with an immature enterohepatic circulation of bile acids. A maturation process occurs within the fetal liver and continues throughout the first year of life, which effectively increases the amount of bile acids available for digestion. The synthesis of bile acids has been demonstrated as early as the 12th week of gestation.[10] The bile acids produced throughout gestation are different from those produced by infants, children and adults. While the primary bile acids, CA and CDCA, make up approximately 75–80% of the biliary bile acids in adults, they make up less than 50% of the total bile acid pool of the fetus.[11] An immature synthetic pathway of bile acids exists in the developing fetus that not only leads to a decreased rate of bile acid synthesis, but also to the production of 'atypical' bile acids not seen in the normal child or adult. These 'atypical' bile acids have additional sites of hydroxylation, which may be important in the development of cholestatic liver disease.[12]

While newborns initially have a decreased synthesis of bile acids and decreased bile acid pool size, both increase during the first several months of life.[13] The decreased bile acid pool size is accompanied by a reduced concentration of intraluminal bile salts. Both term and pre-term normal newborn infants have reduced rates of cholate synthesis and a reduced pool size compared with normal adults when corrected for differences in surface area.[14] A decreased ileal transport of bile acids exists in newborn infants based upon *in vitro* studies.[15] In addition to the impaired synthesis and ileal uptake of bile acids in newborns, the pressure generated by contraction of the newborn gallbladder may be insufficient to overcome the choledochal resistance to bile flow.[16] This insufficient pressure occurs despite normal responsiveness of the term newborn infant's gallbladder to cholecystokinin. For pre-term infants less than 33 weeks gestation, the gallbladder contraction index may be non-existent to less than 50%.[17] Impaired gallbladder contraction may explain why 0.5% of normal neonates have gallstones or gallbladder sludge.[18] A decrease in intraluminal bile salt concentration in the neonate contributes to a phenomenon of decreased fat absorption known as 'physiologic steatorrhea'. Over the first months of life the bile acid synthetic rate increases and the pool expands with concurrent increase in intraluminal bile acid concentrations.[11]

Despite having a decreased rate of bile acid synthesis and decreased bile acid pool size, the serum bile acid concentration is typically increased in normal pre-term and term newborn infants. In fact, the serum bile acid concentration during the first 6 months of life is as high as in adults who have clinical cholestasis.[10] This elevated level of serum bile acids has been termed 'physiologic cholestasis'. The early elevation in serum bile acids relates to a poor hepatic extraction of bile salts from the portal circulation. This hepatic uptake is especially impaired in pre-term infants. An improvement in the hepatic uptake of bile acids occurs over the first year of life and corresponds to a decrease in the peripheral serum bile acid concentration. Levels of serum bile acids in infants decrease into the normal range by approximately 10 months of age.[11]

The bile acid composition in neonates is predominately the primary bile acids, CA and CDCA. An appearance of the secondary bile acids, lithocholic and deoxycholic acid, occurs in both the serum and bile of infants upon intestinal microflora colonization.[11] As the infant matures, primary and secondary bile acids continue to be synthesized and re-circulated. The concentration of bile acids in humans eventually approximates the following: cholic acid (36%), chenodeoxycholic acid (36%), deoxycholic acid (24%) and lithocholic acid (1%) (Fig. 3.3).[19]

ALTERATIONS IN THE ENTEROHEPATIC CIRCULATION

Disruptions in any part of the enterohepatic circulation of bile acids can lead to the development of clinical manifestations ranging from cholestasis to diarrhea. Alterations may occur at the level of primary bile acid synthesis, in the transport of bile acids across the hepatocyte, at the level of secondary bile acid synthesis, or in ileal transport and the recirculation of bile acids.

ALTERATION OF PRIMARY BILE ACID BIOSYNTHESIS

A cascade of enzymatic reactions must occur in the formation of primary bile acids from cholesterol. A deficiency of any of these enzymes will lead to an inborn error of bile acid synthesis.

Δ^4-3-Oxosteroid 5β-reductase deficiency

Δ^4-3-Oxosteroid 5β-reductase is one of the enzymes involved in the synthesis of primary bile acids from cholesterol. A deficiency in this enzyme was first described by Setchell *et al.* in a set of identical twin infants who presented with severe neonatal intrahepatic cholestasis.[20] This enzyme deficiency leads to an impairment of bile acid biosynthesis and low serum bile acids in the presence of conjugated hyperbilirubinemia and normal serum GGT. Fast atom bombardment ionization-mass spectrometry (FAB-MS) of urine from patients with this deficiency yields an elevated level of taurine conjugates of hydroxyl-oxo-bile acids, and gas chromatography-mass spectrometry (GC-MS) can confirm the diagnosis.[20] Findings on liver biopsy reveal a pattern consistent with idiopathic neonatal hepatitis showing lobular disarray, bile stasis and hepatocyte pseudoacinar transformation.[21] Early treatment can prevent development of liver damage and subsequent hepatic failure. Oral replacement therapy with bile acids, such as cholic acid, acts by expanding the bile acid pool and stimulating choleresis. Replacement therapy will prevent formation of the hepatotoxic Δ^4-3-oxo bile acids through feedback inhibition and offer cytoprotection by stimulating bile flow.[21] Ursodeoxycholic acid may also be cytoprotective and expand the bile acid pool but will not inhibit 'toxic' metabolite formation.

3β-Hydroxysteroid dehydrogenase/isomerase deficiency

A second enzymatic deficiency in bile acid synthesis is a defect in the enzyme 3β-hydroxy-Δ^5 steroid dehydrogenase/isomerase. This enzyme deficiency was first identified by Clayton et al. in a 3-month-old boy who presented with cholestatic jaundice.[22] As was demonstrated in this child, this enzyme deficiency can be inherited in an autosomal recessive fashion and can be a result of consanguinity. This defect is now recognized to be the most common of all the inborn errors of bile acid metabolism. The clinical presentation of this enzyme deficiency may vary but can include a conjugated hyperbilirubinemia in the neonate, rickets or consequences of fat soluble vitamin deficiency in older infants and children, or a chronic hepatitis in older children.[21] The conjugated hyperbilirubinemia found in neonates is typically associated with an elevated serum ALT/AST, along with normal serum GGT concentrations. Findings on liver biopsy can vary from those consistent with neonatal hepatitis in infants, to findings of chronic hepatitis or cirrhosis in older children.[23] Diagnosis is suggested by demonstrating increased urinary bile acids on FAB-MS. Confirmation of the diagnosis can be made by using GC-MS on a urine sample which shows the major bile acids to be 3β,7α-dihydroxy- and 3β,7α,12a-trihydroxy-5-cholenoic acids. Treatment is with the oral administration of cholic acid which will increase the bile acid pool and decrease production of the hepatotoxic 3β-hydroxy-Δ^5 bile acids by feedback inhibition of bile acid synthesis.[21]

Oxysterol 7α-hydroxylase deficiency

Deficiency of the bile acid synthetic enzyme oxysterol 7α-hydroxylase was first described by Setchell et al. in a 10-week-old boy whose parents were first cousins.[24] This child presented with intermittent acholic stools at 6 weeks of age and quickly progressed to liver failure requiring liver transplantation. Laboratory studies revealed elevated serum aminotransferases, a conjugated hyperbilirubinemia and prolonged prothrombin time but normal GGT. Primary bile acids were undetectable, but the hepatotoxic, unsaturated monohydroxy-cholenoic bile acids were elevated on urine FAB-MS in urine and serum. Liver biopsy showed bridging fibrosis and cirrhosis, periportal inflammation, intralobular cholestasis and giant cell transformation. Oral replacement of primary bile acids was ineffective in reversing this patient's liver disease, which may make liver transplantation the only treatment option in those patients with advanced liver disease.

Cerebrotendinous xanthomatosis

Cerebrotendinous xanthomatosis is an autosomal recessive lipid-storage disease first characterized by Van Bogaert in 1937. This disease represents the first described defect of bile acid synthesis and is associated with a deficiency in the enzyme 27-hydroxylase. Deficiency of this enzyme leads to deposition of cholesterol throughout various tissues in the body. Patients often present in the first or second decade of life with tendon xanthomas, early atherosclerosis, cataracts, mental retardation, convulsions, myoclonus, pyramidal signs, cerebellar ataxia and spasticity.[25] An increasing number of infants have been identified with this defect through the screening of infants with cholestasis and normal serum bile acids who have FAB-MS analysis of their urine. Diagnosis can be confirmed with urinary capillary gas chromatography, which demonstrates elevated urinary bile alcohols.[26] Chenodeoxycholic acid and, more recently, cholic acid, has been used to decrease serum cholesterol levels and subsequently decrease the excretion of urinary bile acids.[21] It has also been suggested that the use of a statin in combination with chenodeoxycholic or cholic acid may be the preferred therapeutic regimen.

Racemase deficiency

A deficiency in the peroxisomal enzyme 2-methylacyl-CoA racemase[27] was first discovered in an infant who presented at 2 weeks of age with a coagulopathy, elevated transaminases, conjugated hyperbilirubinemia and hematochezia. A previously affected sibling had died because of a

CNS bleed secondary to a coagulopathy. Liver histology revealed periportal inflammation and hemosiderosis along with giant cell transformation and a reduced number of peroxisomes. Elevated levels of cholestanoic acids were detected in the urine, serum and bile using FAB-MS and GC-MS. Oral administration of cholic acid can lead to normalization of liver enzymes and halt progression of the liver disease.

Peroxisomal disorders

Zellweger syndrome (cerebro-hepato-renal syndrome) and neonatal adrenoleukodystrophy are autosomal recessive disorders characterized by an absence of hepatic peroxisomes and can present clinically as seizures, profound developmental delay, blindness, deafness, hypotonia, renal cysts, characteristic facies, and intrahepatic cholestasis.[28] Patients typically present with jaundice and hepatomegaly in the first few weeks of life and progress to death because of central nervous system disease and profound hypotonia or liver failure by 6–12 months of age although survival is variable.[21] Diagnosis can be suggested by the demonstration of very long chain fatty acids in the serum of these patients by GC-MS.[29] Elevated levels of cholestanoic acids can also be detected in the urine, serum and bile using FAB-MS and GC-MS. Current therapy for these patients is directed toward supportive care. Use of cholic acid or ursodeoxycholic acid has not been demonstrated to alter the natural history of the liver disease.

Defects in bile acid conjugation

In the final steps of primary bile acid synthesis, taurine or glycine is added to bile acid intermediates to form the conjugated primary bile acids. A genetic defect in this step of bile acid conjugation has been reported by Setchell et al. in a 14-year-old boy.[30] This child originally presented at 3 months of age with a conjugated hyperbilirubinemia, elevated serum transaminases, and a normal GGT. A liver biopsy revealed periportal fibrosis, proliferation of bile ducts, and cholestasis without signs of hepatitis. A coagulopathy was present but corrected with vitamin K. Anemia, hypocalcemia, and rickets developed by 12 months of age. No further work-up was performed until the age of 14 years when a liver biopsy revealed mild periportal inflammation, minimal fibrosis, and severe hemosiderosis. FAB-MS and GC-MS were used to demonstrate a majority of unconjugated bile acids in urine, serum and bile. Oral administration of the primary conjugated bile acids can likely be used to correct the fat-soluble vitamin malabsorption in these patients.

ALTERATION OF HEPATIC BILE ACID TRANSPORT

Bile acids must be excreted into the canalicular lumen following their synthesis within hepatocytes. It is this excretion of bile acids that serves as the rate-limiting step of bile formation.[31] To maintain a recirculating pool of bile acids, there must also be an efficient uptake of bile acids from portal blood flow. Various bile acid transporters are located within hepatocytes to facilitate flow of bile acids into the canalicular lumen. Defects in any of these bile acid transporters will lead to an impairment of bile flow, interruption of the enterohepatic circulation of bile acids and subsequent cholestasis.

Two bile acid transporters are located on the basolateral surface of hepatocytes in contact with sinusoidal blood. The Na^+-taurocholate cotransporting polypeptide (NTCP) is an ATP driven, sodium-dependent transporter responsible for the uptake of conjugated bile acids from blood into hepatocytes. A sodium independent bile acid transporter, the organic anion transporting polypeptide (OATP), is also located on the basolateral membrane of hepatocytes and aids in the uptake of bile acids. Excretion of bile acids from hepatocytes into the canalicular membrane is dependent on the bile salt export pump (BSEP) and the multidrug resistance protein 2 (MRP2). Other transporters located on the canalicular membrane include the multidrug resistant type 3 protein (MDR3), familial intrahepatic cholestasis type 1 (FIC1) transporter and the SGP transporter. MDR3 is an ATP dependent transporter responsible for the transport of phospholipids into bile. FIC1 is a P-type ATPase which is part of a family of aminophospholipid transporters (Fig. 3.4).[31] Defects in bile acid transport include progressive familial intrahepatic cholestasis (PFIC) types I-3 and Dubin-Johnson syndrome.

Progressive familial intrahepatic cholestasis

Progressive familial intrahepatic cholestasis (PFIC) represents a group of disorders associated with intrahepatic cholestasis that typically presents in the first year of life. Three different genetic mutations in canalicular transport

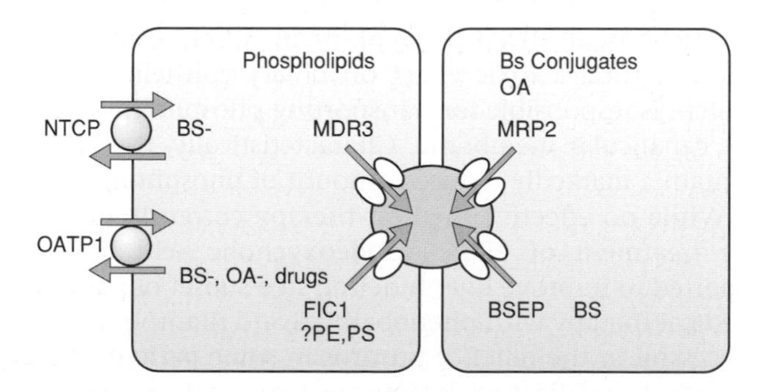

Figure 3.4: Hepatocellular transport of bile acids. The basolateral membranes of hepatocytes express the bile salt (BS) transporters Na^+-taurocholate cotransporting polypeptide (NTCP) and organic anion transporting polypeptides (OATP). Bile salts are then transported into the canalicular lumen by the bile salt export pump (BSEP) and multidrug resistance protein 2 (MRP2). In addition, phospholipids are transported across the canalicular membrane by the multi-drug resistant type 3 protein (MDR3) while aminophospholipids are transported by the familial intrahepatic cholestasis type 1 (FIC1) transporter. Not shown is the SGP transporter at the canalicular membrane whose defect is associated with PFIC-2. (Adapted with permission from Tomer G, Shneider BL. Gastroenterol Clin North Am 2003; 32:839–855.)[31]

proteins lead to the development of the three described forms of PFIC (types 1–3). All forms of PFIC can present clinically with jaundice, pruritus, failure to thrive, cholelithiasis and fat-soluble vitamin deficiency. Cirrhosis typically develops in these patients within 5–10 years, leading to liver failure.

PFIC-1, also known as Byler's disease (for the Amish descendant first described with the mutation), is an autosomal recessive disorder caused by a mutation in the FIC1 gene. Patients with PFIC-1 will present with intrahepatic cholestasis. Serum bile acid concentration will be elevated with an elevated ratio of chenodeoxycholic acid to cholic acid; however, the concentration of biliary bile acids will be low.[10] Other serological markers of this disease will be low or normal gamma glutamyl transpeptidase (GGT) and cholesterol levels. PFIC-1 is a progressive disease that will lead to liver cirrhosis by the second decade of life if left untreated.[10]

PFIC-2 is a disease that has a similar clinical and biochemical presentation to PFIC-1. This defect is known to be related to mutations in the SGP transporter at the canalicular membrane. One difference between the two disorders is that patients with PFIC-2 tend to progress to cirrhosis and liver failure more quickly than patients with PFIC-1. Distinction between the two disorders may be accomplished with a liver biopsy. Patients with PFIC-1 tend to have coarse bile visualized on liver biopsy along with blander intracanalicular cholestasis compared with patients with PFIC-2 who show a filamentous or amorphous bile appearance along with giant cell hepatitis.[32]

A third type of PFIC, PFIC-3, is somewhat different from the first two subtypes. In comparison to PFIC-1 and PFIC-2, PFIC-3 is associated with an elevated serum GGT level. Patients with PFIC-3 will present with a severe intrahepatic cholestasis in infancy and will progress to liver failure within the first few years of life. Liver biopsy of these patients will show bile duct proliferation along with periportal fibrosis. This disorder has been associated with lack of a functional MDR3 p-glycoprotein which results in bile acids exerting a toxic effect on biliary epithelium.[33] This protein is responsible for transporting phospholipids across the canalicular membrane. Characteristically, the bile will contain a markedly reduced amount of phospholipids.

While no effective medical therapy currently exists for the treatment of PFIC, ursodeoxycholic acid has been reported to improve liver function in a subset of patients.[34] Medical therapy with phenobarbital and rifampin has been successful in the relief of pruritus in some patients. Biliary diversion and ileal exclusion are two surgical procedures that have also been shown to relieve symptoms of pruritus while improving the biochemical markers of cholestasis and liver injury.[31] Liver transplantation is the only effective treatment for patients with PFIC who have progressed to end-stage liver disease.

Dubin–Johnson syndrome

Dubin Johnson syndrome is a rare, autosomal-recessive disorder associated with a lack of the MRP2 canalicular transporter.[35] Patients with this disorder may present in the neonatal period but will typically become clinically apparent in early adolescence. Patients will frequently present with an intermittent conjugated hyperbilirubinemia that will occur during times of stress or in association with the use of oral contraceptives. Diagnosis can be made by demonstrating an elevated urinary excretion of coproporphyrin isomer I or by demonstration of an abnormal sulfobromophthalein clearance curve. Liver biopsy is characterized by a dark black pigmentation of hepatocytes. Prognosis is good, as no specific therapy is needed.

ALTERATION OF THE ENTEROHEPATIC CIRCULATION OF BILE ACIDS

Bile acids can serve as mediators of diarrhea in patients with various clinical conditions that result in bile acid malabsorption. The three types of bile acid malabsorption that have been described include primary, secondary and tertiary malabsorption. Such alterations in bile acid circulation can be seen in patients with Crohn's disease, ileal resection, radiation injury, cystic fibrosis and in patients who have undergone a cholecystectomy.[36]

Primary bile acid malabsorption (Type 2) is associated with either an absent or inefficient ileal bile acid transport.[19] A group of patients with intractable diarrhea of infancy have been shown to have this type of bile acid malabsorption with increased secretion of sodium and water into the intestinal lumen.[36] Infants and children with primary bile acid malabsorption have impaired intestinal absorption of bile acids, a contracted bile acid pool size, decreased intraluminal bile acid concentrations, reduced plasma cholesterol and malabsorption of water, electrolytes and lipids.[37] Idiopathic bile acid catharsis in adults has also been associated with a similar type of malabsorption.[36]

Diarrhea has also been associated with secondary bile acid malabsorption (Type 1) where terminal ileal dysfunction leads to delivery of increased amounts of bile acids to the colon which can also induce water and electrolyte secretion.[36] Mild forms of this condition may be seen in cystic fibrosis, radiation induced injury to the ileum, or Crohn's disease affecting the terminal ileum. One of the most common causes of bile acid-induced diarrhea in children is ileal resection. The consequences of such resections are largely dependent on the liver's ability to compensate for fecal bile acid loss. During times of high fecal losses, the liver can increase synthesis of bile acids up to 10-fold.[38] When excess quantities of bile acids are lost in the stool, fewer bile acids are returned to the liver leading to upregulation of hepatic synthesis. With relatively short ileal resections, an increased bile acid synthetic rate is able to adequately compensate for fecal losses.[19] Diarrhea will occur in these patients as a direct effect of the bile acids on colonic mucosa.

McJunkin et al. showed that a cholerrheic enteropathy would be induced if dihydroxylated bile acids were present in the fecal aqueous phase in elevated concentrations (>1.5 mM) and stool pH was alkaline.[39] The dihydroxy-bile acids, chenodeoxycholic and deoxycholic acid, have hydroxyl groups in the alpha positions on the steroid nucleus and are capable of inducing water and electrolyte secretion. However, this is not the case for ursodeoxycholic acid whose 7-OH group is in the beta orientation. Patients with small ileal resections tend to have a normal or slightly alkaline fecal pH and higher fecal aqueous dihydroxy bile acid concentrations. The elevated fecal bile acid concentrations can result in colonic water and electrolyte secretion causing diarrhea with modest steatorrhea.[39] Patients with such bile-induced diarrhea often respond to bile acid binding agents, such as cholestyramine, which act to bind intraluminal bile acids. In young children, the intraluminal concentrations of dihydroxy bile acids may not reach concentrations sufficient to induce water and electrolyte secretion, and bile acid binders may not be helpful; however, with increasing age, the sequestrants may be helpful as the fecal bile acid concentration exceeds the levels associated with diarrhea.

Larger ileal resections in adults can be associated with a bile acid loss of 2.0 to 2.5 g/day. A compensatory increase in the hepatic synthesis of bile acids is unable to compensate for fecal losses.[38] As a result of this bile acid loss, the concentration of intraluminal bile acids falls below the critical micellar concentration (CMC), with associated impaired solubilization of lipolytic products in the upper small intestine. A higher fat concentration will subsequently be delivered to the colon leading to a significant steatorrhea.[19] Despite such a large loss of bile acids, treatment of diarrhea with binding agents such as cholestyramine is ineffective as the fatty acids and hydroxyl fatty acids delivered to the colon mediate the water and electrolyte secretion responsible for the diarrhea. An improvement in the diarrhea may be seen with dietary substitution of long-chain triglycerides (LCT) with medium-chain triglycerides (MCT), which are more easily absorbed with lower concentrations of intraluminal bile acids.[19]

Patients presenting with 'tertiary' bile acid malabsorption (Type 3) include individuals with a history of previous cholecystectomy, diabetes mellitus, or in association with certain drugs. These individuals typically do not have a severe bile acid malabsorption. As with the other types of bile acid malabsorption, these individuals can develop a diarrhea secondary to non-absorbed bile acids entering the colon. These bile acids will draw sodium and water into the colon and can enhance colonic motility.

MECHANISM OF BILE ACID-INDUCED DIARRHEA

Multiple studies have shown various effects of bile acids throughout the large and small bowel which may contribute to the development of diarrhea seen in patients with ileal dysfunction. These effects include the following: reduction in fluid and electrolyte absorption, net fluid secretion, altered mucosal structure, increased mucosal permeability, altered motor activity, decreased nonelectrolyte absorption, and increased mucosal cyclic adenosine monophosphate.[19]

Bile acids can produce a reduction in fluid and electrolyte absorption as well as stimulate secretion of fluid from the colon of humans.[19] Mekhjian et al. showed that chenodeoxycholic acid and deoxycholic acid could inhibit sodium and water absorption in the colon at lower concentrations but actually stimulate water secretion at higher concentrations (5 mM and 3 mM, respectively). In comparison, there was no change in sodium or water absorption from the colon with concentrations of cholic acid as high as 10 mM.[40]

Bile acids have also been shown to produce an altered mucosal structure within the GI tract. Low-Beer et al. showed that deoxycholic acid and chenodeoxycholic acid produced histological changes in the bowel (proximal> distal) and that these changes were more profound than those seen with cholic acid.[41] These mucosal changes can cause a disturbance of fluid and electrolyte absorption contributing to the development of diarrhea in patients with ileal dysfunction.

Bile acids can also cause an increase in intestinal mucosal permeability. In one study, researchers were able to show that deoxycholic and chenodeoxycholic acids could alter colonic structure and subsequently lead to an increased mucosal permeability.[42] This increased mucosal permeability may lead not only to the development of diarrhea but also to increased antigen absorption from the intestinal lumen.

Colonic motor activity has been shown to be stimulated by bile acids. The alterations in motor activity are both species and bile acid dependent. Kirwan et al. showed that chenodeoxycholic acid was more active than cholic acid in humans in stimulating colonic motility when the bile acids were infused directly into the sigmoid colon and rectum.[43] While the increased activity may lead to a decreased colonic transit time, it is unlikely that this is a major contributor to the development of diarrhea in patients with ileal dysfunction.

Bile acids also play a role in the absorption of many nonelectrolytes. In the normal human jejunum, a close correlation exists between dihydroxy bile acid induced net water movement and the fractional absorption of glucose, xylose, and fatty acids.[44] The decreased jejunal absorption of these compounds is likely from a detergent effect of the dihydroxy bile acids on the enterocyte membrane.[19]

A final mechanism by which bile acids may contribute to the development of diarrhea in patients with ileal dysfunction is through the production of cyclic adenosine monophosphate (cAMP). Cyclic AMP likely plays a role in fluid and electrolyte secretion by dihydroxy bile acids. While many studies have shown that dihydroxy bile acids will stimulate the production of cAMP in enterocytes, other studies have not provided support for the role of cAMP in the production of bile acid-induced water secretion. Although a definitive answer has not been reached, evidence would suggest that cAMP does play a significant role in the production of bile acid-stimulated diarrhea.[19]

SUMMARY

Bile acids are vital in the processing and absorption of dietary lipids as well as for the stimulation of bile flow and regulation of sterol metabolism. Multiple enzymatic steps occur in the conversion of cholesterol to the primary and secondary bile acids. A disruption of synthesis in one of the primary bile acids, cholic acid or chenodeoxycholic acid, within the liver will lead to cholestasis as well as fat and fat soluble vitamin malabsorption. If a disruption in the recycling of bile acids occurs at the level of the intestine, diarrhea or steatorrhea can occur depending on the severity of the interruption. Newborns are particularly susceptible to any disruptions in bile acid synthesis or alterations in the enterohepatic circulation of bile acids because of an immature synthetic pathway of bile acid biosynthesis.

References

1. Russell DW, Setchell KD. Bile acid biosynthesis. Biochemistry 1992; 31:4737–4749.
2. Vlahcevic ZR, Pandak WM, Stravitz RT. Regulation of bile acid biosynthesis. Gastroenterol Clin North Am 1999; 28:1–25.
3. Swell L, Gustafsson J, Schwartz CC, et al. An in vivo evaluation of the quantitative significance of several potential pathways to cholic and chenodeoxycholic acids from cholesterol in man. J Lipid Res 1980; 21:455–466.
4. Bove KE. Liver disease caused by disorders of bile acid synthesis. Clin Liver Dis 2000; 4:831–848.
5. Hofmann AF. The continuing importance of bile acids in liver and intestinal disease. Arch Intern Med 1999; 159:2647–2658.
6. Huijghebaert SM, Hofmann AF. Pancreatic carboxypeptidase hydrolysis of bile acid-amino acid conjugates: selective resistance of glycine and taurine amidates. Gastroenterology 1986; 90:306–315.
7. Bahar RJ, Stolz A. Bile acid transport. Gastroenterol Clin North Am 1999; 28:27–58.
8. Nathanson MH, Boyer JL. Mechanisms and regulation of bile secretion. Hepatology 1991; 14:551–566.
9. Dawson PA. Bile secretion and the enterohepatic circulation of bile acids. In: Feldman M, Friedman LS, Sleisenger MH, eds. Gastrointestinal and Liver Disease Pathophysiology/Diagnosis/Management, 7th edn. Philadelphia, PA: Saunders; 2002: 1051–1064.
10. Emerick KM, Whitington PF. Molecular basis of neonatal cholestasis. Pediatr Clin North Am 2002; 49:221–235.
11. Heubi JE. Bile acid metabolism and the enterohepatic circulation of bile acids. In: Gluckman PD, Heymann MA, eds. Pediatrics & Perinatology: The Scientific Basis, 2nd edn. London: Arnold; 1996:663–668.
12. Back P, Walter K. Developmental pattern of bile acid metabolism as revealed by bile acid analysis of meconium. Gastroenterology 1980; 78:671–676.
13. Balistreri WF, Heubi JE, Suchy FJ. Immaturity of the enterohepatic circulation in early life: factors predisposing to 'physiologic' maldigestion and cholestasis. J Pediatr Gastroenterol Nutr 1983; 2:346–354.
14. Watkins JB, Ingall D, Szczepanik P, et al. Bile-salt metabolism in the newborn. N Engl J Med 1973; 288:431–434.
15. Belle RC de, Vaupshas V, Vitullo BB, et al. Intestinal absorption of bile salts: immature development in the neonate. J Pediatr 1979; 94:472–476.
16. Kaplan GS, Bhutani VK, Shaffer TH, et al. Gallbladder mechanics in newborn piglets. Pediatr Res 1984; 18:1181–1184.
17. Lehtonen L, Svedström E, Kero P, et al. Gall-bladder contractility in preterm infants. Arch Dis Child 1993; 68:43–45.
18. Wendtland-Born A, Wiewrodt B, Bender SW, et al. Prevalence of gallstones in the neonatal period. Ultraschall Med 1997; 18:80–83.
19. Heubi JE. Bile acid-induced diarrhea. In: Lebenthal E, Duffey M, eds. Textbook of Secretory Diarrhea. New York, NY: Raven Press; 1990:281–290.
20. Setchell KD, Suchy FJ, Welsh MB, et al. Delta 4-3-oxosteroid 5 beta-reductase deficiency described in identical twins with neonatal hepatitis. A new inborn error in bile acid synthesis. J Clin Invest 1988; 82:2148–2157.
21. Balistreri WF. Inborn errors of bile acid biosynthesis and transport-novel forms of metabolic liver disease. Gastroenterol Clin North Am 1999; 28:145–172.
22. Clayton PT, Leonard JV, Lawson AM, et al. Familial giant cell hepatitis associated with synthesis of 3β,7a,12a-trihydroxy-5-cholenoic acids. J Clin Invest 1987; 79:1031–1038.
23. Ichimiya H, Nazer H, Gunasekaran T, et al. Treatment of chronic liver disease caused by 3β-hydroxy-?^{5}-C27-steroid dehydrogenase deficiency with chenodeoxycholic acid. Arch Dis Child 1990; 65:1121–1124.
24. Setchell KDR, Schwarz M, O'Connell NC, et al. Identification of a new inborn error in bile acid synthesis: Mutation of the oxysterol 7a-hydroxylase gene causes severe neonatal liver disease. J Clin Invest 1998; 102:1690–1703.
25. Bel S, Garcia-Patos V, Rodriguez L, et al. Cerebrotendinous xanthomatosis. J Am Acad Derm 2001; 45:292–295.
26. Bouwes Bavinck JN, Vermeer BJ, Gevers Leuben JA. Capillary gas chromatography of urine samples in diagnosing cerebrotendinous xanthomatosis. Arch Derm 1986; 122:1269–1272.
27. Setchell KDR, Heubi JE, Bove KE, et al. Liver disease caused by failure to racemize trihydroxycholestanoic acid: gene mutation and effect of bile acid therapy. Gastroenterology 2003; 124:217–232.
28. Smith DW, Opitz JM, Inhorn SL. A syndrome of multiple developmental defects including polycystic kidneys and intrahepatic biliary dysgenesis in 2 siblings. J Pediatr 1965; 67:617–624.
29. Takemoto Y, Suzuki Y, Horibe R, et al. Gas chromatography/mass spectrometry analysis of very long chain fatty acids, docosahexaenoic acid, phytanic acid and plasmalogen for the screening of peroxisomal disorders. Brain Dev 2003; 25:481–487.
30. Setchell KDR, Heubi JE, O'Connell NC, et al. Identification of a unique inborn error in bile acid conjugation involving a deficiency in amidation. In: Paumgartner G, Stiehl A, Gerok W, eds. Bile Acids in Hepatobiliary Disease: Basic and Clinical Applications. Boston: Kluwer Academic; 1997:43–47.
31. Tomer G, Shneider BL. Disorders of bile formation and biliary transport. Gastroenterol Clin North Am 2003; 32:839–855.
32. Bull LN, Carlton VE, Stricker NL, et al. Genetic and morphological findings in progressive familial intrahepatic cholestasis (Byler disease [PFIC-1] and Byler syndrome): evidence for heterogeneity. Hepatology 1997; 26:155–164.
33. Deleuze JF, Jacquemin E, Dubuisson C, et al. Defect of multidrug-resistance 3 gene expression in a subtype of progressive familial intrahepatic cholestasis. Hepatology 1996; 23:904–908.
34. Jacquemin E, Hermans D, Myara A, et al. Ursodeoxycholic acid therapy in pediatric patients with progressive familial intrahepatic cholestasis. Hepatology 1997; 25:519–523.

35. Keppler D, Konig J. Hepatic canalicular membrane 5: expression and localization of the conjugate export pump encoded by the MRP2 (cMRP/cMOAT) gene in liver. FASEB 1997; 11:509–516.
36. Balistreri WF, Heubi JE, Suchy FJ. Bile acid metabolism: relationship of bile acid malabsorption and diarrhea. J Pediatr Gastroenterol Nutr 1983; 2:105–121.
37. Heubi JE, Balistreri WF, Partin JC, et al. Refractory infantile diarrhea due to primary bile acid malabsorption. J Pediatr 1979; 94:546–551.
38. Hofmann AF, Poley JR. Role of bile acid malabsorption in pathogenesis on diarrhea and steatorrhea in patients with ileal resection. Gastroenterology 1972; 62:918–934.
39. McJunkin B, Fromm H, Sarva RP, et al. Factors in the mechanism of diarrhea in bile acid malabsorption: fecal pH-a key determinant. Gastroenterology 1981; 80:1454–1464.
40. Mekhjian HS, Phillips SF. Perfusion of the canine colon with unconjugated bile acids. Gastroenterology 1970; 59:120–129.
41. Low-Beer TS, Schneider RE, Dobbins WO. Morphological changes of the small-intestinal mucosa of guinea pig and hamster following incubation in vitro and perfusion in vivo with unconjugated bile salts. Gut 1970; 11:486–492.
42. Chadwick VS, Gaginella TS, Carlson GL, et al. Effect of molecular structure on bile acid-induced alterations in absorptive function, permeability, and morphology in the perfused rabbit colon. J Lab Clin Med 1979; 94:661–674.
43. Kirwan WO, Smith AN, Mitchell WD, et al. Bile acids and colonic motility in the rabbit and the human. Gut 1975; 16:894–902.
44. Wanitschke R, Ammon HV. Effects of dihydroxy bile acids and hydroxyl fatty acids on the absorption of oleic acid in the human jejunum. J Clin Invest 1978; 61:178–186.

Chapter 4
Indigenous flora

Jonathan E. Teitelbaum

INTRODUCTION

Researchers have estimated that the human body contains 10^{14} cells, only 10% of which are not bacteria and belong to the human body proper.[1] The mammalian intestinal tract represents a complex, dynamic and diverse ecosystem of interacting aerobic and anaerobic, non-pathologic bacteria. This complex yet stable colony includes more than 400 separate species.[2]

Within any segment of the gut, some organisms are adherent to the epithelium, while others exist in suspension in the mucus layer overlying the epithelium.[3] Binding to the epithelial surface is a highly specific process. For example, certain strains of lactobacilli and coagulase negative staphylococci adhere to the gastric epithelium of the rat whereas *Escherichia coli* and *Bacteroides* are unable to do so.[4] Bacterial adherence is also modulated by the local environment (i.e. pH), surface charge and presence of fibronectin.[5] Those unbound bacteria within the lumen of the gut represent those organisms shed from the epithelium or swallowed from the oropharynx.

Luminal flora accounts for the majority of organisms within the gut and represents 40% of the weight of feces,[1] however the fecal flora found in stool samples does not necessarily represent the important host-microbial symbiosis of the mucosal bound flora.[6] Since the majority of indigenous species are obligate anaerobes, their culture, identification and quantification are technically difficult, and it is estimated that at least half of the indigenous bacteria cannot be cultured by traditional methods.[2,7] Limitations of conventional microbiological techniques have confounded a detailed analysis of the enteric flora, and led to a shift from traditional culture and phenotyping to genotyping. Modern techniques of ribotyping, pulsed field electrophoresis, plasmid profiles, specific primers and probes for PCR and nucleic acid hybridization and 16S rRNA sequencing have allowed for identification of bacteria without culturing. Furthermore, specific 16S rRNA-based oligonucleotide probes allow detection of bacterial groups by fluorescent *in situ* hybridization (FISH). Such techniques are limited only by the number of probes developed to date to identify the bacteria of interest.

Research efforts analyzing the symbiotic relationship that exists within the gastrointestinal tract of man have been aided by studies of two well-described systems: the symbiosis between *Rhizobium* bacteria and leguminous plants and the cooperative interaction between *Vibrio fischeri* and the light-producing organ of the squid. In each host tissue, modifications are made to allow a favorable niche to be established by the symbiont.[8] The use of newer microbiological techniques has helped to further elaborate the ways in which bacteria affect change within the host. For example, the use of laser capture microdissection and gene array analysis of germ free mice colonized with *Bacteroides thetaiotaomicron* has shown affects on murine genes influencing mucosal barrier function, nutrient absorption, metabolism, angiogenesis and the development of the enteric nervous system.[9]

Of the fungi, only yeasts play a major role in the oro-intestinal tract, with *Candida* being the predominant genus. Various strains are commonly, but not always present in different locations, suggesting that they may only be transient flora. However, some strains of *C albicans* can inhabit the GI tract for longer periods of time as evidenced by the fact that strains isolated from newborns are the same as the mother's.[10] The presence of *Candida* in the GI tract does not indicate candidiasis. The colony counts of *Candida* in normal small and large bowel do not exceed 10^4 colony forming units (cfu/ml).[10] The introduction of *Candida* into a well-developed fecal flora system under continuous flow culture did not lead to multiplication of the yeast. Thus, normal bacterial flora appears to provide protection against pathologic colonization by yeast. However, if the fecal flora was destroyed by antibiotics, then the yeast would multiply.[10,11] The addition of a *Lactobacillus* species to the system was able to reduce the colony counts of the *Candida* significantly.[11] It has been found that up to 65% of individuals harbor fungi in the stool.[12] As opposed to the numerous indigenous bacterial flora and yeast forms, there does not appear to be a normal viral flora.[13]

UNDERSTANDING THE INDIGENOUS FLORA BY STUDYING GERM-FREE ANIMALS

Further understanding of the beneficial effects of developing a normal bacterial flora is achieved by the analysis of germ-free animal models (Table 4.1). Germ-free mice have small intestines that weigh less than their normal counterparts. Their intestinal wall is thinner and less cellular; the villi are thinner and more pointed at the tip; and the crypts are shallower, resulting in a reduced mucosal surface area.[14] Histologically, the mucosal cells are cuboidal rather than columnar and uniform in size and shape. The stroma has sparse concentrations of inflammatory cells under aseptic conditions with only few lymphocytes and macrophages.

- Reduced
  - Mucosal cell turnover
  - Digestive enzyme activity
  - Local cytokine production
  - Mucosa associated lymphoid tissue (MALT)
  - Lamina propria cellularity
  - Vascularity
  - Muscle wall thickness
  - Motility
- Increased
  - Enterochromaffin cell area
  - Caloric intake to sustain body weight

Data from Shanahan F. The host-microbe interface within the gut. Best Pract Res Clin Gastroenterol 2002; 16:915–931.[7]

Table 4.1 Changes in intestinal structure and function in germ-free animals

Plasma cells are absent and Peyer's patches are smaller with fewer germinal centers, and subsequently there is little or no IgA expression.[15,16] The T-cell component of the lamina propria is largely composed of CD4+ lymphocytes; these are reduced in numbers in germ free animals.[17] Furthermore, antigen transport across the intestinal barrier is increased in the absence of intestinal microflora.[18] Cellular turnover is decreased compared with colonized animals, and migration time for 3H-thymidine labeled mucosal cells from crypt to tip is doubled.[15,16] After exposure to enteric bacteria the intestines of germ-free animals take on a conventional appearance within 28 days, as one notes the infiltration of the lamina propria by lymphocytes, histiocytes, macrophages and plasma cells.[15,19]

Functional differences have also been noted in the intestines of germ-free animals including a more alkaline intraluminal pH and a more positive reduction potential (Eh).[20] Intestinal transit time and gastric emptying are also decreased in germ-free states.[21] There is also increased absorption of calcium, magnesium, xylose, glucose and some vitamins and minerals in the germ-free animal.[22] The germ-free animal also has increases in the activity of intestinal cell enzymes, such as alkaline phosphatase, disaccharidases and α-glucosidase.[22]

Without a microflora, the rate of epithelial cell renewal is reduced in the small intestine, the cecum becomes enlarged and the GALT is altered.[23] Studies have revealed that colonization of germ-free mice induces GDP-fucose asialo-GM1 α1,2-fucosyltransferase activity in the epithelium, increased neutral glycolipid, fucosyl asialo-GM1, a decrease in asialo-GM1, and the production of Fuca1, 2Gal structures.[8] These changes occur selectively based on specific bacterial strains and density.[8] In studying the *Rhizobium*-legume symbiosis, researchers have learned that the soluble factors released by the bacteria signal a release of signaling molecules from the host resulting in the expression of bacterial genes required for nodulation (*nod* genes).[24] These same genes have now been noted to be abnormal in Crohn's disease and Blau syndrome.[25]

ESTABLISHING THE INDIGENOUS FLORA

Colonization of the newborn's initially sterile gut with bacteria occurs within the first few days after birth. Such colonization appears to be rapid, indeed bacteria have been found in meconium as early as 4 h of life.[26] Initial inoculation is with diverse flora including Bifidobacteria, Enterobacteria, *Bacteroides*, Clostridia and gram positive cocci.[27,28] *Staphylococcus aureus* has recently been shown to be a major colonizer of the infant gut, perhaps a sign of reduced competition from other microbes.[29] The flora then rapidly changes and is affected by the mode of delivery, gestational age and diet. Some evidence exists that maternal stress can alter the neonatal intestinal microflora.[30]

The study by Long and Swenson analyzed stools from 196 infants and helped to define intestinal bacterial colonization with anaerobes, including *B. fragilis*. Among infants born vaginally, 96% were colonized with anaerobic bacteria within 4–6 days, with 61% harboring *B. fragilis*.[31] In contrast, at 1 week infants born full-term via cesarean section, anaerobes were present in only 59% and *B. fragilis* was found in 9%.[31] A study by Gronlund et al. utilizing standard culture techniques could find no permanent colonization with *B. fragilis* prior to 2 months of age among newborns born via cesarean, with maternal prophylactic antibiotics. At 6 months of age, the colonization rate was 36%, half of that found in a group of vaginally born infants.[32] These studies suggest that the sterile manner in which children are born via cesarean section, as well as the use of perinatal antibiotics, delays intestinal anaerobic colonization. A delay in colonization with aerobic bacteria has also been observed in a study of 70 healthy Swedish newborns, which found that 45% of vaginally delivered *vs* 12% of cesarean delivered infants were colonized with *E. coli* by the 3rd day of life.[33]

As to gestational age, significantly fewer vaginally born pre-term infants had anaerobes found in their stool at the end of 1 week, as compared with their vaginally born full-term counterparts, suggesting that either local conditions in the pre-term infant's intestine, such as lower acidity or the sterile environment of an incubator, affect colonization.[31]

Breast-fed infants born vaginally had similar colonization to vaginally born formula-fed infants at 48 h of age, indicating a similar 'inoculum'. However, by 7 days, only 22% of breast-fed infants have *B. fragilis*, *vs* 61% of the formula-fed infants.[31] Harmsen et al. studied the development of fecal flora in six breast-fed and six formula-fed infants during the first 20 days after birth, using newer molecular techniques and comparing them with traditional culturing.[34] The study supported prior studies in demonstrating an initially diverse colonization that became *Bifidobacterium* predominant in the breast-fed group, whereas the formula-fed group had similar amounts of *Bacteroides* and *Bifidobacterium*. Breast-fed infants also had some lactobacilli and streptococci as colonizers,[34] while formula-fed infants develop a more diverse flora, which also include Enterobacteriacaceae, enterococci and *Clostridia*.[27,28,34] One study found *Lactobacillus* to be more dominant than *Bifidobacterium* in breast-fed babies.[35] The acquisition of aerobic gram-negative bacilli also varied with feeding type, as 62% of formula-fed infants and 82% breast-fed infants were colonized by 48 h of life.[31] After weaning, the flora becomes more diverse with fewer *E. coli* and *Clostridium* and more *Bacteroides* and gram positive anaerobic cocci, and resembles that of adults.[27,36] The differences in fecal flora observed between breast-fed and formula-fed infants has been proposed to be the result of multiple causes including the lower iron content and different composition of proteins in human milk, a lower phosphate content, the large variety of oligosaccharides in human milk and numerous humoral and cellular mediators of immunologic function in breast milk.[37]

Longitudinal studies by Mata et al. of impoverished Guatemalan children born vaginally and breast-fed, documented the prevalence of *Bifidobacterium* in this group. Within the first few hours of life facultative micrococci, streptococci and gram-negative bacilli were more readily cultured than anaerobes.[36] On day of life 2, almost all infants demonstrated *E. coli* in concentrations of 10^5–10^{11} g. Only a few babies had *Bifidobacterium* on the first day of life, while by day 2, 33% were so colonized with concentrations of 10^8–10^{10} g.[36] By 1 week all had *Bifidobacterium* at concentrations of 10^{10}–10^{11} g.[36] By 1 year of age, those that were still breast-fed had bacterial colonization with almost exclusive *Bifidobacterium*.[36]

A study utilizing bacterial enzyme activity as an indirect measure of bacterial colonization found no difference in flora during the first 6 months of life based on the mode of delivery. However, stools collected from formula-fed infants had greater urease activity at 1–2 months and higher β-glucuronidase activity at 6 months compared with breast-fed infants.[38] This is in conflict with a study from Finland, in which no differences were found in enzyme activity based on feeding groups.[39] Examples of urease producing fecal bacteria include *Bifidobacterium, Clostridium, Eubacterium,* and *Fusobacterium*. β-glucuronidase producers include *Lactobacillus, Clostridium, Peptostreptococcus* and *E. coli*.

Despite these differences in colonization with *Bifidobacterium Bacteroides*, as well as differences in the colonization rate with *C. perfringens* (57% in the cesarean group *vs* 17% in the vaginal group), no differences in gastrointestinal signs such as flatulence, abdominal distention, diarrhea, foul-smelling stool, or bloody stools could be detected.[32]

Infants born vaginally have traditionally thought to acquire their fecal flora from the mother's vaginal and intestinal flora. More recently, this has been called into question with nosocomial/environmental spread appearing to be significant contributors. Within maternity wards, nosocomial spread of fecal bacteria among healthy newborns has been documented. Murono et al. studied the plasmid profiles of *E. coli* strains isolated from the stool of maternal and infant pairs to determine the degree of vertical *vs* nosocomial spread. In only 4 of the 29 pairs were shared *Enterobacteriaceae* documented. However, 8 of 10 infants in one hospital did share a single plasmid profile indicating nosocomial acquisition of the fecal flora.[40] Tannock et al. used the same plasmid profiling technique to show that *Lactobacillus* inhabiting the vaginas of mothers did not appear to colonize the infant digestive tract, while *Enterobacteriaceae* and *Bifidobacterium* from the mother's feces could be found to colonize the infant in four out of five cases.[41] The environment appears to play a greater role among infants born via cesarean section and for those separated from their mother for long periods after birth.[40]

As opposed to prior studies in the 1970s that showed colonization rates with *E. coli* in Western countries of at least 70%[42] and in developing countries of nearly 100%[43] by the first week of life regardless of mode of delivery, a more recent Swedish study found less than 50% colonization.[33] The reduction was attributed to decreased nosocomial spread by the practice of 'rooming-in' and early hospital discharge. It took almost 6 months before all infants were colonized with *E. coli*.[33] The turnover rate of individual *E. coli* strains was low, most likely due to a limited circulation of fecal bacteria in the Swedish home. Environmental factors, such as siblings, pets or feeding mode did not affect colonization kinetics.

While some *E. coli* strains appear transient and disappear from the intestine within a few weeks, others become resident for months to years. Resident strains have certain characteristics such as the expression of *P fimbriae* and a capacity to adhere to colonic epithelial cells. *P fimbriae* are composed of a fimbrial rod with a tip adhesion that exists in three papG classes. These recognize the Gal α1-4 Gal glycoproteins, with slight differences in binding.[44] Intestinal persistence of *E. coli* has been linked to the class II variety of the adhesin.[45] The resident strains more commonly have other virulence factors such as the iron chelating compound aerobactin, and capsular types K1 and K5, when compared to the transient strains[45] Within the Swedish study, the P fimbrial class III adhesion gene associated with urinary tract infections was more common in *E. coli* from children who had cats in their home than among *E. coli* from homes without pets.[33] This raises the question as to whether this *E. coli* could be transferred with close contact with a family cat.

The role of diet on the composition of fecal flora in the older child and adult appears to be minimal as individuals fed a standard institutional diet had similar fecal flora to those who consumed a random diet.[46] The ingestion of an elemental diet resulted in reduction of stool weight and frequency but few qualitative changes in the composition of the fecal flora.[47] Furthermore, in analysis of the microorganisms measured in an aliquot of fresh feces, there does not appear to be significant differences in the fecal flora based on a diet's fiber content, or meat content.[20] However, studies of the metabolic activity of the flora via measuring of bacterial enzymes have demonstrated marked differences.[20]

BACTERIAL FLORA WITHIN THE VARIOUS SECTIONS OF THE GASTROINTESTINAL TRACT

Oral flora

Infants with a developing oral ecosystem are amenable to colonization perhaps because specific antibodies capable of inhibiting bacterial adherence are present only in low levels in early infancy.[48] The indigenous microflora of the oral cavity is an integral component of the function of this site. The commensal bacteria help to defend against colonization by pathogens. Secretory immunoglobulin A (S-IgA) represents the main specific defense mechanism of the oral mucosa. The S-IgA of infant saliva and human milk are mainly composed of the IgA1 subclass.[49] IgA proteases are produced by pathogenic bacteria as well as oral commensals. Saliva contains other immunoglobulins and defense factors to inhibit microbial adhesion and growth.[50] After teeth emerge, IgG appears in greater concentrations.[49,50] The early low concentrations of antibodies[49,50] may be beneficial in allowing the invading bacteria to more easily colonize the oral surfaces. Initially only the buccal and palatal mucosa, as well as the crypts of the tongue, allow for colonization, but with the emergence of teeth, new gingival crevices and tooth surfaces become potential niches. Oxygen tension is an important environmental determinant for oral bacteria. The fastidious anaerobic growth even in edentulous mouths is explained by the formation of biofilms. *Fusobacterium nucleatum*, an obligate anaerobe, appears to play a crucial role in the maturation of oral biofilm communities.[48]

The initial colonization of the oral cavity is dependent on mode of delivery, exposure to antibiotics, feedings and gestational age.[48] For example, the establishment of the primary bacterial group viridans streptococci is delayed in pre-term infants and transiently compensated for by less prevalent inhabitants, such as yeast.[48] The initial colonization by streptococci and *Actinomyces* allows for further colonization by other species. Initial bacteria are acquired through direct and indirect salivary contacts during everyday activities, thus the colonies found within the oral cavity of young children often resemble that of the mother.[51] *Streptococcus viridans* are the first persistent oral colonizers. The principal streptococcal species are *Streptococcus mitis* and *salivarius*. Oral actinomycetes (i.e. *A. odontolyticus*) and various anaerobic species (i.e. *Prevotella melaninogenica, F. nucleatum*) are also found during the first year of life. After the first year of life, the versatility among oral microflora increases remarkably. Among infants, there appears to be no stability among the specific clonal populations, and such instability is noted among adults, but to a lesser degree.[52] This stability, or lack of, appears to be variable based on the bacterial species being studied.[48] Pathologic bacteria such as *Streptococci mutans*, the main causative bacteria in caries, appear in the oral cavity only after the primary teeth emerge. Children colonized early by this bacteria are more susceptible to caries than those colonized later.[53]

Stomach flora

The stomach typically contains less than 10^3 cfu/ml. In a limited number of impoverished Guatemalan children, the colony counts ranged from 10^2–10^7 cfu/ml.[36] The lower counts are attributed to gastric juices which destroy most oral bacteria.[20] The microflora of the stomach typically consists of gram-positive and aerobic bacteria with streptococci, staphylococci, *Lactobacillus* and various fungi being most commonly isolated.[54] Indeed, *Candida* can be isolated from the stomach in up to 30% of healthy people.[12]

Small bowel flora

The small intestine represents a transitional zone between the sparsely populated stomach and the exuberant bacterial flora of the colon. Accordingly, the proximal small bowel has bacterial counts similar to that of the stomach, with concentrations ranging between 10^3 and 10^4 cfu/ml in the duodenum[20] and higher concentrations of 10^2–10^6 in the Guatemalan childhood study.[36] Jejunal flora is similar to that of the stomach.[5] The predominant species are streptococci, staphylococci, and *Lactobacillus*. In addition, *Veillonellae* and *Actinomyces* species are also frequently isolated but other anaerobic bacteria are present in lower concentrations.[20] Interestingly, small bowel concentrations are variable among animal species. Normal cats were noted to have relatively high numbers of bacteria (10^5–10^8 cfu/ml) including many obligate anaerobes in the proximal small intestine. This was thought to be secondary to a strictly carnivorous diet.[55] At the end of the transition, within the distal ileum, the gram-negative organisms out-number gram-positive organisms.[20] Here, anaerobic bacteria such as *Bacteroides, Bifidobacterium, Fusobacterium* and *Clostridium* are found at substantial concentrations along with coliforms.[20] The distal ileum has an oxidation-reduction potential (Eh) of –150 mV, which is similar to that of the cecum (–200 mV), thus allowing it to support the growth of anaerobic bacteria.[56]

Colonic flora

Once in the colon, the bacterial concentrations increase dramatically. Colonic bacterial concentrations are typically 10^{11}–10^{12} cfu/ml.[20] Here anaerobic bacteria out-number aerobes by 1000 fold.[20] Predominant species include *Bacteroides, Bifidobacterium* and *Eubacterium*, with anaerobic gram-positive cocci, *Clostridia*, enterococci and various Enterobacteriaceae also being common.[20]

CONTROLLING THE GROWTH OF THE INDIGENOUS POPULATION

Various host defenses are responsible for controlling the proliferation of intestinal bacteria thus limiting the population size (Table 4.2). Such limitation is needed since under optimal conditions *in vitro* coliform bacteria can divide every 20 min.[20] If this were to occur *in vivo* the host would quickly become overwhelmed. Within the gastroin-

Host factors
Intestinal motility/peristalsis
Gastric acid
Antibacterial quality of pancreatic and biliary secretions
Intestinal immunity (IgA, Paneth cell products (defensins), lysozyme, bactericidal permeability increasing protein), epithelial cell products
Mucus layer
Microbial factors
Alteration in redox potential
Substrate depletion
Growth inhibitors (short chain fatty acids, bacteriocins)
Suppression of bacterial adherence
Data from Batt R, Rutgers G, Sancak A. Enteric bacteria: friend or foe? J Small Animal Prac 1996; 37:261–267.[74]

Table 4.2 Regulation of the indigenous microflora

testinal tract, bacterial generation time is longer at one to four divisions per day.[57] Within the small intestine, the major defenses against bacterial overgrowth are gastric acid and peristalsis. The ability of the peristaltic wave to propel bacteria is inferred by Dixon's classic study in which he inoculated ^{51}Cr-labeled red blood cells (RBC) and bacteria into a surgically created subcutaneous loop of rat small intestine. The bacteria and RBCs were noted to be rapidly cleared from the small intestine by the rat's peristaltic activity.[58] The effectiveness of peristalsis in moving bacteria is further emphasized by those circumstances in which one has a loop of intestine with ineffective peristalsis, and bacterial overgrowth is found. Experimental studies show that gastric emptying and intestinal transit are slowed in a germ-free state and restored with re-colonization by normal flora.[59]

Gastric acid has also been shown to contribute to the sparse bacterial colonization of the proximal intestine. Gram-negative organisms are particularly susceptible to the effects of a low pH, and a large inoculum of *Serratia* organisms is eradicated within 1 h when in contact with normal gastric acidity.[5] Indeed, patients with achlorhydria harbor coliforms and anaerobic gram-negative bacilli in the proximal small bowel, as well as increased numbers of streptococci, *Lactobacillus* and fungi.[20] Lowering of gastric acid pharmacologically has been shown to impair host defenses against pathologic bacteria including *Vibrio cholera,*[60] *Candida,*[61] *Campylocacter*[62] and *Strongyloides stercoralis*.[63]

Bile duct ligation in experimental animals results in cecal overgrowth with coliforms, suggesting that bile acids or some other component of bile plays a role in the regulation of the bacterial flora.[64] It is suspected that the deconjugation of bile acids by the indigenous flora to create simple bile acids with the ability to inhibit bacterial growth is a possible mechanism.[5]

Microbial interactions constitute a major factor in regulating the indigenous microflora, particularly within the colon. Various interactions can either promote or inhibit growth of organisms. One mechanism would be competition for substrates. An example is the inhibition of the growth of *Shigella flexneri* by coliform organisms which compete for carbon.[65] Another mechanism would be manipulation of the oxygen content of the environment. The maintenance of a reduced environment by facultative bacteria allows the growth of anaerobic bacteria.[20] By-products of bacterial metabolism can create an intraluminal environment that restricts growth. Short chain fatty acids such as acetic, propionic and butyric acid can inhibit bacterial proliferation.[20] At sufficiently low pH these acids are undissociated and can enter the bacterial cell to inhibit microbial metabolism.[22] *Lactobacillus*, particularly *L. plantatum* are found throughout the GI tract and their ability to adhere to mannose-containing receptors on epithelial cells is important in protecting against colonization by pathogens.[66] Finally, some bacteria can produce antibiotic-like substances termed bacteriocins, enocin and hydrogen peroxide, which can inhibit the growth of other bacterial species or even contribute to self-regulation. Included in this group are colicines produced by strains of *E. coli*.[67]

Mucus provides protection at the mucosal surface with its viscous high molecular weight glycoprotein providing a physiochemical barrier which in concert with secreted immunoglobulins entrap bacteria.[68] The carbohydrate component of mucin can also compete for receptor specific binding proteins of microbes.

Host immunity also plays a role in limiting the growth of the indigenous bacterial population. IgA synthesis by B cells of the gut-associated lymphoid tissue is stimulated by the endogenous flora, and increased further with pathologic colonization as in *Shigella* infection or bacterial overgrowth.[5] Distinct B-cell populations secrete different types of IgA which may help control the volume and composition of the flora.[69] Such IgA is thought to prevent bacterial adhesion to epithelial cells.[70] However, isolated IgA deficiency is not associated with alterations in the pattern of colonization.[71] Moreover, the acquisition and composition of T- or B-cell deficient mice is indistinguishable from that of their immunologically intact littermates.[5] Paneth cells of the small intestine secrete antibacterial peptides called defensins that have antibacterial properties, as well as phospholipase A2, bactericidal permeability-increasing protein and lysozyme.[5]

The pattern of antibodies directed against fecal bacteria appears to be unique for each individual. People tend to make antibodies against both indigenous bacteria as well as transient bacteria. The antibodies include both polyspecific IgM as well as specific IgG and IgA. Relatively more specific IgA antibodies appear to be directed against transient bacteria as apposed to indigenous bacteria.[72]

SYMBIOSIS BETWEEN HOST AND FECAL FLORA

A microflora associated characteristic (MAC) is defined as the recording of any anatomical structure, physiological or biochemical function in a micro-organism that has been influenced by the microflora. When such changes occur in the absence of microflora, they are designated as a germ-free animal characteristic (GAC).[73] The distinction between MAC and GAC helps to define the symbiotic relationship that exists between human and the microbial host, and elucidates those processes which bacteria perform that are advantageous to the host (Table 4.3). Bacterial β-glucuronidase and sulfatase are responsible for the enterohepatic circulation of numerous substances including bilirubin, bile acids, estrogens, cholesterol, digoxin, rifampin, morphine, colchicine and diethylstilbestrol.[20] Microflora also play a role in the degradation of intestinal mucin, conversion of urobilin to urobilinogen, cholesterol to coprostanol, and the production of short chain fatty acids (SCFA).[20,73] Mucin degrading microbes are evident in all children by 20–21 months.[20] This appears to be a gradual acquisition process starting at about 3 months of age.[73] Bacterial synthesis of vitamins such as biotin, Vitamin K, B12, pantothenate and riboflavin and folate help supplement dietary sources.[22,74] Bacterial enzymatic degradation of urea is probably the only source of ammonia in the animal host.[22]

Scheline stressed that the 'gut flora have the ability to act as an organ with a metabolic potential equal to, or sometimes greater than the liver'.[75] A broad spectrum of metabolic reactions have been performed by intestinal flora, including hydrolysis, dehydroxylation, decarboxylation, dealkylation, dehalogenation, deamination, heterocyclic ring fission, reduction, aromatization, nitrosamine formation, acetylation, esterification, isomerization and oxidation.[75,76] Gut flora acts on drugs to result in activation, toxin production or deactivation. One of the earliest examples of activation by micro-organisms is seen with protosil.[77] The bioavailability and pharmacological effect of numerous drugs, such as opiates, digoxin, hormones and antibiotics have been demonstrated to be altered by gut flora.[78] Beta-lyases transform xenobiotic cysteine conjugates to toxic metabolites such as thiols or thiol derivatives.[76] The azoreductase activity of the colonic flora metabolizes the pro-drug sulfasalazine to its active aminosalicylate.

SCFA production is thought to occur in the cecum and ascending colon mainly by the anaerobic flora.[73] It appears that those infants fed breast milk produce fewer SCFA than those fed formula in which there is a more varied, adult like SCFA profile. SCFA produced in the colon may represent up to 70% of the energy available from the ingestion of carbohydrate.[79]

Intestinal microfloral enzymes β-glucuronidase and sulfatase catalyze the deconjugation of estrogens excreted with bile into the intestine to allow for reabsorption as part of the enterohepatic circulation. The presence of estriol-3-glucuronide in the urine is an indicator of estrogen resorption in the intestine.[20] The suppression of the intestinal microflora with antibiotics results in a decrease in the enterohepatic circulation of sex steroids, and can thus lower the concentrations of these hormones significantly. Indeed, reports of failed oral contraception have been linked to concomitant use of antibiotics.[80]

Bile acids are derived from cholesterol in the liver. Within the liver, primary bile acids are conjugated and excreted into the bile. Bile acids undergo enterohepatic circulation several times each day. Most of the absorption takes place by active transport in the terminal ileum. In the intestine, conjugated bile acids are acted upon by bacterial enzymes and converted to secondary bile acids. These secondary bile acids are either excreted into the feces or absorbed and sometimes further metabolized within the liver into tertiary bile acids. Microbial transformation of bile acids includes deconjugation, desulfation, deglucuronidation, oxidation of hydroxyl groups and reduction of oxo-groups.[81] Since humans are born germ-free, primary bile acids can be found in the meconium of newborn babies. Short chain bile acids are elevated in children and adults with cholestasis.[82] In healthy children, the levels of short chain bile acids are undetectable. The ability to hydrolyze taurine and glycine bile acid conjugates has been detected in *Bifidobacterium, Peptostreptococcus, Lactobacillus* and *Clostridium* shortly after birth.[83] The occurrence, substrate specificity and kinetics of this enzyme activity vary among species and bacterial strain.[83] Jonsson et al. observed a decrease in sulfated conjugates within the stool at approximately 6 months of age. This was the same time that sulfate rich mucin disappeared and thus they suspected this was due to the action of microbial desulfanates.[81] Two clostridia strains (*Clostridium sp* S1 and S2) and *Peptostreptococcus niger* H4 desulfate bile acid-3-sulfates.[81] Jonsson also noted that by 24 months of age, all the children studied had an adult pattern of excreted bile acids in that they were lacking a hydroxyl group at C-7.[81] Bacteria that are known to have 7α-dehydroxylation activity include *Eubacterium, Clostridium* and *Lactobacillus.*[83] Cholesterol elimination is accomplished by two major

Beneficial
- Competitive exclusion of pathogens
- Production of short chain fatty acids
- Synthesis of vitamins and nutrients
- Enterohepatic circulation of numerous substances (e.g. bilirubin, bile acids, estrogens, cholesterol, digoxin, rifampin, morphine, colchicines and diethylstilbestrol)
- Degradation of intestinal mucin
- Conversion of urobilin to urobilinogen
- Conversion of cholesterol to coprostanol
- Degradation of urea
- Drug metabolism and activation
- Development of the immune system
- Development of the enteric nervous system

Detrimental effects
- Competition for calories and essential nutrients
- Production of harmful metabolites (carcinogens, deconjugated bile acids, hydroxyl fatty acids)
- Mucosal damage
  - Direct effect of bacteria
  - Exacerbate inflammatory disease

Data from Batt R, Rutgers G, Sancak A. Enteric bacteria: friend or foe? J Small Animal Prac 1996; 37:261–267.[74]

Table 4.3 Effects of enteric bacteria

routs, conversion of cholesterol to coprostanol and 7α-dehydroxylation of bile acids. Infants appear to be unable to perform such elimination during the first several months of life.[81] Thus, during those months sulfation appears to be a compensatory mechanism for the excretion of breakdown products of cholesterol.[84]

BACTERIAL FLORA IN ILLNESS

Pathologic colonization occurs with the same species that predominate in nosocomial infections, and studies suggest that colonization is a risk factor for infection. This is the theory behind prophylactic decontamination of the digestive tract in the critically ill, which has been shown to reduce mortality.[5] Changes in the composition of the gut flora are common in critical illness due to reduced enteral intake, reduced intestinal motility, use of acid blockade therapy and broad spectrum antibiotics.[5] Gram-negative organisms are rarely found in the oropharynx of healthy individuals, yet can be found in up to 75% of hospitalized patients.[85] Similarly, du Moulin et al. documented the effects of antacids on the flora of the stomach. Among 59 critically ill patients, simultaneous colonization of the gastric and respiratory tract was seen with aerobic gram-negative bacteria.[86] This and similar studies have been the basis of the controversy surrounding routine acid blockade therapy for critically ill patients. Overall, it appears as though only in selective patients does the benefit of stress ulcer prophylaxis outweigh the risk of nosocomial pneumonia.[87] Gastric colonization in these patients also appears to be a risk factor for wound infections, urinary tract infections, peritonitis and bacteremia.[88] Studies aimed at decreasing bacterial overgrowth via selective decontamination of the digestive tract using topical, non-absorbed, antimicrobial agents active against aerobic gram negatives (tobramycin and polymyxin) and fungi (amphotericin) but leaving gram positive flora to preserve colonization resistance, have been varied. However, a meta-analysis indicates that this strategy is effective in preventing nosocomial respiratory infection, and reduces ICU mortality.[89]

Total parenteral nutrition given to experimental animals increased the concentration of aerobic gram-negative organisms in the cecum and bacterial translocation into lymph nodes when compared with enterally fed animals.[90] Indeed enteral feeding in the critically ill human is associated with fewer nosocomial infections.[91]

BACTERIAL FLORA AND ALLERGY

Although the exact pathophysiology of allergic disease is incompletely understood, it is thought to represent the end result of disordered function of the immune system. The intestinal barrier in the infant is thought to be immature, and thus vulnerable to allergic sensitization during the first few months of life. The intestinal microflora strengthens the immune defense and stimulates the development of the gut immune system.[69] In newborns the type 2 T helper cell (Th2) cytokines, essential mediators in the formation of allergic inflammation, predominate over Th1 cytokines.[69] Th2 cytokines include IL-4 which induces B-cell differentiation into IgE producing cells, and IL-5 which is important for eosinophil activity. Intestinal bacteria can counterbalance this Th2 activity, promote the development of the Th1 cell lineage, and thus regulate the IgE response.[92] This may be the result of the CpG motif which can induce polyclonal B cell activation and secretion of Th1 cytokines such as IL-6, IL-12, and interferon (IFN).[93] Intestinal bacteria may also modulate allergic inflammation via modification of antigen uptake,[94] presentation[95] and degradation.[96,97] Thus, in those children with an aberrant array or insufficient number of intestinal micro-organisms, there may be an inability to strengthen the gut barrier or counterbalance a Th2 cytokine profile. This inability to reduce the two major risk factors toward developing allergy may lead to sensitization.

The role of bacteria in the formation of allergy is strengthened by clinical studies which demonstrate that there are differences in the microflora between allergic and non-allergic individuals. One study revealed that non-allergic individuals had higher counts of aerobic bacteria during the first week of life, as well as greater numbers of *Lactobacillus* at 1 month and 1 year of age. At age 1 to 2 years the allergic children have greater prevalence of *Staphylococcus aureus* and Enterobacteriaceae and fewer *Bacteroides* and *Bifidobacterium*.[98] Allergic children also appear to have greater number of *Clostridia* at 3 weeks of age.[98,99] *Bifidobacterium* are known to elicit a Th1 type immune response.[100] In another study, allergic infants were found to have high levels of the adult type *Bifidobacterium adolescentis* compared with healthy infants who had greater numbers of *B. bifidum*. Comparison of the adhesive properties of these two strains found that *B. bifidum*'s adhesive abilities was significantly higher. These results suggest that the greater adhesive qualities may help to stabilize the mucosal barrier and prevent absorption of antigenic proteins.[101]

Lifestyles which limit antibiotic use and encourage the ingestion of fermented foods appear to have a decreased risk of developing allergy. Similarly the early use of antibiotics appears to be a risk factor for developing later atopic disease.[102] Inflammation is triggered by toll-like receptors (TLRs), a group of evolutionarily conserved pattern recognition receptors present in intestinal epithelial cells and antigen presenting cells.[102] More than 10 members of the TLR family have been described, each of them possessing specificity towards microbial surface structure elements.[102]

BACTERIAL FLORA AND ANTIBIOTICS

Nearly all antibiotics have an effect on the bacterial flora. The effect is dependent on the intraluminal concentration, as well as the antimicrobial spectrum.[20] Such an effect can be advantageous, and numerous studies have demonstrated the reduction of wound infections following surgery with the use of prophylactic antibiotics.[103,104] Among neutropenic patients, intestinal colonization with gram-negative aerobic bacilli, especially *P. aeruginosa*, frequently precedes infection. Prophylactic antibiotics to modify the intestinal flora have been shown to reduce the incidence of infection in this population.[104]

The use of oral ampicillin or penicillin suppresses the normal aerobic and anaerobic flora including *Bifidobacterium, Streptococcus* and *Lactobacillus* spp and causes overgrowth of *Klebsiella, Proteus* and *Candida* spp.[105,106] However, cefaclor, an oral cephalosporin, and cephalexin administration appear to cause little change, except for a reduction in Enterobacteriaceae.[106] Erythromycin administration results in fewer marked changes than observed with penicillins; however, there is a significant decrease in Enterobacteriaceae.[106] Oral gentamicin administration results in drastic changes including a marked decline in *E. coli*.[106] However, intravenous gentamycin is excreted into the intestine with bile at lower concentrations and thus alter the flora only slightly.[107] Cefpiramide, a parenteral expanded-spectrum cephalosporin, which is excreted in the bile at high concentrations suppresses normal flora so markedly that almost all species of organisms are eradicated and the active growth of yeast is promoted.[106] There appears to be a rapid return of the disturbed flora to normal levels within 3 to 6 days after therapy,[106] although a minority of researchers believe recovery time could be longer, in the order of 2 weeks or greater.[108] Suppression of the normal flora results in lowered colonization resistance and promotes overgrowth of resistant organisms,[109] as well as allowing for colonization with pathogens such as *C. difficile*.

Antibiotics may also affect fecal bulk. Volunteers on a constant diet who were administered ampicillin and metronidazole were noted to have a 97% increase in their fecal bulk. This was accompanied by a 69% increase in fecal fiber. The author suggests that the absence of digestion of the fecal fiber by the indigenous flora was the mechanism by which the antibiotics resulted in increased fecal bulk.[110]

BACTERIAL OVERGROWTH

Bacterial overgrowth is the term used when there are excessive amounts of bacteria inhabiting the small intestine. Those disorders that alter small bowel motility appear to predispose individuals to the greatest extent. These include small bowel diverticula, surgically created blind loops, strictures, pseudo-obstruction, scleroderma, diabetic neuropathy, resection of small bowel including the ileocecal valve, cirrhosis, malnutrition and abdominal radiation.[20] Bacteriologic analysis of the microflora includes aerobic and anaerobic bacteria. Bacterial concentrations can range from 10^7 to 10^9 cfu/ml, and rarely to 10^{11}.[20]

Additional host factors that allow for bacterial overgrowth include defective gastric acid secretion and defective local immunity. The use of acid blockade significantly affects the mean gastric bacterial count, such that as the pH rises above 4, the bacterial count increased from 0 to $10^{6.4}$, and the mean number of bacterial species increased from 0.5 to 4.3.[111]

Clinical manifestations of bacterial overgrowth include diarrhea, steatorrhea, vitamin B12 deficiency, protein malnutrition, weight loss and impaired sugar absorbtion.[22] These effects are mediated via increased deconjugation of bile salts, volatile fatty acids, alcohols, volatile amines, and hydroxyl fatty acids.[22] These products can result in increasing intraluminal osmolarity and subsequent diarrhea. Malabsorption appears more common when colonization includes anaerobes. Some speculate it is the deconjugation of bile acids, specifically by *Bacteroides* strains, that favor the growth of anaerobes.[112] B12 deficiency is thought to be due to uptake of the vitamin by the bacteria, indeed ingested B12 in these patients is found in the feces bound to bacterial cell wall components.[20] Amino acid absorption is also impaired in overgrowth, with increased fecal nitrogen.[20] D-lactic acidosis has also been linked to bacterial overgrowth and the inability of humans to rapidly metabolize D-lactate.[113]

An increased serum folate or reduced cobalamin provides indirect evidence of bacterial overgrowth. Permeability tests may reflect mucosal damage in overgrowth. Histologically, the intestinal mucosa may loose its villous architecture and most of its absorptive surface. The use of hydrogen breath testing has been shown to be useful. Endoscopic collection of duodenal juice for culture and quantification would be the gold standard. Initial treatment should be directed at the cause of the overgrowth. This is often inapparent, and thus oral broad spectrum antibiotic therapy is typically employed.

TROPICAL SPRUE

Tropical sprue is characterized by chronic diarrhea, malaise, weight loss, and malabsorption of carbohydrates, fats, vitamin B12 and folate. The disease effects tropical areas most notably India and the Caribbean area.[20] Onset of symptoms is typically after a gastroenteritis, small bowel overgrowth then ensues and symptoms resolve with treatment including antibiotics.[114] There appears to be significant colonization of the small bowel with Enterobacteriaceae. The fecal flora of affected patients is abnormal in that aerobic organisms outnumber anaerobes.[115] Enterotoxigenic coliforms are thought to colonize the small intestine and contribute to the diarrhea. Histologically, there is villus blunting and infiltration of the lamina propria that are more marked than those found in bacterial overgrowth.[20] Here one also sees delayed small bowel transit.

PROBIOTICS

Documentation of the health benefits of bacteria in food dates back to as early as the Persian version of the Old Testament (*Genesis* 18:8), which states 'Abraham owed his longevity to the consumption of sour milk'.[116] In 1908 Nobel Prize winning Russian scientist Elie Metchnikoff suggested that the ingestion of *Lactobacillus* containing yogurt decreases the number of toxin-producing bacteria in the intestine and thus contributes to the longevity of Bulgarian peasants.[117] The term probiotic was first used in 1965 in contrast to the word antibiotic and defined as 'substances secreted by one micro-organism, which stimulates the growth of another'.[116] A more complete definition would be 'A preparation of or a product containing viable, defined micro-organisms in sufficient numbers, which alter the microflora (by implantation or colonization) in a compartment of the host and by that exert beneficial health effects on the host'.[116] Current criteria for defining probiotics are found in Table 4.4. Effects of probiotics on improving health have been proclaimed in many areas including immunomodulation, cholesterol lowering, cancer prevention, cessation of diarrhea, avoidance of allergy and necrotizing enterocolitis, treatment of *H. pylori* infection and inflammatory bowel disease, although for many these claims remain to be proven scientifically.[118] The potential benefits of probiotics has led industry to consider routine addition of these bacteria to infant formulas.[119]

Although typically considered benign and without pathologic potential, there is a report of a 1-year-old immunocompetent patient who was fungemic after being treated with *Saccharomyces boulardii* for gastroenteritis.[120] The Mayo Clinic reported eight patients immunocompromised after liver transplant who were found to have positive blood cultures for *Lactobacillus*.[121] Recently, two infants with short bowel syndrome were found to be bacteremic with probiotic strains of *Lactobacillus GG*.[122] The Food and Drug Administration (FDA) has no authority to establish a formal regulatory category for functional foods that include either probiotics or prebiotics.[123] As such, there is variability among products, and some studies have found that certain preparations contain no viable bacteria.[124]

Various bacteria have been identified as meeting the diagnostic criteria for probiotics, and include *Bifidobacterium*, a major group of saccharolytic bacteria in the large intestine. It accounts for up to 25% of the bacteria in the adult colon and 95% of that in the breast-fed newborn. They do not form aliphatic amines, hydrogen sulfide or nitrites. They produce vitamins, mainly B group, as well as digestive enzymes such as casein phosphatase and lysozyme.[125] *Bifidobacterium* produce strong acids as metabolic end products such as acetate and lactate to lower the pH in the local environment, which provides antibacterial effects. One study showed that the supplementation of bottle-fed infants with *Bifidobacterium* successfully lowered the fecal pH to 5.38 which was identical to that of breast-fed infants, yet significantly lower than bottle-fed infants whose fecal pH was 6.38.[126] Determination of survivability found that on average, approximately 30% of ingested *B. bifidum*, and 10% *L. acidophilus* can be recovered from the cecum.[127]

Lactobacillus casei GG (LGG) is another common probiotic. *Lactobacillus* have no plasmids, thus antibiotic resistance is stable, and makes only L-lactic acid (not the D-isomer).[128] It inhibits other anaerobic bacteria *in vitro* including *Clostridium, Bacteroides, Bifidoacterium, Pseudomonas, Staphylococcus, Streptococcus* and Enterobacteriaceae.[129] It has also been shown to inhibit the growth of pathogenic bacteria including *Yersinia enterocolitica, Bacillus cereus, E. coli, Listeria monocytogenes* and *Salmonella*.[130] *Lactobacillus* generate hydrogen peroxide, decrease intraluminal pH and redox potential and produce bacteriocins which can inhibit the growth of pathologic bacteria.[131] In general, colonization only lasts as long as the supplement is consumed. A study found that when LGG supplementation was stopped it disappeared from the feces in 67% of volunteers within 7 days.[132]

Saccharomyces boulardii is a patented yeast preparation that has been shown to inhibit the growth of pathogenic bacteria both *in vivo* and *in vitro*. It lives at an optimum temperature of 37° C, and has been shown to resist digestion, and thus reach the colon in a viable state. It appears to be unaffected by antibiotic therapy. However, once therapy is completed, it is rapidly eliminated.[133]

A probiotic should:

1 Be of human origin
2 Be non-pathogenic in nature
3 Be resistant to destruction by technical processing
4 Be resistant to destruction by gastric acid and bile
5 Adhere to intestinal epithelial tissue
6 Be able to colonize the gastrointestinal tract, if even for a short time
7 Produce anti-microbial substances
8 Modulate immune responses
9 Influence human metabolic activities (i.e. cholesterol assimilation, vitamin production etc.)

Table 4.4 Defining criteria of micro-organisms that can be considered probiotics

Probiotics and promotion of health

Immunomodulation

Probiotic's ability to affect the host's immune system remains ill-defined. Good evidence exists for alterations in the humoral system, most notably IgA. However, effects on the cellular immune system and cytokine production are not as well established. Both human and rodent studies have documented an augmentation of the secretory IgA production during probiotic treatment. Intestinal IgA is a dimer that binds antigens and thus prevents their interaction with the epithelial cell.[134] Studies demonstrate that *L. casei* and *L. acidophilus* enhances the IgA production from plasma cells in a dose dependent fashion.[135] Other studies have documented that probiotics can alter cytokine production[136,137] and macrophage phagocytic capacity.[138,139] However, Spanhaak investigated the effects of *Lactobacillus casei* on the immune system in 20 healthy volunteers. In a placebo-controlled trial, the probiotic was found to have no effect on natural killer cell activity, phagocytosis, or cytokine production.[140]

Cholesterol levels

Studies of animals randomized to receive yogurt with or without *Bifidobacterium* found that the total cholesterol of all rats fed yogurt was decreased. The probiotic group had a notable increase in HDL-cholesterol, and a lowering of the LDL-cholesterol by 21–31% compared with those rats fed whole milk.[141,142] The studies of probiotic use among humans appear somewhat mixed, although overall probiotics appeared to have little to no significant cholesterol lowering effect.[143–145]

The mechanism by which probiotics might lower serum cholesterol levels remains unclear. Observations that 3 hydroxy-3-methtlglutaryl coenzyme A reductase in the liver decreased significantly with the consumption of the probiotics points towards a decrease in cholesterol synthesis. Increases in the amounts of fecal bile acids suggests that there is a compensatory increased conversion of cholesterol to bile acids.[146] Others suggest the effect is secondary to precipitation of cholesterol with free bile acids formed by bacterial bile salt hydrolase.[147] A final mechanism by which probiotics may have an effect is via hydrolysis of bile acids. Those bacteria that hydrolyze efficiently would lead to a faster rate of cholesterol conversion to bile acids and thus lower the serum cholesterol concentration.[148]

Probiotics and disease

Diarrhea

The mechanism by which probiotics prevent or ameliorate diarrhea can be through stimulation of the immune system, competition for binding sites on intestinal epithelial cells,[135,149,150] or through the elaboration of bacteriocins such as nisin.[151] These and other mechanisms are thought to be dependent on the type of diarrhea being investigated, and therefore may differ between viral diarrhea, antibiotic-associated diarrhea, or traveler's diarrhea.

The effect of *Lactobacillus* GG on the shortening of rotavirus diarrhea has been well documented. On average, the duration of diarrhea was shortened by 1 day in both hospitalized children[152–159] and those treated at home.[160] As to why LGG appears to be effective for viral diarrhea, but not bacterial, the author speculates that this is due to LGG enhancement of the expression of the elaboration of intestinal mucins. These glycoproteins appear to be protective during intestinal infections. However, the protective qualities are overcome by mucinase-producing bacteria.[161] Probiotics were also proven to increase the number of rotavirus specific IgA secreting cells and serum IgA in the convalescent stage[154–156,162] suggesting that the humoral immune system plays a significant role in the probiotics' effect. Interestingly, a study found equal efficacy of heat inactivated LGG *vs* viable bacteria in the treatment of rotavirus, however the heat inactivated strains did not result in an elevated IgA response at convalescence.[156] Finally, one study revealed that infants fed formula supplemented with probiotics had a lower risk of acquiring rotavirus associated gastroenteritis.[163]

The success of probiotics in reducing or preventing antibiotic-associated diarrhea has also been convincing.[164–166] Large studies of hospitalized patients on antibiotics revealed that 13–22% of placebo and 7–9% of probiotic group developed diarrhea.[167–169] Other studies reveal that probiotics result in firmer stools, and patients have less abdominal pain.[128,170]

The use of probiotics for the treatment of *Clostridium difficile* diarrhea is a logical step, particularly given the historical use of fecal enemas in the treatment of relapsing *C. difficile*.[171,172] Indeed this is supported by an early case report of four children with relapsing *C. difficile* that responded to supplement with LGG.[173] A study in which *Saccharomyces boulardii* was used in conjunction with standard antimicrobial treatment in 124 adult patients with *C. difficile* found that the probiotic group had no effect on those with their first infection, but the probiotic significantly inhibited further recurrence in those patients with prior *C. difficile* disease.[174] Overall, the studies investigating probiotics for use of treatment or prevention of bacterial diarrhea, other than *C. difficile*, appear mixed.[175–181]

Allergy

The use of probiotics in allergic disease is based on their ability to improve gut barrier function and mature the host immune response. Probiotics have been shown to decrease gut permeability in suckling rats exposed to a prolonged cow's milk challenge. This may be achieved via increase in the secretion of antibodies directed against β-lactoglobulin, a major antigen of the cow milk protein.[94]

Studies by Isolauri investigating cow's milk sensitive infants with atopic dermatitis revealed that probiotics greatly improved the extent and intensity of their eczema. Analysis of various inflammatory markers reflected a down regulation of the T-cell mediated inflammatory state and eosinophilic inflammatory activity. The author speculated that the probiotic generated enzymes that can act as a suppressor of lymphocyte proliferation, and generate protein breakdown products that result in IL-4 down regulation. Furthermore, an increase in secretory IgA helps in increasing antigen elimination.[182,183] A study by Kalliomaki provided LGG in a double-blind placebo-controlled fashion to pregnant mothers with a first degree relative that is atopic. The newborn infants were then treated postnatally for 6 months. At 2 years of age, only 23% of the LGG group *vs* 46% of the placebo group were found to have atopic eczema.[184]

Inflammatory bowel disease

It has long been conjectured that bacteria or other infectious agents play a role in the pathogenesis of inflammatory bowel disease (IBD). Indeed, it is well accepted that antibiotics are effective in the treatment of Crohn's disease, and certain animal models of colitis only have phenotypic manifestations when exposed to bacteria. Furthermore, anti-neutrophil cytoplasmic antibody (pANCA) associated with ulcerative colitis has been linked to bacteria which express a pANCA-related epitope.[185] Epidemiologic studies have found that *Bifidobacterium* colony counts are decreased in numbers in the feces of patients with Crohn's disease.[186,187]

Clinical studies of affected patients have demonstrated the efficacy of probiotics in maintaining remission in ulcerative colitis at a rate equivalent to mesalamine.[188,189] Among Crohn's patients, the addition of a probiotic to mesalamine resulted in a greater number of patients maintaining remission.[190] Various probiotic bacteria have also been shown to be useful in the maintenance treatment of chronic pouchitis including *Bifidobacterium, Lactobacillus* and *Streptococcus*.[191] However, a recent study in children showed no beneficial effect of probiotics in the treatment of Crohn's disease.[192]

PREBIOTICS

Evidence of the beneficial effects of certain non-pathologic enteric bacteria, probiotics, gave birth to the concept of prebiotics. Gibson defined a prebiotic in 1995 as a 'nondigestible food ingredient which beneficially affects the host by selectively stimulating the growth of and/or activating the metabolism of one or a limited number of health promoting bacteria in the intestinal tract, thus improving the host's intestinal balance'.[125] Since this concept has only been recently defined, there is not as much data to support their health promoting effects. Examples of prebiotics include the fructooligosaccharides, and complex oligosaccharides in human milk. Each of these satisfies the defining criteria of prebiotics as outlined in Table 4.5.

Evidence suggests that prebiotics improve the bioavailability of minerals such as calcium,[193–195] magnesium,[193,196,197] and iron for absorption.[198] Increased calcium absorption is hypothesized to be mediated by its increased solubility within the colon due to fermentation of the prebiotic and the subsequent decrease in intraluminal pH, through fermentation of fecal products to short chain fatty acids (SCFA),[199] or by an increased expression of calcium binding proteins such as calbindin-D9k.[200] This increase has been thought to be clinically relevant in the treatment and or prevention of diseases such as osteoporosis. However, human studies have been of short duration and therefore have not addressed the more important question of effect on bone mineralization.

Although health benefits are attributed to these compounds they do have potential side-effects. When inulin was given at a dose of 14 g/day, women reported an increase in flatulence, borborygmi, abdominal cramping and bloating.[201] There also appears to be a laxative effect in which these compounds have been shown to increase the daily stool output from 136 g/day to 154 g/day.[202]

SYNBIOTICS

As Gibson introduced the concept of prebiotics he also speculated as to the additional benefits one might see if prebiotics were combined with probiotics to form what he called a 'synbiotic'. He defined this as 'a mixture of probiotics and prebiotics that beneficially effects the host by improving the survival and implantation of live microbial dietary supplements in the gastrointestinal tract by selectively stimulating the growth and/or by activating the metabolism of one or a limited number of health-promoting bacteria, and thus improving host wealthfare'.[125] By virtue of the name it is implied that the prebiotic should offer a selective advantage for the growth of the probiotic it is combined with to provide a synergistic effect. To date, there has been a limited amount of scientific research into this form of supplementation and it is thus unclear whether this theoretical entity will provide any additional health promoting effects above those afforded by the prebiotic or probiotic alone.

A prebiotic should:

1 Neither be hydrolyzed nor absorbed in the upper part of the gastrointestinal tract
2 Be a selective substrate for one or more potentially beneficial commensal bacteria in the large intestine. As such, it should simulate that bacteria to divide, become metabolically active, or both
3 Alter the colonic microenvironment toward a healthier composition
4 Induce luminal or systemic effects that are advantageous to the host

Table 4.5 Defining criteria to classify a food ingredient as a prebiotic

References

1. Savage DC. Microbial ecology of the human gastrointestinal tract. Annu Rev Microbiol 1977; 31:107–133.
2. Moore W, Holdeman L. Human fecal flora: the normal flora of 20 Japanese Hawaiians. Appl Microbiol 1974; 27:961–979.
3. Rozee K, Cooper D, Lam K, Costerton J. Microbial flora of the mouse ilium mucous layer and epithelial surface. Appl Environ Microbiol 1982; 43:1451–1463.
4. Kawai Y, Suegara N. Specific adhesion of lactobacilli to keratinized epithelial cells of the rat stomach in vitro. Am J Clin Nutr 1977; 30:1777–1790.
5. Marshall J. Gastrointestinal flora and its alterations in critical illness. Curr Op Clin Nutr Metabol Care 1999; 2:405–411.
6. Nelson D, Mata L. Bacterial flora associated with the human gastrointestinal mucosa. Gastroenterology 1970; 58:56–61.
7. Shanahan F. The host-microbe interface within the gut. Best Pract Res Clin Gastroenterol 2002; 16:915–931.
8. Hooper L, Bry L, Falk P, Gordon J. Host-microbial symbiosis in the mammalian intestine: exploring an internal ecosystem. BioEssays 1998; 20:336–343.
9. Hooper L, Gordon J. Commensal host-bacterial relationships in the gut. Science 2001; 292:1115–1118.
10. Bernhardt H, Knoke M. Mycological aspects of gastrointestinal microflora. Scand J Gastroenterol 1997; 32:102–106.
11. Payne S, Gibson G, Wynne A, Hudspith B, Brostoff J, Tuohy K. In vitro studies on colonization resistance of the human gut microbiota to Candida albicans and the effects of tetracycline and Lactobacillus plantarum LPK. Curr Issues Intest Microbiol 2003; 4:1–8.
12. Cohen R, Roth F, Delgado E, Ahearn D, Kalser M. Fungal flora of the normal human small and large intestine. N Engl J Med 1969; 280:638–641.
13. Michalski F. Is there an indigenous viral flora in man? J Med Soc NJ 1984; 81:121–123.
14. Gordon H, Bruchorer-Kardoss E. Effect of normal microbial flora on intestinal surface area. Am J Physiol 1961; 201: 175–182.
15. Abrams G, Bauer H, Sprinz H. Influence on the normal flora on mucosal morphology and cellular renewal in the ileum. A comparison of germ-free and conventional mice. Lab Invest 1963; 12:355–364.
16. Lesher S, Walburg H, Sacher G. Generation cycle in the duodenal crypt cells of germ free and conventional mice. Nature 1964; 202:884–886.

17. Macpherson AJ, Martinic MM, Harris N. The functions of mucosal T cells in containing the indigenous commensal flora of the intestine. Cell Mol Life Sci 2002; 59:2088–2096.
18. Heyman M, Corthier G, Petit A, Meslin JC, Morcau C, Desjeux JF. Intestinal absorption of macromolecules during viral enteritis: an experimental study on rotavirus-infected conventional and germ-free mice. Pediatr Res 1987; 22:72–78.
19. McCraken VJ, Lorenz RG. The gastrointestinal ecosystem: a precarious alliance among epithelium, immunity and microbiota. Cellular Microbiol 2001; 3:1–11.
20. Simon G, Gorbach S. The human intestine microflora. Dig Dis Sci 1986; 31:147S–162S.
21. Abrams G. Microbial effects on mucosal structure and function. Am J Clin Nutr 1977; 30:1880–1886.
22. Rolfe R. Interactions among microorganisms of the indigenous intestinal flora and their influence on the host. Rev Inf Dis 1984; 67:S73–S59.
23. Umesaki Y, Okada Y, Matsumoto S, Imaoka A, Setoyama H. Segmented filamentous bacteria are indigenous intestinal bacteria that activate intraepithelial lymphocytes and induce MHC class II molecules and fucosyl asialo GM1 glycolipids on the small intestinal epithelial cells in the ex-germ-free mouse. Microbiol Immunol 1995; 39:555–562.
24. Fisher R, Long S. Rhizobium-plant signal exchange. Nature 1992; 357:655–660.
25. Girardin S, Hugot J, Sansonetti P. Lessons from Nod2 studies: towards a link between Crohn's disease and bacterial sensing. Trends Immunol 2003; 24:652–658.
26. Mata L, Urrutia J. Intestinal colonization of breast-fed children in a rural area of low socioeconomic level. Ann NY Acad Sci 1971; 176:93.
27. Stark P, Lee A. The microbial ecology of the large bowel of breast-fed and formula fed infants during the first year of life. J Med Microbiol 1982; 15:189–203.
28. Sakata H, Yoshioka H, Fujita K. Development of the intestinal flora in very low birth weight infants compared to normal full-term newborns. Eur J Pediatr 1985; 144:186–190.
29. Lindberg E, Nowrouzian F, Adlerberth I, Wold A. Long-time persistence of superantigen producing Staphylococcus aureus strains in the intestinal microflora of healthy infants. Pediatr Res 2000; 48:741–747.
30. Bailey M, Lubach G, Coe C. Prenatal stress alters bacterial colonization of the gut in infant monkeys. J Pediatr Gastroenterol Nutr 2004; 38:414–421.
31. Long S, Swenson R. Development of anaerobic fecal flora in healthy newborn infants. J Pediatr 1977; 91:298–301.
32. Gronlund MM, Lehtonen OP, Eerola E, Kero P. Fecal microflora in healthy infants born by different methods of delivery: permanent changes in intestinal flora after cesarean delivery. J Pediatr Gastroenterol Nutr 1999; 28:19–25.
33. Nowrouzian F, Hesselmar B, Saalman R, et al. Escherichia coli in infants' intestinal microflora: colonization rate, strain turnover, and virulence gene carriage. Pediatr Res 2003; 54:8–14.
34. Harmsen H, Wildeboer-Veloo A, Raangs G, et al. Analysis of intestinal flora development in breast fed and formula-fed infants by using molecular identification and detection methods. J Pediatr Gastroenterol Nutr 2000; 30:61–67.
35. Hall M, Cole C, Smith S. Factors influencing the presence of faecal Lactobacilli in early infancy. Arch Dis Child 1990; 65:185–188.
36. Mata L, Mejicanos M, Jimenez F. Studies on the indigenous gastrointestinal flora of Guatemalan children. Am J Clin Nutr 1972; 25:1380–1390.
37. Kunz C, Rodriguez-Palmero M, Koletzko B, Jensen R. Nutritional and biochemical properties of human milk, Part I: General aspects, proteins, and carbohydrates. Clin Perinatal 1999; 26:307–333.
38. Gronlund M, Salminen S, Mykkanen H, Kero P, Lehtonen O. Development of intestinal bacterial enzymes in infants-relationship to mode of delivery and type of feeding. APMIS 1999; 107:655–660.
39. Mykkanen H, Tikka J, Pitkanen T, Hanninen O. Faecal bacterial enzyme activities in infants increase with age and adoption of adult-type diet. J Pediatr Gastroenterol Nutr 1997; 25:312–316.
40. Murono K, Fujita K, Yoshikawa M, et al. Acquisition of nonmaternal Enterobacteriaceae by infants delivered in hospitals. J Pediatr 1993; 122:120–125.
41. Tannock G, Fuller R, Smith S, Hall M. Plasmid profiling of members of the family Enterobacteriaceae, lactobacilli, and bifidobacteria to study the transmission of bacteria from mother to infant. J Clin Microbiol 1990; 28:1225–1228.
42. Hewitt J, Rigby J. Effect of various milk feeds on numbers of Escherichia coli and Bifidobacterium in the stools of new-born infants. J Hyg (Lond) 1976; 77:129–139.
43. Adlerberth I, Carlsson B, Man Pd, et al. Intestinal colonization with Enterobacteriaceae in Pakistani and Swedish hospital-delivered infants. Acta Paediatr Scand 1991; 80:602–610.
44. Stromberg N, Marklund B, Lund B, et al. Host-specificity of uropathogenic Escherichia coli depends on differences in binding specificity to Gal alpha 1-4Gal-containing isoreceptors. EMBO J 1990; 9:2001–2010.
45. Nowrouzian F, Adlerberth I, Wold AE. P fimbriae, capsule and aerobactin characterize colonic resident Escherchia coli. Epidemiol Infect 2001; 126:11–18.
46. Gorbach S, Nahas L, Lerner P, Weinstein L. Studies of intestinal microflora. I. Effects of diet, age, and periodic sampling on numbers of fecal microorganisms in man. Gastroenterology 1967; 53:845–855.
47. Bornside G, Jr IC. Stability of normal human fecal flora during a chemically defined, low residue diet. Ann Surg 1974; 181:58–60.
48. Kononen E. Development of oral bacterial flora in young children. Ann Med 2000; 32:107–112.
49. Fitzsimmons S, Evans M, Pearce C, Sheridan M, Wientzen R, Cole M. Immunoglobulin A subclasses in infant's saliva and in saliva and milk from their mothers. J Pediatr 1994; 124:566–573.
50. Tenovuo J, Grahn E, Lehtonen O, Hyyppa T, Karhuvaara L, Vilja P. Antimicrobial factors in saliva: ontogeny and relation to oral health. J dent Res 1987; 66:475–479.
51. Redme-Emanuelsson I, Li Y, Bratthall D. Genotyping shows different strains of mutans streptococci between father and child and within parental pairs in Swedish families. Oral Microbiol Immunol 1998; 13:271–277.
52. Kononen E, Saarala M, Karjalainen J, Jousimies-Somer H, Alaluusa S, Asikainen S. Transmission of oral Prevotella melaninogenica between a mother and her young child. Oral Microbiol Immunol 1994; 9:310–314.
53. Alaluusua S, Renkonen O. Streptococcus mutans establishment and dental caries experience in children from 2 to 4 years old. Scand J Dent Res 1983; 91:453–457.
54. Gorbach S, Plaut A, Nahas L, Weinstein L. Studies of intestinal microflora II. Microorganisms of the small intestine and their relations to oral and fecal flora. Gastroenterology 1967; 53:856–867.
55. Johnson K, Lamport A, Batt R. An unexplained bacterial flora in the proximal small intestine of normal cats. Veterinary Record 1993; 132:362–363.
56. Simon G, Gorbach S. Intestinal flora in health and disease. Gastroenterology 1984; 86:174–193.

57. Gibbons R, Kapsimalis B. Estimates of the overall role of growth of the intestinal microflora of hamsters, guinea pigs and mice. J Bact 1967; 93:510–512.
58. Dixon J. The fate of bacteria in the small intestine. J Path Bact 1960; 79:131–140.
59. Abrams G, Bishop J. Effect of the normal microbial flora on gastrointestinal motility. Proc Soc Exp Biol Med 1967; 126:301–304.
60. Cash R, Music S, Libonati J, Snyder M, Wenzel R, Hornick R. Response of man to infection with *V. cholerae*. I. Clinical, serologic and bacteriologic response to a known inoculum. J Infect Dis 1974; 129:45–52.
61. Goenka M, Kochhar R, Chakrabarti A, et al. Candida overgrowth after treatment of duodenal ulcer. A comparison of cimetidine, famotidine, and omeprazole. J Clin Gastroenterol; 23:7–10.
62. Neal K, Slack R. Diabetes mellitus, anti-secretory drugs and other risk factors for campylobacter gastro-enteritis in adults: a case-control study. Epidemiol Infect 1997; 119:307–311.
63. Wurtz R, Mirot M, Fronda G, Peters C, Kocka F. Short report: gastric infection by Strongyloides stercoralis. Am J Trop Med Hyg 1994; 51:339–340.
64. Deitch E, Sittig K, Li M, Berg R, Specian R. Obstructive jaundice promotes bacterial translocation from the gut. Am J Surg 1990; 159:79–84.
65. Freter R. In-vivo and in-vitro antagonism of intestinal bacteria against *Shigella flexneri* II. The inhibitory mechanism. J Infect Dis 1962; 110:38–46.
66. Ahrne S, Nobaek S, Jeppsson B, Adlerberth I, Wold A, Molin G. The normal Lactobacillus flora of healthy human oral and rectal mucosa. J Appl Microbiol 1998; 85:88–94.
67. Luckey T. Bicentennial overview of intestinal microecology. Am J Clin Nutr 1977; 30:1753–1761.
68. Forstner J. Intestinal mucins in health and disease. Digestion 1978; 17:234–241.
69. Kirjavainen P, Gibson G. Healthy gut microflora and allergy: factors influencing development of the microbiota. Ann Med 1999; 31:288–292.
70. Niederman M, Merrill W, Polomski L, Reynolds H, Gee J. Influence of sputum IgA and elastase on tracheal cell bacterial adherence. Am Rev Respir Dis 1986; 133:255–260.
71. Brown W, Savage D, Dubois R, Alp M, Mallory A, Kern F. Intestinal microflora of immunoglobulin deficient and normal human subjects. Gastroenterology 1972; 62:1143–1152.
72. Apperloo-Renkema H, Jagt T, Tonk R, Waaij Dvd. Healthy individuals possess circulating antibodies against their indigenous faecal microflora as well as against allogenous faecal microflora: an immunomorphometrical study. Epidemiol Infect 1993; 111:273–285.
73. Midtvedt A, Carlstedt-Duke B, Norin K, Saxerholt H, Midtvedt T. Development of five metabolic activities associated with the intestinal microflora of healthy infants. J Pediatr Gastroenterol Nutr 1988; 7:559–567.
74. Batt R, Rutgers G, Sancak A. Enteric bacteria: friend or foe? J Small Animal Prac 1996; 37:261–267.
75. Scheline R. Metabolism of foreign compounds by gastrointestinal microorganisms. Pharmacol Rev 1973; 25:451–523.
76. Mikov M. The metabolism of drugs by the gut flora. Eur J Drug Metab Pharmacokinetics 1994; 19:201–207.
77. Spink W, Hurd F, Jermsta J. In vitro conversion of protonsil-soluble to sulfanilamide by various types of microorganism. Proc Soc Exp Biol Med 1940; 43:172–175.
78. Ilett K, Tee L, Reeves P, Minchin R. Metabolism of drugs and other xenobiotics in the gut lumen and wall. Pharmacol Ther 1990; 46:67–93.
79. Cummings J. Fermentation in the human large intestine: evidence and implications for health. Lancet 1983; 2:1206–1209.
80. Dossetar J. Drug interactions with oral contraceptives. Br J Med 1975; 4:467–468.
81. Jonsson G, Midtvedt A, Norman A, Midtvedt T. Intestinal microbial bile acid transformation in healthy infants. J Pediatr Gastroenterol Nutr 1995; 20:394–402.
82. Pyrek JS, Little J, Lester R. Detection of 3-hydroxy-eianic and 3-hydroxy-bisnorcholanoic acids in human serum. J Lipid Res 1984; 25:1324–1329.
83. Midtvedt T. Microbial bile acid transformation. Am J Clin Nutr 1974; 27:1341–1347.
84. Robben J, Caenepeel P, Eldere JV, Eyssen H. Effects of intestinal microbial bile salt sulfatase activity on bile salt kinetics in gnotobiotic rats. Gastroenterology 1988; 94:492–502.
85. Johanson W, Pierce A, Sanford J. Changing pharyngeal bacterial flora of hospitalized patients. N Engl J Med 1969; 281:1137–1140.
86. Moulin Gd, Hedley-Whyte J, Paterson D, Lisbon A. Aspiration of gastric bacteria in antacid treated patients: a frequent cause of postoperative colonization of the airway. Lancet 1982; 1:242–245.
87. Tryba M. Role of acid suppressants in intensive care medicine. Best Pract Res Clin Gastroenterol 2001; 15:447–461.
88. Marshall J, Christou N, Meakins J. The gastrointestinal tract: the undrained abscess of multiple organ failure. Ann Surg 1993; 218:111–119.
89. D'Amico R, Pifferi S, Leonetti C, Torri V, Tinazzi A, Liberati A. Effectiveness of antibiotic prophylaxis in critically ill adult patients: systematic review of randomised controlled trials. BMJ 1998; 316:1275–1285.
90. Alverdy J, Aoys E, Moss G. Total parenteral nutrition promotes bacterial translocation from the gut. Surgery 1988; 104:185–190.
91. Kudsk K, Croce M, Fabian T, et al. Enteral versus parenteral feeding. Effects on septic morbidity after blunt and penetrating abdominal trauma. Ann Surg 1992; 215: 503–513.
92. Sudo N, Sawamura S, Tanaka K, Aiba Y, Kubo C, Koga Y. The requirement of intestinal bacterial flora for the development of an IgE production system fully susceptible to oral tolerance induction. J Immunol 1997; 159:1739–1745.
93. Klinman D, M., Yi AK, Beaucage SL, Conover J, Kreig AM. CpG motifs present in bacterial DNA rapidly induce lymphocytes to secrete interleukin 6, interleukin 12, and interferon g. Proc Natl Acad Sci USA 1996; 93:2879–2883.
94. Isolauri E, Majamaa H, Arvola T, Rantala I, Virtanen E, Arviolmmi H. Lactobacillus casei strain GG reverses increased intestinal permeability induced by cow milk in suckling rats. Gastroenterology 1993; 105:1643–1650.
95. Dahlgren UIH, Wold AE, Hanson LA, Midtvedt T. Expression of a dietary protein in E. coli renders it strongly antigenic to gut lymphoid tissue. Immunology 1991; 73:394–397.
96. Sutas Y, Hurme M, Isolauri E. Down-regulation of anti-CD3 antibody-induced IL-4 production by bovine caseins hydrolysed with Lactobacillus GG-derived enzymes. Scand J Immunol 1996; 43:687–689.
97. Sutas Y, Soppi E, Korhonen H, et al. Suppression of lymphocyte proliferation in vitro by bovine caseins hydrolyzed with Lactobacillus casei GG-derived enzymes. J Allergy Clin Immunol 1996; 98:216–224.

98. Bjoksten B, Sepp E, Julge K, Voor T, Mikelsaar M. Allergy development and the intestinal microflora during the first year of life. J Allergy Clin Immunol 2001; 108:516–520.
99. Kalliomaki M, Kirjavainen P, Eerola E, Kero P, Salminen S, Isolauri E. Distinct patterns of neonatal gut microflora in infants in whom atopy was and was not developing. J Allergy Clin Immunol 2001; 107:129–134.
100. Hessle C, Andersson B, Wold A. Gram-positive bacteria are potent inducers of monocytic interleukin-12 (IL-12) while gram-negative bacteria preferentially stimulate IL-10 production. Infect Immun 2000; 68:3581–3586.
101. He F, Ouwehand AC, Isolauri E, Hashimoto H, Benno Y, Salminen S. Comparison of mucosal adhesion and species identification of bifidobacteria isolated from healthy and allergic infants. FEMS Immunol Med Microbiol 2001; 30:43–47.
102. Kalliomaki M, Isolauri E. Role of intestinal flora in the development of allergy. Curr Op Allergy Clin Immunol 2003; 3:15–20.
103. Clarke J, Condon R, Bartlett J, Gorbach S, Nichols R, Ochi S. Preoperative oral antibiotics reduce septic complications of colon operations: Results of prospective, randomized, double-blind clinical study. Ann Surg 1977; 178:251–259.
104. Dion T, Richards G, Prentis J, Hinchey E. The influence of oral versus parenteral preoperative metronidazole on sepsis following colon surgery. Ann Surg 1980; 192:221–226.
105. Finegold S, Davis A, Miller L. Comparative effect of broad-spectrum antibiotics on non-sporeforming anaerobes and normal bowel flora. Ann NY Acad Sci 1967; 145:268–281.
106. Sakata H, Fujita K, Yoshioka H. The effect of antimicrobial agents of fecal flora in children. Antimicrobial Agents Chemother 1986; 29:225–229.
107. Akita H. The change in intestinal flora by administration of antibiotics. Jpn J Infect Dis 1982; 56:1216–1224.
108. Nakaya R, Chida T, Shibaoka H. Antimicrobial agents and intestinal microflora. Bifidobacteria Microflora 1982; 1:25–37.
109. Wiegertsma N, Jansen G, Waaij D. Effect of twelve antimicrobial drugs on the colonization resistance of the digestive tract of mice and on endogenous potentially pathologic bacteria. J Hyg 1982; 88:221–230.
110. Kurpad A. Effects of antimicrobial therapy on fecal bulking. Gut 1986; 27:55–58.
111. Snepar R, Poporad G, Romana J, Kobasa W, Kaye D. Effect of cimetidine and antacid on gastric microbial flora. Infect Immun 1982; 36:518–524.
112. Gorbach S, Tabaqchali S. Bacteria, bile, and the small bowel. Gut 1969; 10:963–972.
113. Stolberg L, Rolfe R, Gitlin N, et al. d-Lactic acidosis due to abnormal gut flora: diagnosis and treatment of two cases. N Engl J Med 1982; 306:1344–1348.
114. Klipstein G. Tropical sprue. Gastroenterology 1968; 1:946–949.
115. Bhat P, Shantakumari S, Rajan D, et al. Bacterial flora of the gastrointestinal tract in southern Indian control subjects and patients with tropical sprue. Gastroenterology 1972; 62:11–21.
116. Schrezenenmeir J, deVrese M. Probiotics, prebiotics, and synbiotics-approaching a definition. Am J Clin Nutr 2001; 73:361S–364S.
117. Sanders ME. Considerations for use of probiotic bacteria to modulate human health. J Nutr 2000; 130:384S–390S.
118. Teitelbaum J, Walker W. Nutritional impact of pre- and probiotics as protective gastrointestinal organisms. Ann Rev Nutr 2002; 22:107–138.
119. Agostoni C, Axelsson I, Braegger C, et al. Probiotic bacteria in dietetic products for infants: A commentary by the ESPGHAN Committee on Nutrition. J Pediatr Gastroenterol Nutr 2004; 38:365–374.
120. Pletincx M, Legein J, Vandenplas Y. Fungemia with *Saccharomyces boulardii* in a 1-year-old girl with protracted diarrhea. J Pediatr Gastroenterol Nutr 1995; 21:113.
121. Patel R, Cockerill FR, Porayko MK, Osmon DR, Ilstrup DM, Keating MR. Lactobacillemia in liver transplant patients. Clin Infect Dis 1994; 18:207.
122. Kunz A, Noel J, Fairchol M. Two cases of Lactobacillus bacteremia during probiotic treatment of short gut syndrome. J Pediatr Gastroenterol Nutr 2004; 38:557–558.
123. Ross S. Functional foods: the Food and Drug Administration perspective. Am J Clin Nutr 2000; 71:1735S–1738S.
124. Hamilton-Miller JMT, Shah S, Smith CT. 'Probiotic' remedies are not what they seem. Br J Med 1996; 312:55–56.
125. Gibson GR, Roberfroid MB. Dietary modulation of the human colonic microbiota: introducing the concept of prebiotics. J Nutr 1995; 125:1401–1412.
126. Pahwa A, Mathur BN. Assessment of a bifidus containing infant formula. Part II. Implantation of *Bifidobacterium bifidum*. Indian J Dairy Sci 1987; 40:364–367.
127. Marteau P, Minekus M, Havenaar R, Hiuis in't Veld JHJ. Survival of lactic acid bacteria in a dynamic model of the stomach and small intestine: validation and the effects of bile. J Dairy Sci 1997; 80:1031–1037.
128. Vanderhoof JA, Whitney DB, Antonson DL, Hanner TL, Lupo JV, Young RJ. *Lactobacillus GG* in the prevention of antibiotic-associated diarrhea in children. J Pediatr 1999; 135:564–568.
129. Silva M, Jacobs NV, Deneke C, et al. Antimicrobial substance from a human *Lactobacillus* strain. Antimicrob Agents Chemother 1987; 31:1231–1233.
130. Simmering R, Blaut M. Pro- and prebiotics-the tasty guardian angels? Appl Microbiol Biotechnol 2001; 55:19–28.
131. Itoh T, Fujimoto Y, Kawai Y, Toba T, Saito T. Inhibition of food-borne pathogenic bacteria by bacteriocins from *Lactobacillus gasseri*. Lett Appl Microbiol 1995; 21:137.
132. Goldin B, Gorbach SL, Saxelin M, Barakat S, Gualtieri L, Salminen S. Survival of *Lactobacillus* species (strain GG) in human gastrointestinal tract. Dig Dis Sci 1992; 37:121–128.
133. Rolfe RD. The role of probiotic cultures in the control of gastrointestinal health. J Nutr 2000; 130:396S–402S.
134. Erickson KL, Hubbard NE. Probiotic immunomodulation in health and disease. J Nutr 2000; 130:403S–409S.
135. Perdigon G, Alvarez S, Rachid M, Aguero G, Gobbato N. Immune system stimulation by probiotics. J Dairy Sci 1995; 78:1597–1606.
136. Marin ML, Tejada-Simon MV, Lee JH, Murtha J, Ustunol Z, Pestka JJ. Stimulation of cytokine production in clonal macrophage and T-cell models by *Streptococcus thermophilus*: comparison with *Bifidobacteria* sp and *Lactobacillus bulgaricus*. J Food Prot 1998; 61:859–864.
137. Miettinen M, Matikainen S, Vuopio-Varkila J, et al. Lactobacilli and streptococci induce interleukin-12 (IL-12), IL-18, and gamma interferon production in human peripheral blood mononuclear cells. Infect Immun 1998; 66:6058–6062.
138. Schiffrin EJ, Brassart D, Servin AL, Rochat F, Donnet-Hughes A. Immune modulation of blood leukocytes in humans by lactic acid bacteria: criteria for strain selection. Am J Clin Nutr 1997; 66:515S–520S.
139. Schiffrin EJ, Rochat F, Link-Amster H, Aeschlimann JM, Donnet Hughes A. Immunomodulation of human blood cells following the ingestion of lactic acid bacteria. J Dairy Sci 1995; 78:491–497.

140. Spanhaak S, Havenaar R, Schaafsma G. The effect of consumption of milk fermented by *Lactobacillus casei* strain Shirota on the intestinal microflora and immune parameters in humans. Eur J Clin Nutr 1998; 52:1–9.

141. Beena A, Prasad V. Effect of yogurt and bifidus yogurt fortified with skim milk powder, condensed whey and lactose-hydrolyzed condensed whey on serum cholesterol and triacylglycerol concentrations in rats. J Dairy Res 1997; 64:453–457.

142. Akalin AS, Gonc S, Duzel S. Influence of yogurt and acidophilus yogurt on serum cholesterol levels in mice. J Dairy Sci 1997; 80:2721–2725.

143. Thompson LU, Jenkins DJ, Amer MA, Reicher R, Jenkins A, Kamulsky J. The effects of fermented and unfermented milks on serum cholesterol. Am J Clin Nutr 1982; 36:1106–1111.

144. De Roos N, Schouten EG, Katan MB. Yoghurt enriched with *Lactobacillus acidophilus* does not lower blood lipids in healthy men and women with normal to borderline high serum cholesterol levels. Eur J Clin Nutr 1998; 53:277–280.

145. Lin SY, Ayres JW, Winkler W, Sandine WE. *Lactobacillus* effects on cholesterol: in vitro and in vivo results. J Dairy Res 1989; 72:2885–2899.

146. Fukushima M, Nakano M. Effects of a mixture of organisms, *Lactobacillus acidophilus* or *Streptococcus faecalis* on cholesterol metabolism in rats fed on a fat- and cholesterol-enriched diet. Br J Nutr 1996; 76:857–867.

147. De Roos N, Katan MB. Effects of probiotic bacteria on diarrhea, lipid metabolism, and carcinogenesis: a review of papers published between 1988 and 1998. Am J Clin Nutr 2000; 71:405–411.

148. Eyssen H. Role of the gut microflora in metabolism of lipids and sterols. Proc Nutr Soc 1973; 32:59–63.

149. Duffy LC, Zielezny M, Riepenhoff-Talty M, et al. Reduction of virus shedding by *B. bifidum* in experimentally induced MRV infection. Dig Dis Sci 1994; 39:2334–2340.

150. Duffy LC, Zielezny M, Riepenhoff-Talty M, et al. Effectiveness of *Bifidobacterium bifidum* in mediating the clinical course of murine rotavirus diarrhea. Pediatr Res 1994; 35:690–695.

151. Jack RW, Tagg JR, Ray B. Bacteriocins of gram-positive bacteria. Microbiol rev 1995; 59:171–200.

152. Isolauri E, Juntunen M, Rautanen T, Sillanaukee P, Koivula T. A human *Lactobacillus* strain (*Lactobacillus Casei* sp strain *GG*) promotes recovery from acute diarrhea in children. Pediatrics 1991; 88:90–97.

153. Isolauri E, Kaila M, Mykkanen H, Ling WH, Salminen S. Oral bacteriotherapy for viral gastroenteritis. Dig Dis Sci 1994; 39:2595–2600.

154. Kaila M, Isolauri E, Saxelin M, Arviolmmi H, Vesikari T. Viable versus inactivated lactobacillus stain GG in acute rotavirus diarrhea. Arch Dis Child 1995; 72:51–53.

155. Kaila M, Isolauri E, Soppi E, Virtanen E, Laine S, Arviolmmi H. Enhancement of the circulating antibody secreting cell response in human diarrhea by a human *Lactobacillus* strain. Pediatr Res 1992; 32:141–144.

156. Majamaa H, Isolauri E, Saxelin M, Vesikari T. Lactic acid bacteria in the treatment of acute rotavirus gastroenteritis. J Pediatr Gastroenterol Nutr 1995; 20:333–338.

157. Shornikova A-V, Isolauri E, Burnakova L, Lukovnikova S, Vesikari T. A trial in the Karelian Republic of oral rehydration and *Lactobacillus GG* for treatment of acute diarrhea. Acta Paediatr 1997; 86:460–465.

158. Pant AR, Graham SM, Allen SJ, et al. *Lactobacillus GG* and acute diarrhoea in young children in the tropics. J Trop Pediatr 1996; 42:162–165.

159. Guandalini S, Pensabene L, Zikri MA, et al. *Lactobacillus* GG administered in oral rehydration solution to children with acute diarrhea: a multicenter European trial. J Pediatr Gastroenterol Nutr 2000; 30:54–60.

160. Guarino A, Canani RB, Spagnuolo MI, Albano F, DiBenedetto L. Oral bacterial therapy reduces the duration of symptoms and of viral excretion in children with mild diarrhea. J Pediatr Gastroenterol Nutr 1997; 25:516–519.

161. Mack DR, Michail S, S. W, et al. Probiotics inhibit enteropathogenic E. coli adherence in vitro by inducing intestinal mucin gene expression. Am J Physiol 1999; 276:G941–G950.

162. Phuapradit P, Varavithya W, Vathanophas K, et al. Reduction of rotavirus infection in children receiving bifidobacteria-supplemented formula. J Med Assoc Thai 1999; 82: S43–S48.

163. Saavedra JM, Bauman NA, Oung I, Perman JA, Yolken RH. Feeding of *Bifidobacterium bifidum* and *Streptococcus thermophilus* to infants in hospital for prevention of diarrhea and shedding of rotavirus. Lancet 1994; 344:1046.

164. Arvola T, Laiho K, Torkkeli S, et al. Prophylactic *Lactobacillus GG* reduces antibiotic-associated diarrhea in children with respiratory infections: a randomized study. Pediatrics 1999; 104:e64–e68.

165. Wunderlich PF, Braum L, Fumagalli I, et al. Double-blind report on the efficacy of lactic-acid producing *Enterococcus* SF68 in the prevention of antibiotic-associated diarrhoea and in the treatment of acute diarrhoea. J Int Med Res 1989; 17:333–338.

166. Gotz V, Romankiewicz JA, Moss J, Murray HW. Prophylaxis against ampicillin-associated diarrhea with a lactobacillus preparation. Am J Hosp Pharm 1979; 36:754–757.

167. Surawicz CM, Elmer GW, Speelman P, McFarland LV, Chin J, van Belle G. Prevention of antibiotic-associated diarrhea by *Saccharomyces boulardii*: a prospective study. Gastroenterology 1989; 96:981–988.

168. Adam J, Barret A, Barret-Bellet C. Essais cliniques controles en double insu de l'ultra-levure lyophilisee: etude multicentrique par 25 medicins de 388 cases. Gaz Med Fr 1977; 84:2072–2078.

169. MacFarland LV, Surawicz CM, Greenberg RN, et al. Prevention of beta-lactam-associated diarrhea by *Saccharomyces boulardii* compared with placebo. Am J Gastroenterol 1995; 90:439–448.

170. Siitonen S, Vapaatalo H, Salminen S, et al. Effect of *Lactobacillus GG* yoghurt in prevention of antibiotic associated diarrhoea. Ann Med 1990; 22:57–59.

171. Bowden TAJ, Mansberger ARJ, Lykins LE. Pseudomembranous enterocolitis: mechanism for restoring floral homeostasis. Am Surg 1981; 47:178–183.

172. Schwan A, Sjolin S, Trottestam U, Aronsson B. Relapsing *Clostridium difficile* enterocolitis cured by rectal infusion of normal faeces. Scand J Infect Dis 1984; 16:211–215.

173. Biller JA, Katz AJ, Flores AF, Buie TM, Gorbach SL. Treatment of recurrent *Clostridium difficile* colitis with *Lactobacillus GG*. J Pediatr Gastroenterol Nutr 1995; 21:224–226.

174. McFarland LV, Surawicz CM, Greenberg RN, et al. A randomized placebo-controlled trial of *Saccharomyces boulardii* in combination with standard antibiotics for *Clostridium difficile* disease. J Am Med Assoc 1994; 271:1913–1918.

175. Oksanen PJ, Salminen S, Saxelin M, et al. Prevention of traveler's diarrhoea by *Lactobacillus* GG. Ann Med 1990; 22:53–56.

176. Hilton E, Kolakowski P, Singer C, Smith M. Efficacy of *Lactobacillus GG* as a diarrheal preventative in travelers. J Travel Med 1997; 4:41–43.

177. Kollaritsch H, Wiedermann G. Traveller's diarrhoea among Austrian tourists: epidemiology, clinical features and attempts

at nonantibiotic drug prophylaxis. In: Pasini W, ed. Proceedings of the second international conference on tourist health. Rimini: World Health Organization; 1990:74–82.

178. Clements ML, Levine MM, Black RE, Robins-Browne RM, Cisneros LA, Drusano GL. Lactobacillus prophylaxis for diarrhea due to enterotoxigenic Escherichia coli. Antimicrob Agents Chemother 1981; 20:104–108.
179. Gonzalez SN, Cardozo R, Apella MC, Oliver G. Biotherapeutic role of fermented milk. Biotherapy 1995; 8:126–134.
180. Zychowicz C, Surazynska A, Siewierska B, Cieplinska T. Effect of Lactobacillus acidophilus culture (acidophilus milk) on the carrier state of Shigella and Salmonella organisms in children. Pediatr Pol 1974; 49:997–1003.
181. Alm L. The effect of Lactobacillus acidophilus administration upon survival of Salmonella in randomly selected human carriers. Prog Food Nutr Sci 1983; 7:13–17.
182. Majamaa H, Isolauri E. Probiotics: a novel approach in the management of food allergy. J Allergy Clin Immunol 1997; 99:179–185.
183. Isolauri E, Arvola T, Sutas Y, Moilanen E, Salminen S. Probiotics in the management of atopic eczema. Clin Exp Allergy 2000; 30:1604–1610.
184. Kalliomaki M, Salminen S, Arviolmmi H, Kero P, Koskinen P, Isolauri E. Probiotics in primary prevention of atopic disease: a randomised placebo-controlled trial. Lancet 2001; 357:1057–1059.
185. Cohavy O, Bruckner D, Gordon L, et al. Colonic bacteria express an ulcerative colitis pANCA-related protein epitope. Infect Immun 2000; 68:1542–1548.
186. Van de Merwe JP, Schroder AM, Wensinck F, Hazenberg MP. The obligate anaerobic fecal flora of patients with Crohn's disease and their first-degree relatives. Scand J Gastroenterol 1988; 23:1125–1131.
187. Favier C, Neut C, Mizon C, Cortot A, Colombel JF, Mizon J. Fecal b-d-galactosidase production and *Bifidobacteria* are decreased in Crohn's disease. Dig Dis Sci 1997; 42:817–822.
188. Rembacken BJ, Snelling AM, Hawkey PM, Chalmers DM, Axon AT. Non-pathologic Escherichia coli versus mesalamine for the treatment of ulcerative colitis: a randomised trial. Lancet 1999; 354:635–639.
189. Kruis W, Schotz E, Fric P, Fixa B, Judmaier G, Stolte M. Double-blind comparison of an oral Escherichia coli preparation and mesalazine in maintaining remission of ulcerative colitis. Aliment Pharmacol Ther 1997; 11:853–858.
190. Guslandi M, Mezzi G, Sorghi M, Testoni PA. Saccaromyces boulardii in maintenance treatment of Crohn's disease. Dig Dis Sci 2000; 45:1462–1464.
191 Gionchetti P, Rizzello F, Venturi A, et al. Maintenance treatment of chronic pouchitis: a randomized placebo-controlled, double-blind trial with a new probiotic preparation (abstract). Gastroenterology 114; 114:G4037.
192. Group LMS. A multi-center placebo controlled double blind study of Lactobacillus GG in addition to standard maintenance therapy in children with Crohn's disease. J Pediatr Gastroenterol Nutr 2002; 35:406 (abstract).
193. Scholz-Ahrens KE, Schaafsma G, van den Heuvel EGHM, Schrezenenmeir J. Effects of prebiotics on mineral metabolism. Am J Clin Nutr 2001; 73:459S–464S.
194. Ohta A, Ohtsuki M, Baba S, Adachi T, Sakaguchi EI. Calcium and magnesium absorption from the colon and rectum are increased in rats fed fructooligosaccharides. J Nutr 1995; 125:2417–2424.
195. van den Heuvel EGHM, Muys T, van Dokkum W, Schaafsma G. Oligofructose stimulates calcium absorption in adolescents. Am J Clin Nutr 1999; 69:544–548.
196. Ohta A, Baba S, Takizawa T, Adachi T. Effects of fructooligosaccharides on the absorption of magnesium in the magnesium-deficient rat model. J Nutr Sci Vitaminol (Tokyo) 1994; 40:171–180.
197. Ohta A, Ohtsuki M, Baba S, Takizawa T, Adachi T, Kimura S. Effects of fructooligosaccharides on the absorption of iron, calcium, and magnesium in iron-deficient anemic rats. J Nutr Sci Vitaminol (Tokyo) 1995; 41:281–291.
198. Delzenne N, Aertssens J, Verplaetse H, Roccaro M, Roberfroid M. Effect of fermentable fructo-oligosaccharides in mineral, nitrogen and energy digestive balance in the rat. Life Sci 1995; 57:1579–1587.
199. Trinidad TP, Wolever TM, Thompson LU. Interactive effects of calcium and short chain fatty acids on absorption in the distal colon of man. Nutr Res 1993; 13:417–425.
200. Ohta A, Motohashi Y, Ohtsuki M, Hirayama M, Adachi T, Sakuma K. Dietary fructooligosaccharides change the intestinal mucosal concentration of calbindin-D9k in rats. J Nutr 1998; 128:934–939.
201. Pederson A, Sandstrom B, Van Amelsvoort JMM. The effects of ingestion of inulin on blood lipids and gastrointestinal symptoms in healthy females. Br J Nutr 1997; 78:215–222.
202. Gibson GR, Beatty ER, Wang X, Cummings JH. Selective stimulation of bifidobacteria in the human colon by oligofructose and inulin. Gastroenterology 1995; 108:975–982.

Chapter 5
Gastrointestinal motility

Rita Steffen

INTRODUCTION

This chapter discusses gastrointestinal motility – the coordinated motor function of the gastrointestinal (GI) tract from the mouth down to the anorectal area. Developments in technology have allowed the functional assessment of all areas of the GI tract, in both healthy and diseased states. Normal anatomy and physiology is presented, followed by abnormal physiology and particular disease states that can be characterized by manometric and functional tests.

Motility is the function of the bowel that has the endowed and controlled power of spontaneous movement. Manometry is the study of this function by measuring the pressure produced by muscular contraction recorded by a manometer, which typically registers these changes in millimeters of mercury (mmHg).[1] For convenience, the term motility and manometry are used synonymously here. Ongoing efforts to standardize motility protocols in pediatrics and adults are ongoing and evolving.[2]

The basic rule of the gut is that food stimulates contraction above and behind the food bolus and relaxation below or distal to the bolus, forming the peristaltic wave that is probably the most studied phenomenon in the functional assessment of motility of the GI tract. The term 'receptive relaxation' describes the opening of the part of the GI tract ahead of the bolus to receive the incoming ingested material.

The tubular GI tract is functionally separated by specialized sphincters. Circular and longitudinal layers of smooth muscle provide the segmentation for mixing and peristalsis, and motility testing measures the timely contraction and relaxation of these muscles in fasting and the fed states. The outer longitudinal layer is an intact sheath until it separates into three bands or teniae of muscle extending for the length of the colon. A syncytium of ganglion cells (or Meissner's plexus) occupies the submucosal layer of the gut, and yet another is situated anatomically between the two muscle layers (the myenteric or Auerbach's plexus). In recent years, attention has been focused increasingly on the role that interstitial cells of Cajal play on local electrical pacing of bowel contractions.

Smooth muscle contraction is controlled by three things:

- The enteric nervous system (ENS)[3]
- Peptide hormones
- The inherent timing of the myocytes themselves.

Smooth muscle of the intestine is excitable tissue that may be in three states: resting, slow-wave, or action or spike potential. Spike potentials are a result of depolarization of the membrane potential from intracellular accumulation of calcium ions, which causes coupling of smooth muscle excitation–contraction. Local distention or stretch with activation of myenteric neurons and release of acetylcholinesterase results in depolarization of the membrane, which may cause slow waves to convert to action potentials in the myocytes. Bursts of action potentials are associated with muscle contraction, which is the basis of peristalsis from oral to caudal migration of intestinal contents. Neurohumoral modulators may influence this activity to span a segment of bowel.[4] The frequency of slow waves varies according to location in the GI tract. Intricate control mechanisms are evident in the bowel during the fasting and the fed states. Motility measures these events in their temporal and spatial relationships.

The central nervous system receives and sends limited sympathetic and parasympathetic information into the GI tract. The ENS itself is composed of a stunning number of neurons, equal in magnitude to the number present in the spinal cord. The ENS controls motility and secretion, and responds to neuroendocrine peptides, autocrine, paracrine and other transmitters.[5]

The development of normal GI motor activity, besides unfolding according to a predetermined gestational timetable in the fetus, is also nurtured by suckling, swallow-induced esophageal peristalsis and cyclic, triphasic small intestinal motor activity fronts.[6] Segmentation and local retention for optimal contact with brush border enzymes on the microscopic intestinal villi and subsequent transport mechanisms for absorption into the cells is made possible by specialized motor activity that has evolved to sustain nutritional status and growth.

Assessment of motility in pediatric patients is challenging because of the frequently suboptimal cooperation compared with that of adult patients. A spectrum of catheter sizes, spacing between pressure sensors, balloon sizes, other modifications, plus a great deal of patience and interest are all needed to gather reliable information on pediatric patients referred for motility tests.[7]

ESOPHAGEAL MANOMETRY

Esophageal manometry measures the interactive pressures of the pharynx, upper esophageal sphincter (UES), tubular body of the esophagus and the lower esophageal sphincter (LES). Thus, it measures the ability of the esophagus to propel boluses down into the stomach by peristalsis and also measures the integrity of the LES to prevent gastric contents from escaping upward into the esophagus. Several working groups in adult and pediatric gastroenterology have started formally to organize standards for performing esophageal manometry and other types of manometric testing.[2,8–11]

ANATOMY

The upper third of the esophagus is striated muscle, followed by a zone of overlap with smooth muscle, then smooth muscle alone forms the distal two-thirds of the hollow tube. The organization of the muscle layers is constant throughout the GI tract, with the inner circular layer surrounding the hollow viscus, wrapped by the outer longitudinal muscle layer. Neural control of the striated muscle of the upper esophagus originates in the nucleus ambiguus, whereas the ganglia that control the smooth muscle and LES arise in the dorsal motor nucleus. The central nervous system input to esophageal muscle is carried down via the vagus nerve from cell bodies located in the swallowing center of the medulla. Esophageal lengths have been studied from newborns to adult size, and can be estimated by the Strobel formula.[12] Unlike other hollow viscera of the GI traact, the esophagus lacks a serosal lining as it courses through the thoracic cavity.

The UES is the barrier that keeps inspired air out of the GI tract and prevents ingesta from aspirating into the trachea. The UES is tonically contracted between swallows. It relaxes for swallows, for releasing gases during eructation, and for vomiting. The pressures in the UES are not symmetric as posterior pressures are higher than those in anterior plane. The UES is coordinated with pharyngeal propulsive forces and opens normally to accept the food bolus. Multiple cranial nerves transmit afferents (cranial nerves V, IX and X) to the swallowing center in the medulla, and then efferent nerves (cranial nerves V, VII, IX, X and XII) send control information to the oropharynx and upper esophagus to effect a swallow.

PHYSIOLOGY

Primary peristalsis is stimulated by swallowing a bolus; primary peristaltic waves travel at a velocity of 2–4 cm/s. Secondary peristaltic waves are seen following distention of the esophagus by a balloon, refluxate or retained food, and resemble primary peristaltic waves in amplitude and duration. Tertiary peristaltic waves are of lower amplitude, spontaneous and non-peristaltic. They may be seen on barium roentgenography and result from independent depolarization of esophageal smooth muscle, not directed by the swallowing center of the brain. The presence of some 'dropped' peristaltic waves, which begin in the upper esophagus and are not transmitted all the way to the distal esophagus, is also found in normals. Some double-peaked waves may be encountered in normals, but the presence of triple-peaked waves is seen in association with spasm of the esophagus.

In a study of 95 normal adults, Richter et al.[13] concluded that:

- Distal esophageal contractile amplitude and duration after wet swallows increases with age.
- Triple-peaked waves and wet swallow-induced simultaneous contractions should suggest an esophageal motility disorder. Double-peaked waves are a common variant of normal.
- Dry swallows have little current use in the evaluation of esophageal peristalsis.

This study formed the basis of normal values and is a landmark justifying the practice of giving water to the patient to swallow while recording the peristaltic response. When the amplitude of esophageal waves drops below 40 mmHg, the effectiveness of the stripping wave also diminishes. In adults, amplitudes lower than 35 mmHg are hypotensive and those above 180 mmHg are hypertensive,[14] but accumulation of comparable data in normal children has been slower.

Manometric evaluation combined with prolonged 24-h pH testing has shown that low basal LES pressure and transient inappropriate relaxations of the LES have a role in the pathophysiology of gastroesophageal reflux (GER) in children.[15,16] When 49 esophageal manometry studies were done in 27 premature babies, non-peristaltic (either synchronous, incomplete or retrograde) pressure waves were speculated to contribute to poor clearance of refluxed material.[17]

Corroborating evidence from 42 children with gastroesophageal reflux disease (GERD) came from a study with paired esophageal manometry and pH testing that replicated the findings of increased esophageal acid exposure, reduced basal LES pressure and peristalsis, and more drift of basal LES tone observed compared with values in healed patients. Drift in basal LES pressure had the highest predictive value for refractoriness of GERD to therapy.[18] GER may lead to esophagitis and rarely Barrett's esophagus or stricture in children.

The topic of reflux as a motility disorder in itself, and its treatment and complications, is covered in more detail in Chapter 20.

Figures 5.1 and 5.2 demonstrate normal esophageal motor propagation from the pharynx to the LES. Normal relaxation of the LES is shown in Figure 5.1 and normal relaxation of the UES in Figure 5.2.

LES pressure is similar from birth through adulthood, although basal pressure has been variable in studies where it has been measured. As the esophageal length grows with age, so do the UES and LES lengthen from infancy to adulthood. The circular muscle component of the LES is responsible for the tonic end-expiratory pressure. The diaphragmatic component of the LES is responsible for the phasic changes in pressure that occur with respiratory excursions of the chest. The LES measures close to 1 cm in the newborn, and grows to a length of 2–5 cm in the adult.[19] An increase in LES pressure develops in premature infants studied from 27 to 41 weeks' gestational age.[20] Although esophageal peristalsis appears to take longer to mature, LES basal pressure and relaxation have been noted to be well developed even at early postconceptual age. The mean fasting LES pressure in healthy premature infants was 20.5 ± 1.7 mmHg, and 13.7 ± 1.3 mmHg in the fed state.[17] Many factors have been identified to have an

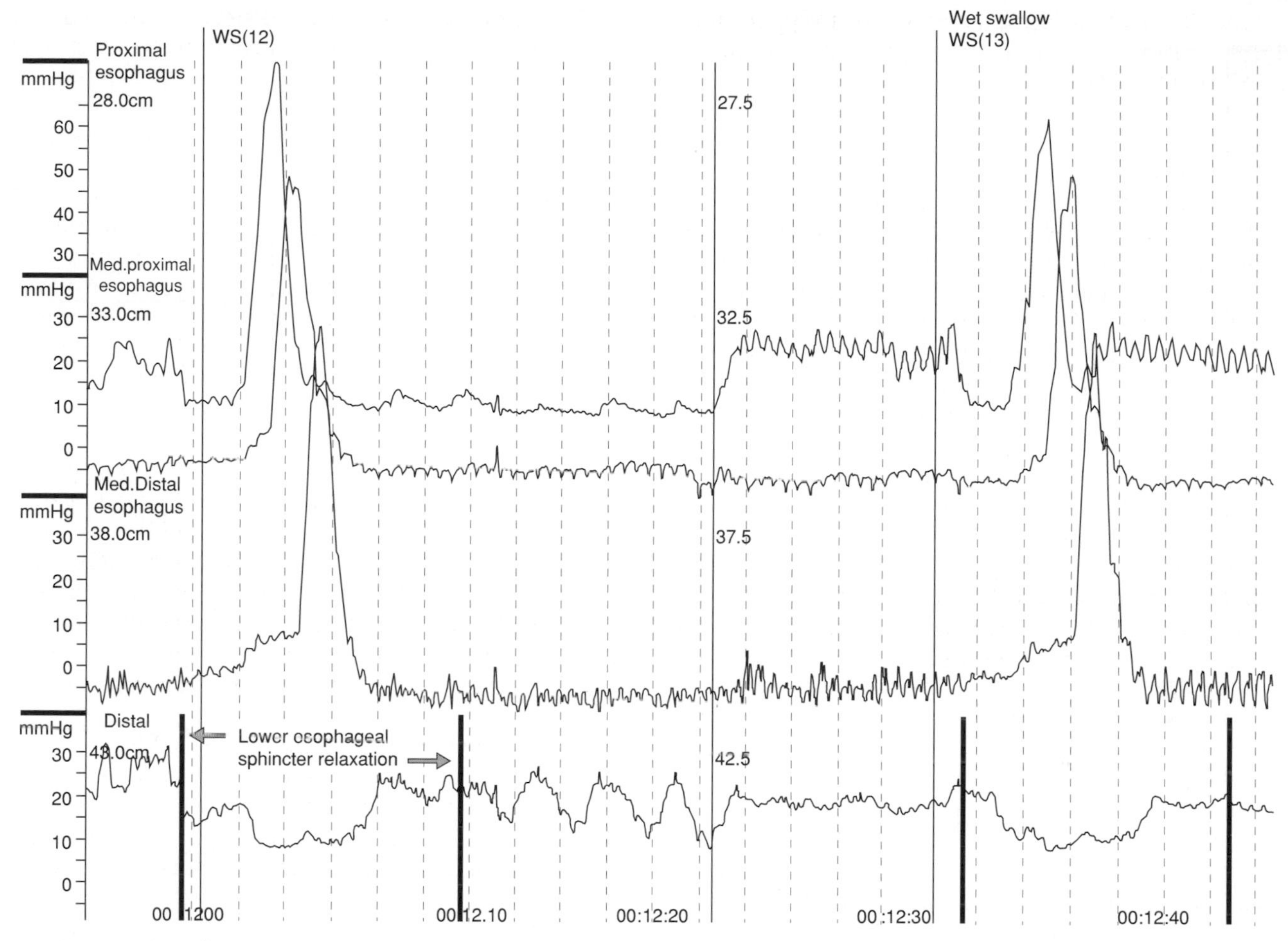

Figure 5.1: Normal esophageal manometry demonstrating sequential peristaltic waves in the first three rows in the esophagus. The tracing at the bottom is from the lower esophageal sphincter, which relaxes from baseline, then returns to baseline, effectively closing the sphincter. A second wet swallow approximately 30 s later provides an almost identical repeated pattern of the waveforms to the right.

influence on LES pressure, including medications, hormones and certain types of food.[21,22]

Tracking the neuromuscular development of the GI tract in the pre-term infant has led to increased understanding of feeding difficulties in this age group. The ontogeny of this maturation process leads to arrival of normal pattern of innervation and contractile activity that can be measured in near-term infants.[23] There are significant differences in performing and analyzing the spectrum of motility disorders in pediatric patients compared with adults. An appreciation of developmental stages of GI function and age-related expression of motility disorders is required to diagnose and treat infants, children and adolescents.[24]

Phasic contractions are isolated peaks of pressure above the baseline that are seen from the pharynx to the rectum. Phasic contractions are important because they represent the activity front of the muscles that serially transmit intestinal secretions and ingested food down the GI tract. Sequential phasic contractions in the esophagus and GI tract are visually recognized as a peristaltic event capable of transmitting a bolus in the aborad direction. Computer software is available to scan manometric tracings for peristaltic sequences and quantitatively measure the amplitude, velocity and duration of the contractions. Thus, phasic contractions are readily recognizable motor events that occur throughout the GI tract and they occur in organized patterns that are characteristic to the segment of digestive tract under investigation. It is the regular occurrence of these patterns that has allowed gastrointestinal manometry to map out normal, and hence abnormal, motility in patients.

THE MANOMETRY PROCEDURE

The act of swallowing is complex, being partly reflexive and partly under voluntary control. Esophageal manometry evaluates the oral, pharyngeal and esophageal phases of swallowing and bolus transfer into the stomach. Relaxation of the UES and LES is almost simultaneous, allowing food to enter the stomach at the end of the propagated wave in the body of the esophagus. Bolus velocity is about 3 cm/s in the esophagus. Deposition into the stomach is accomplished in about 7 s.

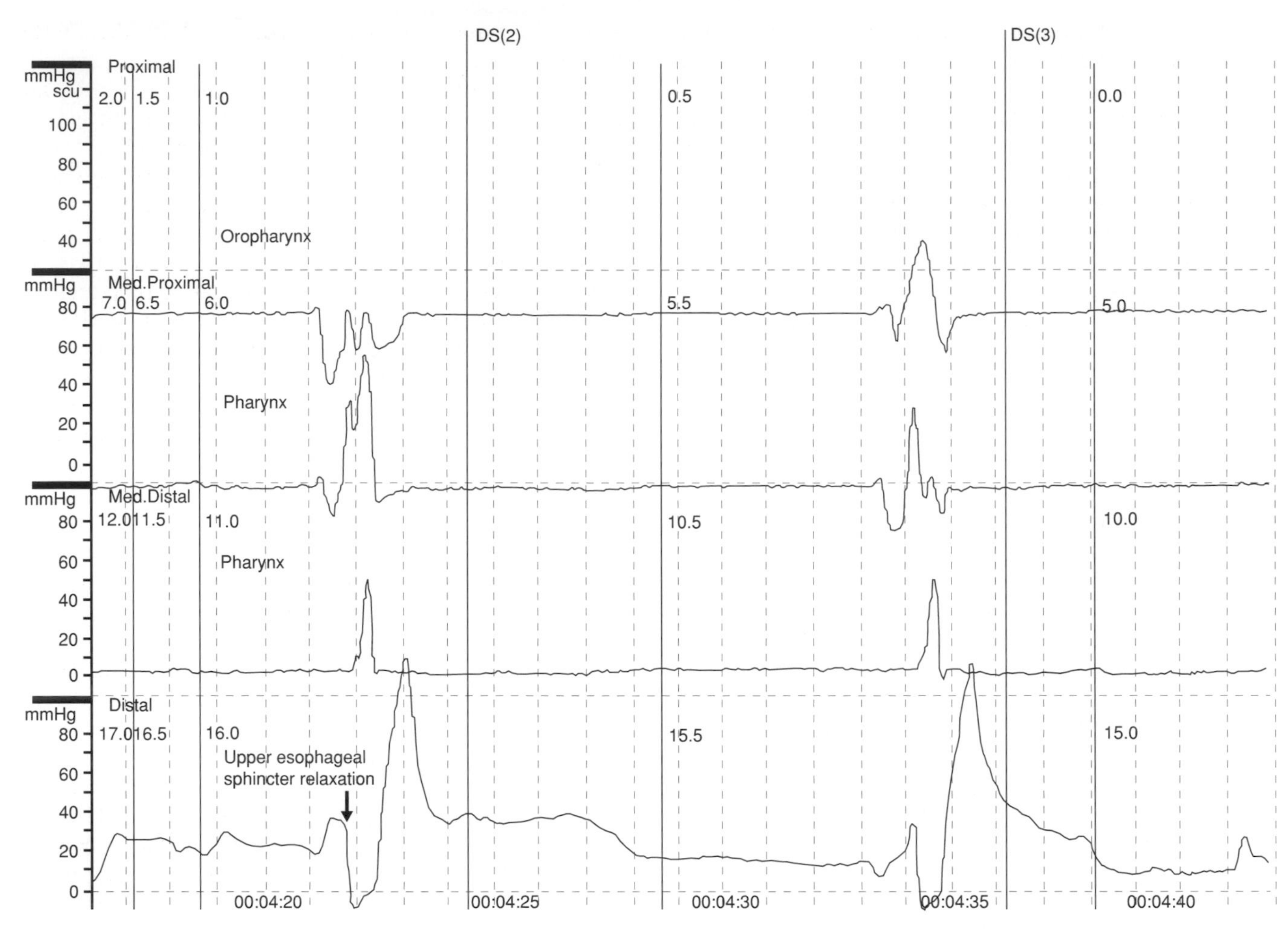

Figure 5.2: Normal esophageal manometry demonstrating oropharyngeal pressure waves in the upper three rows with a swallow. The lowest tracing shows a pressure sensor in the upper esophageal sphincter with baseline tonic pressure approximately 20–40 mmHg. The upper esophageal sphincter relaxes to open, coordinated in timing to receive the bolus from the hypopharynx, then closes by returning the pressure back up to the baseline. Two sequential swallows are shown, separated in time by about 30 s.

Esophageal manometry is the preferred investigation for the diagnosis of esophageal motility disorders, but is usually preceded by a barium swallow or upper endoscopy. Reasons for performing esophageal manometry in children are:[9]

- To evaluate symptoms of dysphagia, odynophagia, noncardiac chest pain, aspiration and recurrent food impaction
- To provide diagnostic information in the workup of achalasia, chronic intestinal pseudo-obstruction (CIPO) and connective tissue disorders such as scleroderma and dermatomyositis
- To locate the UES and LES prior to pH and impedance monitoring for reflux.

Dysphagia and vomiting are frequent abnormalities for which esophageal motility testing is indicated. Esophageal manometry is also helpful in localizing the LES for pH studies, in investigation for CIPO,[25] in presurgical evaluation, in investigation for achalasia and to confirm or evaluate suspicion of abnormal motility on other studies.

Transfer dysphagia relates to problems in the oropharyngeal phase of the swallow, whereas globus refers to a feeling of food being lodged in the esophagus. The timing of pharyngeal waves with the cricopharyngeus protects the airway from aspiration and, if abnormal, may lead to dysphagia and aspiration. Wyllie et al.[26] have demonstrated that medications such as nitrazepam may desynchronize this protective timing sequence and that discontinuation of the medication will result in restoration of normal motility.

The differential diagnosis of dysphagia is broad, including structural causes from an intrinsic or extrinsic process that produces a fixed narrowing. Diseases that cause functional dysphagia include central and peripheral nervous system diseases that can affect any level of nervous control. Neuromuscular disorders, such as the dystrophies, that affect striated skeletal muscle will affect the motility of the upper esophagus and the UES, whereas the lower esophagus and LES will be normal. By contrast, in non-myotonic dystrophies or disorders of smooth muscle, lower esophageal motility and LES will be affected while the upper esophagus and UES are normal. Inflammatory processes and metabolic disorders may also affect the esophagus. Barium radiography is a good first step in the evaluation of dysphagia to exclude stenosis, esophageal dilation and possible involvement of the respiratory tract with aspiration.

There are water-perfused systems and solid-state catheters and, more recently, some that measure both motility and impedance flow. Although solid-state catheters do not use water perfusion, they are significantly more costly to purchase and maintain, so water-perfused systems are much more commonly used by the pediatric gastroenterologist.

A low-compliance system with a rate of infusion as low as 0.1–0.4 ml/min per port will pick up changes in pressure within the lumen without overloading the bowel with water. Physiologic pressure changes are recorded and saved on a computer. Small-diameter flexible tubes with side-holes radially placed 1–5 cm apart are connected to pressure transducers driven by a pneumohydraulic system. Contractions occlude the pressure ports and the resistance to flow is transmitted as pressure change to the strain gauges. Swallowing events and provocative medications, if used, are recorded by the computer for accurate timing analysis when the study is reviewed. The author's department uses a pull-through technique to profile LES pressure, although a sleeve sensor is used in many pediatric centers continuously to monitor a broader expanse of the LES during swallows.

The size of the catheter and spacing of the recording sensors are chosen according to the age and size of the patient. An inventory of three or four different configurations of manometric catheter is recommended for performing motility studies on children, as the spectrum will include infants through adult-sized patients. Premanufactured catheters are commercially available, and it is also possible to custom design one's own catheters to meet the examiner's recording needs.

Esophageal manometry is most often performed unsedated with good nursing preparation to elicit the child's cooperation. The catheter is lubricated and introduced through the nose. Tilting the head downward and swallowing some water before and during this process assists in successful intubation. Some use a numbing agent on a cotton-tipped swab in the back of the nares prior to sliding the tube into the posterior nasopharynx. Sprayed pharyngeal anesthetics are avoided because of the potential inhibition of sensation and motor function in the posterior pharynx and cricopharyngeal areas.

If it is not possible to obtain a successful nasogastric placement, as sometimes occurs when narrow nasal passages are encountered, the tube may be introduced through the oral cavity, but there is a risk that the child may bite the tube if he or she has well developed dentition. Sedation with oral midazolam (Versed) (which has replaced oral chloral hydrate) at a dose of 0.5 mg/kg, to a maximum of 10 mg, may be used.[27] Another option is intranasal application of midazolam if the oral route is not feasible. If pediatric anesthesiology is available, the range recommended is 0.5–1.0 mg/kg to a maximum of 15 mg, administered orally. At times, it is convenient to schedule esophageal manometry immediately after upper endoscopy in which conscious sedation has already been administered.

The catheter is first introduced into the stomach and a baseline gastric pressure is recorded. As the catheter approaches the region of the LES, an increase in respiratory artifact appears in the proximal or 'scout' sensor(s) because it is getting close to the diaphragm. The catheter is then pulled through the LES at 0.5-cm increments, and the length and zone of maximal pressure are recorded. Normally a value 15–25 mmHg greater than gastric pressure is seen. The manometrist should note the transition from positive pressure in the stomach, to the LES basal tone, and thence into the chest where intrathoracic pressure is negative and is a physiologic landmark or 'respiratory inversion point' seen on the tracing. When this sequence is observed, it assures that the catheter has in fact entered the stomach rather than being curled up on itself in the esophagus.

Placing the catheter in the LES to observe its total length and extent of relaxation is done. Any residual pressure seen during maximal relaxation of the LES should be noted, and should normally be only a few millimeters of mercury (<8 mmHg in adults) and close to zero in children. The catheter has ports at different levels to pick up the pressures of the propagated wave through the esophagus and the timing and completeness of LES relaxation. The LES remains open for 7–10 s in anticipation of the bolus, and closes when the wave finishes propagation at the base of the esophagus. The swallowing center in the brain orchestrates the timely relaxation of the UES and LES through vagal nerve inhibition of resting tone. Abnormally low or high pressures, peristalsis and ability of the sphincters to relax are examined systematically.

Characteristics of normal esophageal motility are presented in Table 5.1. The neural control of deglutition and the esophagus are discussed in more detail in Chapter 18.

The manometrist now slowly withdraws the catheter at 1-cm increments, and the serial pressure ports measure the peristaltic waves in the esophagus. Most protocols measure at least 10 wet swallows in the body of the esophagus. During this excursion of the catheter, cardiac artifact may appear as a registration of the patient's pulse as it moves in contiguity with the great vessels in the mediastinum. Respiration temporarily ceases during swallowing. Relaxation of the UES is assessed and the pharyngeal pressure waves of the oral phase of deglutition can be seen.

Modifications and innovation in adapting the equipment and test to the child are part of motility testing in pediatric gastroenterology. Placing the manometry catheter through a plastic nipple is a technique that is sometimes helpful in settling a baby and obtaining less motion artifact. The baby can also be cradled in a parent's arms as long as there is a relatively steady baseline from which to measure esophageal events. In contrast to the controlled timing and volume of wet and dry swallows that can often be achieved in older children, and almost always in cooperative adolescents and adults, infants need to be observed during the recording for spontaneous swallowing activity. A puff of air on the face will cause reflex

Location	Comments
LES	Basal pressure: <1 year, 40–45 mmHg; >1-year 28–33 mmHg Other studies: infant to 2 years, varies from 13 to 27 mmHg 22.4 ± 4.7 mmHg[28] 29.1 ± 2.4 mmHg[29] Relaxation at the time of the swallow almost completely to baseline Relaxation timed to relaxation of UES
Body pressure	Resting pressure: varies with respiration; lower than gastric baseline pressure Amplitude >30–40 mmHg, <180 mmHg; duration 2–4 cm/s Need more data on normal children
UES	Resting pressure: 30–150 mmHg, 18–44 cmH_2O in infants[30] Relaxation at the time of swallow almost completely to baseline; relaxes at same time as LES

LES, lower esophageal sphincter; UES, upper esophageal sphincter.

Table 5.1 Normal esophageal motility values

swallowing to occur (the Santmyer reflex)[31] and is more frequently seen after the postconceptual age of 34 weeks.

Feeding young infants during esophageal manometry is contraindicated because this frequently results in choking, salivation and cough, thereby placing the infant at risk for aspiration and certainly disturbing the desired resting state required to obtain a readable tracing.

Much valuable information on the pathophysiology of the esophagus can be obtained when esophageal manometry is combined with multichannel intraluminal impedance (MII) monitoring and prolonged pH testing. This combination technology is now available to measure both acid and non-acid reflux in the esophagus and pharynx. (The refluxed bolus can be characterized as gas, mixed gas–liquid, or liquid.) It has been used to monitor 17 infants with apnea, bradycardia, aspiration pneumonia, wheezing and failure to thrive. More than 75% of GER events extended to the pharynx, and the use of impedance helped to characterize the volume clearance in the esophagus and to allow symptom correlation with non-acid events that previously were not detected by the pH testing alone. Combination monitoring of acid and non-acid reflux thus has an important role in elucidating the feeding and respiratory problems of infants and pediatric patients on acid-suppressing medications whose reflux would be missed by pH testing alone.[32] Impedance manometry allows simultaneous bolus tracking in the esophagus, which complements the pressure information that is obtained by standard esophageal manometry.

The pressures in the sphincters are asymmetric, and we measure the pressure in four quadrants and calibrate an average. Again, the relaxation of the UES, any residual pressure remaining at maximal relaxation (<8 mmHg is normal) and coordination with the pharyngeal motor activity are assessed. Catheter tubes, fitted with a 'sleeve' type of sensor, measure the maximal pressure over the length of the sleeve, which may be 3–5 cm. An advantage of using the sleeve-type manometry catheter in children is that it can remain in the sphincter; a directional sensor may slip out with motion of the patient, and may therefore shorten the duration of the study for the child. The normal pressures in the UES vary from 30 to 150 mmHg. Concurrent manometric and videofluoroscopic recordings of UES function reveals that the cricopharyngeus muscle assembly moves upwards some 0.9–1.5 cm in adults during deglutition; similar motion is anticipated in UES testing in children. Consequently, this motion of the UES also needs to be anticipated and accounted for in stationary recording in children. Pediatric patients tend to change position more frequently than adults during motility testing, and motion artifacts must be recognized and excluded from analysis. Kahrilas et al.[33] found the larger the swallowed bolus, the greater the magnitude of orad movement of the UES. The duration of UES relaxation was longer with increased volume of the swallowed bolus.

Neurologic diseases affect esophageal motility and may involve autonomic nervous system dysfunction (familial dysautonomia), cerebral palsy, strokes, multiple sclerosis and poliomyelitis. Neuromuscular diseases such as myasthenia gravis and botulism affect swallowing and peristalsis of the esophagus.

ABNORMAL ESOPHAGEAL FUNCTION

Cricopharyngeal achalasia

Beginning with the UES, resting tone may be either hypertensive or hypotensive. As a sphincter, its relaxation is judged by its completeness or lack of adequate relaxation, leaving a barrier of residual pressure, which is sometimes seen as an upper esophageal abnormality in patients with achalasia. The UES and cricopharyngeus muscle are considered a single functional motor unit, composed of striated muscle fibers. The innervation of the UES is therefore different from the nervous control of the distal two-thirds of the esophagus, which is composed of smooth muscle fibers.

Abnormally low UES pressure may disturb the gating function of the sphincter, allowing air to enter the GI tract and potentially refluxed material or swallowed matter to penetrate into the airway.[34] Indeed, fatal aspiration has occurred in pediatric patients with abnormal UES function. Data on UES pressures in normal children is limited, but was reported to range from 18 to 44 cmH_2O in 11 normal infant controls.[30]

Transfer dysphagia and globus sensation have been described in patients with cricopharyngeal achalasia or spasm. Prominent cricopharyngeal impression may be seen radiographically, but it is not always possible to find abnormally high pressures with manometry, although some have noted incomplete relaxation of the UES. Some pediatric gastroenterologists treat patients with one or more dilations, whereas others treat the symptoms supportively and the problem seems to improve over time. Some patients not responding to supportive treatment with nutritional and pulmonary measures have undergone myotomy for cricopharyngeal achalasia.

In a series of 15 children with cricopharyngeal achalasia, 11 had associated central nervous system diseases. Reichert et al.[35] wrote that congenital cricopharyngeal achalasia was more common than previously recognized, and that esophageal manometry was valuable in the assessment of the entire esophagus.

UES dysfunction in five young children as reported by Putnam et al.[36] to be associated with Chiari malformations. All five were evaluated by preoperative and postoperative esophageal manometry, and surgical decompression of the craniocervical lesion led to normal manometric findings and resolution of dysphagia, choking, cough and nasopharyngeal reflux. The authors concluded that esophageal manometry was more valuable than barium swallow in demonstrating the abnormality, and correlated better than radiographic images with symptomatic improvement after surgery.[36] In fact, the correlation was so high as to suggest screening for brainstem malformations in children who present with dysphagia and UES dysfunction.

Achalasia

Abnormal esophageal manometric findings can be pathognomonic for particular disease states. Achalasia is the prime condition that can be detected reliably by motility testing in both children and adults. Criteria for the manometric diagnosis of achalasia are summarized in Table 5.2. Raised resting LES pressure and abnormal LES relaxation may be documented, but the signature manometric sign of achalasia is the absence of progressing peristaltic waves in the body of the esophagus. Hence, if aperistalsis is not found, a diagnosis of achalasia cannot be tendered. That is to say, if 10 wet swallows are performed, and one of them is peristaltic with normal wave progression whereas the other nine are not, achalasia cannot be diagnosed. In advanced cases in which the esophagus is dilated, the pressure within the esophagus exceeds gastric pressure, instead of being negative intrathoracic pressure compared with the stomach. Vomiting of undigested food and weight loss are typical clinical signs of achalasia.

Once the diagnosis of achalasia has been established, serially repeating esophageal manometry is usually unnecessary; however, as an objective clinical tool, some use esophageal manometry for its role in quantitatively assessing severity of achalasia and response to treatment. Some evidence suggests that achalasia may have a mild or subtle onset and may display a spectrum of signs and symptoms as it evolves into the unmistakable cardiospasm and functional obstruction of the distal esophagus. A subgroup with high-amplitude tertiary contractions are described as having 'vigorous achalasia'.

Achalasia is usually suspected from barium esophagraphy showing a dilated esophagus, with only a trickle of barium flowing through a 'bird's beak' or 'rat's tail' distal esophagus in advanced cases (Fig. 5.3). In some patients it may be necessary to truncate the test to obtain the basics for manometric diagnosis. Clinically, these children or adolescents are apprehensive and may begin to vomit or display the symptoms of dysphagia during wet swallows, and the manometric testing is pruned down to obtain the essential evidence for a diagnosis of achalasia. In these cases, the manometrist should focus on the LES baseline pressure, see whether the LES relaxes and to what extent, then go directly to the body of the esophagus to see whether there is peristalsis.

Although less common, achalasia may also present in infancy, usually with feeding and respiratory problems predominating.[37]

Preoperative and postoperative esophageal manometry in 13 children with achalasia revealed motor findings similar to those in adults with achalasia. Partial motor recovery was observed in some children, but the authors concluded that their esophageal peristalsis would be always ineffective. Because splitting the LES eliminates the barrier to acid reflux, a fundoplication is also added so that the partially wrapped gastric fundus can perform the function of being the new valve between the stomach and lower esophagus.[38]

In a larger study of 45 patients with achalasia, researchers attempted to find factors that might predict a return of peristalsis following Heller myotomy. It was determined that earlier detection in patients at a time when they had minimal esophageal dilation was associated with a chance for some preserved contractile capacity. However, the chance of having peristalsis even in a part of the esophagus was still less than 47%.[39]

Treatment of achalasia with medication, balloon dilation and laparoscopic myotomy is discussed in detail in Chapter 21. Figure 5.4 shows simultaneous waves in the esophagus and a non-relaxing LES in a child with achalasia. Figure 5.5 shows the hallmark of achalasia, which is the lack of peristalsis in the esophageal body.

Spasm

Spasm may occur in the smooth muscle of the esophagus, causing chest pain and dysphagia. Esophageal manometry is the preferred diagnostic test for spastic disorders of the esophagus.[40] Abnormalities in propulsive waveforms and their amplitudes and duration are recognized, and are summarized in Table 5.2.

Hypertonic LES and nutcracker esophagus are rare conditions in childhood, but are nevertheless disorders that need to be recognized because their successful treatment with calcium channel blockers or other pharmacologic agents depends on the vigilant manometrist.

Nutcracker esophagus, also rare in childhood, may present with chest pain and/or dysphagia. Nutcracker waves are high-amplitude peristaltic waves (generally >180 mmHg) that have a longer duration than normal. In a study of 1300 adult patients, 4% were found to have hypertension of the LES with a resting pressure above 26.5 mmHg, defined as the upper limit of normal resting LES pressure. Such a large series is not available in the

Condition	Findings
Abnormal esophageal manometry	
Cricopharyngeal achalasia	Dysfunctional, incomplete relaxation of the UES May be suspected by a prominence of cricopharyngeal muscle radiologically UES spasm is often not corroborated manometrically
Low cricopharyngeal/UES pressure	With neuromuscular disorders places child at risk for recurrent aspiration
Achalasia	Absence of peristaltic waves in the body (required for diagnosis) Raised resting pressure in the body may be seen with a 'water balloon' or 'common cavity' type of appearance with simultaneous waves Incomplete LES relaxation, but this is variable Increased LES resting pressure Dilated esophagus will have higher baseline pressure than gastric baseline pressure May have variable abnormalities in UES, such as raised resting pressure
Vigorous achalasia	Subgroup of patients with achalasia who have the above findings, plus tertiary esophageal contractions of high amplitude
Chagas' disease	Some tertiary care centers may see patients from Latin America, or parents may have an adopted child with achalasia secondary to infection with *Trypanosoma cruzi*
Spasm or disorders characterized by increased pressure	
Nutcracker esophagus	High-amplitude (usually >180 mmHg) peristaltic waves High-amplitude non-peristaltic contractions in distal esophagus Common to see increased duration of waves
Non-specific spasm	More common than nutcracker or diffuse esophageal spasm in childhood Multiple contractions of varying amplitude and duration may follow a single swallow Baseline pressure may be raised Contractions may be simultaneous and non-peristaltic Occasionally pressures exceeding 300 mmHg are seen in spastic disorders
Diffuse esophageal spasm	Distal esophageal amplitudes >140 mmHg, duration prolonged >7 s; multiple contractions with these characteristics follow one swallow At least 10% of wet swallows are repetitive, simultaneous (non-peristaltic) contractions Sequences of normal peristalsis Increased duration and amplitude contractions, but some have normal amplitude Most have normal LES, but some demonstrate incomplete LES relaxation or hypertensive LES
Hypertensive LES	Raised LES pressure, >45 mmHg LES relaxes normally and esophageal peristalsis is normal
Non-specific motor disorders	May see dropped peristalsis in patients with esophagitis
Other disorders	
	Simultaneous contractions, double-peaked contractions, tertiary contractions or decreased amplitude ineffective contractions (ineffective esophageal motility) <30 mmHg in distal esophagus
Gastroesophageal reflux	Normal peristalsis, but may show TLESRs Mean LES pressure may be significantly lower than normal
Dermatomyositis	Decreased proximal esophageal pressure Distal esophagus remains normal
Scleroderma	Decreased LES resting pressure Incomplete LES relaxation Absence of peristaltic wave or diminished waves in distal esophagus Proximal esophagus remains normal until later in the disease when striated muscle in the proximal third begins to appear

LES, lower esophageal sphincter; TLESR, transient lower esophageal sphincter relaxation; UES, upper esophageal sphincter.

Table 5.2 Abnormal esophageal manometry

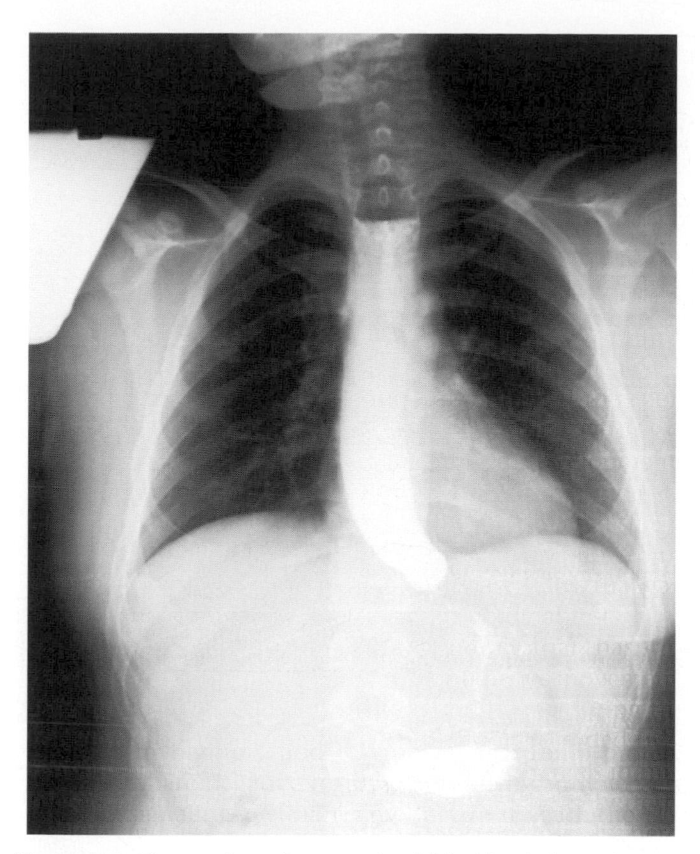

Figure 5.3: Abnormal esophagram of a child with achalasia. The esophagus is dilated and there is an air–fluid level visible within the esophagus near the thoracic inlet. The distal segment narrows down to a thin trickle of barium seen entering the fundus of the stomach. The manometry catheter may coil back upon itself in the distal esophagus in these patients. This patient's manometric highlights are presented in Figs 5.4 & 5.5.

pediatric literature. This represented a heterogeneous group of motility disorders when the esophageal function was then added to the data.

A raised LES pressure can occur by itself, or in achalasia, post-Nissen fundoplication, nutcracker esophagus, diffuse esophageal spasm, GERD and other conditions.[41] Diffuse esophageal spasm is well described in adults but is rarely encountered in pediatric clinical practice or literature. Criteria for manometric diagnosis of diffuse esophageal spasm are included in Table 5.2.[34] Being present during the motility study facilitates pattern recognition and correlation of swallowing behaviors with the tracing, and enables more subtle observations that may be helpful clinically.

There is considerable literature on the topic of the manometric findings that can be encountered following bougienage and myotomy. Lamet et al.[43] noted a return of peristalsis after successful pneumatic dilation in 7 of 34 adults, possibly due to shrinking of the esophagus back to a normal size from the dysfunctional dilated state that preceded therapy. This is the exception rather than the rule in achalasia, for esophageal aperistalsis predominates in most patients, even after treatment. In a study of treated children with achalasia, the authors stated that motor recovery was never complete and that abnormal esophageal function could be expected to last a lifetime.[44]

Primary esophageal motility disorders are therefore:

- Achalasia
- Disorders of spasm, or increased pressure
- Diffuse esophageal spasm
- Nutcracker esophagus
- Non-specific esophageal motor disorders.

Anatomic postsurgical change and congenital atresias

The esophagus is affected secondarily by many disease processes with an etiology that is within the usual spectrum of anatomic postsurgical change and congenital atresia. For example, absent peristalsis and reflux in the esophagus of a child is expected after esophageal atresia and tracheo-esophageal fistula repair. Manometric evaluation of esophageal function has been done with both stationary pull-through testing in the office and prolonged 24-h ambulatory recording.

Esophageal manometric abnormalities are known to persist in the majority of patients with repaired esophageal atresia and tracheo-esophageal fistula, even in the absence of symptoms.[45] Abnormal gastric motility was found in 36% of patients with esophageal atresia and repaired tracheo-esophageal fistula, prompting the authors to recommend subsequent evaluation of stomach function in these patients, particularly because delayed gastric emptying predisposes to GER.[46]

Other disorders

Esophageal motility is also affected by neurologic diseases, including autonomic nervous system dysfunction (familial dysautonomia), cerebral palsy, stroke, multiple sclerosis and poliomyelitis. Neuromuscular diseases such as myasthenia gravis and botulism also affect swallowing and peristalsis of the esophagus. The various subtypes of muscular dystrophy frequently cause abnormal deglutition and esophageal peristalsis, which can be documented radiographically and manometrically.[47]

Inflammation from acid reflux, eosinophil infiltration, connective tissue diseases, neuromuscular diseases and metabolic disorders such as diabetes and hypothyroidism also directly affect detectable esophageal function. Peristaltic dysfunction is known to occur in patients with GERD and esophagitis. When Kahrilas et al.[48] paired simultaneous videofluoroscopic and manometric recordings of patients with non-obstructive dysphagia or heartburn, peristaltic dysfunction led to impaired volume (and presumably acid) clearance from the esophagus. Patients will swallow saliva, which helps to neutralize refluxed gastric acid.[48]

Eosinophils are seen in esophageal biopsy tissue in children with GERD, but are significantly more populous in the disorder of eosinophilic esophagitis (EE). Both patients with GERD and those with EE may demonstrate abnormal motility. However, children with EE were found to be unlikely to have pathologic reflux.[49]

The motility of the esophagus is also affected by injection therapy for varices, residual scarring from caustic

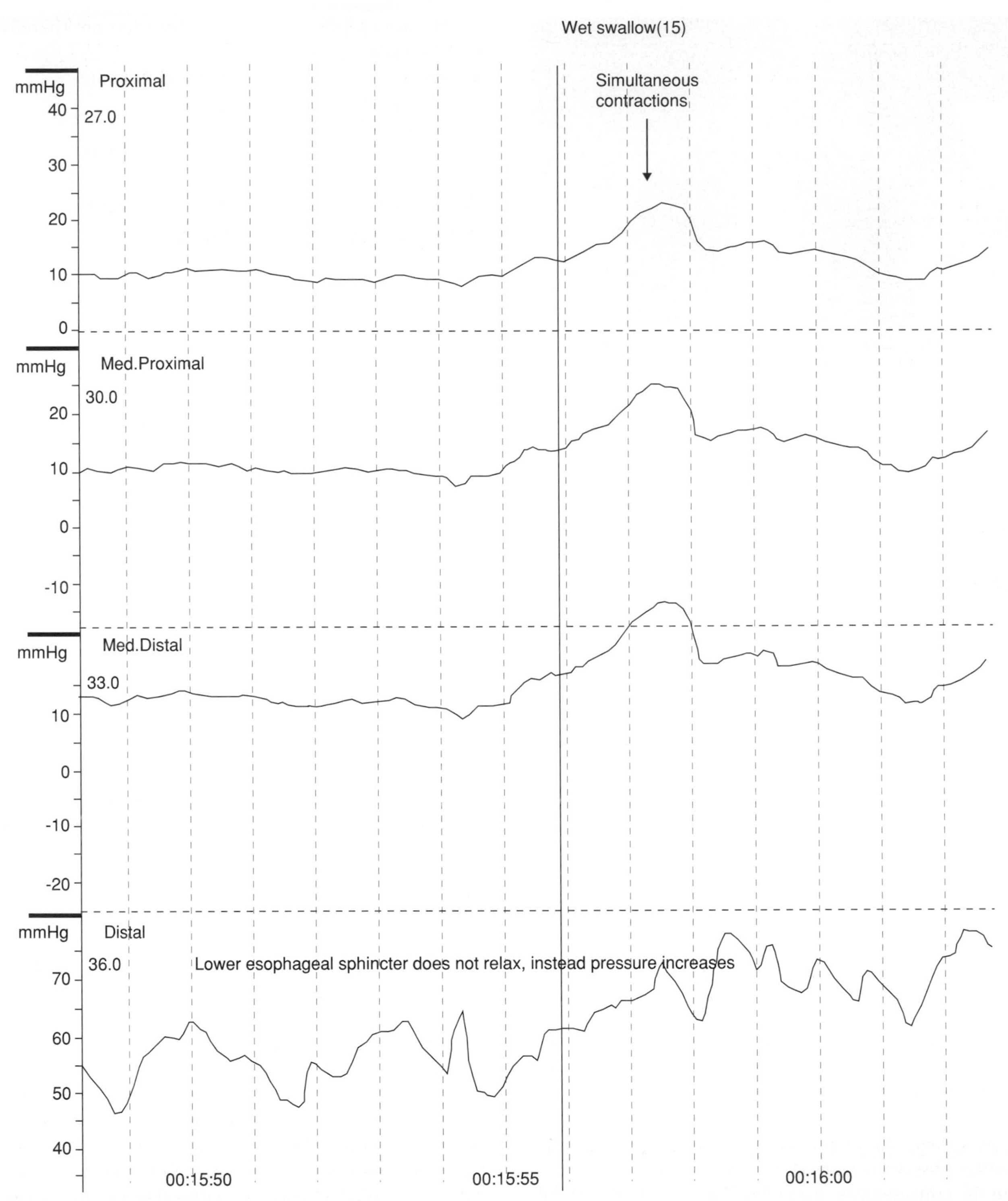

Figure 5.4: Abnormal esophageal manometry in an 11-year-old child with achalasia. The lower esophageal sphincter (LES) in this tracing is located in the bottom row. In response to a wet swallow (marked by the vertical line labeled WS), there are low-amplitude simultaneous contractions in the esophageal body in the three pressure sensors located at 3-cm intervals above the LES. The LES does not relax normally, instead showing an increase in the already raised baseline pressure. Rather than peristaltic waves, simultaneous waves are demonstrated. Contrast this appearance to the normal physiology shown in Figure 5.1.

ingestion, and stricture formation. Motility disorders of other parts of the GI tract may impact esophageal function as well, notably CIPO and Hirschsprung's disease (HD). When HD affects larger areas of the bowel, proximal to the rectosigmoid area, it becomes more likely that abnormalities of esophageal motor function can also be discerned. Specifically, tertiary and double-peaked contractions may be seen in HD. Achalasia was reported to occur concomitantly in two male siblings with HD.[50] Esophageal manometry can be used as a screening test for CIPO, as

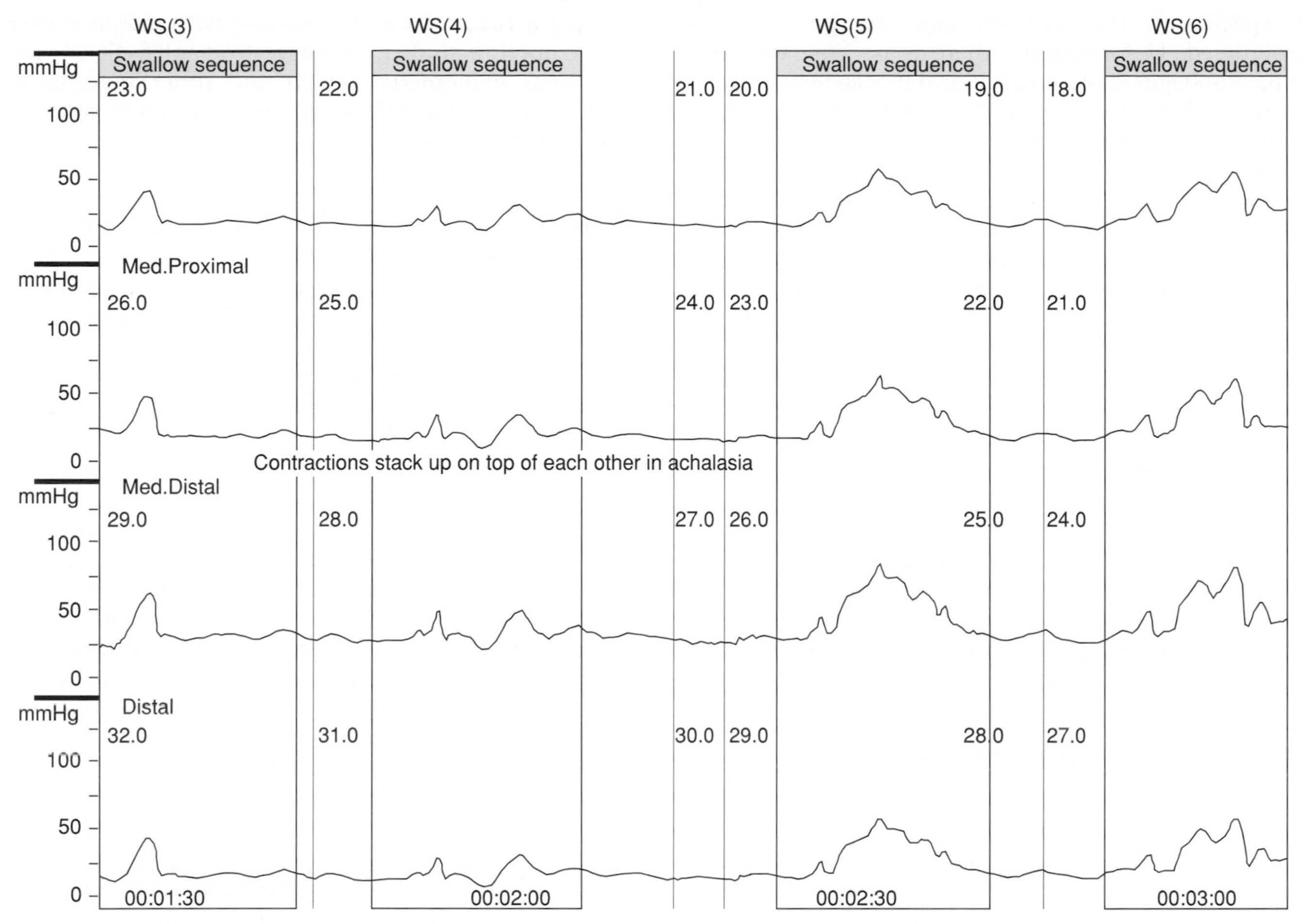

Figure 5.5: Abnormal esophageal manometry. A series of four wet swallows occurring about 30 s apart from one another are recorded from the body of the esophagus of a 12-year-old boy with achalasia. Note that the contractions are weak and of low amplitude, but, more importantly, they lack the peristaltic progression when contrasted to the normal sequential waves seen in Figures 5.1 and 5.2. Simultaneous contractions or the absence of peristalsis is the hallmark of achalasia.

abnormalities can be diagnosed in about half of these patients. Abnormalities of esophageal manometry were reported in up to 85% of children with CIPO in a national survey by Vargas et al.,[25] after which the practice of evaluating pediatric patients with suspected CIPO routinely included manometry of the esophagus.

Non-specific esophageal motor disorders

Non-specific esophageal motor disorders (NEMDs) may be found in pediatric patients. This category is defined as abnormalities discovered on esophageal manometry that do not follow the recognized patterns of the primary esophageal motility disorders. These disorders are more difficult to define in terms of their correlation to symptoms bringing them to manometry. In a study of 154 children (mean age 11.6 ± 2.6 years), GER was found in 71% and, although patients with reflux had normal peristalsis, the mean LES pressure was lower.

Both patients with GER and reflux-free children with upper GI symptoms and dysphagia may demonstrate NEMD. In a study by Rosario et al.,[51] these children were more likely to suffer from food impaction in the esophagus. More subtle findings are frequently identified at the time of testing, and may be recognized in the future in their own categories of esophageal dysfunction.

Recognized characteristics of hiatal hernia and fundoplication can also be seen as the pressure signatures in the distal esophagus to the trained eye of the observer.

Both dermatomyositis and scleroderma have manometric characteristics that are sometimes readily appreciated, yet may sometimes be obscure until the disease has progressed to a well developed state. It is common for these children to present with dysphagia and weight loss, among other signs and symptoms.

A study of 17 pediatric patients (range 5–18 years) with scleroderma and mixed connective tissue disorders seen at a referral center found that 73% had esophageal motor abnormalities, a figure comparable to values reported in adults with these disorders. Specifically, inadequate LES resting pressure and impaired smooth muscle peristalsis were the most frequently seen abnormalities, but several non-specific or transient pressure changes were also encountered. Unfortunately, there is no cure for scleroderma esophagus at present, but acid blockade is employed routinely to treat associated GER. Children with linear scleroderma escaped abnormal esophageal dysfunction.[52]

Other connective tissue diseases, such as lupus, may also be accompanied by a number of esophageal motor abnormalities, most often inadequate LES function and ineffective esophageal body peristaltic waves. Aperistalsis may also be seen with rheumatologic disorders of mixed connective tissue disease, namely progressive systemic sclerosis and systemic lupus erythematosus.

The proximal esophagus is composed of striated muscle, and diseases affecting striated muscle show aperistalsis proximally and normal motility in the distal esophagus. In a variable section of the mid-esophagus, overlap of striated and smooth muscle results in lower-amplitude peristaltic waves; this is a normal and expected finding and is referred to as a 'transition zone' of the esophagus.[53] Conversely, disorders of smooth muscle show normal upper esophageal waves but lack peristalsis distally. Rarely, infiltration of the distal esophagus by a primary malignancy or its effects will result in secondary achalasia.

Ineffective esophageal motility

In adults there is a disorder known as ineffective esophageal motility (IEM), which may also be seen in children. The manometric definition of IEM is low-amplitude contractions of less than 30 mmHg or non-transmitted contractions in 30% or more of 10 swallows in the distal esophagus. In patients with GERD-associated respiratory symptoms, IEM was found to be the most prevalent abnormality of motility.[54] A study of 16 children with GERD requiring fundoplication showed IEM persisting after surgery, prompting the authors to conclude that it may be a primary etiologic factor.[55]

More recently, esophageal manometry has been combined with MII to measure transit of a bolus simultaneously with pressure changes in patients with IEM.[56] Impedance monitoring is done by measuring the resistance to the flow of electrons in the refluxate. In another study, patients with achalasia and scleroderma had dysphagia and abnormal bolus transit compared with patients with normal manometric fundings, IEM, diffuse esophageal spasm, nutcracker esophagus, and hypertensive and hypotensive LES.[57]

GASTRIC MOTILITY

Designed for optimal digestion and absorption, the stomach provides a combination of mixing and forward propulsion of food. The fundus of the stomach dilates to accommodate liquid and gas, and the antrum grinds and triturates food particles before they are propelled into the duodenum. Particles greater than 5 mm are retrojected into the fundus for further milling into smaller pieces. Control of the stomach is diverse in origin and is governed partly by its own inherent electrical control activity.

Gastric function can be measured with radionuclide gastric emptying studies, electrogastrography (EGG), antroduodenal manometry (ADM) and other investigations. Normal and abnormal gastric function and its assessment are discussed in more detail in Chapter 27.

GASTRIC EMPTYING STUDIES

Gastric emptying of solid and liquid phases is estimated from technetium-radiolabeled meal imaging. Most pediatric surgeons obtain a gastric emptying study prior to performing an anti-reflux operation, as it assists in determining whether a pyloroplasty should be done. Nuclear imaging can also provide information on esophageal transit time and GER.

Gastroparesis may occur in children and adolescents as a result of a viral infection. Emptying of solids from the stomach is considered the best screening test for gastroparesis. A stomach that does not empty well may also progress to delayed emptying of liquids and predispose to GER. Gastric emptying combined with antroduodenal manometry confirmed postprandial hypomotility in 10 of 11 children with postviral gastroparesis, and the prognosis was good as all patients recovered within 6–24 months.[58] Adolescents with anorexia nervosa may have abnormalities in esophageal and gastric function, which may normalize with nutritional repletion of the patient.

ELECTROGASTROGRAPHY (EGG)

EGG can be conceptualized as the equivalent of an electrocardiograph of the stomach's electrical activity. Gastric slow waves occur at a basal rate of 3 cycles per minute (cpm). Rhythms greater than 4 cpm are termed tachygastria, and may be associated with dyspepsia. Gastric rhythms in the range of 1.5–2.4 cpm are termed bradygastria, and may be associated with delayed gastric emptying. EGG did not correlate well with radionuclide gastric emptying when both were performed simultaneously in nine children with vomiting, abdominal pain and/or dyspepsia.[59]

The EGG was used to evaluate regurgitation and vomiting in seven infants with cow's milk protein allergy in comparison with nine infants with GER and 10 normal controls. The researchers found that, in sensitized infants, a challenge with cow's milk induced severe gastric dysrhythmia and delayed gastric emptying. The EGG parameters for the normals and the cohort of infants with GER were similar and significantly different from those of the infants allergic to cow's milk.[60] In this clinical setting, the application the EGG seems to hold some promise for separating different subgroups of infants with vomiting, but its role is still evolving.

Sometimes, EGG has been helpful when coupled with ADM in differentiating groups of children with normal manometry from a cohort with myopathic or neuropathic changes. Yet, in the same study it was impossible to interpret the EGG, and the problem of overlap of findings of normal and abnormal EGG rhythms occurred.[61]

The place of EGG in the armamentarium of gastric function tests is still being explored. Research over the past 10 years has established normal EGG values for pediatric patients and developmental changes in the postnatal studies of premature infants.[62–64] Certainly EGG is non-invasive, fulfilling an important criterion for pediatric motility testing, but it must be considered in its formative stages at the present time.

ANTRODUODENAL MOTILITY (ADM)

In the neonate, the length of the small intestine is about 270 cm, growing and developing to a length of 4–5 m in the adult. Intestinal contractions cause mixing and propulsion of ingested food and secretions to bathe the absorptive surface area of the small bowel. There is a complex neural control of this coordinated muscular activity, rendered in concert by the central nervous system, secreted regulatory peptide hormones, and the autonomic nervous system within the gut, which is richly extensive in neurons, ganglia and nerve processes.

In the fasting state, the migrating motor complex (MMC) occurs in three phases in the small bowel. Phase I is characterized by motor quiescence. In phase II, random, intermittent contractions similar to those seen in the fed state are seen. Phase III is characterized by high-amplitude, high-frequency contractions that sweep the intestinal contents toward the ileum. The peristaltic wave of the MMC may start anywhere from the lower esophagus to the small bowel. The antrum contracts at a frequency of 3 cpm and the small intestine at 11–12 cpm in phase III. This interdigestive pattern cleans the bowel of undigested residual food, bacteria and sloughed enterocytes, all of which move ahead of the advancing front of intestinal contraction. In younger children the MMC occurs more frequently, and for older adolescents the interval between MMCs is about 100 min, similar to that in adults.

When the normal housekeeping function of the MMC is altered, stasis of intestinal contents promotes dilation of the small intestine and bacterial overgrowth. Disorders of gastric emptying such as gastroparesis are also evaluated with ADM, although radionuclide gastric emptying for solids and liquids should precede ADM for the evaluation of gastroparesis. Children with abdominal distention, chronic nausea and vomiting, and early satiety may be candidates for ADM. Feeding will abolish the MMC pattern, rendering the pattern back to phase II, which is optimal for mixing and absorption.

The pattern of normal ADM has been established in children with no upper GI or small bowel symptoms, and was found to be similar to that of adults.[65] In a study by Ittmann et al.[66] comparing ADM in 19 pre-term and 9 term infants, fasting antral activity was found to be comparable in the two groups. The data also suggested that the temporal association of antral duodenal motor activity develops in association with progressive changes in duodenal motor activity.[66] Data are available from a group of 95 children with signs and symptoms of motility disorder in contrast to 20 control children.[67] The authors concluded that some manometric features had a clear association with motility disorders in children:

- Absent, abnormal migration of or short interval between phase III of the MMC
- Persistent low-amplitude contractions
- Sustained tonic contractions.

In addition, when controlled for meal composition with standardized upright awake and recumbent sleep periods, circadian variation in ADM is known to occur in normal subjects.[68] The experience with ADM was felt to be best left to the referral center in one study, as the authors encountered a frustratingly large number of non-specific abnormalities in 72% of older patients. However, ADM was helpful in recommending a new therapy (medication, surgery, feeding or referral) in 29% of patients.[69]

It is possible to measure GI tract motility wherever the catheter can be reasonably and safely positioned. An example of this is ileal manometry in children following ileostomies and pull-through operations. In a group of 23 children who had ileal manometry studies (mean age 7 years, range from 2 months to 17 years), some of the patterns were found to be different from those in adults, wheres contractions in infants and toddlers were similar to those in adults.[70] Functioning ileostomies were cannulated and random phasic contractions were the most common feature recorded. Phase III of the MMC was found in only 2 of the 23 children. The ileum was found to have some characteristics in common with the proximal small bowel and the colon. In fact, the origin of the colonic high-amplitude propagating contraction (HAPC) was in the ileum in the form of propagating or clustered contractions in some of the patients.

The technique of antroduodenal motility

In performing antroduodenal manometry, the manometrist first places the catheter across the antrum into the duodenum. This can be accomplished during upper GI endoscopy when the catheter can be dragged alongside the endoscope, or placed over a guidewire once the endoscope has been removed. An interventional radiologist can place the ADM catheter with or without a guidewire in some settings. Some have placed these catheters into the jejunum and recorded data from the proximal part of this section of the small intestine, but this is infrequently done in motility laboratories, making jejunal recording more of a research tool than a practical method in children. Figure 5.6 demonstrates proper placement of the ADM catheter for optimal recording of motor activity in this region.

The pressure transducers of the manometer must straddle the antrum and the duodenum. The number of sensors needed and the optimal distance between them is usually determined by the size of the patient. A minimum number is two in the antrum and three in the duodenum, but more will give information about contractile activity (or lack of it) across a longer expanse of small intestine. Recording takes place later that day and over the following day until sufficient information has been obtained.

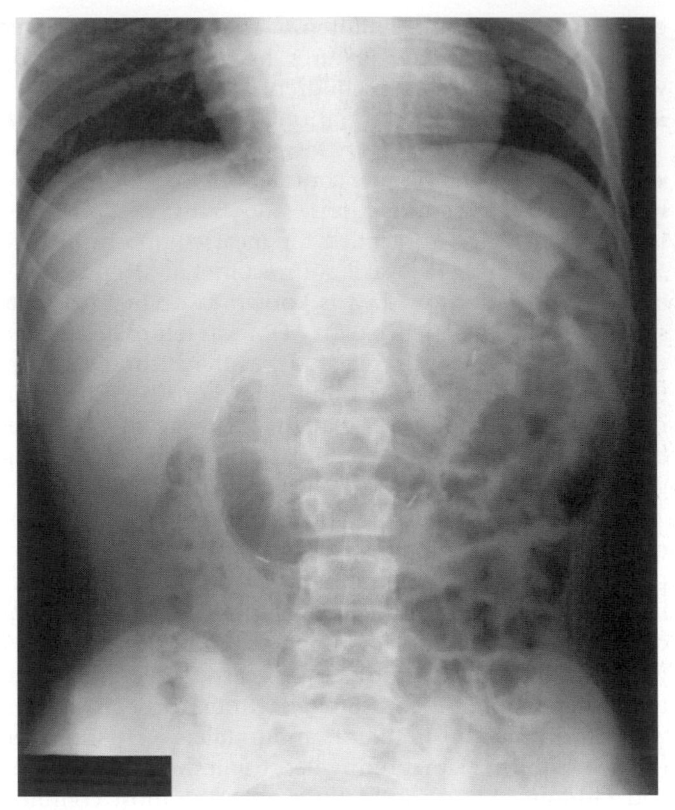

Figure 5.6: Radiograph of the abdomen demonstrating normal placement of the antroduodenal catheter. The outline of the stomach is visible with the proximal pressure sensors in the antrum. The catheter courses through the C loop of the duodenum. The sensors are visible on plain film of the abdomen because there are small radio-opaque metal markers next to the pressure port.

Recording can also be accomplished by taking out a gastrostomy tube and threading the motility catheter through the ostomy and into the duodenum. Fasting motility recording is done for 3–4 h, followed by a meal and/or prokinetic agents. Figure 5.7 demonstrates the pattern seen in normal ADM recording (Table 5.3).

Postoperative adhesions and chronic pseudo-obstruction may cause abdominal distention and small bowel bacterial overgrowth when the MMC is not producing normal peristalsis. Classifying CIPO as myopathic or neuropathic type is done with ADM. If a more generalized motility disorder is suspected, it is recommended that ADM information be obtained before major decisions are made, such as colectomy for colonic inertia. Limitations to ADM are difficulty in intubating the duodenum, catheter migration, and the stressful effects of the procedure itself.[71]

Some recommend ADM as part of the assessment of a child's feeding readiness or for discerning whether enteral feedings will be tolerated. A study of 48 pre-term infants revealed that infants who tolerated feedings changed their pattern of motor activity in response to feeding and infants who did not tolerate feedings had no 'fed response'. The sensitivity of manometry to predict feeding intolerance was 1.0, and the specificity was 0.13.[66]

Provocative medications and ADM

Provocative medications may be administered during ADM, which may take a few hours to an entire day to perform.

Use of the macrolide antibiotic erythromycin at subtherapeutic doses of 1–3 mg/kg will stimulate antral contractions and phase III-like episodes by acting as a motilin receptor agonist on GI tract smooth muscle cells.[72] Some manometrists use a dose of less than one-quarter of the recommended antibiotic doseage and have found a beneficial effect in promoting tolerance of enteral feeds or enhancing a measured index of GI motility in infants and children. A fatal reaction has been reported when giving intravenous erythromycin to neonates in antibiotic doses.[51,73] For ADM, administration may be intravenous, oral or through the tip of the motility catheter directly into the duodenum; in the author's department the last method is used.

Motilin infusion studies have shown that initiation of antral phase III is subject to a refractory period and that the duration is longer than the refractory periods observed following MMCs of pyloric, duodenal or jejunal origin. Motilin did not stimulate MMCs in the pylorus or the intestine. The gallbladder responds to motilin by contracting, and appears to have no refractory period. Thus, motilin has different regional effects as a motility agent.[74]

Conversely, the somatostatin analog octreotide inhibits gastric motility in the antrum and phase III activity, so the choice and timing of administration during small bowel manometry should be planned. When children with chronic bowel disorders were given subcutaneous octreotide at doses of 0.5–1.0μg/kg, MMCs were induced that appeared to be different from spontaneous MMCs. Subsequent administration of a meal abolishes the inhibitory effect of octreotide on the gastric antrum[75] Pretreatment with erythromycin prevents the octreotide-induced antral quieting, suggesting that manipulation of motilin release may be the mechanism controlling antral activity.[76]

A physiologic study of the role of motilin during selective muscarinic or serotonergic pharmacologic blockade in normal subjects was done in 1997. The researchers concluded that in the antrum motilin induces phase III activity via muscarinic pathways, whereas in the duodenum motilin mediates contractions by a non-cholinergic mechanism.[77]

Metaclopramide can also be given during ADM to stimulate MMCs. Early studies have shown enhanced gastric emptying[78] and gastroduodenal motility[79] with this drug.

The clinical response to the limited number of prokinetic medications currently available can be assessed if desired, and the procedure can be tailored to the individual child. A general protocol is applied, but when performing pediatric gastroenterologic motility procedures flexibility, patience and the comfort of the child during the procedure must all be considered. In contrast, motility studies in adults are done in a prescribed sequence the majority of the time and can be more standardized because of the level of cooperation that can be expected.

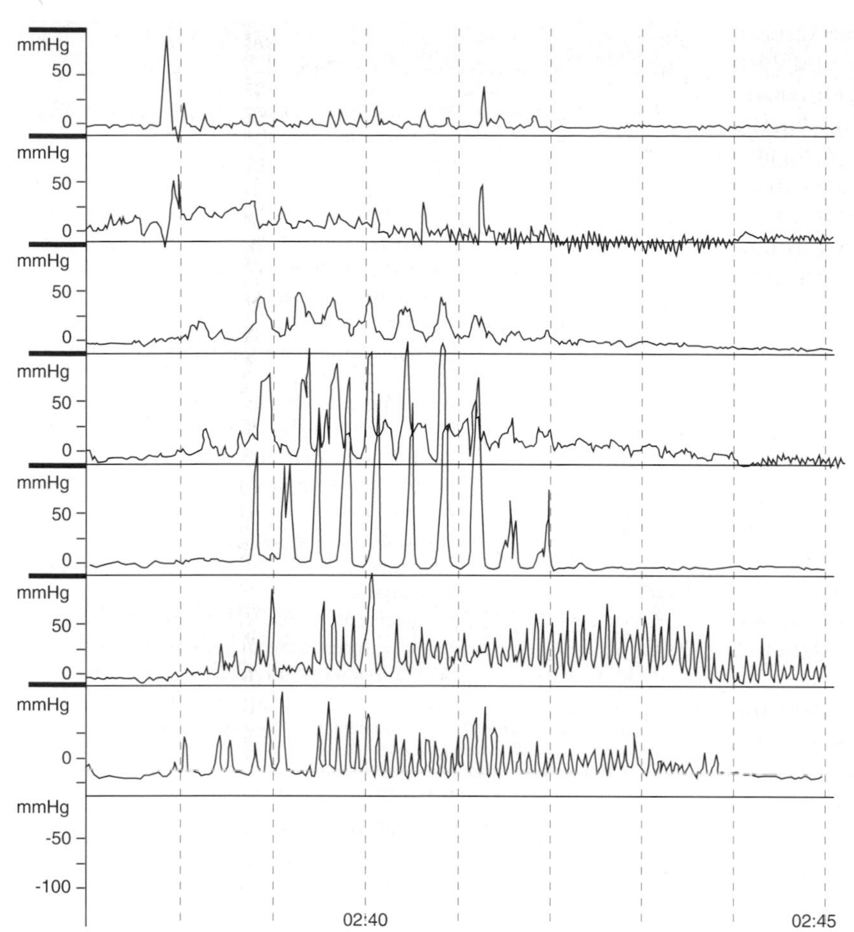

Figure 5.7: Normal antroduodenal manometry. The recording is taken as the catheter migrates upward. The top row is pharyngeal, the second row is in the upper esophageal sphincter, the third and fourth rows are in the esophagus. The fifth row is recording strong phasic antral contractions at a frequency of 3 cpm, and the last rows are picking up the migrating motor complex in the duodenum. The frequency of contractions in the duodenum is 11–14 cpm.

The standardization and order of a protocol may have to be altered according to circumstances, involving a significant difference from performing these procedures in adults. Currently under study is the effect of tegaserod, a partial 5-HT_4 receptor agonist, on antroduodenal motility. Cisapride and alosetron have been taken off the market by the US Food and Drug Administration (FDA) because of potential cardiac dysrhythmogenicity. Tegaserod seems to be devoid of adverse electrocardiographic effects,[80] but recently a warning was issued about intestinal ischemia as an possible adverse event. At this point in time, however, it is not clear whether this prokinetic agent causes this problem in greater than the expected background rate in patients with irritable bowel syndrome (IBS) and in the general population.

Normal – MMC appears in fasting state
Phase I – inactivity or quiescence
Phase II – intermittent contraction activity with random periodicity and amplitude
Phase III – regular contractions in antrum at 3 per min, and in small bowel at 11–13 per min, complete the MMC
An MMC cycle lasts about 100 min, but depends on age (may be more frequent in young children)
A meal is then given, and provocative medications if needed
Fed state – contractions occur irregularly and vary in amplitude
Meal composition affects quality and amplitude of contractions
Abnormal
In CIPO (see Table 5.4)
Retrograde contractions, low-amplitude contractions, absence of phase III, non-propagated bursts of duodenal activity
Myopathic process – low-amplitude contractions, no phase III seen
Neuropathic process – abnormal waveform and propagation

CIPO, chronic intestinal pseudo-obstruction; MMC, migrating motor complex.

Table 5.3 Antroduodenal manometry

Recordings of activity of the ileum in 23 children (age range from 2 months to 17 years) through ileostomies have taught us that there are random intermittent contractions, cluster contractions, tonic contractions and prolonged propagated contractions. These patterns are morphologically different from proximal small bowel recordings. The MMC was rare in the distal ileum, seen only twice in 55 h of fasting recording.[70] This information may be relevant to the 'ileal brake' mechanism of feedback to the proximal small bowel to decrease peristalsis.[81]

The duodenum also has an immediate 'brake' function of restricting gastric outflow; this is dependent upon the composition of contents in the duodenum, whether bilious, lipid or acidic.[82] This regulatory function promotes optimal digestion and absorption, and prevents rapid dumping of stomach contents into the upper small intestine.

Prolonged ambulatory ADM recording has been utilized to study adults with slow-transit constipation,[83] and 24-h recordings have been used to gather more information than can be obtained at stationary manometric testing with esophageal and colonic manometry. For practical purposes, however, this is an investigational tool used by research centers and does not have reimbursement codes beyond the usual test. As such, use of overnight ambulatory manometry is not standard practice in pediatrics.

ADM and chronic intestinal pseudo-obstruction

ADM is central to the diagnosis of CIPO.[84,85] CIPO is a model of abnormal GI motility disorders, as abnormalities may be detected from the esophagus to the anorectum, or they may be localized to one segment of bowel, such as the duodenum, small bowel or colon. Manometric and functional findings seen in CIPO are summarized in Tables 5.3 and 5.4. Pseudo-obstruction is discussed in more detail in Chapter 42.

Feeding difficulties are the most common problem the pediatric gastroenterologist struggles with in patients with CIPO. Using ADM has taught us that the presence of jejunal MMCs in patients who had abnormal ADM findings and intolerance of gastrostomy tube feeds was a predictor of successful adaptation to jejunal feeds.[86] A study of ruminators who had previous extensive GI workup demonstrated normal fasting MMCs. Postprandial results showed brief, simultaneous pressure increases at all recording sites, and 8 of the 12 adolescents studied had associated effortless regurgitation. The utility of ADM in this clinical situation is its characteristic pattern, which excludes motility disorders that may be confused with rumination syndrome.

The diagnosis of CIPO is made clinically with the assured absence of structural obstruction. Patients may present with vomiting, abdominal distention, constipation, abdominal pain and failure to thrive. After anatomic obstruction has been ruled out, ADM is an appropriate step in making a diagnosis of CIPO and provides objective data on intestinal motility.[87]

A normal ADM excludes CIPO in children.[88] Hence, referral back to other sources of symptoms is done if normal activity fronts of MMCs are found. Subgroups of neuropathic and myopathic CIPO can be determined manometrically and have been correlated with histologic findings in children[89] (Table 5.4).

ADM and Munchausen's syndrome by proxy

Chronic motility problems may be the presenting facade of Munchausen's syndrome by proxy, and the diagnosis may emerge with the opportunity to observe the behaviors and psychosocial interactions of parents and children undergoing evaluation.[84]

GI segment	Findings
Esophageal motility	Abnormalities in approximately half of CIPO, although in some series up to 85% demonstrate abnormalities
	Decreased LES pressure
	Failure of LES relaxation
	Esophageal body: low-amplitude waves, poor propagation, tertiary waves, retrograde peristalsis, occasionally aperistalsis
Gastric emptying	May be delayed
EGG	Tachygastria or bradygastria may be seen
ADM	Postprandial antral hypomotility is seen and correlates with delayed gastric emptying
	Myopathic subtype: low-amplitude contractions, <10–20 mmHg
	Neuropathic subtype: contractions are uncoordinated
	Fed response is absent
	Fasting MMC is absent, or MMC abnormally propagated
Colonic	No gastrocolic reflex as there is no increased motility in response to a meal
ARM	Normal rectoanal inhibitory reflex (RAIR)

Findings vary according to the segment(s) of the gastrointestinal tract that are involved. ADM, antroduodenal manometry; ARM, anorectal manometry; CIPO, chronic intestinal pseudo-obstruction; EGG, electrogastrography; LES, lower esophageal sphincter; MMC, migrating motor complex.

Table 5.4 Findings in pseudo-obstruction

MANOMETRIC STUDY OF THE SPHINCTER OF ODDI

Sphincter of Oddi manometry is conducted in conjunction with endoscopic retrograde cholangiopancreatography in the evaluation of chronic abdominal pain. Manometric study of the sphincter of Oddi is challenging, and is still evolving in its role of determining whether a pressure-relieving sphincteroplasty could alleviate symptoms of abdominal pain in children. This topic is discussed in further detail in Chapter 79 in terms of the evaluation of pancreaticobiliary disorders.

COLONIC MANOMETRY

It is possible to study the entire colon with colonic manometry. The colon has been relatively inaccessible to study until recent years, however, and so knowledge of motility of the colon has lagged behind the knowledge of esophageal motility that has been accrued for decades.[90]

The colon has to be prepared for colonoscopy with a thorough cleanout, which can present a challenge to patients with chronic stool retention. In the author's department a water-perfused catheter is placed during colonoscopy and threaded over a guidewire. Ideally the catheter tip will be in the cecum, but occasionally placement is not pancolonic. Catheters of at least three different lengths with port spacing 5, 10 and 15 cm apart are needed to prepare for the range of colon sizes in children and adolescents. Figure 5.8 demonstrates the position of a colonic

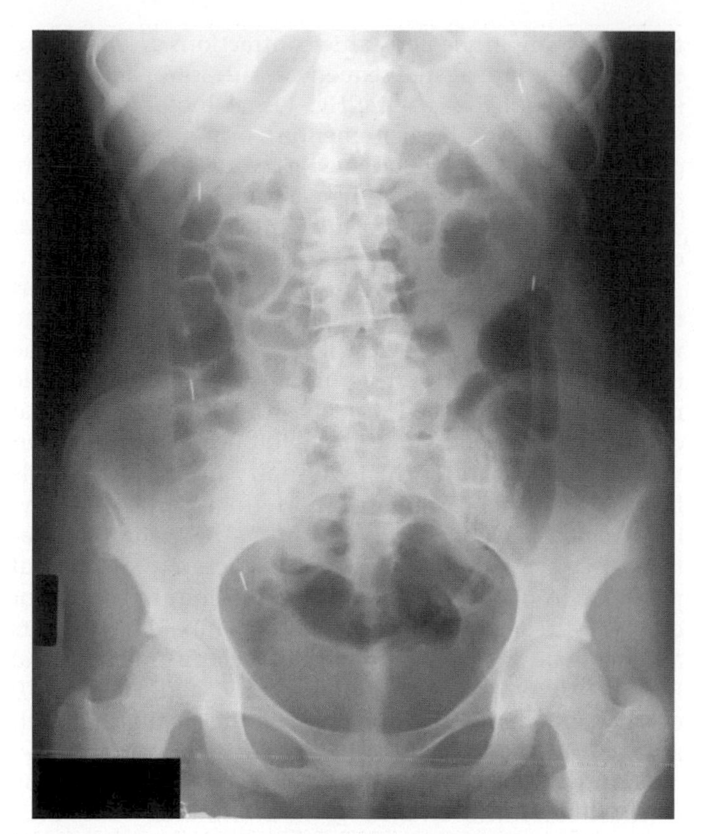

Figure 5.8: Abdominal radiograph demonstrating the position of a colonic motility catheter following the expected course of the colon. The small metal bars indicate the location of the pressure-sensing ports. In this catheter the sensors are 10 cm apart, and the most proximal sensor is in the cecum.

manometry catheter within the colon. Colonic manometry is limited to studying the parts of the colon covered by the catheter; sometimes the catheter will not traverse the entire colon to the cecum, but may end up in the transverse colon or splenic flexure if there are problems with insertion of the tube over the guidewire or if it slides out of position, as may occur with defecation. The manometrist performs a qualitative analysis of the recording; automated analysis will be available soon.[91]

Colonic manometry is now used throughout the world in tertiary medical centers to evaluate colonic disorders and is becoming increasingly popular as a guide in management decisions such as surgical resection for segmental colonic inertia, and placement of colonic antegrade enema ports. It is used to help discriminate functional from organic colonic diseases. It is an invasive test, however, and should be reserved for patients with intractable constipation in whom previous evaluation has proved unrevealing.

Uses with surgery

Pediatric surgeons are using colonic manometry more routinely because the information obtained can be valuable in deciding the need for and timing of diversion, the extent of resection required, and the suitability of restoring bowel continuity in out-of-circuit colon for children with ileostomy or colostomy.[92,93]

In an analysis of 150 studies performed in 146 children, colonic manometry provided information that clarified the pathophysiology of lower GI tract complaints and frequently resulted in new recommendations for medical and/or surgical management. This investigation has come of age in providing information regarding reanastomosis of a diverted colon and for preoperative and postoperative colonic function in patients with HD, CIPO and spinal cord disorders.[94]

Colonic manometry also plays an important role in children with chronic constipation that is recalcitrant to therapy, in determining colonic function before and after surgery in order to predict which patients will benefit from resection or reanastomosis.

Colonic manometry combined with anorectal manometry (ARM) helps to elucidate the pathophysiology of the colon and sphincters in children who have undergone surgical repair of imperforate anus. In a group of 10 patients it was possible to identify the mechanisms of fecal incontinence as being multifactorial: propagation of excessive HAPCs to the neorectum combined with internal anal sphincter (IAS) dysfunction.[95]

The antegrade continence enema procedure was described by Malone et al.[95a] using the appendix as a stoma fashioned to attach to the abdominal wall. The stoma is intubated and enema fluid is given into the right colon while the patient sits on the toilet to evacuate the fecal contents of the colon.

Colonic manometry also plays a role in decision-making on the appropriateness of cecostomy in children with slow-transit constipation.[96] Modification of this method has been done by others who have placed the antegrade enema access directly into the left colon of children, promoting continence by means of regular colonic cleansing.

Of 350 colonic manometry investigations performed over the years for clinical indications, 12 could not be interpreted due to chronic colonic dilation. None of these 12 patients (mean age 4 years, range 2–14 years) was responsive to medical intervention. Surgical colonic diversion was recommended for them: four for intestinal neuronal dysplasia, two had hypoganglionosis, one for hollow visceral myopathy and five with normal histologic findings. All 12 children were restudied 6–30 months later with colonic manometry. Based on the manometric data after temporary diversion, the authors recommended resection of a part of the colon that appeared atonic and aperistaltic, or reanastomosis for decompressed colons in children who exhibited a normal gastrocolonic response and HAPCs. They reported successful resolution of defecation problems in 10 of the 12 patients when seen at follow-up at 5–30 months.[97]

Colonic manometry and Hirschsprung's disease

Persistent symptoms of constipation and fecal incontinence plague children with HD long after resection and pull-through surgery. Even though the possibility of a retained segment of aganglionosis may have been resolved, when the etiopathogenesis is investigated with colonic manometry four patterns are seen, each with its own treatment path. In one, HAPCs, which in the native state terminate at the rectosigmoid part of the colon, now travel to the pelvic floor directly, without the braking function of the resected storage-capacity rectosigmoid colon. In the second pattern, normal colonic manometry with functional withholding occurs. In the third, absent HAPCs and simultaneous contractions may occur. The fourth pattern is hypertensive anal sphincter.

When colonic manometry was used to categorize the type of motility pattern, therapy could be more accurately directed, resulting in a 72% improvement in bowel actions and decreased or resolved abdominal pain in 80% of 46 symptomatic patients with HD (mean age 5.5 ± 3.3 years).[98] Others have substantiated the persistence of abnormal GI motility dysfunction long after corrective surgery.[99] This has led to conceptualizing HD as a risk for systemic motility problems, even in the esophagus. Indeed, the possibility of enterocolitis should be entertained in a child who has suggestive signs and symptoms years after documented resection of aganglionic bowel.[100]

Chronic constipation

Colonic manometry is used in the evaluation of chronic constipation resistant to the known therapeutic maneuvers, such as stool softeners, stimulant laxatives and bowel programs of regular sitting. Combined with other tests, such as marker studies and anorectal manometry, the pathophysiology of constipation becomes clearer. Di Lorenzo et al.[101] studied 23 children with intractable constipation using colonic manometry. All children were screened previously to exclude HD. They concluded that colonic manometry was able to differentiate the causes of chronic constipation accurately by the response to meals. Patients with functional fecal retention, hollow visceral myopathy and neuropathy were distinguished by their motility indexes and by the presence or absence of HAPCs.

The discussion on chronic constipation, functional fecal retention in children and encopresis is found in Chapter 11.

Physiology in colonic motility

In contrast to small bowel motility in which fasting produces the MMC pattern, colonic manometry can demonstrate HAPCs with the stimulus of a meal. Food stimulates phasic and tonic motor activity in the colon, called the gastrocolonic reflex, and this can be seen within 10 min of ingestion. The amplitude of an HAPC varies widely, from 50 to more than 180 mmHg, and is defined as extending at least 30 cm of colon as detected by the pressure sensors. Pressures higher than this are associated with mass movement of colonic contents and defecation. Some definitions vary in amplitude and distance of the colon traversed by the peristaltic sequence. The HAPC has consensus as being rapidly migrating, high-amplitude, long-duration contractions that move the contents of the colon towards the rectum.[4] Low-amplitude peristaltic contractions are also seen; these are also propagated sequences with lower amplitudes in the range of 5 to 40 mmHg. Rectal motor complexes (RMCs) are a local phenomenon, occurring more frequently at night, at a frequency of two to four per minute and an amplitude greater than 5 mmHg and lasting for about 10 min. RMCs are postulated to play a role in fecal continence.[102]

The circular muscle layer produces phasic contractions that are analyzed by their appearance as single pressure waves, the timing of groups of peristaltic waves, and the timing of phases or recurring motility patterns.[103] Colonic motor response has been shown to vary according to meal composition: carbohydrate meals induce a response, but the response is shorter than with fatty meals. Fatty meals induce prolonged, segmental and retrograde phasic activity that may delay colonic transit.[104] Antegrade propagation of sequenced phasic contractions is aboral propagation of the wavefront. In the colon, retrograde or orally directed contractions function to mix fecal contents and facilitate absorption. Figure 5.9 demonstrates normal HAPC activity on colonic manometry, and Figure 5.10 demonstrates abnormal colonic manometric findings with absence of HAPC activity.

During sleep, colonic activity quiets considerably. By contrast, morning awakening is a stimulus to colonic motility, which may contribute to the regularity some individuals experience in the timing of bowel actions. Also recognized are low-amplitude, propagated, phasic contractions, which occur more frequently in a 24-h cycle than HAPCs. Although the significance of these awaits further elucidation, it is speculated that LAPCs play a role in preserving nocturnal fecal continence. The sigmoid colon may have a role in protecting continence as it is here that the flow of fecal contents is considerably slowed before reaching the rectum. In the rectum, a phenomenon termed rectal motor complexes has been identified on prolonged colonic manometry and is also speculated to play a role in preserving nocturnal continence.[102] The infant defecate spontaneously by reflex; the older child learns to withhold bowel movements until a convenient or appropriate time for emptying the colon. Manometric findings in colonic motor studies are presented in Table 5.5.

Colonic distention appears to be a stimulus for contraction to propel stool in a caudad direction, although some retrograde contractions occur and result in mixing and segmentation of stool. In a study combining colonic manometry and urodynamic studies in children with constipation and voiding difficulties, colonic manometry was found to be abnormal in all subjects. In the subgroup of patients in whom neuropathy affecting both the colon and urinary bladder was present, successful treatment of the constipation did not result in resolution of urinary symptoms.[105] This is in contrast to the improvement expected in children with frequent urinary tract infections and vesicoureteral reflux secondary to chronic functional fecal retention with megarectum, fecal impaction and encopresis.

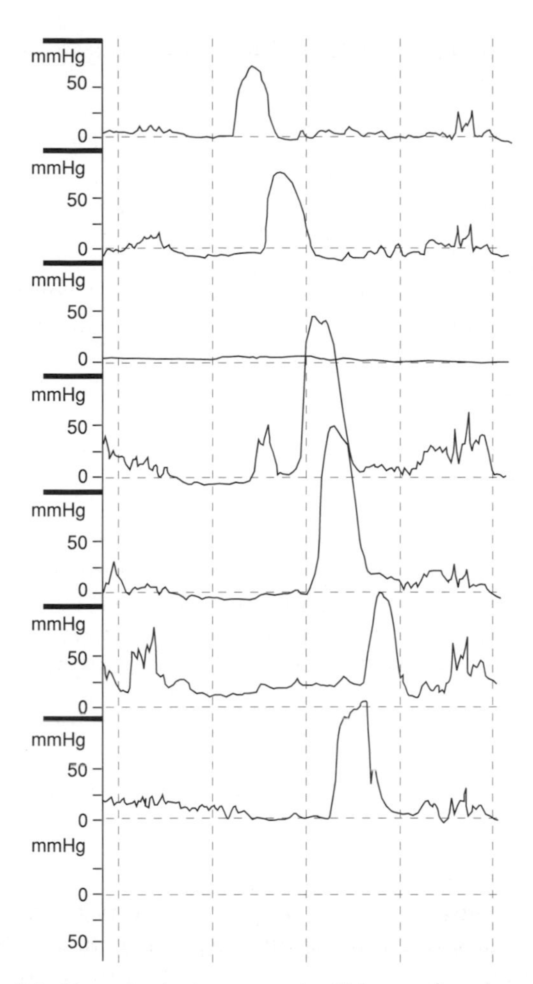

Figure 5.9: Normal colonic manometry. This recording demonstrates normal postprandial high-amplitude peristaltic contractions (HAPCs). These contractions are phasic, or isolated peaks from baseline, and usually more than 100 mmHg. The recording sensors are located 10 cm apart, and the top tracing represents the most proximal port located in the cecum. The lowest tracing represents a pressure port recording from the rectosigmoid junction. On the left a contraction starts in the fourth row down, corresponding to the distal transverse colon near the splenic flexure, and propagates over 30 cm to the rectosigmoid. About 2 min later another HAPC is recorded to the right, this time starting at the ascending colon and propagating down to the rectosigmoid region.

Similar findings and natural history would be expected in children with spinal cord dysfunction, such as myelomeningocele or trauma. In a review of 32 colonic manometric studies of children who were not found to have colonic disease, HAPCs were more frequent in younger children before and after a meal, and colonic contractions that were different in morphology from the HAPCs occurred more commonly with increased age.[106]

Use of provocative medications in colonic manometry

Provocative medications are also commonly administered during colonic manometry to assess the physiologic response to prokinetic agents. Using water-perfused colonic manometry catheters inserted into the right colon, the effect of intracecal bisacodyl was compared to installation of intrarectal bisacodyl in 28 children and to administration of edrophonium. The children had disorders of chronic constipation, and a fraction had known neuromuscular disease. Readings were recorded after patients had fasted for 1 h, 1 h postprandially, then 30 min after a provocative agent. Bisacodyl induced HAPCs in all subjects. The effect of intrarectal bisacodyl was identical, but delayed by 10 min. Bisacodyl was superior to edrophonium in stimulating HAPCs, and the morphology of the waveforms was similar to that of naturally occurring HAPCs seen in 22 of the 28 children prior to stimulant laxative administration. The authors speculated that, for children on total parenteral nutrition or restricted fluid intake, it may be possible to shorten the duration of colonic manometry testing by giving bisacodyl early, rather than waiting for spontaneous HAPCs to occur.[107] The present author routinely uses the stimulant laxative bisacodyl at a dosage of 5–10 mg, instilling the drug directly into the colonic manometry catheter during study. Colonic motor events occur infrequently, so fasting before the procedure is standard practice in order to feed a child as a stimulus.

The author and colleagues are also studying the effect of tegaserod, a selective 5-HT^4 partial receptor agonist during colonic manometry when a child fails to produce HAPCs. Other pharmacologic agents, such as colchicine, which has been studied in small numbers of adults but not in children, are instilled into the colon via the colonic motility catheter.

Colonic transit time

Recently, data on normal values for segmental and total colonic transit time (CTT) have been contributed to the relatively small volume of literature available for pediatric patients. Transit was measured in 22 healthy children of median age 10 (range 4–15) years after they ingested markers daily for six consecutive days. Using Abrahamsson's method, a single abdominal radiography set at low radiation was taken on day 7. The mean total CTT was 40 h, with the upper limit of normal established at the 95th percentile at 84 h. Each segment was found to have the following upper limits: ascending 14 h, transverse 33 h, descending 21 h and rectosigmoid 41 h.[108]

Ingestion of radio-opaque markers followed by abdominal radiography to assess their progression through the colon is used to determine CTT in patients with chronic constipation. This method is simple, convenient for clinical use, and has much to offer in selected patients with chronic constipation.[109]

A collection of markers in the rectosigmoid suggests outlet dysfunction such as anismus or paradoxical puborectalis contraction (PPC). PPC is the act of squeezing the external anal sphincter (EAS) when straining. The patient may or may not be aware of this habit, which may have developed as a conditioned response to prior painful defecation, and may therefore have evolved as a protective response of withholding stool to avoid the discomfort of experiencing stretching of the anal canal by large or hard

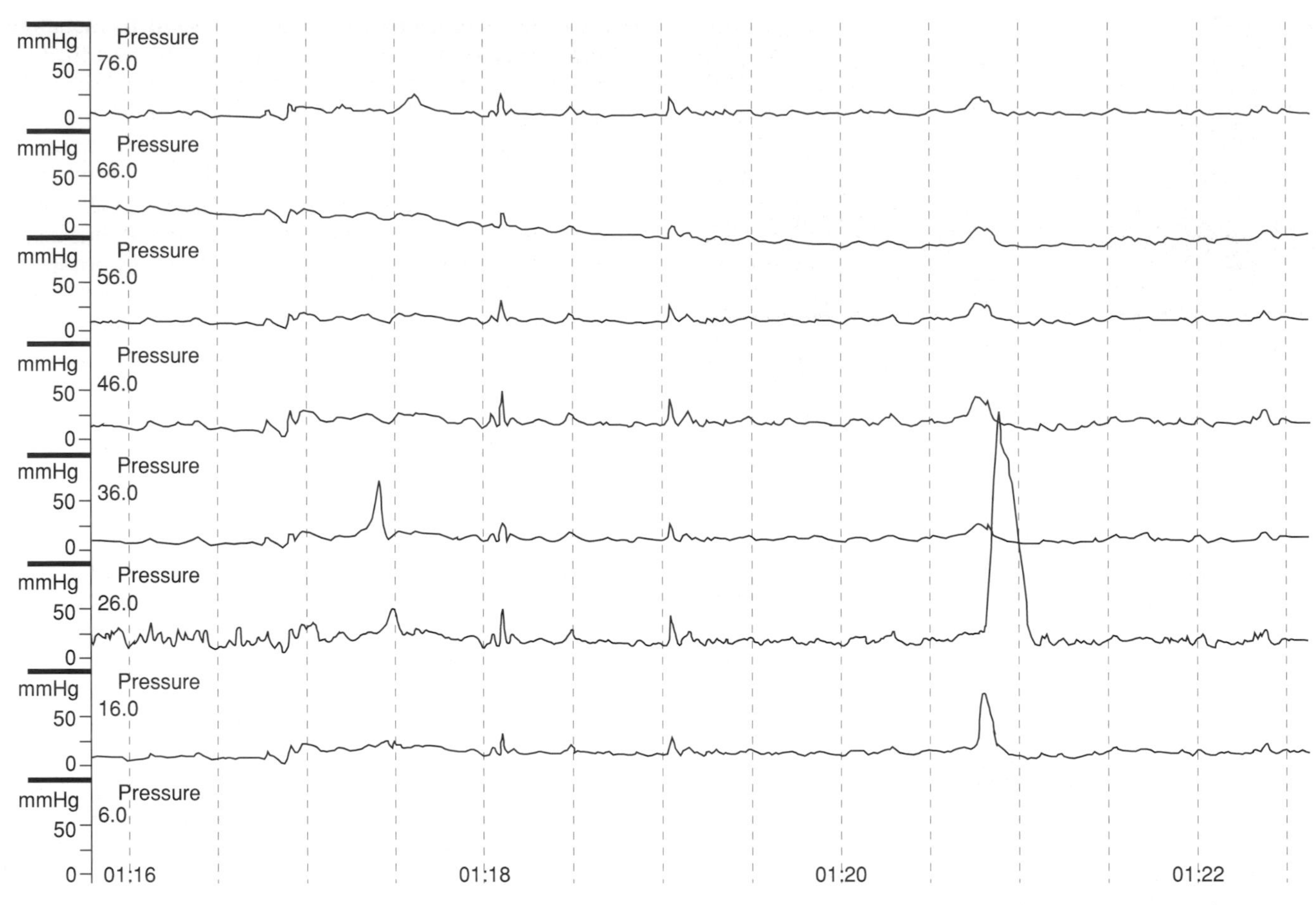

Figure 5.10: Abnormal colonic manometry. No visible high-amplitude peristaltic contractions are seen, even after a meal. Bisacodyl was administered through the colonic manometry catheter to stimulate the colon to contract.

stools. Unfortunately, this creates a vicious cycle in which successfully withheld bowel movements will become larger and drier in the rectal vault (and therefore more painful to void), as the function of the rectum is to absorb water and electrolytes and to store the stool for the appropriate time of evacuation.

Normal values
Some are available; more information on normal children needed
HAPCs – 80–100 mmHg, with meal and/or bisacodyl; last for 10 s and travel at least 30 cm of the colon
LAPCs – 5–40 mmHg, speculated to have role in nocturnal continence
Rectal motor complex seen more frequently at night; also thought to have a role in nocturnal continence. Amplitude >5 mmHg, frequency 2–4 per min[102]
Abormal values
No gastrocolic reflex or augmentation of contractions after a high-fat, high-calorie-density meal
Absent HAPCs

HAPC, high-amplitude peristaltic contraction; LAPC, low-amplitude peristaltic contraction.

Table 5.5 Colonic manometry

Also known as rectoanal dyssynergia and by a number of other synonyms, PPC creates an increased work of straining (or the Valsalva maneuver) to overcome this pressure barrier to passage of stool.

One expects to see a clustering of markers in the rectosigmoid colon in children with PPC, as PPC can be conceptualized as a functional form of pelvic outlet obstruction. This problem is amenable to treatment with various forms of biofeedback therapy utilizing both ARM and electromyography (EMG). Short-term reassessments show promising results in children randomized to receiving biofeedback with manometric techniques. However, the long-term follow-up of children receiving biofeedback has shown a lack of sustained effect of this intervention, prompting some to continue to offer conventional stool softeners and bowel habit training.[110] No additional benefit of adding ARM to conventional treatment was found in chronically constipated children in another randomized controlled trial. An effectiveness rate of 30% was found for conventional treatment of these patients referred to a tertiary hospital. Again, the authors reiterated the importance of adequate long-term laxative treatment.

Others have reported assistance with markers in making decisions in children with chronic constipation because this simple method helps determine total and segmental CTT, which distinguishes dysfunction of the right or left colon from distal outlet obstruction.[112] Figure 5.11 demon

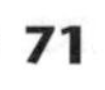

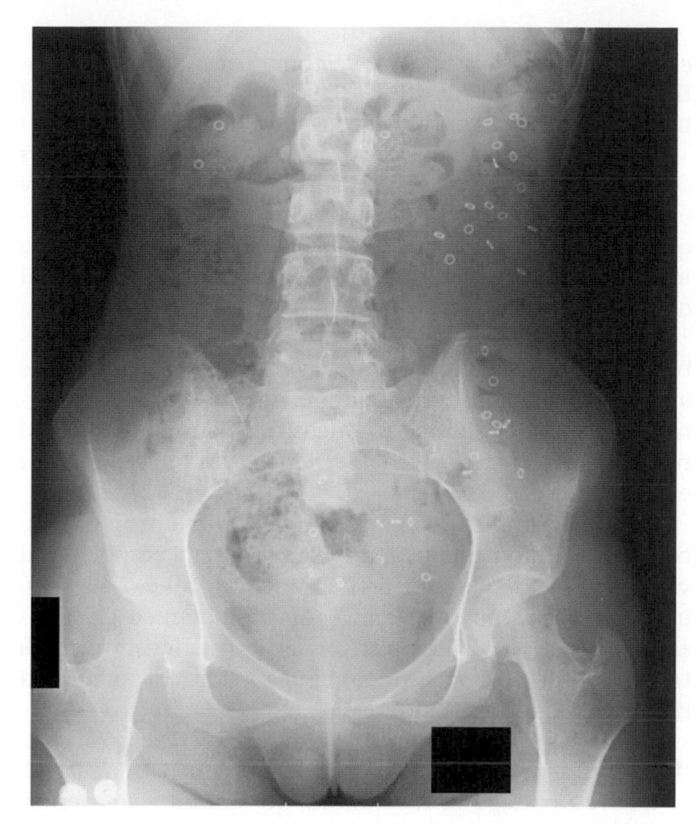

Figure 5.11: Abdominal radiograph demonstrates a collection of radio-opaque circular markers dispersed chiefly in the left side of the colon and rectosigmoid areas in an adolescent with melanosis coli secondary to chronic laxative use.

strates a clustering of ingested circular markers in the left colon and rectosigmoid regions of a patient with melanosis coli secondary to chronic laxative use.

Colonic inertia

Colonic inertia is defined as global delay in transit in all segments of the colon. Using identical methodology for measuring CTT, another study compared 38 children with idiopathic chronic constipation with 30 normal children. Upper reference values were similar: total CTT 45.7 h, ascending colon 19.02 h, left colon 19 h and rectosigmoid colon 32 h. The participants also underwent ARM, which demonstrated abnormal defecation dynamics of PPC in 64% of children of constipated children with distal delay but in none of the patients with colonic inertia.[113] Coupled with colonic manometry, the use of radio-opaque markers may assist in making the diagnosis of segmental colonic inertia of the right or left colon prior to surgical resection of the non-peristaltic segment[112] (Fig. 5.11).

ANORECTAL MANOMETRY

The most frequently performed motility test in infants and children is ARM (Tables 5.6 & 5.7). Constipation is a common problem in infants and children, but the majority do not need to be screened with ARM. A detailed history and physical examination including the perianal area, spine, reflexes in the distal extremities and digital rectal exami-

Normal[128] (limited data)
IAS (smooth muscle) and EAS (striated muscle) are in a state of tonic contraction
75–85% of basal anal canal tone is from the IAS, remaining 15–25% from the EAS
Length of the sphincter may be only 5 mm in a small infant, and vary from 2 to 4 cm in older children. Anal canal length (varies with age): 3.3 ± 0.8 cm
Basal pressure varies from 25 to 85 cmH_2O
Squeeze pressures resulting from voluntary contraction of the EAS should normally double or triple from baseline resting pressure
Rectal pressure rises with filling with stool, balloon distention and straining (Valsalva maneuver)
IAS shows RAIR with drop in pressure in response to rectal distention; amplitude of reflex relaxation increases with increasing balloon distention volume
Threshold volume is the minimal amount of air that will produce the RAIR
Sensory volumes
Volume first sensed (VFS) – threshold of rectal sensation 5 ± 2 to 14 ± 7 ml air
Volume of first urge (VFU; 'critical volume') – minimum volume creating a sensation of urge or call to stool; critical volume: 101 ± 39 ml
Maximum tolerated volume (MTV) – volume of constant relaxation 104 ± 49 ml
Defecation dynamics
Resting anal pressure: 57 ± 10 to 67 ± 12 mmHg
Maximum squeeze pressure: 118 ± 32 to 140 ± 52 mmHg
Strain
Cough
Modification
Modification with biofeedback, coaching maneuvers identified as needing improvement (e.g. recognition of rectal sensation, relaxation of EAS upon straining (corrects PPC), increasing intra-abdominal and intrarectal pressures upon straining)

IAS, internal anal sphincter; EAS, external anal sphincter; PPC, paradoxical puborectalis contraction; RAIR, rectoanal inhibitory reflex.

Table 5.6 Normal anorectal manometry

nation are part of the initial evaluation. Review of medications and exclusion of underlying metabolic or neurologic disease, if suspected, followed by appropriate long-term treatment with stool softeners precedes ARM.

Some indications for ARM testing include exclusion of HD in patients who have been chronically constipated, laxative dependent or laxative unresponsive, in infants who have delayed passage of the meconium stool at birth or prolonged neonatal jaundice, failure to thrive, and in children who have a gush of stool and gas from the rectum upon removal of the examining glove. Other clinical scenarios in which ARM would be helpful include the evaluation of fecal incontinence that is found in children in postoperative states and in those suffering from meningomyelocele, tethered cord and various other types of spinal cord dysfunction. Children with spinal abnormalities have loss of voluntary squeeze or EAS function.

Condition	Findings
HD	RAIR is absent; instead basal pressure may remain the same or even increase with rectal distention stimulus Esophageal motility abnormalities reported: tertiary and double-peaked contractions
Ultrashort-segment HD	Absent RAIR; normal rectal biopsy Also known as anal achalasia
Chronic functional withholding constipation	RAIR is present, but may require higher volumes of rectal distention to elicit Basal pressure may be normal, increased or decreased Sensory threshold volumes may be markedly increased due to chronic rectal distention
Encopresis	Associated with a volume of first sensation ≥120 ml air
Anismus or PPC	RAIR is present, but contraction of EAS occurs on straining. Biofeedback is beneficial in the short term
Meningomyelocele	Depending on the level of the spinal defect, resting pressure of the IAS is decreased Sensory parameters may be not obtainable
Premature infants	May have abnormal RAIR initially, but with maturation a normal RAIR may be detected at follow-up
Irritable bowel syndrome	Hypersensitivity to rectal balloon distention at lower volumes compared with normals Balloon distention may reproduce symptoms of abdominal pain

IAS, internal anal sphincter; EAS, external anal sphincter; HD, Hirschsprung's disease; PPC, paradoxical puborectalis contraction; RAIR, rectoanal inhibitory reflex.

Table 5.7 Abnormal anorectal manometry

Most pediatric patients tolerate the test well. Again, water-perfused systems delivering less than 1 ml water per min and a catheter tip 5 mm or less in diameter are used most frequently owing to their cost-effectiveness compared with solid-state manometry.

Hirschsprung's disease

The primary indication for ARM is to rule out HD in infants and children, although ARM is also used in the evaluation of fecal incontinence. In the absence of ganglion cells, there is no normal reflex relaxation of the IAS when the rectum is distended with air. The presence of the rectoanal inhibitory reflex (RAIR) – an intrinsic reflex mediated by the myenteric plexus – rules out HD.[114] The baseline anal sphincter pressure may remain the same, or may increase, which distinguishes the response from that in normals. If the RAIR is absent or equivocal, ARM can be repeated after an enema. If still equivocal, suction rectal biopsy should be performed.

ARM is also used in pediatric surgical cases to assess the candidacy for anorectal myectomy or a second pull-through operation for HD.[115] The evaluation and surgical treatment are discussed in more detail in Chapter 48.

Manometric testing of anorectal function provides objective measures leading to specific underlying etiology in patients with constipation and incontinence, and frequently provides new information that can influence the management and outcome.[116,117] If constipation is atypical or biofeedback is needed, ARM may be helpful.

ARM is also done in older children in whom the possibility of a short segment of HD is suspected. In general, the longer the segment of aganglionosis, the sooner the diagnosis is made. Therefore, the neonatal period is the usual time for infants to present with signs and symptoms of obstruction.

Clinical features distinguishing HD from chronic functional withholding constipation include an empty rectal vault, increased anal tone and a transition zone of narrowing.[118] An unprepped barium enema is obtained to delineate the extent of the disease and the location of a transition zone between the tight aganglionic segment and the dilated proximal colon.

Researchers have observed the value of repeat ARM in the workup for HD. In a study of 56 patients with a history of delayed passage of meconium, 95 studies were performed. Anorectal manometry was done at weekly intervals for up to a month later, at which time suction rectal biopsy was added in conjunction with an indeterminant or equivocal RAIR. The authors concluded that, although the procedure could provide false-positive results, no false negatives were observed. Five cases of HD were diagnosed by manometry and confirmed by rectal biopsy.[119]

Although rare, some cases of HD still escape detection in infancy and childhood. There is always a history of lifelong constipation, usually with chronic use of stool softeners and laxatives. Five such patients were identified in the author's department by screening initially with ARM; this experience is also supported by other centers.[120] Patients with short-segment HD form the estimated 8–20% of all patients with HD who will be diagnosed above the age of 3 years.[121] This emphasizes the importance of the role of manometric screening for this disease, even in older patients. ARM is useful in this subgroup of patients because it is sensitive and specific, and because the morphology of the RAIR response helps to clarify the diagnosis even in the clinical scenario where the unprepped barium enema and rectal biopsy tissue are equivocal.

Most patients with HD (about 85%) are limited to the rectosigmoid colon and below. The remaining 15% involve more proximal segments, such as total colonic HD, and less commonly involve even the small intestine with absence of ganglion cells. When HD involves the colon more extensively, with or without small intestinal aganglionosis, it becomes more common to see accompanying esophageal motor abnormalities as well.[122] This suggests to some that HD may be conceptualized more as a systemic motility disorder. Alternatively, esophageal motor abnormalities may be secondary to the distal aganglionosis and its effects, so a future study of esophageal manometry after successful treatment of HD may be more illuminating with regard to this phenomenon.

A selective absence of relaxation accompanies HD. In manometric testing, this is evident in the persistence of tonic contraction when the distending stimulus should elicit reflexive relaxation of the IAS. In infants and children without HD, a reflex contraction of the EAS normally follows distention of the rectum with air; this phenomenon is regarded to contribute to the continence mechanism. Furthermore, a 'sampling reflex' of the epithelial cells of the anorectal area permits humans to distinguish among gas, liquid and solid fecal content.

Anorectal manometry procedure

ARM is performed in the following steps. An enema the night before the test is recommended preparation. Some patients may need a 'cleanout' in the 2–3 days beforehand to assure at least a minimally empty rectal vault on arrival for ARM. Fasting for 4–6 h is also prudent to prepare the child in the event that anxiolytic medication needs to be employed. Bringing familiar toys, a blanket or other transition objects is encouraged. The nurse explains the procedure to the child and the parents to help reduce anxiety and promote cooperation. The child lies comfortably in the left lateral decubitus position, keeping the parent(s) in the room to assist in comforting and holding, except for a teenager who may prefer to do the test alone.

The catheter with the balloon attached to its distal segment is inserted into the rectum and the balloon is inflated (smaller-volume balloons are used for infants). Starting 6 cm from the anal verge in older children and at a shorter distance with infants and toddlers, the tube is withdrawn slowly at 1- or 0.5-cm intervals as a 'stationary pull-through' profile of the anal sphincter is obtained. A soft catheter with four to eight tiny openings around its circumference is used to measure pressure. This design provides directional pressure measurements in four quadrants of the anal sphincter.

The catheter is left in the zone of highest pressure (usually 1–2 cm from the anal verge) for serial inflations to document the RAIR. The amplitude of the relaxation is volume dependent, so that rectal distention with 50 ml air is usually expected to bring a longer and lower drop, or relaxation of the internal sphincter, than would be elicited by 20 or 30 ml air.[123] The lowest volume of air inducing the RAIR is called the threshold volume of relaxation; this may be as little as 5 ml in small patients. The threshold volume may be quite high in chronically constipated children; at times 120 ml is needed to demonstrate the reflex. Figure 5.12 shows the appearance of the normal RAIR.

Newborns and infants aged less than 1 year can be tested without sedation, particularly if a fast of 3–4 h precedes the manometry. Infants can feed during manometry and provides sufficient distraction to permit placement and movement of the catheter. In addition, the gastrocolonic reflex frequently sets in with a full stomach to stimulate physiologically normal RAIRs. This is often followed by stooling during the test – some infants even successfully push out the motility catheter. Thus, feeding a hungry infant will add functional information to rectal motility testing. The RAIR is elicited without artificial balloon inflation because the rectum is being filled up with stool and gas, producing normal rectal distention and relaxation of the internal sphincter.

In a study of 16 neonates aged 27–30 weeks' gestation, the RAIR was successfully elicited 81% of the time. The mean anal sphincter pressure was 24.5 ± 11.4 mmHg, and was normal.[124] Sometimes, when the RAIR is equivocal or the maximal resting pressure is too low to demonstrate a RAIR response, it is helpful to reschedule the ARM. At least three reflex drops per study are required to state confidently that the manometry is negative for HD. Ultrashort-segment HD has also been called achalasia of the IAS, and is diagnosed by ARM as absence of the RAIR in the presence of ganglion cells on rectal biopsy. Another aspect of interpretation in infant manometry is the development of the intact continence mechanism and the ability to demonstrate the reflex. It is also the author's experience that an indeterminant RAIR should be reassessed 1–4 weeks later, as it is uncommon not to see a well developed drop reflex on repeat testing.

If a study seems to be suboptimal (perhaps due to inadequate preparation and fecal loading), repeating the ARM is recommended to elicit the RAIR. In the vast majority of cases of indeterminate RAIR, the subsequent manometry will be more productive in demonstrating a normal reflex. This practice also obviates the need to do a rectal biopsy, avoiding the potential complications of that procedure. Corroborating this is a study of 22 healthy neonates with a mean gestational age of 32 (range 30–38) weeks, in which a sleeve catheter was used to evaluate anorectal pressures.[125] Inflation of air without a latex or non-latex balloon, or with a balloon, produced a normal RAIR and the infants had normal resting anal pressures.

Reasons for difficulty in obtaining the RAIR may be fecal loading, artifact from positioning the catheter in the anal sphincter, resting baseline pressure too low to demonstrate a significant drop in pressure, or motion of the child during the test.

Fewer data on normal and abnormal values in children are available compared with those in adults. The information from Nurko et al.[126] and Loening-Baucke[127] is summarized in Tables 5.6 and 5.7.

Sedation

Toddlers and very anxious children may be sedated with oral madazolam (Versed), which has replaced chloral hydrate in the author's motility laboratory. Rarely, intravenous sedation is used. Even under general anesthesia, the RAIR can be reliably detected. Although the anticholinergic glycopyrrolate appeared to inhibit the RAIR, the choice of general anesthetic or neuromuscular blocker made no significant difference to the presence or absence of RAIR.[129] The size of the catheter, the distance between the anal sensors and the balloon, and size of the balloon

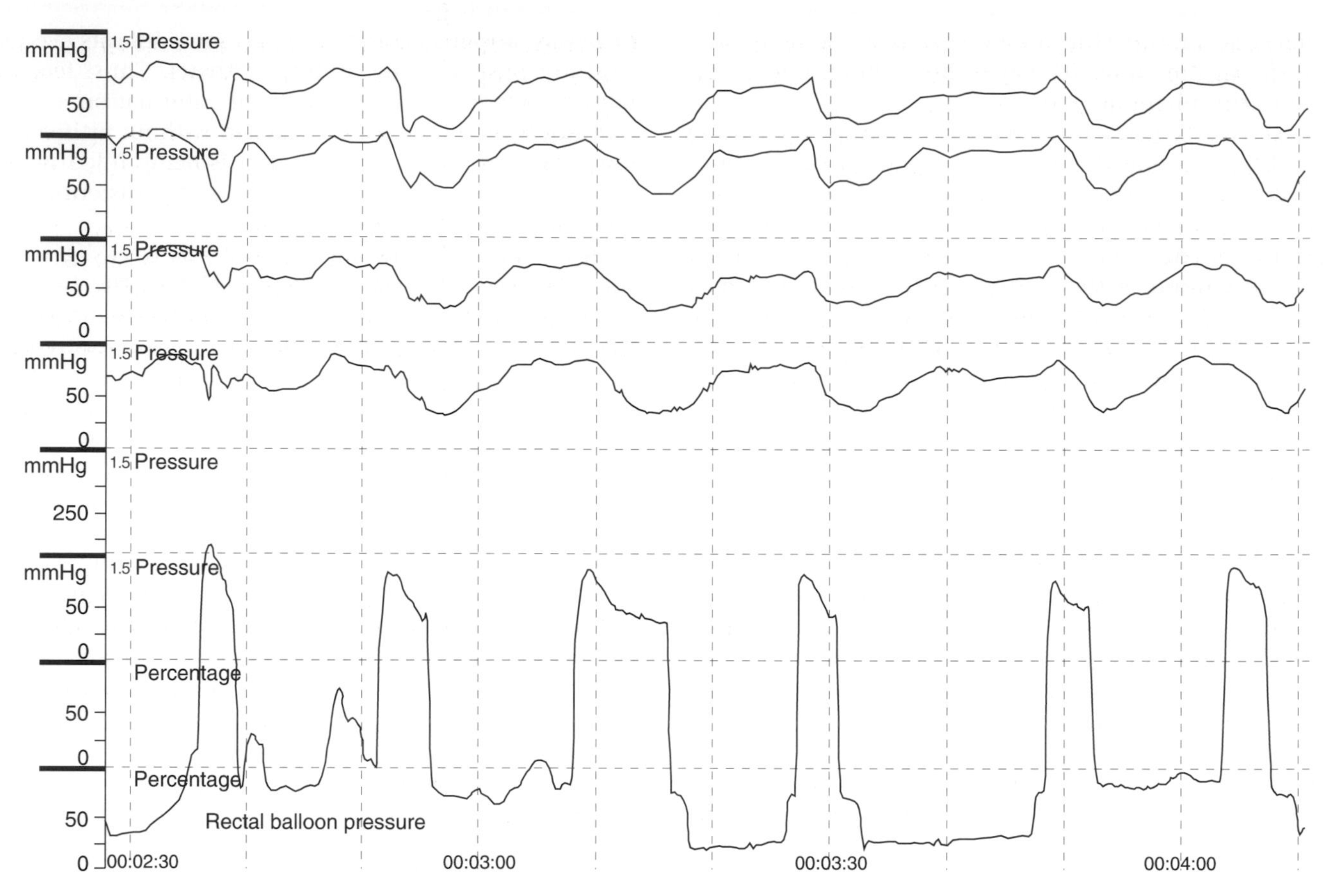

Figure 5.12: Normal anorectal manometry in a 17-month-old child. No sedation was used and the patient sucked on a bottle during the test. The top four tracings measure pressure in four quadrants of the anal sphincter, and the lowest tracing indicates the pressure of air instilled into rectal balloon. Corresponding reflex drops in the baseline smooth muscle of the internal anal sphincter appear in the tracings immediately above the inflation stimulus. Serial inflations show the reflex drop to be easily reproduced with volumes of air ranging from 20 to 40 ml. The tracing demonstrates a well developed rectoanal inhibitory reflex, ruling out Hirschsprung's disease. At the far left, an abrupt drop in pressure is considered to be artifact caused by catheter migration out of the sphincter zone. Artifactual drops in pressure are distinguished from the third reflex relaxation in this series, which is a smooth decline in pressure followed by a smooth recovery to baseline pressure.

dictate that three to four age-appropriate sizes are needed for a practice that sees neonates to adult-sized patients with anorectal disorders.

Functional assessment

In older children, a full functional assessment of the anorectum starts with a pressure profile of the length of the anal sphincter. ARM provides information about the strength of the muscles forming the anal sphincter. The patient is asked voluntarily to squeeze at each 1-cm zone of the pull-through. Figure 5.11 shows normal voluntary squeeze activity. Placing the pressure sensors in the zone of maximal pressure is the first step to measuring the relaxation reflex because the drop in pressure is more readily ascertained from this level. The RAIR is established, as is the threshold volume, which is the lowest amount of air that achieves a reproducible reflex relaxation of the internal sphincter.

Rectal sensitivity is evaluated by measuring the child's response to rectal distention with a balloon attached to the end of the motility catheter. Sensory thresholds are measured to determine:

- The volume of air first sensed, usually correlating with the perception of flatus
- The volume at which the patient first senses the urge to defecate
- The maximal volume tolerated, matching the urgent sensation to pass a stool.

High values for rectal sensation correlate with a distended rectum. Indeed, a rectal distention volume of more than 120 ml air has been shown to correlate with encopresis in children, who start to exhibit fecal incontinence above this volume. Long-term treatment with stool softeners, a regular toilet-sitting schedule and biofeedback training can help restore sensory levels to normal when the rectum recovers to a normal size. On the other hand, Loening-Baucke[130] showed that, in constipated children who recovered, abnormalities in the sensitivity of the rectum and sigmoid persisted when they were restudied 7 months to 3 years later, despite improvement in clinical symptoms and return of the rectum to a normal size. It was concluded that this may explain why these children are so vulnerable to recurrence of constipation and fecal soiling.

Abnormally increased levels of sensation can be primary as in meningomyelocele, spinal cord abnormalities, and diseases of the central and peripheral nervous systems. Secondary sensory impairment is the result of distention of the rectum and sigmoid colon from the fecal impaction or fecal retention that occurs with functional withholding and infrequent evacuation of the rectum. The ability of the rectal wall to contract when stretched to the point of megarectum may also reflect a change in motor function, being dilated, flaccid and therefore atonic. Furthermore, the weight and mass of the stool may cause decreased IAS pressure, shortening of the anal canal and hindrance of the ability to contract the EAS. This results in loss of the continence mechanism. On the other hand, decreased IAS function has also been thought to contribute to the pathogenesis of constipation.[131]

Resting and squeeze pressures are measured. Basal resting anal canal pressure is reflective of IAS tone, as 75–85% of the tone is contributed from its tonic contraction. The remaining 15–25% is contributed by the overlap with part of the EAS. Squeeze pressure indicates the voluntary augmentation of pressure achieved by the EAS. Maximal voluntary squeeze pressures are measured and are normally expected to double the amount of baseline pressure (in mmHg), but often can exceed this. Voluntary recruitment of the squeeze exercise is represented graphically as an upsurge in baseline pressure and represents the phasic EAS contraction, which is important in preserving continence during cough, sneezing, lifting and exercise[132] (Fig. 5.13).

Again, data in children are limited. In a study by Benninga et al.[133] of 13 normal children (age range 8–16 years), resting anal tone was 33–90 mmHg, maximum squeeze pressure was 81–276 mmHg, threshold for rectal sensation (volume first sensed) was 5–50 ml, threshold for eliciting the RAIR was 5–40 ml and the critical volume (volume of first urge or 'call to stool') was 90–180 ml.[133] Cough reflex and the 'wink reflex' (or anocutaneous reflex) are also measured. The anocutaneous reflex can be elicited by scratching the perianal skin, and is mediated by sacral nerves 2, 3 and 4.

Defecatory dynamics of straining are then assessed. Normally, a Valsalva maneuver with abdominal compression, relaxation of the anal sphincter and perineal descent produces a bowel movement. Figure 5.14 shows normal strain activity. The rectal balloon measures the adequacy of abdominal compression during straining. A combination of anal and rectal pressure recording, optimally combined with surface EMG of the anal sphincters and abdominal wall, is used to screen for paradoxical puborectalis contraction (PPC) and adequacy of intrarectal pressures upon straining.[114] (Paradoxical contraction of the EAS and puborectalis has several synonyms documented in the

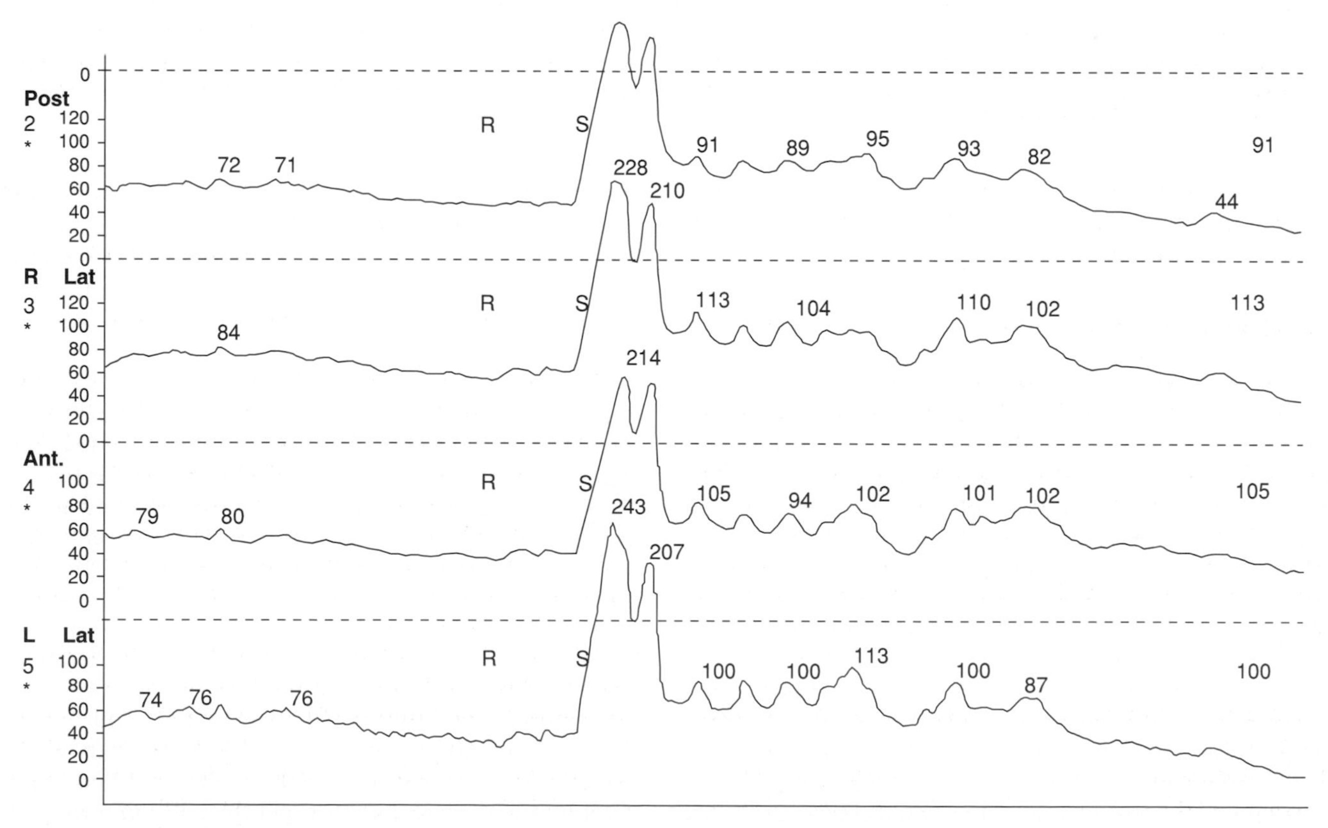

Figure 5.13: Anorectal manometry. Normal voluntary squeeze pattern in the anal canal is demonstrated in all four quadrants as an abrupt rise from resting baseline pressure to form a double-peaked or M-shaped pattern.

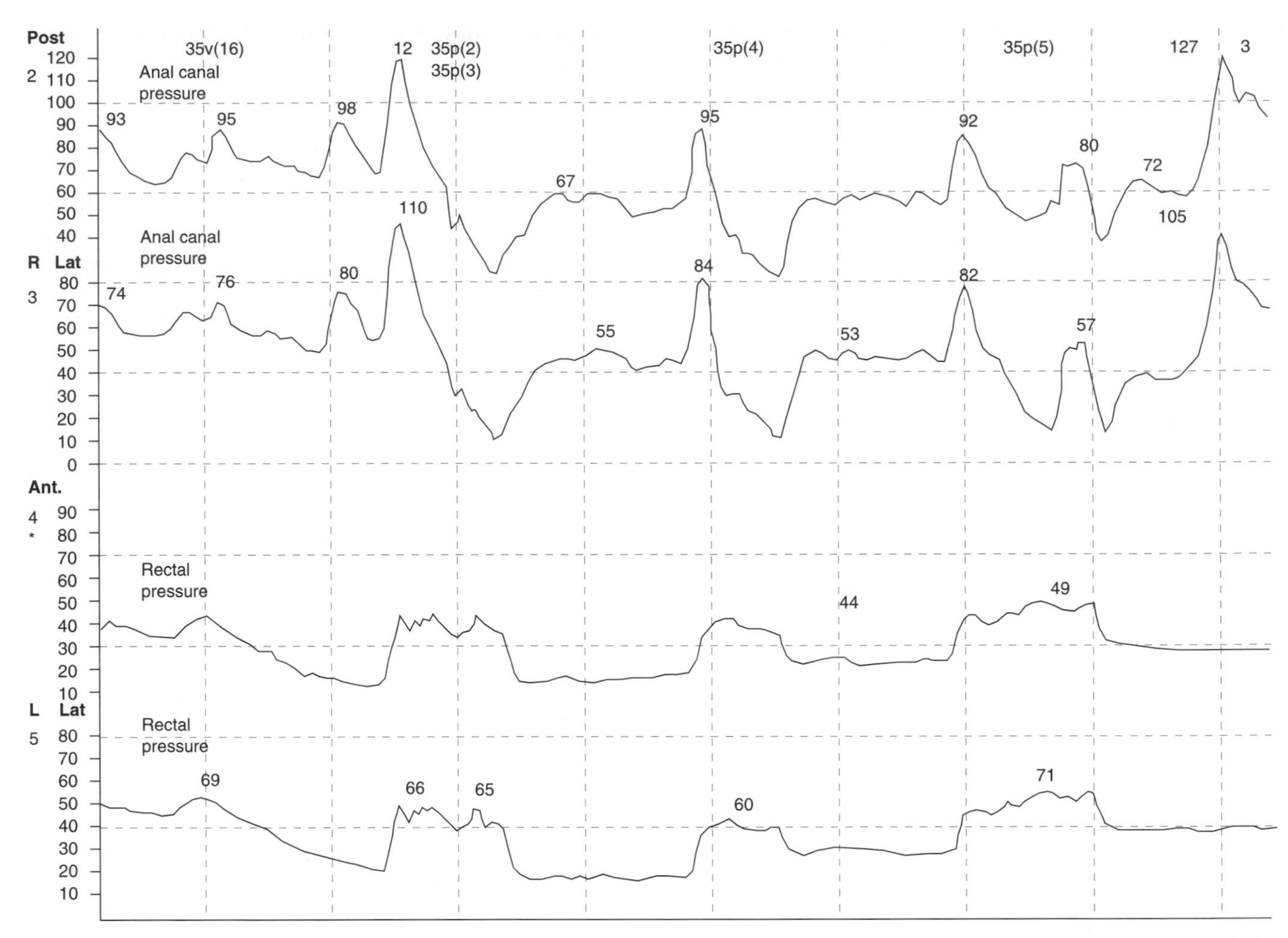

Figure 5.14: Anorectal manometry. Normal strain activity is demonstrated as the intrarectal pressures in the lower two tracings increase during the Valsalva maneuver. Simultaneously, the top two tracings, which have recorded anal canal pressures, demonstrate an initial reflex squeeze but then a marked decrease in pressure, while the anal canal relaxes to open and facilitate defecation.

literature, such as anismus, pelvic floor dyssynergia and functional outlet obstruction.) Figure 5.15 demonstrates PPC. The correlation of manometric recording and EMG is reliable and provides an integrated picture of the abdominal contraction and relaxation of the anal canal.[134]

The combination of anorectal pressure monitoring with EMG recordings from the anal sphincters and abdominal wall provides the most useful information for diagnosing physiologic function and for therapeutic uses. The EMG electrode reads the electrical activity produced by the muscles and amplifies the signals displayed on the screen.

Measurements of compliance of the rectum to balloon distention are commonly performed in adult manometry settings, but can easily be a part of the ARM of older children and adolescents, if desired. Compliance is the pressure–volume relationship during balloon distention of the rectum, and is thus the change in volume divided by the change in pressure; the numerator is the maximum tolerated volume. Compliance affects the size and capacity or dispensability of the rectum. Thus, increased compliance correlates with megarectum, as is seen in children with fecal impaction, and decreased compliance in a stiff rectum puts a patient at risk for fecal incontinence, for example from chronic ulcerative colitis or pelvic irradiation. Decreased compliance means that the reservoir function of the rectum is compromised. The 'barostat', a special kind of balloon designed to measure pressure changes in the rectum, is acknowledged to be the most accurate indicator of rectal compliance, but has not yet found a clinical niche in pediatrics and thus must still be considered a research technology. Attempts at standardizing protocols for manometric assessment of the anorectum in children and adults are under way. Difficulty in obtaining data, especially anorectal norms, on large numbers of normal individuals has imposed some limitation on the ability to compare the values of symptomatic patients.

Balloon expulsion is another functional test of anorectal function and has been evaluated as a predictor of outcome in children with functional constipation and encopresis (FCE). All healthy controls and 47% of patients with FCE were able to defecate a 100-ml water-filled balloon. Children who were able to expel the balloon were twice as likely to recover from their chronic constipation at 1-year follow-up compared with children who could not. The pro

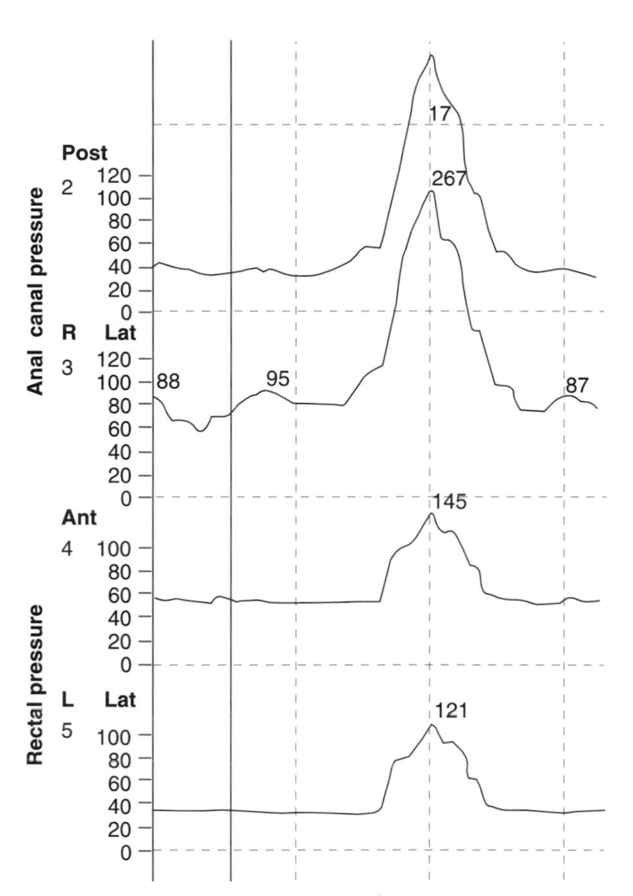

Figure 5.15: Abnormal anorectal manometry. Paradoxical puborectalis contraction of the external anal sphincter is demonstrated. The upper two rows show the pressure in the anal canal rising as the patient is squeezing while straining. This is termed paradoxical because the anal canal should relax during straining. The lower two rows show the pressure in the intrarectal balloon rising as the patient is straining.

dictive values of the test, however, were inadequate to predict recovery.[135] In older patients, the balloon expulsion test has been found to be a simple and useful screening test for excluding constipated patients without PPC. The specificity was 89% and the negative predictive value 97% for balloon expulsion, which may make expensive physiologic tests unnecessary.[136] Thus, balloon expulsion is another way of screening for PPC or functional outlet obstruction.[137]

Biofeedback

Biofeedback may be useful in the individual patient:

- For increasing discrimination of sensation of volumes in the rectal vault
- To teach use of abdominal muscles to increase intrarectal pressure during straining
- To relax the EAS during straining (that is, to overcome PPC).

Use of biofeedback is controversial. Earlier studies indicated that biofeedback was complementary to conventional treatments.[137] Some studies of long-term follow-up after biofeedback, however, showed no increased benefit in the groups treated with anorectal biofeedback over the conventional treatments of stool softeners or bowel training programs in randomized controlled trials.[111,138,139] However, other studies have shown efficacy in older patients at follow-up ranging from 12 to 44 months. These patients had PPC with or without abnormally slow CTT.[140] In a group of children with encopresis, some of whom had undergone surgery for anorectal malformations, biofeedback was helpful, although some patients needed repeat sessions to become continent.[141]

In the author's own experience at the Cleveland Clinic, a series of chronically constipated children with PPC demonstrated the ability to recognize and change PPC-type straining patterns in an average of two biofeedback sessions.[142] Compared with older adults who have received an average of 10 biofeedback sessions for PPC, children exhibited a faster learning curve in changing the habit of contracting the pelvic floor when coached in the proper manner of performing the Valsalva maneuver. Thus, at least in the short term, pediatric patients who are carefully selected to receive biofeedback can display remarkable understanding and flexibility to change their behavior given the opportunity to practice straining, even in the artificial circumstances of the motility laboratory.

'Critical volume' is the minimal amount of water in the rectal balloon that stimulates an urge to defecate (or volume of first urge). This critical volume of water is then instilled in the rectal balloon for straining exercises. Techniques used included a combination of exercises that are intuitive to children:

- Placing a hand over the abdomen while pushing down against the intrarectal balloon filled with a predetermined amount of water based on the sensory threshold information provided by the child to be comfortably 'full'
- Use of the exercise of pretending to blow out candles on a birthday cake
- Blowing against a 'pinwheel' to make it spin while straining
- Some children respond to vocalizing the sound 'Eeeeh' during straining.

These maneuvers are effective in teaching a child to strain because they all recruit the abdominal muscles. Other factors seem to contribute positively to this process, namely:

- Slowing down the entire process to allow focusing and to prevent reflex EAS contraction
- Planning for a period of time (usually 5–10 min) to leave the room and let the patient practice the exercises with the parent(s) present
- Use of pauses for taking deep breaths, as this may contribute to the patient's level of relaxation.

The puborectalis muscle wraps around the rectum and, when contracted, creates an angle (called the anorectal angle, with the two sides of the angle formed by the rectum and the anal canal) that facilitates continence by pulling it posteriorly toward the sacrum. At rest the angle is 85–105°. When the patient learns to relax the pelvic floor upon straining, the anorectal angle also straightens, so facilitating the process of defecation.

The same combined assembly of equipment using manometry and EMG, or the use of either method alone, can also be used for biofeedback training. With attention to proper placement techniques, surface electrode recording of EAS activity at the anal brim has been shown to approach the quality of concentric needle electrodes.[144] Needle EMG has a role in specialized circumstances, such as localization of the EAS on the perineum in imperforate anus or ectopic anus, and the technique is sometimes used during surgery on the perineum. Electrodes applied to the skin surface are connected to a small wire that feeds electrical information from the muscle to a computer. It is ideal to combine this with simultaneous manometric recording of pressures. Thus, surface EMG is a non-invasive method that complements manometry and is suitable for pediatric ARM testing. In 88 children with fecal incontinence or encopresis, ARM showed abnormalities of sphincter spasm and megacolon to be pathophysiologic, distinguishing this group from control children.[145] Measurements of compliance are more commonly performed in adult manometry settings, but could easily be a part of the ARM of older children and adolescents if desired.

Pudendal nerve terminal motor latency

Pudendal nerve terminal motor latency (PNTML) is a test that is used in adult colon and rectal surgery units to evaluate fecal incontinence, but it is not useful with pediatric patients. When PNTML was tested in 23 normal and 23 encopretic children, there was no evidence that abnormal pudendal nerve function was important in the pathogenesis of encopresis.[146] PNTML is not a standard part of pediatric ARM assessment and is being used less because it reflects only the fastest fibers, so is not as reliable as an index of nerve damage as it was once thought to be.[147]

Visceral hyperalgesia

Visceral hyperalgesia is thought to be one of the mechanisms of IBS. Sensory thresholds during colonic[148] and rectal balloon distention have been found to be lower for patients with IBS than in control patients. In positron emission tomography of adults with IBS, alterations in the response to rectal distention resulted in greater activity in the anterior cingulate cortex and thalamus compared with those in controls.[149] Children diagnosed with IBS by the Rome II criteria have been found to have a significantly lowered threshold for pain to balloon distention on ARM and a disturbed contractile response to a meal. Therefore, children with IBS may suffer from visceral hyperalgesia and from the same GI motility abnormalities that are hypothesized to have a role in adult IBS.[150] Other authors support this, noting that many characteristics of IBS are similar, regardless of age of onset, suggesting a uniform pathogenesis.[151]

Although not pathognomonic, the distention volume on ARM in adolescents being investigated for constipation may be noted to reproduce typical symptoms of cramping and abdominal pain at low volumes. This provides a clue that these patients may be hypervigilant to somatic stimuli and may have IBS. Others agree that altered rectal perception is present in almost all patients with IBS and that it represents a reliable biologic marker for the condition.[152]

CONSIDERATIONS FOR STARTING A PEDIATRIC MOTILITY LABORATORY

The pediatric gastroenterology motility laboratory will be set up to measure several bowel functions. Most pediatric gastroenterologists set up breath hydrogen testing for lactose intolerance. The use of breath testing can extend to fructose tolerance, glucose for bacterial overgrowth, and sucrose. In addition *Helicobacter pylori* breath testing is convenient to have available in the office. Lactulose breath hydrogen testing can measure orocecal transit time, if desired, but is seldom needed.

The decision to purchase a manometric system is next. Compare the major and minor vendors, and make a decision about what you want to be able to measure competently in pediatric patients. This decision depends upon having an interest in performing these procedures in infants, children and adolescents, and a comparable amount of patience and flexibility in adapting the procedure and equipment to the individual patient. Certainly, competence in performing manometry procedures is paramount. In addition to training in fellowship programs, further training can be obtained from vendors and meetings, although there seems to be no substitute for on-the-job training with a motility expert. Training guidelines for level 1 competency in pediatric gastroenterology fellowships are a basic understanding of motility disorders and knowledge of the rationale, indications and limitations of tests of GI function. When competent at level II, the physician can perform specialized tests such as ADM and colonic manometry.[153]

Testing with impedance is also now FDA-approved for measuring non-acid reflux, and to combine this with acid reflux testing. However, basic pH testing is currently considered the standard for reflux monitoring, until the value of adding simultaneous non-acid reflux has been further established. The system chosen may have prolonged 24-h esophageal reflux testing, alone or in combination with software modules for esophageal and anorectal manometry. Most choose water-perfused catheters because the system is more cost effective, is usually durable, and requires little maintenance. Solid-state catheters provide reliable tracings of good quality, but are expensive to purchase and maintain. Newer systems that measure manometric pressure combined with multiple intraluminal electrical impedance-metry can provide additional information on bolus transport.[154]

The next decision is to choose the number of transducers that are needed. For esophageal and anorectal manometry, four channels are recommended but more may be used simultaneously to cover more of the distance between the pharynx and stomach, if desired. Six channels are better for anorectal manometry, dedicating four to the anal canal and two to the rectal balloon. Additional channels may be dedicated to EMG recording from the EAS and abdominal wall. Antroduodenal and colonic manometry are recommended for referral centers.

For colonic transit time, both total and segmental, it is recommended that the manometrist keep premanufactured capsules with a defined number of markers in them (usually 20 to 24) available in the office. The first capsule(s) can be given to the patient, observing to see that it is swallowed with fluid in the presence of the healthcare provider. The reason for this vigilance is to assure compliance in patients who may complain of constipation and yet pass markers appropriately. These patients can be referred for counseling to change their perception of what is normal bowel frequency.

SUMMARY

Manometry of the digestive tract from the mouth to the anorectal area, together with the other laboratory techniques such as gastric emptying, marker studies for CTT, impedance monitoring and other tests of functional GI tract information are still evolving as diagnostic tools for digestive motility disorders. Nevertheless, they have already become indispensable tools for the pediatric gastroenterologist.

As the design of the catheter is related to its application, a range of catheter lengths and spacing between sensors is needed for children. In older children, spacing is consequently farther apart to cover more of the intestine. There is a lack of standardization for some of the motility protocols and contraction characteristics; the diversity of sizes and spacing of recording sites contributes to this problem when comparing multiple authors' manuscripts in the literature. Most of these studies involve a combination of qualitative and quantitative analysis. Recognition of artifact is essential to interpreting all motility studies, as artifact must always be excluded from analysis. Artifacts are most often secondary to motion of the child, coughing and movement of the catheter out of the desired zone of interest. Caution is advised in interpreting motility studies to avoid over-reading and to exclude artifact in the analysis.

References

1. Camilleri M, Hasler WL, Parkman HP, Quigley EM, Soffer E. Measurement of gastrointestinal motility in the GI laboratory. Gastroenterology 1998; 115:747–762.
2. Di Lorenzo C, Hillemeier C, Hyman P, et al. Manometry studies in children: minimum standards for procedures. Neurogastroenterol Motil 2002; 14:411–420.
3. Milla PJ. The physiology of gastrointestinal motility. J Pediatr Gastroenterol Nutr 2001; 32(Suppl 1):S3–S4.
4. Scott RB. Motility disorders. In: Walker WA, Durie PR, Hamilton JR, Walker-Smith JA, Watkins JB, eds. Pediatric Gastrointestinal Disease: Pathophysiology, Diagnosis, Management, 3rd edn. Hamilton, Ontario: BC Decker; 2000:103–115.
5. Corazziari E. Neuro-enteric mechanisms of gastrointestinal motor function. J Pediatr Gastroenterol Nutr 1997; 25(Suppl 1):S3–S4.
6. Milla PJ. Intestinal motility during ontogeny and intestinal pseudo-obstruction in children. Pediatr Clin North Am 1996; 43:511–532.
7. Kaul A, Rudolph CD. Gastrointestinal manometry studies in children. J Clin Gastroenterol 1998; 27:187–191.
8. Murray JA, Clouse RE, Conklin JL. Components of the standard oesophageal manometry. Neurogastroenterol Motil 2003; 15:591–606.
9. Gilger MA, Boyle JT, Sondheimer JM, Colletti RB. A medical position statement of the North American Society for Pediatric Gastroenterology and Nutrition. Indications for pediatric esophageal manometry. J Pediatr Gastroenterol Nutr 1997; 24:616–618.
10. Kahrilas PJ, Clouse RE, Hogan WJ. American Gastroenterological Association technical review on the clinical use of esophageal manometry. Gastroenterology 1994; 107:1865–1884.
11. Rao SS, Azpiroz F, Diamant N, Enck P, Tougas G, Wald A. Minimum standards of anorectal manometry. Neurogastroenterology Motil 2002; 14:553–559.
12. Strobel CT, Byrne WJ, Ament ME, Euler AR. Correlation of esophageal lengths in children with height: application to the Tuttle test without prior esophageal manometry. J Pediatr 1979; 94:81–84.
13. Richter JE, Wu WC, Johns DN, et al. Esophageal manometry in 95 healthy adult volunteers. Variability of pressures with age and frequency of 'abnormal' contractions. Dig Dis Sci 1987; 32:583–592.
14. Kahrilas PJ, Clouse RE, Hogan WJ. American Gastroenterological Association technical review on the clinical use of esophageal manometry. Gastroenterology 1994; 107:1865–1884.
15. Kawahara H, Dent J, Davidson G. Mechanisms responsible for gastroesophageal reflux in children. Gastroenterology 1997; 113:399–408.
16. Mittal RK, Holloway RH, Penagini R, Blackshaw LA, Dent J. Transient lower esophageal sphincter relaxation. Gastroenterology 1995; 109:601–610.
17. Omari TI, Miki K, Fraser R, et al. Esophageal body and lower esophageal sphincter function in healthy premature infants. Gastroenterology 1995; 109:1757–1764.
18. Cucchiara S, Campanozzi A, Greco L, et al. Predictive value of esophageal manometry and gastroesophageal pH monitoring for responsiveness of reflux disease to medical therapy in children. Am J Gastroenterol 1996; 91:680–685.
19. Moroz SP, Espinoza J, Cumming WA, Diamant NE. Lower esophageal sphincter function in children with and without gastroesophageal reflux. Gastroenterology 1976; 71:236–241.
20. Newell SJ, Sarkar PK, Durbin GM, Booth IW, McNeish AS. Maturation of the lower oesophageal sphincter in the preterm baby. Gut 1988; 29:167–172.
21. Castell DO. Anatomy and physiology of the esophagus and its sphincters. In: Castel DO, Diederich LL, Castell JA, eds. Esophageal Motility and pH Testing, 3rd edn. Highlands Ranch, CO: Sandhill Scientific; 2000:13–28.
22. Nurko S. Other motor disorders. In: Walker WA, Durie PR, Hamilton JR, Walker-Smith JA, Watkins JB, eds. Pediatric Gastrointestinal Disease: Pathophysiology, Diagnosis, Management, 3rd edn. Hamilton, Ontario: BC Decker, 2004:437–439.
23. Dumont RC, Rudolph CD. Development of gastrointestinal motility in the infant and child. Gastroenterol Clin North Am 1994; 23:655–671.
24. Di Lorenzo C, Hyman PE. Gastrointestinal motility in neonatal and pediatric practice. Gastroenterol Clin North Am 1996; 25:203–224.

25. Vargas JH, Sachs P, Ament ME. Chronic intestinal pseudo-obstruction syndrome in pediatrics. Results of a national survey by members of the North American Society of Pediatric Gastroenterology and Nutrition. J Pediatr Gastroenterol Nutr 1988; 7:323–332.
26. Wyllie E, Wyllie R, Cruse RP, Rothner AD, Erenberg G. The mechanism of nitrazepam-induced drooling and aspiration. N Engl J Med 1986; 314:35–38.
27. Fung KP, Math MV, Ho CO, Yap KM. Midazolam as a sedative in esophageal manometry: a study of the effect on esophageal motility. J Pediatr Gastroenterol Nutr 1992; 15:85–88.
28. Hillemeier AC, Grill BB, McCallum R, Gryboski J. Esophageal and gastric motor abnormalities in gastroesophageal reflux during infancy. Gastroenterology 1983; 84:741–746.
29. Moroz SP, Espinoza J, Cumming WA, Diamant NE. Lower esophageal sphincter function in children with and without gastroesophageal reflux. Gastroenterology 1976; 71:236–241.
30. Sondheimer JM. Upper esophageal sphincter and pharyngoesophageal motor function in infants with and without gastroesophageal reflux. Gastroenterology 1983; 85:301–305.
31. Orenstein SR, Giarrusso VS, Proujansky R, Kocoshis SA. The Santmyer swallow: a new and useful infant reflex. Lancet 1988; i:345–346.
32. Skopnik H, Silny J, Heiber O, Schulz J, Rau G, Heimann G. Gastroesophageal reflux in infants: evaluation of a new intraluminal impedance technique. J Pediatric Gastroenterol Nutr 1996; 23:591–598.
33. Kahrilas PJ, Dodds WJ, Dent J, Logemann JA, Shaker R. Upper esophageal sphincter function during deglutition. Gastroenterology 1988; 95:52–62.
34. Nurko S. Other motor disorders. In: Walker WA, Durie PR, Hamilton JR, Walker-Smith JA, Watkins JB, eds. Pediatric Gastrointestinal Disease: Pathophysiology, Diagnosis, Management, 3rd edn. Hamilton, Ontario: BC Decker; 2000:317–350.
35. Reichert TJ, Bluestone CD, Stool SE, Sieber WK, Sieber AM. Congenital cricopharyngeal achalasia. Ann Otol, Rhinol Laryngol 1977; 86:603–610.
36. Putnam PE, Orenstein SR, Pang D, Pollack IF, Proujansky R, Kocoshis SA. Cricopharyngeal dysfunction associated with Chiari malformations. Pediatrics 1992; 89:871–876.
37. Asch MJ, Liebman W, Lachman RS, Moore TC. Esophageal achalasia: diagnosis and cardiomyotomy in a newborn infant. J Pediatr Surg 1974; 9:911–912.
38. Tovar JA, Prieto G, Molina M, Arana J. Esophageal function in achalasia: preoperative and postoperative manometric studies. J Pediatr Surg 1998; 33:834–838.
39. Parrilla P, Martinez de Haro LF, Ortiz A, Morales G, Garay V, Aguilar J. Factors involved in the return of peristalsis in patients with achalasia of the cardia after Heller's myotomy. Am J Gastroenterol 1995; 90:713–717.
40. Milla P, Cucchiara S, Di Lorenzo C, Rivera NM, Rudolph C, Tomomasa T. Motility disorders in childhood. Working Group Report of the First World Congress of Pediatric Gastroenterology, Hepatology, and Nutrition. J Pediatr Gastroenterol Nutr 2002; 35(Suppl 2):S187–S195.
41. Katada N, Hinder RA, Hinder PR, et al. The hypertensive lower esophageal sphincter. Am J Surg 1996; 172:439–442; discussion 442–443.
42. Fontan JP, Heldt GP, Heyman MB, Marin MS, Tooley WH. Esophageal spasm associated with apnea and bradycardia in an infant. Pediatrics 1984; 73:52–55.
43. Lamet M, Fleshler B, Achkar E. Return of peristalsis in achalasia after pneumatic dilatation. Am J Gastroenterol 1985; 80:602–604.
44. Tovar JA, Prieto G, Molina M, Arana J. Esophageal function in achalasia: preoperative and postoperative manometric studies. J Pediatr Surg 1998; 33:834–838.
45. Dutta HK, Grover VP, Dwivedi SN, Bhatnagar V. Manometric evaluation of postoperative patients of esophageal atresia and tracheo-esophageal fistula. Eur J Pediatr Surg 2001; 11:371–376.
46. Romeo C, Bonanno N, Baldari S, et al. Gastric motility disorders in patients operated on for esophageal atresia and tracheoesophageal fistula: long-term evaluation. J Pediatr Surg 2000; 35:740–744.
47. Fois A. Gastrointestinal disorders in muscular dystrophies. J Pediatr Gastroenterol Nutr 1997; 25(Suppl 1):S20–S21.
48. Kahrilas PJ, Dodds WJ, Hogan WJ. Effect of peristaltic dysfunction on esophageal volume clearance. Gastroenterology 1988; 94:73–80.
49. Cheung KM, Oliver MR, Cameron DJ, Catto-Smith AG, Chow CW. Esophageal eosinophilia in children with dysphagia. J Pediatr Gastroenterol Nutr 2003; 37:498–503.
50. Kelly JL, Mulcahy TM, O'Riordain DS, et al. Coexistent Hirschsprung's disease and esophageal achalasia in male siblings. J Pediatr Surg 1997; 32:1809–1811.
51. Rosario JA, Medow MS, Halata MS, et al. Nonspecific esophageal motility disorders in children without gastroesophageal reflux. J Pediatr Gastroenterol Nutr 1999; 28:480–485.
52. Flick JA, Boyle JT, Tuchman DN, Athreya BH, Doughty RA. Esophageal motor abnormalities in children and adolescents with scleroderma and mixed connective tissue disease. Pediatrics 1988; 82:107–111.
53. Weinstock LB, Clouse RE. Esophageal physiology: normal and abnormal motor function. Am J Gastroenterol 1987; 82:399–405.
54. Fouad YM, Katz PO, Hatlebakk JG, Castell DO. Ineffective esophageal motility: the most common motility abnormality in patients with GERD-associated respiratory symptoms. Am J Gastroenterol 1999; 94:1464–1467.
55. Godoy J, Tovar JA, Vicente Y, Olivares P, Molina M, Prieto G. Esophageal motor dysfunction persists in children after surgical cure of reflux: an ambulatory manometric study. J Pediatr Surg 2001; 36:1405–1411.
56. Tutuian R, Castell DO. Combined multichannel intraluminal impedance and manometry clarifies esophageal function abnormalities: study in 350 patients. Am J Gastroenterol 2004; 99:1011–1019.
57. Tutuian R, Castell DO. Combined multichannel intraluminal impedance and manometry clarifies esophageal function abnormalities: study in 350 patients. Am J Gastroenterol 2004; 99:1011–1019.
58. Sigurdsson L, Flores A, Putnam PE, Hyman PE, Di Lorenzo C. Postviral gastroparesis: presentation, treatment, and outcome. J Pediatr 1997; 131:751–754.
59. Barbar M, Steffen R, Wyllie R, Goske M. Electrogastrography versus gastric emptying scintigraphy in children with symptoms suggestive of gastric motility disorders. J Pediatr Gastroenterol Nutr 2000; 30:193–197.
60. Ravelli AM, Tobanelli P, Volpi S, Ugazio AG. Vomiting and gastric motility in infants with cow's milk allergy. J Pediatr Gastroenterol Nutr 2001; 32:59–64.
61. Di Lorenzo C, Reddy SN, Flores AF, Hyman PE. Is electrogastrography a substitute for manometric studies in children with functional gastrointestinal disorders? Dig Dis Sci 1997; [illegible].
62. Levy J. Use of electrogastrography in children. Curr Gastroenterol Rep 2002; 4:259–265.

63. Riezzo G, Indrio F, Montagna O, et al. Gastric electrical activity and gastric emptying in term and preterm newborns. Neurogastroenterol Motil 2000; 12:223–229.
64. Riezzo G, Chiloiro M, Guerra V. Electrogastrography in healthy children: evaluation of normal values, influence of age, gender, and obesity. Dig Dis Sci 1998; 43:1646–1651.
65. Uc A, Hoon A, Di Lorenzo C, Hyman PE. Antroduodenal manometry in children with no upper gastrointestinal symptoms. Scand J Gastroenterol 1997; 32:681–685.
66. Ittmann PI, Amarnath R, Berseth CL. Maturation of antroduodenal motor activity in preterm and term infants. Dig Dis Sci 1992; 37:14–19.
67. Tomomasa T, Di Lorenzo C, Morikawa A, Uc A, Hyman PE. Analysis of fasting antroduodenal manometry in children. Dig Dis Sci 1996; 41:2195–2203.
68. Bortolotti M, Annese V, Coccia G. Twenty-four hour ambulatory antroduodenal manometry in normal subjects (co-operative study). Neurogastroenterol Motil 2000; 12:231–238.
69. Verhagen MA, Samsom M, Jebbink RJ, Smout AJ. Clinical relevance of antroduodenal manometry. Eur J Gastroenterol Hepatol 1999; 11:523–528.
70. Sood MR, Cocjin J, Di Lorenzo C, Narasimha Reddy S, Flores AF, Hyman PE. Ileal manometry in children following ileostomies and pull-through operations. Neurogastroenterolog Motil 2002; 14:643–646.
71. Quigley EM, Donovan JP, Lane MJ, Gallagher TF. Antroduodenal manometry. Usefulness and limitations as an outpatient study. Dig Dis Sci 1992; 37:20–28.
72. Cucchiara S, Minella R, Scoppa A, et al. Antroduodenal motor effects of intravenous erythromycin in children with abnormalities of gastrointestinal motility. J Pediatr Gastroenterol Nutr 1997; 24:411–418.
73. Curry JI, Lander TD, Stringer MD. Erythromycin as a prokinetic agent in infants and children. Aliment Pharmacol Ther 2001; 15:595–603.
74. Luiking YC, Akkermans LM, van der Reijden AC, Peeters TL, van Berge-Henegouwen GP. Differential effects of motilin on interdigestive motility of the human gastric antrum, pylorus, small intestine and gallbladder. Neurogastroenterol Motil 2003; 15:103–111.
75. Di Lorenzo C, Lucanto C, Flores AF, Idries S, Hyman PE. Effect of octreotide on gastrointestinal motility in children with functional gastrointestinal symptoms. J Pediatr Gastroenterol Nutr 1998; 27:508–512.
76. Di Lorenzo C, Lucanto C, Flores AF, Idries S, Hyman PE. Effect of sequential erythromycin and octreotide on antroduodenal manometry. J Pediatr Gastroenterol Nutr 1999; 29:293–296.
77. Boivin M, Pinelo LR, St-Pierre S, Poitras P. Neural mediation of the motilin motor effect on the human antrum. Am J Physiol 1997; 272:G71–G76.
78. Hyman PE, Abrams C, Dubois A. Effect of metoclopramide and bethanechol on gastric emptying in infants. Pediatr Res 1985; 19:1029–1032.
7.9 Hitch DC, Vanhoutte JJ, Torres-Pinedo RB. Enhanced gastroduodenal motility in children. Am J Dis Child 1982; 136:299–302.
80. Morganroth J, Ruegg PC, Dunger-Baldauf C, Appel-Dingemanse S, Bliesath H, Lefkowitz M. Tegaserod, a 5-hydroxytryptamine type 4 receptor partial agonist, is devoid of electrocardiographic effects. Am J Gastroenterol 2002; 97:2321–2327.
81. Read NW, McFarlane A, Kinsman RI, et al. Effect of infusion of nutrient solutions into the ileum on gastrointestinal transit and plasma levels of neurotensin and enteroglucagon. Gastroenterology 1984; 86:274–280.
82. Rao SS, Lu C, Schulze-Delrieu K. Duodenum as a immediate brake to gastric outflow: a videofluoroscopic and manometric assessment. Gastroenterology 1996; 110:740–747.
83. Penning C, Gielkens HA, Hemelaar M, et al. Prolonged ambulatory recording of antroduodenal motility in slow-transit constipation. Br J Surg 2000; 87:211–217.
84. Hyman PE. Chronic intestinal pseudo-obstruction in childhood: progress in diagnosis and treatment. Scand J Gastroenterol Suppl 1995; 213:39–46.
85. Hyman PE, Bursch B, Beck D, Di Lorenzo C, Zeltzer LK. Discriminating pediatric condition falsification from chronic intestinal pseudo-obstruction in toddlers. Child Maltreat 2002; 7:132–137.
86. Di Lorenzo C, Flores AF, Buie T, Hyman PE. Intestinal motility and jejunal feeding in children with chronic intestinal pseudo-obstruction. Gastroenterology 1995; 108:1379–1385.
87. Watanabe Y, Ito T, Ando H, Seo T, Nimura Y. Manometric evaluation of gastrointestinal motility in children with chronic intestinal pseudo-obstruction syndrome. J Pediatr Surg 1996; 31:233–238.
88. Cucchiara S, Borrelli O, Salvia G, et al. A normal gastrointestinal motility excludes chronic intestinal pseudoobstruction in children. Dig Dis Sci 2000; 45:258–264.
89. Cucchiara S, Annese V, Minella R, et al. Antroduodenojejunal manometry in the diagnosis of chronic idiopathic intestinal pseudoobstruction in children. J Pediatr Gastroenterol Nutr 1994; 18:294–305.
90. Di Lorenzo C, Hillemeier C, Hyman P, et al. Manometry studies in children: minimum standards for procedures. Neurogastroenterol Motil 2002; 14:411–420.
91. De Schryver AM, Samsom M, Akkermans LM, Clemens CH, Smout AJ. Fully automated analysis of colonic manometry recordings. Neurogastroenterol Motil 2002; 14:697–703.
92. Martin MJ, Steele SR, Mullenix PS, Noel JM, Weichmann D, Azarow KS. A pilot study using total colonic manometry in the surgical evaluation of pediatric functional colonic obstruction. J Pediatr Surg 2004; 39:352–359.
93. Martin MJ, Steele SR, Noel JM, Weichmann D, Azarow KS. Total colonic manometry as a guide for surgical management of functional colonic obstruction: preliminary results. J Pediatr Surg 2001; 36:1757–1763.
94. Pensabene L, Youssef NN, Griffiths JM, Di Lorenzo C. Colonic manometry in children with defecatory disorders. role in diagnosis and management. Am J Gastroenterol 2003; 98:1052–1057.
95. Heikenen JB, Werlin SL, Di Lorenzo C, et al. Colonic motility in children with repaired imperforate anus. Dig Dis Sci 1999; 44:1288–1292.
95a. Malone PS, Ransley PG, Kiely EM. Preliminary report: the antegrade continence enema. Lancet 1990; 336: 1217–1218.
96. Marshall J, Hutson JM, Anticich N, Stanton MP. Antegrade continence enemas in the treatment of slow-transit constipation. J Pdiatr Surg 2001; 36:1227–1230.
97. Villarreal J, Sood M, Zangen T, et al. Colonic diversion for intractable constipation in children: colonic manometry helps guide clinical decisions. J Pediatr Gastroenterol Nutr 2001; 33:588–591.
98. Di Lorenzo C, Solzi GF, Flores AF, Schwankovsky L, Hyman PE. Colonic motility after surgery for Hirschsprung's disease. Am J Gastroenterol 2000; 95:1759–1764.
99. Miele E, Tozzi A, Staiano A, Toraldo C, Esposito C, Clouse RE. Persistence of abnormal gastrointestinal motility after

operation for Hirschsprung's disease. Am J Gastroenterol 2000; 95:1226–1230.

100. Marty TL, Matlak ME, Hendrickson M, Black RE, Johnson DG. Unexpected death from enterocolitis after surgery for Hirschsprung's disease. Pediatrics 1995; 96:118–121.

101. Di Lorenzo C, Flores AF, Reddy SN, Hyman PE. Use of colonic manometry to differentiate causes of intractable constipation in children. J Pediatr 1992; 120:690–695.

102. Rao SS, Welcher K. Periodic rectal motor activity: the intrinsic colonic gatekeeper? Am J Gastroenterol 1996; 91:890–897.

103. Scott SM. Manometric techniques for the evaluation of colonic motor activity: current status. Neurogastroenterol Motil 2003; 15:483–513.

104. Rao SS, Kavelock R, Beaty J, Ackerson K, Stumbo P. Effects of fat and carbohydrate meals on colonic motor response. Gut 2000; 46:205–211.

105. Lucanto C, Bauer SB, Hyman PE, Flores AF, Di Lorenzo C. Function of hollow viscera in children with constipation and voiding difficulties. Dig Dis Sci 2000; 45:1274–1280.

106. Di Lorenzo C, Flores AF, Hyman PE. Age-related changes in colon motility. J Pediatr 1995; 127:593–596.

107. Hamid SA, Di Lorenzo C, Reddy SN, Flores AF, Hyman PE. Bisacodyl and high-amplitude-propagating colonic contractions in children. J Pediat Gastroenterol Nutr 1998; 27:398–402.

108. Wagener S, Shankar KR, Turnock RR, Lamont GL, Baillie CT. Colonic transit time – what is normal? J Pediatr Surg 2004; 39:166–169.

109. Metcalf AM, Phillips SF, Zinsmeister AR, MacCarty RL, Beart RW, Wolff BG. Simplified assessment of segmental colonic transit. Gastroenterology 1987; 92:40–47.

110. van der Plas RN, Benninga MA, Redekop WK, Taminiau JA, Buller HA. Randomised trial of biofeedback training for encopresis. Arch Dis Child 1996; 75:367–374.

111. van Ginkel R, Buller HA, Boeckxstaens GE, van Der Plas RN, Taminiau JA, Benninga MA. The effect of anorectal manometry on the outcome of treatment in severe childhood constipation: a randomized, controlled trial. Pediatrics 2001; 108:E9.

112. Zaslavsky C, da Silveira TR, Maguilnik I. Total and segmental colonic transit time with radio-opaque markers in adolescents with functional constipation. J Pediatr Gastroenterol Nutr 1998; 27:138–142.

113. Gutierrez C, Marco A, Nogales A, Tebar R. Total and segmental colonic transit time and anorectal manometry in children with chronic idiopathic constipation. J Pediatr Gastroenterol Nutr 2002; 35:31–38.

114. Steffen R, Loenig-Baucke V. Constipation and encopresis. In: Wyllie R, Hyams J, eds. Pediatric Gastrointestinal Disease: Pathophysiology, Diagnosis and Management, 2nd edn. Philadelphia, PA: WB Saunders; 1999:43–50.

115. Abbas Banani S, Forootan H. Role of anorectal myectomy after failed endorectal pull-through in Hirschsprung's disease. J Pediatr Surg 1994; 29:1307–1309.

116. Rao SS, Patel RS. How useful are manometric tests of anorectal function in the management of defecation disorders? Am J Gastroenterol 1997; 92:469–475.

117. Vaizey CJ, Kamm MA. Prospective assessment of the clinical value of anorectal investigations. Digestion 2000; 61:207–214.

118. Steffen R, Wyllie R. Constipation. In: Kliegman RM, Greenbaum LA, Lye PS, eds. Practical Strategies in Pediatric Diagnosis and Therapy. 2nd ed. Philadelphia, Pennsylvania PA: Elsevier Saunders; 2004:373–381.

119. Lopez-Alonso M, Ribas J, Hernandez A, Anguita FA, Gomez de Terreros I, Martinez-Caro A. Efficiency of the anorectal manometry for the diagnosis of Hirschsprung's disease in the newborn period. Eur J Pediatr Surg 1995; 5:160–163.

120. Wu JS, Schoetz DJ,Jr, Coller JA, Veidenheimer MC. Treatment of Hirschsprung's disease in the adult. Report of five cases. Dis Colon Rectum 1995; 38:655–659.

121. Swenson O, Sherman JO, Fisher JH. Diagnosis of congenital megacolon: an analysis of 501 patients. J Pediatr Surg 1973; 8:587–594.

122. Staiano A, Corazziari E, Andreotti MR, Clouse RE. Esophageal motility in children with Hirschsprung's disease. Am J Dis Child 1991; 145:310–313.

123. Kaur G, Gardiner A, Duthie GS. Rectoanal reflex parameters in incontinence and constipation. Dis Colon Rectum 2002; 45:928–933.

124. de Lorijn F, Omari TI, Kok JH, Taminiau JA, Benninga MA. Maturation of the rectoanal inhibitory reflex in very premature infants. J Pediatr 2003; 143:630–633.

125. Benninga MA, Omari TI, Haslam RR, Barnett CP, Dent J, Davidson GP. Characterization of anorectal pressure and the anorectal inhibitory reflex in healthy preterm and term infants. J Pediatr 2001; 139:233–237.

126. Nurko S, Garcia-Aranda JA, Guerrero VY, Worona LB. Treatment of intractable constipation in children: experience with cisapride. J Pediatr Gastroenterol Nutr 1996; 22:38–44.

127. Loening-Baucke V. Anorectal manometry and biofeedback. In: Hyman PE, ed. Pediatric Gastrointestinal Motility Disorders. New York: Academy Professional Information Systems; 1994:231–252.

128. Nurko S. Gastrointestinal manometry: methodology and indications. In: Walker WA, Durie PR, Hamilton JR, Walker-Smith JA, Watkins JB, eds. Pediatric Gastrointestinal Disease: Pathophysiology, Diagnosis, Treatment, 3rd edn. Hamilton, Ontario: BC Decker; 2000:1485–1510.

129. Pfefferkorn MD, Croffie JM, Corkins MR, Gupta SK, Fitzgerald JF. Impact of sedation and anesthesia on the rectoanal inhibitory reflex in children. J Pediatr Gastroenterol Nutr 2004; 38:324–327.

130. Loening-Baucke VA. Sensitivity of the sigmoid colon and rectum in children treated for chronic constipation. J Pediatr Gastroenterol Nutr 1984; 3:454–459.

131. Loening-Baucke VA, Younoszai MK. Abnormal and sphincter response in chronically constipated children. J Pediatr 1982; 100:213–218.

132. Whitehead WE, Schuster MM. Anorectal physiology and pathophysiology. Am J Gastroenterol 1987; 82:487–497.

133. Benninga MA, Wijers OB, van der Hoeven CW, et al. Manometry, profilometry, and endosonography: normal physiology and anatomy of the anal canal in healthy children. J Pediatr Gastroenterol Nutr 1994; 18:68–77.

134. Azpiroz F, Enck P, Whitehead WE. Anorectal functional testing: review of collective experience. Am J Gastroenterol 2002; 97:232–240.

135. Loening-Baucke V. Balloon defecation as a predictor of outcome in children with functional constipation and encopresis. J Pediatr 1996; 128:336–340.

136. Minguez M, Herreros B, Sanchiz V, et al. Predictive value of the balloon expulsion test for excluding the diagnosis of pelvic floor dyssynergia in constipation. Gastroenterology 2004; 126:57–62.

137. Loening-Baucke V. Modulation of abnormal defecation dynamics by biofeedback treatment in chronically constipated children with encopresis. J Pediatr 1990; 116:214–222.

138. Nolan T, Catto-Smith T, Coffey C, Wells J. Randomised controlled trial of biofeedback training in persistent encopresis with anismus. Arch Dis Child 1998; 79:131–135.
139. Loening-Baucke V. Biofeedback treatment for chronic constipation and encopresis in childhood: long-term outcome. Pediatrics 1995; 96:105–110.
140. Chiotakakou-Faliakou E, Kamm MA, Roy AJ, Storrie JB, Turner IC. Biofeedback provides long-term benefit for patients with intractable, slow and normal transit constipation. Gut 1998; 42:517–521.
141. Hibi M, Iwai N, Kimura O, Sasaki Y, Tsuda T. Results of biofeedback therapy for fecal incontinence in children with encopresis and following surgery for anorectal malformations. Dis Colon Rectum 2003; 46(Suppl):S54–S58.
142. Steffen R, Schroeder TK. Paradoxical puborectalis contraction in children. Dis Colon Rectum 1992; 35:1193–1194.
143. Wald A. Anorectum. In: Schuster MM, ed. Atlas of Gastrointestinal Motility in Health and Disease. Baltimore, MD: Williams & Wilkins; 1993:229–249.
144. O'Donnell P, Beck C, Doyle R, Eubanks C. Surface electrodes in perineal electromyography. Urology 1988; 32:375–379.
145. Sutphen J, Borowitz S, Ling W, Cox DJ, Kovatchev B. Anorectal manometric examination in encopretic-constipated children. Dis Colon Rectum 1997; 40:1051–1055.
146. Sentovich SM, Kaufman SS, Cali RL, et al. Pudendal nerve function in normal and encopretic children. J Pediatr Gastroenterol Nutr 1998; 26:70–72.
147. Diamant NE, Kamm MA, Wald A, Whitehead WE. AGA technical review on anorectal testing techniques. Gastroenterology 1999; 116:735–760.
148. Fukudo S, Kanazawa M, Kano M, et al. Exaggerated motility of the descending colon with repetitive distention of the sigmoid colon in patients with irritable bowel syndrome. J Gastroenterol 2002; 37(Suppl 14):145–150.
149. Ringel Y, Drossman DA, Turkington TG, et al. Regional brain activation in response to rectal distension in patients with irritable bowel syndrome and the effect of a history of abuse. Dig Dis Sci 2003; 48:1774–1781.
150. Van Ginkel R, Voskuijl WP, Benninga MA, Taminiau JA, Boeckxstaens GE. Alterations in rectal sensitivity and motility in childhood irritable bowel syndrome. Gastroenterology 2001; 120:31–38.
151. Staiano A, Corazziari E. Irritable bowel syndrome: contrasts and comparisons between children and adults. J Pediatr Gastroenterol Nutr 2001;32(Suppl 1):S32–S34.
152. Mertz H, Naliboff B, Munakata J, Niazi N, Mayer EA. Altered rectal perception is a biological marker of patients with irritable bowel syndrome. Gastroenterology 1995; 109:40–52.
153. Rudolph CD, Winter HS. NASPGN guidelines for training in pediatric gastroenterology. NASPGN Executive Council, NASPGN Training and Education Committee. J Pediatr Gastroenterol Nutr 1999; 29(Suppl 1):S1–S26.
154. Nguyen HN, Silny J, Matern S. Multiple intraluminal electrical impedancometry for recording of upper gastrointestinal motility: current results and further implications. Am J Gastroenterol 1999; 94:306–317.

Chapter 6
Gastrointestinal mucosal immunology and mechanisms of inflammation

Maya Srivastava

INTRODUCTION

Our understanding of basic mucosal immunology and mechanisms of inflammation in the human gastrointestinal tract has undergone major advances since the last edition of this text. Because of the ongoing revolution in molecular biology in the pharmaceutical industry, we are beginning to target specific components of the immune system for the benefit of our patients. This is a new frontier for all of us, and the pace of discovery in this area continues rapidly. We offer herein an overview of this exciting area of pediatric gastroenterology. It is dedicated to the researchers without whom this chapter could not have been written, and to the investigators of the future who will someday write its conclusions.

FETAL AND NEONATAL DEVELOPMENT OF THE GASTROINTESTINAL MUCOSAL IMMUNE SYSTEM

Early in gestation, leukocytes originating from precursor hematopoietic stem cells in the liver and bone marrow arrive in the fetal gastrointestinal tract. Along with structural components of the developing gut, including the single cell thick epithelium, these leukocytes will make up the future gastrointestinal mucosal immune system.[1] In the normal adult, all leukocytes originate in the bone marrow, including those that traffic to the mature gut. Both fetal and adult T cells undergo a final maturation process in the thymus. Genetic diseases such as *Bruton's agammaglobulinemia*, which affects B-cell development, or *severe combined immunodeficiency* which affects T and B cells, result in defective systemic and mucosal immunity.[2] Fetal dendritic cells, future antigen presenting cells, are the first leukocytes to arrive in the distal small bowel, followed by intraepithelial lymphocytes by 11 weeks. T cells are present in the gut by 14 weeks gestation and CD5 positive B cells by 16 weeks. Specialized epithelial *M cells* that will overlie the *Peyer's patches* in the terminal ileum are identifiable by 11 weeks. Peyer's patches are major sites of antigen uptake and presentation in the gut, as well as favored sites of pathogen invasion, such as by *Salmonella tyhpi*. By 19 weeks gestation, the mucosal immune cells begin to differentiate and organize. Adhesion molecule expression and cytokines, especially IL-7,[3] and TNF family members including lymphotoxin or TNF-β orchestrate this process. For example, as Peyer's patches develop in the ileum, adhesion molecule expression becomes locally intense in that area. The normal gastrointestinal mucosa, then, even before birth, is in a state of controlled or *'physiologic inflammation'*. The absence of any of these immune elements, not just their overabundance, is thereafter abnormal.

Development of the gastrointestinal mucosal immune system is not completed by term, and is influenced by multiple factors. Although all nutrition to the fetus is received from the placenta, beginning at 12–16 weeks gestation, commensurate with fetal swallowing, the gastrointestinal tract is also exposed to *amniotic fluid,* from 16 cc/day at 20 weeks, to 450 cc/day at term. Amniotic fluid is immunologically active, containing high concentrations of growth factors, cytokines, and soluble receptors (Table 6.1).[4] Amniotic fluid epidermal growth factor (EGF) increases intestinal weight, DNA and RNA content, calcium binding protein expression, calcium transport, vitamin D receptor expression, acid secretion, enzyme expression, and crypt cell turnover. *Stem cell factor* (c-kit ligand) is critical for mast cell survival and proliferation. Latent TGF-β2 and TGF-β1 once activated by gastric acid promote IgA production by mucosal B cells, decrease pro-inflammatory cytokine production, and induce further differentiation, matrix deposition, and mesoderm formation in the gut. IL-1RA and soluble IL-2R (p55) in amniotic fluid down regulate cytokine production and influence T cell activation by competing for IL-1 and IL-2, respectively. Other cytokines and chemokines found in amniotic fluid have the potential to greatly influence the formation and activity of the fetal mucosal immune system. Further, high concentrations of placental hormones may influence this process. *In*

Concentration	Immune protein
>10 ng/ml	HGF/SF
1–10 ng/ml	Latent TGF-β2, IL-1RA, IL-6,IL-8, SCF, GRO-α, MIP-1β
100–1000 pg/ml	sFAS, latent TGF-β1, s IL-2Rα, TNF-α, MIP-1α
<100 pg/ml	IL-4, IL-10, free TGF-β2, free TGF-β1, IL-2, TNF-β, LIF, GM-CSF, IFN-γ, IL-11
Not detected	VEGF, sFAS, IL-5

Table 6.1 Cytokines and immune factors in amniotic fluid

vitro, sex steroids directly modulate the production of cytokines, in particular IL-10 by human T cells, and chemokine expression by T, B, myeloid, and epithelial cells. Cortisol and other steroids with glucocorticoid activity, not only inhibit the inflammatory cascade via decreasing the transcription factor NFκB, but also act directly on gut epithelial cells to tighten cellular junctions, lessen edema, and promote maturation.

The maternal immune system itself has a further modulating role on gastrointestinal development.[1] During the third trimester of pregnancy, large quantities of *maternal IgG*, but not IgA, D, E, or M, are actively transported across the placenta, providing passive, temporary, but specific protection to the fetus. This complement of immunoglobulins is the maternal repertoire resulting from infections as distant as the mother's own childhood. Re-exposure or immunization around the time of conception or during pregnancy results in specific maternal memory B cell activation and the production of high titer, highly specific IgG antibodies via *affinity maturation* that would then be provided to the fetus. Such strategies of maternal vaccination are being studied as a method to boost fetal immunity against common neonatal pathogens, including viruses such as rotavirus that target the gut. However, novel IgG *monoclonal antibody* based therapies, such as anti-TNF-a antibodies for maternal Crohn's disease, could also be potentially transferred to the fetus via this pathway, with unknown effects on the developing fetal mucosal and systemic immune systems. Premature infants are at increased risk of *necrotizing enterocolitis,* and *allergic-eosinophilic enterocolitis* to cow milk protein, if exposed by formula feedings after birth, because they have not had the benefit of prolonged exposure to amniotic fluid, they have not received normal amounts of maternal antibodies, and overall, the mucosal epithelial barrier is much more 'leaky', allowing antigens to get through to the leukocytes lying in wait beneath.

Immediately after delivery, the previously sterile gastrointestinal mucosal immune system is exposed to and colonized by microbes for the first time.[5] These new antigens must be tolerated immediately, or else an uncontrolled inflammatory reaction will ensue. The microbes which the newborn gut encounters and the milieu in which they are encountered greatly determine the flora to be found in the gut normally thereafter. Once established, these microbes are a critical protective factor to the host against dangerous, invasive organisms, via *colonization resistance*. Over 10^{14} bacteria of 500–1000 species inhabit the gastrointestinal tract of adults, mostly anaerobes (>99%) in the intestine.[6–8] Loss of tolerance to these organisms, once established, has been implicated in the pathogenesis of Crohn's disease.[9–12]

The microbial flora in the infant gastrointestinal tract differs significantly from the adult, and is influenced by many factors that may promote or inhibit the likelihood of normal future gastrointestinal mucosal immunity.[5] The type of delivery influences the species of bacteria that becomes established in the GI tract. Vaginally delivered infants are colonized by maternal strains encountered in the cervix, vagina, and perianal region, and include *E. coli* and *Enterococcus* (aerobes), followed by *Bifidobacter* and *Bacteroides* (anaerobes) and *Lactobacillus*. C-section, the rate of which is as high as one out of every four births in the USA, results in increased *Klebsiella* and delayed colonization with *Bifidobacter*, a 'good' bacterium. Host genetics, including the expression of specific and polymorphic receptors for microbial products on intestinal epithelia, and local variation in expression within the GI tract may influence this process as well.[13,14] Antibiotic treatment influences the total number of species and relative counts of microbes in the neonatal gut, and could allow the overgrowth of pathogenic resistant bacteria and yeast.[6] This could overwhelm the immature mucosal immune system, resulting in breach of the immature mucosal barrier and systemic infections. The increased use of antibiotics in the newborn for sepsis rule-out and the general overuse of antibiotics in children is therefore a cause for concern due to potential effects on the mucosal immune system. Onset and type of feeding has the most profound influence on the microbial component of the mucosal immune system. Delayed oral feeding delays anaerobic colonization in the neonate. Breast milk, via its immunological components, especially secretory IgA, promotes the establishment and maintenance of *Bacterium bifidus*. Breast-fed infants have approximately equal numbers of aerobic and anaerobic microbes, and 5–10 species in total in their stools, with some fluctuation. These microbes are helpful to the developing mucosa also by providing short chain fatty acids, including acetic acid, that colonocytes use as fuel. Formula-fed infants have more *Bacteroides* and enterobacteria, and stool cultures like those of adults, with increased species complexity, and production of a different complement of short chain fatty acids than breast-fed babies. Introduction of solid foods results in the appearance of *Clostridia*, and thereafter, the bacterial flora and their products progressively resemble that of the adult.

Breast-feeding is arguably the most important postnatal extrinsic modifying factor to the developing gastrointestinal mucosal immune system. Breast milk contains non-immune and immune factors that protect the developing gastrointestinal tract and specifically aid in the development of an effective yet tolerant mucosal immune system.[4,15,16] Even the term infant's mucosa is significantly more 'leaky' than that of the adult. Thus, the antigen exposure to immunocompetent cells beneath the epithelial is much greater, as is the potential for sensitization (allergy) and invasion (infection). In fact, not until age 2 years will barrier function even approach that of the adult. The benefits of breast-feeding may be life-long and include a reduction in the risk of chronic diseases, including inflammatory bowel disease. Although controversial, many studies also suggest a reduction in the risk of atopic disorders in breast-fed infants.[15] Breast-feeding results in substantial reductions in neonatal morbidity, and mortality, especially in the developing world. As little as 1 cc/h reduces the risk of premature infants of necrotizing enterocolitis.[1]

Multiple innate immune system components are present and active in human milk (Table 6.2). Human beta *defensins* 1, 2, alpha defensins 5, 6 and human neutrophil defensins are present in μg/ml quantities.[16] These antimicrobial peptides, which are stable in acid and resistant to proteolysis but inactive at high salt concentrations, protect the developing mucosa against invasion and prevent overgrowth by lysis of targets. As each defensin, even each isoform, has unique antimicrobial targets, this may be an important component in mucosal defense. Most recently, it was shown that defensins can also act as immunomodulators.[17] *In vitro*, HBD-2 treatment of mucosal epithelial cell line CaCo-2 resulted in downregulation of LL-37 and toll-like receptor 7 expression, decreased chemokine (LARC) expression, among other effects.[18] Thus, breast milk defensins could promote tolerance or induce a decreased ability to respond to TLR-7 ligands. Using similar competitive ELISA procedures as for defensins, multiple soluble forms of toll-like receptors, including sTLR-1, sTLR-2, sTLR-4 have recently been identified in human serum and in mature milk (MD Srivastava, unpublished data 2004). Soluble TLRs in human milk, especially sTLR-2, present in higher amounts, may regulate soluble CD14 mediated microbial recognition in the neonatal gut to inhibit excessive local inflammation following bacterial colonization. The effect of other defensins and soluble toll-like receptors in milk, remains to be thoroughly studied.

The amount and type of cytokines in human milk varies between individuals, and for some cytokines, with the duration of breast-feeding, phase of lactation and gestational age of the infant.[15] In general, however, extremely high quantities of latent *TGF-β2* and *TGF-β1* are present.[15] This growth factor is activated, not destroyed by acidification.[15] Further, cytokines are protected against destruction by the buffering capacity of the milk, competition by nutrient proteins casein and whey, the presence of large amounts of protease inhibitors in human milk, and the immaturity of the neonatal digestive tract with low pancreatic chymotrypsin and trypsin production. The free TGF-β is a potent anti-inflammatory factor, decreasing immune activation, promoting epithelial cell differentiation, and promoting the production of sIgA by resident B cells on the mucosal immune system. TGF-β is also a product of T-reg cells, and acts on other T cells to induce IL-10 and promote tolerance. Chemokines IL-8, GRO-α, RANTES, MCP-1 may aid in protection against invasive infection.[15] M-CSF aids in the proliferation and maturation of maternal macrophages in milk, and mucosal dendritic cells and macrophages in the infant, improving innate immune system function. Soluble Fas in milk may influence apoptosis.[4] Soluble receptors to proinflammatory cytokines, including IL-1RA, can act as antagonists and prevent/inhibit an acute inflammatory response. HGF and EGF in milk promote epithelial cell barrier formation and repair, and HGF/SCF mucosal leukocyte proliferation.[4] Nerve growth factor NGF, and neurotransmitters substance P, and vasoactive intestinal peptide, are critical components of the developing enteric nervous system, responsible for normal motility, and also modulate neurogenic inflammation.[1] Leukocytes express receptors for these neurotransmitters, and demonstrate changes in activation state and cytokine/mediator production with ligand binding. *Motility* function is critical in defense of the mucosa, to prevent stasis, overgrowth, attachment and invasion by pathogens. Breast milk hormones, including sex steroids, cortisol, somatomedin C and insulin, promote maturation. Lactoferrin in milk is bactericidal, antiviral, anti-adhesive and inhibits IL-6 production.[19,20] Lysozyme can hydrolyze bacterial cell wall components. K-casein inhibits adhesion, including of *Helicobacter pylori*, to the gastric mucosa. Free fatty acids disrupt membranes of multiple types of microbes, and glycoconjugates act as false receptors for pathogens, preventing interaction with the real receptors on the GI epithelia. Maternal immune cells may take up residence in the wall of the intestinal tract, and migrate to distal sites, including the secondary lymphoid organs, such as the spleen. Maternal immunoglobulins, IgM, D, E, G, A also provide protection.

Concentration	Immune protein
>10 μg/ml	sTLR-2, sTLR-4, HαD1-3, HBD-2
>1 μg/ml	sTLR-1, HαD5, HαD6, HBD-1
>10 ng/ml	VEGF
1–10 ng/ml	HGF, latent TGF-β2, M-CSF, GRO-α, sFAS
100–1000 pg/ml	Latent TGF-β1, IL-8, IL-1RA, sFAS-L
<100 pg/ml	TNF-α, IL-10, MCP-1, IFN-γ, MIP-1β, IL-1β, RANTES, IL-6, IL-5
Not detected	IL-4, free TGF-β2, free TGF-β1, IL-2, sIL-2Rα, TNF-β, LIF, MIP-1α, GM-CSF, SCF, IL-11, IL-12, IL-13, IL-15

Table 6.2 Cytokines, defensins and soluble toll-like receptors in human breast milk

The *entero-broncho-mammary pathway* in the mother results in the provision of very high amounts of sIgA in breast milk, of specificity for pathogens most likely to be encountered by the mucosa. IgA comprises over 90% of the immunoglobulin in milk, over 80% of the protein in colostrum (breast milk produced in the first 0–5 days after delivery).[1] Up to 4 g/day may be received by the breast-fed infant. This is equivalent to adult production, and is critical as the immature mucosal immune system does not produce protective levels of sIgA for several years. The milk sIgA influences the development of the mucosal immune system topically, by decreasing microbial adherence, and also systemically by promoting B cells in the gut to activate, proliferate, and produce immunoglobulin. It functions on gut phagocytes to increase phagocytosis, especially by polymorphonuclear cells, and can also bind toxins. SIgA favors humoral/TH2 responses, preventing the development of a TH1 response, which could be more dangerous and potentially damaging to the gastrointestinal tract. Thus, breast-feeding favors the establishment of tolerance.

In the gastrointestinal tract, epithelial cells and their products are important components of the innate immune system and a barrier to pathogen invasion. The tight junctions between epithelial cells reduce paracellular antigen transport. Salivary lysozyme destroys microbial membranes. *Acid* and *pepsin* in the stomach decrease microbial numbers. Treatment with drugs such as histamine receptor type 2 antagonists or proton pump inhibitors, which decrease gastric acid, permit bacterial proliferation and increase the risk of infection, including pneumonias. Further in the intestine, proteolytic *enzymes* also help keep microbe numbers low in the small bowel. The epithelial cells throughout the digestive tract cells secrete *mucus*, which is actually a complex mix of glycoproteins that can bind to and trap invading pathogens and dietary antigens, preventing their interaction with receptors in the epithelial cells. The ultrastructure of the epithelial cells, especially the microvilli and normal *motility*, also aid in the clearance of bacteria and the prevention of disease.[1] Physical or functional obstruction allows for bacterial overgrowth, increased production of toxic microbial products, and damage to the epithelial cell layer. Other epithelial products act to directly kill the microbes or prevent their growth. The *Paneth cells* of the small intestine produce large amounts of human alpha defensins 5 and 6. These and additional defensins produced by the epithelial cells, beta defensin 1 and beta defensin 2, and the cathelicidin LL-37, are critical to this action.[17,38–48] Defensins are small, acid stable and protease stable antimicrobial peptides, active in low salt environments that act directly on microbe membranes to cause lysis. In humans, alpha defensins 1–4, which are related, alpha defensins 5 and 6, and beta defensins 1,2,3,4, as well as cathelicidin (LL37) have been identified (Table 6.3).[17,38–48] Production of beta defensins 2, 3, and 4 may be induced/upregulated in the presence of inflammation by NFκB, IL-1, or TNF-α.[40–42] Paneth cell metaplasia, as occurs in Crohn's disease, is associated with increased alpha defensins 5 and 6 production in the large bowel. LL-37 is increased in the epithelium and gastric secretions of H. pylori infected patients.[39] Defensins may also have immunomodulatory actions. Beta defensin 2 can bind to the CCR6 receptor, competing with MIP-3α, and acting as a chemokine. High systemic HBD2 and HNP1-3 have been associated with protection against HIV infection not explained by CCR5 mutation.[17] Normal commensal bacteria also, by colonization resistance, competition for nutrition, and the production of substances such as colicins, keep numbers of competing pathogens low.[6,8,49] Cytokines, low molecular weight glycoproteins, that have autocrine, paracrine, and endocrine actions, are components of the innate immune system that are a crucial bridge to the adaptive response.

In addition to secreted proteins, gastrointestinal epithelial cells and other cells of the innate immune system such as granulocytes, monocytes, macrophages, dendritic cells, and NK cells, as well as B cells selectively express transmembrane *toll-like receptors 1–10* (Fig. 6.1).[24–26,50–57] The effector cells, including NK and B cells may also directly recognize and kill microbes via this mechanism.[56,57] Products recognized by the TLRs include bacterial lipoproteins, peptidoglycans (TLR-2), viral dsRNA and poly I:C (TLR-3), lipopolysaccharide (TLR-4), bacterial flagellin (TLR-5), and unmethylated CpG DNA motifs associated with bacterial DNA (TLR-9). TLR-1 and TLR-6 signal only as dimmers with TLR-2. Ligands for TLR-7 and TLR-8 are not known, but antiviral drugs imidazole imiquimod and R848, and recently U-rich viral single stranded RNA have been found to act as agonists.[58] Ligands for TLR-10 are not known. TLR signaling following ligand binding requires other proteins,[25,55] such as MYD88 (except for TLR-3), TRIF, IRAKs, TRAF6, MD1 and MD2, eventually resulting in the activation of NFκB, MAPK, AP-1. TLR-3 and TLR-4 can signal via an MYD88 independent pathway including IRF-3. This leads to induction of effector molecules such as nitric oxide, defensins, enhanced expression of co-stimulatory molecules on APCs, synthesis and release of cytokines including IL-12, TNF-α, IL-6, IL-8 and interferons. These in turn, activate NK cells, and stimulate specific adaptive

Defensin	Expressing cell	Activity
Alpha defensins		
HNP-1,2,3,4	Neutrophils, NK, epithelial cells, monocytes, and CD8+ cells	Anti-HIV; also against *Mycobacteria and other bacteria*
HαD5	Paneth cells; small intestinal epithelial	Antimicrobial against *Salmonella*; expressed in active colonic CD
HαD6	Paneth cells of small intestine	Expressed in active colonic CD
Beta defensins		
β-defensin 1	Constitutive by small bowel and colon	Antimicrobial against gram negatives, e.g. *E. coli*, *Pseudomonas* and *M. catarrhalis*
β-defensin 2	Induced by inflammation in colon, stomach, small bowel	Inducible: antimicrobial against *S. pneumoniae*, HIV
β-defensin 3	Induced in oral epithelial cells	Inducible: antimicrobial against aerobes and strains of *Candida*, HIV
β-defensin 4	Induced in gastric antrum; neutrophils	Antimicrobial against gram positive and gram negative and yeast; chemoattracts monocytes
Cathelicidin (LL-37)	NK cells, neutrophils, gastric and intestinal epithelia	Antimicrobial against Group A *Streptococcus*, *E. coli*, *Listeria*, and Cag A+ *H. pylori*

Table 6.3 The human defensins and cathelicidin

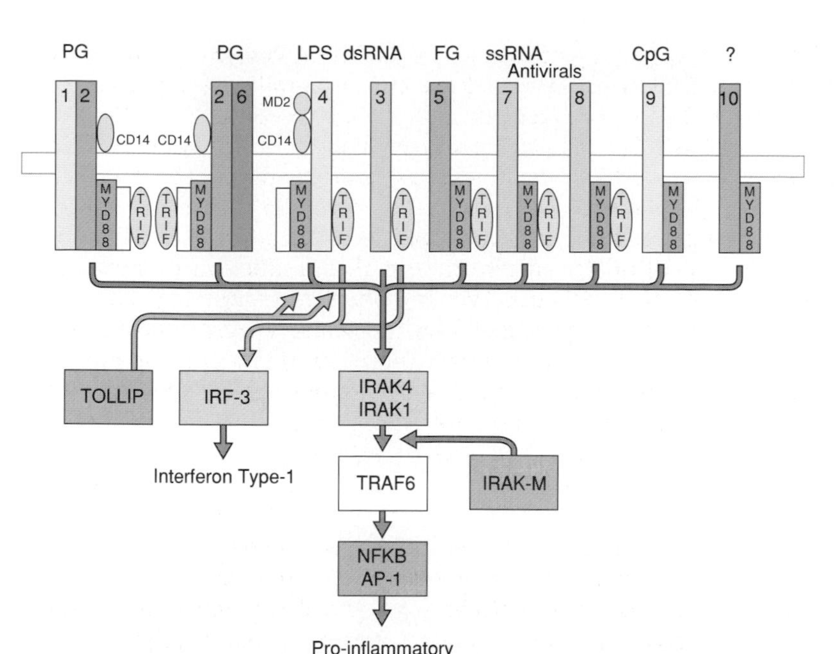

Figure 6.1: The human toll-like receptors and their ligands and signaling pathways. Not all cells express all receptors.

responses involving T and B lymphocytes. Tollip protein and IRAK-M are negative regulators[25] which can downregulate TLR signaling. Cytokines produced vary with the TLR activated. TLR-3 activation is a potent inducer of interferon. TLR 9 ligation skews the cytokine response to that of a TH1 profile, and is being used in trials to improve the efficacy of immunotherapy, and modify an ongoing TH2 immune response. Deceased expression of TLR-1, TLR-2, TLR-4, TLR-6 and MD2 and increased TOLLIP correlate with intestinal epithelial cell protection against dysregulated proinflammatory gene expression in response to commensal bacteria in the gut.[26,52,53] Increased expression of TLR-2 and TLR-4 protein in Paneth cells and in lamina propria cells have been found in patients with Crohn's disease,[50,54] with increased TLR-2, TLR-4, TLR-5 at inflamed sites (Fig. 6.2). Weakness in the TLR system can also be exploited by pathogens. For example, H. pylori flagellins have very low intrinsic activity to stimulate human gastric epithelial cells via TLR-5.[51] The LPS of H. pylori, due to its special structure, is a poor agonist for TLR-4,[7] which is also normally only weakly present in the gastric mucosa. These special features of H. pylori and its ability to cycle between intracellular and extracellular phases gives it capacity to escape host defenses and establish persistent infection,[7] leading to duodenal ulcers, chronic nodular gastritis, and an increased risk of malignant transformation.

Intracellular pathogen pattern recognition receptors also exist (Fig. 6.3),[59] including proteins like NOD2/CARD15,[13,14,59–61] that normally binds muramyl dipeptide, a component of cell wall peptidoglycans of Mycobacteria, gram positive, and gram negative bacteria. NOD2 belongs to a new family of NBS-LRR (nuclear binding site-leucine rich repeat) molecules related to plant disease resistance genes. These may represent the intracellular detectors of pathogen associated molecular patterns. These include also NOD1, NALP-1/CARD7, NALP-2, NAIP and cryopynin.[59] Muramyl dipeptide does not interact with TLR-2, the extracellular receptor for intact peptidoglycan. Muramyl dipeptide has been used clinically to upregulate the immune response to vaccines as Freund's adjuvant. NOD2 is a very polymorphic gene, with well-defined structure, expressed by monocytes, macrophages, dendritic cells, granulocytes and Paneth cells.[13,14] NOD2 contains a bacterial recognition region with leucine rich repeats, a nuclear binding domain that allows for oligomerization, and two caspase activating domains, that lead to NF?B activation and apoptosis. Three specific mutations (substitution of arginine for tryptophan at amino acid 702, substitution of glycine for arginine at amino acid 908, and a frame shift mutation at amino acid 1007 that truncates the end 3% of the protein) have been demonstrated[13,14,60,61] with the development of familial Crohn's disease in Caucasian populations, but not ulcerative colitis (Fig. 6.4). Patients with these mutations may have a compromised response to intracellular bacterial products, leading to impaired clearance, and subsequent inflammation. Mutations at other regions in NOD2 are associated with Blau syndrome.[59] Overall, only 3–15% of Crohn's disease patients are homozygous or compound heterozygous for the mutations, 10–30% of patients are heterozygous for one of the three.[13,14,60,61] Notably, 8–15% of controls are heterozygous, and 1% homozygous, supporting additional genetic and environmental factors in pathogenesis.[13,14,60,61] The cryopyrin gene has also been implicated in human inflammatory diseases, including cold autoinflammatory syndrome and Muckle-Wells syndrome.[59]

The epithelial cells also are capable of producing a myriad of cytokines,[22,23,62] including IL-1, TNF-α, IL-8, exotoxin, MIP-1α, and upregulating production when activated. These cytokines can further activate leukocyte components of the innate immune system, including tissue macrophages, which can engulf and kill the invaders. The

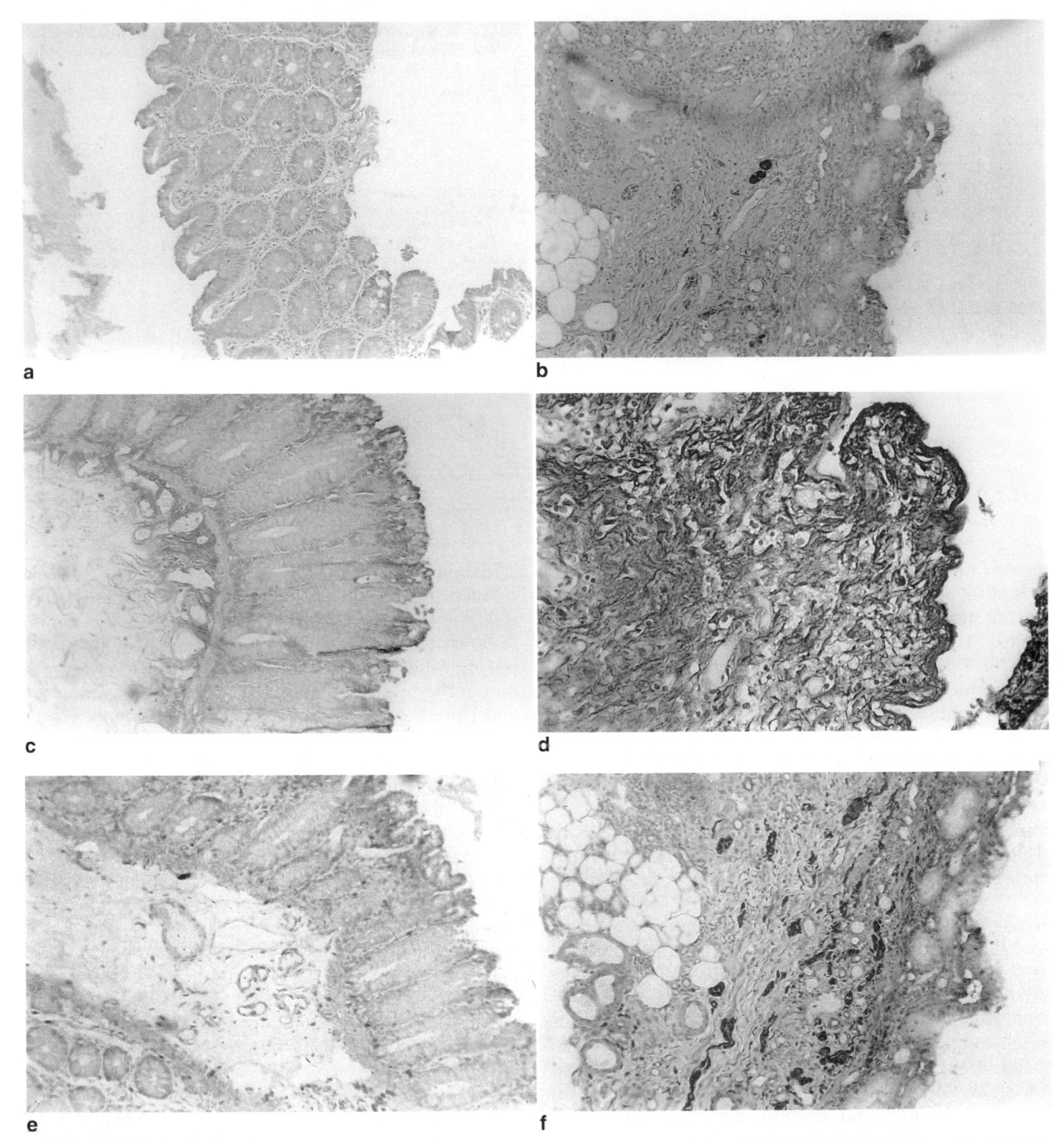

Figure 6.2: Toll-like receptor expression in the colon of patients with Crohn's disease. Note increased (**a,b**) TLR-2, (**c,d**) TLR-4 and (**e,f**) TLR-5 proteins in involved *vs* uninvolved areas by immunohistochemistry (MD Srivastava and M Kulaylat, unpublished data).

chemokines can also lead to the influx of additional effector cell types, and elicit an inflammatory response.[63] The activated macrophages and dendritic cells in the gastrointestinal tract can also then exit into the lymphatics, to the draining nodes, and there present the antigen to naive B and T cells, activating these cells, and causing their differentiation and proliferation, followed by their trafficking back to the damaged gut. This is a mechanism whereby the innate immune system and the specific adaptive immune systems are linked.

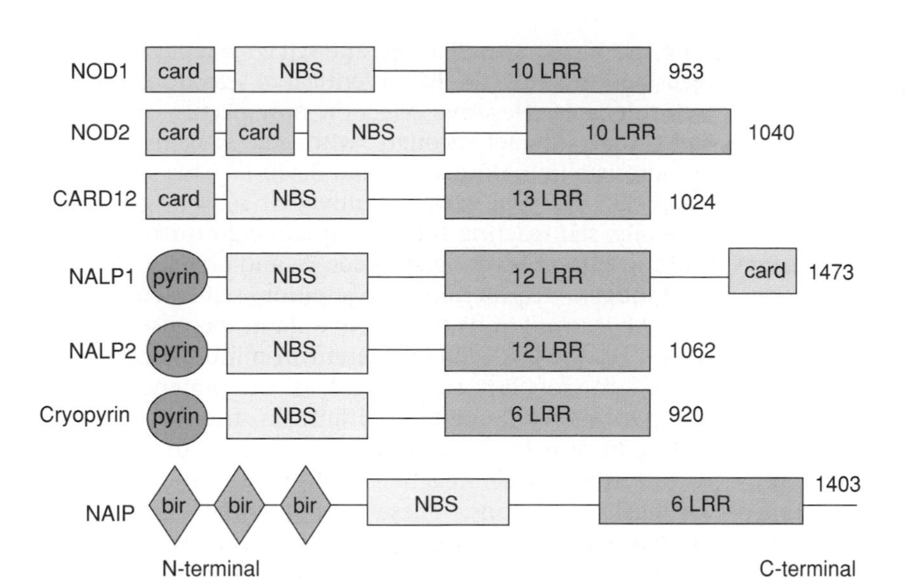

Figure 6.3: Intracellular pathogen recognition receptor family.

THE ADAPTIVE IMMUNE SYSTEM

The most important cells of the adaptive immune cells are T cell and B cells. The adaptive or acquired immune system is evolutionally much younger than innate immune system components. Found phylogenetically first in the ancestors of bony fishes, the adaptive immune system originated from the infection of an ancient immunoglobulin-like gene with a *transposable element* (transposon) able to insert itself in and cut itself out of genomic DNA. The adaptive immune response is delayed, but it is exquisitely specific and can deal with antigens and infections that evade the innate immune system. Receptors on the B and T cells provide the specificity, and are not encoded by the germ line, but require successful somatic gene rearrangements[64] mediated by the *RAG1* and *RAG2 recombinases*, the enzymes remaining from the ancient transposon. Over the lifetime of the individual over 10^{14} different TCR and BCRs can be expressed. Exposure to the specific antigen in the periphery that engages a TCR or a membrane IgM (BCR) leads to activation, proliferation, and further gene rearrangements including isotype switching and affinity maturation in B cells, with the ultimate production of memory B and memory T cells. These long-lived cells can then provide very rapid, specific protection should the antigen ever be encountered again.

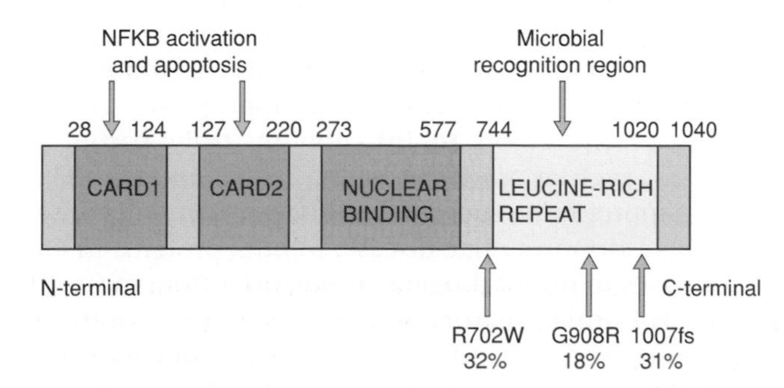

Figure 6.4: NOD-2 protein structure showing common mutations observed in Crohn's disease.

T cells

T cells, as noted above, originate from a common lymphocyte precursor in the bone marrow and then journey to the thymus, a central lymphoid organ present in the chest. The thymus is largest in infancy, and shrinks significantly with age or with corticosteroid treatment. Support cells in the thymus produce hormones and other growth factors that foster the development of T cells. It is in the thymus that effective production of a T-cell receptor must occur. Cells initially express neither the TCR, nor the accessory molecules CD3, CD4 or CD8. These are called *double negative* T cells. Normally, these *double negative* cells are not found outside the thymus in significant numbers, but are increased in the circulation of patients with hereditary defects in the FAS/FAS-ligand genes controlling apoptosis. Subsequently, with the expression of a functionally rearranged TCR usually of the α and β chain heterodimer along with CD3, both CD4 and CD8 are expressed. Eventually, mature T cells expressing the TCR and either CD4 or CD8 in conjunction with CD3 leave the thymus to take up residence in the peripheral lymphoid tissues, including the lymphoid nodes, spleen, and MALT (*mucosa associated lymphoid tissues*) such as in the gut. The thymus is also the site of clonal selection. T cells expressing receptors that recognize self-antigens and bind too strongly to MHC molecules are deleted normally. If this process is defective, then autoimmunity may result. Therapies that interfere with apoptosis, such as those that antagonize the TNF pathway, could potentially increase the generation of self-reactive clones by this mechanism.

In the thymus, the characteristics of the rearranged T cell receptor-CD4/orCD8 complex determine the fate of the developing T cell, and its final phenotype.[64] The AG-*MHC:TCR* and AG-*MHC:CD4/*or *CD8* interactions are both required. As CD interacts with invariant sites on MHC Class 1, and CD4 on the invariant sites on MHC Class 2, this further ensures appropriate co expression and *positive selection* of CD4+TCR+ cells that interact with MHC2, and CD8+TCR+ that interact with MHC1 and express the appropriate 'program.' Immature T cells that express a T cell receptor-CD (TCR:CD) complex that can not interact with self-MHC die in the thymus. These T cells would be useless to the host as they could not recognize antigen and therefore could not be activated. *Negative selection* then further shapes the T-cell repertoire in the thymus. Those immature T cells expressing TCR:CD complexes that strongly engage self antigen:MHC are eliminated. These are the potentially dangerous T cells that could incite immune responses against self. Underlying mechanisms of negative selection may result from too strong an interaction of self antigen:MHC and the TCR-CD due to avidity, or due to differential signaling/clustering of receptors leading to cell deletion in the thymus. In contrast, in the rest of the body, strong signaling activates mature T cells. Not all potentially self-reactive T-cell clones are eliminated depending on the signaling (a weak signal during negative selection could prevent them from undergoing apoptosis). In addition, some self antigens are expressed only outside the thymus and/or only normally during specific times during the human lifespan, or are usually 'hidden' (i.e. non-surface expressed nuclear or cytoplasmic proteins spilled during necrotic cell death), or exposed only during disease. Others may react to neoantigens, such as to gluten-derived peptides that have been acted upon by tissue transglutaminase in the digestive tract. T cells that could interact with these antigens will not have been subjected to the same selection process. Once these potentially dangerous cells leave the thymus, they may never encounter the antigen and also undergo apoptosis. However, preventing their activation in the periphery (peripheral tolerance) is critical.

B cells

The other key arm of the adaptive immune system is the B lineage. These cells undergo development in the bone marrow in humans. B cells express receptors that are in fact membrane-bound forms of the immunoglobulin that will be produced by the cell. These receptors, like the T-cell receptors, are the result of successful somatic cell gene rearrangement,[64] of one (of two) heavy chain genes, and of one (of four) light chain genes mediated by the RAG1 and RAG 2 enzymes. The result is incredible diversity of BCR, and therefore, antibody, protecting against over 10^{15} different antigens. The *immunoglobulin* heavy chain genes are found on chromosome 14, the light chain genes on 2 (κ) and 22 (λ), respectively. In early Pro-B cell development, the heavy chain genes begins to rearrange with rearrangement and joining of D and J segments to the Constant (C) μ region of the heavy chain. This is followed by rearrangement and joining of the V (variable) to the DJ segment. Only after successful heavy chain gene rearrangement will there be similar rearrangement of the κ gene(s), or of the lambda gene (if κ gene rearrangement to an in-frame product is not successful). B-cell receptor rearrangement depends upon the principle of *allelic exclusion*, such that the successful rearrangement of any one allele will prevent further rearrangement of the others. The end result is an immature B cell expressing surface IgM and IgD of only one specificity, as well as Igα and Igβ co-receptors. As for T cells and the TCR, the BCR is critical to selection, and thus self-tolerance. Negative selection now occurs, as those B cells that interact strongly with self-antigens undergo apoptosis/elimination via clonal deletion. This is observed in B cells reacting with a multivalent self antigen. Alternatively, self reacting B cells may undergo further genetic editing of their rearranged receptors, and no longer react to self antigen, *receptor editing*. In addition, self reactive B cells may be *ignorant* of its self-reactive status, because the antigen it reacts to is hidden, present in minute amounts, or unable to cross-link surface IgM. In the presence of high concentrations of soluble self antigen, the self-reactive B cells can also become *anergic,* or resistant to activation. Clearly, though, self-reactive B cells exist in the circulation of healthy persons. These are potential producers of autoantibodies causing tissue damage, such as seen in *autoimmune enteritis* patients, whose B cells make IgG against the enterocyte, leading to inflammation and destruction of the villi. The ignorant clones may be potentially the most dangerous, should they become educated to their antigen. However, if mature B cells fail to enter the nodes, they survive only a few days in circulation; once they enter a node they receive growth and stimulating signals that lead to their selection and they become longer lived. After stimulation by antigen, with T cell help including expression of co-stimulatory molecules such as CD40 ligand, the B cell undergoes activation and isotype switching to IgA, IgE, or IgG and affinity maturation of the receptor to produce antibody of exquisite specificity. In the normal gut, there is preferential expression of IgA, which combined with the secretory component from epithelial cells, becomes secretory IgA and protects the mucosal surfaces.

INFLAMMATION

When tolerance fails to be established, is abrogated, and/or is not reestablished, the result is inflammation of the gastrointestinal tract. The normal mucosa is characterized by a state of *controlled inflammation*, or rather the microscopic evaluation of the layers reveals the presence of multiple types of leukocytes, including *intraepithelial* $\gamma\delta$ *T cells*, scattered plasma cells in the lamina propria, and collections of lymphocytes as lymphoid aggregates throughout the gastrointestinal tract. The absence of such cells is abnormal, and may indicate an immunodeficiency state. The number, type, and activity of these cells and of other cellular and biochemical components of the mucosa is dramatically altered in inflammation. This can be appropriate, as in the response of the colon to invasion by truly pathogenic organisms, such as *Shigella* bacteria or *Entamoeba histolytica*, or inappropriate, such as the inflammatory response to gluten ingestion in Celiac disease, to milk proteins in allergic colitis, or to nonpathogenic indigenous flora in Crohn's disease. The inflammatory response is actually quite heterogeneous, and depends upon specific characteristics of the antigen (i.e. in H. pylori infection is it *Cag A+* or negative),[20] and of the host including genetic susceptibility (i.e.

is there a strong family history or atopy for milk protein allergy, HLA-DQ2 positivity for Celiac disease, or a NOD2 mutation for Crohn's disease)[13] age/developmental stage (i.e. premature infant with necrotizing enterocolitis), and nutritional status/diet (i.e. malnutrition or micronutrient zinc deficiency, inappropriate early feeding) along with modifying environmental factors[65] such as additional exposures to adjuvants/medications (i.e. antibiotics), or systemic (i.e. measles) and gastrointestinal (i.e. rotavirus) infections resulting in a specific cytokine milieu. The duration of the reaction also impacts this process, as remodeling/healing[66,67] with tissue fibrosis (scarring) may require a longer period. The inflammatory response, therefore, is not static over time, does not evolve at the same rate, and is truly a unique occurrence in each patient at each point in time. Genetic expression profiling, performed using gene chip technology, has confirmed this.[23,68–71] Yet, a limited number of critical common pathways and key immunologic players have been identified and are now being successfully and specifically targeted for therapy, such as with anti-TNF-a antibodies (Infliximab) for Crohn's disease.[37] Thus, a more detailed knowledge of these components of the inflammatory response and the underlying molecular mechanisms is required for the pediatric gastroenterologist, and will allow for the individualized management of patients.

Acute inflammation

The acute inflammatory process in the gastrointestinal tract is characterized by the presence of neutrophils. These are polymorphonuclear phagocytes characterized by non-specific (azurophilic) and specific cytoplasmic granules. Contained in the granules are enzymes, such as myeloperoxidase and lysozyme, that aid in bacterial cell killing. Other granule enzymes, like elastase and collagenase, result in the breakdown of tissues, including the supportive connective tissue *matrix*, allowing the neutrophils to enter tissues, and releasing matrix proteins, including cytokines and growth factors and angiogenesis factors. In addition, antimicrobial peptides, such as defensins HNP 1–3 are present in the granules. Neutrophils originate in the bone marrow and migrate to sites of inflammation. They are very short-lived in the bloodstream, surviving only a matter of hours and are post-mitotic they can no longer divide/proliferate. Thus, they must be constantly generated and their numbers are sensitive to bone marrow suppressive agents, such as azathioprine or 6-merceptopurine, which may be used in some patients with Crohn's disease.

Systemic cytokines, including TNF-α, IL-6, and IL-1, produced as part of the acute phase response activate the endothelia, resulting in upregulation of adhesion molecule expression and additional inflammatory mediator production. In response to inflammatory cytokines and especially the CXC chemokine IL-8, neutrophils migrate out of the blood stream towards an inflammatory stimulus in the tissue (Fig. 6.5).[63] This is mediated by a complex family of proteins known as *adhesion molecules*. At first, the neutrophils via *selectins* interact with the endothelium of

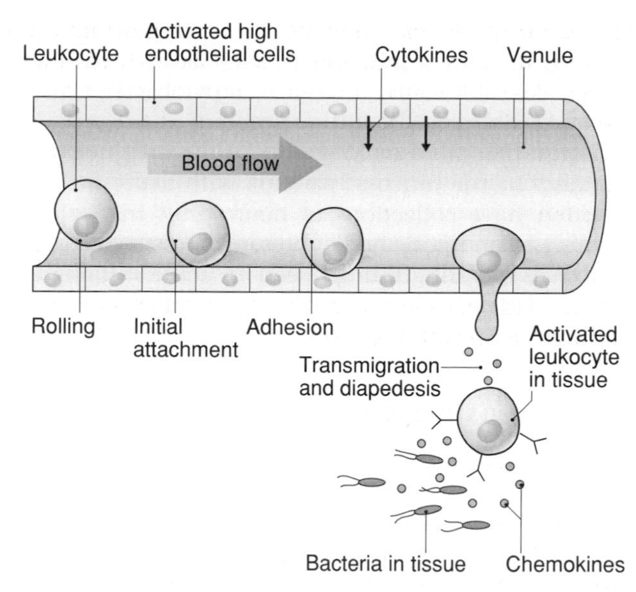

Figure 6.5: Overview of leukocyte trafficking from the vascular space to the tissues in the presence of inflammatory stimuli, such as infection with resultant chemokine expression.

blood vessels at the site of the inflammatory reaction. L-selectin, on the neutrophils binds to sialyl-Lewis^x, a carbohydrate present on the vascular epithelium. In the mucosal blood vessels of the gastrointestinal tract, a special adhesion molecule *MAdCAM-1* on high endothelial venules binds to L-selectin on leukocytes, ensuring their preferential recruitment. This results in the process called *margination*, and rolling and weak attachment of the neutrophil to the endothelium. This is followed by more secure attachment to the endothelium, mediated by *integrins*, specifically LFA-1 on the neutrophil binding to ICAM-1 on the endothelium lining the blood vessel. Interference with this process by the use of antisense oligonucleotides to ICAM-1, preventing its successful synthesis, was attempted as a therapy for Crohn's disease (ISIS 2303). Then, the neutrophils begin to traverse between endothelium cells via diapedesis. This process is mediated by PECAM-1, an adhesion molecule of the Ig superfamily.

The neutrophils in the tissues are activated and secrete granule contents. They also produce additional cytokines and chemokines, like TNF-α and IL-8, amplifying the inflammatory response. Neutrophils have receptors for bacterial products, complement, antibody, and for many chemokines and cytokines. They phagocytose or engulf the invading pathogens, and sequester their catch in a phagosome in the cytoplasm. Lysosomes, containing additional microbicidal enzymes, must fuse with the phagosome for there to be killing of the now intracellular bacteria. Inside the phagolysosome, superoxide and other *radicals* hydrogen peroxide (H2O2) and hypochlorous acid (HOCL-) are generated via the respiratory burst with enzymes of the cytochrome B558 system, ultimately destroying the microbes. Patients with defects in generation of the superoxide radical, such as patients with chronic granulomatous disease, can not effectively kill pathogens and present with recurrent infections and chronic inflammation, abscess, and stricturing in the GI tract. In acute gastrointestinal infections in normal individuals, such as with pathogenic bacteria, like Salmonella, Shigella, Campylobacter, Clostridia difficile, Yersinia, neutrophils are present in the stool 'fecal leukocytes' that are used to screen for the presence of such infections. In the mucosa, patients with acute inflammation often have collections of neutrophils in the crypts, there may be apoptotic bodies present, these collections are called *crypt abscesses* and are seen in acute inflammatory reactions with pathogens, and in active phases of chronic inflammatory bowel diseases.

Allergic-eosinophilic inflammation

Initiators of allergic inflammation depend on the action of *mast cells* that express the high affinity receptor for IgE. Mast cells and basophils are distributed throughout the gastrointestinal tract. These cells are derived from the bone marrow, and not normally found in significant numbers in the bloodstream. Mast cells are typically found in the deeper layers of the digestive tract, often next to blood vessels. They absolutely depend on the growth factor SCF (stem cell factor) the ligand of the receptor c-kit, which has tyrosine kinase activity. Mastocytosis, with huge numbers of mast cells present on gastrointestinal biopsy, results in adults from activating mutations in c-kit, and is being targeted in trial with TK inhibitors, such as *imatinib*. Of course, the IgE that binds to mast cells originates from B lineage cells on re-exposure to antigen presented in a context favoring an allergic/TH-2 predominant response (IL-4, IL-5). This IgE in circulation then binds to the high affinity receptor *FcεR1* present on the mast cell. If two or more molecules of specific IgE bound to FceR1 on mast cells are then cross linked by antigen, the mast cell becomes activated, and in a calcium dependent process, releases preformed mediators, most notably *histamine*, but also TNF-α, heparin, and other enzymes such as tryptase, which can be a useful marker in acute anaphylaxis. Histamine binds to H1 receptors and leads to increased vascular permeability, and smooth muscle contraction. In the GI tract, this leads to diarrhea and abdominal pain. In the stomach, increased histamine binds H2 receptors on parietal cells and increases acid output. In addition to histamine, the mast cell or basophil that is activated releases arachidonic acid from its membrane via phospholipase C and phospholipase A2 enzymes. Cyclo-oxygenase and lipo-oxygenase pathways lead to *de novo* synthesis of prostaglandins (especially PGD2) and leukotrienes, including the cysteinyl leukotrienes CD, D4, E4, which are proinflammatory. NSAIDs and aspirin compounds inhibit the cyclooxygenase pathway. The receptor for the cysteinyl leukotrienes is blocked by drugs such as montelukast, which show promise in treating allergic-eosinophilic disorders of the gut. Mast cells also produce large amounts of cytokine mediators, including IL-4 and IL-13, IL-3, IL-5, MIIP-α, and GM-CSF. Thus, mast cells play a key role in recruiting additional inflammatory cells, most notable the eosinophil, and support a TH2 predominant milieu of the ensuing inflammatory reaction.

The characteristic leukocyte found in the gastrointestinal tract in increased numbers and in an increased activation state in gastrointestinal allergic inflammation is the polymorphonuclear cell the *eosinophil*. The specific granules of the eosinophil contain large amounts of *major basic protein* which gives the cell its characteristic brilliant orange color with acid (eosin) dyes. Other eosinophil granule products, eosinophil peroxidase, eosinophil derived neurotoxic peptide, and eosinophil cationic protein. Increased concentrations of these mediators are found in the stool and in intestinal perfusates in eosinophilic-allergic conditions of the gastrointestinal tract,[72–77] and in early UC and CD, which are also characterized by eosinophilic infiltrate in the mucosa.[78,79] Eosinophils are produced in the bone marrow from myeloid precursors and require IL-3, GM-CSF, and IL-5 as growth factors. Eosinophils express multiple CC and CXC chemokine receptors, but *eotaxin-1* is the most specific chemokine for eosinophils[75] and binds CCR3[77] on the cell membrane. CCR3 binds to additional chemokines, RANTES, MCP-3, 4, and is expressed by TH2 cells,[74] perpetuating the reaction. Other cytokines, including TNF-α can activate eosinophils. Once activated, they express high affinity FcεR1 and increased IG receptors. They also produce cytokines IL-1,3,4,5,6,8,10,16,GM-CSF, RANTES, TNF-α, TNF-β, TGF-β1, and MIP-1α and products of the prostaglandins and leukotriene pathways, such as leukotriene C4, PGE1 and E2, and TXB2.[77] PAF receptors on eosinophils result in degranulation when ligated. They respond to leukotrienes also, including to LTB4, which stimulates the respiratory burst. Eosinophils express receptors for the Fc portion of IgG and IgE (FcεRII or CD23), IgA, and complement (CR1 and CR3). Eosinophils are recruited to sites of allergic inflammation by adhesion molecules. P-selectin is the most important selectin involved in the initial rolling phase of recruitment of eosinophils. Stronger adhesion is then provided by VLA-4 and MAC-1on the eosinophil and VCAM-1 and ICAM-1 on endothelia, respectively. Eosinophils also express *α4β7* which binds to *MADCAM-1*, specifically targeting the eosinophil to exit into the mucosa, such as of the GI tract. Monoclonal antibodies to the a4 subunit, natalizumab, are being investigated for Crohn's disease.[80] Once in the tissues, eosinophils can become activated to release their granules, produce cytokines and lipid mediators, and attack and kill pathogens, in particular parasites. In invasive parasitic infections of the gut, such as with *E. histolytica*, biopsies reveal abscesses in the mucosa composed of large numbers of activated eosinophils. In the absence of parasitic infections, eosinophils have been observed to be critical to inflammatory process in inflammatory bowel disease, graft *vs* host disease, milk-soy protein allergic colitis/enteritis, and in eosinophilic esophagitis/gastroenteritis. In eosinophilic esophagitis, there may be eosinophilic clusters in the squamous mucosa, a ringed appearance on endoscopy, and whitish plaques of eosinophils on biopsy. This condition is resistant to acid blockade, is associated with a negative Ph probe, and possibly is linked to respiratory as well as food allergies. Treatment is with topical steroids, sometimes utilized inhaled steroids that are swallowed and diet restriction. In the future, cytokine antagonists, such as anti-IL-5 (mepolizumab) may be used. Long-term consequences include strictures, Schatzki rings, and food impaction/dysmotility. In eosinophilic gastroenteritis, depending upon the layers and sites of the GI tract involved, symptoms may be due to outlet obstruction/dysmotility (i.e. mimics pylori stenosis) when affecting the muscular layers of the duodenum and antrum, gastrointestinal bleeding/diarrhea, if mucosal such as in the colon are involved, or even ascites, if serosal involvement. Standard therapy was glucocorticoids, which effectively lyse eosinophils, but patients tend to become steroid dependent. In infants with milk protein colitis, eosinophils can be found on biopsy of the rectal mucosa, but strict elimination and use of a hydrolysate or amino acid formula to the age of at least 1 year, usually is sufficient to resolve the eosinophilic inflammation and permit future exposure without reaction.

Chronic inflammation

Chronic inflammatory processes in the digestive tract are characterized by the presence of marked increases in lymphocytes, such as plasma cells, and a more mixed inflammatory infiltrate. Chronic inflammation is never physiologic. It may result if the inciting antigen or antigens are not or can not be eliminated by the host. Characteristically, these pathogens, such as *Mycobacterium tuberculosis*, are taken up by macrophages, but not effectively killed. There is chronic activation of the cell, with cytokine production. In the setting of high interferon-γ, IL-12, and perhaps IL-18,[81] a TH1 skewed milieu, the result is *granuloma* formation. In these structures, there is a fusion of macrophages, to 'giant cells' with several nuclei. Also, the epithelioid macrophages are seen, surrounded by a ring of activated T lymphocytes. This is one attempt by the body to 'wall off' or contain the pathogen; unfortunately, it is very destructive. In Crohn's disease, unlike in tuberculosis, the granulomas do not have a necrotic center, they are *non-caseating*.[82] In addition, activated macrophages produce multiple matrix metalloproteinases[83] which have been associated with *fistula* formation in Crohn's disease. It is presently controversial as to whether infection with atypical *Mycobacteria* (*M. paratuberculosis*) may play a role in CD pathogenesis in some patients,[65,84,85] but antimycobacterial agents have been helpful in some patients.[65,84] This bacteria can be grown in RPMI 1640/10% fetal calf serum. It can also proliferate and co-exist on co-culture with colon carcinoma cell line CaCo-2 or a CD8+ human NK leukemia cell line without killing the cells (Fig. 6.6).[86] This indicates its potential for chronic infection, in contrast to *M. avium subspecies avium*, which killed these cells. Recently, the complete genome sequence of *M. paratuberculosis* has been characterized, and methods to identify substrains have been developed,[87,88] which may clarify the role of this microbe in Crohn's disease. Novel flagellin antigens,[89] bacterial protein 12 from *Pseudomonas fluorescens*[90] and OMP-C from *E. coli*[12] have also been proposed as inflammation inciting agents in Crohn's disease, and antibodies to these are being used as serological markers. Chronicity may also result if the antigen(s) driving the inflammation are inappropriately self-antigens, again because the body will never be able to clear them. This is often an underlying pathologic mechanism in many autoimmune disorders. Alternatively, chronic inflammation can result from the inability to downregulate the immune system normally, even if the inciting agent(s) have been successfully eliminated, or a failure of normal healing. This too, is a complex process. Pathologically, in the colon, chronicity is noted by changes in the morphology of the crypt. Branching or unusually shaped crypts are noted on biopsy. In the chronic inflammatory reactions, T cells, B cells, eosinophils, neutrophils, basophils, mast cells, constituent stroma cells, and epithelial cells all participate in the persistent reaction.[82] There is a complex cytokine milieu present.[21–23,81,91,92] Chronic inflammation can lead to tissue remodeling, and scarring/fibrosis in some cases. This is particularly observed in Crohn's disease. The stricturing that results can lead to small bowel obstruction and may require surgical resection.[82,92] Chronic inflammation also risks *malignancy*, as there is continued expression of growth/healing genes, and cell turnover.

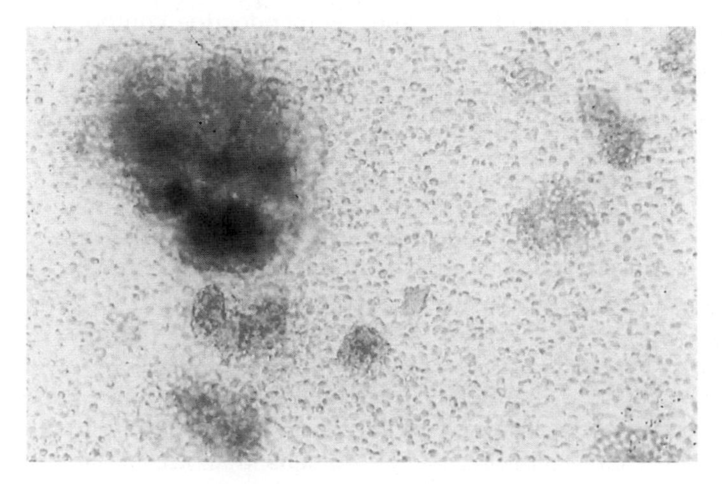

Figure 6.6: *Mycobacterium paratuberculosis* cultured *in vitro* in RPMI 1640 media 10% fetal calf serum along with natural killer cell line SRIK-NKL. The large clumped material represents the bacteria, surrounded by smaller NK cells. These bacteria also can be grown in above media alone.

TH1 *vs* TH2 dichotomy

One of the most widely held theories regarding inflammation categorizes any response into either TH1 or TH2. This is based on studies originating in mice and is based on the predominant cytokine profile. Over the last 20 years, it has been posited that inflammation results from an imbalance between TH1 and TH2 cytokines. It therefore followed that by adjusting this 'see-saw' once would favorably treat the underlying disease. Early trials in animals and humans attempted exactly that. For example, in asthma, a disease process like ulcerative colitis in which TH2 cytokines are more likely detected, it was theorized that treatment of active disease would be ameliorated by use of exogenous TH1 cytokines such as IL-12. Subsequently, it was theorized that the problem was not an imbalance of TH1>TH2 or TH2>TH1, but that favorable, immunosuppressive interleukins were deficient. Indeed, in the mucosa of patients with Crohn's disease, there is a lack of normal IL-10 expression compared to healthy persons. This led to trials with anti-inflammatory cytokines, including recombinant IL-10. Unfortunately, these trials were overall ineffective.[13] Presently, the limitations of focusing on the TH1/TH2 paradigm have come into the forefront, and the utility of strictly applying this classification has been questioned.[93] The evidence suggests that the underlying mechanism of autoimmunity or inflammation depends more upon the concepts presented earlier in this chapter, specifically tolerance, and on regulatory T-cell generation and function. Additional studies regarding the cytokine profiles in humans further supports that the inflammation in the mucosa is not perfectly TH1 or TH2, that it is not static over space and time, and that both TH1 and TH2 cytokine dependent immune reactions can coexist in the same patient at the same time, such as food allergy and Crohn's disease. Studies in *atopic dermatitis* have also supported this. In the early phases of AD, for example, TH2 cytokine profile predominates, but as the lesion becomes chronic, there is shift to a TH1 profile, including the expression of interferon gamma. Pathologic studies in Crohn's disease also support this. Early lesions in the gut are characterized by eosinophil infiltration.[78,79] Eosinophils are classically associated with TH2 cytokines, such as IL-5 and IL-4. Later in established Crohn's Disease, the pathognomonic granulomas are found, and interferon-γ is detected in the mucosa. Gene chip and linkage studies of both AD and CD have identified common susceptibility genes. Demographic studies also support this.[65] Over the last 20 years, the incidence of TH2 diseases, specifically typified by asthma, food allergies, and other allergies has increased dramatically. This has been recognized by immunology/allergy experts for some time. At the same point in time, TH1 diseases, including Crohn's disease of the gastrointestinal tract, have been increasing dramatically. If the TH2-TH1 hypothesis as originally held were correct, the relationship should be inverse. Clearly, as the population is not mutating, and diagnostic ability has not changed significantly, there must be environmental factors, perhaps not previously encountered, that are driving the increased incidence of these disorders.[65,92] Identification of the 'triggers' or predisposing factors that favor the establishment of inflammation, have been and continue to be the focus of much study. The *hygiene hypothesis* has been used to explain the increased occurrence of allergy, asthma and other atopic disorders, due to decreased infections in childhood and a skewing of the immune response. However, this hypothesis is being brought into serious question because it also depends on the TH1 and TH2 dichotomy.

NORMAL DOWNREGULATION OF INFLAMMATION IN THE GASTROINTESTINAL TRACT

Downregulation of an established inflammatory response depends upon the production of both cellular and soluble mediators and complex cellular signaling pathways. *Apoptosis* or programmed cell death of immune cells, such as activated T cells that are no longer needed, is a critical component. Fas is a membrane bound receptor that when activated signals the cell to die (undergo apoptosis via the enzymes known as *caspases*). Expression of its ligand, Fas-L, is tightly controlled, but induced with activation. Therefore, normally, Fas-Fas-L interactions limit the number of activated lymphocytes (by lymphocyte fratricide). Other members of the TNF receptor family can also transmit death signals. The *clearance* of the inciting antigen and removal of *necrotic* debris is critical to down regulation, as the positive driving force of the reaction is removed and loss of positive signals result in decreased growth factor and cytokine expression, decreased cell activation, and increased apoptosis of the inflammatory cells. Anti-inflammatory cytokines, including TGF-β and IL-10, IL-4, IL-13, also play a role in decreasing the immune response. They actively suppress via inducing the synthesis and activation of *SOCS* (suppressor of cytokine signaling) and SMAD signaling pathways and decrease inflammatory cytokine production. Other soluble anti-inflammatory factors include soluble cytokine receptors (IL-1RA, sTNFR1 and 2) acting as competitive inhibitors, nitric oxide which increases blood flow, prostaglandin E2, and neuroendocrine components of the counter-regulatory response (cortisol, epinephrine). The production of *anti-idiotype* antibodies by B cells limits the damage by antibodies. Production of growth factors, including EGF, KGF, HGF by immune cells and stromal cells also reduce inflammation and promote *angiogenesis* and healing. These mediators, however, have the potential for malignancy or for complications, such as scarring, if produced in excess. Actively inhibitory T cells can specifically and non-specifically downregulate the inflammatory process, and decreased co-stimulatory molecule expression (CD80, CD86) or increased inhibitory receptor expression (CTLA-4)[27] are also critical, as discussed above. When these systems fail, damage and chronic inflammation result.

MEDICAL TREATMENT OF GASTROINTESTINAL INFLAMMATION

Treatment of chronic GI inflammation is undergoing a revolution.[13,37,49,80,94–97] Classically, broad spectrum agents that globally affect the immune system have been used to treat inflammatory gastrointestinal diseases. Presently, we have a growing pharmacologic armamentarium of specific agents that target the immune response. We have never before had the ability to alter the function of the human immune system in such a specific manner. Although these drugs offer the promise of improved efficacy and decreased side effects, because our understanding of the human immune system is incomplete, we as practitioners must be vigilant also for the development of novel side effects/diseases due to our interventions. As products of recombinant DNA technology and molecular biology, these *designer drugs*[13,37,80] are also extremely expensive and issues of access to care, beyond the scope of this chapter, will likely become of increasing importance to our practice. Old agents, around for decades, still have great therapeutic efficacy and utility in treating our patients with chronic inflammatory disorders.

Glucocorticoids

With the discovery of cortisol and its synthesis in the laboratory, patients with inflammatory disorders, including of the GI tract had effective therapy. Over the years, much has been learned regarding the mechanism of steroid action, and also of the associated side-effects. Prednisone and methylprednisolone are agents commonly used to treat allergic-eosinophilic inflammation of the GI tract, as well as ulcerative colitis and Crohn's disease.[13,92,94,95] Topical fluticasone developed for inhalant form when swallowed is used for allergic esophagitis. Budesonide, a very potent steroid with high *first pass metabolism*, is available in a formulation specifically designed to act upon the terminal ileum/right colon. All glucocorticoids share similar mechanisms of action. Glucocorticoids are lipid soluble and diffuse through the membrane passively and bind to the widely expressed *glucocorticoid receptor*. This provides their extraordinary efficacy, but also leads to their troublesome side effects. The cytoplasmic receptor or GR is usually bound to heat shock proteins that keep it in the inactive state. Upon binding, HSP fall off, and the GR-hormone complex traverses into the nucleus of the cell. There the complex binds to specific sequences of DNA called *glucocorticoid response elements* or GRE present in the promoter regions of genes sensitive to glucocorticoids. Negative GREs result in decreased gene transcription, while positive GREs increase gene transcription, when bound by liganded GR. The glucocorticoid receptor-hormone complex can also interfere with the function of other transcription factors by direct protein-protein interactions, such as with *AP-1*, critical to the inflammatory response. In some cells, glucocorticoids also increase the synthesis of *IKB-a*, the inhibitor of the potent pro-inflammatory transcription factor *NFκB*. The overall result of glucocorticoid treatment includes improvement of tight junctions on epithelia, downregulation of cytokine and adhesion molecule expression on immune cells, apoptosis induction, inhibition of lipolysis in fat cells, and many other effects. Steroids have multiple side effects, especially if used longer term. Unfortunately, the chronic inflammatory GI disorders have often required this. Long-term side-effects include hypertension, diabetes, growth failure, osteoporosis, *Cushing syndrome*, GI bleeding/ulcers, thinning of the skin, cataracts, and aseptic necrosis of the femoral head (rare).[92,94] High dose, long-term use is particularly dangerous, and many side-effects, including cataracts and severe striae, that do not completely resolve after the drug is discontinued. In addition, patients may become 'dependent' or 'resistant' to steroid action. *Steroid resistance* may be mediated by increased synthesis of the isoform β of the glucocorticoid receptor, or by decreased GR-GRE binding. Overcoming steroid resistance and decreasing side effects are present goals of steroid research. Due to steroid side effects, other broad spectrum agents have been used.

Antimetabolites: 6-MP and azathioprine

These drugs were initially developed for the treatment of childhood leukemia. In large doses they are still used today for induction therapy and in lower doses for maintenance therapy in ALL. At lower doses, they have also been found to have steroid sparing effects, both in transplant, and in inflammatory disorders of the GI tract, especially Crohn's disease. These drugs have a complex metabolism, and there exists in the population various alleles of the enzyme *thiopurine methyltransferase*.[13] Up to 1% of the population is homozygous for the mutant allele which has decreased activity and therefore results in shunting of more of the drug via the HGPRTase enzyme to the active metabolite 6-TG. This leads to excessive 6-TG, irreversible bone marrow failure, and death without a bone marrow transplant. Trials of *6-TG* itself revealed severe hepatotoxicity and had to be discontinued in IBD and even leukemia patients. It is possible now to test for the allele and the activity of TPMT prior to the use of the drug.[13] Indeed, even heterozygotes may need to avoid these agents, due to a heightened risk of *secondary malignancy* (5q- or 11q-AML) as observed in ALL. Azathioprine is non-enzymatically transformed into 6-mercaptopurine. This is then acted upon by several enzymes: xanthine oxidase, thiopurine methyltransferase, and hypoxanthine guanine phosphoribosyl transferase. Inhibition of XO by drugs such as for gout (allopurinol) will also raise levels and require dose adjustment. Metabolism via TPMP leads to generation of 6MMP, which is hepatotoxic. Levels of therapeutic and toxic metabolites have been established and can be followed, as some patients preferentially shunt to this pathway and may not safely receive the drug. Also, other agents, including 5ASA can impact this pathway. Ultimately, the 6TG metabolites inhibit RNA and DNA synthesis, leading to decreased leukocyte production and decreased inflammation. Earlier introduction of these medications for Crohn's disease has resulted in prolonged remission and decreased steroid use and risk of relapse.[13,92,95] However, even with proper attention to metabolites, idiosyncratic reactions to these medications are common, including severe pancreatitis, and hepatitis, resulting in a significant population intolerant to these agents. Long-term studies in adults have been reassuring with regard to risk of secondary malignancy, however detailed immunologic studies in young children, who have not yet had primary exposure to many infections, and may not have completed their immunizations, have not been performed. Secondary exposure, *in utero* or to breast-fed newborns of mothers with IBD being treated with these agents is a matter of some controversy, and is not recommended by pediatricians. However, it has been repetitively shown that fetal and maternal outcome most depends upon activity of the disease at the time of conception, and thus control of the underlying disease during pregnancy is critical.

Calcineurin inhibitors

The drug ciclosporin, developed from soil fungus, revolutionized solid organ transplantation. Ciclosporin and the related FK506 or tacrolimus bind to a group of proteins called immunophilins. There are many of these proteins in a cell. Ciclosporin binds cyclophilin, and FK506 binds FK binding protein 12 (FKB12). The complex then binds to the calcium-dependent phosphatase calcineurin. This inhibits the phosphatase and results in the inactivation of NFATc, a potent transcription factor that can bind and interact with multiple other transcription factors. This decreases IL-2 and other cytokine production and therefore T cell activation. A related compound rapamycin or sirolimus does not bind to immunophilins but instead inhibits MTOR. These agents are extremely potent immunosuppressants, and greatly increase the risk of opportunistic infections. They also have significant side-effects, including renal damage/failure with ciclosporin and diabetes with FK506. Outside of transplant, this class of agents has been helpful in autoimmune enteritis. They have also been used in systemic (IV) form for fulminant ulcerative colitis[94] and in topical form for fistulizing Crohn's disease (FK506). Use in perianal Crohn's must be undertaken with caution, as relapse and worsening of perianal disease to the point of colectomy upon withdrawal has been reported.[13] The use of these potent non-specific agents has decreased significantly with the dawn of the age of biologic response modifiers.

Biologic response modifiers

These are defined as biologic agents, usually made using recombinant DNA technology, used to modulate the function of the immune system. The most important BRM in the treatment of inflammation in the GI tract thus far has been the TNF-α inhibitors, especially *infliximab*, a *humanized monoclonal antibody*.[13,37] TNF inhibitors were not originally developed for use for the GI tract, but rather to treat sepsis. It had been hypothesized in the early 1990s that it was the cytokines of the acute phase response, especially TNF-α that led to capillary leak, multiple organ failure and death. Thus, inhibition of TNF-α would increase survival: unfortunately, this was not observed in clinical trials.[98] However, when this agent was tried in patients with inflammatory conditions that involved TNF, first RA and then Crohn's disease, the results were remarkable.[13,37] Up to two-thirds of the most severely ill, steroid dependent patients responded. Unfortunately, it was not possible to predict response or non-response prospectively. For the first time, there also was an agent that closed anal fistulae, although subsequent MRI studies showed that the tract itself was persistent.

The use of infliximab, first to treat acute disease, and then as maintenance therapy every 8 weeks, decreased hospitalization and was a milestone in pediatric gastroenterology practice. Unfortunately, infliximab, a potent immunosuppressant, did have serious side-effects. In particular, infections with microbes that were intracellular or dependent on macrophages for killing were increased. Specifically, patients with prior *M. tuberculosis* exposure experienced reactivation[13,37,92,94] and uncontrollable infection, leading to death in some cases. Also, some patients developed new autoimmune conditions, including vasculitis (Fig. 6.7), lupus, and demyelination. The neurologic complications have not been shown to reverse in all patients. Patients with known MS are not to receive this agent, and all patients require CXR and PPD prior to exposure. In addition, the longer-term risk of malignancy is not known. Anaphylactic-like infusion reactions are common, but pretreatment with steroids and hydrocortisone decrease this side-effect. Further, the majority of patients not on immunomodulators develop human anti-chimera antibodies, with possible decreased efficacy. This risk may be decreased with concomitant immunomodulatory use. In general, there appears to be a waning of efficacy in a significant number of patients, and they may not be able to successfully use the drug life-long for a presumed life-long disease, such as Crohn's. In up to one-third of UC patients, infliximab may also be helpful, but this remains to be established.[94] Other inhibitors of TNF, including TNFR:Fc (etanercept) and subcutaneous anti-TNF-α antibody (Adalimumab) have been tried in Crohn's disease.[13,92,95] Other small molecule TNF inhibitors are in study. In addition to TNF inhibitors, recombinant IL-10 was tried unsuccessfully for Crohn's,[13] as was antisense oligonucleotides to ICAM-1.[96] G-CSF and GM-CSF are in trial, as are anti-interferon gamma antibodies and anti-adhesion molecule antibodies.[80] There will be many choices of BRM for our patients. However, as noted above, along with great efficacy, there may be new never before seen disease or immunologic derangements and the practitioner of the future will need to be vigilant for their appearance and possibly need to develop new treatments for their management. Further, with the many choices, it will be pressing to be able to determine the most appropriate therapy for each individual patient. This may be based possibly on results of gene chip analysis. Already this is possible for the p450 system of drug metabolic enzymes.[68] In addition,

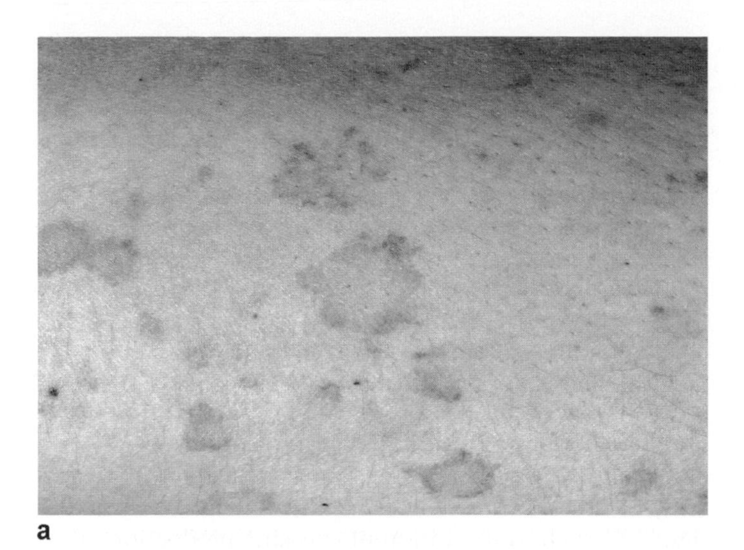
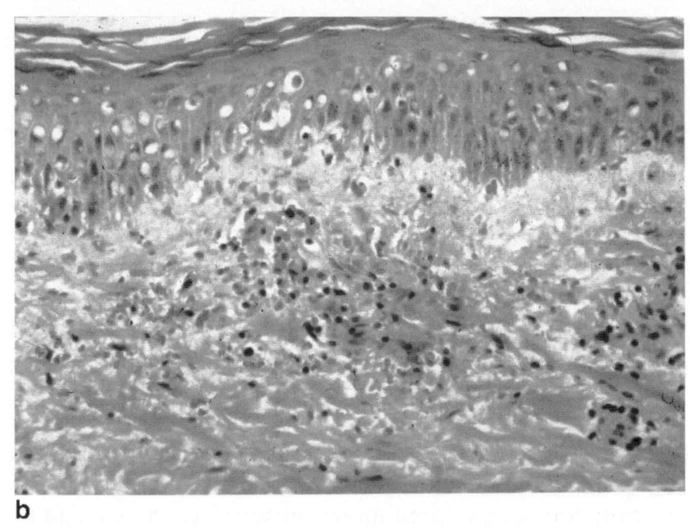

a b

Figure 6.7: Picture of (**a**) vasculitic lesions and (**b**) dermatologic biopsies induced by infliximab treatment in a patient with Crohn's disease. As new biologic agents become available, unusual autoimmune complications may arise.

careful records of different treatments used their duration, dose, and the patients' response will be necessary to detect side-effects, as these agents may be FDA approved and the expected side-effects, such as difference in malignancy rate, could take years to become manifest. These will be challenges for the future management of inflammatory gut disorders.

5-Aminosalicylates

These agents are related to aspirin. They include such compounds as mesalamine and sulfasalazine, used primarily for the treatment of ulcerative colitis, and also Crohn's disease.[13,92,94,95] In the case of mesalamine (or 5-ASA), different formulations exist that control the release of these agents depending on pH, or site in the digestive tract, and some depend on the action of intestinal bacteria (sulfasalazine) to release the active form. The drugs work topically on the mucosa, to inhibit the activation of NFKB and TNF-α production, and also to inhibit prostaglandin synthesis via effects on cyclo-oxygenase pathways. They are remarkably safe agents, but serious side-effects including worsening of colitis/bleeding, pulmonary fibrosis, renal damage are possible and physicians should be aware of these potential side-effects. Also, although commonly used, there are few studies in children that document efficacy in active Crohn's disease that is more than mild, or as a maintenance agent. These agents may also be useful in decreasing the risk of recurrence in Crohn's disease after resection, but larger studies are needed.

Antibiotics

With the identification of *Helicobacter pylori* as the causative agent for ulcers, antibiotics have had an established role in this inflammatory condition. Pending resistance, which is most commonly seen for metronidazole and clarithromycin, a two drug combination with amoxicillin, clarithromycin, metronidazole, tetracycline, and PPI for 1–2 weeks is standard therapy.[13] In the associated tumor or *MALTOMA*, clearance of the infection may be sufficient in some cases to resolve the tumor, supporting the bacterium as a potent human carcinogen. In children, household contacts may also need to be treated in order to reduce the likelihood of reinfection. Otherwise, the role of antibiotics in treatment of gastrointestinal inflammation in children is presently limited to discussion on Crohn's disease, and for *pouchitis* in patients with ulcerative colitis who underwent *ileoanal pouch* construction and anatomists. In Crohn's disease, *metronidazole*, a narrow spectrum agent that is microbicidal for anaerobes, particularly *Bacteroides*, has been shown to be useful in decreasing activity of fistulae.[13] Unfortunately, chronic use is associated with peripheral neuropathy that may not be reversible. Metronidazole is often used for acute abscess in CD, along with other agents. Use of metronidazole as primary therapy for active CD is under investigation. Similarly, ciprofloxacin has been effective in some patients with fistula, alone or in combination with metronidazole, and also has been tried for active disease. It is notable that *Ciprofloxacin* and metronidazole in addition to antibacterial actions, have immunomodulatory effects *in vitro*, and could theoretically be impacting on the basic immunobiology of the inflammatory process. In pouchitis, these antibiotics are standard therapy, presumed to work by decreasing the overgrowth of bacteria or improving the microbial milieu. Rifampin, clarithromycin, and other agents targeting *M. paratuberculosis* have been tried in combination long term, with reported success in some Crohn's disease patients with active disease.[13,65,85] As the use of antibiotics is associated with the growing problem of resistance, studies investigating the mechanism and role of these agents in IBD are needed.

Other immunomodulators

Other various agents have been tried to control chronic inflammation. *Methotrexate* given subcutaneously once per week has been shown in small studies to be efficacious in adults with severe Crohn's disease.[13,95] This agent at high dose is used as chemotherapy, and is very toxic, as it suppresses the bone marrow. At low doses it has been used for years for *rheumatoid arthritis*. Concerns regarding frequent development of *hepatic fibrosis* in RA have not been realized, and surveillance biopsies are no longer required. Yet, there is no data long term with this drug in IBD, in patients who may have been sequentially exposed to other hepatotoxic drugs, such as the immunomodulator 6-MP. Further methotrexate is a *category X* drug, it is never to be used during pregnancy; it is a proven *teratogen*. Not only can methotrexate cause spontaneous miscarriage, it can lead to very severe birth defects, including of the brain, heart and face. This is due in large part to antagonistic actions of the drug on *folic acid* metabolism. Thus, use on a chronic basis in children with IBD is undertaken with care, as efficacy is not established.

Thalidomide, another oral TNF-α inhibitor, has been shown to be helpful in adults, and research on developing related compounds is ongoing,[99–101] but there are major issues with use of this drug in children. Thalidomide is perhaps the most notorious drug of the 1960s. It was used in Europe in pregnancy as an anxiolytic. Tragically, in contrast to rodent studies, thalidomide was a potent *teratogen-category X* and led to the birth of babies with *phocomelia*: children without limbs. Thus it was banned until its efficacy in leprosy in South America was demonstrated in the 1980s, leading to investigations showing it had immunomodulatory activity decreasing TNF-α.[101] It has also been shown to cause severe and *irreversible neuropathy* and still has significant sedating actions. Thalidomide must never be used in patients who are or who may become pregnant, such as teenage females with IBD. Clearly the toxicity of this agent limits its use in chronic intestinal inflammation.

Alternative treatment strategies

As can be concluded from the above discussion, the current drug therapies are limited in efficacy, particularly for Crohn's disease that is not curable by *surgery*. Nonetheless, surgical procedures, including such advancements[102] as *laparoscopic resections* and *stricturoplasty,* and *ileoanal anastomoses* have a clear place in the management of inflammatory diseases of the GI tract, particularly ulcerative colitis and Crohn's disease, and can greatly improve quality of life. Yet, there are long-term side-effects of these procedures, including risk to fertility in pouch procedures requiring *in vitro* fertilization/assisted reproduction technologies in up to one-third of females desiring offspring, and the psychological and social morbidity of a permanent stoma. Thus, in many patients, alternative strategies have been tried. For example: nutritional therapy has been tried with NG or GT elemental *formulas*, and has been successful in remission induction in Crohn's disease of the small bowel, but relapse has occurred with discontinuation and reintroduction of solid diet. *TPN* has been tried, and although improving growth, did not control inflammation. Lactobacilli of various strains and *prebiotics/ probiotics* are still in trial,[49] but a large well-controlled trial of *lactobacillus GG* for active Crohn's did not show efficacy. *IVIG* has been reported useful[97] in case reports and *bone marrow transplant* is being studied. *Heparin* and *ridogrel* were tried in ulcerative colitis, with negative results. Many patients concomitantly have tried elimination diets or alternative medical therapies with *herbal remedies,* which in some cases could interfere with the metabolism/activity of anti-inflammatory agents or with proper nutrition and growth. *Cannabinoids* have been used in the past to treat gastroenteritis and diarrhea and have anti-inflammatory activities,[103–105] such as inhibition of cytokine production.[106] As an endogenous cannabinoid system exists in the gut, including cannabinoid receptors CB-1 and CB-2 and their ligands anandamide and 2-arachidonyl glycerol, synthetic non-psychoactive cannabinoids have potential as therapy for gastrointestinal inflammation.[103–105] It is critical to ensure that treatment strategies do not have a higher morbidity and mortality than the underlying disease process. Supportive therapy in these disorders is of critical importance, but beyond the scope of this chapter.

Treating allergic-eosinophilic disorders

In addition to the steroids discussed above, drug therapy for allergic-eosinophilic disorders of the gastrointestinal tract has also become more diverse.[72–75] In most instances, if the antigen/allergen has been identified by clinical history, RAST testing, or skin-prick testing, it is best to treat by *avoidance* of the antigen without resorting to medications. In cases of infants with milk protein allergy, for example, this will be most likely a temporary condition, and ultimate tolerance is the expected outcome in most babies by 1 year of age, provided there has been strict elimination from the diet. The limitation to this strategy is that there are non-IgE mediated adverse reactions to foods that cannot be tested for by current means. Thus, inflammation with eosinophils may be present, but all RAST testing or skin-prick testing is negative, history unrevealing, and a trial of elimination of the most common suspect or suspects may be unhelpful. In younger children, feeding exclusively a hypoallergenic amino acid-based diet may be tried. However, in older children who are not G tube dependent, and who have had a normal diet previously, this is almost impossible due to non-compliance for any significant length of time. Also, it may not be efficacious, as in many cases of eosinophilic esophagitis or eosinophilic enteritis. Steroids are usually effective, but their use is limited by side-effects. In milder cases, combination antihistamines with *H1 receptor* and *H2 receptor* antagonism has been utilized successfully in some patients, even those with idiopathic anaphylaxis to an unidentified antigen. Also *cromolyn*, which stabilizes mast cell membranes is often tried, although evidence in the literature for efficacy is limited, the agent is extremely safe.

Recent studies have supported the use of *montelukast*, a leukotriene antagonist approved in asthma, in cases with allergic-eosinophilic inflammation. Agents currently under study for allergic-eosinophilic disorders include: *omalizumab* (anti-IgE), which is effective in asthma, allergic rhinitis, and atopic dermatitis; *imantinib* (tyrosine kinase inhibitor including of c-kit), which inhibits mast cell growth factor (SCF) signaling; *mepolizulmab* (anti-IL-5), which inhibits the potent eosinophil growth factor, and *supraplast tosilate*, which inhibits IL-4 and IL-5 dependent responses. Clearly, many choices will exist for this subtype of inflammation, and it will be important to individualize therapy. Studies to improve diagnostic ability and characterization of the immune response in these disorders will further allow for individualized treatment and better outcomes in the future.

THE IMMUNOLOGY OF MUCOSAL HEALING

Healing of injury to the GI mucosa after resolution of an inflammatory process is a complex process that is still not completely understood.[66,67] Normally, the type of repair depends upon the *depth* of injury involved. In cases where only epithelial cells are lost or damaged, *restitution* of the barrier results first from adjacent epithelial cells that undergo a phenotypic change to a migratory cell that spreads out to cover the denuded area. At the same time, *myofibroblasts* contract the wound, and ultimately new *tight junctions* are formed between the epithelial cells. Cell *proliferation* occurs, in the crypts, and differentiating cells migrate up the *crypt-villus axis*. Luminal *trefoil factors*,[107] clover-shaped proteins secreted by goblet epithelial cells, and dietary factors short chain fatty acids and polyamines promote healing. Three trefoil factors (TEF-1, TEF-2, AND TEF-3) are abundant in the GI tract.[107] TEF-1 is mostly produced by the gastric pit cells, TEF-2 by gastric mucus neck cells, and TEF-3 by goblet cells of the intestines. Trefoil factors are rapidly upregulated with inflammation and critical to repair of mucosal injury, and have potential as therapy in Crohn's disease, ulcerative colitis, and other inflammatory GI disorders.[107]

Cytokines, prostaglandins, nitric oxide (made by *iNOS*) and growth factors, including epidermal growth factor (EGF), fibroblast growth factors (FGF), hepatocyte growth factor/scatter factor (HGF), keratinocyte growth factor (KGF), vascular endothelial growth factor (VEGF), transforming growth factors (TGF), and insulin-like growth factor (IGF), made by invading immune cells, platelets, and myofibroblasts promote angiogenesis and tissue repair also in deeper injury. Recombinant forms of KGF have been produced and shown to be efficacious systemically in gastrointestinal mucositis patients.[13] Recombinant EGF administered rectally has shown to heal active ulcerative colitis, but there are legitimate concerns regarding increasing risk of malignant transformation, particularly in a premalignant condition like UC, because EGF, like the other growth factors, is a tumor cell growth and invasion factor. The normal repair process in deeper injury depends to a significant degree on the *extracellular matrix,* which lies beneath the epithelial cells layer, especially prominent in the submucosa. The cellular components include smooth muscle cells, and fibroblasts that produce *fibronectin* and *collagens*, particularly collagen 1 and 4 as well as laminin, crucial support structures. Healing and remodeling depend on the actions also of *metalloproteinases*, which break down the collagen molecules. Metalloproteinase enzymes are produced by invading neutrophils and other inflammatory cells in response to activation, such as by cytokines including TNF-α. The non-cellular components of the matrix, such as heparin sulfate, also function as a vast reserve of bound, pre-synthesized cytokines and angiogenesis factors, released enzymatically by the metalloproteinases and other enzymes also from invading microbes. The normal reconstitution of the damaged mucosa is orchestrated by the ordered expression of various adhesion molecules, specifically the *integrins* (α1, α2, α3, α6), which bind not only immune cell receptors, but also components of the matrix (laminin, collagens) and the cytoskeleton (actinin, vinculin, talin) to mediate cell migration. Ultimately *myosin-actin* activation occurs via intracellular signaling

Sequence	Fold-change	Gene	Function
AI763065	74.03	REG1A	Regenerating islet-derived 1 alpha (pancreatic stone protein, pancreatic thread protein)
U33317	37.79	DEF6	Defensin 6
D17291	24.08	REG1B	Regenerating protein 1 beta
L15533	22.47	PAP	Pancreatitis associated protein
AF097021	4.76	GW112	Differentially expressed in hematopoietic lineages
AJ000342	4.14	DMBT1	Deleted in malignant brain tumors 1
X01683	3.12	SERPINA1	Serine (or cysteine) proteinase inhibitor, clade A (alpha-1 antiproteinase, antitrypsin), member 1
U31511	2.33	NOS2A	nitric oxide synthase 2A (inducible)
M22430	1.91	PLA2G2A	phospholipase A2, group IIA

[a]Most of these are involved in mucosal defense and repair.

Table 6.4 Results of Affymetrix Gene Chip analysis in colonic Crohn's disease identified genes significantly upregulated in involved *vs* uninvolved resected segments in all patients tested[a]

dependent upon changes in intracellular calcium concentrations and G protein signaling. Normally, the balance between tissue breakdown and repair is key. Inadequate collagen synthesis, such as in diabetes or hyperglycemia, leads to poor healing, while excess contributes to scarring and stricturing. Recent *gene chip* studies,[108] performed in patients with severe surgical Crohn's disease, identified additional proteins involved in the healing process that may contribute to the disease process when overexpressed (Table 6.4). *PAP* (pancreatitis associated polypeptide) and *REG-1a* and *REG-1β* mRNA expression were markedly upregulated in diseased *vs* normal appearing adjacent areas of the diseased colon, and levels in the blood stream have been correlated with disease activity/severity.

CONCLUSIONS

Much has been learned of gastrointestinal mucosal immunology and the underlying mechanisms of inflammatory diseases of the GI tract in the last decade. The recognition of the importance of innate immune factors and of tolerance and an appreciation for the complexity of the inflammatory response is particularly noteworthy. Finally, we have begun to realize the promise of molecular biology to improve the lives of children with these serious diseases of the digestive system. Continued advancement in this area over the next 10 years will allow us to tailor treatments to the individual patient, with the promise of improved outcome and fewer side-effects, as we continue to strive towards ultimate disease prevention and cure.

References

1. Srivastava MD, Walker WA. The development of the mucosal immune system in the sick neonate. In: Bellanti JA, ed. Neonatal Hematology and Immunology III. Amsterdam: Elsevier Science; 1997:127–138.
2. Lai Ping So A, Mayer L. Gastrointestinal manifestations of primary immunodeficiency disorders. Sem Gastrointest Dis 1997; 8(1):22–32.
3. Adachi S, Yoshida H, Honda K, et al. Essential role of IL-7 receptor alpha in the formation of Peyer's patch anlage. Int Immunol 1998; 10(1):1–6.
4. Srivastava MD, Lippes J, Srivastava BIS. Hepatocyte growth factor in human milk and reproductive tract fluids. Am J Reprod Immunol 1999; 42:347–354.
5. Zetterstrom R, Bennet R, Nord KE. Intestinal fecal microflora during early infancy. Influence of genetic and environmental factors. In: Bellanti JA, ed. Neonatal Hematology and Immunology III. Amsterdam: Elsevier Science; 1997: 127–138.
6. Glimore MS, Ferretti JJ. The thin line between gut commensal and pathogen. Science 2003; 299:1999–2002.
7. Rhen M, Eriksson S, Clements M, et al. The basis of persistent bacterial infections. Trends Microbiol 2003; 11:80–86.
8. Hooper LV, Gordon JJ. Commensal host bacterial relationships in the gut. Science 2001; 292:1115–1118.
9. Swidsinski A, Ladhoff A, Pernthaler A, et al. Mucosa flora in inflammatory bowel disease. Gastroenterology 2002; 122:44–54.
10. Sartor RB. Therapeutic manipulations of the enteric microflora in inflammatory bowel disease: antibiotic, probiotics, and prebiotics. Gastroenterology 2004; 126:1620–1633.
11. Steidler L. Microbiological and immunological strategies for treatment of inflammatory bowel disease. Microbes Infect 2001; 3:1157–1166.
12. Landers CJ. Selected loss of tolerance evidenced by Crohn's diseased associated immune responses to auto and microbial antigens. Gastroenterology 2002; 123:689–699.
13. Ahmad T, Tamboli CP, Jewell D, et al. Clinical relevance of advances in genetics and pharmacogenetics of IBD. Gastroenterology 2004; 126:1533–1549.
14. Bouma G, Strober W. The immunological and genetic basis of inflammatory bowel disease. Nat Rev Immunol 2003; 3:521–533.
15. Srivastava MD, Srivastava A, Brouhard B, et al. Cytokines in human milk. Res Comm Mol Pathol Pharm 1996; 93(1):263–287.
16. Armogida SA, Yannaras N, Melton AL, et al. The innate immune system in human breast milk. Allergy Asthma Proc 2004; 25(5):297–304.
17. Defensins GT. antimicrobial peptides of innate immunity. Nat Rev Immunol 2003; 3:710–720.
18. Stroinnigg N, Srivastava MD. Effect of human beta defensin-2 (HBD-2) on the innate immune system in Caco-2 colonic and MCF-7 breast epithelial cells. J Allergy Clin Immunol 2004; 113(2):S47.
19. Hamosh M, Hamosh P. Protective function of human milk. In: Bellanti JA, ed. Neonatal Hematology and Immunology III. Amsterdam: Elsevier Science; 1997:109–114.
20. Farnoud S, Evans RW. Lactoferrin – a multifactorial protein with antimicrobial properties. Mol Immunol 2003; 40:395–405.
21. Ajuebor MN, Swain MG. Role of chemokines and chemokine receptors in the gastrointestinal tract. Immunology 2002; 105:137–143.
22. Banks C, Bateman A, Payne R, Johnson P, Sheron N. Chemokine expression in IBD. Mucosal chemokine expression is unselectively increased in both ulcerative colitis and Crohn's disease. J Pathol 2003; 199:28–35.
23. Autschbach F, Giese T, Gassler N, et al. Cytokine/chemokine messenger-RNA expression profiles in ulcerative colitis and Crohn's disease. Virchows Arch 2002; 441:500–513.
24. Lien E, Ingalls RR. Toll-like receptors. Crit Care Med 2002; 30:S1–S11.
25. Akira S. Toll-like receptor signaling. J Biol Chem 2003; 278:38105–38108.
26. Otte JM, Cario E, Podolsky DK. Mechanisms of cross hyporesponsiveness to toll-like receptor bacterial ligands in intestinal epithelial cells. Gastroenterology 2004; 126:1054–1070.
27. Ueda H, Howson JWW, Esposita L, et al. Association of the T-cell regulatory gene CTLA-4 with susceptibility to autoimmune diseases. Nature 2003; 423:506–511.
28. Young NT, Uhrberg M. KIR expression shapes cytotoxic repertoires: a developmental program of survival. Trends Immunol 2002; 23:71–75.
29. Stephens HAF. MHC haplotypes , MICA genes and the wonderland of NK receptor polymorphism. Trends Immunol 2002; 23:385–386.

30. McQueen KL, Parham P. Variable receptors controlling activation and inhibition of NK cells. Curr Opin Immunol 2002; 14:615–621.
31. Jones DC, Young NT. Natural killer receptor repertoires in transplantation. Eur J Immuno Genet 2003; 30:169–176.
32. Leon F, Roldau E, Sanchez L, et al. Human small intestinal epithelium contains functional natural killer lymphocytes. Gastroenterology 2003; 125:345–356.
33. Emoto M, Kaufman SHE. Liver NKT cells: an account of heterogeneity. Trends Immunol 2003; 24:364–369.
34. Brigyl M, Bry L, Kent SC, et al. Mechanism of CD1d-restricted natural killer T cell activation during microbial infection. Nat Immunol 2003; 4:1230–1237.
35. Moretta L, Romagnani C, Pietra G, et al. NK-CTLS, a novel HLA-E restricted T cell subset. Trends Immunol 2003; 24:136–143.
36. Barton LL, Moussa SL, Villar RG, et al. Gastrointestinal complications of chronic granulomatous disease: a case report and literature review. Clin Pediatr 1998; 37(4):231–236.
37. Rutgeerts P, Asche GV, Vermere S. Optimizing anti-TNF treatment in inflammatory bowel disease. Gastroenterology 2004; 126:1593–1610.
38. Scott MG, Hancock EW. Cationic antimicrobial peptides and their multifactorial role in the immune system. Crit Rev Immunol 2000; 20:407–431.
39. Hase K, Murakami M, Imura M, et al. Expression of LL-37 by human gastric epithelial cells as a potential host defense mechanism against Helicobacter pylori. Gastroenterology 2003; 125:1613–1625.
40. Garcia JRC, Krause A, Schulz S, et al. Human β-defensin 4: a novel inducible peptide with a specific salt sensitive spectrum of antimicrobial activity. FASEB J 2001; 15:1819–1821.
41. Harder J, Bartels J, Chrostophers E, et al. Isolation and characterization of human beta defensin 3, a novel human inducible peptide antibiotic. J Biol Chem 2001; 276:5707–5713.
42. Hamanaka Y, Nakashima M, Wada A, et al. Expression of human β-defensin 2 (HBD-2) in Helicobacter pylori induced gastritis: antibacterial effect of HBD-2 against Helicobacter pylori. Gut 2001; 49:481–487.
43. Cunliffe RN. α-defensins in the gastrointestinal tract. Mol Immunol 2003; 40:463–467.
44. Yang D, Chertiv O, Oppenheim JJ. Participation of mammalian defensins and cathelicidins in antimicrobial immunity: receptors and activities of human defensins and cathelicidin (LL-37). J Leukocyte Biol 2001; 69:691–697.
45. Kaiser V, Diamond G. Expression of mammalian defensin genes. J Leukocyte Biol 2000; 68:779–784.
46. Risso A. Leukocyte anti-microbial peptides: multifactorial effector molecules of innate immunity. J Leukocyte Biol 2000; 68:785–792.
47. Yang D, Chen Q, Chertov O, Oppenheim JJ. Human neutrophils defensins selectively chemoattract naïve and immature dendritic cells. J Leukocyte Biol 2000; 68:9–14.
48. Cunliffe RN, Kamal M, Rose FRAJ, James PD, Mahida YR. Expression of antimicrobial neutrophil defensins in epithelial cells of active inflammatory bowel disease mucosa. J Clin Pathol 2002; 55:298–304.
49. Sartor RB. Therapeutic manipulation of the enteric microflora in inflammatory bowel disease: antibiotics, probiotics, and prebiotics. Gastroenterol 2004; 126:1620–1633.
50. Hart A, Al-Hassi HO, Kamm M, et al. Toll-like receptors 2 and 4 are upregulated on human lamina propria dendritic cells in intestinal inflammation. Gastroenterology 2004; 126:A148–A149.
51. Lee SK, Stack A, Katzowitsch E, et al. Helicobacter pylori flagellins have very low intrinsic activity to stimulate human gastric epithelial cells via TLR-5. Microbes Infect 2003; 5:135–136.
52. Melmed G, Thomas LS, Lee N, et al. Human intestinal epithelial cells are broadly unresponsive to toll-like receptor 2 dependent bacterial ligands: implications for host-microbial interactions in the gut. J Immunol 2003; 170:1406–1415.
53. Abreu M, Vora TP, Faure E, et al. Decreased expression of Toll-like receptor 4 and MD2 correlates with intestinal epithelial cell protection against dysregulated proinflammatory gene expression in response to bacterial lipopolysaccharide. J Immunol 2001; 167:1609–1616.
54. Ayabe T, Ashida T, Kobayashi S, et al. Upregulation of toll-like receptor 2 expression in intestinal Paneth cells in patients with Crohn's disease. Gastroenterology 2004; 126:A-3.
55. Yamamoto M, Takeda K, Akira S. TIR domain containing adaptors define the specificity of TLR signaling. Mol Immunol 2004; 40:861–868.
56. Bernasconi NL, Onai N, Lanzavecchia A. A role for Toll-like receptors in acquired immunity: upregulation of TLR-9 by BCR triggering in naïve B cells and constitutive expression in memory B cells. Blood 2003; 101:4500–4504.
57. Bourke E, Bosisio D, Golay J, et al. The toll-like receptor repertoire of human B lymphocytes: inducible and selective expression of TLR9 and TLR10 in normal and transformed cells. Blood 2003; 102:956–963.
58. Heil F, Hemmi H, Hochrein H, et al. Species specific recognition of single stranded RNA via toll-like receptors 7 and 8. Science 2004; 303:1526–1529.
59. Girardin SE, Sansonetti PJ, Philpot DJ. Intracellular vs extracellular recognition of pathogens-common concepts in mammals and flies. Trends Microbiol 2002; 10:193–199.
60. Lesage S, Zouali H, Cezard JP, et al. CARD15/NOD2 mutational analysis and genotype-phenotype correlation in 612 patients with inflammatory bowel disease. Am J Hum Genet 2002; 70:845–857.
61. Cuthbert AP, Fisher SA, Mirza MM, et al. The contribution of NOD2 gene mutations to the risk and site of disease in inflammatory bowel disease. Gastroenterology 2002; 122:867–874.
62. Heshima K. CCL28 has dual roles in mucosal immunity as a chemokine with broad spectrum antimicrobial activity. J Immunol 2003; 170:1452–1461.
63. Moser B, Wolf M, Walz A, et al. Chemokines: multiple levels of leukocyte migration control. Trends Immunol 2004; 25:75–84.
64. Schwartz R. Shattuck Lecture: Diversity of the immune repertoire and immunoregulation. N Engl J Med 2003; 348:1017–1026.
65. Loftus EV. Clinical epidemiology of inflammatory bowel disease: incidence, prevalence, and environmental influences. Gastroenterology 2004; 126:1504–1517.
66. Mamman JM, Matthews JB. Mucosal repair in the gastrointestinal tract. Crit Care Med 2003; 31(8):S532–S537.
67. Mb W, Barbul A. Repair of full-thickness bowel injury. Crit Care Med 2003; 31(8):S538–S546.
68. Basik M, Mousses S, Trent J. Integration of genomic technologies for accelerated cancer drug development. BioTechniques 2003; 35:580–593.

69. Yowe D, Cook WJ, Ramos JCG. Microarrays for studying the host transcriptional response to microbial infection and for the identification of host targets. Microbes Infect 2001; 3:813–821.
70. Dieckgraefe B, Stenson W, Krzenik JR, Swanson P, Harrington C. Analysis of mucosal gene expression in inflammatory bowel disease by parallel oligonucleotide arrays. Phys Genomics 2000; 4:1–11.
71. Lawrence IC, Fiocchi C, Chakravarti S. Ulcerative colitis and Crohn's disease: distinctive gene expression profiles and novel susceptibility candidate genes. Hum Mol Genet 2001; 10:445–456.
72. Teitelbaum JE, Fox VL, Twarog FJ, et al. Eosinophilic esophagitis in children: immunopathological analysis and response to fluticasone propionate. Gastroenterology 2002; 122(5):1216–1225.
73. Rothenberg ME, Mishra A, Collins MH, Putnam PE. Pathogenesis and clinical features of eosinophilic esophagitis. J Allergy Clin Immunol 2001; 108(6):891–894.
74. Straumann A, Bauer M, Fischer B, Blaser K, Simon HU. Idiopathic eosinophilic esophagitis is associated with a TH2-type allergic inflammatory response. J Allergy Clin Immunol 2001; 108(6):954–961.
75. Butt AM, Murch SH, Ng CL, et al. Upregulated exotoxin expression and T cell infiltration in the basal and papillary epithelium in cow's milk associated reflux esophagitis. Arch Dis Child 2002; 87(2):124–130.
76. Mishra A, Hogan SP, Brandt EB, Rothenber ME. IL-5 promotes eosinophil trafficking to the esophagus. J Immunol 2002; 168(5):2464–2469.
77. Bandeira-Melo C, Sugiyama K, Woods LJ, Phoofolo M, Center DM, Cruikshank WW, Weller PF. IL-16 promotes leukotriene C4 and IL-4 release from human eosinophils via CD4 and autocrine CCR3-chemokine mediated signaling. J Immunol 2002; 168(9):4756–4763.
78. Dubucquoi S, Janin A, Klein O, et al. Activated eosinophils and interleukin-5 expression in early recurrence of Crohn's disease. Gut 1995; 37(2):242–246.
79. Levy AM, Gleich GJ, Sandborn WJ, et al. Increased eosinophil granule proteins in gut lavage fluid from patients with inflammatory bowel disease. Mayo Clin Proc 1997; 72(2):117–123.
80. Ghosh S, Goldin E, Gordon F, et al. Natalizumab for active Crohn's disease. N Engl J Med 2003; 348:24–32.
81. Pizarro TT, Michie MH, Bentz M, et al. IL-18 a novel immunoregulatory cytokine is up-regulated in Crohn's disease: expression and localization in intestinal mucosal cells. J Immunol 1999; 162(11):6829–6835.
82. Sands BE. From symptoms to diagnosis: clinical distinctions among various forms of intestinal inflammation. Gastroenterology 2004; 126:1518–1532.
83. Kirkegaard T, Hansen A, Bruun E, et al. Expression and localization of matrix metalloproteinases and their natural inhibitors in fistulae of patients with Crohn's disease. Gut 2004; 53(5):701–709.
84. Hermon-Taylor J, Barnes N, Clarke C, Finlayson C. Mycobacterium paratuberculosis cervical lymphadenitis followed five years later by terminal ileitis similar to Crohn's disease. BMJ 1998; 516:449–453.
85. El-Zaatari F, Osata MS, Graham DY. Etiology of Crohn's disease: the role of Mycobacterium avium paratuberculosis. Trends Mol Med 2001; 7:247–252.
86. Srivastava BIS, Srivastava MD. A novel more rapid method for the detection and discrimination of Mycobacterium avium subspecies avium and Mycobacterium avium subspecies paratuberculosis. FASEB J 2003; 17:A664–A665.
87. Amonsin A, Li LL, Zhang Q, Bannantine JP, et al. Multilocus short sequence repeat sequencing approach for differentiating among Mycobacterium avium subspecies paratuberculosis strains. J Clin Microbiol 2004; 42:1694–1702.
88. Motiwala AS, Amonsin A, Strother M, et al. Molecular epidemiology of mycobacterium avium subspecies paratuberculosis isolates recovered from wild animal species. J Clin Microbiol 2004; 42:1703–1712.
89. Lodes MJ, Cong Y, Elson CO, et al. Bacterial flagellin is a dominant antigen in Crohn's disease. J Clin Invest 2004; 113(9):1296–1305.
90. Dalwadi H, Wei B, Kronenberg M, et al. The Crohn's disease associated bacterial protein 12 is a novel enteric T cell superantigen. Immunity 2001; 15:149–158.
91. Seegert D, Rosenstiel P, Pfahler H, Pfefferkorn P, Nikolaus S, Schreiber S. Increased expression of IL-16 in inflammatory bowel disease. Gut 2001; 48(3):326–332.
92. Kim SC, Ferry GD. Inflammatory bowel disease in pediatric and adolescent patients: clinical, therapeutic and psychological considerations. Gastroenterology 2004; 126:1550–1560.
93. Mocellin S, Panelli M, Wang E, et al. The dual role of IL-10. Trends Immunol 2003; 24(1):36–43.
94. Hanauer SB. Medical therapy of ulcerative colitis. Gastroenterology 2004; 126:1582–1592.
95. Egan LJ, Sandborn WJ. Advances in the treatment of Crohn's disease. Gastroenterology 2004; 126:1574–1581.
96. Gewirtz AT, Sitaram S. Alicaforsen Isis Pharmaceuticals. Curr Opin Invest Drugs 2001; 2(10):1401–1406.
97. Mackay IR, Rosen FS. Immunomodulation of autoimmune and inflammatory diseases with intravenous immune globulin. N Engl J Med 2001; 345(10):747–755.
98. Remick DG. Cytokine therapeutic for the treatment of sepsis: why has nothing worked? Curr Pharm 2003; 9(1):75–82.
99. Dredge K, Marriott JB, Dalgleish G. Immunological effects of thalidomide and its chemical and functional analogs. Crit Rev Immunol 2002; 22:425–437.
100. Baidas S, Tfayli A, Bhargava P. Thalidomide, an old drug with new clinical applications. Cancer Invest 2002; 20:835–848.
101. Dredge K, Marriott JB, Dalgleish AG. Immunological effects of thalidomide and its chemical and functional analogs. Crit Rev Immunol 2002; 22:425–437.
102. Milsom JW, Hammerhofer KA, Bohm B, et al. Prospective, randomized trial comparing laparoscopic vs. conventional surgery for refractory ileocolic Crohn's disease. Dis Colon Rectum 2001; 44(1):1–9.
103. Sugiura T, Waku K. Cannabinoid receptors and their endogenous ligands. J Biochem 2002; 132:7–12.
104. Massa F, Marsicano G, Hermann H, et al. The endogenous cannabinoid system protects against colonic inflammation. J Clin Invest 2004; 113:1202–1209.
105. Ligresti A, Bisogno T, Matias J, et al. Possible endocannabinoid control of colorectal cancer growth. Gastroenterology 2003; 125:677–687.
106. Srivastava MD, Srivastava BIS, Brouhard B. Delta-9-tetrahydrocannabinol and cannabidiol alter cytokine production by human immune cells. Immunopharmacology 1998; 40:179–185.
107. Taupin D, Podolsky DK. Trefoil factors: initiators of mucosal healing. Mol Cell Biol 2003; 4:721–732.

108. Srivastava MD, Kulaylat M. Affymetrix gene chip analysis with RT-PCR confirmation identifies massive upregulation of HD5, HD6, GST, PDECGF, I-BABP, REG-1β, PAP, PreApo A4, Apo A1, and Apo B100 involved versus uninvolved segments of Crohn's Colitis. J Pediatr Gastroenterol Nutr 2001; 33(3):370.

Further Reading

Yuan Q, Walker WA. Innate immunity of the gut: mucosal defense in health an disease. J Pediatr Gastroenterol Nutr 2004; 38(5):463–473.

Mayer L, Shao L. Therapeutic potential of oral tolerance. Nat Rev Immunol 2004; 4(6):407–419.

Lichtenstein GR. Medical therapy of inflammatory bowel disease. Gastroenterol Clin North Am 2004; 33(2):XV–XVI.

SECTION TWO
CLINICAL PROBLEMS

SECTION TWO
CLINICAL PROBLEMS

Chapter 7
Chronic abdominal pain of childhood and adolescence

Lori A. Mahajan and Barbara Kaplan

INTRODUCTION

Despite almost five decades of research, chronic abdominal pain of childhood and adolescence remains a common and oftentimes challenging affliction for patients, their families and healthcare providers. The term 'recurrent abdominal pain' (RAP) was derived from the British pediatrician John Apley's pioneering study of 1000 school children in the 1950s.[1] He characterized abdominal pain as chronic or recurrent if at least one episode of pain occurs per month for three consecutive months and is severe enough to interfere with routine functioning. Initial studies indicated that chronic abdominal pain affects 10–15% of school-age children; however, more recent data suggests that approximately 20% of middle school and high school students experience abdominal pain on a daily to weekly basis.[1,2]

Many classification schemes for recurrent abdominal pain have been proposed over the past several decades. Most commonly, the pain is classified as either organic or non-organic, depending on whether a discrete cause is identified. Non-organic RAP or 'functional' recurrent abdominal pain (FRAP), refers to abdominal pain that cannot be explained on the basis of biochemical or structural abnormalities. FRAP is not synonymous with psychogenic or imaginary abdominal pain, but it is generally accepted to represent genuine pain. Recent efforts have led to the development of a symptom-based diagnostic classification system for the functional gastrointestinal disorders in children and adults, known as the Rome II criteria.[3] Using these criteria, a positive diagnosis of a functional gastrointestinal disorder is made as opposed to the former method of diagnosis in which a functional disorder was only considered as a diagnosis of exclusion. These criteria are detailed later in this chapter.

Early investigators found an organic cause for RAP in only 5%–10% of patients.[1] Progressive refinement of endoscopic techniques and radiologic imaging modalities as well as the advent of newer technologies such as breath hydrogen testing, motility studies and wireless capsule endoscopy have greatly enhanced our ability to identify organic causes of RAP. As a result, the percentage of patients with FRAP appears to be decreasing. A study by Hyams and associates examined 227 children with RAP. A total of 76 patients (33%) were found to have definable causes of RAP such as inflammatory bowel disease, carbohydrate malabsorption, peptic inflammation, or celiac disease.[4]

The possibility of overlooking a serious organic condition is of most concern to the physician and family, oftentimes making the formulation of a credible diagnostic and management strategy quite taxing. In the search for the etiology of the abdominal pain, the pediatric patient is at risk for extensive, possibly invasive and expensive diagnostic testing as well as therapeutic interventions that may not be without side-effects or long-term complications. This chapter offers an approach to the diagnosis and care of pediatric patients with recurrent abdominal pain that emphasizes a basic screening evaluation for possible organic etiologies, the use of new diagnostic strategies that incorporate symptom-based criteria for functional gastrointestinal disorders, and options for symptom monitoring and management.

Epidemiology

Because the precise pathogenesis of recurrent abdominal pain in pediatric patients has remained unclear for decades, many researchers have turned to epidemiology for insight. In Apley's original survey of 1000 unselected children in primary and secondary schools, 10.8% of children were found to have recurrent abdominal pain.[1] There was a slight female predominance with a female-to-male ratio of those affected of 1.3:1. Of note, there were no complaints of pain in children younger than 5 years of age. Between 10% and 12% of males ages 5 to 10 years had recurrent abdominal pain, followed by a decline in incidence with a later peak at age 14 years. In contrast, however, females had a sharp rise in the incidence of recurrent abdominal pain after age 8 years, with more than 25% of all females affected at age 9 years, followed by a steady decline. More recently, Hyams and colleagues studied 507 adolescents in a suburban town in the USA.[2] The researchers found that abdominal pain occurred at least weekly in 13–17% of adolescents, but that only half of these individuals had sought medical attention within the preceding year. Thus, the incidence of RAP is likely higher than clinical experience would lead us to believe. Sociocultural, familial and cognitive-behavioral factors help determine the response of the child and family to the pain and affect the likelihood of seeking medical attention.

Family history

A significantly higher proportion of children with FRAP have relatives with alcoholism, conduct or antisocial disorder, attention deficit disorder, or somatization disorder when compared with children with organically based abdominal pain.[5] The patient often comes from a 'painful family' (i.e. family members have a high frequency of medical complaints).[1,6] The parents and siblings of patients with FRAP have an increased incidence of recurrent abdominal complaints, mental health disorders, and migraines when compared with controls. Stone and Barbero found that 44% of fathers and 56% of mothers of patients with FRAP had been diagnosed with medical illnesses.[6] Approximately 46% of these fathers with medical conditions had gastrointestinal illness and 10% had migraines. Similarly, half of the mothers had gastrointestinal complaints diagnosed as 'functional' by their physician, and 10% carried the diagnosis of migraine headaches. In addition, approximately 25% of the mothers with a child with FRAP have a mild level of psychiatric depression. It is unclear whether the mother's feelings result from having a child with FRAP or whether the mother's emotional state contributes to the child's development of pain.[7]

Perinatal and past medical history

The mothers of patients with FRAP report that their pregnancies were characterized by excessive nausea, emesis, fatigue, or headaches. Difficult labor and delivery with breech presentation or cesarean section is reported in 20–31%. Neonatal difficulty, including respiratory distress, infection, or colic, is reported in 20%. The child's past history may also reveal recurrent nightmares, toilet training difficulties and enuresis.[6,8]

Pathophysiology of functional recurrent abdominal pain

Chronic abdominal pain is a multi-factorial experience currently believed to result from a complex interaction between psychosocial and physiologic factors via the brain-gut axis. Functional recurrent abdominal pain is thought to result from alterations in the neurophysiologic functioning at the level of the gut, spinal afferents, central autonomic relay system and/or brain. Alterations along this pain axis are thought to result in central nervous system amplification of incoming visceral afferent signals resulting in hyper-responsiveness to both physiologic and noxious stimuli. This failure of down regulation and concomitant pain amplification has come to be known as *visceral hypersensitivity*.[9]

The precise cause of visceral hypersensitivity in patients with functional recurrent abdominal pain is not yet clear. Researchers currently believe that transient noxious stimuli, such as mucosal infection or injury, can alter the synaptic efficiency of peripheral and central neurons.[10] This may occur through altered release of serotonin (5-HT) from the enteroenteric cells in the myenteric plexus and/or the release of inflammatory cytokines from activated immune/inflammatory cells following exposure. Through a process known as the *wind up*, neurons can develop a *pain memory* than can persist long after the removal of the noxious stimulus.

For many years, functional abdominal pain was considered a motility disorder. Pineiro-Carrero and colleagues demonstrated that patients with FRAP had more frequent migrating motor complexes with slower propagation velocities compared with healthy controls.[11] In addition, these patients also had high-pressure duodenal contractions that were associated with abdominal pain during the study period. Subsequently, Hyman and co-workers identified manometric abnormalities in 89% of pediatric patients with FRAP undergoing antroduodenal manometry.[12] Years of subsequent research in adult and pediatric patients, however, have led to the conclusion that although patients with functional abdominal pain have motility abnormalities, no specific pattern of motility disturbance is diagnostic for any subgroup of patients.

Psychosocial factors have also been extensively studied with regards to the development and perpetuation of functional recurrent abdominal pain. Early life factors such as family attitude toward illness, abuse history and major loss may significantly influence a person's psychosocial development and thereby their coping skills, social support systems and susceptibility to life stress. Particular personality traits and family psychosocial dynamics have been identified in association with functional recurrent abdominal pain of childhood. Children with FRAP are frequently timid, nervous, or anxious and are often described as perfectionists or overachievers.[8] Measures of intelligence in these children have not been found to differ significantly from those of controls. Birth order has been thought to possibly contribute to the development of symptoms, because children with FRAP are typically the first- or last-born in the family.[6,8]

Research shows that children with FRAP, like behaviorally disordered children, experience more life stressors than healthy controls.[13] Mother, teacher and child self-report questionnaires indicate that children with FRAP have higher levels of emotional distress and internalize problems more often than asymptomatic children.[14] Children with FRAP, however, have not been found to have an increased incidence of depression or other psychological disorders when compared with children with chronic abdominal pain of organic etiology.[7,15] Raymer and colleagues found that psychological distress accompanies both organic and non-organic abdominal pain in pediatric patients and that psychological evaluation does not readily distinguish organic from functional pain.[15]

The child's home environment has also been found to greatly influence the child's FRAP. Parents relate the onset of pain to significant events such as family disturbance, excitement or punishment approximately 70% of the time. Marital discord with excessive arguing and/or violence, separation or divorce is found in almost 40% of affected families. Also, extreme parenting techniques such as excessive punishment or parental oversubmissiveness have been commonly identified in these families.[6,16]

EVALUATION OF THE CHILD WITH CHRONIC ABDOMINAL PAIN

The initial evaluation of the child with chronic abdominal pain should include a comprehensive interview with the child and parents, a thorough physical examination and specific screening laboratory studies. In addition to performing the evaluation, the physician must also convey genuine concern and establish a trusting and supportive environment. The clinician must ensure that adequate time is allotted for this process.

History

As with any other medical condition, a thorough and detailed history is the most important component of the patient's assessment and often leads to the correct diagnosis. Initial questions should be directed at the patient, using a developmentally appropriate technique. It is important to hear the patient's complaints in his or her own words and to minimize parental influence on patient response to questions. Ask the patient to indicate with his or her own hand the location of the pain. It is not helpful when the entire hand is swept diffusely across the abdomen, but it may be helpful when one finger is used to localize an area of pain.

Information should be sought regarding the quality, intensity, duration and timing of the pain. Sharp pain suggests a cutaneous or more superficial structural origin; poorly localized pain is more characteristic of a visceral or functional etiology. Inquire how well the patient sleeps at night. Pain that awakens the patient from sleep usually indicates organic disease. Temporal correlation of the abdominal pain and other symptoms such as emesis, diarrhea, constipation or fever are also suggestive of organic disease. In addition, ask whether there is any relationship between the pain and food consumption, activity, posture or psychosocial stressors.

Medications, including prescription and over-the-counter products, should be accurately recorded. Ask whether the child started taking such products prior to the onset of the abdominal pain. This is of particular importance in patients with conditions such as juvenile rheumatoid arthritis or recurrent headaches who regularly use non-steroidal anti-inflammatory medications for pain relief, because these medications are known to cause both gastritis and mucosal ulceration. Also, ask whether medications have been taken in an attempt to relieve the child's abdominal pain, and if so, how efficacious they were. Transient improvement following a laxative may indicate chronic constipation as the cause of the recurrent pain. Temporary relief following antacids may indicate peptic inflammation as the etiology.

Physical examination

The physical examination should begin during the history gathering process. The physician should carefully note the patient's facial expressions, respiratory pattern, body positioning and movements. Also, it is imperative to carefully note how the child interacts with family members during the interview and how he or she climbs onto and down from the examination table. It is usually reassuring when the patient energetically jumps from the table following the examination.

The importance of performing a meticulous physical examination cannot be overemphasized. To facilitate a thorough examination, all clothing should be removed and the patient placed in a gown. It is important for the examiner to carefully cover the patient to maintain modesty and prevent embarrassment. The physical examination should be performed with the parents present. This often makes the child more comfortable and allows the parents to appreciate the thoroughness of the examination. The older child or adolescent may prefer that only the same-sex parent remain in the room during the examination. It is usually best to ask the patient what would make him or her the most comfortable.

The clinician should carefully review the child's growth parameters using standard charts. Normal growth is reassuring and is a consistent finding in children with functional recurrent abdominal pain. In contrast, growth failure or weight loss is suggestive of an organic etiology. Typically, patients with functional abdominal pain do not exhibit significant autonomic arousal. The presence of diaphoresis, tachycardia or elevated systolic blood pressure may actually suggest an acute organic etiology of the abdominal complaints.

Particular attention should be given to the abdominal examination. It is essential to an adequate examination that the patient is as relaxed as possible, room lighting is adequate, and the abdomen is fully exposed from the xiphoid to the symphysis pubis. Before laying hands on the abdomen, carefully inspect the abdomen for the presence of distention, peristaltic waves, striae, dilated vessels, or scars indicative of previous surgery. Next, the character of the bowel sounds should be assessed. High-pitched, frequent bowel sounds may indicate a partial bowel obstruction; hypoactive bowel sounds are consistent with an ileus. While auscultating the abdomen, slight compression with the stethoscope should be applied over the area of complaint to help grade the severity of the pain.

Detailed palpation of the entire abdomen should then be performed to evaluate organ size, presence or absence of masses, or any areas of tenderness. Carnett's test can be performed to aid in distinguishing visceral or somatic pain from central hypervigilance.[17] Once the region of maximal abdominal pain is identified, the patient is asked to assume a partial sitting position, thereby flexing the abdominal wall musculature. Increased abdominal pain (a positive test) is suggestive of a muscle wall etiology (a hernia or cutaneous nerve entrapment) or a CNS contribution to the pain; whereas, a negative test is consistent with a visceral contribution to the pain. Because frequently identified organic causes of chronic abdominal pain in children are localized to the urinary tract, careful attention must be given to each flank in an attempt to detect tenderness.

Hernial orifices should be carefully examined. The perianal region must be thoroughly inspected for fissures, fistulae or skin tags. Digital rectal examination is mandatory to assess external anal sphincter tone, the size of the rectal vault, volume and consistency of stool present in the rectal vault and hemoccult status of the stool. Because the child is often free of abdominal pain at the time of the initial examination, it is important to re-examine the child during an episode of abdominal pain.

Laboratory and imaging studies

Laboratory, radiologic, endoscopic and ancillary evaluation of the patient with chronic abdominal pain should be individualized according to the information obtained during the history and physical examination. Most authors, however, recommend the following studies as an initial screen for all patients with recurrent abdominal pain: complete blood count with differential, urinalysis with culture, serum aminotransferases, erythrocyte sedimentation rate and fecal examination for ova and parasites.[18–20] It has been suggested that these screening studies, if normal, in combination with a normal physical examination, effectively rule out an organic cause in 95% of cases.[20] Other non-invasive studies such as lactose breath hydrogen testing and abdominal ultrasound should be performed if indicated. Ultrasound has gained a prominent role over the past decade because it is painless and does not involve radiation. Three separate studies to investigate the diagnostic value of routine abdominal ultrasound in children with recurrent abdominal pain, however, have failed to demonstrate its utility in this clinical setting.[21–23] In these studies, a total of 217 patients were evaluated. A total of 16 patients were found to have abnormalities identified by abdominal ultrasound, but in no case could the pain be attributed to the abnormality. Thus, the ultrasound did not influence management. In addition, one author suggested that the ultrasound may have even been detrimental when findings such as accessory uterine horn, a uterus small for age, and absence of an ovary were identified, because these caused anxiety and prompted further unnecessary consultation.[23]

- Gastrointestinal
  - Esophagitis (peptic, eosinophilic, infectious)
  - Gastritis (peptic, eosinophilic, infectious)
  - Peptic ulcer
  - Celiac disease
  - Malrotation (with Ladd's bands or intermittent volvulus)
  - Duplications
  - Polyps
  - Hernias (diaphragmatic, internal, umbilical, inguinal)
  - Inflammatory bowel disease
  - Chronic constipation
  - Parasitic infection
  - Bezoar or foreign body
  - Carbohydrate malabsorption
  - Intussusception
  - Tumor (e.g. lymphoma)
- Hepatobiliary/pancreatic
  - Biliary dyskinesia
  - Sphincter of Oddi dysfunction
  - Chronic hepatitis
  - Cholelithiasis
  - Cholecystitis
  - Choledochal cyst
  - Chronic pancreatitis
  - Pancreatic pseudocyst
- Respiratory
  - Infection, inflammation or tumor near diaphragm
- Genitourinary
  - Ureteropelvic junction obstruction/hydronephrosis
  - Nephrolithiasis
  - Recurrent pyelonephritis/cystitis
  - Hematocolpos
  - Mittelschmerz
  - Endometriosis
- Metabolic/hematologic
  - Porphyria
  - Hereditary angioedema
  - Diabetes mellitus
  - Lead poisoning
  - Sickle cell disease
  - Collagen vascular disease
- Musculoskeletal
  - Trauma, tumor, infection of vertebral column (e.g. leukemia, herpes zoster, discitis)

Table 7.1 Organic causes of chronic abdominal pain

DIFFERENTIAL DIAGNOSIS

More than 100 causes of abdominal pain have been identified in children and adolescents. Table 7.1 lists many of these causes by organ system. The following discussion briefly reviews the more commonly identified organic causes of recurrent abdominal pain of childhood as well as more recent diagnostic considerations, including eosinophilic esophagitis and biliary dyskinesia. Table 7.2 lists 'alarm features' that are suggestive of an organic etiology of symptoms in children with RAP.

Peptic disease

Peptic disease refers not only to ulcer formation in the stomach and duodenum, but also to gastroesophageal reflux disease, gastritis and duodenitis. Ulcers are typically associated with underlying systemic illness in children younger than age 10 years. Gastric ulcers may occur in association with extensive burn injuries, head trauma and ingestion of non-steroidal anti-inflammatory medications, selective COX 2 inhibitors, or corticosteroids. Such ulcers usually do not recur, and there is typically no family history of ulcer disease. In contrast, ulcers in older children usually occur in the absence of underlying illness or medication usage. A positive family history can often be elicited. Such ulcers are often recurrent and have been associated with antral colonization with *H. pylori*.[24] Epidemiologic studies show that the rate of acquisition of *H. pylori* increases with age, is higher in blacks than whites and is inversely proportional to socioeconomic status.[25] Intrafamilial clustering of *H. pylori* infection has been found, suggesting person-to-person spread of the bacteria.[26] Because *H. pylori* IgG seropositivity has a sensitivity and specificity of only 45–50% in children,

History
Patient age <5 years
Constitutional symptoms: fever, weight loss, joint symptoms, recurrent oral ulcers
Emesis, particularly if bile- or blood stained
Nocturnal symptoms that awaken child from sleep
Pain well localized away from the umbilicus
Referred pain to the back, shoulders, or extremities
Dysuria, hematuria, or flank pain
Chronic medication use: NSAIDs, herbals
Family medical history of IBD, peptic ulcer disease, celiac disease, atopy
Physical examination
Growth deceleration, delayed puberty
Scleral icterus/jaundice, pale conjunctivae/pallor
Rebound, guarding, organomegaly
Perianal disease (tags, fissures, fistulae)
Occult or gross blood in stool
Screening laboratory studies
Elevated WBC or ESR
Anemia
Hypoalbuminemia

Table 7.2 Alarm features suggestive of organic etiology in child with RAP

it is not recommended.[27] The 13C-urea breath test is a noninvasive method for diagnosis of *H. pylori*. Although it has been found to have a sensitivity of 100% and specificity of 92% in children, it does not confirm the presence of an ulcer or gastritis. For this reason, endoscopy and antral biopsy remains the preferred method of diagnosis of *H. pylori* infection in pediatric patients.[27] A recent study investigated the accuracy of the *H. pylori* stool antigen test for the detection of infection in children living in the USA. The authors concluded that the polyclonal antibody test has a sensitivity of only 67% for infection in children in the USA and at present cannot replace histologic findings as the gold standard diagnostic test.[28] The breath test remains a valuable tool to monitor eradication of the organism following therapy.

The vast majority of pediatric patients with peptic disease present with RAP. Abdominal pain secondary to peptic ulceration in adult patients is considered classic if it is located in the epigastric region, occurs following meals, and awakens the patient in the early morning hours. Pain experienced by children younger than age 12 years is atypical and occurs anywhere in the middle to upper abdomen, is unrelated to meals, and has no periodicity. The presenting complaints in children older than age 12 years with peptic disease are similar to the classic adult pattern.[29] Endoscopy is the procedure of choice when mucosal abnormalities are suspected, because contrast radiography of the upper gastrointestinal tract has been found to be unreliable for establishing the diagnosis of peptic ulcer disease in children.

Carbohydrate intolerance

Dietary carbohydrates that are malabsorbed serve as substrates for bacterial fermentation in the colon. By-products of bacterial fermentation include hydrogen, carbon dioxide and volatile fatty acids such as acetate, propionate and butyrate. The resultant clinical symptoms include abdominal cramping, bloating with abdominal distention, diarrhea and excessive flatulence.[30]

Malabsorption of lactose is widely recognized as a cause of gastrointestinal distress. The prevalence of lactose malabsorption varies widely among different races, with the lowest prevalence found in Scandinavia and Northwestern Europe. In sharp contrast, between 70–100% of North American Indians, Australian aboriginal populations, and inhabitants of Southeast Asia are lactose intolerant. There is also a high prevalence in those of Italian, Turkish and African descent.[31,32] Historical information regarding the temporal relationship of lactose consumption to clinical symptoms has been found to be a poor predictor of the presence of lactose intolerance.[33] The least invasive means to establish the diagnosis of lactose malabsorption is breath hydrogen testing. If the test is positive, a strict lactose elimination diet for 2 weeks and maintenance of an abdominal pain diary is advised. Complete resolution of abdominal complaints confirms lactase deficiency as the cause. Subsequently, lactose can be reintroduced into the diet and the patient supplemented with lactase during periods of lactose consumption to minimize symptoms.[30]

Fructose and sorbitol are also common dietary carbohydrates that may be malabsorbed. Fructose-containing foods include fruits, fruit juices and honey. The fruits highest in fructose include apples (5 g/100 g of apple) and pears (5–6.5g/100g of pear). The fructose contents of apple and pear juice are comparable (6 g/100 ml of juice). Excessive intake of these products may lead to abdominal pain in susceptible individuals and should be discouraged. Sorbitol is a polyalcohol sugar commonly found in 'sugar-free' gums and confections. It is poorly absorbed by the small intestinal mucosa and has been shown to cause chronic abdominal pain in children.[34]

Celiac disease

Celiac disease or gluten-sensitive enteropathy is becoming an increasingly recognized cause of RAP in both the pediatric and adult populations. It is a chronic inflammatory disorder of the small intestine caused by exposure to dietary gluten in genetically susceptible individuals. Although the typical presentation involves diarrhea, steatorrhea, iron deficiency anemia, abdominal distention and failure to thrive, latent or atypical forms of the disease are becoming more commonplace. Patients may present at any age with nonspecific abdominal complaints. Previous figures from the USA suggested that the condition is relatively rare with a prevalence of 1:6000. In a recent study of 2000 healthy blood donors in Baltimore, MD, who were screened for anti-gliadin (AGA) and IgA endomysial antibodies (EMA), the estimated prevalence of celiac disease was 1:300, suggesting that a large number of Americans with celiac sprue are undiagnosed.[35,36] Known predisposing factors in the pediatric population include trisomy 21 and insulin-dependent diabetes mellitus.

Serologic tests currently available serve as excellent screening tools. IgA antiendomysial antibodies are currently the best serologic test for celiac sprue with a sensitivity greater than 90% and a specificity approaching 100%.[37] Alternatively, a tissue transglutaminase enzyme-linked immunosorbent assay, reported to have a sensitivity of 95% and specificity of 94% may be ordered.[38] Because up to 3% of individuals with celiac sprue have selective IgA deficiency, IgA levels should be measured. In the IgA deficient individual, less specific antigliadin IgG antibodies or tissue transglutaminase IgG antibodies are ordered. Unfortunately, the positive predictive value of gliadin antibodies is relatively poor. In one series, the positive predictive value of gliadin IgG corrected for its expected prevalence in the general population was less than 2%.[39] The gold standard for diagnosis remains upper endoscopy with biopsy of the distal duodenum/proximal jejunum. Diagnostic histologic findings include total or subtotal villous atrophy, lowering of the villous height to crypt depth ratio (normal, 3 to 5:1), an increase in intraepithelial lymphocytes (normal, 10 to 30 per 100 epithelial cells) and extensive surface cell damage and infiltration of the lamina propria with inflammatory cells.

Inflammatory bowel disease

The prevalence of inflammatory bowel disease also appears to be on the rise. This is likely in part due to recent advances in diagnostic technology. Chronic abdominal pain is a common complaint of children with inflammatory bowel disease (IBD). More than 80% of children with ulcerative colitis present with abdominal pain, hematochezia and diarrhea.[40] The onset of Crohn's disease is oftentimes more insidious and presenting complaints are more variable. Symptoms may include RAP, anorexia, weight loss, growth failure and diarrhea. Associated abdominal pain may be intense and frequently awakens the child from sleep. Perianal disease develops in 30–50% of children with Crohn's disease, emphasizing the importance of careful inspection of the perianal region during physical examination.[41]

Laboratory findings suggestive of IBD include anemia, elevated erythrocyte sedimentation rate, thrombocytosis, hypoalbuminemia and heme-positive stool. The perinuclear anti-neutrophil cytoplasmic autoantibodies (pANCA) and anti-Saccharomyces cerevisiae mannan antibodies (ASCA) have also been found over the past several years to be potentially valuable biologic markers for ulcerative colitis and Crohn's disease, respectively. The combination of a positive pANCA test and a negative ASCA assay yielded a sensitivity, specificity and positive predictive value for the diagnosis of ulcerative colitis of 57%, 97% and 93%, respectively. A positive ASCA test combined with a negative pANCA test yielded a sensitivity, specificity and positive predictive value for the diagnosis of Crohn's disease of 49%, 97% and 96%, respectively.[42] Although the tests have a low sensitivity, they may help distinguish one form of IBD from the other and they may serve as further indication to proceed with endoscopy if positive. Wireless capsule endoscopy is another recent medical innovation that enables clinicians to directly visualize the mucosa of the upper gastrointestinal tract and small bowel. This innovative technology is progressively gaining favor and enabling clinicians to determine the health of the small bowel. Despite these technologic advances, accurate diagnosis of IBD relies on a combination of clinical, laboratory, radiologic, endoscopic, and histologic findings.

Intestinal parasites

Giardiasis is an infection of the small intestines with the protozoan parasite *Giardia lamblia*. This organism is found throughout temperate and tropical regions worldwide and is the most common human protozoal enteropathogen.[43] Infection typically follows ingestions of fresh water contaminated with the cysts. Although infection is self-limited in the majority of cases, 30% of patients develop chronic symptoms of abdominal pain, nausea, flatulence, diarrhea and weight loss secondary to malabsorption. Diagnosis is made through identification of the cysts or trophozoites on light microscopy of fresh stool specimens or the more sensitive enzyme-linked immunosorbent assay for Giardia antigen.

Individuals infected with parasitic helminths such as *Ascaris lumbricoides* (roundworm) and *Trichuris trichuria* (whipworm) are often asymptomatic. Heavy infestation, however, may lead to chronic abdominal pain, anorexia, diarrhea, rectal prolapse, or even bowel obstruction.[44] Ova and parasite screening of the stool should be performed when infection is suspected.

Chronic constipation

Chronic constipation is a common cause of RAP in children and accounts for up to 25% of all referrals to the pediatric gastroenterologist.[45] This condition leads to colonic distention, gas formation and painful defecation. There are both functional and organic (myogenic, neurologic, mechanical) forms of chronic constipation.[46] In patients with functional constipation, there is typically voluntary withholding of stool. This may be secondary to such factors as the previous painful passage of stool or refusal to use a public restroom. Such withholding behavior, if prolonged, results in rectal and colonic accumulation of stool, overstretching of anal sphincters, and resultant fecal soiling. Thus, both physical and psychological factors perpetuate this cycle. Diagnosis is often readily made through history and physical examination. A flat plate radiograph of the abdomen is sometimes helpful, especially if the patient's body habitus precludes deep palpation of the abdomen.

Congenital anomalies

Intestinal malrotation occurs when there is incomplete or abnormal rotation of the intestines about the superior mesenteric artery.[47] The majority of symptomatic cases present in infancy, and the diagnosis is readily made by the presence of the 'double bubble' on plain radiograph of the abdomen or malpositioned bowel on upper gastrointestinal series or barium enema.[48] In the older child, the diagnosis may not be readily apparent, as the presentation is not typically duodenal obstruction. Some 50% of older children with intestinal malrotation present with chronic abdominal pain with or without emesis. The associated abdominal pain is usually transient and poorly localized. There are typically no associated abnormal physical or laboratory findings. The pain is most often postprandial and may be accompanied by bilious emesis, diarrhea, or evidence of malabsorption.[49]

Gastrointestinal tract duplications are tubular or cystic structures, attached to the intestine, often sharing a common muscular wall and vascular supply. The most commonly involved site is the ileum. Chronic abdominal pain, gastrointestinal hemorrhage and obstruction due to mass effect have been identified as the most common presenting signs and symptoms of duplications in children. When identified, surgery is recommended.[50]

Genitourinary disorders

Ureteropelvic junction (UPJ) obstruction is an established cause of renal damage in the pediatric population. Early diagnosis allows salvage of renal tissue as well as renal function. UPJ obstruction is more common in males and is most often left-sided.[51] Non-specific RAP may be the only presenting complaint in a child with this condition. Of note, it has been shown that a normal urinalysis and physical examination do not always exclude a genitourinary abnormality as the cause of the recurrent pain and ultrasound is necessary if the diagnosis is suspected.[52] In infancy, the diagnosis of UPJ obstruction is rarely delayed, as the patient usually presents with a palpable abdominal mass or urinary tract infection which prompts imaging studies. As children become older, the diagnosis becomes more difficult because the presenting complaint is often nonspecific RAP. Studies show that approximately 70% of patients older than age 6 years with UPJ obstruction present with RAP.[51] It is especially important to consider this diagnosis when the pain is referred to the groin or flank region, and when it is paroxysmal in nature. Additional diagnostic clues include palpation of an abdominal mass to the left or right of midline or hematuria on urinalysis.

Nephrolithiasis is another diagnostic consideration in the child with RAP. In a recent study of 1440 children with nephrolithiasis, the most common presenting complaint was recurrent abdominal pain, reported in 51%.[53] Dysuria was reported in only 13% of these patients and only 26.7% were found to have hematuria. This condition is more common in males, with a 3:1 ratio. When evaluating a patient with RAP, genitourinary disorders must be kept in mind and further imaging studies performed if clinically indicated.

Eosinophilic esophagitis

Eosinophilic esophagitis (EE) is becoming an increasingly recognized entity in both pediatric and adult patients. The esophagus, which is normally devoid of eosinophils, has been found over the past decade to be an immunologically active organ capable of recruiting eosinophils in response to a variety of stimuli.[54] Eosinophilic esophagitis is characterized by eosinophilic infiltration of the esophagus presumably due to allergic or idiopathic causes. Common presenting symptoms include epigastric pain, nausea, vomiting, growth failure, dysphagia and solid food impaction. The disorder has a slight male predominance. A common finding in children is a history of allergies and peripheral eosinophilia.[55]

This disorder may have a similar endoscopic appearance to reflux esophagitis with circumferential rings and vertical grooves.[56] The rings appear to be caused by lamina propria and dermal papillary fibrosis due to mediators that stimulate the tissue eosinophils or from the eosinophils themselves. An association with Schatzki ring formation has also been described.[57] Strictures are typically located in the proximal or mid-esophagus, as opposed to reflux-induced strictures which are located in the distal esophagus.[55] The presence of white specks adherent to the esophageal mucosa has recently been found to be highly specific for EE. The specks microscopically are composed of eosinophils.[58] The diagnosis of EE is based on finding more than 20 eosinophils per high power field on esophageal biopsies or finding eosinophilic microabscesses on biopsies. As opposed to reflux esophagitis, in which fewer than 7 eosinophils per high power field are seen, patient's with EE have normal 24-h pH probe studies and often do not benefit from acid suppressive therapy. Many patients with EE benefit from food allergy testing with subsequent elimination diets and topical corticosteroid therapy.[59,60]

Biliary dyskinesia

Biliary dyskinesia or hypokinetic gallbladder disease refers to decreased contractility and poor emptying of the gallbladder that leads to symptomatology. In children, presentation has included right upper quadrant or epigastric pain, nausea, vomiting and fatty food intolerance. Diagnosis is made utilizing functional gallbladder emptying studies. Ultrasonography is typically normal. If the diagnosis is suspected, scintigraphy should be performed to measure gallbladder volume before and 30 min after intravenous cholecystokinin (CCK) is injected to stimulate gallbladder emptying. In most centers, a gallbladder ejection fraction of greater than or equal to 35% is considered normal. In a recent pediatric study, 41 of 42 patients diagnosed with biliary dyskinesia became pain-free following laparoscopic cholecystectomy.[61]

DIAGNOSIS OF CHILDHOOD FUNCTIONAL ABDOMINAL PAIN DISORDERS

The diagnosis of functional pediatric disorders has evolved since the turn of the millennium from the exclusion of organic disease to the utilization of positive symptom criteria in combination with a conservative diagnostic approach. This paradigm shift has resulted from the Rome II criteria.[3] An international team of pediatric

of anticipation of pain, increased anxiety, concomitant physiological arousal, lowered pain threshold and increased distress.[64] All therapeutic strategies should be designed to teach the pediatric patient that he or she can cope with the pain. After prolonged school absenteeism, it is advisable to encourage abbreviated attendance at school initially to help the patient build confidence that they can manage an episode of pain while at school.[63] It is best to advise initial return to school for several hours per day with gradual escalation of the time in the classroom. Should a pain episode occur while at school, it is advisable that the patient be permitted to lie down in the nurse's office for a brief period until able to return to class rather than call home or leave school early. The child may also benefit from referral to a specialist for training in relaxation techniques.

The abdominal pain diary: the patient and family take responsibility

The patient and family need to take an active role with a chronic disorder such as recurrent abdominal pain. The patient and family should be encouraged to maintain a symptom diary at the initial medical visit and at anytime a therapeutic measure is initiated. The diary often empowers them with observational skills and insight they would not have had otherwise. As in clinical studies, prospective observations are more reliable than those made retrospectively. Abdominal pain diaries should be customized according to the patient and clinical scenario. At a minimum, the diary should include the following entry columns: (1) date and time when the symptom exacerbation occurred, (2) the location of the pain, (3) the character, severity (on a scale on 1–10), and duration of the pain, (4) factors preceding onset of symptoms (food, activity, psychosocial stressors, school attendance, interactions with friends or family, menses), (5) description of daily stooling pattern and (6) identified relieving factors.[65] Many times, patients and their families are surprised when they identify exacerbating factors such as psychological stressors, excess fat in the diet or stooling irregularities that are amenable to therapy.

Negotiate therapy

To maximize the potential for compliance, the physician, the patient and the family must agree on the plan of therapy. This is done after adequate evaluation and education regarding the patient's condition has taken place. The physician should make inquiries regarding the family's understanding of, personal experience with and interest in a variety of treatments. The physician should then provide choices consistent with the family's wishes and beliefs, rather than mandate a particular course of therapy.[65]

Patients with mild symptoms and little impact on psychosocial functioning usually respond well to reassurance, education and applicable dietary or lifestyle modification. Those patients with moderately severe symptoms require pharmacotherapy and/or behavioral therapy. If abdominal symptoms are severe, continuous and unrelated to changes in gastrointestinal functioning, psychoactive medications for central analgesia (such as tricyclic antidepressants or serotonin re-uptake inhibitors) are indicated in addition to a 'team approach' including psychiatrists, behavioral specialists, dietitians and social workers working in combination with the primary care physician and gastroenterologist.

DIET

Dietary recommendations may be helpful for some patients with FRAP of childhood. If specific dietary triggers are identified such as lactose, caffeine, spicy foods, fatty foods, carbonated beverages, large meals, or gas-forming vegetables, they should be reduced or eliminated from the diet. Excess consumption of artificial sweeteners such as mannitol or sorbitol should also be avoided as this may lead to increased flatus production with concomitant abdominal discomfort and distension.[34]

The role of increased dietary fiber in patients with FRAP remains controversial. Most studies of dietary fiber intake and irritable bowel syndrome in adults have shown that while dietary fiber does improve constipation, it does not appear to consistently improve abdominal pain. A recent meta-analysis concluded that only three previously performed studies in adults were of 'high quality'. The authors determined that even the positive studies showed no significant improvement in stool frequency, abdominal pain and bloating.[66] In one pediatric study, adding 10 g of fiber daily for 6 weeks resulted in a decrease in the number of pain episodes in almost 50% of patients.[67] As a general rule, the number of grams of fiber consumed daily should be at least the age of the patient in years plus five up to the adult recommendation of 30 g/day. The patient should be advised to increase dietary fiber gradually, as a rapid increase may lead to increased colonic gas production, abdominal distension and pain. The importance of regular, well-balanced meals consumed in calm surroundings with minimal distractions should also be emphasized. Potentially dangerous restrictive or fad diets should be discouraged.

PHARMACOTHERAPY

The placebo response rate can be very high in functional gastrointestinal disorders, making it difficult to establish superiority of a new treatment over placebo. In functional dyspepsia, the placebo response has varied from 13–73% while for irritable bowel syndrome, the reported range has been up to 88%.[68] There have been no placebo-controlled trials evaluating the therapeutic effect of pharmacologic agents in pediatric patients with FRAP. As with many disorders, data from adult studies is, therefore, extrapolated and medications judiciously prescribed to the pediatric population.

Patients symptoms that are severe enough to disrupt daily activities will likely benefit from pharmacologic therapy. Such therapy should be individualized and directed toward the predominant symptom.

Acid suppressive therapy

For patients with predominant dyspepsia (discomfort centered in the epigastrium, nausea, early satiety, postprandial fullness, recurrent emesis), a short course of empiric therapy with an H2-histamine receptor antagonist or proton pump inhibitor is acceptable. Failure to respond to such medication or a recurrence of symptoms following discontinuation of the therapy should prompt further evaluation. There are currently no pediatric data to support the long-term benefit of antisecretory therapy in patients with FRAP.

Peppermint oil

Peppermint oil has been used to soothe the gastrointestinal tract for hundreds of years. It relaxes intestinal smooth muscle by decreasing calcium influx into the smooth muscle cells. A meta-analysis of five randomized, double-blinded, placebo-controlled trials performed in adult patients supported the efficacy of peppermint oil in the treatment of irritable bowel syndrome.[69] One randomized, double-blind, controlled trial in pediatric patients with IBS demonstrated the efficacy of enteric-coated peppermint oil capsules (Colpermin) in the reduction of pain during the acute phase of IBS.[70] Children weighing 30 to 45 kg received one capsule (187 mg peppermint oil) while those over 45 kg received two capsules, three times daily. Use of enteric-coated products reduces side effects such as nausea and heartburn.

Anticholinergic agents

Anticholinergic agents such as dicycloverine (dicyclomine) (Bentyl) and hyoscyamine (Levsin, Levbid, NuLev) are commonly used in the USA to treat pain associated with functional intestinal disorders. These agents are smooth muscle relaxants that block the muscarinic effects of acetylcholine on the gastrointestinal tract, thereby relaxing smooth muscle and potentially reducing spasm and abdominal pain, slowing intestinal motility and decreasing diarrhea. Although commonly prescribed, the efficacy of these agents has not been clearly established in adult trials nor have any randomized, double-blind, placebo-controlled trials been conducted in the pediatric population. Potential side-effects if used in high dosages include drowsiness, blurred vision, dry mouth, tachycardia, constipation and urinary retention. In clinical practice, anticholinergic agents are best utilized on an as-needed or episodic basis given up to four times daily. When postprandial symptoms are predominant, they can be most helpful if given before meals. With chronic use, dicyclomine and hyoscyamine become less effective and a low-dose tricyclic antidepressant should be considered should the patient's pain be constant and/or disruptive to daily functioning.

In addition, hyoscyamine is also available in combination with atropine, scopolamine and phenobarbital (Donnatal). Another combination medication available in the USA is Librax which is an antispasmodic medication with anticholinergic properties (clidinium bromide) combined with chlordiazepoxide hydrochloride. These combination medications have gained popularity over the past several years, but have not been well-evaluated in clinical trials. They cannot currently be recommended for use in pediatric patients as they have the potential for unwanted sedative and addictive side-effects.

Tricyclic antidepressants

Tricyclics (TCAs) may offer some relief to patients with FRAP. The neuromodulatory and analgesic effects of these agents result from a combined anticholinergic effect on the gastrointestinal tract, mood elevation and central analgesia. Unfortunately, data from placebo controlled trials of the usefulness of these agents for patients with FRAP is limited. Because antidepressants are used on a continuous basis rather than on an episodic basis when symptoms arise, they should be reserved for those with frequent or continuous abdominal complaints.

Tricyclic antidepressants have been in use for over 40 years. They have a 'quinidine-like' effect, are arrhythmogenic and can lower the seizure threshold. This class of antidepressants has been the most widely studied for the treatment of irritable bowel syndrome in adults and is relatively inexpensive. In a meta-analysis, TCA medications were shown to result in significant improvement in global gastrointestinal symptoms as compared with placebo.[71] The dosage needed to produce relief of recurrent abdominal pain is typically considerably less than that routinely used for the treatment of primary depression and; therefore, potentially serious cardiovascular side-effects are less likely. Due to the potential for development of serious cardiac arrhythmias in patients with prolonged QT syndrome, some advocate obtaining an electrocardiogram prior to initiation of TCA therapy.

Also important to note is that the timing of onset of pain relief may occur almost immediately or take as long as ten weeks.[72] Amitriptyline may promote sleep whereas desipramine and nortriptyline may be preferred when less anticholinergic and sedative effects are desired. There are anecdotal reports of TCA use in pediatric patients with FRAP.[73] Dosing guidelines are not available, though many clinicians start with very low doses (0.2mg/kg/day and slowly titrate up to 0.5mg/kg/day). The medication is usually given as a single bedtime does.

Serotonergic agents

Serotonin is found in high concentrations in enterochromaffin cells located in the epithelial layer of the gastrointestinal tract. At least 14 serotonin receptor subtypes with varying actions in the peripheral and central nervous systems exist. Of these receptors, 5-HT3 and 5-HT4 receptors appear to play a role in the pathophysiology of IBS and recent studies suggest that pharmacologic agents directed toward these receptors improve symptoms in these patients.

3. Hyman PE, Rasquin-Weber A, Fleisher DR, et al. ROME II: Childhood functional gastrointestinal disorders. In: Drossman DA, ed. Rome II. The Functional Gastrointestinal Disorders. Diagnosis, Pathophysiology and Treatment: A Multinational Consensus, 2nd edn. Lawrence, KS: Allen Press, 2000: 533–575.
4. Hyams JS, Treem WR, Justinich CJ, et al. Characterization of symptoms in children with recurrent abdominal pain: resemblance to irritable bowel syndrome. J Pediatr Gastroenterol Nutr 1995; 20:209–214.
5. Routh DK, Ernst AR. Somatization disorder in relatives of children and adolescents with functional abdominal pain. J Pediatr Psychol 1984; 9:427–437.
6. Stone RT, Barbero GJ. Recurrent abdominal pain in childhood. Pediatrics 1970; 45:732–738.
7. Hodges K, Kline J, Barbero G, Flanery R. Depressive symptoms in children with recurrent abdominal pain and in their families. J Pediatr 1985; 107:622–626.
8. Liebman W. Recurrent abdominal pain in children: a retrospective survey of 119 patients. Clin Pediatr 1978:17:149–153.
9. Delvaux M. Role of visceral sensitivity in the pathophysiology of irritable bowel syndrome. Gut 2002; 51(suppl l):i67–i71.
10. Neal KR, Hebden J, Spiller R. Prevalence of gastrointestinal symptoms six months after bacterial gastroenteritis and risk factors for development of the irritable bowel syndrome: postal survey of patients. BMJ 1997; 314:779–782.
11. Pineiro-Carrero VM, Andres JM, Davis RH, et al. Abnormal gastroduodenal motility in children and adolescents with recurrent functional abdominal pain. J Pediatr 1988; 113:820–825.
12. Hyman PE, Napolitano JA, Diego A, et al. Antroduodenal manometry in the evaluation of chronic functional gastrointestinal symptoms. Pediatrics 1990; 86:39–44.
13. Hodges K, Kline J, Barbero G, et al. Life events occurring in families of children with recurrent abdominal pain. J Psychosom Res 1984; 28:185–188.
14. Walker L, Garber J, Greene J. Psychosocial correlates of recurrent childhood pain: a comparison of pediatric patients with recurrent abdominal pain, organic illness and psychiatric disorders. J Abnorm Psychol 1993; 102:248–258.
15. Raymer D, Weininger O, Hamilton JR. Psychological problems in children with abdominal pain. Lancet 1984; 1:439–440.
16. Oster J. Recurrent abdominal pain, headache and limb pains in children and adolescents. Pediatrics 1972; 50:429–436.
17. McGarrity TJ, Peters DJ, Thompson C, et al. Outcome of patients with chronic abdominal pain referred to chronic pain clinic. Am J Gastroenterol 2000; 95:1812–1816.
18. Bain HW. Chronic vague abdominal pain in children. Pediatr Clin North Am 1974; 21:991–1000.
19. Oberlander TF, Rappaport LA. Recurrent abdominal pain during childhood. Pediatr Rev 1993; 14:313–319.
20. Dodge JA. Recurrent abdominal pain in children. BMJ 1976; 1:385–387.
21. Van der Meer SB, Forget PP, Arends JW, et al. Diagnostic value of ultrasound in children with recurrent abdominal pain. Pediatr Radiol 1990; 20:501–503.
22. Shanon A, Martin DJ, Feldman W. Ultrasonographic studies in the management of recurrent abdominal pain. Pediatrics 1990; 86:35–38.
23. Schmidt RE, Babcock DS, Farrell MK. Use of abdominal and pelvic ultrasound in the evaluation of chronic abdominal pain. Clin Pediatr 1983; 22:147–150.
24. Yeung CK, Fu KH, Yeun KY, et al. Helicobacter pylori and associated duodenal ulcer. Arch Dis Child 1990; 65:1212–1216.
25. Fiedorek S, Malaty H, Evans D, et al. Factors influencing the epidemiology of Helicobacter pylori infection in children. Pediatrics 1991; 88:578–582.
26. Drumm B, Perez-Perez GI, Blaser MJ, et al. Intrafamilial clustering of Helicobacter pylori infection. N Engl J Med 1990; 322:359–363.
27. Chelimsky G, Czinn SJ. Helicobacter pylori infection in children: update. Curr Opin Pediatr 2000; 12(5):460–462.
28. Elitsur Y, Lawrence Z, Hill I. Stool antigen test for diagnosis of *Helicobacter pylori* infection in children with symptomatic disease: A prospective study. J Pediatr Gastroenterol Nutr 2004; 39:64–67.
29. Tolia V, Dubois R. Peptic ulcer disease in children and adolescents: a ten-year experience. J Clin Pediatr 1983:22:665–669.
30. Hyams JS. Recurrent abdominal pain in children. Curr Opin Pediatr 1995; 7:529–532.
31. Simoons FJ. The geographic hypothesis and lactose malabsorption: a weighing of the evidence. Am J Dig Dis 1978; 23:963–980.
32. Gudmand-Hoyer E. The clinical significance of disaccharide maldigestion. Am J Clin Nutr 1994; 59(suppl):735S–741S.
33. Barr RG, Levine MD, Watkins JB. Recurrent abdominal pain of childhood due to lactose intolerance. N Engl J Med 1979; 300:1449–1452.
34. Hyams JS. Chronic abdominal pain caused by sorbitol malabsorption. J Pediatr 1982; 100:772–773.
35. Fasano A. Where have all the American celiacs gone? Acta Paediatr Suppl 1996; 412:20–24.
36. Not T, Horvath K, Hill ID, et al. Celiac disease risk in the USA: High prevalence of antiendomysial antibodies in healthy blood donors. Scand J Gastroenterol 1998; 33:494–498.
37. Maki M. The humoral immune system in celiac disease. Baillières Clin Gastroenterol 1995; 9:231–249.
38. Sulkanen S, Halttunen T, Laurila C, et al. Tissue transglutaminase autoantibody enzyme-linked immunosorbent assay in detecting celiac disease. Gastroenterology 1998; 115:1322–1328.
39. Corrao G, Corazza GR, Andreani ML, et al. Serological screening of coeliac disease: Choosing the optimal procedure according to various prevalence values. Gut 1994; 35:771–775.
40. Michener WM. Ulcerative colitis in children. Problems in management. Pediatr Clin North Am 1967; 14:159–163.
41. Markowitz J, Daum F, Aiges H, et al. Perianal disease in children and adolescents with Crohn's disease. Gastroenterology 1984; 86:829–833.
42. Quinton JF, Sendid B, Reumaux D, et al. Anti-Saccharomyces cerevisiae mannan antibodies combined with antineutrophil cytoplasmic autoantibodies in inflammatory bowel disease: prevalence and diagnostic role. Gut 1998; 42(6):788–791.
43. Farthing M. Giardiasis. Gastroenterol Clin North Am 1996; 25:493–514.
44. Salas SD, Heifetz R, Barrett-Connor E. Intestinal parasites in Central American immigrants in the United States. Arch Intern Med 1990; 150:1514–1516.
45. Fleisher DR. Diagnosis and treatment of disorders of defecation in children. Pediatr Ann 1976; 5:71–101.
46. Miglioli M. Constipation physiopathology and classification. Ital J Gastroenterol 1991; 23:10–12.
47. Wang C, Welch GE. Anomalies of intestinal rotation in adolescents and adults. Surgery 1963; 54:839–855.
48. Louw JH, Cywes S. Embryology and anomalies of the intestine. In: Berk JE, Haubrich WS, Kalser MH, eds. Bockus Gastroenterology, 4th edn. Philadelphia: WB Saunders; 1985:1439–1473.

49. Janik JS, Ein SH. Normal intestinal rotation with nonfixation: a cause of chronic abdominal pain. J Pediatr Surg 1979:14:670–674.
50. Bissler JJ, Klein RL. Alimentary tract duplications in children. Clin Pediatr 1988; 27: 152–157.
51. Drake DP, Stevens PS, Eckstein HB. Hydronephrosis secondary to ureteropelvic junction obstruction in children: a review of 14 years of experience. J Urol 1978; 119:649–651.
52. Byrne WJ, Arnold WC, Stannard MW. Ureteropelvic junction obstruction presenting with recurrent abdominal pain: diagnosis by ultrasound. Pediatrics 1985; 76:934–937.
53. Rizvi SAH, Naqvi SAA, Hussain Z, et al. Pediatric urolithiasis: developing nation perspectives. J Urol 2002; 168(4):1522–1525.
54. Ahmad M, Soetikno RM, Ahmed A. The differential diagnosis of eosinophilic esophagitis. J Clin Gastroenterol 2000; 30:242–244.
55. Khan S, Orenstein SR, Di Lorenzo C, et al. Eosinophilic esophagitis: strictures, impactions, dysphagia. Dig Dis Sci 2003; 48:22–29.
56. Siafakas CG, Ryan CK, Brown MR, et al. Multiple esophageal rings: An association with eosinophilic esophagitis: case report and review of the literature. Am J Gastroenterol 2000; 95:1572–1575.
57. Nurko S, Teitelbaum JE, Jusain K, et al. Association of Schatzki Ring With Eosinophilic Esophagitis in Children. J Pediatr Gastroenterol Nutr 2004; 38:38:436–441.
58. Ahmed A, Matsui S, Soetikno R. A novel endoscopic appearance of idiopathic eosinophilic esophagitis. Endoscopy 2000; 32:S33.
59. Orenstein SR, Shalaby TM, Di Lorenzo, et al. the spectrum of pediatric eosinophilic esophagitis beyond infancy: a clinical series of 30 children. Am J Gastroenterol 2000; 95(6):1422–1430.
60. Markowitz JE, Spergel JM, Ruchelli E, et al. Elemental diet is an effective treatment for eosinophilic esophagitis in children and adolescents. Am J Gastroenterol 2003; 98(4):777–782.
61. Dumont RC, Caniano DA: Hypokinetic Gallbladder Disease: A Cause of Chronic Abdominal Pain in Children and Adolescents. J Pediatr Surg 1999; 34(5):858–862.
62. Zeltzer LK, Barr RG, McGrath PA, et al. Pediatric pain: interacting behavioral and physical factors. Pediatrics 1992; 90:816–821.
63. Walker L. Helping the child with recurrent abdominal pain return to school. Pediatric Annals 2004; 33(2): 128–136.
64. Walker LS. The evolution of research on recurrent abdominal pain: history, assumptions, and a conceptual model. In: McGrath PJ, Finley GA, eds. Progress in Pain Research and Management, Vol. 13. Seattle, WA: International Association for the Study of Pain Press; 1999:141–172.
65. Drossman DA. Diagnosing and treating patients with refractory functional gastrointestinal disorders. Ann Intern Med 1995; 123:688–697.
66. Jailwala J, Imperiale TF, Kroenke K. Pharmacologic treatment of the irritable bowel syndrome: a systematic review of randomized, controlled trials. Ann Intern Med 2000; 133:136–147.
67. Feldman W, McGrath P, Hodgson C, et al. The use of dietary fiber in the management of simple, childhood, idiopathic, recurrent abdominal pain. Am J Dis Child 1985; 139:1216–1218.
68. Peck C, Coleman G. Implications of placebo theory for clinical research and practice in pain management. Theor Med 1991; 12(3):247–270.
69. Pittler MH, Ernst E. Peppermint oil for irritable bowel syndrome: a critical review and meta-analysis. Am J Gastroenterol 1998; 93:1131–1135.
70. Kline RM, Kline JJ, Di Palma J, et al. Enteric-coated, pH-dependent peppermint oil capsules for the treatment of irritable bowel syndrome in children. J Pediatr 2001; 138(1):125–128.
71. Jackson JL, O'Malley PG, Tomkins G, et al. Treatment of functional gastrointestinal disorders with anti-depressants: A meta-analysis. Am J Med 2000; 108:65–72.
72. Egbunike IG, Chaffre BJ. Antidepressants in the management of chronic pain syndromes. Pharmacotherapy 1990; 10(4):262–270.
73. Rudolph C, Miranda A. Treatment options for functional abdominal pain. Pediatric Annals 2004; 33(2):105–112.
74. Mayer EA, Bradesi S. Alosetron and irritable bowel syndrome. Expert Opin Pharmacother 2003; 4(11):2089–2098.
75. Camilleri M, Mayer EA, Drossman DA, et al. Improvement in pain and bowel function in female irritable bowel patients with alosetron, a 5-HT3 receptor antagonist. Aliment Pharmacol Ther 1999; 13(9):1149–1159.
76. Camilleri M, Northcutt AR, Kong J, et al. Efficacy and safety of alosetron in women with irritable bowel syndrome: a randomized, placebo-controlled trial. Lancet 2000; 355(9209):1035–1040.
77. Camilleri M, Chey WY, Mayer EA, et al. A randomized controlled clinical trial of the serotonin type 3 receptor antagonist alosetron in women with diarrhea-predominant irritable bowel syndrome. Arch Intern Med 2001; 161(14):1733–1740.
78. Lembo T, Wright RA, Bagby B, et al. Lotronex Investigator Team. Alosetron controls bowel urgency and provides global symptom improvement in women with diarrhea-predominant irritable bowel syndrome. Am J Gastroenterol 2001; 96(9):2662–2670.
79. Camilleri M. Tegaserod. Aliment Pharmacol Ther 2001; 15:277–289.
80. Rivkin A. Tegaserod maleate in the treatment of irritable bowel syndrome: a clinical review. Clin Ther 2003; 25(7):1952–1974.
81. Sanders MR, Shepherd RW, Cleghorn G, et al. The treatment of recurrent abdominal pain in children: a controlled comparison of cognitive-behavioral family intervention and standard pediatric care. J Consult Clin Psychol 1994; 62(2):306–314.
82. Blanchard EB, Greene B, Scharff L, et al. Relaxation training as a treatment for irritable bowel syndrome. Biofeedback Self Regul 1993; 18:125–132.
83. Prior A, Colgan SM, Whorwell PJ. changes in rectal sensitivity after hypnotherapy in patients with irritable bowel syndrome. Gut 1990; 31:896–898.
84. Anbar RD. Self-hypnosis for the treatment of functional abdominal pain in childhood. Clin Pediatr 2001; 40(8):447–451.
85. Apley J, Hale B. Children with recurrent abdominal pain: how do they grow up? BMJ 1973; 3:7–9.
86. Christensen MF, Mortensen O. Long-term prognosis in children with recurrent abdominal pain. Arch Dis Child 1975; 50:110–114.
87. Magni G, Pierri M, Donzelli F. Recurrent abdominal pain in children: a long term follow-up. Eur J Pediatr 1987; 146:72–74.
88. Farrell MK. Abdominal pain. Pediatrics 1984; 74(suppl):955–957.

Chapter 8
Vomiting and nausea

BU.K. Li and Bhanu K. Sunku

INTRODUCTION

It is accepted that the ability to vomit developed as a protective mechanism to rid the body of ingested toxins.[1] Unfortunately, vomiting also frequently occurs unrelated to the ingestion of noxious agents, a circumstance that produces several clinical challenges. First, vomiting is a sign of many diseases that affect different organ systems. Therefore, determining the cause of a vomiting episode can be difficult. Second, vomiting can produce several complications (e.g. electrolyte derangement, prolapse gastropathy, Mallory-Weiss syndrome) that demand diagnosis and treatment. Third, vomiting is a frequent complication of medical therapy (surgical procedures, cancer chemotherapy). Fourth, selection of appropriate therapy for this distressing problem is essential to improve patient comfort and avoid additional medical complications of the vomiting.

THE VOMITING EVENT

Definition

Vomiting (emesis) is a complex reflex behavioral response to a variety of stimuli (see below). The emetic reflex has three phases: (1) a prodromal period consisting of the sensation of nausea and signs of autonomic nervous system stimulation, (2) retching and (3) vomiting or forceful expulsion of the stomach contents through the oral cavity.[2–5] Although the overall sequence of these three phases is stereotypical, each can occur independently of the others. For example, nausea does not always progress to vomiting and pharyngeal stimulation can induce vomiting without a prodrome of nausea. It is important to note that *vomiting* and *regurgitation* (defined as effortless reflux of the intragastric contents into the esophagus) are not synonymous. Clinically, vomiting can be distinguished from regurgitation as regurgitation is not preceded by prodromal events, retching does not occur and gastric contents are not forcibly expelled. The differentiation between vomiting and regurgitation is critical, as each has different causes and is produced by distinctive physiologic mechanisms.

Physical description

The events that herald the onset of the act of vomiting are nausea and several autonomic manifestations.[2,5–6] *Nausea* is a subjective experience that is difficult to define. It is usually described as an unpleasant, but painless, sensation localized to the epigastrium associated with the feeling that vomiting is imminent. The autonomic signs include cutaneous vasoconstriction, sweating, dilation of pupils, increased salivation and tachycardia. Several gastrointestinal (GI) motor events characterize the emetic prodrome.[6–9] There is inhibition of spontaneous contractions within the GI tract and dilation of the proximal stomach. The esophageal skeletal muscle shortens longitudinally, pulling the relaxed proximal stomach (hiatus and cardia) into the thoracic cavity, with loss of the abdominal segment of the esophagus. These changes result in an anatomy that allows the free flow of gastric contents into the esophagus.[10] Soon after, a single large-amplitude contraction is initiated in the jejunum and propagates toward the stomach at 8–10 cm/sec.[8,11] This retropulsive event is termed the *retrograde giant contraction* (RGC). It propels the duodenal contents into the stomach before the onset of retching.[10,12] The RGC is followed by a brief period of moderate-amplitude contractions in the distal small intestine and a second period of inhibition lasting several minutes.[7]

The two major somatic motor components of vomiting (retching and expulsion) are produced by the coordinated action of the respiratory, pharyngeal and abdominal muscles resulting in rhythmic changes in intrathoracic and intra-abdominal pressures.[4,13] During each cycle of retching, the glottis closes and the diaphragm, external intercostal muscles and abdominal muscles contract,[14,15] producing large negative intrathoracic and positive intra-abdominal pressure spikes. The esophagus dilates and the atonic proximal stomach continues to be displaced into the thoracic cavity. The antireflux mechanisms are overcome, and the gastric contents move to and fro into the esophagus with each cycle of retching.[10]

Sometime after the onset of retching, expulsion or vomiting occurs. During this event the external intercostal muscles and the hiatal region of the diaphragm relax and the abdominal muscles and costal diaphragm contract violently,[14,15] producing positive pressures in both abdomen and thorax, resulting in oral propulsion of the gastric contents. Retrograde contraction of the cervical esophagus assists in oral expulsion.[9] After expulsion, antegrade peristalsis in the esophagus clears the lumen of residual material[3]; the proximal stomach returns to its normal intra-abdominal position, restoring the normal antireflux anatomy.

Gastrointestinal motor activity during nausea and vomiting

GI motor activity during the emetic reflex is mediated by the vagus nerve.[7–9] Vagal preganglionic parasympathetic fibers can activate both inhibitory and excitatory pathways in the enteric nervous system. A wide range of stimuli induce nausea and vomiting;[8] however, these GI motor events do not appear to be the cause of the sensation of nausea. Moreover, the stereotypical somatic pattern of retching and vomiting continues even when the GI motor correlates of vomiting are prevented by disruption of the vagal efferents.[8,9]

Although GI motor activity is not necessary for retching and vomiting, the motor changes that do occur may serve a significant role. As a defense against noxious ingested agents,[1] relaxation of the stomach can confine a toxin before it is expelled, and the RCG can move toxins and alkaline duodenal secretions to the stomach to buffer and dilute gastric irritants (e.g. vinegar, hypertonic saline) in preparation for expulsion. The buffering of the gastric contents can also serve to protect the esophagus from acid injury. Finally, changes in the position of the stomach can place it in an advantageous position for compression by the abdominal musculature.[10]

A different pattern of GI motor activity is observed in circumstances in which nausea is induced by motion.[16,17] Before the onset of nausea, an increase occurs in the gastric slow-wave from 3–9 cycles/min.[18] This phenomena, known as *tachygastria*, is controlled by central cholinergic and α-adrenergic pathways.[19] In motion-induced nausea, the GI motor activity appears to play a role in the induction of symptoms.[18]

The emetic reflex

The emetic reflex consists of an afferent limb (receptor and pathway), central integration and control, and an efferent limb (pathway and effector) (Fig. 8.1).[20,21] This reflex can be induced by visceral pain and inflammation, toxins, motion, pregnancy, radiation exposure, postoperative states and unpleasant emotions. The diverse afferent receptors and pathways may originate within the gut, oropharynx, heart, vestibular system, or central nervous system (e.g. area postrema, hypothalamus and cortical regions). These multiple afferent pathways are integrated within the brainstem and the emetic reflex is completed through a common integrated efferent limb consisting of multiple pathways and effectors.

Within the GI tract, multiple receptors are capable of initiating the emetic reflex.[5,22] Mechanoreceptors present within the muscularis are activated by changes in tension and may be stimulated by passive distension or active contraction of the bowel wall. These conditions are present in bowel obstruction, a clinical state in which vomiting is prominent. Chemoreceptors within the mucosa of the stomach and proximal small bowel respond to a wide range of chemical irritants (hydrochloric acid (HCl), copper sulfate, vinegar, hypertonic saline, syrup of ipecac) and

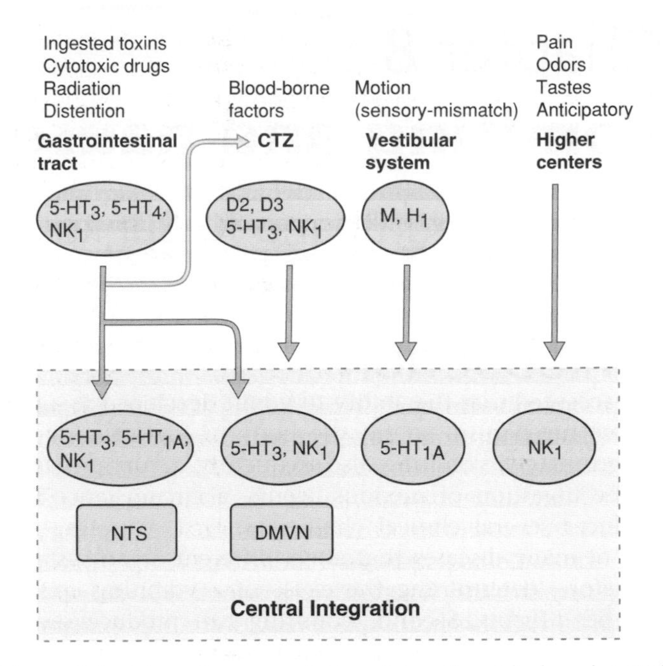

Figure 8.1: Schematic representation of the afferent limb and central integration of the emetic reflex. Receptors known to be involved in each pathway are listed within ovals. The region of central integration is designated by a dashed box to indicate that no single central locus exists as a 'vomiting center'. The nucleus of the solitary tract (NTS) and the dorsal motor vagal nucleus (DMVN) may each play a role in central integration. Receptor abbreviations: 5-HT, 5-hydroxytryptamine (serotonin); D, dopamine; M, acetylcholine muscarinic; H, histamine; NK, neurokinin.

are involved in the emetic reflex induced by radiation and chemotherapeutic agents. The afferent pathways from the GI tract are mediated principally via the vagus nerves; the splanchnic nerves play a minor role.[22] Vagal afferent fibers project centrad principally to the dorsomedial portion of the nucleus of the solitary tract (NTS) and to a lesser extent to the area postrema and the dorsal motor vagal nucleus.[22–24]

Circulating toxins can trigger the emetic reflex. The major detector of blood-borne noxious agents is the chemoreceptor trigger zone (CTZ),[25–27] which is located within the area postrema on the floor of the fourth ventricle, outside of the blood-brain barrier. Substances in the cerebrospinal fluid and blood stream can be detected by the cells of this region. Several types of receptors for endogenous neurotransmitters and neuropeptides have been localized to the CTZ.[26,28] Intravenous infusion or direct application of these neuroactive agents (dopamine, acetylcholine, enkephalin, peptide YY, substance P) to the CTZ can induce vomiting.[29,30] Stimulation of the CTZ is essential for the induction of vomiting by these and other agents (apomorphine, cisplatin), but not for that induced by the stimulation of abdominal vagal afferents or motion. In addition to playing a role in vomiting, the area postrema is involved in taste aversion, the control of food intake, and fluid homeostasis.[27]

Activation of the afferent limb of the vomiting reflex may also occur through real or apparent motion of the body. Motion-induced vomiting is the result of a sensory mismatch involving the visual, vestibular, and proprioceptive systems,[31] although an intact vestibular system is a necessary component.[32] Histamine (H_1) and cholinergic muscarinic receptors are involved in the afferent limb of this pathway.[33] In addition to the above afferent pathways, stimulated by unpleasant situations or in instances of conditioned vomiting (e.g. anticipatory vomiting in chemotherapy) higher cortical centers can activate the emetic reflex.

After activation, the afferent systems project centrad. Although no single central locus has been identified as a 'vomiting center', two models of central coordination of the emetic reflex have been proposed: (1) a group of nuclei (paraventricular system of nuclei, defined by their connection to the area postrema) form a linked neural system whose activation can account for all of the phenomena associated with vomiting;[34,35] (2) vomiting is produced by the sequential activation of a series of discrete effector (motor) nuclei[1] as opposed to being activated in parallel by a single locus. Furthermore, the concept of a localized 'vomiting center' has been refuted by recent anatomic studies implicating a widely distributed area within the medulla as being involved in the organization and control of the emetic reflex.[36,37]

Neurochemical basis

A wide variety of neurotransmitters, neuroactive peptides, and hormones are involved in the emetic reflex. As investigations proceed into the physiology of vomiting and the pharmacology of antiemetic agents, the role of these and other mediators will continue to be defined.

Dopaminergic pathways have long been known to participate in the emetic reflex. Apomorphine, a commonly used experimental emetic agent, acts through the dopamine (D_2 subtype) receptor.[38] Furthermore, several clinically effective antiemetic agents (e.g. metoclopramide) are D_2 receptor antagonists. The site of action of these agents (agonists and antagonists) is the CTZ[25,27] where a high density of D_2 receptors is present.[28] These receptors participate in the emetic reflex induced by several, but not all, noxious agents acting through the CTZ. In addition to this subclass of receptors, recent evidence has implicated D_3 receptors within the area postrema as having a role in the emetic reflex.[39]

The importance of serotonin (5-hydroxytryptamine or 5-HT) and serotonin receptors[40] in the emetic reflex has been demonstrated by the observation that cisplatin-induced vomiting can be prevented by blockade of 5-HT_3 receptors.[41,42] In addition to its involvement in mediating the emetic response to several chemotherapeutic agents, 5-HT_3 receptors play an important role in vomiting induced by radiation therapy[43] and noxious substances in the GI tract.[44,45] The 5-HT_3 receptors are present on vagal afferent fibers in the GI tract and the presynaptic vagal afferent terminals within the central nervous system, specifically in the NTS and CTZ in the area postrema.[46,47] Current evidence indicates that chemotherapeutic agents, irradiation, and various noxious substances act directly on the GI mucosa, inducing release of serotonin from enterochromaffin cells.[42,48] Vagal afferents terminating near these cells are stimulated, producing afferent activation of the emetic reflex. The precise role of the 5-HT_3 receptors on the presynaptic vagal afferents within the central nervous system has not been fully elucidated, but they appear to facilitate the emetic reflex induced by some afferent pathways (e.g. cranial irradiation, chemotherapeutic agents within the cerebrospinal fluid).[43,49] Other members of the 5-HT receptor family also may be involved in the emetic reflex. The 5-HT_4 receptor has been shown to be necessary in the afferent limb of the emetic reflex induced by at least one GI irritant.[50] Blockade of central 5-HT_{1A} receptors, located primarily in the NTS, prevents emesis induced by a broad range of stimuli.[51,52]

Animal studies have convincingly linked physical and psychological stress to gastric stasis via central corticotropin-releasing factor (CRF) acting on CRF-R2 at the dorsomotor nucleus of the vagus.[53] During exposure to stress, CRF initiates the hypothalamic-pituitary-adrenal (HPA) axis and could play an initiating role in emesis. The role of CRF in humans remains to be established but its effects can produce the behavioral, neuroendocrine, autonomic, immunologic and visceral responses to stress.

Substance P (a member of the neurokinin family of peptides) and its receptor neurokinin NK_1 (tachykinin) are widely distributed in the central nervous system and peripheral neural and extraneural tissues.[54,55] Evidence in animal models of vomiting has demonstrated that this ligand and receptor are critical to the emetic response produced by a wide range of stimuli.[56–58] NK_1 receptor antagonists prevent vomiting produced by intravenous (morphine) and intragastric toxins (ipecac, copper sulfate), chemotherapeutic agents (cisplatin), and motion. The site of action of these antagonists is believed to be NK_1 receptors located in the central nervous system (NTS, dorsal motor vagal nucleus).[57–59] Since blockade of this receptor prevents emesis induced by both peripheral and central acting agents, it has been suggested that NK_1 receptors are critical elements in the central integration or effector pathway common to all emesis-inducing stimuli.[57] The first of the tachykinin receptor antagonists has been approved for treatment of chemotherapy-induced vomiting. Given its link between stress and GI motility, CRF may also be responsible for stress induced nausea and dyspepsia.

CINICAL ASPECTS OF VOMITING

Temporal patterns

There are three temporal patterns of vomiting one *acute* and two recurrent, *chronic* and *cyclic* (Fig. 8.2). Because of its frequent association with infections of childhood such as viral gastroenteritis, the *acute* form is the most common and is characterized by an episode of vomiting of moderate to high intensity. Recurrent vomiting is also a common problem encountered by pediatric gastroenterologists. Over a 5-year period, we evaluated 106 consecutive cases

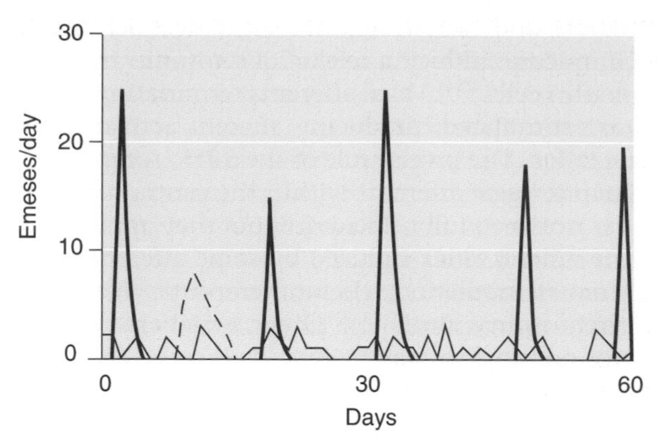

Figure 8.2: Representation of acute, chronic and cyclic patterns of vomiting. Three temporal patterns of vomiting are depicted: *acute* —, *chronic* - - - and *cyclic*—. The number of emeses per day is plotted on the vertical axis over a 2-month period. The *acute* pattern is represented by a single episode of moderate vomiting intensity; the *chronic* pattern by a recurrent low grade vomiting pattern that occurs on a daily basis; and the *cyclic* pattern by recurrent, discrete episodes of high intensity vomiting that occur once every several weeks with normal health in between.

that could be further subclassified: two-thirds as *chronic,* a low grade, daily pattern and one-third as *cyclic*, an intensive, but intermittent one (Table 8.1).[60] Those with the chronic pattern were mildly ill whereas those with the cyclic pattern tended to have severe bouts associated with stereotypic pallor, listlessness and dehydration. Because both the acute and cyclic patterns can produce intense vomiting, until the repetitive nature (>3 episodes) becomes evident, the cyclic pattern is understandably misclassified as an acute one and thus is typically misdiagnosed as a viral gastroenteritis or food poisoning.

Differential diagnosis

The diagnostic profile varies by the temporal pattern of vomiting (Table 8.2).[60–62] The *acute* pattern is dominated by infections both in and outside the GI tract. Other causes include food poisoning, obstruction of the GI tract, and increased intracranial pressure resulting from neurological injury. Among those with the *chronic* pattern, GI disorders outnumbered extraintestinal ones by a ratio of 7:1; the most common were peptic and infectious (*Helicobacter pylori*-induced) inflammation of the upper GI tract.[60] In contrast, the diagnostic profile in those with the *cyclic* pattern was reversed; extraintestinal disorders, exceeded GI ones by a ratio of 5:1. Although the hallmark of idiopathic *cyclic vomiting syndrome* is the cyclic pattern of vomiting, episodic vomiting is also the central manifestation of a number of renal (e.g. acute hydronephrosis from ureteral-pelvic junction obstruction), endocrine (e.g. Addison's disease), and metabolic disorders (e.g. disorders of fatty acid oxidation).

Causes of vomiting also vary with the age of the child (Table 8.3).[63–95] Although most congenital anomalies of the GI tract present in the neonatal period, webs and duplications can be discovered throughout childhood.[64,65] Malrotation or non-fixation of the small intestine complicated by intermittent volvulus can cause episodic vomiting at any age and result in catastrophic necrosis, short bowel syndrome and extended parenteral alimentation.[67,68] Duodenal obstruction from superior mesenteric artery syndrome is associated with acute weight loss from anorexia nervosa, extensive burns, and immobilization in a body cast.[71] Duodenal hematoma typically follows accidental trauma to the abdomen in bicycling children but can result from abuse of toddlers.

Although peptic and infectious injuries of the upper GI tract are most common, allergic (eosinophilic esophagitis) and inflammatory (Crohn's disease) ones also occur. Two unusual forms that affect toddlers include chronic granulomatous disease-induced antral obstruction[72] and cytomegalovirus-associated Ménétrier gastropathy associated with hypoalbuminemia and anasarca.[73] Typhilitis, a necrotizing inflammation of the cecum, principally affects children with acute lymphocytic leukemia during chemotherapy-induced neutropenia.[74] Besides a congenital

Clinical feature	Acute	Chronic recurrent	Cyclic recurrent
Epidemiology	Most common	Two-thirds of recurrent vomiting cohort	One-third of recurrent vomiting cohort
Acuity	Moderate-severe, ± dehydration	Not acutely ill or dehydrated	Severe, dehydrated
Vomiting intensity	Moderate to high	Low, 1–2 emeses/h at the peak	High, ≈6 emeses/h at peak
Recurrence, rate	No	Frequent, >2 episodes/week	Infrequent, ≤2 episodes/week
Stereotypy	Unique – *if child has had three similar episodes, consider cyclic pattern*	No	Yes
Onset	Variable	Daytime	Early morning
Symptoms	Fever, diarrhea	Abdominal pain, diarrhea	Pallor, lethargy, nausea, abdominal pain
Household contacts affected	Usually	No	No
Family history of migraine headache		14% positive	82% positive
Causes	Viral infections	Ratio of *GI* to extra-GI causes 7:1; upper GI tract mucosal injury most common (esophagitis, gastritis)	Ratio of *extra-GI* to GI causes 5:1; cyclic vomiting syndrome most common (also hydronephrosis, metabolic)

Table 8.1 Differentiating acute, chronic and cyclic patterns of vomiting[60]

Category	Acute	Chronic	Cyclic
Infectious	Gastroenteritis* Otitis media* Streptococcal pharyngitis Acute sinusitis Hepatitis Pyelonephritis Meningitis	*H. pylori** *Giardiasis* Chronic sinusitis*	Chronic sinusitis*
Gastrointestinal	Inguinal hernia Intussusception Malrotation with volvulus Appendicitis Cholecystitis Pancreatitis Distal intestinal obstruction syndrome	Anatomic obstruction GERD ± esophagitis* Eosinophilic esophagitis* Gastritis* Peptic ulcer or duodenitis* Achalasia SMA syndrome Gallbladder dyskinesia	Malrotation with volvulus
Genitourinary	Pyelonephritis UPJ obstruction	Pyelonephritis Pregnancy Uremia	Acute hydronephrosis 2° to UPJ obstruction
Endocrine, metabolic	Diabetic ketoacidosis	Adrenal hyperplasia	Diabetic ketoacidosis Addison's disease MCAD deficiency Partial OTC deficiency MELAS syndrome Acute intermittent porphyria
Neurologic	Concussion Subdural hematoma Reye's syndrome	Arnold-Chiari malformation Subtentorial neoplasm	Abdominal migraine* Migraine headaches* Arnold-Chiari malformation Subtentorial neoplasm Reye's syndrome
Other	Toxic ingestion Food poisoning	Rumination Psychogenic Bulimia Pregnancy	Cyclic vomiting syndrome* Munchausen-by-proxy (e.g. Ipecac poisoning)

*Most common disorders. GERD, gastroesophageal reflux disease; MCAD, medium chain acyl-CoA dehydrogenase deficiency; MELAS, mitochondrial myopathy, encephalopathy, lactic acidosis and stroke-like episodes; OTC, ornithine transcarbamylase deficiency; SMA, superior mesenteric artery; UPJ, uretero-pelvic junction.

Table 8.2 Causes of vomiting by temporal pattern[60–62]

form of intestinal dysmotility (chronic idiopathic intestinal pseudoobstruction), acquired viral and diabetes-induced gastroparesis can begin during adolescence.[75] Gallbladder dyskinesia, a cause of nausea, vomiting and right upper quadrant pain, is a newly recognized entity in adolescents.[78]

Addison's disease can mimic cyclic vomiting syndrome at all ages, manifesting itself with recurring bouts of vomiting and hyponatremic dehydration even before hyperpigmentation appears.[79] Pheochromocytoma, as part of a multiple endocrine neoplasia type 2b,[80] carcinoid syndrome[81] and gastrinoma[82] are rare in children and adolescents. Although metabolic disorders usually present in infancy with vomiting and failure to thrive, medium-chain acyl-CoA dehydrogenase deficiency,[83] partial ornithine transcarbamylase deficiency,[84] and acute intermittent porphyria[86] can present with episodic vomiting in older children and adolescents.

Acute hydronephrosis resulting from ureteral pelvic junction obstruction can present as a cyclic vomiting pattern, so called Dietl's crisis.[87] Increased intracranial pressure can result not only from structural subtentorial lesions (brainstem glioma, cerebellar medulloblastoma, and Chiari malformation) but also from pseudotumor cerebri associated with obesity, corticosteroid taper, vitamin A deficit or excess, tetracycline usage, and hypophosphatasia.[88] Both migraine headache and abdominal migraine are associated with vomiting in 40% of affected patients.[96] Epilepsy as a cause of recurrent abdominal pain and vomiting without evident seizure activity remains a controversial entity.[97]

Psychogenic vomiting and Munchausen by proxy (ipecac poisoning) have to be considered when the clinical pattern does not fit known disorders, the laboratory testing is negative, and psychosocial stresses are evident (see Psychogenic vomiting, below). Because of its lipid solubility,

Cause	Neonate (≤1 month)	Infant (1–12 months)	Child (1–11 years)	Adolescent (>11 years)	Reference
Extra-GI infections					
Otitis media		+	+	−	
Acute or chronic sinusitis			+	+	
Streptococcal pharyngitis			+	+	
Pneumonitis		+	+	−	
Pyelonephritis	+	+	+	+	
Meningitis	+	+	+	+	
GI infections					
Gastroenteritis		+	+	+	
Infectious colitis		−	+	+	
Parasitic infections			+	+	
H. pylori gastritis			+	+	
Giardiasis			+	+	
Hepatitis			+	+	
Hepatitic abscess			+	−	
Anatomic insults					
Congenital atresias and stenoses, tracheoesophageal fistula, webs, duplications, imperforate anus	+	+	−	−	63–65
Distal intestinal obstruction syndrome	+	+	+	+	66
Inguinal hernia	+	+	+	+	
Malrotation with volvulus	+	+	+	+	67,68
Intussusception		+	+	−	69
Appendicitis			+	+	70
SMA syndrome				+	71
Bezoar		+	+		
Duodenal hematoma			+	+	
Surgical adhesions			+	+	
Mucosal injuries					
GERD ± esophagitis, stricture	+	+	+	+	
Eosinophilic esophagitis			+	+	
Gastritis ± *H. pylori*			+	+	
Eosinophilic gastroenteropathy			+	+	
Peptic ulcer or duodenitis			+	+	
Cow or soy protein sensitivity	+	+	+		
Celiac disease		−	+	+	
Chronic granulomatous disease		−	+	−	72
Ménétrier disease			+	−	73
Crohn's disease		−	+	+	
Ulcerative colitis			+	+	
Typhilitis			+	−	74
GI motility disorders					
Oropharyngeal discoordination	+	+	+	−	
Achalasia			−	+	
Gastroparesis			−	+	75
Paralytic ileus	+	+	+	+	
Hirschsprung's disease	+	+	−		
Pseudoobstruction	+	+	−		76
Familial dysautonomia	+	+	+	−	77
Visceral GI disorders					
Cholecystitis			−	+	
Cholelithiasis			−	+	
Gallbladder dyskinesia			−	+	78
Choledochal cyst	+	+	−		
Pancreatitis			+	+	
Endocrine derangements					
Adrenal hyperplasia	+	+			
Addison's disease	+	+	+	+	79
Diabetic ketoacidosis		−	+	+	
Pheochromocytoma			−	−	80
Carcinoid syndrome			−	−	81
Zollinger-Ellison syndrome			−	−	82
Metabolic derangements					
Organic acidemias	+	+	−		

(Continued)

Disorders of fatty acid oxidation	−	+	+		83
Amino acidemias	+	+	−		
Urea cycle defects	+	+	−		84
Hereditary fructose intolerance	−	+			
Mitochondriopathies	−	+	+		85
Storage diseases	+	+	−		
Acute intermittent porphyria			−	+	86
Genitourinary disorders					
Hydronephrosis secondary to uteropelvic obstruction		+	+	−	87
Renal stones			+	+	
Uremia			+	+	
Hydrometrocolpos	−	+	+	+	
Pregnancy				+	
Neurologic disorders					
Hydrocephalus with shunt dysfunction	+	+	+	+	
Arnold-Chiari malformation		+	+	+	
Pseudotumor cerebri		−	+	+	88
Concussion	−	−	+	+	89
Subdural hematoma	+	+	+	+	
Subarachnoid hemorrhage			+	+	
Subtentorial neoplasm			+	+	90
Reye's syndrome			+	−	
Migraine headaches			+	+	
Abdominal migraine			+	+	91,92
Epilepsy			+		93
Other causes					
Overfeeding		+			
Rumination			+	+	
Toxic ingestion			+	−	
Lead poisoning			+	−	
Food poisoning			+	+	
Psychogenic vomiting			+	+	
Bulimia				+	
Cyclic vomiting syndrome		+	+	+	60,62,94
Munchausen-by-proxy (Ipecac poisoning)		−	+		95

+, typically presents in this age group; –, occasionally or rarely presents in this age group. GERD, gastroesophageal reflux disease; SMA, superior mesenteric artery.

Table 8.3 Etiology of vomiting by organ system and age at presentation

ipecac can be detected on a toxicology screen as late as 2 months after administration.[95]

Clinical clues to diagnosis

Clinical clues to aid in differential diagnosis are presented in Table 8.4. Hematemesis more commonly results from peptic esophagitis, prolapse gastropathy and Mallory-Weiss injury, and less often from allergic injury, Crohn's disease, and vasculitis involving the upper GI tract. In the face of nonspecific gastric petechiae, vomiting occasionally originates from a bleeding diathesis such as that of von Willebrand disease. Of the causes of morning vomiting upon wakening, the most worrisome is a neoplasm of the posterior fossa. More common causes of early morning nausea and vomiting associated with a history of congestion, postnasal drainage, cough-and-vomit sequence include environmental allergies and chronic sinusitis, and cyclic vomiting syndrome. Vertigo is commonly associated with a migraine headache or middle ear dysfunction (e.g. Ménière syndrome).

Unlike adults, for whom eating often provides pain relief, children more often experience post-prandial exacerbation of their abdominal pain and vomiting. Malodorous breath may be associated with chronic sinusitis, *Helicobacter pylori* gastritis, giardiasis and small bowel bacterial overgrowth. Although seen infrequently, visible peristalsis in infants and a succussion splash in children are indications of a gastric outlet obstruction that is causing gastric distension and retention of fluid. Abdominal masses can be seen in congenital (e.g. mesenteric cyst) or acquired non-neoplastic (e.g. ovarian cysts) and neoplastic (e.g. Burkitt's lymphoma) lesions. In a sexually active female adolescent, pregnancy should always be considered as a cause of an abdominal mass and excluded by a human chorionic gonadotropin level.

Repetitive, stereotypical, intense bouts of vomiting that begin abruptly in the early morning hours and resolve rapidly are characteristic of cyclic vomiting syndrome

Associated symptom or sign	Diagnostic consideration
Systemic manifestations	
Acute illness, dehydration	Infection, ingestion, cyclic vomiting, possible surgical emergency
Chronic malnutrition	Malabsorption syndrome
Temporal pattern	
Low-grade, daily	Chronic vomiting pattern, e.g. upper GI tract disease
Postprandial	Upper GI tract disease (e.g. gastritis), biliary and pancreatic disorders
Relationship to diet	Fat, cholecystitis, pancreatitis; protein allergy; fructose, hereditary fructose intolerance
Early morning onset	Sinusitis, cyclic vomiting syndrome, subtentorial neoplasm
High intensity	Cyclic vomiting syndrome, food poisoning
Stereotypical (well between episodes)	Cyclic vomiting syndrome (See Differential diagnosis in Table 8.2)
Rapid onset and subsidence	Cyclic vomiting syndrome
Character of emesis	
Effortless	Gastroesophageal reflux, rumination
Projectile	Upper GI tract obstruction
Mucous	Allergy, chronic sinusitis
Bilious	Post-ampullary obstruction, cyclic vomiting syndrome
Bloody	Esophagitis, prolapse gastropathy, Mallory-Weiss injury, allergic gastroenteropathy, bleeding diathesis
Undigested food	Achalasia
Clear, large volume	Ménétrier disease, Zollinger-Ellison syndrome
Malodorous	*H. pylori*, giardiasis, sinusitis, small bowel bacterial overgrowth, colonic obstruction
Gastrointestinal symptoms	
Nausea	Absence of nausea can suggest increased intracranial pressure
Abdominal pain	Substernal, esophagitis; epigastric, upper GI tract, pancreatic; right upper quadrant, cholelithiasis
Diarrhea	Gastroenteritis, bacterial colitis
Constipation	Hirschsprung's disease, pseudo-obstruction, hypercalcemia
Dysphagia	Eosinophilic esophagitis, achalasia, esophageal stricture
Visible peristalsis	Gastric outlet obstruction
Surgical scars	Surgical adhesions, surgical vagotomy
Succussion splash	Gastric outlet obstruction with gastric distension
Bowel sounds	Decreased: paralytic ileus, Increased: mechanical obstruction
Severe abdominal tenderness with rebound	Perforated viscera and peritonitis
Abdominal mass	Pyloric stenosis, congenital malformations, Crohn's, ovarian cyst, pregnancy, abdominal neoplasm
Neurologic symptoms	
Headache	Allergy, chronic sinusitis, migraine, increased intracranial pressure
Post-nasal drip, congestion	Allergy, chronic sinusitis
Vertigo	Migraine, Ménière disease
Seizures	Epilepsy
Abnormal muscle tone	Cerebral palsy, metabolic disorder, mitochondriopathy
Abnormal funduscopic exam or bulging fontanelle	Increased intracranial pressure, pseudotumor cerebri
Family history and epidemiology	
Peptic ulcer disease	Peptic ulcer disease, *H. pylori* gastritis
Migraine headaches	Abdominal migraine, cyclic vomiting syndrome
Contaminated water	*Giardia, Cryptosporidium*, other parasites
Travel	Traveler's (*Escherichia coli*) diarrhea, giardiasis

Table 8.4 Clinical clues to diagnosis

(see Cyclic vomiting syndrome and Abdominal migraine, below). Chronic vomiting can be associated with neurological injury such as cerebral palsy or a metabolic disorder that affects muscle tone (e.g. mitochondriopathy).[85] Neurological impairment can be associated with either oropharyngeal discoordination with aspiration or gastroesophageal reflux disease that often does not improve with time.

Evaluation

Evaluation of the child with acute vomiting is usually the purview of the primary care or emergency room physician. The clinical assessment of hydration without laboratory confirmation is usually sufficient basis to begin intravenous rehydration (Table 8.5).[61,98] Viral testing and bacterial cultures in stool in presumed gastroenteritis or colitis can identify the infectious risk to others. If the physical examination reveals acute abdominal signs, abdominal radiographs and surgical consultation are indicated. When the emesis is voluminous and frequent, empiric antiemetic therapy (e.g. promethazine suppositories) may forestall progression to dehydration and the need for intravenous therapy.

In a child presenting with chronic vomiting, screening laboratory tests (e.g. amylase, lipase) and empiric treat-

	Acute	Chronic	Cyclic (*test during the episode!*)
		Studies	
Screening testing	Electrolytes BUN Creatinine	CBC, ESR ALT, AST, GGTP, amylase Urinalysis Stool *Giardia* ELISA	Blood CBC Glucose, electrolytes, ALT, AST, GGTP amylase lipase Ammonia Lactate Carnitine Amino acids Urine Urinalysis Organic acids δ-ALA, porphobilinogen Carnitine
Definitive testing	Rotazyme Stool *Giardia* ELISA Abdominal radiographs Surgical consult	Endoscopy with biopsies Sinus CT UGI/SBFT series Abdominal ultrasound	UGI/SBFT series Endoscopy with biopsies Sinus CT Head MRI Abdominal ultrasound Definitive metabolic testing

ALA, aminolevulinic acid; ALT, alanine transaminase; AST, aspartate aminotransferase; BUN, blood urea nitrogen; CBC, complete blood count; CT, computerized tomography; ESR, erythrocyte sedimentation rate; ELISA, enzyme linked immunosorbent assay; GGTP, γ-glutamyl transpeptidase (gamma); MRI, magnetic resonance imaging; UGI/SBFT, upper gastrointestinal with small bowel follow-through.

Table 8.5 Initial diagnostic evaluation by temporal pattern of vomiting[61,98]

ment with H_2 receptor antagonists or proton pump inhibitors can precede more definitive testing. If the condition does not improve on therapy, definitive tests may be considered: an esophagogastroduodenoscopy to detect suspected peptic, allergic, infectious, and inflammatory mucosal injuries; small bowel radiography to identify possible anatomic lesions and Crohn's disease; an abdominal ultrasound to assess potential cholelithiasis, pancreatic pseudocyst or hydronephrosis, and, sinus computed tomography (CT) to document chronic sinusitis. Sinus evaluation has a 10% yield in chronic vomiting.[60]

In evaluating a child with cyclic or episodic vomiting, laboratory test results are typically abnormal only during the symptomatic attack, therefore blood and urine screening for metabolic disorders must be obtained *during the episode*.[61] The serum chemistry profile can detect hyperglycemia in diabetes mellitus or hypoglycemia in disorders of fatty acid oxidation, hyponatremia in Addison's disease, an anion gap and low bicarbonate in organic acidemias, elevated hepatic transaminases in hepatic and biliary disorders, and elevated lipase in pancreatic disorders. Blood is analyzed for elevations of ammonia in urea cycle defects, lactic acid in mitochondriopathies, amino acids in aminoacidemias and deficiency of carnitine in disorders of fatty acid oxidation. After screening children for pyuria (infection) and hematuria (stones), the urine is analyzed for elevations in organic acids, carnitine esters, δ-aminolevulinic acid and porphobilinogen in organic acidurias, disorders of fatty acid oxidation, and acute intermittent porphyria, respectively. Positive results on screening tests necessitate appropriate definitive testing. For example, the absence of ketones, presence of dicarboxylic aciduria, and elevated urinary esterified:free carnitine ratio of greater than 4:1 implicate a disorder of fatty acid oxidation and diagnosis entails definitive plasma acylcarnitine and urinary acylglycine profiles. Definitive evaluation of GI tract involvement includes small bowel radiography for anatomic lesions, an esophagogastroduodenoscopy for mucosal inflammation, and an abdominal ultrasound for renal, gallbladder, pancreatic and ovarian lesions. With a history suggestive of increased intracranial pressure (e.g. headache, onset upon wakening), magnetic resonance imaging (MRI) of the brain is the best test to visualize the subtentorial region. In the absence of laboratory, radiographic or endoscopic findings, if cyclic vomiting syndrome is suspected, an empiric trial of prophylactic antimigraine may be initiated.

Complications

The two principal complications of acute or cyclic vomiting (during the episode) include dehydration with electrolyte derangement and hematemesis from prolapse gastropathy or Mallory-Weiss injury. The electrolyte disturbance resulting from varying losses of gastric HCl, pancreatic HCO_3, and GI NaCl is generally corrected with standard intravenous replacement. Hypochloremic, hypokalemic alkalosis results from high grade gastric outlet obstruction and predominant loss of gastric H^+ and Cl^- ions. Risk factors for development of alkalosis in pyloric stenosis include female gender, African-American race, longer duration of illness, and more severe dehydration.[99] Preoperative restoration of electrolyte balance reduces the perioperative morbidity.

Prolapse gastropathy occurs more commonly than the Mallory-Weiss injury at the GE junction. The former injury presumably results from repeated severe trauma resulting from herniation of the cardia through the gastroesophageal junction. No therapy or short-term acid suppression suffices.

Complications of persistent peptic injury to the esophagus (e.g. stricture formation and Barrett's metaplasia) and bronchopulmonary aspiration are more likely to occur with long-standing chronic vomiting associated with gastroesophageal reflux disease in which the esophageal mucosa undergoes prolonged acid exposure. Growth failure as a complication of chronic vomiting can be caused by loss of calories, inflammatory burden, or protein-losing enteropathy. Aggressive nutritional rehabilitation may require continuous nasogastric or transpyloric feedings.

Pharmacological treatment

Although the therapy should be directed towards the cause, empiric therapy of the vomiting symptom may be indicated when the severity of the acute or cyclic vomiting places the child at risk of dehydration and other complications. Although laboratory confirmation of cyclic vomiting syndrome is not possible, a positive response to the antimigraine therapy can support the diagnosis. A comprehensive listing of therapeutic agents by pharmacologic category is presented in Table 8.6.[100–102]

Antihistamines (e.g. meclizine) are minimally active antiemetics but have efficacy in motion sickness because of their effects on vestibular function of the middle ear. As a result of D_2 receptor antagonist activity, phenothiazines (e.g. promethazine) have mild to moderate activity in chemotherapy-induced vomiting but carry a substantial risk of extrapyramidal reactions. Butyrophenones (e.g. droperidol) have mild to moderate efficacy when used in chemotherapy and postoperative settings. Their use is limited by extrapyramidal reactions. Benzodiazepines have minimal antiemetic efficacy but are useful adjuncts to other antiemetics. Cannabinoids have mild to moderate potency can be associated with dependence.

The newer serotonergic agonists and antagonists have demonstrated marked antiemetic efficacy. The 5-HT_3 antagonists have demonstrated greater antiemetic efficacy in postoperative and chemotherapy settings than did previous regimens. 5-$HT_{1B/1D}$ agonists (e.g. triptans) have recently shown promise for aborting pediatric migraine headaches[103] and cyclic vomiting.[104,105] Because 5-HT_3 and 5-$HT_{1B/1D}$ agents have both central and peripheral actions, the antiemetic effects may result from a combination of both.

CLINICAL ASPECTS OF NAUSEA

Nausea, a uniquely unpleasant sensation that typically precedes the act of vomiting, is difficult to precisely define. A variety of stimuli, including labyrinth stimulation, visceral pain and unpleasant memories, may induce nausea. Although the precise mechanism of nausea is unknown, evidence suggests that the neural pathways responsible for nausea and vomiting are the same. Nausea may result from less intense activation whereas more intense activation of the same neural pathways triggers vomiting. During nausea, gastric tone and peristalsis are diminished whereas duodenal and proximal jejunal tone tend to be increased.

The major nausea pathways can be activated with chemical, visceral, vestibular and central nervous system stimulation. Chemical stimulation results from the action of blood-born toxins (e.g. chemotherapy) on the CTZ in the area postrema where the blood-brain barrier is virtually nonexistent.[106] The visceral pathway is activated directly by stomach irritation caused by ingested agents (drugs and toxins) or indirectly by enhanced gastric acid secretion resulting from physical and emotional stressors.[107] The vagus and sympathetic nerves, via the nucleus tractus solitarius and nodosum ganglion respectively, mediate the nausea arising from gastric irritants. Antral balloon distention stretching the gastric walls is another mechanism that can evoke nausea.[108] The vestibular pathway involves afferent nerves that project to the vestibular nuclei and lead to activation of the brain stem mediated via histamine H_1 and muscarinic cholinergic pathways. This pathway is most commonly activated when a person is subjected to a novel motion environment.[109] Onset of nausea during motion correlates with gastric dysrhythmias including tachygastria and the release of vasopressin from the posterior pituitary.[108] Nausea can arise in the central nervous system during anticipatory nausea that often precedes recurring chemotherapy. Previous studies have identified motion sickness, trait anxiety, depression, female sex and young age of subject to be predictors of anticipatory nausea and vomiting.[110]

Another area of ongoing investigation is the proposed involvement of neuroendocrine response to stress. In extensive animals studies by Taché's group, secretion of corticotropin-releasing factor atop the hypothalamic-pituitary adrenal axis (HPA) in response to physical or psychological stress, cytokines or ingested noxious substances can cause gastroparesis via sympathetic outflow.[53] Hypothalamic ADH release may also help mediate gastric stasis and symptomatic nausea.[111]

Clinical clues and differential diagnosis

There are distinct autonomic signs that often accompany the symptoms of nausea. Hypersalivation is due to activation of salivary centers that are in close proximity to the medullary vomiting center. Pallor, listlessness, and tachycardia often accompany nausea. Several lines of research implicate the autonomic nervous system (ANS) in the expression of chemotherapy-induced nausea.[112] Bellg measured peak values of heart rate, pulse, pallor, and skin temperature to assess autonomic reactivity over time. These autonomic measures varied in relation to time of emesis but were all associated with the development of nausea.[113] The list of potential causes of nausea is extensive and overlaps known etiologies of vomiting (Table 8.7).

Drug class/generic	Brand name	Dosages[a]	Mechanisms	Side-effects	Indications	Potential applications
Antihistamines (*Minimal* antiemetic activity)						
Diphenhydramine	Benadryl, Benylin	≈1.25 mg/kg q. 6 h PO or i.v.	Vestibular suppression, anti-ACh effect, and H_1 antagonist	Sedation, anticholinergic effects[b]	Motion sickness, mild hemotherapy-induced vomiting	Contraindicated with MAO inhibitors, GI obstruction
Hydroxyzine	Atarax, Vistaril	0.5–0.6 mg/kg q. 6 h PO				
Dimenhydrinate	Dramamine	1.25 mg/kg q 6 h PO or i.m.		Sedation		
Cyclizine	Marezine	1 mg/kg q 8 h PO or i.m. >10 years of age: 50 mg q 4–6 h PO or i.m.	Vestibular suppression, anti-ACh effect			
Meclizine	Antivert	>12 years of age; 25–100 mg/24 h PO divided t.i.d.-q.i.d.				
Phenothiazines (*Mild* to *moderate* antiemetic activity)						
Promethazine	Phenergan	0.25–0.5 mg/kg per dose q 4–6 h PR or i.m.	D_2 receptor antagonist at CTZ and H_1 antagonist	Anticholinergic effects,[b] extrapyramidal reactions	Chemotherapy-induced vomiting	
Prochlorperazine	Compazine	>10 kg: 0.1–0.15 mg/kg per dose i.m. >10 kg: 0.4 mg/kg per 24 h divided t.i.d.-q.i.d. PO or PR Maximum 10 mg/dose	D_2 receptor antagonist at CTZ			
Chlorpromazine	Thorazine	>6 months of age: 0.5–1 mg/kg per dose i.v. or PO q 6–8 h				
Substituted benzamides (*High* antiemetic activity)						
Cisapride	Propulsid	0.2–0.3 mg/kg t.i.d.-q.i.d. PO Adults: 10 mg t.i.d.-q.i.d. PO	$5HT_4$ agonist with ACh release in gut	Diarrhea, abdominal pain, headache	GER, gastroparesis	Arrhythmias with antifungal and macrolide antibiotics, cyclic vomiting
Metoclopramide	Reglan	0.1 mg/kg per dose i.m., i.v., or PO up to q.i.d. The total daily dose should not exceed 0.5 mg/kg. Adults: 10 mg i.m., i.v. or PO 30 min before each meal and at bedtime	D_2 antagonist at CTZ and gut, $5HT_4$ agonist in gut	Irritability and extrapyramidal reactions	GER, gastroparesis, chemotherapy-induced vomiting	
Trimethobenzamide	Tigan	Children <14 kg: 100 mg/dose PR t.i.d.-q.i.d. Children 14–40 kg: 100–200 mg/dose PO or PR t.i.d.-q.i.d. Not recommended for neonates or premature infants.	D_2 antagonist at CTZ			

Table 8.6 Antinausea and antiemetic medications[100–102]

(Continued)

Drug class/generic	Brand name	Dosages[a]	Mechanisms	Side-effects	Indications	Potential applications
$5HT_3$ receptor antagonists (*High* anti-emetic activity)						
Ondansetron	Zofran	0.15 mg/kg i.v. q 8 h or 0.15–0.40 mg/kg Surface area <0.3 m^2: 1 mg/dose PO Surface area 0.3–0.6 m^2: 2 mg/dose PO Surface area 0.6–1.0 m^2: 3 mg/dose PO Surface area >1 m^2: 4 mg/dose PO	$5HT_3$ antagonist at CTZ and vagal afferents in gut	Headache	Chemotherapy, postoperative	Cyclic vomiting
Granisetron	Kytril	Age 2–16 years: 10 µg/kg i.v. q 6 h				Cyclic vomiting
Tropisetron	Navoban	No dose recommendations available.				
Tachykinin receptor antagonists						
Aprepitant	Emend	Adult 3 day regimen: 1st dose 125 mg 1 h prior to chemotherapy and 80 mg q.d. on days 2–3	NK_1 receptor antagonist in CTZ	Fatigue, dizziness, diarrhea	Chemotherapy induced nausea and vomiting	
Anticholinergics (*Minimal* anti-emetic activity)						
Scopolamine	Transderm SCOP	Not recommended for pediatric use. 1 patch is 1 mg scopolamine q 3 days	Vestibular suppression, anti-ACh effect on central pattern generator	Sedation, anticholinergic effects[b]	Prophylaxis of motion sickness	
Benzimidazole derivative (*Mild* to *moderate* anti-emetic activity)						
Domperidone	Motilium	0.6 mg/kg per dose t.i.d.-q.i.d. PO or <2 years: 10 mg PR b.i.d.-q.i.d. 2–4 years: 15 mg PR q.i.d. 4–6 years: 23 mg PR q.i.d. >6 years: 30 mg PR q.i.d.	D_2 antagonist in gut	Headaches	Gastroparesis, chemotherapy	Not available in the USA

Butyrophenone (*Mild* to *moderate* anti-emetic activity)						
Droperidol	Inapsine	0.05–0.075 mg/kg per dose i.m. or i.v. for one dose	D_2 antagonist at CTZ, anxiolytic action and sedation	Hypotension, sedation, extrapyramidal effects	Chemotherapy, postoperative	
Benzodiazepines (*Minimal* anti-emetic activity)						
Lorazepam	Ativan	0.05–0.1 mg/kg per dose i.v.	Enhanced central GABA-ergic inhibition inducing anxiolysis, sedation and amnesia	Sedation, respiratory depression	Chemotherapy adjunct	Cyclic vomiting adjunct
Diazepam	Valium	0.1–0.3 mg/kg i.v. prn Maximum: <0.6 mg/kg per 24 h				
Corticosteroids (*Mild* to *moderate* anti-emetic activity)						
Dexamethasone	Decadron	Initial dose: 5–10 mg/m² i.v., maximum 20 mg, then 5 mg/m² q 12 h i.v.		Unknown	Adrenal suppression	Chemotherapy
Cannabinoids (*Mild* to *moderate* anti-emetic activity)						
Dronabinol	Marinol	>12 years: 5 mg/m² per dose q 4–6 h PO	Unknown	Disorientation, vertigo, hallucinations	Chemotherapy	
Nabilone	Cesamet	<18 kg: 0.5 mg PO b.i.d. 18–30 kg: 1 mg PO b.i.d. >30 kg: 1 mg PO t.i.d.				

[a]Note that these are doses used for anti-emetic effects rather than other indications. [b]Anticholinergic effects – blurred vision, dry mouth, hypotension, palpitations, urinary retention. Within the same drug class, in the blank space, the same attributes apply from the medication above. Ach, acetylcholine; CTZ, chemotrigger zone; D, dopamine; H, histamine; 5HT, 5-hydroxytryptamine; GABA, γ-aminobutyric acid.

Table 8.6 (*Continued*) Antinausea and antiemetic medications[100–102]

Gastrointestinal
- Gastroesophageal reflux disease
- Allergic bowel disease, e.g. eosinophilic esophagitis
- Delayed gastric emptying, e.g. postinfectious gastroparesis
- Intestinal pseudoobstruction and other dysmotility syndromes
- Biliary dysfunction, e.g. biliary dyskinesia
- Food poisoning, e.g. bacillus cereus
- Gastric outlet obstruction, malrotation

Non-gastrointestinal
- Brain and ear, nose and throat
  - Migraine headaches
  - Migraine variants, e.g. abdominal migraines, cyclic vomiting syndrome
  - Chronic sinusitis, allergic rhinitis
  - Motion sickness, e.g. vertigo
  - Autonomic dysfunction, e.g. postural orthostatic tachycardia syndrome
  - Eustachian tube dysfunction, e.g. middle ear infection or Ménière's
  - Arnold-Chiari malformation
  - Brain stem tumor, e.g. brainstem glioma, cerebellar medulloblastoma
- Systemic and behavioral
  - Eating disorders (e.g. anorexia nervosa, bulimia)
  - Thyroid dysfunction
  - Pregnancy and hyperemesis gravidarum
  - Drug-induced (e.g. chemotherapy, ingestion)
  - Postoperative state

Table 8.7 Differential diagnosis of nausea

GI Anatomical	Mucosal	Motility
Contrast UGI/SBFT Abdominal ultrasound Gastric barostat	EGD with biopsies	Solid phase GE scan GB HIDA Scan
Non-GI Autonomic	**Organic (Other)**	**Migraine**
Orthostatic pulse increase	CT sinuses	Historical criteria
Tilt-table testing Stress-induced	MRI subtentorium	Trial of medication

UGI/SBFT, upper gastrointestinal series with small bowel follow through; EGD, esophagogastroduodenoscopy; GE, gastric emptying; GB, gallbladder; HIDA, cholescintigraphy.

Table 8.8 Evaluation of nausea

Evaluation

The evaluation of the symptom of chronic nausea usually involves an investigation that overlaps that of vomiting (Table 8.8). If one suspects an anatomical cause of nausea that is associated with projectile vomiting or bilious emesis, contrast radiography of the stomach and small bowel is indicated. An abdominal ultrasound can be useful in the initial evaluation of symptoms of meal-related nausea with or without right upper-quadrant (RUQ) and left upper-quadrant (LUQ) pain for detecting gallstones or pancreatic pseudocyst respectively. If no gallstones are found but the nausea and RUQ pain persists, a finding on CCK-stimulated gallbladder HIDA scan of less than 30% emptying is compatible with gallbladder dyskinesia.[114]

If mucosal injury is suspected from meal-induced nausea, pain and/or vomiting, an esophagogastroduodenoscopy will detect peptic or allergic esophagitis, gastritis with or without *H. pylori* as well as eosinophilic gastroenteritis. Crohn's disease and celiac disease are unusual organic causes of nausea. If nausea, early satiety, bloating are noted, disordered gastric motility should be suspected. Although a solid phase gastric emptying scan can be useful in this scenario, it unfortunately is a relatively insensitive test. More distal intestinal dysmotility can be suggested by chronically dilated intestinal loops on flat plates and delayed small bowel transit on contrast radiography.

Additional specialized motility tests performed in a few pediatric GI centers include the gastric barostat, antroduodenal motility and electrogastrography (EGG). The gastric barostat is useful in detecting impaired gastric compliance and visceral hypersensitivity in the stomach. Antroduodenal manometry can demonstrate myopathic, neuropathic or obstructive contraction patterns.[108] EGG can demonstrate dysrhythmias (e.g. tachygastria) both in the presence and the absence of altered gastric emptying.[109] The combination of these tests have been used in adults to delineate a full blown gastric neuromuscular disorder with abnormal gastric emptying and EGG results to be treated with prokinetic agents to a visceral hypersensitivity associated with normal results to be tried on tricyclic antidepressants.[108] An important non-gastrointestinal cause of nausea to evaluate includes autonomic dysfunction. In the clinic, one can screen for postural orthostatic tachycardia syndrome (POTS) by looking for a 30 beat/min rise in heart rate following a change in position from supine to upright. A more definitive evaluation includes a tilt-table test to more precisely confirm the postural orthostatic tachycardia response.

There are several important, less appreciated causes of early morning nausea. If post-nasal drip or congestion occurs in the morning, chronic sinusitis or allergic rhinitis should be suspected and if no response to antihistamines, a sinus CT performed. Other common causes include CVS, abdominal migraines or migraine headaches and should be suspected based on the stereotypical pattern, pallor and listlessness; a positive response to a trial of anti-migraine medication can serve as a supporting evidence. However, if the nausea becomes persistent and intractable, an MRI would be indicated exclude a subtentorial neoplasm or Chiari malformation.

Nausea that results from gastric retention from gastroparesis, pseudoobstruction or mechanical obstruction is typically reduced by the action of vomiting. If abdominal pain or altered bowel function are accompanied by nausea, irritable bowel syndrome should be considered.[108] In contrast, nausea of central origin, e.g. that accompanying a migraine, is typically poorly relieved by vomiting. Many patients complain of chronic nausea without full blown retching or vomiting.

In some cases, nausea can persist for months or even years despite an exhaustive evaluation that has excluded numerous organic disorders. On the basis of laboratory exclusion, this can be classified as either functional nausea and/or included under the broader umbrella of functional dyspepsia. As with many incapacitating functional gastrointestinal disorders, it is often difficult to convince the parents that such intractable nausea does not have an organic basis. This concern often propels the parents to seek out more experts and additional laboratory, radiographic and endoscopic testing on behalf of the affected child.

Pharmacologic treatment

Nausea, in part because of the abundance of incapacitating accompanying autonomic symptoms, can become extremely disabling for the child and adolescent. Treatment of chronic nausea requires a multi-disciplinary approach. One must take into account that many of those affected are school-aged children with various stressors related to school, family and friends. For example, prolonged school absenteeism can be self perpetuating and may require the help of a psychologist to acknowledge the validity of the symptoms, modify stress awareness and devise a graded program of reintroducing the child back to school.[111] Stress reduction through a structured program of biofeedback or relaxation therapy can be an essential aid.[111]

A trial of medication can be useful in ameliorating symptoms of nausea and narrowing the possible causes. A positive response to acid suppression or gastric prokinetics can support the possibilities of a peptic disorder or gastric dysmotility. If migraine or migraine equivalent is suspected based on the historical criteria, a trial of β-blockers or tricyclic antidepressants such as amitriptyline may prevent the attacks. Suspected allergies or chronic sinusitis with night-time postnasal drip may respond to a course of antihistamines and/or antibiotics. When no specific cause is discerned, a series of trials of D_2 antagonists, H_1antagonists, and $5HT_3$ antagonists may provide some relief of nausea (Table 8.6).

Dietary modification can be useful when gastric neuromuscular dysfunction is present and the ability of the stomach to triturate and empty meals is compromised.[108] Because liquids require less neuromuscular effort than solids to empty, a staged approach to advance the diet from liquids to soups to starches can be beneficial. Other non-drug treatments include the complementary medicine approaches. Ginger given 1 h before motion sickness has been shown to decrease nausea associated with gastric dysrhythmias in adults.[108] Also, acustimulation via a transcutaneous electrode has been shown to reduce nausea due to pregnancy, chemotherapy and the postoperative state.[108] Although gastric electrical stimulation to the neuromuscular circuitry can reduce the refractory nausea and vomiting by 70%–80% in patients with gastroparesis, the mechanism of action appears to be other than one of improved motility.[108]

Functional nausea is difficult to manage, specifically the relief of discomfort and the return to normal functioning. Some children with functional nausea that we have encountered have been fully bedridden and absent from school for months. Similar to that used in other functional gastrointestinal disorders, in the initial approach it is important to: (1) acknowledge that the child's symptoms are real and are being taken seriously, (2) reassure the parents that the medical evaluation will be thorough in order to exclude serious treatable disorders, (3) note that there will be a series of ongoing empiric treatments used to treat suspected underlying conditions (e.g. acid reflux) as well as relieve the child's discomfort and (4) identify that the principal goal is to rehabilitate the child to normal function even while the nausea persists and its cause remains unclear. Because each treatment may take several weeks (e.g. to achieve therapeutic levels), it is critical to forewarn the parents that this simultaneous evaluative, therapeutic and rehabilitative approach is unlikely to lead to an immediate cure but is more likely to lead to incremental improvement over several months.[111] The return to school may require the medical psychologist to plan a progressively increasing attendance and, if that fails, to exclude the possibility of school phobia.

SPECIFIC VOMITING DISORDERS

Cyclic vomiting syndrome and abdominal migraine

Although cyclic vomiting syndrome is now increasingly recognized, the pathogenesis remains unknown.[60–62] On the basis of its 1.9% prevalence among 5 to 15-year-olds in Aberdeen, Scotland, cyclic vomiting can no longer be considered rare.[115] Both its original description in English by Samuel Gee in 1882[116] and the current consensus on diagnostic criteria in 1994[117] reflect the same emphasis on intermittent, intense, stereotypical episodes of vomiting with normal or baseline health between (Table 8.9).[91,92,117] Although the cyclic *pattern* of vomiting is the key diagnostic feature of cyclic vomiting *syndrome*, the pattern represents a starting point for diagnostic testing and the syndrome refers to those idiopathic cases in whom the diagnostic testing is negative.[118]

Because of similarities in clinical features, overlap with abdominal migraine has been recognized (see Table 8.9).[119–121] The historical criteria for abdominal migraine proposed by Lundberg[91] and Symon and Russell[92] overlap with the consensus criteria for cyclic vomiting syndrome, especially the discrete stereotypical episodes of pain and vomiting associated with symptoms of pallor, listlessness and nausea.[117] Electroencephalographic and autonomic function data support a pathophysiologic overlap between the two entities.[122,123] Other possible pathogenic mechanisms include a hypothalamic discharge with release of CRF and adrenocorticotropin (ACTH) described by Wolff and Sato.[124–127]

In our series of 463 children who presented with the cyclic vomiting syndrome and abdominal migraine, the

Variable	Cyclic vomiting syndrome	Abdominal migraine
Temporal pattern	Recurrent stereotypical episodes of *vomiting* lasting hours–days	Recurrent stereotypical episodes of midline *abdominal pain* lasting >2 h
Associated symptoms	Pallor, lethargy, anorexia, nausea, retching, *abdominal pain*	Pallor, lethargy, anorexia, nausea, *vomiting*
Family history	Family history of migraine	Family history of migraine
Laboratory testing	Negative laboratory, radiographic and endoscopic tests	Negative laboratory, radiographic and endoscopic tests
Therapeutic response	Most respond to antimigraine therapy	Positive response to antimigraine therapy

Table 8.9 Diagnostic criteria for cyclic vomiting and abdominal migraine[91,92,117]

typical patient is a 5–8-year-old girl who has stereotypical, severe (15 emeses) episodes once every 2–4 weeks, yet returns to normal or baseline health between episodes. Although the term *cyclic* is used, because only 49% have regular intervals, *episodic* would be a more precise term. The attacks most frequently begin at 02:00 to 07:00 h, are preceded by a short prodrome (1.5 h), last 24 h, require intravenous (i.v.) hydration (58%) and cause 15 days of school absence per year. Because each episode is accompanied by dehydration, the condition is most often misdiagnosed as acute gastroenteritis. Common symptoms (in more than 70% of the children) include pallor, lethargy, anorexia, nausea, retching and abdominal pain. The parents can usually (72%) identify a proximate event-psychological stress (e.g. birthday, holiday), an infection (e.g. URI), or a food (e.g. chocolate, cheese). However, typical migraine *symptoms* of headaches and photophobia affect only 30–40% of children. Fortunately, this disorder usually resolves during the teenage years but is often replaced by migraine headaches.

Cyclic vomiting *syndrome* remains a diagnosis of exclusion with normal results of laboratory, radiographic, and endoscopic testing (see Table 8.5). The diagnosis of abdominal migraine,[128] in which pain is the primary or more consistent symptom than vomiting, can be made by the historical criteria of stereotypical episodes associated with pallor, listlessness and a family history of migraine headaches (see Table 8.9).[91,92] Although vomiting can occur in the ictal phase,[93] abdominal epilepsy[129] accompanied by electroencephalographic changes[130] now appears to be a rare cause of vomiting.[97]

In the absence of identified underlying causes, treatment remains empiric and includes supportive therapy, antiemetics, antimigraine agents, prokinetic agents and anticonvulsant medications (Table 8.10).[131–133] Promising therapies used during acute treatment include serotonergic agents, both 5-HT_3 antiemetics (e.g. ondansetron) and the $5HT_{1B/1D}$ (e.g. sumatriptan) anti-migraine agent. Consensus treatment guidelines are being written by a North American Society for Pediatric Gastroenterology, Hepatology and Nutrition task force. Supportive therapy, especially intravenous fluids containing 10% dextrose can attenuate the episode by terminating the ketosis.[60] High dose 5-HT_3 antagonist antiemetics (e.g. ondansetron 0.3 mg/kg) have been used as attenuating agents with encouraging results.[132] Antimigraine agents have been used successfully both as prophylactic (e.g. propranolol) and abortive agents (e.g. triptans), further supporting the putative relationship to migraine phenomena.[60,104,105] Blunting the estrogen decline with low estrogen containing birth control pills has been effective for catamenial (menstrual) migraines in teenage girls.[134,135] With its disruptive, unpredictable occurrence, high level of morbidity, lack of definitive diagnosis and established therapy, parental support from the physician may by itself serve to relieve family stress and reduce frequency of episodes.[98]

Postoperative nausea and vomiting

The prevalence of postoperative nausea and vomiting in children is 20 to 24% after elective operations including strabismus repair, tonsillectomy, dental surgery, and inguinal herniorraphy.[136,137] Although the mechanisms have not been elucidated, there appear to be a number of risk factors for the development of postoperative vomiting. These include age greater than 2 years, female gender, certain operations (tonsillectomies, strabismus repair, otoplasties and ureter surgery), anesthetic used (cyclopropane has greater risk than isoflurane, enflurane and halothane), postoperative opioid analgesia, prior postoperative vomiting, and a history of motion sickness.[136,138]

Recent randomized, double-blind, placebo-controlled trials have established that 5-HT_3 antagonists reduce postoperative emesis following general anesthesia in preadolescent children undergoing strabismus correction,[139] tonsillectomy[140] and other elective operations[141] with the exception of craniotomy.[142] Head-to-head comparisons have established the superior efficacy of 5-HT_3 antagonists to droperidol[140,143,144] and metoclopramide.[140] Although single intravenous intraoperative doses of either ondansetron (0.15 mg/kg)[145] and granisetron (0.4 μg/kg) appear equally effective during the first 4 h,[145,146] some studies detect a prolonged effect lasting 24 h.[139,147] A recent randomized, double-blind placebo-controlled trial also demonstrated the efficacy of intraoperative prophylactic use of ondansetron on postoperative nausea and vomiting.[148] Most but not all recent controlled trials using perioperative electroacupuncture point P6 demonstrate significantly reduced postoperative nausea and vomiting as judged by the number of episodes of emeses or the use

Drug class	Brand name	Dosages	Mechanism of action	Side-effects	Comments
Abortive					
Supportive					
i.v. hydration			Stops ketosis, replaces Na^+, K^+ and lost volume		Glucose may be most effective component by terminating ketosis
Lorazepam	Ativan	0.05–0.1 mg/kg i.v. q 6 h	Central enhanced GABA-ergic inhibition inducing sedation, anxiolysis and amnesia	Sedation, respiratory depression	Adjunct to allow child to sleep
Antimigraine					
Isometheptene	Midrin	Age >12 years, 1 capsule/h PO but ≤5 capsules q 24 h	Sympathomimetic vasoconstrictor	Dizziness	Not effective in vomiting child
Sumatriptan	Imitrex	Age >12 years, 6 mg s.c., may repeat in 1 h (maximum dose: 2 injections/24 h) 20 mg nasally	$5HT_{1D}$ agonist induces cerebral vasoconstriction, relaxes gastric fundus	Transient burning in neck and chest, headache	Use s.c. form if child is vomiting. Contraindicated with coronary vasospasm or hemiplegic or basilar artery migraine
Ketorolac	Toradol	0.5–1.0 mg/kg i.v./i.m. × 1, then 0.2–0.5 mg/kg q 6–8 h ≤ 30 mg/dose	Cyclooxygenase inhibitor of prostaglandin synthesis	GI bleeding, contraindicated in ASA sensitivity	Can be given intravenously. Contraindicated with ASA sensitivity
Anti-emetic					
Ondansetron	Zofran	0.15–0.4 mg/kg i.v. q 6–8 h	$5HT_3$ antagonist in CTZ and vagal afferents in gut	Headache	Use i.v. form if child is vomiting
Granisetron	Kytril	0.10 μg/kg q 6–8 h			
Tropisetron					
Prophylactic					
Antimigraine					
Propranolol	Inderal	0.5–1 mg/kg per day maximum PO divided b.i.d. or t.i.d. 10–20 mg t.i.d.	β_1, β_2 adrenergic antagonist	Hypotension, bradycardia, fatigability	Use in small doses. Contraindicated in asthma, heart block. Withdraw gradually, monitor pulse
Atenolol	Tenormin	0.7–1.4 mg/kg per day PO divided b.i.d. or t.i.d.	β_1 adrenergic antagonist H_1 antagonist and $5HT_2$ antagonist	Sedation, anticholinergic effects[a], weight gain due to appetite stimulation	Contraindicated with asthma MAO inhibitors, GI obstruction
Cyproheptadine	Periactin	0.25–0.5 mg/kg per day PO divided b.i.d. or t.i.d.			
Pizotyline	Sandomigran	1.5 mg/day divided q.d. or t.i.d.			Not available in the USA
Amitriptyline	Elavil	0.5–1 mg/kg/day q.hs	Tricyclic antidepressant, increases synaptic norepinephrine and $5HT_2$ antagonist	Sedation, anticholinergic effects[a]	Contraindicated with SVT, MAO inhibitor, GI obstruction.
		1.5–3 mg/kg/day PO divided q.d. or t.i.d.			
		Age <6 years, 10–30 mg/day 6–12 years, 50–100 mg/day >12 years, 100–200 mg/day			Monitor therapeutic levels
Nortriptyline	Pamelor	0.5–1 mg/kg/day q.hs			

Table 8.10 Medications used to treat cyclic vomiting syndrome and abdominal migraine[60–62,100–102,131–133]

(*Continued*)

Drug class	Brand name	Dosages	Mechanism of action	Side-effects	Comments
Neuroleptic					
Phenobarbital	Luminal	2–3 mg/kg per day PO divided q.d. or b.i.d.	$GABA_A$ potentiation of synaptic inhibition	Sedation	Contraindicated with acute intermittent porphyria, abdominal epilepsy
Phenytoin	Dilantin	4–8 mg/kg per day PO divided b.i.d. or t.i.d.	Slows Na^+ and Ca^{++} channel activation	Gingival hyperplasia	Abdominal epilepsy
Carbamazepine	Tegretol	Age <6 years, 10–20 mg/kg per day PO divided b.i.d. or t.i.d. 6–12 years, 400–800 mg/day PO divided b.i.d. or t.i.d. >12 years, 600–1200 mg/day PO divided b.i.d. or t.i.d.	Slows Na^+ channel activation	Sedation, anticholinergics effects[a]	Contraindicated with MAO inhibitors
Prokinetic					
Erythromycin	Erythrocin, Pediamycin, E-mycin	20 mg/kg per day PO divided q.i.d.	Motilin agonist stimulates gastric motility	Gastric cramps in larger doses	Use in small, prokinetic doses 5–20 mg/kg per day, gastroparesis
Cisapride	Propulsid	0.2–0.3 mg/kg dose PO t.i.d. or q.i.d.	$5HT_4$ agonist with ACh release in gut	Diarrhea, abdominal pain, headache	Can cause arrhythmias with imidazole antifungals and macrolide antibiotics, gastroparesis
Birth control					
Norethindrone/ ethinyl estradiol	Loestrin 1.5/30		Attenuates estrogen drop before onset of menses	Estrogen effects	Catamenial migraines

[a]Anticholinergic effects include blurred vision, dry mouth, hypotension, palpitations, urinary retention. Ach, acetylcholine; ASA, acetylsalicylic acid; CTZ, chemotrigger zone; GABA, γ-aminobutyric acid; H, histamine; 5HT, 5-hydroxytryptamine; MAO, monamine oxidase inhibitor; SST, supraventricular tachycardia.

Table 8.10 Medications used to treat cyclic vomiting syndrome and abdominal migraine[60–62,100–102,131–133]

of rescue antiemetics.[149] Ketorolac used for postoperative analgesia provided equivalent pain relief to morphine but with significantly less vomiting.[150]

Chemotherapy-induced emesis

The current theories by which chemotherapy induces emesis include injury to the GI tract with release of serotonin and learned (anticipatory) responses.[151] Factors known to increase the incidence of vomiting in response to chemotherapy include young age (toddlers), female gender, emetogenicity of the agent (high, cisplatin; moderate, cyclophosphamide; mild, methotrexate), dose and higher rate of administration. In one study in children, chemotherapy increased urinary 5-HT and 5 hydroxyindole acetic acid (5-HIAA) excretion whereas 5-HT antagonists diminished the vomiting and 5-HIAA excretion, thus implicating serotonin in the pathophysiologic cascade.[152]

The new 5-HT_3 antagonists are more efficacious than former regimens that included metoclopramide-dexamethasone and chlorpromazine-dexamethasone combinations.[153,154] All three 5-HT_3 antagonists – ondansetron 3 mg/M^2,[155] granisetron 10 μg/kg,[156,157] and tropisetron 0.2 mg/kg[158] – have similar rates (75–96%) of complete or major control of chemotherapy-induced vomiting.[159] Few side-effects were noted except for headache (ondansetron) and constipation (tropisetron). These 5-HT_3 agents appear to be more effective on the early emesis (within the first 24 h) than late (1 to 2 weeks after chemotherapy).[153] These 5-HT_3 agents were effective on repeated cycles of chemotherapy without loss of efficacy, could be potentiated by dexamethasone,[160] and were more effective in larger than standard doses with no additional adverse effects.[161] The 5-HT_3 agents also appear effective in controlling radiotherapy-induced emesis.[162] Lorazepam has been suggested as an adjunctive agent for the treatment of acute chemotherapy-induced nausea and vomiting.[163] New tachykinin receptor antagonists (NK_1) (aprepitant) have just been approved in chemotherapy-induced emesis and may be more effective in the late phase of nausea and vomiting.

Psychogenic vomiting

Although the term *psychogenic vomiting* has been used as a diagnosis of exclusion when no organic cause can be found, the term is not ideal – for several reasons. First, one study demonstrated that all children initially labeled as having psychogenic vomiting were found to have mucosal injuries of the upper GI tract during endoscopic evaluation.[164] The use of more sensitive diagnostic modalities such as endoscopic biopsy, gallbladder emptying scans and GI motility studies enable more of those suspected to have psychogenic vomiting to be diagnosed with organic disease.[165] Second, careful case studies indicate that both organic and psychological factors coexist (e.g. *H. pylori* gastritis associated with anxiety-induced vomiting); thus, individual patients cannot always be classified into either organic or psychogenic categories.[166]

Studies of psychogenic vomiting patients reveal some common predisposing factors including a symbiotic relationship between parent and affected child, a family history of vomiting, and exogenous depression or conversion reaction secondary to the loss of a parent. To make a positive diagnosis of psychogenic vomiting, Gonazlez-Heydrich et al. have suggested that in addition to the absence of positive test results, one of the following psychological criteria be included: (1) vomiting as a somatic expression of anxiety, (2) cultural or family conflict or specific traumatic event with primary or secondary gain and (3) vomiting as manipulative behavior act, including malingering or Munchausen by proxy.[166] Although one group has suggested that varying temporal patterns of vomiting may reflect differing underlying psychopathologies – a cyclic pattern is associated with a higher incidence of conversion reactions and the postprandial pattern is more typical of depression – these associations remain to be confirmed.[167]

Acknowledgements

The authors gratefully acknowledge Abid Kagalwalla for his help in organizing the cyclic vomiting patient database and references, respectively.

References

1. Davis CJ, Harding RK, Leslie RA, et al. The organisation of vomiting as a protective reflex: A commentary on the first day's discussions. In: Davis CJ, Lake-Bakaar GV, Grahame-Smith DG, eds. Nausea and Vomiting: Mechanisms and Treatment. Berlin: Springer; 1986:65.
2. Borison HL, Wang SC. Physiology and pharmacology of vomiting. Pharm Rev 1953; 5:193.
3. Lumsden K, Holden WS. The act of vomiting in man. Gut 1969; 10:173.
4. Brizzee KR. Mechanics of vomiting: A mini review. Can J Physiol Pharm 1990; 68:221.
5. Grundy D, Reid K. The physiology of nausea and vomiting. In: Johnson LR, ed. Physiology of the Gastrointestinal Tract. New York NY: Raven Press; 1994:879–901.
6. Lang IM. Digestive tract motor correlates of vomiting and nausea. Can J Physiol Pharm 1990; 68:242.
7. Lang IM, Marvig J, Sarna SK, et al. Gastrointestinal myoelectric correlates of vomiting in the dog. Am J Physiol 1986; 251:G830.
8. Lang IM, Sarna SK, Condon RE. Gastrointestinal motor correlates of vomiting in the dog: quantification and characterization as an independent phenomenon. Gastroenterology 1986; 90:40.
9. Lang IM, Sarna SK, Dodds WJ. Pharyngeal, esophageal, and proximal gastric responses associated with vomiting. Am J Physiol 1993; 265:G963.
10. Smith CC, Brizzee KR. Cineradiographic analysis of vomiting in the cat. I. Lower esophagus, stomach, and small intestine. Gastroenterology 1961; 40:654.
11. Thompson DG, Malagelada J-R. Vomiting and the small intestine. Dig Dis Sci 1982; 27:1121.
12. Ehrlein H-J. Retroperistalsis and duodenogastric reflux in dogs. Scand J Gastroenterol 1981; 67(Suppl):29.

105. Huang S, Lavine JE. Efficacy of sumatriptan in aborting attacks of cyclic vomiting syndrome. Gastroenterology 1997; 112:A751.
106. Borison HL, Borison R, McCarthy LE. Role of the area postrema in vomiting and related functions. Fed Proc 1984; 43:2955.
107. Fessele KS. Managing the multiple causes of nausea and vomiting in the patient with cancer. Oncol Nurs Forum 1996; 23:1409–1415.
108. Koch KL. Nausea: An approach to a symptom. Clin Perspect Gastro 2001; :285–297.
109. Quigley EM, Hasler WL, Parkman HP. AGA technical review on nausea and vomiting. Gastroenterology 2001; 120:263–286.
110. Challis GB, Stam HJ. A longitudinal study of the development of anticipatory nausea and vomiting in cancer chemotherapy patients: the role of absorption and autonomic perception. Health Psychol 1992; 11:181–189.
111. Issenman RM, Persad R. The queasy teen: A common presentation of gastrointestinal dysmotility in adolescence, in press.
112. Morrow GR, Angel C, Dubeshter B. Autonomic changes during cancer chemotherapy induced nausea and emesis. Brit J Cancer Suppl 1992; 19:S42–S45.
113. Bellg AJ, Morrow GR, Barry M, et al. Autonomic measures associated with chemotherapy-related nausea: techniques and issues. Cancer Invest 1995; 13:313–323.
114. Dumont RC, Caniano DA. Hypokinetic gallbladder disease: a cause of chronic abdominal pain in children and adolescents. J Pediatr Surg 1999; 34:858–861.
115. Abu-Arafeh I, Russell G. Cyclical vomiting syndrome in children: A population based study. J Pediatr Gastroenterol Nutr 1995; 21:454.
116. Gee S On fitful or recurrent vomiting. St. Bart Hosp Rep 1882(18):1.
117. Li BUK, ed. Cyclic Vomiting Syndrome: Proceedings of the International Scientific Symposium. J Pediatr Gastroenterol Nutr 1995; 21(Suppl):Svi.
118. Li BUK. Cyclic vomiting: The pattern and syndrome paradigm. In Li BUK, ed. Cyclic Vomiting Syndrome: Proceedings of the International Scientific Symposium. J Pediatr Gastroenterol Nutr 1995; 21(Suppl):S6.
119. Li BUK. Cyclic vomiting syndrome: A pediatric Rorschach test. J Pediatr Gastroenterol Nutr 1993; 17:351.
120. Smith CH. Recurrent vomiting in children: Its etiology and treatment. J Pediatr 1937; 10:719.
121. Pfau BT, Li BUK, Murray RD, et al. Cyclic vomiting in children: A migraine equivalent? Gastroenterology 1992; 102:A23.
122. Mortimer MJ, Good PA. The VER as a diagnostic marker for childhood abdominal migraine. Headache 1990; 30:642.
123. Rashed H, Abell TL, Cardoso J. Cyclic vomiting syndrome is associated with a distinct adrenergic abnormality. Gastroenterology 1997; 112:A901.
124. Wolff SM, Adler R. A syndrome of periodic hypothalamic discharge. Am J Med 1964; 36:956.
125. Sato T, Igarashi M, Minami S, et al. Recurrent attacks of vomiting, hypertension, and psychotic depression: A syndrome of periodic catecholamine and prostaglandin discharge. Acta Endocrinol 1988; 117:189.
126. Pasricha P, Schuster M, Saudek C, et al. Cyclic vomiting: Association with multiple homeostatic abnormalities and response to Ketorolac. Am J Gastroenterol 1996; 91:2228.
127. Chong SKF, Nowak TV, Goddard M, et al. Abnormal gastric emptying and myoelectrical activity in cyclic vomiting syndrome. Gastroenterology 1997; 112:A712.
128. Mavromichalis I, Zaramboukas T, Giala MM. Migraine of gastrointestinal origin. Eur J Pediatr 1995; 154:406.
129. Douglas EF, White PT. Abdominal epilepsy-a reappraisal. J Pediatr 1971; 78:59.
130. Millichap JH, Lombroso CT, Lennox MD. Cyclic vomiting as a form of epilepsy in children. Paediatrics 1955; 15:705.
131. Igarashi M, May WN, Golden GS. Pharmacological treatment of childhood migraine. J Pediatr 1992; 120:653.
132. Fleisher DR. Management of cyclic vomiting syndrome. In Li BUK, ed. Cyclic Vomiting Syndrome: Proceedings of the International Scientific Symposium. J Pediatr Gastroenterol Nutr 1995; 21(Suppl 1):S52.
133. Vanderhoof JA, Young R, Kaufmann SS, et al. Treatment of cyclic vomiting syndrome in childhood with erythromycin. J Pediatr Gastroenterol Nutr 1993; 17:387.
134. Edelson RN. Menstrual migraine and other hormonal aspects of migraine. Headache 1985; 25:376.
135. Welch KMA, Darnley D, Simkins RT. The role of estrogen in migraine: A review and hypothesis. Cephalalgia 1984; 4:227.
136. Kermode J, Walker S, Webb I. Postoperative vomiting in children. Anaes Intens Care 1995; 23:196.
137. Sossai R, Johr M, Kistler W, et al. Postoperative vomiting in children. A persisting unsolved problem. Eur J Pediatr Surg 1993; 3:206.
138. Kenny GN. Risk factors for postoperative nausea and vomiting. Anaesthesia 1994; 49:6.
139. Rose JB, Martin TM, Corddry DH, et al. Ondansetron reduces the incidence and severity of poststrabismus repair vomiting in children. Anesth Analg 1994; 79:489.
140. Furst SR, Rodarte A. Prophylactic antiemetic treatment with ondansetron in children undergoing tonsillectomy. Anesthesiology 1994; 81:799.
141. Rust M, Cohen LA. Single oral dose ondansetron in the prevention of postoperative nausea and emesis. The European and US study groups. Anaesthesia 1994; 49:16.
142. Furst SR, Sullivan LJ, Soriano SG, et al. Effects of ondansetron on emesis in the first 24 hours after craniotomy in children. Anesth Analg 1996; 83:325.
143. Splinter WM, Rhine EJ, Roberts DW, et al. Ondansetron is a better prophylactic antiemetic than droperidol for tonsillectomy in children. Can J Anaesth 1995; 42:848.
144. Davis PJ, McGowan FX Jr, Lansman I, et al. Effect of antiemetic therapy on recovery and hospital discharge time. A double-blind assessment of ondansetron, droperidol, and placebo in pediatric patients undergoing ambulatory surgery. Anesthesiology 1995; 83:956.
145. Rose JB, Brenn BR, Corddry DH, et al. Preoperative oral ondansetron for pediatric tonsillectomy. Anesth Analg 1996; 82:558.
146. Ummenhofer W, Frei FJ, Urwyler A, et al. Effects of ondansetron in the prevention of postoperative nausea and vomiting in children. Anesthesiology 1994; 81:804.
147. Khalil S, Rodarte A, Weldon BC, et al. Intravenous ondansetron in established postoperative emesis in children. Anesthesiology 1996; 85:270.
148. Sadhasivam S. Prophylactic ondansetron in prevention of postoperative nausea and vomiting following pediatric strabismus surgery: a dose-response study. Anesthesiology 2000; 92:1035–1042.

149. Rusy LM. Electroacupuncture prophylaxis of postoperative nausea and vomiting following pediatric tonsillectomy with or without adenoidectomy. Anesthesiology 2002; 96:300–305.

150. Purday JP, Reichert CC, Merrick PM. Comparative effects of three doses of intravenous ketorolac or morphine on emesis and analgesia for restorative dental surgery in children. Can J Anaes 1996; 43:221.

151. Grunberg SM, Hesketh PJ. Control of chemotherapy-induced emesis. N Engl J Med 1993; 329:1790.

152. Matera MG, DiTullio M, Lucarelli C, et al. Ondansetron, an antagonist of 5-HT_3 receptors, in the treatment of antineoplastic drug-induces nausea and vomiting in children. J Med 1993; 24:161.

153. Dick GS, Meller ST, Pinkerton CR. Randomized comparison of ondansetron and metoclopramide plus dexamethasone for chemotherapy induced emesis. Arch Dis Child 1995; 71:243.

154. Miyajima Y, Numata S, Katayama I, et al. Prevention of chemotherapy-induced emesis with granisetron in children with malignant diseases. Am J Pediatr Hematol Oncol 1994; 16:236.

155. Pinkerton CR, Williams D, Wootton C, et al. 5-HT_3 antagonist ondansetron – an effective outpatient antiemetic in cancer treatment. Arch Dis Child 1990; 65:822.

156. Craft AW, Price L, Eden OB, et al. Granisetron and antiemetic therapy in children with cancer. Med Pediatr Oncol 1995; 25:28.

157. Lemerle J, Amaral D, Southall DP, et al. Efficacy and safety of granisetron in the prevention of chemotherapy-induced emesis in paediatric patients. Eur J Cancer 1991; 27:1081.

158. Benoit Y, Hulstaert F, Vermylen C, et al. Tropisetron in the prevention of nausea and vomiting in 131 children receiving cytotoxic chemotherapy. Med Pediatr Oncol 1995; 25:457.

159. Jacobson SJ, Shore RW, Greenberg M, et al. The efficacy and safety of granisetron in pediatric cancer patients who had failed standard antiemetic therapy during anticancer chemotherapy. Am J Pediatr Hematol Oncol 1994; 16:231.

160. Alvarez O, Freeman A, Bedros A, et al. Randomized double-blind crossover ondansetron-dexamethasone versus ondansetron-placebo study for the treatment of chemotherapy-induced nausea and vomiting in pediatric patients with malignancies. J Pediatr Hematol Oncol 1995; 17:145.

161. Brock P, Brichard B, Rechnitzer C, et al. An increased loading dose of ondansetron: A North European, double-blind randomized study in children, comparing 5 mg/M^2 with 10 mg/M^2. Eur J Cancer 1996; 32:1744.

162. Miralbell R, Coucke P, Behrouz F, et al. Nausea and vomiting in fractionated radiotherapy: A prospective on-demand trial of tropisetron rescue for non-responders to metoclopramide. Eur J Cancer 1995; 31:1461.

163. Dupuis LL. Options for the prevention and management of acute chemotherapy-induced nausea and vomiting in children. Paediatr Drugs 2003; 5:597–613.

164. Stacher G. Differentialdiagnose psychosomatischer Schluckstorungen. Wien Klin Wochenschr 1986;. 98:648.

165. Abell TL, Kim CJ, Malagelada JR. Idiopathic cyclic nausea and vomiting: A disorder of gastrointestinal motility? Mayo Clin Proc 1988; 63:1169.

166. Gonzalez-Heydrich J, Kerner JA, Steiner H. Testing the psychogenic vomiting diagnosis: Four pediatric patients. Am J Dis Child 1991; 145:913.

167. Muraoka M, Mine K, Matsumoto K, Nakai Y. Psychogenic vomiting: The relation between patterns of vomiting and psychiatric diagnoses. Gut 1990; 31:526.

located in the small intestinal crypts. In the colon Na^+ absorption occurs in the crypts, consequently additional hydraulic forces due to a small neck enlarge Na^+ and water absorption enormously.[13]

This Na^+ absorptive state is reversed to a Cl^- secretory state under the influence of cAMP or calcium secretagogues. In the small intestine Cl^- secretion induced by these secretagogues occurs mainly in the crypts.

DEFINITIONS OF DIARRHEA

Feces contain up to 75% water. A relatively small increase in water losses will cause liquid stools. In infants, stool volume in excess of 10g/kg per day is considered abnormal.[3] Diarrhea is the frequent (more than three times a day) evacuation of liquid feces. Fecal composition is abnormal and will often be malodorous and acid due to colonic fermentation and putrefaction of nutrients. Stools may contain blood, mucus, fat or undigested food particles. The urge to evacuate stools may cause incontinence and nocturnal defecation in toilet trained children.

Acute diarrhea is often self-limiting and lasts for a few days. When persisting for over 3 weeks this condition is considered chronic.

CLINICAL OBSERVATIONS OF TYPES OF DIARRHEA

Diarrheic stools may be watery, acid or greasy and may contain blood, mucus or undigested food particles. Parents often worry about the color of their child's feces.

Red (blood) and white (cholestasis) are alarming, but all shades of yellow, brown and green should be tolerated.

Various pathophysiological mechanisms causing diarrhea have been clarified. Often several mechanisms act simultaneously.

Watery diarrhea

Mechanisms of intestinal fluid and electrolytes absorption and secretion have been studied extensively. Oral intake and intestinal secretions account for about 9 l fluid per day at the level of the Treitz ligament in older children and adults.[9] Fluid reabsorption in the small intestine is determined by osmotic gradients. Sodium, potassium, chloride, bicarbonate and glucose are key players. Primarily, sodium creates an osmotic gradient allowing passive water diffusion. The sodium pump, sodium potassium adenosinetriphosphatase (ATPase), located in the basolateral enterocyte membrane, maintains a low intracellular sodium concentration.[14] In adults, the fluid content at the level of the ileocecal valve has decreased to 1 l.[15] Colonic water reabsorption will determine the water content of the stools.

In the case of *osmotic diarrhea* undigested nutrients (e.g. mono- or disaccharides) increase the osmotic load in the distal small intestine and colon leading to decreased water reabsorption.[16,17] The intestinal electrolyte content becomes lower than the serum content. Therefore an 'osmotic gap' can be calculated. The fecal osmotic gap is 290 – 2× (sodium + potassium concentration). In the presence of osmotic molecules, the osmotic gap will be at least 50 units. In *osmotic diarrhea* associated with carbohydrate malabsorption stools are acid with pH under 5 and fasting will improve the symptoms. Milk of magnesia, used as a laxative, causes osmotic diarrhea without pH drop.

In the case of *secretory diarrhea* a noxious agent causes the intestinal epithelium to secrete excessive water and electrolytes into the lumen.[17–19] There is no osmotic gap (less than 50) and food intake does not affect symptoms. Examples are bacterial toxins that turn on adenylate cyclase activity, as well as certain gastrointestinal peptides, bile acids, fatty acids and laxatives.

Steatorrhea

In the case of fat malabsorption, stools may be greasy and stain the toilet bowl. Steatorrhea occurs when fecal fat in a 72 h stool collection exceeds 7% of oral fat intake over 24 h. Isolated fat malabsorption strongly suggests exocrine pancreatic insufficiency due to absence of lipase or colipase.[20] More generalized exocrine pancreatic insufficiencies such as cystic fibrosis and Shwachmann's syndrome cause multiple nutrient malabsorption. Small intestinal damage and villous atrophy lead to malabsorption of all nutrients including fat.

Creatorrhea/azotorrhea

Creatorrhea (azotorrhea) or the excretion of proteins occurs also in pancreatic insufficiency and in protein losing enteropathy.[21] Fecal albumin losses can be demonstrated using intravenously injected ^{51}Cr labeled albumin[22] or indirectly by the amount of fecal $\alpha 1$ antitrypsine.[23] Creatorrhea or azotorrhea in pancreatic insufficiency or subtotal villous atrophy is always accompanied by other obvious clinical signs due to generalized malabsorption.

Mucus and blood

Intestinal inflammation is an important cause of diarrhea. The mucosa is invaded and destroyed by a cellular inflammatory infiltrate secreting numerous cytokines. Normal absorptive processes are impaired, exudative materials (mucus, blood) are excreted and intestinal motility is altered. Intestinal inflammation may be caused by allergic reactions, infections or by idiopathic auto-immune type reactions as seen in inflammatory bowel disease (IBD).

Undigested food particles

In toddlers, undigested food particles are often visible in looser stools. Usually the child thrives and is otherwise free of symptoms. This condition is called chronic nonspecific diarrhea of childhood (CNSD) and is considered a functional problem.[24] An accelerated intestinal transit in this age group may be caused by the failure of nutrients to interrupt the migrating motor complexes and to induce a fed-pattern.[25]

Overflow incontinence

Some children present with foul smelling diarrhea but a careful physical evaluation, including a digital rectal examination, will reveal constipation and rectal impaction. Patients with fecal overflow and often incontinence or encopresis need treatment for chronic constipation. It is important to explain the pathophysiology of the situation to the family. Treatment starts with disimpaction and then promotes more frequent defecation and modifies the child's behavior.

PATHOPHYSIOLOGY OF SECRETORY DIARRHEA

Diarrhea is mainly caused by abnormal fluid and electrolyte transport by decreased absorption or increased secretion. The human colon is capable of absorbing 3–5 l/24 h, but decreased small intestinal absorption of 8–10 l of daily fluid can exceed this colonic capacity. Decrease of small intestinal absorption by more than 50% will lead to diarrhea in this setting. If colonic absorption is diminished due to colonic disease, the normal amount of 1,5 l arriving in the cecum might not be absorbed and then also lead to diarrhea. After the initial discovery that bacterial enterotoxins stimulate chloride and water secretion, it was later found that over 50% of intestinal secretion is controlled by enterochromaffin cells releasing 5-hydroxytryptamine that activates the enteric nervous system, secondary enhancing enterocyte chloride secretion also by signal transport to distant areas of the nervous system. Other inflammatory mediators (histamine, serotonin, prostaglandins) produced by immune cells, intestinal mast cells, eosinophils, macrophages, neutrophils and mesenchymal cells in the lamina propria and submucosa are capable of initiating and enhancing intestinal secretion. These mediators may stimulate enterocytes directly and also activate the enteric nervous system. Moreover, this process of electrogenic chloride and bicarbonate secretion inhibits electrical neutral sodium-chloride absorption in the small intestine and the colon through intercellular messengers. Because of the net fluid movement into the lumen, this is a combined cause of malabsorption of water and electrolytes and enhanced secretion, seen as diarrhea. From a pathophysiological perspective, solitary secretion is rare.

PATHOPHYSIOLOGY OF OSMOTIC DIARRHEA

In osmotic diarrhea, a meal has the same, normal dilution in the duodenum but thereafter, the water content of the intestinal lumen will increase. For instance lactase deficient subjects are unable to re-absorb adequate fluid because lactose is not metabolized to galactose and glucose, which act to help transport water and electrolytes.

Osmotic diarrhea can be induced to alleviate constipation. Healthy normal adults receiving increasing doses of polyethylene glycol 3350 (PEG) or lactulose have been studied. PEG 3350 (lower molecular weights do not bind water as well) is poorly absorbed, not digested by human or bacterial enzymes, carries no electrical charge and causes pure osmotic diarrhea. With daily doses of 50–250 g/day stool weight increases gradually from 364–1539 g/day. Stool water content does not rise above 80% due to high fecal concentration of PEG. PEG attracts water: stool weight, water output and fecal PEG output correlate in a linear fashion.

With lactulose doses increasing from 45–125 g/day, stool weight increases from 254–1307 g/day. Water content percentage increases from 79–90%. With increasing lactulose doses, fecal organic acids content decrease while carbohydrate content increases. This means that with lower dosages up to 95 g/day, organic acids are absorbed and water absorption is co-transported. Only in higher dosages lactulose is no longer fermented and contributes directly to diarrhea. Interestingly, electrolyte concentrations in diarrheal stools are higher with lactulose than PEG and a linear correlation between organic acid output and electrolyte output is obvious. However, conservation of electrolytes is excellent even with water output over 1200 g/d. Diarrhea in lower dosages is mainly caused by unabsorbed organic acids and with higher dosages by a combination of organic acids and undigested carbohydrate. Since there is no correlation between organic acid concentration and rate of individual bowel movements, the argument of rapid colonic emptying or effects on colonic motility are probably not justified.[26]

In lactose intolerant patients with diarrhea, the introduction of 50 g lactose for 14 days was compared with the same amount of sucrose. Interestingly, the fecal weight in both groups did not change and was around 350 g/24 h. On the other hand, the number of stools decreased in both groups as did symptom score; there was less pain, less flatulence, less bloating, less borborygmi. Only in the lactose groups pH dropped, breath hydrogen excretion dropped. This suggests that clinical symptoms in lactose intolerance are subject to psychogenic factors and of limited clinical importance.[27]

In the short bowel syndrome lactulose feeding of 60 g/daily showed lower carbohydrate and organic acid excretion in the stools, carried out in comparison with volunteers fed lactulose for 2 weeks. This experiment demonstrates a spontaneous adaptation of the gut flora in short bowel syndrome patients with intact colon.[28]

The contribution of fat to osmotic diarrhea is still under debate. Triglycerides do not directly contribute to diarrhea, but their fatty acids might. Medium chain fatty acids are absorbed in the colon as are short chain fatty acids or are lost in the feces as are long chain fatty acids. In carbohydrate malabsorption sodium and water stay in the lumen until the colon is reached, where up to 90 g/day sugars are metabolized by bacteria. A considerable amount of short

intestinal levels, villus atrophy could be present through the whole small intestine without causing steatorrhea. This experience challenged the assumption of a gluten dosage-related extent of villus atrophy over a variable length distal to the duodenum. Still the usual presentation of diarrhea is fatty stools with an egg odor. Depending on the severity of the inflammatory infiltrate, chloride secretion might be enhanced and diarrhea presents with a more watery aspect. In rare cases, secretion is abundant leading to dehydration at presentation: the so-called celiac crisis.

Eosinophilic gastroenteritis occurs in children; complaints are in keeping with mild and severe forms of inflammatory bowel disease within 75% peripheral eosinophilia. Symptoms are abdominal pain, nausea, vomiting and weight loss with diarrhea. An eosinophilic infiltrate is present in the mucosa, sometimes extending to muscle layer and serosa of the gut. Depending on the degree of mucosal inflammation, protein losing enteropathy ensues and depending on the degree of villus atrophy steatorrhea occurs. The treatment is comparable with inflammatory bowel disease.[53]

In short bowel syndrome, the intestinal absorptive capacity is insufficient for growth as a consequence of congenital short length of the intestine, surgical resection or dysfunction. Intermittent and more generalized intestinal motility disorders called intestinal pseudo-obstruction lead to small bowel overgrowth and maldigestion. Bacterial overgrowth in the small intestine occurs due to regurgitation of bacteria from the colon or stasis. Bile salts are precipitated or deconjugated and hydroxylated, become less amphiphilic and participate no longer in micelle formation. In pseudo-obstruction syndromes, bacterial overgrowth frequently occurs and children benefit from antibiotics. In short bowel syndrome, steatorrhea is caused by a diminished absorptive surface area, decreased transit time and diminished bile salt pool due to fecal losses. Steatorrhea is aggravated by bacterial overgrowth as mentioned and postoperative temporary gastric hypersecretion. Most children have sufficient small bowel adaptation in a few years to sustain normal growth and development despite persistent diarrhea and steatorrhea.

All conditions causing *exocrine pancreatic insufficiency* cause steatorrhea. The most frequent entity is cystic fibrosis (CF), others are Shwachman's syndrome or chronic pancreatitis. In cystic fibrosis, pancreatic insufficiency develops after more than 90% of exocrine pancreatic secretory capacity has been lost. This explains why a substantial number of infants with CF due to ongoing obstruction of pancreatic ducts become gradually pancreatic insufficient during the first year of life. The high variability of pancreatic insufficiency (10–80% steatorrhea) at the time of diagnosis is in keeping with this diminishing function. With pancreatic enzyme replacement therapy steatorrhea disappears in 50% and improves in the remainder. Malabsorption of medium-chain triglycerides (MCTs) improve with pancreatic enzyme supplements.[54] Insufficient bile salt secretion contributes to steatorrhea and might explain the ongoing malabsorption in 50% of patients. Pancreatic and biliary secretions have a severely diminished bicarbonate content leading to an acidic duodenum and proximal jejunum with less efficient enzyme release from acid-resistant coated granules and precipitation of some bile salts, also contributing to steatorrhea. Despite normalization of steatorrhea with optimal enzyme replacement lean body-mass development lags behind due to chronic anorexia in permanent chronic lung infection and inflammation. Up to the age of 8 years, bodyweight improves with pancreatic enzyme replacement therapy. Afterwards it declines in all cystic fibrosis patients growth is stunted, suggesting insufficient intake. Nutritional support including additional tube-feeding improves bodyweight.

Shwachman's syndrome is another cause of exocrine pancreatic insufficiency in childhood. In this condition, bile salt and bicarbonate secretion are normal, while pancreatic enzyme output is low. Steatorrhea normalizes in many patients after the age of 5 years.[55] Isolated lipase and co-lipase deficiency has been reported.[56,57] Enterokinase deficiency causes lack of activation of pancreatic proenzymes leading to steatorrhea and creatorrhea; besides malnutrition these infants have edema due to low serum proteins. Recently, mutations in the proenteropeptidase gene have been identified as the cause of congenital enterokinase (or enteropeptidase) deficiciency.[58]

All *cholestatic hepatic* conditions cause deficient intestinal fat absorption because of bile salt deficiency. In biliary atresia, congenital biliary stenosis, choledochal cyst, cystic fibrosis, bile salt secretion becomes insufficient to reach the critical micellar concentration in the duodenal lumen (3 mmol/l).[59] Below this concentration, micelles cannot be formed to trap fatty acids and fat soluble vitamins.[60] Within micelles, penetration of the unstirred layer of the mucosa is facilitated and fat absorption is 120 times more efficient. MCTs are less dependent on micelles for digestion and absorption. Steatorrhea still occurs to a variable extent in operated biliary atresias. Addition of MCT to the diet, as energy source is advised, but elongation to long-chain fatty acids does not occur in the human body. MCT cannot therefore replace long-chain fatty acids as fat source in the diet of infants and children with bile salt deficiency. Since long-chain fatty acid malabsorption without any bile salt secretion is about 50%, it is justified keeping long-chain fats in the children's diet.[61]

Congenital absence of the ileal receptor for bile acid uptake (the apical sodium co-dependent bile acid transporter) leads to bile acid losses with a diminished bile acid pool. Affected infants have steatorrhea, failure to thrive and low plasma levels of low-density lipoprotein cholesterol. They lack the postprandial rise in serum bile acids since the gallbladder has not accumulated bile in the fasting periods.[62]

In Zellweger's syndrome, abnormal bile acids are not sufficiently amphiphilic to contribute to micelle formation. The resulting steatorrhea can be somewhat improved with oral bile acids supplementation.[63]

Immune active cells are scattered in the intestinal wall. In the case of congenital *immune deficiencies*, such as severe combined immune deficiency syndrome (SCIDS) or AIDS, diarrhea is often an early warning sign. Poorly understood autoimmune derangements lead to generalized enteropathy. Autoimmune enteropathy in infants and children presents as steatorrhea to watery diarrhea with failure to thrive. Histology of the small intestine shows villus atrophy and an inflammatory infiltrate indistinguishable from celiac disease. A gluten free diet has no effect, but in some infants a hypoallergenic formula controls symptoms. Other children require immuno-suppressive therapy with mixed results. In addition to villus atrophy, these children have other autoimmune diseases such as diabetes mellitus type I, thyroiditis, autoimmune anemia and glomerulonephritis. The onset of diarrhea is within the first 3 months of life, the volume of diarrhea is around 125 ml/kg, sodium content 100 mmol/l, suggesting a combination of malabsorption and inflammation mediated increased secretion of electrolytes.[40]

Inflammatory conditions of the small intestinal or colonic wall manifest themselves by blood and mucus in loose stools. The most frequent chronic inflammatory diseases (IBD) are Crohn's disease and ulcerative colitis. The incidence of Crohn's disease is rising and the age at presentation decreasing. A population study of the incidence in UK and Ireland yielded an alarming incidence of 5.2/100 000 children under 16 years of age per year.[64] In inflammatory bowel disease, diarrhea is caused by decreased sodium, chloride and water absorption, the inflamed mucosa is less tight and more permeable with diminished water absorption and secretion. Diarrhea is not voluminous. Important features are protein loss and with it calcium and magnesium. Malabsorption does not occur until more than 1 m of distal small bowel is resected; steatorrhea is an uncommon feature of inflammatory bowel disease. Inflammatory mediators may induce chloride secretion in proximal not affected small bowel.[65]

Overflow incontinence is often misinterpreted as diarrhea. The differential diagnosis for fecal impaction includes Hirschsprung's disease, congenital anorectal malformations and functional constipation depending on the clinical features and the age of the child.

Dietary mistakes are a frequent cause of diarrhea in a thriving child. Overfeeding or the ingestion of large quantities of indigestible carbohydrates such as sorbitol in fruit juice can easily be corrected.

Toddler's diarrhea or chronic non-specific diarrhea is a benign condition in a thriving, healthy child. Stools are loose and reveal identifiable remains of recent food intake. Rapid intestinal transit may be the cause of this benign condition. It has been shown in small intestinal motility studies that fasting activity was normal, but postprandial motility was abnormal. The initiation of postprandial activity is accompanied by disruption of MMCs. In toddler's diarrhea the MMCs continue and go along with increased intestinal transit.[66] Another mechanism may be the dumping of bile acids and hydroxy fatty acids into the colon leading to cholerrheic diarrhea. This was substantiated by stool examination.[67] The precipitating event of chronic non-specific diarrhea is often an acute episode of gastroenteritis with watery diarrhea. The study of intestinal biopsies revealed normal morphology but increased adenyl cyclase activity and Na/K-ATPase activity, in keeping with the assumption of recovering mucosa.[68] It was also claimed, that correction of a low fat intake leads to resumption of symptoms.[69] Clinically these children have a non-specific diarrheal pattern, grow normally and are obviously well. Some might have their symptoms reduced by diminishing their consumption of fructose, sorbitol and other sugars dependent on facilitated mucosal transport.[24,49,70]

This might hold for an irritable bowel syndrome like picture with predominant diarrhea and without pain in older children, but as in adults distinct mild abnormalities or forms of diseases are found in increasing numbers such as lactose intolerance, microscopic colitis, fructose malabsorption, food hypersensitivities, celiac disease.

Symptoms improve with dietary modifications: increased fat and fiber intake, limited fluid intake and avoidance of fruit juices.[71]

Irritable bowel syndrome (IBS) can be diagnosed in older children and adolescents with alternating stool patterns. By definition organic disease is absent but one should not feel compelled to rule out every possible organic diagnosis using invasive tests. Psychosocial stressors need to be identified and deserve attention.[72] Often IBS is preceded by an infectious episode.[73] The pathways leading to IBS and the relationship between hormonal or mucosal markers and mood remain largely unidentified. Both mucosal changes (increased enterochromaffin cells) and depression have been identified as predictors for post-infectious IBS.[74]

Medications or *toxic substances* may cause diarrhea as a primary or as a side-effect. Some are taken by prescription, some accidentally, some intentionally. *Melanosis coli* or the presence of pigmented colonocytes on sigmoid biopsy strongly suggests laxative abuse.[75]

In the case of contradictory findings and severe persistent diarrhea of unclear etiology, suspicion of *Polle syndrome* or *Munchausen by proxy* may arise. Observation of the child in isolation is useful in such case.[76]

Finally a number of non-gastrointestinal conditions cause diarrhea by hormonal or neuro secretory pathways, e.g. hyperthyroidism. Rare *tumors* cause true secretory diarrheas. The gastrinoma syndrome is reported from the age of 7 years. In children, the presentation is with abdominal pain, rarely with typical ulcer pain, hematemesis, vomiting and melena. A small intestinal biopsy showing goblet cell transformation in a patient with persistent diarrhea and unexplained steatorrhea should lead to investigation of gastrinoma. High acid output into the proximal small bowel leads to precipitation of bile salts with a diminished critical micellar concentration causing steatorrhea. Calcium binding to malabsorbed fatty acids leads to free oxalate absorption and kidney stone formation. Vipoma syndrome presents at all ages as profuse watery diarrhea with fecal losses between 20–50 ml/kg per day. The culprit usually is a ganglioneuroblastoma producing VIP, although the exact mechanism causing diarrhea is unknown.[77] Hypokalemia is often present and may be clue to the presence of a tumor based diarrhea.

APPROACH OF THE CHILD WITH DIARRHEA

The approach to a child presenting with diarrhea will first consist of a careful history and physical examination (see Table 9.6). Diagnostic work-up will be performed depending on this first evaluation, on the age of the child and on the duration of diarrhea. One should favor non-invasive tests and keep in mind that a diagnosis of functional or factitious diarrhea is not necessarily an exclusion diagnosis.

History taking includes perinatal course (constipation, cystic fibrosis), previous surgery (short bowel, terminal ileum) and family history (celiac disease, IBD). The severity of the diarrhea, the type of stools and the presence of associated symptoms should be assessed. The physician should examine a stool sample. A dietary history should be obtained at the first visit. Prior weight and the child's growth chart are of great importance to evaluate the presence of weight loss or failure to thrive.

The *physical examination* should include all systems with specific attention for growth and development, head and neck region and obviously abdomen and rectum. The assessment of pubertal stage is useful to assess malnutrition with delayed puberty (Table 9.3).

Based on history and clinical examination, one should attempt to establish the likelihood that symptoms are organic (as opposed to functional), to distinguish malabsorptive from colonic or inflammatory forms of diarrhea and to assess the need for further examinations (Table 9.4).[78]

Red flags (Table 9.5), such as severe continuous and nocturnal diarrhea, blood and mucus in the stools, very acid stools, weight loss or failure to thrive and associated symptoms strongly suggest a specific organic cause.

Some typical descriptions of the different types of diarrhea are given below.

Growth chart		
Vital signs		
Muscle mass		
Subcutaneous fat		
Pubertal stage		
Psychomotor development		
Skin (perianal)		
ENT region		
Abdomen		
Organomegaly		
Tenderness		
Rectal exam		
Stool sample		
Color		
Consistency		
? Occult blood	→	Hemoccult
? pH	→	Indicator
? Fermentation	→	Clinitest

Table 9.3 Essential elements of the physical examination of the child with diarrhea

Watery and inflammatory diarrheas present with nocturnal diarrhea and occasionally incontinence. With carbohydrate malabsorption the dietary connection may be present in the medical history. In true *secretory* diarrhea fasting may cause some degree of amelioration because food also stimulates secretion but diarrhea persists, including nocturnal diarrhea, incontinence and sometimes dehydration. In the case of *malabsorptive* diarrhea signs of steatorrhea with flatulence, bulky greasy foul-smelling stools and weight loss may be discrete or even absent. Steatorrhea is much more frequent in exocrine pancreatic insufficiency (10–80%) than in mucosal disease such as celiac disease (12–15%). In *inflammatory* diarrheas, children usually have longstanding anorexia, stunted growth and weight loss. Inflammation causes diarrhea and fecal protein losses. Stools are usually not abundant but contain mucus and sometimes blood. Dehydration is lacking. Abdominal pain is localized with a palpable infiltrate, diffuse pain and tenderness. Systemic manifestations of inflammatory disease such as aphthous ulcers in the buccal mucosa, uveitis and arthralgia or erythema nodosum need to be sought.

Investigations are frequently needed to better direct the differential diagnosis or to confirm the suspicion of a specific disease (Table 9.6). Initial investigations are *laboratory tests* and stool cultures. The blood tests can indicate the presence of inflammation, allergy, nutritional deficiencies, immune or endocrine disorders.

A meaningful screening test for celiac disease is IgA anti-endomysium antibody or human transglutaminase assay.[79] Note that the patient may be Ig A deficient and that a firm diagnosis of celiac disease is still based on small bowel biopsy.[80] However, an excellent correlation of a new serological marker, anti-actin filament antibody Ig A, with the degree of intestinal villous atrophy was recently reported.[81]

Stool cultures are not needed in benign acute diarrhea as most cases are viral and self-limiting. In the presence of 'red flags' or protracted diarrhea cultures including microscopic examination for ova, cysts and parasites of at least three fresh stool samples are in order. Malabsorption is usually generalized, meaning that (fermented) carbohydrates, fat and protein are excreted. Carbohydrate fermentation lowers fecal pH below 5.

Stool fat can be identified with various methods. Single stool samples can be analyzed for fat using the Sudan III stain[82] or the acid steatocrit.[83]

Qualitative examinations for fat content in stools consist of heating a mixture of feces, alcohol and water. The Sudan stain reveals neutral fat and triglycerides but not the fatty acids soaps, these are remaining dietary triglycerides and phospholipids from endogenous sources (bile, enterocytes, bacteria).

The quantitative 72 h fecal fat collection is cumbersome but widely used. Stool collection has to be done for 3 days, because bowel movements vary from day to day in children. Fat intake needs to be constant prior to and during the collection. Because of lack of standardization between laboratories and limited diagnostic value of a positive result the relevance of this method is being questioned, at least in

Data collection	Differential
Step 1: History	
Duration >3 weeks	
Defecation frequency – pattern (?nocturnal)	Hypersecretion – inflammation
Fecal aspect: watery – foamy – floating – mucous – blood – undigested particles	Congenital absorption defects – steatorrhea – inflammation – Toddler's diarrhea
Associated symptoms: abdominal cramping – flatulence – fever – extra intestinal symptoms	Carbohydrate malabsorption – IBD
Dietary history	Toddler's diarrhea – undigestible carbohydrates
Step 2: Physical examination	
Biometry: normal growth	Functional, dietary
failure to thrive	Malabsorption
Mucous membranes (oral sores)	IBD
Distended abdomen	Fermentation (CH malabsorption), fecal impaction, inflammation
Abdominal mass	IBD – tumor – fecal impaction
Rectal anomalies	IBD
Extra intestinal symptoms: pulmonary, joints, eye, skin	CF, IBD, celiac disease
Step 3: Laboratory tests	
Rise in inflammatory parameters	IBD
Electrolyte disturbances	Hypersecretive state
Anemia	Mixed malabsorption: celiac disease, IBD
Low fat soluble vitamins	Steatorrhea: CF, $\alpha\beta$ lipoproteinemia mixed malabsorption: celiac disease, IBD
Elevated transaminases	IBD
Elevated bilirubin, bile acids	Cholestasis, CF
Elevated pancreatic enzymes	IBD
Low albumin	Protein losing enteropathy: IBD
Low cholesterol, triglycerides	$\alpha\beta$ lipoproteinemia
Elevated human tissue transglutaminase or IgA anti-endomysium	Celiac disease
Stool cultures	R/o bacterial or parasitic infection

Table 9.4 Initial assessment of chronic diarrhea

adults.[84,85] Normal values up to the age of 6 months are a mean of 7.5 g fat/100 g of stool and afterwards of 5 g fat/100 g of stool. The upper limits are up to the age of 6 months: 15 g/100 g of stool, up to the age of 4 years: 9 g and afterwards 7 g. This translates into 15% of ingested fat up to the age of 6 months, 10% up to the age of 3 years and 5% afterwards.[86,87] A useful and sensitive test is the fecal elastase 1[88] in a single stool. Be aware of normal fat excretion in celiac disease in 30% of children, despite severity of the disease and that in Shwachman's syndrome, steatorrhea disappears after the age of 5 years for unknown reasons.

The presence of protein in stools due to intestinal losses or *creatorrhea* can be reflected by fecal alpha 1 antitrypsin.[23]

Stools
Blood
Mucus
Acid (perianal excoriation)
Nocturnal
Weight loss or failure to thrive
Associated symptoms
Fever
Rash
Arthritis

Table 9.5 Red flags or warning signals in the patient with chronic diarrhea suggesting more serious pathology

Fecal calprotectin, a neutrophil product, is a promising marker for gastrointestinal inflammation but is not widely introduced yet.[89,90]

Measurement of stool electrolytes for calculation of the *osmotic gap* is useful as a guideline for classification of watery diarrhea. The normal plasma osmolality of 290 mmol/kgH_2O is essentially isotonic with plasma. Na+ and K+ concentration must be measured in stool and multiplied by two, to account for the obligate (mainly organic) anions in the stool. The osmotic gap or the difference between stool osmolality (290 mmol/l) and (NA+K+ × 2) concentrations should normally be less than 125 and is usually less than 50. In secretory diarrhea, twice the sum of stool Na+K+ approximates stool osmolality, stool weight is minimally or moderately reduced during fasting and remains above 200 g/24 h. In general, if stool Na+ concentrations are greater than 90 mmol and the osmotic gap is less than 50, secretory diarrhea is present. Conversely, if stool Na+ is less than 60 mmol and the osmotic gap is greater than 125, osmotic diarrhea is likely. Osmotic diarrhea is caused by non-absorbable luminal constituents that displace Na+. Osmotic diarrhea improves during fasting and stool weight returns to values under 200 g/24 h. In most cases, stool sodium concentration is between 60 to 90 mmol and the calculated osmotic gap between 50 and 100 mmol, indicating that both secretory and malabsorptive pathophysiological elements are present.

Investigation		
Non-invasive		
Observe, document		
Historical food intake		
Laboratory parameters		
Inflammation	ESR, CRP, liver function	
Allergy	IgE, RAST	
Nutrition	CBC, urea and electrolytes, PT, Vit A,E,D,B12,Ca, ferritin, folate ac, triglycerides, cholesterol	
Immunity	IgA, anti endomysium IgA, human tissue transglutaminase	
Toxicology		
Thyroid function		
Stool		
Cultures		
Steatocrit		
Sudan III stain		
Elastase		
72^{h} fecal fat collection		
α1 Antitrypsin		
Osmotic gap		
Breath tests evaluating absorption		
^{13}C lactose breath test		
H^2 lactose breath test		
^{13}C mixed triglyceride breath test		
Sweat Cl test		
Plain abdominal X-ray		
Small bowel follow through		
White blood cell scan		
Invasive		
Esophagogastroduodenoscopy with small bowel biopsy	To rule out villous atrophy, celiac disease, histological abnormalities	To perform enzyme assays
Sigmoidoscopy with biopsy	To rule out allergic or inflammatory colitis	
Ileocolonoscopy with biopsy	To rule out IBD	
Duodenal intubation	To rule out exocrine pancreatic insufficiency	
Anorectal manometry/deep rectal biopsy	To rule out Hirschsprung's disease	

Table 9.6 Investigations

Hydrogen breath tests are widely used to assess carbohydrate maldigestion. The lactose hydrogen breath test is easily performed and is as sensitive and specific as the mucosal lactase assay.[91] A dose of lactose (2 g/kg) is given after overnight fast and hydrogen exhalation is monitored. In the absence or reduced presence of lactase, lactose will be fermented by intestinal bacteria and a hydrogen peak will appear. A rise of 10 ppm above baseline is considered positive by some[92] but most require a rise of 20 ppm. Symptoms are also monitored during the test. However, some children harbor a flora that does not produce hydrogen yielding false negative tests (up to 25%). Therefore a trial of lactose free diet should be considered when the diagnosis is suspected.[78] A high baseline or a double peaked curve may be caused by bacterial overgrowth. The ^{13}C xylose breath test has also been proposed to diagnose small bowel overgrowth in children.[93]

^{13}C carbohydrate breath tests indicate the absorption of the tested ^{13}C labeled carbohydrate. ^{13}C lactose breath test can be used in children to assess lactose absorption.[94] ^{13}C sucrose test similarly, to test sucrase activity. Stable isotope breath tests are harmless, non-invasive and child friendly but require more specialized laboratory equipment for analysis.

Another useful ^{13}C breath test is the ^{13}C mixed triglyceride breath test to measure lipase activity.[95] In addition to being an excellent alternative to duodenal aspirate for pancreatic enzyme analysis, this test can assess the efficacy of exogenous lipase supplementation in cystic fibrosis.[96]

The *Sweat chloride* test is indicated in any case of infantile chronic diarrhea and suspicion of cystic fibrosis. It is the first step in the differential diagnosis of steatorrhea (Table 9.7).

Radiological examinations are contributive to rule out sub-obstruction (plain X-ray in the upright position) and fecal impaction and to document small intestinal lesions (enteroclysis). Sonography, when performed by an experienced radiologist, is helpful to document intestinal wall thickening.[97] White blood cell scanning[98] and MRI techniques[99] have been proposed as non-invasive methods to evaluate intestinal inflammation especially in Crohn's disease. These methods do not allow a diagnosis but a follow-up of documented lesions.

In the case of chronic diarrhea and a strong suspicion of intestinal damage or inflammation *endoscopic* and *histological examinations* are warranted. Except for flexible rectosigmoidoscopy endoscopic procedures are performed under general anesthesia or with conscious sedation.[100]

Situation:	Chronic, foul smelling, foamy stools in a child with failure to thrive
	↓
	Laboratory tests: fat soluble vitamins, triglycerides, cholesterol
	Hb, albumin, inflammatory parameters
	↓
	Rule out cystic fibrosis: Cl sweat test
	If dubious results: genetic analysis of D508 and alleles
	↓
	72 h fecal fat collection with stable fat intake:
	Normal → Reconsider diagnosis
	Elevated → Small bowel biopsy → R/o celiac disease
	Special fat staining → R/o αβ lipoproteinemia
	↓
	If normal: assess pancreatic secretion fecal elastase 1
	^{13}C mixed triglyceride breath test
	Or secretin test with duodenal fluid collection

Table 9.7 Differential diagnosis of steatorrhea

A small bowel biopsy is essential for the diagnosis of celiac disease (Fig. 9.1). Other causes of villous atrophy can be demonstrated such as allergic enteropathy (Fig. 9.2). Ileo-colonoscopy with biopsies is diagnostic for various types of colitis and Crohn's' disease.[101,102]

Duodenal tubage and analysis of pancreatic secretions before and after stimulation with secretin is the classical test to document pancreatic exocrine deficiency.[103] A somewhat simplified technique was described in which duodenal fluid is aspirated through an endoscope after stimulation with pancreozymin and secretin.[104] Valuable indirect tests that might replace the secretin test are the ^{13}C mixed triglyceride breath test and fecal chymotrypsin and elastase 1. The ^{13}C mixed triglyceride breath test is very sensitive in severe cases of pancreatic insufficiency, but fails to detect mild cases whereas the fecal elastase 1 test has a high sensitivity, specificity and a lower cost.[105]

In the case of fecal impaction with fecal incontinence, a history of early constipation and a suggestive digital rectal examination, *anorectal manometry* and *deep rectal biopsies* are indicated to rule out Hirschsprung's disease.

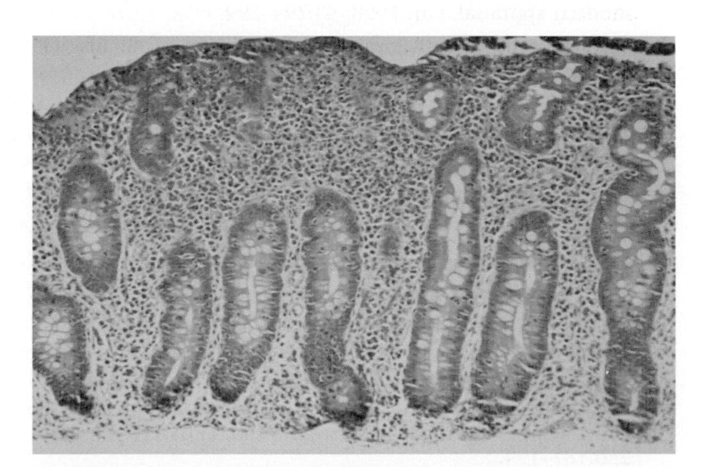

Figure 9.1: Small bowel biopsy from patient with celiac disease demonstrating villous atrophy and increased number of intraepithelial lymphocyte (*see plate section for color*).

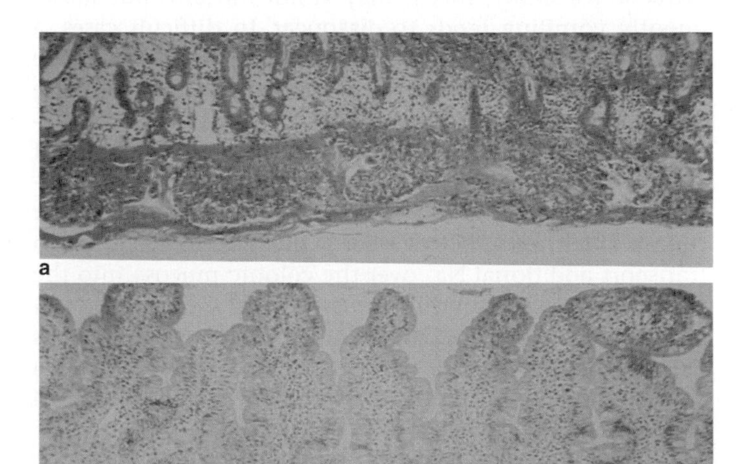

Figure 9.2: Small bowel biopsy (**a**) prior to and (**b**) after soy challenge in child with soy allergy. After the challenge the epithelium is damaged: villi are destroyed and the mucosa is invaded by a dens cellular infiltrate (*see plate section for color*).

CLINICAL MANAGEMENT

The diagnosis will obviously guide therapeutic management of a patient with diarrhea.[106] Acute self-limiting diarrhea necessitates little intervention besides some dietary adjustments.

Treatment of acute infectious diarrhea

Profuse diarrhea with signs or risk for dehydration necessitates oral rehydration with the adapted Oral-Rehydration-Solutions (ORS). Despite its proven efficacy and widespread use in developing countries, oral rehydration therapy is insufficiently applied in the USA.[107] Current recommendations are to re-feed early on after a short period of rehydration.[108,109]

In bacterial diarrheas, the glucose-sodium transporter and the basolateral Na-K-ATPase are always preserved and functional. Using this pathway, equimolar luminal glucose and sodium can transport sodium to the extracellular space. ORS with sodium in a range between 50 and 90 mmol/l are capable to rehydrate children in 3–4 h. This was also proven in viral diarrheas, where the glucose sodium transporter is not fully expressed on immature enterocytes on partially atrophic villi. The patchy nature of villus atrophy and preservation of sufficient normal villi explain the efficacy of ORS in this condition. The recommended quantity of ORS if offered on demand is 10–45 ml/kg bodyweight. Thirst is an important guide to limit rehydration time. Not the degree of dehydration, nor the child's age, influences the efficacy of rehydration. Parenteral rehydration is equally effective but is only indicated when the child has such abundant quantities of diarrhea that it cannot drink enough ORS and gets too tired, which is rare. The child might have enormous thirst and drink so forcefully, that it may vomit initially, but subsequently vomiting tends to disappear. In difficult cases, a nasogastric tube can be used to rehydrate. The advantage of immediate maximal rehydration is that after 3–4 h, the child might start to eat its normal food (breast feeding, bottle feeding or toddler food) with maintenance of ORS at 10 ml/kg bodyweight/watery stool.

The addition of soluble fiber to ORS has its benefits for the treatment of Cholera. Fiber is digested to SCFA which transport additional Na^+ over the colonic mucosa into the extracellular space. In milder diarrheas a benefit could not be demonstrated. The addition of a probiotic, Lactobacillus GG to ORS in a European multicenter trial resulted in shorter duration of diarrhea, less chance of a protracted course and faster hospital discharge.[110]

Treatment of chronic diarrhea

Chronic diarrhea is caused by malabsorption (as in osmotic diarrhea), secretory or inflammatory diarrhea. Luminal nutrients, such as protein, trigger mucosal mediators inducing increased secretion.[111] Fasting therefore diminishes secretory diarrhea somewhat as it does in malabsorptive osmotic and inflammatory diarrheas. In diseases, all three mechanisms are frequently involved, consequently for pathophysiologic, diagnostic and therapeutic purposes a separation is not clear-cut. Hydrolyzed formulas cause less secretion and are therefore indicated in mucosal disease.[112] Long chain triglycerides should be tried in most chronic diarrheas since they are osmotically inert, calory dense and absorbed to a variable extent in biliary obstruction, pancreatic insufficiency with enzyme supplements and mucosal disease. MCT are absorbed in the small and large bowel, constitute an excellent energy source but do not replace long chain fat. Poly- and disaccharides may increase diarrhea and should be titrated monitoring fecal reducing substances and stool frequency. This supports the approach of an oral regimen with normal constituents and caloric density and with limited place for special ingredients. Treatment of specific disease entities will be discussed in related chapters.

Other measures

Probiotics may lower the risk for infectious gastroenteritis but their efficacy in acute diarrhea was not demonstrated.[113]

Oral or enteral feeding is essential to stimulate mucosal recovery and avoid protracted diarrhea. Elemental, semi-elemental formulas and modular diets[114] allow early re-feeding despite a damaged mucosa with impaired digestive capacity.

Parents should be encouraged to normalize their child's diet as soon as possible, since restricted diets lead to chronic non-specific diarrhea.[115] Parenteral nutrition should be avoided and if needed, combined with minimal enteral feeding.

In unusual and unclear situations, the possibility of factitious diarrhea or Munchausen by Proxy should be considered. Observing the child in isolation should be preferred to a useless escalation of diagnostic tests and therapeutic interventions.

References

1. Boehm G, Lidestri M, Casetta P, et al. Supplementation of a bovine milk formula with an oligosaccharide mixture increases counts of faecal bifidobacteria in preterm infants. Arch Dis Child Fetal Neonatal Ed 2002; 86(3):F178–F181.
2. Goy J, Eastwood M, Mitchell W, et al. Fecal characteristics contrasted in the irritable bowel syndrome and diverticular disease. Am J Clin Nutr 1976; 29:1480.
3. Weaver L. Bowel habit from birth to old age. J Pediatr Gastroenterol Nutr 1988; 7:637.
4. Fontana M, Bianchi C, Cataldo F, et al. Bowel frequency in healthy children. Acta Paediatr Scand 1989; 78:682.
5. Myo-Khin, Thein-Win-Nyunt, Kyaw-Hla S, et al. A prospective study on defecation frequency, stool weight, and consistency. Arch Dis Child 1994; 71:311.
6. Weaver L, Steiner H. The bowel habit of young children. Arch Dis Child 1984; 59:649.
7. Yamada T, Powell D. Approach to the patient with diarrhea. Textbook of Gastroenterology. Ch. 40, 3rd edn. Philadelphia, PA: Lippincott; 2003.
8. Review SG. Salt and water absorption in the human colon: a modern appraisal. Gut 1998; 43:294–299.
9. Fordtran J, Locklear T. Ionic constituents and osmolality of gastric and small intestinal fluids after eating. Am J Dig Dis 1966; 11:503.
10. Wright E, Hirsch J, Loo D, Zampighi G. Regulation of Na+/glucose cotransporters. J Exp Biol 1997; 200:287–293.
11. Loo D, Zentlen T, Chandy G, Wright E. Cotransport of water by the Na+/glucose cotransporter. Proc Nat Acad Sci 1996; 93:B367–B370.
12. Ramaswamy K, Harig J, Soergel K. Short chain fatty acid transport by human intestinal apical membranes. In: Binder HJCJ, Soergel K, eds. Short chain fatty acids. Vol Falk Symposium 73. Lancaster, UK: Kluwer; 1994:93–103.
13. Naftalin RJPK. Video enhanced imaging of the fluorescent Na+ probe SBFI indicates that colonic crypts absorb fluid by generating a hypertonic interstitial fluid. FEBS Lett 1990; 260:187–194
14. Diamond JM. Solute-linked water transport in epithelia. In: Hoffman F, ed. Membrane Transport Processes. New York, NY: Raven Press; 1978.

15. Phillips S, Giller J. The contribution of the colon to electrolyte and water conservation in man. J Lab Clin Med 1973; 81:733.
16. Christopher N, Bayless T. Role of the small bowel and colon in lactose-induced diarrhea. Gastroenterology 1971; 60:845.
17. Branski D, Lerner A, Lebenthal E. Chronic diarrhea and malabsorption. Pediatr Clin North Am 1996; 43(2):307.
18. Levine M, Edelman R. Enteropathic Escherichia coli of classic serotypes associated with infant diarrhea: epidemiology and pathogenesis. Epidemiol Rev 1987; 6:31.
19. Moriarty K, Turnberg L. Bacterial toxins and diarrhoea. Clin Gastroenterol 1986; 15:529.
20. Gaskin K, Durie PR, Lee L, Hill R, Forstner GG. Colipase and lipase secretion in childhood onset pancreatic insufficiency: delineation of patients with steatorrhoea secondary to relative colipase deficiency. Gastroenterology 1984; 86:1.
21. Jeffries G, Holman H, Sleisinger M. Plasmaproteins and the gastrointestinal tract. N Engl J Med 1962; 266:652.
22. Waldman T. Gastrointestinal protein loss demonstrated by ^{51}Cr labeled albumin. Lancet 1961; 11:121.
23. Magazzu, Jacono G, Di Pasquale G, et al. Reliability and usefulness of random α1 antitrypsin concentration: further simplification of the method. J Pediatr Gastroenterol Nutr 1985; 4:402.
24. Kneepkens C, Hoekstra J. Chronic nonspecific diarrhea of childhood: Pathophysiology and Management. Pediatr Clin North Am 1996; 43(2):375.
25. Fenton T, Harries J, Milla P. Disordered small intestinal motility: A rational basis for toddlers' diarrhoea. Gut 1983; 24:897.
26. Hammer H, Santa Ana C, Schiller L, Fordrean J. Studies of osmotic diarrhea induced in normal subjects by ingestion of polyethylene glycol and lactulose. J Clin Invest 1989; 84:1056–1062.
27. Briet F, Pochart P, Marteau P, Flourie B, Arrigoni E, Rambaud J. Improved clinical tolerance to chronic lactose ingestion in subjects with lactose intolerance: a placebo effect? Gut 1997; 41:632–635.
28. Briet F, Flourie B, Achour L, Maurel M, Rambaud J, Messing B. Bacterial adaptation in patients with short bowel and colon in continuity. Gastronenterology 1995; 109:1446–1453.
29. Jeppesen P, Mortensen P. The influence of preserved colon on the absorption of medium chain fat in patients with small bowel resection. Gut 1998; 43:478–483.
30. Beeken W. Absorptive defects in young people with regional enteritis. Pediatrics 1973; 52:69–74.
31. Ball J, Tian P, Zeng C-Y, Morris A, Estes M. Age dependent diarrhea is induced by a viral non-structural glycoprotein. Science 1996; 272:101–104.
32. Hirshorn N. The treatment of acute diarrhea in children. A historical and physiological perspective. Am J Clin Nutr 1980; 33:637–663.
33. Mackenzie A, Barnes G, Shann F. Clinical signs of dehydration in children. Lancet 1989; 28(2(8670)):1038.
34. Guerrant R, Thielman N, Steiner T. Types of Escherichia coli enteropathogens. In: Blaser Mne, ed. Infections of the gastrointestinal tract. Philadelphia, PA: Lippincott; 2002:573–577.
35. Saavedra J. Probiotics and infectious diarrhea. Am J Gastroenterol 2000; 95(suppl 1):S16.
36. Guarino A, Spagnuolo MI, Russo S, et al. Etiology and risk factors of severe and protracted diarrhea. Pediatr Gastroenterol Nutr 1995; 20(2):173.
37. Hill D, Davidson F, Cameron D, et al. The spectrum of cow's milk allergy in childhood. Acta Paediatr Scand 1979; 68:847.
38. Kerner J. Formula allergy and intolerance. Ped Gastroenterol 1995; 24:1.
39. Catassi C, Fabiani E, Spagnuolo MI, Barera G, Guarino A. Severe and protracted diarrhea: results of the 3-year SIGEP multicenter survey. J Pediatr Gastroenterol Nutr 1999; 29:63.
40. Goulet O, Brousse N, Canioni D, et al. Syndrome of intractable diarrhoea with persistent villous atrophy in early childhood: a clinicopathological survey of 47 cases. J Pediatr Gastroenterol Nutr 1998; 26:151–161.
41. Rhoads J, Vogler R, Lacey S, et al. Microvillus inclusion disease. Gastroenterology 1991; 100:811–817.
42. Phillips A, Schmitz J. Microvillus atrophy. J Pediatr Gastroenterol Nutr 1992; 14:380–396.
43. Reifen R, Cutz E, Griffiths A, et al. Tufting enteropathy: a newly recognized clinicopathological entity associated with refractory diarrhea in infants. J Pediatr Gastroenterol Nutr 1994; 18:379–385.
44. Girault D, Goulet O. Deist le F, et al. Intractable infant diarrhea associated with phenotypic abnormalities and immunodeficiency. J Ped 1994; 125:36–42.
45. Aichbichler B, Zer C, Santa Ana C, et al. Proton pump inhibition of gastric chloride secretion in congenital chloridorrhea. N Engl J Med 1997; 336:106–109.
46. Canani R, Terrin G, Cirillo P, et al. Butyrate as an effective treatment of congenital chloride diarrhea. Gastroenterology 2004; 127:630–634.
47. Muller T, Wijmenga C, Phillips A, et al. Congenital sodium diarrhea is an autosomal recessive disorder of sodium/proton exchange but unrelated to known candidate genes. Gastroenterology 2000; 119:1506–1513.
48. Wright E. Genetic disorders of membrane transport I. glucose galactose malabsorption. Am J Physiol 1998; 275:G879–G882.
49. Hoekstra J. Fructose breath hydrogen testing in infants with chronic non-specific diarrhea. Eur J Pediatr 1995; 154:362–364.
50. Sarvilahti E, Laminda K, Kuitunen P. Congenital lactase deficiency. A clinical study on 16 patients. Arch Dis Child 1983; 58:246–252.
51. Jarvela I, Sabri Enattah N, Kokkonen J, Varilo T, Savilahti E, Peltonen L. Assignment of the locus for congenital lactase deficiency to 2q21, in the vicinity of but separate from the lactase-phlorizin hydrolase gene. Am J Hum Genet 1998; 63(4):1078–1085.
52. Lebenthal E, Khin-Maung-U, Zheng BY, Lu RB, Lerner A. Small intestinal glucoamylase deficiency and starch malabsorption: a new recognized alpha-glucosidase deficiency in children. J Pediatr 1994; 124:541–546.
53. Steffen R. Wyllier, Petras R, et al. The spectrum of eosinofilic gastroenteritis. Report of 6 pediatric cases and review of the literature. Clin Pediatr 1991; 30:404.
54. Durie P, Hamilton J, Forstner G. Malabsorption of medium chain triglycerides in infants with cystic fibrosis, correction with pancreatic enzyme supplements. J Pediatr 1980; 96:862–864.
55. Hill REDP, Gaskin KJ, Davidson GP, Forstner GG. Steatorrhea and pancreatic insufficiency in Shwachman syndrome. Gastroenterology 1982; 83:22–27.
56. Ghishan F, Moran J, Durie P, Green E. Isolated congenital lipase-colipase deficiency. Gastroenterology 1984; 86:1580–1582.
57. Ligumsky M, Granot E, Branski D, Stankiewicz H, Goldstein R. Isolated lipase and colipase deficiency in two brothers. Gut 1990; 31(12):1416–1418.
58. Holzinger A, Maier E, Buck C, et al. Mutations in the proenteropeptidase gene are the molecular cause of

congenital enteropeptidase deficiency. Am J Hum Genet 2002; 70(1):20–25.

59. Zentler-Munroe P, Fitzpatrick W, Battem J, Dorthfield T. Effect of intrajejunal acidity on the aqueous phase bile acid and lipid concentration in pancreatic steatorrhea due to cystic fibrosis. Gut 1984; 25:500–507.
60. Watkins J, Tercyak A. Sczepani K, et al. Bile salts kinetics in cystic fibrosis: influence of pancreatic enzyme replacement. Gastroenterology 1977; 73:1023–1028.
61. Glasgow J, Hamilton J, Sass Kortsak A. Fat absorption in congenital obstructive liver disease. Arch Dis Child 1973; 48:601–607.
62. Oelkers P, Kirby L, Heubi J. Primary bile acid malabsorption caused by mutations in the ileal sodium-dependent bile acid transporter gene (SLC19A2). J Clin Invest 1997; 99:1880–1887.
63. Setchell K, Borgetti P. Zimmer-Nechimias L, et al. Oral bile acid treatment and the patient with Zellweger syndrome. Hepatology 1992; 15:198–207.
64. Sawczenko A, Sandhu BK, Logan RF, et al. Prospective survey of childhood inflammatory bowel disease in the British Isles. Lancet 2001; 357(9262):1093.
65. Binder H, Prak T. Jejunal absorption of water and electrolytes in inflammatory bowel disease. J Lab Clin Med 1970; 76:915.
66. Fenton TRHJ, Milla PJ. Disordered small intestinal motility: a rational basis for toddlers' diarrhoea. Gut 1983; 24(10):897–903.
67. Jonas A, Diver-Haber A. Stool output and composition in the chronic non-specific diarrhoea syndrome. Arch Dis Child 1982; 57(1):35–39.
68. Tripp J, Manning J, Muller D, et al. Mucosal adenylate cyclase and sodium-potassium stimulated adenosine triphosphatase in jejunal biopsies of adults and children with coeliac disease. In: McNicholl B, ed. Perspectives in coeliac disease. Proceedings of the 3rd International Coeliac Symposium. Lancaster: MTP Press; 1978:461.
69. Cohen S, Hendricks K, Mathis R, et al. Chronic nonspecific diarrhea: dietary relationships. Pediatrics 1979; 64:402–407.
70. Kneepkens C, Hoekstra J. Chronic nonspecific diarrhea of childhood. Pediatr Clin North Am 1996; 43:375–389.
71. Hyams J. Diet and gastrointestinal disease. Curr Opin Pediatr 2002; 14(5):567–569.
72. Hyams J. Irritable bowel syndrome, functional dyspepsia, and functional abdominal pain syndrome. Adolesc Med Clin 2004; 15(1):1–15.
73. Parry S, Stansfield R, Jelley D, et al. Does bacterial gastroenteritis predispose people to functional gastrointestinal disorders? A prospective, community-based, case-control study. Am J Gastroenterol 2003; 98(9):1970–1975.
74. Dunlop S, Jenkins D, Neal K, Spiller R. Relative importance of enterochromaffin cell hyperplasia, anxiety, and depression in postinfectious IBS. Gastroenterology 2003; 125(6):1651–1659.
75. Badiali D, Marcheggiano A, Pallone F, et al. Melanosis of the rectum in patients with chronic constipation. Dis Colon Rectum 1985; 28(4):241–245.
76. Ackerman N, Strobel C. Polle syndrome: chronic diarrhea in Munchausen's child. Gastroenterology 1981; 81:1140.
77. Long R. Vasoactive intestinal polypeptide-secreting tumors (VIPomas) in childhood. J Pediatr Gastroenterol Nutr 1983; 2(1):122–126.
78. Thomas PD, Forbes A, Green J, et al. Guidelines for the investigation of chronic diarrhoea. Gut 2003; 52:v1.
79. Laadhar LBN, Ben Ayed M, Chaabouni M, et al. Determination of anti-transglutaminase antibodies in the diagnosis of coeliac disease in children: results of a five year prospective study. Ann Biol Clin 2004; 62(4):431–436.
80. Catassi C, Ratsch IM, Fabiani E, et al. High prevalence of undiagnosed celiac disease in 5280 Italian students screened by antigliadin antibodies. Acta Paediatr Scand 1995; 84:672.
81. Clemente MGMM, Troncone R, Volta U, Congia M, Ciacci C, Neri E. Enterocyte actin autoantibody detection: a new diagnostic tool in celiac disease diagnosis: results of a multicenter study. Am J Gastroenterol 2004; 99(8): 1551–1556.
82. Fine K, Ogunji F. A new method of quantitative fecal fat microscopy and its correlation with chemically measured fecal fat output. Am J Clin Pathol 2000; 113:528.
83. Van den Neucker AM, Kerkvliet EM, Theunissen PM, Forget PP. Acid steatocrit: a reliable screening tool for steatorrhoea. Acta Paediatr Scand 2001; 90(8):873.
84. Duncan A, Hill P. A UK survey of laboratory based gastrointestinal investigations. Ann Clin Biochem 1998; 35:492.
85. Hill P. Faecal fat: time to give it up. Ann Clin Biochem 2001; 38:164.
86. Rivero-Marcotegui A, Oliveira-Olmedo J, Sanches Valverde-Fisus F, et al. Water, fat, nitrogen and sugar contents in faeces: reference intervals in children. Clin Chem 1998; 44:1540–1544.
87. Hernell O. Assessing fat absorption. J Pediatr 1999; 135:407–409.
88. Soldan W, Henker J, Sprossig C. Sensitivity and specificity of quantitative determination of pancreatic elastase 1 in feces of children. J Pediatr Gastroenterol Nutr 1997; 24(1):53.
89. Fagerberg UL, Loof L, Merzoug RD, Hansson LO, Finkel Y. Fecal calprotectin levels in healthy children studied with an improved assay. J Pediatr Gastroenterol Nutr 2003; 37(4):468.
90. Nissen AC, van Gils CE, Menheere PP, Van den Neucker AM, van der Hoeven MA, Forget PP. Fecal calprotectin in healthy term and preterm infants. J Pediatr Gastroenterol Nutr 2004; 38(1):107.
91. Brummer R, Karibe M, Stockbrugger R. Lactose malabsorption. Optimalization of investigational methods. Scand J Gastroenterol Suppl 1993; 200:65.
92. Barr R, Watkins J, Perman J. Mucosal function and breath hydrogen excretion: comparative studies in the clinical evaluation of children with non-specific abdominal complaints. Pediatrics 1981; 68:526.
93. Dellert SF, Nowicki MJ, Farrell MK, Delente J, Heubi JE. The ^{13}C-xylose breath test for the diagnosis of small bowel bacterial overgrowth in children. J Pediatr Gastroenterol Nutr 1997; 25:153.
94. Vonk RJ, Stellaard F, Hoekstra H, Koetse HA. ^{13}C carbohydrate breath tests. Gut 1998; 43 (Suppl)(3):S20.
95. van Dijk-van Aalst K, Van Den Driessche M, van Der Schoor S, et al. The ^{13}C mixed triglyceride breath test: a non-invasive method to assess lipase activity in children. J Pediatr Gastroenterol Nutr 2001; 32:579.
96. De Boeck K, Delbeke I, Eggermont E, Veereman-Wauters G, Ghoos Y. Lipid digestion in cystic fibrosis: comparison of conventional and high-lipase enzyme therapy using the mixed triglyceride breath test. J Pediatr Gastroenterol Nutr 1998; 26:408.
97. Siegel M, Friedland J, Hildebolt C. Bowel wall thickening in children: differentiation with US. Radiology 1997; 203(3):631.
98. Bruno I, Martelossi S, Geatti O, et al. Antigranulocyte monoclonal antibody immunoscintigraphy in inflammatory bowel disease in children and young adolescents. Acta Paediatr 2002; 91(10):1050.

99. Magnano G, Granata C, Barabino A, et al. Polyethylene glycol and contrast-enhanced MRI of Crohn's disease in children: preliminary experience. Pediatr Radiol 2003; 33(6):385.
100. Tolia V, Peters J, Gilger M. Sedation for pediatric endoscopic procedures. J Pediatr Gastroenterol Nutr 2000; 30(5):477.
101. Xin W, Brown P, Greenson J. The clinical significance of focal active colitis in pediatric patients. Am J Surg Pathol 2003; 27(8):1134.
102. Chang JW, Wu TC, Wang KS, Huang IF, Huang B, Yu IT. Colon mucosal pathology in infants under three months of age with diarrhea disorders. J Pediatr Gastroenterol Nutr 2002; 35:386.
103. Gislon J, Lefevre R, Fiesse-Vandale P, Bonfils S. Pancreatic functional exploration by duodenal tubage after ceruleine and secretinic stimulation. Arch Fr Mal App Dig 1976; 65(6):463–472.
104. Madrazo-de la Garza J, Gotthold M, Lu R, Hill I, E L. A new direct pancreatic function test in pediatrics. J Pediatr Gastroenterol Nutr 1991; 12(3):356–360.
105. Loser C, Brauer C, Aygen S, Hennemann O, Folsch U. Comparative clinical evaluation of the 13C-mixed triglyceride breath test as an indirect pancreatic function test. Scand J Gastroenterol 1998; 33(10):1118–1120.
106. Lee W, Boey C. Chronic diarrhoea in infants and young children: causes, clinical features and outcome. J Paediatr Child Health 1999; 35:260.
107. Santosham M, Keenan EM, Tulloch J, Broun D, Glass R. Oral rehydration therapy for diarrhea: an example of reverse transfer of technology. Pediatrics 1997; 100(5):E10.
108. Sandhu B. European Society of Paediatric Gastroenterology HaNWGoAD. Rationale for early feeding in childhood gastroenteritis. J Pediatr Gastroenterol Nutr 2001; 33(Suppl 2):S13.
109. Sandhu B. European Society of Paediatric Gastroenterology HaNWGoAD. Practical guidelines for the management of gastroenteritis in children. J Pediatr Gastroenterol Nutr 2001; 33(Suppl 2):S36.
110. Guandelini S, Pensabene L. Zikri MA, et al. Lactobacillus GG administered in oral rehydration solution to children with acute diarrhea: a multicenter European trial. J Pediatr Gastroenterol Nutr 2000; 30(2):214–216.
111. Heyman M, Desjeux J. Significance of intestinal food protein transport. J Pediatr Gastroenterol Nutr 15(1):48–57.
112. Walker Smit J. Nutritional management of enteropathy. Nutrition 1998; 14:775–779.
113. Costa-Ribeiro H, Ribeiro TC, Mattos AP, et al. Limitations of probiotic therapy in acute, severe dehydrating diarrhea. J Pediatr Gastroenterol Nutr 2003; 36(1):112.
114. Kolacek S, Grguric J, Percl M, Booth IW. Home-made modular diet versus semi-elemental formula in the treatment of chronic diarrhoea of infancy: a prospective randomized trial. Eur J Pediatr 1996; 155:997.
115. Boehm P, Nassimbeni G, Ventura A. Chronic non-specific diarrhoea in childhood: how often is it iatrogenic? Acta Paediatr 1998; 87:268.

Chapter 10
Colic and gastrointestinal gas

Sandeep K. Gupta

GASTROINTESTINAL GAS

Complaints related to increased gastrointestinal air load, or 'gassiness', are encountered both in the pediatric population and adult patients though often for different reasons. For example, the new mother may be concerned that increased gastrointestinal gas is making her infant colicky, while an adult may be more worried about excessive belching, and socially unacceptable, frequent passage of flatus especially if of offensive odor. On the contrary, abdominal bloatiness and distension may be a source of discomfort in both children and adults with lactose intolerance or irritable bowel syndrome.

It is important to appreciate the physiology of gastrointestinal gas in order to understand its relationship to disease. Excessive gas production may be cited, inaccurately, as the cause of symptoms associated with irritable bowel syndrome. Additionally, patients with complaints of excessive gastrointestinal gas are at risk of being subjected to expensive and unnecessary diagnostic tests in an effort to 'cure' a non-existent problem. The vast numbers of unscientific notions and home-remedies available for gassiness further challenge effective and efficient management of such patients.

In this chapter, the physiology of gastrointestinal gas will be reviewed along with a discussion of the clinical manifestations of excessive gastrointestinal gas and infantile colic.

Composition of gastrointestinal gas

Gastrointestinal gas may originate from three sources: (1) swallowed air, (2) intraluminal production, i.e. bacterial production, and reaction of acid and bicarbonate and (3) diffusion from the blood (Fig. 10.1). Gas may be lost from the gastrointestinal tract via eructation/belching, passage of flatus, bacterial consumption and diffusion into the blood stream. While there are no published data on the gas content of the gastrointestinal tract of an infant or a child, studies in healthy adults indicate that the normal gastrointestinal tract contains less than 200 ml of gas.[1]

Over 99% of gastrointestinal gas is comprised of five gases, namely carbon dioxide (CO_2), hydrogen (H_2), methane (CH_4), nitrogen (N_2) and oxygen (O_2), in varying percentages (Table 10.1). Two of these, H_2 and CH_4, are combustible and can be explosive in a proper mixture with O_2. All these gases are odorless. Odoriferous gases are present in trace amounts, i.e. less than 1% of flatus, and are sulfur based. Hence, while the most anxiety and embarrassment is often generated by odoriferous flatus, the culprit gases are present only in miniscule amounts. Most of the symptoms from excessive gastrointestinal gas are attributable to the five odorless gases.

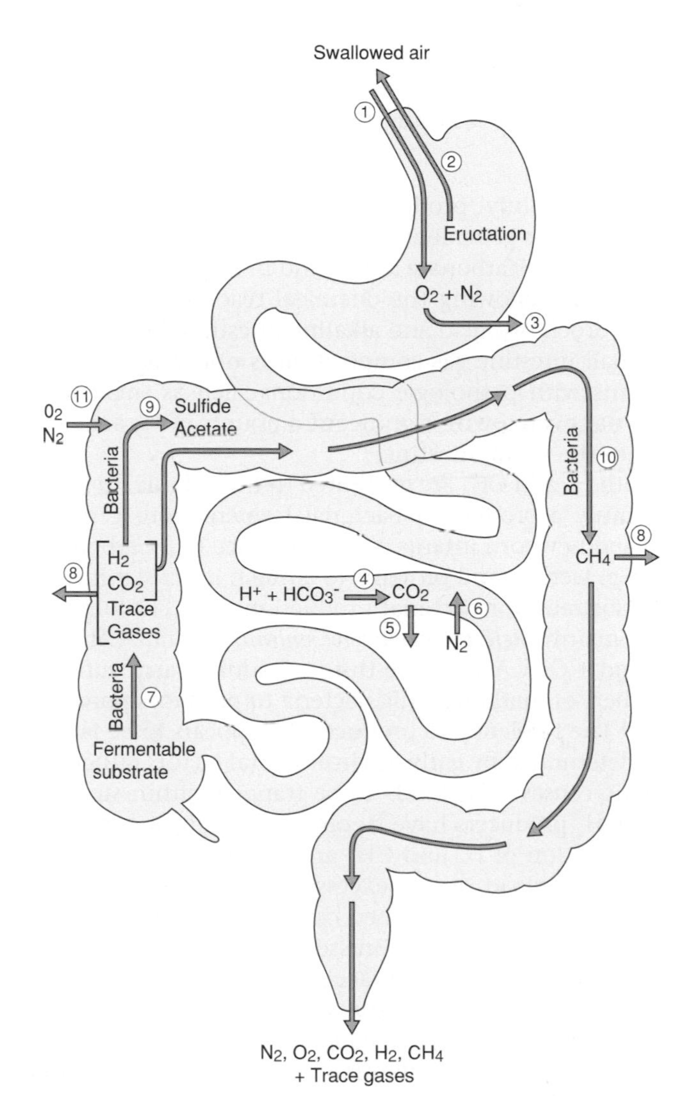

Figure 10.1: Physiology of gastrointestinal gas production (from Feldman M, Friedman L Sleisenger M (2002) Sleisenger & Fordtran's Gastrointestinal and Liver Disease, 7th edn Philadelphia, PA. Saunders, with permission).[1]

Sources and relative distribution of gastrointestinal gases

The main source of N_2 is swallowed air. An adult ingests over half an ounce (15 ml) of air with each swallow, the main components of which are N_2 and O_2. As such, gastric luminal gas is composed mainly of N_2 and O_2. CO_2, H_2 and

Composition
Odorless gases (99%)
Carbon dioxide
Hydrogen[a]
Methane[a]
Nitrogen
Oxygen
Odoriferous gases (<1%)
Dimethylsulfide
Hydrogen sulfide
Methanethiol

[a]Combustible

Table 10.1 Composition of intestinal gas

CH_4 are mainly produced within the gastrointestinal lumen. CO_2 is generated through the interaction of hydrogen ion and bicarbonate and found in large volumes in the duodenum following the chemical reaction between gastric hydrochloric acid and alkaline intestinal fluid. The distal small intestine gas composition is not well defined. In patients with pathologic conditions such as small bowel bacterial overgrowth, significant amounts of H_2 are generated in the small intestine.[2]

Both H_2 and CH_4 are generated in the colonic lumen. H_2 is mainly a product of bacterial fermentation; germ free rats and newborn infants do not produce H_2.[1] Carbohydrates, e.g. lactose, and proteins to a much lesser significance, are substrates for bacterial production of H_2. Colonic bacteria, mainly *Methanobrevibacter smithii*, generate CH_4 using H_2 and CO_2.[3] About one-third of adults carry sufficient numbers of methanogenic bacteria to produce appreciable CH_4.[4] The tendency to produce CH_4 appears to be familial and determined by early environmental factors rather than genetic causes. CH_4 tends to be trapped within stool and large CH_4 producers have stools that float in water.

Generation of H_2 and CH_4 are also enhanced by carbohydrate overload, as in excessive intake of fruit juices, ingestion of poorly absorbed carbohydrates such as cauliflower, cabbage, broccoli, Brussel sprouts and beans, or disaccharidase deficiency. Disaccharidase deficiency may be primary, as noted in primary lactose intolerance, or secondary, as in a variety of maladies including celiac disease, allergic enteropathy, inflammatory bowel disease, giardiasis and viral gastroenteritis.

Symptoms attributable to gastrointestinal gas

Excessive gastrointestinal gas may contribute to a number of symptoms including eructation, abdominal distension and bloating, excessive flatulence and infantile colic.

Eructation

This behavior, also referred to as belching or burping, is often considered normal in infants. In fact, infants are encouraged to burp during and after feeds in the hope of minimizing gastroesophageal reflux and feeding intolerance. As in infants who are liable to swallow air during normal periods of crying and feeding, excessive eructation in older children and adults is almost always secondary to aerophagia.[5] Undue aerophagia may result from excessive gum chewing, use of a straw, imbibing of carbonated beverages, clenching on a pencil, or oral breathing as in adeno-tonsillar hypertrophy, or unrecognized H-type tracheo-esophageal fistula; patients should be counseled on chewing the food slowly and not gulp the food. Rare patients with excessive belching have been found to have allergic (eosinophilic) esophagitis (personal observation). In adults, chronic eructation is generally thought to be a functional disorder.[1]

Gas-bloat syndrome, seen in children following gastric surgery such as Nissen fundoplication, results from an inability of the patient to belch/eructate effectively. While this can be a source of significant patient discomfort and family distress, the condition is generally transient and self-resolves.

Abdominal distension

Abdominal distension, or bloating, may result from excessive aerophagia and increased gastrointestinal gas production, as in malabsorption syndromes. Children with aerophagia often have a non-distended abdomen upon rising, which progressively distends over the day and may be accompanied by crampy abdominal pain. The physical examination may be impressive for abdominal distension and tympany. Plain abdominal films reveal gaseous distension of the bowel. Symptoms and signs may be so intense as to mimic intestinal obstruction[5] or Celiac disease. Fatal tension pneumoperitoneum has been reported secondary to aerophagia.[6]

Abdominal distention is also part of the symptom constellation of irritable bowel syndrome.[7] The discomfort associated with bloating in patients with irritable bowel syndrome is more due to dysmotility and heightened perception.[8] No appreciable differences were found in the volume of intragastrointestinal gas in adults with complaints of bloating *vs* controls, although there was an increased symptomatic response to gas infusion in patients with bloating.[9]

Flatulence

An adult passes flatus an average of 10 times per day with an upper limit of 20 times a day. The frequency of flatus does not correlate with age or gender[1] though data on children are lacking. While flatulence can be a social embarrassment, comfort should be derived from the fact that over 99% of the flatus consists of odorless gases. Increased gastrointestinal gas production, rather than aerophagia, is usually responsible for flatulence in adults, though it is not known if the same can be extrapolated to children.[5] The source of the flatus may be assessed by gas chromatographic analysis of flatus collected via a rectal tube. Aerophagia should be considered the main contributor if N_2 is the leading component; predominance of H_2, CO_2 and CH_4 would suggest increased intraluminal production, e.g. secondary to bacterial fermentation of malabsorbed carbohydrates.

An extensive radiological and endoscopic evaluation of a patient with excessive flatulence alone is generally

Symptom or sign	Air swallowing	Bacterial fermentation
Increased eructation	Yes	No
Increased salivation	Yes	No
Gas is stress related	Yes	No
Gas is meal related	No	Yes
Abdominal bloating	Yes	No
Malodorous gas	No	Yes
Nocturnal gas	No	Yes

Adapted from Suarez and Levitt 2000[10] (Reproduced with permission).

Table 10.2 Symptoms and signs suggesting air swallowing or bacterial fermentation as the cause of excessive flatulance

fruitless and should be avoided.[10] Efforts should instead be directed at eliciting a detailed history (Table 10.2). Appropriate investigation should be considered if the flatulence is accompanied by other symptoms such as diarrhea, hematochezia/melena, abdominal pain, or weight loss. Otherwise, dietary modifications directed towards limiting intake of fruit juices and poorly absorbed carbohydrates, such as cabbage and legumes, may need enforced. Excessive consumption of high-carbohydrate containing beverages is more apt to be a culprit in children than high intake of cruciferous vegetables like cabbage. A detailed inquiry into intake of liquid medications and sugar-free drinks should be undertaken as these products contain sorbitol. Sorbitol is an artificial sweetener that is poorly absorbed and readily fermented by colonic bacteria.

If the patient is bothered by odoriferous flatus, a commercially-available charcoal-lined cushion (TooT TrappeR®; Ultratech, Houston, TX) has been shown to effectively absorb over 90% of the sulfur gases.

COLIC

The word 'colic' refers to acute and unexpected abdominal pain, independent of age. In infants, 'colic' takes on a different connotation that is often associated with a reaction of frustration and helplessness on the part of the caregiver and the healthcare provider. Infantile colic refers to excessive bursts of crying in otherwise healthy infants that are not relieved by routine comfort measures. The classical and most often cited definition of infantile colic is based on the rule of threes: 'periods of crying that last for 3 hours or more per day for 3 or more days per week for a minimum of 3 weeks'.[11] Another 'three' to add would be that the condition generally resolves by the age of 3 months.[12,13] The crying often begins suddenly and is loud, piercing and high-pitched. It has a rapid crescendo and the infant is inconsolable. The infant may exhibit a tense abdomen, lift the head, clench the fists, flex the legs to the abdomen and appear flushed. The episodes are most common in the late afternoon and evening hours and tend to peak at age 6 weeks.[14] These characteristics help differentiate colic, which affects about 700 000 infants each year in the USA, from other more serious medical conditions. Infantile colic may be graded as mild, moderate or severe, but there are no set definitions.[12] Infantile colic equally affects infants of all socioeconomic strata and there are no reported differences in prevalence between boys and girls, nursed and formula-fed babies, and absence and presence of allergies in the family.[15]

Although understanding of this disease process has advanced over the decades, the gains have been limited. Despite the salience of infantile colic in terms of its prevalence, affecting between 9 and 26% of infants,[16] it frustrates the healthcare provider, produces parental anxiety and reduces confidence in parents' infant-caring capabilities. It would be most helpful to elucidate the etiopathogenesis which would lend better understanding of the condition and permit more effective, scientifically-sound management of the afflicted infant (and his/her exasperated caregiver). The proposed etiologies of infantile colic are shown in Table 10.3.[17]

Is colic a gastrointestinal disorder?

The fact that a pediatric gastroenterologist is often consulted for the colicky infant supports the notion that parents and pediatricians/primary-care providers perceive colic to be a disturbance of the gastrointestinal tract. This belief is further substantiated by the infant's behavior, i.e. grimacing and drawing up of legs and excessive passage of flatus.

Excessive gastrointestinal gas

This may result from aerophagia secondary to the inconsolable crying exhibited by the colicky infant, or from increased gas generation from colonic fermentation. The latter may be due to altered (increased) intestinal bacterial load and/or the presence of malabsorbed carbohydrates. There is, however, a paucity of data to support the notion that excessive gastrointestinal gas incites a colicky episode. Harley[18] demonstrated radiographically normal gastric outlines during a colic episode. Measures to prevent aerophagia, such as upright positioning, are of little benefit in the management or prevention of infantile colic.[19,20] A recent randomized, placebo-controlled, multicenter trial of the

- Gastrointestinal
  - Nutritive
    - Excessive intraintestinal air load:
      - Aerophagia
      - Colonic fermentation/malabsorption
    - Mode of feeding
    - Protein allergy/intolerance
  - Non-nutritive:
    - Motility
    - Gastroesophageal reflux
    - Gut hormones
- Non-gastrointestinal

From Gupta 2002[17] (Reproduced with permission).

Table 10.3 Proposed etiologies of infantile colic

use of simethicone in the treatment of infantile colic failed to detect an efficacy difference between simethicone and placebo, thereby refuting, albeit indirectly, the hypothesis that increased gastrointestinal gas has a major role in the pathogenesis of infantile colic.[21] Lehtonen et al.[22] did not detect any differences in the intestinal microflora between colicky and non-colicky infants.

A subset of normal infants may partially malabsorb dietary carbohydrate in the early postnatal period.[23–25] The malabsorbed sugars undergo colonic fermentation with generation of gas, including H_2. This phenomenon of 'physiological malabsorption' generally resolves around the age of 3 months, which is when colicky behavior also generally subsides.[23,24] Two studies have detailed an association between elevated breath H_2 levels and infantile colic, but the range of values was wide.[26,27] As many as one-third of the colicky infants had low breath H_2 levels and one-third of the non-colicky infants had elevation of their breath H_2 levels. Hyams et al.[28] did not note a difference in breath H_2 levels between colicky and non-colicky infants when fed a standardized non-absorbable carbohydrate. Data on the role of lactose consumption in infantile colic is controversial. Lack of symptom improvement was demonstrated by two studies that examined the effects of lactase supplementation in infants with colic[29,30] or one study that used low-lactose containing formula in infants with colic.[31] Kanabar et al., however, found symptomatic improvement in a subset of colicky infants following pre-treatment of feeds with lactase.[32] Investigations aimed at uncovering evidence of malabsorption, such as stool alpha-1-antitrypsin levels, pH, reducing substances and occult blood, have been unrewarding and no significant differences have been found between colicky and non-colicky infants.[19]

Mode of feeding

The prevalence, pattern and amount of crying associated with infantile colic are reportedly similar in both human milk- and formula-fed infants.[15,33–35] One study reported an earlier peak of colicky behavior in formula-fed infants compared with human milk-fed infants (age 2 weeks *vs* 6 weeks).[36]

Protein allergy/intolerance

Allergy to human- and cow milk-proteins has been implicated in the etiopathogenesis of infantile colic, but convincing, reproducible evidence is lacking or, controversial at best.[31,37–40] Scientific methodology would dictate that appropriate diagnostic tests be conducted to substantiate (or refute) an allergy causality. The diagnostic tests, including endoscopic studies with mucosal biopsies for histological examination, are cumbersome and difficult to access.

Jakobsson and Lindberg[37] reported in 1978 that exclusion of cow milk-protein from the diet of mothers of nursed infants with colic resulted in colic resolution. Campbell[38] too tended to favor a role of cow milk-protein in the pathogenesis of infantile colic. Some 68% (13/19) of infants studied had resolution of colic with dietary modifications that consisted of switching from a cow milk-protein-based formula to soy protein-based formula, or switching from the latter to a protein-hydrolysate formula. Forsyth[39] found a similar initial result which was not sustained. He alternated the feedings of 17 colicky infants between a casein hydrolysate formula and a cow milk-protein-containing formula. Infants fed the hydrolysate formula had less crying and colic initially, but the effects diminished over time. More recently, Lucassen et al.[41] randomized Dutch infants with colic to either a whey-hydrolysate formula or a standard formula; the former group demonstrated a decrease in crying duration of 63 min/day (95% confidence interval: 1–127 min/day). Lindberg[42] opines that about 25% of infants with moderate or severe colic respond favorably to a diet free of cow milk-protein. On the contrary, Thomas et al.[33] noted the prevalence of colic to be similar between infants fed human milk, formula and formula-supplemented human milk. They concluded that dietary protein hypersensitivity is probably not the cause of colic in most healthy infants. These results are supported by a more recent study of prevalence of colic among breast-fed, formula-fed and complementary-fed infants.[43] No associations were noted between the source of infant nutrition and development of colic in this questionnaire-based study. Leibman[44] also failed to uncover objective evidence of protein allergy in his study of 56 infants with colic. He found the complete blood cell count, sedimentation rate, quantitative serum IgE level and fecal occult blood to be normal in these infants. He also reported normal results for radioallergosorbent tests for cow milk-protein in the 15 infants tested. In spite of these, a recent article suggests the use of pancreatic enzyme supplements by lactating mothers in the treatment of infantile colic.[45] The authors theorize that hydrolysis of human milk-protein by pancreatic enzyme supplements benefits colicky infants with cow milk allergy.

Motility

Altered intestinal motility may lead to abdominal cramping and colicky behavior. Jorup[46] stated that most cases of infantile colic could be explained by colonic hyperperistalsis and increased rectal pressure. This may be supported by the documented beneficial effects of dicyclomine hydrochloride on infantile colic.[47–48] The actions of dicyclomine may be central or peripheral, where it decreases gastrointestinal motility by a direct relaxant effect on the colonic smooth muscle. The utility of this drug, however, is limited due to its central effects and potential for respiratory depression; death associated with its use has been seen. In a controlled trial, a herbal tea preparation containing some antispasmodics (chamomile, fennel and balm mint) was shown to benefit colicky infants.[49] It should be cautioned that fennel tea was recently reported to have mutagenic effects on bacteria and a carcinogenic effect in mice.[50]

Italian researchers evaluated the use of cimetropium bromide in a placebo-controlled trial of 86 colicky infants.[51] Cimetropium bromide is a quaternary ammonium semi-synthetic derivative of the belladonna alkaloid scopolamine with two main actions: a competitive antagonism of muscarinic receptors of the visceral smooth muscles and direct myolytic activity. The drug reduced the duration of crying in the treated group compared with controls. The treated infants did have more sleepiness compared with controls, but no respiratory distress or apnea were observed.

Use of chiropractic spinal manipulation in treatment of colicky infants has been examined in a number of studies.[52–54] While the earlier data showed a favorable response,[52,53] a more recent study did not.[54] In the latter study, 46 infants with colic and 40 controls underwent chiropractic spinal manipulation in a randomized, blinded, placebo control manner. A similar degree of improvement was noted between the treatment and the placebo groups.

Gastroesophageal reflux

Much attention has been given to a possible cause-effect relationship between gastroesophageal reflux (GER) and infantile colic. Though GER may present with excessive crying, as does infantile colic, the crying is generally less intense in GER.[19] Few studies have examined the role of pathologic GER in colicky infants and the results are contentious. Berkowitz et al.[55] performed 24-h continuous intraesophageal pH monitoring studies ('pH probe') in 26 infants with persistent, excessive crying, who had been labeled colicky. They detected pathologic GER in 16 of these 26 (61%) infants. While the data appear compelling, it is difficult to establish a cause–effect relationship, as these infants did not exhibit classic symptoms of GER, like regurgitation and emesis. Additionally, 12 of the 16 (75%) infants with pathologic GER were aged 4 months or older, by which age infantile colic generally resolves. In another study of 24 infants under the age of 3 months, who had excessive crying and presumed GER, only one infant had pathologic GER on pH probe studies.[56] Hence, is pathologic GER, if present, a culprit or an innocent sojourner in infants with colic? The available data would suggest that pathologic GER may be implicated at most in a small subset of young infants with colicky symptoms. Some clinicians suggest a limited duration empiric trial of anti-reflux pharmacotherapy in selected colicky infants.[57–58]

Gut hormones

The gastrointestinal tract contains a repertoire of hormones, transmitters and other biologically-active proteins, such as prostaglandins. Of these, motilin appears to be a lead contender to play a role in the etiopathogenesis of infantile colic. Basal motilin levels are raised in colicky infants independent of their diet and are higher at birth in infants who later develop colic.[59] It is speculated that motilin promotes gastric emptying, which increases small bowel peristalsis and decreases transit time. These could contribute to perceived intestinal pain and lend substance to the hyperperistalsis theory.[60]

Is colic due to non-gastrointestinal pathology?

This aspect of infantile colic has long been proposed, widely studied and passionately debated. Nearly 6 decades ago, Spock[61] had suggested that infantile colic could be due to transmission of anxiety and tension from the mother to the infant. Various studies, many with methodological deficiencies, have since attempted to further this observation.[62] Stewart et al.[63] reported in 1954, that mothers of excessive criers experienced more psychological conflicts regarding their maternal role and displayed more hostility towards their child. Rautava et al.[64] suggested important roles for maternal distress during pregnancy and childbirth and unsatisfactory sexual relationships, but not for socioeconomic factors, in the cause of colic in Finnish infants. Reijneveld et al.[65] examined the relationship between maternal behavior and colic by studying the association of maternal smoking and type of feeding with colic in 3345 Dutch infants between the ages of 1 and 6 months. They found the prevalence of colic to be two-fold higher in infants of smoking mothers. Similar results were reported in a study of maternal smoking and colic in Danish infants.[66] A more recent Canadian study found increased likelihood of colic with higher levels of maternal anxiety, maternal alcohol consumption at 6 weeks and shift-work during pregnancy.[43] On the other hand, being married or having a common-law partner and being employed full-time during the pregnancy were associated with a reduced risk of colic. In contrast, Paradise[15] found that maternal emotional factors do not play a role in infantile colic. The incidence of colic in this study was independent of family socioeconomic status, maternal age, birth order, infant gender, weight gain, type of feeding or family history of allergic or gastrointestinal disorder. Superior maternal intelligence and higher education were associated with higher incidences of infantile colic. There was no correlation with maternal emotional factors, whether estimated clinically or measured using standardized psychological tests like Minnesota Multiphasic Personality Inventory (MMPI). Similar conclusions were reached in a recent Canadian study of 547 mother–infant dyads.[13] The authors found that colic remitted in over 85% of infants by the age of 3 months. More importantly, no residual effects on levels of maternal distress were noted on resolution of the colic. The study did not find any significant relationships between persistent cases of colic and birth order, source of infant nutrition, parental education, or maternal age.

The effects of caregiving practices have been studied, though the data are often contradictory, and their interpretation hindered by methodological limitations.[40,62] Taubman[67] counseled parents of colicky infants on behavior modification in a randomized clinical study. He showed that parental counseling reduced distressed behavior to an extent similar to the introduction of a cow milk-protein free diet. In a follow-up phase to this study, he found that the distressed behavior of infants with diet-responsive colic further decreased with parental counseling. A central,

55. Berkowitz D, Naveh Y, Berant M. 'Infantile colic' as the sole manifestation of gastroesophageal reflux. J Pediatr Gastroenterol Nutr 1997; 24:231–233.
56. Heine RG, Jaquiery A, Lubitz L, et al. Role of gastro-esophageal reflux in infant irritability. Arch Dis Child 1995; 73:121–125.
57. Sutphen JL. It is colic or is it gastroesophageal reflux? J Pediatr Gastroenterol Nutr 2001; 33:110–111.
58. Putnam PE. GERD and crying: cause and effect or unhappy coexistence? J Pediatr 2002; 140:3–4.
59. Lothe L, Ivarsson A, Lindberg T. Motilin, vasoactive intestinal peptide and gastrin in infantile colic. Acta Paediatr Scand 1987; 76:316–320.
60. Barr RG. Colic and gas. In: Walker WA, Durie PR, Hamilton JR, Walker-Smith JA, Watkins JB, eds. Pediatric Gastrointestinal Disease. Pathophysiology, Diagnosis, Management, 3rd edn. Hamilton, Ontario: BC Decker; 2000:116–128.
61. Spock B. Etiological factors in hypertrophic pyloric stenosis and infantile colic. Psychosom Med 1944; 6:162–165.
62. Miller AR, Barr RG. Infantile colic. Is it a gut issue? Pediatr Clin N Am 1991; 38:1407–1423.
63. Stewart AH, Weiland IH, Leider AR, et al. Excessive infant crying (colic) in relation to parent behavior. Am J Psychiatry 1954; 110:687–694.
64. Rautava P, Helenius H, Lehtonen L. Psychosocial predisposing factors for infantile colic. Brit Med J 1993; 307:600–604.
65. Reijneveld SA, Brugman E, Hirasing RA. Infantile colic: maternal smoking as potential risk factor. Arch Dis Child 2000; 83:302–303.
66. Sondergaard C, Henriksen TB, Obel C, et al. Smoking during pregnancy and infantile colic. Pediatrics 2001; 108:342–346.
67. Taubman B. Parental counseling compared with elimination of cow's milk or soy milk protein for the treatment of infant colic syndrome: a randomized trial. Pediatrics 1988; 81:756–761.
68. Raiha H, Lehtonen L, Huhtala V, et al. Excessively crying infant in the family: mother-infant, father-infant and mother-father interaction. Child Care Health Dev 2002; 28:419–429.
69. Ellett MLC. What is known about infant colic? Gastroenterol Nurs 2003; 26:60–65.
70. St James-Roberts I, Goodwin J, Peter B, et al. Individual differences in responsivity to a neurobehavioural examination predict crying patterns of 1-week-old infants at home. Develop Med Child Neurol 2003; 45:400–407.
71. Canivet C, Jakobsson I, Hagander B. Infantile colic. Follow up four years age: still more 'emotional'. Acta Paediatr 2000; 89:13–17.
72. Rautava P, Lehtonen L, Helenius H, et al. Infantile colic: child and family three years later. Pediatrics 1995; 96:43–47.
73. Neu M, Robinson J. Infants with colic: their childhood characteristics. J Pediatr Nurs 2003; 18:12–20.
74. Wolke D, Rizzo P, Woods S. Persistent infant crying and hyperactivity problems in middle childhood. Pediatrics 2002; 109:1054–1060.
75. Jan MMS, Al-Buhairi AR. Is infantile colic a migraine-related phenomenon? Clin Pediatr 2001; 40:295–297.
76. Kalliomaki M, Laippala P, Korvenranta H, et al. Extent of fussing and colic type crying preceding atopic disease. Arch Dis Child 2001; 84:349–350.
77. Castro-Rodriguez JA, Stern DA, Halonen M, et al. Relation between infantile colic and asthma/atopy: a prospective study in an unselected population. Pediatrics 2001; 108:878–882.

Chapter 11
Constipation and encopresis

Vera Loening-Baucke

INTRODUCTION

Constipation and encopresis represent common problems in children. As a symptom, constipation can be caused by many different disorders (Table 11.1). Constipation is a complaint that is frequently heard by those providing healthcare to children. As many as 3% of visits to primary care pediatricians and 25% of visits to pediatric gastroenterologists are for the treatment of this condition. Constipation was defined by a group of pediatric gastroenterologists from the North American Society of Gastroenterology and Nutrition as a delay or difficulty in defecation, present for ≥2 weeks, and sufficient to cause significant distress to the patient.[1] Constipation is most common due to functional constipation, which is constipation not due to organic and anatomical causes or intake of medication.

In North America, Issenman reported that 16% of 22-month-old children were thought by their parents to be constipated.[2] In England, Yong and Beattie[3] reported that 34% of otherwise healthy 4–11-year-old school children had constipation. Most often, constipation is short-lived and of little consequence; however, chronic constipation often follows an inadequately managed acute problem. Only 5% of the otherwise healthy 4- to 11-year-old school children in Great Britain had chronic constipation lasting for more than 6 months.[3] Publications from Brazil report that 18% to 37% of children suffer from constipation.[4–6]

Encopresis is the involuntary loss of formed, semiformed, or liquid stool into the child's underwear in the presence of functional constipation after the child has reached a developmental age of 4 years.[7] In less than 10% of children, the fecal soiling is not due to constipation or underlying disease and is called non-retentive fecal soiling. Rare organic conditions for fecal soiling should be considered and ruled out. The list of causes for diseases causing fecal soiling is long (Table 11.1), but more than 90% of children with fecal soiling have encopresis with functional constipation as the cause.

The aims of this chapter are to describe functional constipation, functional constipation with encopresis and non-retentive fecal soiling in children, to present the differential diagnosis of constipation, to describe the evaluation and treatment of these children, and to report on short-term and long-term treatment outcome.

- Functional constipation in >90%
- Neurogenic constipation:
  - Hirschsprung's disease
  - Disorders of the spinal cord, such as myelomeningocele, tumor
  - Neuronal intestinal dysplasia
  - Cerebral palsy, hypotonia
  - Chronic intestinal pseudo-obstruction
- Constipation secondary to anal lesions:
  - Anal fissures
  - Anterior location of the anus
  - Anal stenosis
  - Anal atresia with fistula
  - Anal atresia
- Constipation secondary to endocrine and metabolic disorders:
  - Hypothyroidism
  - Renal acidosis
  - Diabetes insipidus
  - Hypercalcemia
  - Cystic fibrosis
- Constipation secondary to neuromuscular disorders:
  - Myotonic dystrophy
  - Muscular dystrophy
  - Chronic intestinal pseudo-obstruction
- Constipation due to abnormal abdominal musculature:
  - Prune belly syndrome
  - Gastroschisis
  - Down syndrome
- Constipation induced by drugs:
  - Methylphenidate
  - Phenytoin
  - Imipramine hydrochloride
  - Antidepressants
  - Antacids
  - Codeine-containing medication

Table 11.1 Diseases that cause constipation with or without fecal soiling

ANATOMY AND PHYSIOLOGY

Very special control mechanisms are developed in the body to prevent loss of gas, stool and urine. Unconscious regulation of bowel movements is the normal phenomenon after birth. Conscious regulation of bowel movements is achieved at an average age of 28 months. Fecal continence is the body's ability to recognize when the rectal ampulla fills; to discriminate whether the content is formed stool, liquid stool, or gas; and to retain the content until emptying is convenient.

The major structures responsible for continence and defecation are the external anal sphincter, the puborectalis muscle, the internal anal sphincter and the rectum. The external sphincter is a skeletal muscle and is innervated by the pudendal nerve (S2–4). It contracts together with the pudendal nerve when the rectum is full. Part of the levator muscle is the puborectalis muscle. It forms a U-shaped sling around the anorectal junction, pulling it forward to create the anorectal angle. During defecation, this angle becomes straighter. The internal anal sphincter is the continuation of the circular smooth muscle of the rectum. It is tonically contracted and is controlled by the sympathetic nerves of the sacral plexus and the parasympathetic fibers from the thoraco-lumbar plexus.[8] The rectum is normally empty and collapsed, but has distensible walls. It contains the valves of Houston, which produce a series of kinks.

The factors which are responsible for maintaining fecal continence and which also facilitate defecation are the high pressure zone in the anal canal, the anal and rectal sensory and reflex mechanisms, the viscoelastic properties of the rectum and stool volume and consistency. Fecal material can be retained by contraction of the external sphincter and puborectalis muscle. Fecal material can be expelled by the combination of increased intra-abdominal pressure produced by closure of the glottis, fixation of the diaphragm, contractions of the abdominal muscles and rectal wall, and relaxation of the internal and external anal sphincters.

ROME II CRITERIA

A set of diagnostic guidelines, known as the ROME II criteria, was published in 1999.[9] The criteria describe three types of constipation in children: infant dyschezia, functional constipation, and functional fecal retention. Fecal soiling can occur with functional constipation, functional fecal retention and non-retentive fecal soiling.

Dyschezia

Some otherwise healthy infants less than 6 months of age appear to have significant discomfort and excessive straining associated with passing soft stools. If an infant exhibits straining and crying for over 10 min, followed by successful passage of soft stool, the infant meets the Rome II criteria for infant dyschezia. This defecation disorder is seen in the first few months of life and can occur several times a day for up to 20 min at a time. Very little research has been done to actually characterize the physiology of this disorder. The etiology of dyschezia is not understood. It is speculated that this disorder occurs when neonates fail to coordinate increased intra-abdominal pressure with relaxation of the pelvic floor. Symptoms improve without intervention in most cases. Parents need to be reassured that this phenomenon is part of the child's learning process and that there is no intervention necessary.

Functional constipation

Functional constipation is defined in infants and preschool children by the ROME II criteria as at least 2 weeks of: scybalous, pebble-like, hard stools for a majority of stools or firm stools two or less times per week and no structural, endocrine, or metabolic disease.[9] ROME II criteria for constipation in school-aged children were not established.

Functional fecal retention

Functional fecal retention is a more severe form of constipation. Functional fecal retention is defined by the ROME II criteria [9] as: passage of large diameter stools less than two times per week and retentive posturing (avoiding defecation by contracting the pelvic floor and gluteal muscles). The ROME II criteria for functional retention are quite restrictive in requiring less than two bowel movements per week and retentive posturing, as counting bowel movements can be an inaccurate process. Should only bowel movements defecated into the toilet be counted, or should the tally include bowel movements evacuated into the underwear as well? How should one account for small and large bowel movements? The main reason against using a defined number of bowel movements per week is that fecal retention is not a result of the number of bowel movements which are defecated but a result of the amount of stool retained. Thus, frequency of bowel movements cannot be considered in isolation. The consistency and size of the bowel movement and the accompanying abdominal pain are at least as important.

FUNCTIONAL CONSTIPATION

Infants and toddlers

Constipation in early life is a special situation because of the possibility of a serious congenital disorder. If meconium passage is delayed for more than 24 h, Hirschsprung's disease must be considered. Evaluation of Hirschsprung's disease usually includes plain abdominal radiographs, barium enema, anorectal manometry, and rectal suction biopsy. Anatomical defects of the spinal cord or anorectum must also be ruled out by examination and, if necessary, by appropriate imaging studies. Common anatomic defects include anal atresia, anal atresia with fistula, anal stenosis, high obstructive lesions, such as colonic strictures, and spinal cord anomalies. Meconium plugs may also cause neonatal constipation, and may be associated with either Hirschsprung's disease or cystic fibrosis. The different congenital causes are described in more detail elsewhere in this book.

The overwhelming majority of constipated infants and toddlers have functional constipation, resulting from factors other than anatomic or congenital abnormalities.

Pre-school and school-aged children

Constipation is usually defined in terms of alterations in the frequency, size, consistency or the ease in passage of stool. Constipation in school-aged children can be defined by a stool frequency of less than three per week, or passage of painful bowel movements, or stool retention with or without encopresis, even when the stool frequency is more than three per week.[10–19]

Functional constipation may be thought of as a maladaptive response of overcontrol. In children, if defecation is painful, the pain-producing activity may be avoided by stool withholding. When the child decides not to have a bowel movement, the external anal sphincter and pelvic floor muscles are tightened. The rectum adjusts to the contents and the urge to defecate gradually passes. As the cycle is repeated, successively greater amounts of stool build-up in the rectum with longer exposure to its drying action, and a vicious cycle is started. Children may ignore the call to stool, which results in fecal retention and leads to suppression of rectal sensation. In others, pain and fear prevent the relaxation of the pelvic floor muscles during defecation. Stool retention results when stool expulsion has not occurred for several days.

When stool retention persists, the formed, soft or semi-liquid stools can leak to the outside around the accumulated firm stool mass. Fecal soiling in the presence of constipation in children 4 years and older is called encopresis. When stool retention remains untreated for a prolonged period of time, the rectal wall becomes stretched and a megarectum develops. The intervals between bowel movements become increasingly longer and the rectum becomes so large that the stored stool can be felt as an abdominal mass that reaches up to the umbilicus, above the umbilicus, and occasionally up to the sternum. Functional fecal retention is a more severe form of constipation and is characterized by the presence of an abdominal fecal mass on abdominal examination, or by a rectal impaction on rectal examination, or by a history of passing bowel movements which obstruct the toilet, and may be a history of abdominal pain relieved by enema and laxative. Often the need for retentive behavior has disappeared.

Some children will have no stool palpable through the abdominal wall. They may have recently passed a large bowel movement or have soft fecal loading of their megarectum which is sometimes not recognized by an inexperienced examiner, except if a rectal examination is performed.

No single mechanism is responsible for functional constipation. The most common cause of constipation in children is an acquired behavior that occurs when a child begins to delay defecation after experiencing a painful or frightening defecation. Then fear of defecation leads to voluntary withholding of stool. There are two peaks for worsening of constipation. The first is during toilet training and the second occurs when a child begins to attend school, when toilet use is regulated to special times and toilets may not be clean and private. Constitutional and inherited factors, such as intrinsic slow motility contribute to constipation.

Constipation is also present in some children with irritable bowel syndrome (IBS). These children have functional abdominal pain or abdominal discomfort as their main complaint. IBS by ROME II criteria is defined as abdominal discomfort for at least 12 weeks or more, which need not be consecutive, in the preceding 12 months. This abdominal pain must have at least two of three features; it is relieved with defecation; the onset is associated with a change in the frequency of stool; and/or the onset is associated with a change in the stool appearance.[9] Several other symptoms such as less than three bowel movements per week, lumpy or hard bowel movements, straining for defecation, or feeling of incomplete evacuation support the diagnosis of IBS with constipation. No structural or metabolic abnormalities are present to explain the symptom.

FUNCTIONAL CONSTIPATION WITH ENCOPRESIS

In the USA, only 25% to 30% of children are reliably toilet trained by 2 years of age and 80% by 3 years. The relatively wide range in age for achieving bowel control among normal children influences the definition of encopresis to children who are at least 4 years of age.[7] Encopresis is the involuntary loss of formed, semi-formed, or liquid stool into the child's underwear in the presence of functional constipation. Encopresis is involuntary, although it can be prevented for short periods of time if the child concentrates carefully on closing the external anal sphincter. Encopresis is reported to affect 2.8% of 4-year-old children, 1.5% of 7- to 8-year-old children, and 1.6% of 10- to 11-year-old children. The male to female ratio for encopresis ranges from 2.5:1 to 6:1.

The clinical features of constipation with encopresis are listed in Table 11.2. Some children will have intermittent soiling. A period free of soiling may occur after a huge bowel movement, which may obstruct the toilet, and soiling will resume only after several days of stool retention. Usually, the consistency of stool found in the underwear is loose or clay-like. Sometimes the core of the impaction breaks off and is found as a firm stool in the underwear. Occasionally, a full bowel movement is passed into the underwear. Many children display or have displayed retentive posturing. Instead of using the bathroom and sitting down for defecation and relaxing the pelvic floor at times when an urge to defecate is felt, the retentive child will

- Difficulties with defecation began early in life, in 50% of children prior to 1 year of age
- Passage of enormous stools
- Obstruction of the toilet by the stools
- Symptoms due to the increasing accumulation of stool:
  - Retentive posturing
  - Encopresis
  - Abdominal pain and irritability, anal or rectal pain
  - Anorexia
  - Urinary symptoms:
    - Daytime urinary incontinence
    - Nighttime urinary incontinence
    - Urinary tract infection
- Unusual behaviors in an effort to cope with the encopresis:
  - Nonchalant attitude regarding the encopresis
  - Hiding of soiled underwear
  - Lack of awareness of an encopretic episode
- Dramatic disappearance of most symptoms following the passage of a huge stool

Table 11.2 Clinical features of constipation with encopresis in children

seizures, or death. Children with megarectum or megacolon who do not respond to phosphate enemas can be disimpacted with a hyperosmolar milk of molasses enema (1:1 milk and molasses) with the infusion stopped when the child indicates discomfort (200–600 ml). The milk of molasses enema may need to be repeated. Cardiopulmonary compromise associated with milk of molasses enema in children with serious underlying medical conditions have been reported.[28]

Disimpaction can also be achieved with oral lavage using polyethylene glycol-electrolyte solution[29] and the new electrolyte-free polyethylene 3350 (PEG).[30] When taken orally, PEG increases water content and can both soften and expel the fecal impaction. The oral lavage solution with electrolytes is given orally or by nasogastric tube due to poor taste and the refusal of the children to drink it in large quantities. Large volumes were necessary for bowel cleanout, the average was 12 l given over 23 h at a rate of 14–40 ml/kg per h, till clear fluid was excreted through the anus.[29] It is recommended to give 5–10 mg metoclopramide by mouth 15 min prior to the lavage solution to reduce nausea and vomiting. The electrolyte-free PEG has no taste and is effective at treating impaction. A recent study by Youssef et al.[30] demonstrated that 1.5 g/kg bodyweight/day for 3 days was efficient in removing the rectal fecal impaction within 5 days from children without the use of enemas. Only children with a palpable fecal mass in the lower rectum and/or a dilated rectum were included in this study. The fecal impaction can also be softened and liquefied with large quantities of oral mineral oil or other osmotic laxatives with the oral administration continued daily until the fecal mass is passed. Fecal soiling, abdominal pain, and cramping may increase during the oral treatment of the fecal impaction. Manual disimpaction is an extreme technique and should be performed rarely and if necessary under anesthesia.

Prevention of re-accumulation of stools

Behavior modification

The child needs to be reconditioned to normal bowel habits by regular toilet use. The child is encouraged to sit on the toilet for up to 5 min, three to four times a day following meals. The gastrocolic reflex, which goes into effect during and shortly after a meal, should be used to his or her advantage. The children and their parents need to be instructed to keep a daily record of bowel movements, fecal soiling, urinary incontinence and medication use. This helps to monitor compliance and helps to make appropriate adjustments in the treatment program by parents and physician. If necessary positive reinforcement and rewards for compliant behavior are given for effort and later for success, using star charts, little presents or television viewing or computer game time as rewards.

Fiber

In the early 1970s, Burkitt et al. had observed a relationship between stool volume and fiber ingestion in Africans.[31] Burkitt et al. speculated that the frequent occurrence of constipation among Western societies was the result of reduced dietary fiber intake. Dietary fiber increases water retention, provides substrate for bacterial growth with increase of colonic flora and gas production during colonic fermentation of fiber. Treatment programs for the majority of children with chronic constipation have included increase in dietary fiber, in addition to scheduled toilet sittings and daily laxatives.[11–15,21]

The dietary recommendation for children older than 2 years of age is to consume an amount of dietary fiber equivalent to age in years plus 5 g/day.[32] The dietary fiber should come preferably from food rather than from supplements. Recommended are several servings daily from a variety of fiber-rich foods such as whole grain breads and cereals, fruits, vegetables and legumes. Most children, healthy as well as constipated children, do not eat an adequate amount of fiber. McClung et al.[33] found that even in health-conscious families, about half of the children did not receive the recommended daily grams of fiber. Several studies reported that the fiber intake is lower in constipated children than in controls.[34,35] Zaslavsky et al.[36] did not detect significant differences in daily fiber intake between healthy and constipated adolescents in Brazil.

Dietary fiber treatments have ranged from raw foods such as fruits and vegetables, to synthetic preparations such as guar gum and pectin fiber. However, to be effective, these fiber agents have to be ingested in large quantities, which most children find unacceptable. Recent reports have shown that glucomannan, a fiber gel polysaccharide (composed of β-1,4-linked D-glucose and D-mannose) prepared from the tubers of the Japanese Konjac plant, is a soluble fiber, can be taken in much smaller quantities than guar gum or pectin, and has no unpleasant smell or taste.[37,38]

Laxative

In most constipated patients, daily defecation is maintained by the daily administration of laxatives beginning in the evening of the clinic visit. Magnesium hydroxide (milk of magnesia), mineral oil, lactulose, sorbitol and polyethylene glycol 3350 without electrolytes (MiraLax®) have been used for long-term treatment. Laxatives should be used according to bodyweight and severity of the constipation. Suggested dosages of commonly used laxatives are given in Table 11.6. The choice of medication for functional constipation does not seem as important as the children's and parents' compliance with the treatment regimen. There is no set dosage for any laxative. There is only a starting dosage for each child (Table 11.6) that must be adjusted to induce one to two bowel movements per day that are loose enough to ensure complete daily emptying of the lower bowel and to prevent soiling and abdominal pain.

The mechanism of action of milk of magnesia is the relative non-absorption of magnesium and the resultant increase in luminal osmolality. For severe constipation with rock-hard stools, the starting dosage of milk of magnesia is 2 to 3 ml/kg bodyweight per day, given with the evening meal. For children who have retention of mostly soft formed stools, usually 1 ml/kg bodyweight daily is adequate.

Medication	Age	Dose
For long-term treatment (years):		
Milk of magnesia	>1 month	1–3 ml/kg body weight/day, divide in 1–2 doses
Mineral oil	>12 months	1–3 ml/kg body weight/day, divided in 1–2 doses
Lactulose or sorbitol	>1 months	1–3 ml/kg body weight/day, divide in 1–2 doses
Polyethylene glycol 3350 (MiraLax®)	>1 month	0.7 g/kg body weight/day, divide in 1–2 doses
For short-term treatment (months):		
Senna (Senokot®) syrup/tablets	1–5 years	5 ml (1 tablet) with breakfast, max 15 ml daily
	5–15 years	2 tablets with breakfast, maximum 3 tablets daily
Glycerin enemas	>10 years	20–30 ml/day (1/2 glycerin and 1/2 normal saline)
Bisacodyl suppositories	>10 years	10 mg daily

Table 11.6 Suggested medications and dosages for maintenance therapy of constipation

Mineral oil is converted into hydroxy fatty acids, which induce fluid and electrolyte accumulation. Dosages are 1–3 ml/kg bodyweight/day. A major concern about long-term mineral oil use had been its action as a lipid solvent, which could interfere with the fat-soluble vitamins. This concern has been dismissed by a study showing negligible reduction of plasma levels of vitamins A and E after 6 months of mineral oil use.[39] Mineral oil should never be force-fed or given to patients with dysphagia or vomiting because of the danger of aspiration pneumonia. Anal seepage of the mineral oil, often causing an orange stain, is an undesirable side-effect, especially in children going to school.

Lactulose or sorbitol, are non-absorbable carbohydrates. They cause increased water content by the osmotic effects of lactulose, sorbitol and their metabolites. They are fermented by colonic bacteria, thereby producing gas and sometimes causing abdominal discomfort. Both are easily taken by the children when mixed in soft drinks.

Polyethylene glycol 3350 without added electrolytes (MiraLax®, Braintree Laboratories, Inc., Braintree, MA) has been developed and now tested for long-term daily use as a laxative in children, toddlers and infants.[16,40–45] MiraLax® (PEG) is a chemically inert polymer, a powder, tasteless, odorless, colorless and has no grit when stirred in juice, Kool-aid or water for several minutes. PEG is not degraded by bacteria, is not readily absorbed and thus, acts as an excellent osmotic agent, and is safe.[16,43]

Senna has an effect on intestinal motility as well as on fluid and electrolyte transport and will stimulate defecation. We use senna when liquid stools produced by osmotic laxatives are retained and in children with fecal incontinence and constipation due to organic or anatomic causes. The North American Society for Pediatric Gastroenterology, Hepatology and Nutrition recommended senna products for short-term therapy.[1]

Occasionally, the author uses a 10-mg bisacodyl suppository or either a phosphate or a glycerin enema daily as initial treatment for several months in an older child who would like immediate control of the encopresis.

Once an adequate dosage is established, it is continued for approximately 6 months to help the distended bowel to regain some of its function. Usually, regular bowel habits are established by that time. Then, the dosage may be reduced in small decrements, while maintaining a daily bowel movement without soiling or abdominal pain. Laxatives need to be continued for many months sometimes years at the right dose to induce daily soft stools and prevent fecal soiling and abdominal pain. The laxative needs to be restarted when relapse occurs.

Psychological treatment

Adherence to the treatment program will improve the constipation and encopresis in all children. The presence of coexisting behavioral problems often is associated with poor treatment outcome. If the coexisting behavior problem is secondary to constipation and/or encopresis then it will improve with treatment. Children who do not improve should be referred for further evaluation, because continued problems can be due to noncompliance or control issues by the child and/or the parent. Psychological intervention, family counseling, and occasional hospitalization of a child for two to four weeks to get a treatment program started have helped some of these unfortunate children.

It has been suggested that children with non-retentive fecal soiling may also benefit from psychological intervention.[9,46]

Follow-up visits and weaning from medication

Since the management of functional constipation with or without encopresis requires considerable patience and effort on the part of the child and parents, it is important to provide necessary support and encouragement through frequent office visits. Progress should be initially assessed monthly, later less frequently by reviewing the stool records and repeating the abdominal and rectal examination to assure that the problem is adequately managed. If necessary, dosage adjustment is made and the child and parents are encouraged to continue with the regimen. After regular bowel habits are established, the frequency of toilet sitting is reduced and the medication dosage is gradually decreased to a dosage that maintains one bowel movement daily and prevents encopresis. Once the child feels the urge to defecate and initiates toilet use on his/her own, then the scheduled toilet times are discontinued. Fiber intake is stressed at that time. After 6–12 months, reduction with discontinuation of the medication is attempted. Treatment needs to resume if constipation recurs.

What can go wrong in the treatment?

Physicians, as well as the parents and children, make frequent mistakes (Table 11.7). Frequent mistakes by physicians are: treating with stool softeners and laxatives, but not removing the fecal impaction; removing the fecal impaction, but failing to prescribe a laxative; giving too low a dose; not controlling the adequacy and success of therapy with follow-up visits; stopping the laxative too soon; and not providing education, anticipatory guidance, continuing support and regular follow-up. Frequent mistakes by the parents and children are: not insisting that the child use the toilet at regular times for defecation trials; not giving the medication daily, or worse, discontinuing the laxatives as soon as the encopresis has disappeared; not restarting the laxative after the child has a relapse. Occasionally, the constipation is well treated, but the child continues to complain of abdominal pain or discomfort. Evolving therapies for irritable bowel syndrome are probiotics, prokinetic agents such as the group of serotonin receptor partial agonists (tegaserod, prucalopride, mosapride), neurothrophins and prostaglandin analog such as misoprostol. They show early promise in adult patients, but have not been tested in children.

Non-retentive fecal soiling

The treatment of children with non-retentive fecal soiling has not been well defined. Most children will benefit from a precise, well-organized plan. Treatment suggestions include various forms of behavioral therapy and psychological approaches and is designed to promote regular bowel habits. The treatment includes education, reconditioning to normal bowel habits with regular toilet use, and fiber.

Mistakes by physicians:
- Not removing the fecal impaction
- Removing the fecal impaction, but failing to prescribe a laxative
- Giving too low a dose
- Not controlling the adequacy and success of therapy with a rectal examination
- Stopping the laxative too soon
- Not providing continuing support and follow-up

Mistakes by parents and children:
- Not insisting that the child uses the toilet at regular times for defecation trials
- Not giving the medication daily, or worse
- Discontinuing the laxatives as soon as the encopresis has disappeared
- Not restarting the laxative after the child has relapsed
- Not returning for follow-up

Table 11.7 Frequent therapy mistakes made by physicians, parents and children

OUTCOME

Constipation with and without encopresis

Outcome in most publications of constipated children with or without encopresis was assessed by rates of successful treatment and recovery. The constipation was rated as successfully treated if the child had, in the last month, three or more bowel movements per week, two or less smears per month and suffered no abdominal pain, independent of laxative use.[47,48] Recovery was defined by the same criteria, except that the child was off laxatives for at least 1 month.[10–21,47,48]

Behavior modification

The only study to examine behavior modification as monotherapy for children with constipation and encopresis was by Nolan et al. from Australia.[18] In this randomized study, they found that 1 year after start of behavior modification, 36% of 86 children had recovered and more children, 51% of 83 children, had recovered with behavior modification and additional laxative treatment ($p<0.08$).

Fiber

Olness and Tobin[49] reported that constipation resolved in 60 constipated children within an average of 4.3 weeks when given raw unprocessed bran and a very restricted diet, excluding all milk products. The addition of bran alone was not adequate to control the constipation.

The effect of glucomannan, a fiber prepared from the tubers of the Japanese Konjac plant, and placebo, were evaluated in 31 children, 5–12 years of age, with chronic functional constipation with and without encopresis in a double-blind, randomized, crossover study.[38] A total of 18 constipated children had encopresis when recruited. Fiber and placebo were given as 100 mg/kg bodyweight daily (maximal 5 g/day) with 50 ml fluid/500 mg for 4 weeks each. If children were on laxatives at the time of recruitment, they remained on the same laxative and dose during the fiber and placebo periods. While on fiber, significantly fewer children complained of abdominal pain as compared with placebo (10% *vs* 42%) and more children were successfully treated (45% *vs* (13%). Duration of constipation and initial low (71%) or acceptable fiber intake did not predict response to fiber treatment. Children with constipation only were significantly more likely to be successfully treated with additional fiber (69%) than those with constipation and encopresis (28%). Fiber was beneficial in the treatment of constipation and therefore the recommendation to increase the fiber in the diet of constipated children should be continued.

Laxatives and behavior modification

1-year outcome At least eight well-designed studies have looked at 1-year outcome (Table 11.8). Laxative treatment with behavior modification dramatically improved constipation, abdominal pain and encopresis. Four of these studies looked at children who had constipation with or without encopresis.[17,48,50,51] They showed that 47% of these children in the USA,[50] 47% in Italy[51] and 31–59% in The Netherlands,[17,48] had recovered 1 year after start of treatment, see Table 11.8. The largest study by van Ginkel et al.,[48] involved 399 Dutch children, 83% were successfully treated with lactulose and 59% had recovered 1 year after start of treatment.

The 1-year recovery rates in constipated children with encopresis ranged from 39– 51%.[13,18,52,53] They showed that 39–51% of the children in the USA[13,52,53] and 51% of these children in Australia[18] had recovered 1 year after start of therapy.

Significantly better recovery rates were reported in constipated children without encopresis,[48,50] in children with secondary encopresis (previously toilet trained for at least one month),[18,50,51] and in children who presented initially with abdominal pain.[50]

Long-term outcome Many studies have followed children for years after start of treatment (Table 11.9). One study specifically targeted younger children (4 years of age or less) to examine whether early intervention might improve outcome.[54] Of 90 children who were followed for a mean of 7 years after beginning treatment, 63% recovered. The recovery rate of children two years of age or less was higher than the rate of the children 2 to 4 years of age. Staiano et al.[51] followed 62 children, 1 to 11 years of age, and found that 48% had recovered after 5 years. Early age of onset of constipation and family history of constipation were predictive of persistence, they found. Loening-Baucke reported that 53% of 129 children with chronic constipation and encopresis, who were 5 years of age or older at the initiation of treatment, had recovered after a mean follow-up period of 4 years.[55]

The largest study is by van Ginkel et al.[48] They initially enrolled 418 constipated children; two-thirds with and one-third without encopresis. All were older than 5 years of age at initiation of therapy. Some of the children were followed for as long as 8 years, with a median follow-up of 5 years. A total of 59% had recovered at the 1-year follow-up.

Author	Subjects (*n*)	Laxative	Recovery rate (%)
Constipation with or without encopresis:			
Abrahamian et al.[50]	68	Muliple laxatives	47
Staiano et al.[51]	31	Lactulose	47
van Ginket et al.[17]	212	Lactulose	31
van Ginket et al.[48]	399	Lactulose	59
Constipation with encopresis:			
Levine and Barkow[52]	110	Mineral oil	51
Loening-Baucke[13]	97	Milk of magnesia	43
Nolan et al.[18]	83	Multiple laxatives	51
Loening-Baucke[53]	181	Milk of magnesia	39

Table 11.8 1-year recovery rates in children with constipation

Three-year data showed a decline in the recovery rate, to about 50%, as some children relapsed and were not restarted on laxative therapy. The recovery rate of 193 children was 63% after 5 years, 69% of 120 children had recovered after 7 years and 68% of 48 children had recovered after 8 years.[48] However, 50% of recovered children had at least one relapse and approximately 30% of children, who had reached adolescence, were still having problems with constipation or encopresis. These findings suggest that this is not a problem children will eventually outgrow.

Outcome using other treatments

Biofeedback treatment as adjunct therapy

The concept of applying biofeedback to certain anorectal function is logical because anorectal function is regulated by physiologic processes; some are under cortical influence. These cortical influenced processes include the ability to sense rectal distention and impending defecation and the ability to relax and contract the striated muscles of the pelvic floor. Patients can be taught to enhance the recognition of rectal distention, to contract and relax the external anal sphincter and puborectalis muscle, and to coordinate these functions.

Previous research has shown that from 25% to 56% of constipated children have abnormal defecation dynamics, an abnormal contraction of the external anal sphincter and pelvic floor muscles during attempted defecation.[11–13,56] These muscles are amenable to biofeedback

Author	Subjects (*n*)	Age (years)	Laxative	Follow-up (years)	Recovery rate (%)
Constipation only:					
Loening-Baucke[54]	90	1–4	Milk of magnesia	7 (mean)	63
Constipation with and without encopresis:					
Staiano et al.[51]	62	1–11	Lactulose	5	48
van Ginket et al.[48]	193	>5	Lactulose	5	69
Constipation with encopresis:					
Loening-Baucke[55]	129	>5	Milk of magnesia	4 (mean)	53

Table 11.9 Long-term recovery rates in children with constipation with and without encopresis

childhood constipation: a randomized, controlled trial. http://www.pediatrics.org/cgi/content/full/108/1/e9. Assessed July 21, 2005.

18. Nolan TM, Debelle G, Oberklaid F, et al. Randomised trial of laxatives in treatment of childhood encopresis. Lancet 1991; 338(8766):523–527.
19. Nolan T, Catto-Smith T, Coffey C, et al. Randomised controlled trial of biofeedback training in persistent encopresis with anismus. Arch Dis Child 1998; 79(2):131–135.
20. Benninga MA, Taminiau JAJM. Diagnosis and treatment efficacy of functional non-retentive fecal soiling in childhood. J Pediatr Gastroenterol Nutr 2001; 32(suppl 1):42–43.
21. van Ginkel R, Benninga MA, Blommaart PJE, et al. Lack of benefit of laxatives as adjunctive therapy for functional nonretentive fecal soiling in children. J Pediatr 2000; 137(6):808–813.
22. Loening-Baucke V. The ROME II criteria for functional pediatric disorders of defecation: are they adequate for children with fecal soiling? Gastroenterology 2004; 126:375.
23. van der Plas RN, Benninga MA, Redekop WK. Randomized trial of biofeedback training for encopresis. Arch Dis Child 1996; 75(5):367–374.
24. Loening-Baucke V. Urinary incontinence and urinary tract infection and their resolution with treatment of chronic constipation of childhood. Pediatrics 1997; 100(2):228–232.
25. Beach RC Management of childhood constipation. Lancet 1996; 348(9030):766–767.
26. Gold DM, Levine J, Weinstein TA et al. Frequency of digital rectal examination in children with chronic constipation. Arch Pediatr Adolesc Med 1999; 153(4):377–379.
27. Harrington L, Schuh S. Complications of Fleet® enema administration and suggested guidelines for use in the pediatric emergency department. Pediatr Emergency Care 1997; 13(3):225–226.
28. Walker M, Warner BW, Brilli RJ, et al. Cardiopulmonary compromise associated with milk of molasses enema use in children. J Pediatr Gastroenterol Nutr 2003; 36(1):144–148.
29. Ingebo KB, Heyman MB. Polyethylene glycol-electrolyte solution for intestinal clearance in children with refractory encopresis. Am J Dis Child 1988; 142(3):340–342.
30. Youssef NN, Peters JM, Henderson W, et al. Dose responses of PEG 3350 for the treatment of childhood fecal impaction. J Pediatr 2002; 141(3):410–414.
31. Burkitt DP, Walker AR, Painter NS. Dietary fiber and disease. JAMA 1974; 229(8):1068–1074.
32. Williams CL, Bollella M, Wynder EL. A new recommendation for dietary fiber in childhood. Pediatrics 1995; 96(5):985–988.
33. McClung HJ, Boyne L, Heitlinger L. Constipation and dietary fiber intake in children. Pediatrics 1995; 96(5):999–1001.
34. Roma E, Adamidis D, Nikolara R, et al. Diet and chronic constipation in children: the role of fiber. J Ped Gastroenterol Nutr 1999; 28(2):169–174.
35. Morais MB, Vitolo MR, Aquirre ANC, et al. Measurement of low dietary fiber intake as a risk factor for chronic constipation in children. J Ped Gastroenterol Nutr 1999; 29(2):132–135.
36. Zaslavsky C, Reverbel da Silveira T, Maguilnik I. Total and segmental colonic transit time with radio-opaque markers in adolescents with functional constipation. J Ped Gastroenterol Nutr 1998; 27(2):138–142.
37. Staiano A, Simeone D, Del Giudice E, et al. Effect of the dietary fiber glucomannan on chronic constipation in neurologically impaired children. J Pediatr 2000; 136(1):41–45.
38. Loening-Baucke V, Miele E, Staiano A. Fiber (glucomannan) is beneficial in the treatment of childhood constipation. http://www.pediatrics.org/cgi/content/full/113/3/e258. Assessed July 21, 2005.
39. Clark JK, Russel GJ, Fitzgerald JF, et al. Serum beta-carotene, retinol, and alpha-tocopherol levels during mineral oil therapy for constipation. Am J Dis Child 1987; 141:1210–1212.
40. Pashankar DS, Bishop WP. Efficacy and optimal dose of daily polyethylene glycol 3350 for treatment of constipation and encopresis in children. J Pediatr 2001; 139(3):428–432.
41. Gremse DA, Hixon J, Crutchfield A. Comparison of polyethylene glycol 3350 and lactulose for treatment of chronic constipation in children. Clin Pediatr 2002; 41(4):225–229.
42. Pashankar DS, Bishop WP, Loening-Baucke V. Long-term efficacy of polyethylene glycol 3350 for the treatment of chronic constipation in children with and without encopresis. Clin Pediatr 2003; 42:815–819.
43. Pashankar DS, Loening-Baucke V, Bishop WP. Safety of polyethylene glycol 3350 for the treatment of chronic constipation in children. Arch Pediatr Adolesc Med 2003; 157(7):661–664.
44. Erickson BA, Austin JC, Cooper CS, et al. Polyethylene glycol 3350 for constipation in children with dysfunctional elimination. J Urol 2003; 170(4):1580–1582.
45. Loening-Baucke V, Krishna R, Pashankar DS, et al. Polyethylene glycol 3350 without electrolytes for the treatment of functional constipation in infants and toddlers. J Ped Gastroenterol Nutr 2004; 39:536–539.
46. Di Lorenzo C. Pediatric anorectal disorders. Gastroenterol Clin 2001; 30(1):269–287.
47. Loening-Baucke V. Urinary incontinence and urinary tract infection and their resolution with treatment of chronic constipation of childhood. Pediatrics 1997; 100(2):228–232.
48. van Ginkel R, Reitsma JB, Büller HA, et al. Childhood constipation: longitudinal follow-up beyond puberty. Gastroenterology 2003; 125(2):357–363.
49. Olness K, Tobin S. Chronic constipation in children. Can it be managed by diet alone? Postgrad Med 1982; 72(4):149–154.
50. Abrahamian FP, Lloyd-Still JD. Chronic constipation in childhood: a longitudinal study of 186 patients. J Pediatr Gastroenterol Nutr 1984; 3(3):460–467.
51. Staiano A, Andreotti MR, Greco L, et al. Long-term follow-up of children with chronic idiopathic constipation. Dig Dis Sci 1994; 39(3):561–564.
52. Levine MD, Bakow H. Children with encopresis: a study of treatment outcome. Pediatrics 1976; 58(6):845–852.
53. Loening-Baucke V. Functional fecal retention with encopresis in childhood. J Pediatr Gastroenterol Nutr 2004; 38(1):79–84.
54. Loening-Baucke V. Constipation in early childhood: patient characteristics, treatment, and longterm follow up. Gut 1993; 34(10):1400–1404.
55. Loening-Baucke V. Biofeedback treatment for chronic constipation and encopresis in childhood: long-term outcome. Pediatrics 1995; 96(1):105–110.
56. Wald A, Chandra R, Gabel S, Chiponis D. Evaluation of biofeedback in childhood encopresis. J Pediatr Gastroenterol Nutr 1987; 6(4):554–558.
57. Loening-Baucke V. Modulation of abnormal defecation dynamics by biofeedback treatment in chronically constipated children with encopresis. J Pediatr 1990; 116(2):214–222.
58. van der Plas RN, Benninga MA, Büller HA, et al. Biofeedback training in treatment of childhood constipation: A randomised controlled study. Lancet 1996; 348(9030):776–780.
59. Staiano A, Cucchiara S, Andreotti MR, et al. Effect of cisapride on chronic idiopathic constipation in children. Dig Dis Sci 1991; 36(6):733–736.
60. Odeka EB, Sagher F, Miller V, et al. Use of cisapride in treatment of constipation in children. J Ped Gastroenterol Nutr 1997; 25(2):199–203.

61. Nurko S, Garcia-Aranda JA, et al. Cisapride for the treatment of constipation in children: a double-blind study. J Pediatr 2000; 136(1):35–40.
62. Bishop JM, Hill DJ, Hosking CS. Natural history of cow milk allergy: clinical outcome. J Pediatr 1990; 116(6):862–867.
63. Iacono G, Carroccio A, Cavataio F, et al. Chronic constipation as a symptom of cow milk allergy. J Pediatr 1995; 126(1):34–39.
64. Iacono G, Cavataio F, Montalto G, et al. Intolerance of cow's milk and chronic constipation in children. N Engl J Med 1998; 339(16):1100–1104.
65. Shah N, Lindley K, Milla P. Cow's milk and chronic constipation in children. N Engl J Med 1999; 340(11):891–892.
66. Daher S, Tahan S, Solé D, et al. Cow's milk protein intolerance and chronic constipation in children. Pediatr Allergy Immunol 2001; 12(6):339–342.
67. Vanderhoof JA, Perry D, Hanner TL, et al. Allergic constipation: association with infantile milk allergy. Clin Pediatr 2001; 40(7):399–402.
68. Miele E, Boccia G, Auricchio R, et al. Chronic constipation and atopy. Acta Gastro-Enterologica Belgica 2003(suppl); April:65.
69. Malone PS, Ransley PG, Kiely EM. Preliminary report: the antegrade continence enema. Lancet 1990; 336(8725):1217–1218.
70. Chait PG, Shandling B, Richards HF. The cecostomy button. J Pediatr Surg 1997; 32(6):849–851.
71. Youssef NN, Barksdale E, Griffiths JM, et al. Management of intractable constipation with antegrade enemas in neurologically intact children. J Pediatr Gastroenterol Nutr 2002; 34(4):402–405.

Chapter 12
Failure to thrive

Vasundhara Tolia

'It didn't take elaborate experiments to deduce that an infant would die from want of food. But it took centuries to figure out that infants can and do perish from want of love'.

Louise J. Kaplan, 1995

INTRODUCTION

Growth is one of the most important indicators of child's well-being. The growth pattern is the result of the complex interaction between genetic and environmental factors.[1] It is generally expected that infants and children will grow and thrive to resemble the beautiful baby seen in infant advertisements. When children do not grow and meet the expectations that their families and society hold, there are implications for both the child and family. Growth monitoring is most useful in identifying conditions that are not diagnosed easily and growth patterns that deviate substantially from normal.

EPIDEMIOLOGY

Failure to thrive, labeled as FTT, is due to a set of heterogenous conditions affecting growth. The term FTT originated in industrialized countries in the last century, and is best defined as inadequate physical growth diagnosed by observation of growth over time using a standard growth chart. Terms such as growth failure, failure to gain weight and growth faltering are synonymous with FTT.[2,3] Commonly, the pediatrician first detects that a child is not thriving as parents often do not recognize the subtle slowing of growth in their child.

The prevalence of FTT has been reported as 1–5% of all referrals to pediatric hospitals and from 10–20% of all children who are treated in ambulatory care settings.[4] In personal experience, the frequency of the diagnosis of FTT in the gastroenterology outpatient clinic at Children's Hospital of Michigan varied between 2.76–6.63% annually during the years 1998 to 2003, with an average incidence of 3.97% during these 6 years. Children with neurologic compromise were not included in this analysis.

FTT has crucial implications for the child which include physical and developmental retardation with emotional and behavioral problems.[5] The causes of FTT were previously categorized as organic, non-organic and mixed, however the organic failure to thrive (OFTT) and non-organic failure to thrive (NOFTT) dichotomy in diagnosis is inadequate as there is a significant overlap in the spectrum of growth failure. This classification has limited usefulness because multiple factors may contribute towards FTT in a patient. There are three basic mechanisms for occurrence of FTT: (1) insufficient nutritional intake because of the child's inability to feed properly, e.g. neurological disabilities, oropharyngeal malformations, anorexia; (2) proper amount of nutrition consumed but inadequately absorbed and/or utilized, e.g. malabsorption syndromes; (3) abnormal utilization of calories, or increased metabolic requirements as in chronic diseases or hypermetabolic states. It is not uncommon for FTT to be the first clue to an active disease process, such as celiac disease or Crohn's disease.

DEFINITION

There is no consensus regarding the definition and criteria of FTT.[6] Failure to thrive is a term used by pediatricians to describe infants and toddlers, under 3 years of age, with an abnormally low weight for age and gender. 'Failure to thrive' implies failure, not only of growth, but also of other aspects of a child's well-being. Identification of FTT and an assessment of the severity of the nutritional state is important to identify children at risk, and to provide appropriate intervention. It is surprising, therefore, that such a common and important problem lacks a consistent definition.[7] In older children, it is commonly referred to as growth failure. Commonly used criteria include children who are less than 75% of median weight-for-height for age in children under the age of 2 years *or* weight (or weight for height) less than 2 standard deviations below the mean for sex and age *or* if the weight curve has crossed more than two percentile lines using the National Center for Health Statistics (NCHS) growth charts after having achieved a previously stable pattern.

Accurate assessment of the child's height, weight and head circumference is essential. These should be plotted on the NCHS growth charts and related to previous measurements. The NCHS growth charts are gender specific and appropriate for all races and nationalities. A single assessment of height and weight may have limited usefulness because it does not provide any indication of whether the child's growth pattern is deviating from the percentile. Genetic growth expectation should be kept in perspective while assessing growth status.

Alternative criteria include calculating Z scores, which are standard deviation scores that express anthropometric data normalized for age and sex, and can be calculated with software available from the Centers for Disease Control and Prevention. Z scores are used in research studies as they allow more precise description of anthropometric status than percentile curves.

One in three low-weight children is not identified as a possible problem if the child has professional parents, if the child appears well-cared for, if there is no reported feeding difficulty, if growth charts are not used and if there are no treatment facilities, so parents and healthcare providers need to be vigilant to identify such children at risk.[8] The value of any index of FTT lies in its usefulness in identifying the child at risk and in predicting the severity of other coexisting nutrition related problems. In a recent prospective study, a comparison of five anthropometric methods of classifying FTT validated weight for age as the simplest and most reasonable marker for FTT.[9] An anthropolometric classification of FTT using all three growth parameters weight, height and head circumference for practical use is shown in Table 12.1 dividing the diagnosis into three major categories with the disease groups associated with each type. Attention to the percentile curves of length, weight and head circumference give valuable clues to the etiology of FTT. When all measurements are decreased, the incidence of organic disease is about 70%. Gastrointestinal disorders are more common when only the weight is below the 5th percentile. Table 12.2 shows a partial list of various diseases in which FTT can occur.

PATHOGENESIS

FTT affects growing children in many important ways regardless of its etiology. FTT is associated with persistently small stature. Severe malnutrition has been shown to cause permanent structural aberrations in the central nervous system.[10] Even mild malnutrition in the absence of significant growth failure has been associated with developmental impairment and disability.[11] Moreover, undernourished children with FTT are more likely to have infectious diseases.[12,13] They are more prone to changes in cell-mediated immunity, complement levels and opsonization that increase susceptibility to various infections.[14] Severe FTT can be associated with secondary changes in cardiovascular and gastrointestinal functioning.[15]

CAUSES AND CONTRIBUTORY FACTORS

FTT is most commonly caused by inadequate calorie intake, which can arise when food is not available or from insufficient food intake due to feeding and behavioral problems. Table 12.3 depicts potential risk factors for the development of this type of FTT. Low birthweight and prematurity appear to be risk factors in the development of eating problems.[16] While the origin of FTT can be complex, the most common time for FTT problems to emerge is at the time of weaning.[17] Food acceptance patterns develop early in life and this is a time of particular sensitivity for imprinting food preferences. This is when a child's oral motor skills develop, which allow the child to accept new flavors and textures. For some young children, the progression through weaning and the acceptance of more solid textures can be difficult. Many parents of children who fail to thrive report feeding difficulties in their child such as spitting food out, vomiting and refusal of solid food.[18] There can be many reasons for food refusal, including excessive food temperature, inappropriate-sized pieces and insensitive or forceful feeding techniques. In some cases where this does occur, a child can later refuse new textures and/or solids leading to an overdependence on milk with resultant insufficient calorie intake for normal growth.[19]

Initial problems with coordinating swallowing, breathing and sucking can establish problematic feeding interactions with the mother. Later refusal to progress onto mixed or more solid textures of food because of problems coordinating chewing and swallowing can create a significant problem, even though weight is being maintained.[20] A further problem can be the reluctance of parents to allow the young child to self-feed and make the inevitable 'mess'. The nature of the interaction between the child and the parent can affect the child's behavior at mealtimes and consequently the child's food intake.[21] Although FTT is seen in all socioeconomic groups, its incidence is especially high among poor urban and rural families. Poverty by itself is the single greatest risk factor for undernutrition.[22]

Psychosocial factors contributing to FTT are the emotional neglect of the child or a lack of appropriate attachment, a lack of education and knowledge about parenting, poverty and abuse of the child. When caregivers do not spend enough time with or neglect feeding the infant correctly because of personal problems such as depression or isolation, inappropriate attachment is formed leading to a disturbed pattern of interactions between the infant and caregiver.[23] A schema for classification of these disorders by age of onset is depicted in Figure 12.1. A few of the factors that increase the likelihood of poor attachment are poor social supports within the family and the presence of mental illness.[24] Many mothers of children with FTT have been reported to have

	Weight	Height	Head circumference	Associated diseases
Type I	Decreased	Decreased/normal	Normal	Malnutrition of organic or non-organic etiology usually secondary to intestinal, pancreatic, liver diseases or systemic illness or psychosocial factors.
Type II	Decreased	Decreased	Normal	Endocrinopathies, bony dystrophy, constitutional short stature
Type III	Decreased	Decreased	Decreased	Chromosomal, metabolic disease, intrauterine and perinatal insults, severe malnutrition

Table 12.1 Three major anthropologic categories of failure to thrive

- Decreased caloric intake
  - Neurologic disorders with impaired swallowing
  - Injury to mouth and esophagus
    - Trauma
    - Infections
    - Neoplasms
  - Congenital anomalies affecting oro-naso-pharyngeal and upper gastrointestinal tract
  - Chromosomal abnormalities
  - Genetic diseases
    - IGF-1 receptor abnormality
  - Metabolic diseases
  - Diseases leading to anorexia
    - malignancy
    - Renal diseases
    - Cardiac diseases
    - Liver diseases
    - Inflammatory bowel disease
    - Psychologic
    - Neglect/abuse
    - Acquired immunodeficiency syndrome
    - Gastroesophageal reflux disease with esophagitis
  - Accidental or inadvertent
    - Decreased breast milk
    - Improper formula preparation
    - Bizarre diets
  - Psychosocial
    - maternal and/or infant related factors
  - Iatrogenic
    - Food allergy diets
    - Special diets from misdiagnosis
- Increased requirements
  - Sepsis
  - Trauma
  - Burns
  - Chronic respiratory disease
  - Hyperthyroidism
  - Congenital heart disease
  - Diencephalic syndrome
  - Hyperactivity
  - Chronic infections
- Impaired utilization
  - Inborn errors of metabolism
- Excessive caloric losses
  - Persistent vomiting
  - Pyloric stenosis
  - Gastroesophageal reflux
  - Malabsorptive states
  - Pancreatic insufficiency
  - Celiac disease
  - Enzyme deficiency
  - Short bowel
  - Anatomic gut lesions
  - Microvillus inclusion disease
  - Protein losing enteropathy
  - Chronic inflammatory bowel disease
  - Chronic immunodeficiency
  - Allergic gastroenteropathy
  - Parasitic infestations
  - Chronic enteric infections
  - Postenteritis syndrome
  - Chronic cholestasis
  - Diabetes mellitus

Table 12.2 Major causes of failure to thrive

- Infant related
  - IUGR
  - Anemia
  - Prematurity
  - Acute illnesses
  - Neurologic diseases
  - Lead poisoning
  - Anatomic abnormalities
  - Oral motor dysfunction
  - Malabsorptions states
  - Other chronic diseases
  - Chromosomal or genetic diseases
  - Developmental delay
- Maternal
  - Lower education
  - Lack of support
  - Depression
  - Single parent
  - Abuse/neglect
- Family
  - Lower income
  - Family dysfunction
  - Aberrant beliefs
  - Abuse/neglect
  - Less enriched environment
  - Disordered feeding techniques
  - Substance abuse
  - Factitious disorders

Table 12.3 Risk factors for FTT

aberrant responses to show appropriate physical or emotional concern or care because their parental role models often were inappropriate and faulty.[25] The age of the parent also may be a factor because FTT occurs more commonly among children of younger mothers.[26] Parents may make accidental errors in food preparation or may not know basic child-care practices.[27] Deliberate starvation and food restriction is a contributing factor to cases of FTT. Although these severe cases are few, they do occur and, according to the law, all cases of FTT resulting from underfeeding or neglect by caregivers must be reported to child protective services (CPS).[28] The most common cause for CPS involvement occurs when the parents do not provide the child with appropriate care despite efforts made by medical staff and

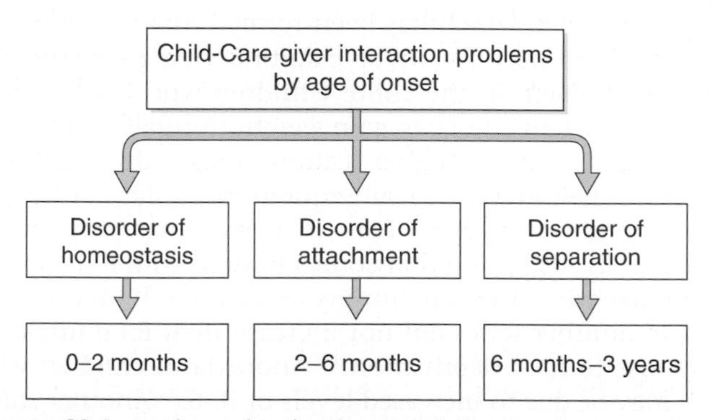

Figure 12.1: A schema for classification of disorders: homeostasis, attachment and separation, by age of onset.

social workers. Earlier reports on mothers of infants with FTT having been more deprived, abused and neglected than controls have not been substantiated in later studies.[29]

While undernutrition may result from failure to offer adequate calories, it may also occur because of inadequate ingestion of food by the infant. Historically, non-organic FTT was considered to be secondary to the mother's role in providing adequate nutrition, and treatment approaches have primarily focused on family dysfunction. As a result, few attempts have been made to ascertain whether the child is able to ingest the nutrients provided. Recent studies suggest that the role of deprivation and neglect has been overstated and that undemanding behavior, low appetite and poor feeding skills in infants themselves may contribute to the onset and persistence of FTT.[30] Moreover, feeding disorders are now commonly recognized in the pediatric population, with prevalence estimates ranging from 25–35% in developmentally normal children. Severe feeding problems are more prevalent (40–70%) in children with developmental disabilities and chronic disease.[31] Feeding problems may be due to many etiologies including neurodevelopmental disorders, disorders of appetite regulation, metabolic diseases, sensory defects, conditioned dysphagia and anatomic abnormalities. Many feeding disorders initially develop as a result of organic diseases which are further exacerbated by behavioral factors.

The presence of oral-motor dysfunction (OMD) may prevent some children from achieving a satisfactory nutritional intake.[32] Sucking, chewing and swallowing difficulties could contribute to FTT in infancy by leading to prolonged mealtimes and inappropriate parental reaction. Children with OMD might have a subtle neurodevelopmental disorder. In a prospective study to identify infants with non-organic FTT, a subgroup of infants with OMD was identified in whom cognitive stimulation within the home and cognitive-growth fostering during mealtimes by caretakers was much poorer. It is speculated that children with OMD may be 'biologically' more vulnerable from birth to develop FTT, however, this study did not support the co-existence of a subtle neurodevelopmental disorder. The identification of an as yet unappreciated organic component to the disorder may eventually classify these children differently than non-organic FTT.[32]

Some children with FTT have been suggested to have an eating disorder, which has been termed infantile anorexia nevosa.[33] FTT may also involve an underlying appetite regulation problem in the child. Children who fail to thrive take insufficient energy to gain weight normally, and when challenged with a higher calorie meal, they did not decrease their intake at a subsequent meal, like controls in a randomized study.[34] This is consistent with earlier hypothesis suggesting that some children who FTT 'do not recognize when they are hungry or satiated'.[33] Infants with FTT in another series did not increase their food intake in response to food deprivation.[35] Anorexia in children with FTT may be due to increased levels of IL-6.[36] Another study has provided further indications of the role of diminished appetite and vigor of eating style in the child.[37] It also suggested that children with FTT eat a reduced number and variety of foods, and progress onto feeding solids more slowly. What cannot be elucidated from either of these studies is whether these characteristics are a cause or an effect of their FTT, or indeed whether they genuinely reflect the child's behavior or simply the parental interpretation of it. However, children who receive intervention go on to have a better appetite, as well as better weight gain.[37]

It is important to understand the pattern of growth in specific circumstances. Breast-fed infants grow more slowly than bottle-fed infants. Despite their slower growth rate, nursed infants eventually reach the same final height by 2 years of age.[38] This early growth pattern can be alarming to healthcare personnel, to the point of considering alternative modalities of nutrition. Another situation is that of premature infants where corrected age should be used to plot the growth percentiles.

Growth from birth to maturity has been described as occurring in three additive phases: infancy, childhood and puberty, i.e. the ICP-model.[39] The infancy phase starts in mid-gestation and continues in a similar fashion during the first months after birth. Thereafter, it rapidly decreases and ends at approximately 4 years of age. The onset of the second growth period, the childhood phase, normally occurs during the second half of the first postnatal year and is characterized by an increase in height gain. Among pre-term newborns, the term small for gestational age (SGA) usually refers to infants born with a birthweight <10th percentile, based on population curves. Pre-term SGA newborns comprise a heterogeneous group. The majority of these SGA infants have intrauterine growth restriction.[40] Symmetrical SGA refers to both body weight and head circumference of <10th percentile for gestational age in relation to standard curves and is considered to begin in early pregnancy. Asymmetrical SGA refers to birthweight of <10th percentile for gestational age.[41] A population-based study to characterize longitudinal growth in a group of pre-term children born at <29 weeks gestational age (GA) showed that it takes the very pre-term child up to 7 years to catch up what is lost in weight and length during the first months of extrauterine life.[42] However, nearly all children were close to normal in height and weight when they started school. This study showed a distinct linear catch-up growth starting at the same time as the childhood component in the ICP model, if age corrected for GA is used. It may be speculated that preterm birth disturbs the normal regulation of the infancy growth period, resulting in a poor growth outcome during the first years, whereas the childhood growth period remains normal.[42] SGA status seems to have only modest independent effects on learning, cognition, and attention in adolescence. Severity but not symmetry of growth restriction predicted learning difficulties.[43]

EVALUATION OF FAILURE TO THRIVE

Despite the common emphasis on the search for an underlying pathology, major organic causes are unusual. Exhaustive investigations for organic causes and prolonged hospitalizations to evaluate family dynamics and poor infant weight gain often are costly and frequently fail to yield a definitive diagnosis. A full detailed pediatric assessment including physical examination and psychosocial evaluation will usually exclude organic disease. The past medical history and review of systems can provide important clues. Table 12.4 depicts some of these factors which aid in such assessment.

Some of the medical problems that may cause FTT are listed in Table 12.2.[3] Eosinophilic esophagitis is also a cause of dysphagia, which can contribute to decreased appetite and may mimic reflux in its presentation.[44] In addition, neurological difficulties that manifest as oral motor delay or dysfunction impact on how able the child is to cope with changing textures of foods.[32] A complete developmental assessment including careful evaluation should be made for dysmorphic features and for signs of neurologic, pulmonary, cardiac, gastrointestinal disorders and nutritional deficiency. Isolated defects in the soft or hard palate may indicate a feeding problem. Other genetic and chromosomal defects, intrauterine growth retardation (IUGR), and fetal alcohol syndrome may also have characteristic physical findings. In these infants, presenting symptoms and signs of regurgitation, vomiting, poor feeding, diarrhea, dysphagia, coughing, abdominal distension, wasting and those of primary pathology contributing to FTT may be obvious. However, eosinophilic esophagitis and celiac disease may have subtle presentations. When there is a clear medical explanation for the growth deficit the diagnosis is not difficult. Depending on the age of the child, the severity and length of the condition at diagnosis with FTT, children may present with a range of physical symptoms from mild weight loss and diminished height to weakness and gluteal muscle wasting so severe that folds of skin hang loose. Signs of neglect may be indicated by a diaper rash, impetigo, flat occiput, poor hygiene, protuberant abdomen, lack of appropriate behavior and inappropriate infantile postures.[45] Some children with non-organic FTT may exhibit listlessness, expressionless facies, hypervigilance, and/or self-stimulatory, stereotypical movements of their bodies and hands.[46] Observation of the child for drooling and assessment of bowel habits is essential.

A comprehensive nutritional assessment has five components: dietary history, medical and medication history, physical examination, growth and anthropometric measurements, and laboratory tests. Neurological abnormalities put children at very high risk of developing feeding problems that increase the likelihood of poor development.[22,47] Mutations in the insulin like growth factor 1 receptor have been recently added to the list of genetic defects leading to intrauterine growth retardation (IUGR) which persists postnatally.[48]

Birth history
Low birthweight
IUGR
Prematurity
Postnatal complications
Tube feeding
Dietary
Type of food eaten
Time spent over a meal
Number of meals and snacks
Does the child self-feed?
If nursed, is there enough milk?
Formula or special diets
Food or other supplements
Medications
Presence of food allergies, intolerances
Unusual feeding behaviors
Recurrent infections
Otitis media
Gastroenteritis
Persistent vomiting
Gastroesophageal reflux
Food intolerances
Eosinophilic esophagitis
Persistent diarrhea
Malabsorption syndrome
Presence of blood
Difficulty swallowing
Behavior
Interactions with caretakers
Child left alone
Sleep patterns
Family history
Parental heights
Sibling heights
Any other close relative with similar problems
Specific disease including mental illness
Structural abnormalities
Dysmorphism
Congenital anomalies
Systemic diseases
Asthma
Anemia
Others
Social history
Family members
Employment status
Caregivers
History of neglect in family
Abuse of drugs/alcohol
Stressful events in family
Child's temperament

Table 12.4 Important parameters (past and current symptom history)

INVESTIGATIONS

Necessary laboratory testing to search for an organic disease should be guided by the history and physical examination. Laboratory studies not suggested on the basis of the initial examination are rarely helpful. One study revealed that less than 2% of the laboratory studies performed in evaluating children with FTT were useful diagnostically.[49] A few routine screening tests, such as a complete blood count, BUN, creatinine, serum electrolytes, albumin, calcium, phosphorus, alkaline phosphatase, urinalysis and urine culture help in excluding systemic diseases. Some of the special investigations needed for further testing in selected patients are shown in Table 12.5. It is important to construct a complete picture of all aspects of and influences on the child's feeding. Dietary assessment is complex and involves taking a dietary recall, completion of a food diary and, if possible, feeding observation. A 24-h recall may not reflect the 'normal' eating pattern and cannot be used for accurate calculation of nutrient intake, so a 3-day diet diary is used to assess the calorie intake. Any use of alternative or complementary medications should always be asked. Observation of feeding will also provide important information about how the baby feeds, parent-child interaction and the emotions surrounding feeding (Table 12.6). Observing a meal-time, together with information from the diaries, allows discussion with the parents on appropriate interventions.[50]

MANAGEMENT

The physician must be an advocate for the child and his/her family without becoming an adversary of the parents. If an organic disease is diagnosed, appropriate drug and/or dietary intervention must be started. Parents should be counseled about the disease, its outcomes and be made aware of any available support groups. Close follow-up with growth monitoring will help to restore the child's well-being. A multidisciplinary team approach requires close liaison between the pediatrician, pediatric gastroenterologist, psychologist, speech and language therapists as well as dieticians.[51,52] Hospitalization may not be helpful or necessary unless the child is seriously ill or is at risk of physical or sexual abuse or admission is warranted because of parental concern and anxiety. Moreover, separation of the child from the family by hospitalization may promote anxiety.[53] Helping parents can be difficult and must be done in a sensitive way without blaming or criticizing parenting skills. Only in rare instances of suspected neglect or abuse, the child needs to be removed from its environment. The possibility that calorie deprivation in infancy will produce severe, irreversible developmental deficits is the reason that treatment should begin expeditiously. The overall aims of intervention are to increase nutritional intake, to induce catch-up growth, to resolve feeding difficulties and improve feeding style, to create positive interactions between the mother and the child and to create a positive feeding environment.[54]

The main goal of dietary intervention in the management of undernutrition is to increase calorie intake to enable 'catch-up' weight gain at a rate that is greater than average for age so that the weight deficit is repaired or overcome. Nutritional requirements for the healthy infant at birth are 110 kcal/kg per day and at 1 year are an average of 100 kcal/kg per day. A child who fails to gain weight normally and whose weight is below the 5th percentile will not experience 'catch-up' unless calorie intake is higher than basal requirement for age. A common regimen is to increase caloric intake by 50% greater than basal requirement (e.g. 150/kcal/kg per day in a 1-year-old child).[54] Another way to determine caloric requirements for infants with poor growth is to determine the calories required by using the following formula:

$$\text{(RDA for age (kcal/kg)} \times \text{ideal weight for height (kg))/actual weight (kg)}$$

where ideal weight for height is the median weight for the patient's height (as read from the NCHS weight for height curves).

High calorie intake is difficult to achieve as many toddlers eat small food portions and are not able to consume large quantities at any one time. Energy intake can be increased by: frequent meals, use of energy-dense foods and adding extra calories to foods. During the catch-up growth phase, existing stores of vitamins may not be sufficient. A multivitamin preparation including iron and zinc is recommended. Close follow-up and frequent contact with the healthcare team are essential for reinforcing nutritional recommendations and psychosocial support. Involvement with the family by community social service workers, visiting nurses, and nutritionists is important to ensure a nurturing environment for the children.[52] During nutritional recovery, some malnourished children experience the symptoms of a nutritional recovery syndrome,

Quantitative immunoglobulins, *Helicobacter pylori*, IgG
Antigliadin, anti-reticulin and anti-endomysial antibodies
Serum vasoactive intestinal peptide
Urine organic acids, catecholamines, amino acids
Chromosomal studies, growth hormone levels
Human immunodeficiency virus antibody, liver function tests, thyroid studies
Serology for inflammatory bowel disease
Stool cultures, ova and parasites, α_1-antitrypsin in stool
Barium contrast studies
Abdominal ultrasound
Head CT/MRI
Sweat chloride
Breath testing
Extended intraesophageal pH monitoring
Small intestinal biopsy
Upper and lower endoscopy
Electrocardiogram
Chest radiograph, bone age, skeletal survey
Other specific tests as indicated

Table 12.5 Optional investigations for organic Failure to Thrive

Observe the child for:	Observe the parents for:
Interest in own and other's food	Awareness of child's needs and demands
Quantity, type and texture of food eaten	Quantity, type and texture of food offered
Ability to concentrate and persevere	Management style, e.g. force, encouragement
Ability to communicate needs	Emotional style, e.g. frustration, anxiety
Reaction to parents' behavior	Control over child's behavior
Desire to feed or drink by itself	Ability to tolerate mess

Table 12.6 Assessment of a feeding session

including sweatiness, hepatomegaly (caused by increased glycogen deposition in the liver), widening of the sutures (the brain growth is greater than the growth of the skull in infants with open sutures) and irritability or mild hyperactivity.[55] If weight gain does not occur in 4–6 weeks, oral feedings should be supplemented with feeding by a nasogastric tube. Feeding assessment by occupational therapist to improve sucking and swallowing may be needed. If weight gain is inadequate after nasogastric tube feeding or if prolonged nasogastric tube feeding will be required (more than 2 months), gastrostomy tube placement may be appropriate.[35] The use of tube feeding as part of the medical management of many children's illnesses can create problems as well as ameliorate others.[56] The psychological management of long-term tube feeding is an important element in reducing the anxiety and concern about a child who cannot or will not eat. In most children with neurologic compromise, it is required on a long-term basis, especially in those at risk for aspiration with swallowing. Figure 12.2 provides an algorithm for management of calorie intake in a child with FTT.

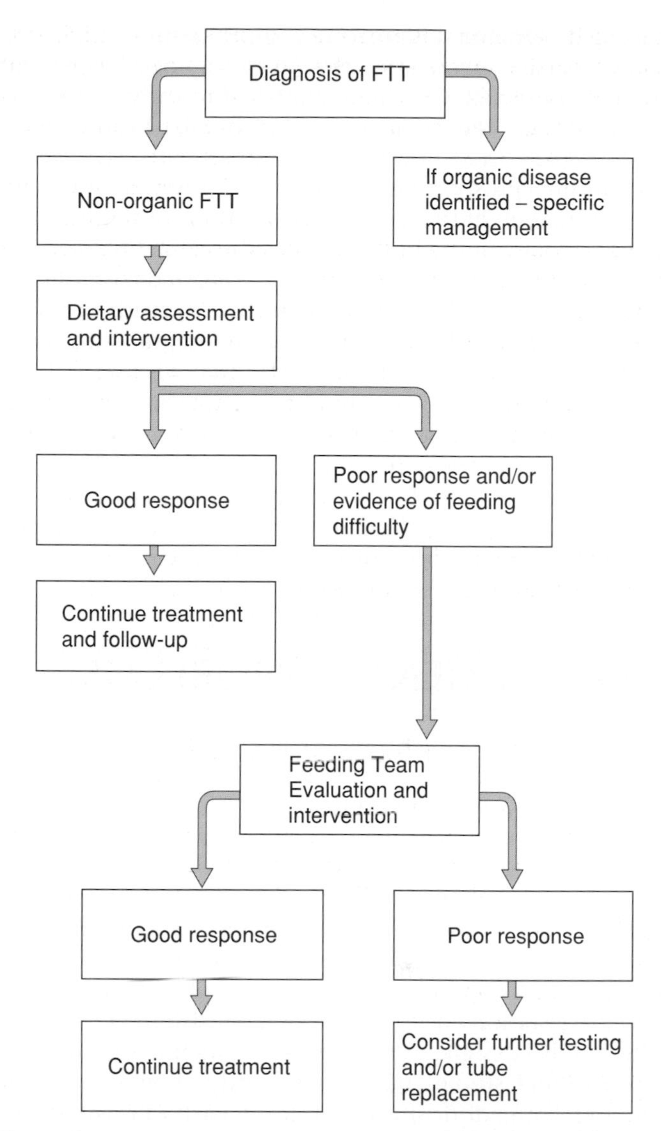

Figure 12.2: Algorithm for management of a child with Failure to Thrive (FTF).

OUTCOME

Development of the brain and cognitive processes take place during the first three years of a child's life.[57] Because of the accelerated cerebral growth during this period, any significant reduction in nutrition that results in FTT carries a high risk for negative effects for intellectual development later in life.[58] A recent study suggests that brain growth during infancy and early childhood is more important than growth during fetal life in determining cognitive function.[59] The fact that children who fail to thrive have poorer head growth is not surprising considering that human brain growth is rapid in the early childhood years and insults during this time may impact permanently on developmental and intellectual outcome. These findings emphasize the importance of early and intensive intervention for children with or at risk for FTT to prevent permanent growth retardation. Although the prognosis with respect to weight gain and growth is good, between 25 to 60% of infants with FTT remain small (weight or height <20th percentile). Cognitive function is below normal in one-half of the children with FTT, and a high frequency of behavior problems and learning difficulties is found on follow-up of children with FTT. Whether these findings are a direct result of the failure to thrive or are the result of continued adverse social circumstances is not known. Maternal IQ was the strongest predictor of reading scores and other cognitive abilities in two studies.[60,61] It may be that the extent and quality of cognitive stimulation and the style of parenting provided by such mothers help promote brain growth and intellectual development. Several studies have demonstrated that provision of a cognitively enriched environment in early life can lead to improvements in intellectual performance.[62–64]

While previous data from long-term studies in children with poor nutrition suggest lower mean IQ scores and a high incidence of attention deficit disorder in comparison to a control group, more recent studies show better results with increases in cognitive development that appear to be related to growth recovery.[65] The cognitive recovery experienced by children with a history of FTT is consistent with their growth recovery. When children with a history of FTT participated in an interdisciplinary specialty clinic by age 6, only 3% were wasted or stunted,[63] although they were shorter than children who had not experienced FTT. Two other studies that found no significant differences in the IQ scores of children with and without histories of FTT.[5,65] However, these results differ from two studies that found long-lasting deficits in cognitive development at age 11 and in adolescence.[66,67] These differences may be partially explained by differences in sampling.

GROWTH ABNORMALITIES

Growth failure is the most obvious and persistent symptom and sequelae of FTT. Depending on the age of the child when growth failure occurred and the length of time it existed before it was corrected, short stature commonly always persists even after the child is once again adequately nourished. Children who failed to thrive from 1 to 5 years of age were smaller and had smaller head circumferences than their non-FTT counterparts at school age.[65] In another prospective, longitudinal outpatient study, weight and height for age were shown to be of significantly slower velocity in the FTT group despite catch up growth.[68] A longitudinal 5-year follow-up study showed a significant difference within the FTT group with the severity of poor growth (weight and height) and developmental outcome.[69] Overall, these studies comparing children who were thriving with those who were undernourished in both developed and developing countries show that children with FTT are at substantial risk for continued poor growth in weight, height, and head circumference, and that this growth disturbance is difficult to reverse despite appropriate interventions. Earlier diagnosis and intervention leads to potentially better long-term outcome.

DEVELOPMENTAL PROBLEMS

There is a consistent trend for children with a history of FTT to score lower than their social class peers on developmental/cognitive test scores. It is difficult to ascertain whether the deficits identified are attributable to FTT in early life or to concurrent undernutrition and environmental stressors at the time the outcome is measured. There is a consistent association between FTT in early life and lower developmental test scores in the pre and primary school years. While the studies are methodologically disparate and conducted with samples of diverse ethnicities and gestational age, the effect is consistent across multiple study designs. Prospective, epidemiological, and observational studies have consistently shown increased rates of feeding difficulties in children with FTT, with additional non-specified 'neurological' findings in some of them.[32] Slow feeding and delayed acquisition of age-appropriate feeding skills are commonly observed.

CONCLUSION

There is persuasive evidence pointing to the potential adverse effects of infant growth faltering for subsequent child development,[22,70] although long-term developmental deficits have not been consistently observed among children with a history of FTT.[65] Poor weight gain in infancy has also been associated with an increased risk of cardiovascular disease in adult life,[71] developmental delay, emotional and social problems.

Recent research has led to a radical shift in our understanding of the condition since the 1940s. FTT is now seen as a form of malnutrition that develops through the complex interaction of subtle oral-motor dysfunction and psycho-social factors. Increasingly infants are diagnosed to have subtle physical conditions like OMD which may physically hinder suckling. Such OMD is also now thought to be an important cause of malnutrition in a variety of organic disease states, and effectively reduces the infant's ability to signal hunger. Maternal deprivation is very rare. Successful behavioral intervention is possible to address the children's feeding problems even if they result from a combination of organic diseases and parental mismanagement of meal time. Removal of blame from the family, their close involvement as part of management team and respect is an integral part of this long-term process.

Acknowledgements

I would like to thank Vicky Yoas for expert secretarial assistance and Kirit, Vinay and Sanjay for their patience, support and understanding.

References

1. Pampanich R, Garner P. Growth Monitoring in Children (Cochrane review), issue 1. Update Software. Oxford: The Cochrane Library; 1999.
2. Wilcox WD, Nieburg P, Miller DS. Failure to thrive: A continuing problem of definition. Clin Pediatr 1989; 28:391–394.
3. Zenel J. Failure to thrive: A general pediatrician's perspective. Pediatr Rev 1997; 18:371–378.
4. Mitchell W, Gorrell R, Greenberg R. Failure to thrive: a study in a primary care setting epidemiology and follow-up. Pediatrics 1980; 65:971–977.
5. Boddy J, Skuse D, Andrews B. The developmental sequelae of nonorganic failure to thrive. Psychol Psychiatr 2000; 414:1003–1014.
6. Gahagan S, Holmes R. A stepwise approach to evaluation of undernutrition and failure to thrive. Pediatr Clin North Am 1998; 45:169–187.
7. Casey PH. Failure to thrive. In: Levine MD, Carey WB, Crocker AC, eds. Developmental Behavioral Pediatrics. Philadelphia, PA: Saunders; 1992:379–383.
8. Batchlor J, Kerslake A. Failure to Thrive: The Case for Improving Screening, Prevention and Treatment in Primary Care. London: Whiting and Birch; 1990.
9. Raynor P, Rudolf MC. Anthropometric indices of failure to thrive. Arch Dis Child 2000; 82:364–365.
10. Skuse DH, Pickles A, Wolke D, et al. Postnatal growth and mental development: Evidence for a sensitive period. Child Psychol Psychiatry 1996; 35:521–545.
11. Dawson G, Fischer KW. Human Behavior and the Developing Brain. New York, NY: Guilford; 1994.
12. Pandey A, Chakraborty AK. Undernutrition, vitamin A deficiency and ARI morbidity in under fives. Indian J Public Health 1996; 40:13–16.
13. Friedland LR. Bacteraemia in severely malnourished children. Ann Trop Paediatr 1992; 12:433–440.
14. Neves C, Forte W, Martins Campos JV, Carneiro Leao R. Nonspecific immunological response in moderate malnutrition. Allergol Immunopathol (Madr) 1984; 12(6):489–496.
15. Kothari SS, Patel TM, Shetalwad A, et al. Left ventricular mass and function in children with severe protein energy malnutrition. Int J Cardiol 1992; 35:19–25.
16. Douglas JE, Bryon M. Interview data on severe behavioural eating difficulties in young children. Arch Dis Child 1996; 74:304–308.
17. Ramsey M, Gisel EG, Boutry M. Non-organic failure to thrive, growth failure secondary to feeding-skills disorder. Dev Med Child Neurol 1993; 35:285–297.

18. Selley WG, Boxall J. A new way to treat sucking and swallowing difficulties in babies. Lancet 1986; 1:1182–1184.
19. Wright C, Loughridge J, Moore G. Failure to thrive in a population context: two contrasting studies of feeding and nutritional status. Proc Nutrition Soc 2000; 59:37–45.
20. Babbitt RL, Hoch TA, Coe DA, et al. Behavioral assessment and treatment of pediatric feeding disorders. Develop Behav Pediatr 1994; 15(4):278–291.
21. Crist W, Napier-Phillips A. Mealtime behaviors of young children: a comparison of normative and clinical data. Develop Behav Pediatr 2001; 22(5):279–286.
22. Raynor P, Rudolf MC. What do we know about children who fail to thrive? Child Care Health Develop 1996; 22:241–250.
23. Chattor I. Infantile anorexia nervosa, a development disorder of separation and individuation. Am Acad Psychoanal 1989; 17:43–64.
24. Schwartz ID. Failure to thrive: an old nemesis in the new millennium. Pediatrics 2000; 21:257–264.
25. Drotar D, Eckerle D, Satola J, et al. Maternal interactional behavior with nonorganic failure to thrive infants: A case comparison study. Child Abuse Neglect 1990; 14:41–51.
26. Stier S, Leventhal J, Berg A, et al. Are children born to young mothers at increased risk of maltreatment? Pediatrics 1995; 91:642–647.
27. Pugliese M, Weyman-Daum M, Moses N, et al. Parental health beliefs as a cause of nonorganic failure to thrive. Pediatrics 1988; 12:327–339.
28. Wright C, Talbot E. Screening for failure to thrive – What are we looking for? Child Care Health Dev 1996; 22:223–234.
29. Skuse D, Gill D, Reilly S, et al. Failure to thrive and the risk of child abuse; a prospective population study. J Med Screen 1995; 2:1145–149.
30. Burklow KA, Phelps AN, Schultz JR, et al. Classifying complex pediatric feeding disorders. Pediatr Gastroenterol Nutr 1998; 27:143–147.
31. Kerwin ME. Empirically supported treatments in pediatric psychology: severe feeding problems. Pediatr Psychol 1999; 24:193–214.
32. Reilly SM, Skuse DH, Wolke D. Oral-motor dysfunction in children who fail to thrive: Organic or non-organic? Dev Med Child Neurol 1999; 41:115–122.
33. Chatoor I, Egan J, Getson P, et al. Mother-infant interaction in infantile anorexia nervosa. Am Acad Child Adoles Psychiatr 1987; 27:535–540.
34. Kases-Hara M. Wright, Drewett R. Energy compensation in young children who fail to thrive. Child Psychol Psychiatry 2002; 43:449–456.
35. Tolia V. Very early onset nonorganic failure to thrive in infants. J Pediatr Gastroenterol Nutr 1995; 20:73–80.
36. Shaval R, Kessel A, Toubi E, et al. Leptin and cytokines levels in children with failure to thrive. J Pediatr Gastroenterol Nutr 2003; 37:487–491.
37. Wright CM. Identification and management of failure to thrive: a community perspective. Arch Dis Child 2000; 82:5–9.
38. Zadik Z, Borondukov E, Zung A, et al. Adult height and weight of breast-fed and bottle-fed Israeli infants. J Pediatr Gastroenterol Nutr 2003; 37(4):462–467.
39. Karlberg J. Modeling of human growth. Thesis, 1987. Goteborg University, Sweden.
40. Wilcox AJ. Intrauterine growth retardation: beyond weight criteria. Early Human Dev, 1983, 8, 189–193.
41. Lin CC, Su SJ, River LP. Comparison of associated high-risk factors and perinatal outcome between symmetric and asymmetric fetal intrauterine growth retardation. Am J Obst Gynecol 1991; 164:1535–1542.
42. Niklasson A, Engstrom E, Hard AL, et al. Growth in very preterm children: A longitudinal study. Pediatr Res 2003; 54:899–905.
43. O'Keefe MJ, O'Callaghan M, Williams GM, et al. Learning, cognitive and attention problems in adolescents born small for gestational age. Pediatrics 2003; 112:301–307.
44. Markowitz JE. Liacouras CA. Gastorenterol Clin North Am 2003; 32(3):949–966.
45. Kempe R, Cutler C, Dean J. The infant with failure to thrive. In: Kempe CH, Helfer R, eds. The Battered Child, 3rd edn. Chicago: The University of Chicago Press; 1980:56–76.
46. Altemeier W, O'Connor S, Sherrod K, et al. A prospective study of antecedents for nonorganic failure to thrive. J Pediatr 1985; 106:360–365.
47. Bauchner H. Children with special health needs – failure to thrive. In: Behrman R, ed. Nelson Textbook of Pediatrics, 15th edn. Philadelphia, PA: Saunders; 1996:122–123.
48. Abuzzahab MJ, Schneider A, Goddard A, et al. IGF-1 receptor mutations resulting in intrauterine and postnatal growth retardation. NEJM 2003; 249:2211–2222.
49. Sills RH. Failure to thrive: The role of clinical and laboratory evaluation. Am J Dis Child 1978; 132:967–969.
50. Linscheid TR. Behavioral treatment of feeding disorders in children. In: Watson TS, Gresham FM, eds. Behavioral Treatment of Childhood Disorders. New York, NY: Plenum Press; 1998:357–368.
51. Bithoney WG, McJunkin J, Michalek J, et al. Prospective evaluation of weight gain in both non-organic and organic failure to thrive children: an outpatient trial of a multidisciplinary team intervention strategy. J Develop Behav Pediatr 1989; 10:27–31.
52. Wright C, Callum J, Birks E, et al. Community based management of failure to thrive; a randomized control trial. Br Med J 1998; 317:571–574.
53. Berwick D, Levy J, Kleinerman R. Failure to thrive: diagnostic yield of hospitalization. Arch Dis Child 1982; 7:347–351.
54. Magioni A, Lifshitz F. Nutritional management of failure to thrive. Pediatr Clin North Am 1995; 42:791–810.
55. Dunn RL, Stettler N, Mascarenhas MR. Refeeding syndrome in hospitalized pediatric patients. Nutrition Clin Pr 2003; 18:327–332.
56. Bazyk S. Factors associated with the transition to oral feedings in infants fed by nasogastric tubes. Am J Occup Ther 1990; 44:1070–1078.
57. McCall RB, Hogarty PS, Hulbert N. Transitions in infants sensorimotor development and the prediction of childhood IQ. Am Psychol 1972; 27:728–748.
58. Politt E. The relationship between nutrition and behavioral development in children. J Nutr 1995; 25:2211S–2284S.
59. Gale CR, O'Callaghan FJ, Godfrey KM, et al. Critical periods of brain growth and cognitive function in children. Brain 2003; 127:321–329.
60. Anderson LM, Shinn C, Fulliove MT, et al. The effectiveness of early childhood development programs. A systematic review. Am J Prev Med 2003; 24:32–46.
61. Eickmann SH, Lima AC, Guerra MQ, et al. Improved cognitive and motor development in a community-based intervention of psychosocial stimulation in Northeast Brazil. Develop Med Child Neurol 2003; 45:536–541.
62. Hill JL, Brooks-Gunn J, Waldfogel J. Sustained efforts of high participation in an early intervention for low birth-weight premature infants. Devel Psychol 2003; 39:730–744.

63. Black MM, Krishnakumar A. Predicting longitudinal growth curves of height and weight using ecological factors for children with and without early growth deficiency. J Nutr 1999; 129:5395–5435.

64. Grantham-McGregor S, Schefield W, Powell C. Development of severely malnourished children who received psychosocial stimulation: six-year follow-up. Pediatarics 1998; 79: 247–254.

65. Drewett R, Corbett S, Wright C. Cognitive and educational attainments at school age of children failed to thrive in infancy: a population based study. J Child Psychol Psychiatry 1999; 40:551–561.

66. Dowdney I, Skuse D, Morrik et al. Short normal children and environmental disadvantage: a longitudinal study of growth and cognitive development from 4–11 years. J Child Psychol Psychiatry 1998; 39:1017–1030.

67. Oates K. Child abuse and nonorganic failure to thrive: similarities and differences in parents. Aust Paediatr J 1984; 20:177–780.

68. Reif S, Belor B, Villa Y, et al. Long-term follow-up and outcome of infants with non-organic failure to thrive. Isr J Med Sci 1995; 31:483–489.

69. Corbett SS, Drewett RF, Wright CM. Does a fall down centile chart matter? The growth and developmental sequelae of mild failure to thrive. Acta Paediatr 1996; 85:1278–1283.

70. Mackner LM, Starr RH Jr, Black MM. The cumulative effect of neglect and failure to thrive on cognitive functioning. Child Abuse Neglect 1997; 21:691–700.

71. Barker DJP. Early growth and cardiovascular disease. Arch Dis Child 1999; 80:305–310.

Chapter 13
Gastrointestinal hemorrhage

Marsha Kay and Robert Wyllie

INTRODUCTION

Gastrointestinal hemorrhage is a common problem encountered by pediatric gastroenterologists and those caring for children. Hemorrhage can be from a variety of etiologies. The disorders causing gastrointestinal (GI) bleeding can range from minor problems to severe life threatening conditions. Parents are often alarmed with any type of unexpected bleeding and will appropriately seek immediate medical attention. Patients who are seriously ill require timely, focused and appropriate assessment and treatment. In contrast, patients with trivial bleeding of readily discernible etiology who are not seriously ill still require assessment, but may require little if any further testing or therapy.[1] Balancing these extremes can be challenging. This chapter describes an approach to the patient with gastrointestinal bleeding that will assist the physician in determining the urgency with which to proceed with an evaluation and reviews the utility of diagnostic tests, the differential diagnosis and therapeutic modalities available for use. The pathophysiology of disorders associated with gastrointestinal blood loss is reviewed elsewhere, in the text.

Historical information
Present illness
Source of bleeding
Magnitude of bleeding
Duration of bleeding
Associated gastrointestinal symptoms (vomiting, diarrhea, pain)
Associated systemic symptoms (fever, rash, joint pains)
Review of systems
Gastrointestinal disorders
Liver disease
Bleeding diatheses
Anesthesia reactions
Medications (NSAIDs, warfarin, hepatotoxins, recent antibiotic use)
Recent travel, ill contacts and contacts with animals
Family history
Gastrointestinal disorders (polyps, ulcers, colitis)
Liver disease
Bleeding diatheses
Anesthesia reactions

NSAIDs, non-steroidal anti-inflammatory drugs.

Table 13.1 Historical information

Definitions

Melena is the passage of black, tarry stools. *Hematochezia* is the passage of bright or dark red blood per rectum. *Hematemesis* is the passage of vomited material that is black ('coffee grounds') or contains frank blood.

Initial assessment

Patients with symptoms of GI bleeding may contact the physician by phone, present to the physician's office or present to the emergency room for evaluation. Office personnel who are triaging calls from patients with GI bleeding must be trained to gather enough information to determine whether the patient is seriously ill and should undergo immediate examination (in the office or in the ER) or if the patient may undergo elective evaluation.[1] Historical information that should be obtained in any patient with acute GI bleeding is indicated in Table 13.1. The source, magnitude and duration of bleeding must be documented. If a parent or caregiver has not witnessed the bleeding and if the child is old enough they may be able to provide an estimate of the amount of bleeding. The presence of other gastrointestinal symptoms (e.g. diarrhea, cramping, abdominal pain, constipation, vomiting) should be determined. The presence of systemic symptoms (e.g. fever, rash, dizziness, shortness of breath, pallor, palpitations, cool extremities) should also be determined. In the acutely ill child, an abbreviated review of systems, pertinent medical history and family history that includes gastrointestinal disorders, liver disease, bleeding diatheses and medication use should be obtained. In patients who are stable, a complete review of systems, past and family history should be obtained. For patients who are calling the office, if the interviewer suspects severe bleeding is occurring, instructions should be given to immediately access local emergency services. Patients who appear to be critically ill in the office or emergency room should undergo immediate stabilization.

Phone intake from patients known to the physician's practice who are chronically ill represent a special case.[2] A patient with long-standing ulcerative colitis who describes tenesmus and liquid stools that are almost all blood requires a different approach from a toddler with painless, intermittent small volume bright red rectal bleeding. The approach to patients with chronic medical conditions must be individualized based on their diagnosis, current medication regimen and recent changes in their medicines.

In evaluating the child with GI hemorrhage, physicians must make several rapid determinations: (1) Has the child been bleeding? (2) Was/is the bleeding of sufficient magnitude to result in actual or impending circulatory compromise? (3) Is the child bleeding now? (4) What actions are required? In some instances, caregivers or children will report 'blood' in their stool or emesis when blood was not actually present. Foods and medications that can alter the color of stool or vomitus and result in unnecessary diagnostic testing or therapy are indicated in Table 13.2.[3–5] Red foods and medications and deeply pigmented foods such as blueberries can all result in stools or vomitus that can fool even the experienced observer into believing that blood is present. Although it is reassuring to find that a child with black stools recently ingested a bismuth preparation, it is imperative to determine whether the stools are guaiac-positive. If the test is rapidly positive, the child has been passing blood until proven otherwise. If a single test is negative and the stools have been only intermittently dark, then serial stool examinations, determination of the blood count and observation may be indicated. In the case of vomitus, a test kit for gastric fluid (e.g. Gastroccult) should be used rather than the routine stool kits, because they are more reliable at an acid pH.[1,6]

The questions of duration and magnitude of bleeding are more difficult to answer. Children beyond the age of toilet training do not routinely share their bowel habits with their parents. In addition, they do not know the range of normal or what is abnormal. Frank blood makes children alarmed regardless of the source, but melena may be ignored for some time. Lay persons routinely overestimate the amount of blood passed in the stool or in vomited material. In practice, comparison with the first day of a menstrual period provides a useful guide to the amount of blood passed. If the water of the commode is opacified with blood, the bleeding is likely to be significant.

Physical examination and laboratory evaluation

On physical examination (Table 13.3), the presence or absence of signs of anemia (e.g. pallor) is useful to confirm whether a significant amount of blood has been lost. Typically, gradual blood loss is better tolerated than rapid blood loss and has a lower likelihood of cardiovascular decompensation. In both acute and chronic blood loss, decompensation eventually occurs. The presence of resting tachycardia or orthostatic changes in blood pressure and heart rate indicates actual or impending decompensation of circulatory status regardless of the duration of bleeding.

Red	Black
Candies	Bismuth
Fruit punch	Activated charcoal
Beets	Iron
Laxatives	Spinach
Phenytoin	Blueberries
Rifampin	Licorice

Table 13.2 Substances that commonly color emesis or stools

- Skin
  - Pallor
  - Jaundice
  - Ecchymoses
  - Abnormal blood vessels
  - Hydration
  - Rash
- Head, eyes, ears, nose and throat
  - Nasopharyngeal injection, oozing
  - Tonsillar enlargement, bleeding
- Cardiovascular
  - Heart rate: lying, sitting, upright
  - Pulse pressure: lying, sitting, upright
  - Gallop rhythm
  - Capillary filling
- Abdomen
  - Organomegaly
  - Tenderness
- Perineum
  - Fissure
  - Fistula
  - Rash
  - Induration
  - External hemorrhoids or vascular lesion
- Rectum
  - Gross blood
  - Melena
  - Tenderness

Table 13.3 Physical examination

Laboratory studies can assist the physician in assessing the magnitude and duration of blood loss. For chronic loss, reductions in the red blood cell (RBC) count, hemoglobin and hematocrit are the most useful indices of the magnitude of loss. With acute bleeding, values must be interpreted in light of the hydration status. The presence of anemia with normal RBC volume is indicative of rapid loss of circulating volume; conversely, the presence of anemia with reduced RBC volume is suggestive of chronic loss. Caveats to these last points include folate or vitamin B_{12} deficiency in the former case and hemoglobinopathies in the latter.

The question of whether the child is actively bleeding at the time of the examination can be difficult to answer. Placement of a nasogastric tube is often employed to evaluate complaints of hematemesis and melena, symptoms most often associated with sources of bleeding in the upper gastrointestinal tract. If the lavage aspirate is clear and contains neither coffee grounds nor fresh blood, bleeding proximal to the ligament of Treitz is less likely.[7] If the aspirate contains coffee grounds and then rapidly clears, the bleeding probably originated in the upper intestinal tract but may have ceased. If the aspirate contains fresh blood or a mixture of fresh and old blood that does not rapidly clear, the bleeding probably originated in the proximal gastrointestinal tract and continues to be active. Some physicians prefer not to place NG tubes in a patient with known or suspected varices. Irrigation may also dislodge or 'wash off' a clot that is tamponading a visible vessel in an acute ulcer. Although the likelihood of this is small, physicians must be prepared to deal with a potential increase in bleeding if nasogastric lavage is performed.

Regarding more distal sources, the best assessment of active bleeding is observation of stool output and character combined with serial hemoglobin, or hematocrit measurements. Although hematochezia usually signifies a more distal bleeding source, patients with severe upper tract bleeding may present with hematochezia and diarrhea, as blood acts as a cathartic within the GI tract.

The actions to be taken are dictated by the history and the findings on physical examination. The initial focus of the history should be to identify the patient at risk for circulatory compromise. Questions should initially be brief and should be asked while the initial physical assessment proceeds. The initial physical assessment must include the following: vital signs, including orthostatic maneuvers; examination of the skin for signs of pallor, jaundice, pruritus, spider hemangiomata, ecchymoses and prominent vessels on the abdomen; examination of the abdomen for organomegaly, masses and tenderness; examination of the oropharynx for signs of bleeding from the nasopharynx, tonsils or buccal mucosa; examination of the perineum for fissures, fistulae, or indurations; rectal examination for tenderness and blood; and, in the case of hematemesis, consideration of nasogastric aspiration. If the patient has signs of actual or impending circulatory compromise, resuscitation should be prompt and thorough. Resuscitation should be completed before radiographic or endoscopic studies are considered. Resuscitation should include establishment of intravenous access, fluid resuscitation either crystalloid or colloid depending on the estimated degree of blood loss, blood typing if transfusion may be required and medication administration as necessary and transport to the appropriate location for ongoing stabilization and management such as a pediatric intensive care unit if necessary.

If the initial physical examination does not demonstrate the presence of actual or impending circulatory compromise, then a complete history of the present illness, along with a review of systems, a family history and the physical examination should be completed as would be appropriate for any consultation.

LABORATORY ASSESSMENT

The history and physical examination should guide the use of laboratory tests in patients with gastrointestinal bleeding. In general, laboratory tests should be limited to those that are appropriate to the clinical setting. For some patients, testing may be extensive, but for most, the initially indicated studies are decidedly fewer (Table 13.4).

Patients with hematemesis, melena, or both, require limited laboratory testing if they do not show signs of cardiovascular compromise, systemic disease, or portal hypertension. A complete blood count with platelet quantification and possibly prothrombin and partial thromboplastin times and type and screen or crossmatch may be indicated in this setting. Patients with signs and symptoms suggestive of isolated portal hypertension or chronic liver disease with cirrhosis require an extensive evaluation to assess the magnitude of altered hepatic synthetic, metabolic and excretory function. In addition, studies are needed to identify the cause of liver disease. Imaging studies including abdominal ultrasound, hepatic Doppler flow studies and possibly CT or MRI imaging of the abdomen and likely later elective liver biopsy are also a part of the evaluation for almost all patients in this situation.[8] Patients with signs and symptoms of other chronic diseases, such as decreased muscle mass, subcutaneous tissue mass, fever, or fatigue, may require more extensive testing appropriate to the age of the patient and suspected underlying condition.

Signs of shock, systemic or liver disease absent	Signs of shock, systemic or liver disease present
Complete blood count	Complete blood count
Erythrocyte sedimentation rate	Erythrocyte sedimentation rate
BUN	Prothrombin time
Prothrombin time	Partial thromboplastin time
Partial thromboplastin time	Guaiac stool, emesis
Guaiac stool, emesis	Blood typing and crossmatch
	Aspartate aminotransferase
	Alanine aminotransferase
	γ-Glutamyl transpeptidase
	BUN
	Creatinine
	Albumin
	Total protein

Table 13.4 Initial laboratory studies

Patients who present with hematochezia also may require a variable number of tests.[9] Children with painless rectal bleeding consistent with polyps should have a complete blood count. Children with massive, paroxysmal, painless rectal bleeding require a blood count and a nuclear medicine scan to rule out the presence of a Meckel's diverticulum. Infants with a history and physical examination consistent with functional constipation, anal fissure, or allergic colitis require little if any laboratory testing. Flexible sigmoidoscopy with biopsy can usually be performed in the office and will quickly establish the diagnosis in infants suspected of having allergic colitis, allowing for rapid dietary modification. Children with signs of an acute illness including fever and joint pains require a complete blood count, erythrocyte sedimentation rate, stool examination for culture for enteric pathogens, ova and parasite examination and *Clostridium difficile* toxin assay. If there is concern that the patient is dehydrated or that hemolytic-uremic syndrome is present, or if it is unclear whether the bleeding is occurring in the upper or the lower portion of the intestinal tract, serum bicarbonate, blood urea nitrogen, (BUN) and creatinine should be measured and urine output must be monitored. The BUN/creatinine ratio may be useful in assessing whether the blood is arising high or low in the intestinal tract as children with a significant elevation of their BUN with a normal serum creatinine for age likely have an upper tract source for their bleeding.[10,11] A ratio of 30 or above is 98% sensitive and 69% specific for upper GI bleeding in

colon, which is made even more difficult by fresh blood in the GI tract. In patients who require rapid preparation of the colon, polyethylene glycol solutions have become the standard of care. These solutions can be administered either orally or via a nasogastric tube (50–80 ml/kg, usual maximal volume 4 l).[23,24] Children younger than 10 years of age are unlikely to orally ingest sufficient volume at a rate adequate to evacuate the colon and may require nasogastric administration. In patients who do not require preparation for an urgent examination, a variety of options are available including a combination of oral stimulants (e.g. magnesium citrate, senna, bisacodyl, oral phosphate containing preparations and polyethylene glycol) in combination with a clear liquid diet and enemas or suppositories can be given. Patients with significant bleeding and diarrhea such as those with a new diagnosis of ulcerative colitis or Crohn's disease may need minimal preparation to remove stool before the examination can proceed although in almost all cases they should still receive a bowel preparation.

In the case of upper intestinal bleeding, newer guidelines suggest that a patient requires only 2–3 h of fasting after a clear liquid meal before sedation or anesthesia.[25,26] Longer times are often required to clear solid foods, barium, antacids, or sucralfate to allow adequate visualization of the mucosa. Longer fasting times may also be required in patients with suspected strictures, gastroesophageal reflux disease or delayed gastric emptying, Unless there is an emergency situation, it is better to allow adequate time to clear the stomach before examination. In an emergency, gastric lavage with large-bore tubes is often helpful to provide clearance of the stomach contents to a degree sufficient to allow adequate examination of the mucosa. Use of smaller-bore tubes in young patients is often insufficient to provide adequate clearance of the stomach for a complete examination of the gastric mucosa. Gastric lavage can also be performed during the endoscopic procedure using irrigation and suction through the endoscope channel.

The concept of urgent *vs* semi-elective endoscopy has been one of considerable debate. Urgent endoscopy allows prompt diagnosis and the ability to guide or perform therapy to hasten cessation of bleeding. On the other hand, urgent endoscopy carries the risk of rapid decompensation in an unstable patient and poor visualization of the field due to inadequate preparation. Therefore, the trend has been to perform urgent endoscopy only for patients who cannot be stabilized, in those in whom surgery to provide emergency therapy is contemplated or if therapeutic intervention can be performed that would be expected to terminate the bleeding episode (i.e. injection or cauterization of a visible vessel or actively bleeding vessel, ligation or sclerotherapy of a bleeding varix or a Dieulafoy's lesion). In this setting, the increased risks become appropriate; one will either attempt to stop the bleeding with endoscopic treatment or provide guidance to the surgeon who will do so by other operative means.

Our opinion is that the standard of care has evolved in favor of therapeutic endoscopy; that is, the endoscopist should be prepared to proceed with therapy if a bleeding lesion such as a varix or ulcer is encountered. Pediatric endoscopists should be familiar with techniques such as injection therapy, thermocoagulation and band ligation and know appropriate solutions and volumes for injection and appropriate coagulation settings as well as endoscope and equipment limitations in the young patient.[12] At some centers, an attempt has been made to have a limited number of practitioners perform therapeutic endoscopy so that they can accumulate the necessary experience.[12,27] At other centers, surgeons or adult gastroenterologists are asked to assist with such patients. In the latter setting, it is critical that the pediatric gastroenterologist collaborates with other practitioners to ensure that lesions are interpreted in the appropriate context. Furthermore, although the surgeon or adult gastroenterologist may be expert with the techniques required to achieve hemostasis, he or she is not likely to be expert in pediatric endoscopy. These issues remain controversial and will undoubtedly evolve in the coming years.

The selection of the endoscopic examination to be performed is relatively straightforward. For patients with melena or hematemesis in whom the source of bleeding is likely to be proximal to the ligament of Treitz, the first examination is typically esophagogastroduodenoscopy (EGD). In patients with hematochezia, colonoscopy is usually the first examination, although EGD may be required as indicated above in patients with significant upper tract bleeding and rapid transit. Colonoscopy has replaced flexible sigmoidoscopy as the first line examination for a number of reasons, but primarily due to improved technique and the widespread availability of appropriately sized pediatric endoscopes and well-trained pediatric endoscopists. In pediatric patients with juvenile polyps, in up to one-third of these patients the polyps will be located proximal to the splenic flexure requiring full colonoscopic examination and in a similar percentage of patients more than one polyp will be found if a complete colonoscopy is performed.[28,29] In patients with inflammatory bowel disease it is often helpful to assess the extent of upper tract involvement at initial endoscopy as well as performing a colonoscopy. Many centers perform both examinations at the time of diagnosis, especially in children suspected of having Crohn's disease. In patients with blood loss and anemia, when esophagogastroduodenoscopy and colonoscopy fail to identify the cause or site of bleeding, small bowel enteroscopy and video capsule endoscopy are adjunctive tools being increasingly performed in pediatric patients.[30] Intraoperative endoscopy can also be used to localize GI bleeding and can be used to resect lesions such as polyps or perform endoscopic therapy.[31]

THERAPY

Initial therapy for the pediatric patient with GI bleeding depends on the severity of the bleeding and the patient's underlying illness. Patients who are ill or with significant bleeding require supportive care: fluids including administration of blood products and drugs are used in resuscitation. For patients who are not critically ill, these approaches are not required. In the patient who has signs of cardiovascular compromise, appropriate supportive treatment and monitoring must be provided. In many cases, this requires the assistance of pediatric intensivists. When the patient has been adequately stabilized, diagnostic and therapeutic studies can proceed to allow more specific therapy to begin (Tables 13.6, 13.7).

In the past, gastric lavage and vasopressin administration were the initial therapies for patients with suspected stress ulcers, varices and diffuse gastritis. These therapies have assumed a secondary supportive role with advances in pediatric endoscopy and therapeutic endoscopy. Some pediatric gastroenterologists use gastric lavage not as a therapy but rather as a means to prepare the patient for endoscopy or to assess whether the patient is continuing to bleed. The literature is replete with multiple citations but few controlled studies that support the efficacy of iced lavage with or without epinephrine; these techniques are not without risks and are probably of little benefit.[32] Vasopressin is an effective agent to decrease splanchnic blood flow and thereby decrease gastrointestinal bleeding; it is also known to have significant side-effects including bowel ischemia that have significantly limited its use. Since the long-acting somatostatin analog Octreotide (Sandoz Pharma Ltd, Basel, Switzerland) has became available, vasopressin use has steadily declined. Somatostatin also decreases splanchnic blood flow and decreases gastric acid secretion. Somatostatin is at least as effective as vasopressin, has less effect on systemic blood flow and has a reduced frequency and severity of side effects compared with vasopressin although it must still be used with caution.[33–35] The mechanism by which Octreotide reduces splanchnic blood flow is not known.[34] Doses for acute GI bleeding are typically in the range of an initial i.v. bolus of 1 μg/kg bolus up to 50 μg and then 1–2 μg/kg per h, as a continuous infusion.[34,36] Usually the dose is gradually tapered after cessation of bleeding or endoscopic therapy rather than being abruptly stopped and Octreotide may be re-administered if rebleeding occurs.

Techniques available during therapeutic endoscopy are numerous but can be grouped.[37] The merits of each technique are beyond the scope of this chapter but can be obtained elsewhere and are also discussed elsewhere in the text.[12] Thermal energy can be used to cauterize a bleeding site.[38] Methods include monopolar cautery, bipolar cautery, heater probe, argon plasma coagulation and laser techniques.[5,39–41] Pressure can be used to tamponade a bleeding site.[42] When used in combination with application of thermal energy this is known as coaptive coagulation. Ulcers with a visible vessel or active bleeding can be injected with a variety of regimens usually including a combination of a 'sclerosing or hemostatic agent' and an agent that results in tamponade such as epinephrine thereby prolonging the contact time of the hemostatic agent. Epinephrine should be used only with caution with sclerosant medications and with established dosing regimens. For all injection methods, injection volumes should be precise and endoscopists must be familiar with appropriate dosing of injection medications including their possible adverse effects. For patients with esophageal varices, techniques to achieve hemostasis include intravariceal injection, paravariceal injection and band ligation.[43–47] Techniques can be modified for bleeding gastric varices. Hemostatic clips passed via the endoscopic channel can also be used in cases of bleeding due to ulcers.[41] The recent development of preloaded easily deployable clips will likely lead to increasing application of this technique for acute bleeding.[45] Band ligation of a bleeding Dieulafoy (submucosal) vessel has been reported.[48] Polyps that are the source of bleeding can be removed with electrocautery using monopolar hot biopsy forceps or bipolar snares. Patient grounding is required with monopolar techniques. The merits of each technique can be found in the appropriate citations and in the chapter on gastrointestinal endoscopy.

- Supportive care
  - Intravenous fluids (normal saline, Ringer's lactate)
  - Blood products (whole blood, packed RBCs, fresh-frozen plasma)
  - Vasopressors
- Specific care
  - Barrier agents (sucralfate)
  - H_2 antagonists (cimetidine, ranitidine, famotidine, nizatidine)
  - Proton pump inhibitors (omeprazole, lansoprazole, esomeprazole, pantoprazole)
  - Somatostatin analogue
- Endoscopic therapy
  - Injection (sclerosant, epinephrine, normal saline, hypertonic saline)
  - Coagulation (bipolar coagulation, heater probe, laser, argon plasma coagulator)
  - Variceal injection or ligation
  - Band ligation
  - Polypectomy

Table 13.7 Therapy

DIFFERENTIAL DIAGNOSIS

Upper GI bleeding: neonate and infants

The diagnosis of gastrointestinal bleeding in the newborn (Table 13.8) presents special challenges. Significant bleeding in the newborn is uncommon.[49] When significant bleeding does occur, the limited reserve of neonates makes them prone to decompensate quickly. The most common cause of blood in the stool or emesis of newborns is swallowed blood, either from amniotic fluid or from a fissure in the nipple of the breast-feeding mother. The Apt test[50–52] can be used to determine whether the blood is of maternal origin. This test is based on the premise that fetal hemoglobin (HbF) has a greater resistance to alkaline denaturation than adult hemoglobin (HbA). Fetal blood remains pink with addition of sodium hydroxide whereas adult blood turns brown.[49] Spectrophotometric assay also distinguishes the hemoglobin types and may also be useful for a number of maternal hemoglobin variants.[52] Gastric or duodenal ulceration may occur in newborn infants related

Chapter 14
Eating disorders and obesity

Dean L. Antonson, Douglas G. Rogers and James K. Madison

ANOREXIA NERVOSA

Historical perspective

The first clinical description of anorexia nervosa in the medical literature was published by Richard Morton, physician to James II, in his textbook of medicine in 1689.[1] Significant time then elapsed before further descriptions of anorexia nervosa were noted in the literature, with Robert Whytt reporting a case in 1767 and Louis-Victor Marce of Paris reporting his observations in 1859.[2] In almost simultaneous reports in 1873 and 1874, Charles Laseque and William W. Gull laid the foundation for our current understanding of this disorder. In several reports in 1873, Laseque provided insight into the emotional etiology of this illness, and in 1874 William W. Gull further detailed the clinical findings of starvation, amenorrhea, loss of appetite, decreased vital signs, constipation and emaciation.[2] In 1914, Simmonds described a case of cachexia associated with pituitary infarction and suggested that the common cause for anorexia nervosa may well be pituitary insufficiency.[3] However, in 1949 Sheehan clearly established that pituitary insufficiency was rare, concluding that the majority of patients with anorexia nervosa did not have this dysfunction.[4] It was not until the 1960s that significant advancements in the understanding of anorexia nervosa occurred, led by the pioneering work of Hilde Bruch, who began to unravel the psychologic basis and identified three common hallmarks of the anorexic patient: a distorted body image, an inability to interpret hunger and satiety, and a paralyzing sense of ineffectiveness.[2] More recent contributions have been added by the extensive work of Gerald Russell, who also was the first to describe and define bulimia nervosa.[5]

Epidemiology

Five well controlled, multinational studies have examined the incidence of anorexia nervosa over sequential decades in a single population.[5] In Sweden, the incidence increased from 0.08 to 0.45 per 100 000 population from 1940 to 1960; in Monroe County, New York, it increased from 0.37 to 0.64 per 100 000 population from 1960 to 1976; and in Rochester, Minnesota, it increased from 4.63 to 14.2 per 100 000 population from 1950 to 1984.[5] Several investigators have normalized these rates to look at the specific at-risk population of young women aged between 15 and 25 years. They reported incidences ranging from 30 to as high as 156 per 100 000 population, making anorexia nervosa the third most common illness in female adolescents and young adults, after obesity and asthma.[6] Because patients with eating disorders are often very secretive about their behaviors and significant underreporting can be anticipated, the higher incidence rate may be more accurate. Several additional surveys indicate that anorexia nervosa may occur in as many as 1–5% of high-school and college-age females.[7,8] The incidence for males with anorexia nervosa is 5–10% of that for females.

The most commonly quoted prevalence rates for anorexia nervosa are between 0.5% and 1%, including the rates identified by the American Psychiatric Association in 1994.[9] A 1996 study from Sweden determined the prevalence rates for 15-year-olds to be 0.84% for girls and 0.09% for boys.[6]

In examining the lifetime prevalence of eating disorders in adolescents of both sexes, a 2004 study reported that the overall prevalence of all eating disorders for girls was 17.9%, for anorexia nervosa 0.7%, bulimia nervosa 1.2%, binge-eating disorders 1.5% and eating disorders not otherwise specified 14.6%. For boys, the corresponding prevalence for all eating disorders was 6.5%, anorexia nervosa 0.2%, bulimia nervosa 0.4%, binge-eating disorders 0.9% and eating disorders not otherwise specified 5.0%.[6,10,11]

More common is the pervasive presence of dieting behaviors in Western societies and the simultaneous presence of a distorted body image. A survey from Canada found that, by the age of 18 years, 50% of adolescent girls perceived themselves as being too fat, even though 80% of this group had normal bodyweights. Eighty per cent of this same female population desired to lose weight.[12] In a similar US study, one-half of all underweight female adolescents desired to lose weight and 80% claimed that they were unhappy with their present weight.[12] In a study from the Centers for Disease Control and Prevention, 44% of all adolescent girls were involved with dieting, whereas only 15% of boys were similarly concerned.[9] Forty per cent of the adolescent girls felt very negative about their body image, with their greatest displeasure being focused on their hips, waist and thighs.[9]

Although most early reports described anorexia nervosa as occurring primarily in white, middle- to upper-class females, more recent studies have demonstrated that anorexia nervosa is present at all socioeconomic levels and is seen in minority as well as white populations.[6,10,13] Anorexia nervosa is now also being reported from other countries, including Japan, China, Spain, Argentina and Fiji.[14] Rates in Japan now equal that in the USA.[14] Anorexia nervosa is especially prominent in appearance-related sports and occupations such as acting, modeling, ballet

Epidemiology

Like anorexia nervosa, bulimia nervosa is a disorder that occurs primarily in adolescent girls or young adult women. The male:female ratio is between 1:10 and 1:20, similar to that for anorexia nervosa. The overall incidence of bulimia nervosa is significantly higher than that of anorexia nervosa – between 3% and 10% for high-school and college-age females, with some series reporting an incidence as high as 20%.[37,38] The lifetime risk rates for bulimia nervosa were calculated by Fombonne to be 1.9% for women and 0.2% for men.[39] Fifty percent of patients with bulimia nervosa develop the condition before the age of 18 years.[12]

Prevalence rates for bulimia nervosa range from 3% to 10% in most studies.[9,12,37] The American Psychiatric Association places the prevalence of bulimia nervosa at 1–3% of the general population.[9]

The incidence of the partial syndrome of bulimia nervosa, in which the patient manifests many but not all of the symptoms of bulimia, is further increased, with many studies reporting that 17–19% of college-age women engage in bulimic behaviors.[25,40]

Development and clinical presentation

Bulimia nervosa generally begins with initiation of a diet by a teenager or young adult, again in reaction to the perception of being fat and overweight. After a relatively short period, dieting is deemed unsuccessful and too difficult to maintain. A means of short-circuiting the process to achieve a more rapid weight loss is then sought. The patient experiments with various means of purging, such as vomiting, use of diuretics or use of laxatives to eliminate the calories ingested. The loss of calories resulting from the purging behavior (or from restricted caloric intake after a binge) produces increasing hunger. The patient developing bulimia is unable to control her desire for food and initiates a binge-eating episode. The average intake of a binge episode has been estimated to be 4000 calories.[12] Severe guilt, resulting from the consumption of large amounts of food and superimposed on an impulsive behavioral pattern with poor self-control, culminates in an intense desire to eliminate the food, and purging then recurs. An initial sense of relief often follows the purging episode, and some patients with bulimia transfer this feeling to situations of stress. Purging may then become a mechanism of stress relief as well. While this process is developing, the bulimic individual remains very secretive about her behaviors, often concealing them from friends and family for years. Unlike the patient with anorexia nervosa, the bulimic patient ultimately perceives her difficulties as problematic and often seeks help or assistance, particularly when the disorder progresses to the point that most of her daily thoughts and actions are controlled by this process.

Early in the process, bulimic individuals may seek medical attention, but not because of the difficulties or guilt associated with bingeing and purging. Rather, they present with requests for information on weight loss and dieting, or requests for diuretics and treatment of fluid retention.

Etiology

The pathogenesis of bulimia nervosa, like that of anorexia nervosa, is multifactorial and encompasses familial, developmental, social, cultural, physiologic and genetic factors. Familial factors are supported by the strong association of bulimia with affective disorders (depression and dysthymia) and a strong family history of affective disorders in first-degree relatives. Depression has been reported to be present in as many as 50% of first-degree family members of bulimics.[41] Additionally, alcoholism and drug addiction are prevalent, alcoholism being reported in 50–60% of first- and second-degree family members.[42] Common behavioral patterns within families include high levels of family conflict, unstructured and ambivalent lines of authority, high achievement orientation and low expressivity.[43] Affective instability and low self-esteem are the hallmark personality features of bulimia nervosa.[43] Marked ineffectiveness, significant self-criticism, learned helplessness and a high achievement orientation all are significant predisposing factors. Significant body dissatisfaction, body image distortion and difficulties with sexual identification are also present. Studies have shown that the incidence of sexual abuse in bulimia nervosa is no higher than that seen in adolescents presenting with other psychiatric disorders.[44]

Dieting in the bulimic individual rarely progresses to the point of fully disrupting hunger and satiety. The poorly self-controlled, impulsive individual developing bulimia cannot override the strong urge of hunger, loses control and binges on food. The subsequent sense of loss of control resulting from this behavior further intensifies the desire to diet. When rapid results are not achieved by dieting, a means to short-circuit the process by purging is sought. Although initially this is followed by relief, the bulimic individual begins to loathe once again the loss of self-control resulting from the purging and attempts to intensify dieting, thereby establishing a positive reinforcing loop that results in repetitive cycles of bingeing and purging.

Clinical and laboratory features

Most bulimic individuals are of normal weight, and their behavior remains quite secretive until their difficulties with loss of control lead to their desire to confront it. Before this, however, it is not uncommon for the bulimic individual to seek medical care for one of the many associated signs or symptoms of this disorder, including fluid retention, abdominal fullness, frequent headaches, chest pain, constipation, hematemesis and dental problems (Table 14.3). On physical examination, three distinct abnormalities may be recognized that are pathognomonic for bulimia nervosa:

- Calluses or scarring over the dorsum of the hand or fingers used to induce vomiting (Russell's sign)
- Hypertrophy of the salivary glands (sialoadenitis)
- Erosion of the dental enamel (perimolysis).

Up to 70% of bulimics have dental caries, and an even greater percentage demonstrate perimolysis on careful

Gastrointestinal	
Constipation	Dyspepsia
Cathartic colon	Barrett's esophagus
Esophagitis	Gastroparesis
Esophageal ulcer, stricture, rupture	Pancreatitis
Mallory–Weiss tear	Gastric rupture
Dysphagia	Abdominal pain
Oral/Dental	
Perimolysis – lingual and occlusal surfaces	Cheilosis
Dental caries	Sialadenosis 10–50%
Pharyngeal erythema/soreness	Salivary hyperamylasemia
Dermatologic	
Russell's sign (calluses over fingers)	
Cardiovascular	
Arrhythmias	Ipecac toxicity
Hypotension	Palpitations
Mitral valve prolapse	
Pulmonary	
Aspiration pneumonia	Pneumothorax
Pneumomediastinum	
Neurologic	
Seizures (diet pill toxicity)	Increased ventricular size
Neuromyopathy (ipecac toxicity)	Widened sulci
Renal	
Failure	Proteinuria
Hematuria	Azotemia
Dehydration	
Fluid and Electrolytes	
Dehydration	Metabolic alkalosis
Hypokalemia	Metabolic acidosis
Hyponatremia	Pseudo-Bartter's syndrome
Hypochloremia	Hypomagnesemia
Endocrinologic	
Increased cortisol	Irregular menses
Hypoglycemia	Increased miscarriage rates
Increased birth complications	

Table 14.3 Clinical and laboratory complications of bulimia nervosa

examination.[45] A chronic sore throat is frequently reported, and on physical examination the posterior pharyngeal areas are erythematous. Occasionally, Mallory–Weiss tears and esophageal rupture occur with persistent and frequent vomiting. Esophageal rupture (Boerhaave's tear) continues to carry a mortality rate of 20%.[37] Although amenorrhea is uncommon, menstrual irregularities are frequently noted.[26]

On laboratory testing, the bulimic individual is often found to have electrolyte abnormalities, most commonly hypokalemia, hyponatremia and hypochloremic alkalosis.[46] Profound electrolyte abnormalities, with potassium levels lower than 3.0 mEq/l, can occur with laxative or diuretic abuse. Chronic dehydration is frequently present as well (see Table 14.3).

Medical complications

Table 14.3 lists the common medical complications seen in association with bulimia nervosa. The majority of these complications are caused by the abnormal bingeing and purging behaviors used by the patient. Gastrointestinal side-effects remain the most common, including abdominal and epigastric pain, hematemesis, persistent sore throat and constipation. Gastrointestinal and electrolyte abnormalities are frequently seen with laxative abuse and may be quite prominent. Over-the-counter laxatives containing phenolphthalein are usually used. The amount of laxatives taken varies from 3 to 4 doses per day up to 150 doses per day. Long-term chronic use of stimulant cathartics may ultimately result in a cathartic colon requiring extensive medical and possibly surgical management.

ECG abnormalities are again common in patients with bulimia nervosa. Particularly worrisome are the ECG abnormalities occurring in association with profound hypokalemia, which can result in arrhythmias and sudden death. Cardiac arrhythmias are the leading cause of death among patients with bulimia nervosa.[12] As with anorexia nervosa, central nervous system changes, with an increase in sulcal spaces and ventricular size, have been noted for bulimia nervosa, in spite of maintaining a normal weight.[26,29] Again, these structural changes appear to be only partially reversible after treatment of the disorder. Recently, reduced thalamic and hypothalamic serotonin transporter availability has been reported, and increases the longer the bulimia persists.[29] Erosion of the dental enamel, particularly involving the lingual and occlusal surfaces, may be severe. Complete loss of teeth may occur as early as the third decade.

Diagnostic criteria

Table 14.4 details the revised diagnostic criteria for bulimia nervosa as listed in the features of both anorexia and bulimia nervosa. The purging type of bulimic patient uses laxatives, diuretics, enemas or vomiting, whereas the non-purging type uses other compensatory behaviors, such as fasting or excessive exercise.

Treatment

If electrolyte abnormalities are severe, and particularly if potassium levels are below 3.0 mEq/l, potassium supple-

1. Recurrent episodes of binge-eating. An episode of binge-eating is characterized by both of the following: (1) eating, in a discrete period of time (e.g. within any 2-h period), an amount of food that is definitely larger than most people would eat in a similar period of time and under similar circumstances; and (2) a sense of lack of control over eating during the episode (e.g. a feeling that one cannot stop eating or cannot control what or how much one is eating)
2. Recurrent inappropriate compensatory behavior to prevent weight gain, such as self-induced vomiting; misuse of laxatives, diuretics, enemas or other medications; fasting; or excessive exercise
3. These behaviors both occur, on average, at least twice a week for 3 months
4. Self-evaluation is unduly influenced by body shape and weight
5. The disturbance does not occur exclusively during episodes of anorexia nervosa

Purging type: During the current episode of bulimia nervosa, the person has regularly engaged in self-induced vomiting or the misuse of laxatives, diuretics or enemas

Non-purging type: During the current episode of bulimia nervosa, the person has engaged in other inappropriate compensatory behaviors, such as fasting or excessive exercise

Table 14.4 Diagnostic criteria for bulimia nervosa

mentation may be required during the first few days of treatment. Dental consultation should be obtained for the majority of individuals who have used vomiting as a means of purging. The most troublesome medical problem is pseudo-Bartter's syndrome, which can occur after the abrupt discontinuation of diet pills or laxatives in patients who have had significant abuse of these medications.[47] Chronic laxative and diuretic abuse leads to a chronic state of dehydration, activating the renin–angiotensin–aldosterone system and resulting in hyperaldosteronism. Significant fluid retention and peripheral edema can occur within 2–7 days after cessation of the use of laxatives or diuretics in these patients. Diuretic therapy is frequently required for fluid mobilization, after which a slow tapering of diuretic medication can be achieved over the course of 4–12 weeks, while aldosterone levels slowly normalize. Potassium supplementation is frequently required during this period. Nutritional rehabilitation of the patient with bulimia nervosa focuses on stopping the purging behaviors; dispelling the myths and inaccuracies regarding food, calories and fat; and improving the body image distortion.

Prognosis: morbidity and mortality

Mortality rates for bulimia nervosa within 2–5 years of diagnosis continue to remain at 5%.[12] Some 50–60% of patients demonstrate recovery over this same period, with a relapse rate of 30–50%.[12] A review by Woodside[12] of four follow-up studies in patients 2 years after treatment demonstrated that 20–25% were well, 10–15% had minor slips, 15% had major slips, 15% were ill most of the time and 20–25% were ill continuously. The most prominent factor resulting in failure to remain well was co-morbidity with alcohol or drug use.[12]

PSYCHOTHERAPY AND PSYCHOTROPIC MEDICATIONS FOR ANOREXIA NERVOSA AND BULIMIA NERVOSA

Pretreatment assessment issues

A careful evaluation of the patient's psychologic status is warranted. Goals include excluding other explanations of the eating disturbance, assessing for the presence of other psychopathology, and developing clinical hypotheses about the psychologic processes that initiated and maintain the disorder. Some of the most common psychologic causes for disturbed eating, aside from anorexia and bulimia and related disorders, are depression, somatoform disorders, conditioned aversion and obsessive–compulsive disorder. These disorders can produce patterns of behavior very similar to those seen in eating disorders. All of these conditions can coexist with an eating disorder and may interact with symptoms of eating disorders in complex ways.

Failure to identify and treat concomitant psychologic disorders results in poorer long-term adaptation and decreased likelihood of successful treatment for the eating disorder. Malnutrition is known to produce depressive symptoms. Because rates of depression are high among people with eating disorders (69% in a University of Nebraska clinical sample), this is a particularly important diagnostic category of which the treatment team must be aware. Rates of obsessive–compulsive disorder as high as 69% have been found in a sample of anorexic patients.[48] The differential for this disorder again becomes important in that many patients with eating disorders have obsessions and compulsions regarding food or weight. These do not justify the additional diagnosis of obsessive–compulsive disorder unless there is evidence of manifestations that are not part of the typical patterns of thought and action seen in patients with eating disorders. When both disorders are present, the treatment plan must be modified to account for this great complexity. Anxiety disorders and addictive behaviors also are highly prevalent among patients with eating disorders and warrant careful attention during the evaluation. The frequent presence of a history of sexual abuse among such patients also indicates the need for screening for post-traumatic stress disorder.

Treatment should begin with consideration of why this particular person developed an eating disorder at this particular time in her life. Issues that have been identified as common among people with eating disorders, such as perfectionism, mistrust, poor awareness of internal cues and ineffectiveness, should be addressed. Additionally, the specific forms of eating-related thoughts and beliefs to which the patient subscribes should be identified. General patterns of behavior and attitudes toward self and others also are relevant, with particular attention to significant personality disorders, impulsivity and deficits in self-concept. Sources of stress should be identified. Family factors such as adaptability, cohesiveness, conflict resolution, openness to expressed emotion and emotional support are particularly relevant to treatment planning for children and adolescents.

Hospitalization

The most fundamental decision when treating a patient with a newly diagnosed eating disorder is whether hospitalization is necessary. One factor in this decision is the bodyweight of the patient. Anorexic patients who are at less than 70–75% of their ideal bodyweight are typically too compromised physically and psychologically to engage effectively in outpatient care. The authors have found that some long-term anorexic patients who are ready to commit to treatment are stable enough to make use of partial hospital programs rather than requiring full hospitalization. Conversely, younger patients with more recent onset tend to show signs of medical instability at higher weights than do older patients with more chronic conditions. Combined with the stronger denial that is common among young patients, they become poor candidates for outpatient approaches at higher weights. Because these younger patients also have the greatest opportunity to recover from such potential long-range problems as osteoporosis, the authors advocate more aggressive treatment, often considering hospitalization at 80% of ideal bodyweight.

For patients with bulimia, medical stability is a key issue in determining hospitalization. However, a very intense symptom such as vomiting six or more times per day also leads to consideration of hospitalization. Among both anorexic and bulimic patients, failure to achieve appropriate eating patterns and weight on an outpatient basis should be regarded as grounds to move the patient to more intensive care, such as partial hospital, residential or inpatient treatment. The presence of suicidal thoughts or serious self-injurious behavior also favors inpatient treatment, as it would for any patient. Finally, the coexistence of other significant mental health disorders (e.g. major depression, substance abuse or dependency) also indicates that outpatient care will be very difficult or not practical.

Treatment modalities

Psychopharmacology

At this time, no psychotropic medication has been shown to treat effectively the core symptoms of anorexia. Clinically, some anorexic patients do improve with administration of an antidepressant or other medication. Unpublished observations have suggested that the use of antidepressant medications may affect the rate of relapse among anorexics, but these data remain preliminary at this time.

There has been strong interest in using atypical antipsychotic medications such as olanzapine and carbamazepine for treating anorexia. Malina et al.[49] found that anorexic patients reported reduced anxiety about eating and weight gain during an open-label trial of olanzapine. Powers et al.[50] also reported that a majority of their patients in an open-label trial gained weight during a 10-week treatment, but there was no control group or extended follow-up. Weight gain also was moderate, averaging 8.75 lbs for the patients who gained weight.[50] Boachie et al.[51] reported more weight gain (0.99 kg/week) in a group of four patients with whom olanzapine was used to supplement inpatient treatment. However, this rate of weight gain is the standard expectation in inpatient treatment. Also, until broader controlled trials have been conducted, caution is warranted beause olanzapine has been implicated in inducing bulimic symptoms in patients without eating disorders.[52] Although no large-scale trials indicate effectiveness with eating disorders, Banas et al.[53] found that 32% of a diverse sample of patients whom they studied for clinical outcome was being treated with carbamazepine. However, its effectiveness has been studied only in studies of small sample size.[54]

Antidepressant medications have demonstrated effectiveness with bulimia. Significant reductions in frequency of bingeing and purging, and a variety of other measures of bulimic behavior, have been shown with the use of imipramine,[55] desipramine[56] and fluoxetine.[57] Goldbloom and Olmsted[58] showed that 8 weeks of treatment with a dose of 60 mg/day fluoxetine (Prozac) was more effective than either placebo or a 20-mg dose. Agras et al.[59] showed that 24 weeks' treatment with desipramine was more effective than 16 weeks. Other studies have demonstrated decreasing effectiveness with single medications over time, necessitating multiple sequential medication trials.[60] Although antidepressants are effective in the treatment of bulimia, a recent review of 19 trials has shown no differential effect of the efficacy of the various classes of antidepressants (tricyclic antidepressants, selective serotonin-reuptake inhibitors, monoamine oxidase inhibitors (MAOIs), and other classes).[61] The proportion of patients showing complete symptom remission tends to be lower with medication alone than when medication is combined with other treatments (see below). Mitchell et al.[55] noted that few studies of antidepressants show more than one-third of patients in remission at the end of the medication trial. Goldstein et al.[57] reported only 19% complete symptom remission among their patients treated with Prozac. Walsh et al.'s studies indicate that phenelzine was effective in reducing the frequency of binge-eating and produced a higher frequency of abstinence than placebo.[62–64] As in most studies of antidepressant effect on bulimia, the effect was not confined to patients with depression. None of Walsh et al.'s patients experienced hypertensive crisis,[63] but in a long term follow-up study of bulimic patients Fallon et al.[65] found three accounts of clinically significant hypertensive episodes, one of which was fatal. The MAOIs are not frequently used with bulimia owing to the difficulty in regulating food intake, which could increase the risk for adverse food–drug interactions.

Family therapy

Minuchen et al.[66] emphasized family processes of enmeshment, poor conflict resolution and difficulty adapting to change in their seminal volume on family therapy for patients with eating disorders. They were able to demonstrate the effectiveness of structural family therapy for patients with anorexia. Systemic[67] and behavioral[68] methods also have been prominent in the treatment of eating disorders. Shugar and Krueger[69] demonstrated significant correlation between family communication of aggression and improvement in patients' symptoms using systemic interventions. Their findings particularly implicated covert expression of aggression as a factor that may maintain anorexic behavior and thought patterns. VanFurth et al.[70] found that reduced maternal hostility correlated with improvement in anorexic patients during treatment. Humphrey[71] studied ratings of parent behavior and found that parents of anorexic patients tended to engage more in passive forms of hostility such as negating and ignoring their children, whereas parents of bulimics were more blaming and belittling than parents of adolescents without eating disorders.

Recent advances in family therapy have shown impressive promise in the treatment of anorexia nervosa[72] and, more recently, bulimia.[73] One method relies on a three-phase approach in which the family initially take control over the child's eating, then gradually returns control of eating to the patient after she has begun weight restoration, and finally actively teaches and encourages age-appropriate autonomy. This method has demonstrated good initial results with younger patients and is being tested further in multisite clinical trials. Eisler et al.[74] have shown effectiveness for two related forms of family therapy, conjoint family therapy (CFT) and separated family therapy (SFT), with some indication that SFT is more effective than CFT when there is a high level of maternal criticism toward the patient. Family therapies for anorexia have shown superior effectiveness to individual therapies primarily in patients with a short duration of illness (less than 3 years) and less than 18 years of age.[75,76] However, a recent study by Dare et al.[77] demonstrated relative effectiveness for a form of family therapy for outpatient anorexic adult patients compared with a placebo control treatment.

Cognitive behavioral therapy

Cognitive behavioral therapy (CBT) seeks to alter behavioral patterns, distortions in beliefs and dysfunctional self-perceptions that promote eating-disorder behaviors. The therapist assumes that the patient's beliefs about weight and body size trigger and maintain such behaviors. Initially, the therapist helps the patient challenge the dysfunctional beliefs by using corrective information, logic and experiential tests that the patient conducts as a form of homework. Ultimately, the patient learns to challenge mistaken beliefs and to correct other distortions such as negative self-evaluation, black-and-white thinking and perfectionistic attitudes. Fairburn et al.[78] provided a detailed explanation of the treatment model and methods for treating bulimia. Garner and Bemis[79] described modifications applicable to anorexia, but most of the research continues to focus on bulimia.

At the present time, CBT has the strongest research support of any intervention for eating disorders. Fairburn[80] demonstrated that this approach can produce success rates as high as 70% in outpatient treatment of bulimia. Fairburn et al.[81] monitored a group of patients who had received 18 weeks of treatment and found that almost 66% had no eating disorder after a mean follow-up of 5.8 years. Wilson and Fairburn[82] pooled data from 19 comparable controlled trials of CBT and demonstrated an 84% reduction in purging and a 79% reduction in binge-eating. The average complete abstinence rates were 48% and 62% for purging and binge-eating, respectively. Mitchell et al.[83] demonstrated similarly impressive results using group CBT. CBT was shown to be superior to either behavioral therapy or placebo.[83] Mitchell and co-workers[84] also presented evidence that twice-weekly therapy sessions may be more effective than traditional once-weekly schedules, at least in the context of group CBT.

CBT typically is superior to antidepressants alone. There seems to be little advantage in treating bulimic symptoms with antidepressants plus CBT rather than CBT alone.[85] Herzog and Sacks[86] found some indications that the combined treatment is more effective in earlier phases of therapy. Mitchell et al.[83] also noted that depressive symptoms improved more with combined CBT and imipramine treatment than with CBT alone, even though symptoms of the eating disorder were equally improved with either intervention. Walsh et al.[87] demonstrated some advantage in controlling binge-eating and depressive symptoms with a two-step antidepressant intervention that was used for patients who did not respond to an initial intervention with desipramine.

Interpersonal therapy

Interpersonal therapy (IPT) was originally developed as a treatment for depression and has had well documented success in that context.[88] Fairburn et al.[89] included IPT as a treatment control in a study of the effectiveness of CBT. The therapist helps the patient to evaluate interpersonal skills, conflicts with significant people, difficulty in role transitions, and resolution of any significant loss. The emphasis is on solving interpersonal problems and patterns of relating to others rather than on changing thoughts.

Although initial assessment indicated that IPT did not affect patients' concerns about weight and preoccupation with dieting, at 12 and 24 months of follow-up patients treated with IPT could not be differentiated from those treated with CBT.[89] Even on early post-treatment assessment, overt behavioral symptoms were not significantly different between the two groups of patients, although results in both cases were superior to those in untreated controls. The care with which these studies were conducted and the clarity of the results suggest that IPT should be given serious consideration in the treatment of bulimia, even though more research must be conducted. Wilfley[90] modified IPT for administration in a group format and reported good initial success in reducing binge-eating with this method.

Psychodynamic psychotherapy

Although the American Psychiatric Association practice guidelines[91] imply that psychodynamic therapy is appropriate for treating eating disorders and may be particularly useful with patients who are refractory to other treatments, there is sparse evidence to support this viewpoint. Garner et al.[92] demonstrated a 62% reduction in purging with the use of an 18-week psychodynamically oriented treatment. CBT produced reductions of 81.9% in their study. More significant was the discrepancy in abstinence rate: 12% for the dynamically treated group compared with 36% for those treated with CBT. Walsh et al.[87] evaluated the effectiveness of a supportive, psychodynamically based treatment for bulimia in a double-blind, placebo-controlled study including medications and CBT. CBT produced results superior to those achieved with supportive therapy or antidepressants alone. Supportive therapy combined with antidepressants was no more effective than antidepressants alone.

OBESITY IN CHILDREN

Childhood obesity is epidemic in the USA, and all indications are that it is getting worse. Using the 95th percentile for weight derived from the National Health and Nutrition Evaluation I (NHANES I), there has been a dramatic increase in the number of children above the 95th percentile in both the NHANES II (1976–1980) and especially the NHANES III (1988–1994).[93] Because of this, weight data only from NHANES I and NHANES II were used to create the currently available growth charts.[94] This explains such arithmetically impossible statements as '12% of boys age 12–17 years are above the 95th percentile for weight'.[93]

Obesity in childhood is defined as being abnormally heavy and having an abnormal amount of body fat. Most children with a body mass index (BMI) above the 95th percentile for age are considered obese. The BMI is a good estimate of body fat in all but the most well trained athletes.[95] Thus, a 'rock solid' football player who has a BMI over the 95th percentile would not be considered obese. BMI is easily calculated:

$$\text{BMI} = \text{weight (kg)}/\text{height}^2\ (\text{m}^2)$$

Multiple factors contribute to the development of obesity in children. However, the root cause is the sustained intake of more calories than the child's body requires. The family must accept the notion that when their child is gaining weight abnormally, he or she is consuming too many calories. Until the family accepts this, attempts at controlling weight gain are doomed to failure. You can estimate the amount of excess calories a child is taking in on an average daily basis by calculating how many pounds per year a child is gaining excessively, and multiplying this by 10. Doing this reinforces the fact that small, sustained imbalances between calories consumed and calories burned will result in abnormal weight gain. Thus, changes in the rate of weight gain (and not just loss of weight) should be used to judge whether changes in feeding behavior have had any effect on a child's weight gain.

As an example, an obese child who is gaining 50 lbs per year is taking in about 500 more calories per day than are required by their body. The family then eliminates all beverages that contain sugar from their household, including all soda pop, fruit juices and fruit punches. The child's rate of weight gain falls to 20 lbs per year (200 excess calories per day). This should be viewed as a good response to the changes the family has made, even though the child continues to gain weight.

Factors that contribute to the risk of becoming obese include genetics, environment, prenatal environment, activity level and feeding behavior. Of these, factors that healthcare providers may be able to influence are limited to activity level and feeding behavior.

The initial laboratory evaluation of an obese child should look for underlying conditions that may contribute to the development of obesity, as well as medical conditions that may result from the obesity (Table 14.5). If no underlying condition is discovered, behavioral changes as outlined below should be initiated.

Healthcare providers must be familiar with the 'Stages of Change' approach to help patients and families change their behavior (Table 14.6).[96,97] Programs that involve the family and apply behavior modification to feeding, food choices and activity have the best chance of long-term success.[98] When changing a child's behavior, all households that provide any care to the child must be identified, and the desired behavior change must be complete within each household to have any impact on the child. A separated or divorced parent may use abundant unhealthy foods to curry favor with the obese child versus the parent who is trying to implement changes within their household. Grandparents are notorious for sabotaging the good intentions of parents. Before embarking on a treatment plan for an obese child, the motivating factors for the child and their family must be discussed. Families who have been referred for treatment, but do not believe there is a problem, are in the stage of precontemplation (see Table 14.6). Just getting the family to appreciate the potentially lethal and debilitating consequences of severe childhood obesity is a step in the right direction. For families who are genuinely worried about their child's obesity, a treatment plan should be formulated that corresponds to the family's expectations and what co-morbidities exist as a result of the obesity. A child with pickwickian syndrome (obstructive sleep apnea and hypoventilation) requires much more aggressive intervention than a child with milder or no comorbidity. Realistic expectations must be set with the child and family before embarking on a treatment plan. An

Fasting glucose and insulin levels
Free T4, thyroid-stimulating hormone
Free testosterone (in adolescent girls)
Fasting lipid panel
ALT, AST levels
Other tests as indicated by the history or examination

Table 14.5 Laboratory evaluation of an obese child

Stage in transtheoretical model of change	Patient stage
Precontemplation	Not thinking about change May be resigned Feeling of no control Denial: does not believe it applies to self Believes consequences are not serious
Contemplation	Weighing benefits and costs of behavior Proposed change
Preparation	Experimenting with small changes
Action	Taking a definitive action to change
Maintenance	Maintaining new behavior over time
Relapse	Experiencing normal part of process of change Usually feels demoralized

From Prochaska et al., 1992.[97]

Table 14.6 'Stages of Change' model

adolescent who expects to lose 30 lbs in 30 days on a 'diet' is doomed to failure. That adolescent may lose 8 lbs in 1 month – a very good response to any feeding behavior change – but be so disappointed that they just give up and resume their previous feeding behaviors.

Feeding behaviors that may need to be changed in every household caring for the obese child who wishes to try to control their rate of weight gain are listed in Table 14.7. Each of these feeding behaviors should be dealt with separately, completely and permanently before attempting to make another behavior change. In most cases portion control and 'dieting' should be one of the last steps taken to control a child's rate of weight gain.

Some of these changes (see Table 14.7) deserve further consideration. Beverages that contain a high concentration of sugars provide excess calories that will not be compensated for by eating less solid food.[99] Many obese children rarely eat breakfast; this may lead to increased calorie intake in the late afternoon, when children are returning home from school, snacking and often unsupervised. The consumption of more than 3 g dietary fiber in the morning may decrease food-seeking behavior at lunchtime and possibly in the late afternoon.[100] Many cereals, oatmeal, breakfast bars and breads, if carefully selected, can provide 3 g or more of fiber per serving. Those individuals who do the family's food shopping must read nutrition labels and provide breakfast foods that contain more fiber to their family. Eating at 'fast food' restaurants is commonplace, and for some families difficult to avoid. Booklets are available that itemize the calories and other nutrients in most of the items offered at the most popular fast-food restaurants. Using this information, individuals can pick ahead of time those foods that are less calorically dense.

Patients and their families frequently misunderstand the role of activity and exercise in controlling an obese child's rate of weight gain. Many think that the activity is burning up extra calories. However, when a child exercises vigorously for 30 min they will burn off only about 180 calories. If the child then rewards itself by drinking a 12-oz can of unsweetened orange juice (180 calories), there is no net change in calorie intake. The major benefit of activity and exercise is due to the increase in muscle mass, and the resulting increase in an individual's resting metabolic rate.

Most children who are obese due to excess calorie consumption are tall for their age and genetic height potential. Obese children who are not tall for their age should be aggressively evaluated for possible underlying medical conditions that could be contributing to the obesity. Specific physical examination findings may suggest the presence of syndromes or medical conditions associated with obesity (Table 14.8). More often, physical examination findings detect medical conditions that have been caused by the obesity (Table 14.9). Many patients and families seek help to deal with abnormal weight gain solely for esthetic reasons. However, obese children and adolescents are much more prone to becoming obese adults than children of normal weight. In addition, prevention of the conditions listed in Table 14.9 provides even more reason for trying to decrease a child's rate of abnormal weight gain.

Some of the complications of childhood obesity are of particular interest to the pediatric gastroenterologist. Nonalcoholic fatty liver disease (NAFLD) is the most common form of liver disease in the USA. An alanine aminotransferase concentration four times greater than normal, and higher than the aspartate aminotransferase level, suggests NAFLD in the obese child. The prevalence of

Unhealthy feeding behavior	Desired behavior
Consuming large amounts of beverages that contain sugar	Complete elimination of beverages that contain sugar, including but not limited to all: fruit juice (sweetened and unsweetened), soda pop, fruit punches, sports drinks, iced tea
Eating calorically dense snacks after school and between meals	Providing air popped popcorn, fresh fruit or snacks cooked with Olestra
Drinking whole milk	Drinking fat-free milk
Skipping or not eating any fiber for breakfast	Eating a minimum of 3 g fiber every morning
Eating in front of the television	Eating meals with the family at table
Eating school lunches	Providing child with a healthy lunch to take to school every day
Rewarding accomplishments with food	Rewarding accomplishments with special activities
Eating at 'fast food' restaurants	Planning ahead what foods may be eaten at 'fast food' restaurants
Eating at buffet restaurants	Never eating at buffet restaurants

Table 14.7 Unhealthy feeding behaviors for obese children

Down syndrome
Prader–Willi syndrome
Cohen syndrome
Alstrom syndrome
Lawrence–Moon–Bardet–Beidel syndrome
Pseudohypoparathyroidism
Hypothyroidism
Cushing syndrome
Hypothalamic brain injury
Leptin deficiency (extremely rare)

Table 14.8 Examples of syndromes and medical conditions associated with obesity in children

Potentially life-threatening
Obstructive sleep apnea
Non-alcoholic fatty liver disease
Hypertriglyceridemia and pancreatitis
Type 2 diabetes mellitus
Depression
Potentially debilitating
Metabolic syndrome – central obesity, insulin resistance, low high-density lipoprotein levels, hypertriglyceridemia, hypertension
Polycystic ovary syndrome
Hypertension
Legg–Calve–Perthes disease
Slipped capital femoral epiphysis
Blounts disease
Hyperlipidemia
Gallstone formation
Gastroesophageal reflux disease (GERD)
Pseudo-tumor cerebri
Other conditions
Intertriginous irritation or infection
Acanthosis nigricans
Impaired glucose tolerance

Table 14.9 Co-morbidities and medical conditions caused by obesity in children

NAFLD in children can be expected to rise as a result of the increase in obesity and insulin resistance in children. Hyperinsulinemia causes increased triglyceride formation in the liver cell, and lower rates of hydrolysis and export of free fatty acids from the liver cell. Increased lipid peroxidation within the liver cell contributes to an inflammatory reaction that can eventually lead to steatohepatitis and fibrosis. Weight loss and improved insulin sensitivity are the only known treatments for NAFLD. However, rapid weight loss can exacerbate steatohepatitis and should be avoided.[101] Obesity accounts for the majority of gallstones in children who do not have another underlying medical condition that predisposes to gallstones. Obeisty causes increased biliary excretion of cholesterol relative to bile acid and phospholipid secretion, thus increasing the likelihood of gallstone formation. Rapid weight loss in an obese individual also increases the risk of gallstone formation.[102] Gastroesophageal reflux disease is also considered to be more common in obese than in non-obese children.

The use of medications to change the rate of weight gain in obese children has not been studied extensively. Available medications aim to decrease food-seeking (sibutramine) or block the absorption of nutrients (orlistat). The use of metformin has proven beneficial in children with polycystic ovary syndrome, insulin resistance and type 2 diabetes.[103]

Obese children are often depressed. The use of cognitive psychotherapy and bupropion can be particularly beneficial for treating the depression without any increase in food-seeking. Ultra-low-calorie, protein-sparing modified fasts have been used in adolescents with good success. This should be attempted only in those adolescents who are very motivated and have very supportive households. Complications from this diet are numerous, and careful medical supervision is required.[104] Bariatric surgery for obese children is now being offered at a few centers. It should be reserved for those individuals with serious co-morbidities who have failed to respond to feeding behavior changes, increased activity, portion control and medications.

Healthcare providers often neglect the prevention of obesity in at-risk children. A child born to two obese parents has a 12-fold greater risk of becoming obese than a child born to parents of normal weight. Because of this, the feeding behaviors of the family with two obese parents should be evaluated (see Table 14.6) and changed systematically where necessary to prevent the child from ever becoming obese. The obese parents should plan to award their children's achievements with special activities and not with food. Instead of taking their child to the local ice-cream parlor after the child hits a home run, consider taking them roller skating, horseback riding, swimming, to a water park, go-cart racing, canoeing, etc.

CONCLUSION

Obesity in children is increasing. This is due to many factors, including genetics, environment, prenatal environment, feeding behaviors and activity level. Every household that cares for an obese child must be assessed for the presence of behaviors that can contribute to abnormal weight gain. Each identified behavior must be dealt with individually using the 'Stages of Change' model for behavior change. The use of medications to help control weight gain in children has not been studied systematically. Despite this, the use of medications may be appropriate in some children. Portion control and 'dieting' are used only after changing the individual behaviors listed in Table 14.6 has been tried. Bariatric surgery in children should be used only as a last resort.

References

1. Bemporad JR. Self-starvation through the ages: reflections on the pre-history of anorexia nervosa. Int J Eat Disord 1996; 19:217–237.

2. Blinder BE, Chad K. Eating disorders: a historical perspective. In: Alexander-Mott L, Lumsden DB, eds. Understanding Eating Disorders: Anorexia Nervosa, Bulimia Nervosa, and Obesity. Washington, DC, Taylor & Francis; 1994:3–35.
3. Lucas AR. Anorexia nervosa: historical background and bio-psychosocial determinants. Semin Adolesc Med 1986; 2:1–9.
4. Slaby AE, Dwenger R. History of anorexia nervosa. In: Giannini AJ, Slaby AE, eds. The Eating Disorders. New York: Springer; 1993:1–17.
5. Russell GFM. Anorexia nervosa through time. In: Szmukler G, Dare C, Treasure J, eds. Handbook of Eating Disorders. New York: John Wiley; 1995:5–17.
6. Wakeling A. Epidemiology of anorexia nervosa. Psychiatr Res 1996; 62:3–9.
7. Hill OW. Epidemiologic aspects of anorexia nervosa. Adv Pschysom Med 1977; 9:45–62.
8. Kurtzman FD, Yaher J, Landsverk J, et al. Eating disorders among selected female student populations at UCLA. J Am Diet Assoc 1989; 39:45–53.
9. Thompson JK. Introduction. Body image, eating disorders, and obesity: an emerging synthesis. In: Thompson JK, ed. Body Image, Eating Disorders, and Obesity. Washington, DC: American Psychological Association; 1996:1–20.
10. Mehler PS. Eating disorders: 1. Anorexia nervosa. Hosp Pract 1996; 31:109–117.
11. Kjelsas E, Bjornstrom C, Gotestam KG. Prevalence of eating disorders in female and male adolescents (14–15 years). Eat Behav 2004; 5:13–25.
12. Woodside DB. A review of anorexia nervosa and bulimia nervosa. Curr Probl Pediatr 1995; 25:67–89.
13. Crago M, Shisslak CM, Estes LS. Eating disturbances among American minority groups: a review. Int J Eat Disord 1996; 19:239–248.
14. American Psychiatric Association Work Group of Eating Disorders. Practice guideline for the treatment of patients with eating disorders (revision). Am J Psychiatry 2000; 157(Suppl):1–39.
15. Drake MA. Symptoms of anorexia nervosa in female university dietetic majors. J Am Diet Assoc 1989; 39:97–98.
16. Sundgot-Borgen J, Torstveit MK. Prevalence of eating disorders in elite athletes is higher than in the general population. Clin J Sport Med 2004; 14:25–32.
17. Rayworth BB, Wise LA, Harlow BL. Childhood abuse and risk of eating disorders in women. Epidemiology 2004; 15:271–278.
18. Sokol MS. Infection-triggered anorexia nervosa in children: clinical description of four cases. J Child Adolesc Psychopharmacol 2000; 10:133–145.
19. Kuboki T, Nomura S, Ide M, et al. Epidemiological data on anorexia nervosa in Japan. Psychiatr Res 1996; 62:11–16.
20. Garner DM, Garfinkel PE. Socio-cultural factors in the development of anorexia nervosa. Psychol Med 1980; 10:647–656.
21. Vandereycken W, Meerman R. What are the causes? In: Anorexia Nervosa. A Clinician's Guide to Treatment. Berlin: Walter de Gruyter; 1984:43–64.
22. Brewerton TD, Jimerson DC: Studies of serotonin function in anorexia nervosa. Psychiatr Res 1996; 62:31–42.
23. Pirke KM. Central and peripheral noradrenalin regulation in eating disorders. Psychiatr Res 1996; 62:43–49.
24. Kaye WH. Neuropeptide abnormalities in anorexia nervosa. Psychiatr Res 1996; 62:65–74.
25. Zerbe KJ. Anorexia nervosa and bulimia nervosa: when the pursuit of bodily perfection becomes a killer. Postgrad Med 1996; 99:161–184
26. Treasure J, Szmukler G. Medical complications of chronic anorexia nervosa. In: Szmukler G, Dare C, Treasure J, eds. Handbook of Eating Disorders. New York: John Wiley; 1995:197–220.
27. Russell GFM. Premenarchal anorexia nervosa and its sequelae. J Psychiatr Res 1985; 19:363–369.
28. Herholz K. Neuroimaging in anorexia nervosa. Psychiatr Res 1996; 62:105–110.
29. Stamatakis EA, Hetherington MM. Neuroimaging in eating disorders. Nutr Neurosci 2003; 6:325–334.
30. American Psychiatric Association. Eating disorders. In: American Psychiatric Association: Diagnostic and Statistical Manual of Mental Disorders, 4th edn. Washington, DC: American Psychiatric Association; 1994:539–550.
31. Herzog DB, Greenwood DN, Dorer DJ, et al. Mortality in eating disorders: a descriptive study. Int J Eat Disord 2000; 28:20–26.
32. Keel PK, Dorer DJ, Eddy KT, et al. Predictors of mortality in eating disorders. Arch Gen Psychiatry 2003; 60:179–183.
33. Steinhausen HC. The outcome of anorexia nervosa in the 20th century. Am J Psychiatry 2002; 159:1284–1293.
34. Russell GFM. Bulimia nervosa: an ominous variant of anorexia nervosa. Psychol Med 1979; 9:429–448.
35. Giannini AJ. A history of bulimia. In: Giannini AJ, Slaby AE, eds. The Eating Disorders. New York: Springer; 1993:18–21.
36. Ziolko HU. Bulimia: a historical outline. Int J Eat Disord 1996; 20:345–358.
37. Mehler PS. Eating disorders: 2. Bulimia nervosa. Hosp Pract 1996; 31:107–126.
38. Crowther JH, Wolf EM, Sherwood NE. Epidemiology of bulimia nervosa. In: Crowther JH, Tennenbaum DL, HobFoll SE, Stephens MA, eds. The Etiology of Bulimia Nervosa. Washington, DC: Hemisphere; 1992:1–26.
39. Fombonne E. Is bulimia nervosa increasing in frequency? Int J Eat Disord 1996; 19:287–296.
40. Heatherton TF, Nichols P, Mahamedi F, Keel P. Body weight, dieting, and eating disorder symptoms among college students, 1982 to 1992. Am J Psychiatry 1995; 152:1623–1629.
41. Laessle RG. Affective disorders and bulimic syndromes. In: Fichter MM, ed. Bulimia Nervosa: Basic Research, Diagnosis, and Therapy. New York: John Wiley; 1990:112–125.
42. Bulik CM. Drug and alcohol abuse by bulimic women and their families. Am J Psychiatry 1987; 144:1604–1606.
43. Wonderlich S. Relationship of family and personality factors in bulimia. In: Crowther JH, Tennenbaum DL, HobFoll SE, Stephens MA, eds. The Etiology of Bulimia Nervosa. Washington, DC: Hemisphere; 1992:103–126.
44. Pope HG, Hudson JI. Is childhood sexual abuse a risk factor for bulimia nervosa? Am J Psychiatry 1992; 149:455–463.
45. McComb RJ. Dental aspects of anorexia nervosa and bulimia nervosa. In: Kaplan AS, Garfinkel PE, eds. Medical Issues and the Eating Disorders: The Interface. New York: Brunner/Mazel; 1993:101–122.
46. Mitchell JE, Pyle RL, Eckert ED, et al. Electrolyte and other physiological abnormalities in patients with bulimia. Psychol Med 1983; 13:273–278.
47. Mitchell JE, Pomeroy C, Seppala M, Huber M. Pseudo-Bartter's syndrome, diuretic abuse, idiopathic edema, and eating disorders. Int J Eat Disord 1988; 7:225–237.
48. Thiel A, Brooks A, Ohlmeier M, et al. Obsessive–compulsive disorder among patients with anorexia nervosa and bulimia nervosa. Am J Psychiatry 1995; 152:72–75.

49. Malina A, Gaskill J, McConaha C, et al. Olanzapine treatment of anorexia nervosa: a retrospective study. Int J Eat Disord 2003; 33:234–237.
50. Powers PS, Santana CA, Bannon TS. Olanzapine in the treatment of anorexia nervosa: an open label trial. Int J Eat Disord 2002; 32:146–154.
51. Boachie A, Goldfiled GS, Spettigue W. Olanzapine use as an adjunctive treatment for hospitalized children with anorexia nervosa: case reports. Int J Eat Disord 2003; 33:98–103.
52. Theisen FM, Linden A, Konig IR, et al. Spectrum of binge eating symptomatology in patients treated with clozapine and olanzapine. J Neural Transm 2003; 110:111–121
53. Banas A, Januszkiewicz-Grabias A, Radziwillowicz P, Smoczynski S. Follow-up study of quality of life and treatment of eating disorder: dynamics of the depressive and anxiety symptoms. Psychiatr Pol 2002; 36(Suppl):323–329.
54. Kaplan AS, Garfinkel PE, Darby PL, Garner DM. Carbamazepine in the treatment of bulimia. Am J Psychiatry 1983; 140:1225–1226.
55. Mitchell JE, Pyle RL, Eckert E, et al. A comparison study of antidepressants and structured intensive group psychotherapy in the treatment of bulimia nervosa. Arch Gen Psychiatry 1990; 47:149–157.
56. Walsh BT, Wilson GT, Loeb KL, et al. Medication and psychotherapy in the treatment of bulimia nervosa. Am J Psychiatry 1997; 154:523–531.
57. Goldstein DJ, Wilson MG, Thompson VL, et al. Long-term fluoxetine treatment of bulimia nervosa. Br J Psychiatry 1995; 166:660 666.
58. Goldbloom DS, Olmsted MP. Pharmacotherapy of bulimia nervosa with fluoxetine: assessment of clinically significant attitudinal change. Am J Psychiatry 1993; 150:770–774.
59. Agras WS, Rossiter EM, Arnow B, et al. One year follow-up of psychosocial and pharmacologic treatments for bulimia nervosa. J Clin Psychiatry 1994; 55:179–183.
60. Pope HG, Hudson JI. Biological treatment of eating disorders. In: Emmett SW, ed. Theory and Treatment of Anorexia Nervosa and Bulimia. New York: Brunner/Mazel; 1985:73–92.
61. Bacaltchuk J, Hay P. Antidepressants versus placebo for people with bulimia nervosa. Cochrane Database Syst Rev 2003(4):CD003391.
62. Walsh BT, Stewart JW, Roose SP, Gladis M, Glassman AH. A double-blind trial of phenelzine in bulimia. J Psychiatr Res 1985; 19485–489.
63. Walsh BT, Gladis M, Roose SP, Stewart JW, Stetner F, Glassman AH. Phenelzine *vs* placebo in 50 patients with bulimia. Arch Gen Psychiatry 1988; 445:471–475.
64. Walsh BT, Stewart JW, Roose SP, Gladis M, Glassman AH. Treatment of bulimia with phenelzine. A double-blind, placebo-controlled study. Arch Gen Psychiatry 1984; 41:1105–1109.
65. Fallon BA, Walsh BT, Sadik C, Saoud JB, Lukasik V. Outcome and clinical course in inpatient bulimic women: a 2- to 9-year follow-up study. J Clin Psychiatry 1991; 52:272–278.
66. Minuchen S, Roseman BL, Baker L. Psychosomatic Families: Anorexia Nervosa in Context. Cambridge, MA: Harvard University Press; 1978.
67. Selvini-Palazzoli M. Self-starvation: From Individual to Family Therapy in Treatment of Anorexia Nervosa, 2nd edn. New York: Jason Aronson; 1978.
68. Robin AL, Siegel PT, Moye A. Family versus individual therapy for anorexia: impact on family conflict. Int J Eat Disord 1995; 17:313–322.
69. Shugar G, Krueger S. Aggressive family communication, weight gain, and improved eating attitudes during systemic family therapy for anorexia nervosa. Int J Eat Disord 1995; 17:23–31.
70. VanFurth EF, VanStrein DC, Martina LM, et al. Expressed emotion and the prediction of outcome in adolescent eating disorders. Int J Eat Disord 1996; 20:19–31.
71. Humphrey LL. Family process in anorexia and bulimia. Address to the Thirteenth National Conference on Eating Disorders, Columbus, Ohio, October 1994.
72. Lock J, LeGrange D. Can family-based treatment of anorexia nervosa be manualized? J Psychother Pract Res 2001; 10:253–261.
73. LeGrange D, Lock J, Dymek M. Family-based therapy for adolescents with bulimia nervosa. Am J Psychother 2003; 57:237–251.
74. Eisler I, Dare C, Hodes M, Russell G, Dodge E, Le Grange D. Family therapy for adolescent anorexia nervosa: the results of a controlled comparison of two family interventions. J Child Psychol Psychiatry 2000; 41:727–736.
75. Russell GF, Szmukler GI, Dare C, Eisler I. An evaluation of family therapy in anorexia nervosa and bulimia nervosa. Arch Gen Psychiatry 1987; 44:1047–1056.
76. Eisler I, Dare C, Russell GF, Szmukler G, le Grange D, Dodge E. Family and individual therapy in anorexia nervosa. A 5-year follow-up. Arch Gen Psychiatry 1997; 54:1025–1030.
77. Dare C, Eisler I, Russell G, Treasure J, Dodge L. Psychologoical therapies for adults with anorexia nervosa: randomized controlled trial of out-patient treatments. Br J Psychiatry 2001; 178:216–221.
78. Fairburn CG, Marcus MD, Wilson GT. Cognitive behaviour therapy for binge eating and bulimia nervosa: a comprehensive treatment manual. In: Fairburn G, Wilson GT, eds. Binge Eating: Nature, Assessment and Treatment. New York: Guilford Press; 1993:361–404.
79. Garner DM, Bemis KM. Cognitive therapy for anorexia nervosa. In: Garner DM, Garfinkel PE, eds. Handbook of Psychotherapy for Anorexia Nervosa and Bulimia. New York: Guilford Press; 1985:107–146.
80. Fairburn CG. Cognitive behavioral treatment for bulimia. In: Garner DM, Garfinkel PE, eds. Handbook of Psychotherapy for Anorexia Nervosa and Bulimia. New York: Guilford Press; 1985:160–192.
81. Fairburn CG, Norman PA, Welch SL, et al. A prospective study of outcome in bulimia nervosa and the long-term effects of three psychosocial treatments. Arch Gen Psychiatry 1995; 52:304–312.
82. Wilson GT, Fairburn CG. Treatment of eating disorders. In: Nathan PE, Gorman JM, eds. Psychotherapies and Drugs That Work: A Review of the Outcome Studies. New York: Oxford University Press 2007 (in press).
83. Mitchell JE, Pyle RL, Eckert ED, et al. Antidepressant *vs*. group therapy in the treatment of bulimia. Psychopharmacol Bull 1987; 23:41–44.
84. Mitchell JE, Pyle RL, Pomeroy C, et al. Cognitive behavioral group psychotherapy of bulimia nervosa: importance of logistical variables. Int J Eat Disord 1993; 14:277–287.
85. Wilson GT. Cognitive behavioral treatment of bulimia nervosa. Clin Psychol 1997; 50:10–12.
86. Herzog DB, Sacks NR. Bulimia nervosa: comparison of treatment responders *vs*. nonresponders. Psychopharmacol Bull 1993; 29:121–125.
87. Walsh BT, Wilson GT, Loeb KL, et al. Medication and psychotherapy in the treatment of bulimia nervosa. Am J Psychiatry 1997; 154:523–531.

88. Klerman GL, Weissman MM, Rounsaville BJ, Chevron ES. Interpersonal Therapy of Depression. New York: Basic Books; 1984.
89. Fairburn CG, Peveler RC, Jones R, et al. Predictors of 12-month outcome in bulimia nervosa and the influences of attitudes to shape and weight. J Consult Clin Psychol 1993; 61:696–698.
90. Wilfley DE. Interpersonal psychotherapy adapted for group and for the treatment of binge eating disorder. Presented at the Thirteenth National Conference on Eating Disorders, Columbus, Ohio, October 1994.
91. Yager J, Andersen A, Devlin M, et al. Practice guidelines for eating disorders. Am J Psychiatry 1993; 150:207–223.
92. Garner DM, Rockert W, Davis R, et al. Comparison between cognitive behavioral and supportive–expressive therapy for bulimia nervosa. Am J Psychiatry 1993; 150:37–46.
93. Troiano RP, Flegal KM, Kuczmarski RJ, Campbell SM, Johnson CL. Overweight prevalence and trends for children and adolescents. The National Health and Nutrition Examination Surveys, 1963 to 1991. Arch Pediatr Adolesc Med 1995; 149:1085–1091.
94. National Center for Health Statistics. Growth charts. Online. Available: http://www.cdc.gov/growthcharts/ 22 March 2005
95. Himes JH, Dietz WH. Guidelines for overweight in adolescent preventive services: recommendations from an expert committee. Am J Clin Nutr 1994; 59:307–316.
96. Zimmerman GL, Olsen CG, Bosworth MF. A 'Stages of Change' approach to helping patients change behavior. Am Fam Physician 2000; 61:1409–1416.
97. Prochaska JO, DiClementecc, Norcross JC. In search of how people change. Am Psychol 1992; 47:1102–1104.
98. Epstein LH, Valaski A, Wing RR, McCurley J. Ten-year follow up of behavioral family-based treatment for obese children. JAMA 1990; 264:2519–2523.
99. Ludwig DS, Peterson KE, Gortmaker SL. Relation between consumption of sugar-sweetened drinks and childhood obesity: a prospective, observational analysis. Lancet 2001; 357:505–508.
100. Warren JM, Henry JK, Simonite V. Low glycemic index breakfasts and reduced food intake in preadolescent children. Pediatrics 2003; 112:e414–e419.
101. Charlton M. Nonalcoholic fatty liver disease: a review of current understanding and future impact. Clin Gastroenterol Hepatol 2004; 2:1048–1058.
102. Gungor N, Arslanian SA. Nutritional disorders: integration of energy metabolism and its disorders in childhood. In: Sperling M, ed. Pediatric Endocrinology. Philadelphia, PA: WB Saunders; 2002:689–724.
103. Freemark M, Bursey D. The effects of metformin on body mass index and glucose tolerance in obese adolescents with fasting hyperinsulinemia and a family history of type 2 diabetes. Pediatrics 2001; 107:E55.
104. Styne, D. Obesity. In: Pediatric Endocrinology. Philadelphia: Lippincott Williams & Wilkins; 2004:248–265.

Chapter 15
Jaundice

Glenn R. Gourley

INTRODUCTION

The term *jaundice* originated from the French *jaune,* which means 'yellow'. Jaundice, or icterus (from the Greek *ikteros*), refers to the yellow discoloration of the skin, sclerae and other tissues caused by deposition of the bile pigment bilirubin. Jaundice is a sign that the serum bilirubin concentration has risen above normal levels (approximately 1.4 mg/dl after 6 months of age; 1 mg/dl = 17 μmol/l). The intensity of the yellow color is directly related to the level of serum bilirubin and the related degree of deposition of bilirubin into the extravascular tissues. The yellow skin of hypercarotenemia is not associated with yellow sclerae.

BILIRUBIN METABOLISM

The term *bilirubin* is derived from Latin (*bilis*, bile; *ruber*, red) and was used in 1864 by Städeler[1] to describe the red-colored bile pigment. Bilirubin is formed from the degradation of heme-containing compounds (Fig. 15.1). The largest source for the production of bilirubin is hemoglobin. However, other heme-containing proteins are also degraded to bilirubin, including the cytochromes, catalases, tryptophan pyrrolase and muscle myoglobin.

The formation of bilirubin is accomplished by cleavage of the tetrapyrrole ring of protoheme (protoporphyrin IX), which results in a linear tetrapyrrole. The first enzyme system involved in the formation of bilirubin is microsomal heme oxygenase.[2] It is located primarily in the reticuloendothelial tissues and to a lesser degree in tissue macrophages and intestinal epithelium. This enzyme system results in reduction of the porphyrin iron (Fe^{3+} to Fe^{2+}) and hydroxylation of the α methine (=C–) carbon. This α-carbon is then oxidatively excised from the tetrapyrrole ring, yielding carbon monoxide. This excision opens the ring structure and is associated with oxygenation of the two carbons adjacent to the site of cleavage. The cleaved α-carbon is excreted as carbon monoxide and the released iron can be reused by the body. The resultant linear tetrapyrrole is biliverdin IXα. The *IX* designation is a result of Fischer's grouping of the protoporphyrin isomers, group IX being the physiologic source of bilirubin.

The stereospecificity of the enzyme produces cleavage almost exclusively at the α-carbon of the tetrapyrrole. This is unlike *in vitro* chemical oxidation, which results in

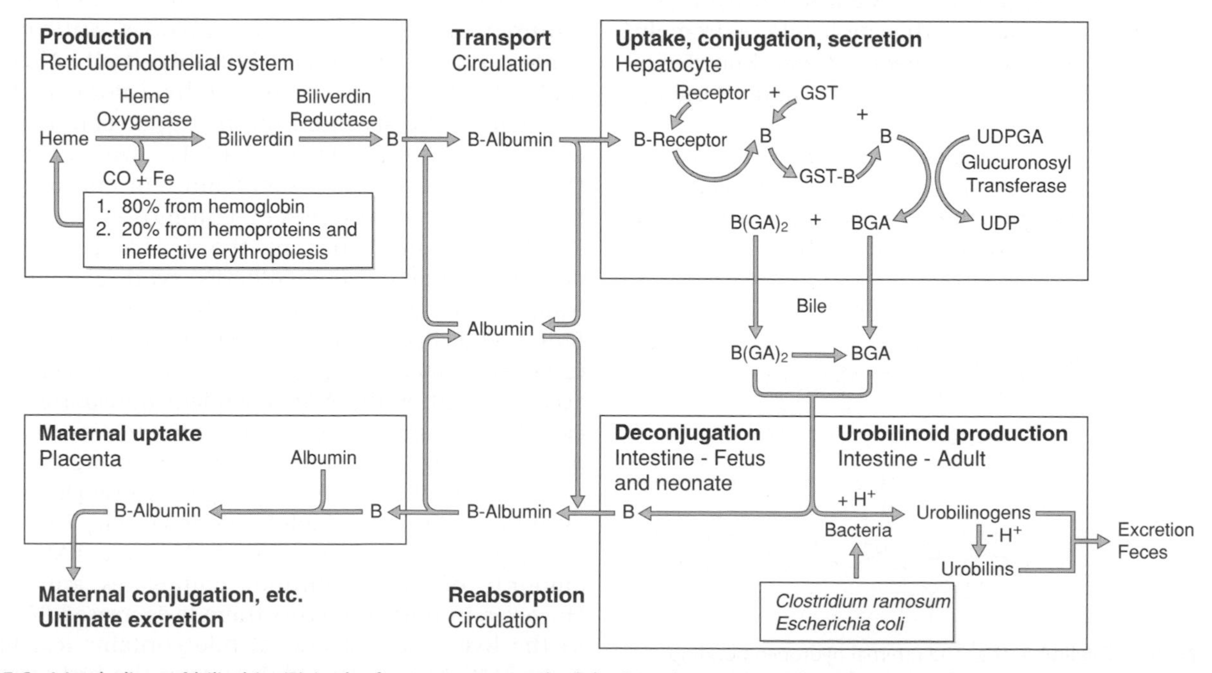

Figure 15.1: Metabolism of bilirubin (B) in the fetus, neonate and adult. GA, glucuronic acid; UDP, uridine diphosphate; GST, glutathione-S-transferase.

cleavage at any of the four carbons (α, β, γ and δ) linking the four pyrrole rings and produces equimolar amount of the α, β, γ and δ isomers. The central (C10) carbon on biliverdin IXα is then reduced from a methine to a methylene group ($-CH_2-$), thus forming bilirubin IXα. This is accomplished by the cytosolic enzyme biliverdin reductase.[3] The proximity of this enzyme results in very little biliverdin ever being present in the circulation.

Bilirubin formation can be assessed by measurement of carbon monoxide production. Such assessments indicate that the daily production rate of bilirubin is 6–8 mg/kg per 24 h in healthy, full-term infants and 3–4 mg/kg per 24 h in healthy adults.[4,5] In mammals, approximately 80% of bilirubin produced daily originates from hemoglobin.[6] Degradation of hepatic and renal heme appears to account for most of the remaining 20%, reflecting the very rapid turnover of certain of these heme proteins. Although the precise fate of myoglobin heme is unknown, its turnover appears to be so slow as to be relatively insignificant.

Catabolism of hemoglobin occurs very largely from the sequestration of erythrocytes at the end of their life span (120 days in adult humans, 90 days in newborns, 50–60 days in rats). A small fraction of newly synthesized hemoglobin is degraded in the bone marrow. This process, termed *ineffective erythropoiesis*, normally represents less than 3% of daily bilirubin production but may be substantially increased in persons with hemoglobinopathies, vitamin deficiencies, or heavy metal intoxication. Infants produce more bilirubin per unit body weight because their red blood cell (RBC) mass is greater and their RBC life span is shorter. Additionally, hepatic heme proteins represent a larger fraction of total body weight in infants.

Bilirubin requires biotransformation to more water-soluble derivatives before excretion from the body.[7] Bilirubin is not linear but rather has extensive internal hydrogen bonding, as shown in Figure 15.2. The internal hydrogen bonding of bilirubin makes the molecule extremely hydrophobic and insoluble in aqueous media. Knowledge of this stereochemistry is important for understanding phototherapy.

When bilirubin is transported from its sites of production to the liver for excretion, a carrier molecule is necessary. Albumin serves this purpose and has very high affinity for bilirubin (affinity constant $\sim 10^8$).[8]

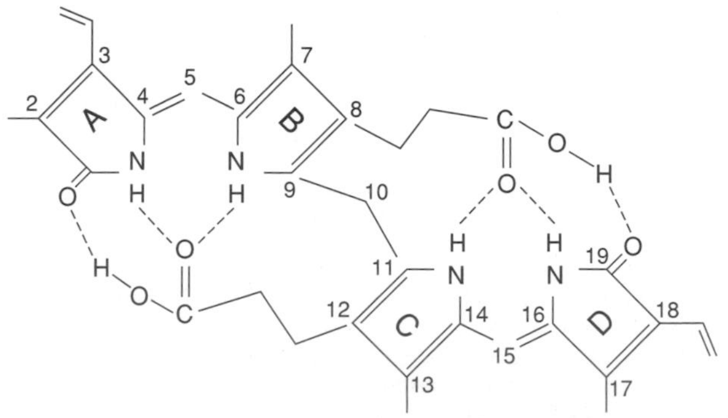

Figure 15.2: 4Z,15Z-Bilirubin IXa. The internal hydrogen bonding which shields the polar propionic acid groups is responsible for the hydrophobic nature of bilirubin.

Bilirubin is taken up into the hepatocyte from the hepatic sinusoids by either passive diffusion or a carrier molecule in the plasma membrane, which also transports other organic anions such as bromsulfophthalein.[9] This carrier protein is competitively inhibited by simultaneous exposure to bromsulfophthalein or indocyanine green. Some refer to this liver plasma membrane carrier as bilitranslocase. Review of this uptake mechanism has shown it to meet the necessary kinetic criteria for carrier-mediated transport in a number of experimental models ranging from intact patients to isolated hepatocytes and sinusoidal membrane vesicles.

Once within the aqueous environment of the hepatocyte, bilirubin is again bound by a protein carrier, glutathione *S*-transferase, traditionally referred to as ligandin. This is a family of cytosolic proteins that have enzymatic activity and also bind non-substrate ligands. Although the affinity of purified glutathione *S*-transferase for bilirubin (acid dissociation constant = 10^6) is less than that of albumin, this compound is believed to be of importance in preventing bilirubin and its conjugates from refluxing back into the circulation.[10]

Bilirubin is conjugated with glucuronic acid within the endoplasmic reticulum of the hepatocyte. The glucuronic acid donor is uridine diphosphate glucuronic acid (UDP-glucuronic acid). The enzyme responsible for this conjugation is bilirubin glucuronosyltransferase (BGT). Several different classes of glucuronosyltransferases, with different substrate specificity (e.g. thyroxine, steroids, bile acids and xenobiotics), have been described. Catalysis of bilirubin by BGT results in both monoglucuronides and diglucuronides of bilirubin (BMGs and BDGs, respectively). This conjugation disrupts the internal hydrogen bonding of bilirubin and the resulting glucuronide conjugates are more water-soluble. Depletion of hepatic UDP-glucuronic acid results in decreased BDGs and increased BMGs. BGT activity for bilirubin can be induced by narcotics, anticonvulsants, contraceptive steroids and bilirubin itself. Alternatively, BGT activity can be decreased by caloric and protein restriction. The specific isoform responsible for bilirubin conjugation is UGT1A1 (EC 2.4.1.17), which is part of the UDP glycosyltransferase superfamily of enzymes encoded by the *UGT1* gene complex on chromosome 2.[11] More than 30 different mutations in the *UGT1* gene have been described which cause Gilbert's syndrome and Crigler Najjar syndromes I and II. After bilirubin conjugation, the BMGs and BDGs are excreted through the hepatocyte canalicular membrane into the bile canaliculi. This is accomplished by the ATP-dependent transporter known as canalicular multispecific organic anion transporter (cMOAT) or multidrug resistance-associated protein (MRP2).[12] Mutations in the cMOAT/MRP2 gene cause Dubin Johnson syndrome.[13] In normal adult duodenal bile, 70–90% of the bile pigments are BDGs and 7–27% are BMGs. Smaller amounts of other bilirubin conjugates are also seen. However, in normal infants there is decreased BGT activity in the liver,[14] and duodenal bile contains less BDG and more BMG than in the adult.[15] After the first week of life, the rate-limiting step in bilirubin clearance is secretion of bilirubin conjugates by the hepatocyte.[16] Canalicular secretion of bilirubin conjugates can be increased by choleretic agents (e.g. phenobarbital) and decreased by cholestatic agents (e.g. estrogens, anabolic steroids) or pathologic conditions (e.g. liver disease).

Under normal conditions, there is evidence that bilirubin conjugates equilibrate across the sinusoidal membrane of hepatocytes. This results in the presence of small amounts of bilirubin conjugates in the systemic circulation. If there is diminished hepatic glucuronidation of bilirubin (e.g. in the neonate), there will be a decreased amount of bilirubin conjugates present in the serum.[17]

In many pathologic circumstances, BMGs and BDGs are not excreted from the hepatocyte fast enough to prevent reflux back into the circulation. The increased serum levels of bilirubin conjugates result in the spontaneous (non-enzymatic) transesterification of bilirubin glucuronide with an amino group on albumin, producing a covalent bond between albumin and bilirubin. This product is known as delta bilirubin or bilirubin-albumin.[18] Delta bilirubin is not formed in hyperbilirubinemic conditions unless there is elevation of the conjugated bilirubin fraction. Delta bilirubin is direct-reacting (Van den Bergh's test) and is cleared from the circulation slowly owing to the long (~20-day)[19] half-life of albumin.

When bilirubin conjugates enter the intestinal lumen, several possibilities for further metabolism arise. In adults, the normal bacterial flora hydrogenate various carbon double bonds in bilirubin to produce assorted urobilinogens. Subsequent oxidation produces the related urobilins. The large number of unsaturated bonds in bilirubin results in a large family of related reduction-oxidation products known as urobilinoids, which are excreted in the feces. The conversion of bilirubin conjugates to urobilinoids is important because it blocks the intestinal absorption of bilirubin, known as the enterohepatic circulation.[20] Neonates lack an intestinal bacterial flora and are more likely to absorb bilirubin from the intestine. This difference in bile pigment excretion between adults and neonates is demonstrated in Figures 15.3 and 15.4. Bilirubin conjugates in the intestine can also act as substrate for either bacterial or endogenous tissue β-glucuronidase. This enzyme hydrolyzes glucuronic acid from bilirubin glucuronides. The unconjugated bilirubin produced is more rapidly absorbed from the intestine.[21] After birth, increased intestinal β-glucuronidase can increase the neonate's likelihood of experiencing higher serum bilirubin levels.[22] The ability of endogenous tissue β-glucuronidase to deconjugate bilirubin glucuronides has been demonstrated in germ-free animals.

Neonates are at risk for the intestinal absorption of bilirubin because (1) their bile contains increased levels of BMG, which allows easier conversion to bilirubin; (2) they have within the intestinal lumen significant amounts of β-glucuronidase, which hydrolyzes bilirubin conjugates to more easily absorbed bilirubin; (3) they lack an intestinal flora to convert bilirubin conjugates to urobilinoids; and (4) meconium, the intestinal contents accumulated during gestation, contains significant amounts of bilirubin and

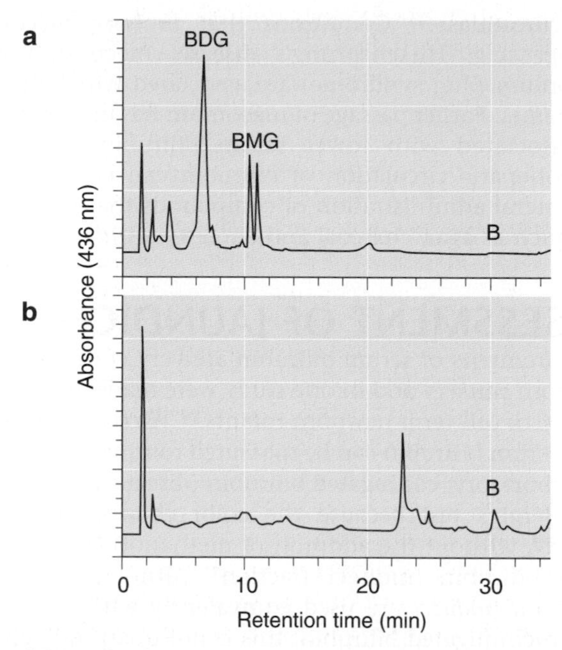

Figure 15.3: Bile pigment excretion in an adult as assessed by HPLC. (**a**) Duodenal bile (20 μl) from a normal man (GG). (**b**) Fecal extract equivalent to 50 mg of wet stool from the same normal man (GG). The BDGs and BMGs that predominate in adult bile are not present in adult stool because they are converted to urobilinoids by intestinal bacteria. Small amounts of bilirubin (B) are present in adult feces. (From Gourley, 1997, with permission.)[65]

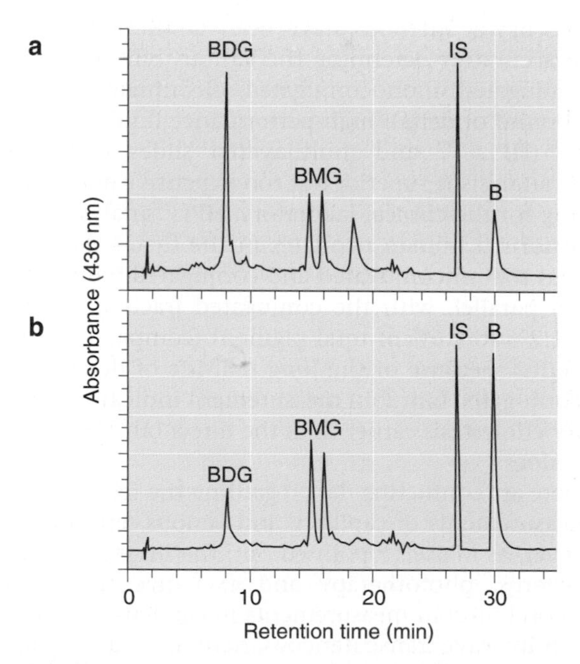

Figure 15.4: (**a**) The analysis of a sample of duodenal bile (20 μl) from a full-term, jaundiced, 6-day-old infant. (**b**) The analysis of a sample of fecal extract equivalent to 4 mg wet stool from the same infant. Neonates lack an intestinal bacterial flora and hence large quantities of BDGs, BMGs and bilirubin (B) are present in feces. The deglucuronidation action of intestinal β-glucuronidase is evident from the relatively decreased amounts of BDG and the increased amounts of BMG and B. IS, internal standard. (From Gourley, 1997, with permission.)[65]

β-glucuronidase.[23] Conditions that prolong meconium passage (e.g. Hirschsprung's disease, meconium ileus, meconium plug syndrome) are associated with hyperbilirubinemia. Earlier passage of meconium has been shown to be associated with lower serum bilirubin levels. The enterohepatic circulation of bilirubin can be blocked by the enteral administration of compounds that bind bilirubin, such as agar, charcoal and cholestyramine.

ASSESSMENT OF JAUNDICE

Measurements of serum bilirubin are very common in the newborn nursery and in one study were made at least once in 61% of full-term newborn infants.[24] Two components of total serum bilirubin can be measured routinely in the clinical laboratory: conjugated bilirubin (direct fraction in Van den Bergh's test because the color change takes place directly, without the addition of methanol) and unconjugated bilirubin (indirect fraction). Although the terms *direct* and *indirect* are used equivalently with conjugated and unconjugated bilirubin, this is not quantitatively correct, because the direct fraction includes both conjugated bilirubin and delta bilirubin. Elevation of either of these fractions can result in jaundice. There is a long history of undesirable variability in the measurement of serum bilirubin fractions.[25] Of the various laboratory methods, the Jendrassik-Grof procedure is the method of choice for total bilirubin measurement, although this method also has problems.[26] When the total serum bilirubin level is high, factitious elevation of the direct fraction has been reported.

Two newer methods have been developed which can more accurately determine the various bilirubin fractions (unconjugated, monoconjugated, diconjugated and albumin-bound or delta): high-performance liquid chromatography (HPLC)[27] and multilayered slides (Ektachem).[28] HPLC analysis is superior but too expensive and time-consuming for the clinical laboratory. HPLC analysis of serum from normal human neonates in the first 4 days of life[29] showed that unconjugated and conjugated bilirubin levels rise in parallel, with the conjugated fraction making up only 1.2% to 1.6% of total pigment (compared with 3.6% in adults). Because of the long half-life of delta bilirubin, the conjugated bilirubin measurement indicates relief from biliary cholestasis earlier than the direct bilirubin measurement does.

There are conflicting data regarding the relative accuracy of measurements of capillary and venous serum bilirubin. However, as Maisels[30] pointed out, the literature regarding kernicterus, phototherapy and exchange transfusion is based on bilirubin measurements in capillary samples.

Non-invasive transcutaneous methods to assess jaundice at the point of care are available and include: Bilicheck (Respironics, Pittsburgh, PA)[31,32] and Jaundice Meter (Minolta/Air Shields, Air-Shields Vickers, Hatboro, PA).[33] A neonatal hour-specific total serum bilirubin nomogram has been developed that can predict the risk of subsequent hyperbilirubinemia based on total serum bilirubin[34] (see Fig. 15.5) or transcutaneous bilirubin,[31] thus facilitating follow-up and intervention for infants.

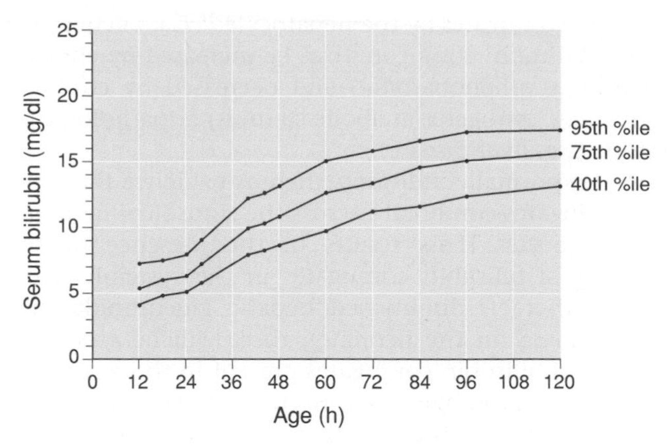

Figure 15.5: Risk designation of term and near-term well newborns based on their hour-specific serum bilirubin values. The high-risk zone is designated by the 95th percentile. The intermediate-risk zone is subdivided to upper- and lower-risk zones by the 75th percentile. The low-risk zone has been electively and statistically defined by the 40th percentile track (Reproduced from Bhutani VK, Johnson L, Sivieri EM Predictive ability of a predischarge hour-specific serum bilirubin for subsequent hyperbilirubinemia in healthy term and near-term newborns. Reproduced with permission from *Pediatrics* 1999; 103: 6–14).[34]

NEONATAL JAUNDICE

Infants usually are not jaundiced at the moment of birth, because the placenta has the ability to clear bilirubin from the fetal circulation. However, during the first week of life, most if not all infants have elevated serum bilirubin concentrations (>1.4 mg/dl). As the serum bilirubin rises, the skin becomes more jaundiced in a cephalopedal manner. Icterus is first appreciated in the head and progresses caudally to the palms and soles. Kramer[35] found the following serum indirect bilirubin levels as jaundice progressed: head and neck, 4–8 mg/dl; upper trunk, 5–12 mg/dl; lower trunk and thighs, 8–16 mg/dl; arms and lower legs, 11–18 mg/dl; palms and soles, more than 15 mg/dl. When the bilirubin was higher than 15 mg/dl, the entire body was icteric. Jaundice is best appreciated by blanching the skin with gentle digital pressure under well-illuminated (white light) conditions. Moderate jaundice (>12 mg/dl) occurs in at least 12% of breast-fed infants and 4% of formula-fed infants and severe jaundice (>15 mg/dl) occurs in 2% and 0.3% of these respective feeding groups.[36]

Fundamentally, jaundice has only two causes: increased production or decreased excretion of bilirubin. These mechanisms are not mutually exclusive; specific examples are listed in Table 15.1. One possible clinical approach to arrive at these diagnoses is presented in Figure 15.6.

The high incidence of jaundice in otherwise completely normal neonates has resulted in the term physiologic jaundice. However, physiologic jaundice is merely the result of a number of factors involving increased bilirubin production and decreased excretion. Jaundice should always be considered to be a sign of possible disease and not routinely explained as physiologic. Specific characteristics of neonatal jaundice to be considered abnormal until proved otherwise include (1) development of jaundice before 36 h of age, (2) persistence of jaundice beyond 10 days of age, (3) a serum bilirubin concentration higher than 10 mg/dl

Causes
Increased production of bilirubin
Fetal-maternal blood group incompatibilities
Extravascular blood in body tissues
Polycythemia
Red blood cell abnormalities (hemoglobinopathies, membrane and enzyme defects)
Induction of labor
Decreased excretion of bilirubin
Increased enterohepatic circulation of bilirubin
Breast feeding
Inborn errors of metabolism
Hormones and drugs
Prematurity
Hepatic hypoperfusion
Cholestatic syndromes
Obstruction of the biliary tree
Combined increased production and decreased excretion of bilirubin
Sepsis
Intrauterine infection
Congenital cirrhosis

Table 15.1 Causes of neonatal hyperbilirubinemia

at any time and (4) elevation of the direct-reacting fraction of bilirubin to more than 2 mg/dl at any time.

Factors associated with increased neonatal bilirubin levels are low birth weight; certain races (Oriental, Native American, Greek); maternal medications (e.g. oxytocin); premature rupture of the membranes; increased weight loss after birth; delayed meconium passage; breast feeding; and neonatal infection. Factors associated with decreased neonatal bilirubin levels include maternal smoking, black race and certain drugs given to the mother (e.g. phenobarbital).

Neonatal jaundice caused by increased production of bilirubin

The most common cause of severe early jaundice, is fetal-maternal blood group incompatibility with resulting isoimmunization. Maternal immunization develops because of leakage of erythrocytes from the fetal to the maternal circulation. When the fetal erythrocytes carry different antigens, they are recognized as foreign by the maternal immune system, which forms antibodies against them (maternal sensitization). These antibodies (immunoglobulin G) cross the placental barrier into the fetal circulation and bind to fetal erythrocytes. In Rh incompatibility, sequestration and destruction of the antibody-coated erythrocytes takes place in the reticuloendothelial system of the fetus. In ABO incompatibility, hemolysis is intravascular, complement-mediated and usually not as severe as in Rh disease. Significant hemolysis can also result from incompatibilities between minor blood group antigens (e.g. Kell). These conditions are associated predominately with elevation of unconjugated bilirubin, but occasionally the conjugated fraction is also increased.

Rh incompatibility usually does not develop until the second pregnancy. Therefore, prenatal blood typing and serial testing of Rh-negative mothers for the development of Rh antibodies provide important information to guide possible intrauterine care. If maternal Rh antibodies develop during pregnancy, potentially helpful measures include serial amniocentesis (with bilirubin measurement),[37] ultrasound assessment of the fetus, intrauterine transfusion and premature delivery. The prophylactic administration of anti-D gammaglobulin has been most helpful in preventing Rh sensitization. The newborn infant with Rh incompatibility presents with pallor, hepatosplenomegaly and a rapidly developing jaundice in the first hours of life. If the problem is severe, the infant may be born with generalized edema (fetal hydrops). Laboratory findings in the neonate's blood include reticulocytosis, anemia, a positive direct Coombs' test and a rapidly rising serum bilirubin level. Exchange transfusion continues to be an important therapy for seriously affected infants.[38]

ABO incompatibility usually manifests clinically with the first pregnancy. ABO hemolytic disease is largely limited to infants with blood group A or B who are born to group O mothers. ABO hemolytic disease is relatively rare in type A or B mothers. Development of jaundice is not as rapid as with Rh disease; a serum bilirubin concentration higher than 12 mg/dl on day 3 of life would be typical. Laboratory abnormalities include reticulocytosis (>10%) and a weakly positive direct Coombs' test, although this is sometimes negative. Spherocytes are the most prominent feature seen in the peripheral blood smear of neonates with ABO incompatibility.

When extravascular blood is present within the body, the hemoglobin can be rapidly converted to bilirubin by tissue macrophages. Examples of this type of increased bilirubin production include cephalohematoma; ecchymoses; petechiae; occult intracranial, intestinal, or pulmonary hemorrhage; and swallowed maternal blood. The Apt test can be used to distinguish blood of maternal or infant origin because of differences in alkali resistance between fetal and adult hemoglobin.[39]

Polycythemia (venipuncture hematocrit >65%) can cause hyperbilirubinemia because the absolute increase in RBC mass results in elevated bilirubin production through normal rates of erythrocyte breakdown. A number of mechanisms can result in neonatal polycythemia, including maternal-fetal transfusion, a delay in cord clamping, twin-twin transfusions, intrauterine hypoxia and maternal diseases (e.g. diabetes mellitus). Therapy for symptomatic polycythemia is partial exchange transfusion; therapy for asymptomatic polycythemia remains controversial.

A number of specific abnormalities related to the RBC can result in neonatal jaundice, including hemoglobinopathies and RBC membrane or enzyme defects. Hereditary spherocytosis is not usually a neonatal problem, but hemolytic crises can occur and can manifest with a rising bilirubin level and a falling hematocrit. The characteristic spherocytes seen in the peripheral blood smear may be impossible to distinguish from those seen with ABO hemolytic disease. Other hemolytic anemias associated with neonatal jaundice include drug-induced hemolysis, deficiencies of the erythrocyte enzymes (e.g. glucose-6-phosphate dehydrogenase deficiency, pyruvate kinase deficiency) and hemolysis induced by vitamin K or

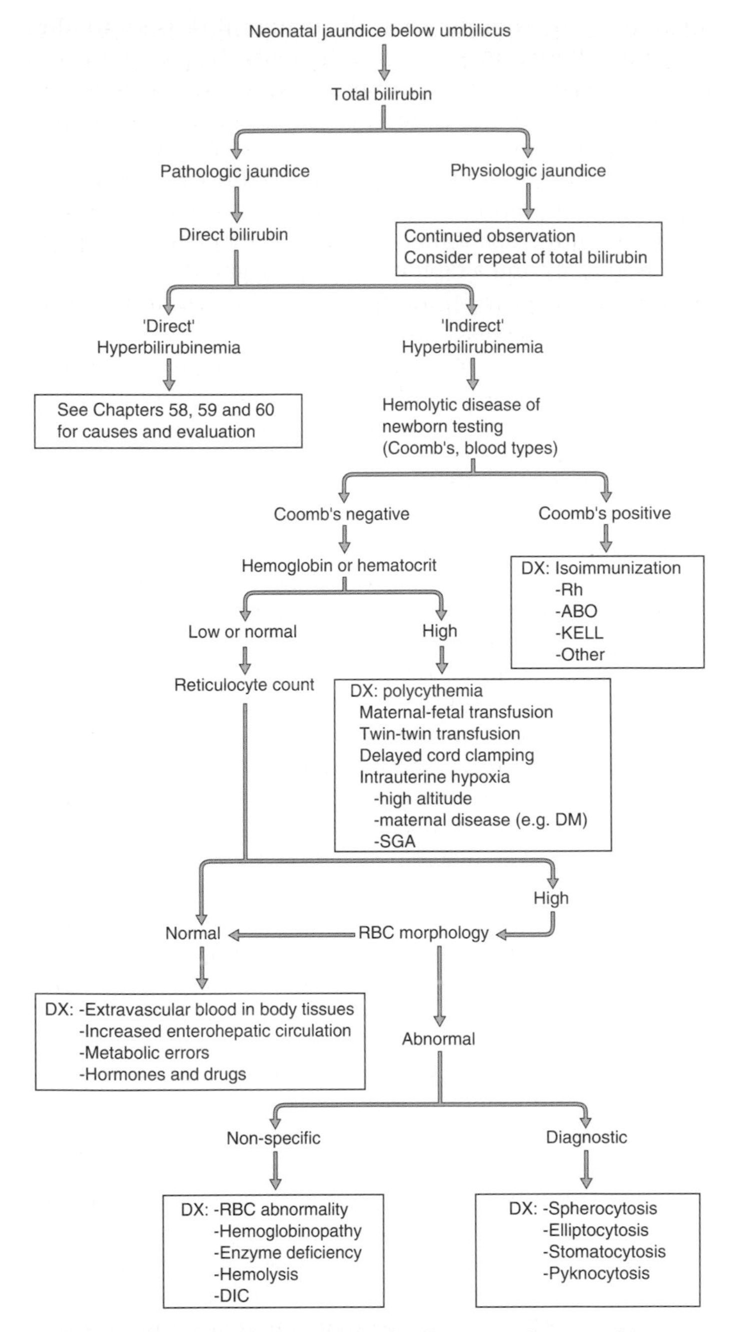

Figure 15.6: A clinical approach to the diagnosis of neonatal jaundice.

bacteria. α-Thalassemia can result in severe hemolysis and lethal hydrops fetalis. γ β-Thalassemia may also occur, with hemolysis and severe neonatal hyperbilirubinemia. Drugs or other substances responsible for hemolysis can be passed to the fetus or neonate across the placenta or via the breast milk. Co-inheritance of Gilbert's syndrome along with the above hematologic abnormalities is associated with an increased incidence of hyperbilirubinemia in neonates and older individuals.[40]

Induction of labor with oxytocin has been shown to be associated with neonatal jaundice. There is a significant association between hyponatremia and jaundice in infants of mothers who received oxytocin to induce labor. The explanation for this observation is not clear.

Neonatal jaundice caused by decreased excretion of bilirubin

Increased enterohepatic circulation of bilirubin is an important factor in neonatal jaundice. Conditions that prolong meconium passage (e.g. Hirschsprung's disease, meconium ileus, meconium plug syndrome) are associated with hyperbilirubinemia, presumably by allowing more time for intestinal bilirubin absorption. Earlier passage of meconium is associated with lower serum bilirubin levels. The enterohepatic circulation of bilirubin can be blocked by enteral administration of compounds that bind bilirubin, such as agar, charcoal and cholestyramine.

Breast-feeding has been identified as a significant factor related to neonatal jaundice.[36,41,42] Breast-fed infants have significantly higher serum bilirubin levels than formula-fed infants on each of the first 5 days of life and this unconjugated hyperbilirubinemia can persist for weeks to months. Research has shown that bilirubin is a significant antioxidant which is possibly of physiologic benefit in protecting against cellular damage by free radicals. During the first week of life some distinguish this early jaundice as 'breast-feeding jaundice' to differentiate it from the later breast milk jaundice syndrome, which occurs after the first week of life and in which the breast milk supply is well established. There is probably overlap between these conditions and physiologic jaundice. Early reports linking breast milk and jaundice with a steroid (pregnane-3α,20β-diol) in some milk samples[43] have not been confirmed by subsequent, larger studies employing more sensitive methods.[44] There are conflicting data regarding the association of this jaundice with increased lipase activity in the breast milk, which results in increased levels of free fatty acids that could inhibit hepatic BGT. The enterohepatic circulation of bilirubin might be facilitated by the presence of β-glucuronidase[22] or some other substance in human milk. Other factors possibly related to jaundice in breast-fed infants include caloric intake, fluid intake, weight loss, delayed meconium passage, intestinal bacterial flora and inhibition of BGT by an unidentified factor in the milk. It has been suggested that a healthy, breast-fed infant with unconjugated hyperbilirubinemia, normal hemoglobin concentration, normal reticulocyte count, normal blood smear, no blood group incompatibility and no other abnormality on physical examination may be presumed to have early breast-feeding jaundice.[45]

Because there is no specific laboratory test to confirm a diagnosis of breast milk jaundice, it is important to rule out treatable causes of jaundice before ascribing the hyperbilirubinemia to breast milk. The 2004 American Academy of Pediatrics Clinical Practice Guideline provides recommendations for the evaluation and treatment of neonatal jaundice.[46] The age of the infant is important in assessing the severity of neonatal jaundice and the need for evaluation and treatment. If the bilirubin level is rising, published recommendations support encouraging mothers to breast feed more frequently, with an average suggested interval between feeds of 2 h and no feeding supplements. More frequent nursing may not increase intake, but it has been suggested to increase peristalsis and stool frequency, thus promoting bilirubin excretion. However, one study comparing 'frequent' (9 feedings per day) *vs* 'demand' (6.5 feedings per day) feeding schedules during the first 3 days of life showed no significant relation between the frequency of breast-feeding and infant serum bilirubin levels in 275 infants.[47] The point at which breast-feeding should be discontinued is controversial; recommendations include total bilirubin levels of 14,[48] 15,[49] 16 to 17,[50] and 18–20 mg/dl.[51] When breast-feeding is interrupted, formula-feeding may be initiated for 24–48 hours, or breast- and formula-feeding can be alternated with each feeding. A fall in the serum bilirubin level of 2–5 mg/dl[52] is consistent with a diagnosis of breast milk jaundice. Breast-feeding may then be resumed; although the serum bilirubin levels may rise for several days, they will gradually level off and decline.[45,49] In one study, interruption of breast-feeding for approximately 50 h (during which time a formula was given) was shown to have the same bilirubin-lowering effect as a similar duration of phototherapy.[53] If formula is substituted for breast milk for several days, it is not clear which formula would be most cost effective in lowering serum bilirubin. However, it has been shown that neonates fed a casein hydrolysate have less jaundice than neonates fed a routine formula,[54,55] that casein hydrolyate formula inhibits β-glucuronidase[56] and that the majority of the β-glucuronidase inhibition in hydrolyzed casein is due to l-aspartic acid.[57]

There is much controversy about the potential dangers of hyperbilirubinemia in full-term and near-term newborns who do not have hemolytic disease. Regardless of whether hyperbilirubinemia in these infants causes mild neurodevelopmental or intellectual handicaps, there is no doubt that Frank kernicterus in this population is rare. However, it appears that in the USA we are currently experiencing a re-emergence of classic kernicterus[58,59] and warnings from the Centers for Disease Control and Prevention, the American Academy of Pediatrics and the Joint Commission on Accreditation of Healthcare Organizations indicate that otherwise healthy full-term and near-term infants are at risk. Since 1992 there has been a kernicterus registry in the USA that, as of March, 2004, contains more than 165 individuals.[60] Although G6PD deficiency is present in approximately one-third of these individuals with kernicterus, another third had no obvious etiology and appeared to be healthy breast-feeding infants.

Several inborn errors of metabolism can cause neonatal hyperbilirubinemia. Crigler-Najjar syndrome (CN), or congenital nonhemolytic jaundice,[61] is characterized by a hereditary deficiency of hepatic BGT. This syndrome may be divided into CN1 and CN2 (Arias' syndrome) according to the response to phenobarbital – a significant decrease of serum bilirubin in CN2 and no response in CN1. In CN1, serum bilirubin levels typically range from approximately 15–45 mg/dl and there is a risk of both neonatal and later kernicterus. Hyperbilirubinemia is less severe in CN2 patients, varying from approximately 8–25 mg/dl. CN2 is associated with a much lower incidence of kernicterus, although such damage has been documented. Bile pigment analysis has been reported to aid in the differentiation of CN1 from CN2 and in the differential diagnosis of unconjugated hyperbilirubinemia. In both forms of CN, traces of monoconjugates can be detected in serum and bile, but no diconjugates are present. Whereas phenobarbital can increases the level of serum monoconjugated bilirubin even in patients with CN1, the diagnosis of CN1 *vs* CN2 is based on finding a substantial decrease of unconjugated bilirubin in the serum after administration of phenobarbital in CN2. In the first months of life, a phenobarbital trial can still be unsuccessful in the presence of CN2. Therapy for CN1 has included lifelong phototherapy, bilirubin binders (agar, cholestyramine, calcium phosphate) to interrupt the enterohepatic circulation, plasmapheresis for acute episodes of severe hyperbilirubinemia related to intercurrent illness and, rarely, heme oxygenase inhibition to prevent bilirubin production. In CN1, orthotopic liver transplantation has been performed, even though liver function is otherwise normal, because of concern about kernicterus. Several mutations in the bilirubin UDP-glucuronosyltransferase (UGT 1) gene of CN1 and CN2 patients have been identified which result in complete inactivation of this enzyme in CN1 patients and markedly reduced glucuronidation in CN2 patients. A third type of CN has also been reported; it resembles CN1 in that there is no biliary excretion of bilirubin glucuronide. However, patients with CN3 do excrete monoglucoside and diglucoside conjugates of bilirubin. It has been speculated that CN3 patients lack the long-proposed permease, which has been hypothesized to transport UDP-glucuronic acid to the luminal side of the endoplasmic reticulum, where glucuronosyltransferase is located. This absence forces utilization of a very inefficient substrate for conjugation to bilirubin, UDP-glucose.

Various hormones and drugs may cause development of neonatal unconjugated hyperbilirubinemia. Congenital hypothyroidism can manifest with serum bilirubin higher than 12 mg/dl before the development of other clinical findings. Similarly, hypopituitarism and anencephaly may be associated with jaundice caused by inadequate thyroxine, which is necessary for hepatic clearance of bilirubin.

Infants of diabetic mothers have prolonged and higher serum bilirubin levels than control patients. Explanations include prematurity, polycythemia, substrate deficiency for glucuronidation (secondary to hypoglycemia) and poor hepatic perfusion (secondary to either respiratory distress, persistent fetal circulation, or cardiomyopathy).

The Lucey-Driscoll syndrome[62] consists of neonatal hyperbilirubinemia within families in whom there is *in vitro* inhibition of BGT by both maternal and infant serum. It is presumed that this is caused by gestational hormones.

Drugs may interfere with the metabolism of bilirubin and result in hyperbilirubinemia or displacement of bilirubin from albumin.[63] Such displacement increases the risk of kernicterus and can be caused by sulfonamides, moxalactam, or ceftriaxone (independent of its sludge-producing effect). The popular Chinese herb, Chuen-Lin, given to

approved for use and a clinical trial gathering data for Food and Drug Administration evaluation is currently on hold.[82]

Another experimental therapy for neonatal hyperbilirubinemia is hemoperfusion. Research into this method has employed hemoperfusion with ion exchange, bilirubin oxidase and sorbents.

JAUNDICE IN INFANTS AND OLDER CHILDREN

A brief list of the causes of jaundice in infants and older children is presented in Table 15.3. Several hereditary hyperbilirubinemia syndromes may manifest in infants or older children.[83] These include Gilbert's syndrome, Dubin-Johnson syndrome and Rotor's syndrome.

Gilbert's syndrome usually is not recognized until after puberty. It is characterized by a hereditary, chronic, mild, unconjugated hyperbilirubinemia with otherwise normal liver function test results. Gilbert's syndrome appears to be a heterogeneous group of disorders that share a decrease in hepatic BGT activity of at least 50%. Based on plasma clearance of other organic anions (bromsulfophthalein and indocyanine green), there appear to be at least four subtypes of Gilbert's syndrome. Mild hemolysis can be seen. Patients with this disorder show a pronounced increase of serum bilirubin concentration in response to fasting. The clinical manifestations of Gilbert's syndrome are commonly associated with a DNA polymorphism in the promoter region of *UGT1A1*, the gene that encodes bilirubin UDP-glucuronosyltransferase, although more rare heterozygous missense mutations in the coding region of *UGT1A1* have also been reported.[84] Odell[85] speculated that some infants with neonatal jaundice are manifesting Gilbert's syndrome because of the transient hormonal milieu (estrogenization) of the fetus. Data show that infants homozygous for this DNA polymorphism have a more rapid rise in jaundice during the first 2 days of life.[86] Although some individuals with Gilbert's syndrome complain of fatigue or abdominal pain, rigorous study suggests symptoms do not differ significantly from controls[87] and, in general there are no negative implications for health or longevity. Limited data raises concern about metabolism of xenobiotics metabolized by BGT which might be impaired in Gilbert's syndrome.[84]

- Metabolic disorders
  - Hereditary hyperbilirubinemias
    - Gilbert's syndrome; Dubin-Johnson syndrome; Rotor's syndrome; Crigler-Najjar syndrome
  - Alpha$_1$-antitrypsin deficiency
  - Cystic fibrosis
  - Hemochromatosis
  - Wilson's disease
- Viral hepatitis
  - Hepatitis A, B, C, D, E; Epstein-Barr virus; Cytomegalovirus
- Autoimmune hepatitis
- Biliary tract disease
  - Cholecystitis; cholelithiasis; Caroli's disease; choledochal cyst
- Tumor
  - Hepatic; biliary; pancreatic; peritoneal; duodenal
- Red blood cell abnormalities
  - Sickle cell disease
  - Thalassemia
  - Hemolysis
- Drugs/toxins
  - Acetaminophen; Valproate; Chlorpromazine; Amanita toxin; Sepsis; Others
- Sclerosing cholangitis
  - Primary; Secondary to inflammatory bowel disease
- Veno-occlusive disease
  - Pyrrolidizine alkaloids; bone marrow transplantation; Chemotherapy
- Impaired delivery of bilirubin to liver
  - Congestive heart failure; cirrhosis

Table 15.3 Causes of jaundice in infants and older children

Dubin-Johnson syndrome[88] and Rotor's syndrome[89] are two distinct but similar hyperbilirubinemia syndromes with autosomal recessive inheritance. In both syndromes the direct and indirect fractions of bilirubin are elevated but the results of other liver function tests, including serum bile acid concentrations, are normal. Rotor's syndrome can be seen in early childhood, whereas Dubin-Johnson syndrome manifests from birth to 40 years of age. In both conditions total serum bilirubin levels usually range from approximately 2 to 7 mg/dl, with at least half present as conjugated bilirubin, but can reach 20 mg/dl under certain conditions (e.g. intercurrent illness).

Dubin-Johnson syndrome is more common than Rotor's syndrome and the hyperbilirubinemia is often exacerbated by pregnancy and the use of oral contraceptives. Liver histology is completely normal in Rotor's syndrome. In Dubin-Johnson syndrome, liver examination may reveal a distinctive brown-black pigmentation that is visible grossly, with storage located in the lysosomes microscopically. This pigment is believed to originate from melanin or from metabolites of epinephrine. Dubin-Johnson syndrome is more common in males, but there is no male predominance in Rotor's syndrome. Oral cholecystography is normal in Rotor's syndrome but often fails to visualize the gallbladder in Dubin-Johnson syndrome.

An important pathophysiologic finding in Rotor's syndrome is the marked reduction in hepatic anion storage. This is consistent with the finding of deficient glutathione *S*-transferase activity in a patient with Rotor's syndrome.[90] Decreased storage allows both direct and indirect bilirubin fractions to reflux back into the circulation, explaining the elevation of both in serum. Hepatic anion storage is normal in Dubin-Johnson syndrome, but there is a marked decrease in secretion by the biliary canaliculus, allowing reflux of conjugated bilirubin back into the circulation. This is due to a defect in the ATP-binding cassette (ABC) transporter located in the apical canalicular membrane. This transporter, originally known as canalicular multispecific organic anion transporter (cMOAT), also called multidrug resistance-associated protein 2 (MRP2) is encoded by the gene, *ABCC2*, located on chromosome 10q24. Mutations of this gene can produce a defective, nonfunctional or absent cMOAT/MRP2 resulting in Dubin Johnson Syndrome.[91]

Also useful in differentiating these two syndromes is the difference in total urinary excretion of coproporphyrins I and III. Urinary coproporphyrin excretion is 2.5 to 5 times higher than normal in Rotor's syndrome but is usually normal or slightly elevated in Dubin-Johnson syndrome. Further, there are significant differences in the distribution of total urinary coproporphyrins I and III, with isomer I less than 80% of the total in Rotor's syndrome[92] and more than 80% of the total in Dubin-Johnson syndrome (normal, 25%).[93]

Patients with Rotor's syndrome are asymptomatic and require no therapy. Although jaundice is life-long, there is no associated morbidity or mortality. Although Dubin-Johnson syndrome is also associated with normal health and longevity, a significant number of patients have nonspecific abdominal complaints and hepatomegaly. Diagnosis can be made by confirming conjugated hyperbilirubinemia and otherwise normal liver function tests. Coproporphyrin excretion in the urine or hepatic scintigraphy[94] allows differentiation of the two syndromes.

The other causes of jaundice listed in Table 15.3 are described elsewhere in this volume.

Acknowledgement

The author gratefully acknowledges the assistance of Jeri Sager-Roach.

References

1. Städeler G. Ueber die farbstoffe der galle. Justus Liebigs Ann Chem 1864; 132:323–354.
2. Tenhunen R, Marver HS, Schmid R. Microsomal heme oxygenase. Characterization of the enzyme. J Biol Chem 1969; 244:6388–6394.
3. Colleran E, O'Carra P. Enzymology and comparative physiology of biliverdin reduction. In: Berk PD, Berlin NE, editors. International symposium on chemistry and physiology of bile pigments. Washington, DC: US Government Printing Office, 1977:69.
4. Maisels MJ, Pathak A, Nelson NM, et al. Endogenous production of carbon monoxide in normal and erythroblastotic infants. J Clin Invest 1971; 50:1–8.
5. Bloomer JR, Berk PD, Howe RB, Waggoner JG, Berlin NI. Comparison of fecal urobilinogen excretion with bilirubin production in normal volunteers and patients with increased bilirubin production. Clin Chim Acta 1970; 29:463.
6. Ostrow JD, Jandle JG, Schmid R. The formation of bilirubin from hemoglobin in vivo. J Clin Invest 1962; 41:1628–1637.
7. Bonnett R, Davies JE, Hursthouse MB. Structure of bilirubin. Nature 1976; 262:327–328.
8. Jacobsen J. Binding of bilirubin to human serum albumin-determination of the dissociation constants. FEBS Lett 1969; 5:112–114.
9. Berk PD, Potter BJ, Stremmel W. Role of plasma membrane ligand-binding proteins in the hepatocellular uptake of albumin-bound organic anions. Hepatology 1987; 7:165–176.
10. Wolkoff AW, Goresky CA, Sellin J, Gatmaitan Z, Arias IM. Role of ligandin in transfer of bilirubin from plasma into liver. Am J Physiol 1979; 236:E638–E648.
11. Ritter JK, Chen F, Sheen Y, Tran HM, Kimura S, Yeatman MT et al. A novel complex locus *UGT1* encodes human bilirubin, phenol and other UDP-glucuronosyltransferase isozymes with identical carboxyl termini. J Biol Chem 1992; 267:3257–3261.
12. Keppler D, Konig J. Hepatic canalicular membrane 5: Expression and localization of the conjugate export pump encoded by the MRP2 (cMRP/cMOAT) gene in liver. FASEB J 1997; 11:509–516.
13. Borst P, Evers R., Kool M, Wijnholds J. A family of drug transporters: the multidrug resistance-associated proteins. J Natl Cancer Inst 2000; 92:1295–1302.
14. Kawade N, Onishi S. The prenatal and postnatal development of UDP-glucuronyltransferase activity towards bilirubin and the effect of premature birth on this activity in the human liver. Biochem J 1981; 196:257–260.
15. Blumenthal SG, Taggart DB, Rasmusseen RD, et al. Conjugated and unconjugated bilirubins in humans and Rhesus monkeys. Structural identity of bilirubins from biles and meconiums of newborn humans and Rhesus monkeys. Biochem J 1979; 179:537–547.
16. Natzschka JC, Odell GB. The influence of albumin on the distribution and excretion of bilirubin in jaundiced rats. Pediatrics 1966; 37:51–61.
17. Rubaltelli FF, Muraca M, Vilei MT, Largajolli G. Unconjugated and conjugated bilirubin pigments during perinatal development. III. Studies on serum of breast-fed and formula-fed neonates. Biol Neonate 1991; 60:144–147.
18. Brett EM, Hicks JM, Powers DM, Rand RN. Delta bilirubin in serum of pediatric patients: Correlations with age and disease. Clin Chem 1984; 30:1561–1564.
19. Berson SA, Yalow RS, Schreiber SS. Tracer experiments with I^{131} labeled human serum albumin: distribution and degradation studies. J Clin Invest 1953; 32:746–768.
20. Poland RL, Odell GB. Physiologic jaundice: the enterohepatic circulation of bilirubin. N Engl J Med 1971; 284:1–6.
21. Lester R, Schmid R. Intestinal absorption of bile pigments. I. The enterohepatic circulation of bilirubin in the cat. J Clin Invest 1963; 42:736–746.
22. Gourley GR, Arend RA. β-glucuronidase and hyperbilirubinemia in breast-fed and formula-fed babies. Lancet 1986; i:644–646.
23. Odell GB. Normal metabolism of bilirubin during neonatal life. Neonatal Hyperbilirubinemia. New York: Grune & Stratton; 1980:35–49.
24. Newman TB, Easterling MJ, Goldman ES, Stevenson DK. Laboratory evaluation of jaundice in newborns -frequency, cost and yield. Am J Dis Child 1990; 144:364–368.
25. Schreiner RL, Glick MR. Interlaboratory bilirubin variability. Pediatrics 1982; 69:277–281.
26. Schlebusch H, Axer K, Schneider C, Liappis N, Rohle G. Comparison of five routine methods with the candidate reference method for the determination of bilirubin in neonatal serum. J Clin Chem Clin Biochem 1990; 28:203–210.
27. Blanckaert N, Kabra PM, Farina FA. Measurement of bilirubin and its monoconjugates and diconjugates in human serum by alkaline methanolysis and high-performance liquid chromatography. J Lab Clin Med 1980; 96:198–212.
28. Wu TW, Dappen GM, Spayd RW. The EKTACHEM Clinical Chemistry slide for simultaneous determination of unconjugated and sugar conjugated bilirubin. Clin Chem 1984; 30:1304–1309.
29. Muraca M, Rubaltelli FF, Blanckaert N, Fevery J. Unconjugated and conjugated bilirubin pigments during perinatal development. II. Studies on serum of healthy newborns and of neonates with erythroblastosis fetalis. Biol Neonate 1990; 57:1–9.

Chapter 16
Ascites

Michael J. Nowicki and Phyllis R. Bishop

Ascites is defined as the pathologic accumulation of fluid within the peritoneal cavity. The word ascites is derived from the Greek *askites* and *askos*, meaning 'bag', 'bladder' or 'belly'. Ascites is found in patients of all age groups, and has even been described *in utero*. The major causes of ascites in the pediatric age group are related to diseases of the liver and kidneys. However, ascites can result from heart disease, malignancy, pancreatitis, disruption of the urinary or biliary tract, and abdominal trauma.

ETIOLOGY

The etiology of ascites differs considerably according to the age of the patient. Similarly, the composition of the ascitic fluid varies dependent upon the cause. In addition, there are certain intra-abdominal processes that mimic ascites, including omental cysts, intestinal duplications, fluid-filled intestinal loops and large ovarian cysts.[1–3]

Fetal ascites

Fetal ascites has been associated with a myriad of conditions and may occur with hydrops, both immune and non-immune. In the fetus, isolated ascites – fluid accumulation in the peritoneal cavity without fluid accumulation in other body cavities or subcutaneous tissue – is less commonly described (Fig. 16.1). The majority of reports are of single cases or small case series. In one large series, isolated ascites accounted for nearly one-third of all fetal ascites.[4] Regardless of the underlying associated disease, the pathogenesis of fetal ascites is the same as that for the post-term infant.

Isolated fetal ascites can be due to gastrointestinal abnormalities, genitourinary abnormalities, cardiovascular abnormalities, congenital infections, metabolic disease and genetic abnormalities. In addition, isolated ascites may be a harbinger of impending hydrops fetalis. The use of high-resolution ultrasonography and a structured investigative protocol has led to a decrease in the proportion of fetal ascites defined as idiopathic to 4%, from rates in previous series of 15–45%.[4–8] A list of some causes of fetal ascites is presented in Tables 16.1 and 16.2.

The causes of gastrointestinal abnormalities associated with isolated fetal ascites may be intestinal or hepatic. Intrauterine bowel perforation with subsequent meconium peritonitis is the cause most commonly reported.[4,5] Bowel obstruction without perforation has also been implicated, including obstruction due to intrauterine intussusception, malrotation and jejunal atresia.[4,5,9,10]

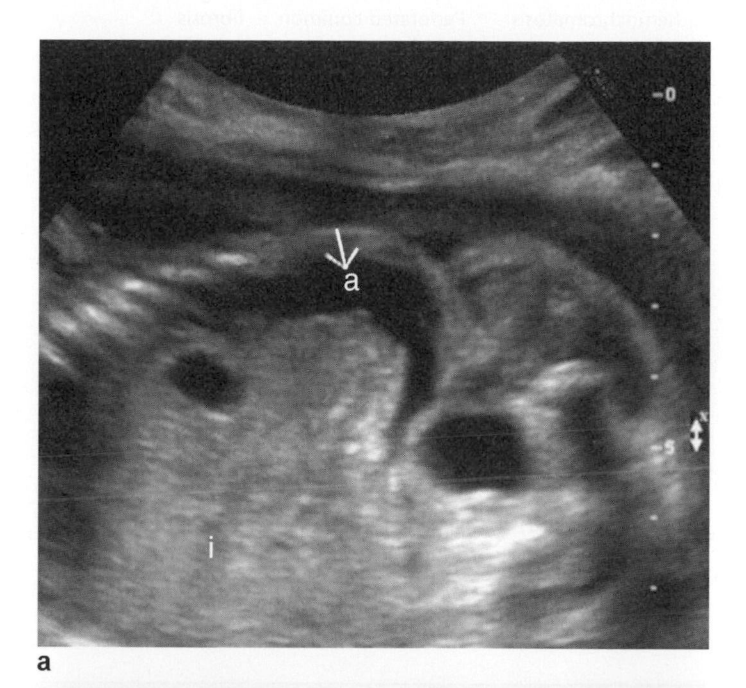

a

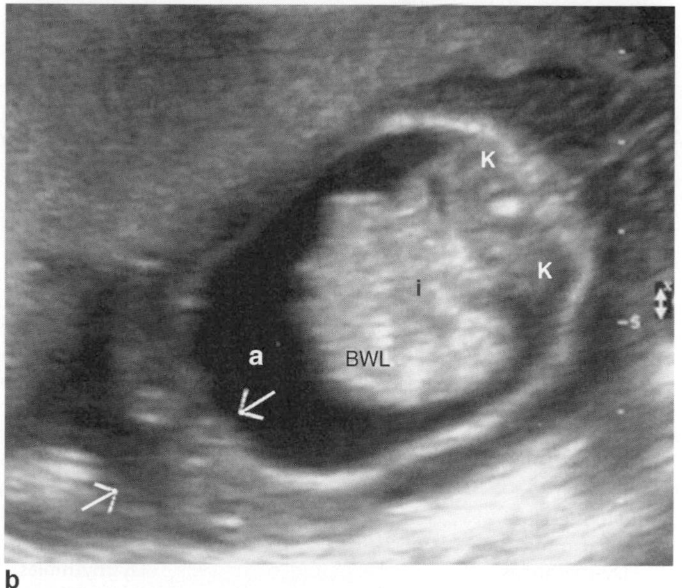

b

Figure 16.1: Fetal ascites can be seen by ultrasonography as an isolated finding (**a**) or complicating hydrops (**b**). In isolated fetal ascites no other fluid collections or edema is demonstrable; ascites (a) is seen surrounding the intestines (i). When accompanying hydrops, fetal ascites is associated with body wall edema (the area between the arrows). (BWL), bowel; (K) kidney.

Fetal	Neonatal	Infant and child
Biliary atresia	$Alpha_1$-antitrypsin deficiency	$Alpha_1$-antitrypsin deficiency
Cytomegalovirus	Budd–Chiari syndrome	Budd–Chiari syndrome
Niemann–Pick disease type C	Cirrhosis	Cirrhosis
Neonatal hemochromatosis	Hepatitis	Congenital hepatic fibrosis
	Perforated common bile duct	Hepatitis
		Perforated common bile duct

Table 16.1 Hepatobiliary causes of ascites

Primary intestinal lymphangiectasia and omphalocele have been reported as causes of isolated fetal ascites.[5] Rare hepatic causes include biliary atresia, ductal plate malformation, neonatal iron storage disease and Niemann–Pick disease type C.[5,11–13]

Genitourinary causes of fetal ascites include hydronephrosis, multicystic kidney, cloacal dysgenesis, hydrometrocolpos and urinary obstruction with subsequent perforation.[4,5,14,15] Cardiac anomalies that lead to cardiac failure and resultant increased hepatic pressure can cause isolated ascites, including structural abnormalities (tetralogy of Fallot, coarctation of the aorta and AV canal) and dysrhythmias.[4,5]

Congenital infections that lead to hydrops have also been reported to cause isolated fetal ascites, probably related to hepatic injury. However, as a group, congenital infection accounts for a small proportion (8–11.5%) of fetal ascites.[4,5] The list of infections includes cytomegalovirus, toxoplasmosis, syphilis, enterovirus, varicella, hepatitis A virus and parvovirus B19. In one series parvovirus B19 accounted for nearly 50% of all congenital infections causing ascites.[5] It can lead to ascites by causing intestinal perforation or by inducing anemia, and resulting high-output cardiac failure.

The list of metabolic causes of fetal ascites includes Wolman disease, sialic acid storage disease, Niemann–Pick disease type C, Gaucher's disease, infantile galactosialidosis, Sly disease and infantile GM gangliosidosis.[5,16–18] Chromosomal abnormalities that have been associated with fetal ascites include Turner syndrome, Down syndrome and trisomy-18. Other causes include pulmonary (laryngeal atresia, cystic adenomatosis malformation), hematologic (anemia), neoplastic and ovarian causes, as well as fetal abuse.[19–23]

The prognosis of fetal ascites varies widely, reflecting the underlying etiology. Fetuses with isolated ascites have a higher rate of survival (52%) than those with ascites associated with other anomalies (43%) or hydrops (33%).[5] Age at diagnosis of ascites appears to be a reasonable prognostic indicator. In one series, diagnosis of ascites at less than

Fetal	Neonatal	Infant and child
Gastrointestinal disorders	Gastrointestinal disorders	Pancreatitis
Meconium peritonitis	Malrotation of the intestines	Chylous ascites
Malrotation of the intestines	Intestinal perforation	Post-traumatic
Intussusception	Jejunal atresia	Non-traumatic
Jejunal atresia	Cystic fibrosis	Urinary tract
Cystic fibrosis	Acute appendicitis	Nephrotic syndrome
Infection	Uroascites	Peritoneal dialysis
Parvovirus	Obstructive uropathy	Heart failure
Syphilis	Bladder rupture	Ventriculoperitoneal shunts
Cytomegalovirus	Renal rupture	Liver transplantation
Toxoplasmosis	Renal extravasation	Neoplasm
Genitourinary tract disorders	Bladder rupture	Serositis
Hydronephrosis	Spontaneous	Henoch–Schönlein purpura
Multicystic kidney	Umbilical artery catheter	Eosinophilic gastroenteritis
Urinary tract obstruction	Urinary catheter	Other
Ovarian cyst	Nephrotic syndrome	Vitamin A intoxication
Chylous ascites	Chylous ascites	Central hyperalimentation
Cardiac disorders	Cardiac disorders	Chronic granulomatous disease
Dysrhythmias	Dysrhythmias	
Heart failure	Heart failure	
Neoplasm	Pancreatitis	
Other	Other	
Inborn error of metabolism	Metabolic storage diseases	
Trisomy	Lysosomal storage disease	
Turner's syndrome	Wolman's disease	
Hemolytic anemia	Central hyperalimentation	
Idiopathic	Intravenous vitamin E	

Table 16.2 Nonhepatic causes of ascites

24 weeks' gestation had a higher fetal loss (79%) than diagnosis at more than 24 weeks' gestation (45%).[5] In another series, diagnosis in the second trimester was associated with a higher mortality rate (63%) than diagnosis in the third trimester (10%), even when elective termination of pregnancy was excluded.[4]

Treatment of fetal ascites has been accomplished with intrauterine paracentesis and abdomino-amniotic shunting. Paracentesis typically leads to short-term improvement in ascites, often requiring repeated procedures. It has been used to improve neonatal pulmonary function,[24] and to avoid dystocia if performed just prior to vaginal delivery.[25] Abdomino-amniotic shunting is not used for isolated uncomplicated fetal ascites alone because of the risk of preterm labor. However, it has been successfully employed for ascites associated with polyhydramnios and hydrops.[26,27] The risk of treatment must be balanced against the risk of fetal loss and pre-term labor, keeping in mind that fetal ascites may resolve spontaneously.[8,15,28–30]

Neonatal ascites

Ascites in the neonate is caused by many of the same disorders that cause fetal ascites, often simply reflecting persistence of fetal ascites (Tables 16.1 and 16.2).[13,14,16,31] Similar to fetal ascites, neonatal ascites has been associated with a number of conditions, most reported as single cases. Neonatal liver diseases, such as alpha$_1$-antitrypsin deficiency, biliary atresia, congenital hepatic fibrosis and hepatitis, infrequently produce ascites in the first month of life.[32–34] However, severe hepatic injury due to metabolic liver disease is frequently accompanied by ascites. Ascites can be a presenting sign of Budd–Chiari syndrome.[35–36] A well described cause of neonatal ascites is perforation of the common bile duct. Usually reported as 'spontaneous', perforation of the common bile duct can result from abuse (Fig. 16.2). Most cases of spontaneous bile duct perforation occur in the neonatal period, most frequently between the ages of 4 and 12 weeks.[37] Clinically these infants have ascites and hyperbilirubinemia, without significant increase in aminotransferase levels;[38] ultrasonography may demonstrate ascites or fluid around the gallbladder without bile duct dilation, suggesting perforation.[39] Biliary leakage can be demonstrated by HIDA scanning, but definitive diagnosis is made by laparotomy.[38] Treatment consists of prompt surgical intervention with intraoperative cholangiography, drainage of the spilled bile, and surgical correction with cholecystostomy or T-tube drainage.[38,40] The typical location for spontaneous bile duct perforation is the junction of the cystic and common bile ducts.[41] Hypotheses for this condition include embryologic weakness of the wall of the bile duct with resulting diverticulum, focal ischemia and perforation.[42,43]

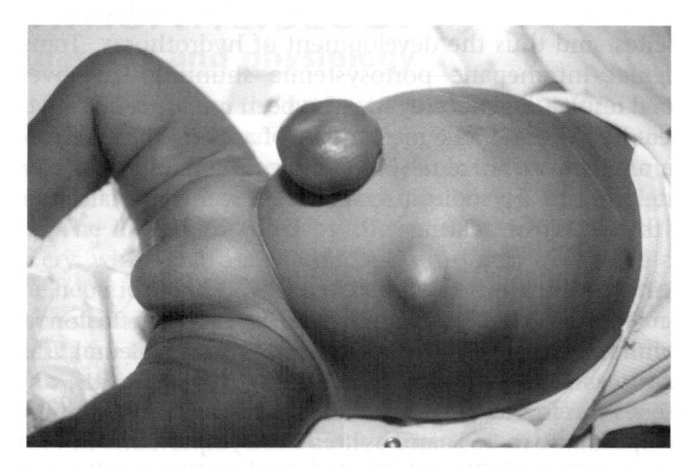

Figure 16.2: Ruptured bile duct secondary to physical abuse in a 4-month-old baby. Tense ascites is seen with resulting marked umbilical hernia and bilateral inguinal hernias. A ventral wall hernia is also present, providing an important clue to abuse.

Uroascites accounts for nearly 30% of all cases of neonatal ascites.[44] Most cases of neonatal uroascites result from obstructive uropathy due to posterior urethral valves;[45] however, ureterocele, lower ureteral stenosis and ureteral atresia have also been implicated. Rarely, neonatal rupture of the bladder occurs without a demonstrable anatomic urinary obstruction.[46] In the face of obstructive uropathy, rupture of the urinary system and resulting uroascites provides decompression and better renal function.[47] With uroascites, the intraperitoneal urine is 'autodialyzed' by the peritoneal membrane, resulting in a characteristic serum biochemical profile including marked hyponatremia, hyperkalemia and raised serum creatinine levels.[48] The presence of these serum findings and a low protein content of the ascitic fluid strongly support the diagnosis of uroascites.

Iatrogenic causes of ascites have been reported, particularly with placement of umbilical vein catheters. These catheters may erode through the liver or perforate the peritoneum and result in TPN-ascites or lead to uroascites by eroding through the bladder or causing rupture of a patent urachus.[48–53] Rupture of the urinary bladder following catheterization has also been associated with uroascites.[54] The use of an intravenous vitamin E preparation, E-Ferol, caused outbreaks of liver injury with ascites in premature infants.[55]

Gastrointestinal causes of neonatal ascites include intestinal malrotation with malposition of the portal vein, intestinal perforation, gastroschisis and acute appendicitis.[56,57] Neonatal ascites has been reported in cases of a ruptured corpus luteum cyst and hydrometrocolpos.[58,59] Neoplastic processes that have presented with neonatal ascites include transient myeloproliferative disorder associated with Down syndrome, ruptured hepatic mesenchymal hamartoma and myofibromatosis of the ovary.[60–62] Metabolic conditions that have been described in association with neonatal ascites include GM$_1$ gangliosidosis, Salla disease, Gaucher disease, mucopolysaccharidosis type VII, infantile galactosialidosis and free sialic acid storage disease.[16,17,63–66]

Ascites in infants and children

Hepatobiliary

Cirrhosis is the most common cause of hepatic ascites in infants and children; it may be caused by a number of

97% of the time, compared with 56% for total protein concentration.[107]

Fluid obtained at paracentesis should at a minimum be sent for cell count and differential, Gram stain and culture, and albumin concentration (serum albumin should also be obtained). These studies will determine whether peritonitis or portal hypertension is the cause of the ascites. Other studies on the ascitic fluid should be directed by historic and clinical features in an attempt to confirm clinical suspicion as to the cause of ascites.

Complications from paracentesis are uncommon, although bleeding is seen occasionally. With the exception of Frank disseminated intravascular coagulopathy, paracentesis can be performed despite a prolonged prothrombin time.

TREATMENT

Most, but not all, patients with ascites require treatment. Small quantities of ascites that do not produce symptoms or have no clinical sequelae may require little or no therapy. Tense ascites typically requires prompt treatment because of symptoms such as severe abdominal pain and respiratory embarrassment. The etiology of ascites should also be considered when a treatment plan is being developed. For example, in the majority of patients, pancreatic ascites is self-limiting and needs no specific therapeutic intervention, whereas cirrhotic ascites requires treatment in the majority of cases. The treatment options for cirrhotic ascites are outlined below.

Sodium and fluid restriction

Because of the significant role of sodium homeostasis in the development of ascites, a major goal of treatment is to limit sodium intake. Restriction of sodium to 2 mEq per kg bodyweight is usually suggested, although a 'no added sodium' diet has also been used. Sodium restriction is sufficient as a lone therapy in a minority of patients; most require a combination of sodium restriction and diuretic therapy. Water restriction is typically initiated when the serum sodium level decreases to 125 or 130 mEq/l or less.

Diuretics

The goal of diuretic therapy is to reduce bodyweight by about 0.5–1% (up to 300–500 g) each day until ascites is resolved and then to prevent reaccumulation (Table 16.3). The cornerstone of treatment for cirrhotic ascites is diuretic therapy, in particular agents that combat the hyperaldosteronism characteristic of this form of ascites. Spironolactone has proved to be the most effective diuretic because of its ability to block the binding of aldosterone to specific receptors in the cortical and medullary collecting tubules (Fig. 16.6). Because of its action distally, spironolactone inhibits the resorption of only 2% of filtered sodium. In patients with ascites, the bioactive metabolites of spironolactone have prolonged half-lives, ranging from 24 to 58 h; as a result, more than 5 days is required to achieve steady state. Administration of medication more than once daily is unnecessary; adjustment of dose should take into account the prolonged half-life.

Pretreatment weight (kg)	Desired daily weight loss (g)[a]
5–10	25–100
11–20	50–200
21–30	100–300
31–40	150–400
41–50	200–500
> 50	250–500

[a]0.5–1.0% of bodyweight per day.

Table 16.3 Goal of diuretic therapy

In non-azotemic cirrhotic patients with avid sodium retention, head-to-head comparison showed a superior response in those treated with spironolactone (95%) compared with patients receiving furosemide (52%). Patients who did not respond to furosemide had higher plasma levels of renin and aldosterone; when subsequently treated with spironolactone, 90% of these patients responded.[108] Failure of patients with cirrhotic ascites to respond to spironolactone can be tied to enhanced sodium resorption in the proximal tubule and resulting decreased fractional sodium delivery to the distal renal tubule.

Furosemide is the other commonly used diuretic for cirrhotic ascites. It exerts its effect on the thick ascending limb of the loop of Henle (Fig. 16.6), increasing the fractional excretion of sodium by as much as 30% of filtered sodium. Furosemide has no effect on the distal and collecting tubules. In contrast to spironolactone, furosemide is absorbed rapidly and has a fast onset of activity; peak activity is seen at 1–2 h and duration of activity is 3–4 h.[109]

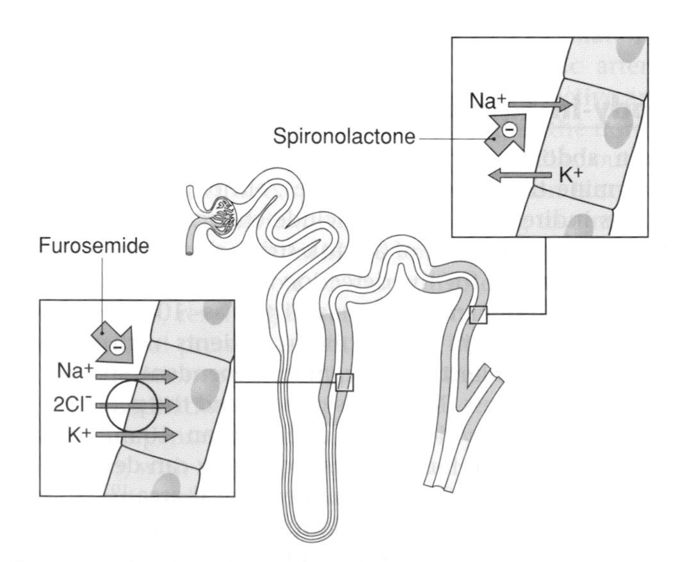

Figure 16.6: Metabolites of spironolactone act on the cortical and medullary collecting tubule by inhibiting the binding of aldosterone to a specific receptor protein there, resulting in impairment of sodium absorption and potassium excretion. Furosemide acts on the renal epithelial cells of the thick ascending loop of Henle by inhibiting the sodium chloride potassium carrier co-transport system.

Diuretic therapy should be guided by the severity of the ascites. In less severe ascites a stepwise approach can be used, whereas in severe ascites combination therapy should be started from the beginning. When a stepwise approach is employed, spironolactone is started as a single morning dose of 2–3 mg per kg bodyweight (up to 100 mg; Table 16.4). In the absence of response, the dose is increased by 2 mg/kg (up to 100 mg) every 5–7 days up to a maximum of 4–6 mg/kg/day (up to 200–400 mg). If there is still not an adequate response, furosemide is added, the initial dose being 1 mg/kg (up to 40 mg). The dose of furosemide can be increased every 5–7 days by 1 mg/kg (up to 40 mg) until a response is seen or a maximum dose of 4 mg/kg (up to 160 mg) is reached. In severe ascites combination therapy with both spironolactone and furosemide can be initiated. The starting dose is similar to that for the medications when used sequentially; spironolactone at 2 mg/kg (up to 100 mg) and furosemide at 1 mg/kg (up to 40 mg) each morning.

The doses are increased every 5–7 days by 2 mg/kg (up to 100 mg) for spironolactone and 1 mg/kg (up to 40 mg) for furosemide until a response is seen or maximum doses are reached.

Diuretic therapy is not without complications. Treatment with spironolactone can lead to hyperkalemic acidosis, and furosemide therapy can lead to hypokalemic alkalosis. When used in combination, disturbances of potassium and pH occurs less commonly. Over-aggressive diuretic therapy, particularly intravascular furosemide, can lead to intravascular volume depletion and resulting renal failure. Other complications include hyponatremia, hepatic encephalopathy, antiandrogenic effects and muscle cramps.

Therapeutic paracentesis

Paracentesis is used to treat ascites that has not responded to medical therapy, to give rapid relief from large-volume ascites and periodically to treat refractory ascites. Therapeutic paracentesis of medically resistant tense ascites is safe, rapid and effective. Paracentesis is superior to diuretics in eliminating ascites, shortening the duration of hospitalization and reducing the complication rate.[110] Total large-volume paracentesis is as safe as repeated partial paracentesis. Removal of large volumes of ascitic fluid is accompanied by increased cardiac output and decreased systemic vascular resistance, leading to a decrease in blood pressure. Resulting effective hypovolemia potentiates the neurohumoral and renal abnormalities as evidenced by increased serum norepinephrine, plasma renin activity and aldosterone levels, elevation of serum creatinine and blood urea nitrogen levels, and a reduction in serum sodium concentration. These physiologic changes, although not clinically apparent, can be prevented by the administration of albumin as a volume expander at the time of paracentesis. In the only reported experience of large-volume paracentesis in children, albumin was administered to provide hemodynamic stability and as a replacement for removed ascitic albumin. Albumin infusion was begun at the beginning of paracentesis; 0.5–1.0 g 5% albumin per kg dry bodyweight was infused over 1–2 h. In this report all procedures were well tolerated, with only a single episode of decreased urine output which responded to volume expansion; no bleeding or infectious complications were seen.[111]

	Spironolactone	Furosemide
Starting dose	2–3 mg/kg, up to 100 mg	1 mg/kg, up to 40 mg
Incremental dose	2 mg/kg, up to 100 mg	1 mg/kg, up to 40 mg
Maximum dose	4–6 mg/kg, up to 400 mg	2–4 mg/kg, up to 160 mg

Table 16.4 Diuretic treatment

The use of albumin in conjunction with large-volume paracentesis has potential drawbacks including downregulation of the albumin synthesis gene, cost and risk of infection.[110] Synthetic plasma expanders, such as dextran and polygeline, are as effective as albumin in preventing clinical complications of paracentesis (i.e. hyponatremia and renal impairment). However, albumin is more effective than synthetic plasma expanders in preventing post-paracentesis hypovolemia, defined by an increase in plasma renin activity or aldosterone concentration.[112] Patients receiving albumin after total paracentesis have a longer time before rehospitalization, and a longer survival time than those receiving synthetic plasma expanders.[112] Albumin infusion, in conjunction with adequate oral protein intake, may counter the depletion of protein associated with repeated large-volume paracenteses.

Despite total paracentesis being superior to diuretics in eliminating ascites, it does not negate the need for diuretics. Recurrence of ascites after paracentesis is much higher (93%) in patients receiving placebo than in those receiving diuretics (18%).[113]

A major drawback of paracentesis is early recurrence of ascites, because paracentesis does not address the mechanisms resulting in formation of ascites.[114]

Transjugular intrahepatic portosystemic stent shunting

Transjugular intrahepatic portosystemic stent (TIPS) shunting was developed in order to provide a means to lower portal pressure, without the need for invasive vascular surgery. A TIPS provides a direct, intrahepatic, connection between the portal and systemic circulations, resulting in a decrease in sinusoidal pressure and hepatic lymph production. As such, TIPS placement has been shown to prevent rebleeding from varices and to alleviate cirrhotic ascites. In adults, a TIPS is indicated when there is a need for large-volume paracentesis more than three times per month.[110] There are no such guidelines for children; however, for the child with cirrhosis and refractory ascites a TIPS can be useful as a treatment bridge to transplantation. A TIPS can reverse some of the renal abnormalities arising from cirrhosis, leading to increased urinary sodium excretion and free water clearance, and an improved glomerular filtration rate. The renal response to diuretics also improves. Compared with adults, a TIPS procedure can be technically more difficult in children, due in part to the small vessel size. Another major contributing factor may be the underlying cause; biliary atresia is a major cause of cirrhosis in children. The periportal fibrosis characteristic of biliary atresia has been associated with a reduced size of the portal veins and a higher resistance during portal vein puncture.[115] In biliary atresia the hepatic veins tend to be on the periphery and follow a tortuous course. Although technically difficult, a 94% 'technical success' rate has been reported.[115] Complications associated with the TIPS procedure include bleeding (due to puncture of the hepatic capsule, inferior vena cava and portal veins), perforation of a local organ (kidney, gallbladder and colon) and problems with the contrast material (allergic reactions and renal failure). The most common post-procedure complication is re-stenosis or re-occlusion of the stent. Early (< 30 days) re-stenosis is reported in nearly 25% of children having a TIPS placed. Shunt obstruction can arise from intimal hyperplasia or by stent migration due to growth. It has been suggested that periodic sonography be performed every 3–6 months to follow stent patency.[116] Hepatic encephalopathy can follow TIPS placement, although it is less common in children than in adults. Worsening liver failure due to inadequate hepatic perfusion is reported even less frequently. In reported children with TIPS placement, nearly 60% have had liver transplantation; no failed attempts at transplantation following a TIPS have been reported.[115,116]

Other treatments

Peritoneovenous shunts were developed to shunt ascitic fluid back into the central circulation. Although superior to diuretics in relieving ascites, peritoneovenous shunts are fraught with complications, including shunt obstruction, coagulopathy, superior vena caval thrombosis and obstruction, pulmonary embolization and sepsis. These shunts have been all but abandoned, being replaced by large-volume paracentesis;[117] peritoneovenous shunting may be useful in patients who are not candidates for liver transplantation, TIPS placement or repeated large-volume paracentesis.[110] Attempts at ultrafiltration of ascitic fluid and reinfusion into the blood have not been successful in supplanting other treatments. Liver transplantation may be the only effective treatment for some patients.

SPONTANEOUS BACTERIAL PERITONITIS

Spontaneous bacterial peritonitis (SBP) is defined as an infection of ascitic fluid without evidence of an intra-abdominal source. Secondary bacterial peritonitis is defined as an intra-abdominal infection caused by a problem that requires surgical treatment.

The true incidence of SBP in children is unknown, but is thought to be similar to that in adults. In adult patients with cirrhosis and ascites, the incidence of SBP per hospital admission is 8–27%. About half of the infections are community acquired and the other half nosocomial. The incidence of SBP in patients with fulminant hepatic failure and ascites is significantly higher (40%). Presenting signs and symptoms of SBP may be subtle and variable; in some cases the patient is asymptomatic. Findings in SBP include abdominal pain, abdominal distension, fever, vomiting, worsening liver disease, worsening encephalopathy or renal failure. Diffuse abdominal pain is the rule, with rebound tenderness present less often.

The pathogenesis of SBP is not definitely known but is most likely multifactorial. The typical patient has cirrhosis and ascites, although ascites alone for any reason predisposes to SBP. SBP has been reported with nephrotic syndrome, fulminant hepatic failure and cardiac ascites. Translocation of bacteria from the intestine to peritoneal fluid via peritoneal lymph nodes is thought to be the most common source of the infection. Other implicated sites are the pulmonary tract, urinary tract and skin. Factors contributing to successful infection of the peritoneal fluid are depressed reticuloendothelial phagocytic activity and decreased antibacterial opsonization. Low complement levels and low protein levels in ascitic fluid further increase the risk of SBP. Patients with ascites fluid protein concentration of 1 g/dl are ten times more likely to develop SBP than those with protein levels greater than 1 g/dl. Cirrhotics with SBP are more likely to have defective opsonization (100%) than cirrhotics without SBP (14%). Similarly, cirrhotics with SBP are more likely to have decreased complement levels (89–100%) than those without SBP (14–59%).

The most common cause of SBP in adult patients is Gram-negative aerobic organisms; *Escherichia coli* and *Klebsiella pneumoniae* are most often isolated. In children, the causative organisms differ somewhat different, with *Streptococcus pneumoniae* being most commonly cultured; other common organisms include *E. coli*, *K. pneumoniae* and *Staphylococcus aureus*. *Neisseria meningitidis* (serogroup Z) has also been reported as the etiology of SBP in children.

Diagnosis of SBP is made with a high degree of clinical suspicion and analysis of ascitic fluid. A polymorphonuclear leukocyte (PMN) count of 250 cells/ml is the threshold considered diagnostic of ascitic fluid infection. Lactate levels, pH and total protein levels are less reliable in determining whether or not infection exists. Gram stain is usually negative because of the low concentration of organisms, but may be helpful in discriminating between SBP and secondary peritonitis. Bedside inoculation of blood culture bottles with ascitic fluid is superior to delayed inoculation in the lab. Culture of 2–10 ml ascitic fluid detects 80–93% of organisms. Based on cell count and culture results, SBP is classified as: (1) culture-positive neutrocytic (PMN count 250 cells/ml with positive culture); (2) culture-negative neutrocytic (PMN 250 cells/ml with negative culture); or (3) monomicrobial non-neutrocytic bacterascites (PMN count < 250 cells/ml and positive culture for a single organism). Some data suggest that culture-negative neutrocytic ascites could resolve spontaneously and may be less severe than culture-positive neutrocytic SBP. Other studies have found similar short-term outcomes in culture-negative compared with culture-positive cases, including a mortality rate of 16–50%. Therefore, culture-negative neutrocytic ascites must be considered a true infection and treated aggressively. Monomicrobial non-neutrocytic bacterascites resolves spontaneously in 62–86% of cases. Patients with symptoms at the time of paracentesis are more likely to go on to develop SBP and should receive antibiotic treatment. Empiric antibiotic therapy should be instituted if the ascitic fluid PMN count is 250 cells/ml; a complete antibiotic course should be completed even if culture results are negative.

In adults, third-generation cephalosporins are the recommended first-line therapy for SBP, having been found to be superior to ampicillin–tobramycin combination. Cefotaxime (2 g every 8–12 h) and ceftriaxone (2 g daily) yielded a cure rate of 80–90% and 95–100% respectively. In a randomized trial of 100 adults with SBP, a 5-day course of cefotaxime (2 g every 8 h) was as effective as a 10-day course. In a multicenter randomized study of cirrhotic adults with SBP, oral ofloxacin (400 mg every 12 h) resulted in the same 84% cure rate as intravenous cefotaxime. When clinical response is good, repeat paracentesis is not necessary. If response is suboptimal or secondary peritonitis is suspected, follow-up paracentesis is recommended 48 h after the first.

Attempts at prophylaxis against spontaneous bacterial peritonitis have focused on avoiding exposure to pathogens by selective bowel decontamination. Short-term selective bowel decontamination with oral antibiotics has been effective in adults. Norfloxin (400 mg daily) has been show to lower the incidence of SBP in cirrhotic patients with ascites and gastrointestinal bleeding from 37% to 10%. Daily norfloxin has also been shown to decrease the recurrence rate of SBP from 35% to 12%. Ciprofloxacin (750 mg once weekly) has been shown to decrease the incidence of SBP from 22% to 3.6%. Trimethoprim–sulfamethoxazole has also been effective in decreasing the incidence of SBP and bacteremia from 27% to 3%. Side-effects of antibiotic therapy include candidal esophagitis and selection of resistant organisms. For these reasons, long-term prophylaxis with antibiotics is debatable. Diuretics, a mainstay of ascites treatment, have been shown to increase opsonic activity and complement levels in ascitic fluid, making it less susceptible to infection. The mechanism is thought to be simple concentration.

References

1. Purohit DM, Lakin CA, Othersen HB Jr. Neonatal pseudoascites: an unusual presentation of long tubular duplication of small bowel. J Pediatr Surg 1979; 14:193–194.
2. Granot E, Decklebaum RJ. 'Pseudoascites' as a presenting physical sign of celiac disease. Am J Gastroenterol 1983; 78:730–731.
3. Prasad KK, Jain M, Gupta RK. Omental cyst in children presenting as pseudoascites: report of two cases and review of the literature. Indian J Pathol Microbiol 2001; 44:153–155.
4. Favre R, Dreaux S, Dommergues M, et al. Nonimmune fetal ascites: a series of 79 cases. Am J Obstst Gynecol 2004; 190:407–412.
5. Schmider A, Henrich W, Reles A, et al. Etiology and prognosis of fetal ascites. Fetal Diagn Ther 2003; 18:230–236.
6. Sarno AP Jr, Bruner JP, Southgate WM. Congenital chyloperitoneum as a cause of isolated fetal ascites. Obstet Gynecol 1990; 76:955–957.
7. Winn HN, Stiller R, Grannum PA, et al. Isolated fetal ascites: prenatal diagnosis and management. Am J Perinatol 1990; 7:370–373.
8. Zelop C, Benacerraf BR. The causes and natural history of fetal ascites. Prenat Diagn 1994; 14:941–946.
9. Hertel J, Volsted-Pedersen P. Congenital ascites due to mesenteric vessel constriction caused by malrotation of the intestines. Acta Paediatr Scand 1979; 68:281–283.
10. Woodall DL, Birken GA, Williamson K, Lobe TE. Isolated fetal–neonatal abdominal ascites: a sign of intrauterine intussusception. J Pediatr Surg 1987; 22:506–507.
11. Maconochie IK, Chong S, Meili-Vergani G, et al. Fetal ascites: an unusual presentation of Niemann–Pick disease type C. Arch Dis Child 1989; 64:1391–1393.
12. Singh S, Sills JH, Waffarn F. Interesting case presentation: neonatal hemochromatosis as a cause of ascites. J Perinatol 1990; 10:214–216.
13. Rosgaard A, Mertz H, Skavbo P, Ebbesen F. Intra-uterine ascites associated with ductal plate malformation of the liver. J Pediatr 1996; 155:990–991.
14. Jacquemyn Y, De Catte L, Vaerenberg M. Fetal ascites associated with an imperforate hymen: sonographic observation. Ultrasound Obstet Gynecol 1998; 12:67–69.
15. Hecher K, Henning K, Spernol R, Szalay S. Spontaneous remission of urinary tract obstruction and ascites in a fetus with posterior urethral valves. Ultrasound Obstet Gynecol 1991; 1:426–430.
16. Clayes M, van der Hoeven M, de Die-Smulders C, et al. Early-infantile type of galactosialidosis as a cause of heart failure and neonatal ascites. J Inhert Metab Dis 1999; 22:666–667.
17. Ben-Haroush A, Yogev Y, Levit O, et al. Isolated ascites caused by Wolman disease. Ultrasound Obstet Gynecol 2003; 21:297–298.
18. Carbillon L, Largillière C, Bucourt M, et al. Ultrasound assessment in a case of sialic acid storage disease. Ultrasound Obstet Gynecol 2001; 18:272–274.
19. Greenberg F, Stein F, Gresik MV, et al. The Perlman familial nephroblastomatosis syndrome. Am J Med Genet 1986; 24:101–110.
20. Machin GA. Disease causing fetal and neonatal ascites. Pediatr Pathol 1985; 4:195–211.
21. Shweni PM, Kambaran SR, Ramdial K. Fetal ascties. S Afr Med J 1984; 66:616–618.
22. Lienhardt A, Aubard Y, Laroche C, et al. A rare cause of fetal ascites: a case report of Gunther's disease. Fetal Diagn Ther 1999; 14:257–261.
23. Akduman EI, Luisiri A, Launius GD. Fetal abuse: a cause of fetal ascites. AJR Am J Roentgenol 1997; 169:1035–1036.
24. Yamashita Y, Iwangaga R, Goto A, et al. Congenital cytomegalovirus infection associated with fetal ascites and intrahepatic calcifications. Acta Paediatr Scand 1989; 78:965–967.

25. de Crespigny LCH, Robinson HP, McBain JC. Fetal abdominal paracentesis in the management of gross fetal ascites. Aust N Z J Obstet Gynaecol 1980; 20:228–230.
26. Seeds JW, Herbert WN, Bowes WA Jr, Cefalo RC. Recurrent idiopathic fetal hydrops: results of prenatal therapy. Obstet Gynecol 1984; 64(Suppl):30S–33S.
27. Fung TY, Fung HYM, Lau TK, Chang AMZ. Abdomino-amniotic shunting in isolated fetal ascites with polyhydramnios. Acta Obstet Gynecol Scand 1997; 76:706–707.
28. Wloch A, Respondek M, Wlock S, et al. Fetal functional pulmonary atresia with ascites resolving spontaneously before birth. A case report. Fetal Diagn Ther 1997; 12:43–45.
29. Horng SG, Chao AS, Cheng PJ, Soong YK. Isolated fetal ascites: five cases report. Changgeng Yi Xue Za Zhi 1998; 21:72–77.
30. Chou YY, Huang HC, Liu HC, et al. Isolated fetal and neonatal ascites: report of two cases. Acta Paediatr Taiwan 2001; 42:166–168.
31. Chye JK, Lim CT, Van der Heuvel M. Neonatal chylous ascites – report of three cases and review of the literature. Pediatr Surg Int 1997; 12:296–298.
32. Ghishan FK, Gray GF, Greene HL. Alpha-1 antitrypsin deficiency presenting with ascites and cirrhosis in the neonatal period. Gastroenterology 1983; 85:435–438.
33. Ghishan FK, Nau S, Younoszai MK. Portal hypertension in a neonate with congenital hepatic fibrosis. South Med J 1981; 74:243–244.
34. Decklebaum RJ, Weizman CMZ, Bauer CR. Ascites in the newborn associated with hepatitis. Clin Pediatr 1980; 19:374–376.
35. Jaffe R, Yunis EJ. Congenital Budd–Chiari syndrome. Pediatr Pathol 1983; 1:187–192.
36. Gilanz V, Emons D, Hansmann M, et al. Hydrothorax, aascites, and right diaphragmatic hernia. Radiology 1986; 158:243–246.
37. Lilly DA, Mickel RE. Spontaneous rupture of the extrahepatic ducts and bile peritonitis in neonates and infants. Br J Surg 1980; 67:621–623.
38. Niedbala A, Lankford A, Boswell WC, Rittmeyer C. Spontaneous perforation of the bile duct. Am Surg 2000; 66:1061–1063.
39. Banani SA, Bahador A, Nezakatogoo N. Idiopathic perforation of the extrahepatic bile duct in infancy: pathogenesis, diagnosis, and management. J Pediatr Surg 1993; 28:950–952.
40. Hammoudi SM, Alauddin A. Idiopathic perforation of the biliary tract in infancy and childhood. J Pediatr Surg 1988; 23:185–187.
41. Karrer FM, Hall RJ, Stewart BA, Lilly JR. Congenital biliary tract disease. Surg Clin North Am 1990; 70:1403–1418.
42. Davenport M, Heaton ND, Howard ER. Spontaneous perforation of the bile duct in infants. Br J Surg 1991; 78:1068–1070.
43. Lloyd DA, Mickel RE. Spontaneous perforation of the extra-hepatic bile ducts in neonates and infants. Br J Surg 1980; 67:621–623.
44. Avery G, Fletcher M, Macdonald M, eds. Neonatology: Pathophysiology and Management of the Newborn, 5th edn. Philadelphia, PA: JP Lippincott; 1999:989.
45. Garrett RA, Franken EA. Neonatal ascites: perirenal urinary extravasation with bladder outlet obstruction. J Urol 1969; 102:627–632.
46. Murphy D, Simmons M, Guiney EJ. Neonatal urinary ascites in the absence of urinary tract obstruction. J Pediatr Surg 1978; 13:529–531.
47. Claahsen-van der Grinten HL, Monnens LA, de Gier RP, Feitz WF. Perinatal rupture of the uropoietic system. Clin Nephrol 2002; 57:437–438.
48. Oei J, Garvey PA, Rosenberg AR. The diagnosis and management of neonatal urinary ascites. J Paediatr Child Health 2001; 37:513–515.
49. Mohan MS, Patole SK. Neonatal ascites and hyponatremia following umbilical venous catheterization. J Paediatr Child Health 2002; 38:612–614.
50. Coley BD, Seguin J, Cordero L, et al. Neonatal total parenteral nutrition ascites from liver erosion by umbilical vein catheters. Pediatr Radiol 1998; 28:923–927.
51. Nakstad B, Naess PA, deLange C, Schistad O. Complications of umbilical vein catheterization: neonatal total parenteral nutrition ascites after surgical repair of congenital diaphragmatic hernia. J Pediatr Surg 2003; 37:1–3.
52. Sayan A, Demircan M, Erikci VS, et al. Neonatal bladder rupture: an unusual complication of umbilical catheterization. Eur J Pediatr Surg 1996; 6:378–379.
53. Hepworth RC, Milstein JM. The transected urachus: an unusual cause of neonatal ascites. Pediatrics 1984; 73:397–400.
54. Basha M, Subhani M, Mersal A, et al. Urinary bladder perforation in a premature infant with Down syndrome. Pediatri Nephrol 2003; 18:1189–1190.
55. Arrowsmith JB, Faich GA, Tomita DK, et al. Morbidity and mortality among low birth weight infants exposed to an intravenous vitamin E product, E-Ferol. Pediatrics 1989; 83:244–249.
56. Puvabanditsin S, Garrow E, Vizarra R. An unusual cause of congenital ascites. Acta Paediatr 1995; 84:829–830.
57. Lloyd DA. Gastroschisis, malrotation, and chylous ascites. J Pediatr Surg 1991; 26:106–107.
58. Vyas ID, Variend S, Dickson JAS. Ruptured ovarian cyst as a cause of ascites in a newborn infant. Z Kinderchir 1984; 39:143–144.
59. Hu MX, Methratta S. An unusual case of neonatal peritoneal calcifications associated with hydrometrocolpos. Pediatr Radiol 2001; 31:742–744.
60. Shiffer J, Natarajan S. Transient myeloproliferative disorder in Down syndrome presenting with ascites: a case report. Acta Cytol 2001; 45:610–612.
61. George JC, Cohen MD, Tarver RD, Rosales RN. Ruptured cystic mesenchymal hamartoma: an unusual cause of neonatal ascites. Pediatr Radiol 1994; 24:304–305.
62. Ng WT, Book KS, Ng WF. Infantile myofibromatosis of the ovary presenting with ascites. Eur J Pediatr Surg 2001; 11:415–418.
63. Gillan JE, Lowden JA, Gasskin K, Cutz E. Congenital aascites as a presenting sign of lysosomal storage disease. J Pediatr 1984; 104:225–231.
64. Groener J, Maaswinkel-Mooy P, Smit V, et al. New mutations in two Dutch patients with early infantile galactosialidosis. Mol Genet Metab 2003; 78:222–228.
65. Lemyre E, Russo P, Melancon SB, et al. Clinical spectrum of infantile free sialic acid storage disease. Am J Med Genet 1999; 82:385–391.
66. Saxonhouse MA, Behnke M, Williams JL, et al. Mucopolysaccharidosis type VII presenting with isolated neonatal ascites. J Perinatol 2003; 23:73–75.
67. Gómez-Cerezo J, Cano AB, Suárez I, et al. Pancreatic ascites: study of therapeutic options by analysis of case reports and case series between the years 1975 and 2000. Am J Gastroenterol 2003; 98:568–577.
68. Athow AC, Wilkinson ML, Saunders AJ, Drake DP. Pancreatic ascites presenting in infancy, with review of literature. Dig Dis Sci 1991; 36:245–250.
69. Saps M, Slivka A, Khan S, et al. Pancreatic ascites in an infant. Lack of symptoms and normal amylase. Dig Dis Sci 2003; 48:1701–1704.

70. Lebenthal E, Lee PC. Developmental functional responses in human exocrine pancreas. Pediatrics 1980; 66:556–560.
71. Haas LS, Gates LK Jr. The ascites to serum amylase ratio identifies two distinct populations in acute pancreatitis with ascites. Pancreatology 2002; 2:100–103.
72. Runyon BA. Amylase levels in ascitic fluid. J Clin Gastroenterol 1987; 9:172–174.
73. Akriviadis EA, Kapnias D, Hadjigavriel M, et al. Serum/ascites albumin gradient: its value as a rational approach to the differential diagnosis of ascites. Scand J Gastroenterol 1996; 31:814–817.
74. Maringhini A, Ciambra M, Patti R, et al. Ascites, pleural and pericardial effusions in acute pancreatitis. Dig Dis Sci 1996; 41:848–852.
75. Browse NL, Wilson NM, Russo F, et al. Aetiology and treatment of chylous ascites. Br J Surg 1992; 79:1145–1150.
76. Olazagasti JC, Fitzgerald JF, White SJ, Chong SK. Chylous ascites: a signs of unsuspected child abuse. Pediatrics 1994; 94:737–739.
77. Vasko JS, Tapper RI. The surgical significance of chylous ascites. Arch Surg 1967; 95:355–368.
78. Goodman GM, Gourley GR. Ascites complicating ventriculo-peritoneal shunts. J Pediatr Gastroenterol Nutr 1988; 7:780–782.
79. West GA, Berger MS, Geyer JR. Childhood optic pathway tumors associated with ascites following ventriculoperitoneal shunt placment. Pediatr Neurosurg 1994; 21:254–258.
80. Trigg ME, Swanson JD, Letellier MA. Metastasis of an optic glioma through a ventriculoperitoneal shunt. Cancer 1983; 52:599–601.
81. Fernbach SK. Ascites produced by peritoneal seeding of neuroblastoma. Pediatr Radiol 1993; 23:569.
82. Berry PJ, Favara BE, Odom LF. Malignant peritoneal mesothelioma in a child. Pediatr Pathol 1986; 5:397–409.
83. Chung CJ, Bui V, Fordham LA, et al. Malignant intraperitoneal neoplasms of childhood. Pediatr Radiol 1998; 28:317–321.
84. Barabino AV, Castellano E, Gandullia P, et al. Chronic eosinophilic ascites in a very young child. Eur J Pediatr 2003; 162:666–668.
85. Venuta A, Bertolani P, Garetti E, et al. Hemorrhagic ascites in a child with Henoch–Schönlein purpura. J Pediatr Gastrentol Nutr 1999; 29:358–359.
86. Rosenberg HK, Berezin S, Heyman S, et al. Pleural effusion and ascites: unusual presenting features in a pediatric patient with vitamin A intoxication. Clin Pediatr 1982; 21:435–440.
87. Morrow CS, Kantor M, Armen RN. Hepatic hydrothorax. Ann Intern Med 1958; 49:193–203.
88. Alberts WM, Salem AJ, Soloman DA, Boyce G. Hepatic hydrothorax. Cause and management. Arch Intern Med 1991; 151:2382–2388.
89. Strauss RM, Boyer TD. Hepatic hydrothorax. Sem Liver Dis 1997; 17:227–232.
90. Kakizaki S, Katakai K, Yoshinaga T, et al. Hepatic hydrothorax in the absence of ascites. Liver 1998; 18:216–220.
91. Jefferies MA, Kazanjian S, Wilson M, et al. Transjugular intrahepatic portosystemic shunts and liver transplantation in patients with refractory hepatic hydrothorax. Liver Transpl Surg 1998; 4:416–423.
92. Dumortier J, Leprêtre J, Scalone O, et al. Successful treatment of hepatic hydrothorax with octreotide. Eur J Gastroenterol Hepatol 2000; 12:817–820.
93. Gonwa TA, Klintmalm GB, Levy M, et al. Impact of pretransplant renal function on survival after liver transplantation. Transplantation 1995; 59:361–365.
94. Dudley F. Pathophysiology of ascites formation. Gastroenterol Clin North Am 1992; 21:216–236.
95. Henriksen JH. Cirrhosis: ascites and hepatorenal syndrome. Recent advances in pathogenesis. J Hepatol 1995; 23(Suppl 1):25–30.
96. Schrier RW, Arroyo V, Bernardi M, et al. Peripheral arterial vasodilation hypothesis: a proposal for the initiation of renal sodium and water retention in cirrhosis. Hepatology 1988; 8:1151–1157.
97. Alam I, Bass NM, Bacchetti P, et al. Hepatic tissue endothelin-1 levels in chronic liver disease correlate with disease severity and ascites. Am J Gastroenterol 2000; 95:199–203.
98. Martin P-Y, Ginès P, Schrier RW. Nitric oxide as a mediator of hemodynamic abnormalities and sodium and water retention in cirrhosis. N Engl J Med 1998; 339:533–541.
99. Ginès P, Cárdenas A, Arroyo V, Rodés J. Management of cirrhosis and ascites. N Engl J Med 2004; 350:1646–1654.
100. Schrier RW. Pathogenesis of sodium and water retention in high-output and low-output cardiac failure, nephrotic syndrome, cirrhosis, and pregnancy. N Engl J Med 1988; 319:1065–1072.
101. Nguyen KT, Sauerbrei EE, Nolan RL. The peritoneum and the diaphragm. In: Rumack CM, Wilson SR, Charboneau JW, eds. Diagnostic Ultrasound. St Louis, MO: Mosby-Year Book; 1991.
102. Bichet D, Szatalowicz V, Chaimovitz C, Schrier RW. Role of vasopressin in abnormal water excretion in cirrhotic patients. Ann Intern Med 1982; 96:413–417.
103. Dinkle E, Lehnart R, Troger J, et al. Sonographic evidence of intraperitoneal fluid. Pediatr Radiol 1984; 14:299–303.
104. Hibbeln JF, Wehmueller MD, Wilbur AC. Chylous ascites: CT and ultrasound appearance. Abdom Imag 1995; 20:138–140.
105. Pare P, Talbot J, Hoefs JC. Serum ascites albumin concentration gradient: a physiological approach to the differential diagnosis of ascites. Gastroenterology 1983; 85:240–244.
106. Harjai KJ, Kamble MS, Ashar VJ, et al. Portal venous pressure and the serum–ascites albumin concentration gradient. Cleve Clin J Med 1995; 62:62–67.
107. Runyon BA, Montano AA, Akriviadis EA, et al. The serum–ascites albumin gradient is superior to the exudate–transudate concept in the differential diagnosis of ascites. Ann Intern Med 1992; 117:215–220.
108. Perez-Ayuso RM, Arroyo V, Planas R, et al. Randomized comparative study of efficacy of furosemide versus spironolactone in nonazotemic cirrhosis with ascites. Gastroenterology 1983; 84:961–968.
109. Arroyo V, Ginès P, Planas R. Treatment of ascites in cirrhosis: diuretics, peritoneovenous shunt, and large-volume paracentesis. Gastroenterol Clin North Am 1992; 21:237–256.
110. Moore KP, Wong F, Ginès P, et al. The management of ascites in cirrhosis: report on the consensus conference of the international ascites club. Hepatology 2003; 38:258–266.
111. Kramer RE, Sokol RJ, Yerushalmi B, et al. Large-volume paracentesis in the management of ascites in children. J Pediatr Gastroeterol Nutr 2001; 33:245–249.
112. Ginès P, Fernandez-Esparrach G, Monescillo A, et al. Randomized trial comparing albumin, dextran 70, and polygeline in cirrhotic patients with ascites treated by paracentesis. Gastroenterology 1996; 111:1002–1010.
113. Fernandez-Esparrach G, Guevara M, Sort P, et al. Diuretic requirements after therapeutic paracentesis in non-azotemic patients with cirrhosis. A randomized double-blind trial of spironolactone versus placebo. J Hepatol 1997; 26:614–620.
114. Ginès P, Cárdenas A, Arroyo V, Rodés J. Management of cirrhosis and ascites. N Engl J Med 2004; 350:1646–1654.

115. Hupert PE, Goffette P, Astfalk W, et al. Transjugular intraheptic portosystemic shunts in children with bilairy atresia. Cardiovasc Intervent Radiol 2002; 25:484–493.

116. Heyman MB, LaBerge JM. Role of transjugular intrahepatic portosystemic shunt in the treatment of portal hypertension in pediatric patients. J Pediatr Gastroenterol Nutr 1999; 29:240–249.

117. Ginès P, Arroyo V, Vargas V, et al. Paracentesis with intravenous infusion of albumin as compared with peritoneovenous shunting in cirrhosis with refractory ascites. N Engl J Med 1991; 325:829–835.

Chapter 17

Caustic ingestion and foreign bodies: damage to the upper gastrointestinal tract

Adrian Jones

INTRODUCTION

Virtually anything that can be swallowed by a child will be swallowed – by some child somewhere, somehow. Our responsibility as parents and as healthcare advocates is to minimize the opportunities and the damage that ingestion may cause. Infants and children in the first 3 years of life explore their environment using all senses, including taste and smell. Thus, any foreign materials, including coins, toys, nails and pins, pebbles and anything else lying around the house or yard, are fair game for ingestion. In addition, anything in bottles or cups may be tasted or swallowed. This includes dangerous substances stored in unsafe containers.

Adolescents and young adults may suffer from self-destructive feelings. If caustic materials are readily available, they may use such materials to attempt suicide. The bimodal curve of ingestion of potentially dangerous materials peaks in the toddler and in the teenager/young adult age groups.

CAUSTIC INGESTION AS A COMMON WORLDWIDE PROBLEM

Ingestion of caustic materials is a worldwide challenge. Large series from India, Spain, South America, sub-Saharan Africa, Europe and North America attest to the inadequate storage of these products, or the intent on suicide by teenagers and young adults. However, in countries with a well developed public health service and a strong emphasis towards preventive strategies, caustic ingestion is becoming less frequent and damage less common.[1,2] This reduction is the result of political pressure and legislation that have limited the type and concentration of caustic materials sold to the public, improved labeling laws, advocated public safety messages in regard to safe storage, and caused a greater public awareness of the danger of these products. However, in less developed countries strong caustic agents may be stored, or even sold in bazaars and open marketplaces in inappropriate containers such as soft drink bottles, jars or cans originally used for other purposes. Similarly, in industrial and farm operations, caustic agents may be transferred to generic containers without adequate safety closures. Up to 75% of accidental ingestions may occur from secondary containers.[3] Under these circumstances, children remain extremely vulnerable.[4,5] In other cases, known caustic agents may be employed for 'therapeutic' use. One example is lead battery acid (sulfuric acid), which is ubiquitous, has been tragically used for suicide attempts[6] and is prescribed orally by traditional healers in sub-Saharan Africa, with catastrophic results to the recipients.[5]

MECHANISMS OF DAMAGE TO THE UPPER GASTROINTESTINAL TRACT

Caustic materials damage by direct chemical or osmotic reaction on tissue (Table 17.1). The degree of damage has been classified by a number of scales which are useful in determining the likelihood of complications following ingestion. A frequently used classification is indicated in Table 17.2.

Strong alkaline materials (usually drain cleaner, oven and grill cleaner, dishwasher detergent designed to liquefy animal and food products, milking-machine pipe cleaners)[7] liquefy tissue by dissolving and saponifying lipid, producing liquefaction necrosis. Damage varies from minor erythema to deep ulceration, which can lead to perforation of a viscus.

Strong acids (such as lead battery acid, concentrated vinegar, toilet and industrial cleaners) coagulate proteins. After contact an eschar forms that partially inhibits deeper damage, but deep ulceration and perforation can occur if a sufficiently large volume has been ingested.

Bleaches, usually sodium hypochlorite, but including sodium perborate, hydrosulfite and hydrogen peroxide, cause tissue damage by oxidation.[8] Hydrogen peroxide ingestion has more commonly caused gas embolization with particular damage to the central nervous system,[9] although there are very occasional reports of gastric ulceration. 'Hair relaxer' is a common household liquid in many cultures. Hair relaxers, which are alkali products, may contain any of a number of different chemicals, each designed to break the disulfide bonds in hair. These include sodium or calcium hydroxide, guanidine carbonate, dimethylsulfone and thioglycolic acid salts. Several studies have confirmed that ingestion of hair relaxer does not result in significant tissue injury, although pain and minor erythema in the mouth may occur.[10,11]

	Most damaging agents	Other agents
Alkaline drain cleaners, milking-machine pipe cleaners	Sodium or potassium hydroxide	Ammonia Sodium hypochlorite Aluminum particles
Acidic drain openers	Hydrochloric acid Sulfuric acid	
Toilet cleaners	Hydrochloric acid Sulfuric acid Phosphoric acid Other acids	Ammonium chloride Sodium hypochlorite
Oven and grill cleaners	Sodium hydroxide Perborate (borax)	
Denture cleaners	Persulfate (sulfur) Hypochlorite (bleach)	
Dishwasher detergent	Sodium hydroxide	
Liquid	Sodium hypochlorite	
Powdered	Sodium carbonate	
Bleach	Sodium hypochlorite	Ammonia salt
Swimming pool chemicals	Acids, alkalis, chlorine	
Battery acid (liquid)	Sulfuric acid	
Disk batteries	Electric current	Zinc or other metal salts
Rust remover	Hydrofluoric, phosphoric, oxalic and other acids	
Household de-limers	Phosphoric acid Hydroxyacetic acid Hydrochloric acid	
Barbeque cleaners	Sodium and potassium hydroxide	
Glyphosate surfactant (RoundUp®) acid	Glyphosate herbicide	Surfactants

Source: National Library of Medicine. Health and safety information on household products. http://householdproducts.nlm.nih.gov/

Table 17.1 Ingestable caustic materials around the house

The herbicide glyphosate surfactant (RoundUp®) is a mild acid, but ingestion of a large volume (usually suicide attempts) has resulted in Zargar's grade 1–2 damage[12] (see Table 17.2) to the esophageal and gastric mucosa. The systemic toxicity and pulmonary complications following ingestion of this agent are generally of greater consequence to survival.[13]

Medication in pill form may lodge and disintegrate in the esophagus, resulting in 'pill esophagitis' (Fig. 17.1). The pill may be acid (e.g. tetracycline, ferrous sulfate), alkaline (e.g. phenytoin) or have a high osmolality when dissolved. The mucosal damage may be deep enough to produce ulceration and subsequent scarring.[14,15]

Solid foreign bodies, such as coins, toy parts or sharp objects (Fig. 17.2), damage by perforation or pressure necrosis. In addition, some coins contain a high concentration of zinc, which itself is toxic to tissues.[16] However, zinc toxicity

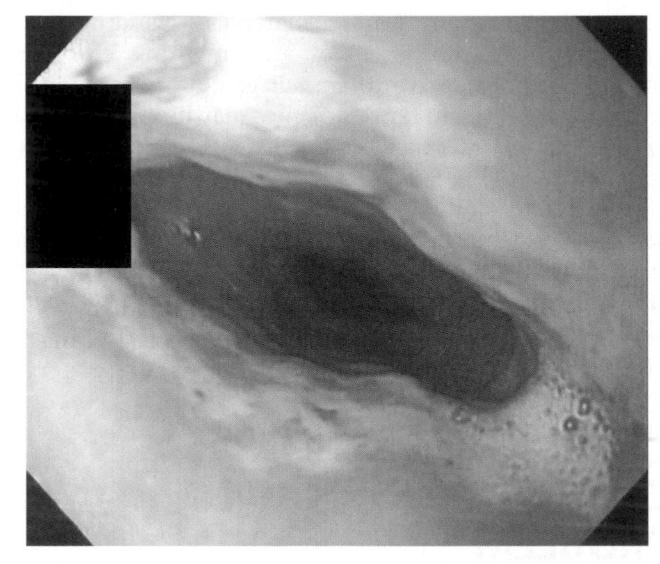

Figure 17.1: 'Pill esophagitis' in a teenage girl on doxycycline (*See plate section for color*).

Grade	Visible appearance	Clinical significance
Grade 0	History of ingestion, but no visible damage or symptoms	Able to take fluids immediately
Grade 1	Edema, loss of normal vascular pattern, hyperemia. No transmucosal injury	Temporary dysphagia, able to swallow within 0–2 days. No long-term sequalae
Grade 2a	Transmucosal injury with friability, hemorrhage, blistering, exudate, scattered superficial ulceration	Scarring. No circumferential damage = no stenosis. No long-term sequalae
Grade 2b	Grade 2a *plus* deep discrete ulceration and/or circumferential ulceration	Small risk of perforation. Scarring that may result in later stenosis
Grade 3a	Scattered deep ulceration with necrosis of tissue	Risk of perforation. High risk of later stenosis
Grade 3b	Extensive necrotic tissue	High risk of perforation and death. High risk of stenosis

Source: Zargar et al., 1991.[11]
Other classifications vary slightly in detail from this one and may include 'grade 4' to indicate perforation.

Table 17.2 Classification of caustic injury

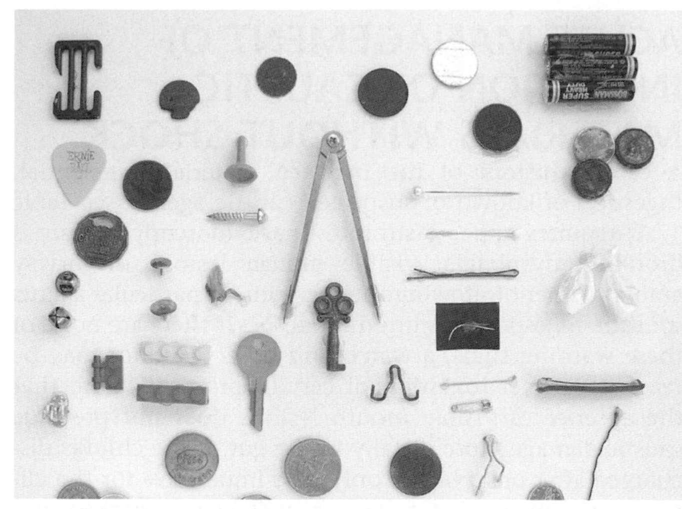

Figure 17.2: What did your child eat today? A small collection of objects removed endoscopically in a single practice.

has not been reported following coin ingestion. Live disk batteries ('button batteries') used, for example, for electronic toys and watches discharge their current across tissue or liquid. If impacted in the esophagus, they can produce a bilateral burn as the edge of the battery is wedged into the tissue (Figs 17.3 & 17.4). In the stomach, batteries (disk batteries and dry cell batteries) discharge their current through the gastric fluid without damaging the mucosa. Regular dry cell batteries ('alkaline batteries') (e.g. for penlights) may contain manganese dioxide, zinc and potassium hydroxide. Rechargeable and disk batteries may contain lithium and/or cadmium.[17] Information from major battery manufacturers (Duracell®, EverReady®) suggests that the risk of leakage is very small with modern cylindrical alkaline batteries; however, it is suggested that they be removed if still in the gastric lumen after 72 h.[18,19] Details may be found in technical sections of the various manufacturers' web pages, or through poison control centers.[20]

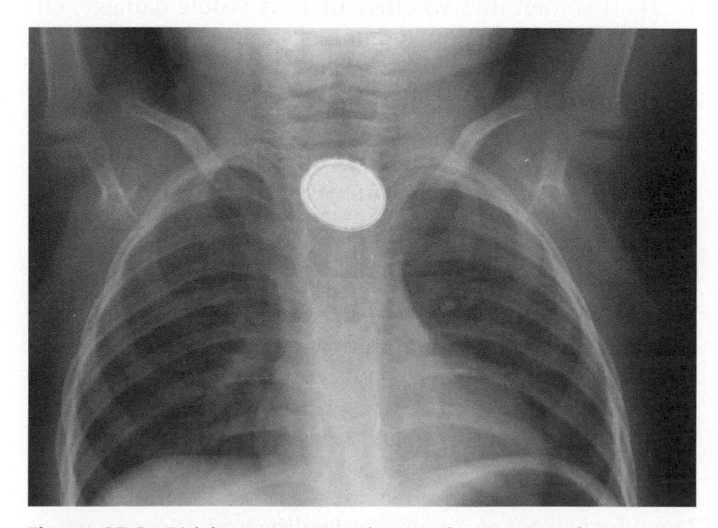

Figure 17.3: Disk battery impacted in esophagus. Note the 'double rim'.

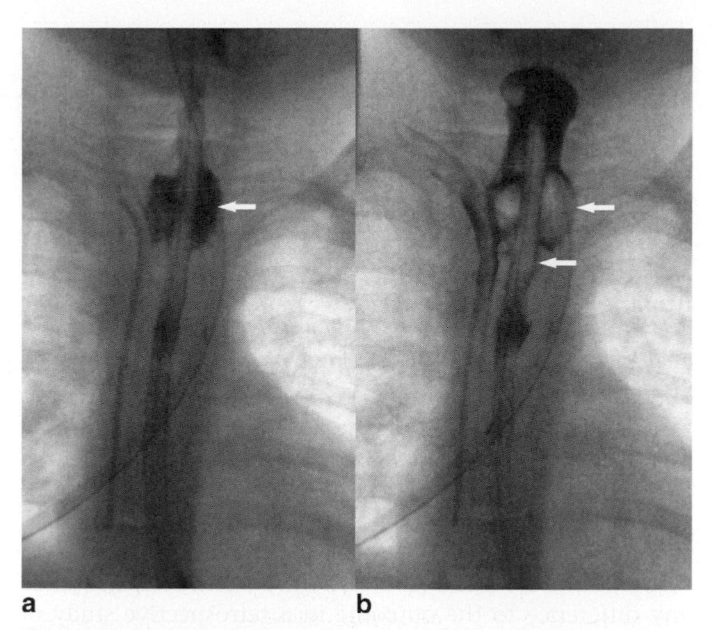

Figure 17.4: Esophageal perforation and leak on upper gastrointestinal radiograph due to disk battery impaction and secondary electrical burn. (**a**) Contrast media in the mediastinum. (**b**) Air in the mediastinum, with air and contrast media leaking superiorly and inferiorly subsequent to 'button battery' impaction and electrical burn.

COMPLICATIONS IMPOSED BY ANATOMY

The lips, mouth and oropharynx may be damaged by caustic liquids, but lack of visible damage in the mouth does *not* preclude damage lower in the gut.[21,22] Caustic material may pool in the hypopharynx due to upper esophageal sphincter spasm, and granulated caustic materials such as dishwasher detergent or denture cleaner will stick onto the mucosa in the oropharynx and upper esophagus. Profound damage then occurs to the periglottic tissues. This can result in severe contraction and scarring, leading to partial or complete obstruction of the airway and upper esophageal sphincter.[23]

Perforation of the esophagus by either caustic materials or foreign bodies results in profound illness due to mediastinitis. In addition, the ulceration may extend into the tracheobronchial tree resulting in an esophagobronchial fistula, or into a major blood vessel resulting in life-threatening hemorrhage. Perforation of the stomach (usually resulting from large-volume alkali ingestion) results in damage to surrounding tissues including the pancreas and bowel.

A large-volume ingestion – at least one tablespoon (15 ml) of granulated lye for an adult[24] – is required to produce serious damage in the duodenum. As caustic ingestion into the stomach results in pylorospasm, the duodenum is often spared. However, this pylorospasm results in more severe damage to the antrum and may cause profound scarring, contraction of the antrum and later gastric obstructive symptoms.

PRESENTATION

Children and teenagers who have ingested a caustic material are usually brought to the hospital very quickly because of pain, dysphagia or observation of the event by a caregiver, and fear of the consequences. If emergency personnel have the opportunity to speak to the caregiver before leaving home, it is useful to arrange to bring the container of caustic material if this can be done safely. This allows confirmation of the type of ingested material and enables the teaching process with regard to safe storage to be started.

Although antidotes such as milk, water, or dilute acid or alkali have been recommended in the past, their use following the ingestion of caustic agents is not supported by any controlled trials of antidotes. A study in animals with a controlled alkali skin burn using either water or neutralization with 5% acetic acid (weak vinegar) showed clear superiority of the weak acid neutralization over water.[25] Mamede and De Mello Filho[26] found no antidote that made any difference to the outcome in a retrospective study of 215 patients presenting over a 37-year period. Until controlled studies have been published, antidotes are best avoided.

LARGE-VOLUME INGESTIONS WITH SHOCK AND PERFORATION

For the patient who presents in shock, the ABCs of resuscitation are instituted, as for any life-threatening illness. Although pulmonary complications are rare, tracheal intubation may be required. Patients in shock or with pulmonary signs that may advance to adult respiratory distress syndrome (ARDS) will require full intensive care unit support. An indwelling venous catheter is placed to provide fluids, broad-spectrum antibiotic coverage and, if the patient survives, total parenteral nutrition until enteral feeding is possible. The presence of shock, fever or prostration indicates profound tissue damage and requires immediate surgical consultation. Gastric perforation is almost invariably fatal, as a result of the toxic and septic effects of acute hemorrhagic pancreatitis, multiple bowel perforations and peritonitis. Urgent and aggressive surgical debridement of all necrotic tissue in the chest and abdomen has been shown significantly to improve survival. This may include complete esophagectomy and partial to complete gastrectomy, as well as excision of all necrotic tissue in the abdominal cavity, thorough peritoneal lavage and postoperative drainage.[27,28] Endoscopy in the setting of a suspected perforation should be performed only in concert with the surgeon, and if required for planning of the surgical approach. If the patient survives, a psychiatric consultation is required once the patient is healing to manage the ongoing stress associated with the consequences of the major surgery, as well as to deal with prior suicidal ideation if that had precipitated the ingestion.

ACUTE MANAGEMENT OF INGESTION OF CAUSTIC MATERIALS WITHOUT SHOCK

A careful history of the ingested material is essential. Ingestion of known or suspected caustic agents (see Table 17.1) requires upper gastrointestinal endoscopy if there is drooling, dysphagia, visible mouth lesions or airway embarrassment following the ingestion of particular agents or if the ingestion was intentional.[29,30] If there are none of these warning signs, a watch and observe stance may be reasonable after ingestion of certain products. Note that the absence of visible mouth lesions does not preclude caustic damage more distally in the gut. If the child is discharged after observation only, it is imperative for the clinician to ensure that follow-up will be undertaken and that preventive teaching is provided.

When endoscopy is warranted it should be performed immediately. In the past there was debate regarding 'early' *vs* 'late' endoscopy, but this has now been resolved in favor of early endoscopy. Endoscopes with a diameter as small as 3–6 mm can be passed safely through a severely inflamed and narrowed lumen to identify the extent of the injury. In the past, endoscopy usually stopped at the first evidence of severe injury, but some centers now consider it appropriate to identify the full extent of injury, at least down to the duodenum. The endoscopic procedure is terminated if a perforation is suspected or encountered. Air insufflation is minimized to decrease the risk of a 'blowout' through a deeply ulcerated area. Physicians from otorhinolaryngology, pediatric surgery and pediatric gastroenterology may be in attendance at the first endoscopy to perform a complete examination of the upper airway and gastrointestinal tract as necessary.

Endoscopy is performed with adequate intravenous access, anesthesia and airway protection (orotracheal or nasotracheal intubation). The objective of the endoscopy is to categorize the extent and grade of injury (see Table 17.2). This identifies whether there is visible damage, circumferential ulceration (grade 2b or greater), and which organs are involved. This information will guide treatment and indicate prognosis. In the case of severe ulceration in a viscus, computed tomography is useful to examine the deeper tissues Although endoscopic ultrasonography has been proposed, before it can be generally recommended further evidence is required of both its practicality and usefulness in this situation.[31,32] In the face of extensive damage of Zarger's grade 2b or higher in the esophagus, a nasogastric or nasointestinal tube should be left in place. This can be passed over a guidewire left in as the scope is removed. If the tube is to be nasointestinal, the guidewire can initially be brought back through the mouth, then passed retrogradely through the nasally placed tube until the guidewire exits the hub of the tube, at which time the tube can be advanced down into the stomach (Fig. 17.5). The tube will act as a route for feeding and, if necessary, as a stent. Although individual practitioners have designed stents of various types,[33,34] there is no generally accepted stent management protocol except to place a nasogastric tube as soon as possible, with as large a diameter as is practical in the child. The tube can initially be used for enteral feeding. As the swelling decreases, the child can feed around the tube. As soon as the child is able to swallow saliva adequately, oral feedings can be started. Total parenteral nutrition will be required if intestinal feeding is not possible initially. Antibiotics should be used only if there is fever or evidence of deep ulceration on endoscopic examination (grade 2b or greater).

Corticosteroids, specifically prednisone and hydrocortisone, *have no beneficial effect* in decreasing scar formation and stricture.[35,36] Dexamethasone 1 mg/kg daily may be of benefit. However, this is supported by only a single controlled trial.[35] The use of high-dose steroids for the several weeks that collagen is being laid down is unlikely to be an effective therapy, and may increase the incidence of complications.

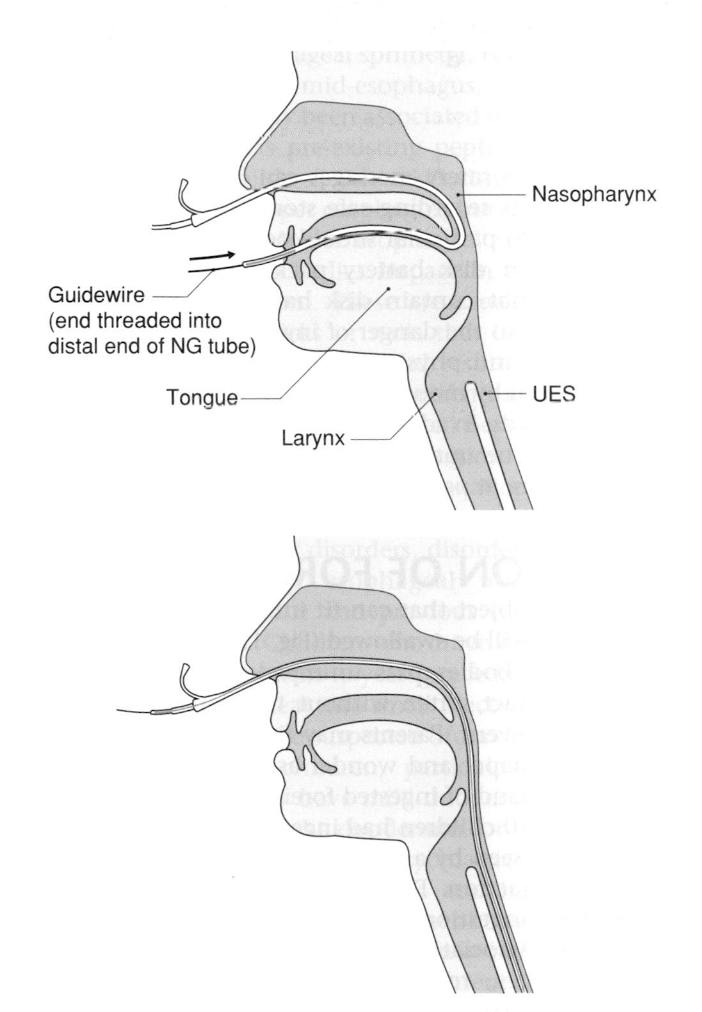

Figure 17.5: Placement of a nasogastric (NG) tube over guidewire for feeding and/or stenting. Guidewire exits mouth, NG tube is pulled out of mouth, guidewire is inserted into distal end of tube and passed retrogradely up tube until it exits hub end; tube is pulled out until distal end is in oropharynx, then advanced down esophagus over guidewire.

If the damage is of grade 2a or less, management consists of adequate nutrition, by mouth if possible, with repeat endoscopy at 2–3 weeks to ensure that there is no evidence of developing stricture, and that healing is progressing well.

Normal acid reflux can impair the healing process and intensify damage.[37] All subjects with grade 2 or higher esophageal lesions should be maintained on acid reduction therapy, ideally a proton pump inhibitor twice daily, until ulcerations have healed over completely. Subsequent to complete healing, a pH probe should be performed to identify the quantity of acid reflux. If it is excessive, or if there is abnormally slow clearance of acid (episodes greater than 5 min on repeated occasions, or single episodes longer than 30 min), then long-term prophylactic acid-suppressing therapy should be considered.

FOLLOW-UP OF CAUSTIC INGESTION DAMAGE

Every child who has suffered grade 2 damage or greater from a caustic ingestion should be endoscoped 3 weeks after the ingestion to assess healing and the development of a stricture. If a stricture is present, dilation should be started at this time, using bougies of graduated size or, for a long stricture, a balloon. There is no difference in complications between balloon and Savary–Gilliard bougie dilation.[38] Significant strictures may require repeated dilations over a period of 1–2 years, at gradually decreasing intervals.[39] There is a small risk of severe complications during esophageal dilation, including mediastinitis, pneumothorax, peritoneal soiling and brain abscess.[40,41]

Once any deep ulcerations have healed over, there is empirical evidence that dilation followed immediately by the application of mitomycin C solution to the scarred area may impede scar tissue regeneration and decrease the number of dilations required[42,43] (Fig. 17.6). Other agents (e.g. halofuginone, which inhibits collagen type 1 synthesis) are being investigated for topical or systemical use immediately after the injury to inhibit scarring and stenosis.[44] Recently, laser-assisted remodeling of stenotic areas has been reported, with good to excellent results.[45]

As the scar tissue matures, the esophagus may be shortened as well as narrowed. Shortening of the esophagus wedges apart the diaphragmatic crura as the stomach is pulled up. This produces a so-called 'sliding hiatus hernia', which increases the risk of pathologic gastroesophageal reflux. Acid-suppressing therapy may then be needed indefinitely.

Motility in the injured viscus is affected, and is permanent after deep injury to the tissue. Alkaline injury appears to cause a serious and long-term change in motility more frequently than acid injury. The initial injury results in delayed esophageal clearance with low-caliber and simultaneous waves.[46] Depending on the depth of this scar, the myenteric plexus may be damaged, and the normal syncitium of smooth muscle cells will have been interrupted.

References

1. Christesen HB. Epidemiology and prevention of caustic ingestion in children. Acta Paediatr 1994; 83:212–215.
2. Nuutinen M, Uhari M, Karvali T, Kouvalainen K. Consequences of caustic ingestions in children. Acta Paediatr 1994; 83:1200–1205.
3. Bautista CA, Estevez ME, Varela CR, et al. A retrospective analysis of ingestion of caustic substances by children. Ten-year statistics in Galicia. Eur J Pediatr 1997; 156:410–414.
4. Dabadie A, Roussey M, Oummal M, et al. Accidental ingestion of caustics in children. Apropos of 100 cases. Arch Fr Pediatr 1989; 46:217–222.
5. Ogunleye AO, Nwaorgu GB, Grandawa H. Corrosive oesophagitis in Nigeria: clinical spectrums and implications. Trop Doct 2002; 32:78–80.
6. Wilson DA, Wormald PJ. Battery acid – an agent of attempted suicide in black South Africans. S Afr Med J 1995; 85:529–531.
7. Edmonson MB. Caustic alkali ingestions by farm children. Pediatrics 1987; 79:413–416.
8. Trabelsi M, Loukhil M, Boukthir S, Hammami A, Benneceur B. Accidental ingestion of caustics in Tunisian children. Report of 125 cases. Pediatrie 1990; 45:801–805.
9. Cina SJ, Downs JC, Conradi SE. Hydrogen peroxide: a source of lethal oxygen embolism. Case report and review of the literature. Am J Forensic Med Pathol 1994; 15:44–50.
10. Cox AJ 3rd, Eisenbeis JF. Ingestion of caustic hair relaxer: is endoscopy necessary? Laryngoscope 1997; 107:897–902.
11. Zargar SA, Kochhar R, Mehta S, et al. The role of fiberoptic endoscopy in the management of corrosive ingestion and modified endoscopic classification of burns. Gastrointest Endosc 1991; 37:165–169.
12. Ahsan S, Haupert M. Absence of esophageal injury in pediatric patients after hair relaxer ingestion. Arch Otolaryngol Head Neck Surg 1999; 125:953–955.
13. Chang CY, Peng YC, Hung DZ, Hu WH, Yang DY, Lin TJ. Clinical impact of upper gastrointestinal tract injuries in glyphosate-surfactant oral intoxication. Hum Exp Toxicol 1999; 18:475–478.
14. Kirkendall JM. Pill esophagitis. J Clin Gastroenterol 1999; 28:298–305.
15. Jasperson D. Drug-induced oesophageal disorders: pathogenesis, incidence, prevention and management. Drug Saf 2000; 22:237–249.
16. O'Hara SM, Donnelly LF, Chuang E, Briner WH, Bisset GS 3rd.Gastric retention of zinc-based pennies: radiographic appearance and hazards. Radiology 1999; 213:113–117.
17. Gillette Company. Technical information for Original Equipment Manufacturers. Online. Available: http://www.duracell.com/oem/ 23 March 2005.
18. Litovitz T, Schmitz BF. Ingestion of cylindrical and button batteries: an analysis of 2382 cases. Pediatrics 1992; 89:747–757.
19. Rebhandl W, Steffan I, Schramel P, et al. Release of toxic metals from button batteries retained in the stomach: an *in vitro* study. J Pediatr Surg 2002; 37:87–92.
20. American Association of Poison Control Centers. Poison help. Online. Available: http://www.aapcc.org/ 23 March 2005.
21. DiCostanza J, Noirclerc M, Jougland J, et al. New therapeutic approach to corrosive burns of the upper gastrointestinal tract. Gut 1980; 21:370–375.
22. Kay M, Wyllie R. Caustic ingestions and the role of endoscopy (editorial). J Pediatr Gastroenterol Nutr 2001; 32:8–10.
23. Kynaston JA, Patrick MK, Shepherd RW, Raivadera PV, [illegible]. The hazards of automatic-dishwasher detergent. Med J Aust 1989; 151:5–7.
24. Mamede RC, de Mello Filho FV. Ingestion of caustic substances and its complications. Sao Paulo Med J 2001; 119:10–15.
25. Andrews K, Mowlavi A, Milner SM The treatment of alkaline burns of the skin by neutralization. Plast Reconstr Surg 2003; 111:1918–1921.
26. Mamede RC, De Mello Filho FV. Treatment of caustic ingestion: an analysis of 239 cases. Dis Esophagus 2002; 15:210–213.
27. Berthet B, Castellani P, Brioche MI, et al. Early operation for severe corrosive injury of the upper gastrointestinal tract. Eur J Surg 1996; 162:951–955.
28. Andreoni B, Farina ML, Biffi R, et al. Esophageal perforation and caustic injury: emergency management of caustic ingestion. Dis Esophagus 1997; 10:95–100.
29. Christesen HB. Prediction of complications following unintentional caustic ingestion in children. Is endoscopy always necessary? Acta Paediatr 1995; 84:1177–1182.
30. Gupta SK, Croffie JM, Fitzgerald JF. Is esophagogastroduodenoscopy necessary in all caustic ingestions? J Pediatr Gastroenterol Nutr 2001; 32:50–53.
31. Kamijo Y, Kondo I, Soma K, et al. Alkaline esophagitis evaluated by endoscopic ultrasound. J Toxicol Clin Toxicol 2001; 39:623–625.
32. Bernhardt J, Ptok H, Wilhelm L, Ludwig K.Caustic acid burn of the upper gastrointestinal tract: first use of endosonography to evaluate the severity of the injury. Surg Endosc 2002; 16: 1004.
33. Mutaf O.Treatment of corrosive esophageal strictures by long-term stenting. J Pediatr Surg 1996; 31:681–685.
34. DePeppo F, Zaccara A, Dall'Oglio LM, et al. Stenting for caustic strictures: esophageal replacement replaced. J Pediatr Surg 1998; 33:54–57.
35. Bautista A, Varela R, Villanueva A, et al. Effects of prednisolone and dexamethasone in children with alkali burns of the oesophagus. Eur J Pediatr Surg 1996; 6:198–203.
36. Ulman I, Mutaf O. A critique of systemic steroids in the management of caustic esophageal burns in children. Eur J Pediatr Surg 1998; 8:71–74.
37. Mutaf O, Genc A, Herek O, et al. Gastroesophageal reflux: a determinant in the outcome of caustic esophageal burns. J Pediatr Surg 1996; 31:1494–1495.
38. Hernadez LJ, Jacobson JW, Harris MS. Comparison among the perforation rates of Maloney, balloon, and savary dilation of esophageal strictures. Gastrointest Endosc 2000; 51:460–462.
39. Broto J, Asensio M, Jorro CS, et al. Conservative treatment of caustic esophageal injuries in children: 20 years of experience. Pediatr Surg Int. 1999; 15:323–325.
40. Karnak I, Tanyel FC, Buyukpamukcu N, et al. Esophageal perforations encountered during the dilation of caustic esophageal strictures. J Cardiovasc Surg (Torino) 1998; 39:373–377.
41. Appignani A, Trizzino V. A case of brain abscess as complication of esophageal dilation for caustic stenosis. Eur J Pediatr Surg 1997; 7:42–43.
42. Rahbar R, Jones DT, Nuss RC, et al. The role of mitomycin in the prevention and treatment of scar formation in the pediatric aerodigestive tract: friend of foe? Arch Otolaryngol Head Neck Surg 2002; 128:401–406.
43. Afzal NA, Albert D, Thomas AL, Thomson. A child with oesophageal strictures. Lancet 2002; 359:1032.
44. Ozcelik MF, Pekmzci S, Saribeyoglu K, et al. The effect of halofuginone, a specific inhibitor of collagen type 1 synthesis, in the prevention of esophageal strictures related to caustic injury. Am J Surg 2004; 187:257–260.
45. Saetti R, Silvestrini M, Cutrone C, Barion U, Mirri L, Narne S. Endoscopic treatment of upper airway and digestive tract

lesions caused by caustic agents. Ann Otol Rhinol Laryngol 2003; 112:29–36.

46. Genc A, Mutaf O. Esophageal motility changes in acute and late periods of caustic esophageal burns and their relation to prognosis in children. J Pediatr Surg 2002; 37:1526–1528.
47. Dantas RO, Mamede RCM. Esophageal motility in patients with esophageal caustic injury. Am J Gastroenterol 1996; 91:1157–1161.
48. Conners GP, Chamberlain JM, Weiner PR. Pediatric coin ingestion: a home-based survey. Am J Emerg Med 1995; 13:638–640.
49. Narla LD, Hingsbergen EA, Jones JE. Adult diseases in children. Pediatr Radiol 1999; 29:244–254.
50. Cheung KM, Oliver MR, Cameron DJ, et al. Esophageal eosinophilia in children with dysphagia. J Pediatr Gastroenterol Nutr 2003; 37:498–503.
51. Eisen GM, Baron TH, Dominitz JA, et al. Guideline for the management of ingested foreign bodies. Gastrointest Endosc 2002; 55:802–806.
52. Applegate KE, Dardinger JT, Lieber ML, et al. Spiral CT scanning technique in the detection of aspiration of LEGO foreign bodies. Pediatr Radiol 2001; 31:836–840.
53. Soprano JV, Fleisher GR, Mandl KD. The spontaneous passage of esophageal coins in children. Arch Paediatr Adolesc Med 1999; 153:1073–1076.
54. Sharieff GQ, Brousseau TJ, Bradshaw JA, et al. Acute esophageal coin ingestion: is immediate removal necessary? Pediatr Radiol 2003; 33:859–863.
55. Mehta D Attia M, Quintana E, et al. Glucagon use for esophageal coin dislodgment in children: a prospective, double-blind, placebo-controlled trial. Acad Emerg Med 2001; 8:200–203.
56. Harned RK 2nd, Strain JD, Hay TC, et al. Esophageal foreign bodies: safety and efficacy of Foley catheter extraction of coins. AJR Am J Roentgenol 1997; 168:443–446.
57. Soprano JV, Mandl KD. Four strategies for the management of esophageal coins in children. Pediatrics 2000; 105:e5.
58. Emslader HC, Bonadio W, Klatzo M. Efficacy of esophageal bougienage by emergency physicians in pediatric coin ingestion. Ann Emerg Med 1996; 27:726–729.
59. Berthold LD, Moritz JD, Sonksen S, Alzen G. Esophageal foreign bodies: removal of the new euro coins with a magnet tube. Rofo Fortschr Geb Rontgenstr Neuen Bildgeb Verfahr 2002; 174:1096–1098.
60. Kao LS, Nguyen T, Dominitz J, et al. Modification of a latex glove for the safe endoscopic removal of a sharp gastric foreign body. Gastrointest Endosc 2000; 52:127–129.
61. Cauchi JA, Shawis RN. Multiple magnet ingestion and gastrointestinal morbidity. Arch Dis Child 2002; 87:539–540.
62. Aldrighetti L, Paganelli M, Giacomelli M, et al. Conservative management of cocaine-packet ingestion: experience in Milan, the main Italian smuggling center of South American cocaine. Panminerva Med 1996; 38:111–116.
63. Beerman R, Nunez D Jr, Wetli CV.Radiographic evaluation of the cocaine smuggler. Gastrointest Radiol 1986; 11:351–354.
64. June R, Aks SE, Keys N, et al. Medical outcome of cocaine bodystuffers. J Emerg Med 2000; 18:221–224.
65. Tenenbein M. Position statement: whole bowel irrigation. American Academy of Clinical Toxicology; European Association of Poison Centres and Clinical Toxicologists. J Toxicol Clin Toxicol 1997; 35:753–762.
66. DuBose TM 5th, Southgate WM, Hill JG. Lactobezoars: a patient series and literature review. Clin Pediatr (Phil) 2001; 40:603–606.
67. Gaya J, Barranco L, Llompart A, Reyes J, Obrador A. Persimmon bezoars: a successful combined therapy. Gastrointest Endosc 2002; 55:581–583.
68. Bonilla F, Mirete J, Cuesta A, Sillero C, Gonzalez M. Treatment of gastric phytobezoars with cellulase. Rev Esp Enferm Dig 1999; 91:809–814.
69. Ladas SD, Triantafyllou K, Tzathas C, Tassios P, Rokkas T, Raptis SA. Gastric phytobezoars may be treated by nasogastric Coca-Cola lavage. Eur J Gastroenterol Hepatol 2002; 14:801–803.
70. Gockel I, Gaedertz C, Hain HJ, et al. The Rapunzel syndrome: rare manifestation of a trichobezoar of the upper gastrointestinal tract. Chirurg 2003; 74:753–756.
71. Purcell L, Gremse DA Sunflower seed bezoar leading to fecal impaction. South Med J 1995; 88:87–88.
72. Karjoo M, A-Kader H. A novel technique for closing and removing an open safety pin from the stomach. Gastrointest Endosc 2003; 57:627–629.

SECTION THREE
THE ESOPHAGUS

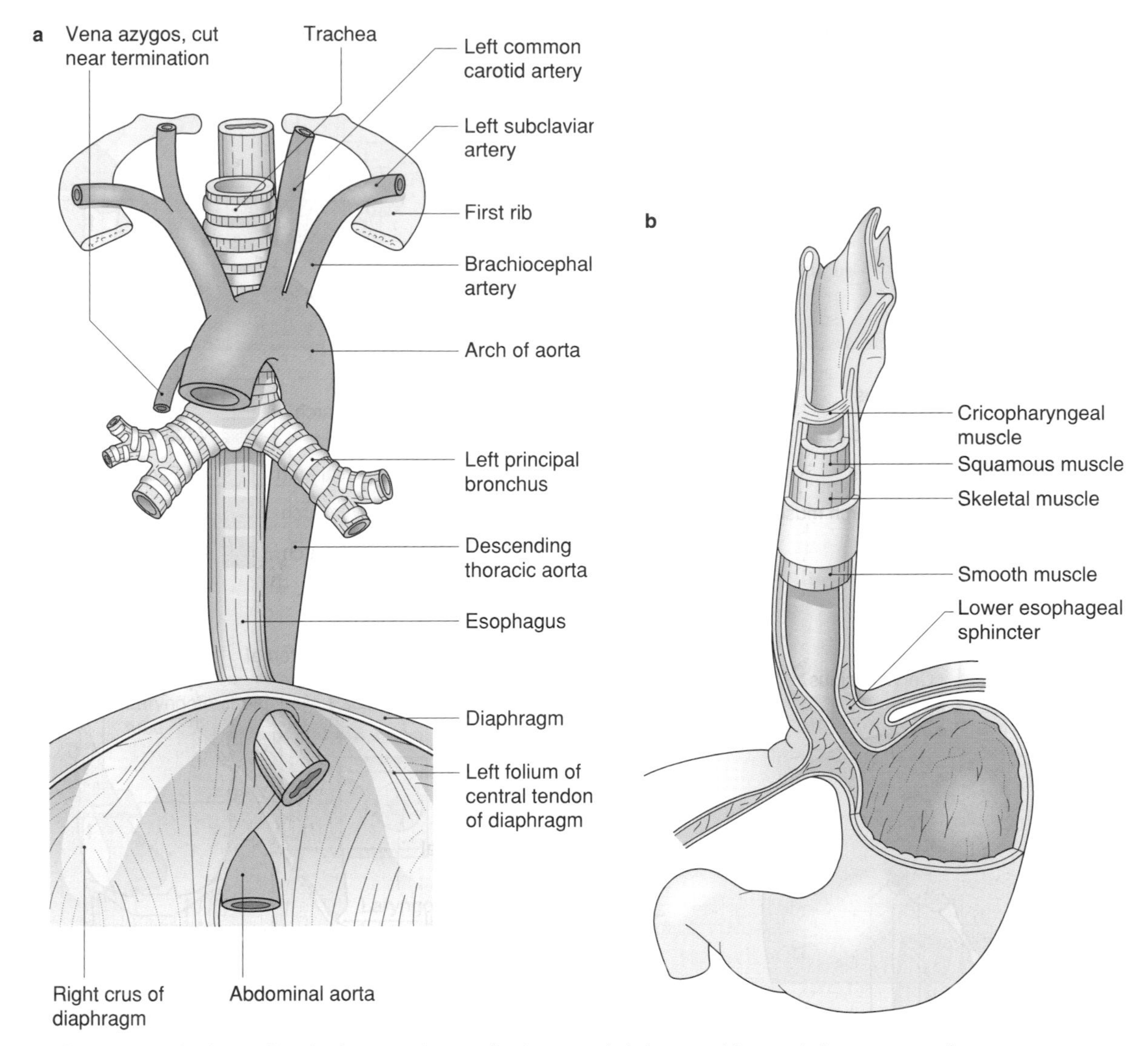

Figure 18.5: a,b Esophageal relationships in the posterior mediastinum and abdomen with muscle layers exposed.

fibers at the junction of the esophagus and diaphragm (a factor not supported by one group);[3] the phrenicoesophageal ligament, which is a layer of connective tissue extending from the inferior diaphragmatic surface and blending with the interfascicular septa and submucosa of the esophagus; the effects of spiral and longitudinal muscle, and various mucosal folds at the gastroesophageal junction. Hence some structures may exert a 'physiologic sphincteric' control that may be compromised in the infant as anatomy matures; however, this remains poorly understood and the main mechanism for infantile GER is thought more likely to be due to inappropriate relaxation of the gastroesophageal junction (see below). It is therefore interesting to postulate how anti-reflux procedures such as open, laparoscopic or even now endoscopic fundoplications work, given the lack of clear understanding of the reasons for GER.[4]

Vasculature supply is from the regional arteries such as the inferior thyroid branch of the thyrocervical trunk, descending aorta, bronchial arteries, left gastric branch of the celiac artery and left phrenic artery. Veins drain in a similar longitudinal way to the inferior thyroid veins, the azygos vein and left gastric vein. The left gastric vein is the most important of the portosystemic communications, and raised portal pressure will therefore lead to esophageal varices.

Nerve supply is considered further in the secion on physiology below. In short, the parasympathetic is from the vagal, and the sympathetic from the cervical and thoracic sympathetic trunks, and greater splanchnic nerves. These form plexi between the two layers of the muscular coat and a second submucous plexus. This is shown in the cross-sectional diagram along with the layers of the esophagus that roughly translate to those in the rest of the gut (Fig. 18.9) – except that the upper third of the esophagus has a striated muscle layer, and the epithelium of the esophagus is non-keratinized stratified compared with that in other parts of the gut – leading to comparisons being drawn between cutaneous eczema and allergic esophagitis.[5] The recent development of endosonography has allowed differentiation of these seven layers at endoscopy (Fig. 18.10), with identification of submucosal and muscle layer pathology in entities such as eosinophilic esophagitis.[6] At endoscopy, it is normally possible to biopsy only the mucosa and part of the submucosa, unless jumbo biopsy forceps are used as is advocated in the Seattle pro-

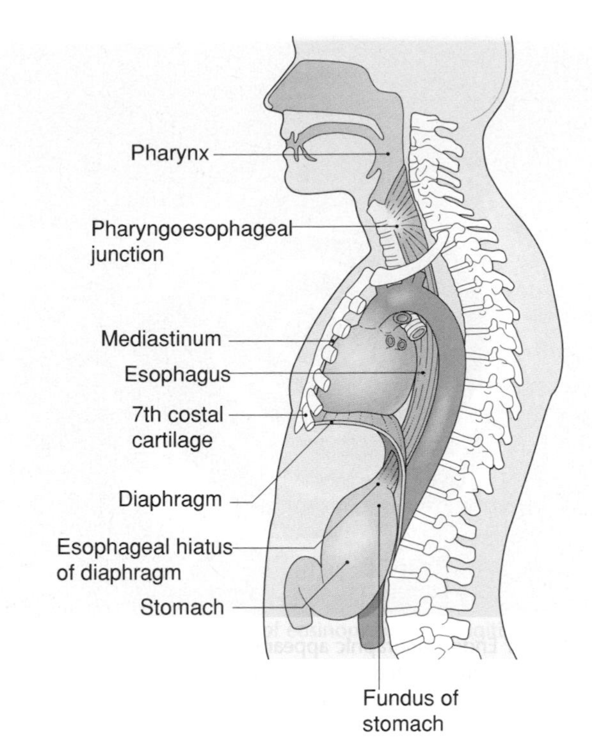

Figure 18.6: The esophagus descends posterior to the trachea and bends in a posterior and then anterior fashion to follow the contours of the cervical and thoracic vertebral columns.

tocol for the accurate detection of intestinal metaplasia signifying Barrett's esophagus.[7] Macroscopically the mucosa shows thickened folds that disappear on distension, except in the presence of edema, and this appearance may alert the endoscopist to the possibility of chronic esophagitis (Fig. 18.11). If circumferential furrows on abnormally pale mucosa are detected, this may point to eosinophilic esophagitis (Fig. 18.12). Histologic examination of the mucosal biopsy may allow conclusions to be drawn regarding the presence of GER and esophagitis. The

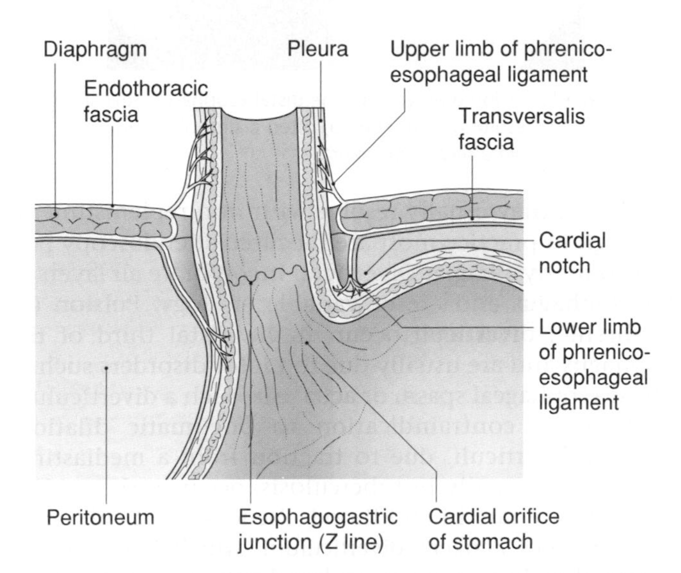

Figure 18.7: The upward movement of the esophagus is limited by the upper limb of the phrenicoesophageal ligament, which connects the esophagus flexibly to the diaphragm. The intra-abdominal portion of the esophagus is much shorter in the infant.

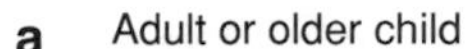

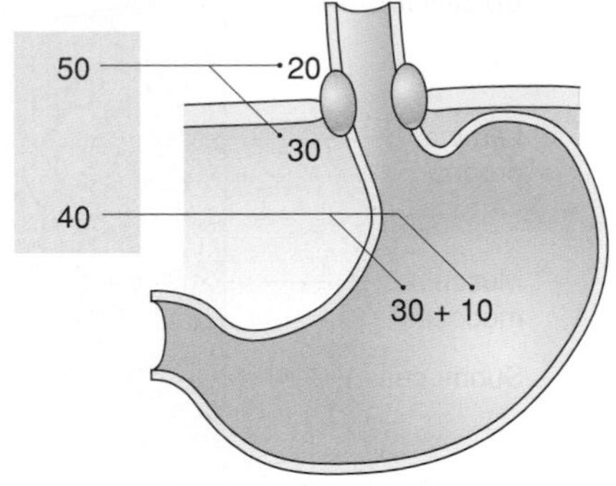

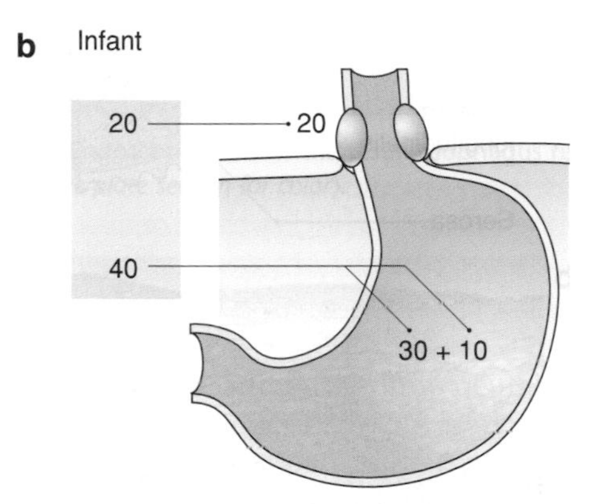

Figure 18.8: (**a**) Importance of the intra-abdominal portion of the esophagus in the maintenance of a pressure gradient to aid in the anti-reflux barrier. (**b**) The absence of this in an infant can be seen to predict the possibility of reflux.

site of biopsy should be above the distal 15% of the esophagus to avoid confusion with normal variation.[8] Biopsies should include epithelium, lamina propria and muscularis mucosae, and be oriented in a perpendicular plane in order to maximize diagnostic yield, such as evaluating properly the thickness of the basal zone, vascular ingrowth and elongation of the stromal papillae. For definitive diagnosis, the presence of two of these three features is preferable; this will not be possible with poorly oriented tissue.[9,10] In an adult study, failure to use well defined histologic criteria resulted in only 50% sensitivity for diagnosing esophagitis.[11] Elongation of stromal papillae is a useful indicator of reflux, and basal zone hyperplasia is defined when the papillae are more than 25% of the entire thickness of the epithelium; when more than 50%, the papillae are considered to be elongated[10,12,13] (Fig. 18.13).

Anatomic variations from normal were partly dealt with in the section above on development of the esophagus. Tracheo-esophageal fistulae, esophageal stenoses and atresia, and congenital webs are explained above, but other abnormalities may occur, for instance rings. Two types of ring occur: the Schatzki ring, which is a submucosal

activity and enteric nerve fetal/neonatal development.[25] Nevertheless the influence of non-nutritive sucking on esophageal and intestinal motor activity, and consequent enteral feeding tolerance, suggests that this can be manipulated, at least partially, by learnt experience.[26]

Lower esophageal sphincter development

Intraluminal pressure and postconceptional age are linked, and a number of perfused manometric systems have been used to produce data in support of this.[27] Effective sphincter pressure was shown to rise by a factor of 4 between 27 weeks' gestation and term. Interestingly resting esophageal pressure does not change, but the effective sphincter pressure of the LES (difference between pressure in the fundus of the stomach and that in the high-pressure area of the lower esophagus) rises significantly in line with postconceptional age: 3.8 mmHg at 27 weeks' gestation, 8.5 mmHg at 31 weeks, 12.2 mmHg at 35 weeks and 18.1 mmHg at 37 weeks and above.[27] This suggests that the resting esophageal pressure itself is not the rate-limiting factor for the problem of GER. This study was undertaken with nasogastric tubes *in situ*; this may or may not have influenced the results. More recently, combined low-volume water perfusion manometric, pH, intraluminal esophageal impedance techniques have been employed in this population, and similar results have been obtained. This elegant experiment in a small number of pre-term neonates (35–37 weeks' postmenstruation), combined with assessment of gastric emptying by ^{13}C-Na octanoate breath test, showed unequivocally that transient lower esophageal relaxation episodes (TLESRs) are the factor that allows GER to occur; indeed, GER was also shown to be worse in the left lateral position than the right lateral position, in keeping with previous clinical studies. In addition, this work showed that gastric emptying was faster in the right lateral position, leading to the conclusion that gastric emptying has little or no influence on GER in this population.[28]

Development of effective gastric emptying, especially from the fundus, may have an influence on esophageal clearance; this is dealt with in Chapter 23.

Swallowing in the normal infant and child

The process of swallowing consists of four phases for liquids and solids alike: oral preparatory, oral, pharyngeal and esophageal. Only the latter two are considered here (Fig. 18.18).

Pharyngeal phase

The pharyngeal phase begins with the production of a swallow and the elevation of the soft palate to close off the nasopharynx, and consists of peristaltic contraction of the pharyngeal constrictors to propel the bolus through the pharynx. Simultaneous closure of the larynx protects against airway penetration of the bolus. Simultaneously there is complete and automatic closure of the glottis, and the epiglottis is brought down over the glottis, thereby deflecting the bolus laterally and posteriorly towards the upper esophageal sphincter (UES). With high-speed videofluoroscopy, four sequential events associated with laryngeal closure have been noted:

1. Adduction of the true vocal cords associated with the horizontal approximation of the arytenoids cartilages
2. Vertical approximation of the arytenoids to the base of the epiglottis
3. Laryngeal elevation
4. Epiglottic descent.

The other major function of the laryngopharyngeal space is in eliciting a protective cough reflex, precipitated by a number of vagally mediated receptors (chemo-, thermo-, etc.) that detect the presence of potentially damaging noxious stimuli and cause laryngeal closure and a cough. This is becoming increasingly important to gastroenterologists as a phenomenon, with the recent appreciation of the pathologic importance of laryngopharyngeal reflux from the stomach in symptoms such as recurrent cough, hoarseness and dysphonia. An increased resting pressure of the cricopharyngeal muscle is necessary to prevent pharyngeal penetration of the retrograde esophageal bolus.

The dynamics of UES function have been shown to be dependent on bolus size in adults, with increased opening size and prolongation of opening occurring with increase in bolus size.[29] Once complete bolus transfer through the UES, policed by coordinated cricopharyngeal relaxation and laryngeal closure, has occurred and the bolus has been transported into the esophagus by continuation of the peristaltic stripping action of the pharyngeal muscles, the esophageal phase of swallowing begins.

Esophageal phase

Swallow-induced automatic esophageal peristalsis usually propagates at 2–4 cm/s and will traverse the pediatric esophagus in around 6–10 s.[30,31] The peristalsis is more likely to traverse the entire esophageal length if the bolus is solid.[32] Peristalsis in the striated upper third of the esophageal muscular wall seems to be similar to that in the distal two-thirds, which is smooth muscle, and the esophageal phase of swallowing is controlled by the swallowing center. Once the bolus has passed the UES, a reflex action causes the sphincter to constrict, then the primary peristaltic wave begins just below the UES. If this primary peristaltic wave does not clear the bolus completely, the continued distension of the esophagus initiates another peristaltic wave, termed secondary peristalsis (Fig. 18.19). Real-time assessment of swallowed bolus transport is now possible with a new technique called intraluminal impedance; this can be combined with pH analysis and now even long-term manometry with low-flow water perfusion as part of the catheter.[33]

Lower esophageal sphincter function

Differences in the function of the LES have been investigated.[34,35] This is an area that is tonically contracted at rest, at a pressure of about 20 mmHg, and mediated mainly by

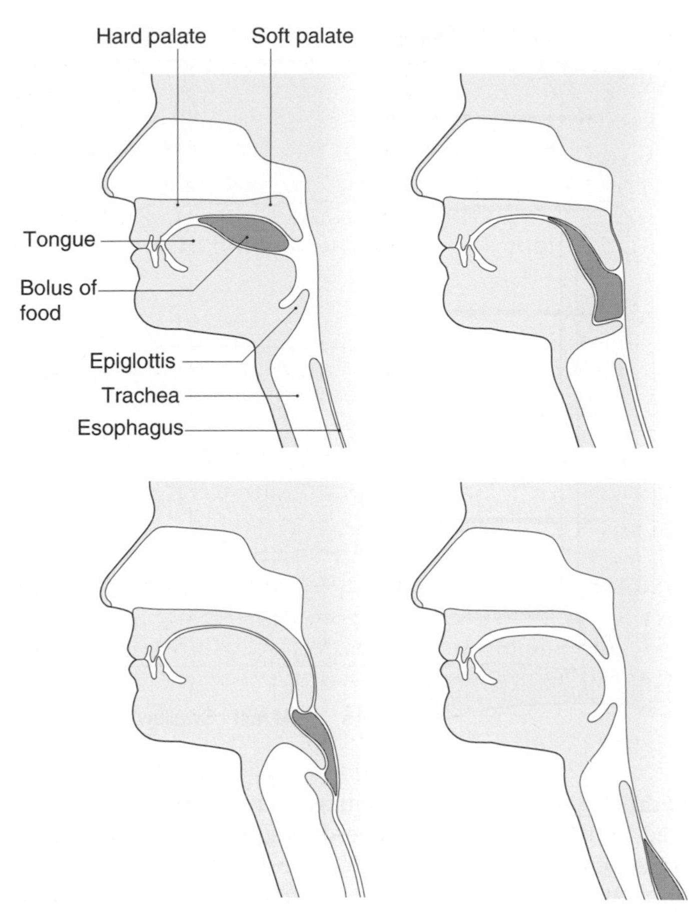

Figure 18.18: A bolus being transported through the four phases of swallowing.

vagal cholinergic fibers (Fig. 18.8) (although stimulation of the sympathetic nerves to the sphincter also causes contraction). Relaxation occurs consequent to an esophageal peristaltic wave. Hence the LES is innervated by both vagal excitatory fibers and vagal inhibitory fibers; increased activity of the inhibitory fibers and decreased activity of the excitatory fibers is associated with LES relaxation, and the opposite occurs as the LES regains its tone (Fig. 18.20). Inhibitory neurotransmitter production is integral to LES relaxation, and the NANC neurotransmitter NO has received attention in animal[16] and human[17,18] studies. VIP is another candidate undergoing investigation, and the importance of the ontogeny of neuropeptides in the human fetus and infant is becoming increasingly apparent. [19] Rather than a 'weak' LES in infants, it is more likely that a combination of anatomic relationships of the LES precluding effective pressure generation, and inappropriate LES relaxation, is responsible for infantile GER and its subsequent age-related improvement.[36,37] In adults, 90% of the refluxate is cleared in seconds and the remainder is neutralized by subsequent swallows.[38] Efficiency of esophageal clearance is therefore vitally important in the genesis of esophagitis. Propagation of a peristaltic wave in the esophagus with pressure generation and the contemporaneous LES relaxation is shown in Figure 18.19. The LES opens with the initiation of esophageal peristalsis. The intricacies of esophageal motility are considered in greater depth in Chapter 21.

Work exists suggesting that acid exposure of the distal esophagus induces dysmotility in pediatric patients,[39] allowing the potential for a 'vicious cycle' of LES dysfunction to GER to LES dysmotility to further GER to esophagitis and back to LES dysmotility (Fig. 18.21), but it is still not clear how an inflamed esophagus further impairs esophageal tone or motility. However emerging work suggests a role for IL-5 and eotaxin in allergic neurohumoral modification and possible inappropriate relaxation of the gastroesophageal junction, with an interrelationship with mast cell degranulation and histamine release to afferent, then efferent, neurons that control TLESRs.[40] iNOS, which is markedly upregulated in gastrointestinal inflammatory conditions such as Crohn's disease, is important in relaxation of the LES during TLESRs – which are the single most common mechanism underlying GER – but in one study was not upregulated in the inflamed pediatric esophagus.[41] However, other workers have suggested an increased release of NO in the inflamed esophagus in children.[42] Other factors that affect clearance are posture–gravity interactions, volume, size and content of a meal, for example breast milk,[43,44] defective peristalsis of the esophagus, gastric emptying and increased noxiousness of refluxate.

PATHOPHYSIOLOGY

Mucosal immunology and inflammation

From the anatomic and physiologic discussion in this chapter it can be seen that the esophagus is relatively quiescent in the non-pathologic state from the immunologic standpoint, not having a major function as part of the largest immune organ in the body – the gut. The esophagus has no Brunner's glands or Peyer's patches involved in antigen recognition and presentation, for instance, but if the epithelial barrier is breached then immunologic functions can occur. Equally, in the pathologic state induced by T cell-mediated allergy in the small bowel, homing of inflammatory cells to the esophagus can occur in the absence of luminal or epithelial damage.[5]

Acid, particularly when combined with pepsin which, it is now realized, is still active up to around pH 5.5–6, is known to cause severe esophagitis in animals and humans.[38–41] Even an infant of 24 weeks' gestation in an intensive care setting has the ability to reduce intragastric pH to less than 2.[42] Pepsin plays a critical role in esophagitis as a result of acidic and possibly non-acidic refluxate. Animal work in dogs and rabbits has shown that the infusion of hydrochloric acid alone caused no damage, but that in combination with low concentrations of pepsin at pH <2 severe esophagitis resulted.[43,44] Proteolysis may allow deeper penetration of harmful refluxate, and the simple notion that acid causes epithelial damage must therefore be questioned in favor of a more complex interplay of a

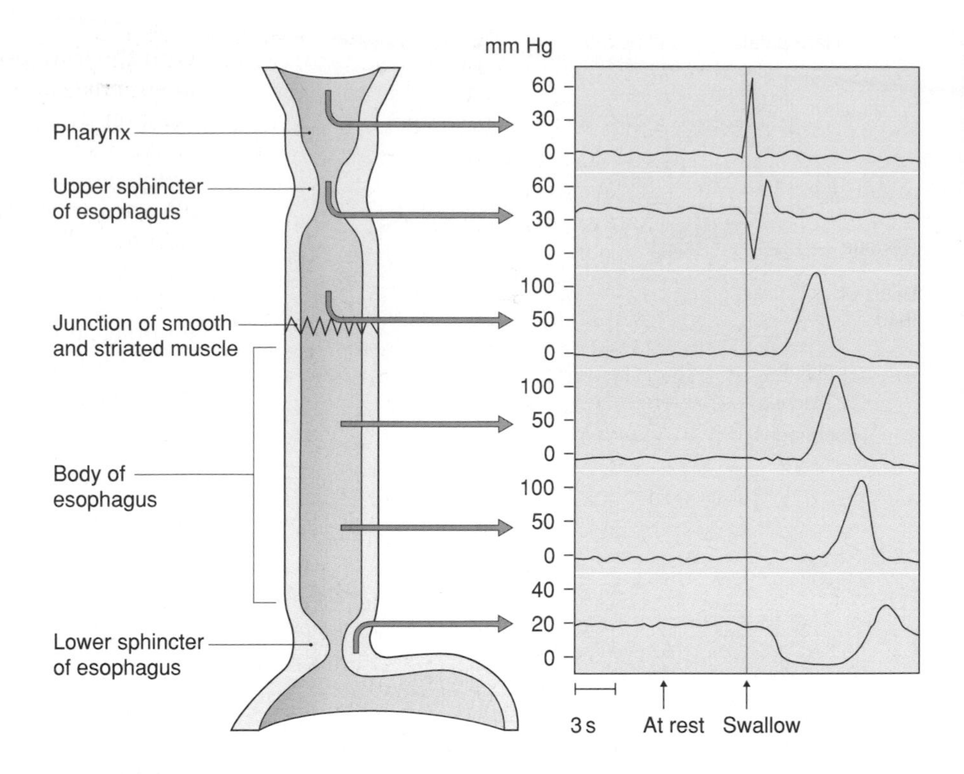

Figure 18.19: Swallowing pressures with timed relaxation of the upper and lower esophageal sphincters.

number of noxious stimuli in the pathogenesis of reflux esophagitis in infants and children.

Furthermore, the role of duodenogastroesophageal reflux (DGER) remains controversial[45,46] and has not, to date, been studied adequately in the pediatric population. What is clear from adult studies is that alkaline reflux does not correlate well with bile reflux, the former being attributable to reasons other than DGER, such as saliva, food, oral infection or an obstructed esophagus.[47] In fact, in one study, bile acid DGER correlated well with acid reflux, and those with more severe esophagitis had greater exposure to the simultaneously damaging effects of acid and bile acids.[45] Perfusion studies of the rabbit esophagus have shown that conjugated bile acids in an acidic environment produce mucosal injury, whereas unconjugated bile acids and trypsin are more harmful at more neutral pH values (pH 5–8).[43] It is further suggested by animal work that the hydrochloric acid–pepsin damage may actually be attenuated by the presence in the esophagus of conjugated bile acids, but that if damage is done to the squamous epithelium the un-ionized forms of conjugated bile acids at low pH may be allowed access to mucosal cells and cause damage by the dissolution of cell membranes and mucosal tight junctions.

Recently, however, the place of intraluminal ambulant esophageal pH measurement as the 'gold standard' for investigation of GER has been challenged. Mainly because pH-directed GER diagnosis is obscured by postprandial neutralization of gastric contents after milk ingestion and

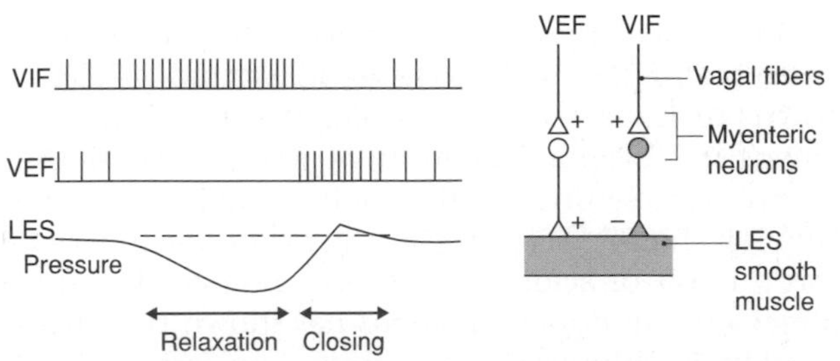

VIF
VEF
LES Pressure
Relaxation
Closing
VEF
VIF
Vagal fibers
Myenteric neurons
LES smooth muscle

Figure 18.20: The lower esophageal sphincter (LES) is innervated by excitatory (VEF) and inhibitory (VIF) fibers from the vagus. Relaxation of the LES occurs with an increased activity of inhibitory fiber action potentials and a corresponding decrease in the action potential frequency from the excitatory fibers. The opposite occurs as the LES returns to resting tone.

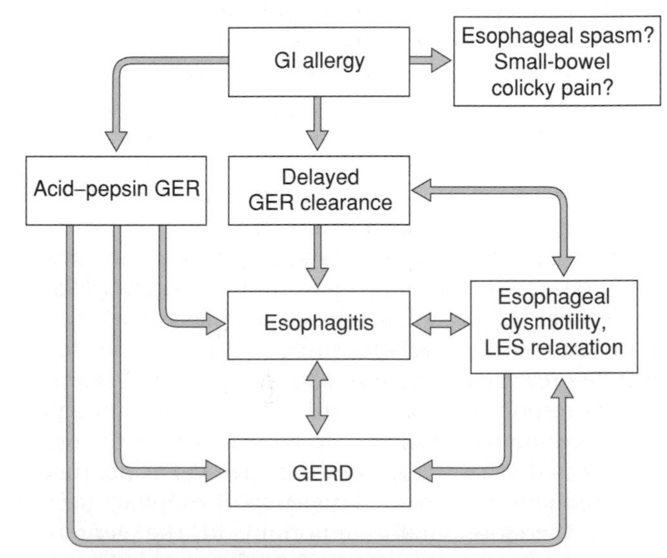

Figure 18.21: The relationships of gastroesophageal reflux (GER), physiology, allergy and esophagitis in the child. GERD, gastroesophageal reflux disease; LES, lower esophageal sphincter.

by drugs,[48–50] other tests have been developed to detect pH-independent GER (e.g. ultrasonography, barium radiography, scintigraphy, external electrical impedance tomography and manometry).[51–56] However, disadvantages of these methods include short-term applicability, high incidence of artefact due to body movement and the need for unphysiologic non-ambulant body positioning. A new pH-independent intraluminal esophageal impedance technique, which relies on the higher conductivity of a liquid bolus compared with esophageal muscular wall or air, has been validated in adults.[57,58] When applied to GER in infants with simultaneous pH measurement over prolonged periods, this intraluminal impedance technique has shown that 73% of all GER occurs during or in the first 2 h after feeding; furthermore, it is pH neutral and will therefore be missed by pHmetry. Even during so-called fasting, 34% of reflux events were missed by pHmetry. Some 75% of GER reached proximally as far as the pharyngeal space, and this has far-reaching implications for the study of GER-associated respiratory phenomena.[50] The intraluminal technique may also allow evaluation of GER in conditions associated with gastric hypoacidity or in infants receiving antacid therapy; at present, H_2 antagonists and proton pump inhibitors must be stopped for 2 and 5 days respectively before pHmetry can be performed reliably.

The clinical importance of DGER may become evident with the recent advent of a spectrophotometric device that detects bilirubin in the esophageal refluxate.

Although it is now clear that multiple food antigens may induce esophagitis,[59] the most common precipitant is cow's milk protein. Standard endoscopic biopsy and histology do not distinguish reliably between primary reflux esophagitis and the emerging clinical entity of cow's milk-associated reflux esophagitis. This variant of cow's milk allergy appears to be a particularly common manifestation in infancy, with symptoms indistinguishable from those of primary GER, but settling on an exclusion diet.[60] Some differentiation from primary reflux has been suggested on the basis of the esophageal pH testing pattern and β-lactoglobulin antibody response, although the former has not been substantiated by more than one center.[5,61,62]

Esophageal mucosal eosinophilia has been described in both suspected cow's milk-associated[5,60] and primary[63] reflux esophagitis, as well as in other conditions such as primary eosinophilic esophagitis.[64,65] Primary eosinophilic esophagitis has a reported prevalence of up to 40 per 100 000 population in parts of the USA, with other countries reporting similar figures.[66] The clinical significance of eosinophils and their role in the pathogenesis of mucosal injury is poorly understood and the subject of recent debate.[63,67,68] Some have suggested an active role for eosinophils in the inflammatory process of esophagitis, and have supported this with the observation of activation of the eosinophils by electron-microscopic criteria.[69] In addition to dietary exclusion of cow's milk,[45,60–62] oral steroids can induce remission of symptoms with decreased mucosal eosinophilia,[64,65] suggesting a pathoetiologic role for eosinophils. In addition, mepolizumab, a monoclonal anti-IL-5 antibody, has been used with success in a person with eosinophilic esophagitis, suggesting a pivotal role for IL-5 in recruitment, trafficking and possible activation of eosinophils in mucosal eosinophilic conditions such as this.[70] As well as eosinophils, intraepithelial T lymphocytes, known as cells with irregular nuclear contours (CINCs), have been implicated as markers of reflux esophagitis.[71,72] In adults, such cells are of memory phenotype and display activation markers, although little is known of their pediatric equivalents. Mast cells may also serve as markers of allergic-type reflux.

A variety of immunohistochemical markers have been used to examine the esophageal mucosa, including eotaxin, a recently described eosinophil-specific chemokine,[67] and markers of T-cell lineage and activation. Despite the mild histologic abnormality in cow's milk protein-associated esophagitis, an increased expression of eotaxin co-localized with activated T lymphocytes to the basal and papillary epithelium has been shown,[5] distinguishing this from primary reflux esophagitis. The molecular basis of the eotaxin upregulation in cow's milk-sensitive enteropathy (CMSE) is unknown. However, there is evidence from murine models of asthma that antigen-specific upregulation of eotaxin expression can be induced by T cells and blocked by anti-CD3 monoclonal antibodies. This suggests the possibility of a distinct mechanism in CMSE, in which mucosal homing to the esophagus occurs for lymphocytes activated within the small intestine.[72–74] This may explain the seemingly counterintuitive finding of basal, as opposed to superficial, chemokine expression and the common occurrence of mucosal eosinophilia in this condition.[5] The esophageal motility disturbance of CMSE-associated esophagitis is thus suggested to occur as a neurologic consequence of the inflammatory infiltration induced from lamina propria vessels into the epithelial compartment.[20,68] This proposed mechanism contrasts with the current concept of luminally induced inflammation found in primary reflux esophagitis, and is consistent with the characteristically delayed onset and chronic nature of cow's milk-associated reflux esophagitis.

SUMMARY

At first glance, this part of the gut is different in many respects from its cousins in the gastrointestinal tract, and may be thought to be fairly uninspiring. However, if one takes the time to look more closely, the esophagus can clearly be seen as a more complex organ with many more responsibilities than simply acting as a conduit for bolus passage from pharynx to stomach. We are now in possession of a much greater understanding of many of the etiologic mechanisms that cause pathology in the esophagus, and with that acquisition of knowledge has come the realization that apparently simple pathologies such as esophagitis may have contributions from many different avenues – abnormal anatomy, disordered physiology, induction of newly identified neurohumoral pathways, presence of excess inflammatory cytokines such as IL-5 and excess chemoattractants such as eotaxin, and complex interactions of all of these and others. The conditions affecting the esophagus are increasingly common in children and this is not merely acquisition bias: clearly, the explosion in allergic conditions has had an impact on this and, indeed, other diseases of apparently idiopathic etiology, such as eosinophilic esophagitis, are rapidly rising in incidence and hence prevalence. In some studies, eosinophilic esophagitis is now reportedly more common than Crohn's disease. Adding to this the increasing disease burden of GER, and considering the high and increasing prevalence of esophageal diseases in general, a sound and up-to-date comprehension of the embryology, development, anatomy and physiology of the esophagus in the normal non-pathologic state is the cornerstone on which can be built knowledge of the increasingly complex interactions in the esophagus that lead to abnormality or disease. This fundamental understanding can then be used in the diagnosis and appropriate therapy of infants and children with esophageal problems to our, and their, greatest advantage.

References

1. Gray S, Skanadalakis J. Embryology for Surgeons. The Embryological Basis for the Treatment of Congenital Defects. Philadelphia, PA: WB Saunders; 1972:63–281.
2. Ingram M, Arregui M. Endoscopic ultrasonography. Surg Clin North Am 2004; 84:1035–1059.
3. Atkinson M, Edwards D, Honour A, Rowlands E. Comparison of cardiac and pyloric sphincters: a manometric study. Lancet 1957; ii:918–922.
4. Endoscopic fundoplication for the treatment of paediatric gastro-oesophageal reflux disease. Thomson M, Fritscher-Ravens A, Afsal N, Hall S, Swain P. Gut. 2004;53(12): 1745-50.
5. Butt A, Murch S, Ng CL, et al. Upregulated eotaxin expression and T-cell infiltration in the basal and papillary epithelium in cows' milk associated reflux oesophagitis. Arch Dis Child 2002; 87:124–130.
6. Fox VL, Nurko S, Teitelbaum JE, Badizadegan K, Furuta GT. High-resolution EUS in children with eosinophilic 'allergic' esophagitis. Gastrointest Endosc 2003; 57:30–36.
7. Sampliner RE. Practice guidelines on the diagnosis, surveillance, and therapy of Barrett's esophagus. The Practice Parameters Committee of the American College of Gastroenterology. Am J Gastroenterol 1998; 93:1028–1032.
8. Hyams J, Ricci A, Leichtner A. Clinical and laboratory correlates of esophagitis in young children. J Pediatr Gastroenterol Nutr 1988; 7:52–56.
9. Thomson M. The pediatric esophagus comes of age. J Pediatr Gastroenterol Nutr 2002; 34:S40–S45.
10. Vandenplas Y. Reflux esophagitis in infants and children: a report from the working group on gastro-oesophageal reflux disease of the European Society of Paediatric Gastroenterology and Nutrition. J Pediatr Gastroenterol Nutr 1994; 18:413–422.
11. Wienbeck M. Cisapride acts as a motor stimulation in the esophagus. Gastroenterology 1984; 86:1298.
12. Mangano MM, Antonioli DA, Schnitt SJ, Wang HH. Nature and significance of cells with irregular nuclear contours (CINC) in esophageal mucosa. Mod Pathol. 1992 Mar;5(2):191-6.
13. Cucchiara S, D'Armiento F, Alfieri E, et al. Intraepithelial cells with irregular nuclear contours as a marker of esophagitis in children with gastroesophageal reflux disease. Dig Dis Sci 1995; 40:2305–2311.
14. Bisset W. The development of motor control systems in the gastrointestinal tract of the preterm infant. In: Milla P, ed. Disorders of Gastrointestinal Motility in Childhood, vol. 2. Chichester, UK: Wiley; 1988:17–28.
15. Del Buono R, Wenzl T, Rawat D, Ball G, Thomson M. Acid and non-acid gastro-oesophageal reflux in neurologically impaired children: investigation with the multiple intraluminal impedance procedure. J Pediatr Gastroenterol Nutr (in press).
16. Murray J, Du C, Ledlow A, Bates J, Conklin J. Nitric oxide: mediator of nonadrenergic noncholinergic responses of opossum esophageal muscle. Am J Physiol 1991; 261:G401–G406.
17. Hitchcock R, Pemble M, Bishop A, Spitz L, Polak J. Quantitative study of the development and maturation of human oesophageal innervation. J Anat 1992; 180:175–183.
18. Preiksaitis H, Tremblay L, Diamant N. Nitric oxide mediates inhibitory nerve effects in human esophagus and lower esophageal sphincter. Dig Dis Sci 1994; 39:770–775.
19. Hitchcock R, Pemble M, Bishop A, Spitz L, Polak J. The ontogeny and distribution of neuropeptides in the human fetal and infant esophagus. Gastroenterology 1992; 102:840–848.
20. Subba Rao G et al. Can eosinophil-derived neurotoxin (EDN) act as a surrogate marker for disease activity in children with allergic eosinophilic esophagitis (AEE)? Am J Gastroenterol 2004; Suppl:Abstract 103867.
21. Furuta G T. Eosinophils in the esophagus: acid is not the only cause. J Pediatr Gastroenterol Nutr 1998; 26:468–471.
22. Pritchard J. Fetal swallowing and amniotic fluid volume. Obstet Gynecol 1966; 28:606–610.
23. Crump EP, Gore PM, Horton CP. The sucking behavior in premature infants. Hum Biol 1958; 30:128–141.
24. Gryboski J. The swallowing mechanisms of the neonate: 1. Esophageal and gastric motility. Pediatrics 1965; 35:445–452.
25. Herbst J. Development of suck and swallow. J Pediatr Gastrointest Nutr 1983; 2(Suppl 1):S131–S135.
26. Bernbaum J, Gilberto R, Watkins J, Peckham J. Non-nutritive sucking during lavage feeding enhances growth and maturation in premature infants. Pediatrics 1983; 71:41–45.
27. Newell S, Sarkar P, Booth I, McNeish A. Maturation of the lower oesophageal sphincter in the pre-term neonate. Pediatr Res 1986; 20:692.
28. Omari T, Rommel N, Staunton E, et al. Paradoxical impact of body positioning on gastroesophageal reflux and gastric emptying in the premature neonate: new insights revealed by combined intraluminal impedance and micromanometry. J Pediatr Gastroenterol Nutr 2004; 39(Suppl 1):S17.
29. Kahrilas P, Dodds W, Dent J, Logemann J, Shaler R. Upper esophageal function during deglutition. Gastroenterology 1988; 95:52–62.
30. Dodds W, Hogan W, Reid D, Stewart E, Arndorfer R. A comparison between primary esophageal peristalsis following wet and dry swallows. J Appl Physiol 1973; 35:851–857.
31. Ingelfinger F. Esophageal motility. Physiol Rev 1958; 38:533–584.
32. Miller A. Deglutition. Physiol Rev 1982; 62:129–184.
33. Wenzl T. Investigating esophageal reflux with the intraluminal impedance technique. J Pediatr Gastroenterol Nutr 2002; 34:261–268.
34. Cucchiara S, Staina A, Di Lorenzo C et al. Pathophysiology of gastroesophageal reflux and distal esophageal motility in children with gastroesophageal reflux disease. J Pediatr Gastroenterol Nutr 1988; 7:850–856.

35. Dent J, Holloway R, Toouli J, Dodds W. Mechanisms of lower oesophageal sphincter incompetence in patients with symptomatic gastrooesophageal reflux. Gut 1988; 29:1020–1028.
36. Cucchiara S, Bortolotti M, Minella R, Auricchio S. Fasting and post-prandial mechanisms of gastroesophageal reflux in children with gastroesophageal reflux disease. Dig Dis Sci 1993; 38:86–92.
37. Hillemeier A, McCallum R, Biancani P. Developmental characteristics of the lower esophageal sphincter in the kitten. Gastroenterology 1985; 89:760–766.
38. Helm J, Dodds W, Riedel D. Determinant of esophageal acid clearance in normal subjects. Gastroenterology 1983; 85:607–612.
39. Ganatra JV, Medow MS, Berezin S, et al. Esophageal dysmotility elicited by acid perfusion in children with esophagitis. Am J Gastroenterol 1995; 90:1080–1083.
40. Torrente F, Fitzhenry R, Heuschkel R, Thomson M, Murch S. Cow's milk induces T cell proliferation and mucosal mast cell degranulation with neural tropism in an *in vitro* organ culture model. J Pediatr Gastroenterol Nutr 2003; 36:527.
41. Gupta S, Fitzgerald J, Chong S, Croffie J, Garcia J. Expression of inducible nitric oxide synthase (iNOS) mRNA in inflamed esophageal and colonic mucosa in a pediatric population. Am J Gastroenterol 1998; 93:795–798.
42. Zicari A, Corrada G, Cavaliere M, et al. Increased levels of prostaglandins and nitric oxide in esophageal mucosa of children with reflux esophagitis. J Pediatr Gastroenterol Nutr 1998; 26:194–199.
43. Harman J, Johnson L, Maydonovitch C. Effects of acid and bile salts on the rabbit esophageal mucosa. Dig Dis Sci 1981; 26:65–72.
44. Lillemoe K, Johnson L, Harman J. Taurodeoxycholate modulates the effects of pepsin and trypsin in experimental esophagitis. Surgery 1985; 97:662–667.
45. Marshall R, Anggiansah A, Owen W, Owen W. The relationship between acid and bile reflux and symptoms in gastro-oesophageal reflux disease. Gut 1997; 40:182–187.
46. Orel R, Markovich S. Bile in the esophagus: a factor in the pathogenesis of reflux esophagitis in children. J Pediatr Gastroenterol Nutr 2003; 36:266–273.
47. Singh S, Bradley L, Richter J. Determinants of oesophageal 'alkaline' pH environment in controls and patients with gastro-oesophageal reflux disease. Gut 1993; 34:309–316.
48. Booth I. Silent gastro-oesophageal reflux: how much do we miss? Arch Dis Child 1992; 67:1325–1327.
49. Byrne W. Reflux and related phenomena. J Pedieatr Gastroenterol Nutr 1989; 8:283–285.
50. Skopnik H, Silny J, Heiber O, Schulz J, Rau G, Heimann G. Gastroesophageal reflux in infants: evaluation of a new intraluminal impedance technique. J Pedieatr Gastroenterol Nutr 1996; 23:591–598.
51. Höllwarth M, Uray E, Pesendorfer P, Rosanelli K, Rosegger H. Esophageal manometry. Pediatr Surg Int 1986; 1:177–183.
52. Ravelli A, Milla P. Detection of gastroesophageal reflux by electrical impedance tomography. J Pediatr Gastroenterol Nutr 1994; 18:205–213.
53. Riccabona M, Maurer U, Lackner H, Uray E, Ring E. The role of sonography in the evaluation of gastro-oesophageal reflux: correlation to pH-metry. Eur J Pediatr 1992; 14:655–657.
54. Tolia V, Kuhns L, Kauffman R. Comparison of simultaneous esophageal pH monitoring and scintigraphy in infants with gastroesophageal reflux. Am J Gastroenterol 1993; 88:661–664.
55. Vandenplas Y, Derde M, Piepsz A. Evaluation of reflux episodes during simultaneous esophageal pH monitoring and gastroesophageal reflux scintigraphy in children. J Pediatr Gastroenterol Nutr 1992; 14:256–260.
56. Westra S, Derkx H, Taminiay J. Symptomatic gastroesophageal reflux: diagnosis with ultrasound. J Pediatr Gastroenterol Nutr 1994; 19:58–64.
57. Fass J, Silny J, Braun J, et al. Measuring esophageal motility with a new intraluminal impedance device. Scand J Gastroenterol 1994; 29:693–702.
58. Silny J, Rau G. A novel procedure to study bolus movement by intraluminal electrical impedance measurements. In: Janssens J, ed. Progress in Understanding and Management of Gastrointestinal Motility Disorders. Leuven: Department of Medicine, Division of Gastroenterology, K U Leuven; 1993:197–208.
59. Hill DJ, Hosking CS. Emerging disease profiles in infants and young children with food allergy. Pediatr Allergy Immunol 1997; 8:S21–S26.
60. Kelly KJ, Lazenby AJ, Rowe PC, et al. Eosinophilic esophagitis attributed to gastroesophageal reflux: improvement with an amino acid-based formula. Gastroenterology 1995; 109:1503–1512.
61. Iacono G, Caroccio A, Cavataio F, et al. Gastroesophageal reflux and cow's milk allergy in infants: a prospective study. J Allergy Clin Immunol 1996; 97:822–827.
62. Cavataio F, Iacono G, Montalto G, et al. Clinical and pH-metric characteristics of gastro-oesophageal reflux secondary to cows' milk protein allergy. Arch Dis Child 1996; 75:51–56.
63. Winter HS, madara JL, Stafford RJ, et al. Intraepithelial eosinophils: a new diagnostic criterion for reflux esophagitis. Gastroenterology 1982; 83:818–823.
64. Liacouras CA, Wenner WJ, Brown K, Ruchelli El. Primary eosinophilic esophagitis in children: successful treatment with oral corticosteroids. J Pediatr Gastroenterol Nutr 1998; 26:380–385.
65. Liacouras CA Eosinophilic esophagitis in children and adults. J Pediatr Gastroenterol Nutr. 2003; 37(Suppl 1):S23–S28.
66. Rothenberg M. Eosinophilic gastrointestinal disorders (EGID). J Allergy Clin Immunol 2004; 113:11–28.
67. Garcia-Zepeda EA, Rothenberg ME, Ownberg RT, et al. Human eotaxin is a specific chemoattractant for eosinophil cells and provides a new mechanism to explain tissue eosinophilia. Nat Med1996; 2:449–456.
68. Collins SM. The immunomodulation of enteric neuromuscular function: implications for motility and inflammatory disorders. Gastroenterology 1996; 111:1683–1699.
69. Justinich CJ, Ricci A Jr, Kalafus DA, et al. Activated eosinophils in esophagitis in children: a transmission electron microscopic study. J Pediatr Gastroenterol Nutr 1997; 25:194–198.
70. Garrett J, Jameson S, Thompson B, et al. Anti-IL-5 (mepolizumab) therapy for hypereosinophilic syndromes. J Allergy Clin Immunol 2004; 113:115–119.
71. Wang HH, Mangano MM, Antonioli DA. Evaluation of T-lymphocytes in esophageal mucosal biopsies. Mod Pathol 1994; 7:55–58.
72. Pérez-Machado M, Ashwood P, Thomson M, et al. Reduced transforming growth factor-beta1-producing T cells in the duodenal mucosa of children with food allergy. Eur J Immunol 2003; 33:2307–2315.
73. Walker-Smith JA, Murch SH. Gastrointestinal food allergy. In: Diseases of the Small Intestine in Childhood, 4th edn. Oxford: Isis Medical Media; 1999:205–234.
74. Pérez-Machado M, Ashwood P, Torrente F, et al. Spontaneous T_H1 cytokine production by intraepithelial but not circulating T cells in infants with or without food allergies. Allergy 2004; 59:346–353.

Chapter 19
Congenital malformations of the esophagus

Steven W. Bruch and Arnold G. Coran

Congenital lesions of the esophagus fall into three categories: congenital esophageal stenosis, the variants of esophageal atresia and tracheoesophageal fistula, and laryngotracheoesophageal clefts.

CONGENITAL ESOPHAGEAL STENOSIS

Congenital esophageal stenosis presents in three variants: esophageal webs or diaphragms, fibromuscular stenosis, and stenosis due to cartilaginous tracheobronchial remants. Collectively, these lesions are quite rare, occurring in 1 in 25 000–50 000 live births.[1] Most often, congenital esophageal stenosis presents as an isolated finding, but in 15–30% of cases it is associated with other congenital anomalies.[2] Up to 8% of babies with esophageal atresia and tracheo-esophageal fistula have an associated distal congenital esophageal stenosis.[3] Other associated anomalies include cardiac defects, intestinal atresias, imperforate anus and chromosomal abnormalities.

Clinical manifestations and diagnosis

Congenital esophageal stenosis may not manifest in the newborn period as liquid breast milk or formula passes through the stenotic area without difficulty. Symptoms often start at around 6 months of age when semisolid and solid foods are introduced into the diet. The babies then begin to regurgitate undigested foods and may develop recurrent respiratory infections due to aspiration. In unrecognized cases, the babies may present later with growth retardation. When these symptoms occur, babies are often studied by esophagraphy, which reveals the stenotic area and may show dilation of the esophagus proximal to the stenosis. The three variants give a different radiologic appearance. The esophageal diaphragms or webs are thin layers of tissue causing stenosis in the upper portion of the esophagus. The fibromuscular stenoses are thicker than the webs and tend to occur in the middle to lower esophagus. Cartilaginous remnants occur in the distal portion of the esophagus, as shown in Figure 19.1. In a child with these radiologic findings and the appropriate clinical picture, the differential diagnosis would include achalasia and a stricture from gastroesophageal reflux disease. In order to make the distinction between these entities, additional work-up including endoscopy, manometrics and 24-h pH probe studies are useful. Recently, endoscopic ultrasonography has been used to differentiate stenosis due to cartilaginous rests from that due to fibromuscular stenosis.[4]

Treatment

Therapy is dictated by the type of stenosis encountered. The thin proximal esophageal membrane or web can often be dilated at the time of endoscopy.[5] On occasion, these membranes require partial resection with electrocautery or laser through the endoscope followed by dilation.[6] The stenoses with cartilaginous remnants require resection and primary anastomosis, because dilation is not effective in this type of stenosis.[7] Fibromuscular stenosis can be dilated in most cases. A series from Japan used endoscopic ultrasonography to differentiate fibromuscular stenosis from cartilaginous rests. Patients with cartilaginous rests went on to surgery, and the children with fibromuscular stenosis

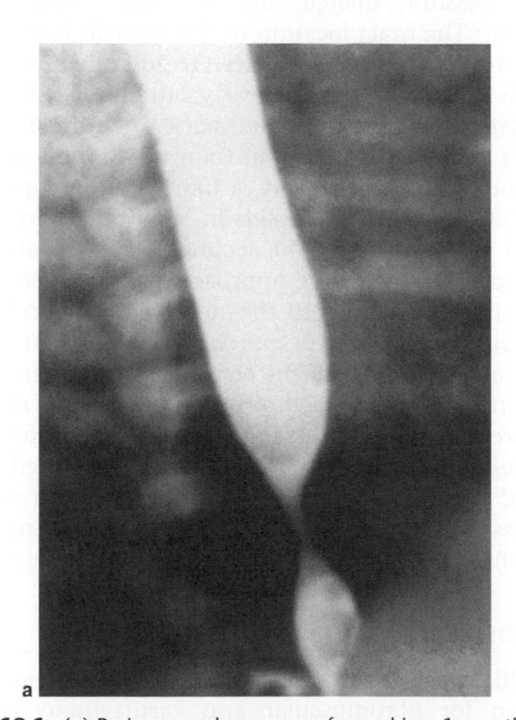

Figure 19.1: (**a**) Barium esophagram performed in a 1-month-old baby with dysphagia shows a congenital esophageal stenosis in the distal esophagus and proximal esophageal dilation. This is characteristic of a fibromuscular stenosis or a stenosis from a persistent cartilaginous remnant.

(*continued*)

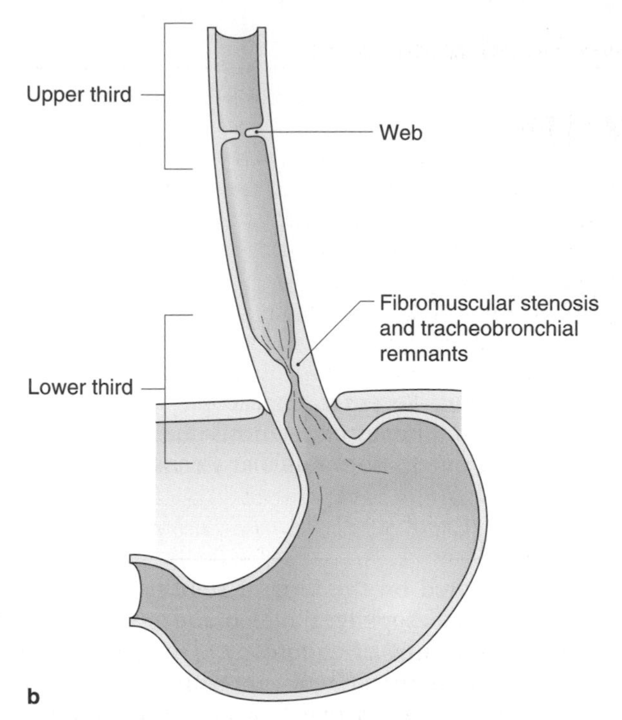

Figure 19.1: Cont'd (b) The usual location of the common forms of congenital esophageal stenosis: esophageal webs in the upper third of the esophagus, and fibromuscular stenosis or persistent cartilaginous tracheobronchial remnants in the distal third. (From O'Neill, 2003, with permission).[55]

were dilated. Ten of 13 children with fibromuscular stenoses were successfully dilated, and the other three required resection.[4] The exact location of the stenosis is often difficult to find on contrast studies. To identify the stenotic area it is helpful to place a Fogarty catheter past the stenosis, inflate the balloon and pull back the catheter. Placing contrast in the esophagus will then verify the location of the stenosis. Intraoperatively, a lighted endoscope placed at the level of the stenosis aids in locating a stenosis that is often impossible to find accurately by palpation and inspection. The operative approach varies depending on the level of the stenosis. If the stenotic area is in the mid esophagus, the operative approach should be through a right thoracotomy, but if the stenosis is located in the distal esophagus a left thoracotomy will provide the necessary exposure. The stenotic area of the esophagus is excised and a single-layer end-to-end anastomosis performed. If the stenotic lesion is close to the gastroesophageal junction and resection may alter the anti-reflux mechanism, then a fundoplication should be added to the procedure.[1]

Outcome

Both dilation for webs and fibromuscular stenosis, and resection for fibromuscular and cartilaginous remnant stenosis, provide adequate relief of the stenosis. Compared with membranes or webs, fibromuscular stenosis required more frequent dilation over a longer period of time.[4] Postoperative dilations following resection of esophageal stenosis were required to prevent anastomotic stricture.[4,8]

ESOPHAGEAL ATRESIA AND TRACHEO-ESOPHAGEAL FISTULA

The treatment of esophageal atresia and tracheo-esophageal fistula, which occurs in about 1 in 4000 live births, remains a challenge.[9] Since the first successful primary anastomosis by Haight in 1941,[10] improvements in surgical technique and neonatal care have increased the survival rate of babies born with esophageal atresia and tracheo-esophageal fistula to nearly 100%, exept when the baby is small and premature (birthweight less than 1500 g) or has associated complex anomalies, usually cardiac in nature. If the baby is small or has associated anomalies, the survival rate approaches 60%, and if the baby is both small and has associated anomalies the survival rate decreases to around 25%.[11]

Anatomy

An understanding of the anatomy involved with each case of esophageal atresia and tracheo-esophageal fistula is important when devising a treatment strategy. There have been several classification systems, but a description of each type is the easiest and most practical way to classify the five different types of esophageal atresia and tracheo-esophageal fistula, as shown in Figure 19.2. The most common configuration is esophageal atresia with a distal tracheo-esophageal fistula. This configuration occurs in 86% of cases.[12] The proximal esophagus ends blindly in the upper mediastinum. The distal esophagus is connected to the tracheobronchial tree, usually just above or at the carina. The second most common type is the isolated esophageal atresia without a tracheo-esophageal fistula. This configuration occurs in 8% of cases.[12] The proximal esophagus ends blindly in the upper mediastinum, and the distal esophagus is also blind-ending and protrudes a varying distance above the diaphragm. The distance between the two ends is often too far to bring together shortly after birth. The third most common configuration, occurring in 4% of cases,[12] is a tracheo-esophageal fistula without esophageal atresia. The esophagus extends in continuity to the stomach, but there is a fistula between the esophagus and the trachea. The fistula is usually located in the upper mediastinum, running from a proximal orifice in the trachea to a more distal orifice in the esophagus. This is also known as an 'H'- or 'N'-type tracheo-esophageal fistula. Two more forms of esophageal atresia and tracheo-esophageal fistula exist, both of which occur about 1% of cases.[12] These are the esophageal atresia with both a proximal and distal tracheo-esophageal fistula, and esophageal atresia with a proximal tracheo-esophageal fistula. These two forms correspond to the first two forms described, with the addition of a proximal fistula between the upper pouch and the trachea. Again the esophageal atresia with proximal tracheo-esophageal fistula, similar to its counterpart without the proximal fistula, will have a long gap between the two ends of the esophagus, making it difficult to repair shortly after birth.

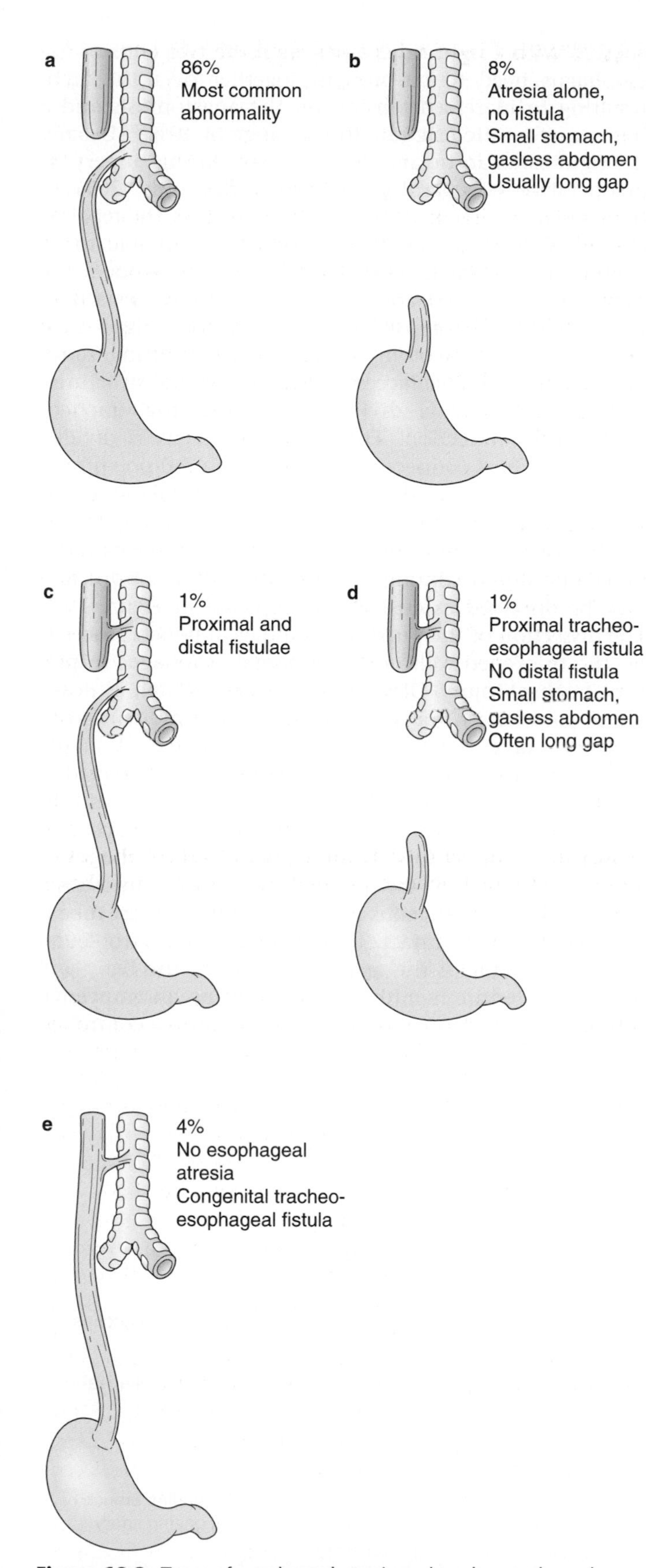

Figure 19.2: Types of esophageal atresia and tracheo-esphageal fistula with rates of occurrence. (**a**) Esophageal atresia with distal tracheo-esophageal fistula. (**b**) Isolated esophageal atresia. (**c**) Esophageal atresia with proximal and distal tracheo-esophageal fistulae. (**d**) Esophageal atresia with proximal tracheo-esophageal fistula. (**e**) H-type tracheo-esphageal fistula.

Associated anomalies

As alluded to above, the main determinants of outcome in babies with esophageal atresia and tracheo-esophageal fistula are how prematurely the baby is born and the associated anomalies, especially cardiac and chromosomal anomalies. Babies with esophageal atresia and tracheo-esophageal fistula have a higher incidence of prematurity than the general population, most likely related to the polyhydramnios resulting from the fetal esophageal obstruction.[13] More than half of babies with esophageal atresia and tracheo-esophageal fistula have one or more associated anomalies.[14] The majority of these anomalies are included in the VACTERL syndrome, which includes abnormalities in the following areas: *v*ertebral, *a*norectal, *c*ardiac, *t*racheal, *e*sophageal, *r*enal and *l*imb. A breakdown of the individual incidences of anomalies in babies with esophageal atresia and tracheo-esophageal fistula is presented in Table 19.1.[15] In addition, chromosomal abnormalities are more common in children with esophageal atresia and tracheo-esophageal fistula than in the general population, including trisomies 13, 18 and 21. Other syndromes associated with esophageal atresia and tracheo-esophageal fistula are the CHARGE syndrome,[16] Potter's syndrome[17] and the SCHISIS syndrome.[11] Infants with esophageal atresia and tracheo-esophageal fistula also have a higher incidence of pyloric stenosis than expected in the general population.[18]

Clinical presentation and diagnosis

Babies with esophageal atresia and tracheo-esophageal fistula present with inability to handle their saliva and will often cough and choke, and possibly develop cyanosis, especially with the first attempt to feed. The baby will spit up undigested formula after the feeding attempt. This usually leads to the placement of a tube in the esophagus that does not go in as far as expected and meets resistance. Plain films of the chest and abdomen will show the tube coiled in the proximal mediastinum. This confirms the presence of esophageal atresia. The bowel gas pattern, or lack of bowel gas in the abdomen, determines whether a distal tracheo-esophageal fistula is present (gas throughout the intestines), or whether there is a pure esophageal atresia

Associated anomaly	Occurrence (%)
Cardiac	30
Anorectal	14
Renal	14
Musculoskeletal	15
Chromosomal	2
Other	25
Overall	53

Table 19.1 Incidence of anomalies associated with esophageal atresia and tracheo-esophageal fistula (Reproduced from Deurloo JA, Ekkelkamp S, Schoorl M, et al. Esophageal atresia: historical evaluation of management and results of 371 patients 2002; 73: 267–272, with permission from The Society of Thoracic Surgeons).

without a distal fistula (gasless abdomen). The remainder of the preoperative evaluation targets the associated anomalies, and seeks to determine the presence of a proximal fistula between the trachea and esophagus. The associated anomalies of the VACTERL syndrome can be identified with four quick simple evaluations. A physical exam evaluates limb and anorectal abnormalities. The plain film that demonstrated the esophageal and tracheal abnormalities is used to look for the vertebral and limb abnormalities. Ultrasonography of the abdomen will delineate renal abnormalities. Echocardiography is required to evaluate for cardiac anomalies and to determine the position of the aortic arch, which helps plan the surgical approach. If suspicious, a chromosome analysis can be obtained. The presence of a proximal fistula may be evaluated in one of three ways. A contrast evaluation of the esophageal pouch will often show a proximal fistula if it is present. An experienced radiologist should do this exam to decrease the risk of aspiration. Bronchoscopy just prior to the surgical repair to look for a proximal fistula may be useful. The last strategy is to look for a fistula during the proximal pouch dissection. A clue that a proximal fistula is present is that the proximal pouch will not be as dilated as usual, because the fistula relieves the distending pressure in the proximal pouch both before and after birth. Tracheo-esophageal fistula without esophageal atresia (H-type fistula) may not present in the initial neonatal period, and is more difficult to diagnose. The tube goes into the stomach when originally passed, but persistent coughing and choking with feeds by mouth should prompt a search for an isolated fistula. Prone pull-back esophagraphy, or bronchoscopy with esophagoscopy, is used to find the isolated fistula.

Treatment

After the diagnosis is confirmed, plans for operative repair should be made. In healthy newborns, the operation can take place within the first 24 h of life to minimize the risk of aspiration and resulting pneumonitis. Prior to the operation the baby should be kept supine with the head elevated 30–45°. A tube should be in the proximal pouch to suction saliva constantly and prevent aspiration. Intravenous access should be established and fluids instilled along with broad-spectrum antibiotics and vitamin K.

The goal of operative therapy for esophageal atresia and tracheoesophageal fistula is to establish continuity of the native esophagus and repair the fistula in one setting. Most of the time, primary repair can be achieved. There are special situations where this may not be possible or advisable, described below. In the usual situation, the baby is stable both hemodynamically and from a pulmonary standpoint, is brought to the operating room and is placed under general anesthesia. Rigid bronchoscopy may be performed to locate the distal fistula, usually at or near the carina, and to look for a proximal fistula. The baby is then placed in the left lateral decubitus position in preparation for a right posterolateral thoracotomy. If the preoperative echocardiogram reveals a right-sided aortic arch, which occurs in 2% of cases, the repair should be approached from the left chest.[19] With a right-sided aortic arch the two ends of the esophagus need to be brought together over the arch, resulting in increased tension on the anastomosis and a high anastomotic leak rate in the range of 40%.[20] Usually the right-sided aortic arch is discovered during surgery, as preoperative echogardiography identifies only 20% of right-sided arches correctly.[20] In this situation, the repair is attempted through the right chest and, if unable to be completed, the tracheo-esophageal fistula is divided, the right chest is closed and a left thoracotomy is used to complete the anastomosis. In the typical case, a right-sided posterolateral thoracotomy using a muscle splitting, retropleural approach gives access to the mediastinal structures. The azygus vein is divided, revealing the tracheo-esophageal connection. The distal esophagus is divided and the tracheal connection is closed with 5-0 polypropylene (Prolene) suture. Manipulation of the distal esophagus is minimized to protect the segmental blood supply to this portion of the esophagus. The proximal esophagus has a rich blood supply coming from the thyrocervical trunk and may be dissected extensively, as depicted in Figure 19.3. The dissection of the proximal esophageal pouch proceeds on the thickened wall of the proximal esophagus to prevent tracheal injury. Dissection is carried as high as possible to gain length for a tension-free anastomosis, and to look for a proximal fistula, which occurs rarely. A single-layered end-to-end anastomosis is performed as depicted in Figure 19.4. A tube placed through the anastamosis into the stomach allows decompression of the stomach and eventual enteral feeding. A chest tube placed in the retropleural space next to the anastomosis controls any subsequent leak. Some surgeons prefer not to use a chest tube if the pleura remains intact. The advantage of a retropleural approach is that, if the anastomosis leaks, the baby will not soil the entire hemithorax and develop an empyema. A leak into the retropleural space will result in a controlled

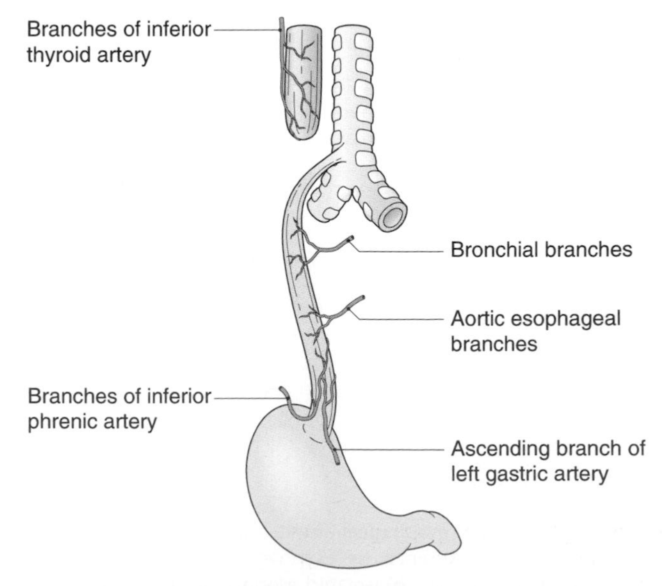

Figure 19.3: Vascular supply of the esophagus in esophageal atresia and tracheo-esophageal fistula

esophagocutaneous fistula, which almost always closes spontaneously. Recently, several authors have described a thoracoscopic approach to the repair of esophageal atresia and tracheo-esophageal fistula.[21,22] Thoracoscopic repair requires advanced laparoscopic skills to perform the intracorporeal anastamosis, and requires a transpleural approach. Advantages include a smaller, less traumatic incision, and better visualization. Whether thoracoscopy becomes the preferred approach for esophageal atresia and tracheo-esophageal fistula repair remains to be seen. These two studies showed that it can be done safely with similar outcomes in the short term, but both series evaluated only eight children.

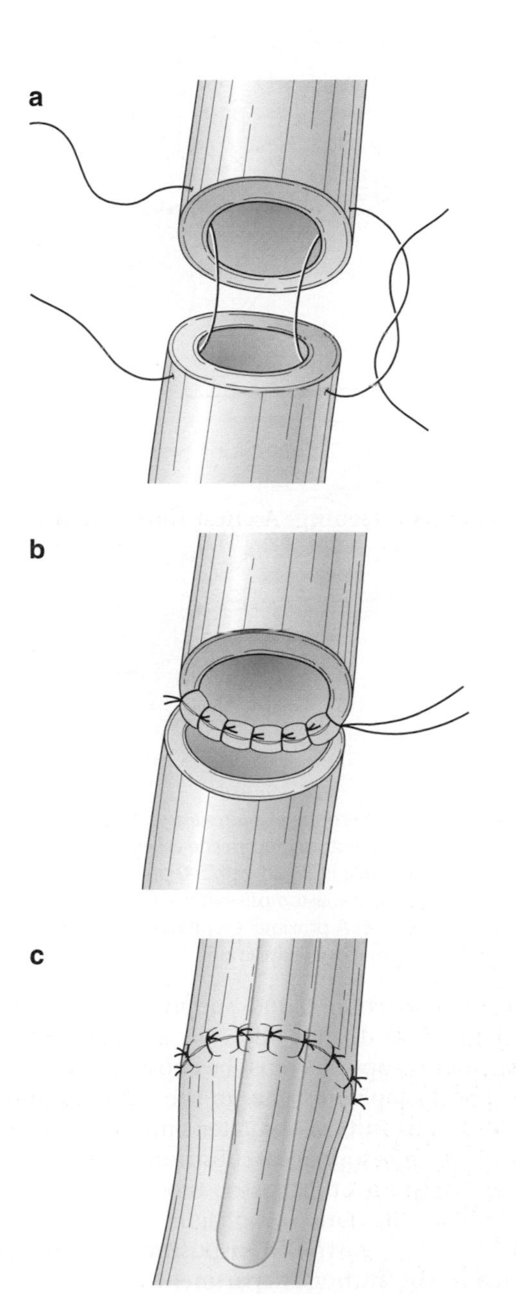

Figure 19.4: Single-layer end-to-end esophageal anastomosis. (**a**) Corner sutures are placed. (**b**) Posterior row sutures are placed. A tube is then passed through the anastomosis into the stomach. (**c**) Anterior row sutures complete the anastomosis.

After surgery the baby is returned to the intensive care unit, and continued on intravenous nutrition and antibiotics. Special care should be directed toward preventing aspiration with frequent oropharyngeal suctioning and elevation of the head of the bed by 30–45°. Feedings may be started through the transanastomotic tube into the stomach 2–3 days after the operation. Acid suppressive therapy should be instituted to prevent acid irritation of the anastomosis and subsequent stricture. On postoperative days 5–7 esophagraphy is performed to check the integrity of the anastomosis. If there is no leak, the chest tube is removed and feeding is started orally. If a leak is present, it is treated conservatively with intravenous antibiotics and nutrition, and chest tube drainage. Another esophagram is ordered in a week. These leaks invariably close without further operative intervention.[23] Only a complete disruption of the anastomosis necessitates further operative procedures. In that case the proximal esophagus should be brought out of the left neck as a cervical esophagostomy, the distal esophagus tied off, and the mediastinum and chest adequately drained.

Special situations

The majority of patients with esophageal atresia and tracheo-esophageal fistula can be treated as described above. There are three variations that require further discussion: (1) babies with esophageal atresia and tracheo-esophageal fistula who have severe respiratory disease where the fistula is contributing to the ventilatory insufficiency; (2) babies with long-gap esophageal atresia; and (3) babies with the H-type tracheo-esophageal fistula. Babies with significant respiratory insufficiency and a tracheo-esophageal fistula are usually premature neonates with lung immaturity requiring significant ventilatory support. The connection between the trachea and the distal esophagus may be the preferred path for air provided by the ventilator. The stiff lungs have a higher resistance than the fistulous tract, allowing a significant portion of each ventilation to go into the esophagus and then into the abdomen, resulting in abdominal distension and elevation of the hemidiaphragms, further impeding ventilation. Different strategies have been developed to deal with this situation. A change to high-frequency ventilation decreases the portion of tidal volume lost to the fistula. Advancing the endotracheal tube past the fistula opening prevents further loss of ventilation into the fistula.[24] Bronchoscopically placed Fogarty catheters positioned in the fistula and inflated temporarily occlude the fistula, but have a tendency to become dislodged.[25] If a gastrostomy tube is present, the tube can be placed to underwater seal to increase the resistance of the tract and reduce airflow through the fistula.[12] However, to prevent further respiratory decompensation, and to ameliorate the risk of gastric perforation, these babies often require an urgent thoracotomy and control of the tracheo-esophageal fistula. If the baby stabilizes, the remainder of the repair can proceed at that time, as is the usual case.[26] However, if the baby remains unstable, the chest is closed, a gastrostomy tube is placed and the definitive repair completed when the baby is stabilized.

The second special situation occurs when there is a long gap between the two ends of the esophagus. This often occurs with the pure esophageal atresia, or the esophageal atresia with a proximal tracheo-esophageal fistula. Both of these situations present with a radiographic picture of a gasless abdomen. On occasion, a baby with esophageal atresia and distal tracheo-esophageal fistula may have a long gap between the two ends of the esophagus, and so belongs to this special group. If the baby presents with a gasless abdomen, a long gap should be suspected. The baby is brought to the operating room for a gastrostomy tube placement to allow enteral feedings while waiting for the two ends of the esophagus to grow adequately so that a primary anastomosis can be attempted. The stomach is quite small in these babies because it was unused during fetal life and has not yet stretched to its full capacity. Care must be taken to avoid injury to the small stomach and its blood supply while placing the gastrostomy tube. Careful placement will not compromise use of the stomach for an esophageal replacement if necessary. During gastrostomy tube placement, an estimate of the distance between the two ends of the esophagus is made using metal sounds and fluoroscopy. If the two ends of the esophagus are more than three vertebral bodies apart, they will not be easily connected. The baby is then nursed with a tube in the proximal pouch to remove the saliva, and is fed via the gastrostomy tube. During the first several months of life, the gap between the two ends of the esophagus shortens owing to spontaneous growth of the atretic esophagus.[27] The upper pouch may or may not be serially dilated to try to stretch the pouch, depending on the surgeon's discretion.[28] The distance between the proximal and distal ends of the esophagus is measured every 2–4 weeks and, if the two ends are within two to three vertebral bodies, a thoracotomy and attempt at anastomosis is performed. If the gap remains greater than three vertebral bodies and the two ends of the esophagus are no longer approaching each other, the baby will require a cervical esophagostomy and esophageal replacement. Waiting longer than 4 months rarely provides extra growth of the esophageal ends resulting in primary anastomosis. The esophagostomy will allow the baby to take sham feeds to prevent oral aversion and subsequent feeding problems without the risk of aspiration while awaiting esophageal replacement. The replacement operation takes place between 9 and 12 months of age and consists of a gastric transposition, creation of a gastric tube, or a colonic interposition to replace the esophagus. If the gap reduces to two or three vertebral bodies, as occurs in about 70% of babies,[29] there are several techniques that can be used to gain length on the esophageal ends during surgery. These include complete dissection of the upper pouch to the thoracic inlet. A circular myotomy of Livaditis performed on the upper pouch produces about 1 cm of length for each myotomy.[30] Use of a circular myotomy is shown in Figure 19.5. A tubularization graft of the upper pouch can be created and connected to the distal esophagus.[31] If these techniques do not allow an adequate anastomosis, the distal esophagus is mobilized,

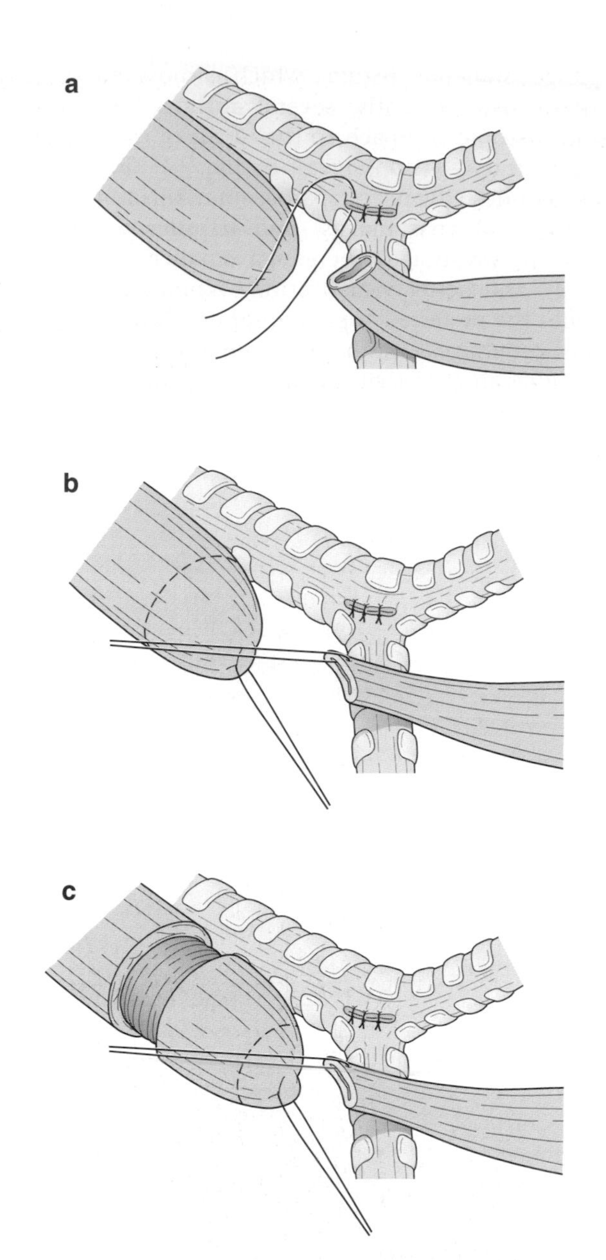

Figure 19.5: Repair of esophageal atresia and distal tracheo-esophageal fistula using a circular myotomy to provide adequate length. (**a**) The tracheo-esophageal fistula is closed with 5-0 polypropylene (Prolene). (**b**) The feasibility of primary anastomosis between the two esophageal segments is assessed. (**c**) A proximal esophagomyotomy provides extra length to allow for a primary anastomosis.

despite its segmental blood supply, to gain length.[12] If these maneuvers do not allow an adequate anastomosis, then one of two options must be chosen. The first is to create a cervical esophagostomy in the left neck and plan an esophageal substitution at a later time. The second option is to perform the esophageal substitution at the time, using a gastric transposition, a gastric tube or a colon interposition to replace the native esophagus. Currently, the second option using a gastric transposition is the preferred approach in the author's department.

The third special situation that demands discussion is the H-type tracheo-esophageal fistula without esophageal atresia. An H-type fistula often escapes discovery in the neonatal period, but is found later during evaluation of coughing and choking episodes with feeds. Often the fistula is identified by contrast studies, usually prone pull-back esophography as shown in Figure 19.6. However, it is not unusual to require bronchoscopy and esophagoscopy to make the diagnosis. To repair this fistula, rigid bronchoscopy and esophagoscopy are used to find the fistula and place a Fogarty catheter through the fistula to aid in its identification during the exploration. The right neck is then explored through an incision just above the clavicle. The fistula is identified and divided. If possible, muscle or other available vascularized tissue is placed between the two suture lines to help prevent a recurrent fistula.

Postoperative complications

Complications following repair of esophageal atresia and tracheo-esophageal fistula relate to the anastomosis and to the underlying disease. The anastomotic problems include anastomotic leaks, anastomotic strictures and recurrent tracheo-esophageal fistulae. The issues related to the underlying disease include gastroesophageal reflux and tracheomalacia.

The number of anastomotic problems that occur after repair varies directly with the amount of tension used to create the anastomosis. The incidence of leak at the anastomosis varies from 5% to 20%.[32] The majority of these leaks seal within 1–2 weeks with conservative management, including withholding oral feeds, intravenous antibiotics, parenteral nutrition and chest tube drainage. Complete disruption of the anastomosis, a rare complication occurring in less than 2% of cases, presents with a tension pneumothorax and significant salivary drainage from the chest tube. This scenario requires a cervical esophagostomy and gastrostomy for feeding with subsequent esophageal replacement.

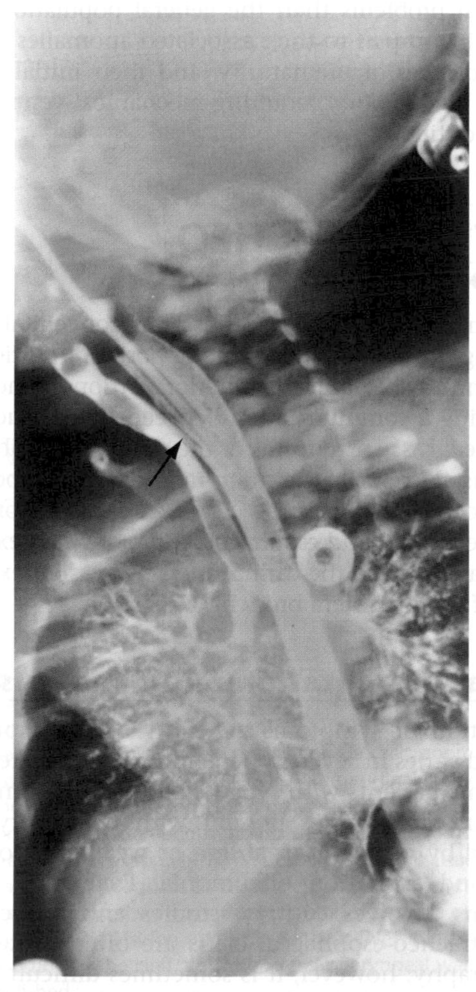

Figure 19.6: H-type fistula (arrow) demonstrated in an infant after barium swallow on frontal-oblique chest X-ray. The tracheal aspect of the fistula is characteristically superior to the esophageal aspect. Barium is seen to outline the tracheobronchial tree.

Anastomotic strictures occur in one-third to one-half of the repairs.[33] All repairs will show some degree of narrowing at the anastomosis, but dilations are not instituted unless the stricture is symptomatic causing dysphagia, associated respiratory difficulties or foreign body obstruction. Most strictures respond to repeated dilation carried out every 3–6 weeks over a 3–6 month period. Strictures that are recalcitrant to dilation are often related to gastroesophageal reflux disease, and will not resolve until the reflux is controlled.

The incidence of recurrent tracheo-esophageal fistula formation ranges from less than 1% to 12% in various series.[32,34–36] These children present with coughing, choking and occasional cyanotic episodes with feeding, and with recurrent pulmonary infections. Recurrent fistulae are often associated with anastomotic leaks, but a missed proximal fistula must also be entertained. Prone pull-back esophagraphy, and bronchoscopy with esophagoscopy, are useful to diagnose recurrent fistulae. A repeat right thoracotomy with closure of the fistula is a difficult operation. Identification of the fistula tract is improved with placement of a ureteral catheter in the fistula at bronchoscopy just prior to opening the chest. After the fistula is identified and divided, a viable piece of tissue, usually a vascularized muscle flap, or a portion of pleura or pericardium should be placed between the suture lines to prevent recurrence of the fistula, which occurs in up to 20% of these repairs.[37] Other means to close these fistulae have been attempted including endoscopic diathermy[38] and Nd:YAG lasar obliteration of the fistula,[39] injection of sclerosing agents[40] and injection of fibrin glue,[41] but surgical closure remains the treatment of choice.

Gastroesophageal reflux is commonly associated with esophageal atresia and tracheo-esophageal fistula. This stems from the abnormal clearance of the distal esophagus due to poor motility, and the altered angle of His that occurs due to tension on the distal esophagus and proximal stomach to allow for an adequate anastomosis. Significant gastroesophageal reflux occurs in 30–60% of children following repair of esophageal atresia and tracheo-esophageal fistula.[32,34,42] The reflux is treated medically with acid-reducing drugs and a prokinetic agent. Often a fundoplication is required to control the reflux, especially when a stricture develops at the anastomosis and is resistant to dilation, or when repeated pulmonary aspiration associated with reflux complicates the postoperative course. Careful consideration should be given to a partial fundoplication in these children owing to their abnormal distal esophageal motility. The choice of complete *vs* partial fundoplication is left to the surgeon, with proponents of both in the literature.[36,43,44]

Tracheomalacia occurs in 10–20% of children after repair of esophageal atresia and tracheo-esophageal fistula.[32,45] Tracheomalacia refers to collapse of the trachea

8. Vasudevan SA, Kerendi F, Lee H, et al. Management of congenital esophageal stenosis. J Pediatr Surg 2002; 37:1024–1026.
9. Harris J, Kallen B, Robert E. Descriptive epidemiology of alimentary tract atresia. Teratology 1995; 52:15–29.
10. Haight C, Towsley H. Congenital atresia of the esophagus with tracheoesophageal fistula: extrapleural ligation of the fistula and end-to-end anastomosis of esophageal segments. Surg Gynecol Obstet 1943; 76:672–688.
11. Spitz L, Kiely EM, Morecroft JA, et al. Esophageal atresia: at risk groups for the 1990s. J Pediatr Surg 1994; 29:723–725.
12. Harmon CM, Coran AG. Congenital anomalies of the esophagus. In: O'Neill JA Jr, Rowe MI, Grosfeld JL, et al., eds. Pediatric Surgery, 5th edn. St Louis, MO: Mosby; 1998:941–967.
13. Losty PD, Baillie CT. Esophageal atresia and tracheo-esophageal fistula. In: Puri P, ed. Newborn Surgery, 2nd edn. New York: Oxford University Press; 2003:337–352.
14. Holder TM, Cloud DT, Lewis JE, et al. Esophageal atresia and tracheoesophageal fistula: a survey of its members by the surgical section of the American Academy of Pediatrics. Pediatrics 1964; 34:542–549.
15. Deurloo JA, Ekkelkamp S, Schoorl M, et al. Esophageal atresia: historical evaluation of management and results of 371 patients. Ann Thorac Surg 2002; 73:267–272.
16. Kutiyanawala M, Wyse RK, Brereton RJ, et al. CHARGE and esophageal atresia. J Pediatr Surg 1992; 27:558–560.
17. Poenaru D, Laberge JM, Neilson IR. A new prognostic classification for esophageal atresia. Surgery 1993; 113:426–432.
18. Spitz L, Hitchcock RJ. Oesophageal atresia and tracheo-oesophageal fistula. In: Freeman NV, ed. Surgery of the Newborn, 1st edn. New York: Churchill Livingstone; 1994:353–373.
19. Bonkett B, Beasly SW, Myers NA. The frequency, significance, and management of a right aortic arch in association with esophageal atresia. Pediatr Surg Int 1999; 15:28–31.
20. Babu R, Pierro A, Spitz L, et al. The management of oesophageal atresia in neonates with right-sided aortic arch. J Pediatr Surg 2000; 35:56–58.
21. Bax KM, van Der Zee DC. Feasibility of thoracoscopic repair of esophageal atresia with distal fistula. J Pediatr Surg 2002; 37:192–196.
22. Rothenberg SS. Thoracoscopic repair of tracheoesophageal fistula in newborns. J Pediatr Surg 2002; 37:869–872.
23. Nambirajan L, Rintala RJ, Losty PD, et al. The value of early postoperative oesophagography following repair of oesophageal atresia. Pediatr Surg Int 1998; 13:76–78.
24. Salem MR, Wong AY, Lin YH, et al. Prevention of gastric distension during anesthesia for newborns with tracheoesophageal fistulas. Anesthesiology 1973; 38:82–83.
25. Filston HC, Chitwood WR Jr, Schkolne B, et al. The Fogarty balloon catheter as an aid to management of the infant with esophageal atresia and tracheoesophageal fistula complicated by severe RDS or pneumonia. J Pediatr Surg 1982; 17:149–151.
26. Templeton J Jr, Templeton JJ, Schnaufer L, et al. Management of esophageal atresia and tracheoesophageal fistula in the neonate with severe respiratory distress syndrome. J Pediatr Surg 1985; 20:394–397.
27. Ein SH, Shandling B, Heiss K. Pure esophageal atresia: outlook in the 1990s. J Pediatr Surg 1993; 28:1147–1150.
28. Mahour GH, Woolley MM, Gwinn JL. Elongation of the upper pouch and delayed anastomotic reconstruction in esophageal atresia. J Pediatr Surg 1974; 9:373–383.
29. Nakayama DK. Congenital abnormalities of the esophagus. In: O'Neill JA Jr, Grosfeld JL, Fonkalsrud EW, et al., eds. Principles of Pediatric Surgery, 2nd edn. St Louis, MO: Mosby; 2003:385–394.
30. Livaditis A, Radburg L, Odensjo G. Esophageal end-to-end anastomosis, reduction of anastomotic tension by circular myotomy. Scand J Thorac Cardiovasc Surg 1972; 6:206–214.
31. Gough MH. Esophageal atresia – use of an anterior flap in the difficult anastomosis. J Pediatr Surg 1980; 15:310–311.
32. Engum SA, Grosfeld JL, West KW, et al. Analysis of morbidity and mortality in 227 cases of esophageal atresia and/or tracheoesophageal fistula over two decades. Arch Surg 1995; 130:502–508.
33. Chittmittrapap S, Spitz L, Kiely EM, et al. Anastomotic stricture following repair of esophageal atresia. J Pediatr Surg 1990; 25:508–511.
34. Konkin DE, O'Hali WA, Weber EM, et al. Outcomes in esophageal atresia and tracheoesophageal fistula. J Pediatr Surg 2003; 38:1726–1729.
35. Vos A, Ekkelkamp S. Congenital tracheoesophageal fistula: preventing recurrence. J Pediatr Surg 1996; 31:936–938.
36. Spitz L, Kiely E, Brereton RJ. Esophageal atresia: five year experience with 148 cases. J Pediatr Surg 1987; 22:103–108.
37. Spitz L. Recurrent tracheoesophageal fistula. In: Spitz L, Coran AG, eds. Pediatric Surgery. London: Chapman & Hall Medical; 1995:128–131.
38. Rangecroft L, Bush GH, Irving IM. Endoscopic diathermy of recurrent tracheoesophageal fistula. J Pediatr Surg 1994; 19:41–43.
39. Bhatnagar V, Lal R, Sriniwas M, et al. Endoscopic treatment of tracheoesophageal fistula using electrocautery and Nd:YAG laser. J Pediatr Surg 1999; 34:464–467.
40. Willetts IE, Dudley NE, Tam PKH. Endoscopic treatment of recurrent tracheo-oesophageal fistula: long-term results. Pediatr Surg Int. 1998; 13:256–258.
41. Gutierrez C, Barrios JE, Lluna J, et al. Recurrent tracheoesophageal fistula treated with fibrin glue. J Pediatr Surg 1994; 29:1567–1569.
42. Little DC, Rescorla FJ, Grosfeld JL, et al. Long term analysis of children with esophageal atresia and tracheoesophageal fistula. J Pediatr Surg 2003; 38:852–856.
43. Snyder CL, Ramachandron V, Kennedy AP, et al. Efficiency of partial wrap fundoplication for gastroesophageal reflux after repair of esophageal atresia. J Pediatr Surg 1997; 32:1089–1092.
44. Wheatley MJ, Coran AG, Wesley JR. Efficacy of the Nissen fundoplication in the management of gastroesophageal reflux following esophageal atresia repair. J Pediatr Surg 1993; 28:53–55.
45. Filler RM, Rossello PJ, Lebowitz RL. Life threatening anoxic spells caused by tracheal compression after repair of esophageal atresia: correction by surgery. J Pediatr Surg 1976; 11:739–748.
46. Schwartz MZ, Filler RM. Tracheal compression as a cause of apnea following repair of tracheoesophageal fistula: treatment by aortopexy. J Pediatr Surg 1980; 15:842–848.
47. Filler RM, Forte V, Fraga JC, et al. The use of expandable metallic airway stents for tracheobronchial obstruction in children. J Pediatr Surg 1995; 30:1050–1056.
48. Chetcuti P, Phelan PD. Respiratory morbidity after repair of oesophageal atresia and tracheo-oesophageal fistula. Arch Dis Child 1993; 68:167–170.
49. Ure BM, Slaney E, Eypasch EP, et al. Quality of life more than 20 years after repair of esophageal atresia. J Pediatr Surg 1998; 33:511–515.

50. Lindahl H, Rintala R, Sariola H. Chronic esophagitis and gastric metaplasia are frequent late complications of esophageal atresia. J Pediatr Surg 1993; 28:1178–1180.

51. Bouman NH, Koot HM, Hazebrock FWJ. Long term physical, psychological, and social functioning of children with esophageal atresia. J Pediatr Surg 1999; 34:399–404.

52. Petterson G. Inhibited separation of the larynx and the upper part of the trachea from the esophagus in a newborn: report of a case successfully operated upon. Acta Chir Scand 1955; 110:250–254.

53. DuBois JJ, Pokorney WJ, Harberg FJ, et al. Current management of laryngeal and laryngotracheoesophageal clefts. J Pediatr Surg 1990; 25:855–860.

54. Donahoe PK, Hendren WH. The surgical management of laryngotracheoesophageal cleft with tracheoesophageal fistula and esophageal atresia. Surgery 1972; 71:363–368.

55. O'Neill JA Jr. Esophageal stenosis, stricture and replacement. In: O'Neill JA Jr, Grosfeld JL, Fonkalsrud EW, et al., eds. Principles of Pediatric Surgery, 2nd edn. St Louis, MO: Mosby; 2003:395–403

Chapter 20
Gastroesophageal reflux

Yvan Vandenplas

INTRODUCTION

Gastroesophageal reflux (GER) is one of the most frequent and commonly occurring phenomena in humans. Episodes of GER occur in normal children and adults. GER disease (GERD) is a highly prevalent gastrointestinal disorder and is one of the most common gastrointestinal diseases encountered in clinical practice. As GER is both a physiologic event and a manifestation of disease, there is considerable controversy on the topic.

DEFINITIONS

GER is the involuntary passage of gastric contents into the esophagus. It is a physiologic event occurring in every individual several times during the day, particularly after meals. Most reflux episodes are asymptomatic, brief and limited to the distal esophagus. 'Physiologic GER' is GER associated with absence of symptoms, or during the first months of life with regurgitation, accompanied only occasionally with vomiting. Physiologic GER is a normal esophageal function, that also serves a protective role during meals or in the immediate postprandial period. If the stomach becomes overdistended, GER of liquid and air serves to decompress it (for instance burping to eliminate gas). Healthy and sick individuals do not differ in the presence or absence of reflux, but in the frequency, duration and intensity of reflux and its association with symptoms or complications. Pathologic GER occurs when the reflux episodes happen too often or when the clearance of the refluxate is poor, and when it causes other symptoms than regurgitation. GERD is reflux associated with mucosal damage or symptoms severe enough to impair quality of life.[1,2]

'Regurgitation' and 'spitting up' are synonyms that are best defined as the passage of refluxed gastric contents into the oral pharynx and mouth, normally accompanied by gastric contents drooling out of the mouth. Because regurgitant reflux is evident without diagnostic testing, this type of reflux received the earliest attention in children. Only a minority of reflux episodes are accompanied by regurgitation. In infants with reflux, less than 20% of scintigraphically or pH probe-detected reflux episodes produce emesis. When regurgitation occurs in healthy, thriving, happy infants, it is nearly always physiologic. Regurgitation occurs more frequently in infants because of developmental problems of the esophagus and stomach, the higher liquid intake of infants, and the small capacity of the esophagus (10 ml in newborn infants).

When infants 'regurgitate frequently', parents often seek medical advice. 'Excessive regurgitation' is one of the symptoms of GERD, but the terms regurgitation and GERD should not be used synonymously. Physiologic GER becomes GERD when reflux increases in frequency and intensity, and is associated with other symptoms such as chronic respiratory disease. Many infants with GERD, but not all, present with (frequent) regurgitation. GERD should be suspected if the regurgitating infant shows one or more other symptoms such as excessive crying, refusal to feed, failure to thrive or hematemesis. The older the infant becomes, the more likely that persisting regurgitation is a symptom of GERD. Frequent regurgitation beyond 3 months of life has been identified as a risk factor for GERD later in childhood.

'Vomiting' is defined as expulsion with force of the refluxed gastric contents from the mouth.[3,4] 'Rumination' is characterized by the voluntary, habitual regurgitation of recently ingested food that is subsequently spat up or reswallowed. Gagging, regurgitation, mouthing and swallowing of refluxed material is identified as rumination. In clinical practice it may be difficult to distinguish cause and consequence: frequent reflux and regurgitation may cause behavioral problems, or the reflux and regurgitation may be the clinical expression of a primary behavioral problem. Neurobehavioral manifestations of reflux are exemplified by the posturing of Sandifer's syndrome: the movements are of varying type and severity, involving the head and neck, and sometimes the upper part of the trunk, but not the limbs. It has been hypothesized that Sandifer posturing may enhance esophageal clearance. Back arching, staring associated with obstructive apnea, periods of cyanosis suggesting neonatal seizures, irritable stretching or neck extension may be less specific neurobehavioral manifestations of GER.

Primary GER results from a primary disorder of function of the upper gastrointestinal tract, due to an insufficiency at the level of the lower esophageal sphincter (LES) function. Secondary GER is caused by disease within or outside the gastrointestinal tract. Examples of diseases that commonly cause secondary GER in infants are cow's milk protein (CMP) allergy and idiopathic pyloric hypertrophy. Treatment of the primary cause – elimination of CMP from the diet and pyloromyotomy respectively – will resolve the symptoms. Secondary GER also results from mechanical factors at play in chronic lung disease or upper airway obstruction (e.g. chronic tonsillitis). Other causes of secondary GER include systemic or local infection (urinary tract infection, gastroenteritis), food allergy, metabolic disorders, intracranial hypertension and medications such as chemotherapy. In some cases, secondary reflux results from stimulation of the vomiting center by afferent impulses from circulating bacterial toxins, or stimulation from sites such as the eye, olfactory epithelium, labyrinths, pharynx, testes, etc.[3,4] These stimuli usually cause vomiting. The symptoms of primary and secondary reflux are similar, but a distinction is conceptually helpful in determining the therapeutic approach. Secondary GER is not discussed further here.

Children with neurologic impairment, cystic fibrosis and repair of esophageal atresia have the most severe reflux. Children with esophageal atresia have abnormal peristalsis of the distal esophagus, whch may be congenital – perhaps the result of morphologic abnormalities of Auerbach's plexus in the distal esophagus. Chronic respiratory disease often follows repair of esophageal atresia. Neurologically impaired children accumulate many risk factors known to cause reflux (horizontal position, constipation, muscular tone disorder).

PREVALENCE

Determination of the exact prevalence of GER and GERD at any age is virtually impossible because most reflux episodes are asymptomatic, because of self-treatment and because of lack of medical referral. Many factors influence the number of reflux episodes (Table 20.1). In normal 3–4-month-old infants, three to four episodes of GER are detectable during 5 min of intermittent fluoroscopic evaluation,[5] and 31 ± 21 acid reflux episodes are recorded within a 24-h period with pH monitoring.[6]

Daily regurgitation is present in 50% of infants younger than 3 months and in more than 66% at 4 months, but in only 5% at 1 year of age.[7,8] In the majority of these infants regurgitation is not accompanied by other manifestations and should be regarded as physiologic. The incidence of regurgitation in unselected populations is comparable in breast-fed and formula-fed infants. Frequent regurgitation, defined as regurgitation that occurs more than three times a day, is found in about 20–30% of all infants during the first months of life. Worldwide, about 20–25% of parents seek medical advice because of infantile regurgitation. The frequency of regurgitation decreases after the age of 4–6 months. Complete resolution of regurgitation is frequent and expected by 10 months in 55%, by 18 months in 60–80% and by 24 months in 98%.[9] A prospective follow-up study reported disappearance of regurgitation in all subjects before 12 months of age, although an increased prevalence of feeding refusal, duration of meals, parental feeding-related distress and impaired quality of life was noticed, even after disappearance of symptoms.[10]

About 5–9% of infants have GERD.[6] In a Western population, GERD affects 4–30% of adults.[11,12] According to parents, heartburn is present in 1.8% of 3–9-year-old healthy children and in 3.5% of 10–17-year-old adolescents; regurgitation is said to occur in 2.3% and 1.4% respectively, and 0.5% and 1.9% need antacid medication. In self-reports, 5.2% of adolescents complain of heartburn and up to 8.2% of regurgitation; antacids are taken by 2.3% and H_2-receptor antagonists by 1.3%, suggesting that symptoms of GER are not rare during childhood and are underreported by parents or overestimated by adolescents.[13] In adults, heartburn and regurgitation resolve within 3–10 years in only 12–33%, regardless of the presence of esophagitis at diagnosis.[1,14]

Reflux esophagitis is reported to occur in 2–5% of the population. Children with GER symptoms undergoing evaluation present with esophagitis in 15–62% of cases, Barrett's esophagus in 0.1–3% and refractory GERD requiring surgery in 6–13%.[15–17] In adults undergoing endoscopy, esophagitis is diagnosed with an incidence of 15–80%.[1,14,15] The large differences in incidence are determined by patient recruitment and availability of self-treatment.

As regurgitation is more frequent in the first 6 months of infancy than in childhood and adulthood, it is frequently postulated that the prevalence of GER and GERD is higher in infants than in children or adults. However, data on the prevalence of GER and GERD during childhood are scarce. This controversy is due to the confusion and mixing of the definitions of regurgitation, GER, GERD and esophagitis. The prevalence of 'severe GERD' seems to be comparable throughout the different age groups.

Mastication, saliva secretion
Swallowing
Esophageal clearance
Esophageal innervation and receptors
Mucosal resistance
LES pressure
Sphincter relaxation
Abdominal esophagus
Sphincter position
Angle of His
Gastric volume, gastric accommodation
Gastric emptying
Gastric acid output
Gastric acid feed buffering
Feeding regimen: type, frequency, volume
Pepsin/trypsin/bile salts
Helicobacter pylori
Intra-abdominal pressure
GER
Genetic factors
Environmental factors
Posture
Physical activity
Sleep state
Respiratory disease
Medication (e.g. xanthines)

Table 20.1 Parameters influencing the pathogenesis of GER

ENVIRONMENTAL AND GENETIC FACTORS

Alcohol, smoking, drugs and dietary components are among the many factors that influence the incidence of

GER. The impact of lifestyle was demonstrated by showing that esophagitis and hiatus hernia were more common in a population with dyspeptic symptoms with the same genetic background living in England than in Singapore.[18] The use of low-dose aspirin and non-steroidal anti-inflammatory drugs available over the counter has a major impact on the incidence of severe GERD.[19] As the lifestyle of women becomes more similar to that of men, the difference in incidence in GERD between the sexes is disappearing. Using pH monitoring, we could not demonstrate a male predominance of pathologic acid GER in children. In adults, GERD affects Caucasians more often than African Americans or Native Americans.[11] Barrett's esophagus is partially genetically determined;[20] however, the same prevalence of troublesome infant regurgitation was found in Caucasian and Indonesian infants.[21]

Race, sex, body mass index and age are independently associated with hiatus hernia and esophagitis, with race being the most important risk factor.[18] Carre et al.[22] described autosomal dominant inheritance of hiatus hernia by discovering the condition in five generations of a large family, but did not demonstrate a link to GERD. The genetic influence on GERD is supported by increased GER symptoms in the relatives of patients with GERD.[23] Moreover, the concordance for GER is higher in monozygotic than in dizygotic twins.[24] The genes in question have been localized to chromosomes 9 and 13. A locus on chromosome 13q, between microsatellite D13S171 and D13S263, has been linked with severe GERD in five multiply affected families.[25] This could not be confirmed in a further five families, probably because of genetic heterogeneity of GERD and the different clinical presentation of patients.[26]

PATHOPHYSIOLOGY

The most important pathophysiologic mechanism causing GER at any age, from prematurity into adulthood, is transient lower esophageal sphincter relaxations (TLESRs).[27,28] However, GER is influenced by genetic, environmental (e.g. diet, smoking), anatomic, hormonal and neurogenic factors (Fig. 20.1).[27,29] Three major tiers of defense serve to limit the degree of GER and to minimize the risk of reflux-induced injury to the esophagus. The first line of defense is the anti-reflux barrier, consisting of the LES and the diaphragmatic pinchcock and angle of His; this barrier serves to limit the frequency and volume of refluxed gastric contents. When this line of defense fails, the second – esophageal clearance – assumes greater importance in limiting the duration of contact between luminal contents and esophageal epithelium. Gravity and esophageal peristalsis serve to remove volume from the esophageal lumen, whereas salivary and esophageal secretions (the latter from esophageal submucosal glands) serve to neutralize acid. The third line of defense, tissue or esophageal mucosal resistance, comes into play when acid contact time is prolonged, for instance when esophageal clearance is defective or not operative (motility disorders, during sleep).[27] Esophageal mucosal defense can be divided in pre-epithe-

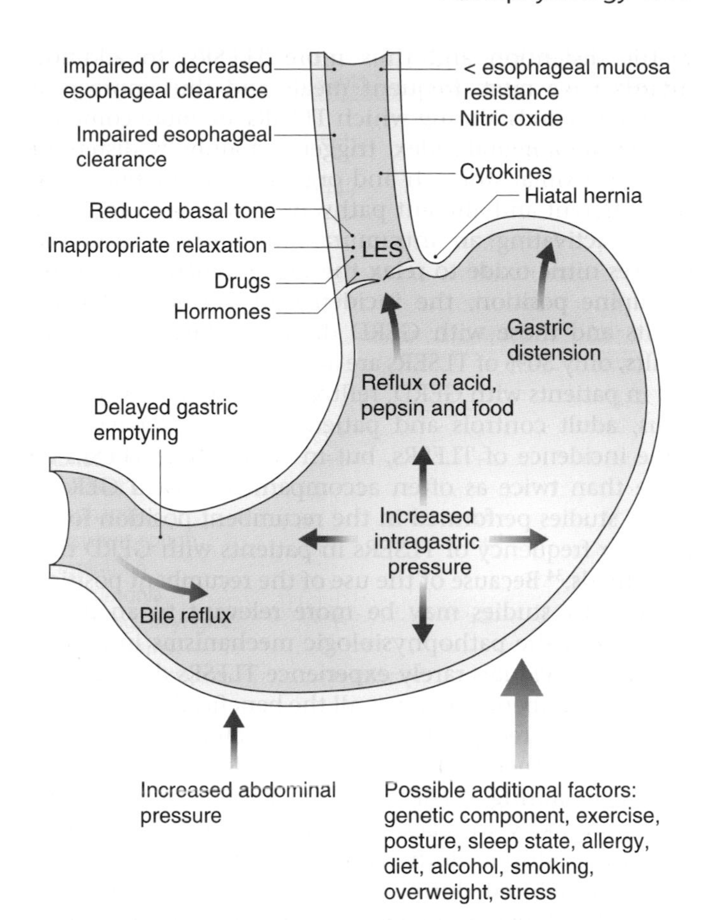

Figure 20.1: Pathophysiologic mechanisms for GER. The major pathophysiologic mechanism of GER at any age is inappropriate transient relaxations of the lower esophageal sphincter (LES).

lial (protective factors in swallowed saliva and esophageal secretions containing bicarbonate, mucin, prostaglandin E_2, epidermal growth factor, transforming growth factor), epithelial (tight junctions, intercellular glycoprotein material) and post-epithelial factors.[27] There is important interindividual variation of reflux perception, suggesting different esophageal-sensitive thresholds. The esophageal mucosa contains acid-, temperature- and volume-sensitive receptors. A widening of the intercellular spaces has been found in patients with esophagitis and in those with endoscopy-negative disease. When esophagitis heals, esophageal sensitivity to acid decreases. The presence of fat in the duodenum increases the sensitivity to reflux. Hyposensitivity, as occurs in patients with Barrett's esophagus, is a secondary phenomenon.[30]

GER occurs during episodes of TLESR or inadequate adaptation of the sphincter tone to changes in abdominal pressure. Not all of the factors responsible for maintaining LES tone have been determined, but nitric oxide likely plays an important role. The incompetent LES mechanism present in most newborn infants, combined with the increased abdominal pressure from crying or straining, commonly becomes a much less frequent cause of regurgitation or vomiting after the age of 4 months.[31] Infants have a short intra-abdominal esophagus. They ingest more than twice the volume compared with adults on a per kilogram basis (100–150 *vs* 30–50 ml/kg daily), causing more

69 children with GERD, regurgitation and vomiting occurred in 72%, symptoms attributed to the esophagus (epigastric or abdominal pain, feeding difficulties, irritability and Sandifer–Sutcliffe syndrome) in 68%, failure to thrive in 28%, chronic respiratory symptoms in 13% and recurrent apnea in 12%, with more feeding difficulties in toddlers and more irritability in infants.[16] The relation between chronic respiratory disease and GERD has been best described in children (this association is discussed below).

Belching or eructation occurs during transient relaxation of the LES and is an important method of venting air from the stomach. The upper esophageal sphincter relaxes in response to esophageal body distention by gas, in contrast to its contractile response to esophageal body distention by fluid. Hiccups or singulti are involuntary reflex contractions of the diaphragm followed by laryngeal closure. In some cases, hiccups cause GER. GERD in adolescents is more adult-like. Heartburn has become the predominant GER symptom, occurring weekly in 15–20%[12,56] and daily in 5–10%[57] of subjects. Atypical symptoms, such as epigastric pain, nausea, flatulence, hiccups, chronic cough, asthma, chest pain, hoarseness and earache, account for 30–60% of presentations of GERD.[1,57] GERD is diagnosed in 50% of adult patients with chest pain and in 80% presenting with chronic hoarseness and asthma.[58] The incidence of GERD in this group with atypical symptoms is determined by selection (bias) of the patients.

The reason for the differences in presentation of GERD according to age remains unclear. The persistence of symptoms and progression to complications are unpredictable for a group of patients and for an individual patient. Alarm symptoms are similar in adults and children: weight loss, dysphagia, bleeding, anemia, chest pain and choking.[57,58] Additional alarm symptoms in infants and children are failure to thrive, irritability or crying, feeding or sleeping difficulties, apnea and apparently life-threatening events.[59]

Peptic strictures represent an undesirable endpoint of reflux esophagitis. The primary symptom of the stricture is dysphagia.

Barrett's esophagus is not infrequent in adolescent children with chronic GER, particularly when *H. pylori* is present.[31] During the past three decades, hospital discharge and mortality rates for gastric cancer, gastric ulcer and duodenal ulcer have declined, whereas those for esophageal adenocarcinoma and GERD have risen markedly.[60] The opposing time trends suggest that corpus gastritis secondary to *H. pylori* infection protects against GERD.[60]

The influence on GERD of gastric colonization by *H. pylori* and its eradication is controversial. It has been suggested that *H. pylori* colonization, especially with the more virulent *cagA*-positive strains, may be protective against severe esophagitis and Barrett's esophagus.[61,62] Increased intragastric ammonia production and pangastritis with gastric atrophy and intestinal metaplasia, both promoting hypoacidity, are the most likely mechanisms.[41] Thus, it has been suggested that eradication of *H. pylori* may 'bring GER back to normal' in some susceptible subjects. However, eradication of *H. pylori* is not associated with increased symptoms of GER in children and adolescents.[63] Improvement in epigastric pain in children is significantly correlated with the improvement in GER symptoms, but not with eradication of *H. pylori*. An inverse association between esophagitis and *H. pylori* in the course of asthma in pediatric patients has been suggested recently.[63]

Symptomatic GER is estimated to occur in 30–80% of children who have undergone repair of esophageal atresia.[31] Children with congenital abnormalities, or following major thoracic or abdominal surgery, are at risk of developing severe GERD. Children with neurologic impairment have more frequent and more severe GER and GERD than neurologically normal children, for obvious reasons – spasticity or hypotonicity, supine position, constipation, etc.

GERD affects quality of life in adults, and probably also in children and their parents. The infant esophagus exposed to acid seems to be susceptible to pain hypersensitivity, despite the absence of tissue damage.[64] In adults, non-erosive reflux disease (NERD) is a generally accepted entity. NERD may exist in infants and children. Impaired quality of life, notably regarding pain, mental health and social function, has been demonstrated in adult patients with GERD, regardless of the presence of esophagitis.[14] In an unselected population, 28% of adults reported heartburn, almost half of them weekly, with a significant impact on quality of life in 76%, especially when the symptoms were frequent and long-lasting. Despite this, only half of the heartburn complainers sought medical help, although 60% were taking medications.[65] Thus, some adults 'learn to live' with their symptoms and acquire tolerance to long-lasting symptoms, whereas others accept an impaired quality of life. Infants and young children may just demonstrate irritability.

GERD AND RESPIRATORY DISEASE

Symptoms differ according to age.[55] Reflux may result in respiratory disease when the protective mechanisms fail (Table 20.3). Although apnea may be the presenting symptom of GER in some infants, in most infants apnea is unrelated to GER.[53,66] The same is true for bradycardia.[67] There is currently insufficient evidence to justify the apparently widespread practice of treating GER in infants with symptoms such as recurrent apnea, without proper diagnosis of GERD.[53] There are some infants, however, with a classic presentation of GER-induced obstructive apnea. These infants often demonstrate a startled 'bug-eyed' look, get red-faced, and appear to struggle to breathe.

A relationship between chronic airway problems and GER has not been demonstrated in pre-term infants.[53] The infant is at particular risk for supraesophageal complications of GER.[66] Many patients with chronic cough have gastrohypopharyngeal reflux.[27] An association of GER with awake apnea, reactive airway disease and recurrent pneumonia has been demonstrated. In a series of 46 children with persistent moderate asthma despite bronchodilata-

Pneumonia
Bronchitis
Wheezing (non-allergic asthma)
Cough
Hoarseness
Pharyngonasal regurgitation
Chronic subglottic stenosis
Sinusitis
Otitis
Obstructive apnea

Table 20.3 Respiratory symptoms that may be associated with GER

tors, inhaled corticosteroids and leukotriene antagonists, 59% (27 of 46) had abnormal pHmetry findings.[68] Reflux treatment resulted in a significant reduction in asthma medication. Patients with a normal pHmetry result were randomized to placebo or reflux treatment: two of eight of the treated patients could reduce their asthma medication, whereas this was not possible for any patient receiving placebo.[68]

Reflux may cause respiratory symptoms via different pathways, such as (micro)aspiration or vagally mediated bronchospasm (Fig. 20.2). Some patients with respiratory disease may have delayed clearance of esophageal reflux, and thus abnormal secondary peristalsis.[69] A consequence of pulmonary aspiration of refluxed material may be the presence of an increased number of lipid-laden macrophages. Although simply observing the presence of lipid-laden alveolar macrophages is non-specific, it has been suggested that quantification is a useful marker of silent aspiration.[70] Data are lacking and thus needed on the diagnostic accuracy, sensitivity and specificity of the detection and quantification of other substances in tracheal aspirates, such as lactose, pepsin, intrinsic factor and others.

Aspiration may be macroscopic, as occurs in aspiration pneumonia, or microscopic, as possibly occurs in some cases of chronic non-specific respiratory disease and apnea. However, aspiration is not mandatory to explain the mechanism, as the relationship may be neurally mediated from esophageal afferents. This may occur in reflex bronchospasm, reflex laryngospasm (obstructive apnea, stridor) and reflex central responses (central apnea, bradycardia). However, the clinician should first look for 'classic' etiologies that may be causing these symptoms; only when these etiologies are not found, should GER be sought.

In some patients it may not be GER that is causing respiratory disease, but the reverse. Respiratory difficulties need greater efforts to breathe and thus cause a more pronounced negative intrathoracic pressure. However, the incidence of a direct temporal relation between cough episodes and reflux is relatively low.[71] Forced expiration, as occurs in cough and wheeze, and forced inspiration, as occurs in stridor and hiccups, may cause GER. Some types of chest physiotherapy may cause or aggravate reflux. Hyperinflation and chronic coughing, as occurs in cystic fibrosis, may predispose to GER. Most patients with cystic fibrosis have more reflux than non-affected siblings. The relationship between GER and bronchopulmonary dysplasia is not well established, but it is likely that the increased respiratory efforts in patients with bronchopulmonary dysplasia predispose to reflux.

The relationship between respiratory disease and GER may also be neurogenic, and in this case designated 'gastric asthma'.[72] The tracheobronchial tree and esophagus have common embryonic foregut origins and share autonomic innervation through the vagus nerve.[73] It can be speculated that GER increases the irritability of the vagal nerve endings in the esophagus, and that as a result these nerve endings hyperreact together with the nerve endings in the airways because they have the same embryonic origin.

ESOPHAGEAL COMPLICATIONS OF GERD

GERD is associated with severe complications such as esophagitis, Barrett's esophagus, strictures and esophageal

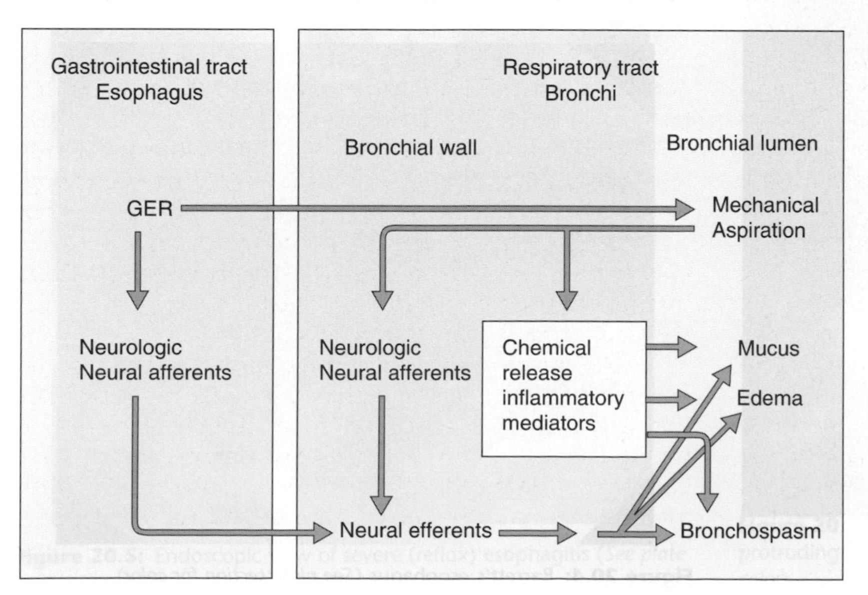

Figure 20.2: Pathophysiologic mechanisms of GER causing respiratory disease.

the presence of acid in the esophagus, but not all reflux causing symptoms are acidic. However, it is likely that the majority of patients with GERD suffer from acid reflux. Esophageal pHmetry is useful in evaluating the effect of a therapeutic intervention to reduce esophageal acid exposure (Fig. 20.8). Medical treatment is directed at reducing gastric acid secretion; the technique offers the possibility of recording intragastric and esophageal pH simultaneously. Results of pH monitoring depend on the hardware and software used.[87] The correlation between results obtained with different type of electrodes, glass and antimony is extremely poor.[88]

Intraluminal esophageal acid perfusion provoking chest pain (Bernstein test) or using other endpoints has been used increasing in practice and research in the USA, but not in Europe.

Manometry does not demonstrate reflux, but is of interest in showing the pathophysiologic mechanisms causing the reflux (by measuring the frequency and duration of TLESRs if the manometry is performed long term), and is indicated in specific situations such as achalasia. Ambulatory 24-h esophageal manometry, in combination with pHmetry, is technically feasible. Lengthy investigations offer the opportunity to measure events in upright and recumbent position, awake and asleep.

Impedance-metry is a technique that is gaining more and more interest. The technique measures electrical potential differences and is therefore not pH dependent. It offers the possibility of distinguishing between acid and non-acid reflux (in combination with pHmetry), and between liquid and gas reflux. Interpretation of the recording is at present quite laborious, and requires sufficient experience. Impedance-metry is of particular interest in patients with negative or normal endoscopic or pHmetric findings.

Because reflux is common in infants, because there is no 'gold standard' investigation and because investigations are invasive and expensive, interest has been focused on the development of an 'infant GER questionnaire'.[7,89] Recently, an improved questionnaire was developed[90] that offers the advantage of an objective, validated and repeatable quantification of symptoms suggestive of GERD, and the possibility of measuring the impact of therapeutic intervention. However, although correlation between the questionnaire and symptoms appears to be fair, that between the questionnaire and results of investigations for reflux is poor. Many studies have suggested a poor correlation between symptoms and the severity of reflux (esophagitis). In the author's unit, the results of a questionnaire did not correlate with the results of pH monitoring and endoscopy.

Investigative techniques for GER all measure different aspects of the mechanisms and characteristics of reflux. Therefore, it is not unexpected that the correlation between different techniques is extremely poor: non-acid reflux can cause esophagitis, severe heartburn can exist without esophagitis, etc.

There is no university optimal investigation technique for GER(D) because the questions being asked differ. 'Logical thinking' (but not evidence-based medicine) suggests that, if the question being asked is 'Does this patient have esophagitis', endoscopy with biopsy will be the best technique. If one is interested in the best method for measuring acid GER episodes, 24-h pHmetry will be the preferred technique. However, if one is interested in quantification of GER episodes, then impedance-metry may be best. As the generally accepted definitions separate GER and GERD on clinical grounds, a validated questionnaire may be the best way of identifying patients with GER and GERD. However, it is well known that esophageal strictures can develop as a consequence of GERD in patients with few or no symptoms. The most logical approach seems to be to adapt the therapeutic approach to the spectrum of symptoms for a given patient. Even this approach is not free of risk for overtreatment or undertreatment, however, as strictures occur in almost asymptomatic patients, and patients with severe heartburn may have NERD.

TREATMENT OPTIONS

Because symptoms suggestive of GERD are frequent and non-specific, especially during infancy, and because there is no 'gold standard' diagnostic technique, many infants are exposed to anti-reflux treatment. Physiologic GER does not need treatment. For 'frequent regurgitation', non-pharmacologic and dietary treatments such as thickened feeds are often used. In infants, hydrolysates are indicated when CMP allergy is suspected. In 'more severe GERD', medical treatment is recommended, and surgery is indicated for patients with the 'most severe reflux' (Table 20.4). In the

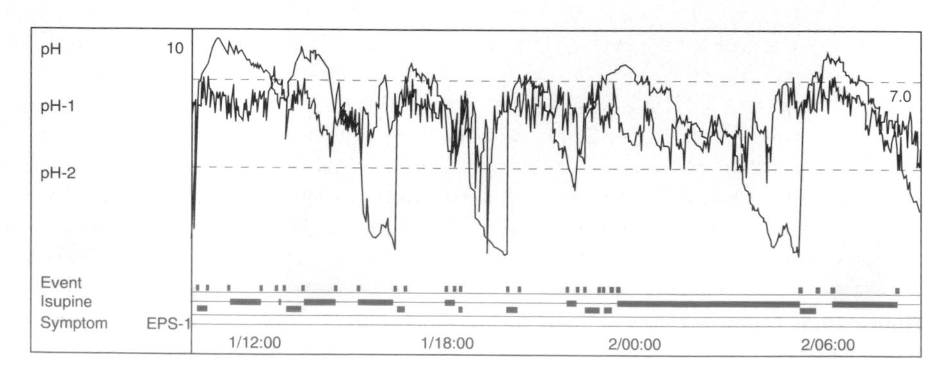

Figure 20.8: Two-channel pH monitoring. Esophageal tracing (pH 1): within normal range, but shows some acid reflux during one of the periods when gastric acid is not buffered. Gastric tracing (pH 2): every time the infant is fed there is a significant rise in gastric pH, buffering gastric acidity for 75% of the registration time. (This may be an example of a false-negative pH recording because of prolonged postprandial buffering of gastric acidity.) 'Events' (episodes of coughing) are both related and unrelated to acid reflux. Other event lines denote periods of sleeping

Phase	Treatment
1	Parental reassurance. Observation. Lifestyle changes. Exclude overfeeding
2	Dietary treatment (decrease regurgitation, no decrease in GER). Thickened formula, thickening agents, hydrolysates in cow's milk allergy
3	Alginates (some efficacy in moderate GERD, relatively safe). Antacids only in older children
4	Prokinetics (products available differ from country to country). Treats pathophysiologic mechanism of GERD, but no commercialized drug can be recommended
5	Proton pump inhibitors (drug of choice in severe GERD). H_2-receptor antagonists less effective than PPIs
6	Laparoscopic surgery (endoscopic procedures under evaluation)

Efficacy and safety data for most anti-reflux drugs in infants and young children are limited.

Table 20.4 Schematic therapeutic approach in 2005

discussion of therapeutic possibilities, attention is focused on safety aspects.

Therapeutic intervention should always be a balance between intended improvement of symptoms and risk of side-effects. It is difficult to recommend a 'best therapeutic approach' because of differences from country to country.

Complications of non-intervention

It is hard to know the true natural history of GERD in infants and children because most patients receive treatment. Knowledge of the natural history in untreated patients from the initial studies, when effective treatment was unavailable, is limited because of the poor description and identification of patients. The paucity of long-term reports, the presence of multiple pathogenic factors and the absence of pathognomonic symptoms for complications make it currently impossible to predict, on individual basis, which child will continue to have GERD into and during adult life. However, we know that untreated GERD may be associated with severe complications such as esophagitis, failure to thrive in children, esophageal stricture and Barrett's esophagus.

Recent observations suggest a decreased quality of life in regurgitating infants and their parents, even when the regurgitation has disappeared. A 10-year follow-up of esophagitis showed that over 70% had persisting symptoms and 2% developed strictures.[91] Untreated or uncontrolled GERD may be associated with severe complications such as esophagitis, Barrett's mucosa, stricture formation and esophageal adenocarcinoma. The frequency, severity and duration of reflux symptoms are related to the risk of esophageal cancer. It is not known whether mild esophagitis or GERD symptoms persisting from childhood into adulthood carries an increased risk for severe complications in adult life. Spontaneous improvement and healing of non-ulcerated esophagitis may occur. Nevertheless, complications and side-effects of medication have to be considered in relation to the natural evolution of untreated GERD.

Non-pharmacologic and non-surgical therapies for GER

The first approach should be careful observation of feeding and handling of the child during and after feedings.[92] Reassurance, showing comprehension for the comfort problems and impaired quality of life of the infant and parents, is of importance. Many infants are overfed or fed with an inappropriate technique.

The data from 10 randomized controlled trials of non-pharmacologic and non-surgical GERD in healthy infants were reviewed recently.[93] Non-pharmacologic (and non-surgical) therapies for reflux do not have proven efficacy on reflux, although some may decrease the incidence of regurgitation. Lifestyle changes (in adults) are rarely beneficial.[90] Despite gravity, the upright seated position leads to significantly more and longer reflux episodes than the simple prone and 30° elevated prone position, when the infant is both awake and asleep.[94] This is likely due to increased abdominal or intragastric pressure. The supine (lying on back) and right lateral positions are associated with the highest incidence of GER, the prone position with the lowest, and the left lateral position with intermediate GER.[94,95] The prone anti-Trendelenburg position (head elevated 30°) is the position with the lowest incidence of GER. However, there is now ample evidence that the prone sleeping position is a risk factor for sudden infant death, independent of overheating, smoking or method of feeding. The impact of pacifier use on reflux frequency was equivocal and dependent on infant position. The lower the osmolality of a feeding, the less the acid reflux. Larger food volumes and osmolality increase the rate of TLESRs; a reduction of the food volume results in a decreased amount of regurgitation but no change in acid reflux.[96]

Feed thickeners and anti-regurgitation formula

Milk thickeners have been reported to reduce regurgitation in infants.[94] Milk-thickening agents include bean gum preparations prepared from St John's bread, a galactomannan, carboxymethylcellulose, a combination of pectin and cellulose, cereals and starch from rice, potato, corn, etc. One study reported better efficacy for carob bean gum than rice cereal. There are as many different compositions of anti-regurgitation formula as there are companies: casein predominance, protein hydrolysates, etc. Although there is consistency in the finding of significant reduction in regurgitation, there is no evidence for a significant reflux-reducing benefit of thickened formula or thickening agents.[97] Studies applying pHmetry or impedance-metry have concluded that the effect of thickened feeds on (acid) reflux is not convincing. The height of reflux episodes is not significantly reduced with thickened feeds, and esophageal acid exposure time is not reduced. The effects of thickened formula on esophageal acid exposure show that in about one-third of infants there is some improvement, in one-third there is no difference and in one-third acid esophageal exposure is increased. One exception may be corn starch: two independent studies of corn starch-thickened formula from two companies indicated a decrease of esophageal acid exposure time. These observations need confirmation. Commercialized thickened formula is preferred to thickening agents added to formula at home; the nutritional content of the thickening agent and its effect on osomolality has been considered in the commercialized formula.

Increased coughing has also been demonstrated in infants receiving milk thickeners.[94] *In vitro* models testing the effect on one meal suggested that bean gum might be associated with malabsorption of minerals and micronutrients.[98] Studies of various thickening agents, including guar gum, carob bean gum and soybean polysaccharides, indicate the potential for decreased intestinal absorption of carbohydrates, fats, calcium, iron, zinc and copper.[99] Abdominal pain, colic and diarrhea may ensue from fermentation of bean gum derivatives in the colon. In some, but not all, animal studies, adding carob bean gum to the diet decreased the growth rate.[99] However, growth and nutritional parameters in infants receiving a casein-predominant formula thickened with bean gum were normal, and no different from those of a control group receiving standard infant formula.[100] Although rare, serious complications such as acute intestinal obstruction in newborns and pre-term babies have been reported.[94] Milk thickeners are often wrongly considered as 'inexpensive'. Allergic reactions to carob bean gum have been reported in adults exposed to it at their workplaces and in infants exposed to formula thickened with carob bean gum.[99] Nevertheless, in view of their safety and efficacy in decreasing regurgitation, milk thickeners remain a valuable first-line measure in relieving regurgitation in many infants. In contrast, their efficacy in GER is questionable.

Prokinetics

Prokinetic agents such as metoclopramide, domperidone and cisapride act on regurgitation via their effects on LES pressure, esophageal peristalsis or clearance and/or gastric emptying. Metoclopramide and domperidone also have antiemetic properties owing to their dopamine receptor-blocking action, whereas cisapride is a prokinetic acting mainly via indirect release of acetylcholine from the myenteric plexus.

Metoclopramide

Data supporting the efficacy of metoclopramide are limited to observations with intravenous administration.[101] Application in infants is limited because of the severe adverse events that occur in more than 20% of patients, including central nervous system (CNS) effects and interactions with the endocrine system.[101] The adverse CNS effects are related mainly to the dopamine receptor-blocking properties in the substantia nigra, and include extrapyramidal effects (dystonic reactions, irritability) and drowsiness, but also asthenia and sleepiness. Isolated cases of methemoglobinemia and sulfhemoglobinemia have been reported.[101,102] Neuroendocrine side-effects such as galactorrhea occur.[103] In addition, metoclopramide has been reported to induce torsade de pointes.[104] Extrapolation from adult data makes it unlikely that 'efficacy data' in infants and young children will be convincing.

Domperidone

Studies supporting the efficacy of domperidone in improving GER in infants and young children are limited.[101] The ability of oral domperidone to increase the pressure of the LES or to promote healing of reflux esophagitis has not been demonstrated in placebo-controlled trials. Most studies have been performed in older children, or have investigated the effects of domperidone co-administered with other anti-reflux agents.[101] Domperidone is better tolerated than metoclopramide: dystonic reactions (tremors) and anxiety are infrequent.[105] Somnolence was acknowledged by 49% of adult patients after 4 weeks of metoclopramide treatment *vs* 29% of patients after 4 weeks' treatment with domperidone.[105] A reduction in mental acuity was reported by 33% of patients, compared with 20% in the domperidone group. Akathisia, asthenia, anxiety and depression were also reported less often and at a lower severity after 4 weeks of domperidone, although the differences were not significant. Prolactin plasma levels may increase as a result of pituary gland stimulation.[106] Domperidone possesses cardiac electrophysiologic effects similar to those of cisapride and class III antiarrhythmic drugs.[101] Intravenous domperidone produces QT prolongation and ventricular fibrillation.[107,108]

There is a striking paucity of clinical trials assessing domperidone in infants and children with GERD. The pediatric studies with domperidone are old and of poor methodology. There are some data available on side-effects, and case reports of cardiac toxicity. These cardiac effects should be evaluated with priority because, in many countries, cisapride has been replaced by domperidone. Because of the widespread use of domperidone in many countries, the absence of pediatric data and the unconvincing data in adults, a well designed comparative trial with another prokinetic molecule is needed.

Erythromycin

Erythromycin has prokinetic activity when it is administered intravenously. Some efficacy has been suggested on gastric emptying, but not on GER or reflux symptoms. Systemic administration of erythromycin in young infants increases the risk of development of hypertrophic pyloric stenosis.[109] Similarly, a possible association exists with maternal macrolide therapy in late pregnancy.[109] Intravenous erythromycin is reported to cause QT prolongation and ventricular fibrillation.[94,110] The use of erythromycin at doses far below the concentrations necessary for an inhibitory effect on susceptible bacteria provides close to ideal conditions for the induction of bacterial mutation and selection.[111]

Cisapride

Critical consensus evaluations of published reports on the efficacy of different prokinetic agents (cisapride, domperidone and metoclopramide) concluded that cisapride is the preferred agent.[112] According to these assessments, the majority of clinical trials on the efficacy of cisapride demonstrated that at least one of the endpoints changed favorably as a result of the intervention.[112] A Cochrane review on cisapride in children analyzed data from seven trials including 236 patients that compared cisapride with placebo in terms of symptoms and improvement.[113] It was concluded that there was a statistically significant difference for the parameter symptoms 'present/absent', but no difference for 'symptom change' between placebo and cisapride. The Cochrane review also concluded that cisapride significantly reduced the number and duration of acid reflux episodes compared with placebo, as there was a significant decrease in the reflux index (the percentage time for which esophageal pH is below 4).[113] Cisapride is the only prokinetic with some evidence of efficacy, although the evidence is weak.

In general, cisapride is well tolerated. The most common adverse events are transient diarrhea and colic (in about 2%). The effect of cisapride on relevant cardiac events such as QT prolongation and arrhythmia is dose and risk factor related. Isolated reports of more serious adverse events (e.g. extrapyramidal reactions, seizures in epileptic patients and cholestasis in very premature infants) have been reported. The relationship between cisapride, the P450 cytochrome and cardiac effect was first considered in 1996.[114] Cisapride possesses class III antiarrhythmic properties and prolongs the action potential duration, delaying cardiac repolarization.[115] Torsades de pointes have been reported with cisapride.[116] Co-treatment of cisapride with macrolides such as clarithromycin and erythromycin prolongs the QT duration.[117] Underlying cardiac disease, drug interactions and electrolyte imbalance are exacerbating factors.[118] Cytochrome P4503A4, which is involved in the metabolism of cisapride, is immature at birth and reaches adults activity by the age of 3 months.[119] A significant QTc prolongation occurs, especially in infants younger than 3 months, but not in older infants.[120,121] This effect is related to higher plasma levels. A more frequent administration of lower doses (resulting in a recommended daily dose of 0.8 mg/kg daily) in premature babies results in lower peak levels.[121] Consumption of grapefruit juice also affects cisapride metabolism.[122]

Other agents

From the pathophysiologic point of view, prokinetics seem a logical therapeutic approach in the treatment of GERD in infants and children. Prucalopride, a $5HT_4$ agonist, seems effective in adult constipation,[123] but its use was forbidden in children because of extrapyramidal side-effects. Mosapride has limited effect, comparable to that of cisapride, on acid reflux variables and esophageal motor function in patients with GERD. However, it has also cardiac side-effects and was reported to induce torsades de pointes. Clebopride, another prokinetic agent, has not

c... m... Itop... not ... recep... placebo-controlled trials published inhibit... itopride, an open-label non- colonic ... patients showed improve- adverse ... with non-ulcer dyspepsia. headache, ... chemothera...ation, because it does mostly been ...ansetron is a $5HT_3$ bowel syndro...ic emptying and accelerate sma... but prolongs proximal coloni... ...y reported tric emptying and ... moderate ing drug. Howeve... ...eiving pediatric GER have ... has aminobutyric acid (... reduce spasticity in ... Given orally, it has ...le healthy adults.[127] Adr... patients was reported to ... eight neurologically imp... months to 16 years) and ... Baclofen significantly decrea... episodes, but did not change ... of esophageal acid exposure ... esophageal acid clearance time ... the eight children.[129]

Antacids

Experience with antacids in infants ... include carbonate and bicarbonate salts ... bonate, and calcium or magnesium carbo... plexes of aluminum and/or magnesium ... and magnesium hydroxides), aluminum a... phosphates, magnesium trisilicate and algin... forming formulations. Antacids do not chan... of GERD, as their only effect is chemically t... gastric acid. These products are used main... symptomatic treatment of heartburn and esop... adults. The key therapeutic advantage of antacid... rapid onset of action, which is limited by their ... to maintain an increased pH in the presence of acid... tion and gastric emptying. Their efficacy in buff... the gastric acidity is strongly influenced by the tim... administration.

Alginate-based raft-forming formulations have a qui... different mode of action. In the presence of gastric aci... alginates precipitate, forming a gel. Alginate-based raf... forming formulations usually contain sodium or potassiu... bicarbonate; in the presence of gastric acid, the bicarbon... ate is converted to carbon dioxide, which becomes entrapped within the gel precipitate, converting it into a foam that floats on the surface of the gastric content, providing a relatively pH-neutral barrier.[130] As alginate-based

patients wit
neous reactio
nemia, leuco
subacute myo
especially fatigue, dizz atulence, const
hepatic disease and epsia and naus-
generally rash a in; hepatic diso d
and agranulo els of aminotran he
gastrointesti s.[94,150,151] Last, bu ct'.
diarrhea though not a med and
2%), zole, lansoprazole ions
cial exhibit clinically im pH-
e:[152] ally metabolized to gas-
is over-
socomial
period of hypochlo has been
overgrowth. The clin te the pro-
nains unclear, althoug mach sec-
ory) infections in cr pounds are
ed. Long-term acid sup nal gastroin-
ion of N-nitrosamine his may have
dary to bacterial ove ls can result in
considered carcinogenic f the impaired
testinal flora and a de d environment.
nutritional conseque er treated for at
vitamin B_{12} deficie PI treatment, had
release of vitamin trols.[153]
However, patie n of acid-blocking
least 2 years w d includes not only
higher vitam o enterochromaffin-
The safe a occurs in nearly all
medicati orn rats raise concern
abnorm levels on the gastric
like ce in level lead to stimula-
pati ell (ECL) population and
of cell mass. Fundic polyps
rted in children taking
nths. Adult patients receiv-
n-8 years remained without
hyperplasia, gastric atrophy,
sia or neoplastic change.[154]
cacy profile, these drugs tend
uld delay the diagnosis of gas-
controlled use of these drugs
l, long-term use of PPIs in chil-
y safe, although these drugs have
de-effects.

ate-b
ge the c
o neutralize
y for the
hagitis in
is their
apacity
secre-
ering
of

ndoscopic procedures

ears, new endoscopic techniques that
function of the anti-reflux barrier have been
. The first results of endoscopic gastroplasty
nch® system), radiofrequency delivery at the cardia
cta® system) and injection therapy (Enteryx® proce-
re) in adults have been reported.[156–159] The first series in
adolescents have been performed; although experience is
too limited to recommend wide usage, the theoretical concept of these procedures is interesting. Further improvements to the techniques are still being introduced.

Peptic strictures are usually about one-third of the esophageal length above the diaphragm. Strictures are best treated with balloon dilation. If the strictures permits passage of an endoscope, biopsies under the stenosis should be taken to exclude Barrett's esophagus. Treatment of peptic strictures has two goals: dilating the stricture and arresting the reflux. Transendoscopic balloon dilators have the advantages of endoscopic visualization and safer radial forces, but, at a given diameter, mercury-weighted bougies may dilate more effectively. Occasionally, refractory strictures benefit from the injection of corticosteroids during endoscopic dilation. Perforation and significant hemorrhage are the most common complications.

Surgery

Gastroesophageal fundoplication is currently one of the three most common major operations on infants and children in the USA.[31] Anti-reflux surgery is performed much more frequently in the USA than in Europe. The reasons for this different approach are likely to be related to differences in healthcare costs and legal consequences. Although anti-reflux surgery in certain groups of children may be of considerable benefit, surgery also has a mortality and failure rate.[160–163] Some 90% of patients remain free from significant reflux symptoms after laparoscopic Nissen fundoplication, although side-effects occur in up to 22%.[164,165] After a median follow-up of 16 years, the Nissen–Rosetti procedure in 24 consecutive children without congenital or acquired anomalies of the esophagus, except GERD, the result was considered excellent in 75%, good in 21% and poor in 4%.[166] Failure rates of 5–20% have been found after objective postoperative follow-up.[165,166] A protective anti-reflux surgical procedure in neurologically impaired children needing a gastrostomy increased the morbidity and mortality rates of the gastrostomy procedure itself.[167] Surgery was also beneficial in those rare (even pre-term) infants with severe life-threatening GERD.[168] In Europe, surgery is mostly restricted to infants with life-threatening GERD and children older than 2–3 years with GERD needing lifelong treatment, or those in whom medical treatment has failed. Although more long-term follow-up data would be welcomed on laparoscopic anti-reflux surgery, it appears that this approach is currently preferred to an open procedure.

CONCLUSION

GER and GERD are common conditions in infants, children and adolescents. Symptomatology differs with age, although the main pathophysiologic mechanism, transient relaxations of the LES associated with reflux, is identical at all ages. Primary GERD is mainly a motility disorder. Although infant regurgitation is likely to disappear with age, little is known about the natural evolution of GER and GERD. The majority of symptomatic reflux episodes are acidic, but non-acidic and gas reflux can also cause symptoms. Complications of reflux disease, such as esophageal stenosis and Barrett's esophagus. may be severe and even life-threatening.

There is no 'gold standard' diagnostic technique. A simple questionnaire may be among the best diagnostic aids for diagnosing GERD in infants. The best investigation in the diagnosis of esophagitis is endoscopy with biopsies. In children with atypical reflux symptoms, pHmetry is still the recommended technique. Impedance-metry needs to be studied further, but is a promising technique that may possibly replace pHmetry.

Guidelines for treatment are difficult to establish, because there is no prokinetic drug with a convincing efficacy profile and the drugs available on the market differ from country to country. Treatment of regurgitation and moderate reflux disease focuses on reassurance, dietary treatment and gastric acid reduction therapy. PPIs are the drug of choice in severe reflux. Laparoscopic surgery is the recommended surgical procedure.

References

1. de Caestecker J. Oesophagus: heartburn. BMJ 2001; 323:736–739.
2. Dent J, Brun J, Fendrick AM. An evidence-based appraisal of the reflux disease management – the Genval Workshop Report. Gut 1999; 44:S1–S16.
3. Rudolph CD, Mazur LJ, Liptak GS, et al. Guidelines for evaluation and treatment of gastroesophageal reflux in infants and children. Recommendations of the North American Society for Pediatric Gastroenterology and Nutrition. J Pediatr Gastroenterol Nutr 2001; 32(Suppl2):S1–S31.
4. Vandenplas Y. Oesophageal pH Monitoring for Gastro-oesophageal Reflux in Infants and Children. Chichester, UK: John Wiley; 1992:27–36.
5. Cleveland RH, Kushner DC, Schwartz AN. Gastroesophageal reflux in children: results of a standardized fluoroscopic approach. AJR Am J Roentgenol 1983; 141:53–56.
6. Vandenplas Y, Goyvaerts H, Helven R. Gastroesophageal reflux, as measured by 24-hour pH-monitoring, in 509 healthy infants screened for risk of sudden infants death syndrome. Pediatrics 1991; 88:834–840.
7. Orenstein SR, Shalaby TM, Cohn J. Reflux symptoms in 100 normal infants: diagnostic validity of the Infant Gastroesophageal Reflux Questionnaire. Clin Pediatr 1996; 35:607–614.
8. Nelson SP, Chen EH, Syniar GM. Prevalence of symptoms of gastroesophageal reflux in infancy. Arch Pediatr Adolesc Med 1997; 151:569–572.
9. Shepherd R, Wren J, Evans S. Gastroesophageal reflux in children. Clinical profile, course and outcome with active therapy in 126 cases. Clin Pediatr 1987; 26:55–60.
10. Nelson SP, Chen EH, Syniar GM. One year follow-up of symptoms of gastroesophageal reflux during infancy. Pediatrics 1998; 102:e67.
11. Sonnenberg A, El-Serag HB. Clinical epidemiology and natural history of gastroesophageal reflux disease. Yale J Biol Med 1999; 72:81–92.
12. Isolauri J, Laippala P. Prevalence of symptoms suggestive of gastro-oesophageal reflux disease in an adult population. Ann Med 1995; 27:67–70.
13. Nelson SP, Chen EH, Syniar GM, Christoffel KK. Prevalence of symptoms of gastroesophageal reflux during childhood. Pediatric Practice Research Group. Arch Pediatr Adolesc Med 2000; 154:150–154.
14. Nandurkar S, Talley NJ. Epidemiology and natural history of reflux disease. Baillieres Clin Gastroenterol 2000; 14:743–757.
15. El-Serag HB, Bailey NR, Gilger M, Rabeneck L. Endoscopic manifestations of gastroesophageal reflux disease in patients between 18 months and 25 years without neurological deficits. Am J Gastroenterol 2002; 97:1635–1639.
16. Lee WS, Beattie RM, Meadows N, Walker-Smith JA. Gastro-oesophageal reflux: clinical profiles and outcome. J Paediatr Child Health 1999; 35:568–571.
17. Treem W, Davis P, Hyams J. Gastroesophageal reflux in the older child: presentation, response to treatment, and long-term follow-up. Clin Pediatr 1991; 30:435–440.
18. Kang JY, Ho KY. Different prevalences of reflux oesophagitis and hiatus hernia among dyspeptic patients in England and Singapore. Eur J Gastroenterol Hepatol 1999; 11:845–850.
19. Kim SL, Hunter JG, Wo JM, Davis LP, Waring JP. NSAIDs, aspirin, and esophageal strictures: are over-the-counter medications harmful to the esophagus? J Clin Gastroenterol 1999; 29:32–34.
20. Hassall E. Co-morbidities in childhood Barrett's esophagus. J Pediatr Gastroenterol Nutr 1997; 25:255–260.
21. Hegar B, Boediarso A, Firmansyah A, Vandenplas Y. Investigation of regurgitation and other symptoms of gastroesophageal reflux in Indonesian infants. World J Gastroenterol 2004; 10:1795–1797.
22. Carre IJ, Johnston BT, Thomas PS, Morrisson PJ. Familial hiatal hernia in a large five generation family confirming true autosomal dominant inheritance. Gut 1999; 45:649–652.
23. Trudgill NJ, Kapur KC, Riley SA. Familial clustering of reflux symptoms. Am J Gastroenterol 1999; 94:1172–1178.
24. Cameron AJ, Lagergren J, Henriksson C. Gastroesophageal reflux disease in monozygotic and dizygotic twins. Gastroenterology 2002; 122:55–59.
25. Hu FZ, Preston RA, Post JC. Mapping of a gene for severe pediatric gastroesophageal reflux to chromosome 13q14. JAMA 2000; 284:325–334.
26. Orenstein SR, Shalaby TM, Barmada MM, Whitcomb DC. Genetics of gastroesophageal reflux disease: a review. J Pediatr Gastroenterol Nutr 2002; 34:506–510.
27. Vandenplas Y, Hassall E. Mechanisms of gastroesophageal reflux and gastroesophageal reflux disease. J Pediatr Gastroenterol Nutr 2002; 35:119–136.
28. Omari TI, Benninga MA, Barnett CP, Haslam RR, Davidson GP, Dent J. Characterization of esophageal body and lower esophageal sphincter motor function in the very premature neonate. J Pediatr 1999; 135:517–521.
29. Sifrim D, Holloway R, Silny J, et al. Acid, non-acid and gas reflux in patients with gastroesophageal reflux disease during 24hr ambulatory pH-impedance recordings. Gastroenterology 2001; 120:1588–1598.
30. Niemantsverdriet EC, Timmer R, Breumelhof R, Smout AJ. The role of excessive gastro-oesophageal reflux, disordered oesophageal motility and decreased mucosal sensitivity in the pathogenesis of Barrett's oesophagus. Eur J Gastroenterol Hepatol 1997; 9:515–519.
31. Fonkalsrud EW, Ament ME. Gastroesophageal reflux in childhood. Curr Probl Surg 1996; 33:1–70.
32. Hirsch DP, Hollowy RH, Tytgat GNJ, Boeckxstaens GE. Involvement of nitric oxide in human transient lower esophageal sphincter relaxations and esophageal primary peristalsis. Gastroenterology 1998; 115:1374–1380.

33. Sifrim D, Tack J, Lerut T, Janssens J. Transient lower esophageal sphincter relaxations and esophageal body muscular contractile response in reflux esophagitis. Dig Dis Sci 2000; 45:1293–1300.
34. Holloway RH, Kocyan P, Dent J. Provocation of transient lower esophageal sphincter relaxations by meals in patients with symptomatic gastroesophageal reflux. Dig Dis Sci 1991; 36:1034–1039.
35. Penagini R, Hebbard G, Horowitz M, et al. Motor function of the proximal stomach and visceral perception in gastro-oesophageal reflux disease. Gut 1998; 42:251–257.
36. Stacher G, Lenglinger J, Bergmann H. Gastric emptying: a contributory factor in gastro-oesophageal reflux activity? Gut 2000; 47:661–666.
37. Van Zanten SJ, Dixon MF, Lee A. The gastric transitional zones: neglected links between gastroduodenal pathology and *Helicobacter* ecology. Gastroenterology 1999; 116:1217–1229.
38. Kuiken S, Van Den Elzen B, Tytgat G, Bennink R, Boeckxstaens G. Evidence for pooling of gastric secretions in the proximal stomach in humans using single photon computed tomography. Gastroenterology 2002; 123:2157–2158.
39. Sifrim D, Holloway R Transient lower esophageal sphincter relaxations: how many or how harmful? Am J Gastroenterol 2001; 96:2529–2532.
40. ela MF, Camacho-Lobato L, Srinivasan R, Tutuian R, Katz PO, Castell DO. Simultaneous intraesophageal impedance and pH measurement of acid and non-acid gastroesophageal reflux: effect of omeprazole. Gastroenterology 2001; 120:1599–1606.
41. McNamara D, O'Morain C. Gastro-oesophageal reflux disease and *Helicobacter pylori*: an intricate relation. Gut 1999; 45(Suppl 1):S13–S17.
42. Graham DY, Yamaoka Y. Disease-specific *Helicobacter pylori* virulence factors: the unfulfilled promise. Helicobacter 2000; 5(Suppl 1):S3–S9.
43. Levine A, Milo T, Broide E, et al. Influence of *Helicobacter pylori* eradication on gastroesophageal reflux symptoms and epigastric pain in children and adolescents. Pediatrics 2004; 113:54–58.
44. Pollet S, Gottrand F, Vincent P, et al. Gastroesophageal reflux disease and *Helicobacter pylori* infection in neurologically impaired children: inter-relations and therapeutic implications. J Pediatr Gastroenterol Nutr 2004; 38:70–74.
45. Salvatore S, Vandenplas Y. Gastroesophageal reflux and cow's milk allergy: is there a link? Pediatrics 2002; 110:972–984.
46. Hill DJ, Heine RG, Cameron DJ, et al. Role of food protein intolerance in infants with persistent distress attributed to reflux esophagitis. J Pediatr 2000; 136:641–647.
47. Mathisen B, Worall L, Masel J, Wall C, Shepherd RW. Feeding problems in infants with gastro-oesophageal reflux disease: a controlled study. J Pediatr Child Health 1999; 35:163–169.
48. Hamilton AB, Zeltzer LK. Visceral pain in infants. J Pediatr 1994; 125(Suppl):S95–S102.
49. Black MM, Dubowitz H, Huctheson J. A randomized clinical trial of home intervention for children with failure to thrive. Pediatrics 1995; 95:807–814.
50. Burklow KA, Phelps AN, Schultz JR, Mc Connel K, Rudolph C. Classifying complex pediatric feeding disorders. J Pediatr Gastroenterol Nutr 1998; 27:143–147.
51. Heine RG, Jaquiery A, Lubitz L, et al. Role of gastro-oesophageal reflux in infant irritability. Arch Dis Child 1995; 73:121–125.
52. Snel A, Barnett CP, Cresp TL. Behavior and gastroesophageal reflux in the premature neonate. J Pediatr Gastroenterol Nutr 2000; 30:18–21.
53. Poets CF. Gastroesophageal reflux: a critical review of its role in preterm infants. Pediatrics 2004; 113:e128–e132.
54. Orenstein SR, Izadnia F, Khan S. Gastroesophageal reflux disease in children. Gastroenterol Clin N Am 1999; 28:947–969.
55. Salvatore S, Hauser B, Vandenplas Y. The natural course of gastro-oesophageal reflux. Acta Paediatr 2004; 93:1063–1069.
56. Locke GR, Talley NJ, Fett SL. Prevalence and clinical spectrum of gastroesophageal reflux: a population based study in Olmsted Country, Minnesota. Gastroenterology 1997; 112:1448–1456.
57. The Jury of the consensus conference. French–Belgian consensus conference on adult gastro-oesophageal reflux disease 'Diagnosis and Treatment'. Paris, France, 21–22 January 1999. Eur J Gastroenterol Hepatol 2000; 12:129–137.
58. De Vault KR, Castell DO. Updated guidelines for the diagnosis and treatment of gastroesophageal reflux disease. Am J Gastroenterol 1999; 94:1434–1442.
59. Vandenplas Y. Reflux esophagitis in infants and children. A report from the Working Group of the European Society of Pediatric Gastroenterology and Nutrition on Gastro-oesophageal Reflux Disease. J Pediatr Gastroenterol Nutr 1994; 18:413–422.
60. Sonnenberg A, El-Serag HB. Clinical epidemiology and natural history of gastroesophageal reflux disease. Yale J Biol Med 1999; 72:81–92.
61. Graham DY, Yamaoka Y. Disease-specific *Helicobacter pylori* virulence factors: the unfulfilled promise. Helicobacter 2000; 5(Suppl 1):S3–S9.
62. Wu JC, Sung JJ, Chan FK, et al. *Helicobacter pylori* infection is associated with milder gastro-oesophageal reflux disease. Aliment Pharmacol Ther 2000; 14:427–432.
63. Sontag SJ. *Helicobacter pylori* infection and reflux esophagitis in children with chronic asthma. J Clin Gastroenterol 2004; 38:3–4.
64. Hyman PE. Gastroesophageal reflux: one reason why baby won't eat. J Pediatr 1994; 125:S103–S109.
65. Louis E, DeLooze D, Deprez P. Heartburn in Belgium: prevalence, impact on daily life, and utilization of medical resources. Eur J Gastroenterol Hepatol 2002; 14:279–284.
66. Rudolph CD. Supraesophageal complications of gastroesophageal reflux in children: challenges in diagnosis and treatment. Am J Med 2003; 115(Suppl3A):150S–156S.
67. Suys B, De Wolf D, Vandenplas Y. Bradycardia and gastroesophageal reflux in term and preterm infants: is there any relation? J Pediatr Gastroenterol Nutr 1994; 19:187–190.
68. Khoshoo V, Le T, Haydel RM Jr, Landry L, Nelson C. Role of GER in older children with persistent asthma. Chest 2003; 123:1008–1013.
69. Gorenstein A, Levine A, Boaz M, Mandelberg A, Serour F. Severity of acid gastroesophageal reflux assessed by pHmetry: is it associated with respiratory disease? Pediatr Pulmonol 2003; 36:333–334.
70. Ahrens P, Noll C, Kitz R, Willigens P, Zielen S, Hofmann D. Lipid-laden alveolar macrophages: a useful marker of silent aspiration in children. Pediatr Pulmonol 1999; 28:83–88.
71. Paterson WG, Murat BW. Combined ambulatory esophageal manometry and dual-probe pHmetry in the evaluation of patients with chronic unexplained cough. Dig Dis Sci 1994; 39:1117–1125.
72. Bruno G, Graf U, Andreozzi P. Gastric asthma: an unrecognized disease with an unsuspected frequency. J Asthma 1999; 36:315–325.
73. Cunningham ET Jr, Ravich WJ, Jones B, Donner MW. Vagal reflexes referred from the upper aerodigestive tract: an

infrequently recognized cause of common cardiorespiratory responses. Ann Intern Med 1992; 116:575–582.

74. Wienbeck M, Barnert J. Epidemiology of reflux disease and reflux esophagitis. Scand J Gastroenterol 1989; 156:7–13.
75. Carre I. The natural history of the partial thoracic stomach ('hiatal hernia') in children. Arch Dis Child 1959; 34:344–353.
76. Karnak I, Senocak ME, Tanyel FC, Buyukpamukcu N. Achalasia in childhood: surgical treatment and outcome. Eur J Pediatr Surg 2001; 11:223–229.
77. Liacouras CA, Wenner WJ, Brown K, Ruchelli E. Primary eosinophilic esophagitis in children: successful treatment with oral corticosteroids. J Pediatr Gastroenterol Nutr 1998; 26:380–385.
78. Orenstein SR, Shalaby TM, Di Lorenzo C. The spectrum of pediatric eosinophilic esophagitis beyond infancy: a clinical series of 30 children. Am J Gastroenterol 2000; 95:1422–1430.
79. Ruchelli E, Wenner W, Voytek T, et al. Severity of esophageal eosinophilia predicts response to conventional gastroesophageal reflux therapy. Pediatr Dev Pathol 1999; 2:15–18.
80. Hassall E. Barrett's esophagus: new definitions and approaches in children. J Pediatr Gastroenterol Nutr 1993; 16:345–364.
81. Krug E, Bergmeijer JH, Dees J. Gastroesophageal reflux and Barrett's esophagus in adults born with esophageal atresia. Am J Gastroenterol 1999; 94:2825–2828.
82. Oberg S, Peters JH, DeMeester TR, et al. Determinants of intestinal metaplasia within the columnar-lined esophagus. Arch Surg 2000; 135:651–656.
83. Sonnenberg A, El-Serag HB. Clinical epidemiology and natural history of gastroesophageal reflux disease. Yale J Biol Med 1999; 72:81–92.
84. Lagergren J, Bergstrom R, Lindgren A, Nyrén O. Symptomatic gastroesophageal reflux as a risk factor for esophageal adenocarcinoma. N Engl J Med 1999; 340:825–831.
85. Al-Khawari HA, Sinan TS, Seymour H. Diagnosis of gastro-oesophageal reflux in children. Comparison between oesophageal pH and barium examinations. Pediatr Radiol 2002; 32:765–770.
86. Aksglaede K, Pedersen JB, Lange A, Funch-Jensen P, Thommesen P. Gastro-esophageal reflux demonstrated by radiography in infants less than 1 year of age. Comparison with pH monitoring. Acta Radiol 2003; 44:136–138.
87. Vandenplas Y, de Pont S, Vandemaele C, et al. Dependability of esophageal pH monitoring data on software. J Pediatr Gastroenterol Nutr 1996; 23:203–204.
88. Vandenplas Y, Helven R, Goyvaerts H. Comparative study of glass and antimony electrodes for continuous oesophageal pH monitoring. Gut 1991; 32:708–712.
89. Orenstein SR, Cohn JF, Shalaby T. Reliability and validity of an infant gastroesophageal questionnaire. Clin Pediatr 1993; 32:472–484.
90. Kaynard A, Flora K. Gastroesophageal reflux disease. Control of symptoms, prevention of complications. Postgrad Med 2001; 110:42–44, 47, 48, 51–53.
91. McDougall NJ, Johnston BT, Kee F. Natural history of reflux oesophagitis: a 10 year follow up of its effect on patient symptomatology and quality of life. Gut 1996; 38:481–486.
92. Arguin Al, Swartz MK. Gastroesophageal reflux in infants: a primary care perspective. Pediatr Nurs 2004; 30:45–51.
93. Carroll AE, Garrison MM, Christakis DA. A systematic review of nonpharmacological and nonsurgical therapies for gastroesophageal reflux in infants. Arch Pediatr Adolesc Med 2002; 156:109–113.
94. Vandenplas Y, Belli D, Benhamou P, et al.. A critical appraisal of current management practices for infant regurgitation – recommendations of a working party. Eur J Pediatr 1997; 156:343–357.
95. Ewer AK, James ME, Tobin JM. Prone and left lateral positioning reduce gastro-oesophageal reflux in preterm infants. Arch Dis Child Fetal Neonatal Ed 1999; 81:F201–F205.
96. Khoshoo V, Ross G, Brown S, Edell D. Smaller volume, thickened formulas in the management of gastroesophageal reflux in thriving infants. J Pediatr Gastroenterol Nutr 2000; 31:554–556.
97. Huang RC, Forbes DA, Davies MW. Feed thickener for newborn infants with gastro-oesophageal reflux. Cochrane Database Syst Rev 2002; CD003211.
98. Bosscher D, van Caillie-Bertrand M, van Dyck K. Thickening of infant formula with digestible and indigestible carbohydrate availability of calcium, iron and zinc *in vitro*. J Pediatr Gastroenterol Nutr 2000; 30:373–378.
99. Aggett PJ, Agostoni C, Goulet O, et al. Antireflux or antiregurgitation milk products for infants and young children : a commentary by the ESPGHAN Committee on Nutrition. J Pediatr Gastroenterol Nutr 2002; 34:496–498.
100. Levtchenko E, Hauser B, Vandenplas Y. Nutritional value of an 'anti-regurgitation' formula. Acta Gastroenterol Belg 1998; 61:285–287.
101. Vandenplas Y. Clinical use of cisapride and its risk–benefit in paediatric patients. Eur J Gastroenterol Hepatol 1998; 10:871–881.
102. Aravindhan N, Chisholm DG. Sulfhemoglobinemia presenting as pulse oximetry desaturations. Anesthesiology 2000; 93:883–884.
103. Cinquetti M, Bonetti P, Bertamini P. Current role of antidopaminergic drugs in pediatrics. Pediatr Med Chir 2000; 22:1–7.
104. Chou CC, Wu D. Torsade de pointes induced by metoclopramide in an elderly woman with preexisting complete left bundle branch block. Chang Gung Med J 2001; 24:805–809.
105. Patterson D, Abell T, Rothstein R, Koch K, Brnett J. A double-blind multicenter comparison of domperidone and metoclopramide in the treatment of diabetic patients with symptoms of gastroparesis. Am J Gastroenterol 1999; 94:1230–1234.
106. Lu F, Wu H, Zhang K, Li D. Domperidone and hyperprolactinemia. Hunan Yi Ke Da Xue Xue Bao 1998; 23:100–102.
107. Drolet B, Rousseau G, Daleau P, Cardinal R, Turgeon J. Domperidone should not be considered a no-risk alternative to cisapride in the treatment of gastrointestinal motility disorders. Circulation 2000; 102:1883–1885.
108. Cameron HA, Reyntjes AJ, Lake-Bakaar G. Cardiac arrest after treatment with intravenous domperidone. BMJ 1985; 290:160.
109. Mahon BE, Rosenman MB, Kleiman MB. Maternal and infant use of erythromycin and other macrolides antibiotics as risk factors for infantile hypertrophic pylori stenosis. J Pediatr 2001; 139:380–384.
110. Mishra A, Friedman HS, Sinha AK. The effects of erythromycin on the electrocardiogram. Chest 1999; 115:983–986.
111. Guerin JM, Leibinger F. Why not use erythromycin in GI motility? Chest 2002; 121:301.
112. Vandenplas Y and the ESPGHAN Cisapride Panel. Current pediatric indications for cisapride. J Pediatr Gastroenterol 2000; 31:480–489.

113. Augood C, MacLennan S, Gilbert R, Logan S. Cisapride treatment for gastro-oesophageal reflux in children. Cochrane Database Syst Rev 2000; (3)CD002300.
114. Shulman RJ. Report from the NASPGN therapeutics subcommittee. Cisapride and the attack of the P-450s. J Pediatr Gatsroenterol Nutr 1996; 23:395–397.
115. Tonini M, De Ponti F, Di Nucci A, Crema F. Cardiac adverse effects of gastrointestinal prokinetics. Aliment Pharmacol Ther 1999; 13:1585–1591.
116. Hill SL, Evangelista JK, Pizzi AM, Mobassaleh M, Furton DR, Berul CI. Proarrhythmia associated with cisapride in children. Pediatrics 1998; 101:1053–1056.
117. Ward RM, Lemons JA, Molteni RA. Cisapride: a survey of the frequency of use and adverse events in premature newborns. Pediatrics 1999; 103:469–472.
118. Levy J, Hayes C, Kern J, et al. Does cisapride influence cardiac rhythm? Results of a US multicenter, double-blind, placebo controlled pediatric study. J Pediatr Gastroenterol Nutr 2001; 32:458–463.
119. Semama DS, Bernardini S, Louf S, Laurent-Atthalin B, Guyon JB. Effects of cisapride on QTc interval in term neonates. Arch Dis Child Fetal Neonat Ed 2001; 84:F44–F46.
120. Benatar A, Feenstra A, De Craene T, Vandenplas Y. QTc interval in infants and serum concentrations. J Pediatr Gastroenterol Nutr 2001; 33:41–46.
121. Cools F, Benatar A, Bruneel E, Theyskens C, Bougatef A, Casteels A, Vandenplas Y. A comparison of the pharmacokinetics of two dosing regimens of cisapride and their effects on corrected QT interval in premature infants. Eur J Clin Pharmacol 2003; 59:17–22.
122. Kivisto KT, Lilja JJ, Backman JT, Neuvonen PJ. Repeated consumption of grapefruit juice considerably increases plasma concentrations of cisapride. Clin Pharmacol Ther 1999; 66:448–453.
123. Coremans G, Kerstens R, De Pauw M, Stevens M. Prucalopride is effective in patients with severe chronic constipation in whom laxatives fail to provide adequate relief. Results of a double-blind, placebo-controlled clinical trial. Digestion 2003; 67:82–89.
124. Culy CR, Bhana N, Plosker GL. Ondansetron: a review of its use as an antiemetic in children. Paediatr Drugs 2001; 3:441–479.
125. Wagstaff A, Frampton J, Croom K. Tegaserod: a review of its use in the management of irritable bowel syndrome with constipation in women. Drugs 2003; 63:1101–1120.
126. Kahrilas PJ, Quigley EM, Castell DO, Spechler SJ. The effects of tegaserod (HTF 919) on oesophageal acid exposure in gastro-oesophageal reflux disease. Aliment Pharmacol Ther 2000; 14:1503–1509.
127. Ciccaglione AF, Marzio L. Effect of acute and chronic administration of the GABA(B) agonist baclofen on 24 hour pHmetry and symptoms in control subjects and in patients with gastro-oesophageal reflux disease. Gut 2003; 52:464–470.
128. Wiersma HE. Pharmacokinetics of a single oral dose of baclofen in pediatric patients with GERD. Ther Drug Monitor 2003; 25:93–98.
129. Kawai M. Effect of baclofen on emesis and 24-hr esophageal pH in neurologically impaired children with GER-disease. J Pediatr Gastroenterol Nutr 2004; 38:317–323.
130. Mandel KG, Daggy BP, Brodie DA, Jacoby HI. Alginate-raft formulations in the treatment of heartburn and acid reflux. Aliment Pharmacol Ther 2000; 14:669–690.
131. Winterberg B, Bertram H, Rolf N, et al. Differences in plasma and tissue aluminum concentration due to different aluminum-containing drugs in patients with renal insufficiency and with normal renal function. J Trace Elem Electrolytes Health Dis 1987; 1:69–72.
132. Flockhart DA, Desta Z, Mahal SK. Selection of drugs to treat gastro-oesophageal reflux disease: the role of drug interactions. Clin Pharmacokinet 2000; 39:295–309.
133. Bachmann KA, Sullivan TJ, Jauregui L, Reese J, Miller K, Levine L. Drug interactions of H_2-receptor antagonists. Scan J Gastroenterol Suppl 1994; 206:14–19.
134. Moayyedi P, Soo S, Deeks J, et al. Antacids, H_2-receptor antagonists, prokinetics, bismuth and sucralfate therapy for non-ulcer dyspepsia. Aliment Pharmacol Ther 2003; 17:1215–1227.
135. Sabesin SM. Safety issues relating to long-term treatment with histamine H_2-receptor antagonists. Aliment Pharmacol 1993; 7(Suppl 2):S35–S40.
136. Kelly DA. Do H_2 receptor antagonist have a therapeutic role in childhood? J Pediatr Gastroenterol 1994; 19:270–276.
137. Adachi N, Seyfried FJ, Arai T. Blockade of central histaminergic H_2-receptors aggravates ischemic neuronal damage in gerbril hippocampus. Crit Care Med 2001; 29:1189–1194.
138. Alliet P, Devos E. Ranitidine-induced bradycardia in a neonate – secondary to a congenital long QT interval syndrome Eur J Pediatr 1993; 152:933–934.
139. Hu WH, Wang KY, Hwang DS, Ting CT, Wu TC. Histamine 2 receptor blocker-ranitidine and sinus mode dysfunction. Zhonghua Yi Xue Za Zhi (Taipei) 1997; 60:1–5.
140. Nault MA, Milne B, Parlow JL. Effects of the selective H_1 and H_2 histmaine receptor antagonists loretadine and ranitidine on autonomic control of the heart. Anesthesiology 2002; 96:336–341.
141. Ooie T, Saaikawa T, Hara M, Ono H, Seike M, Sakata T. H_2-blocker modulates heart rate variability. Heart Vessels 1999; 14:137–142.
142. Basit AW, Newton JM, Lacey LF. Susceptibility of the H_2-receptor antagonists cimetidine, famotidine and nizatidine, to metabolism by the gastrointestinal microflora. Int J Pharm 2002; 237:23–33.
143. Cothran DS, Borowitz SM, Sutphen JL, Dudley SM, Donowitz LG. Alteration of normal gastric flora in neonates receiving ranitidine. J Perinatol 1997; 17:383–388.
144. Messori A, Trippoli S, Vaiani M, Gorini M, Corrado A. Bleeding and pneumonia in intensive care patients given ranitidine and sucralfate for prevention of stress ulcer: meta-analysis of randomised controlled trials. BMJ 2000; 321:1103–1106.
145. Huang JQ, Hunt RH. Pharmacological and pharmacodynamic essentials of H(2)-receptor antagonists and proton pump inhibitors for the practising physician. Best Pract Res Clin Gastroenterol 2001; 15:355–370.
146. Zimmermann AE, Walters JK, Katona BG, Souney PE, Levine D. A review of omeprazole use in the treatment of acid-related disorders in children. Clin Ther 2001; 23:660–679.
147. Vakil NB, Shaker R, Johnson DA, et al. The new proton pump inhibitor esomeprazole is effective as a maintenance therapy in GERD patients with healed erosive esophagitis: a 6-month, randomized, double-blind, placebo-controlled study of efficacy and safety. Aliment Pharmacol Ther 2001; 15:927–935.
148. Jones R, Bytzer P. Acid suppression in the management of gastro-oesophageal reflux disease – an appraisal of treatment options in primary care. Aliment Pharmacol Ther 2001; 16:765–771.
149. Andersson T, Hanssan-alin M, Hasselgren G, Rohss K. Drug interaction studies with esomeprazole, the (*S*)-isomer of omeprazole. Clin Pharmacokinet 2001; 40:523–537.
150. Leufkans H, Claessens A, Heerdink E, van Eijk J, Lamers CB. A prospective follow-up study of 5669 users of lansoprazole in daily practice. Aliment Pharmacol Ther 1997; 11:887–897.

151. Castot A, Bidault I, Dahan R, Efthymiou ML. Evaluation of unexpected and toxic effects of omeprazole A90 – reported to the regional centers of pharmacovigilance during the first 22 postmarketing months. Therapie 1993; 48:469–474.
152. Berardi RR. A critical evaluation of proton pump inhibitors in the treatment of gastroesophageal reflux disease. Am J Manag Care 2000; 6(Suppl):S491–S505.
153. ter Heide H, Hendriks HJ, Heijmans H, et al. Are children with cystic fibrosis who are treated with a proton-pump inhibitor at risk for vitamin B_{12} deficiency? J Pediatr Gastroenterol Nutr 2001; 33:342–345.
154. Singh P, Indaram A, Greenberg R, Visvalingam V, Bank S. Long term omeprazole therapy for reflux esophagitis: follow-up in serum gastrin levels, EC cell hyperplasia and neoplasia. World J Gastroenterol 2000; 6:789–792.
155. Naunton M, Peterson GM, Bleasel MD. Overuse of proton pump inhibitors. J Clin Pharm Ther 2000; 25:333–338.j1
156. Mahmood Z, McMahon BP, Arfin Q, et al. Endocinch therapy for gastro-oesophageal reflux disease: a one year prospective follow up. Gut 2003; 52:34–39.
157. Wolfsen HC, Richards WO. The Stretta procedure for the treatment of GERD: a registry of 558 patients. J Laparoendosc Adv Surg Tech A 2002; 12:395–402.
158. Johnson DA, Ganz R, Aisenberg J, et al. Endoscopic, deep mural implantation of enteryx for the treatment of GERD: 6-month follow-up of a multicenter trial. Am J Gastroenterol 2003; 98:250–258.
159. Galmiche JP, Bruley des Varannes S. Endoluminal therapies for gastro-oesophageal reflux disease. Lancet 2003; 361:1119–1121.
160. Fonkalsrud EX, Bustorff-Silva J, Perez CA, Quintero R, Martin L, Atkinson JB. Antireflux surgery in children under three months of age. J Pediatr Surg 1999; 34:527–531.
161. Pearl RH, Robie DK, Ein SH, et al. Complications of gastroesophageal reflux surgery in neurologically impaired versus neurologically normal children. J Pediatr Surg 1990; 25:1169–1173.
162. Alexander F, Wyllie R, Jirousek K, Secic M, Porvasnik S. Delayed gastric emptying affects outcome of Nissen fundoplication in neurologically impaired children. Surgery 1997; 122:690–697.
163. Spitz L, Roth K, Kiely EM, Brereton RJ, Drake DP, Milla PJ. Operation for gastro-oesophageal reflux associated with severe mental retardation. Arch Dis Child 1993; 68:347–351.
164. Booth MI, Jones L, Stratford J, Dehn TC. Results of laparoscopic Nissen fundoplication 8 years after surgery. Br J Surg 2002; 89:476–481.
165. Norrashidad AW, Henry RL. Fundoplication in children with gastro-oesophageal reflux disease. J Paediatr Child Health 2002; 38:156–159.
166. Bergmeijer JH, Harbers JS, Molenaar JC. Function of pediatric Nissen–Rosetti fundoplication follwed up into adolescence and adulthood. J Am Coll Surg 1997; 184:259–261.
167. Burd RS, Price MR, Whalen TV. The role of protective antireflux procedures in neurologically impaired children: a decision analysis. J Pediatr Surg 2002; 37:500–506.
168. Barnes N, Robertson N, Lakhoo K. Anti-reflux surgery for the neonatal intensive care-dependent infant. Early Hum Dev 2003; 75:71–78.

Chapter 21
Achalasia and other motor disorders

Manu R. Sood and Colin D. Rudolph

The esophagus is a conduit with sphincters at both ends. Its main function is to transport food, fluids and oropharyngeal secretions to the stomach and prevent regurgitation of gastric contents. The term esophageal motor disorder is commonly used to describe abnormal motility patterns demonstrated during esophageal manometry studies. Some of these disorders, such as achalasia, have well defined abnormalities of esophageal motility that correlate well with clinical symptoms. However, other esophageal motility disorders have a typical abnormal contraction pattern on manometry, but the clinical significance is not always clear. Thus, the classification of these disorders has been the subject of some controversy. Owing to differences in the neuromuscular anatomy of the proximal and distal esophagus, the illnesses affecting these regions also differ. We have therefore separated the motor disorders affecting the proximal and distal esophagus into two sections (Table 21.1). Normal esophageal function and development are discussed in Chapter 18. In this chapter, we focus on specific esophageal motility disorders and discuss their clinical presentation, pathophysiology and management.

Disorders affecting proximal esophagus
Primary
Cricopharyngeal achalasia
Cricopharyngeal incoordination
Cricopharyngeal hypotension
Secondary
Central nervous system
Meningocele
Arnold Chiari malformation
Cerebrovasular accidents
Multiple sclerosis
Autonomic nervous system
Familial dysautonomia
Motor neurons
Bulbar poliomyelitis
Neuromuscular junction
Myasthenia gravis
Botulism
Striated muscle
Polymyositis
Dermatomyositis
Muscular dystrophy
Diseases affecting distal esophagus
Primary
Achalasia
Diffuse esophageal spasm
Nutcracker esophagus
Non-specific esophageal motility disorder
Secondary esophageal motility disorders
Gastroesophageal reflux
Hirschsprung's disease
Intestinal pseudo-obstruction
Diabetes mellitus
Scleroderma and CREST
Inflammatory myopathies
Esophageal scaring
Tracheo-esophageal fistula
Esophageal atresia

Table 21.1 Classification of esophageal motor disorders

DISORDERS OF THE PROXIMAL ESOPHAGUS

The upper esophageal sphincter (UES) is a manometrically defined high-pressure zone distal to the hypopharynx. It is formed primarily by the cricopharyngeal muscle with contributions from the lower fibers of the pharyngeal constrictor and the upper striated fibers lining the esophagus. The cricopharyngeal muscle is innervated by the vagus nerve and sensory information is provided by the glossopharyngeal and sympathetic nervous system. Relaxation of the UES with swallowing is initiated in the swallowing center located in the brain stem, and the programmed inhibition travels via the vagus nerve. Normal deglutition requires synchronized pharyngeal contraction, complete relaxation of the UES muscles and traction by the neck muscles. This sequence of events pulls the larynx upward and forward, opening the sphincter as the pharyngeal contractions propel the bolus through the sphincter. When the sequence is uncoordinated or the UES sphincter fails to relax, the bolus is is mishandled. Disorders affecting the UES are usually part of a generalized neurodevelopment problem, and oral and pharyngeal phases of swallowing may also be affected.

Upper esophageal sphincter achalasia

Incomplete relaxation or failure of the cricopharyngeal muscle to relax during swallowing was first described by Utian and Thomas in 1969.[1] Primary cricopharyngeal achalasia usually presents with symptoms from birth.[2,3] As the condition is not well recognized, there is usually a delay in establishing the diagnosis. Choking, coughing, nasal regurgitation of feeds, tracheal aspiration and dysphagia are common presenting symptoms.[2,3]

A prominent posterior indentation is identified on a lateral radiograph in the pharyngoesophageal segment during a contrast swallow study.[2,3] A dilated pharynx with holdup of the contrast, to and fro movement of contrast,[2] aspiration and nasal reflux may also be noted. Videofluoroscopic study using different consistencies of food may be helpful to evaluate the swallowing mechanism further. Manometric studies have confirmed incomplete relaxation of the UES in some patients with radiographic abnormalities; in others, complete relaxation is seen.[2,4,5] This discrepancy in radiographic and manometric findings is not well understood, but could be related to the inherent difficulty in performing manometric studies in this region, especially in an uncooperative infant. Maintaining the position of the transducers in the UES during swallowing can be difficult, but use of a sleeve sensor may overcome this problem to some extent.[6] It is imperative to recognize that a prominent cricopharyngeal muscle during radiographic studies can be seen in normal infants and has been observed in up to 5% of adults having barium swallow studies for various reasons, in the absence of cricopharyngeal achalasia.

Several neuromuscular disorders have been associated with cricopharyngeal achalasia (Table 21.2). In patients with Chiari malformation, swallowing difficulty usually precedes other signs of brain stem compromise.[7] In a study of 15 patients with Chiari malformation, swallowing difficulty was the first symptom in more than half of the patients.[7] Seven of the nine patients in this study who underwent a preoperative barium swallow had cricopharyngeal achalasia, also confirmed by manometry. Two patients with normal findings on contrast study had cricopharyngeal incoordination on manometric studies. Associated esophageal motility abnormalities, such as spontaneous esophageal contractions and non-propagation of swallows, were also noted.[7] In 80% of patients normal swallowing returned following craniocervical decompression. Severity of the preoperative brain stem dysfunction was the only significant predictor of poor outcome following surgery. Other investigators have also reported UES dysfunction in children with Chiari malformation.[8,9]

With time, symptoms of UES achalasia may improve spontaneously in some children, so an initial conservative approach with aggressive pulmonary and nutritional support may be adequate. However, one must be vigilant and aware of the associated risk of aspiration, which can be life threatening. When spontaneous recovery does not happen, dilation[5] or cricopharyngeal myotomy[10] should be considered. In children, unlike adults, a single dilation may be sufficient and is effective in babies as young as 5 months of age. One study of adults with radiographic findings suggestive of cricopharyngeal achalasia used a combination of pharyngeal manometry and fluoroscopy to evaluate the pressure generated in the bolus prior to passage through the UES.[11] Cricopharyngeal myotomy was more likely to benefit those capable of generating high pressures, indicating that the pharyngeal constrictors were able to generate contractions that resulted in bolus transit when the obstruction by the contracted UES was relieved.

Myoneural junction defect
Myasthenia gravis
Muscular abnormality
Dermatomyositis and polymyositis
Systemic lupus erythematosus
Muscular dystrophy
Acrosclerosis
Thyrotoxic myopathy
Paroxysmal hemoglobinuria
Werdnig–Hoffman
Tetanus
Neural defect
Cerebral palsy
Amytrophic lateral sclerosis
Syringobulbia
Poliomyelitis
Posterior inferior cerebellar artery syndrome
Prematurity
Meningomyelocele and hydrocephalus
Arnold–Chiari malformation
Other
Down syndrome

Table 21.2 Conditions associated with cricopharyngeal dysfunction

Cricopharyngeal incoordination

Cricopharyngeal incoordination is characterized by a delay in pharyngeal contraction in relation to cricopharyngeal relaxation. It usually presents with swallowing difficulties. Neonates with 'transient cricopharyngeal incoordination' have a normal suck, but suffer from repeated choking and aspiration episodes. These symptoms can easily be confused with tracheo-esophageal fistula or laryngotracheo-esophageal cleft. Repeated choking and aspiration episodes can be life threatening, and early diagnosis is therefore important. The clinical course is variable and spontaneous improvement has been reported. Nutritional support and feeding advice is essential. The aim should be to minimize the risk of aspiration, which can be life threatening.

UES achalasia and incoordination have been reported in patients with central nervous system dysfunction[8] such as Chiari malformation.[7] UES dysfunction may also result from cervical inflammation and constrictive processes, which restrict laryngeal and hyoid bone movement. In Pierre Robin sequence, sucking-swallowing electromyography and esophageal manometry reveal dysfunction in the motor organization of the tongue, pharynx and esophagus.[12] Patients with familial dysautonomia (Riley–Day syndrome) have delayed, but complete, relaxation of the UES and associated esophageal motility disorders.[13] Wyllie et al. reported two children with drooling following nitrazepam; both had delayed relaxation of the UES in relation to pharyngeal contractions.[14] Cricopharyngeal incoordination with high-peaked esophageal peristalsis was reported in four patients with resistant myoclonic epilepsy being treated with nitrazepam. One patient required ventilation and improved following discontinuation of nitrazepam therapy.[15] UES dysfunction has also been reported in patients with Russell–Silver syndrome, 5p⁻ (cri-du-chat) syndrome and minimal change myopathy.[16]

Upper esophageal sphincter hypotension

Reduced UES resting pressure is seen in a variety of neuromuscular disorders such as myasthenia gravis, polymyositis, oculopharyngeal muscular dystrophy and amytrophic lateral sclerosis.[17] It is a manometric diagnosis, but the clinical significance is not clear. The condition may predispose to regurgitation of esophageal contents into the oropharynx and the respiratory tract.

DISORDERS OF THE DISTAL ESOPHAGUS

Achalasia

Achalasia is a motor disorder of the esophagus characterized by loss of esophageal peristalsis, increased lower esophageal sphincter (LES) pressure and absent or incomplete relaxation of the LES with swallows. The estimated incidence of achalasia is 0.4–1.1 per 100 1000 and the prevalence is 7.9–12.6 per 100 000.[18] Mayberry and Mayell, in a study of 120 children, determined an incidence rate of 0.1–0.3 cases per 100 000 children per year in the UK.[19]

Etiology

Patients with achalasia may present at any time between birth and the ninth decade; most of these cases are sporadic. Reports of familial achalasia represent less than 1% of all patients with achalasia.[20] Most cases of familial achalasia are horizontally transmitted, presenting in the pediatric age group and in siblings. Most of the horizontally transmitted cases result from consanguineous relationships, suggesting an autosomal recessive inheritance.[21,22] Concordance in monozygotic twins has also been reported.[23] It must, however, be remembered that familial achalasia represents a very small proportion of patients. Mayberry and Atkinson studied 167 families of patients with achalasia; 447 siblings were contacted and none had achalasia, suggesting that familial inheritance is rare.[24]

Autoimmune, infectious and environmental causes have been implicated in studies of idiopathic achalasia. Identification of round cell infiltration of ganglion cells of the myenteric plexus and association with class II histocompatibility antigen, Dqw1, supports the autoimmune hypothesis.[25,26] It has been suggested that infectious or toxic inflammatory processes stimulate interferon-γ release, thereby inducing the class II antigen expression on neural tissue.[20] Recognized as foreign antigens, T lymphocytes ultimately destroy the neural tissue. Two separate studies have reported serum antibodies to neurons of the myenteric plexus in 39% and 64% of patients with achalasia.[27,28]

Jones et al. noted significantly higher antibody titers to measles virus in patients with achalasia compared with controls, suggesting a viral etiology.[29] Likewise, Robertson et al. reported higher varicella-zoster complement fixation titers in patients with achalasia.[30] Subsequent studies using DNA hybridization techniques identified varicella-zoster in the esophageal tissue; three of nine specimens from patients with achalasia were positive, compared with 20 negative controls.[31] However, in studies that employed more sensitive and specific polymerase chain reaction techniques to examine 13 achalasia myotomy specimens for herpes, measles and human papillomavirus, no evidence of viral particles was found.[32]

Achalasia has also been reported in association with neurodegenerative disorders such as hereditary cerebellar ataxia and myoneural disorders.[20] Degenerating ganglion cells of the myenteric plexus and vagal dorsal motor nucleus in patients with achalasia in association with Parkinson disease have also been reported.[33]

Associations

Esophageal achalasia has been associated with adrenocorticotropic hormone insensitivity and alacrima in triple A or Allgrove syndrome.[34] The gene for triple A syndrome has been localized to chromosome 12q13[35,36] in the *AAAS* gene. Alacramia is usually present from birth, and hypoglycemia due to adrenocortical deficiency develops within the first 5 years of life. Children with Rozycki syndrome have achalasia associated with autosomal recessive deafness, short stature, vitiligo and muscle wasting.[17] Other associations with achalasia include Chagas disease,[37] sarcoidoisis,[38] Hirschsprung disease,[39] Down syndrome,[40] pyloric stenosis, paraneoplastic syndromes[41] and Hodgkin disease.[42]

Pathology

There may be minimal esophageal dilation in early stages of the disease; full-thickness esophageal biopsies show inflammation of the myenteric plexus, with no reduction in the number of ganglion cells.[43] Later, reduced ganglion cell number,[44–46] decrease in varicose nerve fibers in the myenteric plexus[47] and degenerative changes in the vagus nerve[44] are usually seen. However, it is not unusual for muscle biopsies obtained during surgery to be entirely normal with adequate numbers of ganglion cells. Quantitative and qualitative changes in the dorsal motor nucleus of the vagus, as well as a decrease in vasoactive intestinal peptide (VIP) and neuropeptide Y levels, have been reported in achalasia.[47,48] VIP is postulated as the major inhibitory transmitter released at the intramural postganglionic neurons of the LES, and low levels may be responsible for the lack of LES relaxation during swallowing.[49,50] The intermediate mechanism by which VIP induces LES relaxation is not completely understood. In animal studies VIP and dopamine have been shown to activate adenylate cyclase and increase intracellular 3′5′-cyclic adenosine monophosphate (cAMP) concentration, which results in LES relaxation.[20,51–53] In guinea-pig gastric fundic muscle cells, VIP released presynaptically stimulates intracellular nitric oxide synthase (NOS) and the production of nitric oxide (NO), resulting in muscle relaxation.[17] Human studies have demonstrated the absence of NOS in the LES of patients with achalasia, and physiologic studies showed LES relaxation when NO was added to the muscle strips.[54,55] Similar pathologic findings are present in patients with triple A syndrome.[56]

Clinical presentation

The clinical presentation depends on the duration of the disease and age of the child. The onset is usually gradual. In a review of 12 published studies, the mean duration of symptoms before the diagnosis was 23 months and the mean age at diagnosis 8.8 years.[17] In a worldwide survey of 175 children with achalasia, only 6% presented in infancy.[57] The youngest reported patient is a 900-g 14-day-old premature baby.[58]

Infants and toddlers present with choking, cough, recurrent chest infections, feeding aversion and failure to thrive. Older children usually present with vomiting, dysphagia, weight loss, respiratory symptoms and slow eating (Table 21.3). Dysphagia may initially be confined to solids, but usually progresses to involve both liquids and solids.[59] Stress is known to aggravate the symptoms. The child usually complains of food getting stuck in the chest; repeated attempts at swallowing or washing the food down with liquid helps to relieve the symptom.[60] Owing to swallowing difficulty and discomfort, oral intake may be reduced, resulting in weight loss. Once the esophagus is dilated, the patient may regurgitate undigested, non-bilious and generally non-acidic food, eaten hours or days earlier.[61] A large quantity of saliva can accumulate, especially at night when the patient is lying flat. Early morning waking with choking episodes, bouts of coughing due to aspiration of esophageal contents, and vomiting of whitish frothy saliva may be reported. Sudden death from aspiration is a serious risk.[59] The patient may be aware of the gurgling sound from the fluid sloshing in the dilated esophagus. Some patients may induce vomiting to relieve retrosternal discomfort, and this can be mistaken for bulimia.

Symptom	Percentage of children
Vomiting	80
Dysphagia	76
Weight loss	61
Respiratory symptoms	44
Chest pain or odinophagia	38
Failure to thrive	31
Nocturnal regurgitation	21

Table 21.3 Symptoms of achalasia in children[17]

Diagnosis

Radiography In most instances, the diagnosis of achalasia is considered after a barium swallow study, showing a variable degree of esophageal dilation with tapering at the gastroesophageal junction[62,63] (Fig. 21.1). As the barium fills the dilated esophagus and the height of the barium column generates sufficient pressure to exceed the LES pressure, partial emptying of the barium column may be seen. Later in the disease process the esophagus is grossly dilated and tortuous, with an S-shape described as the 'sigmoid esophagus'. Plain chest radiography shows a widened mediastinum, an air–fluid level and an absent gastric air bubble.[64] Radiography is also useful to evaluate the response to therapy. In adults, measurement of the height of the barium column 5 min after barium ingestion in the upright position predicts a successful outcome following therapeutic intervention.[65]

Manometry Manometry is the most sensitive and specific method for establishing the diagnosis of achalasia.[66] The characteristic manometry findings include increased LES pressure, absent peristalsis, incomplete or absent LES relaxation, and raised intraesophageal pressure. The LES pressure may be normal to twice the normal value.[66] No esophageal contractions are seen with wet or dry swallows, and this usually involve the entire length of the esophagus.[67] Abnormal or incomplete LES relaxation is seen in more than 70% of patients.[67] Maintaining the position of the transducer in the LES can be difficult; therefore, sleeve sensors may be helpful. Owing to distal obstruction, the

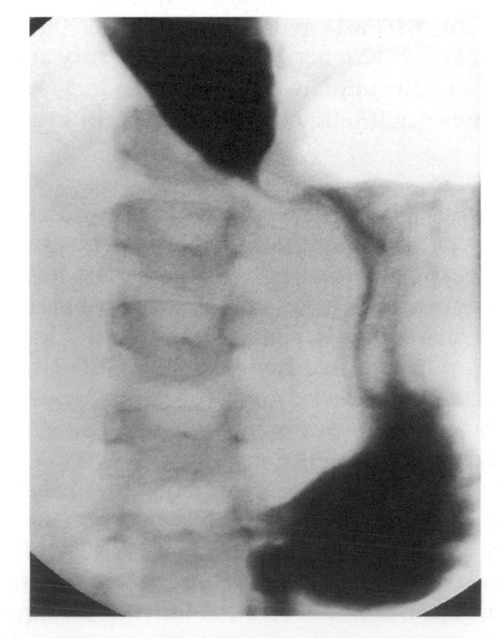

Figure 21.1: Barium swallow study in a child with achalasia showing esophageal dilation and beak-like appearance.

luminal pressure of the esophagus may be higher than the gastric fundal pressure.[68] Manometric abnormalities may be seen in babies as young as 2 weeks old.[69] UES dysfunction, including increased pressure, a short duration of relaxation with swallows and a more rapid onset of pharyngeal contractions after UES relaxation, have been reported.[70] The clinical significance of these findings is not clear.

Endoscopy The esophagus appears patulous, and esophagitis secondary to food stasis and fermentation may be seen. The LES does not open with insufflation of air into the distal esophagus. Often resistance is noted with passage of the endoscope through the gastroesophageal junction, which yields to gentle pressure. Particular attention should be paid to the presence of a hiatal hernia, as this may increase the risk of perforation during dilation.[20] Endoscopy also helps to exclude esophageal mucosal infection, carcinoma and leiomyoma of the esophagus.

Radionuclide tests A solid or liquid meal labeled with technetium-99m sulfur colloid can be used to measure esophageal emptying.[71] Patients with achalasia retain the tracer longer in the upright position.[72] The test may help to differentiate achalasia from other conditions such as scleroderma, because of the differing retention pattern. However, the usefulness of the test to assess patient response to therapy is debatable.

Differential diagnosis

It is important to differentiate achalasia from other causes of esophageal obstruction (Table 21.4). Leimyomas of the distal esophagus have been confused with achalasia in children.[73] Reluctance to eat because of difficulty in swallowing and associated weight loss may be confused with anorexia nervosa.[74] Regurgitation of undigested food may mimic rumination symptoms in adolescents.[75] Esophageal motility abnormalities in Chagas disease result from infection with *Trypanosoma cruzi*. The trypanosome causes destruction of the myenteric plexus, resulting in clinical and manometric findings similar to those of achalasia. This must be excluded in patients who have lived or traveled to Latin America.[76] A transient achalasia-like motility disorder has been reported in a patient with underlying chronic granulomatous disease and candidal esophagitis.[77] In adults, gastric carcinoma of the distal esophagus, oat cell carcinoma of the lung and pancreatic carcinoma may mimic the radiologic and manometric findings of achalasia.[20]

Esophageal stricture
Leiomyomas
Anorexia nervosa
Rumination
Chagas disease
Candidal esophagitis in chronic granulomatous disease
Adenocarcinoma of the stomach, oat cell carcinoma of the lung and pancreatic carcinoma

Table 21.4 Differential diagnosis of esophageal achalasia

Twenty-four-hour pH studies can be abnormal in patients with achalasia.[20] A gradual decrement in the pH, at times below 4, may result from fermentation of retained esophageal contents. This must be taken into account when interpreting the pH study; only sudden drops in intraesophageal pH should be considered gastroesophageal reflux.

Treatment

Pneumatic dilation The objective of forceful esophageal dilation is to stretch and rupture sufficient LES muscle to allow the passage of solids and liquids, without causing complete rupture of the esophagus or inducing post-dilation gastroesophageal reflux. In a review of all published studies that employed dilation therapy, 58% of patients had an excellent or good outcome.[17] The rate of improvement varied from 35% to 100%.[17] Eight studies examining the clinical outcome after esophageal dilation have been published since 1980 (Table 21.5); there is a general trend towards improvement in the number of patients with a 'good' outcome with each succeeding study.[78]

Although balloon dilation techniques vary, several basic principles for successful dilation have emerged over the years:

- Positioning of the balloon in the sphincter is important and should be confirmed radiographically.
- In patients with a dilated, tortuous esophagus, passing the balloon dilator over an endoscopically placed guidewire reduces the risk of perforation.
- Balloon position should be checked intermittently throughout the procedure as the balloon has a tendency to migrate into the stomach.
- The diameter of the balloon when inflated should be known. Newer dilators with plastic balloons that are not elastic ensure a specific diameter and are safer.[79,80] The Brown–McHardy dilator uses a mesh over the balloon to control the diameter. Use of a larger-diameter balloon may increase the risk of perforation.
- The pressure applied during dilation differs between published studies.

The bag is inflated once or twice per session, and the inflation period may last from 15 to 20 s to several minutes. One study evaluated brief (6 s) with more prolonged (60 s) dilation, and found no difference.[81]

Successful dilation allows the patient to eat regular meal without dysphagia. Very few studies have reported the long-term outcome following dilation, and it is not known what proportion of patients are able to avoid surgery completely. In a review of all published series, 25% of 151 patients required myotomy following unsuccessful dilation.[17] If symptoms recur quickly or there is partial improvement, surgery is generally required. Some studies have suggested that children older than 9 years respond best to dilation. If symptoms reappear within 6 months, surgery is eventually needed. With the introduction of minimally invasive surgical techniques, the role of dilation therapy with its inherent risk of perforation has been challenged as first-line treatment for achalasia.

The main complications of pneumatic dilation are esophageal perforation,[82–86] fever and pleural effusion.[20,84]

Reference	Year	No. of patients	No. with good outcome (%)	Comment
Dilation				
Azizkhan et al.[18]	1980	20	5 (25)	Average of two dilations each in patients who improved
Boyle et al.[60]	1981	10	8 (80)	Pain in one patient, fever in two
Seo & Winter[87]	1987	10	4 (40)	GER (pH study) in one patient
Nakayama et al.[63]	1987	15	11 (73)	Eight patients needed two or more dilations and four myotomies
Perisic et al.[140]	1996	12	10 (83)	
Hamza et al.[141]	1997	11	10 (90)	Mean of two dilations
Upadhyaya et al.[142]	2002	12	10 (83)	Repeat dilations in two patients who improved
Khan et al.[143]	2002	12	12 (100)	
Heller's open myotomy				
Buick & Spitz[97]	1985	15	12 (80)	Six had fundoplication; three without fundoplication developed GER
Vane et al.[98]	1988	21	18 (86)	Three required a second myotomy
Nihoul-Fekete et al.[99]	1989	35	34 (97)	Perforation in three patients
Emblem et al.[101]	1993	12	10 (83)	Subphrenic abscess in four patients
Illi & Stauffer[100]	1994	16	14 (88)	Dilations required in four patients
Myers et al.[57]	1994	164	116 (71)	Results not reported in 10; five required a second myotomy; one death
Morris-Stiff et al.[102]	1997	10	9 (90)	Chest infection in two; wound infection in one patient

Values in parentheses are percentages. GER, gastroesophageal reflux.

Table 21.5 Comparison of studies of children with achalasia treated with dilation or open myotomy

Rare complications include persistent esophageal pain, aspiration pneumonia and bleeding.[20] Gastroesophageal reflux is a late complication in 5–12% of children.[87] The incidence of perforation in adults after pneumatic dilation varies form 1% to 5%,[82,84] and the estimated incidence in children is around 5.3%.[17] Most perforations occur at the distal left lateral aspect of the esophagus, usually 5–10 mm proximal to or 5 mm distal to the squamocolumnar junction,[85] suggesting that the LES muscle is fairly resistant to complete tearing.[20] Esophageal perforation is accompanied with severe chest pain, fever, dysphagia, mediastinal and subcutaneous emphysema, or a pleural effusion. Post-dilation water-soluble contrast studies can identify perforation, and some units perform this routinely. In a careful radiographic study, Adams et al.[88] noted four major post-dilation findings: (1) linear mucosal tears, (2) a contained perforation penetrating beyond the muscular wall, (3) diverticular mucosal outpouching just proximal to, within, or below the LES, and (4) free perforation into the mediastinum, pleural space or peritoneal cavity. In this study patients with asymptomatic linear tears required no therapy; when symptomatic, conservative treatment with intravenous antibiotics and nothing by mouth was adequate. Patients with confined perforation beyond the muscular wall were treated conservatively. Immediate surgery and drainage was recommended for free perforation; however, medical treatment with intravenous antibiotics and parenteral nutrition has also been used successfully.

Botulinum toxin injection Botulinum toxin is a neurotoxin that binds to the presynaptic cholinergic terminals, thereby inhibiting the release of acetylcholine at the neuromuscular junction and creating a chemical denervation. It has been used therapeutically in humans, including children, for various neurologic and ophthalmologic disorders. In achalasia, loss of inhibitory neurons in the myenteric plexus results in unopposed excitation of the smooth muscles of the lower esophageal sphincter. This excitatory effect mediated through acetylcholine and anticholinergic drugs has been shown to reduce LES pressure.[89] In adults, botulinum toxin for treatment of achalasia is reported as a safe and simple therapeutic option. The toxin is injected endoscopically into the LES and adult studies have reported a good initial response in 90% of the patients. However, sustained response beyond 2–3 months was reported in only 64% and subsequent therapy was not as effective.[90] Khoshoo et al. reported results of botulinum toxin treatment in three children; all had immediate resolution of symptoms, but only one had a sustained response beyond 10 months.[91] Hurwitz et al. treated 23 children with botulinum toxin; 19 responded to initial treatment for a mean of 4.2 ± 4 months.[92] Seventy-four percent of patients in this study ultimately needed dilation and/or myotomy. More information is required before botulinum therapy can be recommended as first-line treatment for achalasia in children; the limited data indicate that, like drug therapy, botulinum treatment may be a temporizing measure rather than a definitive treatment.

Surgery Surgical treatment for achalasia in children has been reserved for patients who developed perforation during dilation or residual dysphagia after multiple dilations, or those who are poor candidates for dilation.

Most modern surgical procedures are variations of the Heller myotomy, which was first performed in 1914.[93] The length of the myotomy is debatable. In principle, it must be long enough to relieve the obstruction but not so long as to promote excessive gastroesophageal reflux. The incidence of postmyotomy reflux in adult studies ranges from 10% to 60%,[86, 94–96] and 7–50% in pediatric series.[17] Introducing an anti-reflux procedure may reduce the risk of acid reflux, but dysphagia may recur due to a tight wrap, especially as there is no esophageal peristalsis. Good or excellent outcomes with symptom relief in 74–92% of patients has been reported in all but one study.[97–102] In a worldwide survey of 164 children with achalasia who underwent myotomy by a variety of approaches, a good outcome was reported in 74%.[101] The best results followed transabdominal myotomy with an anti-reflux procedure, with 91% of 66 patients achieving long-term symptom improvement. Current data support transabdominal myotomy with a concomitant anti-reflux procedure as the preferred surgery for the treatment of achalasia in children.

With the advent of laparascopic techniques, the morbidity of achalasia surgery has reduced significantly, and the majority of operations in adults are now performed laparoscopically. In a multicenter survey of 22 children who underwent minimally invasive myotomy either laparoscopically ($n = 18$) or via a transthoracic route ($n = 4$), the mean hospital stay was less than 2 days and the majority were able to restart oral feeding within 2 days of surgery.[78] These results are better than those after open surgery. Adult studies show similar complication rates following laparoscopic surgery and open surgery.[20] One study suggested that the use of intraoperative esophageal manometry to document a complete reduction in LES pressure may be useful.[103] The decreased morbidity and more rapid discharge from the hospital support the laparoscopic approach as the preferred method in children and adults.

Drug therapy Isosorbide dinitrate, a smooth muscle relaxant, decreases LES pressure and improves esophageal emptying in achalasia.[104] However, headache and hypotension are common side-effects and drug resistance may develop with prolonged use. Nifedipine, a calcium channel blocker, also reduces LES pressure[105,106] and decreases the amplitude of esophageal contractions.[107] The pediatric experience is rather limited, but in one study of four adolescents with achalasia LES pressure dropped by more than 50% after nifedipine therapy.[105] In one adult study good long-term response was reported in two-thirds of patients.[108] It is generally accepted that drug treatment is a temporizing measure, and definitive therapy by either dilation or surgical myotomy is generally required.

Diffuse esophageal spasm

Diffuse esophageal spasm (DES) is a clinical syndrome characterized by symptoms of substernal distress, dysphagia or both, and an increased incidence of non-peristaltic esophageal contractions on manometry. Simultaneous contractions are rare in healthy individuals, and are usually seen with less than 10% of wet swallows. Manometry criteria for diagnosing DES include simultaneous esophageal contractions in 20% or more of wet swallows intermixed with some normal peristalsis.[109] If all contractions are simultaneous, the diagnosis is achalasia. A prevalence rate for DES ranging from 3% to 18% has been reported in adults with chest pain.[110–114]

Very few studies have looked at DES as a possible explanation of chest pain in children. Milov et al. reported DES in five adolescents with chest pain; two had associated dysphagia.[115] Endoscopy was normal in all five. Three were treated successfully with sublingual isosorbide, and one with diltiazem. Berezin et al. studied 27 children with chest pain; every child had an endoscopy, esophageal manometry and the Bernstein test.[116] Esophageal manometry abnormalities were present in four patients: three had simultaneous esophageal contractions and associated esophagitis and one had DES with normal endoscopic findings. Esophageal spasm has also been reported in a 22-month-old severely handicapped child who had significant acid reflux on pH study but no esophagitis on endoscopic examination.[117] Esophageal manometry, performed on three different occasions, showed DES that coincided with spells of crying and irritability and improved with verapamil, a calcium channel blocker. The etiology of DES is not known, but it has been suggested that it could be due to a defective deglutitive inhibitory reflex. Patients with DES show a hypersensitive response to cholinergic and hormonal stimulation, which may be related to a defect in neural inhibition due to decreased available nitric oxide.[110,118]

DES is a dynamic disorder and the same manometric features were reported in only 33% of patients in an adult study where manometry was repeated at a later time.[119] The prognosis is generally good and transition to achalasia occurs in only 3–5% of adults.[120,121]

Nutcracker esophagus

The typical manometric finding of nutcracker esophagus is high-amplitude peristaltic contractions in a patient presenting with chest pain.[122] The amplitude of esophageal contractions should be at least two standard deviations above the normal. Contractions of prolonged duration have also been described.[110] The manometric features may vary with time, and in one adult study only 54% of patients with an initial diagnosis of nutcracker esophagus had the abnormality on subsequent manometry.[123] The psychologic profile of patients with nutcracker esophagus resembles that of patients with irritable bowel syndrome,[124] and associated symptoms include anxiety, depression and somatization. Lower pain threshold to esophageal balloon distension, suggesting visceral hypersensitivity, has also been reported.[125] Barium studies are normal; tertiary waves or hiatal hernia are observed occasionally.[110] Some patients with nutcracker esophagus may go on to develop achalasia.[122,126] The place of nutcracker esophagus in the spectrum of esophageal motility disorders needs further clarification.

Non-specific esophageal motility disorder

Patients with abnormal esophageal motility who do not fit any of the features described above are categorized as having a non-specific esophageal motility disorder (NEMD). This would include patients with low-amplitude peristalsis (less than 12 mmHg), non-transmitted contractions with more than 20% of wet swallows, and spontaneous, prolonged duration, retrograde and triple-peaked contractions. Presenting symptoms include chest pain, dysphagia and gastroesophageal reflux. In one adult study 600 consecutive manometric recordings were reviewed and 61 patients were classified as having NEMD.[127] The commonest abnormality recorded was non-transmitted esophageal contractions, observed in 40% of the wet swallows, followed by low-amplitude contractions in 22%; only 2% of wet swallows showed retrograde propagation or triple-peaked contractions.

NEMD is commonly seen in association with gastroesophageal reflux disease.[128] Hillemeier et al.[129] reported non-peristaltic esophageal contractions in infants with reflux-related esophagitis.[129] Cucchiara et al.[130] also reported a high incidence of tertiary contractions and double-peaked peristaltic waves, and a decreased amplitude of esophageal contractions, in children with severe esophagitis. These manometric abnormalities improved after effective treatment of esophagitis.

Treatment of non-achalasia esophageal motility disorders

There is very little published data on the treatment of children with non-achalasia esophageal motor disorders. Reassurance and explanation of the underlying disorder responsible for the child's symptoms helps to relieve patient and parent anxiety. Advice regarding chewing food well, utilizing liquid chasers to assure passage of solid food boluses, and avoiding food with extremes of temperature may be helpful. Nitrates may be useful in reducing the amplitude of esophageal contraction, and may improve dysphagia and chest pain. Sublingual nifedipine, a calcium channel blocker, has also been shown to reduce the amplitude and frequency of simultaneous esophageal contractions. In adults, a placebo-controlled trial using trazodone[131] (an antidepressant) and imipramine[132] (a tricyclic antidepressant) reported improvement in chest pain associated with esophageal motility disorders. However, no similar pediatric trials have been published.

Secondary motility disorders of the distal esophagus

Intestinal pseudo-obstruction

Low or absent LES pressure and low-amplitude tertiary esophageal contractions have been reported in children with intestinal pseudo-obstruction.[133]

Hirschsprung's disease

Tertiary esophageal contractions and double- or multi-peaked contractions and non-propagating contractions with more than 20% of swallows have been reported in children with Hirschsprung's disease.[134,135] Abnormal esophageal motility persists after surgical correction. The clinical significance of the manometry findings is unclear as majority of the patients have no symptoms as a result of this esophageal dysmotility.

Connective tissue disease

Scleroderma is a systemic disorder characterized by excessive connective tissue deposition in the skin and gastrointestinal tract. Esophageal motility disorders are common in adults and have also been reported in children.[136,137] These include low-amplitude contractions, tertiary contractions and low LES resting pressure. Regurgitation, heartburn and dysphagia are common symptoms,[138] and are usually worse in patients with Raynaud's phenomenon. Abnormal esophageal motility is detected on barium swallow and manometric studies. Scintiscan studies demonstrate poor esophageal clearance.

Similar but less severe problems have also been reported in patients with polymyositis, dermatomyositis, systemic lupus erythematosus, the CREST syndrome, and mixed connective tissue disease. Corticosteroid treatment to control systemic symptoms may also improve esophageal symptoms. In Sjögren's syndrome, dysphagia due to lack of saliva is commonly noted. Decreased esophageal contraction time and an increased rate of propagation of esophageal contractions has been reported, but this is probably not clinically significant.

Esophageal atresia and tracheo-esophageal fistula

Abnormal esophageal motility is common and present from birth. Absent esophageal propagating contractions, tertiary contractions, low LES pressure and gastroesophageal reflux with prolongation of acid clearance in the distal esophagus have been reported.

Dysmotility due to esophageal scar formation

Ingestion of corrosive poisons results in esophageal chemical burns that heal with scarring. Sclerotherapy for esophageal variceal bleeding may also lead to scarring and stricture formation. Dysphagia may result from stricture formation as well as a lack of esophageal propulsive activity in the area of narrowed region.[139]

References

1. Utian HL, Thomas RG. Cricopharyngeal incoordination in infancy. Pediatrics 1969; 43:402–406.
2. Brooks A, Millar AJ, Rode H. The surgical management of cricopharyngeal achalasia in children. Int J Pediatr Otorhinolaryngol. 2000; 56:1–7.
3. Muraji T, Takamizawa S, Satoh S, et al. Congenital cricopharyngeal achalasia: diagnosis and surgical management. J Pediatr Surg 2002; 37:E12.

4. Dinari G, Danziger Y, Mimouni M, et al. Cricopharyngeal dysfunction in childhood: treatment by dilatations. J Pediatr Gastroenterol Nutr 1987; 6:212–216.
5. Kilman WJ, Goyal RK. Disorders of pharyngeal and upper esophageal sphincter motor function. Arch Intern Med 1976; 136:592–601.
6. Castella JA, Dalton CB, Castella DO. Pharyngeal and upper esophageal sphincter manometry in humans. Am J Physiol 1990; 258:G173.
7. Pollack IF, Pang D, Kocoshis S, Putnam P. Neurogenic dysphagia resulting from Chiari malformations. Neurosurgery 1992; 30:709–719.
8. Putnam PE, Orenstein SR, Pang D, et al. Cricopharyngeal dysfunction associated with Chiari malformations. Pediatrics 1992; 89:871–876.
9. Gendell HM, McCallum JE, Reigel DH. Cricopharyngeal achalasia associated with Arnold–Chiari malformation in childhood. Childs Brain 1978; 4:65–73.
10. De Caluwe D, Nassogne MC, Reding R, et al. Cricopharyngeal achalasia: case reports and review of the literature. Eur J Pediatr Surg 1999; 9:109–112.
11. Dantas RO, Cook IJ, Dodds WJ, et al. Biomechanics of cricopharyngeal bars. Gastroenterology 1990; 99:1269–1274.
12. Baudon JJ, Renault F, Goutet JM, et al. Motor dysfunction of the upper digestive tract in Pierre Robin sequence as assessed by sucking-swallowing electromyography and esophageal manometry. J Pediatr 2002; 140:719–723.
13. Margulies SI, Brunt PW, Donner MW, Silbiger ML. Familial dysautonomia. A cineradiographic study of the swallowing mechanism. Radiology 1968; 90:107–112.
14. Wyllie E, Wyllie R, Cruse RP, et al. The mechanism of nitrazepam-induced drooling and aspiration. N Engl J Med 1986; 314:35–38.
15. Lim HC, Nigro MA, Beierwaltes P, et al. Nitrazepam-induced cricopharyngeal dysphagia, abnormal esophageal peristalsis and associated bronchospasm: probable cause of nitrazepam-related sudden death. Brain Dev 1992; 14:309–314.
16. Staiano A, Cucchiara S, De Vizia B, et al. Disorders of upper esophageal sphincter motility in children. J Pediatr Gastroenterol Nutr 1987; 6:892–898.
17. Nurko S: Other motor disorders. In: Walker WA, Durie PR, Hamilton JR, et al., eds. Pediatric Gastrointestinal Disease: Pathophysiology, Diagnosis and Management, 3rd edn. St Louis, MO: CV Mosby; 2000:317–350.
18. Azizkhan RG, Tapper D, Eraklis A. Achalasia in childhood: a 20-year experience. J Pediatr Surg 1980; 15:452–456.
19. Mayberry JF, Mayell MJ. Epidemiological study of achalasia in children. Gut 1988; 29:90–93.
20. Wong RKH, Maydonovitch CL. Achalasia. In: Castella DO, Richter JE, eds. The Esophagus, 3rd edn. Philadelphia, PA: Lippincott Williams & Wilkins; 1999:185–213.
21. Dayalan N, Chettur L, Ramakrishnan MS. Achalasia of the cardia in sibs. Arch Dis Child 1972; 47:115–118.
22. Hernandez A, Reynoso MC, Soto F, et al. Achalasia microcephaly syndrome in a patient with consanguineous parents: support for A.M. being a distinct autosomal recessive condition. Clin Genet 1989; 36:456–458.
23. Stein DT, Knauer CM.Achalasia in monozygotic twins. Dig Dis Sci 1982; 27:636–640.
24. Mayberry JF, Atkinson M. A study of swallowing difficulties in first-degree relatives of patients with achalasia. Thorax 1985; 40:391.
25. Misiewicz JJ, Waller SL, Anthony PP, Gummer JW. Achalasia of the cardia: pharmacology and histopathology of isolated cardiac sphincteric muscle from patients with and without achalasia. Q J Med 1969; 38:17–30.
26. Lendrum FC. Anatomic features of the cardiac orifice of the stomach with special reference to cardiospasm. Arch Intern Med 1937; 59:474.
27. Verne GN, Sallustio JE, Eaker EY. Anti-myenteric neuronal antibodies in patients with achalasia. A prospective study. Dig Dis Sci 1997; 42:307–313.
28. Storch WB, Eckardt VF, Junginger T. Complement components and terminal complement complex in oesophageal smooth muscle of patients with achalasia. Cell Mol Biol 2002; 48:247–252.
29. Jones DB, Mayberry JF, Rhodes J, Munro J. Preliminary report of an association between measles virus and achalasia. J Clin Pathol 1983; 36:655–657.
30. Robertson CS, Martin BAB, Atkinson M. Possible role of herpes viruses in the etiology of achalasia of the cardia. Gut 1990; 30:A371.
31. Robertson CS, Martin BA, Atkinson M. Varicella-zoster virus DNA in the oesophageal myenteric plexus in achalasia. Gut 1993; 34:299–302.
32. Birgisson S, Galinski MS, Goldblum JR, et al. Achalasia is not associated with measles or known herpes and human papilloma viruses. Dig Dis Sci 1997; 42:300–306.
33. Qualman SJ, Haupt HM, Yang P, Hamilton SR. Esophageal Lewy bodies associated with ganglion cell loss in achalasia. Similarity to Parkinson's disease. Gastroenterology 1984; 87:848–856.
34. Grant DB, Barnes ND, Dumic M, et al. Neurological and adrenal dysfunction in the adrenal insufficiency/alacrima/achalasia (3A) syndrome. Arch Dis Child 1993; 68:779–782.
35. Weber A, Wienker TF, Jung M, et al. Linkage of the gene for the triple A syndrome to chromosome 12q13 near the type II keratin gene cluster. Hum Mol Genet 1996; 5:2061–2066.
36. Yuksel B, Braun R, Topaloglu AK, Mungan NO, Ozer G, Huebner A. Three children with triple A syndrome due to a mutation (R478X). Horm Res 2004; 61:3–6.
37. Herbella FA, Oliveira DR, Del Grande JC. Are idiopathic and chagasic achalasia two different diseases? Dig Dis Sci 2004; 49:353–360.
38. Lukens FJ, Machicao VI, Woodward TA, DeVault KR. Esophageal sarcoidosis: an unusual diagnosis. J Clin Gastroenterol 2002; 34:54–56.
39. Kelly JL, Mulcahy TM, O'Riordain DS, et al. Coexistent Hirschsprung's disease and esophageal achalasia in male siblings. J Pediatr Surg 1997; 32:1809–1811.
40. Zarate N, Mearin F, Hidalgo A, Malagelada JR. Prospective evaluation of esophageal motor dysfunction in Down's syndrome. Am J Gastroenterol 2001; 96:1718–1724.
41. Liu W, Fackler W, Rice TW, Richter JE, Achkar E, Goldblum JR. The pathogenesis of pseudoachalasia: a clinicopathologic study of 13 cases of a rare entity. Am J Surg Pathol 2002; 26:784–788.
42. Buyukpamukcu M, Buyukpamukcu N, Cevik N. Achalasia of the oesophagus associated with Hodgkin's disease in children. Clin Oncol 1982; 8:73–76.
43. Goldblum JR, Rice TW, Richter JE. Histopathologic features in esophagomyotomy specimens from patients with achalasia. Gastroenterology 1996; 111:648–654.
44. Cassella RR, Brown AL Jr, Sayre GP, Ellis FH Jr. Achalasia of the esophagus: pathologic and etiologic considerations. Ann Surg 1964; 160:474–487.
45. Csendes A, Smok G, Braghetto I, et al. Gastroesophageal sphincter pressure and histological changes in distal

esophagus in patients with achalasia of the esophagus. Dig Dis Sci 1985; 30:941–945.

46. Csendes A, Smok G, Braghetto I, et al. Histological studies of Auerbach's plexuses of the oesophagus, stomach, jejunum, and colon in patients with achalasia of the oesophagus: correlation with gastric acid secretion, presence of parietal cells and gastric emptying of solids. Gut 1992; 33:150–154.
47. Wattchow DA, Costa M. Distribution of peptide-containing nerve fibres in achalasia of the oesophagus. J Gastroenterol Hepatol 1996; 11:478–485.
48. Friesen DL, Henderson RD, Hanna W. Ultrastructure of the esophageal muscle in achalasia and diffuse esophageal spasm. Am J Clin Pathol 1983; 79:319–325.
49. Biancani P, Walsh J, Behar J. Vasoactive intestinal peptide: a neurotransmitter for relaxation of the rabbit internal anal sphincter. Gastroenterology 1985; 89:867–874.
50. Guelrud M, Rossiter A, Souney PF, et al. The effect of vasoactive intestinal polypeptide on the lower esophageal sphincter in achalasia. Gastroenterology 1992; 103:377–382.
51. Gidda GS. Control of esophageal peristalsis. Viewpoint Dig Dis 1985; 17:13.
52. Murray JA, Du C, Ledlow A, et al. Guanylate cyclase inhibitors: effect on tone, relaxation, and cGMP content of lower esophageal sphincter. Am J Physiol 1992; 263:G97–101.
53. Torphy TJ, Fine CF, Burman M, et al. Lower esophageal sphincter relaxation is associated with increased cyclic nucleotide content. Am J Physiol 1986; 251:G786– 793.
54. Preiksaitis HG, Tremblay L, Diamant NE. Nitric oxide mediates inhibitory nerve effects in human esophagus and lower esophageal sphincter. Dig Dis Sci 1994; 39:770–775.
55. Anand N, Paterson WG. Role of nitric oxide in esophageal peristalsis. Am J Physiol 1994; 266:G123–131.
56. Khelif K, De Laet MH, Chaouachi B, Segers V, Vanderwinden JM. Achalasia of the cardia in Allgrove's (triple A) syndrome: histopathologic study of 10 cases. Am J Surg Pathol 2003; 27:667–672.
57. Myers NA, Jolley SG, Taylor R. Achalasia of the cardia in children: a worldwide survey. J Pediatr Surg 1994; 29:1375–1379.
58. Polk HC, Burford TH. Disorders of the distal esophagus in infancy and childhood. Am J Dis Child 1964; 108:243–251.
59. Singh H, Gupta HL, Sethi RS, Khetarpal SK. Cardiac achalasia in childhood. Postgrad Med J 1969; 45:327–335.
60. Boyle JT, Cohen S, Watkins JB. Successful treatment of achalasia in childhood by pneumatic dilatation. J Pediatr 1981; 99:35–40.
61. Moersch HJ. Cardiospasm in infancy and childhood. Am J Dis Child 1929; 38:294–298.
62. Lemmer JH, Coran AG, Wesley JR, et al. Achalasia in children: treatment by anterior esophageal myotomy (modified Heller operation). J Pediatr Surg 1985; 20:333–338.
63. Nakayama DK, Shorter NA, Boyle JT, et al. Pneumatic dilatation and operative treatment of achalasia in children. J Pediatr Surg 1987; 22:619–622.
64. Orlando RC, Call DL, Bream CA. Achalasia and absent gastric air bubble. Ann Intern Med 1978; 88:60–61.
65. Vaezi MF, Baker ME, Achkar E, Richter JE. Timed barium oesophagram: better predictor of long term success after pneumatic dilation in achalasia than symptom assessment. Gut 2002; 50:765–770.
66. Eckardt VF, Aignherr C, Bernhard G. Predictors of outcome in patients with achalasia treated by pneumatic dilation. Gastroenterology 1992; 103:1732–1738.
67. Cohen S, Parkman HP. Treatment of achalasia– whalebone to botulinum toxin. N Engl J Med 1995; 332:815–816.
68. Uribe P Jr, Csendes A, Larrain A, Ayala M. Motility studies in fifty patients with achalasia of the esophagus. Am J Gastroenterol 1974; 62:333–336.
69. Asch MJ, Liebman W, Lachman RS, Moore TC. Esophageal achalasia: diagnosis and cardiomyotomy in a newborn infant. J Pediatr Surg 1974; 9:911–912.
70. Dudnick RS, Castell JA, Castell DO. Abnormal upper esophageal sphincter function in achalasia. Am J Gastroenterol 1992; 87:1712–1715.
71. Holloway RH, Krosin G, Lange RC, et al. Radionuclide esophageal emptying of a solid meal to quantitate results of therapy in achalasia. Gastroenterology 1983; 84:771–776.
72. Russell CO, Bright N, Schmidt G, Sloan J. Achalasia of the oesophagus: results of treatment. Aust N Z J Surg 1991; 61:43–48.
73. Payne WS, Ellis FH, Olsen AM. Treatment of cardiospasm (achalasia of esophagus) in children. Surgery 1961; 50:731–735.
74. Duane PD, Magee TM, Alexander MS, et al. Oesophageal achalasia in adolescent women mistaken for anorexia nervosa. BMJ 1992; 305:43.
75. MacKalski BA, Keate RF. Rumination in a patient with achalasia. Am J Gastroenterol 1993; 88:1803–1804.
76. Csendes A, Strauszer T, Uribe P. Alterations in normal esophageal motility in patients with Chagas' disease. Am J Dig Dis 1975; 20:437–442.
77. Bode CP, Schroten H, Koletzko S, et al. Transient achalasia-like esophageal motility disorder after candida esophagitis in a boy with chronic granulomatous disease. J Pediatr Gastroenterol Nutr 1996; 23:320–323.
78. Mehra M, Bahar RJ, Ament ME, et al. Laparoscopic and thoracoscopic esophagomyotomy for children with achalasia. J Pediatr Gastroenterol Nutr 2001; 33:466–471.
79. Stark GA, Castell DO, Richter JE, Wu WC. Prospective randomized comparison of Brown–McHardy and microvasive balloon dilators in treatment of achalasia. Am J Gastroenterol 1990; 85:1322–1326.
80. Kadakia SC, Wong RK. Graded pneumatic dilation using Rigiflex achalasia dilators in patients with primary esophageal achalasia. Am J Gastroenterol 1993; 88:34–38.
81. Khan AA, Shah SW, Alam A et al. Pneumatic dilatation in achalasia: a prospective comparison of balloon distension time. Am J Gastroenterol 1998; 93:1064–1067.
82. Parkman HP, Reynolds JC, Ouyang A, et al. Pneumatic dilatation or esophagomyotomy treatment for idiopathic achalasia: clinical outcomes and cost analysis. Dig Dis Sci 1993; 38:75–85.
83. Olsen AM, Harrington SW, Moersch JH, et al. The treatment of cardiospasm: analysis of a twelve year experience. J Thorac Surg 1951; 22:164–187.
84. Mandelstam P, Sugawa C, Silvis SE, et al. Complications associated with esophagogastroduodenoscopy and with esophageal dilation. Gastrointest Endosc 1976; 23:16–19.
85. Miller RE, Tiszenkel HI. Esophageal perforation due to pneumatic dilation for achalasia. Surg Gynecol Obstet 1988; 166:458–460.
86. Okike N, Payne WS, Neufeld DM, et al. Esophagomyotomy versus forceful dilation for achalasia of the esophagus: results in 899 patients. Ann Thorac Surg 1979; 28:119–125.
87. Seo JK, Winter HS. Esophageal manometric and clinical response to treatment in children with achalasia (abstract). Gasteroenterology 1987; 92:1634.
88. Adams H, Roberts GM, Smith PM. Oesophageal tears during pneumatic balloon dilatation for the treatment of achalasia. Clin Radiol 1989; 40:53–57.

89. Nurko S. Botulinum toxin for achalasia: are we witnessing the birth of a new era? J Pediatr Gastroenterol Nutr 1997; 24:447–449.
90. Pasricha PJ, Rai R, Ravich WJ, et al. Botulinum toxin for achalasia: long-term outcome and predictors of response. Gastroenterology 1996; 110:1410–1415.
91. Khoshoo V, LaGarde DC, Udall JN Jr. Intrasphincteric injection of botulinum toxin for treating achalasia in children. J Pediatr Gastroenterol Nutr 1997; 24:439–441.
92. Hurwitz M, Bahar RJ, Ament ME, et al. Evaluation of the use of botulinium toxin in children with achalasia. J Pediatr Gastroenterol Nutr 2000; 30:509–514.
93. Heller E. Extramukose Kardioplastix beim chronischen Kardiospasmus mit Dilatation Oesophagus. Mitt Grenzgeb Med Chir 1914; 27:141.
94. Ellis FH Jr, Gibb SP. Reoperation after esophagomyotomy for achalasia of the esophagus. Am J Surg 1975; 129:407–412.
95. Agha FP, Keren DF. Barrett's esophagus complicating achalasia after esophagomyotomy. A clinical, radiologic, and pathologic study of 70 patients with achalasia and related motor disorders. J Clin Gastroenterol 1987; 9:232–237.
96. Jara FM, Toledo-Pereyra LH, et al. Long-term results of esophagomyotomy for achalasia of esophagus. Arch Surg 1979; 114:935–936.
97. Buick RG, Spitz L. Achalasia of the cardia in children. Br J Surg 1985; 72:341–343.
98. Vane DW, Cosby K, West K, Grosfeld JL. Late results following esophagomyotomy in children with achalasia. J Pediatr Surg 1988; 23:515–519.
99. Nihoul-Fekete C, Bawab F, Lortat-Jacob S, et al. Achalasia of the esophagus in childhood: surgical treatment in 35 cases with special reference to familial cases and glucocorticoid deficiency association. J Pediatr Surg 1989; 24:1060–1063.
100. Illi OE, Stauffer UG. Achalasia in childhood and adolescence. Eur J Pediatr Surg 1994; 4:214–217.
101. Emblem R, Stringer MD, Hall CM, Spitz L. Current results of surgery for achalasia of the cardia. Arch Dis Child 1993; 68:749–751.
102. Morris-Stiff G, Khan R, Foster ME, Lari J. Long-term results of surgery for childhood achalasia. Ann R Coll Surg Engl 1997; 79:432–434.
103. Chapman JR, Joehl RJ, Murayama KM, et al. Achalasia treatment: improved outcome of laparoscopic myotomy with operative manometry Arch Surg 2004; 139:508–513.
104. Gelfond M, Rozen P, Gilat T. Isosorbide dinitrate and nifedipine treatment of achalasia: a clinical, manometric and radionuclide evaluation. Gastroenterology 1982; 83:963–969.
105. Maksimak M, Perlmutter DH, Winter HS. The use of nifedipine for the treatment of achalasia in children. J Pediatr Gastroenterol Nutr 1986; 5:883–886.
106. Smith H, Buick R, Booth I, et al. The use of nifedipine for the treatment of achalasia in children. J Pediatr Gastroenterol Nutr 1988; 7:146.
107. Richter JE, Dalton CB, Buice RG, Castell DO. Nifedipine: a potent inhibitor of contractions in the body of the human esophagus. Studies in healthy volunteers and patients with the nutcracker esophagus. Gastroenterology 1985; 89:549–554.
108. Thomas E, Lebow RA, Gubler RJ, Bryant LR. Nifedipine for the poor-risk elderly patient with achalasia: objective response demonstrated by solid meal study. South Med J 1984; 77:394–396.
109. Katz PO, Castell JA. Nonachalasia motility disorders. In: Castella DO, Richter JE, eds. The Esophagus, 3rd edn. Philadelphia, PA: Lippincott Williams & Wilkins; 1999:215–234.
110. Dalton CB, Castell DO, Hewson EG, Wu WC, Richter JE. Diffuse esophageal spasm. A rare motility disorder not characterized by high-amplitude contractions. Dig Dis Sci 1991; 36:1025–1028.
111. Clouse RE, Staiano A. Contraction abnormalities of the esophageal body in patients referred to manometry. A new approach to manometric classification. Dig Dis Sci 1983; 28:784–791.
112. Richter JE, Castell DO. Gastroesophageal reflux. Pathogenesis, diagnosis, and therapy. Ann Intern Med 1982; 97:93–103.
113. Patterson DR. Diffuse esophageal spasm in patients with undiagnosed chest pain. J Clin Gastroenterol 1982; 4:415–417.
114. Behar J, Biancani P. Pathogenesis of simultaneous esophageal contractions in patients with motility disorders. Gastroenterology 1993; 105:111–118.
115. Milov DE, Cynamon HA, Andres JM. Chest pain and dysphagia in adolescents caused by diffuse esophageal spasm. J Pediatr Gastroenterol Nutr 1989; 9:450–453.
116. Berezin S, Medow MS, Glassman MS, Newman LJ. Chest pain of gastrointestinal origin. Arch Dis Child 1988; 63:1457–1460.
117. Wyllie E, Wyllie R, Rothner AD, Morris HH. Diffuse esophageal spasm: a cause of paroxysmal posturing and irritability in infants and mentally retarded children. J Pediatr 1989; 115:261–263.
118. Murray JA, Ledlow A, Launspach J, Evans D, Loveday M, Conklin JL. The effects of recombinant human hemoglobin on esophageal motor functions in humans. Gastroenterology 1995; 109:1241–1248.
119. Rhoton AJ et al. The natural history of diffuse esophageal spasm (DES): a long term follow up study. Am J Gastroenterol 1992; 87:A1256.
120. Kramer P, Fleshler B, McNally E, Harris LD. Oesophageal sensitivity to Mecholyl in symptomatic diffuse spasm. Gut 1967; 8:120–127.
121. Vantrappen G, Janssens J, Hellemans J, Coremans G. Achalasia, diffuse esophageal spasm, and related motility disorders. Gastroenterology 1979; 76:450–457.
122. Benjamin SB, Gerhardt DC, Castell DO. High amplitude, peristaltic esophageal contractions associated with chest pain and/or dysphagia. Gastroenterology 1979; 77:478–483.
123. Dalton CB, Castell DO, Richter JE. The changing faces of the nutcracker esophagus. Am J Gastroenterol 1988; 83:623–628.
124. Richter JE, Obrecht WF, Bradley LA, et al. Psychological comparison of patients with nutcracker esophagus and irritable bowel syndrome. Dig Dis Sci 1986; 31:131–138.
125. Richter JE, Barish CF, Castell DO. Abnormal sensory perception in patients with esophageal chest pain. Gastroenterology 1986; 91:845–852.
126. Anggiansah A, Bright NF, McCullagh M, Owen WJ. Transition from nutcracker esophagus to achalasia. Dig Dis Sci 1990; 35:1162–1166.
127. Leite LP, Johnston BT, Barrett J, Castell JA, Castell DO. Ineffective esophageal motility (IEM): the primary finding in patients with nonspecific esophageal motility disorder. Dig Dis Sci 1997; 42:1859–1865.
128. Kahrilas PJ, Dodds WJ, Hogan WJ, Kern M, Arndorfer RC, Reece A. Esophageal peristaltic dysfunction in peptic esophagitis. Gastroenterology 1986; 91:897–904.
129. Hillemeier AC, Grill BB, McCallum R, Gryboski J. Esophageal and gastric motor abnormalities in gastroesophageal reflux during infancy. Gastroenterology 1983; 84:741–746.

130. Cucchiara S, Staiano A, Di Lorenzo C, et al. Esophageal motor abnormalities in children with gastroesophageal reflux and peptic esophagitis. J Pediatr 1986; 108:907–910.
131. Clouse RE, Lustman PJ, Eckert TC, Ferney DM, Griffith LS.Low-dose trazodone for symptomatic patients with esophageal contraction abnormalities. A double-blind, placebo-controlled trial. Gastroenterology 1987; 92:1027–1036.
132. Cannon RO 3rd, Quyyumi AA, Mincemoyer R, et al. Imipramine in patients with chest pain despite normal coronary angiograms. N Engl J Med 1994; 330:1411–1417.
133. Boige N, Faure C, Cargill G, et al. Manometrical evaluation in visceral neuropathies in children. J Pediatr Gastroenterol Nutr 1994; 19:71–77.
134. Faure C, Ategbo S, Ferreira GC, et al. Duodenal and esophageal manometry in total colonic aganglionosis. J Pediatr Gastroenterol Nutr 1994; 18:193–199.
135. Staiano A, Corazziari E, Andreotti MR, Clouse RE. Esophageal motility in children with Hirschsprung's disease. Am J Dis Child 1991; 145:310–313.
136. Flick JA, Boyle JT, Tuchman DN, et al. Esophageal motor abnormalities in children and adolescents with scleroderma and mixed connective tissue disease. Pediatrics 1988; 82:107–111.
137. Tiddens HA, van der Net JJ, de Graeff-Meeder ER, et al. Juvenile-onset mixed connective tissue disease: longitudinal follow-up. J Pediatr 1993; 122:191–197.
138. Weber P, Ganser G, Frosch M, et al. Twenty-four hour intraesophageal pH monitoring in children and adolescents with scleroderma and mixed connective tissue disease. J Rheumatol 2000; 27:2692–2695.
139. Ghoshal UC, Dhar K, Chaudhuri S, et al. Esophageal motility changes after endoscopic intravariceal sclerotherapy with absolute alcohol. Dis Esophagus 2000; 13:148–151.
140. Perisic VN, Scepanovic D, Radlovic N. Nonoperative treatment of achalasia. J Pediatr Gastroenterol Nutr 1996; 22:45–47.
141. Hamza AF, Awad HA, Hussein O. Cardiac achalasia in children. Dilatation or surgery? Eur J Pediatr Surg. 1999; 9:299–302.
142. Upadhyaya M, Fataar S, Sajwany MJ. Achalasia of the cardia: experience with hydrostatic balloon dilatation in children. Pediatr Radiol 2002; 32:409–412.
143. Khan AA, Shah SW, Alam A, et al. Efficacy of Rigiflex balloon dilatation in 12 children with achalasia: a 6-month prospective study showing weight gain and symptomatic improvement. Dis Esophagus 2002; 15:167–170.

Chapter 22
Other diseases of the esophagus

Shehzad A. Saeed and John T. Boyle

ESOPHAGEAL SYMPTOMS

Esophageal symptoms include heartburn, chest pain, dysphagia and odynophagia, with or without associated vomiting or oral regurgitation. The differential diagnosis includes anatomical, infectious and inflammatory disorders. Gastroesophageal reflux disease, eosinophilic esophagitis, structural abnormalities of the esophagus and chest, esophageal foreign body, caustic ingestion and esophageal motility disorders are discussed in other chapters in this volume. This chapter will address esophageal infections, chemotherapy/neutropenia-induced esophagitis, graft-*vs*-host disease, radiation esophagitis, medication-induced esophagitis, esophageal involvement by systemic immune-mediated disorders and esophageal tumors.

ESOPHAGEAL INFECTIONS

Symptomatic esophageal infections are rare in healthy children. The most common infectious etiology in an immunocompetent host is herpes simplex.[1] Rarely, colonization and infection by candida may be a complication of prolonged aggressive acid reduction therapy or chronic broad spectrum antibiotic therapy. Colonization and infection by candida may also complicate chronic disorders that alter esophageal anatomy, disorders that impair esophageal motility, or disorders that disrupt the esophageal mucosal barrier such as injury, radiation, or ulceration.

Most patients who develop infections of the esophagus have impaired immune function, particularly patients infected with human immunodeficiency virus (HIV), bone marrow or solid organ transplant recipients, patients with hematologic malignancies managed with cytotoxic drugs and patients with immunodeficiency disorders that affect cellular immunity and/or granulocyte function.[2,3] Risk factors for esophageal infection also include conditions associated with alteration in cellular immunity including chronic corticosteroids usage (systemic or inhaled), radiation, severe burns and generalized debilitation. Opportunistic esophageal infection by *Candida albicans*, herpes simplex virus and cytomegalovirus (CMV) are most common, although a wide variety of other pathogens have been reported to cause esophageal infection in immunocompromised patients (Table 22.1).

Candida albicans	Mucormycosis
Herpes simplex virus	Varicella-zoster
Cytomegalovirus	Epstein-Barr virus
Miscellaneous Candida species	Papillomavirus
Tuberculosis	Cryptococcus
Miscellaneous bacterial species	Pneumocystis carinii
Aspergillosis	Leishmaniasis
Histoplasmosis	Bacillary angiomatosis
Blastomycosis	Cryptosporidiosis
Human herpes virus 6	Actinomycosis
Enterovirus	Mycobacterium avium

Table 22.1 Pathogens that have been reported to cause esophageal infection

Dysphagia, odynophagia and chest pain are the most common symptoms of all causes of esophageal infection. Clinical presentation in immunocompromised patients may, however, be deceptive. Anorexia, nausea, heartburn, fever, or bleeding may be the predominant clinical presentation in immunocompromised children. Endoscopy with brushings and biopsy is the gold standard for diagnosis of esophageal infection. Radiographic studies lack sensitivity to pick up early esophageal involvement and are of limited value in establishing an etiologic diagnosis of esophageal infection. An esophageal contrast study is most useful to exclude mechanical obstruction and to evaluate for the presence of perforation or fistula which may complicate esophageal infection.

Candida esophagitis

The most common infection of the esophagus is caused by *Candida albicans*, a yeast found in normal oral flora. Colonization entails superficial adherence and proliferation of *Candida* on the esophageal mucosa. Defenses against colonization include normal salivation, esophageal motility, a healthy esophageal epithelia and a balance between oral bacterial and fungal flora. Infection results when Candida invades into esophageal epithelial cell layer, a process that usually requires defective mucosal immunity.[4] Candida esophagitis is an opportunistic infection that complicates disorders associated with granulocyte and /or lymphocyte numbers and dysfunction. Recent antibiotic exposure in such patients is a prominent risk factor. In a large pediatric study of HIV positive patients, low CD4 counts and antibiotic exposure were the most prominent risk factors for development of esophageal *Candidiasis*.[5] Fungal virulence factors have also been implicated in the pathogenesis of infection including ability of the specific species to colonize and adhere to esophageal mucosa by undergoing morphogenesis to hyphal form or ability to express proteinases to lyse host cell membranes.

Oral thrush, a frequent finding among patients with esophageal infection, is often an indicator of an underlying pathologic esophageal process. In a large pediatric

obtained from the margins of ulcers are more likely to show characteristic changes including multinucleated giant cells, cellular 'ballooning' and the presence of eosinophilic intranuclear inclusions. Immunohistochemical stains for debris obtained from brushing ulcers may be useful in identifying sloughed infected HSV infected cells. Culture of HSV from esophageal biopsies is considered diagnostic and has been reported to have a higher yield than histologic techniques.

Decision to treat HSV esophagitis in immunocompetent patients is determined by the severity of the disease. HSV in healthy individuals tends to be self-limiting and most require only supportive care. Resolution of symptoms may be gradual and take up to 2 weeks. The drug of choice for treatment in immunocompromised hosts is acyclovir[11] (oral, 80 mg/kg per day, up to 1000 mg/day in 3–5 doses for 7–14 days; i.v., 15–30 mg/kg per day in three divided doses for 7–14 days). Decision to use parenteral therapy is based on ability to take oral medication and severity of disease. Relapse may occur in immunocompromised patients, being reported in up to 15% of HIV-infected individuals. Such patients may require prolonged suppressive therapy. Acyclovir-resistant HSV infections have been described, especially in immunocompromised patients maintained on long term therapy. Acyclovir-resistant mutant strains of HSV are usually susceptible to other systemic antivirals including foscarnet[12] (i.v. 80–120 mg/kg per day in 2–3 divided doses).

As with Candida, strategies for prevention of HSV infection have been incorporated into treatment protocols for patients with HSV positive antibody status undergoing intensive immunosuppression regimens prior to bone marrow or solid organ transplant. Many of these regimens have started to use ganciclovir, which is effective against both HSV and CMV.

CMV esophagitis

Unlike HSV esophagitis, which is found in a wide range of immunocompromised and healthy patients, CMV esophagitis tends to be a complication of advanced HIV disease or iatrogenic immunosuppression in bone marrow and solid organ transplant recipients. Esophageal disease can occur as a primary infection or from reactivation of latent infection. Esophageal infection occurs in the setting of systemic viral dissemination. Thus, symptoms of fever, nausea, epigastric pain, diarrhea and weight loss may be seen.

The gold standard for diagnosis is upper endoscopy. The gross endoscopic appearance of HSV is nonspecific. Shallow or deep ulcers against a background of normal mucosa are usually located in the mid-to-distal esophagus. Large ulcers greater than 1 cm in size suggest CMV. Because CMV-infected fibroblasts and endothelial cells are found in the base of esophageal ulcers and never in squamous epithelium, multiple biopsies should be taken from the center of the ulcer crater. Characteristic histologic features of CMV infection include large cells with amphophilic intranuclear inclusions, halo surrounding the nucleus and multiple small cytoplasmic inclusions (Fig. 22.3). A biopsy of the ulcer base should also be obtained, although culture positive for CMV alone is poorly predictive of esophageal infection in that CMV viremia and viral shedding are common in the absence of clinical disease.

Both intravenous ganciclovir and foscarnet appear to be very effective as initial therapy for CMV esophagitis. The dose of ganciclovir is 5 mg/kg per dose i.v. q12 h for 2–3 weeks with dosage adjustments for renal insufficiency. The primary toxicity of ganciclovir is marrow suppression, particularly neutropenia. This was an almost universal complication in HIV patients simultaneously receiving zidovudine requiring the addition of granulocyte colony stimulating factors. Recently, the wider choice of antiretroviral agents has reduced the need to maintain patients on zidovudine while being treated with ganciclovir. Other toxicities of ganciclovir include rash, nausea, vomiting, hepatotoxicity and central nervous system toxicities. In patients who fail to respond to ganciclovir, the option is to switch to foscarnet (60 mg/kg per dose i.v. q8 h for 2–3 weeks), or to add foscarnet to ongoing ganciclovir therapy. The primary toxicity of foscarnet is nephrotoxicity. In several adult studies, only 50% of patients with gastrointestinal disease who respond to the initial course of therapy have relapse of symptoms.[13] All patients who do relapse should receive long-term maintenance therapy (ganciclovir, 5 mg/kg i.v. once daily) after acute treatment of their relapse.

All pediatric patients with HIV or candidates for bone marrow or solid organ transplant should be tested for prior exposure to CMV. In seronegative patients, every effort should be made to limit exposure to CMV-infected body fluids and blood products. A prophylaxis regimen, employing either acyclovir or ganciclovir, is now commonly used to treat transplant recipients who are either CMV seropositive to prevent disease reactivation, or are seronegative

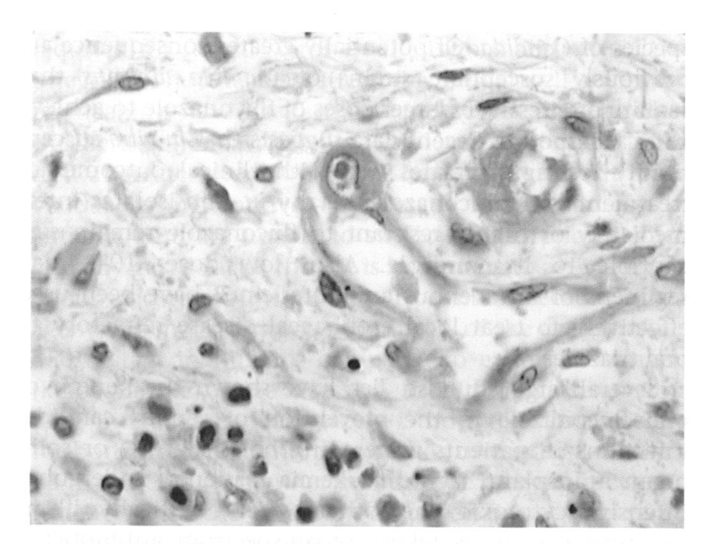

Figure 22.3: CMV esophagitis. This virus typically is characterized by a prominent eosinophilic intranuclear inclusion and displays vascular tropism (H&E, ×330). (Courtesy David R. Kelly, MD, Children's Hospital of Alabama and University of Alabama) (*See plate section for color*).

and receiving an organ from a CMV seropositive donor. Routine primary prophylaxis is currently not recommended for HIV patients. Oral ganciclovir has been shown to be of benefit in decreasing the incidence of CMV infection in this population; but, the cost is high and no effect on overall mortality has been demonstrated.

Other esophageal pathogens

All additional esophageal pathogens listed in Table 22.1 are unusual and would need to be diagnosed specifically by culture, histopathological findings, or serology. Bacterial esophagitis is a possibility in severely immunocompromised neutropenic patients. Most reported infections are due to gram positive pathogens. Endoscopic findings include diffuse esophageal inflammation, pseudomembranes and ulcers. Histopathologic findings include evidence of deep bacterial invasion of mucosal layers without evidence of other pathogens. Culture of esophageal biopsies may or may not be specific, but at least guides therapy.

The esophagus is the gastrointestinal organ least likely to be infected by tuberculosis. Histoplasmosis and blastomycosis should be suspected in immunocompromised patients in areas where these organisms are endemic. Because itraconazole has increased activity against histoplasmosis and filamentous fungi including Aspergillus, this triazole should be considered for treatment of suspected superinfection with multiple opportunistic organisms.

Other inflammatory causes of 'esophageal symptoms'

HIV associated esophageal ulcers

Patients with advanced HIV may develop single or multiple large ulcers in the mid to distal esophagus without evidence of specific infection. Onset is generally subacute. Patients may have coincident oropharyngeal aphthous ulceration. Patients generally have severe odynophagia and dysphagia. In the absence of a specific etiology, treatment is empiric. Some patients respond to high dose systemic corticosteroids, sucralfate and aggressive treatment of the underlying HIV infection.

Non-infectious post-chemotherapy esophagitis

Leukopenic cancer patients or patients being conditioned for bone marrow transplant, especially those with hematologic malignancies, receiving intensive chemotherapy may develop fever, oropharyngeal mucositis or ulcers, odynophagia, dysphagia and retrosternal chest pain. These symptoms often prevent adequate oral intake. The major differential diagnosis is candida esophagitis *vs* chemotherapy induced esophagitis.[14] The latter requires neutropenia and may represent a combination of immunosuppression and chemotherapy-induced cytotoxic mucosal injury or inhibition of mucosal cellular regeneration. Recovery from this severe complication is dependent on restoration of the leukocyte population. At endoscopy the esophageal mucosa is friable, appear desquamated, or contain multiple mucosal ulcerations, raised white plaques, or thick confluent velvety whitish plaques. The appearance may be indistinguishable from that of candida esophagitis. Because at least 50% of patients will have evidence of candida in brushings or mucosal biopsies, strategies for the management of this clinical scenario have not been subjected to the same rigorous analysis as in patients with HIV disease. Fearing the high risk of systemic dissemination of mucosal infection, most pediatric oncologists will forego endoscopic diagnosis and treat patients with this syndrome with broad spectrum antibiotics and aggressive intravenous antifungal therapy.

Graft *vs* host disease

The sudden onset of anorexia, dyspepsia, heartburn, nausea and vomiting may be the earliest manifestation of acute graft *vs* host disease (GVHD). Onset is usually 3–4 weeks after transplantation when the mucositis of conditioning chemotherapy have typically resolved. Gross esophageal involvement is rare, though biopsies of the esophageal mucosa may show characteristic intraepithelial cells with apoptotic keratinocytes diagnostic of GVHD. Diagnosis is more consistently achieved by biopsy of the gastric antrum, which is typically edematous and erythematous. Biopsy of this minimally abnormal mucosa may show the characteristic histologic findings of apoptosis of crypt epithelial cells, crypt dropout and patchy lymphocytic infiltrates diagnostic of acute GVHD. Initial therapy for most patients consists of high dose steroids with bowel rest.

A total of 25 to 40% of long-term survivors of bone marrow transplantation may develop chronic GVHD 3–12 months after engraftment.[15] Some 10% of these may manifest esophageal disease as dysphagia, odynophagia and chest or retrosternal pain.[16] Radiology may reveal webs, ulcers and strictures. Esophagogastroduodenoscopy reveals desquamation, vesicobullous lesions,[17] esophagitis, or normal appearing mucosa. The procedure carries higher than normal risk of bleeding and perforation. The treatment of chronic GVHD is usually with prednisone and immunosuppression with imuran, ciclosporin and tacrolimus.

Medication-induced esophagitis

Drug-induced esophagitis is an under diagnosed entity. The commonest drugs implicated in drug-induced esophagitis are doxycycline, tetracycline, slow-release potassium chloride, quinidine, alendronate and non-steroidal anti-inflammatory agents. Isolated reports have also implicated ferrous sulfate, clindamycin, rifampin, cromolyn sodium, oral theophylline, captopril and ascorbic acid. Although patients with structural abnormalities and motility disorders of the esophagus are most at risk, drug-induced injury can develop in a normal esophagus. Symptoms are usually acute and follow immediately after ingestion of medication to several hours later. Most patients present with heartburn, odynophagia and dysphagia, although hematemesis and melena have been reported from drug-induced esophageal damage. Single contrast X-rays will show changes only in severe cases

SECTION FOUR
THE STOMACH

Chapter 23

Developmental anatomy and physiology of the stomach

Steven J. Czinn, Samra S. Blanchard and Sundeep Arora

INTRODUCTION

The gastrointestinal tract begins as a primitive tubular system and is one of the first organs to polarize the embryo by forming an entry and exit with an anterior and posterior axis, also known as the craniocaudal axis, extending from the mouth to the cloaca (Fig. 23.1). The non-neural elements of the gut are derived from endodermal and mesodermal cells. Bilateral folding of these layers forms the intestinal lumen, which is surrounded by concentric endodermal and splanchnic epithelia, creating a tubular gut. Cells from the outer epithelium migrate outward and form a loose mesenchyme, which later forms the muscle and connective tissue, while neural elements migrate from the neural crest at vagal and sacral levels to form the enteric nervous system.

The tubular gut has three distinct sections: the foregut, midgut and hindgut. One of the first gross morphologic distinctions is the rotation and distention of the posterior foregut to begin differentiating the stomach just distal to esophagus. The stomach is also separated from the esophagus by the newly formed diaphragm from the developing abdominal cavity. At the end of the fourth and beginning of the fifth week, the stomach can be recognized as a fusiform dilation, which is initially oriented in the median plane. This primordial stomach soon enlarges and broadens ventrodorsally. During the next 2 weeks, the dorsal border of the primordial stomach grows faster than its ventral border (lesser curvature), demarcating the greater curvature of the stomach. As the stomach enlarges, it slowly rotates 90° in clockwise direction around its longitudinal axis.[1] The ventral border moves to the right, and the dorsal border (greater curvature) moves to the left, changing the position of stomach. The original left side moves to the ventral surface, and right side moves to the dorsal surface. During rotation and growth of the stomach, the cranial region moves to the left and slightly inferiorly, and its caudal region moves to the right and superiorly. After rotation, the stomach assumes its final position in the upper abdomen, with its long axis almost transverse to the long axis of the body. The rotation and growth of the stomach explains why the left vagus nerve supplies the anterior wall of the adult stomach and the right vagus nerve innervates the posterior wall of the stomach.[2]

Arterial blood supply to the distal esophagus, stomach and proximal duodenum is derived from the branches of celiac axis. The stomach is drained by the left gastric vein, right gastric vein, right and left gastroepiploic veins, and short gastric veins. These veins have no valves and can provide collateral blood flow when any portion of the portal system is obstructed. Esophageal and gastric varices usually involve the left gastric and short gastric veins.

The lymphatic drainage from the stomach enters the thoracic duct via the celiac nodes. Ultimately, the lymphatic drainage enters the venous system in the neck at the junction of the left internal jugular and left subclavian vein. Because of this anatomic relationship, gastric malignancies in adults may present with left supraclavicular lymph node metastasis.

Vagal and sympathetic fibers innervate the entire stomach by about 9 weeks of gestation.[3] Two major networks of nerve fibers are intrinsic to the gastrointestinal tract: the myenteric plexus (Auerbach's plexus), which can be found between the outer longitudinal and middle circular layers of muscle, and the submucus plexus (Meissner's plexus), located between the middle circular muscular layer and the mucosa. Collectively, these neurons constitute the enteric nervous system. Catecholamines have been demonstrated in sympathetic fibers in Auerbach's plexus by week 10 and in Meissner's plexus by week 13.[4]

HISTOLOGY

Development of fetal human gastric mucosa occurs very early during fetal life. The first pit/gland structures are observed at 11–12 weeks of gestation. Between 11 and 17 weeks, the stratified surface epithelium is replaced by a simple mucous columnar epithelium, and gastric glands develop further. At this stage, the progenitor zone of the pit/gland structure is already localized in the isthmus,[5] as in adult mucosa.[1,6]

The gastric mucosa is organized in vertical tubular units consisting of an apical pit region, an isthmus and the actual gland region that forms the lower part of the vertical unit. The progenitor cell of the gastric unit gives rise to all epithelial cells. The mucus-producing pit cells migrate up toward the gastric lumen, and acid-secreting parietal cells (oxyntic; *oxys* is Greek for acid) migrate downward to the middle and lower regions of the gland. Chief (zymogenic) cells secrete pepsinogen and predominate at the base of glands. Neuroendocrine cells, including enterochromaffin cells (serotonin), enterochromaffin-like cells (histamine) and D cells (somatostatin), are also present at the base of the gland.

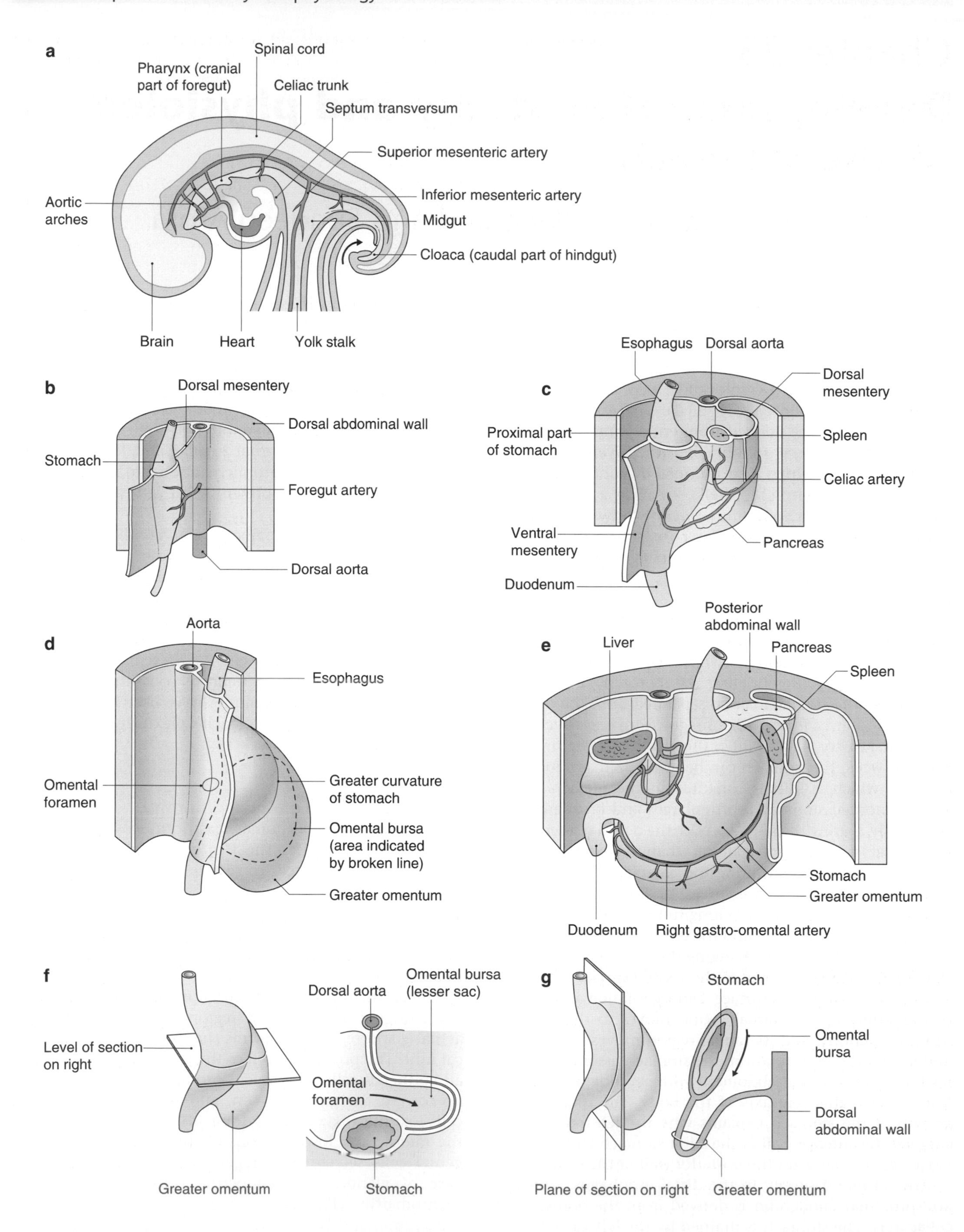

Figure 23.1: Development and rotation of the stomach and formation of the omental bursa (i.e. the lesser sac) and greater omentum. (**a**) 28 days. (**b**) Anterior lateral view at 28 days. (**c**) 35 days. (**d**) 40 days. (**e**) 48 days. (**f**) Lateral view at 52 days with a transverse section of the omental foramen and omental bursa. (**g**) Sagittal section of the omental bursa and greater omentum. (Adapted from Moore and Persaud, 1998, with permission).[45]

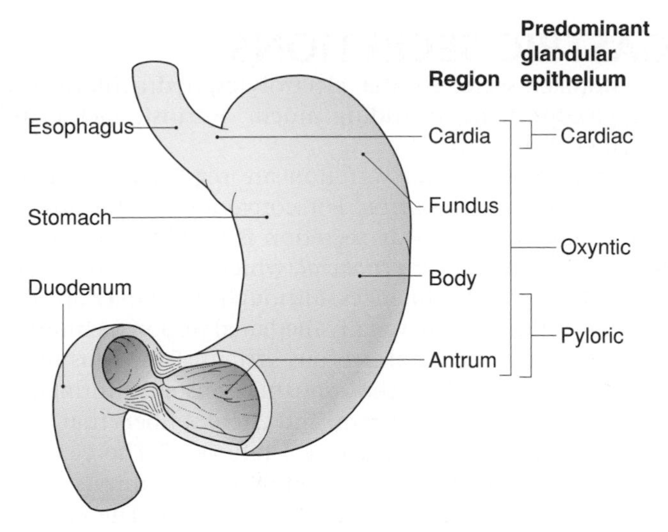

Figure 23.2: Anatomy of the stomach.

The glands of the different anatomic parts of stomach are lined with different types of cell (Fig. 23.2). The cardiac glands are mostly populated by mucus-secreting or endocrine cells. The cardiac pits are irregular and shallow; the ratio of the length of pits:glands is approximately 1:1. In the body of the stomach, including the fundus, the glands are long and deep with straight pits. The ratio of the length of pits:glands is approximately 1:4. The gastric gland has parietal (oxyntic) cells that secrete hydrochloric acid and intrinsic factor, chief (zymogen, peptic) cells that secrete pepsinogens, endocrine and mucous neck cells. The antrum and pylorus contain the pyloric glands, composed of mainly mucus, endocrine and G cells. There are very few parietal or chief cells. The glands here are characterized by deep pits but short glands, with a pit:gland ratio close to 1:1. Mucus is also secreted along with bicarbonate ($HCO3^-$) by the surface mucous cells between glands. Surface mucous cells secrete neutral mucus, rather than the sulfated mucus secreted by mucous neck cells, which reside in close proximity to parietal cells. The surface mucous cells are cytoprotective, whereas the mucous neck cell functions as a stem cell precursor for surface mucous, parietal, chief and endocrine cells.

NEUROMUSCULAR FUNCTIONS

Gastric motility is controlled centrally as well as by local neurohormonal control of the muscle layers, which include outer longitudinal, middle circular and inner oblique fibers. Neuronal control involves the intrinsic myenteric plexus, the extrinsic postganglionic sympathetic fibers of the celiac plexus, and the preganglionic parasympathetic fibers of the vagus nerve. The vagal afferents are both relaxatory and excitatory.

Functionally the stomach can be divided into two parts: the proximal stomach and the antrum. The proximal stomach, consisting of the cardia, fundus and a portion of the body, is responsible for the storage of food and is capable of accommodating a large volume of nutrients with receptive relaxation and no dramatic rise in intragastric pressure.[5] Di Lorenzo et al,[7] demonstrated that the receptive relaxation of the proximal stomach is negligible in infants; this might explain in part the increased incidence of reflux in newborns.

The rate at which the stomach empties into the duodenum also depends on the type and components of food ingested. Liquids and solids have different mechanisms of emptying. An increased tonic intraluminal pressure in the fundus is necessary for the emptying of liquids. Liquid emptying has an exponential pattern of emptying that is dependent on the volume ingested as well as the osmolarity of the liquid. This is determined largely by the pressure differences between the stomach and duodenum, and is modulated by receptors in the duodenum that slow gastric emptying when the caloric density or volume load reaching the duodenum is excessive.[8]

Solid food emptying has an initial lag phase followed by a linear phase. The distal stomach, which consists of the antrum and pylorus, is responsible for grinding and emptying solid food. Gastric peristaltic waves originating in the body of the stomach propagate toward the pylorus. The antral contractions allow only the small particles and liquids to pass into the duodenum, and drive the larger particles (greater than 0.2 mm) back into the body of the stomach by retrograde propulsion. Food rich in carbohydrate leaves the stomach within a few hours. However, protein-rich food leaves more slowly, and emptying is slowest after a meal containing a significant amount of fat.[9] Finally, the rate of emptying also depends on antral distention (gastrogastric reflex), concentration of lipid, protein and acid in the duodenum (duodenogastric reflex), and colonic distention (cologastric reflex).[10,11]

As a result of ingesting a meal, gastric distention stimulates 'gastric mechanoreceptors'; hyperosmolality of the duodenal contents sensed by 'duodenal osmoreceptors' initiate both enterogastric neural reflexes. Cholecystokinin (CCK) is released in response to this reflux and binds to CCK_a receptors on gastric afferents, producing inhibition of the excitatory vagal efferents to the fundus. The primary inhibitory neurotransmitter is nitric oxide, which controls transpyloric flow, antral motility and pyloric contraction. Serotonin is also involved in the inhibitory pathway. Appropriate propagation of gastric contractions or antroduodenal coordination is of great importance to the emptying of the stomach. Gastric motility is regulated by gastric myoelectric activity, and consists of gastric slow waves and spike or second potentials. The gastric slow wave determines the propagation and maximum frequency of gastric contractions. It is generated in an area of the greater curvature that has the fastest rate of inherent rhythmicity and acts as a pacemaker controlling the rate and direction of propagation of gastric electrical activity. The normal frequency of gastric slow waves is 3 cycles per minute (cpm) in healthy humans. Abnormalities in the frequency of the gastric slow waves have been reported in a number of clinical settings, associated with gastric motor disorders and gastrointestinal symptoms. Gastric slow-wave activity can be measured non-invasively using the technique of electrogastrography (EGG).[12–14] Gastric motor activity initially appears between the gestational ages of 14 and 24 weeks.[15] EGG patterns at 35 weeks' gestation are similar to that of a full-term infant.[16] EGG patterns continue to mature over the first 6–24 months, reaching a stable pattern.[17]

A characteristic feature of fasting motor activity in the older child is the migrating motor complex (MMC), a highly organized propagated sequence of contractions that migrates from the stomach into the intestine and towards the ileum every 90–120 min. Three distinctive phases appear in sequence. Phase 1 is a pattern of quiescence that always follows phase 3. Phase 2 is a period of irregular contractions, varying in amplitude and periodicity. Because of this variation, some contractions are not propagated. Phase 3 is a distinctive pattern of regular high-amplitude contractions repeating at a maximal rate for 3–10 min and migrating from proximal to distal. The MMC begins in anywhere from the esophagus to the ileum. About half of these contractions begin in the esophagus or the gastric body and migrate downwards. Motilin is responsible for initiating phase 3 contractions that begin in the stomach. Gastric MMCs are present in newborns and pre-term infants older than 32 weeks' gestational age. In younger pre-term infants, only uncoordinated, non-migrating contractions are present. The clinical implications of non-migrating phase 3 contractions in very pre-term infants are unknown. Theoretically, non-migrating phase 3 contractions should not cause feeding intolerance, because liquid gastric emptying is related to the function of fundus and not to antral peristalsis.

GASTRIC SECRETIONS

The stomach secretes water, electrolytes, hydrochloric acid and glycoproteins, including mucin, intrinsic factor and enzymes (Fig. 23.3).

Gastric motility and secretion are regulated by neural and humoral mechanisms. For convenience, the physiologic regulation of gastric secretion is usually discussed as being either *cephalic* or *peripheral*, which includes both gastric and intestinal influences, although these overlap. The cephalic influences are vagally mediated responses induced by activity in the central nervous system. The vagus nerve contains afferent fibers that transmit sensory information from the gut to the brainstem, and efferent fibers that form the motor limb of the vagovagal reflexes.[18] The cephalic phase of acid secretion is induced by sensory inputs of the thought, smell, sight and taste of the food. The efferent fibers for this reflex are in the vagus nerves. Cephalic influences are responsible for one-third to one-half of the acid secreted in response to a normal meal, and are abolished by vagatomy. Vagal stimulation increases gastrin secretion by release of gastrin-releasing peptide (GRP), or bombesin. Other vagal fibers release acetylcholine, which acts directly on the cells in the glands in the body and the fundus of the stomach. Acetylcholine binds to M_3 muscarinic receptors on the parietal cell and stimulates gastric acid secretion via calcium and phosphoinositol pathways.

The peripheral mechanisms include gastric influences, consisting of local reflex responses to gastrin, and intestinal influences, reflex and hormonal feedback effects on gastric secretion initiated from the mucosa of the small

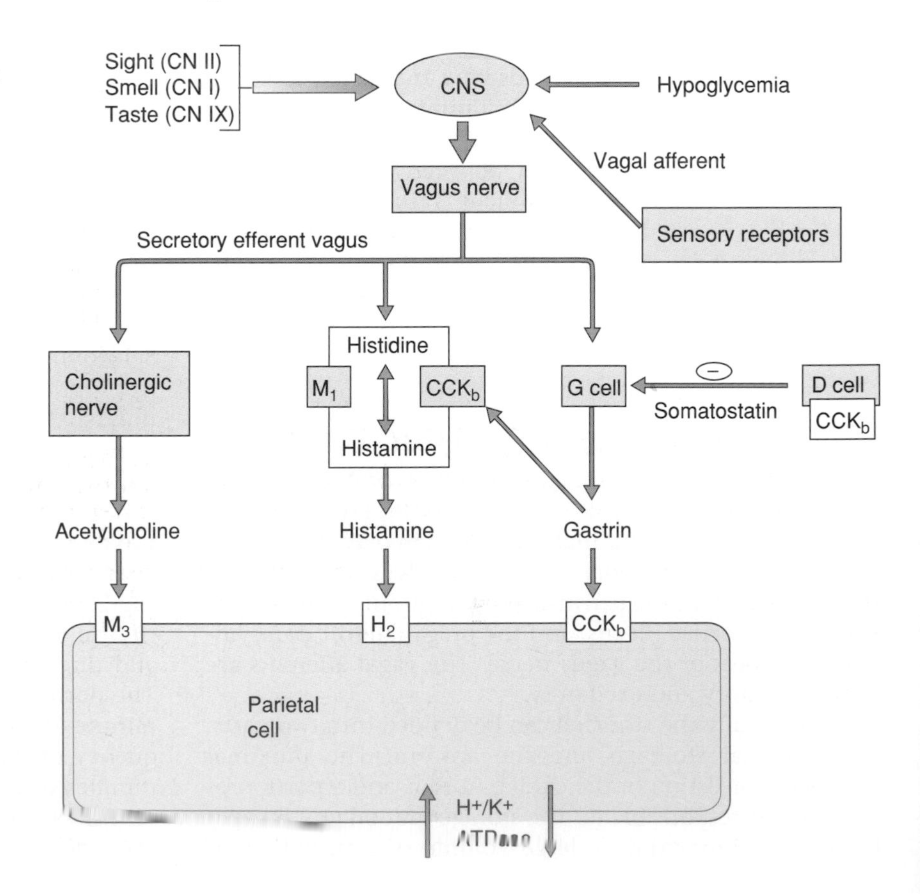

Figure 23.3: Secretory influences and hormones involved in the synthesis and secretion of hydrochloric acid by parietal cells. CCK, cholecystokinin; CNS, central nervous system.

intestine. Finally, the stomach also contains exocrine epithelial cells and endocrine-like neural regulatory cells.

GASTRIC ACID SECRETION

Hydrochloric acid secretion

Golgi first proposed that the parietal cell was the source of gastric acid and that it was formed within the surface invaginations, which he termed secretory canaliculi.[19] The ultrastructure of the parietal cell has numerous large mitochondria to provide adenosine triphosphate (ATP) for acid secretion. The H^+,K^+-ATPase (gastric acid pump, or proton pump) is a membrane-embedded protein identified and isolated in the 1970s. Parietal cells express receptors for acetylcholine, gastrin and histamine (Fig. 23.4). The binding of these ligands to receptors on the surface of the parietal cell starts changes in second messengers that regulate the movement and location of the gastric proton pump. The H^+,K^+-ATPase exchanges protons for potassium and is responsible for gastric luminal acidification. In the resting state, the enzyme is stored in the cytoplasmic tubulovesicles. When the parietal cells are stimulated, the tubulovesicular structures fuse with the apical membrane to form secretory canaliculus, and the proton pumps start actively pumping H^+ ions in exchange for K^+. Pumping H^+ out of the parietal cells in exchange for K^+ requires appreciable energy, and this is provided by hydrolysis of ATP. Cl^- is also extruded down its electrochemical gradient through channels that are activated by cyclic adenosine monophosphate (cAMP) in the apical membrane. Ultimately, acid is generated from the dissociation of two molecules of water to form H_3O^+ and OH^-. The H_3O^+ is secreted via the proton pump in exchange for K^+, while the corresponding OH^- combines in the cell with carbon dioxide to form HCO_3^-. This reaction is catalyzed by carbonic anyhydrase, and the parietal cells are particularly rich in this enzyme. The formed HCO_3^- is extruded by a conductance pathway on the basolateral membrane in exchange for Cl^- ions.

The H^+,K^+-ATPase is a hetrodimer composed of two noncovalently linked subunits, α and β. The α subunit contains the catalytic site of the enzyme, which is important for functioning of the H^+,K^+-ATPase. It contains the cysteine residues where proton pump inhibitors bind. The β subunit appears to play a role in formation of tubulovesicle membranes and the transfer of enzyme to the apical membrane, and may protect the enzyme from degradation.

Stimulants of gastric acid secretion

Gastrin

Gastrin, produced by the antral G cell, is the most potent endogenous stimulant of gastric acid secretion during ingestion of a meal. The major stimulant of G cells in pyloric and duodenal glands are luminal amino acids derived from peptic hydrolysis of dietary proteins. Gastrin stimulates the parietal cells directly, acting via CCK_b receptors, and indirectly by stimulating enterochromaffin-like cells to secrete histamine. Histamine induces acid secretion by activating parietal cell H_2 receptors. The action of gastrin is mediated by an increase in intracellular calcium concentration compared with that of histamine, which is mediated by an increase in both calcium and cAMP levels.

As well as stimulating gastric acid secretion, gastrin has trophic effects on gastric oxyntic mucosa.[20] Gastrin stimulates the migration of gastric epithelial cells directly and indirectly via multiple pathways that include the release of fibroblast growth factor, activation of the epidermal growth factor receptor, and activation of the mitogen-activated protein kinase pathway.

Gastrin is also found in the pancreatic islets in fetal life. This may explain why gastrin-secreting tumors, called gas-

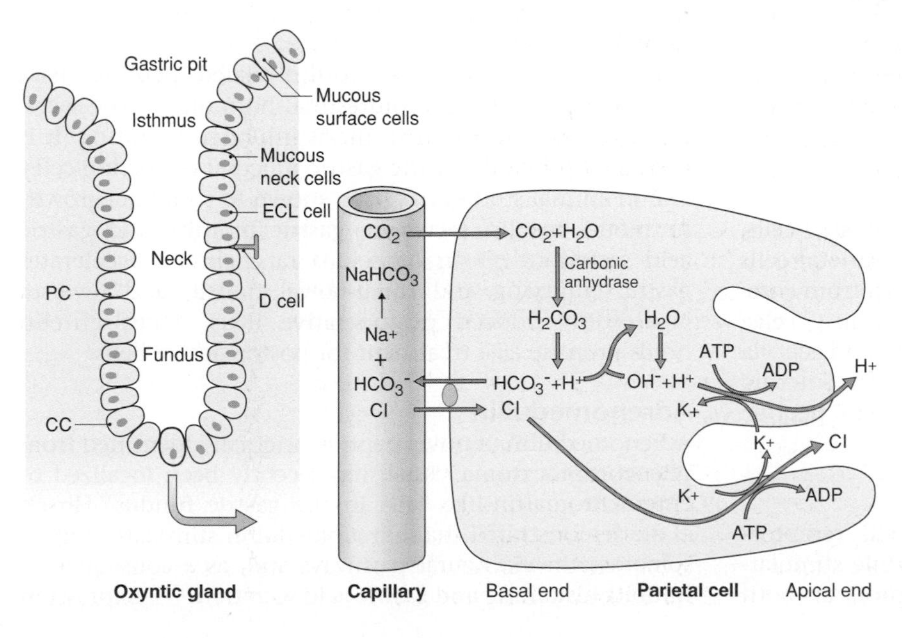

Figure 23.4: Steps involved in the secretion of hydrochloric acid into the gastric lumen. CC, chief cells; D cell, somatostatin-containing D cells; ECL, enterochromaffin-like cells; PC, parietal cell.

trinomas, occur in the pancreas. It is uncertain whether any gastrin is present in the pancreas of normal adults.

Histamine

Histamine is stored primarily in the enterochromaffin-like cells that reside in the basal half of the oxyntic gland.[21] It is formed by the decarboxylation of histidine by histidine decarboxylase. Histamine receptors have been classified into four major subclasses: H_1, H_2, H_3 and, most recently, H_4.[22] Histamine, released from enterochromaffin-like cells, stimulates acid secretion primarily by interacting with H_2 receptors on parietal cells. H_3 receptor agonists have been reported to stimulate acid secretion *in vitro* and to inhibit acid secretion *in vivo*. The former is caused by inhibition of gastric somatostatin secretion, whereas the latter is more than likely caused by the central effects of these agents.[22–24] Gastrin, aspirin, indometacin, dexamethasone, interleukin 1 and tumor necrosis factor stimulate histidine decarboxylase activity. Antisecretory agents also stimulate histidine decarboxylase as a result of hypochlorhydria-induced gastrin secretion.

Acetylcholine

Acetylcholine is released from postganglionic nerves in Meissner's plexus and binds to muscarinic M_3-type receptors. Acetylcholine also stimulates the release of histamine from the enterochromaffin-like cells binding M_1 receptors. Activation of M_3 receptors on the parietal cell leads to an increase in intracellular calcium levels. Calcium and cAMP then activate a set of protein kinases, stimulating activation of the proton pump.

Other stimulating factors

Hypoglycemia acts via the brain and vagal efferents to stimulate acid and pepsin secretion. Other stimulants include alcohol and caffeine, both of which act directly on the mucosa.

Inhibitors of gastric acid secretion

Gastric acid secretion is also regulated by inhibitory mechanisms that are triggered by the stimulation of certain peptides as a result of the presence of nutrients in the intestine.

Somatostatin

In the stomach, somatostatin, which is present in D cells, inhibits acid secretion directly by acting on parietal cells and indirectly by inhibiting histamine secretion from enterochromaffin-like cells and gastrin secretion from G cells. Most of the somatostatin in the stomach is S14 and acts via a paracrine mechanism, whereas the somatostatin entering the circulation after a meal is mostly the S28 peptide derived from the small intestine.

Cholecystokinin

CCK inhibits acid secretion by binding to CCK_a receptors on the gastric mucosal somatostatin cells, while stimulating acid secretion by binding to CCK_b receptors on both parietal and enterochromaffin-like cells. Inhibitory function is more dominant.[18]

Prostaglandins

Prostaglandin E_2 protects the gastric mucosa and inhibits acid secretion. The physiologic effects of prostaglandin E_2 on the gut are mediated by activation of four receptor subtypes that are expressed in parietal cells and one receptor on gastric mucous cells.

Secretin

Secretin-containing cells are located mainly in the upper small intestine. Secretin is released into the circulation from duodenal cells in response to gastric acid delivered into the lumen of the duodenum. In addition, bile salts and digested products of fat and protein can stimulate secretin release.

Physiologic actions of secretin include stimulation of pancreatic exocrine secretion of water and bicarbonate, and inhibition of gastric acid secretion.

Structurally, secretin has sequence homology with other regulatory peptides that inhibit gastric acid, such as gastric inhibitory peptide (GIP), vasointestinal peptide (VIP), pituitary adenylate cyclase-activating polypeptide (PACAP) and glucagon-like peptide (GLP) 1 and 2.

OTHER HORMONES AND PEPTIDES

Leptin

Leptin is a hormone produced mainly by the adipose tissue and plays a role in regulation of energy balance. Leptin has been detected in the fundic glands, both in the pepsinogen granules of chief cells and in the inhibitory peptide granules of endocrine-type cells. It is sensitive to the nutritional state and is rapidly mobilized in response to food ingestion following a fast, and may play a role in the regulation of short-term satiety.[25,26]

Ghrelin

Ghrelin, also known as motilin-related peptide, is a recently discovered gastrointestinal hormone whose secretion increases with fasting and is inhibited by eating. It is expressed primarily in the gastric mucosal endocrine cells, and in animal studies has been shown to stimulate growth hormone, insulin secretion, gastric motility and gastric acid secretion.[27–30] In conscious rats, ghrelin accelerates gastric emptying and small-bowel transit, and reverses laparotomy-induced postoperative ileus. Thus, ghrelin holds promise as a treatment for postoperative ileus.

Adrenomedullin

Adrenomedullin, a novel peptide originally identified from pheochromocytoma tissue, has recently been localized to enterochromaffin-like cells in the gastric fundus. Hirsch et al. demonstrated that adrenomedullin stimulates fundic somatostatin via neural pathways and, as a consequence, inhibits histamine and gastric acid secretion.[31,32] Expression of adrenomullin has also been reported as increased after mucosal injury, suggesting that it can promote epithelial restitution and support mucosal defense.[33,34]

PEPSINOGEN

Pepsinogen is a powerful and abundant protein digestive enzyme secreted by the gastric chief cells as a proenzyme and then converted by gastric acid in the gastric lumen to the active enzyme pepsin. The role of pepsin and its precursor in protein digestion was first described in the nineteenth century. Pepsinogens consist of a single polypeptide chain with a molecular weight of approximately 42 000 Da. Pepsinogens are synthesized and secreted primarily by the gastric chief cells of the human stomach before being converted into the proteolytic enzyme pepsin, which is crucial for digestive processes in the stomach. Furthermore, pepsin can activate additional pepsinogen autocatalytically. Pepsinogens belong to the endopeptidase family of aspartic proteinases. The aspartic proteinases are also called acid proteinases because they act between pH 1.5 and 5.0. The mucosal lining of human gastric mucosa produces four types of pepsinogen: pepsinogen I (PGA or PGI), pepsinogen II (PGC or PGII), cathepsin E and cathepsin D. It has been reported that the moment of the first appearance of measurable pepsinogen in the fetal stomach varies considerably between species. In the human fetus, granules appear in the peptic cells at week 32–36. Cephalic vagal stimulation strongly stimulates pepsinogen secretion. Anticholinergics, histamine H_2-receptor antagonists and vagotomy decrease pepsinogen secretion. Raised serum levels of type 1 pepsinogen have been associated with duodenal ulcer and gastrinoma, whereas atrophic gastritis (with or without pernicious anemia) has been associated with low levels of type 1 pepsinogen.

MUCUS AND BICARBONATE SECRETION

Mucus is a highly hydrated gel that consists of 95% water, 5% mucin glycoprotein and minor components such as electrolytes. Mucins are high-molecular-weight glycoproteins with 80% carbohydrate content; the remaining 20% is constituted by protein core. Mucin is the most important structural component of the mucus gel layer.

The integrity of gastric mucosa is maintained by multiple mechanisms. The mucus barrier forms a continuous gel into which a bicarbonate-rich fluid is secreted, forming a protective pH gradient. Gastric acid is secreted in a pulsatile manner through the mucus gel, allowing the formation of short-lived channels within the mucus gel that rapidly close to prevent the back-diffusion of luminal acid. This mechanism maintains the pH at the mucosa near neutrality, despite the low luminal pH.[35] The hydrophobicity of mucus is important for protection of gastric mucosa by preventing back-diffusion of hydrogen ions. Phospholipids secreted into mucus by gastric mucous cells also contribute to the hydrophobic effect. Dipalmitoylphosphatidylcholine, the predominant surface-active phospholipid found in pulmonary surfactant, is also found in high levels in the stomach and has been proposed to play a major role in mucosal defense.[36]

To date, nine human epithelial mucin genes have been identified and designated *MUC1–4*, *MUC5B*, *MUC5AC* and *MUC6–8*. The secretory mucins MUC5AC and MUC6 are expressed in the gastric epithelium. The superficial epithelium and the cells in the upper part of gastric pits produce MUC5AC. MUC6 expression is confined to the lower mucous neck cells of the antral glands.[37]

A group of small cysteine-rich peptides, trefoil factor (TFF) peptides, also have an important role in the mucus layer. TFF1 is found in the foveolar cells of the stomach, and TFF2 in the distal stomach and lower portion of Brunner's glands of the duodenum.[38,39] Trefoils seem to play a role in gastric epithelial protection and mucosal healing, and may play a part in mucus stabilization by crosslinking with mucins to aid the formation of the gel layer. When mucosal injury occurs, trefoils can stimulate repair by a process known as epithelial restitution.[40]

In the adult stomach, the gastric epithelium displays two well characterized populations of mucus-secreting cells. Superficial epithelium synthesizes MUC5AC, and cells in the deep glands produce MUC6.[41]

GASTRIC LIPASE

The human stomach is also involved in the digestion of fat. Gastric lipase initiates the digestion of dietary fat and hydrolyzes about 20% of the triglycerides in a meal. It is resistant to the acidic environment of the stomach and does not require bile salts or co-factors for triglyceride hydrolysis. Gastric lipase has an important role in lypolysis in the perinatal period and in conditions where there is decreased pancreatic lipase activity. It is secreted by the chief cells located in the fundus. Gastric lipase activity is detectable at 10 weeks' gestation in gastric tissues and steadily increases until 20 weeks, correlating with gastric gland development.

INTRINSIC FACTOR

In addition to hydrochloric acid, the parietal cells in the gastric mucosa secrete intrinsic factor, a 49-kDa glycoprotein that binds to vitamin B_{12} (cyanacobalamin) and is necessary for its absorption from the small intestine. Intrinsic factor is a glycoprotein that contains 15% carbohydrate and is secreted by the parietal cells of the body and fundus of the stomach. The average daily diet in Western countries contains 5–30 μg vitamin B_{12}, of which 1–5 μg is absorbed. The total body stores of the vitamin in adults range from 2 to 5 mg, of which approximately 1 mg is found in the liver. Human foods that contain the vitamin are of animal origin (meat, liver, fish, eggs and milk). Dietary vitamin B_{12} is released from protein and peptide complexes in the stomach as a result of pepsin and an acidic environment; it attaches to both intrinsic factor and a second vitamin B_{12}-binding protein called R-binder.

As well as intrinsic factor, another vitamin B_{12}-binding protein is secreted into the stomach – R-binder. R-binder is degraded by pancreatic trypsin, and the released vitamin B_{12} released further binds to the intrinsic factor. This step is impaired in patients with pancreatic insufficiency, leading to reduced vitamin B_{12} absorption. The intrinsic factor–vitamin B_{12} complex then binds to a specific receptor, cubilin, in the ileal mucosa and is absorbed by endocytosis. An autosomal recessive mutation of the cubulin receptor can cause intrinsic factor–vitamin B_{12} malabsorption and megaloblastic anemia, also known as Imerslund–Graesbeck syndrome.[42] In enterocytes, cyanacobalamin is transferred from intrinsic factor to transcobalamin II, another cyanacobalamin-binding protein that transports cyanacobalamin in plasma. Cells then convert cobalamin to its active forms, metylcobalamin and 5-deoxyadenosyl cobalamin. Even small amounts of intrinsic factor secretion are sufficient for vitamin B_{12} absorption, preventing pernicious anemia in patients with hypochlorhydria due to acid blocker therapy.[43] Intrinsic factor deficiency, bacterial overgrowth, pancreatic insufficiency, ileal resection or disease can cause vitamin B_{12} malabsorption with megaloblastic anemia.[44]

References

1. Grand RJ, Watkins JB, Torti FM. Development of the human gastrointestinal tract. A review. Gastroenterology 1976; 70:790–810.
2. Moore KL. The Developing Human, 6th edn. USA: Elsevier Science; 1998:271–278.
3. Indir J. The development of the nerve supply of the human esophagus and stomach. J Anat Soc India 1955; 4:55–68.
4. Read JB, Burnstock G. Development of adrenergic innervation and chromaffin cells in the human fetal gut. Dev Biol 1970; 22:513–534.
5. Read NW, Houghton LA. Physiology of gastric emptying and pathophysiology of gastroparesis. Gastroenterol Clin North Am 1989; 18:359–373.
6. Deren JS. Development of structure and function in the fetal and newborn stomach. Am J Clin Nutr 1971; 24:144–159.
7. Di Lorenzo C, Mertz H, Alvarez S, Mori C, Mayer E, Hyman P. Gastric receptive relaxation is absent in newborn infants. Gastroenterology 1993; 104:A498.
8. Minami H, McCallum RW. The physiology and pathophysiology of gastric emptying in humans. Gastroenterology 1984; 86:1592–1610.
9. Siegel M, Lebenthal E, Krantz B. Effect of caloric density on gastric emptying in premature infants. J Pediatr 1984; 104:118–122.
10. Lu YX, Owyang C. Duodenal acid-induced gastric relaxation is mediated by multiple pathways. Am J Physiol 1999; 276:G1501–G1506.
11. Quigley E. Gastric motor and sensory function, and motor disorders of the stomach. In: Gastrointestinal and Liver Disease, 7th edn. USA: Elsevier Science; 2002:691–713.
12. Wingate DL. Backwards and forwards with the migrating complex. Dig Dis Sci 1981; 26:641–666.
13. Wingate DL. Complex clocks. Dig Dis Sci 1983; 28:1133–1140.
14. Stern RM, Koch KL, Stewart WR, Vasey MW. Electrogastrography: current issues in validation and methodology. Psychophysiology 1987; 24:55–64.
15. Sase M, Tamura H, Ueda K, Kato H. Sonographic evaluation of antepartum development of fetal gastric motility. Ultrasound Obstet Gynecol 1999; 13:323–326.
16. Cucchiara S, Salvia G, Scarcella A, et al. Gestational maturation of electrical activity of the stomach. Dig Dis Sci 1999; 44:2008–2013.
17. Patterson M, Rintala R, Lloyd DA. A longitudinal study of electrogastrography in normal neonates. J Pediatr Surg 2000; 35:59–61.
18. Schubert ML. Gastric secretion. Curr Opin Gastroenterol 2003; 19:519–525.
19. Golgi C. Sur la fine organization des glandes peptiques des mammiferes. Arch Ital Biol 1893; 19:448.
20. Bjorkqvist M, Dornonville de la Cour C, Zhao CM, Gagnemo-Persson R, Hakanson R, Norlen P. Role of gastrin in the development of gastric mucosa, ECL cells and A-like cells in newborn and young rats. Regul Pept 2002; 108:73–82.
21. Bechi P, Romagnoli P, Panula P. Gastric mucosal histamine storing cells: evidence for different roles of mast cells and enterochromaffin-like cells in humans. Dig Dis Sci 1995; 40:2207–2213.
22. Leurs R, Watanabe T, Timmerman H. Histamine receptors are finally 'coming out'. Trends Pharmacol Sci 2001; 22:337–339.
23. Ballabeni V, Calcina F, Bosetti M. Different role of the histamine H_3-receptor in vagal-, bethanechol-, pentagastrin-induced gastric acid secretion in anaesthetized rats. Scand J Gastroenterol 2002; 37:754–758.
24. Vuyyuru L, Harrington L, Arimura A. Reciprocal inhibitory paracrine pathways link histamine and somatostatin secretion in the fundus of the stomach. Am J Physiol Gastrointest Liver Physiol 1997; 273:G106–G111.
25. Pico C, Oliver P, Sanchez J, Palou A. Gastric leptin: a putative role in the short-term regulation of food intake. Br J Nutr 2003; 90:735–741.
26. Bado A, Levasseur S, Attoub S, et al. The stomach is a source of leptin. Nature 1998; 394:790–793.
27. Gomez G, Englander EW, Greeley GH Jr. Nutrient inhibition of ghrelin secretion in the fasted rat. Regul Pept 2004; 117:33–36.
28. Date Y, Kojima M, Hosoda H, et al. Ghrelin, a novel growth hormone-releasing acylated peptide, is synthesized in a distinct endocrine cell type in the gastrointestinal tracts of rats and humans. Endocrinology 2000; 141:4255–4261.
29. Lee HM, Wang G, Englander EW, Kojima M, Greeley GH Jr. Ghrelin, a new gastrointestinal endocrine peptide that stimulates insulin secretion: enteric distribution, ontogeny, influence of endocrine, and dietary manipulations. Endocrinology 2002; 143:185–190.
30. Wang G, Lee HM, Englander E, Greeley GH Jr. Ghrelin – not just another stomach hormone. Regul Pept 2002; 105:75–81.
31. Hirsch AB, McCuen RW, Arimura A, Schubert ML. Adrenomedullin stimulates somatostatin and thus inhibits histamine and acid secretion in the fundus of the stomach. Regul Pept 2003; 110:189–195.
32. Kitamura K Kangawa K, Kawamoto M, et al. Adrenomedullin: a novel hypotensive peptide isolated from human pheochromocytoma. Biochem Biophys Res Commun 1993; 192:553–560.
33. Fukuda K, Tsukada H, Oya M, et al. Adrenomedullin promotes epithelial restitution of rat and human gastric mucosa *in vitro*. Peptides 1999; 20:127–132.
34. Wang H, Tomikawa M, Jones MK, Sarfeh IJ, Tarnawski AS. Ethanol injury triggers activation of adrenomedullin and its receptor genes in gastric mucosa. Dig Dis Sci 1999; 44:1390–1400.

35. Flemstron G, Garner A. Gastroduodenal HCO_3^- transport: characteristics and proposed role in acidity regulation and mucosal protection. Am J Physiol 1982; 242:G183–G193.

36. Scheiman J, Kraus E, Bonnville L. Synthesis and prostaglandin E_2-induced secretion of surfactant phospholipid by isolated gastric mucous cells. Gastroenterology 1991; 100:1232–1240.

37. Ho S, Roberton A, Shekels L. Expression cloning of gastric mucin complementary DNA and localization of mucin gene expression. Gastroenterology 1995; 109:735–747.

38. Sands BE, Podolsky DK. The trefoil peptide family. Annu Rev Physiol 1996; 58:253–273.

39. Hanby AM, Poulsom R, Singh S, Elia G, Jeffery RE, Wright NA. Spasmolytic polypeptide is a major antral peptide: distribution of the trefoil peptides human spasmolytic polypeptide and pS2 in the stomach. Gastroenterology 1993; 105:1110–1116.

40. Tanaka S, Podolsky DK, Engel E, Guth PH, Kaunitz JD. Human spasmolytic polypeptide decreases proton permeation through gastric mucus *in vivo* and *in vitro*. Am J Physiol 1997; 272:G1473–G1480.

41. De Bolos C, Garrido M, Real FX. MUC6 apomucin shows a distinct normal tissue distribution that correlates with Lewis antigen expression in the human stomach. Gastroenterology 1995; 109:723–734.

42. Aminoff M, Carter JE, Chadwick RB, et al. Mutations in *CUBN*, encoding the intrinsic factor–vitamin B_{12} receptor, cubilin, cause hereditary megaloblastic anaemia 1. Nat Genet 1999; 21:309–313.

43. Kittang E, Aadland E, Schjonsby H. Effect of omeprazole on the secretion of intrinsic factor, gastric acid and pepsin in man. Gut 1985; 26:594–598.

44. Sutter PM, Golner BB, Goldin BR. Reversal of protein-bound vitamin B_{12} malabsorption with antibiotics in atrophic gastritis. Gastroenterology 1991; 101:1039.

45. Moore KL, Persaud TVN. The Developing Human, 6th edn. Philadelphia, PA: WB Saunders; 1998.

Pathogenesis

The exact cause of hypertrophic pyloric stenosis is unknown. In most instances, the condition presents with vomiting after 3 weeks of age; however, about 20% of patients with a classic type are symptomatic from birth.[15,16] Rollins et al.[17] showed prospectively, using sonography, that pyloric muscle hypertrophy is not present during the early newborn period in infants who later develop infantile pyloric stenosis. Sonography has also been used to show that subclinical disease may cause minor degrees of vomiting, with gradual subsequent resolution.[18] Late development of hypertrophic pyloric stenosis is rare, but may occur in association with transpyloric feeding tubes.[19]

Lynn[20] proposed in 1960 that milk curds propelled by gastric peristalsis against a closed pyloric canal produce edema that narrows the pyloric canal and causes work hypertrophy of the pyloric and gastric musculature. Whether the initial cause is edema or an unexplained spasm of the antropyloric muscle, it seems clear that a vicious cycle is established that progresses to high-grade obstruction of the pyloric canal. Hypergastrinemia associated with hyperacidity has been suggested as a possible cause of pyloric stenosis.[21] In addition, increased levels of prostaglandins E_2 and $F_{2\alpha}$, both potent smooth muscle constrictors, have been found in infants with pyloric stenosis.[22] However, these findings may represent a secondary phenomenon caused by chronic gastric retention and distention.

A recent study[23] have demonstrated a selective absence of nerve growth factor receptors (NGFRs) and acetylcholine esterase (AChE)-positive nerve fibers in the circular and longitudinal muscle of hypertrophic pyloric stenosis compared with controls. This suggests that a NFGR deficiency may result in defective cholinergic innervation of pyloric muscle. Again, it is not known whether this is pathogenic or a secondary phenomenon.

Clinical presentation

Non-bilious vomiting is the initial sign of infantile hypertrophic pyloric stenosis. The vomiting may or may not be projectile, is usually progressive, and may become brownish owing to gastritis in later stages. Prolonged vomiting may lead to dehydration, weight loss and failure to thrive.

The onset of vomiting may occur as early as the first week or as late as 5 months of age.[24] As vomiting continues, hydrogen ion loss leads to an increase in serum levels of bicarbonate, followed by a decrease in serum chloride concentration and the development of hypochloremic alkalosis.[25] Serum potassium levels usually remain normal; however, when potassium depletion does occur, it may lead to paradoxical aciduria owing to the preferential loss of hydrogen ions across the distal renal tubules in exchange for sodium reabsorption.[26]

Jaundice occurs in association with pyloric stenosis in approximately 2–5% of infants.[27,28] About 50% of jaundiced infants with pyloric stenosis have a serum bilirubin level between 5 and 10 mg/dl that is mostly unconjugated.[29] Such increases in the serum unconjugated bilirubin levels have been seen in certain infants with neonatal bowel obstruction and were ascribed in the past to the effects of acute starvation on an immature liver. Woolley et al.[30] found decreased levels of glucuronyltransferase in infants with hypertrophic pyloric stenosis. Labrune et al.[31] found abnormally low levels of glucuronyl transferase in several infants 4–5 months after pyloromyotomy, suggesting that the jaundice associated with pyloric stenosis may be an early manifestation of Gilbert's syndrome. The role of caloric deprivation remains unclear, as a reduction in bilirubin levels occurs within 6–24 h after surgery, long before adequate caloric intake resumes.

Although there is no defined relationship between pyloric stenosis and other abnormalities, associated anomalies may be present in 6–20% of infants.[32] Many surgeons have noted an association between esophageal atresia, malrotation and pyloric stenosis in approximately 5% of infants with these anomalies.[33]

Diagnostic evaluation

The diagnosis of pyloric stenosis is best made by physical examination with palpation of a pyloric mass. This firm movable mass is similar to the size and shape of an olive and is located in the mid-epigastrium. A pyloric mass is pathognomonic and is palpable in 80% of patients by experienced examiners. To optimize the physical examination it is important first to empty the stomach of all air and fluid using a 10-Fr Replogle oral gastric tube. The catheter may then be removed, and the infant comforted with 5% glucose in water given orally. Occasionally, small doses of a sedative, such as morphine sulfate 0.1 mg/kg, may be given to facilitate the examination.

Imaging procedures are indicated for infants with bilious vomiting and those with non-bilious vomiting who do not have a palpable pyloric mass. In the latter group of infants, the differential diagnosis includes gastroenteritis, gastroesophageal reflux, pylorospasm, allergic gastroenteropathy and, rarely, antral or pyloric webs. These entities may be distinguished by either an upper gastrointestinal series (UGIS) or pyloric ultrasonography.

UGIS is still the 'gold standard' for the diagnosis of gastric outlet obstruction and has a 100% sensitivity and specificity for pyloric stenosis. The characteristic findings of pyloric stenosis on UGIS are a constant elongation of the pyloric channel,[34] a double tract of barium along the pyloric channel due to folding of compressed mucosa[35] and a prepyloric bulge into the distal antrum that produces a shouldering effect[36] (Fig. 24.1). UGIS may distinguish between most causes of non-bilious vomiting, but requires the administration of barium and exposure to radiation.

Ultrasonography is now the primary means of confirming a diagnosis of pyloric stenosis.[37,38] First described by Teele and Smithf,[39] sonography displays the hypertrophic pyloric musculature as a broad ring with low echo density surrounding an inner layer of high echo density mucosa. In addition to this characteristic overall appearance of the pylorus, strict criteria for pyloric stenosis have been developed including muscle thickness greater or equal to 4 mm[40]

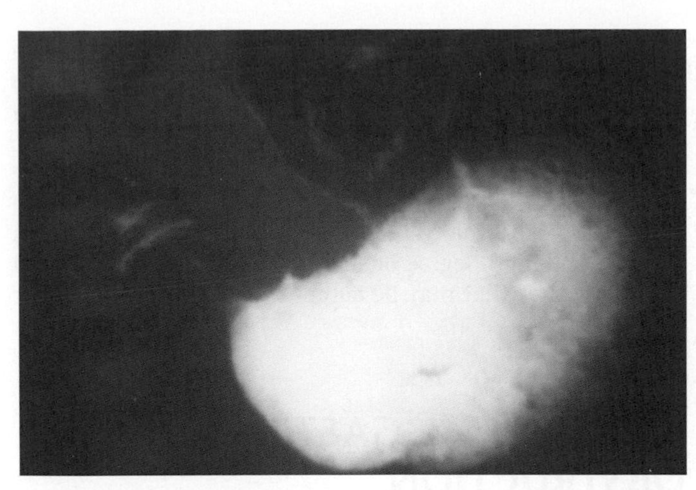

Figure 24.1: UGIS showing elongated pyloric channel and double-tract sign with shouldering of antrum characteristic of hypertrophic stenosis.

or a pyloric length greater than 16 mm,[41] or both (Fig. 24.2). Using this criteria, Forman et al.[42] found that sonography had 100% specificity and 89% sensitivity. Repeat sonography or UGIS is required in 10% of patients if a mass is not identified on physical examination. Sonography is less expensive than UGIS and some have advocated the combined expense would appear to make a primary UGIS more cost effective in this setting.[43] An even more cost-effective approach is to aspirate the stomach beforehand with a nasogastric tube. If the aspirate is greater than 5 ml, the probability of pyloric stenosis is greater than 90%. However, if the aspirate is less than 5 ml, the probability of gastroesophageal reflux is greater than 90%. This algorithm would then stipulate sonography for aspirates greater than 5 ml and UGIS for aspirates of less than 5 ml.[44]

Treatment

Initial treatment of pyloric stenosis is directed toward correction of dehydration and hypochloremic alkalosis.

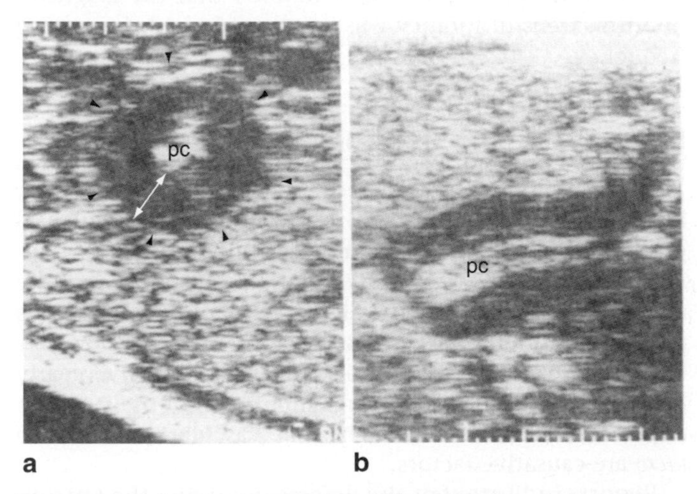

Figure 24.2: (**a**) Cross-sectional and (**b**) transverse sonograms of hypertrophic pyloric stenosis showing increased thickness and length of pyloric muscle. pc, pyloric channel.

Although serum potassium levels are usually normal, it should be recognized that total body potassium may be markedly depleted before serum samples reflect hypokalemia. The degree of dehydration may be assessed according to the usual clinical parameters, but is often reflected by the degree of hypochloremic alkalosis. Although most infants may be prepared for surgery within a 24-h period, advanced dehydration and alkalosis may require preoperative preparation over several days.

For infants with minimal dehydration and a normal electrolyte pattern, many surgeons advocate oral institution of a balanced electrolyte solution once the stomach has been lavaged with normal saline to remove obstructing milk curds and barium. Because vomiting may be persistent and the serum chloride and bicarbonate levels may be unreliable indices of the extent of fluid and electrolytes losses, it is prudent to begin intravenous fluid using 5% dextrose and 0.45% saline with 5 mmol potassium chloride added to each 250-ml intravenous bottle, even for infants with apparently minimal dehydration.

Infants with moderate to severe fluid and electrolyte disturbances, in whom serum bicarbonate levels may range from 25 to 60 mmol/l, are best treated with 5% dextrose in 0.45–0.9% saline given initially as a bolus of 10–20 ml/kg as required, and then at one and one half times maintenance for as long as required, until serum electrolytes have approached normal levels and total body water is judged to be sufficient. Once the stomach has been emptied, most infants stop vomiting. Only in rare cases is continued nasogastric drainage required, and then intravenous rates and electrolyte concentration must be adjusted to cover ongoing losses. Finally, after the infant has voided, it is important to add 5–10 mmol potassium chloride to each 250-ml bottle to help correct the hypochloremic alkalosis.

Correction of alkalemia prior to surgery is essential to prevent postanesthetic apnea, which may occur as a result of alkalemic depression of the respiratory center.[45] Several reports have indicated the incidence of postoperative apnea to range between 1 and 3%.[46,47] Rapid induction of general endotracheal anesthesia is not required; however, the stomach should be drained with an oral gastric tube before induction, to prevent aspiration.

The Ramstedt pyloromyotomy remains the surgical procedure of choice (Fig. 24.3). It is usually performed through a short subcostal incision placed at the liver edge. Whether the oblique muscles or the rectus abdominis muscles are split is a matter of personal preference. The pyloric mass is delivered into the wound and then serosally incised, and the underlying muscle is bluntly split, allowing the mucosa to pout up into the cleft, indicating a release of the obstructive process. Important technical features of this operation include avoidance of a mucosal tear in the region of the pyloric vein, where the risk is greatest, and extension of the pyloromyotomy to the antrum, where recurrence is most likely. Mucosal disruption is inconsequential as long as it is recognized and treated by repair

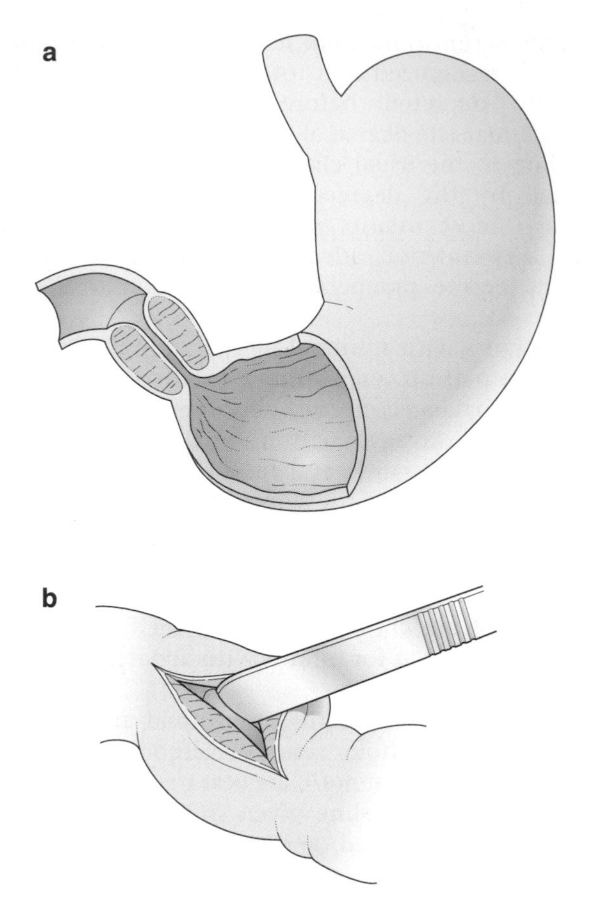

Figure 24.3: **(a)** Cross-section of the elongated, narrow pyloric channel typical of pyloric stenosis. **(b)** Pyloromyotomy is begun by bluntly separating muscle fibers on the anterior surface of the pylorus.

with absorbable suture and decompression of the stomach for 48 h.

Pyloromyotomy may be performed laparoscopically using 5- and 3-mm trocars. This procedure offers a superior cosmetic appearance compared with open pyloromyotomy, but does not result in a shortened hospital stay and may carry an increased risk of unrecognized mucosal perforation.

Results

The surgical treatment of pyloric stenosis is curative,[48] and the prognosis for infants with pyloric stenosis depends on the associated anomalies. Reports[49–51] indicate a mortality rate of 0–0.5%, an incidence of recurrence of 1–3%, and an incidence of wound infection and adhesions between 1% and 5%. Postoperative vomiting is a well recognized phenomenon, occurring in as many as 50% of infants, and is most likely caused by persistent local edema, delayed gastric emptying and gastroesophageal reflux.[52] In most cases, however, diluted feedings may be initiated within 6–12 h after surgery, and most infants may be advanced to maintenance oral feedings within 24–36 h after operation. If vomiting continues, antacids and prokinetic medications may be administered. Serial sonography afater surgery may reveal initial swelling of the muscles with rapid involution over the next 3 weeks, attaining normal thickness by 6 weeks.[53] Persistent hypertrophic pyloric stenosis due to an incomplete pyloromyotomy appears as persistent gastric outlet obstruction with muscle hypertrophy, but may have a tapered appearance.[54] Postoperative bleeding is rare and transfusion is virtually never required. These percentages indicate the high degree of success and low morbidity and mortality rates that may be achieved with skilled pediatric surgical care.

CONGENITAL GASTRIC OUTLET OBSTRUCTION

History

Atresia limited to the pyloric antrum was first described by Calder in 1733.[55] Subsequently, Crooks[56] in 1828 reported the first incomplete prepyloric membrane.[57] The first description of an antral web in the English literature was made by Parsons and Barding[58] in 1933. Since then, approximately 127 cases of congenital outlet obstruction have been reported involving the pylorus and antrum in three general forms: complete segmental defects, fibrous cords and webs.[59]

Incidence

Congenital gastric outlet obstruction due to pyloric atresia or prepyloric or antral webs is rare, representing fewer than 1% of all atresias and diaphragms of the alimentary tract.[60,61] Cook and Rickham[57] reported an incidence of 0.003% over a period of 25 years at the Liverpool Regional Neonatal Centre. Pyloric webs are by far the commonest of these reported; according to Bell et al.,[62] only 32 cases of antral webs were reported in children 16 years of age or younger. The rarity of these lesions notwithstanding, Tunnell and Ide Smith[63] stated in 1980 that the diagnosis of antral webs in infancy was being made with increasing frequency.

Etiology and pathology

The etiology of these defects is unknown. However, because the antrum and pylorus do not undergo mucosal proliferation, the etiology is not related to failure of canalization. Instead, it is speculated that discontinuation of the endodermal tube before the eighth week of gestation leads to segmentation defects, and endodermal redundancy after the eighth week leads to antral web formation. Given early fixation and excellent collateral circulation of the stomach and duodenum, it is unlikely that vascular accidents *in utero* are causative factors.

Reports indicate that the defects involving the antrum or pylorus may be of several types (Fig. 24.4).[64] Antral defects are least common, with antral gap atresia occur-

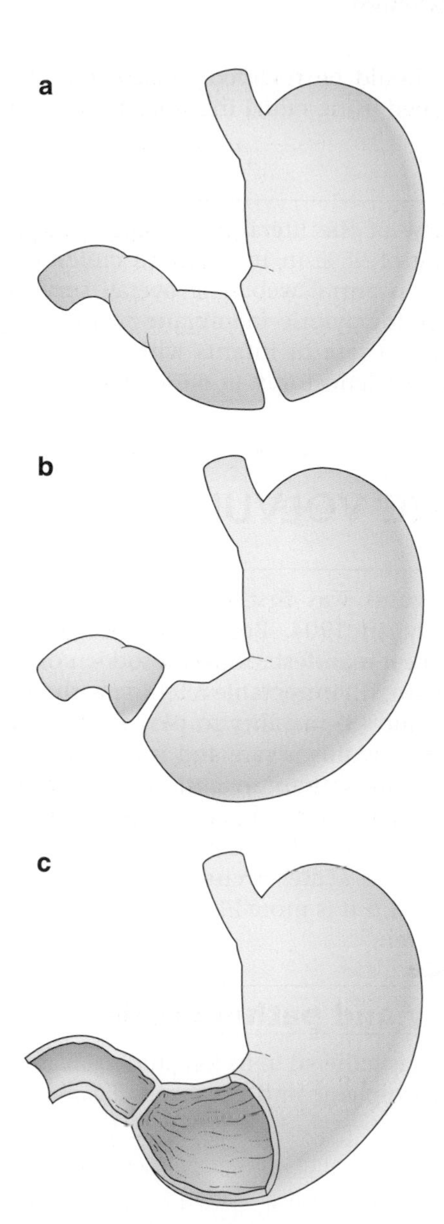

Figure 24.4: Congenital gastric outlet obstruction. (**a**) Antral gap atresia – 1% of cases. (**b**) Pyloric gap atresia – 27% of cases. (**c**) Pyloric web – 67% of cases.

ring in 1% and antral membranes with partial openings occurring in 5% of patients. Pyloric gap atresias with complete or cord separation of the pylorus account for approximately 27% of cases. Pyloric webs are commonest, occurring in 67% of cases, and include single and double membranes and solid atresias 1–2 cm in thickness.

Pyloric atresia may occur in an autosomal recessive mode in association with epidermolysis bullosa lethalis.[65–67] Eighteen cases of pyloric atresia–epidermolysis bullosa syndrome have been reported since Korder and Glasson's initial report in 1977.[68] Gedde-Dahl and Lambrecht[69] have shown that families with pyloric atresia–epidermolysis bullosa syndrome are of two ethnic groups, American Indian and Lebanese–Turkish, thus favoring genetic linkage between two autosomal recessive genes.

Clinical manifestations

Infants with antral or pyloric webs present quite differently from older children with the disorder.[57] Infants present with non-bilious vomiting, usually within the first days of life, along with feeding difficulties and distention of the stomach. Older children tend to present with epigastric pain, weight loss, nausea and vomiting, or symptoms compatible with peptic ulcer disease. Distribution by sex is nearly equal.[62] Polyhydramnios is reported in 61% of neonatal cases, and there is a high percentage of infants with a low birthweight.[66,70,71] Rupture of the stomach in pyloric atresia may occur as early as 12 h after birth.[72]

Diagnosis

The diagnosis of congenital outlet obstruction may be suggested by the non-specific findings of a large dilated stomach with a single gas bubble. As a dilated stomach with no gas in the distal bowel may also be seen in gastric hypotonia of the newborn,[73] it is important to proceed to UGIS. Bell et al.[62] reported that UGIS is 90% accurate in the diagnosis of congenital outlet obstruction. The typical UGIS finding of pyloric atresia is a pyloric dimple sign formed by the shallow pyloric cavity at the proximal point of the atresia[74] in the absence of a beak sign (seen in hypertrophic pyloric stenosis or pyloric duplication). In pyloric atresia, sonographic examination may reveal an absence of the typical echolucent pattern of the pyloric muscle. An antral web may appear on an upper gastrointestinal radiograph as a thin septum projecting into the antral lumen perpendicular to its longitudinal axis several centimeters proximal to the pyloric canal (Fig. 24.5). In older infants and children, gastroscopy may be helpful when UGIS is unclear. Failure to pass the gastroscope into the duodenum is diagnostic of congenital gastric obstruction.

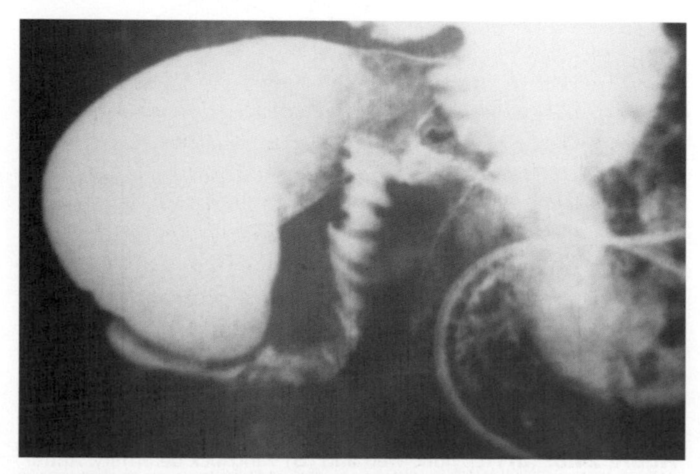

Figure 24.5: UGIS showing weblike filling defect of distal antrum and partial gastric outlet obstruction characteristic of antral web.

Treatment

As with hypertrophic pyloric stenosis, correction of dehydration and hypochloremic alkalosis is essential. Persistent vomiting should be treated with nasogastric suction and lavage if there has been previous feeding.

Operative repair should be approached through a transverse supraumbilical incision. The stomach is opened and a Foley catheter passed to exclude a windsock diaphragm, which is a membranous septum that has prolapsed through the pyloric canal[75] (Fig. 24.6). Standard treatment of an antral web is simple excision. Pyloric webs or septa are best treated by Heineke–Mikulicz pyloroplasty. For gap-type atresia, gastrojejunostomy and gastroduodenostomy have both been performed; however, gastroduodenostomy appears to offer superior results.[62,76]

Antral webs or membranes would seem to be ideal lesions for endoscopic management, as they consist mainly of mucosa and submucosa. A few such attempts have been reported; one infant who underwent endoscopic resection of an antral web later developed stricture and required subsequent surgical management.[77] Endoscopic treatment should be reserved for selected older children and performed using radial incisions to prevent stenosis.[78]

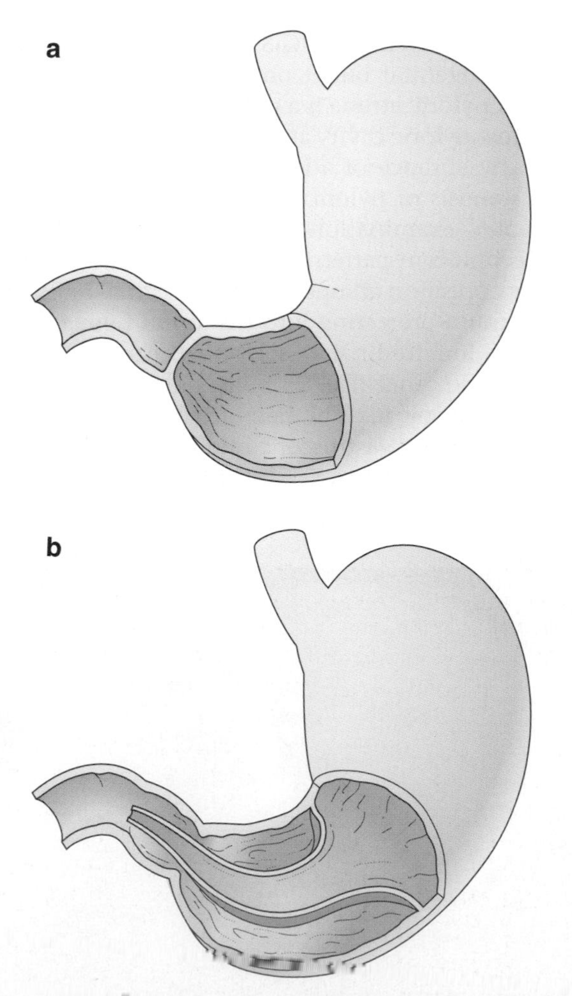

Figure 24.6: (**a**) Prepyloric web and (**b**) windsock deformity. Antral webs with partial openings account for 5% of all cases of congenital outlet obstruction.

Results

In his review of the literature, Moore[59] found an overall survival rate of 95% in infants and children undergoing excision of an antral web. The overall survival rate after pyloroplasty for pyloric membrane was 85%. Finally, the overall survival rate in infants with gap atresia was 84% after gastroduodenostomy *vs* 66% after posterior gastrojejunostomy.

GASTRIC VOLVULUS

History

Gastric volvulus was first described by Berti in 1866.[79] Subsequently, in 1904, Borchardt[80] described the classic triad of clinical manifestations: (1) sudden onset of violent epigastric pain, (2) intractable retching without production of vomitus and (3) inability to pass a tube into the stomach. Gastric volvulus is rare and is encountered more frequently in adults than in children. Only five cases in children younger than 10 years of age were reported in a review of 260 cases between 1914 and 1971.[81] Gastric volvulus may be acute or chronic, but according to Cole and Dickerson,[82] it is more likely to be acute in infants and young children.

Anatomy and pathogenesis

The stomach is tethered in its longitudinal axis by the gastrohepatic, gastrosplenic and gastrocolic ligaments (Fig. 24.7).

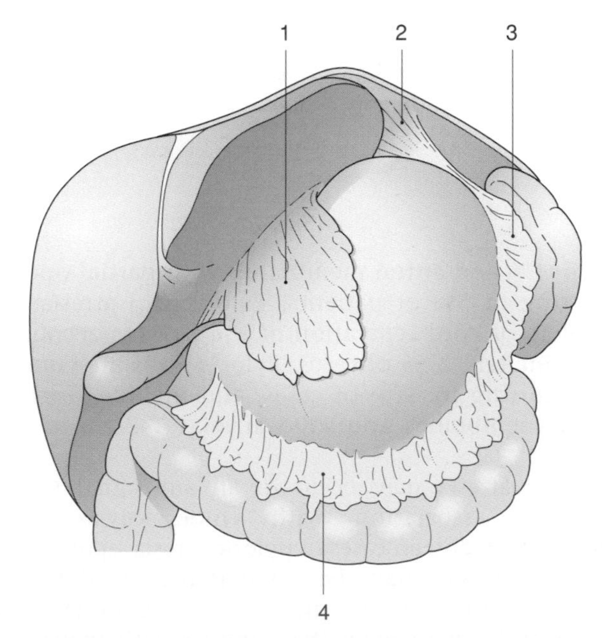

Figure 24.7. Peritoneal attachments of the stomach include the gastrohepatic ligament (1), gastrophrenic ligament (2), gastrosplenic ligament (3) and gastrocolic ligament (4).

It is tethered in its transverse axis by the gastrophrenic ligament and the retroperitoneal attachments of the second portion of the duodenum. For a volvulus to occur, these ligaments must be absent or stretched. In most cases there are associated mesenteric abnormalities, such as malrotation[83] and abnormal mobility at the hiatus.[84] Cole and Dickerson[82] reported eventration or herniation of the diaphragm to be present in 65% of patients with gastric volvulus up to 10 years of age. Idowu et al.[85] reported an even higher incidence of diaphragmatic abnormalities in infants up to 1 month of age with gastric volvulus. Recently, several cases of acute gastric volvulus have been reported in infants and smaller children with asplenia syndrome.[86] Approximately one-third of patients with gastric volvulus have no associated abnormality, and in this group the etiology may be related to gastric distention.[83,84]

Gastric volvulus occurs when one part of the stomach rotates abnormally around another part. Rotation may occur along the longitudinal axis of the stomach to produce organoaxial volvulus (Fig. 24.8), or along the transverse axis to produce mesenteroaxial volvulus (Fig. 24.9). Organoaxial volvulus is commoner in children, occurring in approximately two-thirds of reported cases.[84] Rarely, mixed volvulus may occur if the stomach is rotated in both planes. Torsion beyond 180° results in complete gastric obstruction and strangulation of the vasculature.

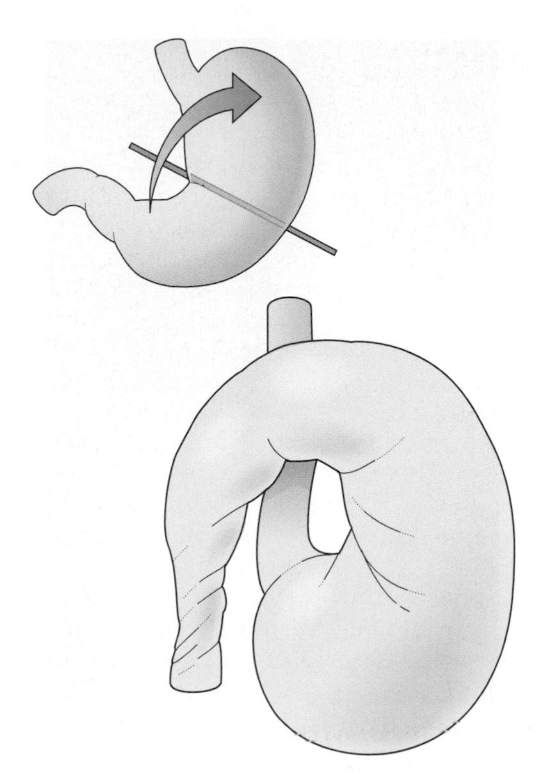

Figure 24.9: Mesenteroaxial volvulus occurs in the transverse axis of the stomach

Clinical presentation

The clinical features of acute gastric volvulus are non-specific but suggest high obstruction of the gastrointestinal tract.[87] The triad of epigastric pain, retching and failure to pass a nasogastric tube may not always apply in children. For example, pain in the newborn period is difficult to assess. Second, gastric volvulus in infants may produce bilious or non-bilious vomiting. Third, not all infants with gastric volvulus exhibit abdominal distention, and in many infants a nasogastric tube may be passed relatively easily.[82] Acute volvulus may advance rapidly to gastric strangulation, perforation and cardiovascular collapse, and should be treated as a surgical emergency. Chronic gastric volvulus, commoner in older children, unusually presents with postprandial pain, belching, vomiting and early satiety. Rarely does chronic volvulus lead to vascular compromise.

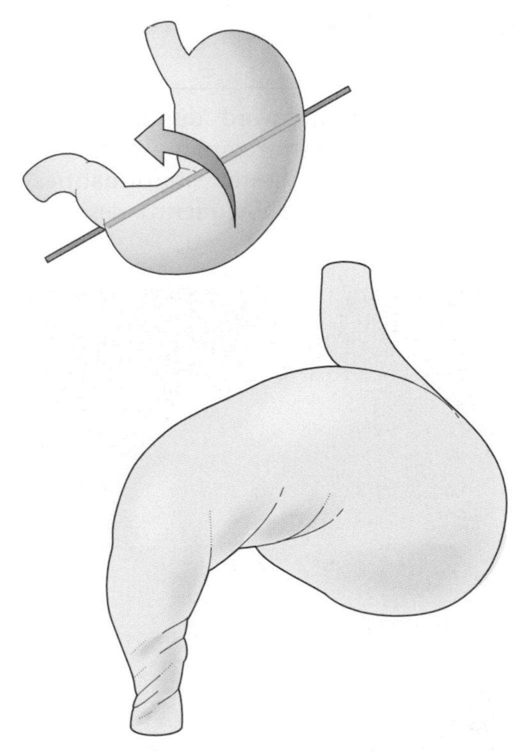

Figure 24.8: Organoaxial volvulus occurs in the longitudinal axis of the stomach.

Gastric volvulus may be suggested on plain radiography by a dilated stomach. In mesenteroaxial volvulus, erect radiographic films often show a double fluid level and a 'beak' located near the esophagogastric junction, which is caused by gaseous distention of the inverted antrum.[83] In erect films, organoaxial volvulus shows just one air–fluid level and no characteristic beak. If a nasogastric tube is passed, the gastroesophageal junction is seen inferior to its normal position with respect to the fundus. On UGIS the gastroesophageal junction is in the normal position; the stomach is visualized upside down and often apparently located within the left chest when associated with a hiatal hernia or other diaphragmatic defect (Fig. 24.10).

Treatment

Acute gastric volvulus requires surgery as soon as adequate resuscitation has been performed. The stomach should be

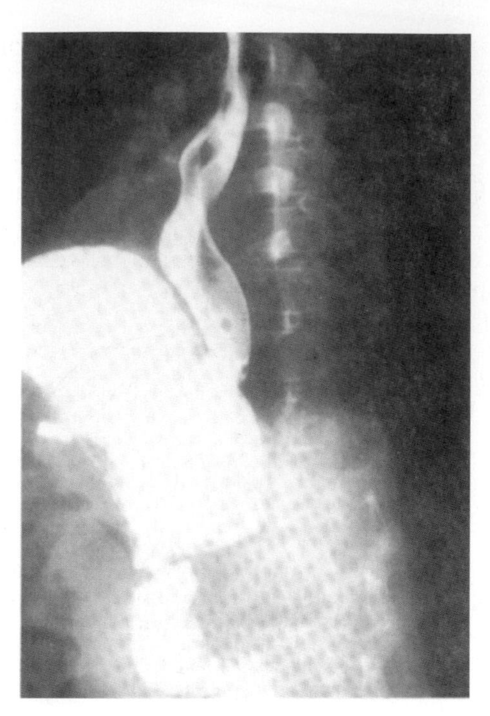

Figure 24.10: UGIS showing characteristic appearance of stomach in mesenteroaxial gastric volvulus.

decompressed by nasogastric suction or, alternatively, by needle aspiration. Once the volvulus is reduced, predisposing causes should be investigated. Hiatus hernia, diaphragmatic eventration or diaphragmatic hernia should be corrected surgically; anterior gastrostomy along with gastropexy is usually curative. A fundoplication or other antireflux procedure should be performed only if there is evidence of severe reflux.[83]

In certain cases of chronic gastric volvulus, endoscopic correction has been advocated.[88] With air insufflation at a minimum, the endoscope is turned into a loop and rotated 180° in a clockwise or anticlockwise direction. Endoscopic examination after this maneuver may reveal the stomach to be in a normal position. Although dual percutaneous endoscopic gastrostomy has been used in the management of chronic gastric volvulus in adults, this technique would seem to offer little advantage in children, who usually require a general anesthetic for repair of acute gastric volvulus.

CONGENITAL MICROGASTRIA

History

Microgastria was first described at necropsy of an adult by Dide in 1894.[89] Blank and Chisholm[90] reported a 26-year follow-up of a patient with congenital microgastria first seen in 1947.

Etiology

Microgastria is a rare congenital anomaly characterized by a small tubular stomach, megaesophagus and incomplete gastric rotation.[91] Multiple associated anomalies have been described, including malrotation, situs inversus and splenia.[92] Skeletal anomalies are common and include micrognathia, radial and ulnar hypoplasia, and hypoplastic nails.

Clinical presentation

The most frequent symptoms of microgastria are vomiting and failure to thrive.[92] These symptoms generally result from associated gastroesophageal reflux, which may also cause aspiration, esophageal erosion and hemorrhage, as well as a dilated esophagus.

Diagnosis

The diagnosis of microgastria is usually made by UGIS (Fig. 24.11). Endoscopy and esophageal pH studies may be helpful in the setting of severe gastroesophageal reflux.

Treatment

Treatment is usually medical and consists of continuous gastrostomy or jejunostomy tube feedings. Gastroesophageal reflux should be treated conservatively with acid blockers and prokinetic agents, such as metoclopramide. When gastroesophageal reflux cannot be managed medically, anti-reflux procedures using the Hill or Thal repair may be considered. In most instances, the stomach will gradually dilate to accommodate oral feedings. In certain protracted cases, construction of a jejunal reservoir has been recommended.[93]

GASTRIC AND DUODENAL DUPLICATION

History

Reginald Fitz[94] coined the word 'duplication' to describe what he thought were cystic remnants of the omphalomesenteric duct. Various cystic abnormalities of the gastrointestinal tract were subsequently described, and in

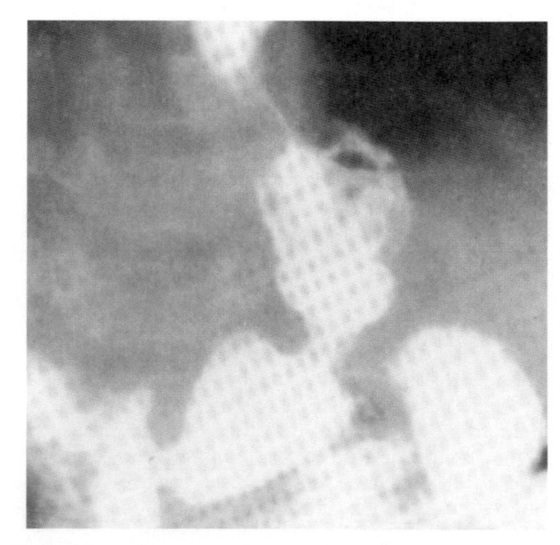

Figure 24.11: UGIS showing typical appearance of microgastria with gastroesophageal reflux.

1952 Gross et al.[95] suggested that the term duplication be used for all such anomalies, irrespective of their site, morphology or embryologic derivation. Gastroduodenal duplications account for less than 10% of all alimentary tract duplications and were classified by Rowling in 1959[96] according to the following criteria: (1) the cyst wall is contiguous with the stomach wall; (2) the cyst is surrounded by smooth muscle contiguous with stomach muscle; and (3) the cyst wall is lined by alimentary epithelium. In 1979 Schwartz et al.[97] described a gastric duplication that was ectopic and separate from the stomach, taking issue with the requirement for continuity of the cyst wall with the stomach.

Embryogenesis and pathology

Bremer[98] proposed that gastroduodenal duplications result from an error of recanalization in which there is coalescence of vacuoles within the embryonic duct wall or fusion of the longitudinal epithelial folds to form a hollow tube. Although this description may apply to duodenal duplications, the embryonic stomach does not go through a stage of mucosal proliferation and recanalization. McLetchie et al.[99] proposed an alternative therapy in which abnormal adhesions between the notochord and the embryonic endoderm form a traction diverticulum, disorganizing endoderm as the embryo grows. Torma[100] has pointed out that this theory may explain the frequent association of gastric duplications with esophageal and pancreatic duplications. Gastric duplications are closed, spherical structures on the greater curvature of the stomach and may be associated with enterogenous cysts in the posterior mediastinum, the esophagus or the duodenum.[101,102] Gastric duplications may be tubular or cystic, and most are smaller than 12 cm in diameter. Wieczorek et al.[103] found that 82% of gastric duplications are cystic and do not communicate with the stomach, whereas 18% are tubular and do communicate. Several cases have been described in which ectopic pancreatic tissue lines the cyst along with gastric mucosa.[100] Rarely, gastroduodenal duplications may be extensive tubular structures that traverse the diaphragm and are associated with anomalous upper cervical and thoracic vertebrae.[104,105]

Associated congenital anomalies occur in 35% of patients with gastric duplications.[106] The commonest anomaly is another cyst, especially of the esophagus or duodenum, although vertebral anomalies and ectopic pancreas are frequently found.

Presentation

Gastric duplications are uncommon and are reported most frequently in children. Wieczorek et al. [103] reviewed the literature in 1984 and found a total of 109 reported gastric duplications. More than half of gastroduodenal duplications are diagnosed within the first year of life; the condition is twice as common in females. The clinical presentation depends on the size and location of the cyst as well as the presence or absence of communication with the alimentary tract. The commonest presentation is that of gastric outlet obstruction, but in 65% of cases there is a palpable abdominal mass.[103] In many cases there is abdominal pain, weight loss and failure to thrive. Occasionally, a large duplication cyst may perforate secondary to ulceration caused by stasis of gastric enzymes and hydrochloric acid with the cyst.[107] Non-communicating duplications may cause gastric irritation, leading to gastritis or peptic ulceration. Thus, hematemesis or melena may be seen in approximately 30% of older children.[103] Finally, when there is a coexistent gastric and pancreatic duplication, pancreatitis or erosion into a contiguous viscus (e.g. the transverse colon) may occur.[108,109]

Diagnosis

Usually, a gastric duplication is revealed by UGIS as an extrinsic defect located on the greater curve of the stomach. A more distal cyst may distort the pyloric or duodenal channel, or both, and usually causes delayed gastric emptying. Sonography or computed tomography may be helpful in demonstrating contiguous cystic structures. Technetium-99m scanning can localize ectopic gastric mucosa but, because of overlapping uptake, is of little help in demonstrating structures adjacent to the stomach.[109]

Treatment

In most instances, the treatment of gastroduodenal duplications is excision of the cyst either by dissection from a common wall or with a margin of normal stomach and primary closure.[103,110] When there is a coexistent pancreatic duplication, the accessory pancreatic lobe can be ligated and transected at its origin.[108,109] When the aberrant pancreatic lobe is adherent to the stomach, an attempt should be made to dissect it free before a more extensive resection is undertaken. Similarly, it may be possible to avoid an extensive resection in the region of the gastroesophageal junction or pyloric channel by performing a partial excision of the gastroduodenal duplication and stripping the mucosa along the common wall to prevent subsequent ulceration.[111] The stomach should then be distended with air to detect any unsuspected perforation. When either complete resection or partial resection with mucosal stripping is not technically possible, marsupialization can be accomplished with internal drainage either into the duodenum or using a Roux-en-Y loop of jejunum.

Results

In their review, Wieczorek et al.[103] found an overall mortality rate of approximately 3%. In more than 10% of patients, perforation of the duplication cyst had occurred either freely into the peritoneal cavity or with fistula formation into adjacent structures. However, there has been only one reported death as a complication of cyst perforation.[112]

7. Laron Z, Horne LM. The incidence of infantile pyloric stenosis. Am J Dis Child 1957; 94:151–154.
8. Jed MB, Melton J, Griffin MR, et al. Factors associated with infantile hypertrophic pyloric stenosis. Am J Dis Child 1988; 142:334–337.
9. Kerr AM. Unprecedented rise in incidence of infantile hypertrophic pyloric stenosis. BMJ 1980; 13:714–715.
10. Knox EG, Armstrong E, Hanes R. Changing incidence of infantile hypertrophic pyloric stenosis. Arch Dis Child 1983; 58:582–585.
11. Martin J, Monk J. Infant Feeding in 1980. Social Survey Division, Office of Population Censuses and Surveys, London: HMSO; 1982.
12. Carter CO, Evans KA. Inheritance of congenital pyloric stenosis. J Med Genet 1969; 6:233–239.
13. Dodge JA. Infantile hypertrophic pyloric stenosis in Belfast. Arch Dis Child 1975; 50:171–178.
14. McKeown T, MacMahon B. Infantile hypertrophic pyloric stenosis in parent and child. Arch Dis Child 1955; 30:497–500.
15. Andrassy RJ, Haff RC, Larsen GL. Infantile hypertrophic pyloric stenosis during the first week of life. Approaches to diagnosis, based on observations of a newborn whose vomiting began on the first day. Clin Pediatr 1977; 16:475–476.
16. Geer LL, Gaisie G, Mandell VS, et al. Evolution of pyloric stenosis in the first week of life. Pediatr Radiol 1985; 15:205–206.
17. Rollins MD, Shields, MD, Quinn RJM, et al. Pyloric stenosis: congenital or acquired? Arch Dis Child 1989; 64:137–138.
18. Stunden RJ, LeQuesne GW, Little KET. The improved ultrasound diagnosis of hypertrophic pyloric stenosis. Pediatr Radiol 1986; 16:200–205.
19. Latchaw LAC, Jacir NN, Harris BH. The development of pyloric stenosis during transpyloric feeding. J Pediatr Surg 1989; 24:823–824.
20. Lynn H. The mechanism of pyloric stenosis and its relationship to preoperative preparation. Arch Surg 1960; 81:453–459.
21. Spitz L, Zail SS. Serum gastrin levels in congenital hypertrophic pyloric stenosis. J Pediatr Surg 1976; 11:33–35.
22. Laferla G, Watson J, Fyfe AHB, et al. The role of prostaglandins E2 and F2α in infantile hypertrophic pyloric stenosis. J Pediatr Surg 1986; 21:410–412.
23. Kobayashi H, Obriain DS, Puri P. Defective cholinergic innervation in pyloric muscle of patients with hypertrophic pyloric stenosis. Pediatr Surg 1994; 9:338–341.
24. Rendle-Short J, Zachary RB. Congenital pyloric stenosis in older babies. Arch Dis Child 1955; 30:70–71.
25. Touloukin RJ, Higgins E. The spectrum of serum electrolytes in hypertrophic pyloric stenosis. J Pediatr Surg 1983; 18:394–397.
26. Winters RW. Metabolic alkaloses of pyloric stenosis: the body fluid in pediatrics. Boston, MA: Little, Brown; 1973:402–414.
27. Benson CD. Infantile hypertrophic pyloric stenosis. In: Welsh KJ, Randolph JG, Ravitch MM, et al., eds. Pediatric Surgery, 4th edn. Chicago: Yearbook Medical; 1986:811–815.
28. Mackay AJ, Mackellar A. Infantile hypertrophic pyloric stenosis: a review of two-hundred and twenty-two cases. Aust N Z J Surg 1986; 56:131–133.
29. Chaves-Carbello E, Harris LE, Lynn HB. Jaundice associated with pyloric stenosis and neonatal small bowel obstruction. Clin Pediatr 1968; 7:198–202.
30. Woolley MM, Felsher BF, Asch MJ, et al. Jaundice, hypertrophic pyloric stenosis, and hepatic glucuronyl transferase. J Pediatr Surg 1974; 9:359–363.
31. Labrune T, Myara A, Huguet P, et al. Jaundice with hypertrophic pyloric stenosis: a possible early manifestation of Gilbert syndrome. J Pediatr 1989; 15:93–95.
32. Ahmed S. Infantile pyloric stenosis associated with major anomalies of the alimentary tract. J Pediatr Surg 1970; 5:660–666.
33. Ziedan B, Wyatt J, Mackersie A, et al. Recent results of treatment of infantile hypertrophic pyloric stenosis. Arch Dis Child 1988; 63:1060–1064.
34. Meuwissen T, Sloof JP. Roentgenologic diagnosis of congenital hypertrophic pyloric stenosis. Acta Pediatr 1932; 14:19–48.
35. Herran PJ, Darling DB, Sciamma F. The value of the double tract sign of the differentiating factor between pyloric spasm and hypertrophic pyloric stenosis. Radiology 1966; 86:723–725.
36. Shopfner CE, Kalmon EH, Coin CG. The diagnosis of hypertrophic pyloric stenosis. AJR Am J Roentgenol 1964; 91:796–800.
37. Ball TI, Atkinson GO, Gay BB. Ultrasound diagnosis of hypertrophic pyloric stenosis: real-time application and demonstration of new sonographic sign. Radiology 1983; 147:499–502.
38. Godbole P, Sprigg A, Dickson JA, et al. Ultrasound compared with clinical examination in infantile hypertrophic pyloric stenosis. Arch Dis Child 1996; 75:335–337.
39. Teele RL, Smith EH. Ultrasound and the diagnosis of idiopathic hypertrophic pyloric stenosis. N Engl J Med 1977; 296:1149–1150.
40. Blumhagen JD, Nobel HG. Muscle thickness in hypertrophic pyloric stenosis: sonographic determination. AJR Am J Roentgenol 1983; 140:221–223.
41. Wilson DA, VanHoutte JJ. The reliable sonographic diagnosis of hypertrophic pyloric stenosis. J Clin Ultrasound 1984; 12:201–204.
42. Forman HP, Leonidas JC, Kronfeld GD. A rational approach to diagnosis of hypertrophic pyloric stenosis: do the results match the claims? J Pediatr Surg 1990; 25:262–266.
43. Olson AD, Hernandez R, Hirsch RB. The role of ultrasonography in the diagnosis of pyloric stenosis: a decision analysis. J Pediatr Surg 1998; 33:676–681.
44. Mandell GA, Wolfson PJ, Adkins ES, et al. Cost-effective imaging approach to the non-bilious vomiting infant. Pediatrics 1999; 103:1198–1202.
45. Kumar V, Bailey WC. Electrolyte and acid–base problems in hypertrophic pyloric stenosis in infancy. Indian Pediatr 1935; 12:839.
46. Steven IM, Allen TH, Sweeny DB. Congenital hypertrophic pyloric stenosis – the anaesthetist's view. Anaesth Intensive Care 1973; 1:544–546.
47. Conn AW. Anaesthesia for pyloromyotomy in infancy. Can Anaesth Soc J 1963; 10:18–29.
48. Scharli A, Sieber WK, Kiesewetter WB. Hypertrophic pyloric stenosis at the Children's Hospital of Pittsburgh from 1912 to 1967. J Pediatr Surg 1969; 4:108–114.
49. Bell MJ. Infantile pyloric stenosis: experience with three hundred and five cases at the Louisville Children's Hospital. Surgery 1968; 64:983–989.
50. Benson CD. Infantile pyloric stenosis: historical aspects and current surgical concepts. Prog Pediatr Surg 1971; 1:63–88.

51. Gibbs MK, vanHeerden JA, Lynn HB. Congenital hypertrophic pyloric stenosis: surgical experience. Mayo Clin Proc 1975; 50:312–316.
52. Scharli AF, Leditschke JF. Gastric motility after pyloromyotomy in infants: a reappraisal of postoperative feeding. Surgery 1968; 64:1133–1137.
53. Sauerbrei EE, Paloschi GGB. The ultrasonic features of hypertrophic pyloric stenosis, with emphasis on the postoperative appearance. Radiology 1983; 147:503–506.
54. Jamroz GA, Blocker SH, McAlister WH. Radiographic findings after incomplete pyloromyotomy. Gastrointest Radiol 1986; 11:139–141.
55. Calder J. Two examples of children preternatural conformation of the guts. Med Essays and Obs (Edinb) 1733; 1:205.
56. Crooks. Estomac se terminant en cude sac. Arch Gen Med 1828; 17:264.
57. Cook RCM, Rickham PP. In: Gastric Outlet Obstruction in Neonatal Surgery, 2nd edn. London: Butterworth; 1978:335–338.
58. Parsons LG, Barding S. Disease of Infancy and Childhood. London: Oxford University Press; 1933.
59. Moore CM. Congenital gastric outlet obstruction. J Pediatr Surg 1989; 24:1242–1246.
60. Gerber BC, Aberdeen SO. Pre-pyloric diaphragm, an unusual abnormality. Arch Surg 1965; 90:472–475.
61. Simstein NL. Congenital gastric anomalies. Am Surg 1986; 52:264–268.
62. Bell MJ, Ternberg JL, McAlister W, et al. Antral diaphragm – a cause of gastric outlet obstruction in infants and children. J Pediatr 1977; 90:196–202.
63. Tunnell WP, Ide Smith E. Antral web in infancy. J Pediatr Surg 1980; 15:152–155.
64. Kume K, Ikeda K, Hayashida Y, et al. Congenital pyloric atresia: a report of three cases and review of the literature. J Pediatr Surg 1980; 16:259–268.
65. El Shafie M, Stidham LG, Klippel CH, et al. Pyloric atresia epidermolysis bullosa letalis: a lethal combination in two premature newborn siblings. J Pediatr Surg 1979; 14:446–449.
66. Bar-Maor Ja, Nissan S, Nero S. Pyloric atresia. J Med Genet 1972; 9:70–72.
67. Pearson RW, Potter B, Strauss F. Epidermolysis bullosa hereditaria lethalis. Arch Dermatol 1974; 109:349–355.
68. Korder JS, Glasson MJ. Pyloric atresia associated with epidermolysis bullosa. J Pediatr 1977; 90:600–601.
69. Gedde-Dahl T Jr, Lambrecht IA. Principles and Practices in Medical Genetics. New York: Churchill-Livingstone; 1981.
70. Ducharme JC, Bensoussan AL. Pyloric atresia. J Pediatr Surg 1975; 10:149–150.
71. Sloop RD, Montagne ACW. Gastric outlet obstruction due to congenital pyloric mucosal membrane. Am Surg 1967; 165:598–604.
72. Burnett HA, Halpert B. Perforation of the stomach of a newborn infant with pyloric atresias. Arch Pathol 1947; 44:318.
73. Franklin EA. Gastrointestinal Imaging in Pediatrics, 2nd edn. Philadelphia, PA: Harper & Row; 1982:131–142.
74. Gruenbaum M, Kornreich L, Ziv N. The imaging diagnosis of pyloric atresia. Z Kinderchir 1985; 40:308–311.
75. Bell MH, Ternberg JL, Keating JP, et al. Prepyloric gastric antral web: a puzzling epidemic. J Pediatr Surg 1978; 13:307–313.
76. Talwalker VC. Pyloric atresia: a case report. J Pediatr Surg 1967; 2:458–460.
77. Brandt LJ, Boley SJ, Dom F, et al. Endoscopic resection of an obstructing antral web in an infant. Dig Dis Sci 1978; 5:65–85.
78. Al-Kawas FH. Endoscopic laser treatment of an obstructing antral web. Gastrointest Endosc 1988; 34:349–351.
79. Berti A. Singolare attortigliamento dell' esofago duodeno sequito da rapida morte. Gass Med Ital 1966; 9:139.
80. Borchardt M. Zur patologie und terapie des magenvolvuls. Arch Klin Chir 1904; 74:243.
81. Wastell C, Ellis H. Volvulus of the stomach: a review with a reported eight cases. Br J Surg 1971; 58:557–562.
82. Cole BC, Dickerson SJ. Acute volvulus of the stomach in infants and children. Surgery 1971; 70:707–717.
83. Ziprkowski MN, Teele RL. Gastric volvulus in childhood. AJR Am J Roentgenol 1979; 132:921–925.
84. Cammeron AEP, Howard ER. Gastric volvulus in childhood. J Pediatr Surg 1987; 22:944–947.
85. Idowu J, Aitken DR, Gorgeson KE. Gastric volvulus in the newborn. Arch Surg 1980; 115:1046–1049.
86. Aoyama K, Tateishi K. Gastric volvulus in three children with asplenia syndrome. J Pediatr Surg 1986; 21:307–310.
87. Campbell JB. Neonatal gastric volvulus. AJR Am J Roentgenol 1979; 132:723–725.
88. Eckhauser ML, Ferron JP. The use of dual percutaneous endoscopic gastrostomy in the management of chronic intermittent gastric volvulus. Gastrointest Endosc 1985; 31:340–342.
89. Dide M. Sur un estomac d'adulte type foetal. Bull Soc Anat Paris 1894; 69:669.
90. Blank E, Chisholm AJ. Congenital microgastria: a case report with a 26-year follow-up. Pediatrics 1973; 51:1037.
91. Campbell JR. Congenital microgastria. In: Pediatric Surgery. Chicago, IL: Yearbook Medical, 1986: 827–828.
92. Kessler H, Smulewicz JJ. Microgastria associated with agenesis of the spleen. Radiology 1973; 107:393–396.
93. Neifeld JP, Berman WF, Lawrence W Jr, et al. Management of congenital microgastria with a jejunal reservoir pouch. J Pediatr Surg 1980; 15:882–885.
94. Fitz RH. Persistent omphalo-mesenteric remains: their importance in the causation of intestinal duplication, cyst formation, and obstruction. Am J Med Sci 1884; 88:30–57.
95. Gross RE, Holcomb GW Jr, Farber S. Duplications of the alimentary tract. Pediatrics 1952; 9:449–468.
96. Rowling JT. Some observations of gastric cysts. Br J Surg 1959; 46:441–445.
97. Schwartz DL, So HB, Becker JM. An ectopic gastric duplication arising from the pancreas and presenting with pneumoperitoneum. J Pediatr Surg 1979; 14:187–188.
98. Bremer JL. Diverticula and duplications of the intestinal tract. Arch Pathol Lab Med 1944; 38:132–140.
99. McLetchie NGB, Purves JK, Saunders RL. The genesis of gastric and certain intestinal diverticula and enterogenous cysts. Surg Gynecol Obstet 1954; 99:135–141.
100. Torma MJ. Of double stomachs. Arch Surg 1974; 109:155–157.
101. Alschibija T, Putnam TC, Yablin BA. Duplication of the stomach simulating hypertrophic pyloric stenosis. Am J Dis Child 1974; 127:120–122.
102. Bowmen M, Singh MP. Pyloric duplication in a preterm neonate. J Pediatr Surg 1984; 19:158–159.
103. Wieczorek RL, Seidman I, Ranson JH, et al. Congenital duplication of the stomach: case report and review of the English literature. Am J Gastroenterol 1984; 79:597–602.

determine whether this mucosa is gastric or Barrett's specialized metaplasia. Whether an 'extension' or 'prominence' of the Z-line is a variant of normal stomach with gastric cardiac or transitional mucosa, or short-segment Barrett's esophagus, can be determined only by biopsy.[65,74,83–85]

Inflammation of the gastric cardia is an area of considerable interest because of the increasing incidence of cancer of the cardia and esophagus, and the potential for detecting preneoplastic changes (intestinal metaplasia). Although some studies in adults have indicated that carditis and intestinal metaplasia are due to *H. pylori* infection as part of a pangastritis,[73,76,86,87] others have indicated the cause as GERD[77,78] and yet others have suggested that both may be etiologies.[74,79] The difference may lie in the definition of cardia, and the sites from which biopsies were taken. A study in children has indicated that *H. pylori* infection is the most important cause of carditis (although GERD may also be a cause), and that the cardia may be the most sensitive area for detecting *H. pylori*.[65]

When endoscopic findings are puzzling or a lesion is present, more biopsies should be taken randomly and from the lesion or its edge. The size of biopsies is also important. Biopsies taken with 'pediatric' forceps often are of little value: they are tiny, difficult to mount, and the amount of useful interpretable tissue is very limited. In most children over 2 or 3 months of age, an endoscope with a 2.8-mm biopsy channel can usually be used, and biopsies with these forceps are often adequate, if several are taken. In contrast, each biopsy taken with 'jumbo' or large cup forceps offers at least two or three times the amount of mucosa for diagnosis; these can often be obtained in older children. The enhanced tissue yield with jumbo biopsy forceps must be compared to the risk of complications when large forceps are used; decisions should be made on a case-by-case basis. Issues regarding mucosal biopsy in children are considered in more detail elsewhere.[6]

On occasion, usually with rare disorders, even large endoscopic biopsies may be insufficient to make a diagnosis, and endoscopic mucosal resection or full-thickness surgical biopsies are required. This may be the case in the infiltrative disorders, which can present with 'thick folds', mass or ulceration, such as cancer, lymphoma, plasmacytoma,[88] or leiomyoma/leiomyosarcoma, or with certain gastric polyposes.[89] These disorders are not discussed in this chapter.

APPROACH TO GASTRITIS

Histologic

There are many ways to approach the histologic description or classification of gastritis. The diversity of approaches reflects the fact that no single one can meet all the descriptive needs of pathologists, and the diagnostic or 'action plan' goals of endoscopists/clinicians.

The Sydney 'classification' of gastritis has been widely accepted in adults. The original approach had an endoscopic[66] as well as a histologic arm,[68] but the former is no longer used. The current Sydney system incorporates topographic, morphologic and etiologic information,[70,90] that is, location (antrum or body) and histologic parameters – inflammation, activity, atrophy, intestinal metaplasia and *H. pylori* infection. Each of these is graded semiquantitatively as mild, moderate or marked. Although often referred to as the 'Sydney classification', it is actually termed the Sydney *system* by its creators.[68,70] It is just that – a system for grading the severity and distribution of histologic changes. It is based on the findings in endoscopic biopsies taken on protocol from specified areas of the stomach – two biopsies from the antrum within 2–3 cm of the pylorus, two from the gastric body and one from the incisura.

The major purpose of the Sydney system is to quantitate the degree of atrophy and intestinal metaplasia in patients with *H. pylori* gastritis, the main risk factor for these preneoplastic changes. Although atrophy and intestinal metaplasia do occur in children, and are both over- and under-called, they remain rare compared with their incidence in adults. The Sydney system is far from perfect in assessing atrophy and metaplasia (see Atrophy below); in addition, it does not classify non-inflammatory conditions.

For these reasons, the Sydney system has little broad application to children. With recently suggested modifications to improve the rate of pick-up of metaplasia (see Atrophy below), it may be useful for study purposes in populations of children with a high prevalence of early-acquired *H. pylori* infection, and in areas of the world with a high prevalence of gastric cancer.

However, it is the authors' opinion that no histologic system will be ideal in children until pediatric gastroenterologists routinely obtain the material needed for reliable histologic analysis (i.e. map the stomach in children with *H. pylori* gastritis or those at risk of atrophy and metaplasia from other causes). It would be better to focus on getting good tissue in individual patients and carefully analyzing the findings with an experienced GI pathologist, than worrying about which classification system to use.

The Sydney system should therefore be used to quantitate histologic changes in individual pediatric patients who have been shown to have atrophy and intestinal metaplasia.

Other ways to approach the histology are descriptive, and semiquantitative, as discussed below.

Inflammation

One approach is to describe the types of cell present and their distribution in the mucosa. 'Acute' or 'active' refers to the presence of neutrophils, 'chronic' refers to the presence of round cells (lymphocytes, monocytes, plasma cells) and 'chronic active' refers to a combination of a chronic process with some neutrophils present.

There are no precise definitions for chronic gastric inflammation because the 'normal' number of mononuclear 'allowable' is unknown.[68,70,90] Although adult 'normal' or asymptomatic volunteers sometimes undergo endoscopy and biopsy as a baseline for studies, their histology even in 'health' may reflect many variables, such as normal aging, smoking, intake of alcohol, NSAIDs, etc.

These findings cannot be extrapolated to children, who should have 'virgin' mucosa, unaffected by aging or toxins.

Nevertheless, a working definition of chronic inflammation in adults that is widely accepted is the presence of more than a few lymphocytes, plasma cells and/or macrophages per high-power field.[70] In children, some acceptable numbers are available from 'retrospective normals'. The information is summarized elsewhere,[7] but in cells per mm^2.

Unlike the presence of round cells in the mucosa, the presence of any number of neutrophils is regarded as abnormal, indicating acute or active inflammation.

The presence of lymphoid follicles is strongly suggestive of active *H. pylori* infection in children[46,55,91] and adults,[58,90] and although initially considered to be a feature of *H. pylori* only in children, if specifically sought, they are said to be present in 100% of adult patients with *H. pylori*.[90] If lymphoid follicles and inflammation are present in the absence of *H. pylori*, it is likely that the organism has been missed. In *H. pylori* infection, lymphoid follicles may be absent if biopsies of sufficient size and number are not taken. The distinction between a lymphoid follicle (active germinal center) and a lymphoid aggregate (no active germinal center) is important – the former are generally found only in active gastritis due to *H. pylori* or other causes, whereas the latter may be found in non-inflamed, non-infected gastric mucosa.[55,58,91]

In addition to the types of cells and lymphoid collections, descriptive terminology also includes the extent or depth of inflammation in the mucosa. This may be described as 'superficial', 'deep' or 'pan-mucosal', and as 'diffuse' or 'focal'. These terms can be combined, to provide an overall description, for instance 'chronic active, pan-mucosal'. The severity of gastritis can be quantitated by a scoring system[55] for comparison of effect of treatment.

Atrophy and intestinal metaplasia

Gastric atrophy (also known as 'atrophic gastritis') is an important consequence of gastritis. It is considered to be a pre-neoplastic lesion when a certain type of intestinal metaplasia develops in the atrophic mucosa.[92–95] That atrophy is far more prevalent in adults follows from the fact that chronicity of inflammation is a contributor. However, there is little information on atrophic gastritis in children. This is likely due to its truly much lower prevalence, as well as to underdiagnosis because, unfortunately, multi-zone multi-biopsy of the stomach is seldom performed by pediatric gastroenterologists. Atrophic gastritis of the stomach is a patchy lesion and may be missed by sampling error, if sufficient tissue from multiple sites is not obtained.[96] In addition, atrophy is traditionally regarded as a disease of adults, so pediatric gastroenterologists may fail to recognize that it may be present in a given child, or subset of patients.

Gastric atrophy has been described as a loss of normal gland components and/or the presence of intestinal metaplasia. It is widely accepted that intestinal metaplasia *per se* consititutes a form of atrophic gastritis, even if gland loss is not striking.[97] More recently, some have expanded the definition to include the presence of pseudo-pyloric metaplasia of the corpus, which is identified by the presence of pepsinogen I in mucosa that is topographically corpus but phenotypically antrum.[98] Atrophy may be missed if pseudopyloric mucosa is not sought, and recognized to be metaplastic.

Considerable caution should be exercised in interpreting or acting on reports of 'atrophic gastritis' and 'intestinal metaplasia'. There is some subjectivity in calling gland loss, even among experts. In addition, when active inflammation is present, inflammatory cells and edema may push glands apart, and give an appearance of atrophy that is reversible by treatment of the underlying *H. pylori* infection, so-called 'pseudo-atrophy'.[99] Thus, atrophy can be overcalled. True atrophy occurs when gland loss has occurred, regeneration is not present, and fibrosis has occurred, with or without metaplasia. In advanced atrophy there may be relatively little inflammation, as the acute and chronic injury may have passed and left a 'quiescent' damaged mucosa. For all of these reasons, interobserver reliability in calling atrophy is less than ideal.[98,100]

Atrophic gastritis and intestinal metaplasia do occur in children, although apparently not often.[94] Although *H. pylori* infection is far and away the most important cause of atrophic gastritis worldwide, atrophy may result from any severe, chronic mucosal injury to the gastric mucosa. In children, the authors have seen it occur with intestinal metaplasia in severe chronic varioliform gastritis and in autoimmune disease (scleroderma) with GI tract involvement. Severity appears to be a factor in addition to chronicity.

Focal intestinal metaplasia may be found very rarely as a congenital occurrence, as has been observed in an autopsy study of neonatal stomachs.[101] If a single focus of a few intestinalized cells is found on random biopsy (usually antrum), this may be congenital or could represent evidence of healing of some previous focal injury. However, if more than a few cells are metaplastic, or more than one focus are found, this may represent a more widespread mucocal disorder. Such findings cannot be interpreted in the absence of detailed mucosal mapping.

Patterns of chronic atrophic gastritis are discussed further under *H. pylori* gastritis.

Endoscopic/clinical

Categorization of entities into gastritides and gastropathies can be helpful in narrowing the diagnostic possibilities in a given case. Further classification of gastritides and peptic ulcer disease according to underlying cause may help to understand the natural history of a lesion.

In Table 25.2, gastritis and gastropathy have been classified primarily by their endoscopic appearance into *erosive* and *hemorrhagic* or *non-erosive* types. The classification cannot be considered absolute, because the same disorder can sometimes present with erosive gastritis, sometimes non-erosive. The purpose is to give the endoscopist a conceptual framework for approaching the patient.

Each disorder is classified by its commonest presentation in the practice of the authors. For example, although Crohn's disease and CMV gastritis are most often non-

Erosive and hemorrhagic gastritis or gastropathy
'Stress' gastropathy
Neonatal gastropathies
Traumatic gastropathy
Aspirin and other NSAIDs
Other drugs
Portal hypertensive gastropathy
Uremic gastropathy
Chronic varioliform gastritis
Bile gastropathy
Henoch–Schönlein gastropathy
Corrosive gastropathy
Exercise-induced gastropathy/gastritis
Radiation gastropathy
Non-erosive gastritis or gastropathy
'Non-specific' gastritis
Helicobacter pylori gastritis
Crohn's gastritis
Allergic gastritis
Proton pump inhibitor gastropathy
Celiac gastritis
Gastritis of chronic granulomatous disease
Cytomegalovirus gastritis
Eosinophilic gastritis
Collagenous gastritis
Graft *vs* host disease
Ménétrièr's disease
Pernicious anemia
Gastritis with autoimmune diseases
Plasmacytoma
Cancer
Gastric lymphoma (MALT lymphoma)
Other granulomatous gastritides
Cystinosis
Phlegmonous and emphysematous gastritis
Other infectious gastritides

Note: Although some disorders can present as either erosive or non-erosive gastritis/gastropathy, each is classified by its most common presentation.

Table 25.2 Classification of gastritis/gastropathy in children

erosive, they often progress to erosions and ulcers. *H. pylori* gastritis is classified as non-erosive, because it most often presents with normal or nodular mucosa, with abnormalities seen only on histologic examination, but it can cause erosions or ulcers in the stomach (and duodenum).

These examples also serve to illustrate the key point that gastritis and ulcer disease are part of a continuum of response to injury.

GASTRITIS

Erosive and/or hemorrhagic gastritis or gastropathy

'Stress' gastropathy

Stress erosions are typically asymptomatic, multiple, superficial and do not perforate; however, when they do present, they do so with overt upper GI hemorrhage. They usually involve the oxyntic mucosa, with early lesions predominantly in the fundus and proximal body, later spreading to the antrum to produce a diffuse erosive and hemorrhagic appearance; antral involvement alone is uncommon. They are not usually associated with significant underlying mucosal inflammation. Stress lesions usually occur within 24 h of the onset of critical illness in which physiologic stress is present, such as shock, hypoxemia, acidosis, sepsis, burns, major surgery, multiple organ system failure or head injury. These stressors cause a reduction of gastric blood flow with subsequent mucosal ischemia,[102,103] and breakdown of mucosal defenses due to local acidosis and decreased production of mucus and bicarbonate.[104,105] As a result 'back diffusion' of gastric acid causes mucosal injury. Gastric acid is important in the pathogenesis of stress erosions, but actual hypersecretion is seen only in cases of sepsis and central nervous system trauma.[106] Risk factors for hemorrhage include gastric hypersecretion, mechanical ventilation and use of corticosteroids.[104,107] Newborns and infants appear to be more prone to perforation.[108]

Neonatal gastropathies

Upper GI endoscopy is infrequently required in the neonatal period as this procedure is unlikely to reveal specific lesions that alter the infant's supportive management. Most neonatal gastropathies are due to physiologic stress, including prematurity, hypoxemia, prolonged ventilatory support, sepsis and acid–base imbalance. Although hemorrhagic gastropathy has been reported in otherwise healthy full-term infants presenting with severe upper GI hemorrhage,[109] and also in one patient as antenatal hemorrhage,[110] most cases of hemorrhagic gastropathy are reported in sick neonates in the intensive care unit. Fatal hemorrhagic gastropathy has been reported in neonates treated with sulindac for patent ductus arteriosus[111] or with dexamethasone for bronchopulmonary dysplasia.[112] A high prevalence of hemorrhagic gastropathy was found in asymptomatic sick neonates who underwent endoscopy as part of a research protocol.[113] Of note, in that series newborns without symptoms,[113] and in other series[114,115] those with upper GI symptoms or signs, seemed to have a high prevalence of hemorrhagic lesions described as 'esophagitis' associated with gastropathy. These lesions are probably due to mechanical suctioning at the time of delivery, or later. A retrospective study of 107 neonates who underwent upper GI endoscopy for irritability during feeds and hematemesis showed that 95% of those with hematemesis had endoscopically identifiable lesions.[115] In addition, endoscopy in sick small infants is not without risk. More often than not, a conservative approach will better serve the patient.

Endoscopy may be helpful in the rare instances of neonatal upper GI bleeding that is unresponsive to medical therapy, such as an actively or recurrently bleeding ulcer that may be amenable to endoscopic hemostasis,[116] or to guide surgery, or for diagnosis and hemostasis in the extremely rare case of a gastric Dieulafoy lesion.[117]

An unusual gastropathy may occur in infants with congenital heart disease receiving prolonged infusions of prostaglandin E to maintain patency of the ductus arteriosus. This consists of antral mucosal thickening or a focal mass due to foveolar cell hyperplasia, presenting as gastric outlet obstruction.[118] This entity has also been described in a 6-week-old infant who received no medications.[119]

Traumatic gastropathy

Forceful retching or vomiting produces typical subepithelial hemorrhages in the fundus and proximal body of the stomach. This is due to 'knuckling' or trapping of the proximal stomach into the distal esophagus, resulting in vascular congestion, and is also known as *prolapse gastropathy*.[120–122] Mallory–Weiss tears immediately above or below the gastroesophageal junction also may occur. Although both prolapse gastropathy and tears tend to resolve quickly, they can result in significant blood loss. By a similar mechanism of trauma, linear erosions may occur in the herniated gastric mucosa of patients with a large hiatal hernia, resulting in chronic blood loss anemia.[123] Gastric erosions may result from trauma secondary to long-term nasogastric tube placement. Aggressive continuous suction through nasogastric tubes, especially in children who are receiving anticoagulants, can cause severe subepithelial hemorrhage and bleeding. Ingestion of foreign bodies, gastrostomy feeding devices and endoscopic procedures such as diathermy[124–126] are also common causes of subepithelial hemorrhage, erosion and ulcer. Figure 25.2 shows a gastric ulcer associated with a migrating gastric feeding device ('buried bumper syndrome').

Aspirin and other NSAIDs

NSAIDs are the most commonly prescribed drugs in the world.[127,128] Although invaluable for the treatment of many disorders, the usefulness of NSAIDs is limited largely by their adverse effects on the GI tract. NSAIDs can result in mucosal damage, ranging from histologic changes alone to Frank ulceration; patients may be asymptomatic or suffer life-threatening ulcer bleeding or perforation. Less frequent but well recognized effects occur in the small and large bowel, and esophagus.

The beneficial and deleterious effects of NSAIDs arise primarily through their ability to inhibit the cyclo-oxygenase (COX)-catalyzed conversion of arachidonic acid to prostaglandins,[129] although it is the topical action of NSAIDs on gastric mucosa that most likely causes acute hemorrhage and erosions within hours of ingestion, even with low doses of NSAID.[130] These early lesions are often asymptomatic and *per se* are not predictive of clinically significant ulcer formation.[131,132] Prostaglandins produced by the COX-1 pathway are largely 'constitutive' (i.e. responsible for mucosal integrity and hemostasis). Inhibition of COX-1 compromises mechanisms of mucosal protection, such as mucus and bicarbonate production, epithelial integrity and regenerative capacity, and microvascular supply. In contrast, prostaglandins produced by the COX-2 ('inducible') pathway mediate pain, inflammation and fever. There is overlap, however, and dual suppression of COX-1 and COX-2 is necessary for GI mucosal damage to occur. Aspirin and other NSAIDS such as ibuprofen, naproxen, sulindac, diclofenac, indometacin, mefenamic acid and meloxicam are non-selective COX inhibitors (i.e. they inhibit both pathways). Aspirin has an additional effect: the inhibition of thromboxane production by platelets.[133,134] As platelets are anuclear, the effect is permanent for the life of the platelet. Although this property is of benefit in primary or secondary cardiovascular prophylaxis, it does enhance bleeding from the GI tract.

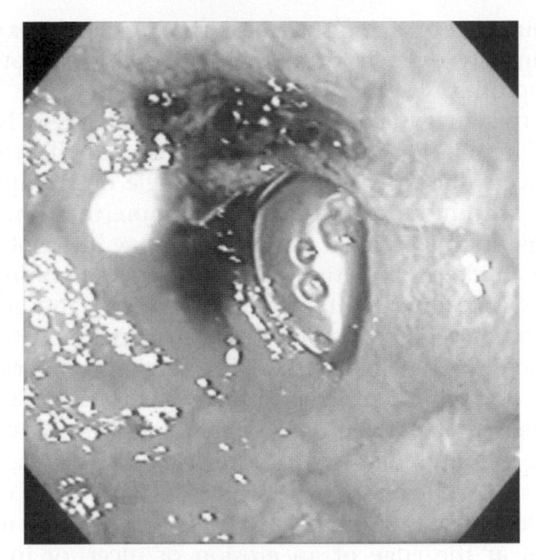

Figure 25.2: The intragastric balloon component of a gastrostomy button is seen migrating through the stomach wall. The device is surrounded by ulceration and blood clots. This patient with cerebral palsy had presented with acute hematemesis and irritability (*See plate section for color*).

Some adverse effects may result from topical action of ingested NSAIDs on the gastroduodenal mucosa, but the systemic presence alone of an NSAID compromises mucosal integrity and may produce severe ulceration of the mucosa. Although many patients report that enteric-coated ('buffered') aspirin is associated with fewer symptoms, enteric-coating of aspirin does not prevent complications.[129,130] Factors that place patients at higher risk for severe gastroduodenal ulceration and complications of NSAIDs include a history of ulcer (complicated or uncomplicated), drug dose, comcomitant use of aspirin and another NSAID, use of a corticosteroid, age over 65 years, use of an anticoagulant and, possibly, *H. pylori* infection.[127,128,134,135] Although gastric acid does not appear to be a primary causative factor in NSAID mucosal injury, acid suppression with PPIs does reduce the risk of gastroduodenal ulceration and bleeding. This suggests that some acid appears to be required for lesions to develop, but not much, as NSAID lesions do occur in achlorhydric subjects.[129]

The newer (selective) COX-2 inhibitors, or 'coxibs', such as celecoxib, rofecoxib and valdecoxib produce fewer adverse GI effects in adults, but these drugs are expensive and not free of such effects. Concerns regarding safety and adverse effects, especially myocardial infarction and stroke, have recently resulted in withdrawal of some of these agents from the United States drug market. Rates of upper GI symptoms ('dyspepsia') are only slightly lower on these drugs than on traditional non-selective NSAIDs.

Combination of a coxib with aspirin – even in low dose – substantially detracts from their otherwise improved GI safety profile.[136]

There are few data on the adverse GI effects of NSAIDs in children, but they do occur.[137–143] As in adults, erosions and ulcers due to NSAIDs may be single or multiple; the gastric antrum tends to be involved more than the body, but any or all regions of the stomach may be involved. In young children, ulceration of the incisura presenting with upper GI bleeding is a typical NSAID lesion, and bleeding may occur after just one or two doses of drug, or with more chronic use. The characteristic histologic NSAID lesion in adults and children is a reactive gastropathy, that is, epithelial hyperplasia, mucin depletion, enlarged (reactive) nuclei, fibromuscular (smooth muscle) hyperplasia, vascular ectasia and edema.[144] Less often, NSAIDs may cause a reactive gastritis. Reactive gastropathy or gastritis may be present at the edge of an erosion or ulcer, or in endoscopically normal mucosa distant from such lesions, but it may also be absent even in the presence of severe NSAID lesions. Reactive gastropathy is not specific to NSAID injury; rather it is a non-specific feature of 'chemical' injury of the gastric mucosa.[5,144]

In children presenting with abdominal pain, blood loss, anemia or upper GI lesions at endoscopy, it is particularly important actively to solicit a history of use of over-the-counter NSAIDs, as parents and children often fail to mention non-prescription drugs in the medication history. For this reason, adverse effects due to NSAIDs in children likely are under-recognized. Use of NSAIDs has increased among children, for example for management of fever in infants. In a recent prospective randomized short-term clinical trial in children under 2 years of age treated for fever,[141] there was no significant difference in the incidence of acute GI bleeding between ibuprofen ($n = 17\,938$) and acetaminophen ($n = 9127$). Only seven of the children receiving ibuprofen (dosage 5 and 10 mg/kg, 6–10 doses over 3 days) had symptoms of vomiting or hematemesis; minor bleeding occurred in three children, not requiring transfusion, and related to forceful vomiting in some. Based on this study, short-term use in this age group appears to be relatively benign, but more data are required.

However, the main area of concern is long-term use of NSAIDs. Upper GI bleeding following NSAID ingestion in children has been well documented.[137–141] Naproxen is the most commonly used NSAID in pediatric rheumatologic practice.[143] In one study, 75% of children with juvenile rheumatoid arthritis who had taken one or more NSAIDs for over 2 months had endoscopic evidence of gastropathy, antral erosions or ulcers;[139] of these, 64% had anemia and abdominal pain. Another study in children with rheumatoid disease showed a relative risk for gastroduodenal injury of 4.8 in those taking NSAIDs *vs* those not taking these drugs.[140] In that study, abdominal pain was present in 28% of patients taking NSAIDs compared with 15% in those not.

Because NSAIDs are protein-bound, and hypoalbuminemia may occur in systemic juvenile rheumatoid arthritis, there is potential for greater NSAID toxicity due to higher levels of free drug.[143] This specific aspect has not been studied in children.

Strategies for minimization of risk in NSAID use include use of selective COX-2 inhibitors and/or concurrent use of PPIs or misoprostol.[128,129,134,135] Although both PPIs and misoprostol are effective in preventing morbidity, the adverse effects (abdominal cramps, diarrhea) of misoprostol limit its use, so that PPIs are likely to be much better accepted in children, as in adults. At present, however, there are no data on this indication in children.

Risk reduction also involves consideration of *H. pylori* status. Although gastropathy induced by NSAIDs does not require the presence of *H. pylori* for its development,[145] there are conflicting and confusing data regarding the role and timing of *H. pylori* eradication in healing NSAID ulcers in adults. For example, studies on omeprazole healing of NSAID ulcers showed higher healing rates with PPIs in *H. pylori*-positive than in *H. pylori*-negative patients.[146,147] Similar results were obtained from an analysis combining the Food and Drug Administration trials for both lansoprazole and NSAID ulcers.[148] This has led some to argue that *H. pylori* infection should not be treated until after the PPI has healed the ulcer; however, there is no consensus on this issue. In *H. pylori*-infected adults with no ulcer disease, evidence for the effectiveness of *H. pylori* eradication as ulcer prophylaxis in chronic NSAID users is also contradictory.[149–151] Nevertheless, the weight of evidence seems to suggests that when there is a history of *H. pylori* ulcer disease eradication of *H. pylori* is indicated before instituting NSAID use.[134,149,151] Until data indicate otherwise, it seems prudent to eradicate *H. pylori* in children requiring high-dose or long-term NSAIDs.

Use of NSAIDs in children may continue to increase, but will likely follow the trends in adults based on the availability and side-effect profile of the newer coxibs. Pediatric patients considered for NSAID therapy may include those with premalignant intestinal polyposis syndromes, and perhaps those with premalignant conditions such as chronic inflammatory bowel disease and Barrett's esophagus. Data on NSAID use in children are much needed.

Other drugs

Although many drugs can cause non-ulcer dyspepsia, erosive or hemorrhagic gastropathies have been described with valproic acid, dexamethasone, chemotherapeutic agents, alcohol, potassium chloride, iron, long-term fluoride ingestion and cysteamine.[112,152–161]

Portal hypertensive gastropathy (PHG)

This congestive gastropathy is common in children with both cirrhotic and non-cirrhotic portal hypertension, but is not related to the severity of underlying liver disease, the size of esophageal varices, the presence of hypersplenism or a previous history of bleeding and variceal sclerotherapy.[162,163] The endoscopic findings of PHG vary from a mild gastropathy with a mosaic pattern of 2–5-mm erythematous patches separated by a fine white lattice, to a severe gastropathy typified by the presence of cherry-red spots or even a confluent hemorrhagic appearance.[162,164,165] (Fig. 25.3). Although hem-

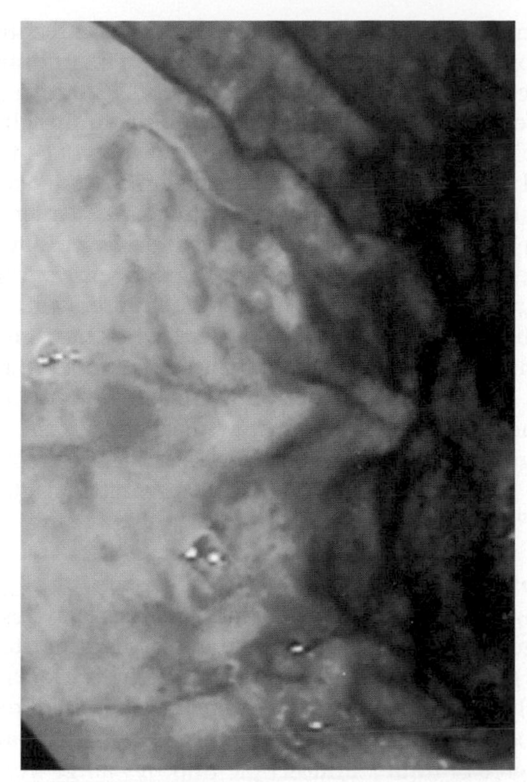

Figure 25.3: Endoscopic view of the stomach demonstrates cherry-red spots overlying a mildly swollen erythematous gastric body mucosa in a patient with portal hypertensive gastropathy and esophageal varices secondary to biliary atresia (*See plate section for color*).

orrhage from PHG is not usually catastrophic, bleeding may occur and result in severe blood loss anemia. In adults, congestive gastropathy is more frequently associated with large gastroesophageal varices than with esophageal varices alone,[165,166] and sclerotherapy of esophageal varices may exacerbate PHG and gastric varices. In contrast, PHG, which develops only after variceal obliteration therapy, is more likely to be transient and less severe.[166,167]

The histologic findings in PHG are ectasia of mucosal capillaries and venules, and submucosal venous dilation, without any significant inflammatory infiltrate.[163,165] However, PHG is an endoscopic diagnosis; biopsy is not required and is potentially dangerous.

Uremic gastropathy

In acute renal failure, gastropathy may be due to physiologic stress rather than renal failure itself. When GI bleeding occurs in acute renal failure, it is associated with erosions and/or ulcers in 71% of cases in adults and with an increased risk of death and duration of hospital stay; additional factors that predispose to bleeding are use of corticosteroids and concurrent disease such as liver cirrhosis.[168]

Chronic renal failure (CRF) is associated with increased densities of parietal, chief and gastrin-producing cells.[169] Despite this, gastric pH may be less acid than expected; this may reflect neutralization of gastric acid with ammonia, a breakdown product of urea which is very high in the gastric juice of patients with chronic renal failure.[169,170] This may explain why patients are more likely to suffer acid–pepsin complications after treatment, that is, lowering the urea/gastric nitrogen levels may remove their neutralizing effect on gastric acid. Hypergastrinemia associated with CRF is likely to be secondary to the gastric acid neutralization as well as reduced gastrin clearance.[169–171]

There are few data on the effects of CRF on the stomach of children. In adults, although active peptic ulcer disease does not seem to be more common in CRF, hemorrhagic gastropathy is quite prevalent in patients receiving chronic hemodialysis.[170] In such patients, gastroduodenal lesions occur in 67–82%, the predominant lesion being antral gastropathy in some 50%.[171] When peptic ulcers do occur in patients with CRF, their presentation is somewhat atypical; they are more often multiple and *H. pylori* negative, and less likely to present with pain – rather, patients tend to be symptom-free or present with bleeding.[171–173] Bleeding may be exacerbated by gastritis associated with CRF, but this is unlikely to be the primary cause. Other factors, such as *H. pylori* infection and NSAID use, should be considered.[174] Although angiodysplastic lesions in the stomach may account for some 13% of cases of upper GI bleeding in CRF, it is unclear whether they are more common in this population or simply more likely to bleed, because of uremic platelet dysfunction or hemodialyisis.[175–177] Patients with recombinant human erythropoietin-resistant anemia should be evaluated for angiodysplastic lesions.[177] In one series endoscopic 'gastritis' was reported in 10 of 17 children with CRF, with only 4 having findings localized to the gastric antrum,[178] but 'gastritis' was not defined endoscopically or histologically.

Chronic varioliform gastritis

Also known as chronic erosive gastritis, CVG is an uncommon disorder of unknown etiology that is associated with a dense lymphocytic infiltrate. Although occurring largely in middle-aged and elderly men of European decent,[60,179–181] CVG has also been reported in a few children[61,62,182,183] who present with varying combinations of upper GI symptoms, anemia, protein-losing enteropathy, peripheral eosinophilia and raised serum IgE levels. Endoscopically, the gastric folds appear thickened, but the most striking features are the innumerable prominent nodules in the fundus and proximal body of the stomach. The nodules, which are located on the crests of the folds, may have an umbilicated central crater or erosion, and are said to resemble the skin lesions of chickenpox, hence the name. Histologic features include edema, foveolar hyperplasia, plasma cell and lymphocytic inflammation, with some eosinophilic infiltrates. Focal superficial subepithelial collagen deposition may represent fibrosis at points of previous surface erosions. The authors have observed variable degrees of collagen deposition with active inflammation and gland atrophy in three adolescents (see Collagenous gastritis, below). In adults, CVG is one cause of a 'lymphocytic gastritis' in which the surface and foveolar epithelium is infiltrated with darkly staining T cells, as in celiac disease.[180,181,184] The lymphocytic infiltrate is much heavier than that seen in association with *H. pylori* infection, and is more prominent in the gastric body.[184] Other causes of lymphocytic gastritis are shown in Table 25.3.

Bile gastropathy

Bile reflux or duodenogastroesophageal reflux (DGER) is well documented following gastric surgery such as Bilroth I and II, and after selective vagotomy with pyloroplasty.[185] Reports of DGER in the intact stomach, however, are confined mainly to the adult literature.[186,187] Bile reflux is reported in normal adolescents who present with reflux-type symptoms that do not respond to conventional acid-suppressing therapy. Gastric bile exposure, measured by means of bile absorbance studies, was 30–75%, compared with 31% in healthy adult controls.[188] The mere finding of bile in the stomach at endoscopy is common and unlikely to be of any significance. Typical endoscopic features of DGER include 'beefy' redness or erythema, bile staining of the gastric mucosa, and occasionally erosions. Despite this, there is little or no increased cellular infiltrate in the lamina propria, the main histologic features of this condition being epithelial – foveolar hyperplasia (occasionally with a corkscrew appearance), lamina propria edema and venous congestion.[185] These changes constitute the entity of a so-called *reactive gastropathy*.[3,144] After srugery they are found more commonly in the stomach than at the anastomosis. Other features include anastomotic erosions, lipid islands and mucosal cysts; the latter are sometimes grossly visible and are known as *gastritis cystica profunda/polyposa*. Some studies report a high prevalence of intestinal metaplasia, although this may reflect sampling from the anastomotic region, which normally contains a mosaic of gastric and intestinal mucosa. Fortunately, nowadays, there are hardly any indications for partial gastrectomy in children, and pyloroplasty in children[189] is seldom recognized to be associated with the above problems.

Henoch–Schönlein gastritis

Henoch–Schönlein purpura (HSP) is a frequently recognized multisystem disorder due to an immune complex-mediated vasculitis. It can present in children and adults of all ages with involvement of skin, GI tract, kidneys and joints. GI symptoms and signs include colicky abdominal pain, nausea and vomiting, and gastrointestinal tract bleeding. Less common serious abdominal complications include intramural hematoma, intussusception, bowel infarction, bowel perforation, pancreatitis, appendicitis and cholecystitis. In HSP, endoscopic findings in the stomach include erythematous or hemorrhagic mucosa, mucosal edema, with erosions or ulcers. Raised blebs may be seen with associated punctate hemorrhages, central erosions or an ulcer with a yellow base.[63,64] The findings may be patchy, antral predominant, or diffuse.[190] Similar lesions are often present in the duodenum and jejunum. Although gastric mucosal biopsies are usually too superficial to show typical histologic changes, they may show a leukoclastic vasculitis similar to that seen in the skin.[63] Patients may have a raised serum IgA and reduced factor XIII levels.[63,64] Endoscopy is seldom required for the diagnosis of this condition, although it may be helpful in children with persistent abdominal pain or vomiting who have not yet demonstrated the typical non-thrombocytopenic rash of HSP. A few may never develop the rash.[191–193] All children with hematemesis, even those with the HSP rash, should undergo endoscopy to diagnose complications or other causes of upper GI bleeding, such as duodenal ulcer disease.[190]

Celiac disease
Ménétrièr's disease in adults
Cytomegalovirus infection
Chronic varioliform gastritis
Helicobacter pylori infection
Idiopathic

Table 25.3 Causes of lymphocytic gastritis

Corrosive gastropathy

The ingestion of strong acids and alkalis usually results in damage to the esophagus, but may involve the stomach. When gastric injury does occur, the pre-pyloric area is particularly vulnerable,[194,195] probably because of pylorospasm and pooling of secretions. The presence of food may limit the degree of injury. Endoscopic findings range from mild friability and erythema to necrosis, ulcers, exudates, hemorrhage and gastric outlet obstruction with perforation rarely occurring. Chronic cicatrization is relatively infrequent and may take several months to become apparent, hence the need for serial imaging or evaluation. Transabdominal ultrasonography was reported to be useful in one series in localizing injury and in determining its depth and the presence of peristalsis, thereby reducing repeated radiation exposure.[196] Iron poisoning, especially with ferrous sulfate, is common in children in some areas of the world, and may cause a corrosive gastropathy with stricture.[197] Therapeutic administration of oral ferrous sulfate can cause mild endoscopic abnormalities in the stomach; these are of uncertain clinical significance.[198] Pine oil cleaner ingestion may also cause cause gastric injury.[199] Failure of button batteries to transit the stomach may cause ulceration from chemical or thermal damage, and possibly even increased blood levels of toxic metals.[200] Caustic ingestons and their management are discussed in more detail in Chapter 17.

Exercise-induced gastropathy or gastritis

This condition is well recognized in long-distance runners, usually presenting with blood loss anemia, with or without upper GI symptoms. Symptoms often occur post-exercise and include abdominal cramps or epigastric pain, nausea, gastroesophageal reflux and vomiting.[201] These symptoms may arise following altered blood circulation and also altered motility occurring in marathon runners.[202] Both erosive gastropathy and non-erosive gastritis have been described with mucosal lesions, occurring almost equally in the gastric antrum, body and fundus.[203,204] Gastritis is usually acute, with hemorrhagic inflammation on biopsy. Postulated mechanisms include splanchnic ischemia with reports of up to 80% reduction in visceral blood flow compared with pre-exercise level.[205] Strenuous exercise does not appreciably affect postprandial gastric secretion or gastric emptying.[206]

Cystinosis

This rare autosomal recessive lysosomal storage disorder is characterized by the deposition of cystine within macrophages of most body organs. Studies have shown that daily cysteamine therapy can reduce the rate of renal and thyroid deterioration, and improve growth and life expectancy.[207] At high doses cysteamine is extremely ulcerogenic and has been used to induce duodenal ulcers in laboratory animals.[208] Cysteamine is a potent secretagog, causing hypergastrinemia and gastric acid hypersecretion, which occur for 1–2 h after drug ingestion.[28,207] Its additional ulcerogenic effects are due to delayed gastric emptying and inhibition of gastric bicarbonate and mucus production.

At endoscopy, 2 of 11 poorly controlled children with cystinosis had a distinctive diffuse fine nodular appearance throughout the stomach.[28] In contrast to the gastric nodularity seen in *H. pylori* gastritis, the nodules of cystinosis are much smaller; their distribution is pangastric and is not associated with underlying inflammatory infiltrate. Under electron microscopic magnification, crystalline structures representing cystine are seen within lysosomes of macrophages of the lamina propria in gastric biopsies.[28]

Radiation gastropathy

This uncommon condition, described primarily in adults, is associated with abdominal irradiation of patients with malignancy, and causes erosions or ulcers particularly in the gastric antrum and pre-pyloric regions,[209] as well as severe diffuse hemorrhagic gastritis or gastropathy.[210,211] Fibrosis and stricture formation may occur and lead to gastric outlet obstruction. Although a high total radiation dose and, perhaps more importantly, a high daily fraction appear to be the main risk factors, hemorrhagic gastritis can occur even with low total radiation dosages of 40 Gy.[210,211] Treatment of hemorrhagic gastritis can be difficult, but there has been some success using argon plasma coagulation at the time of esophagogastroduodenoscopy. In other cases surgical resection may be required.[212–214]

Non-erosive gastritis or gastropathy

Some of the entities in this section may also present as an erosive gastropathy or gastritis, but are included here as they more commonly present without erosions.

In non-erosive gastritis, there is usually poor correlation between endoscopic appearance and histologic findings, that is, the diagnosis is usually established on the basis of histology. Lymphocytic gastritis is a type of gastritis deserving special mention; it may be seen in disorders as diverse as celiac disease, CMV gastritis, Ménétrièr's disease, *H. pylori* infection and chronic varioliform gastritis (Table 25.3). Because ours is an endoscopic classification, lymphocytic gastritis is mentioned under each of those disease entities.

Helicobacter pylori gastritis

H. pylori is the most common cause of gastritis in the world. In addition, given its association with peptic ulcer disease, atrophic gastritis and adenocarcinoma, and with the rare entity of gastric lymphoma, it is the most important.[55,56,215–217] The majority of individuals with *H. pylori* gastritis are asymptomatic, unless they develop ulcer disease, adenocarcinoma or lymphoma.[44–46] The prevalence of *H. pylori* varies widely between socioeconomic classes and countries. This and other aspects pertinent to the infection itself are addressed in Chapter 26.

Acute infection In infected adults and children *H. pylori* induces an acute neutrophilic followed by a chronic gastritis,[55,215,216] which remains present for the duration of the infection. Acute infection has been studied in a number of individuals,[218–221] some of whom infected themselves for study purposes.

The acute infection may cause epigastric pain, nausea, vomiting, halitosis and headache.[218–221] An early consequence of acute infection appears to be increased gastric acid secretion followed by achlorhydria within a week or so, lasting for 6 weeks or more. The decrease in acid secretion seems to correlate with the timing and degree of inflammation of the gastric oxyntic mucosa. In the 1970s and 1980s, before the discovery of *H. pylori*, a puzzling neutrophilic gastritis with transient hypochlorhydria occurred in several research laboratories.[222,223] Patients participating in acid secretory studies were affected by profound hypochlorhydria, including a patient with Zollinger–Ellison syndrome. Normal acid secretion returned by around 4 months. The likely cause was *H. pylori* infection, recognized only much later;[224,225] this was established by antibody and histologic study of stored sera and biopsies. The intensity of inflammation and/or hypochlorhydria may have inhibited organism proliferation, and as the host and organism reached a state of equilibrium the intensity of inflammation likely decreased, as it does with return of acid secretion.

Chronic infection Some studies have suggested that acute infection with *H. pylori* quite often clears spontaneously in children,[226] although this does not appear to be the case in adults[225] in whom infection likely is lifelong if untreated. Most infected individuals develop a chronic, active, non-atrophic gastritis, which is typically asymptomatic. There is focal epithelial cell damage and an inflammatory infiltrate in the lamina propria, consisting of neutrophils, eosinophils and monocytes, largely B and T lymphocytes. There is also development of lymphoid follicles and a plasma cell infiltrate.[58]

In children and adults, the gastric antrum appears to be the commonest site of bacterial colonization and active gastritis.[55,56,97,227–230] A study in adults showed the next most prevalent area to be the gastric cardia, then the gastric body.[73] One study in children showed the gastric cardia to have a higher yield of *H. pylori*-positive biopsies than the antrum and body;[65] although this finding may be anomalous, there are no other studies in children examining the prevalence of histologic yield in different zones. The main point, however, is that the antrum is not the only repository of infection, and so multi-zone sampling is advisable. Even when inflammation is present in the body, the intensity is generally much less than that in the antrum.

In children, the antral-predominant chronic active gastritis is usually superficial, although pan-mucosal involvement does occur.[55] The cellular infiltrate is predominantly lymphocytic with neutrophils, although the latter may not be as abundant as seen in adults.[55,215,231,232] The intensity of inflammation present may vary between different countries, possibly related to the strain of *H. pylori* involved. Infected individuals in South America and Asia appear to have more marked neutrophilic infiltrates, possibly due to infection with *cagA*-positive strains.[233,234] Regional differences in patterns or severity of inflammation may also be due to socioeconomic status, age at time of infection, and exposure to other organisms.

In some individuals, chronic *H. pylori* gastritis progresses with time to atrophic gastritis, with an annual increase in prevalence among otherwise normal subjects of 1–3%.[235] This progression leads to three patterns of atrophic gastritis: body predominant, antral predominant and multifocal.[71,72,90] As the degree of atrophy progresses, the presence of active *H. pylori* infection decreases, owing to the loss of *H. pylori*-friendly acid-secreting superficial gastric mucosa, to intestinal metaplasia which does not harbor *H. pylori*. The supervention of hypochorhydria is also somewhat hostile to *H. pylori* colonization, because in the absence of acid other organisms can proliferate and offer competition for *H. pylori*. The acid–*H. pylori* relationship, and mechanisms of development of atrophy, have been well described elsewhere.[235]

Different patterns of inflammation are associated with different 'disease states' that *H. pylori* may cause. Duodenal ulcer disease is usually accompanied by an antral-predominant gastritis and very little involvement of the corpus; thus, a high acid-output state is maintained. In contrast, gastric ulcer, atrophic gastritis and cancer risk are associated with a pan-mucosal or body-predominant gastritis; this gives rise to a low acid-output state. The two patterns appear to be largely mutually exclusive: the duodenal ulcer disease state appears to 'protect' against atrophic gastritis and cancer or, perhaps more accurately, is simply unassociated with these conditions.[235]

The chronic atrophic gastritis that may result from chronic *H. pylori* infection can give rise to 'pernicious anemia', a hypochlorhydric state with megaloblastic anemia but without the autoantibodies associated with the 'classic' condition of pernicious anemia (see Pernicious anemia, below).

Endoscopy and biopsy Upper GI endoscopy and biopsies is the most reliable way to diagnose *H. pylori* infection in children.[44–46] A striking, diffuse and continuous nodularity of the antrum is the endoscopic feature of *H. pylori* infection.[55,229,236] When *H. pylori* gastritis is associated with duodenal ulcer in children, the nodularity is always present; however, when *H. pylori* causes gastritis alone ('primary gastritis'), the nodularity is seen in only some 50–60% of cases.[55] The authors have not seen this nodularity in cases of true non-*H. pylori* duodenal ulcer disease,[80] nor in any of 8000 upper GI endoscopies performed at their institution; neither ulcer disease nor *H. pylori* was present over an 18-year period. Absence of nodules, however, does not have a high negative predictive value for *H. pylori* infection or ulcer disease. Eradication of the infection results in healing of the gastritis in children, but the mucosal nodularity and histologic lymphoid hyperplasia may persist for months or years,[55,215,237,238] so the presence of nodules at endoscopy does not mean that *H. pylori* or active gastritis is present. Histologic examination is always required to determine this.

Biopsies taken from the antrum often demonstrate organisms in the layer between mucous and gastric epithelium, often in the crypts of the glands. The organisms may be seen on routine hematoxylin and eosin staining, but can be missed if a special stain such as silver (e.g. Steiner), Genta and Giemsa is not used.[239] A chronic active gastritis is present in almost all patients. If active gastritis is present and *H. pylori* is not found, there should be suspicion that the organisms may have been missed; this may occur because of sampling error (too few biopsies), the recent use of antibiotics or bismuth causing 'partial' treatment with a decreased number of organisms, or coccoid forms of the organism that may not be recognized as *H. pylori*. Use of acid-suppressing therapy may change the pattern of inflammation, causing a preferential colonization and inflammation in other zones of the stomach. Often a history of acid-suppressing medications is not obtained, especially as these, including PPIs, are available over-the-counter. Given this, in order to maximize the potential of finding *H. pylori*, and of determining whether atrophic gastritis is present, some centers (including the authors') advocate that biopsies should be taken from all zones of the stomach, including the transitional zone of gastric cardia.

Non-specific gastritis

In the authors' experience, a significant number of children have chronic gastritis for which no cause can be identified.[7] In these cases, the inflammation is chronic, lymphoplasma cellular, more focal than diffuse within the biopsy, and usually superficial. Although it appears to be more prevalent in the antrum than the corpus, this may reflect sampling bias.

Inflammatory bowel disease

Crohn's disease is the commonest cause of granulomatous disease of the stomach.[7] Although gastroduodenal involvement is relatively common, Crohn's disease is rarely isolated to the stomach and usually also involves more distal intestinal disease.[240] If disease is isolated to the upper GI tract, particularly in younger children, other conditions such as chronic granulomatous disease of childhood should be considered and excluded. Reported symptoms are similar to those of acid peptic disease and delayed gastric emptying, with hematemesis and melena occurring less frequently.[241–244] Diagnosis cannot be made reliably by any means other than endoscopy with biopsy; ^{99m}Tc-labeled HMPAO (hexa-methyl-propylene-amine-oxine) leukocyte scintigraphy often results in false-negative findings.[245] Macroscopic and/or histologic abnormalities are present in the esophagus, stomach or duodenum in up to 80% of children with Crohn's disease.[1,7] However, some of these changes are non-specific. The figure becomes 30% if features specific to Crohn's disease, such as giant cells and non-caseating granulomas, are considered; if focal deep gastritis is included, the figure becomes about 50–100%.[7,246–250] As would be expected, the figures quoted for these studies depend largely on the number of biopsy specimens taken, and whether serial sections of those specimens are examined carefully. In one study of *H. pylori-negative* adults, the focal gastritis in 80% of patients with Crohn's disease was characterized by perifoveolar or periglandular accululation of CD3+ lymphocytes and CD68+ and CD68R+ histiocytes, together with granulocytes. This characteristic gastritis was found in the antrum in 48% (36 of 75) and in the body in 24% of patients.[250]

In the appropriate clinical context, the identification of non-caseating granuloma is diagnostic of Crohn's disease, but differentiation from other granulomatous gastritides (Table 25.4) is important.[5,7] Endoscopic and/or histologic evidence of Crohn's disease of the stomach may occur in the absence of upper GI symptoms, and sometimes precedes diagnostic features in the colon.

In the authors' experience, 67 (29%) of 229 patients with Crohn's disease who underwent upper GI endoscopy had histologic evidence of gastritis;[1,7] only one-third of these had endoscopic features including loss of vascular pattern, mucosal swelling, aphthous ulcers or luminal narrowing. Deep ulceration in the duodenum can also occur, and may mimic primary peptic ulcer disease. Histologic features range from focal chronic active inflammation to more typical non-necrotizing granulomas. For both endoscopic and histologic findings, the antrum is the commonest repository of disease, but granulomas are also present in the corpus and cardia. In the authors' experience, gastric Crohn's disease is second overall to *H. pylori* as a cause of gastritis in children.[2]

Not infrequently, histologic findings of chronic antral gastritis result in a change of diagnosis from ulcerative colitis to Crohn's disease, even in absence of granuloma. However, mild chronic gastric inflammation is also seen in ulcerative colitis. Whether or not this represents a greater prevalence than in normal children is still unclear. In a recent study of 39 children with colitis but normal small bowel radiographic findings, non-specific antral gastritis was found almost equally in Crohn's disease and ulcerative colitis (92% *vs* 75%), but focal antral gastritis was more common in patients with Crohn's colitis than in those with ulcerative colitis (52% *vs* 8%).[250] In two other reports, in which 5 and 14 children respectively were said to have ulcerative colitis, gastric inflammation was typically chronic active and mild.[249,251] In the larger of the two studies, although none of the patients had moderate–severe gastritis, 69% did have mild antral gastritis. This, however, did not reach statistical significance when compared with 'control' patients who were endoscoped for possible reflux esophagitis.[251] In another retrospective study, antral focal gastritis was reported in 65% (28 of 43) of children with Crohn's disease, in 21% (5 of 24) with ulcerative colitis and in 2% (3 of 129) of patients without inflammatary bowel disease; it was not considered reliable in differentiating between the two conditions.[252]

Treatment of upper GI Crohn's disease is often challenging but may be responsive to therapy with corticosteroids, 6-mercaptopurine and infliximab.[240,253] Diagnosis and management of Crohn's disease is discussed further in Chapter 40.

Non-infectious causes
Crohn's disease
Chronic granulomatous disease
Vasculitis associated
Sarcoidosis
Infectious causes
Tuberculosis
Syphilis
Histoplasmosis
Parasites
Isolated granulomatous gastritis
Foreign body granulomas
Idiopathic

Table 25.4 Causes of gastric granulomas

Allergic and eosinophilic gastritis

Food allergies are common in the pediatric population but most often present with mild cutaneous eruptions.[254] More recently, and perhaps through the extensive use of endoscopy, other more localized diseases resulting from food interaction have been described, such as eosinophilic gastritis and esophagitis. Allergic and eosinophilic gastritis have common features and may both be part of more extensive diseases, namely allergic and eosinophilic gastroenteropathy. Allergic gastritis usually presents in infancy, but may arise at any age including pre-term infants.[255,256] Allergic gastroenteritis is a relatively benign disease of limited duration; endoscopic findings are mild, and histologic abnormalities are confined to the mucosa and often patchy. A temporal relationship between characteristic symptoms and the ingestion of certain foods is particularly helpful in establishing the diagnosis, with symptoms such as growth failure in infants, irritability, abdominal pain and vomiting occurring within 1–2 h of ingestion.[256–258] Allergic gastritis is usually associated with a specific allergen. In children, cow's or soy milk protein, egg and wheat are the most frequently identified antigens.[257,258] Vomiting may be due to allergen-induced gastric dysrhythmia and delayed gastric emptying in sensitized infants.[259] Unlike eosinophilic gastroenteropathy, in which some patients remain symptomatic into later childhood and even adulthood, in allergic gastritis reintroduction of the antigen is almost always possible by 24 months of age or earlier, although some allergies such as that to peanuts, tree nuts and seafood may persist.[256] The histologic features include an eosinophilic infiltrate in the lamina propria and the surface and foveolar epithelium; occasionally lymphocytes, plasma cells and neutrophils are present. Endoscopy may show normal mucosa, or changes similar to those of eosinophilic gastritis, but usually not so marked. However, erosions have been described in children.[254] Peripheral eosinophilia, raised serum IgE levels and positive radioallergosorbent testing for specific allergens may be observed.

Eosinophilic gastritis/gastroenteropathy is a chronic, severe disease and is often difficult to diagnose. All layers of the gastric wall may be involved; the eosinophilic infiltrate may be patchy, and there may be selective predominance of eosinophilic infiltrates in the mucosa, muscle layer or subserosa.[260] Therefore, diagnosis by endoscopy with biopsies may not always be possible; sometimes, surgical full thickness biopsy is necessary. When present, gastroscopic features are non-specific and include friability and erythema, erosions, swollen mucosal folds and scattered mucosal blebs or nodular lesions, particularly in the gastric antrum. Other causes of eosinophilic infiltration such as inflammatory bowel disease, collagen vascular disease such as scleroderma, parasite infection and and also with acute infections with the parasite Anisakis should be excluded.[261,262] The etiology of this condition is unclear as is its relationship to specific food allergens, which are often never identified. It is characterized by the presence of upper GI symptoms/signs, as well as poor growth, gastrointestinal bleeding, and often, diarrhea. Iron deficiency anemia and hypoproteinemia with protein-losing enteropathy commonly are present.[256,260,263,264] In most, but not all patients, serum IgE is elevated and peripheral eosinophilia is present.[263] A subset of the eosinophilic gastroenteropathies, however, will be food-responsive and these most likely will be due to cell-mediated and/or IgE antibody-mediated process.[258] All age groups may be affected. Treatment can often be difficult and may include dietary elimination, corticosteroids and even elemental diets.

Proton pump inhibitor gastropathy and gastric polyps

Long-term or high-dose PPI therapy often causes a characteristic hyperplasia of parietal cells, with a thickened parietal cell zone, and lingular pseudohypertrophy of individual parietal cells. Endoscopic evidence of polyps and/or nodules has been reported in children within 10–48 months of PPI therapy. Whereas some of the nodules were reported to have disappeared spontaneously, all polyps persisted during the 31-month follow-up.[265] Cystic changes often occur in the glands. In some cases, benign fundic gland polyps may be present. The parietal cell changes regress to normal some weeks after cessation of acid-suppressing therapy.[266–270] In a study of patients on long-term (mean 7.9 years) PPI therapy, ECL cell hyperplasia was reported in more than 50% of patients and was thought to be a trophic effect of the associated hypergastrinemia; no evidence of dysplasia was reported, even after 10 years of therapy.[271]

Gastric polyps unrelated to PPI therapy, although uncommon in pediatrics, should be considered in the differential diagnosis.[92] They can arise in conditions such Peutz–Jehger syndrome.

Celiac gastritis

Celiac disease exists when an immune reaction to gluten occurs. Over 95% of patients are HLA DQ2 positive and, although symptoms may appear during infancy, more typical features will occur afterwards. Although gastroscopy is usually normal, if looked for, a lymphocytic gastritis is often detected;[272–277] this is characterized by the intraepithelial location of the lymphocytic infiltrate. In one study this gastritis was present in 10 (45%) of 22 adults with celiac sprue.[275] It was characterised by a striking mononuclear infiltrate (primarily T cells), mainly in the surface and pit epithelium of the antrum and body, with sparing of the deeper glandular epithelium; the lamina propria was expanded by an infiltrate of plasma cells, lymphocytes and rare neutrophils. Children and adults with this pattern of gastritis have a mean of some 40–46 lymphocytes per 100 epithelial cells, compared with means of 3–5 in normal controls or those with the lymphocytic form of *H. pylori* gastritis.[275,276] In the latter, the infiltrate is predominantly in the lamina propria.[274] A milder lymphocytic gastritis was seen in another pediatric study.[277] The pattern of gastric lymphocytic inflammation in celiac disease resembles that seen in the small bowel and colon; this gastritis is associated with increased gastric permeability[278] and resolves in some patients following treatment of celiac disease.

In one pediatric study,[276] 15 of 25 children with celiac disease had chronic gastritis; 9 of these had lymphocytic gastritis and 6 had mild non-specific inflammation. A more recent study in children reported intraepithelial lymphocytic gastritis (antrum > body) in 29 of 33 children with untreated celiac disease; 15 of these also had evidence of focal or diffuse chronic gastritis within the lamina propria.[277] Mucin depletion was often seen when increased intraepithelial lymphocytes were associated with chronic gastritis. None of the patients had endoscopic evidence of varioliform gastritis, mucosal swelling or ulceration. The number of intraepithelial lymphocytes returned to normal with a gluten-free diet.[277] The variation in severity and prevalence of lymphocytic gastritis between studies may reflect varying amounts of dietary gluten intake as well as the lack of uniformity in the targeting of biopsies.[279] In one study, dyspeptic symptoms, such as epigastric pain and vomiting, were significantly more frequent in celiac children with lymphocytic gastritis than in those without;[276] however, no such correlation was found in another study.[277] The present authors have seen three childhood cases of celiac disease with multiple duodenal erosions, and a case of severe bleeding from multiple gastric ulcers has been described in an adult with celiac disease and lymphocytic gastritis.[280] It has been suggested that patients with *H. pylori*-negative antral-predominant lymphocytic gastritis should be evaluated for celiac disease.[279]

Chronic granulomatous disease

Chronic granulomatous disease is a rare inherited immune deficiency disorder, occurring more frequently in boys, in which granulomatous gastric wall involvement is common. This disease should be differentiated from Crohn's disease. When present, symptoms of delayed gastric emptying occur, with a narrowed, poorly mobile antrum on contrast radiography.[281–283] There are no specific endoscopic findings, but often the antral mucosa is pale, lusterless and swollen. Histologic findings include focal, chronic active inflammation in the antrum, with granulomata or multinuclear giant cells. In the authors' experience of six cases, the diagnostic lipochrome-pigmented histiocytes were absent in gastric biopsies, but were found in the lower gastrointestinal tract.[7]

Cytomegalovirus gastritis

CMV infection occurs most often in immunosuppressed children and adults, such as those with acquired immune deficiency syndrome (AIDS) or following solid organ or bone marrow transplant.[283] It has been associated in childhood with Ménétrièr's disease. CMV infection is so uncommon in apparently immunocompetent adults[284] that its finding suggests an occult malignancy or early immune deficiency.[285] In such patients, this compounds the diagnostic difficulty in distinguishing between gross or histologic lesions caused by infection, graft *vs* host disease (GVHD) and physiologic stress, or that due to chemotherapy. However, if the highly distinctive pattern of injury is present, it is more likely that CMV is the cause. The infection tends to occur in the gastric fundus and body, and may cause wall thickening, ulceration, hemorrhage and perforation.[286,287] Histologic findings include acute and chronic inflammation with edema, necrosis and cytomegalic inclusion bodies in epithelial and endothelial cells, as well as in ulcer bases and mucosa adjacent to ulcers.[288] In contrast to herpes virus infection, which tends to be superficial, CMV usually affects deeper portions of the mucosa, and the active inflammation may be focal or pan-mucosal. The diagnostic yield is increased by viral culture of mucosal biopsies and immunohistochemical detection of CMV early antigen. Treatment with ganciclovir may be beneficial in immunosuppressed patients, but otherwise spontaneous recovery usually occurs within 1–2 months.[289]

Collagenous gastritis

This rare entity, characterized by subepithelial collagen deposition and an associated gastritis, may not itself comprise a distinct disorder, but rather a consequence of inflammation or a local immune response in the stomach, or as one histologic feature of a more diffuse disease process. For example, collagenous gastritis has been described in association with the histologically similar conditions of collagenous sprue and collagenous colitis, lymphocytic colitis and celiac disease.[290–295] In some of these reports it appears to be a 'stand alone' disorder. It has also been described as a prominent histologic feature in some children with the typical endoscopic features of chronic varioliform gastritis, including diffuse gastric erythema, erosions and hemorrhage.[62,296] The pattern of mucosal fibrosis in collagenous gastritis, colitis or sprue is subepithelial in the lamina propria, and quite different from the much deeper (usually circular muscle) involvement seen in scleroderma.[297] In children, collagenous gastritis most often presents with upper abdominal pain, gastrointestinal bleeding and anemia.[62,252,297,298] None of these children had endoscopic or histologic improvement at follow-up, although symptoms may resolve with acid-suppressing treatment. In a single child who was followed for 12 years, histologic evidence of chronic active gastritis, smooth muscle hyperplasia, glandular atrophy and subepithelial collagen deposition was noted in the gastric body.[299] Adults may have profound weight loss,[300] but more often present with diarrhea, which most likely represents associated lymphocytic or collagenous colitis, or even celiac disease.[301] Symptomatic improvement has been reported with therapies including gluten-free diet, corticosteroids and aminosalicylic acid preparations.[292,293,301]

Graft *vs* host disease

Acute GVHD occurs between 21 and 100 days after transplantation, with varying degrees of mucositis, dermatitis, enteritis and hepatic dysfunction.[209] GVHD occurs most often after allogeneic bone marrow transplantation and only occasionally after solid organ transplantation. Although acute GVHD more often involves the small and large intestine, when the stomach and/or esophagus are involved, symptoms such as nausea, vomiting and upper abdominal pain are commonly reported. The stomach is an important area for the histologic diagnosis of gastrointestinal GVHD, even when diarrhea is the main symptom.[302,303] The gastric endoscopic and histologic findings, however, may also underestimate the severity of GVHD elsewhere in the gut. Endoscopy with biopsies is not routinely required for the diagnosis of GVHD, but when performed for investigation of abdominal pain or bleeding, or to exclude opportunistic infection, the findings vary considerably. They range from normal, or subtle changes, even when most or all of the epithelium is lost, to patchy erythema with erosions, to extensive mucosal sloughing. The early biopsy findings are unique to GVHD, consisting of crypt epithelial cell apoptosis and drop-out. In more severe cases, whole crypts may drop out. There is variable lymphocytic infiltration of the epithelium and lamina propria. In advanced cases, there may be ulceration, edema, fibrosis and perforation. When acute GVHD is suspected, the duodenum and esophagus should be biopsied, in addition to the proximal and distal stomach, but with recognition that duodenal biopsy carries higher risk in these patients.[302–304] Histologic distinction between GVHD, CMV infection, human immunodeficiency virus and other immunodefi-

Helicobacter heilmanii (previously *Gastrospirillum hominis*) is probably transmitted from cats and dogs,[356,357] and may cause chronic active gastritis similar to that of *H. pylori*, but with less severe inflammation, which is focal and usually restricted to the antrum.[357–360] Gastric ulceration has been reported in one teenager, and antral nodularity in another.[305,307] However, as yet, a definite association between *H. heilmanii* infection and ulcer disease has not been established.[360] Associated gastritis responds to therapy.[361]

Herpes simplex virus is a rare cause of gastritis and erosions in immunosuppressed patients, with biopsy showing the characteristic intranuclear inclusion bodies.[361,362] Evidence of herpes simplex virus type 1 was identified in 4 of 22 gastric or duodenal ulcers by means of immunohistochemistry and molecular probes.[363] The herpes zoster-varicella virus is a very rare cause of gastritis in adults and possibly in children.[364,365]

Influenza A is a rare cause of bleeding from hemorrhagic gastropathy in children, and is sometimes fatal.[366] In that series, serology was positive in all cases, but gastric biopsies were negative for virus. Bleeding may have been due to a stress gastropathy resulting from a severe systemic illness, rather than directly due to virus.

A gastropathy with hypertrophic gastric folds and protein-losing enteropathy has been described in a 3-year-old with a rising titer of IgM to *Mycoplasma pneumoniae* and no evidence of recent CMV infection.[367] Epstein–Barr virus has been associated with gastritis and diffuse lymphoid hyperplasia within the gastric mucosa.[368]

Mycobacterium tuberculosis involvement of the stomach is very rare, and usually associated with tuberculosis elsewhere or with immune deficiency.[369–371] Syphilis involving the stomach is very rare.[372]

Fungal infections of the stomach, such as candidiasis, histoplasmosis and mucormycosis, may occur, especially in sick neonates, malnourished children and those with burns or immune deficiency.[373–378] If gastric ulceration is seen in immunodeficient patients, fungal infection should be sought and, if present, treated, along with peptic ulcer therapy.

Infection with fungi of the Mucoraceae family (*Rhizopus*, *Mucor* and *Absidia*) can cause the systemic disease mucormycosis, which is fatal in malnourished or immunosuppressed children, and pre-term neonates.[379,380] Mucoraceae are ubiquitous organisms occurring in bread, fruit and decaying material. Bleeding, gastric ulcers and perforation may occur in the rare cases with involvement of the stomach.

Fungal infection of the stomach with *Histoplasma* and *Aspergillus* or the parasite *Strongyloides stercoralis* occurs rarely.[381] *Ascaris lumbracoides* was reported to cause bleeding duodenal ulcer with perforation in an infant.[382]

Acute gastric anisakiasis simplex occurs frequently in Japan and in areas of high consumption of raw fish. Gastric symptoms may occur within 3 h of ingestion and in sensitized people systemic allergic symptoms may arise within 5 h. Peripheral leukocytosis and eosinophilia may also occur. Endoscopy shows one or more worms protruding into the lumen a couple of millimeters off the gastric mucosa, surrounded by a ring of intense erythema, mucosal swelling and sometimes gastric erosions. The worms can be in the antrum or body, but tend to favor the greater curvature of the stomach. Early endoscopy is diagnostic and therapeutic, allowing for removal of worms and relief of symptoms.[263,383–385]

PEPTIC ULCER DISEASE

Peptic ulcers can be classified as primary or secondary (Table 25.5). Secondary ulcers are those occurring in the presence of systemic underlying disease, whereas in primary ulcer disease this is usually not present.

The categorization is essentially based on etiology, but there are other general qualities that are consistent with this approach. For example, *primary* peptic ulcers are usually chronic, with fibrinopurulent debris overlying active inflammatory infiltrate, granulation tissue and fibrosis.[386] In contrast, *secondary* peptic ulcers are usually more acute in onset, often induced by physiologic stress or drug ingestion, and not generally fibrotic. Primary peptic ulcers are more often duodenal, whereas secondary ulcers are more often gastric. In children, primary ulcers may be single, with a punched-out appearance, raised rolled edges, sometimes with satellite erosions, or may be multiple and shallower. Most primary peptic ulcers in children occur between the ages of 8 and 17 (mean 11.5) years,[2,55,56] whereas secondary ulcer disease occurs at all ages, depending on the cause of the underlying gastritis.

Historic perspective

There have been a number of important milestones in the development of our understanding and the treatment of peptic ulcer disease. In the early part of the twentieth century, psychologic stress and diet were regarded as the key pathogenetic factors for peptic ulceration. Therefore, patients with peptic ulcers were hospitalized for bedrest and prescribed unpalatable 'bland diets'. In the 1950s, attention was focused on the major pathogenetic role of

Primary peptic ulcers
H. pylori associated
H. pylori negative or idiopathic
Zollinger–Ellison syndrome
G-cell hyperplasia or hyperfunction
Systemic mastocytosis
Cystic fibrosis
Short bowel syndrome
Hyperparathyroidism
Secondary peptic ulcers
Most causes of gastritis and gastropathy, as listed in Table 25.2

Table 25.5 Classification of peptic ulcer disease in children

gastric acid, and buffering of acid with antacids, or with continuous milk feeds, was in vogue. When Dragsted introduced surgical acid reduction with vagotomy, such was the unpleasantness of the 'bland' or 'alkali diet' that even surgery appeared an attractive option. Even though surgery was attended by high failure rates and significant morbidity, it remained a mainstay of therapy for recalcitrant or recurrent ulcer disease. The advent of the H_2-receptor antagonist cimetidine in the 1970s ushered in the era of acid suppression, replacing buffering. In the 1980s, the introduction of PPIs allowed for more potent acid suppression and better ulcer healing rates. However, studies showed that some 90% of healed ulcers relapsed within a year if treatment with acid-suppressing agents was discontinued. Therefore, until the late twentieth century, peptic ulcer disease was regarded as a chronic relapsing, largely incurable, disorder. By the mid to late 1980s, it had been recognized that most primary duodenal ulcers were associated with gastric infection by a bacterium, *Helicobacter pylori*, the eradication of which resulted in cure of ulcer disease in most cases. Despite the scepticism with which the bacterial etiology was initially greeted, once it had been embraced virtually all chronic duodenal ulcers were considered to be *H. pylori* related. However, more recently, it has been recognized that approximately 20–40% of chronic duodenal ulcers are not related to *H. pylori*, or to NSAIDs or other identifiable causes. This is the current state of play, as described below.

Given the success of medical treatment of peptic ulcer disease with either *H. pylori* eradication and/or PPIs, acid-reducing operations are now hardly ever performed for peptic ulcer disease.

Epidemiology

The prevalence of peptic ulcer disease is so low in children that it is not possible to comment on time trends in the frequency of this disorder in the pediatric age group. However, in adults, there has been a profound decline in the frequency of uncomplicated peptic ulcer disease, but little change or a relative increase in that of complicated disease. The latter may be due to increasing use of NSAIDs.

A number of factors are alleged to cause or predispose to peptic ulcer disease. Current evidence is discussed and referenced in an excellent review,[8] and mentioned here only in brief.

Diet Although spicy foods may cause dyspepsia in some individuals, there is no evidence that they cause peptic ulceration. There is no evidence that any dietary factors contribute to peptic ulcer disease. Coffee, tea and cola are potent acid secretagogs, but no link to peptic ulceration has been established. Decaffeinated coffee is as potent a secretagog as caffeinated coffee. Bland diets have not been shown to be of benefit in treatment.

Genetics Some familial clustering of peptic ulcer disease may be due to *H. pylori* infection, but there appears to be a genetic predisposition independent of this, for example among concordant twins, HLA subtypes and in carriers of blood group antigens. These factors may be important in non-*H. pylori* peptic ulcer disease (see below).

Emotional stress Emotional stress alone, without the contribution of *H. pylori* and NSAIDs, is unlikely to cause ulceration. However, even modern studies have suggested that emotional distress may be a contributing factor to the occurrence of peptic ulcer complications; for example, after an earthquake in Kobe, Japan in the 1990s, the incidence of bleeding gastric ulcers increased. Emotional stress may well play a role in genetically susceptible individuals.

Smoking Cigarette smoking predisposes to ulcer formation and complications, probably by inhibiting prostaglandin synthesis and thereby compromising pre-epithelial or mucosal integrity. In addition, cigarette smoking is a gastric acid secretagog and inhibitor of duodenal bicarbonate secretion.

Alcohol Absolute alcohol (200-proof) causes severe damage to gastric mucosa in experimental animals, but there is little evidence that alcohol in the concentration found in commercially available alcoholic beverages causes peptic ulceration, although it may cause petechiae of uncertain significance. There is no increased incidence of peptic ulceration in non-cirrhotic humans. Modest alcohol ingestion may be protective of gastric mucosa, via stimulation of prostaglandin synthesis.

Associated diseases A strong association exists between chronic pulmonary disease in adults and peptic ulceration. This is poorly understood, but may be related to cigarette smoking. Peptic ulcer disease is associated with hepatic cirrhosis and chronic renal disease, although studies on the latter are contradictory.

Primary peptic ulcer disease

Helicobacter pylori associated

Although *H. pylori* infection is the commonest cause of peptic ulcer disease in children, these ulcers are rare in children under 10 years of age.[44–46] Peptic ulcers that are *H. pylori* related cannot be distinguished by their endoscopic appearance from *H. pylori*-negative ulcers – it is the presence of *H. pylori* gastritis that makes the distinction.

Exactly how many patients with chronic gastritis actually go on to develop ulcer disease is not known in children, but the lifetime risk of an infected patient developing peptic ulcer disease is estimated as 15–20% in adults.[387,388]

How *H. pylori*-associated gastritis causes duodenal ulcer remains unclear. There appears to be a complex interplay between infection, acid production, gastric metaplasia, pro-inflammatory cytokine production and bacterial virulence factors that has yet to be fully explained. Gastric metaplasia refers to the presence of gastric columnar

gastrostomy tubes. J Pediatr Gastroenterol Nutr 1997; 24:75–78.

127. Fitzgerald GA, Patrono C. The coxibs, selective inhibitors of cyclooxygenase-2. N Engl J Med 2001; 345:433–442.

128. Peura DA. Gastrointestinal safety and tolerabity of non-selective nonsteroidal anti-inflammatory agents and cyclooxygenase-2-selective inhibitors. Cleve Clin J Med 2002; 69:S31–S39.

129. Wallace JL. Pathogenesis of NSAID-induced gastroduodenal mucosal injury. Best Pract Res Clin Gastroenterol 2001; 15:691–703.

130. Lanza FL, Royer GL, Nelson RS. Endoscopic evaluation of the effects of aspirin, buffered aspirin, and enteric-coated aspirin on gastric and duodenal mucosa. N Engl J Med 1980; 303:136–138.

131. O'Laughlin JC, Hoftiezer JW, Ivey KJ. Effect of aspirin on the human stomach in normals: endoscopic comparison of damage produced one hour, 24 hours, and 2 weeks after administration. Scand J Gastroenterol 1981; 16:211– 214.

132. Soll AH, Kurata J, McGuigan JE. Ulcers, non-steroidal anti-inflammatory drugs and related matters. Gastroenterology 1989; 96:561–568.

133. Feldman M, Shewmake K, Cryer B. Time course inhibition of gastric and platelet COX activity by acetylsalicylic acid in humans. Am J Gastrointest Liver Physiol 2000; 279:G1113–G1120.

134. Hawkey CJ, Langman MJS. Non-steroidal anti-inflammatory drugs: overall risks and management. Complementary roles for COX-2 inhibitors and proton pump inhibitors. Gut 2003; 52:600–608.

135. Lanza FL and the members of the Ad Hoc Committee on Practice Parameters of the American College of Gastroenterology. A guideline for the treatment and prevention of NSAID-induced ulcers. Am J Gastroenterol 1998; 93: 2037–2046.

136. Silverstein FE, Faich G, Goldstein JL, et al. Gastrointestinal toxicity with celecoxib *vs* nonsteroidal anti-inflammatory drugs for osteoarthritis and rheumatoid arthritis: the CLASS study. A randomized controlled trial. Celecoxib Long-term Arthritis Safety Study. JAMA 2000; 284:1247–1255.

137. Cox K, Ament ME. Upper gastrointestinal bleeding in children and adolescents. Pediatrics 1979; 63:408–413.

138. Newman LJ, Yu WY, Halata M, et al. Peptic ulcer disease in children: aspirin induced. New York State J Med 1981; 81:1099–1101.

139. Mulberg AE, Linz C, Bern E, et al. Identification of non-steroidal anti-inflammatory drug-induced gastroduodenal injury in children with juvenile rheumatoid arthritis. J Pediatr 1993; 122:647–649.

140. Dowd JE, Cimaz R, Fink CW. Nonsteroidal anti-inflammatory drug-induced gastroduodenal injury in children. Arthritis Rheum 1995; 38:1225–1231.

141. Lesko ML, Mitchell AA. The safety of acetaminophen and ibuprofen among children younger than two years old. Pediatrics 1999; 104:e39.

142. Pashankar DS, Bishop WP, Mitros FA. Chemical gastropathy: a distinct histopathologic entity in children. J Pediatr Gastroenterol Nutr 2002; 35:653–657.

143. Laxer RM, Gazarian M. Pharmacology and drug therapy. In: Cassidy JT, Petty RE, eds. Textbook of Pediatric Rheumatology, 4th edn. Philadelphia, PA: Saunders; 2001:90–135.

144. DeNardi FG, Riddell RH. Reactive (chemical) gastropathy and gastritis. In: Graham DY, Genta RM, Dixon F, eds. Gastritis. Philadelphia, PA: Lippincott Williams & Wilkins; 1999:125–146.

145. Laine L, Marin-Sorensen M, Weinstein WM. Nonsteroidal antiinflammatory drug-associated gastric ulcers do not require *Helicobacter pylori* for their development. Am J Gastroenterol 1992; 87:1398–1402.

146. Yeomans ND, Tulassay Z, Juhasz L, et al. A comparison of omeprazole with ranitidine for ulcers associated with nonsteroidal antiinflammatory drugs. Acid Suppression Trial: Ranitidine *versus* Omeprazole for NSAID-associated Ulcer Treatment (ASTRONAUT) Study Group. N Engl J Med 1998; 338:719–726.

147. Hawkey CJ, Karrasch JA, Szczepanski L, et al. Omeprazole compared with misoprostol for ulcers associated with nonsteroidal antiinflammatory drugs. Omeprazole *versus* Misoprostol for NSAID-induced Ulcer Management (OMNIUM) Study Group. N Engl J Med. 1998; 338:727–734.

148. Campbell DR, Haber MM, Sheldon E, Collis, Lukasik N, Huang B, Goldstein JL. Effect of *H. pylori* status on gastric ulcer healing in patients continuing nonsteroidal anti-inflammatory therapy and receiving treatment with lansoprazole or ranitidine. Am J Gastroenterol 2002; 97:2208–2214.

149. Hawkey CJ. What consideration should be given to *Helicobacter pylori* in treating nonsteroidal anti-inflammatory drug ulcers? Eur J Gastroenterol Hepatol 2000; 12:S17–S20.

150. Graham DY. Critical effect of *Helicobacter pylori* infection on the effectiveness of omeprazole for prevention of gastric or duodenal ulcers among chronic NSAID users. Helicobacter 2002; 7:1–8.

151. Chan FK, Sung JJ, Chung SC, et al. Randomized trial of eradication of *Helicobacter pylori* before non-steroidal anti-inflammatory drug therapy to prevent peptic ulcers. Lancet 1997; 350:975–979.

152. Marks WA, Morris MP, Bodensteiner JB, et al. Gastritis with valproate therapy. Arch Neurol 1988; 45:903–905.

153. Wolf YG, Reyna T, Schropp KP, Harmel RP Jr. Steroid therapy and duodenal ulcer in infants. J Pediatr Gastroenterol Nutr 1991; 12:269–271.

154. Tarnawski A, Hollander D, Stachura J, et al. Alcohol injury to the normal human gastric mucosa: endoscopic, histologic and functional assessment. Clin Invest Med 1987; 10:259–263.

155. Laine L, Weinstein WM. Histology of alcoholic hemorrhagic gastritis: a prospective evaluation. Gastroenterology 1988; 94:1254–1262.

156. Trier JS, Szabo S, Allan CH. Ethanol-induced damage to mucosal capillaries of rat stomach. Gastroenterology 1987; 92:13–22.

157. Moore JG, Alsop WR, Freston JW, Tolman KG. The effect of oral potassium chloride on upper gastrointestinal mucosa in healthy subjects: healing of lesions despite continuing treatment. Gastrointest Endosc 1986; 32:210–212.

158. Strasser SI, McDonald GB. Gastrointestinal and hepatic complications. In: Thomas ED, Blume KG, Forman SJ, eds. Hematopoietic Cell Transplantation, 2nd edn. Cambridge, MA: Blackwell Scientific; 1999:627–658.

159. Canioni D, Vassall G, Donadieu J, et al. Toxicity induced by chemotherapy mimicking cytomegalovirus gastritis. Histopathology 1995; 26:473–475.

160. Laine L, Bentley E, Chandrasoma P, et al. Effect of oral iron therapy on the upper gastrointestinal tract. A prospective evaluation. Dig Dis Sci 1988; 33:172–177.

161. Das TK, Susheela AK, Gupta IP, et al. Toxic effects of chronic fluoride ingestion on the upper gastrointestinal tract. J Clin Gastroenterol 1994; 18:194–199.

162. Hyams JS, Treem WR. Portal hypertensive gastropathy in children. J Pediatr Gastroenterol Nutr 1993; 17:13–18.

163. McCormack TT, Sims J, Eyre-Brooke I, et al. Gastric lesions in portal hypertension: inflammatory gastritis or congestive gastropathy. Gut 1985; 26:1226–1232.

164. Vigneri S, Termini R, Piraino A, et al. The stomach in liver cirrhosis. Endoscopic, morphological, and clinical correlations. Gastroenterology 1991; 101:472–478.

165. Viggiano TR, Gostout CJ. Portal hypertensive intestinal vasculopathy: a review of the clinical, endoscopic, and histopathologic features. Am J Gastroenterol 1992; 87:944–954.

166. Sarin SK, Shahi HM, Jain M, et al. The natural history of portal hypertensive gastropathy: influence of variceal eradication. Am J Gastroenterol 2000; 95:2888–2893.

167. Goncalves ME, Cardoso SR, Maksoud JG. Prophylactic sclerotherapy in children with esophageal varices: long-term results of a controlled prospective randomized trial. J Pediatr Surg 2000; 35:401–405.

168. Fiaccadori E, Maggiore U, Clima B, et al. Incidence, risk factors, and prognosis of gastrointestinal hemorrhage complicating acute renal failure. Kidney Int 2001; 59:1510–1519.

169. Paronen I, Ala-Kaila K, Rantala I, et al. Gastric, parietal, chief, and G-cell densities in chronic renal failure. Scand J Gastroenterol 1991; 26:696–700.

170. Ala-Kaila K. Upper gastrointestinal findings in chronic renal failure. Scand J Gastroenterol 1987; 22:372–376.

171. Ravelli AM. Gastrointestinal function in chronic renal failure. Pediatr Nephrol 1995; 9:756–762.

172. Nakajima F, Sakaguchi M, Amaemoto K, et al. *Helicobacter pylori* in patients receiving long-term dialysis. Am J Nephrol 2002; 22:468–472.

173. Kang JY, Ho KY, Yeoh KG, et al. Peptic ulcer and gastritis in uraemia, with particular reference to the effect of *Helicobacter pylori* infection. J Gastroenterol Hepatol 1999; 14:771–778.

174. Fabbian F, Catalano C, Bordin V, et al. Esophagogastroduodenoscopy in chronic hemodialysis patients: 2-year clinical experience in a renal unit. Clin Nephrol 2002; 58:54–59.

175. Zuckerman GR, Cornette GL, Clouse RE, Harter HR. Upper gastrointestinal bleeding in patients with chronic renal failure. Ann Intern Med 1985; 102:588–592.

176. Chalasani N, Cotsonis G, Wilcox CM. Upper gastrointestinal bleeding in patients with chronic renal failure. Am J Gastroenterol 1996; 91:2329–2332.

177. Tomori K, Nakamto H, Kotaki S, et al. Gastric angiodysplasia in patients undergoing maintenance dialysis. Adv Perit Dial 2003; 19:136–142.

178. Emir S, Bereket G, Boyacroglu S, et al. Gastroduodenal lesions and *Helicobacter pylori* in children with end-stage renal disease. Pediatr Nephrol 2000; 14:837–840.

179. Lambert R, Andre C, Moulinier B, Bugnon B. Diffuse varioliform gastritis. Digestion 1978; 17:159–167.

180. Haot J, Jouret A, Willette M, et al. Lymphocytic gastritis: a prospective study of its relationship with varioliform gastritis. Gut 1990; 31:282–285.

181. Rutgeerts L, Stuer A, Vandenborre K, et al. Lymphocytic gastritis: clinical and endoscopic presentation and long-term follow-up. Acta Gastroenterol Belg 1995; 58:238–242.

182. Caporali R, Luciano S. Diffuse varioliform gastritis. Arch Dis Child 1986; 61:405–407.

183. Vinograd I, Granot E, Ron N, et al. Chronic varioliform gastritis in a child. J Clin Gastroenterol 1993; 16:40–44.

184. Wu TT, Hamilton SR. Lymphocytic gastritis: association with etiology and topology. Am J Surg Pathol 1999; 23:153–158.

185. Bechi P, Amorosi A, Mazzanti R, et al. Gastric histology and fasting bile reflux after partial gastrectomy. Gastroenterology 1987; 93:335–343.

186. Sobala GM, King RF, Axon AT, et al. Reflux gastritis in the intact stomach. J Clin Pathol 1990; 43:303–306.

187. Keane FB, Dimagno EP, Malagelada JR. Duodenogastric reflux in humans: its relationship to fasting antroduodenal motility and gastric, pancreatic and biliary secretion. Gastroenterology 1981; 81:726–731.

188. Hermans D, Sokal EM, Collard JM, et al. Primary duodenogastric reflux in children and adolescents. Eur J Pediatr 2003; 162:598–602.

189. Buchmiller TL, Curr M, Fonkalsrud EW. Assessment of alkaline reflux in children after Nissen fundoplication and pyloroplasty. J Am Coll Surg 1994; 178:1–5.

190. Mozrzymas R, d'Amore ES, Montino G, Guariso G. Schönlein–Henoch vasculitis and chronic *Helicobacter pylori* associated gastritis and duodenal ulcer: a case report. Pediatr Med Chir 1997; 19:467–468.

191. Gunasekaran TS, Berman J, Gonzalez M. Duodenojejunitis: is it idiopathic or is it Henoch–Schönlein purpura without the purpura? J Pediatr Gastroenterol Nutr 2000; 30:22–28.

192. Chesler L, Hwang L, Patton W, Heyman MB. Henoch–Schönlein purpura with severe jejunitis and minimal skin lesions. J Pediatr Gastroenterol Nutr 2000; 30:92–95.

193. Fitzgerald JF. HSP – without P. J Pediatr Gastroenterol Nutr 2000; 30:5–7.

194. Byrne WJ. Foreign bodies, bezoars, and caustic ingestion. Gastrointestinal Clin N Am 1994; 4:99–120.

195. Ragheb MI, Ramadan AA, Khalil MAH. Corrosive gastritis. Am J Surg 1977; 134:343–345.

196. Aviram G, Kessler A, Reif S, et al. Corrosive gastritis: sonographic findings in the acute phase and follow-up. Pediatr Radiol 1997; 27:805–806.

197. Gezernik W, Schmaman A, Chappell JS. Corrosive gastritis as a result of ferrous sulphate ingestion. S Afr Med J 1980; 57:151–154.

198. Laine LA, Bentley E, Chandrasoma P. Effect of oral iron therapy on the upper gastrointestinal tract. A prospective evaluation. Dig Dis Sci 1988; 33:172–177.

199. Brook MP, McCarron M, Muellar JA. Pine oil cleaner ingestion. Ann Emerg Med 1989; 18:391–395.

200. Rebhandl W, Steffen I, Schramel P, et al. Release of toxic metals from button batteries retained in the stomach: an *in vitro* study. J Pediatr Surg 2002; 37:87–92.

201. Choi SC, Choi SJ, Kim JA, et al. The role of gastrointestinal endoscopy in long distance runners with gastrointestinal symptoms. Eur J Gastroenterol Hepatol 2001; 13:1089–1094.

202. Simons SM, Kennedy RG. Gastrointestinal problems in runners. Curr Sports Med Rep 2004; 3:112–116.

203. Cooper BT, Douglas SA, Firth LA, et al. Erosive gastritis and gastrointestinal bleeding in a female runner. Gastroenterology 1987; 92:2019–2021.

204. Mack D, Sherman P. Iron deficiency anemia in an athlete associated with *Campylobacter pylori*-negative chronic gastritis. J Clin Gastroenterol 1989; 11:445–447.

205. Qamar M, Read A. Effects of exercise on mesenteric blood flow in man. Gut 1987; 28:583–587.

206. Feldman M, Nixon JV. Effect of exercise on postprandial gastric secretion and emptying in humans. J Appl Physiol 1982; 53:851–854.

207. Gahl WA, Thoene JG, Schneider JA. Cystinosis. N Engl J Med 2002; 347:111–121.

376. Gotlieb-Jensen K, Andersen J. Occurrence of *Candida* in gastric ulcers. Significance for the healing process. Gastroenterology 1983; 85:535–537.

377. Neeman A, Avidor I, Kadish U. Candidal infection of benign gastric ulcers in aged patients. Am J Gastroenterol 1981; 75:211–2113.

378 DiFebo G, Miglioli M, Calo G, et al. *Candida albicans* infection of gastric ulcer frequency and correlation with medical treatment: results of a multicentre trial. Dig Dis Sci 1985; 30:178–181.

379. Michalak DM, Cooney DR, Rhodes KH, et al. Gastrointestinal mucormycosis in infants and children: a cause of gangrenous intestinal cellulitis and perforation. J Pediatr Surg 1980; 15:320–324.

380. Dennis JE, Rhodes KH, Cooney DR, et al. Nosocomial *Rhizopus* infection (zygomycosis) in children. J Pediatr 1980; 96:824–828.

381. Cappell MS, Mandell W, Grimes MM, Neu HC. Gastrointestinal histoplasmosis. Dig Dis Sci 1988; 33:353–360.

382. Sangkhathat S, Patrapinyokul S, Wudhisuthimethawee P, et al. Massive gastrointestinal bleeding in infants with ascariasis. J Pediatr Surg. 2003; 38:1696–1698.

383. Hsui JG, Gamsey AJ, Ives CE, et al. Gastric anisakiasis: report of a case with clinical, endoscopic, and histologic findings. Am J Gastroenterol 1986; 81:1185–1187.

384. Ikeda K, Kumashiro R, Kifune T. Nine cases of acute gastric anisakiasis. Gastrointest Endosc 1989; 35:304–308.

385. Lopez-Serrano MC, Gomez AA, Daschner A, et al. Gastroallergic anisakiasis: findings in 22 patients. J Gastroenterol Hepatol 2000; 15:503–506.

386. Magnus HA. The pathology of peptic ulceration. Postgrad Med J 1954; 30:131–134.

387. Fennerty MB. Is the only good *H. pylori* a dead *H. pylori*? Gastroenterology 1996; 111:1773–1774.

388. Blaser MJ. Not all *H. pylori* strains are created equal: should all be eliminated? Lancet 1997; 349:1020–1022.

389. Wyatt JI, Rathbone BJ, Dixon MF, Heatley RV. *Campylobacter pyloridis* and acid induced gastric metaplasia in the pathogenesis of duodenitis. J Clin Pathol 1987; 40:841–848.

390. Gormally SM, Kierce BM, Daly LE, et al. Gastric metaplasia and duodenal ulcer disease in children infected by *Helicobacter pylori*. Gut 1996; 38:513–517.

391. Savarino V, Mela GS, Zentilin P, et al. Effect of *Helicobacter pylori* eradication on 24-hour gastric pH and duodenal gastric metaplasia. Dig Dis Sci 2000; 45:1315–1321.

392. El-Omar EM, Penman ID, Ardill JE, et al. *Helicobacter pylori* infection and abnormalities of acid secretion in patients with duodenal ulcer disease. Gastroenterology 1995; 109:681–691.

393. Graham DY, Dore MP. Perturbations in gastric physiology in *Helicobacter pylori* duodenal ulcer: are they all epiphenomena? Helicobacter 1997; 2:S44–S49.

394. McGowan CC, Cover TL, Blaser MJ. *Helicobacter pylori* and gastric acid: biological and therapeutic implications. Gastroenterology 1996; 110:926–938.

395. Beales I, Blaser MJ, Srinivasan S, et al. Effect of *Helicobacter pylori* products and recombinant cytokines on gastrin release from cultured canine G cells. Gastroenterology 1997; 113:465–471.

396. Beales IL, Calam J. *Helicobacter pylori* infection and tumour necrosis factor-alpha increase gastrin release from human gastric antral fragments. Eur J Gastroenterol Hepatol 1997; 9:773–777.

397. Shimizu T, Haruna H, Ohtsuka Y, et al. Cytokines in the gastric mucosa of children with *Helicobacter pylori* infection. Acta Paediatr 2001; 90:322–326.

398. Moss SF, Legon S, Bishop AE, et al. Effect of *Helicobacter pylori* on gastric somatostatin in duodenal ulcer disease. Lancet 1992; 340:930–932.

399. Queiroz DM, Moura SB, Mendes EN, et al. Effect of *Helicobacter pylori* eradication on G-cell and D-cell density in children. Lancet 1994; 343:1191–1193.

400. Queiroz DM, Mendes EN, Rocha GA, et al. Effect of *Helicobacter pylori* eradication on antral gastrin- and somatostatin-immunoreactive cell density and gastrin and somatostatin concentrations. Scand J Gastroenterol 1993; 28:858–864.

401. Savarino V, Mela GS, Zentilin P, et al. 24-hour gastric pH and extent of duodenal gastric metaplasia in *Helicobacter pylori*-positive patients. Gastroenterology 1997; 113:741–745.

402. Atherton JC, Peek RM Jr, Tham KT, et al. Clinical and pathological importance of heterogeneity in *vacA*, the vacuolating cytotoxin gene of *Helicobacter pylori*. Gastroenterology 1997; 112:92–99.

403. Loeb M, Jayaratne P, Jones N, et al. Lack of correlation between vacuolating cytotoxin activity, *cagA* gene in *Helicobacter pylori*, and peptic ulcer disease in children. Eur J Clin Microbiol Infect Dis 1998; 17:653–656.

404. Mitchell HM, Ally R, Wadee E, et al. Major differences in the IgG subclass response to *Helicobacter pylori* in the first and third worlds. Scand J Gastroenterol 2002; 37:517–522.

405. Tsuji H, Kohli Y, Fukumitsu S. *Helicobacter pylori*-negative gastric and duodenal ulcers. J Gastroenterol 1999; 34:455–460.

406. Bytzer P, Stubbe Teglbjaerg P and the Danish Ulcer Study Group. *Helicobacter pylori*-negative duodenal ulcers: prevalence, clinical characteristics, and prognosis – results from a randomized trial with 2-year follow-up. Am J Gastroenterol 2001; 96:1409–1416.

407. Demir H, Gurakan H, Ozen H, et al. Peptic ulcer disease in children without *Helicobacter pylori* infection. Helicobacter 2002; 7:111.

408. Hassall E, Hiruki T, Dimmick JE. *Helicobacter pylori*-negative duodenal ulcer in children. Gastroentereology 1993; 104:A96.

409. Wilson SD. Zollinger–Ellison syndrome in children: a 25-year follow-up. Surgery 1991; 110:696–702.

410. De Giacomo C, Fiocca R, Villani L, et al. Omeprazole treatment of severe peptic disease associated with antral G cell hyperfunction and hyperpepsinogenemia I in an infant. J Pediatr 1990; 117:989–993.

411. Zaatar R, Younoszai MK, Mitros F. Pseudo-Zollinger–Ellison syndrome in a child presenting with anemia. Gastroenterology 1987; 92:508–512.

412. Buchta RM, Kaplan JM. Zollinger–Ellison syndrome in a 9 year old child: case report and review of this entity in childhood. Pediatrics 1971; 47:594–598.

413. Roy PK, Venzon DJ, Shojamanesh H, et al. Zollinger–Ellison syndrome. Clinical presentation in 261 patients. Medicine (Baltimore) 2000; 79:379–411.

414. Peghini PL, Annibale B, Azzoni C, et al. Effect of chronic hypergastrinemia on human enterochromaffin-like cells: insights from patients with sporadic gastrinomas. Gastroenterology 2002; 123:68–85.

415. Zollinger RM, Ellison EH. Primary peptic ulcerations of the jejunum associated with islet cell tumours of the pancreas. Ann Surg 1955; 142:709–713.

416. Meko JB, Norton JA. Management of patients with Zollinger–Ellison. Ann Rev Med 1995; 46:395–411.

417. Maton PN. Zollinger–Ellison syndrome: recognition. Drugs 1996; 52:33–44.

418. Friesen ST, Tomita T. Hypergastrinemia, hyperchlorhydria without tumour. Ann Surg 1981; 194:481–493.

419. Euler AR, Lechago J, Byrne W, France GL. Transient hypergastrinemia of 2 years' duration in a young pediatric patient. J Pediatr Gastroenterol Nutr 1984; 3:300–303.

420. Carlei F, Caruso U, Lezoche E, et al. Hyperplasia of antral G cells in uraemic patients. Digestion 1984; 29:26–30.

421. Miner PB. The role of the mast cell in clinical gastrointestinal disease with special reference to systemic mastocytosis. J Invest Dermatol 1991; 96:S40–S44.

422. Ammann RW, Vetter D, Deyhle P, et al. Gastrointestinal involvement in systemic mastocytosis. Gut 1976; 17:107–112.

423. Cherner JA, Jensen RT, Dubois A, et al. Gastrointestinal dysfunction in systemic mastocytosis. A prospective study. Gastroenterology 1988; 95:657–667.

424. Johnson GJ, Silvis SE, Roitman B, et al. Long-term treatment of systemic mastocytosis with histamine H_2 receptor antagonists. Am J Gastroenterol 1980; 74:485–489.

425. Tang SJ, Nieto JM, Jensen DM, et al. The novel use of an intravenous proton pump inhibitor in a patient with short bowel syndrome. J Clin Gastroenterol 2002; 34:62–63.

426. Williams NS, Evans P, King RF. Gastric acid secretion and gastrin production in the short bowel syndrome. Gut 1985; 26:914–919.

427. Hyman PE, Everett SL, Harada T. Gastric acid hypersecretion in short bowel syndrome in infants: association with extent of resection and enteral feeding. J Pediatr Gastroenterol Nutr 1986; 5:191–197.

428. Cadiot G, Houillier P, Allouch A, et al. Oral calcium tolerance test in the early diagnosis of primary hyperparathyroidism and multiple endocrine neoplasia type 1 in patients with the Zollinger–Ellison syndrome. Groupe de Recherche et d'Etude du Syndrome de Zollinger–Ellison. Gut 1996; 39:273–278.

429. Gardner EC Jr, Hersh T. Primary hyperparathyroidism and the gastrointestinal tract. South Med J 1981; 74:197–199.

430. McColley SA, Rosenstein BJ, Cutting GR. Differences in expression of cystic fibrosis in blacks and whites. Am J Dis Child 1991; 145:94–97.

431. Fiedorek SC, Shulman RJ, Klish WJ. Endoscopic detection of peptic ulcer disease in cystic fibrosis. Clin Pediatr 1986; 25:243–246.

432. Cox KL, Isenberg JN, Ament ME. Gastric acid hypersecretion in cystic fibrosis. J Pediatr Gastroenterol Nutr 1982; 1:559–565.

433. Barraclough M, Taylor CJ. Twenty-four hour ambulatory gastric and duodenal pH profiles in cystic fibrosis: effect of duodenal hyperacidity on pancreatic enzyme function and fat absorption. J Pediatr Gastroenterol Nutr 1996; 23:45–50.

434. Miller V, Doig CM. Upper gastrointestinal tract endoscopy. Arch Dis Child 1984; 59:1100–1102.

435. Gyepes MT, Smith LE, Ament ME. Fiberoptic endoscopy and upper gastrointestinal series: comparative analysis in infants and children. AJR Am J Roentgenol 1977; 128:53–56.

436. Miner P Jr, Katz PO, Chen Y, Sostek M. Gastric acid control with esomeprazole, lansoprazole, omeprazole, pantoprazole, and rabeprazole: a five-way crossover study. Am J Gastroenterol 2003; 98:2616–2620.

437. Israel DM, Hassall E. Omeprazole and other proton pump inhibitors: pharmacology, efficacy and safety, with special reference to use in children. J Pediatr Gastroenterol Nutr 1998; 27:568–579.

438. Tolia V, Ferry G, Gunasekaran T, Huang B, Keith R, Book L. Efficacy of lansoprazole in the treatment of gastroesophageal reflux disease in children. J Pediatr Gastroenterol Nutr 2002; 35:S308–S318.

439. Hassall E, Israel DM, Shepherd R, et al. and the International Pediatric Omeprazole Study Group. Omeprazole for treatment of chronic erosive esophagitis in children: a multicenter study of efficacy, safety, tolerability and dose requirements. J Pediatr 2000; 137:800–807.

440. Tolia V, Fitzgerald J, Hassall E, et al. Safety of lansoprazole in the treatment of GERD in children. J Pediatr Gastroenterol Nutr 2002; 35:S300–S307.

441. Hyman PE, Garvey TQ III, Abrams CE. Tolerance to intravenous ranitidine. J Pediatr 1987; 110:794–796.

442. Knight DA, Stewart GA, Thompson PJ. Histamine tachyphylaxis in human airway smooth muscle. The role of H_2-receptors and the bronchial epithelium. Am Rev Respir Dis 1992; 146:137–140.

443. Szabo S, Hollander D. Pathways of gastrointestinal protection and repair: mechanism of action of sucralfate. Am J Med 1989; 83:91–94.

444. McCarthy DM. Sucralfate. N Engl J Med 1991; 325:1017–1025.

445. Szabo S. The mode of action of sucralfate: the $1 \times 1 \times 1$ mechanism of action. Scand J Gastroenterol 1991; 185:7–12.

446. Thorburn K, Samuel M, Smaith EA, Baines P. Aluminum accumulation in critically ill children on sucralfate therapy. Pediatr Crit Care Med 2001; 2:247–249.

447. Chiang BL, Chiang MH, Lin MI, et al. Chronic duodenal ulcer in children: clinical observation and response to treatment. J Pediatr Gastroenterol Nutr 1989; 8:161–165.

448. McArthur K, Hogan D, Isenberg JI. Relative stimulatory effects of commonly ingested beverages on gastric acid secretion in humans. Gastroenterology 1982; 83:199–203.

449. Huang FC, Chuang Jh, Ko SF. Clinical experience in the treatment of ulcer-induced gastric outlet obstruction in seven children. Acta Paediatr Taiwan 2000; 41:189–192.

450. Winkelstein JA, Marino MC, Johnston RB, et al. Chronic granulomatous disease. Report on a national registry of 368 patients. Medicine (Baltimore) 2000; 79:155–169.

451. Yamamoto T, Allan RN, Keighley MR. An audit of gastroduodenal Crohn disease: clinicopathologic features and management. Scand J Gastroenterol 1999; 34:1019–1024.

452. Erdogan E, Eroglu E, Tekant G, et al. Management of esophagogastric corrosive injuries in children. Eur J Pediatr Surg 2003; 13:289–293.

453. Bell EAA, Grothe R, Zivkovich V, et al. Pyloric channel stricture secondary to high-dose ibuprofen therapy in a patient with cystic fibrosis. Ann Pharmacother 1999; 33:693–696.

Country, reference	Study population, year study conducted, design, no. of children	Diagnostic method	Prevalence of H. pylori infection
Scotland, Patel et al.[391] (1994)	School children, aged 7–11 years, conducted ?, cross-sectional, *n* = 554	Anti-*H. pylori* IgG in saliva	Overall 11%
Finland, Ashorn et al.[392] (1995)	Children aged 1–12 years, conducted 1980, cohort study, *n* = 461	Anti-*H. pylori* IgG in serum	3 years, 5%; 6 years, 6%; 12 years, 13%
Sweden, Granström et al.[393] (1997)	Serum samples of a vaccine study, children followed from 6 months to 11 years, started in 1984, cohort study, *n* = 294	Anti-*H. pylori* IgG in serum	Overall 14%; 6 months, 1%;, 2 years, 10%
Italy, Perri et al.[270] (1997)	School children, aged 3–14 years, conducted 1994–95, cross-sectional study, *n* = 216	^{13}C-urea breath test	Overall 23%; 3–4 years, 0%; 13–14 years, 33%
Finland, Rehnberg-Laiho et al.[394] (1998)	Serum samples of a vaccine trial started in 1982 (up to 1995), aged 2–20 years, cohort study, *n* = 337	Anti-*H. pylori* IgG in serum	Overall 6%
Germany, Rothenbacher et al.[395] (1998)	Pre-school children, aged 5–8 years, conducted 1996, cross-sectional study, *n* = 945	^{13}C-urea breath test	Overall 13%; German, 5%; German immigrants, 40%; Turkish, 45%; other Europeans, 29%
Switzerland, Boltshauser and Herzog[396] (1999)	Pre-school children, aged 5–7 years. conducted 1998, cross-sectional study, *n* = 432	^{13}C-urea breath test	Overall 7%; Swiss, 4%; other, 19%; immigrants, 70%
Germany, Rothenbacher et al.[397] (1999)	Pre-school children, aged 5–8 years, conducted 1997, cross-sectional study, *n* = 1221	^{13}C-urea breath test	Overall 11%; German, 5%; German immigrants, 47%; Turkish, 44%; others, 23%
Germany, Roltenbacher et al.[398] (2000)	Turkish children who underwent health screening examinations, aged 1–4 years, conducted 1997–98, cross-sectional study, *n* = 189	Stool test	1-year-olds, 9%; 2-year-olds, 36%; 4-year-olds, 32%
Sweden, Daugule et al.[18] (2001)	Children visiting their doctor for a general health check-up, aged 1–12 years, conducted 1998–99, cross-sectional study, *n* = 142	^{13}C-urea breath test	Overall 21%; 1–2 years, 12%; 9–12 years, 32%
Italy, Dore et al.[49] (2002)	School-aged children aged 5–16 years from Sardinia, conducted 1996–98, cross-sectional study, *n* = 2810	Anti-*H. pylori* IgG in serum	Overall 22%; 2–5 years, 20%; 14–16 years, 26%
Germany, Rothenbacher et al.[48] (2002)	Pre-school children, aged 5–8 years, conducted 1998, cross-sectional study, *n* = 305	^{13}C-urea breath test	Overall 13%; German, 2%; German immigrants, 40%; Turkish, 45%; other, 31%
Germany, Bode et al.[399] (2002)	School children, aged 10–13 years, conducted 1999–2000, cross-sectional study, *n* = 824	Anti-*H. pylori* IgG in serum	Overall 19%; German, 13%; German immigrants, 42%; Turkish, 38%; other European, 31%

From Rothenbacher and Brenner, 2003.[28]

Table 26.1 Prevalence of *H. pylori* infection in children as determined in population-based studies conducted in Europe. (Reproduced from Rothenbacher D, et al. Burden of *Helicobacter pylori* and *H. pylori*-related diseases in developed countries: recent developments and future implications 2003; 5(8):693–703, with permission).

months to 17 years. Seroprevalence increased with age from 17% at 6 months to 78% by 16 years of age. Disease was inversely correlated to family income. Parents of infected children were frequently infected, mothers more so than fathers (85% *vs* 76%). Almost half of the offspring of seropositive mothers were seropositive, compared with

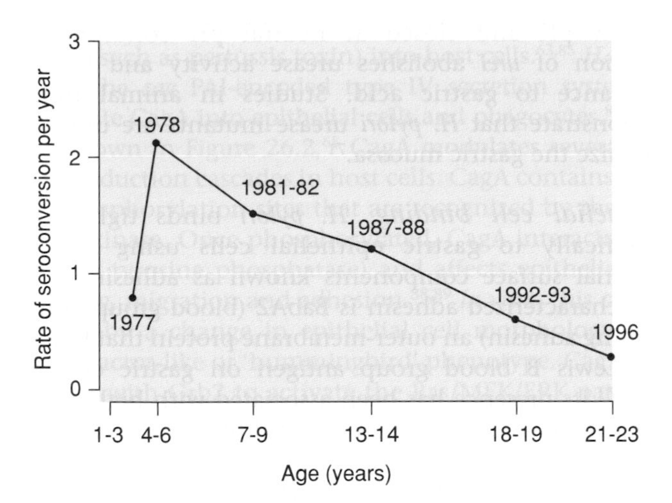

Figure 26.1: Age-specific rate per year of seroconversion for *H. pylori* among 206 children who were seronegative in 1975–1976 at age 1–3 years. (From Malaty et al., 2002, with permission.)[31]

less than one-quarter of the offspring of seronegative mothers. In contrast, Mitchell et al.[33] found no such relationship between maternal infection and the seroprevalence of their children in a study of 166 children and 39 mothers from a Brazilian shantytown.

Cohort effect

The persisting increase in disease prevalence with age seen in developed countries, despite the marked reduction in acquisition rate over many years, is consistent with a birth cohort effect. This reflects a much higher rate of transmission during the childhood of earlier birth cohorts.[34,35] Rupnow et al.,[36] utilizing a dynamic transmission model, suggested that the reduction in *H. pylori* transmission in the US population is the result of markedly improved sanitation in the second half of the nineteenth century. The authors predict that this will eventually lead to the elimination of *H. pylori* from the US population. In the absence of any intervention, however, they predict that it will remain endemic for at least another century.

Spontaneous bacterial clearance

Spontaneous clearance of *H. pylori* infection in early childhood has been reported. Clearance of IgG seen in very young infants is more likely to represent the detection and then clearance of maternal antibodies.[37,38] However, more recent investigative data suggest that spontaneous elimination of *H. pylori* in childhood may be related to antibiotic use in childhood.[31,39–41] Further studies are required to clarify this issue.

Transmission of infection

A full understanding of *H. pylori* disease transmission is hindered by the great difficulties encountered when attempting to culture the bacteria. The detection of DNA by polymerase chain reaction (PCR) has proved to be a very sensitive system for the detection of *H. pylori* in clinical samples. However, it does not differentiate viable from non-viable organisms. Furthermore, false-positive results can occur in the presence of other unidentified *Helicobacter* species.

Person-to-person transmission

H. pylori is yet to be consistently isolated from any reservoir other than humans. This supports the belief that transmission is by direct person-to-person contact. Data supporting this come from numerous studies examining prevalence rates either within families, within residential institutions or within particular workplaces.[15,42–44]

In childhood, the relative importance of various environmental risk factors appear to vary both between countries and within communities. A number of studies have focused on the role that daycare attendance *vs* the *H. pylori* status within the home plays in the acquisition of infection.[18,45–47] Within developed communities, intrafamilial transmission generally predominates over transmission from within the community.[15] For example, in a cross-sectional study of Swedish children, a seroprevalence rate of 2% was detected among children whose parents both originated from regions of low prevalence, compared with a rate of 55% when at least one parent originated from a high-prevalence area.[47] In another study of 305 children and their parents, intrafamilial clustering was demonstrated, with infected mothers playing a key role in transmission of *H. pylori* to the child. There was an increased risk of infection for the child if the father was infected, but the association was not as strong as when the mother was infected.[48]

Several studies have identified no increased risk of infection among children attending daycare.[45,46] However, this finding is not universal. In a study of Hispanic and black children in Houston, USA, a much higher rate of acquisition among children attending the most crowded daycare institutions was identified.[20] Similarly, Dore et al.[49] found a higher seroprevalence in urban Sardinian children who attended daycare in comparison with children who did not.

There is also controversy regarding the role that breast-feeding may play in disease acquisition and/or protection. A variety of studies have confirmed a protective role for breast-feeding,[20,50] which may be due to high levels of lactoferrin[50] or the presence of *H. pylori* antibodies.[51] However, in a study of 946 preschool children in Germany, a higher prevalence of *H. pylori* was detected among children who were breast-fed.[52] The authors concluded that, in industrialized countries, breast-feeding was not protective against *H. pylori* infection. Kitagawa et al.[53] suggested that maternal failure to wash hands and nipples prior to breast-feeding could lead to horizontal transmission.

Route of transmission

If the passage of infection is from person to person, then the routes of transmission are limited to oral–oral, gastric–oral and fecal–oral. The fastidious growth requirements of the organism have frustrated attempts to determine the relative importance of each of these routes. The most probable route is gastro–oral (by vomitus) and/or fecal–oral.[54] In support of this contention, a study by Parsonnet et al.[55] demonstrated that *H. pylori* could be

response to *H. pylori* infection, an uncommon finding in Western countries.[148] This response may be induced by endemic helminth infection, or may reflect a genetic predisposition.[63]

Cytokine polymorphisms Gastric cancer and duodenal ulceration are mutually exclusive outcomes of *H. pylori* infection.[149] However, various *H. pylori* strains are equally associated with both diseases, suggesting that host factors may play a role. Current evidence indicates that cytokine polymorphisms are important host factors that can alter disease outcome. Pro-inflammatory polymorphisms of the IL-1β gene have been associated with the development of gastritis predominantly involving the body of the stomach (corpus gastritis), hypochlorhydria, gastric atrophy and gastric adenocarcinoma, with a reduced risk of duodenal ulceration.[150–154] In the absence of these polymorphisms, *H. pylori* gastritis predominantly involves the antrum and is associated with normal to high acid secretion.[154] Polymorphisms of the TNF-α and IL-10 genes demonstrate a similar but less pronounced association with the development of gastric cancer.[63]

Gastric epithelial cell damage and apoptosis *H. pylori* induces apoptosis both *in vitro* and *in vivo*.[155] Several mechanisms are involved. *H. pylori* or its products may induce apoptosis directly. For example, VacA induces the release of cytochrome *c* from mitochondria.[156,157] Alternatively, the bacterium may induce host immune responses which then mediate apoptosis. For instance, Th1 cell cytokines (TNF-α and IFN-γ) markedly potentiate *H. pylori*-induced epithelial cell apoptosis.[158,159] *H. pylori* also upregulates expression of the Fas death receptor.[160,161] The absence of Fas signaling has been associated with less apoptosis and enhanced premalignant gastric mucosal changes.[162,163]

Gastric epithelial cell apoptosis and carcinogenesis

The mechanisms of *H. pylori*-related carcinogenesis are unclear and are likely the result of both bacterial and host factors, as mentioned previously, and/or environmental factors such as smoking, high-salt diet and antioxidant ingestion.[149]

Carcinomas occur with pangastritis. The more common type occurs following progressive atrophy, hypochlorhydria, intestinal metaplasia and dysplasia. The diffuse type may arise *de novo* in *H. pylori*-colonized mucosa.[63,164] Disturbance of the balance between epithelial cell proliferation and apoptosis is considered a risk factor for gastric atrophy and, later, neoplastic transformation. Studies in humans demonstrate that, in the absence of premalignant lesions or gastric cancer, *H. pylori*-induced apoptosis is associated with increased epithelial proliferation. However, in the presence of metaplasia and *H. pylori* infection, apoptosis returns to normal levels, while proliferation remains increased.[158,163,165]

Carcinogenesis requires DNA damage, which may be caused directly through a variety of *H. pylori* products, or indirectly through the host's response to that infection, such as by the generation of oxygen free radicals released by neutrophils. *H. pylori* infection is associated with a reduction in ascorbic acid, which helps to reduce the effect of oxygen free radicals. In addition, *H. pylori* disrupts the DNA mismatch repair system.[156,166,167] By leading to gastric atrophy, *H. pylori* may be permitting its own replacement by more genotoxic bacteria.[63]

Effect of *H. pylori*-induced inflammation on acid homeostasis

H. pylori infection can cause hypergastrinemia by both reducing D-cell somatostatin production and increasing G-cell gastrin production. Removal of *H. pylori* reverses these effects.[63] However, the ultimate effect of infection on acid homeostasis depends on the topographic distribution of *H. pylori*-induced inflammation within the stomach. In antral-predominant gastritis, gastrin release leads to higher acid levels, and persistently high gastrin levels increase the parietal cell mass.[168,169] This in turn results in increased acid delivery to the duodenum, inducing gastric metaplasia. *H. pylori* can colonize gastric metaplasia,[63] resulting in inflammation and, possibly, ulceration.[169–172]

With pangastritis or corpus-predominant gastritis, *H. pylori* infection suppresses acid production both directly and indirectly. Inflammatory mediators inhibit parietal cell acid secretion and enterochromaffin-like cell histamine production.[173,174] Reduced acid secretion further increases gastrin levels, promoting gastric epithelial cell proliferation. Epithelial cell characteristics become altered, leading to progressive gastric gland loss, and thus gastric atrophy. Gastric atrophy increases the risk of gastric ulceration and non-cardia gastric adenocarcinoma.[155,175]

Putative hormonal effects of *H. pylori* infection

Recent data suggest that *H. pylori* infection affects the expression of the appetite- and satiety-controlling hormones leptin and ghrelin.[176,177] Gastric leptin is produced by chief and parietal cells, and is released in response to meals and associated hormones. Leptin signals satiety to the hypothalamus. Within the stomach, it reduces gastrin and acid secretion, and increases gastric mucosal cell proliferation. Ghrelin is produced in oxyntic glands and is released during fasting and suppressed by feeding and leptin.[178–180] Gastric leptin levels are higher in *H. pylori*-colonized adults than in non-colonized adults, and are reduced following *H. pylori* eradication.[177] Conversely, ghrelin levels increase with *H. pylori* eradication.[176] These initial findings are intriguing and need to be confirmed in additional studies. If confirmed, these results may have implications for growth and obesity in humans.[63]

DISEASE ASSOCIATIONS

A large variety of diseases have been purported to be associated with *H. pylori* infection. The evidence for some is compelling if not conclusive. For others it is highly suggestive. For many, conclusive evidence of association is notably sparse. The spectrum of *H. pylori*-related disease encountered in childhood varies somewhat from that recognized in the adult population.

Gastrointestinal manifestations

Gastritis, recurrent abdominal pain and non-ulcer dyspepsia

Infection with *H. pylori* is associated with chronic gastritis in both children and adults. Early evidence for this came from two adult volunteers who ingested the organism and subsequently developed gastritis.[181] All children colonized with *H. pylori* have chronic gastritis.[182–184] Eradication of *H. pylori* results in the healing of gastritis.[185–187] An area of enormous contention is whether this gastritis, in the absence of ulcer disease, has any manifest symptoms; specifically, does it cause abdominal pain in children? Reports have been conflicting.[188–190] Investigation into the association (or lack thereof) between *H. pylori* infection and either recurrent abdominal pain (RAP) or non-ulcer dyspepsia (NUD) has been conducted along two lines. The first has been to investigate a possible association between *H. pylori* infection and RAP; the other is to examine whether the eradication of *H. pylori* infection results in the resolution of such symptoms.[54,191] To date, the evidence suggests that *H. pylori* gastritis remains largely asymptomatic in children; a relationship between RAP or NUD and *H. pylori* infection has not been demonstrated.[192] However, it remains possible that *H. pylori* infection may be associated with an as yet unrecognized subpopulation of patients with RAP or NUD. An appropriate prospective, well structured, double-blind, randomized, placebo-controlled trial that includes children matched for both age and socioeconomic class would be beneficial to answer these questions.[54]

Duodenal and gastric ulcer disease

H. pylori infection plays a causal role in the development of duodenal and gastric ulcers, and should be eradicated when detected in such settings.[188–190] In adults, the lifetime risk of peptic ulcer disease in the setting of *H. pylori*-positive gastritis varies geographically. In the USA it is reported to be as low as 3%, whereas in Japan the rate is 25%.[28] Previous data in adults attributed up to 95% of duodenal ulcers and 70% of gastric ulcers to *H. pylori* infection.[193] However, a recent population-based study from Denmark in 2003 estimated the attributable risk for peptic ulcer disease to be only 44%, with other risk factors, including smoking, being important contributors.[194] Reinfection with *H. pylori* in adults is a rare event after successful eradication. Thus cure is persistent, and the recurrence rate of *H. pylori*-associated peptic ulcers after successful eradication therapy is very low.[193] This applies even in geographic regions where *H. pylori* is highly prevalent.[195]

In children, however, ulcer disease is rare. A European retrospective cohort of 2550 symptomatic children undergoing upper gastrointestinal endoscopy over a 9-year period demonstrated peptic ulcer in only 2% of subjects. *H. pylori* was identified in 54% of children with peptic ulcer, more frequently in duodenal than in gastric ulcer (60% *vs* 20%, $P<0.001$).[196] The pattern of *H. pylori* gastritis and the age of *H. pylori* acquisition both appear to be important determinants of future sequelae.[65] Antral-predominant gastritis has a higher risk of duodenal ulcer, whereas subjects with corpus-predominant gastritis are more prone to gastric ulcers and gastric malignancy.

Gastroesophageal reflux (disease)

Various epidemiologic studies have demonstrated an inverse relationship between rates of *H. pylori* infection and the prevalence of gastroesophageal reflux disease (GERD) and/or the aggravation of esophagitis with *H. pylori* eradication.[197–202] Conversely, many studies have found no relationship between reflux symptoms and *H. pylori* eradication.[203–209] The first prospective evaluation of the effect of *H. pylori* eradication on GER symptoms in pediatric patients was published in 2004.[210] Ninety-five of 119 children and adolescents completed the study. Thirty-five had symptoms of GER at baseline, 55 were *H. pylori* positive and 84 had epigastric pain. Both symptoms of GER and epigastric pain were unrelated to *H. pylori* status and eradication outcome. In conclusion, there is currently no convincing clinical data in children that *H. pylori* status or eradication affects GER(D).

Gastric cancer

Gastric cancer is the second most frequent cause of cancer-related death in the world,[65] although it is only the eighth most common cause of cancer death in North America.[211] In 1994, *H. pylori* was classified by the International Agency for Research on Cancer as a class I (definite) carcinogen in humans.[5] However, only cancers located distal to the cardia (non-cardia adenocarcinomas) are related to *H. pylori* infection.[5] The initial seroepidemiologic evidence for this association came from three nested case–control studies which all showed that patients with cancer had a higher *H. pylori* seroprevalence compared with controls. The attributable risk with positive serology ranged from 2.1 to 8.7.[164,212,213] Several subsequent studies, including a meta-analysis of 19 studies in 1998, have placed the relative risk of gastric cancer in infected individuals between 2- and 3-fold. The relationship varies with age, with a much stronger relationship among younger subjects.[214–217] A prospective study of 1526 Japanese subjects conducted over an 8-year period reported in 2001 that, during follow-up, gastric cancer developed in infected patients only; no cases were detected in eradicated or uninfected patients.[217]

Again, both bacterial and host factors appear to affect the sequelae of infection. Gastric cancer has been more strongly linked to *cagA*$^{+}$ strains as well as specific polymorphisms within the host's IL-1gene.[154,218–220] In further support of both environmental factors (such as smoking) as well as bacterial and host genetic factors playing an important role in determining disease risk, there is the previously referred to 'African enigma'. This is characterized by a large population with a high prevalence of *H. pylori* infection but a low rate of gastric cancer.[221,222] The putative pathophysiologic mechanisms behind this have already been discussed.

The age at which a subject acquires their infection appears to play a role in the subsequent development of gastric cancer. Acquisition of infection at a very early age has been related to a much higher gastric cancer risk, with an especially high risk in the setting of a positive family history of gastric cancer.[223,224] The familial aggregation of stomach cancer may, in part, be explained by familial aggregation of *H. pylori* infection.[223,224] The implications this has on diagnosis and treatment in the pediatric setting has yet to be determined. An important question that remains unanswered is whether or not *H. pylori* eradication will alter the risk for the development of gastric cancer. The results from ongoing intervention trials examining the effect of *H. pylori* eradication on gastric cancer rates may have a major impact on future approaches to *H. pylori* infection treatment and prevention.[65] A recent prospective, randomized, placebo-controlled, population-based primary prevention study involving 1630 otherwise healthy adults in China with asymptomatic *H. pylori* infection demonstrated that at 7.5 years of follow-up the incidence of gastric cancer was not statistically significantly different after eradication therapy (0.86% *vs* 1.35%, P=0.3).[225] Unfortunately, the study was not powered adequately to demonstrate such a difference. Subgroup analysis suggests that subsequent cancer risk might be reduced in only those carriers without precancerous lesions. As highlighted by Parsonnet and Forman,[226] this is the first experimental evidence in humans that *H. pylori* infection causes cancer; the question of whom to treat, however, remains unanswered.

Mucosa-associated lymphoid tissue lymphoma

Primary malignant tumors of the stomach are uncommon in children and usually consist of lymphoma and sarcoma.[227,228] Primary gastric lymphoma can be divided histopathologically into mucosa-associated lymphoid tissue (MALT) lymphoma and non-MALT lymphoma. Primary gastric lymphoma is a very rare malignancy in children.[229] The risk of gastric MALT lymphoma is significantly increased with *H. pylori* infection.[230] Some 72–98% of patients with gastric MALT lymphoma are infected with *H. pylori*. The eradication of *H. pylori* alone induces regression (and remission) of gastric MALT lymphoma in 70–80% of cases.[231] Failure of the lymphoma to respond to eradication therapy has been associated with certain genetic abnormalities within the host, including the presence of the specific genetic translocations t(11;18)(q21;q21). Such cases usually progress to high-grade tumors.[232–234] Most subjects who respond to eradication therapy remain in remission for many years. However, the experience with treating such patients with antibiotics alone is still quite limited.[233,235,236] There are a few reports of childhood MALT lymphoma in the literature,[229] including a case of a 14-year-old girl with MALT lymphoma that responded to *H. pylori* eradication.[237]

Extraintestinal manifestations

Iron deficiency anemia

Most of the published studies describing anemia in the setting of *H. pylori* infection have been within pediatric populations.[238,239] In general, within developed countries, iron deficiency anemia (IDA) is seen more frequently in children and adolescents, and is a rare problem in adults.[240] Thus, if *H. pylori* infection does lead to IDA, then children would be more likely to be affected than adults.[241]

Epidemiologic studies in both adults and children have indicated an association between *H. pylori* seropositivity and both low serum ferritin and low hemoglobin levels.[242–244] A seroepidemiologic study of 937 children found iron deficiency to be twice as common in *H. pylori*-positive children compared with *H. pylori*-negative ones.[245] A number of case reports have demonstrated IDA, previously resistant to iron replacement therapy, responding to the eradication of *H. pylori*, with a few reports of *H. pylori* eradication resulting in improvement of anemia even without iron supplementation.[238–240,246–251] Both of these findings have been supported in a recent double-blind, placebo-controlled, randomized trial of 22 preadolescent children and adolescents with concurrent IDA and *H. pylori* infection in Korea.[250]

Several mechanisms responsible for *H. pylori*-mediated iron-deficiency anemia have been postulated.[252,253] Chronic gastrointestinal bleeding due to gastritis, erosions or ulceration may be to blame. However, most studies have not detected occult gastrointestinal blood loss in infected patients with anemia.[254] The levels of gastric acidity and gastric ascorbic acid (GAA) are important for the absorption of dietary iron.[255] Ascorbic acid chelates iron, protects its stability in the duodenum, and increases its absorption. Gastric acidity maintains ferric iron in its soluble form and enhances its absorption.[256] Thus, processes that result in hypochlorhydria or decreased GAA levels may impair the bioavailability of iron. *H. pylori* gastritis in adults causes hypochlorhydria and decreased GAA levels.[257,258] Acid production and its regulation during bacterial colonization is not well understood in children; however, it is doubtful whether children with mild pangastritis have functional changes identical to those seen in adults.[241] In most children, the mucosal and glandular structure within the gastric body remains completely normal during chronic *H. pylori* infection, with atrophy being an unusual late phenomenon.[241,259] A recent study of 52 Turkish children undergoing upper gastrointestinal endoscopy demonstrated that *H. pylori*-associated pangastritis was more common in the setting of concurrent IDA.[252] The final postulated mechanism involves scavenging of iron or heme by the organism. It is hypothesized that IDA is related to the sequestration of iron by antral *H. pylori* infection. *H. pylori* is known to possess genes with an iron-scavenging function, thus enabling the bacterium to extract iron from its host.[260,261] Barabino et al.[238] demonstrated that iron was diverted away from the bone marrow in patients with IDA and *H. pylori* infection.

Children with low iron intake or increased iron requirements form an obvious risk group for IDA. In this vulnerable group, it is possible that even minor disturbances in the iron absorption mechanisms that may occur due to *H. pylori* infection might quickly lead to a deficiency state.[241] There is a significant body of evidence linking iron deficiency states in young children with impaired cognitive development, and its potential reversibility with iron store replenishment.[262] The implications that this has in regard to appropriate investigation and therapy in the setting of isolated therapy-resistant iron deficiency anaemia are yet to be determined. However, recently updated Canadian Consensus Guidelines for *H. pylori* infection in children suggest that children presenting with unexplained iron deficiency anemia that is refractory to therapy may warrant investigation for *H. pylori* infection.[263]

Short stature

A number of studies have suggested that *H. pylori* infection may have a negative effect on growth, although reports are conflicting.[254,264–269] Most studies are longitudinal in design, utilizing either serology or UBT for diagnosis, and include children over a fairly wide age range.[270–272] In 2001, Richter et al.[268] conducted a cross-sectional population-based study in Germany involving 3315 children aged 5–7 years. This group represented 88% of all preschool and school-aged children born in the area over a 12-month period. Diagnosis of *H. pylori* was made by the ^{13}C urea test. The overall prevalence of *H. pylori* infection was about 7%. A small, but statistically significant, difference in height (before and after age and sex adjustment) was detected between *H. pylori*-positive and -negative children, and was more pronounced in males.[268] In contrast to other studies,[273] no significant difference in socioeconomic status was found between the two groups. The observed association of *H. pylori* infection and lower height may be explained in a variety of ways. It may be the generic result of a chronic infective process. Alternatively, it has been suggested that growth retardation could be a result of either gastritis[274] or a co-morbidity such as anemia.[275] Alternatively, *H. pylori* infection and growth retardation may be caused coincidentally by the same confounding factors, such as a variety of social factors.[276] All current evidence considered, it is probably premature to recommend a systematic search for *H. pylori* infection in children with growth retardation.

Other suggested associations

A wide variety of other extraintestinal manifestations have been suggested to have an association with *H. pylori* infection. These range in diversity from dermatologic/autoimmune problems such as chronic urticaria and idiopathic thrombocytopenia (ITP) to sudden infant death syndrome (SIDS). Data examining the role that *H. pylori* may play in ITP is currently limited to observational findings and basic science hypotheses.[277] An association in distinct subpopulations appears plausible; however, more investigative data are required. A critical assessment of the evidence on a relationship with SIDS has concluded that a causal association is very unlikely.[278] Current evidence for other putative associations is also not compelling.

Benefits of disease

It is postulated that there may be potential benefits to *H. pylori* infection. This has led some to suggest that complete eradication of the bacterium may not be in the best interests of all human hosts.[279,280] *H. pylori* may stimulate specific local and systemic immunoglobulin secretion and thus participate in host defense against exogenous pathogens. There is a suggestion that *H. pylori* can synthesize antibacterial peptides to which it is resistant, but which would prevent other faster-growing bacteria from colonizing the gastric mucosa and other parts of the gastrointestinal tract.[28,281] Some, but not all, studies suggest that *H. pylori* may be associated with protection from diarrheal diseases in both children and adults from developed countries.[282,283] Given that only a small proportion of *H. pylori* carriers develop clinically related disease, it may well be that there are benefits to colonization. However, the potential positive final consequences of *H. pylori* elimination for human health should not be overlooked.[28]

DIAGNOSIS

The ideal test for *H. pylori* would be non-invasive, highly accurate, inexpensive and readily available. The test would differentiate between active and past infection, and discriminate between *H. pylori* infection and *H. pylori*-associated disease. No such test currently exists. Thus it is important to appraise the advantages and disadvantages of the tests that are available and assess their suitability for use in children.[190]

Amongst all the diagnostic tests currently available, there is no single 'gold standard' for the diagnosis of *H. pylori* infection. The positive and/or negative predictive value of a test (PPV and NPV respectively) depend on the characteristics of both the test and of the population in which it is performed. A variety of studies have now been completed confirming the accuracy of the various diagnostic methods in children. There are only a few data, however, validating these methods in diverse populations.

Two categories of test are available to diagnose *H. pylori* infection: invasive (requiring endoscopy) and non-invasive (or non-endoscopic). Within each broad category there are a variety of different options.

Invasive tests

Endoscopy and biopsy

Upper gastrointestinal endoscopy and biopsy remains the 'gold standard' in the diagnosis and identification of *H. pylori* infection and its consequences in childhood.[188–190] It allows visualization of the upper gastrointestinal tract and also facilitates the diagnosis of diseases other than those related to *H. pylori* infection. Gastric inflammation caused by *H. pylori* is not always observed macroscopically.[284,285] Nodularity within the stomach is seen more frequently in children than in adults. It was first described by Hassall and Dimmick in 1991.[183] The mucosa is irregular in appearance, resembling a cobblestone pavement. Nodules measure 1–4 mm in diameter, have a smooth surface and are the same color as the surrounding mucosa. Seen most often within the gastric antrum, it is frequently referred to as antral nodular gastritis. Recent data demonstrate a positive correlation with antral nodularity and the severity of histologic gastritis.[284] Nodules are often best appreciated following biopsy, when blood from the biopsy site surrounds and highlights them. Endoscopy facilitates the collection of mucosal biopsies, upon which a variety of direct tests can then be performed. Procedural risk, anesthetic/sedation requirements, relative expense and limited access to appropriate pediatric expertise all remain disadvantages, with endoscopy being considered the diagnostic test of choice.

Culture

Culture is a potential 'gold standard' for the diagnosis of suspected *H. pylori* infection. However, the bacterium is fastidious. Under adverse conditions its morphology transforms.[286] Cultivation requires a micro-aerophilic environment and complex media. Undoubtedly the most specific way to establish a diagnosis, its sensitivity has been reported to vary greatly between laboratories,[287] with even experienced laboratories recovering the organism from only 50–70% of infected biopsies.[288] Diagnostic yield is improved when multiple biopsies are collected.[289–291] Yanez et al.[292] studied a variety of invasive and non-invasive diagnostic tests in a group of 59 Mexican children presenting consecutively for upper gastrointestinal endoscopy. The study's derived diagnostic gold standard was three or more positive tests. Some 37% of the children were *H. pylori* positive. The authors collected two biopsies from both the antrum and the body for culture. Although the specificity was 100%, the sensitivity was 77%, resulting in a NPV for this population of 88%. *H. pylori* lacks regulatory genes, making its survival for long periods outside the gastric environment poor.[64] Thus, it is important that specimens be processed within 2–3 h of collection.[287,291,293–295]

In summary, culture of *H. pylori* is a tedious but reliable procedure with a high degree of sensitivity if performed carefully. Its major advantage is in the ability to perform antibiotic sensitivity testing on the isolates, which can influence the outcome of therapy.[296] Both phenotypic and genotypic methods are available for antimicrobial susceptibility testing. However, phenotypic methods are generally easier to perform and more economic.[291]

Rapid urease test

The realization that *H. pylori* possessed an active urease enzyme led to the development of a variety of diagnostic tests, including the rapid urease test (RUT). Urease catalyzes the hydrolysis of urea into ammonia and carbon dioxide. The production of ammonia leads to an increase in the local pH. Samples are placed within a gel containing urea and a pH indicator. A color change occurs as urea is broken down by the bacteria.[190] Although widely used within the adult population, the use of RUTs in pediatrics is limited by a significantly lower sensitivity compared with that of histology; this appears to be related to a lower mucosal bacterial load.[297,298] A variety of studies have validated this method in children. Elitsur and Neace[299] examined a group of 94 children in West Virginia. Using histology as the gold standard (demonstration of *H. pylori* with Giemsa staining), 19% of their study population was *H. pylori* positive. RUT had a sensitivity of about 45% and a specificity of virtually 100%. In their population, the test thus had a PPV about 95% and a NPV of about 89%. When utilizing a combination rather than a single investigation as the comparative gold standard, the demonstrated sensitivity of the RUT in childhood is significantly improved, with the PPV approaching 100%.[292,299–302] In a study of 59 Mexican children with a disease prevalence of 37%, of the three invasive techniques (culture, histologic examination of antrum and corpus biopsies with hematoxylin and eosin (H&E) and Giemsa staining, and RUT), RUT was the most sensitive and had the best NPV (100%).[292]

Histopathology

On H&E staining of gastric mucosal biopsies obtained from *H. pylori*-infected patients, a superficial infiltrate is usually seen with substantial numbers of plasma cells and lymphocytes within the mucosa.[182,303] Biopsies obtained from children infected with *H. pylori* generally have less neutrophil infiltration compared with tissue obtained from infected adults.[182,183,303]

Detection of the *H. pylori* bacterium can be accomplished by utilizing a variety of different stains.[304] The organism can be identified in routinely stained H&E slides.[304] Sensitivity can be enhanced by utilizing special stains, including modified Romanovsky methods (Giemsa, Diff-3), Sayeed stains or silver stains (Dieterle, Warthin-Starry, Steiner, Genta).[304] Silver stains are very sensitive, but also stain a wide variety of bacteria besides *H. pylori*. In addition, they rely on demonstrating the typical morphology of the bacterium.[305] Immunohistochemical techniques utilizing anti-*H. pylori* antibodies have also been shown to be quite effective.[306,307] In the study of 59 Mexican children referred to previously,[292] histology utilizing H&E and Giemsa stains had a sensitivity of 82% and specificity of 95%, resulting in a PPV and NPV of approximately 90%.

Although *H. pylori* colonization results in chronic gastritis, not all chronic gastritis is due to *H. pylori*.[300] However, the special techniques for identifying *H. pylori* can be both time consuming and expensive.[305] Eshun et al.[305] retrospectively reviewed 37 patients and 12 controls in an attempt to determine the optimal combination of histologic tests for confirming *H. pylori* infection in pediatric patients with gastric lymphocytic inflammation and a negative urease test. They found that urease-positive patients tended to have more severe gastritis, a greater abundance of organisms and a greater likelihood of organisms being found on routine staining. In addition, higher grades of gastritis were associated with greater numbers of organisms.[305] These authors concluded that, in children, a positive urease test obviates the need for special histologic staining (anything more than H&E staining). However, when biopsies display chronic inflammation and a negative urease test result, immunohistochemical stains should be utilized to further investigate for *H. pylori* infection.[305]

The site from which the biopsy is taken can affect the accuracy of diagnosis. Elitzur et al.[308] studied 206 children to determine the optimal biopsy location. After sampling six different sites they concluded the mid-antrum at the lesser curvature was the best location for detecting *H. pylori* histologically in children. Biopsies collected from this site had a sensitivity of 100%, compared with a sensitivity of approximately 90% for other sites within the antrum and 73% for sites tested within the gastric body. More recently, Borrelli et al.[300] examined biopsies from 89 consecutive children undergoing upper gastrointestinal endoscopy for symptoms suggestive of acid peptic disease. Some 25% were *H. pylori* positive. All *H. pylori* cases had a positive RUT and positive histology (*H. pylori* demonstrated with Giemsa staining) on biopsies from the cardia (a region defined as the anatomic zone from the squamocolumnar junction to 0.5 cm below it). However, in only 30% of these patients was *H. pylori* also detected in the antral and/or corpus biopsies. This is an unusual finding that requires further investigation. Notably, adult studies have demonstrated the cardia to be second only to the antrum in yield of *H. pylori* on biopsy.[309]

Non-invasive tests

It cannot be assumed that non-invasive diagnostic tests for *H. pylori* infection perform as well in children as they do in adults. Further, methods that perform well in older children will not necessarily produce valid results in younger children. A variety of non-invasive tests are currently available. However, availability does not imply suitability.

Serologic tests

H. pylori infection induces both cellular and humoral immune responses, resulting in an early increase in specific IgM, and a later and persistent increase in specific IgA and IgG.[310] In children, IgA-based tests detect only 20–50% of *H. pylori*-infected patients.[311,312] Serologic tests based on the detection of specific anti-*H. pylori* IgG antibodies in the serum offer a better sensitivity than IgA-based tests. Their most important limitation is the inability to distinguish active from past infection. A number of different techniques are available, including ELISA, agglutination tests and western blotting. The duration of infection and the ability of the host to mount an immune response influence the results of this test. Thus, in some children, the duration and degree of infection may not have been present long enough to generate an immune response in all cases.[292] The accuracy of these tests is no longer adequate to justify their clinical use on either clinical or economic grounds except, perhaps, in high-prevalence situations (prevalence greater than 60%).[313] In general, their utility is restricted to large epidemiology studies.[292] Given the low sensitivity in infants and toddlers, epidemiologic studies based on antibody testing may underestimate the prevalence and transmission of *H. pylori* infection in the very young.[58,314,315] 'Near patient tests' (tests that allow an infection to be diagnosed on the spot, without the need to send samples to a laboratory) cannot be recommended at present due to low sensitivity and specificity.[313,316–322]

Tests on saliva and urine

Results with salivary antibody tests have been disappointing (sensitivity 81%, specificity 73%).[323] Urine antibody results have been variable. A pilot study of 132 adult patients demonstrated a sensitivity of 86% and a specificity of 91%. A follow-up European multicenter trial using the same assay had a sensitivity and specificity of 89% and 69%.[324,325] Thus, these non-invasive methods are not currently recommended.

Urea breath test

The UBT is based on the presence of *H. pylori* urease. Urea is labeled with either ^{13}C (non-radioactive) or ^{14}C (radioactive) isotopes, and then ingested. Labeled urea comes into contact with the mucosa and diffuses through the mucus. Here, urea hydrolysis by *H. pylori* produces ammonia and labeled carbon dioxide. Urea rapidly passes down its concentration gradient into the epithelial blood supply, and within minutes appears in the breath (Fig. 26.5). Labeled urea is usually given with a test meal to delay gastric emptying. Breath samples are collected at variable times postingestion.[325] For optimal results, the gastric environment should be acidic.[326,327]

If using ^{14}C, the radioactivity of each sample is measured by a scintillation counter, and the results expressed either as a percentage of the administered dose or directly as counts per minutes.[325] The cumulative lifetime radiation exposure from this test is calculated as being equal to the background radiation that a person is exposed to in 1 day.[328] However, in general, the ^{14}C UBT is not used in children or women of childbearing age.

^{13}C is a naturally occurring non-radioactive isotope. It can be safely used in even very young infants, and can be repeated without risk to the child.[329] Its detection requires a mass spectrometer rather than a scintillation counter. Results are traditionally reported as delta over baseline (DOB) values for the measured ratio $^{13}CO_2/^{12}CO_2$. DOB values exceeding a fixed cutoff value are considered indicative of *H. pylori* infection.[58] Since it was first described in 1987,[330] a variety of modifications have been made, includ-

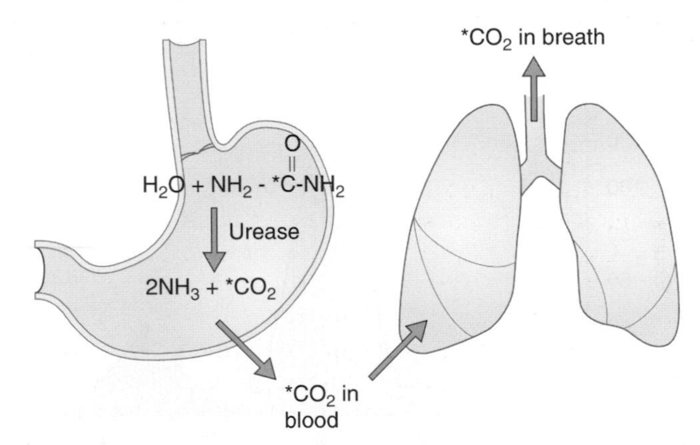

Figure 26.5: Schematic representation of urea breath testing. Following ingestion, labeled urea comes into contact with the mucosa and diffuses through the mucus. It is hydrolyzed by *H. pylori* urease, producing ammonia and labeled carbon dioxide, which passes rapidly into the blood supply and into the breath, within minutes. The expired concentration of labeled carbon dioxide is then measured. For optimal results, the gastric environment should be acidic. (From Fischer et al., 2004, with permission.)[390]

ing dose, sampling time, test meal and cutoff values. These changes are in an effort to reduce the duration of the test, improve its accuracy or reduce the amount of expensive substrate (^{13}C) used. Recently a method utilizing a tablet formulation of [^{13}C]urea has been described. This administration method avoids interference from urease-producing bacteria in the oropharynx, a potential cause of false-positive results.[331] In adults, the quoted overall sensitivity and specificity of the ^{13}C UBT is 94.7% and 95.7% respectively.[313,332–335]

There is increasing validation of this technique in childhood.[336–341] However, comparative evaluations of different protocols are scarce. In particular, data determining the [^{13}C]urea dose, the appropriate type of test meal, the need for a test meal, the number and time interval for breath sampling, and the appropriate cutoff dose is minimal. A multicenter trial in 2000 attempted to address these issues.[333] The authors demonstrated that the DOB cutoff value varied with changes in [^{13}C]urea dose, type of test meal and time of breath collection, and thus needs to be calculated by the receiver–operator characteristic (ROC) curve for any protocol. Test meals that contain citric acid result in higher DOB values in *H. pylori*-positive patients[342,343] and thus may improve the sensitivity of the test in children. A study by Kindermann et al.[339] of 1499 German children confirmed its utility in children over 6 years of age. The researchers demonstrated two very distinct subpopulations of DOB results when plotting the natural logarithms of the DOB (Fig. 26.6). The optimal cutoff value that would be expected to misclassify only 2.2% of patients was then calculated. Utilizing these values, 149 cases were validated with histology and RUT. The sensitivity and specificity for children over 6 years of age in this group were 100% and 98% respectively, with a PPV and NPV of 98% and 100%. In younger age groups, accuracy was compromised by false-positive results. For children under the age

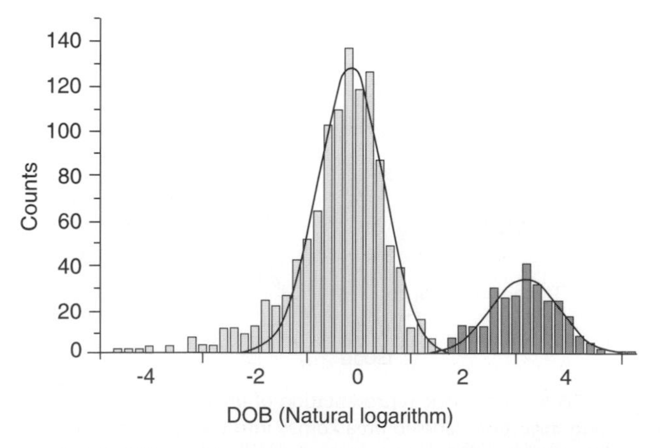

Figure 26.6: ^{13}C-urea breath test delta over baseline (DOB) values in a group of 1499 symptomatic children aged from 2 months to 18 years. The distribution of logarithms of DOB values after [^{13}C]urea intake identified two populations considered to represent children with negative (hatched bars) and positive (solid bars) test results. (From Kindermann A et al., 2000, with permission.)[339]

of 6 years, although the sensitivity remained at 100%, the specificity fell to 88% and the PPV to 69%. The NPV remained at 100%. Koletzko and Feydt-Schmidt[58] have demonstrated a significant inverse relationship between DOB values and age in both infected and non-infected children. Kindermann's analysis demonstrates that UBT accuracy can be improved for patients aged less than 6 years by increasing the DOB cutoff; however, the false-positive rate at best remains at about 8%.[339] There is some evidence to suggest that this age dependence could be eliminated by normalizing the results for estimated carbon dioxide production.[344] All findings support the concept that the DOB cutoff value needs to be calculated by the ROC curve for each protocol in each patient population. Test accuracy may also be compromised by recent use of either antibiotics[345] or acid suppression.[326,346,347] Based on adult data, it is advisable to cease antibiotic therapy at least 4 weeks and proton pump inhibitor (PPI) therapy at least 2 weeks before conducting a UBT. Recently, infrared spectroscopy rather than mass spectroscopy has been tried.[348] If successful, this would reduce the cost of the technique. UBT has not been validated in developing countries.

Stool antigen test

H. pylori antigen can be detected in the stool. Stool testing is a potentially inexpensive, non-invasive method for determining *H. pylori* infection. Two types of enzyme immunoassay are now available to detect *H. pylori* antigen in stool. A polyclonal capture antibody has been used most commonly in the past; a monoclonal test has also been developed recently and tested in children.[349]

The utility of the polyclonal test has been investigated extensively in both the pre- and post-therapy setting for adults, with increasing pediatric data becoming available. In a large review of studies from 1999 to 2001, evaluating 3419 patients in the pretreatment setting, the mean sensitivity and specificity were 93.2% and 93.2% respectively.[313] These results suggest that the polyclonal test is not as reliable as the UBT. Kato et al.[350] studied 264 children aged 2–17 years and demonstrated an overall sensitivity of 96%, specificity of 96.8%, PPV of 93.2% and NPV of 98.4%. Results were independent of age. Results of post-therapy studies are variable, with more recent studies noting a significant inter-test variation, with sensitivity in some studies reported as low as 63%.[325,351,352]

In contrast, results from studies utilizing the monoclonal antibody test look very promising. A recently published multicenter study evaluated the test in 302 symptomatic children and compared it with UBT, RUT, histologic examination and biopsy.[349] The manufacturer's recommended optical density of 0.150 was used as the cutoff value. Figure 26.7 demonstrates the clear demarcation between positive and negative results. Results were independent of age, processing laboratory and production lot. With only two false-positive and two false-negative results, the sensitivity, specificity, PPV and NPV were 98%, 99%, 98% and 99% respectively. Similar findings have been demonstrated pre-

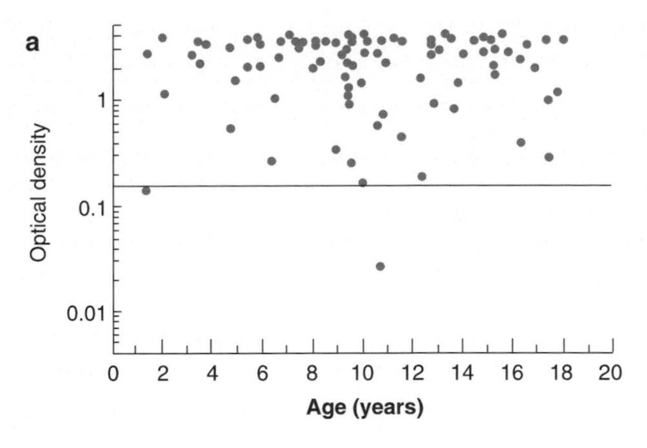

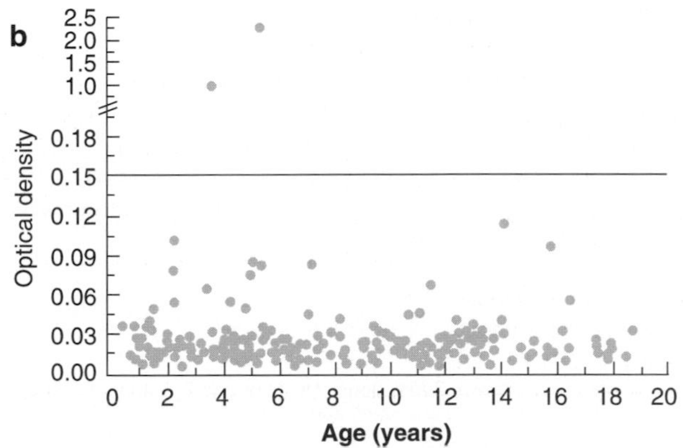

Figure 26.7: Results of monoclonal stool antigen testing in children with known *H. pylori* status (optical density values on a log scale in relation to age). (**a**) Positive *H. pylori* status ($n = 92$). (**b**) Negative *H. pylori* status ($n = 210$). (Reproduced from Koletzko S, Konstantopoulos N, Bosman D, et al. Evaluation of a novel monoclonal enzyme immunoassay for detection of *Helicobacter pylori* antigen in stool from children. Gut 2003; 52:804–806, with permission.)[349]

viously in a pediatric group,[351] and subsequently in an adult population.[353] Although promising, more data are needed before this investigation can be recommended as a replacement to UBT in the post-therapy setting.

When comparing the cost–effectiveness of this method against UBT, the capital equipment involved must be considered. UBT requires a mass spectrophotometer, which in turn requires dedicated personnel and high annual service charges. The stool test requires an optical spectrophotometer, usually present in any laboratory, has negligible maintenance costs and does not require dedicated personnel.[325]

Summary

Although some non-invasive methods are particularly promising for the accurate diagnosis of *H. pylori* infection, currently there is insufficient evidence to recommend them as they cannot be used reliably to diagnose *H. pylori*-associated diseases in children.[58] Current guidelines recommend treatment only in children with *H. pylori*-related peptic ulcer disease, or other complications of the infection.[188–190] However, with further knowledge on the measurable health risks for *H. pylori*-infected children, or with the availability of vaccination and other treatment options, the risk–benefit relationship and thus the recommendations regarding non-invasive testing may change.[58]

When is testing indicated?

At present, the primary goal of testing is to diagnose the cause of clinical symptoms and not simply to detect the presence of *H. pylori*. As in many clinical scenarios, testing is not helpful unless it will alter the management of the disease.[190] As knowledge of the intestinal and extraintestinal manifestations of *H. pylori* expands, so too will the appropriate indications for *H. pylori* testing in children. Table 26.2 summarizes the current indications for testing developed by the 2004 Canadian *Helicobacter pylori* Paediatric Consensus Conference. A summary of recommendations generated from this conference is given in Table 26.3.

TREATMENT

The optimal therapeutic approach to *H. pylori* infection in children is yet to be elucidated. Children with peptic ulcer disease and *H. pylori* infection should receive treatment; the treatment endpoint should be the eradication of infection. However, as previously discussed, the majority of children infected with *H. pylori* do not have peptic ulcer disease. For many, the diagnosis of *H. pylori* infection is incidental. The management of these children remains controversial.

Specific regimens

Adult literature suggests that clinically relevant *H. pylori* eradication regimens must have cure rates of at least 80% (according to intention-to-treat analysis), be without major side-effects and induce minimal bacterial resistance.[65] Antibiotics alone have not achieved this. Luminal acidity influences both the effectiveness of some antimicrobial agents and the survival of the bacterium; thus antibiotics have been combined with acid suppression such as PPIs, bismuth or H_2 antagonists. So-called 'triple therapies' are a combination of one antisecretory agent with two antimicrobial agents for 7–14 days. This therapy has been investigated extensively in adult populations. A number of regimens have been approved by the various pharmaceutical licensing boards.[65] The 'classic' regimen is treatment twice daily for 7 days with omeprazole and clarithromycin plus either amoxicillin or metronidazole.[354]

Endoscopically diagnosed peptic ulcer disease	Yes
Recurrent abdominal pain or non-ulcer dyspepsia	No
Gastroesophageal reflux	No
Iron deficiency anemia refractory to therapy	Yes
Asymptomatic children	No
Family history of gastric cancer	Yes
Documented MALT lymphoma	Yes
Following eradication therapy	Yes

Table 26.2 When is testing for *H. pylori* indicated?

Whom to investigate
• The symptoms of *H. pylori*-related disease are non-specific. The aim of investigating children presenting with persistent abdominal complaints should be directed at diagnosing their cause, and not focused on proving *H. pylori* infection. • There is no role in specifically investigating for *H. pylori* infection following either the diagnosis of gastroesophageal reflux and/or commencing long-term proton pump inhibitor therapy. • Neither recurrent abdominal pain nor functional dyspepsia is an indication to test for *H. pylori* infection. • Investigation of children with unexplained iron deficiency anemia refractory to therapy may warrant investigation for *H. pylori* infection. • Investigation for *H. pylori* infection in children with a family history of gastric cancer should be considered. • Population screening for *H. pylori* in asymptomatic children is not warranted.
How to investigate
• Upper GI endoscopy with multiple biopsies is the optimal approach to the investigation of the pediatric patient with upper abdominal symptoms or suspected peptic ulcer disease. • ^{13}C-urea breath testing is the recommended non-invasive diagnostic method for *H. pylori* in children. • There is currently insufficient evidence to recommend a role for stool antigen tests in the diagnosis of *H. pylori* infection. • Serologic, urinary or salivary antibody tests are not recommended as diagnostic tools for *H. pylori* infection in children.
How to treat
• The first-line treatment for *H. pylori* infection is a twice-daily triple-drug regimen comprising a proton pump inhibitor (PPI) , clarithromycin, and either amoxicillin or metronidazole. PPI with amoxicillin and metronidazole is an acceptable alternative. • The optimal treatment period is 10–14 days. • Antibiotic sensitivity testing should be performed in cases where eradication therapy has failed. • Antibiotic resistance patterns should be monitored, and treatment choices modified accordingly.

Adapted from guidelines generated at the Canadian *Helicobacter pylori* Paediatric Consensus Conference, Ottawa, 2004. (Jones NL, Sherman P, Fallone CA et al. for the Canadian Helicobacter Study Group. Canadian Helicobacter Study Group Consensus Conference. *Can J Gastroenterol* 2005; 19(7):399–408).

Table 26.3 Recommendations on the approach to *H. pylori* infection in children and adolescents

A meta-analysis in 1999 of 666 studies in 53 228 adult subjects demonstrated parity between all regimens that included a PPI plus any two of the three antibiotics (clarithromycin, amoxicillin and a nitroimidazole), with cure rates ranging from 79% to 83%.[355]

Bismuth has been used in the treatment of peptic ulcer disease for many years. The exact mechanism of action in *H. pylori* eradication is not known. A variety of regimens involving bismuth have been described in both the pediatric and adult literature. Concern has been expressed about the potential toxic effects of bismuth salts in children. However, there appears to be no more risk than that seen in adults. Chronic ingestion of high-dose bismuth associated with encephalopathy and/or acute renal impairment has been reported, but not in children being treated for *H. pylori* disease.[182,356] In Europe, colloidal bismuth subcitrate is available and in North America bismuth subsalicylate is used; a further concern about the risk of Reye's syndrome has thus been raised. Finally, it has been suggested that the strong taste of ammonia associated with liquid bismuth may reduce compliance.[357] Treatment regimens utilizing PPIs are often felt to be more attractive in the pediatric setting.

Most of the treatment studies in children have been open trials with small numbers of participants. In 2000, Oderda et al.[358] performed a systematic review of all published eradication treatment schedules in children. Given the limited number of adequate studies, the small numbers in each study and the marked heterogeneity, it was difficult to make any definitive statements from the data. Recommendations for eradication therapy outlined in the various pediatric consensus statements are based on the extrapolation of adult data. To date, only one randomized controlled double-blind trial has been reported.[359] Published in 2001, this compared 1 week of triple therapy with omeprazole, amoxicillin and clarithromycin (OAC) against dual antibiotic therapy with amoxicillin and clarithromycin (AC). Eradication was 75% *vs* 9.4% respectively; a finding in keeping with adult data.[359] An open Brazilian study of 25 children in 2001 demonstrated eradication rates of only 50% after 7 days' therapy, improving to 73% after 10 days.[360] In the same year, an open randomized study of 106 Russian children demonstrated eradication rates of 80–89% after 7 days' therapy with omeprazole, amoxicillin and metronidazole (OAM).[361] A prospective study of quadruple therapy for 1 week, utilizing omeprazole, amoxicillin, clarithromycin and metronidazole (OACM), demonstrated an eradication rate of 94%.[362] Table 26.4 summarizes the *H. pylori* treatment guidelines currently recommended by the North American Society of Pediatric Gastroenterology and Nutrition. The recently updated Canadian Consensus guidelines have re-endorsed these recommendations.

Treatment failure

A variety of factors contribute to treatment failure. The important ones include bacterial factors such as antibiotic resistance, virulence and bacterial load, and traditional host factors such as patient adherence to therapy and ade-

	Medications	Dosage
First-line options		
1	Amoxicillin	50 mg/kg/day up to 1 g bid
	Clarithromycin	15 mg/kg/day up to 500 mg bid
	PPI: omeprazole[a]	1 mg/kg/day up to 20 mg bid
2	Amoxicillin	50 mg/kg/day up to 1 g bid
	Metronidazole	20 mg/kg/day up to 500 mg bid
	PPI: omeprazole[a]	1 mg/kg/day up to 20 mg bid
3	Clarithromycin	15 mg/kg/day up to 500 mg bid
	Metronidazole	20 mg/kg/day up to 500 mg bid
	PPI: omeprazole[a]	1 mg/kg/day up to 20 mg bid
Second-line options		
4	Bismuth subsalicylate	1 tablet (262 mg) qid *or* 15 ml (17.6 mg/ml) qid[b]
	Metronidazole	20 mg/kg/day up to 500 mg bid
	PPI: omeprazole[a]	1 mg/kg/day up to 20 mg bid
	Plus an additional antibiotic:	
	Amoxicillin	50 mg/kg/day up to 1 g bid
	or tetracycline[c]	50 mg/kg/day up to 1 g bid
	or clarithromycin	15 mg/kg/day up to 500 mg bid
5	Ranitidine bismuth citrate[b]1 tablet qid[b]	
	Clarithromycin	15 mg/kg/day up to 500 mg bid
	Metronidazole	20 mg/kg/day up to 500 mg bid

Initial treatment should be provided in a twice-daily regimen (to enhance compliance) for 7–14 days.
[a] Or comparable acid inhibitory doses of another proton pump inhibitor (PPI).
[b] This is the dose recommended for adults.
[c] Only for children 12 years of age or older.
bid, twice daily; qid, four times daily.
Source: North American Society for Pediatric Gastroenterology and Nutrition. Medical position statement. J Pediatr Gastroenterol Nutr 2000; 31:490–497.

Table 26.4 Recommended eradication therapies for *H. pylori* disease in children

quacy of drug delivery as well as, possibly, specific genotypic factors including the recently recognized *CYP2C19* genotype (extensive and poor PPI metabolizers).[363–366] There are few data available on many of these factors in pediatric populations.

Antibiotic resistance

The chief antimicrobial agents used are amoxicillin, clarithromycin, metronidazole and tetracycline. *H. pylori* resistance to these is an important variable in successful eradication. In general, rates of resistance are increasing with time, with pronounced geographic variation.[367] Antibiotic resistance may be primary (present before therapy) or secondary (developing during therapy).

The activity of metronidazole against *H. pylori* is dependent on reduction of its nitro moiety to highly reactive compounds that in turn cause DNA strand breakage. *H. pylori* resistance is caused primarily by a variety of mutational inactivations of the nitroreductase genes (these include *rdxA*, *frxA* and *fdxB*).[65] Table 26.5 documents the variable metronidazole resistance rates recently seen in isolates from children throughout Europe and Japan.[367]

Clarithromycin's activity against *H. pylori* depends on its binding to ribosomes and thus disrupting protein synthesis. It is thought that clarithromycin needs effective acid control to achieve high eradication rates. Resistance to clarithromycin was first reported in 1996.[368] It is caused by point mutations at two sites along the 23S ribosomal RNA gene sequence. These mutations can be

	Amoxicillin (%)	Metronidazole (%)	Clarithromycin (%)
Western Europe			
Austria	0	25	–
Belgium	0	18	17
France	0	43	21
Germany	0	32	22
Portugal	0	19	45
Spain	0	23	21
Eastern Europe	0.9	31	9.5
Japan	0	24	29
North America	4.6	–	41
Mexico	15.7	–	22

Adapted from Dupont et al., 2003.[367]

Table 26.5 Levels of antibiotic resistance documented in *H. pylori* isolates from infected children in Europe, America and Japan prior to eradication therapy

detected by a variety of molecular methods including fluorescence *in situ* hybridization (FISH).[369] PCR-restriction fragment length polymorphism (RFLP) (with a sensitivity of 92% and specificity of 100%) can rapidly detect clarithromycin-resistant strains within 24 h.[370] A European multicenter survey in 2001 demonstrated that clarithromycin resistance was much higher in children and adolescents (17.3% and 13.6% respectively) than in all other age groups (8.2%).[371] Numerous studies have demonstrated a rapid increase in resistance over time.[367,372] Table 26.5 documents the current geographic variability in clarithromycin resistance seen in pediatric populations. The markedly higher level of resistance seen in strains isolated from children compared with adults suggests the potentially noxious effect of macrolide overusage in children.[54]

H. pylori was previously thought not to develop resistance to amoxicillin. Recently, *H. pylori* strains resistant to amoxicillin have been isolated from children in Mexico, the USA and eastern Europe.[367,373] Antimicrobial susceptibilities are summarized in Table 26.5.[367]

The antibiotics used in the treatment of *H. pylori* are also used to treat a variety of other common infections. It is likely that *H. pylori* organisms will have unintentionally come into contact with the agents previously when they were given for another indication. Thus, local therapeutic trends and official guidelines are likely to have an effect on emerging resistance patterns, particularly in childhood.[374] Perez Aldana et al.[375] demonstrated that the regional prevalence of clarithromycin and metronidazole resistance was related to the annual consumption of these antimicrobial agents.[375] A prospective study of 23 infected children treated with triple therapy containing metronidazole indicated that eradication rates were dependent on metronidazole susceptibility (83% *vs* 17% for metronidazole-resistant strains).[376] In a group of 61 children whose treatment included clarithromycin, eradication was achieved in all those with clarithromycin-sensitive strains and in none of those with clarithromycin-resistant ones (P=0.0001).[377] Subsequent meta-analysis has demonstrated that primary resistance to either macrolides or imidazoles is an independent predictor of eradication failure, with the effect more pronounced in primary macrolide (clarithromycin) resistance.[296]

The current consensus statements on *H. pylori* infection in children[188–190] do not recommend susceptibility testing prior to initial therapy. Guidelines recommend that eradication is confirmed in all patients post-therapy. It is recommended that children who remain infected undergo a second endoscopy with culture and resistance testing at that time to adapt treatment based on antimicrobial susceptibility. As resistance patterns change, so too may this recommendation. The importance of monitoring resistance rates in children is thus highlighted.

Vaccination

The race between *H. pylori* adaptation to a host and the host's development of effective immunity implies the eventual feasibility of a vaccine. Vaccination offers probably the most cost-effective and successful approach in the prevention of infectious disease.[378–380] Given the evolving problems with antimicrobial resistance, the concept of a therapeutic vaccine is enticing. A variety of lines of evidence from various animal models have demonstrated the feasibility of both a therapeutic and a prophylactic vaccine against *H. pylori*.[378,381–385] Preliminary results on single-component, mucosally delivered vaccines in human studies have shown limited results thus far.[386,387] However, promising immunogenicity and safety profiles are now being obtained for parenterally delivered multicomponent vaccines in animal studies.[378,388,389] Studies demonstrating the reproducibility of these results in humans are eagerly awaited.[378]

CONCLUSIONS

Our understanding of *H. pylori* and its interactions with its human host is constantly evolving. Current clinical recommendations will no doubt change as our knowledge of the basic science and its clinical applicability continues to develop. *H. pylori* has proven to be a good model for the potential interactions between bacteria and the gastrointestinal system. It may well help us in the future to understand better some of the other perplexing chronic inflammatory conditions of the gastrointestinal system, such as the inflammatory bowel diseases.

References

1. Warren JR, Marshall B. Unidentified curved bacilli on gastric epithelium in active chronic gastritis. Lancet 1983; i:1275.
2. Marshall B, Warren JR. Unidentified curved bacilli in the stomach of patients with gastritis and peptic ulceration. Lancet 1984; i:1311–1314.
3. Sobel RK, Marshall B. A gutsy gulp changes medical science. US News World Report 2001; 131:59.
4. NIH Consensus Conference. *Helicobacter pylori* in peptic ulcer disease. NIH Consensus Development Panel on *Helicobacter pylori* in Peptic Ulcer Disease. JAMA 1994; 272:65–69.
5. International Agency for Research on Cancer, WHO. Infection with *Helicobacter pylori*, schistosomes, liver flukes and *Helicobacter pylori*. Monogr Eval Carcinog. Risks Hum 1994; 60:177–240.
6. Solnick JV, Schauer DB. Emergence of diverse *Helicobater* species in the pathogenesis of gastric and enterohepatic diseases. Clin Microbiol Rev 2001; 14:59–97.
7. Dubois A. Spiral bacteria in the human stomach: the gastric *Helicobacters*. Emerg Infect Dis 1995; 1:79–85.
8. Versalovic J. *Helicobacter pylori*. Pathology and diagnostic strategies. Am J Clin Pathol 2003; 119:403–412.
9. Bumann D, Meyer TF, Jungblut PR. Proteome analysis of the common human pathogen *Helicobacter pylori*. Proteomics 2001; 1:473–479.
10. Jungblut PR, Bumann D, Haas G, et al. Comparative proteome analysis of *Helicobacter pylori*. Mol Microbiol 2000; 36:710–725.
11. Bjorkholm B, Oh JD, Falk PW, Engstrand L, Gordon JI. Genomics and proteomics converge on *Helicobacter pylori*. Curr Opin Microbiol 2001; 4:237–245.

12. Nilsson C, Larsson T, Gustafsson E, Karlsson KA, Davidsson P. Indentification of protein vaccine candidates from *Helicobacter pylori* using a preparative two-dimensional electrophoretic procedure and mass spectrometry. Anal Chem 2000; 72:2148–2153.
13. Nilsson I, Utt M, Nilsson H, Ljungh A, Wadstrom T. Two-dimensional electrophoretic and immunoblot analysis of cell surface proteins of spiral-shaped and coccoid forms of *Helicobacter pylori*. Electrophoresis 2000; 21:2670–2677.
14. Utt M, Nilsson I, Ljungh A, Wadstrom T. Identification of novel immunogenic proteins of *Helicobacter pylori* by proteome technology. J Immunol Methods 2002; 259:1–10.
15. Mitchell H, Megraud F. Epidemiology and diagnosis of *Helicobacter pylori* infection. Helicobacter 2002; 7(Suppl 1):8–16.
16. Bazzoli F, Palli D, Zagari RM, et al. The Loiano-Monghidoro population-based study of *Helicobacter pylori* infection: prevalence by ^{13}C-urea breath test and associated factors. Aliment Pharmacol Ther 2001; 15:1001–1007.
17. Giannuzzi F, Giannuzzi U, Bianciardi L, et al. Risk factors for acquiring *Helicobacter pylori* infection in a group of Tuscan teenagers. New Microbiol 2001; 24:165–170.
18. Daugule I, Rumba I, Lindkvist P, Bergström M, Ejderhamn J. A relatively low prevalence of *Helicobacter pylori* infection in a healthy pediatric population in Riga, Latvia. A cross-sectional study. Acta Paediatr 2001; 90:1199–1201.
19. Yamashita Y, Fujisawa T, Kimura A, Kato H. Epidemiology of *Helicobacter pylori* infection in children: a serologic study of the Kyushu region in Japan. Pediatr Int 2001; 43:4–7.
20. Malaty HM, Logan ND, Graham DY, Ramchatesingh JE. *Helicobacter pylori* infection in preschool and school-aged minority children: effect of socioeconomic indicators and breast-feeding practices. Clin Infect Dis 2001; 32: 1387–1392.
21. Reshetnikov OV, Haiva VM, Granberg C, Kurilovich SA, Babin VP. Seroprevalence of *Helicobacter pylori* infection in Siberia. Helicobacter 2001; 6:331–336.
22. Fernando N, Perera N, Vaira D, Holton J. *Helicobacter pylori* in school children from the Western province of Sri Lanka. Helicobacter 2001; 6:169–174.
23. Broutet N, Sarasqueta AM, Sakarovitch C, Cantet F, Lethuaire D, Megraud F. *Helicobacter pylori* infection in patients consulting gastroenterologists in France: prevalence is linked to gender and region of residence. Eur J Gastroenterol Hepatol 2001; 13:677–684.
24. Goh KL, Parasakthi N. The racial cohort phenomenon: seroepidemiology of *Helicobacter pylori* infection in a multiracial South-East Asian country. Eur J Gastroenterol Hepatol 2001; 13:177–183.
25. You WC, Zhang L, Pan KF, et al. *Helicobacter pylori* prevalence and CagA status among children in two counties of China with high and low risks of gastric cancer. Ann Epidemiol 2001; 11:543–546.
26. Park IS, Lee YC, Park HJ, et al. *Helicobacter pylori* infection in Korea. Yonsei Med J 2001; 42:457–470.
27. Kim JH, Kim HY, Kim NY, et al. Seroepidemiological study of *Helicobacter pylori* infection in asymptomatic people in South Korea. J Gastroenterol Hepatol 2001; 16:969–975.
28. Rothenbacher D, Brenner H. Burden of *Helicobacter pylori* and *H. pylori*-related diseases in developed countries: recent developments and future implications. Microb Infect 2003; 5:693–703.
29. Rehnberg-Laiho L, Rautelin H, Koskela P, et al. Decreasing prevalence of helicobacter antibodies in Finland, with reference to the decreasing incidence of gastric cancer. Epidemiol Infect 2001; 126:37–42.
30. Seo JK, Ko JS, Choi KD. Serum ferritin and *Helicobacter pylori* infection in children: a sero-epidemiologic study in Korea. J Gastroenterol Hepatol 2002; 17:754–757.
31. Malaty HM, El-Kasabany A, Graham DY, et al. Age at acquisition of *Helicobacter pylori* infection: a follow-up study from infancy to adulthood. Lancet 2002; 359:931–935.
32. Yilmaz E, Dogan Y, Gurgoze MK, Unal S. Seroprevalence of *Helicobacter pylori* infection among children and their parents in eastern Turkey. J Paediatr Child Health 2002; 38:183–186.
33. Mitchell A, Silva TM, Barrett LJ, Lima AA, Guerrant RL. Age-specific *Helicobacter pylori* seropositivity rates of children in an impoverished urban area of northeast Brazil. J Clin Microbiol 2003; 41:1326–1328.
34. Banatvala N, Mayo K, Megraud F, Jennings R, Deeks JJ, Feldman RA. The cohort effect and *Helicobacter pylori*. J Infect Dis 1993; 168:219–221.
35. Roosendaal R, Kuipers EJ, Buitenwerf J, et al. *Helicobacter pylori* and the birth cohort effect: evidence of a continuous decrease of infection rates in childhood. Am J Gastroenterol 1997; 92:1480–1482.
36. Rupnow MF, Shachter RD, Owens DK, Parsonnet J. A dynamic transmission model for predicting trends in *Helicobacter pylori* and associated diseases in the United States. Emerg Infect Dis 2000; 6:228–237.
37. Blecker U, Vandenplas Y. *Helicobacter pylori* serology. J Clin Microbiol 1993; 31:173.
38. Gold BD, Khanna B, Huang LM, Lee CY, Banatvala N. *Helicobacter pylori* acquisition in infancy after decline of maternal passive immunity. Pediatr Res 1997; 41:641–646.
39. Tindberg Y, Blennow M, Granstrom M. Clinical symptoms and social factors in a cohort of children spontaneously clearing *Helicobacter pylori* infection. Acta Paediatr 1999; 88:631–635.
40. Rothenbacher D, Bode G, Brenner H. Dynamics of *Helicobacter pylori* infection in early childhood in a high-risk group living in Germany: loss of infection higher than acquisition. Aliment Pharmacol Ther 2002; 16:1663–1668.
41. Glynn MK, Friedman CR, Gold BD, et al. Seroincidence of *Helicobacter pylori* infection in a cohort of rural Bolivian children: acquisition and analysis of possible risk factors. Clin Infect Dis 2002; 35:1059–1065.
42. Wallace RA, Schluter PJ, Forgan-Smith R, Wood R, Webb PM. Diagnosis of *Helicobacter pylori* infection in adults with intellectual disability. J Clin Microbiol 2003; 41:4700–4704.
43. Nessa J, Chart H, Owen RJ, Drasar B. Human serum antibody response to *Helicobacter pylori* whole cell antigen in an institutionalized Bangladeshi population. J Appl Microbiol 2001; 90:68–72.
44. Morad M, Merrick J, Nasri Y. Prevalence of *Helicobacter pylori* in people with intellectual disability in a residential care centre in Israel. J Intellect Disabil Res 2002; 46:141–143.
45. Taneike I, Tamura Y, Shimizu T, Yamashiro Y, Yamamoto T. *Helicobacter pylori* intrafamilial infections: change in source of infection of a child from father to mother after eradication therapy. Clin Diagn Lab Immunol 2001; 8:731–739.
46. Wizla-Derambure N, Michaud L, Ategbo S, et al. Familial and community environmental risk factors for *Helicobacter pylori* infection in children and adolescents. J Pediatr Gastroenterol Nutr 2001; 33:58–63.
47. Tindberg Y, Bengtsson C, Granath F, Blennow M, Nyren O, Granstrom M. *Helicobacter pylori* infection in Swedish school children: lack of evidence of child-to-child transmission outside the family. Gastroenterology 2001; 121:310–316.
48. Rothenbacher D, Winkler M, Gonser T, Adler G, Brenner H. Role of infected parents in transmission of *Helicobacter pylori* to their children. Pediatr Infect Dis J 2002; 21:674–679.

49. Dore MP, Malaty HM, Graham DY, Fanciulli G, Delitala G, Realdi G. Risk factors associated with *Helicobacter pylori* infection among children in a defined geographic area. Clin Infect Dis 2002; 35:240–245.
50. Okuda M, Miyashiro E, Koike M, Okuda S, Minami K, Yoshikawa N. Breast-feeding prevents *Helicobacter pylori* infection in early childhood. Pediatr Int 2001; 43:714–715.
51. Roma-Giannikou E, Shcherbakov PL. *Helicobacter pylori* infection in pediatrics. Helicobacter 2002; 7(Suppl 1):50–55.
52. Rothenbacher D, Bode G, Brenner H. History of breastfeeding and *Helicobacter pylori* infection in pre-school children: results of a population-based study from Germany. Int J Epidemiol 2002; 31:632–637.
53. Kitagawa M, Natori M, Katoh M, et al. Maternal transmission of *Helicobacter pylori* in the perinatal period. J Obstet Gynaecol Res 2001; 27:225–230.
54. Wewer V, Kalach N. *Helicobacter pylori* infection in pediatrics. Helicobacter 2003; 8(Suppl 1):61–67.
55. Parsonnet J, Shmuely H, Haggerty T. Fecal and oral shedding of *Helicobacter pylori* from healthy infected adults. JAMA 1999; 282:2240–2245.
56. Forbes GM, Glaser M, Cullen DJ, et al. Duodenal ulcer treated with *Helicobacter pylori* eradication: seven-year follow-up. Lancet 1994; 343:258–260.
57. Rowland M, Kumar D, Daly L, O'Connor P, Vaughan D, Drumm B. Low rates of *Helicobacter pylori* reinfection in children. Gastroenterology 1999; 117:336–3341.
58. Koletzko S, Feydt-Schmidt A. Infants differ from teenagers: use of non-invasive tests for detection of *Helicobacter pylori* infection in children. Eur J Gastroenterol Hepatol 2001; 13:1047–1052.
59. Hildebrand P, Bardhan P, Rossi L, et al. Recrudescence and reinfection with *Helicobacter pylori* after eradication therapy in Bangladeshi adults. Gastroenterology 2001; 121:792–798.
60. Blaser MJ, Berg DE. *Helicobacter pylori* genetic diversity and risk of human disease. J Clin Invest 2001; 107:767–773.
61. Ghose C, Perez-Perez GI, Dominguez-Bello MG, Pride DT, Bravi CM, Blaser MJ. East Asian genotypes of *Helicobacter pylori*: strains in Amerindians provide evidence for its ancient human carriage. Proc Natl Acad Sci USA 2002; 99:15107–15111.
62. Falush D, Wirth T, Linz B, et al. Traces of human migration in *Helicobacter pylori* populations. Science 2003; 299:1582–1585.
63. Blaser MJ, Atherton JC. *Helicobacter pylori* persistence: biology and disease. J Clin Invest 2004; 113:321–333.
64. Tomb JF, White O, Kerlavage AR, et al. The complete genome sequence of the gastric pathogen *Helicobacter pylori*. Nature 1997; 388:539–547 [erratum appears in Nature 1997; 389:412].
65. Suerbaum S, Michetti P. *Helicobacter pylori* infection. N Engl J Med 2002; 347:1175–1186.
66. Falush D, Kraft C, Taylor N, et al. Recombination and mutation during long-term gastric colonization by *Helicobacter pylori*: estimates of clock rates, recombination size, and minimal age. Proc Natl Acad Sci USA 2001; 98:15056–15061.
67. Suerbaum S, Smith J, Bapumia K, et al. Free recombination within *Helicobacter pylori*. Proc Natl Acad Sci USA 1998; 95:12619–12624.
68. Josenhans C, Suerbaum S. The role of motility as a virulence factor in bacteria. Int J Med Microbiol 2002; 291:605–614.
69. Mobley HL. *Helicobacter pylori* factors associated with disease development. Gastroenterology 1997; 113(Suppl):S21–S28.
70. Weeks DL, Eskandari S, Scott DR, Sachs G. A H+-gated urea channel: the link between *Helicobacter pylori* urease and gastric colonization. Science 2000; 287:482–485.
71. Mollenhauer-Rektorschek M, Hanauer G, Sachs G, Melchers K. Expression of UreI is required for intragastric transit and colonization of gerbil gastric mucosa by *Helicobacter pylori*. Res Microbiol 2002; 153:659–666.
72. Gerhard M, Rad R, Prinz C, Naumann M. Pathogenesis of *Helicobacter pylori* infection. Helicobacter 2002; 7(Suppl 1):17–23.
73. Ilver D, Arnqvist A, Ogren J, et al. *Helicobacter pylori* adhesin binding fucosylated histo-blood group antigens revealed by retagging. Science 1998; 279:373–377.
74. Gerhard M, Lehn N, Neumayer N. Clinical relevance of the *Helicobacter pylori* gene for blood-group antigen-binding adhesin. Proc Natl Acad Sci USA 1999; 96:12778–12783.
75. Yu J, Leung WK, Go MY. Relationship between *Helicobacter pylori* babA2 status with gastric epithelial cell trunover and premalignant gastric lesions. Gut 2002; 51:480–484.
76. Pride D, Blaser MJ. Concerted evolution between duplicated genetic elements in *Helicobacter pylori*. J Mol Biol 2002; 316:629–642.
77. Xu Q, Morgan R, Roberts R, Blaser MJ. Identification of type II restrction and modification systems in *Helicobacter pylori* reveals their substantial diversity among strains. Proc Natl Acad Sci USA 2000; 97:9671–9676.
78. Pride D, Meinersmann R, Blaser MJ. Allelic variation within *Helicobacter pylori* babA and babB. Infect Immun 2001; 69:1160–1171.
79. Mahdavi J, Sonden B, Hurtig M. *Helicobacter pylori* SabA adhesin in persistent infection and chronic inflammation. Science 2002; 297:573–578.
80. Clyne M, Dillon P, Daly S, et al. *Helicobacter pylori* interacts with the human single-domain trefoil protein TFF1. Proc Natl Acad Sci USA 2004; 101:7409–7414.
81. Bjorkholm B, Sjolund M, Falk PG, Berg OG, Engstrand L, Andersson DI. Mutation frequency and biological cost of antibiotic resistance in *Helicobacter pylori*. Proc Natl Acad Sci USA 2001; 98:14607–14612.
82. Aras RA, Kang JC, Tschumi AI, Harasaki Y, Blaser MJ. Extensive repetitive DNA facilitates prokaryotic genome plasticity. Proc Natl Acad Sci USA 2003; 100:13579–13584.
83. Suerbaum S. Genetic variability within *Helicobacter pylori*. Int J Med Microbiol 2000; 290:175–181.
84. Bjorkholm B, Zhukhovitsky V, Lofman C, et al. *Helicobacter pylori* entry into human gastric epithelial cells: a potential determinant of virulence, persistence, and treatment failures. Helicobacter 2000; 5:148–154.
85. Ricci V, Ciacci C, Zarrilli R, et al. Effect of *Helicobacter pylori* on gastric epithelial cell migration and proliferation *in vitro*: role of VacA and CagA. Infect Immun 1996; 64:2829–2833.
86. Odenbreit S, Puls J, Sedlmaier B, Gerland E, Fischer W, Haas R. Translocation of *Helicobacter pylori* CagA into gastric epithelial cells by type IV secretion. Science 2000; 287:1497–1500.
87. Segal ED, Cha J, Lo J, Falkow S, Tompkins LS. Altered states: involvement of phosphorylated CagA in the induction of host cellular growth changes by *Helicobacter pylori*. Proc Natl Acad Sci USA 1999; 96:14559–14564.
88. Yamazaki S, Yamakawa A, Ito Y, et al. The CagA protein of *Helicobacter pylori* is translocated into epithelial cells and binds to SHP-2 in human gastric mucosa. J Infect Dis 2003; 187:334–337.
89. Higashi H, Tsutsumi R, Muto S, et al. SHP-2 tyrosine phosphatase as an intracellular target of *Helicobacter pylori* CagA protein. Science 2002; 295:683–686.

90. Mimuro H. Grb2 is a key mediator of *Helicobacter pylori* CagA protein activities. Mol Cell 2002; 10:745–755.

91. Tsutsumi J, Higashi H, Higuchi M, Okada M. Attenuation of *Helicobacter pylori* CagA x SHP-2 signaling by interaction between CagA and C-terminal Src kinase. J Biol Chem 2003; 278:3664–3670.

92. Selbach M, Moese S, Hurwitz R, Hauck CR, Meyer TF, Backert S. The *Helicobacter pylori* CagA protein induces cortactin dephosphorylation and actin rearrangment by c-Src inactivation. EMBO J 2003; 22:515–528.

93. Higashi H, Tsutsumi R, Fujita A, et al. Biological activity of the *Helicobacter pylori* virulence factor CagA is determined by variation in the tyrosine phosphorylation sites. Proc Natl Acad Sci USA 2002; 99:14428–14433.

94. Nomura AM, Lee J, Stemmermann GN, Nomura RY, Perez-Perez GI, Blaser MJ. *Helicobacter pylori* CagA seropositivity and gastric carcinoma risk in a Japanese American population. J Infect Dis 2002; 186:1138–1144.

95. Nomura AM, Perez-Perez GI, Lee J, Stemmermann G, Blaser MJ. Relation between *Helicobacter pylori* cagA status and risk of peptic ulcer disease. Am J Epidemiol 2002; 155:1054–1059.

96. Blaser MJ. Role of *vacA* and the *cagA* locus of *Helicobacter pylori* in human disease. Aliment Pharmacol Ther 1996; 10(Suppl 1):73–77.

97. Harris PR, Godoy A, Arenillas S, et al. CagA antibodies as a marker of virulence in Chilean patients with *Helicobacter pylori* infection. J Pediatr Gastroenterol Nutr 2003; 37:596–602.

98. Ashour AA, Collares GB, Mendes EN, et al. *iceA* genotypes of *Helicobacter pylori* strains isolated from Brazilian children and adults. J Clin Microbiol 2001; 39:1746–1750.

99. Day AS, Jones NL, Lynett JT, et al. cagE is a virulence factor associated with *Helicobacter pylori*-induced duodenal ulceration in children. J Infect Dis 2000; 181:1370–1375.

100. Benenson S, Halle D, Rudensky B, et al. *Helicobacter pylori* genotypes in Israeli children: the significance of geography. J Pediatr Gastroenterol Nutr 2002; 35:680–684.

101. Hofreuter D, Odenbreit S, Haas R. Natural transormation competence in *Helicobacter pylori* is mediated by the basic components of a type IV secretion system. Mol Microbiol 2001; 41:379–391.

102. Alm R, Ling L, Trust T, et al. Genomic-sequence comparison of two unrelated isolates of the human gastric pathogen *Helicobacter pylori*. Nature 1999; 397:176–180.

103. Santos A, Queiroz DM, Menard A, et al. New pathogenicity marker found in the plasticity region of the *Helicobacter pylori* genome. J Clin Microbiol 2003; 41:1651–1655.

104. de Jonge R, Kuipers EJ, Langeveld S, et al. A *Helicobacter pylori* plasticity region is associated with duodenal ulcer disease and interleukin-12 production in monocyte cells. Gastroenterology 2004; 126(Suppl 2):A108.

105. Kersulyte D, Velapatino B, Mukhopadhyay AK, et al. Cluster of type IV secretion genes in *Helicobacter pylori*'s plasticity zone. J Bacteriol 2003; 185:3764–3772.

106. Atherton JC, Cao P, Peek RM Jr, Tummuru MK, Blaser MJ, Cover TL. Mosaicism in vacuolating cytotoxin alleles of *Helicobacter pylori*: association of specific vacA types with cytotoxin production and peptic ulceration. J Biol Chem 1995; 270:17771–17777.

107. Letley DP, Atherton JC. Natural diversity in the N terminus of the mature vacuolating cytotoxin of *Helicobacter pylori* determines cytotoxin activity. J Bacteriol 2000; 182:3278–3280.

108. Letley DP, Rhead JL, Twells RJ, Dove B, Atherton JC. Determinants of non-toxicity in the gastric pathogen *Helicobacter pylori*. J Biol Chem 2003; 278:26734–26741.

109. Fischer W, Gebert B, Rainer H. Novel activities of the *Helicobacter pylori* vacuolating cytotoxin: from epithelial cells towards the immune system. Int J Med Microbiol 2004; 293:539–547.

110. Szabo I, Brutsche S, Tombola F, et al. Formation of anion-selective channels in the cell plasma membrane by the toxin VacA of *Helicobacter pylori* is required for its biological activity. EMBO J 1999; 18:5517–5527.

111. Papini E, Satin B, Norais N, et al. Selective increase of the permeability of polarized epithelial cell monolayers by *Helicobacter pylori* vacuolating toxin. J Clin Invest 1998; 102:813–820.

112. Zheng PY, Jones NL. *Helicobacter pylori* strains expressing the vacuolating cytotoxin interrupt phagosome maturation in macrophages by recruiting and retaining TACO (coronin 1) protein. Cell Microbiol 2003; 5:25–40.

113. Molinari M, Salio M, Galli C, et al. Selective inhibition of Ii-dependent antigen presentation by *Helicobacter pylori* toxin VacA. J Exp Med 1998; 187:135–140.

114. Gebert B, Fischer W, Weiss E, Hoffmann R, Haas R. *Helicobacter pylori* vacuolating cytotoxin inhibits T lymphocyte activation. Science 2003; 301:1099–1102.

115. Pai R, Cover TL, Tarnawski A. *Helicobacter pylori* vacuolating cytotoxin (VacA) disorganizes the cytoskeletal architecture of gastric epithelial cells. Biochem Biophys Res Commun 1999; 262:245–250.

116. Kuck D, Kolmerer B, Iking-Konert C, Krammer PH, Stremmel W, Rudi J. Vacuolating cytotoxin of *Helicobacter pylori* induces apoptosis in the human gastric epithelial cell line AGS. Infect Immun 2001; 69:5080–5087.

117. Cover TL, Krishna U, Israel DA, Peek RM. Induction of gastric epithelial cell apoptosis by *Helicobacter pylori* vacuolating cytotoxin. Cancer Res 2003; 63:951–957.

118. Salama NR, Otto G, Tompkins L, Falkow S. Vacuolating cytotoxin of *Helicobacter pylori* plays a role during colonization in a mouse model of infection. Infect Immun 2001; 69:730–736.

119. Atherton JC. The clinical relevance of strain types of *Helicobacter pylori*. Gut 1997; 40:701–703.

120. Athman R, Philpott DJ. Innate immunity via Toll-like receptors and Nod proteins. Curr Opin Microbiol 2004; 7:25–32.

121. Bauer S, Kirschning CJ, Hacker H, et al. Human TLRp confers responsiveness to bacterial DNA via species-specific CpG motif recognition. Proc Natl Acad Sci USA 2001; 98:9237–9242.

122. Lee SK, Stack A, Katzowitsch E, et al. *Helicobacter pylori* flagellins have very low intrinsic activity to stimulate human gastric epithelial cells via TLR5. Microb Infect 2003; 5:1345–1356.

123. Medzhitov R, Preston-Hurlburt P, Janeway CA Jr. A human homologue of the *Drosophila* Toll protein signals activation of adaptive immunity. Nature 1997; 388:394–397.

124. Backhed F, Rokbi B, Torstensson E, et al. Gastric mucosal recognition of *Helicobacter pylori* is independent of Toll-like receptor 4. J Infect Dis 2003; 187:829–836.

125. Girardin SE, Boneca IG, Carneiro LA, et al. Nod1 detects a unique muropeptide from Gram-negative bacterial peptidoglycan. Science 2003; 300:1584–1587.

126. Allen LA, Schlesinger LS, Kang B. Virulent strains of *Helicobacter pylori* demonstrate delayed phagocytosis and stimulate homotypic phagosome fusion in macrophages. J Exp Med 2000; 191:115–128.

127. Ramarao N, Gray-Owen SD, Backert S, Meyer TF. *Helicobacter pylori* inhibits phagocytosis by professional phagocytes involving type IV secretion components. Mol Microbiol 2000; 37:1389–1404.

128. Menaker RJ, Ceponis PJ, Jones N. *Helicobacter pylori* induces apoptosis of macrophages in association with alterations in the mitochondrial pathway. Infect Immun 2004; 72:2889–2898.
129. Gobert AP, Cheng Y, Wang JY, et al. *Helicobacter pylori* induces macrophage apoptosis by activation of arginase II. J Immunol 2002; 168:4692–4700.
130. Bamford KB, Fan X, Crowe SE, et al. Lymphocytes in the human gastric mucosa during *Helicobacter pylori* have a T helper cell 1 phenotype. Gastroenterology 1998; 114:482–492.
131. Wang J, Brooks EG, Bamford KB, Denning TL, Pappo J, Ernst PB. Negative selection of T cells by *Helicobacter pylori* as a model for bacterial strain selection by immune evasion. J Immunol 2001; 167:926–934.
132. Ceponis PJ, McKay DM, Menaker RJ, Galindo-Mata E, Jones NL. *Helicobacter pylori* infection interferes with epithelial Stat6-mediated interleukin-4 signal transduction independent of cagA, cagE, or VacA. J Immunol 2003; 171:2035–2041.
133. Mitchell DJ, Huynh HQ, Ceponis PJ, Jones NL, Sherman PM. *Helicobacter pylori* disrupts STAT1-mediated gamma interferon-induced signal transduction in epithelial cells. Infect Immun 2004; 72:537–545.
134. Wirth HP, Yang M, Peek RM, Tham KT, Blaser MJ. *Helicobacter pylori* Lewis expression is related to the host Lewis phenotype. Gastroenterology 1997; 113:1091–1098.
135. Blaser MJ. The versatility of *Helicobacter pylori* in the adaptation to the human stomach. J Physiol Pharmacol 1997; 48:307–314.
136. Dooley CP, Cohen H, Fitzgibbons P. Prevalence of *Helicobacter pylori* infection and histologic gastritis in asymptomatic persons. N Engl J Med 1989; 321:1562–1566.
137. Goodwin CS, Mendall MM, Northfield TC. *Helicobacter pylori* infection. Lancet 1997; 349:265–269.
138. Yamaoka Y, Kita M, Kodama T, et al. *Helicobacter pylori cagA* gene and expression of cytokine messenger RNA in gastric mucosa. Gastroenterology 1996; 110:1744–1752.
139. Negrini R, Savio A, Appelmelk BJ. Autoantibodies to gastric mucosa in *Helicobacter pylori* infection. Helicobacter 1997; 2(Suppl 1):S13–S16.
140. Mohammadi M, Czinn S, Redline RW, Nedrud JG. *Helicobacter*-specific cell-mediated immune response display a predominant Th1 phenotype and promote a delayed-type hypersensitivity response in the stomaches of mice. J Immunol 1996; 156:4729–4738.
141. Mattapallil J, Dandekar S, Canfield DR, Solnick JV. A predominant Th1 type of immune response is induced early during acute *Helicobacter pylori* infection in rhesus macaques. Gastroenterology 2000; 118:307–315.
142. Tomita T, Jackson AM, Hida N, et al. Expression of interleukin-18, a Th1 cytokine, in human gastric mucosa is increased in *Helicobacter pylori* infection. J Infect Dis 2001; 183:620–627.
143. Luzza F, Parrello T, Sebkova L, et al. Expression of proinflammatory and Th1 but not Th2 cytokines is enhanced in gastric mucosa of *Helicobacter pylori* infected children. Dig Liver Dis 2001; 33:14–20.
144. Fox JG, Beck P, Dangler CA, et al. Concurrent enteric helminth infection modulates inflammation and gastric immune responses and reduces helicobacter-induced gastric atrophy. Nat Med 2000; 6:536–532.
145. Kamradt A, Greiner M, Stefan H, et al. *Helicobacter pylori* infection in wild-type and cytokine-deficient C57BL/6 and BALB/c mouse mutants. Microbes Infect 2000; 2:593–597.
146. Smythies LE, Waites KB, Lindsey JR, Harris PR, Ghiara P, Smith PD. *Helicobacter pylori*-induced mucosal inflammation is Th1 mediated and exacerbated in IL-4, but not IFN-gamma, gene-deficient mice. J Immunol 2000; 165:1022–1029.
147. Segal I, Ally R, Sitas F, Walker AR. Co-screening for primary biliary cirrhosis and coeliac disease. *Helicobacter pylori*: the African enigma. Gut 1998; 43:300–301.
148. Mitchell HM, Ally R, Wadee A, Wiseman M, Segal I. Major differences in the IgG subclass response to *Helicobacter pylori* in the first and third worlds. Scand J Gastroenterol 2002; 37:517–522.
149. Hansson LE, Nyren O, Hsing AW, et al. The risk of stomach cancer in patients with gastric or duodenal ulcer disease. N Engl J Med 1996; 335:242–249.
150. El-Omar EM, Oien K, El-Nujumi A, et al. *Helicobacter pylori* infection and chronic gastric acid hyposecretion. Gastroenterology 1997; 113:15–24.
151. El-Omar EM, Oien K, Murray LS, et al. Increased prevalence of precancerous changes in relatives of gastric cancer patients: critical role of *H. pylori*. Gastroenterology 2000; 118:22–30.
152. El-Omar EM, Rabkin CS, Gammon MD, et al. Increased risk of noncardia gastric cancer associated with proinflammatory cytokine gene polymorphisms. Gastroenterology 2003; 124:1193–1201.
153. Machado JC, Figueiredo C, Canedo P, et al. A proinflammatory genetic profile increases the risk for chronic atrophic gastritis and gastric carcinoma. Gastroenterology 2003; 125:364–371.
154. el-Omar E, Carrington M, Chow WH, et al. Interleukin-1 polymorphisms associated with increased risk of gastric cancer. Nature 2000; 404:398–402.
155. Peek RM Jr, Blaser MJ. *Helicobacter pylori* and gastrointestinal tract adenocarcinomas. Nat Rev Cancer 2002; 2:28–37.
156. Maeda S, Yoshida H, Mitsuno Y, et al. Analysis of apoptotic and antiapoptotic signalling pathways induced by *Helicobacter pylori*. Gut 2002; 50:771–778.
157. Willhite DC, Blanke SR. *Helicobacter pylori* vacuolating cytotoxin enters cells, localizes to the mitochondria, and induces mitochondrial membrane permeability changes correlated to toxin channel activity. Cell Microbiol 2004; 6:143–154.
158. Xia H, Talley N. Apoptosis in gastric epithelium induced by *Helicobacter pylori* infection: implications in gastric carcinogenesis. Am J Gastroenterol 2001; 96:16–26.
159. Lehmann F, Terracciano L, Carena I, et al. *In situ* correlation of cytokine secretion and apoptosis in *Helicobacter pylori*-associated gastritis. Am J Physiol 2002; 283:G481–G488.
160. Rudi J, Kuck D, Stremmel W, et al. Involvement of the CD95 (APO-1/Fas) receptor and ligand system in *Helicobacter pylori*-induced gastric epithelial apoptosis. J Clin Invest 1998; 102:1506–1514.
161. Jones NL, Day AS, Jennings HA, Sherman PM. *Helicobacter pylori* induces gastric epithelial cell apoptosis in association with increased Fas receptor expression. Infect Immun 1999; 67:4237–4242.
162. Houghton J, Bloch L, Goldstein M, Von Hagen S, Korah RM. *In vivo* disruption of the fas pathway abrogates gastric growth alterations secondary to *Helicobacter* infection. J Infect 2000; 182:856–864.
163. Jones N, Day AS, Jennings HA, Shannon P, Galindo-Mata E, Sherman P. Enhanced disease severity in *Helicobacter pylori* infected mice deficient in Fas signaling. Infect Immun 2002; 70:2591–2597.
164. Nomura A, Stemmermann G, Chyon PH, et al. *Helicobacter pylori* infection and gastric carcinoma among Japanese Americans in Hawaii. N Engl J Med 1991; 325:1132–1136.
165. Scotiniotis IA, Rokkas T, Furth EE, Rigas B, Shiff SJ. Altered gastric epithelial cell kinetics in *Helicobacter pylori*-associated

intestinal metaplasia: implications for gastric carcinogenesis. Int J Cancer 2000; 85:192–200.

166. Go MF, Smoot DT. *Helicobacter pylori*, gastric MALT lymphoma, and adenocarcinoma of the stomach. Semin Gastrointest Dis 2000; 11:134–141.
167. Kim JJ, Tao H, Carloni E, Leung WK, Graham DY, Sepulveda AR. *Helicobacter pylori* impairs DNA mismatch repair in gastric epithelial cells. Gastroenterology 2002; 123:542–553.
168. el-Omar EM, Penman ID, Ardill JE, et al. *Helicobacter pylori* infection and abnormalities of acid secretion in patients with duodenal ulcer disease. Gastroenterology 1995; 109:681–691.
169. Gillen D, el-Omar EM, Wirz AA, Ardill JE, McColl KE. The acid response to gastrin distinguishes duodenal ulcer patients from *Helicobacter pylori*-infected healthy subjects. Gastroenterology 1998; 114:50–57.
170. Olbe L, Hamlet A, Dalenback J, Fandriks L. A mechanism by which *Helicobacter pylori* infection of the antrum contributes to the development of duodenal ulcer. Gastroenterology 1996; 110:1386–1394.
171. Ohkusa T, Okayasu I, Miwa H, Ohtaka K, Endo S, Sato N. *Helicobacter pylori* infection induces duodenitis and superficial duodenal ulcer in Mongolian gerbils. Gut 2003; 52:797–803.
172. Gormally S, Bourke B, Drumm B, et al. Gastric metaplasia and duodenal ulcer disease in children infected by *Helicobacter pylori*. Gut 1996; 38:513–517.
173. Beales IL. *H. pylori*-associated hypochlorhydria. Gastroenterology 1998; 114:618–621.
174. Beales IL, Calam J. Interleukin-1 beta and tumour necrosis factor alpha inhibit acid secretion in cultured rabbit parietal cells by multiple pathways. Gut 1998; 42:227–234.
175. Kuipers EJ, Uyterlinde AM, Pena AS, et al. Long-term sequelae of *Helicobacter pylori* gastritis. Lancet 1995; 345:1525–1528.
176. Nwokolo CU, Freshwater DA, O'Hare P, Randeva HS. Plasma ghrelin following cure of *Helicobacter pylori*. Gut. 2003; 52:637–640.
177. Azuma T, Suto H, Ito Y, et al. Gastric leptin and *Helicobacter pylori* infection. Gut 2001; 49:324–329.
178. Sobhani I, Buyse M, Goiot H, et al. Vagal stimulation rapidly increases leptin secretion in human stomach. Gastroenterology 2002; 122:259–263.
179. Goiot H, Attoub S, Kermorgant S, et al. Antral mucosa expresses functional leptin receptors coupled to STAT-3 signaling which is involved in the control of gastric secretions in the rat. Gastroenterology 2001; 120:1417–1427.
180. Asakawa A, Inui A, Kaga T, et al. Ghrelin is an appetite-stimulatory signal from stomach with structural resemblance to motilin. Gastroenterology 2001; 120:337–345.
181. Morris AJ, Ali MR, Nicholson MI, et al. Long-term follow-up of voluntary ingestion of *Helicobacter pylori*. Ann Intern Med 1991; 114:662–663.
182. Drumm B. *Helicobacter pylori* in the pediatric patient. Gastroenterol Clin North Am 1993; 22:169–182.
183. Hassall E, Dimmick JE. Unique features of *Helicobacter pylori* disease in children. Dig Dis Sci 1991; 36:417–423.
184. Bourke B, Jones N, Sherman P. *Helicobacter pylori* infection and peptic ulcer disease in children. Pediatr Infect Dis J 1996; 15:1–13.
185. Goggin N, Rowland M, Imrie C, Walsh D, Clyne M, Drumm B. Effect of *Helicobacter pylori* eradication on the natural history of duodenal ulcer disease. Arch Dis Child 1998; 79:502–505.
186. O'Connor HJ, Stewart C, Walsh R, McGee CN, Flynn B. Six-year follow-up after *Helicobacter pylori* eradication in peptic ulcer disease. Irish J Med Sci 2001; 170:24–27.
187. Walsh D, Drumm B. *Helicobacter pylori*: challenges for the paediatrician. J Paediatr Child Health 1997; 33:469–470.
188. Sherman P, Hassall E, Hunt RH, Fallone CA, Veldhuyzen Van Zanten S, Thomson AB. Canadian *Helicobacter* Study Group Consensus Conference on the Approach to *Helicobacter pylori* Infection in Children and Adolescents. Can J Gastroenterol 1999; 13:553–559.
189. Drumm B, Koletzko S, Oderda G. *Helicobacter pylori* infection in children: a consensus statement. European Paediatric Task Force on *Helicobacter pylori*. J Pediatr Gastroenterol Nutr 2000; 30:207–213.
190. Gold BD, Colletti RB, Abbott M, et al. *Helicobacter pylori* infection in children: recommendations for diagnosis and treatment. J Pediatr Gastroenterol Nutr 2000; 31:490–497.
191. Splawski JB. *Helicobacter pylori* and nonulcer dyspepsia: is there a relation? J Pediatr Gastroenterol Nutr 2002; 34:274–277.
192. Gottrand F. *Helicobacter pylori* infection: what are the specific questions in childhood? Gastroenterol Clin Biol 2003; 27:484–487.
193. Hopkins RJ, Girardi LS, Turney EA. Relationship between *Helicobacter pylori* eradication and reduced duodenal and gastric ulcer recurrence: a review. Gastroenterology 1996; 110:1244–1252.
194. Rosenstock S, Jorgensen T, Bonnevie O, Andersen L. Risk factors for peptic ulcer disease: a population based prospective cohort study comprising 2416 Danish adults. Gut 2003; 52:186–193.
195. Mitchell HM, Hu P, Chi Y, Chen MH, Li YY, Hazell SL. A low rate of reinfection following effective therapy against *Helicobacter pylori* in a developing nation (China). Gastroenterology 1998; 114:256–261.
196. Roma E, Kafritsa Y, Panayiotou J, Liakou R, Constantopoulos A. Is peptic ulcer a common cause of upper gastrointestinal symptoms? Eur J Pediatr 2001; 160:497–500.
197. Labenz J, Malfertheiner P. *Helicobacter pylori* in gastro-oesophageal reflux disease: causal agent, independent or protective factor? Gut 1997; 41:277–280.
198. Fallone CA, Barkun AN, Friedman G, et al. Is *Helicobacter pylori* eradication associated with gastroesophageal reflux disease? Am J Gastroenterol 2000; 95:914–920.
199. Vakil N, Hahn B, McSorley D. Recurrent symptoms and gastro-oesophageal reflux disease in patients with duodenal ulcer treated for *Helicobacter pylori* infection. Aliment Pharmacol Ther 2000; 14:45–51.
200. Koike T, Ohara S, Sekine H, et al. Increased gastric acid secretion after *Helicobacter pylori* eradication may be a factor for developing reflux oesophagitis. Aliment Pharmacol Ther 2001; 15:813–820.
201. Wu J, Sung J, Chan FK, et al. *Helicobacter pylori* infection is associated with milder gastro-esophageal reflux disease. Aliment Pharmacol Ther 2000; 14:427–432.
202. Malfertheiner P, O'Connor HJ, Genta RM, Unge P, Axon AT. Symposium: *Helicobacter pylori* and clinical risks – focus on gastro-oesophageal reflux disease. Aliment Pharmacol Ther 2002; 16(Suppl 3):1–10.
203. Moayyedi P, Bardhan C, Young L, Dixon MF, Brown L, Axon AT. *Helicobacter pylori* eradication does not exacerbate reflux symptoms in gastroesophageal reflux disease. Gastroenterology 2001; 121:1120–1126.
204. Laine L, Sugg J. Effect of *Helicobacter pylori* eradication on development of erosive esophagitis and gastroesophageal reflux disease symptoms: a *post hoc* analysis of eight double blind prospective studies. Am J Gastroenterol 2002; 97:2992–2997.

205. Schwizer W, Thumshirn M, Dent J, et al. *Helicobacter pylori* and symptomatic relapse of gastro-oesophageal reflux disease: a randomised controlled trial. Lancet 2001; 357:1738–1742.
206. Rosioru C, Glassman MS, Halata MS, Schwarz SM. Esophagitis and *Helicobacter pylori* in children: incidence and therapeutic implications. Am J Gastroenterol 1993; 88:510–513.
207. Labenz J, Blum AL, Bayerdorffer E, Meining A, Stolte M, Borsch G. Curing *Helicobacter pylori* infection in patients with duodenal ulcer may provoke reflux esophagitis. Gastroenterology 1997; 112:1442–1447.
208. Werdmuller BF, Loffeld RJ. *Helicobacter pylori* infection has no role in the pathogenesis of reflux esophagitis. Dig Dis Sci 1997; 42:103–105.
209. Befrits R, Sjostedt S, Odman B, et al. Curing *Helicobacter pylori* infection in patients with duodenal ulcer does not provoke gastroesophageal reflux disease. Helicobacter 2000; 5:202–205.
210. Levine A, Milo T, Broide E, et al. Influence of *Helicobacter pylori* eradication on gastroesophageal reflux symptoms and epigastric pain in children and adolescents. Pediatrics 2004; 113:54–58.
211. GLOBOCAN. Cancer Incidence, Mortality and Prevalence Worldwide, Version 1.0. IARC CancerBase No. 5. Lyons: IARC; 2000–2001.
212. Forman D, Newell D, Fullerton JW, et al. Association between infection with *Helicobabter pylori* and risk of gastric cancer: evidence from a prospective investigation. BMJ 1991; 302:1302–1305.
213. Parsonnet J, Friedmann GD, Vandersteen DP, et al. *Helicobabter pylori* infection and the risk of gastric carcinoma. N Engl J Med 1991; 325:1127–1131.
214. Huang JQ, Sridhar S, Chen Y, Hunt RH. Meta-analysis of the relationship between *Helicobacter pylori* seropositivity and gastric cancer. Gastroenterology 1998; 114:1169–1179.
215. Eslick GD, Lim LL, Byles JE, Xia HH, Talley NJ. Association of *Helicobacter pylori* infection with gastric carcinoma: a meta-analysis. Am J Gastroenterol 1999; 94:2373–2379.
216. Danesh J. *Helicobacter pylori* infection and gastric cancer: systematic review of the epidemiological studies. Aliment Pharmacol Ther 1999; 13:851–856.
217. Uemura N, Okamoto S, Yamamoto S, et al. *Helicobacter pylori* infection and the development of gastric cancer. N Engl J Med 2001; 345:784–789.
218. Kikuchi S. Epidemiology of *Helicobacter pylori* and gastric cancer. Gastric Cancer. 2002; 5:6–15.
219. de Figueiredo Soares T, de Magalhaes Queiroz DM, Mendes EN, et al. The interrelationship between *Helicobacter pylori* vacuolating cytotoxin and gastric carcinoma. Am J Gastroenterol 1998; 93:1841–1847.
220. Figueiredo C, Machado JC, Pharoah P, et al. *Helicobacter pylori* and interleukin 1 genotyping: an opportunity to identify high-risk individuals for gastric carcinoma. J Natl Cancer Inst 2002; 94:1680–1687.
221. Campbell DI, Warren BF, Thomas JE, Figura N, Telford JL, Sullivan PB. The African enigma: low prevalence of gastric atrophy, high prevalence of chronic inflammation in West African adults and children. Helicobacter 2001; 6:263–267.
222. Brenner H, Arndt V, Bode G, Stegmaier C, Ziegler H, Stumer T. Risk of gastric cancer among smokers infected with *Helicobacter pylori*. Int J Cancer 2002; 98:446–449.
223. Brenner H, Arndt V, Sturmer T, Stegmaier C, Ziegler H, Dhom G. Individual and joint contribution of family history and *Helicobacter pylori* infection to the risk of gastric carcinoma. Cancer 2000; 88:274–279.
224. Blaser MJ, Chyou PH, Nomura A. Age at establishment of *Helicobacter pylori* infection and gastric carcinoma, gastric ulcer, and duodenal ulcer risk. Cancer Res 1995; 55:562–565.
225. Wong BC, Lam SK, Wong WM, et al. *Helicobacter pylori* eradication to prevent gastric cancer in a high-risk region of China: a randomized controlled trial. JAMA 2004; 291:187–194.
226. Parsonnet J, Forman D. *Helicobacter pylori* infection and gastric cancer – for want of more outcomes. JAMA 2004; 291:244–245.
227. Mahour GH, Isaacs H, Chang I. Primary malignant tumors of the stomach in children. J Pediatr Surg 1980; 15:603–608.
228. Bethel CA, Bhattachayya N, Hutchinson C, et al. Alimentary tract malignancies in children. J Pediatr Surg 1997; 32:1004–1009.
229. Kurugoglu S, Mihmanli I, Celkan T, Aki H, Aksoy H, Korman U. Radiological features in paediatric primary gastric MALT lymphoma and association with *Helicobacter pylori*. Pediatr Radiol 2002; 32:82–87.
230. Wotherspoon AC, Dogan A, Du MQ. Mucosa-associated lymphoid tissue lymphoma. Curr Opin Hematol 2002; 9:50–55.
231. Bayerdorffer E, Miehlke S, Neubauer A, Stolte M. Gastric MALT-lymphoma and *Helicobacter pylori* infection. Aliment Pharmacol Ther 1997; 11(Suppl 1):89–94.
232. Liu H, Ye H, Ruskone-Fourmestraux A, et al. T(11;18) is a marker for all stage gastric MALT lymphomas that will not respond to *H. pylori* eradication. Gastroenterology 2002; 122:1286–1294.
233. Du MQ, Isaccson PG. Gastric MALT lymphoma: from aetiology to treatment. Lancet Oncol 2002; 3:97–104.
234. Isaacson PG. Gastric MALT lymphoma: from concept to cure. Ann Oncol 1999; 10:637–645.
235. Morgner A, Bayerdorffer E, Neubauer A, Stolte M. Gastric MALT lymphoma and its relationship to *Helicobacter pylori* infection: management and pathogenesis of the disease. Microsc Res Tech 2000; 48:349–356.
236. Wundisch T, Kim TD, Thiede C, et al. Etiology and therapy of *Helicobacter pylori*-associated gastric lymphomas. Ann Hematol 2003; 82:535–545.
237. Blecker U, McKeithan TW, Hart J, Kirschner BS. Resolution of *Helicobacter pylori*-associated gastric lymphoproliferative disease in a child. Gastroenterology 1995; 109:973–977.
238. Barabino A, Dufour C, Marino CE, Claudiani F, De Alessandri A. Unexplained refractory iron-deficiency anemia associated with *Helicobacter pylori* gastric infection in children: further clinical evidence. J Pediatr Gastroenterol Nutr 1999; 28:116–119.
239. Ashorn M, Ruuska T, Makipernaa A. *Helicobacter pylori* and iron deficiency anaemia in children. Scand J Gastroenterol 2001; 36:701–705.
240. Choe YH, Kwon YS, Jung MK, Kang SK, Hwang TS, Hong YC. *Helicobacter pylori*-associated iron-deficiency anemia in adolescent female athletes. J Pediatr 2001; 139:100–104.
241. Ashorn M. Acid and iron disturbances related to *Helicobacter pylori* infection. J Pediatr Gastroenterol Nutr 2004; 38:137–139.
242. Parkinson AJ, Gold BD, Bulkow L, et al. High prevalence of *Helicobacter pylori* in the Alaska native population and association with low serum ferritin levels in young adults. Clin Diagn Lab Immunol 2000; 7:885–888.
243. Yip R, Limburg PJ, Ahlquist DA, et al. Pervasive occult gastrointestinal bleeding in an Alaska native population with prevalent iron deficiency. Role of *Helicobacter pylori* gastritis. JAMA 1997; 277:1135–1139.

244. Berg G, Bode G, Blettner M, Boeing H, Brenner H. *Helicobacter pylori* infection and serum ferritin: a population-based study among 1806 adults in Germany. Am J Gastroenterol 2001; 96:1014–1018.
245. Choe YH, Kim S, Hong YC. The relationship between *Helicobacter pylori* infection and iron deficiency: seroprevalence study in 937 pubescent children. Arch Dis Child 2003; 88:178.
246. Dufour C, Brisigotti M, Fabretti G, Luxardo P, Mori PG, Barabino A. *Helicobacter pylori* gastric infection and sideropenic refractory anemia. J Pediatr Gastroenterol Nutr 1993; 17:225–227.
247. Marignani M, Angeletti S, Bordi C, et al. Reversal of long-standing iron deficiency anaemia after eradication of *Helicobacter pylori* infection. Scand J Gastroenterol 1997; 32:617–622.
248. Konno M, Muraoka S, Takahashi M, Imai T. Iron-deficiency anemia associated with *Helicobacter pylori* gastritis. J Pediatr Gastroenterol Nutr 2000; 31:52–56.
249. Choe YH, Lee JE, Kim SK. Effect of *Helicobacter pylori* eradication on sideropenic refractory anaemia in adolescent girls with *Helicobacter pylori* infection. Acta Paediatr 2000; 89:154–157.
250. Choe YH, Kim SK, Son BK, Lee DH, Hong YC, Pai SH. Randomized placebo-controlled trial of *Helicobacter pylori* eradication for iron-deficiency anemia in preadolescent children and adolescents. Helicobacter 1999; 4:135–139.
251. Annibale B, Marignani M, Monarca B, et al. Reversal of iron deficiency anemia after *Helicobacter pylori* eradication in patients with asymptomatic gastritis. Ann Intern Med 1999; 131:668–672.
252. Baysoy G, Ertem D, Ademoglu E, et al. Gastric histopathology, iron status and iron deficiency anemia in children with *Helicobacter pylori* infection. J Pediatr Gastroenterol Nutr 2004; 38:146–151.
253. Barabino A. *Helicobacter pylori*-related iron deficiency anemia: a review. Helicobacter 2002; 7:71–75.
254. Sherman PM, Macarthur C. Current controversies associated with *Helicobacter pylori* infection in the pediatric population. Frontiers Biosci 2001; 6:E187–E192.
255. Annibale B, Capurso G, Martino G, Grossi C, Delle Fave G. Iron deficiency anaemia and *Helicobacter pylori* infection. Int J Antimicrob Agents 2000; 16:515–519.
256. Benito P, Miller D. Iron absorption and bioavailability: an updated review. Nutr Res 1998; 18:581–603.
257. Rokkas T, Liatsos C, Petridou E, et al. Relationship of *Helicobacter pylori* CagA(+) status to gastric juice vitamin C levels. Eur J Clin Invest 1999; 29:56–62.
258. Capurso G, Lahner E, Marcheggiano A, et al. Involvement of the corporal mucosa and related changes in gastric acid secretion characterize patients with iron deficiency anaemia associated with *Helicobacter pylori* infection. Aliment Pharmacol Ther 2001; 15:1753–1761.
259. Ganga-Zandzou PS, Michaud L, Vincent P, et al. Natural outcome of *Helicobacter pylori* infection in asymptomatic children: a two-year follow-up study. Pediatrics 1999; 104:216–221.
260. Velayudhan J, Hughes NJ, McColm AA, et al. Iron acquisition and virulence in *Helicobacter pylori*: a major role for FeoB, a high-affinity ferrous iron transporter. Mol Microbiol 2000; 37:274–286.
261. Dhaenens L, Szczebara F, Husson MA. Identification, characterization, and immunogenicity of the lactoferrin-binding protein from *Helicobacter pylori*. Infect Immun 1997; 65:514–518.
262. Saloojee H, Pettifor JM. Iron deficiency and impaired child development. BMJ 2001; 323:1377–1378.
263. Jones NL, Sherman P, Fallone CA, et al. on behalf of the Canadian Helicobacter Study Group. Consensus guidelines on *H. pylori* infection in children and adolescents. Can J Gastroenterol 2005 (in press).
264. Takahashi M, Kimura H, Watanabe K. *Helicobacter pylori* infection in patients with idiopathic short stature. Pediatr Int 2002; 44:277–280.
265. Ertem D, Pehlivanoglu E. *Helicobacter pylori* may influence height in children independent of socioeconomic factors. J Pediatr Gastroenterol Nutr 2002; 35:232–233.
266. Demir H, Saltik IN, Kocak N, Yuce A, Ozen H, Gurakan F. Subnormal growth in children with *Helicobacter pylori* infection. Arch Dis Child 2001; 84:89–90.
267. Ozcay F, Demir H, Ozen H, et al. Normal growth in young children with *Helicobacter pylori* infection. J Pediatr Gastroenterol Nutr 2002; 35:102.
268. Richter T, List S, Muller DM, et al. Five- to 7-year-old children with *Helicobacter pylori* infection are smaller than *Helicobacter*-negative children: a cross-sectional population-based study of 3315 children. J Pediatr Gastroenterol Nutr 2001; 33:472–475.
269. Buyukgebiz A, Dundar B, Bober E, Buyukgebiz B. *Helicobacter pylori* infection in children with constitutional delay of growth and puberty. J Pediatr Endocrinol Metab 2001; 14:549–551.
270. Perri F, Pastore M, Leandro G, et al. *Helicobacter pylori* infection and growth delay in older children. Arch Dis Child 1997; 77:46–49.
271. Oderda G, Palli D, Saieva C, Chiorboli E, Bona G. Short stature and *Helicobacter pylori* infection in italian children: prospective multicentre hospital based case–control study. The Italian Study Group on Short Stature and *H. pylori*. BMJ 1998; 317:514–515.
272. Herbarth O, Krumbiegel P, Fritz GJ, et al. *Helicobacter pylori* prevalences and risk factors among school beginners in a German urban center and its rural county. Environ Health Perspect 2001; 109:573–577.
273. Sauve-Martin H, Kalach N, Raymond J, et al. The rate of *Helicobacter pylori* infection in children with growth retardation. J Pediatr Gastroenterol Nutr 1999; 28:354–355.
274. Dale A, Thomas JE, Darboe MK, Coward WA, Harding M, Weaver LT. *Helicobacter pylori* infection, gastric acid secretion, and infant growth. J Pediatr Gastroenterol Nutr 1998; 26:393–397.
275. Choe YH, Kim SK, Hong YC. *Helicobacter pylori* infection with iron deficiency anaemia and subnormal growth at puberty. Arch Dis Child 2000; 82:136–140.
276. Vaira D, Menegatti M, Salardi S, et al. *Helicobacter pylori* and diminished growth in children: is it simply a marker of deprivation? Ital J Gastroenterol Hepatol 1998; 30:129–133.
277. Franchini M, Veneri D. *Helicobacter pylori* infection and immune thrombocytopenic purpura. Haematologica 2003; 88:1087–1090.
278. Rowland M, Drumm B. *Helicobacter pylori* and sudden-infant-death syndrome. Lancet 2001; 357:327.
279. Blaser MJ. *Helicobacter pylori* eradication and its implications for the future. Aliment Pharmacol Ther 1997; 11(Suppl 1):103–107.
280. Blaser MJ. Hypothesis: the changing relationships of *Helicobacter pylori* and humans: implications for health and disease. J Infect Dis 1999; 179:1523–1530.
281. Putsep K, Branden CI, Boman H, Normark S. Antibacterial peptide from *H. pylori*. Nature 1999; 398:671–672.

282. Rothenbacher D, Blaser MJ, Bode G, Brenner H. Inverse relationship between gastric colonization of *Helicobacter pylori* and diarrheal illnesses in children: results of a population-based cross-sectional study. J Infect Dis 2000; 182:1446–1449.
283. Bode G, Rothenbacher D, Brenner H. *Helicobacter pylori* colonization and diarrhoeal illness: results of a population-based cross-sectional study in adults. Eur J Epidemiol 2002; 17:823–827.
284. Bahu Mda G, da Silveira TR, Maguilnick I, Ulbrich-Kulczynski J. Endoscopic nodular gastritis: an endoscopic indicator of high-grade bacterial colonization and severe gastritis in children with *Helicobacter pylori*. J Pediatr Gastroenterol Nutr 2003; 36:217–222.
285. Bujanover Y, Reif S, Yahav J. *Helicobacter pylori* and peptic disease in the pediatric patient. Pediatr Clin North Am 1996; 43:213–234.
286. Owen RJ. Bacteriology of *Helicobacter pylori*. Baillieres Clin Gastroenterol 1995; 9:415–440.
287. Glupczynski Y. Microbiological and serological diagnostic tests for *Helicobacter pylori*: an overview. Acta Gastroenterol Belg 1998; 61:321–326.
288. Grove DI, Koutsouridis G, Cummins AG. Comparison of culture, histopathology and urease testing for the diagnosis of *Helicobacter pylori* gastritis and susceptibility to amoxicillin, clarithromycin, metronidazole and tetracycline. Pathology 1998; 30:183–187.
289. Genta RM, Graham D. Comparison of biopsy sites for the histopathologic diagnosis of *Helicobacter pylori*: a topographic study of *H. pylori* density and distribution. Gastrointest Endosc Clin North Am 1994; 40:342–345.
290. Karnes WE, Samloff IM, Siurala M, et al. Positive serum antibody and negative tissue staining for *Helicobacter pylori* in subjects with atrophic gastritis. Gastroenterology 1991; 101:167–174.
291. Ndip RN, MacKay WG, Farthing MJ, Weaver L. Culturing *Helicobacter pylori* from clinical specimens: review of microbiologic methods. J Pediatr Gastroenterol Nutr 2003; 36:616–622.
292. Yanez P, la Garza AM, Perez-Perez G, Cabrera L, Munoz O, Torres J. Comparison of invasive and noninvasive methods for the diagnosis and evaluation of eradication of *Helicobacter pylori* infection in children. Arch Med Res 2000; 31:415–421.
293. Kjoller M, Fischer A, Justesen T. Transport conditions and number of biopsies necessary for culture of *Helicobacter pylori*. Eur J Clin Infect Dis 1991; 10:166–167.
294. Soltesz V, Zeeberg B, Wadstroom T. Optimal survival of *Helicobacter pylori* under various transport conditions. J Clin Microbiol 1992; 30:1453–1456.
295. Veenendaal RA, Lichtendahl-Bernards AT, Pena A. Effect of transport medium and transport time on culture of *Helicobacter pylori* from gastric biopsy specimens. J Clin Pathol 1993; 46:561–563.
296. Jenks PJ. Causes of failure or eradication of *Helicobacter pylori*, antibiotic resistance is the major cause, and susceptibility testing may help. BMJ 2002; 325:3–4.
297. Drumm B, Sherman P, Cutz E, Karmali M. Association of *Campylobacter pylori* on the gastric mucosa with antral gastritis in children. N Engl J Med 1987; 316:1557–1561.
298. McNulty CA, Dent JC, Uff JS, Gear MW, Wilkinson SP. Detection of *Campylobacter pylori* by the biopsy urease test: an assessment in 1445 patients. Gut 1989; 30:1058–1062.
299. Elitsur Y, Neace C. Detection of *Helicobacter pylori* organisms by Hp-fast in children. Dig Dis Sci 1999; 44:1169–1172.
300. Borrelli O, Hassall E, D'Armiento F, et al. Inflammation of the gastric cardia in children with symptoms of acid peptic disease. J Pediatr 2003; 143:520–524.
301. Chong S, Lou Q, Asnicar M. *Helicobacter pylori* infection in recurrent abdominal pain in childhood: comparison of diagnostic tests and therapy. Pediatrics 1995; 96:211–215.
302. Elitsur Y, Hill I, Lichtman SN, Rosenberg AJ. Prospective comparison of rapid urease tests (PyloriTek, CLO test) for the diagnosis of *Helicobacter pylori* infection in symptomatic children: a pediatric multicenter study. Am J Gastroenterol 1998; 93:217–219.
303. Mitchell HM, Bohane TD, Tobias V, et al. *Helicobacter pylori* infection in children: potential clues to pathogenesis. J Pediatr Gastroenterol Nutr 1993; 16:120–125.
304. Genta RM, Robason GO, Graham D. Simultaneous visualization of *Helicobacter pylori* and gastric morphology:a new stain. Hum Pathol 1994; 25:221–226.
305. Eshun JK, Black DD, Casteel HB, et al. Comparison of immunohistochemistry and silver stain for the diagnosis of pediatric *Helicobacter pylori* infection in urease-negative gastric biopsies. Pediatr Dev Pathol 2001; 4:82–88.
306. Ashton-Key M, Diss TC, Isaacson PG. Detection of *Helicobacter pylori* in gastric biopsy and resection specimens. J Clin Pathol 1996; 49:107–111.
307. Toulaymat M, Marconi S, Garb J, Otis C, Nash S. Endoscopic biopsy pathology of *Helicobacter pylori* gastritis: comparison of bacterial detection by immunohistochemistry and Genta stain. Arch Pathol Lab Med 1999; 123:778–781.
308. Elitzur Y, Lawrence Z, Triest WE. Distribution of *Helicobacter pylori* organisms in the stomachs of children with *Helicobacter pylori* infection. Hum Pathol 2002; 33:1133–1135.
309. Genta RM, Huberman RM, Graham D. The gastric cardia in *Helicobacter pylori* infection. Hum Pathol 1994; 25:915–919.
310. Thomas JE, Dale A, Harding M, Coward WA, Cole TJ, Weaver LT. *Helicobacter pylori* colonization in early life. Pediatr Res 1999; 45:218–223.
311. Kindermann A, Konstantopoulos N, Lehn N, Demmelmair H, Koletzko S. Evaluation of two commercial enzyme immunoassays, testing immunoglobulin G (IgG) and IgA responses, for diagnosis of *Helicobacter pylori* infection in children. J Clin Microbiol 2001; 39:3591–3596.
312. Czinn SJ. Serodiagnosis of *Helicobacter pylori* in pediatric patients. J Pediatr Gastroenterol Nutr 1999; 28:132–134.
313. Vaira D, Vakil N. Blood, urine, stool, breath, money, and *Helicobacter pylori*. Gut 2001; 48:287–289.
314. Pelser HH, Househam KC, Joubert G, et al. Prevalence of *Helicobacter pylori* antibodies in children in Bloemfontein, South Africa. J Pediatr Gastroenterol Nutr 1997; 24:135–139.
315. Kumagai T, Malaty HM, Graham DY, et al. Acquisition versus loss of *Helicobacter pylori* infection in Japan: results from an 8-year birth cohort study. J Infect Dis 1998; 178:717–721.
316. Hawthorne AB, Morgan S, Westmoreland D, Stenson R, Thomas GA, Newcombe RG. A comparison of two rapid whole-blood tests and laboratory serology, in the diagnosis of *Helicobacter pylori* infection. Eur J Gastroenterol Hepatol 1999; 11:863–865.
317. Chey WD, Murthy U, Shaw S, et al. A comparison of three fingerstick, whole blood antibody tests for *Helicobacter pylori* infection: a United States, multicenter trial. Am J Gastroenterol 1999; 94:1512–1516.
318. Laine L, Knigge K, Faigel D, et al. Fingerstick *Helicobacter pylori* antibody test: better than laboratory serological testing? Am J Gastroenterol 1999; 94:3464–3467.
319. Faigel DO, Magaret N, Corless C, Lieberman DA, Fennerty MB. Evaluation of rapid antibody tests for the diagnosis of *Helicobacter pylori* infection. Am J Gastroenterol 2000; [illegible]

320. Wong BC, Wong W, Tang VS, et al. An evaluation of whole blood testing for *Helicobacter pylori* infection in the Chinese population. Aliment Pharmacol Ther 2000; 14:331–335.

321. Ladas SD, Malamou H, Giota G, et al. Prospective evaluation of a whole-blood antibody test (FlexPack HP) for in-office diagnosis of *Helicobacter pylori* infection in untreated patients. Eur J Gastroenterol Hepatol 2000; 12:727–731.

322. Duggan AE, Elliott C, Logan RF. Testing for *Helicobacter pylori* infection: validation and diagnostic yield of a near patient test in primary care. BMJ 1999; 319:1236–1239.

323. Luzza F, Imeneo M, Marasco A, et al. Evaluation of a commercial serological kit for detection of salivary immunoglobulin G to *Helicobacter pylori*: a multicentre study. Eur J Gastroenterol Hepatol 2000; 12:1117–1120.

324. Miwa H, Hirose M, Kikuchi S, et al. How useful is the detection kit for antibody to *Helicobacter pylori* in urine (URINELISA) in clinical practice? Am J Gastroenterol 1999; 94:3460–3463.

325. Gatta L, Ricci C, Tampieri A, Vaira D. Non-invasive techniques for the diagnosis of *Helicobacter pylori* infection. Clin Microbiol Infect 2003; 9:489–496.

326. Graham DY, Opekun AR, Hammoud F, et al. Studies regarding the mechanism of false negative urea breath tests with proton pump inhibitors. Am J Gastroenterol 2003; 98:1005–1009.

327. Rektorschek M, Weeks DL, Sachs G, Melchers K. Influence of pH on metabolism and urease activity of *Helicobacter pylori*. Gastroenterology 1998; 115:628–641.

328. Goddard AF, Logan R. Urea breath tests for detecting *Helicobacter pylori*. Aliment Pharmacol Ther 1997; 11:641–649.

329. Koletzko S, Sauerwald T, Demmelmair H. Safety of stable isotope use. Eur J Pediatr 1997; 156(Suppl 1):12–17.

330. Graham D, Klein PD, Evans DJ. *Campylobacter pylori* detected non-invasively by the ^{13}C-urea breath test. Lancet 1987; i:1174–1177.

331. Hamlet A, Stage L, Lonroth H, Cahlin C, Nystrom C, Pettersson A. A novel tablet-based ^{13}C urea breath test for *Helicobacter pylori* with enhanced performance during acid suppression therapy. Scand J Gastroenterol 1999; 34:367–374.

332. Vaira D, Malfertheiner P, Megraud F, et al. Diagnosis of *Helicobacter pylori* infection with a new non-invasive antigen-based assay. HpSA European Study Group. Lancet 1999; 354:30–33.

333. Bazzoli F, Cecchini L, Corvaglia L, et al. Validation of the ^{13}C-urea breath test for the diagnosis of *Helicobacter pylori* infection in children: a multicenter study. Am J Gastroenterol 2000; 95:646–650.

334. Cave DR, Zanten SV, Carter E, et al. A multicentre evaluation of the laser assisted ratio analyser (LARA): a novel device for measurement of $^{13}CO_2$ in the ^{13}C-urea breath test for the detection of *Helicobacter pylori* infection. Aliment Pharmacol Ther 1999; 13:747–752.

335. Van Der Hulst RW, Lamouliatte H, Megraud F, et al. Laser assisted ratio analyser ^{13}C-urea breath testing, for the detection of *H. pylori*: A prospective diagnostic European multicentre study. Aliment Pharmacol Ther 1999; 13:1171–1177.

336. Cadranel S, Corvaglia L, Bontems P, et al. Detection of *Helicobacter pylori* infection in children with a standardized and simplified ^{13}C-urea breath test. J Pediatr Gastroenterol Nutr 1998; 27:275–280.

337. Kalach N, Briet F, Raymond J, et al. The ^{13}carbon urea breath test for the noninvasive detection of *Helicobacter pylori* in children: comparison with culture and determination of minimum analysis requirements. J Pediatr Gastroenterol Nutr 1998; 26:291–296.

338. Rowland M, Lambert I, Gormally S, et al. Carbon 13-labeled urea breath test for the diagnosis of *Helicobacter pylori* infection in children. J Pediatr 1997; 131:815–820.

339. Kindermann A, Demmelmair H, Koletzko B, Krauss-Etschmann S, Wiebecke B, Koletzko S. Influence of age on ^{13}C-urea breath test results in children. J Pediatr Gastroenterol Nutr 2000; 30:85–91.

340. Herold R, Becker M. ^{13}C-urea breath test threshold calculation and evaluation for the detection of *Helicobacter pylori* infection in children. BMC Gastroenterol 2002; 2:12.

341. Kato S, Ozawa K, Konno M, et al. Diagnostic accuracy of the ^{13}C-urea breath test for childhood *Helicobacter pylori* infection: a multicenter Japanese study. Am J Gastroenterol 2002; 97:1668–1673.

342. Dominguez Munoz JE, Leodolter A, Sauerbruch T, Malfertheiner P. A citric acid solution is an optimal test drink in the ^{13}C-urea breath test for the diagnosis of *Helicobacter pylori* infection. Gut 1997; 40:459–462.

343. Graham DY, Runke D, Anderson SY, Malaty HM, Klein PD. Citric acid as the test meal for the ^{13}C-urea breath test. Am J Gastroenterol 1999; 94:1214–1217.

344. Sauerwald T, Demmelmair H, Tasch C, Konstantopoulos N, Weigand H, Koletzko S. Imroving accuracy of the ^{13}C-urea breath test in children by normalizing results for CO_2 production rates. Gut 2000; 47(Suppl 1):A93.

345. Leung WK, Hung LC, Kwok CK, Leong RW, Ng DK, Sung JJ. Follow up of serial urea breath test results in patients after consumption of antibiotics for non-gastric infections. World J Gastroenterol 2002; 8:703–706.

346. Laine L, Estrada R, Trujillo M, Knigge K, Fennerty MB. Effect of proton-pump inhibitor therapy on diagnostic testing for *Helicobacter pylori*. Ann Intern Med 1998; 129:547–550.

347. Gatta L, Ricci C, Tampieri A. Noninvasive tests to diagnose *Helicobacter pylori* infection. Curr Gastroenterol Rep 2003; 5:351–352.

348. Kawakami E, Machado RS, Reber M, Patricio FR. ^{13}C-urea breath test with infrared spectroscopy for diagnosing *Helicobacter pylori* infection in children and adolescents. J Pediatr Gastroenterol Nutr 2002; 35:39–43.

349. Koletzko S, Konstantopoulos N, Bosman D, et al. Evaluation of a novel monoclonal enzyme immunoassay for detection of *Helicobacter pylori* antigen in stool from children. Gut 2003; 52:804–806.

350. Kato S, Ozawa K, Okuda M, et al. Accuracy of the stool antigen test for the diagnosis of childhood *Helicobacter pylori* infection: a multicenter Japanese study. Am J Gastroenterol 2003; 98:296–300.

351. Makristathis A, Barousch W, Pasching E, et al. Two enzyme immunoassays and PCR for detection of *Helicobacter pylori* in stool specimens from pediatric patients before and after eradication therapy. J Clin Microbiol 2000; 38:3710–3714.

352. Gisbert JP, Pajares JM. Diagnosis of *Helicobacter pylori* infection by stool antigen determination: a systematic review. Am J Gastroenterol 2001; 96:2829–2838.

353. Weingart V, Russmann H, Koletzko S, Weingart J, Hochter W, Sackmann M. Sensitivity of a novel stool antigen test for detection of *Helicobacter pylori* in adult outpatients before and after eradication therapy. J Clin Microbiol 2004; 42:1319–1321.

354. Lind T, Veldhuyzen van Zanten S, Unge P, et al. Eradication of *Helicobacter pylori* using one-week triple therapies combining omeprazole with two antimicrobials: the MACH I Study. Helicobacter 1996; 1:138–144.

355. Laheij RJ, Rossum LG, Jansen JB, Straatman H, Verbeek AL. Evaluation of treatment regimens to cure *Helicobacter pylori*

infection – a meta-analysis. Aliment Pharmacol Ther 1999; 13:857–864.

356. Gorbach SL. Bismuth therapy in gastrointestinal diseases. Gastroenterology 1990; 99:863–875.
357. Rowland M, Imrie C, Bourke B, Drumm B. How should *Helicobacter pylori* infected children be managed? Gut 1999; 45(Suppl 1):I36–I39.
358. Oderda G, Rapa A, Bona G. A systematic review of *Helicobacter pylori* eradication treatment schedules in children. Aliment Pharmacol Ther 2000; 14(Suppl 3):59–66.
359. Gottrand F, Kalach N, Spyckerelle C, et al. Omeprazole combined with amoxicillin and clarithromycin in the eradication of *Helicobacter pylori* in children with gastritis: a prospective randomized double-blind trial. J Pediatr 2001; 139:664–668.
360. Kawakami E, Ogata SK, Portorreal AC, Magni AM, Pardo ML, Patricio FR. Triple therapy with clarithromycin, amoxicillin and omeprazole for *Helicobacter pylori* eradication in children and adolescents. Arq Gastroenterol 2001; 38:203–206.
361. Shcherbakov PL, Filin VA, Volkov IA, Tatarinov PA, Belousov YB. A randomized comparison of triple therapy *Helicobacter pylori* eradication regimens in children with peptic ulcers. J Int Med Res 2001; 29:147–153.
362. Chan KL, Zhou H, Ng DK, Tam PK. A prospective study of a one-week nonbismuth quadruple therapy for childhood *Helicobacter pylori* infection. J Pediatr Surg 2001; 36:1008–1011.
363. Sagar M, Seensalu R, Tybring G, Dahl ML, Bertilsson L. *CYP2C19* genotype and phenotype determined with omeprazole in patients with acid-related disorders with and without *Helicobacter pylori* infection. Scand J Gastroenterol 1998; 33:1034–1038.
364. Furuta T, Shirai N, Watanabe F, et al. Effect of cytochrome P4502C19 genotypic differences on cure rates for gastroesophageal reflux disease by lansoprazole. Clin Pharmacol Ther 2002; 72:453–460.
365. Lin CJ, Yang JC, Uang YS, Chern HD, Wang TH. Time-dependent amplified pharmacokinetic and pharmacodynamic responses of rabeprazole in cytochrome P450 2C19 poor metabolizers. Pharmacotherapy 2003; 23:711–719.
366. Kawabata H, Habu Y, Tomioka H, et al. Effect of different proton pump inhibitors, differences in *CYP2C19* genotype and antibiotic resistance on the eradication rate of *Helicobacter pylori* infection by a 1-week regimen of proton pump inhibitor, amoxicillin and clarithromycin. Aliment Pharmacol Ther 2003; 17:259–264.
367. Dupont C, Kalach N, Raymond J. *Helicobacter pylori* and antimicrobial susceptibility in children. J Pediatr Gastroenterol Nutr 2003; 36:311–313.
368. Versalovic J, Shortridge D, Kibler K, et al. Mutations in 23S rRNA are associated with clarithromycin resistance in *Helicobacter pylori*. Antimicrob Agents Chemother 1996; 40:477–480.
369. Russmann H, Adler K, Haas R, et al. Rapid and accurate determination of genotypic clarithromycin resistance in cultured *Helicobacter pylori* by fluorescent *in situ* hydridization. J Clin Microbiol 2001; 39:4142–4144.
370. Yang YJ, Yang JC, Jeng YM, et al. Prevalence and rapid identification of clarithromycin-resistant *Helicobacter pylori* isolates in children. Pediatr Infect Dis J 2001; 20:662–666.
371. Glupczunski Y, Megraud F, Lopez-Brea M, Andersen L. European multicenter survey of *in vitro* antimicrobial resistance in *Helicobacter pylori*. Eur J Microbiol Infect Dis 2001; 20:820–823.
372. Crone J, Granditsch G, Huber WD, et al. *Helicobacter pylori* in children and adolescents: increase of primary clarithromycin resistance, 1997–2000. J Pediatr Gastroenterol Nutr 2003; 36:368–371.
373. Boyanova L, Koumanova R, Gergova G, et al. Prevalence of resistant *Helicobacter pylori* isolates in Bulgarian children. J Med Microbiol 2002; 51:786–790.
374. Megraud F. Resistance of *Helicobacter pylori* to antibiotics and its impact on treatment options. Drug Resist Updat 2001; 4:178–186.
375. Perez Aldana L, Kato M, Nakagawa S, et al. The relationship between consumption of antimicrobial agents and the prevalence of primary *Helicobacter pylori* resistance. Helicobacter 2002; 7:306–309.
376. Raymond J, Kalach N, Bergeret M, et al. Effect of metronidazole resistance on bacterial eradication of *Helicobacter pylori* in infected children. Antimicrob Agents Chemother 1998; 42:1334–1335.
377. Kalach N, Benhamou PH, Campeotto F, Bergeret M, Dupont C, Raymond J. Clarithromycin resistance and eradication of *Helicobacter pylori* in children. Antimicrob Agents Chemother 2001; 45:2134–2135.
378. Ruggiero P, Peppoloni S, Rappuoli R, Del Giudice G. The quest for a vaccine against *Helicobacter pylori*: how to move from mouse to man? Microb Infect 2003; 5:749–756.
379. Rupnow MF, Owen DA, Shachter RD, Parsonnet J. *Helicobacter pylori* vaccine development and use: a cost-effectiveness analysis using the Institute of Medicine methodology. Helicobacter 1999; 4:272–280.
380. Rupnow MF, Shachter RD, Owens DK, Parsonnet J. Quantifying the population impact of a prophylactic *Helicobacter pylori* vaccine. Vaccine 2002; 20:879–885.
381. Marchetti F, Rossi M, Giannelli V, et al. Protection against *Helicobacter pylori* infection in mice by intragastric vaccination with *H. pylori* antigens is achieved using a non-toxic mutant of *E. coli* heat-labile enterotosin (LT) as adjuvant. Vaccine 1998; 16:33–37.
382. Del Giudice G, Covacci A, Telford J, Montecucco C, Rappuoli R. The design of vaccines against *Helicobacter pylori* and their development. Annu Rev Immunol 2001; 19:523–563.
383. Del Giudice G. Towards the development of vaccines against *Helicobacter pylori*: status and issues. Curr Opin Invest Drugs 2001; 2:40–44.
384. Kleanthous H, Tibbitts TJ, Gray HL, et al. Sterilizing immunity against experimental *Helicobacter pylori* infection is challenge-strain dependent. Vaccine 2001; 19:4883–4895.
385. Garhart CA, Redline RW, Nedrud JG, Czinn S. Clearance of *Helicobacter pylori* infection and resolution of posimmunization gastritis in a kinetic study of prophylactically immunized mice. Infect Immun 2002; 70:3529–3538.
386. Banerjee S, Medina-Fatimi A, Nichols R, et al. Safety and efficacy of low dose *Escherichia coli* enterotoxin adjuvant for urease based oral immunisation against *Helicobacter pylori* in healthy volunteers. Gut 2002; 51:634–640.
387. Sougioultzis S, Lee CK, Alsahli M, et al. Safety and efficacy of *E. coli* enterotoxin adjuvant for urease-based rectal immunization against *Helicobacter pylori*. Vaccine 2002; 21:194–201.
388. Rossi G, Rossi MR, Vitale G, et al. A conventional beagle dog model for acute and chronic infection with *Helicobacter pylori*. Infect Immun 1999; 67:3112–3120.
389. Malfertheiner P, Schultze V, Del Giudice G, et al. Phase 1 safety and immunogenicity of a three-component *H. pylori* vaccine. Gastroenterology 2002; 122(Suppl):A585.
390. Fischer W, Gebert B, Haas R. Novel activities of the *Helicobacter pylori* vacuolating cytotoxin: from epithelial cells

towards the immune system. Int J Med Microbiol 2004; 293:539–547.

391. Patel P, Mendall MA, Khulusi S, Northfield TC, Strachan DP. *Helicobacter pylori* infection in childhood: risk factors and effect on growth. BMJ 1994; 309:1119–1123.

392. Ashorn M, Mäki M, Hällström M, et al. *Helicobacter pylori* infection in Finnish children and adolescents. A serologic cross-sectional and follow-up study. Scand J Gastroenterol 1995; 30:876–879.

393. Granström M, Tindberg Y, Blennow M. Seroepidemiology of *Helicobacter pylori* infection in a cohort of children monitored from 6 months to 11 years of age. J Clin Microbiol 1997; 35:468–470.

394. Rehnberg-Laiho L, Rautelin H, Valle M, Kosunen TU. Persisting *Helicobacter* antibodies in Finnish children and adolescents between two and twenty years of age. Pediatr Infect Dis J 1998; 17:796–799.

395. Rothenbacher D, Bode G, Berg G, et al. Prevalence and determinants of *H. pylori* infection in preschool children: a population based epidemiological study from Germany. Int J Epidemiol 1998; 27:135–141.

396. Boltshauser S, Herzog D. Prevalence of *Helicobacter pylori* infection in asymptomatic 5–7-year-old children of St Gallen canton. Schweiz Med Wochenschr 1999; 129:579–584.

397. Rothenbacher D, Bode G, Berg G, et al. *Helicobacter pylori* among pre-school children and their parents: evidence for parent–child transmission. J Infect Dis 1999; 179:398–402.

398. Rothenbacher D, Inceoglu J, Bode G, Brenner H. Acquisition of *Helicobacter pylori* infection in a high risk population occurs within the first 2 years of life. J Pediatr 2000; 136:744–748.

399. Bode G, Piechotowski I, Rothenbacher D, Brenner H. *Helicobacter pylori*-specific immune responses of children: implications for future vaccination strategy. Clin Diagn Lab Immunol 2002; 9:1126–1128.

Chapter 27
Gastric motility disorders

Frances L. Connor and Carlo Di Lorenzo

NORMAL GASTRIC MOTILITY

The stomach is a complex electromechanical chamber with multiple functions including the storage, physical breakdown, mixing and controlled delivery of ingesta to the small intestine. Gastric emptying rate is tailored to the nutrient content of the meal, with differential handling for solids and liquids. The stomach also participates in protective reflexes in response to ingested toxins and pathogens, when the vomiting reflex empties the upper small intestine and antrum. These complex activities are regulated by both neural and hormonal mechanisms.

Gastric motor physiology and gastric emptying

Anatomically, the stomach consists of four main areas, the cardia, fundus, body (corpus) and antrum. Functionally, however, there are two major zones, the proximal stomach, comprising the cardia and fundus and the distal stomach, made up of corpus and antrum. Within these zones, three basic motility functions are present, smooth muscle tone, peristaltic contractions and retrograde giant contractions associated with vomiting. Through alterations in gastric smooth muscle tone the proximal stomach expands to receive and store the ingested meal, then gradually transfers nutrients to the distal stomach for peristaltic grinding and delivery to the duodenum. The gastric motility responses to solid food ingestion are summarized in Figure 27.1.[1]

Proximal stomach

Gastric accommodation Gastric accommodation to a meal allows the fundus to expand to receive ingested food without increasing wall tension (Fig. 27.1a). Fundic relaxation initiates upon swallowing and may be activated by duodenal nutrient infusion or distension. It is mediated via vagal pathways and involves serotonin and nitric oxide as neurotransmitters.[2] Gastric accommodation is absent after vagotomy and is defective in almost half the adult patients with functional dyspepsia. Associated symptoms include early satiety and weight loss. Pharmacological inhibition of gastric accommodation induces early satiety in normal controls.[3] Fundic relaxation may be enhanced or restored by several drugs including 5-HT_1 receptor agonist sumatriptan,[4] buspirone, clonidine and nitrates.

Tonic contraction After the initial period of relaxation, a gradual increase in smooth muscle tone in the proximal stomach results in transfer of the meal to the distal stomach (Fig. 27.1a). Maldistribution in meal contents within the stomach has been identified in adults[5] and children[6–8] with functional dyspepsia. Different dyspeptic symptoms are associated with different patterns of abnormality, early satiety is associated with early distal redistribution of the liquid phase (possibly due to poor fundal relaxation) and fullness was associated with late proximal retention.[5]

Distal stomach

Immediately after feeding, antral contractions are suppressed, whereas isolated pyloric contractions and duodenal activity increase, regulating the flow of liquids to the duodenum.[9,10] Liquid meals are transferred rapidly from proximal to distal stomach and emptied into the duodenum by a series of strong peristaltic contractions. Gastric emptying of neutral, isosmolar and calorically inert solutions (e.g. normal saline) is rapid, in the range of 10–20% per min, reaching a simple exponential rate.[11] This results in almost log linear emptying kinetics when measured by nuclear scintigraphy. In contrast, there is a significant lag phase in the delivery of solids to the duodenum (Fig. 27.1d). In response to a meal containing solids, the distal stomach purees solid and liquid nutrients, gastric acid and pepsin into a suspension, or chyme, suitable for delivery to the small intestine, a process called trituration. Ingested solids are ground into particles of 1–2 mm diameter by repeated antral peristaltic contractions, driving food towards the partially closed pylorus. Small jets of a few milliliters of chyme pass through the pylorus with each wave of contraction (Fig. 27.1c). Solids that cannot be broken down by trituration are cleared during fasting.

Antral contractions occur at a typical rate of 3 cycles/min, governed by electrical slow waves that originate in the pacemaker region on the greater curvature at the junction of the fundus and corpus. Recently, the intrinsic pacemaker cells have been identified as specialized mesenchymal cells, the interstitial cells of Cajal (ICC) that are closely associated with both gastric smooth muscle and enteric nerves. Electrical slow waves propagate distally through the circular muscle layer of the stomach via gap junctions between individual smooth muscle cells, facilitating coordinated peristaltic contractions through the gastric corpus, antrum and pylorus. However, the slow waves themselves are insufficient for the generation of peristaltic contractions. Local neural and hormonal stimuli, especially acetylcholine, stimulate additional plateau and spike potentials. Superimposed on the slow wave depolarizations, these potentials exceed the electrical threshold required to generate forceful peristaltic contractions.

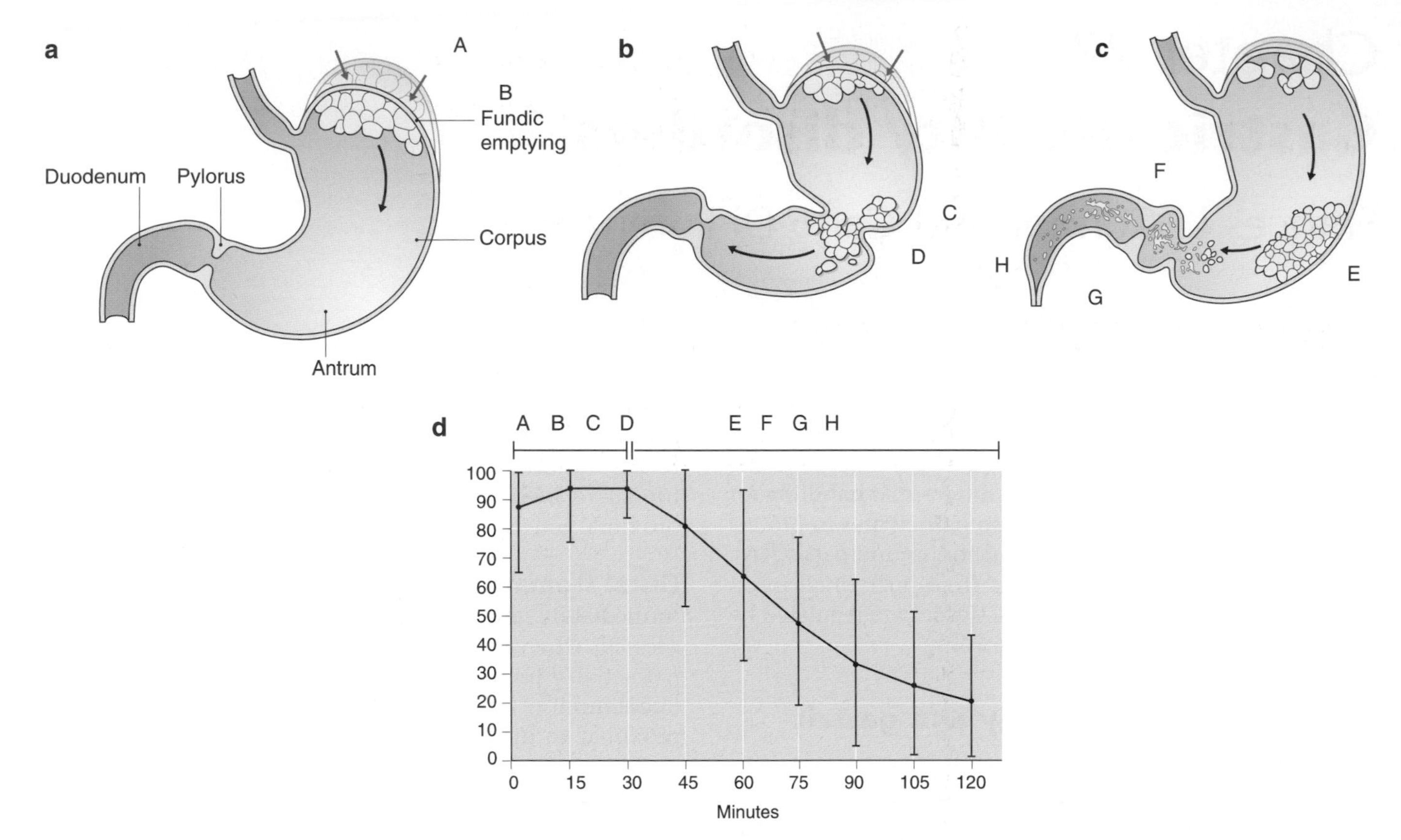

Figure 27.1: Gastric motility responses to solid food. (**a**) Ingested food is received in the gastric fundus, which relaxes as the food bolus enters the proximal stomach (i.e. receptive relaxation, A). Receptive relaxation is a property of the proximal stomach-the fundus and proximal gastric body (corpus). Relaxation of the fundus allows for the accommodation of large volumes of food without a concomitant increase in pressure within the stomach. The ingested food is subsequently emptied from the fundus (B) into the corpus and antrum. Slow (0.3–1/min) contractions force the ingested food into the more distal stomach, where mixing begins. (**b**) The corpus and the antrum fill (C) as the food is received from the fundus. Recurrent and gentle peristaltic waves mix the food with secreted acid and pepsin and move the food toward the pylorus (D). The peristaltic waves break the food into tiny pieces (1 mm) and mix them into a suspension suitable for emptying. Antral peristalses normally occur at 3 cpm, the rate of the pacesetter potentials. (**c**) When the food particles in suspension are less than 1 mm and caloric content and viscosity are appropriate, then antral peristaltic contractions (E) occurring at three peristalses per minute sweep aliquots of the nutrient suspension through the pylorus. The pyloric sphincter may offer variable resistance or may close (F) during the antral peristaltic wave. Pyloric closure results in retropulsion of larger food particles back into the stomach for further mixing. Normal antroduodenal coordination (G) ensures that antral peristalsis is coordinated with decreased duodenal pressure and resistance (H) to ensure efficient emptying with each antral peristalsis. Abnormalities in any of these postprandial phases of gastropyloroduodenal muscular relaxations or contractions may lead to symptoms (epigastric fullness, epigastric pain, nausea) or altered gastric emptying of the solid foods. (**d**) When gastric motility is normal (as outlined in A though H), ingested meals are emptied in a normal fashion. This figure shows the gastric emptying rate for two technetium-labeled scrambled eggs as recorded by scintigraphy. The lag phase represents the time of redistribution of food from fundus to antrum and mixing of the contents (A to D) before the linear phase of emptying of gastric contents into the duodenum takes place (E, F, and G). During the linear emptying period, recurrent gastric peristaltic contractions empty small aliquots, or gushes, of the suspended nutrients into the duodenum. Extragastric factors such as duodenal resistance (H) also affect the rate of gastric emptying. Thus, gastric emptying rates are produced by complex myoelectrical and mechanical (contractile) events coordinated by extrinsic and intrinsic neural activity of the stomach in concert with hormonal, duodenal, and small bowel influences on the rate of gastric emptying. (Reproduced with permission of BC Decker, Inc from Lacy BE, Crowell MD, Koch KL. Manometry. In: Schuster M, Crowell M, Koch K, eds. Schusters Atlas of Gastrointestinal Motility: In Health and Disease, 2nd edn. Hamilton, ON: BC Decker; 2002: 135–150).[1]

During fasting, the stomach, small intestine and biliary smooth muscle follow a stereotyped motility pattern, the migrating motor complex (MMC) (Fig. 27.2). Beginning in the antrum or proximal small intestine, waves of contractions traverse the upper gastrointestinal tract sweeping it clean of dietary residues and bacteria. During phase one of the MMC, there is complete motor quiescence. Phase II is characterized by contractions of variable amplitude and frequency. In phase III of the MMC, contractions occur at maximal frequency and amplitude for that specific site of the gastrointestinal tract. This frequency is governed by the local electrical slow wave frequency and is 3/min in the antrum (as discussed above) and 11/min in the duodenum. Feeding interrupts this pattern.

Regulation of gastric emptying

Although the basic motility functions of smooth muscle tone and peristaltic contractions are generated by smooth muscle, ICC and local neurons of the enteric nervous system (ENS), gastric motility is subject to extensive extrinsic neural and hormonal regulation. The rate of gastric

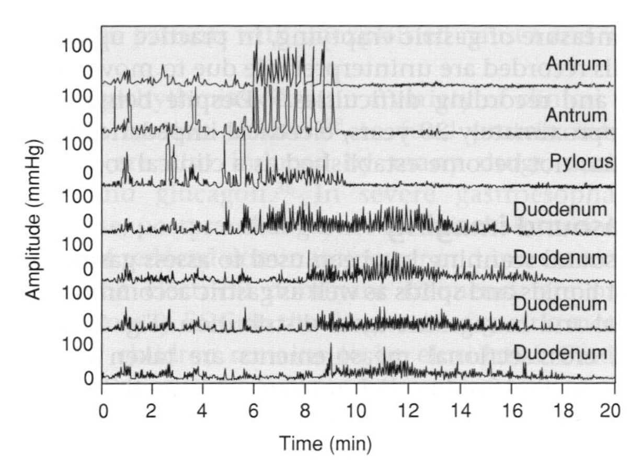

Figure 27.2: Antroduodenal manometry showing normal fasting motility: the migrating motor complex, using GiPC™ software.

emptying is modulated by hormones such as cholecystokinin released from the duodenum in response to chemical contents of the chyme, such as lipid, protein and carbohydrate, pH, osmolality and caloric density (Table 27.1). In studies of infant formula feeding, formulas based on medium chain triglycerides empty faster than those with long chain and those utilizing glucose polymers as a carbohydrate source empty faster than lactose based formulas.[12] The nature of the protein is also important, with whey-based milk formulas emptying more rapidly than those based on casein and hydrolyzed formulas emptying more rapidly than whole proteins.[13,14] Overall, the energy content of a meal, irrespective of its composition, has been shown to be the most important factor that affects the gastric emptying of a meal.[15,16] Duodenal distension also slows gastric emptying via a vagal reflex. Sympathetic nervous system activity also inhibits gastric emptying as part of the 'fight or flight response',[17] emphasizing the importance of the 'gut-brain axis' between central nervous system (CNS) and ENS in the regulation of motility in health and disease.

Stimulus	Effect on gastric emptying
Luminal contents in duodenum	
Acid	Slows
Osmolar load	Slows
Lipids (fatty acids, monoglycerides, diglycerides)	Slows
Amino acids (L-tryptophan)	Slows
Caloric density	Slows
Distension/volume	Rate proportionate to volume
Other factors	
Hypoglycemia	Accelerates
Hyperglycemia	Slows
Ileal fat	Slows (ileal brake)
Ileal/colonic short chain fatty acids	Slows
Rectal/colonic distension	Slows
Pregnancy	Slows
Psychological stress	Slows

Table 27.1 Factors influencing rate of gastric emptying in health

Development of gastric motility

There is evidence that gastric emptying occurs *in utero* from 30 weeks.[18] After delivery, postprandial duodenal feedback mechanisms and antropyloric mechanisms regulating gastric emptying can function normally in premature infants as young as 30 weeks.[10] However, gastric emptying in premature infants is slower than in term infants.[19] Maturation of gastrointestinal motility is promoted by early introduction of enteral feedings.[20]

Fasting antral motility in term and pre-term infants consists of isolated single contractions and clustered phasic contractions. Between 25 and 30 weeks, contractions may be identified in the gastric antrum but not duodenum. The temporal association of antral and duodenal activity develops in association with progressive changes in duodenal motor activity.[21] Fasting duodenal motility is characterized by clusters of contractions, which become less frequent and longer in duration with advancing postmenstrual age.[22] The mature MMC appears at 32 weeks postmenstrual age.[23]

ASSESSMENT OF GASTRIC MOTOR AND SENSORY FUNCTIONS

Currently, there is a wide range of specialized investigations to detect motor dysfunction of the stomach, including transit studies, volumetric measurements, electrogastrography and manometry.

Tests of gastric emptying

Barium contrast studies

In the context of gastric motility disorders, barium contrast studies are only useful to exclude mechanical obstruction, and visualize retained food particles and bezoars. Because barium itself delays gastric emptying, barium studies are not a useful assessment of gastric emptying rate.

Nuclear scintigraphy

Nuclear scintigraphy is currently the most popular method of assessment of gastric emptying rate, because it is widely available and gives relatively rapid results (Fig. 27.3).[24,25] A variety of foods may be labeled with radioisotopes, usually technetium (^{99m}Tc). In infants, formula may be labeled. For older children emptying of labeled solids is a more sensitive test of impaired gastric motility. The lag phase of the solid emptying curve (Fig. 27.1d) represents gastric trituration and reflects antral contractile function. After administration of the test meal, images are acquired with the patient in the supine position every 10 min for up to 2 h. Note that the supine position may artefactually increase emptying time. Results are usually expressed as the percentage of emptying over a defined time period or as the gastric half emptying time ($T_{1/2}$), the time needed to empty half of the radioactive material. Normal ranges are available for adults and children,[25,26] but due to regional differences in technique, local reference ranges are preferred.

Similarly, in adults and children with functional abdominal pain or dyspepsia, one or more of the following mechanisms may contribute to symptoms in an individual patient: impaired receptive relaxation (associated with early satiety), delayed emptying, pylorospasm, visceral hypersensitivity and maldistribution of gastric contents, resulting in antral distension and contributing to abdominal pain and nausea.[4,38,105]

Research using the ever-expanding range of gastric motility investigations available aims to develop therapies specifically targeted to the pathophysiology in individual patients and disease groups.

FUTURE DIRECTIONS

Investigations

Tests of gastric emptying

SPECT Another non-invasive test to assess gastric volume, accommodation to a meal, regional distension and emptying rate is single photon emission computed tomography (SPECT) (Fig. 27.6). This method requires intravenous injection of (99m) Technetium pertechnetate to label the stomach mucosa, followed by volume estimations using computerized gastric reconstruction from tomographic images.[106] Current experience with this technique consists of adult series, although SPECT may also represent an attractive noninvasive test for use in pediatric patients in future. Gastric volumes estimated with SPECT are less than those obtained from intragastric barostat balloon measurements.[107]

Tests of hypersensitivity and gastric accommodation

Several tests are being developed for evaluation of sensation, baseline tone and the accommodation reflex (gastric relaxation in response to a meal). In addition to SPECT and ultrasound tests mentioned above, both of which assess gastric accommodation, drink tests and gastric barostat studies are increasingly employed in research settings.

Drink tests Drink tests utilizing water or nutrient drinks evaluate total volume and caloric intake. They are proposed as indicators of gastric hypersensitivity and/or impaired accommodation. Drink tests evaluate intake and can precipitate symptoms, potentially making them a simple and valuable tool in clinical assessment. However, their correlation with gastric physiology is still being elucidated.[38]

Barostat The gastric barostat test uses a highly compliant intragastric balloon attached to an air pump. The system adjusts the volume of air in the balloon to maintain constant distending pressure. Thus changes in gastric tone are reflected as alterations in balloon volume (Fig. 27.7). This method is used to assess gastric accommodation and hypersensitivity to distension.[4,108] Although extensively used in adults, data from children remain sparse[108,109] and this is currently considered a research technique.

Management

Enhancement of gastric accommodation

Pharmacological relaxation of the stomach was associated with symptomatic improvement in some patients with functional dyspepsia.[4] Drugs such as buspirone, sumatriptan and clonidine show promise as fundic relaxants in this context. One mechanism of action of gastric pacemakers may be enhancement of gastric fundic relaxation, reducing symptoms in patients with gastroparesis without affecting gastric emptying rate.[110]

Gastric pacemakers

Implantable electrical devices capable of stimulating the gastrointestinal tract via serosal wires have been investigated for the treatment of gastrointestinal disorders including severe gastroparesis. Recently, the Medtronic Enterra™ Therapy device was licensed by the United States Food and Drug Administration as a humanitarian device for use in adults with medically intractable gastroparesis. Based on the frequency of the electrical stimulus used for chronic treatment of gastroparesis, gastric electrical stimulation can be classified into low-frequency stimulation (LFS) and

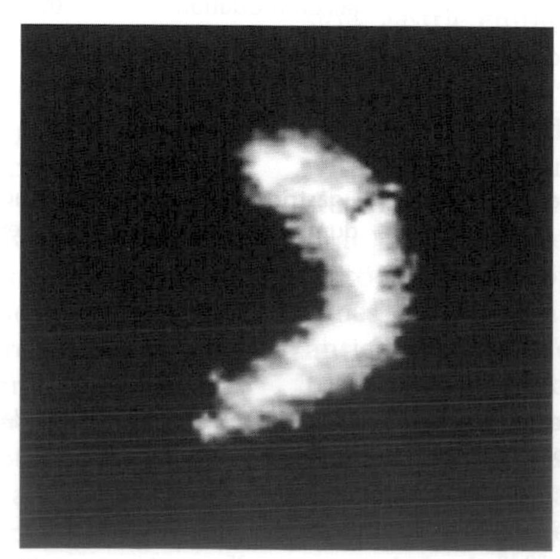

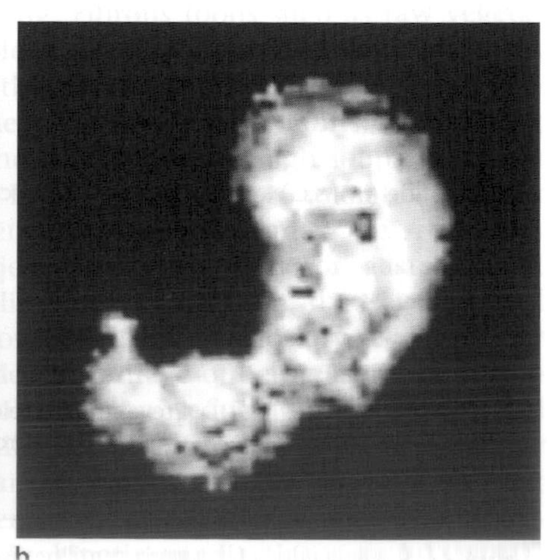

Figure 27.6: Gastric accommodation to a meal as measured by SPECT. Outlines of fasting (**a**) and postprandial (**b**) stomach constructed from transaxial SPECT images, after intravenous injection of ^{99m}Tc (99m Technetium) pertechnetate to label the stomach mucosa. (Reproduced from Kuiken SD, et al. Development of a test to measure gastric accomodation in humans. AJP 1999; 277: 1217–1221, with permission.)

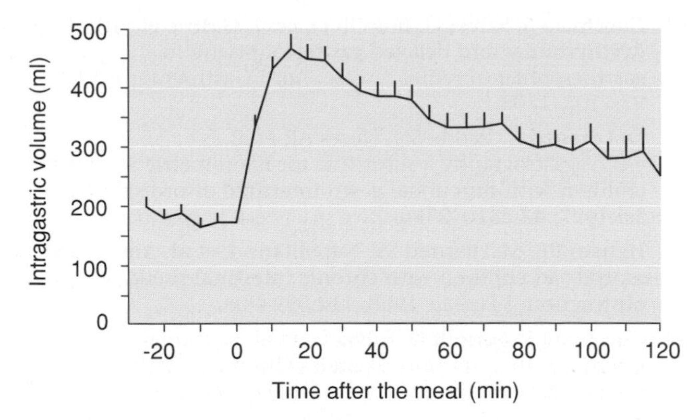

Figure 27.7: Gastric accommodation to a meal as measured by barostat. Mean intragastric volume at 5-min intervals as measured by a gastric barostat in healthy volunteers before and after administration of a mixed liquid meal (time 0). Ingestion of the meal induces a rapid and sustained increase in intragastric volume, reflecting a relaxation of the gastric fundus. (Reproduced from Tack J, Piessevaux H, Coulie B, Caenepeel P, Janssens J. Role of impaired gastric accommodation to a meal in functional dyspepsia. Gastroenterology 1998; 115:1346–1352. Copyright (1998), with permission from the American Gastroenterological Association.)[4]

high-frequency stimulation (HFS). Evidence from adult studies shows that LFS seems to normalize gastric dysrhythmias and entrain gastric slow waves, accelerating gastric emptying. On the other hand, HFS has no effect on gastric emptying, but is able to significantly reduce symptoms of nausea and vomiting in gastroparetic patients,[110] possibly by enhancing accommodation or decreasing hyperalgesia.[111] Gastric electrical stimulation is associated with improvements in symptom relief, nutritional status, health resource utilization and costs and offers new hope to patients with gastroparesis unresponsive to conventional medical management.[110]

Botulinum toxin

Pylorospasm is associated with epigastric pain and delayed gastric emptying and is present in some patients with gastroparesis.[38] In addition, even normal pyloric contractions could theoretically provide a functional obstruction in patients with ineffective antral and/or fundic motility. Recent trials of botulinum toxin, injected into the pylorus, have improved gastric emptying and reduced symptoms in adult and pediatric patients with gastroparesis.[112,113]

Psychological factors

As a group, adults and children with functional gastrointestinal disorders have increased anxiety and depression.[108] However, there is no direct correlation between anxiety and sensory thresholds and reduced sensory thresholds are regional, depending on predominant symptoms.[108] Thus it is likely that visceral hypersensitivity is not due to generalized sensory hypervigilance. A multidisciplinary biopsychosocial approach to functional gastrointestinal disorders has been advocated as the most effective means of addressing all contributing factors.

References

1. Lacy B, Crowell M, Koch K. Manometry. In: Schuster M, Crowell M, Koch K, eds. Schuster's Atlas of Gastrointestinal Motility: In Health and Disease, 2nd edn. Hamilton, ON: BC Decker; 2002:135–150.
2. Coulie B, Tack J, Sifrim D, et al. Role of nitric oxide in fasting gastric fundus tone and in 5-HT_1 receptor-mediated relaxation of gastric fundus. Am J Physiol 1999; 276:G373–G377.
3. Tack J, Demedts I, Meulemans A, et al. Role of nitric oxide in the gastric accommodation reflex and in meal induced satiety in humans. Gut 2002; 51:219–224.
4. Tack J, Piessevaux H, Coulie B, Caenepeel P, Janssens J. Role of impaired gastric accommodation to a meal in functional dyspepsia. Gastroenterology 1998; 115: 1346–1352.
5. Piessevaux H, Tack J, Walrand S, et al. Intragastric distribution of a standardized meal in health and functional dyspepsia: correlation with specific symptoms. Neurogastroenterol Motil 2003; 15:447–455.
6. Cucchiara S, Minella R, Iorio R, et al. Real-time ultrasound reveals gastric motor abnormalities in children investigated for dyspeptic symptoms. J Pediatr Gastroenterol Nutr 1995; 21:446–453.
7. Olafsdottir E, Gilja OH, Aslaksen A, et al. Impaired accommodation of the proximal stomach in children with recurrent abdominal pain. J Pediatr Gastroenterol Nutr 2000; 30:157–163.
8. Olafsdottir E, Gilja OH, Tefera S, et al. Intragastric maldistribution of a liquid meal in children with recurrent abdominal pain assessed by three-dimensional ultrasonography. Scand J Gastroenterol 2003; 38:819–825.
9. Berseth CL, Ittmann PI. Antral and duodenal motor responses to duodenal feeding in preterm and term infants. J Pediatr Gastroenterol Nutr 1992; 14:182–186.
10. Hassan BB, Butler R, Davidson GP, et al. Patterns of antropyloric motility in fed healthy preterm infants. Arch Dis Child Fetal Neonatal Ed 2002; 87:F95–F99.
11. Hunt JN. Some properties of an alimentary osmoreceptor mechanism. J Physiol 1956; 132:267–288.
12. Siegel M, Krantz B, Lebenthal E. Effect of fat and carbohydrate composition on the gastric emptying of isocaloric feedings in premature infants. Gastroenterology 1985; 89:785–790.
13. Billeaud C, Guillet J, Sandler B. Gastric emptying in infants with or without gastro-oesophageal reflux according to the type of milk. Eur J Clin Nutr 1990; 44:577–583.
14. Tolia V, Lin CH, Kuhns LR. Gastric emptying using three different formulas in infants with gastroesophageal reflux. J Pediatr Gastroenterol Nutr 1992; 15:297–301.
15. Hunt JN, Stubbs DF. The volume and energy content of meals as determinants of gastric emptying. J Physiol 1975; 245:209–225.
16. Hunt JN, Smith JL, Jiang CL. Effect of meal volume and energy density on the gastric emptying of carbohydrates. Gastroenterology 1985; 89:1326–1330.
17. Monnikes H, Tebbe JJ, Hildebrandt M, et al. Role of stress in functional gastrointestinal disorders. Evidence for stress-induced alterations in gastrointestinal motility and sensitivity. Dig Dis 2001; 19:201–211.
18. McLain C. Amniographic studies of the gastrointestinal activity of the human fetus. Am J Obstet Gynecol 1963; 85:1079–1087.
19. Gupta M, Brans YW. Gastric retention in neonates. Pediatrics 1978; 62:26–29.

20. Berseth CL, Nordyke C. Enteral nutrients promote postnatal maturation of intestinal motor activity in preterm infants. Am J Physiol 1993; 264:G1046–G1051.
21. Ittmann PI, Amarnath R, Berseth CL. Maturation of antroduodenal motor activity in preterm and term infants. Dig Dis Sci 1992; 37:14–19.
22. Berseth CL. Gestational evolution of small intestine motility in preterm and term infants. J Pediatr 1989; 115:646–651.
23. Jadcherla SR, Berseth CL. Effect of erythromycin on gastroduodenal contractile activity in developing neonates. J Pediatr Gastroenterol Nutr 2002; 34:16–22.
24. Smout A, Horowitz M, Armstrong D. Methods to study gastric emptying. Frontiers in gastric emptying. Dig Dis Sci 1994; 39:130S–132S.
25. Heyman S. Gastric emptying in children. J Nucl Med 1998; 39:865–869.
26. Montgomery M, Escobar-Billing R, Hellstrom PM, et al. Impaired gastric emptying in children with repaired esophageal atresia: a controlled study. J Pediatr Surg 1998; 33:476–480.
27. Perri F, Clemente R, Festa V, et al. 13C-octanoic acid breath test: a reliable tool for measuring gastric emptying. Ital J Gastroenterol Hepatol 1998; 30:211–217.
28. Barnett C, Snel A, Omari T, et al. Reproducibility of the 13C-octanoic acid breath test for assessment of gastric emptying in healthy preterm infants. J Pediatr Gastroenterol Nutr 1999; 29:26–30.
29. Gatti C. di Abriola FF, Dall'Oglio L, et al. Is the 13C-acetate breath test a valid procedure to analyse gastric emptying in children? J Pediatr Surg 2000; 35:62–65.
30. Maes BD, Ghoos YF, Geypens BJ, et al. Combined carbon-13-glycine/carbon-14-octanoic acid breath test to monitor gastric emptying rates of liquids and solids. J Nucl Med 1994; 35:824–831.
31. Cavell B. Gastric emptying in preterm infants. Acta Paediatr Scand 1979; 68:725–730.
32. Lange A, Funch-Jensen P, Thommesen P, et al. Gastric emptying patterns of a liquid meal in newborn infants measured by epigastric impedance. Neurogastroenterol Motil 1997; 9:55–62.
33. Brown BH. Electrical impedance tomography (EIT): a review. J Med Engl Technol 2003; 27:97–108.
34. Bateman DN, Whittingham TA. Measurement of gastric emptying by real-time ultrasound. Gut 1982; 23:524–527.
35. Ewer AK, Durbin GM, Morgan ME, et al. Gastric emptying in preterm infants. Arch Dis Child Fetal Neonatal Ed 1994; 71:F24–F27.
36. Cucchiara S, Raia V, Minella R, et al. Ultrasound measurement of gastric emptying time in patients with cystic fibrosis and effect of ranitidine on delayed gastric emptying. J Pediatr 1996; 128:485–488.
37. Levy J. Use of electrogastrography in children. Curr Gastroenterol Rep 2002; 4:259–265.
38. Koch KL. Diagnosis and treatment of neuromuscular disorders of the stomach. Curr Gastroenterol Rep 2003; 5:323–330.
39. Parkman HP, Hasler WL, Barnett JL, et al. Electrogastrography: a document prepared by the gastric section of the American Motility Society Clinical GI Motility Testing Task Force. Neurogastroenterol Motil 2003; 15:89–102.
40. Ravelli AM, Tobanelli P, Volpi S, et al. Vomiting and gastric motility in infants with cow's milk allergy. J Pediatr Gastroenterol Nutr 2001; 32:59–64.
41. Cucchiara S, Salvia G, Borrelli O, et al. Gastric electrical dysrhythmias and delayed gastric emptying in gastroesophageal reflux disease. Am J Gastroenterol 1997; 92:1103–1108.
42. Di Lorenzo C, Reddy SN, Flores AF, et al. Is electrogastrography a substitute for manometric studies in children with functional gastrointestinal disorders? Dig Dis Sci 1997; 42:2310–2316.
43. Hyman PE, McDiarmid SV, Napolitano J, et al. Antroduodenal motility in children with chronic intestinal pseudo-obstruction. J Pediatr 1988; 112:899–905.
44. Cucchiara S, Borrelli O, Salvia G, et al. A normal gastrointestinal motility excludes chronic intestinal pseudoobstruction in children. Dig Dis Sci 2000; 45:258–264.
45. Tomomasa T, DiLorenzo C, Morikawa A, et al. Analysis of fasting antroduodenal manometry in children. Dig Dis Sci 1996; 41:2195–2203.
46. Sigurdsson L, Flores A, Putnam PE, et al. Postviral gastroparesis: presentation, treatment, and outcome. J Pediatr 1997; 131:751–754.
47. Uc A, Hoon A, Di Lorenzo C, et al. Antroduodenal manometry in children with no upper gastrointestinal symptoms. Scand J Gastroenterol 1997; 32:681–685.
48. Di Lorenzo C, Flores AF, Buie T, et al. Antroduodenal manometry predicts success of jejunal feeding in children with chronic intestinal pseudoobstruction. Gastroenterology 1993; 104:A497.
49. Hyman PE, Di Lorenzo C, McAdams L, et al. Predicting the clinical response to cisapride in children with chronic intestinal pseudo-obstruction. Am J Gastroenterol 1993; 88:832–836.
50. Hveem K, Sun WM, Hebbard G, et al. Relationship between ultrasonically detected phasic antral contractions and antral pressure. Am J Physiol Gastrointest Liver Physiol 2001; 281:G95–G101.
51. Berseth CL. Chronic therapeutic morphine administration alters small intestinal motor patterns and gastroanal transit in preterm infants. Pediatr Res 1996; 39:305A.
52. Omari TI, Barnett C, Snel A, et al. Mechanisms of gastroesophageal reflux in healthy premature infants. J Pediatr 1998; 133:650–654.
53. Omari TI, Benninga MA, Barnett CP, et al. Characterization of esophageal body and lower esophageal sphincter motor function in the very premature neonate. J Pediatr 1999; 135:517–521.
54. Berseth CL. Effect of early feeding on maturation of the preterm infant's small intestine. J Pediatr 1992; 120:947–953.
55. Berseth CL. Feeding methods for the preterm infant. Semin Neonatology 2001; 6:417–424.
56. Cavell B. Gastric emptying in infants fed human milk or infant formula. Acta Paediatr Scand 1981; 70:639–641.
57. Driessche M Van Den, Peeters K, Marien P, et al. Gastric emptying in formula-fed and breast-fed infants measured with the 13C-octanoic acid breath test. J Pediatr Gastroenterol Nutr 1999; 29:46–51.
58. Ville K de, Knapp E, Al-Tawil Y, et al. Slow infusion feedings enhance duodenal motor responses and gastric emptying in preterm infants. Am J Clin Nutr 1998; 68:103–108.
59. Pezzati M, Dani C, Biadaioli R, et al. Randomised controlled trial of the effect of cisapride on the pyloric muscle in preterm infants. Eur J Pediatr 2001; 160:572–575.
60. Hyman PE, Abrams CE, Dubois A. Gastric emptying in infants: response to metoclopramide depends on the underlying condition. J Pediatr Gastroenterol Nutr 1988; 7:181–184.

61. Ng SC-Y, Gomez JM, Rajadurai VS, et al. Establishing enteral feeding in preterm infants with feeding intolerance: A Randomized Controlled Study of Low-dose Erythromycin. J Pediatr Gastroenterol Nutr 2003; 37:554–558.
62. ElHennawy AA, Sparks JW, Armentrout D, et al. Erythromycin fails to improve feeding outcome in feeding-intolerant preterm infants. J Paediatr Gastroenterol Nutr 2003; 37:281–286.
63. Bonthala S, Sparks JW, Musgrove KH, et al. Mydriatics slow gastric emptying in preterm infants. J Pediatr 2000; 137:327–330.
64. Parkman HP, Harris AD, Krevsky B, et al. Gastroduodenal motility and dysmotility: an update on techniques available for evaluation. Am J Gastroenterol 1995; 90:869–892.
65. Nimmo WS, Heading RC, Wilson J, et al. Inhibition of gastric emptying and drug absorption by narcotic analgesics. Br J Clin Pharmacol 1975; 2:509–513.
66. Lydon AM, Cooke T, Duggan F, et al. Delayed postoperative gastric emptying following intrathecal morphine and intrathecal bupivacaine. Can J Anaesth 1999; 46:544–549.
67. Bardhan PK, Salam MA, Molla AM. Gastric emptying of liquid in children suffering from acute rotaviral gastroenteritis. Gut 1992; 33:26–29.
68. Meeroff JC, Schreiber DS, Trier JS, et al. Abnormal gastric motor function in viral gastroenteritis. Ann Intern Med 1980; 92:370–373.
69. Kebede D, Barthel JS, Singh A. Transient gastroparesis associated with cutaneous herpes zoster. Dig Dis Sci 1987; 32:318–322.
70. Neild PJ, Nijran KS, Yazaki E, et al. Delayed gastric emptying in human immunodeficiency virus infection: correlation with symptoms, autonomic function, and intestinal motility. Dig Dis Sci 2000; 45:1491–1499.
71. Vassallo M, Camilleri M, Caron BL, et al. Gastrointestinal motor dysfunction in acquired selective cholinergic dysautonomia associated with infectious mononucleosis. Gastroenterology 1991; 100:252–258.
72. Oh JJ, Kim CH. Gastroparesis after a presumed viral illness: clinical and laboratory features and natural history. Mayo Clin Proc 1990; 65:636–642.
73. Kassander P. Asymptomatic gastric retention in diabetes (gastroparesis diabeticorum). Ann Intern Med 1958; 48:797.
74. Horowitz M, O'Donovan D, Jones KL, et al. Gastric emptying in diabetes: clinical significance and treatment. Diabetic Med 2002; 19:177–194.
75. Reid B, DiLorenzo C, Travis L, et al. Diabetic gastroparesis due to postprandial antral hypomotility in childhood. Pediatrics 1992; 90:43–46.
76. Cucchiara S, Franzese A, Salvia G, et al. Gastric emptying delay and gastric electrical derangement in IDDM. Diabetes Care 1998; 21:438–443.
77. Perri F, Pastore M, Zicolella A, et al. Gastric emptying of solids is delayed in celiac disease and normalizes after gluten withdrawal. Acta Paediatr 2000; 89:921–925.
78. Franco VH, Collares EF, Troncon LE. Gastric emptying in children. IV. Studies on kwashiorkor and on marasmic kwashiorkor. Arq Gastroenterol 1986; 23:42–46.
79. Rigaud D, Bedig G, Merrouche M, et al. Delayed gastric emptying in anorexia nervosa is improved by completion of a renutrition program. Dig Dis Sci 1988; 33:919–925.
80. Laskin BL, Choyke P, Keenan GF, et al. Novel gastrointestinal tract manifestations in juvenile dermatomyositis. J Pediatr 1999; 135:371–374.
81. Alexander F, Wyllie R, Jirousek K, et al. Delayed gastric emptying affects outcome of Nissen fundoplication in neurologically impaired children. Surgery 1997; 697:690–698.
82. Chitkara DK, Nurko S, Shoffner JM, et al. Abnormalities in gastrointestinal motility are associated with diseases of oxidative phosphorylation in children. Am J Gastroenterol 2003; 98:871–877.
83. McArthur CJ, Gin T, McLaren IM, et al. Gastric emptying following brain injury: effects of choice of sedation and intracranial pressure. Intensive Care Med 1995; 21:573–576.
84. Krausz Y, Maayan C, Faber J, et al. Scintigraphic evaluation of esophageal transit and gastric emptying in familial dysautonomia. Eur J Radiol 1994; 18:52–56.
85. Cucchiara S, Bortolotti M, Colombo C, et al. Abnormalities of gastrointestinal motility in children with nonulcer dyspepsia and in children with gastroesophageal reflux disease. Dig Dis Sci 1991; 36:1066–1073.
86. Hillemeier AC, Lange R, McCallum R, et al. Delayed gastric emptying in infants with gastroesophageal reflux. J Pediatr 1981; 98:190–193.
87. Papaila JG, Wilmot D, Grosfeld JL, et al. Increased incidence of delayed gastric emptying in children with gastroesophageal reflux. A prospective evaluation. Arch Surg 1989; 124:933–936.
88. Byrne WJ, Cipel L, Euler AR, et al. Chronic idiopathic intestinal pseudo-obstruction syndrome in children – clinical characteristics and prognosis. J Pediatr 1977; 90:585–589.
89. Romeo C, Bonanno N, Baldari S, et al. Gastric motility disorders in patients operated on for esophageal atresia and tracheoesophageal fistula: long-term evaluation. J Pediatr Surg 2000; 35:740–744.
90. Grill BB, Lange R, Markowitz R, et al. Delayed gastric emptying in children with Crohn's disease. J Clin Gastroenterol 1985; 7:216–226.
91. Yamataka A, Pringle KC, Wyeth J. A case of zinc chloride ingestion. J Pediatr Surg 1998; 33:660–662.
92. Ravelli AM. Gastrointestinal function in chronic renal failure. Pediatr Nephrol 1995; 9:756–762.
93. Barczynski M, Thor P. Reversible autonomic dysfunction in hyperthyroid patients affects gastric myoelectrical activity and emptying. Clin Auton Res 2001; 11:243–249.
94. Jonderko G, Jonderko K, Marcisz C, et al. Gastric emptying in hypothyreosis. Isr J Med Sci 1997; 33:198–203.
95. Koch KL. Approach to the patient with nausea and vomiting. In: Yamada T, ed. Textbook of Gastroenterology. Philadelphia, PA: Lippincott; 1995:731–749.
96. Michaud L, Guimber D, Carpentier B, et al. Gastrostomy as a decompression technique in children with chronic gastrointestinal obstruction. J Pediatr Gastroenterol Nutr 2001; 32:82–85.
97. Smith DS, Williams CS, Ferris CD. Diagnosis and treatment of chronic gastroparesis and chronic intestinal pseudo-obstruction. Gastroenterol Clin North Am 2003; 32:619–658.
98. Hauben M, Amsden GW. The association of erythromycin and infantile hypertrophic pyloric stenosis: causal or coincidental? Drug Saf 2002; 25:929–942.
99. Chial HJ, Camilleri M, Burton D, et al. Selective effects of serotonergic psychoactive agents on gastrointestinal functions in health. Am J Physiol Gastrointest Liver Physiol 2003; 284:G130–G137.
100. Gui D, Gaetano A De, Spada PL, et al. Botulinum toxin injected in the gastric wall reduces body weight and food intake in rats. Aliment Pharmacol Ther 2000; 14:829–834.

101. Samuk I, Afriat R, Horne T, et al. Dumping syndrome following Nissen fundoplication, diagnosis, and treatment. J Pediatr Gastroenterol Nutr 1996; 23:235–240.
102. Khoshoo V, Roberts PL, Loe WA, et al. Nutritional management of dumping syndrome associated with antireflux surgery. J Pediatr Surg 1994; 29:1452–1454.
103. Li-Ling J, Irving M. Therapeutic value of octreotide for patients with severe dumping syndrome – a review of randomised controlled trials. Postgrad Med J 2001; 77:441–442.
104. Di Lorenzo C, Orenstein S. Fundoplication: friend or foe? J Pediatr Gastroenterol Nutr 2002; 34:117–124.
105. Ladabaum U, Koshy SS, Woods ML, Hooper FG, Owyang C, Hasler WL. Differential symptomatic and electrogastrographic effects of distal and proximal human gastric distension. Am J Physiol Gastrointest Liver Physiol 1999; 275:G418–G424.
106. Kuiken SD, Samsom M, Camilleri M, et al. Development of a test to measure gastric accommodation in humans. Am J Physiol 1999; 277:G1217–G1221.
107. Elzen BD van den, Bennink RJ, Wieringa RE, et al. Fundic accommodation assessed by SPECT scanning: comparison with the gastric barostat. Gut 2003; 52:1548–1554.
108. Di Lorenzo C, Youssef NN, Sigurdsson L, et al. Visceral hyperalgesia in children with functional abdominal pain. J Pediatr 2001; 139:838–843.
109. Zangen T, Ciarla C, Zangen S, et al. Gastrointestinal motility and sensory abnormalities may contribute to food refusal in medically fragile toddlers. J Pediatr Gastroenterol Nutr 2003; 37:287–293.
110. Lin Z, Forster J, Sarosiek I, et al. Treatment of gastroparesis with electrical stimulation. Dig Dis Sci 2003; 48:837–848.
111. Tack J, Coulie B, Cutsem E Van, et al. The influence of gastric electric stimulation on proximal gastric motor and sensory function in severe idiopathic gastroparesis. Gastroenterology 1999; 116:A1090.
112. Lacy BE, Zayat EN, Crowell MD, et al. Botulinum toxin for the treatment of gastroparesis: a preliminary report. Am J Gastroenterol 2002; 97:1548–1552.
113. Woodward MN, Spicer RD. Intrapyloric botulinum toxin injection improves gastric emptying. J Pediatr Gastroenterol Nutr 2003; 37:201–202.

Chapter 28
Bezoars

Daniel L. Preud'Homme and Adam G. Mezoff

INTRODUCTION

The term *bezoar* comes from the Persian word *badzehr,* which refers to the material found in sacrificed animals such as goats. In ancient times, this material was thought to have magical or medicinal powers and was used as an antidote to poisons from snake bites, infections, diverse diseases, and even as a means of combating aging.[1,2] The Indian physician Charak reported the presence of bezoars in his work in the 2nd and 3rd centuries BC.[3] Baudamant was the first to describe bezoars in the western world, in an autopsy performed in 1779.[4] Matas performed the first extensive review in 1915; subsequently Debakey and Oschner published their landmark review in 1938.[1,2] Schonbon first published a description of the surgical removal of bezoars in the 19th century.[3]

DEFINITIONS

Bezoars are defined as aggregates of undigested or inedible material found anywhere in the gastrointestinal tract, although most commonly found in the stomach. Plant fiber, hair and medication bezoars have all been well described.

ETIOLOGY AND PATHOGENESIS

Phytobezoars

Phytobezoars are the most frequently observed type and account for approximately 40% of the total number of reported bezoars. They are composed of indigestible vegetable fibers, most commonly from pulpy fruits, orange pits, seeds, roots or leaves. Predisposing factors are indicated in Table 28.1. A case of a 'cotton' bezoar was reported in a heroin addict who swallowed the cotton ball used to filter a water-methadone pill preparation for intravenous infusion.[5] These bezoars are usually found in the stomach (78%), although up to 17% may occur in the small intestine.[6] Sunflower seed concretions have been described in the colons of children.[7]

Factor	Prevalence in patients (%)
Poor mastication	80
Gastric surgery with vagotomy	56
Gastroparesis	20
Histamine H_2 receptor antagonists	12
Diabetes mellitus	6
Excessive intake of fibers	44

Table 28.1 Factors predisposing to the formation of phytobezoars

Diospyrobezoar (Persimmon bezoar)

Although made of vegetable matter, persimmon bezoars represent a class by themselves and account for up to 29% of all bezoars in some series.[1] Persimmon bezoars are named for a Native American tree that also is present in Iran and the Middle East, *Diospyros virginiana.* Its fruit, a berry, contains a material called shiboul or phobatanin. This substance is present in the unripened fruit and under the skin of the ripe fruit.[8]

Trichobezoar

Trichobezoars occur predominantly (up to 90%) in females under the age of 20, and often in children.[1] They have been described in children as young as 1 year old. They consist of an aggregation of hair and foodstuff and are black regardless of the patient's hair color, because of the chemical reaction of hair with gastric acid (Fig. 28.1). The hair in the trichobezoar is usually from the patient, although hair from animals, carpet, or toys is occasionally recovered.[9] Trichobezoars are usually the site for intense

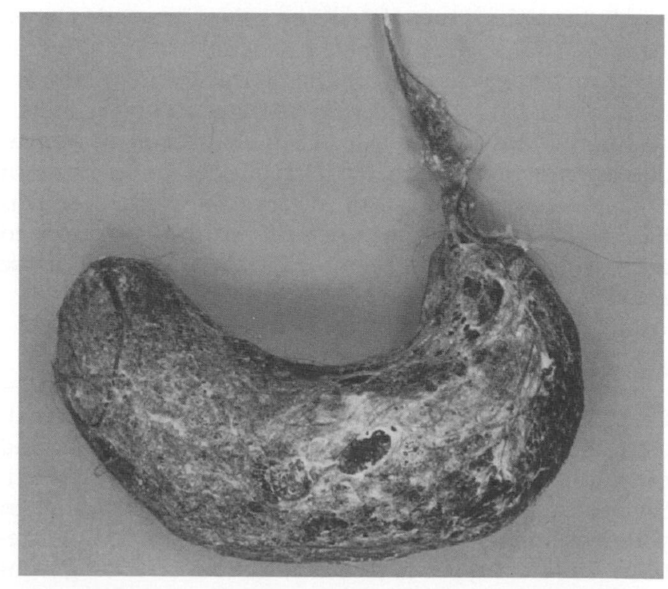

Figure 28.1: Hair cast of the stomach. (Courtesy of D. Mirkin, MD, Children's Medical Center, Dayton, OH.)

food putrefaction and can generate a very foul-smelling odor and halitosis. The act of hair swallowing is thought to be akin to pica or nail biting. Only about 9% of patients with trichobezoars have proven psychiatric problems.[10] Trichobezoars usually are present in the stomach but may have very long tails. These tails can invade the esophagus proximally and extend to the small intestine. Involvement from the stomach extending to the entire length of the small intestine is referred to as Rapunzel syndrome.[3] Trichobezoars may weigh up to 6.5 pounds.

Lactobezoar

Lactobezoars are gastric masses made of milk protein. They occur primarily in premature, low-birthweight infants. Although the exact cause remains unclear, formation is thought to be related to formula composition, protein flocculation, thickening agents, immature gastric motility and rapidity of feeding.[11] Most reported cases have occurred in infants fed high-calorie formula for premature babies.[12] However, human milk bezoars have also been described.[13] The formation of lactobezoars may be precipitated by the addition of thickening agents, such as gel of pectin, to the infant's formula.[14] Lactobezoars have also been reported in adults fed Osmolite (Ross Nutritionals, Columbus, Ohio).[15]

Paper bezoars

At least two case reports of paper bezoars, one in a child and one in an adult, have been described. The undigested material was toilet paper, ingested over several days.[16]

Medication bezoar

A large number of case reports have documented the formation of concretions from various medications, leading to gastric bezoars. The medications implicated include nifedipine XL,[17] sucralfate,[18] bromide,[19] enteric-coated aspirin,[20] iron,[21] meprobamate,[22] slow-release theophylline [23] and antacids.[24] Along with the typical obstructive symptoms of bezoars, these foreign bodies may also induce symptoms based on their intrinsic pharmacologic effects. Bezoar formation is probably related to the composition of the inert compound in the medication (e.g. cellulose). This has been a particular problem with medications packaged in insoluble material for long, continuous delivery of the active drug.[17]

Cement bezoars

Cement contains oxides of silica, aluminum, iron and calcium, sulfuric anhydroxide, magnesium hydroxide and calcium carbonate. It is easily accessible to children. Several cases of cement bezoars have been reported in young children, with the formation of solidified concretions. Different types of cement require various lengths of time to 'set'. After this time has elapsed, attempts at gastric lavage are futile and surgery is required.

Yeast Bezoars

Yeast bezoars have been reported primarily in patients undergoing gastric surgery, particularly vagotomy, although one was described in a newborn and was composed of *Candida albicans* and polystyrene resin.[25] Of the 43 patients with yeast bezoars reported in a Finnish study in 1974, 48% had undergone a Billroth I procedure and vagotomy. The most common species of fungus noted were *C. albicans* and *Torulopsis glabrata*.[26] Yeast bezoars are usually asymptomatic and are discovered incidentally. They have a tendency to recur.

Shellac bezoars

Although glue bezoars have been described in experimenting adolescents, most shellac bezoars occur in adult alcoholics who drink shellac to intensify the effect of their alcohol. Shellac can be found in furniture polish and is readily available to children.[1]

Polybezoars

The term *polybezoars* refers to bezoars composed of multiple objects (metallic, plastic, or even wood) encased in trichobezoars. These usually are found in children or in neurologically impaired adults. Polybezoars often contain a large number of metal pins or clips.[27] Table 28.2

CLINICAL PRESENTATION

A summary of the clinical manifestations of bezoars is shown in Table 28.2.[1,28–32] The initial presentation of many bezoars depends on their type. In premature infants and newborns, the most common bezoar is the lactobezoar. The most common symptom is feeding intolerance.[11] With time, symptoms may include abdominal distension, irritability and vomiting. Physical examination often discloses a palpable mid-abdominal mass.

Trichobezoars and phytobezoars are more common in older children and adults. Trichobezoars form over long periods (several years), and early in their course, their signs and symptoms can be subtle such as early satiety or nau-

Characteristic	Incidence in patients (%)
Halitosis	20–40
Abdominal/epigastric pain	40–70
Fullness after meal	20–60
Nausea/vomiting	10–50
Abdominal mass	10–88
Perforation/pneumatosis/acute abdomen	7–10
Dysphagia	5
Intestinal obstruction, partial or complete	≤75
Weakness/weight loss	6–30
Peptic ulcer disease	10–24
Hematemesis	≤71

Table 28.2 Clinical manifestation of bezoars

sea.[1] These bezoars can grow to a substantial size and mass, causing pressure necrosis of the gastric mucosa, ulceration, gastrointestinal bleeding, and even gastric perforation.[31] Most trichobezoars have 'tails,' either up into the esophagus, or distally into the small intestine, which can lead to partial or complete obstruction. Trichobezoars can often be identified by abdominal palpation. Crepitus, caused by putrefaction and bacterial growth, may be elicited. Phytobezoars are formed much more rapidly than trichobezoars. Symptoms include nausea, vomiting and signs of gastric outlet obstruction, which may persist even after the bezoar has been removed. Serious complications such as gastric perforation are rare but have been the subject of case reports in both adult and pediatric patients.[31] Pharmacobezoars not only may induce symptoms as a result of their gastric mass, but they also carry the potential for drug intoxication.[17–23,33] Concretion of foreign objects in the duodenum and in the biliary tract can cause pancreatitis (toxic 'sock' syndrome).[34] Symptoms such as malabsorption and protein-losing enteropathy can also arise from bezoars in these locations.[1]

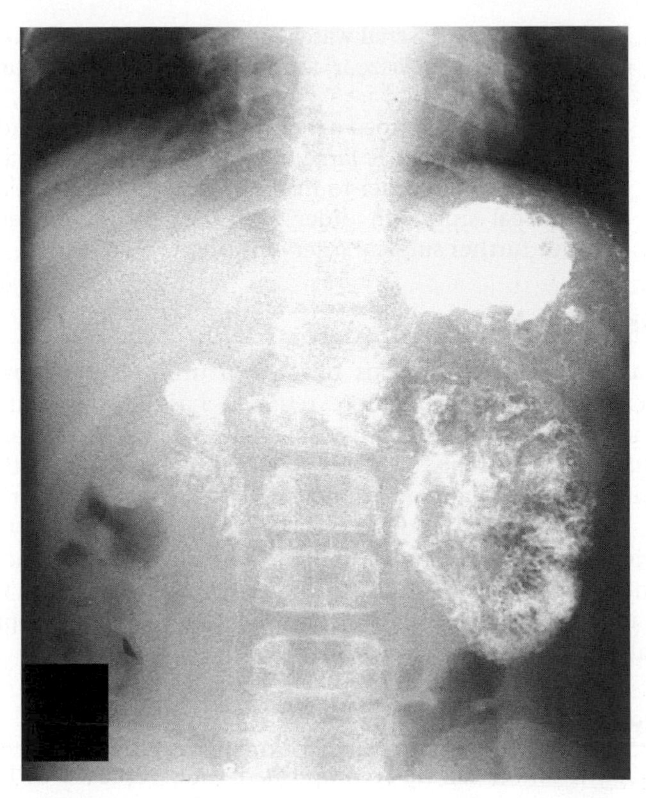

Figure 28.2: Barium swallow, showing a mass effect in the body of the stomach. This mass was a trichobezoar that had to be removed surgically. (Courtesy of F. Unger, MD, Children's Medical Center, Dayton, OH.)

DIAGNOSIS

The diagnosis of bezoars in adult patients can often be made by history and physical examination. Knowledge of predisposing factors may heighten clinical suspicion. Laboratory studies are of limited value, although occasionally, a mild microcytic anemia or leukocytosis may develop. Imaging studies such as plain abdominal radiographs are the initial diagnostic modality identifying most bezoars. Barium studies may be useful to identify the bezoar and to determine the extent of the mass (Fig. 28.2). However, upper gastrointestinal series may fail to diagnose bezoars in 36–50% of patients.[24,34] Moreover, in a reported case of enteric-coated aspirin bezoar, the use of barium changed the acid environment, leading to its distribution and a subsequent increase in the salicylate level.[20] Other methods, such as ultrasound or computed tomography, have also been used to document gastric bezoars.[35,36] These studies do not add to the diagnostic accuracy. Endoscopy remains the diagnostic modality of choice for identifying the type of gastric bezoar. Endoscopy also allows further therapeutic interventions.[23]

TREATMENT

Various methods have been used to both dissolve and/or retrieve the bezoar mass. Often they are used in concert depending on the type of bezoar and its location in the GI tract. They can be divided into categories based on an attempt at either (1) lavaging or dissolving the bezoar, (2) retrieval, or (3) fragmentation.

Lavage/dissolution

Instillation of various pharmacologic agents have been attempted to chemically dissolve bezoars. This may require direct access to the GI tract via nasogastric tube, endoscope or even laparotomy. Various solutions have been attempted:

1 *Acetylcysteine*. Schlang described lavaging with 15 ml of an acetylcysteine solution diluted in normal saline. This was instilled per nasogastric tube and the bezoar was successfully dissolved.[37]
2 *Papain*. This enzyme, while no longer available in tablet form, is found in high concentrations in commercial meat tenderizers, along with high concentrations of sodium (1880 mg/5 ml).[38] It has been used successfully to enzymatically break protein bonds in phytobezoars, and can be administered in a lavage solution.[39] Care must by used with this modality as complications such as hypernatremia and perforation of the esophagus or stomach have been reported.[40,41]
3 *Cellulase*. It is believed that this enzyme cleaves the bond between leukoanthocyanidine-hemicellulose-cellulose. Several cases of successful dissolution of a bezoar with the use of a 3–5 g cellulose solution diluted with up to 500 ml water administered orally for 2–5 days have been reported.[39,42]
4 *Coca-Cola*. Phytobezoars have been successfully dissolved using nasogastric installation of 3 l of Coca-Cola over a 12-h period.[43]
5 *Polyethylene-glycol*. This is often reported as an adjunct in the removal of colonic bezoars, along with colonoscopy and attempts at retrieval.[44]
6 *Enemas*. Various enema preparations have been utilized to help soften and dissolve colonic bezoars. Koneru et al.

describe the use of serial water-soluble contrast enemas to dissolve a colonic bezoar found in a 532 g premature infant.[45]

7 Steinberg et al. described a method whereby they laparoscopically discovered a large bezoar, then performed an appendectomy in order to insert a catheter through the appendiceal stump in order to lavage the hard mass without further surgical intervention.[46]

Retrieval

Various retrieval methods have been utilized to remove bezoars *en-bloc*. Endoscopic retrieval has been the first choice for treatment in this category, however often times surgical enterotomy is necessary to remove large, or difficult to dissolve bezoars such as shellac or cement bezoars.

Kanetaka et al. reported on a dual technique whereby a trichobezoar was fragmented by accessing the stomach with a laparoscope, and utilizing laparoscopic scissors to fragment the bezoar so it could be retrieved endoscopically.[47]

Fragmentation

Fragmentation can be accomplished endoscopically or by extracorporeal means.

1 *Endoscopically*. This is the procedure of choice, often utilizing a snare to help break the large hard bezoar into smaller pieces, which can pass through the intestinal tract. Lavage solutions or metoclopramide have been utilized to augment the passage of gastric bezoars that have been fragmented endoscopically.[48] Gaya et al. described the successful removal of persimmon bezoars with a combination of snare fragmentation and administration of cellulase, cysteine, and metaclopramide.[49] The authors cautioned that large fragments may not pass the pylorus and may lead to obstruction.

2 *Electrohydraulic lithotripsy*. Kuo et al. reported on 11 patients successfully undergoing lithotripsy to fragment gastric phytobezoars.[50]

PREVENTION

Gastric motility disorders, previous gastric surgery, poor mastication and hypochlorhydria are major risk factors for the development and recurrence of many forms of gastric phytobezoars. Dietary counseling to avoid pulpy and fiber rich foods should be provided to patients with these problems. Prokinetic agents such as metoclopramide or cisapride may be useful in preventing recurrences in certain patient populations. Identification of pica-like behavior in children should initiate counseling to prevent the ingestion of foreign substances. A history of significant trichotillomania may prompt psychological evaluation.

References

1. Debakey M, Ochsner A. Bezoars and concretions. Surgery 1938; 4:934–963.
2. Debakey M, Ochsner A. Bezoars and concretions. Part 2. Surgery 1939; 5:132–160.
3. Deslypere JP, Praet M, Verdonk G. An unusual case of trichobezoar; the Rapunzel syndrome. Am J Gastroenterol 1982; 7:467–470.
4. Baudmant WW. Memoire sur des cheveux trouves dans l'estomac et dans les intestins greles. J Med Chir Pharm 1979(52):507–514.
5. Tebar TC, Robles Campos R, Parilla Paricio, et al. Gastric surgery and bezoars. Dig Dis Sci 1992; 11:1694–1696.
6. Kaden W. Phytobezoar in an addict: the cottonpicking stomach syndrome. JAMA 1969; 209:1367.
7. Tsou VM, Bishop PR, Nowicki MJ. Colonic sunflower seed bezoars. Pediatrics 1997; 6:896–897.
8. Izumi S, Isida K, Iwamoto M. Mechanism of formation of phytobezoar with special reference to a persimmon ball. Jpn J Med Sc Tr, II Biochemistry 1933; 2:21.
9. Sidhu BS, Singh G, Khanna S. Trichobezoar. J Indian Med Assoc 1993; 4:100–101.
10. Bhatnagar V, Mitra DK. Childhood trichobezoar. Indian J Pediatr 1984; 51:489–492.
11. Schreiner RL, Brady MS, Franken EA, et al. Increased incidence of lactobezoars in low birth weight infant. Am J Dis Child 1979; 133:936–939.
12. Schreiner RL, Brady MS, Ernst JA, et al. Lack of lactobezoars in infants given predominantly whey containing formula. Am J Dis Child 1982; 136:437–439.
13. Yoss B. Human milk bezoars. J Pediatr 1984; 5:819–822.
14. Faverge B, Gratecos LA. Lactobezoar gastrique du nourrisson induit par Gelopectose. Pediatrie 1987; 42:685–686.
15. Chintapalli KN. Gastric bezoar causing intramural pneumatosis. J Clin Gastroenterolo 1994; 3:264–266.
16. Majeski JA. Paper bezoars in the stomach. South Med J 1985; 12:1520.
17. Stack PE, Patel NR, Young MF, et al. Pharmacobezoars: the irony of the antidote. First case report of nifedipine XL bezoars. J Clin Gastroenterol 1994; 3:264–265.
18. Strozik KS, Walele AH. HoffmanH: Bezoar in a preterm baby associated with sucralfate. Clin Pediatr 199(8):423–424.
19. Iberti TJ, Patterson BK, Fisher CJ. Prolonged bromide intoxication resulting from a gastric bezoar. Arch Intern Med 1984; 144:402–403.
20. Boghacz K, Caldron P. Enteric coated aspirin: elevation of the serum salicylate level by barium study. Case report and review of the medical management. Am J Med 1987; 83:783–787.
21. Landsman I, Bricker JT, Reid BS, et al. Emergency gastrectomy: treatment of choice for iron bezoar. J Pediatr Surg 1987; 22:184–185.
22. Schwartz HS. Acute meprobamate poisoning with gastrostomy and removal of drug containing mass. N Eng J Med 1976; 295:1177–1178.
23. Cereda JM, Scott J, Quigley EM. Endoscopic removal of a pharmacobezoar of slow release theophylline. BMJ1986;. 293:1143–1144.
24. Lee J. Bezoars and foreign bodies of the stomach. Gastrintest Endosc Clin North Am 1966; 6:605–619.
25. Metlay L, Klionsky B. An unusual gastric bezoar in a newborn: polystyrene resin and *Candida albicans*. J Pediatr 1983; 1(1):121–123.
26. Perttala Y, Peltokallio P, Leiviska T, et al. Yeast bezoar formation following gastric surgery. Am J Roentgenol Radium Ther Nucl Med 1975; 2:365–373.
27. Bitar D. Polybezoar and gastrointestinal foreign bodies in the mentally retarded. Am Surg 1975; 41:497–499.

28. Raffin SB. Bezoars. In: Slesienger MH, Fortran JS, eds. Gastrointestinal Disease: Pathophysiology, Diagnosis, Management, 4th edn. Philadelphia, PA: WB Saunders; 1989:741–745.
29. Towsend C, Remmers A, Sarles H, et al. Intestinal obstruction from a medication bezoar in patients with renal failure. N Engl J Med 1973; 288:1058–1059.
30. Zarling EJ, Thompson L. Nonpersimmon gastric phytobezoar, a benign recurrent condition. Arch Intern Med 1994; 144:959–961.
31. Robles R, Parrilla P, Escamilla C, et al. Gastrointestinal bezoars. Br J Surg 1994; 81:1000–1001.
32. Lagios MD. Emphysematous gastritis with perforation complicating phytobezoar. Am J Dis Child 1968; 116:202–204.
33. Brady PG. Gastric phytobezoar consequent to delayed gastric emptying. Gastrointest Endosc 1978; 24:159–161.
34. Adler AI, Olscamp A. Toxic 'sock' syndrome: bezoar formation and pancreatitis associated with iron deficiency and pica. West J Med 1995; 163:480–481.
35. Naik DR, Bolia A, Boon AW. Demonstration of a lactobezoar by ultrasound. Br J Radiol 1987; 60:506–508.
36. Tamminen J, Rosenfeld D. CT diagnosis of a gastric trichobezoar. Comput Med Imaging Graph 1988; 6:339–341.
37. Schlang HA. Acetylcysteine in the removal of a bezoar. JAMA 1970; 214:1329.
38. Zarling EJ, Moeller DD. Bezoar therapy: complications using Adolph meat tenderizer and alternatives from literature review. Arch Intern Med 1981; 141:1669–1670.
39. Walker-Renard P. Update on the medical management of phytobezoar. Am J Gastroenterol 1993; 10:1663–1666.
40. Dugan FA, Lilly JO, McCaffey TD. Dissolution of a phytobezoar with short term medical management. South Med J 1972; 65:313–316.
41. Holsinger JW, Fuson RL, Sealy WC. Esophageal perforation following meat impaction and papain ingestion. JAMA 1968; 204:188–189.
42. Lee P, Holloway WD, Nicholson GI. The medicinal dissolution of phytobezoar using cellulose. Br J Surg 1977; 64:403–405.
43. Ladas SD, Triantafyllou K, Tzathas C, Tassios P, Rokkas T, Raptis SA. Gastric phytobezoars may be treated by nasogastric Coca-Cola lavage. Eur J Gastroenterol Hepatol 2001; 14:801–803.
44. Chae HS, Kim SS, Han SW, et al. Endoscopic removal of a phytobezoar obstructing the distal small bowel. Gastrointest Endosc 2001; 54:264–6.
45. Koneru PJ, Kaufman RA, Talati AJ, Jenkins MB, Korones SK. Successful treatment of sodium polystyrene sulfonate bezoars with serial water-soluble contrast enemas. J Perinatal 2003; 23:431–433.
46. Steinberg R, Schwartz E, Gelber E, Lerner A, Zer M. A rare case of colonic obstruction by 'cherry tomato' phytobezoar: A simple technique to avoid enterotomy. J Pediatr Surg 2002; 37:794–795.
47 Kanetaka K, Azuma T, Ito S, et al. Two-channel method for retrieval of gastric trichobezoar: Report of a case. J Pediatr Surg 2003; 38(2):e7.
48. Delpre G, Kadish U, Glanz I. Metoclopramide in the treatment of gastric bezoar. Am J Gastroenterol 1984; 79:739–740.
49. Gaya J, Barranco L, Llompart A, Reyes J, Obrador A. Persimmon bezoars: A successful combined therapy. Gastrointest Endosc 2002; 55:581–3.
50. Kuo JY, Mo LR, Tsai CC, Chou CY, Lin RC, Chang KK. Nonoperative treatment of gastric bezoars using electrohydraulic lithotripsy. Endoscopy 1999; 31:386–388.

SECTION FIVE
THE SMALL AND LARGE INTESTINE

Chapter 29
Anatomy and physiology of the small and large intestine

Bankole Osuntokun and Samuel A. Kocoshis

INTRODUCTION

The small and large intestines are contiguous and occupy most of the abdominal cavity. Working in concert, and with remarkable efficiency, they are responsible for several complex functions involving the digestion, secretion and absorption of nutrients, including vitamins and trace elements. Other functions include fluid and electrolyte transport, excretion, physical and immunologic defense mechanisms.

The intestines are morphologically adapted to serve these functions, with unique regional and anatomic variations. The digestion and absorption of nutrients is almost solely restricted to the small intestine. Fluid and electrolyte transport occur along the entire length of small and large intestines, with most of it taking place in the small intestine.

The mucosal surface of the small intestine is anatomically and physiologically designed to provide extensive surface area for nutrient absorption. However, this remarkable adaptation unfortunately also serves as a double-edged sword, providing a massive interface for possible antigenic interaction with the environment. This interface is modulated via the activity of the immunoendocrine system and the integrative functions of the enteric nervous system. The enteric nervous system is an independent nervous system within the wall of the digestive tract, now often referred to as the second brain, because of its ability to generate and modulate essential gastrointestinal tract functions without input from the autonomic or central nervous system.

There is a growing understanding of the complex processes of nutrient digestion and absorption, and the roles of hormones and neurotransmitters in intestinal motility regulation, as well as the vast field of enteric neuroimmunophysiology; these are all beyond the scope of this chapter. This chapter focuses on the morphology of the small and large intestines along with the physiologic roles of fluid and electrolyte transport.

INTESTINAL ANATOMY

Gross anatomy

The small intestine is a convoluted tubular organ, extending from the pylorus to the ileocecal valve, occupying the central and lower parts of the abdominal cavity. Mostly confined by the larger intestines, it is divided into three segments: duodenum, jejunum and ileum. The average length of the small intestine is between 250 and 300 cm in the newborn,[1,2] increasing to as much as 600–800 cm in the adult. The caliber of the small intestine gradually diminishes from its origin to its termination. The duodenum constitutes approximately the first 25 cm of the small intestine in adults; the remaining length is arbitrarily divided into the proximal two-fifths, designated as the jejunum, and the distal three-fifths, designated as the ileum. The transition from jejunum to ileum is arbitrary, as there are no histologic or gross anatomic demarcations between these segments.

The duodenum is derived from the distal foregut during embryologic development. It is partly retroperitoneal. The proximal 2–5 cm of the duodenum are occasionally supported on a short mesentery and the remainder lies firmly fixed in a retroperitoneal position, forming an incomplete circle around the head of the pancreas, where it is devoid of mesenteric cover. The duodenum emerges from this retroperitoneal position at the ligament of Treitz in the left upper quadrant. The duodenum is arbitrarily divided into four segments:

- The first portion of the duodenum, which begins at the pylorus and ends at the neck of the gallbladder, is the most mobile segment.
- The second portion, often referred to as the descending portion, descends from the neck of the gallbladder along the right side of the vertebral column to the level of the third lumbar vertebra.
- The third portion, or the horizontal part, courses over the lower boarder to the third lumbar vertebra, passing from right to left, with a slight inclination upwards, lying just inferior to the origin of the superior mesenteric artery in front of the aorta
- The fourth portion, or ascending part, usually ascends immediately to the left of the aorta, up to the level of the second lumbar vertebra, where it makes a ventral turn to unite with jejunum (duodenojejunal flexure or ligament of Treitz).

The biliary and pancreatic ducts drain into the second portion of the duodenum. In most children, both ducts join together approximately 1–2 cm from the outer margins of the duodenal wall, and thereafter transverse the posteromedial aspect of the duodenal wall to empty into the lumen of the second part of the duodenum at the ampulla of Vater. In 5–10% of individuals, an accessory pancreatic duct also enters 1–2 cm proximal to the ampulla of Vater, as the duct of Santorini.[3]

The jejunum and ileum are derived from the endodermal midgut. There is no distinct demarcation between them, but progressive structural differences are present from the proximal jejunum to the distal ileum. The jejunum is thicker and more vascular than the ileum, diminishing in size with distal progression. The intestinal luminal diameter is also greatest in the jejunum, shrinking in diameter as it progresses distally.

Lastly, the plicae circulares, which are crescentic luminal protrusions of the submucosa covered by mucosa, running almost circumferentially in a circular fashion along the inside diameter of the intestinal wall, are most prominent in the distal duodenum and proximal jejunum, decreasing in number and size with progression through the ileum. They are permanent structures and do not smooth out when the intestine is distended.[3] Consequently there is a four-fold reduction in the surface area, occurring over the course of the small intestine from distal duodenum and jejunum to the ileum.

The intestines are overall quite rich in lymphoid tissue; the Peyer's patches are small aggregates of lymphoid tissue located along the antimesenteric border of the small intestine. They are most abundant in the region of the mid-ileum to the ileocecal valve. The Peyer's patches are more prominent during childhood and regress in size and number with advancing age.

The junction of the small intestines with the large intestines is referred to as the ileocecal valve, partly because of its structural appearance in most individuals and partly because the end of the terminal ileum (being wedged into the wall of the cecum) functions like a flutter valve. The ileocecal valve (sphincter) opens when a peristaltic wave strong enough to overcome the resistance of the valve arrives at the terminal ileum. The cecum, in concert, will manifest reflexive relaxation. Overdistention or peristaltic contraction of the cecum causes a reflexive contraction of the sphincter. This protective mechanism prevents overfilling of the cecum or cecoileal reflux. This is an important factor to be remembered by endoscopists when attempting to intubate the terminal ileum during colonoscopy. Reflexive contraction of the sphincter due to overdistention with air will often thwart successful intubation of the ileum.

The jejunum and ileum, attached to and loosely suspended from the posterior abdominal wall by the mesentery, are freely mobile, enabling each coil to accommodate easily to changes in form and position with propulsive peristaltic contractions.

The mesentery begins as an anterior reflection of the posterior peritoneum, attached to the posterior abdominal wall along a line extending from the left side of the body of the lumbar vertebra to the right sacroiliac joint, where it crosses over the duodenum along with other retroperitoneal structures, enveloping the jejunum, ileum, the jejunal and ileal branches of the superior mesenteric blood vessels, nerves, lacteals, lymph nodes and a variable amount of fat.[3] The mesentery is fan-shaped, with the breadth greater in the middle than at its upper and lower ends. The entire length of the jejunum and the ileum is suspended in the mesentery, with the exception of the very distal ileum, which is retroperitoneal along with the cecum.

The duodenum derives its arterial supply from the right gastric, supraduodenal, right gastroepiploic, and superior and inferior pancreaticodoudenal arteries, whereas the venous drainage is via the superior mesenteric, splenic and portal veins. The jejunal and ileal branches of the superior mesenteric artery form the arterial arcade that courses through the mesentery to supply the jejunum and ileum. The main venous drainage of the jejunum and ileum is through the portal and superior mesenteric veins.

Lymphatic drainage, coursing through the mesentery from the villous lacteals and the lymph follicles, converges to the preaortic lymph nodes around the superior mesenteric and celiac arteries. Approximately 70% of the lymph passes via the intestinal trunk and about 25% via the thoracic duct to the main subclavian vein.[4]

Intestinal structure and cellular morphology

The small intestinal wall is made up of four layers. From outside inwardly, these consist of the serosa, the muscularis propria, the submucosa and the mucosa. The mucosa is further subdivided into distinct layers, again starting from the outside inwardly: the muscularis mucosa, lamina propria and epithelial cell layer (Fig. 29.1).

The serosa, or the outermost layer, is a simple extension of the visceral peritoneum and mesentery as it envelops the tubular intestines. It consists of a single layer of flattened mesothelial cells supported by a small amount of

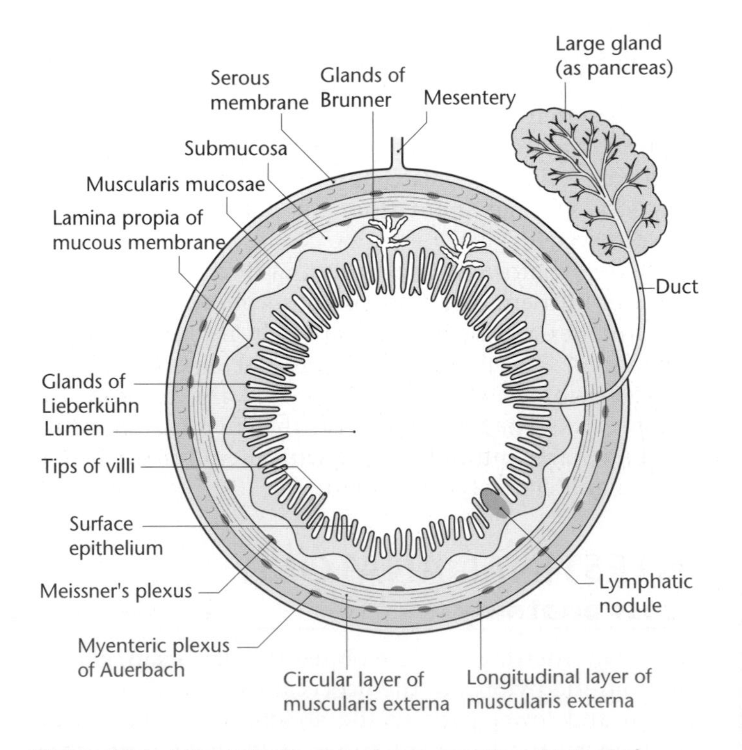

Figure 29.1: Schematic diagram of a cross-section of intestinal mucosa. (Adapted from Bloom and Fawcett, 1968.)[70]

connective tissue, the adventitia. All segments of the small intestine are fully invested in the serosal coat with the exception of the retroperitoneal portions (the duodenum and the very terminal portion of the ileum), which have serosa covering only on their anterior or anterolateral surfaces.

The muscularis propria is made up of two distinct layers of smooth muscle: the thinner outer longitudinal layer and the thicker inner circular layer.

There are two major ganglionated enteric nervous system plexi embedded within the wall of the intestines, the submucosal (Meissner's) plexus and the myenteric (Auerbach's) plexus. Meissner's plexus is found within the submucosa, and the myenteric plexus is located in the plane between the longitudinal and circular layers of the muscularis. The numerous ganglia and localized collection of nerve cell bodies that make up the submucosal and myenteric plexi are extensively interconnected by nerve bundles, giving the appearance of a flat meshwork. Some of the nerve bundles do not connect to ganglia; they ramify over the smooth muscles within the plane of the myenteric plexus to contact individual smooth muscle cells.[4]

The plexi extend without discontinuity within the circumference of the intestinal wall throughout the gastrointestinal tract. The ganglia of the myenteric plexus are more prominent and contain more nerve cell bodies than those of the submucosal plexus.

Interstitial cells of Cajal, present within the myenteric plexus at the interface between the circular muscle and the submucosa, are now recognized as pacemakers of intestinal contractile activity, regulating intestinal tone.[5,6] Abnormalities of the interstitial cells of Cajal have been demonstrated in several intestinal motility disorders.[7,8]

The submucosa consists of a band of loose connective tissue bounded below by the muscularis and above by the outermost layer of the mucosa, the muscularis mucosa. The submucosa, lying next to the mucosa, supports it in its specialized function of nutrient, fluid and electrolyte absorption by carrying a rich network of blood vessels, lymphatics and nerves. The rich vascular supply and lymphatic drainage ensures efficient handling of absorbed nutrients and fluids following a meal. The extensive nerve network, working via the enteric nervous system, ensures adequate agitation and propulsion of the ingesta, and hormonal secretion and control necessary for efficient digestion and absorption. Brunner's glands are located almost exclusively in the submucosa of the duodenum; they begin at the pylorus, where they are most numerous, and extend for a variable length within the walls of the proximal jejunum (Fig. 29.2). They form an array of extensively branched epithelial tubules that contain mainly mucus and serous secretions. Brunner's glands secrete a layer of mucus, forming a slippery viscoelastic gel that lubricates the mucosal lining of the proximal intestinal tract.[9] The mucous layer also possesses the capacity to protect the delicate epithelia surface from peptic digestion. This unique property is due primarily to the gel-forming properties of the glycoprotein molecules (Pb1), class III mucin glycopro-

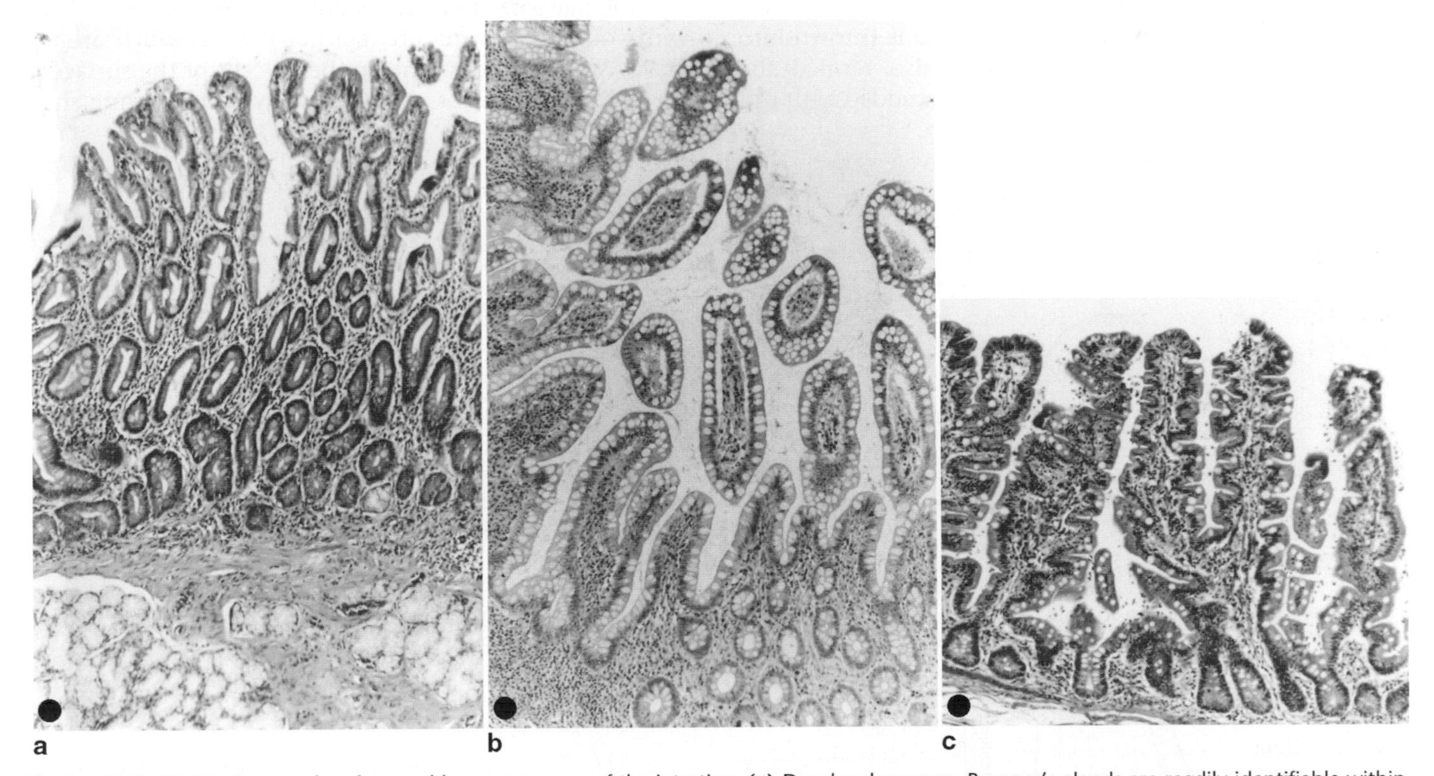

Figure 29.2: Light micrographs of normal human mucosa of the intestine. **(a)** Duodenal mucosa. Brunner's glands are readily identifiable within the submucosa. **(b)** Jejunal mucosa. Villi are tall, thin and most prominently developed within the jejunum. **(c)** Ileal mucosa. Villi are broader and shorter, goblet cells are prominent, and the lamina propria contains more lymph follicles and lymphoid cells. Hematoxylin and eosin stain, ×100. (Courtesy of R. S. Markin MD.)

teins, and is thought to be the product of mucin gene *MUC6*, assigned to chromosome 11.[10]

Brunner's glands interconnect and drain into the base of the duodenal crypts, where they secrete mucin and bicarbonate to a limited extent, along with a host of additional factors including epidermal growth factor, trefoil peptides, bactericidal factors, proteinase inhibitor and surface-active lipids.[9] These factors are said to guard against the degradation of the mucin-protective barrier coat and the underlying mucosa by digestive enzymes and other surface-active agents produced in this region. Some of these factors also play important roles in passive and active immunologic defense mechanisms. Brunner's gland secretion, along with bicarbonate, contributes to the increased luminal pH of the region by promoting pancreatic secretion and gallbladder contraction.

The muscularis mucosae is the deepest layer of mucosa, lying next to the submucosa. It consists of an outer longitudinal and inner circular layer of smooth muscle cells. It is a fairly thin layer, being only three to ten cells thick, extending into the circular folds.

Lying above the muscularis mucosae, the lamina propria provides structural support for the basement membrane of the epithelium. It is composed of a thin layer of connective tissue that embraces the crypts and extends into the villous protusions. The lamina propria is rich in arterioles, veins, lacteals, nerve fibrils and fibroblasts, as well as various cell types, including lymphocytes, macrophages, eosinophils, mast cells and neutrophils.

The mucosa is thick and highly vascularized in the proximal portion of the small intestine, but thinner and less vascular in the distal portions. The mucosa is thrown into crescentic folds, the plicae circulares (also termed the valves of Kerckring), and whole surface is studded with finger-like or leaf-like protrusions, the intestinal villi. These two striking morphologic and physiologic features, along with the formation of microvilli on the epithelial surface, combine to produce a 400–500-fold increase in the surface area of the mucosa.[11]

The luminal surface of small intestine is covered by millions of tiny hair-like, highly vascularized structures called villi (Fig. 29.3). The villi project for about 0.5–1.5 mm into the lumen, giving it a velvety appearance and feel. The height of the villi decreases progressively from the duodenum to the ileum. Villi are larger and denser in the duodenum and jejunum, and smaller and fewer in the ileum.[12] They are wider and ridge-shaped in the proximal duodenum, whereas in the distal duodenum and proximal jejunum they are predominantly leaf-shaped and only occasionally finger-shaped. Finger-shaped villi predominate in the distal jejunum and ileum. Villi are covered primarily with mature absorptive enterocytes, interspersed with a few mucus-secreting goblet cells. Each villus contains a central artery, a vein and a central lacteal. A cascading capillary bed is formed at the tips of the villi in close proximity to the basal surfaces of the epithelium, allowing for rapid clearance of absorbed nutrients, fluids and electrolytes into the systemic circulation. The capillary walls are fenestrated with diaphragmatic covers, greatly facilitating the absorptive process.[13] The core of the villus also contains some small nerve fibers, plasma cells, macrophages, mast cells, lymphocytes, eosinophils and fibroblasts The bases of the villi are surrounded by several pit-like crypts, the crypts of Liberkuhn, extending down through the lamina propria to the muscularis mucosa. The crypts are lined with younger, less mature, epithelial cells, which are primarily secretory cells. The epithelial cells of the surface of the villi are viable for only a few days before being shed,

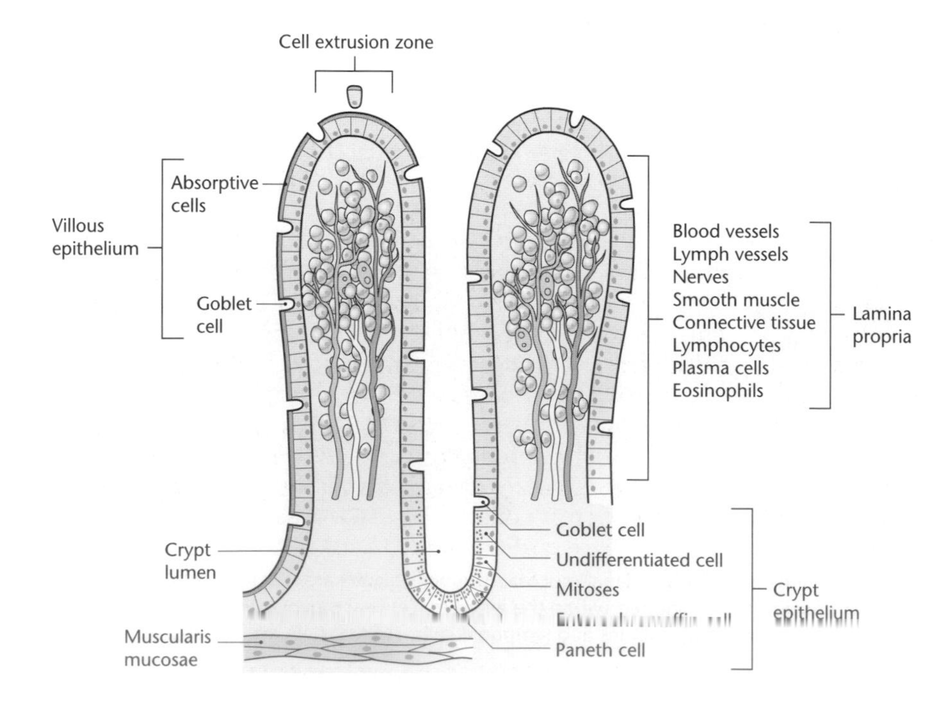

Figure 29.3: Schematic diagram of two sectioned villi and a crypt illustrating the histologic organization of the small intestinal mucosa. (Adapted from Sleisenger and Fordtran, 1989.)[71]

digested and absorbed along with the ingesta. The bases of the crypts are occupied by stem cells, which steadily replenish epithelial cells of both the villi and the crypts.

The epithelial cell lining of the small intestine is continuous, but the cell population differs between the villi, the crypts and the epithelium overlying the Peyer's patches. The crypts are populated primarily by undifferentiated columnar epithelial cells, with a minor scattering of goblet cells, Paneth cells, tuft cells, cup-like cells and enteroendocrine cells. The villous epithelium contains the same array of cells, with the exception of Paneth cells. The undifferentiated cells are replaced with mature enterocytes. The epithelial cells overlying the Peyer's patches contain all of the above-mentioned cells plus functionally and structurally distinct membranous cells (M cells), which are thought to be key sites of antigen and luminal bacteria sampling for the mucosa-associated lymphoid system.[14] M cells are responsible for transepithelial transport, delivering foreign antigens and micro-organisms to the mucosal lymphoid tissue for recognition and handling, an attribute currently being exploited in vaccine production.[15] Structurally distinct, the M cells usually assume an oval or globular configuration, but with a widened base and narrowed apex. Some enteroinvasive pathogens are known to exploit these features of M cells to bridge the intestinal epithelial barrier.[16] The M cells are also found in other parts of the body, especially where there is an interface between the mucosal and the external environment; these sites include, but are not limited to, the tonsils, adenoids, airways and ocular mucosa.[17] The apical microvilli overlying Peyer's patches are randomly shortened and occasionally fused into folds or ridges.

The mucosal epithelial cells are turned over every 5–7 days, hence intense mitotic activity occurs within the intestinal crypts; the stem cells are continuously differentiated, producing a constant supply of enterocytes and other cellular types including Paneth cells, cup cells, tuft cells, enteroendocrine cells and M cells. Further differentiation occurs as most of the cells migrate upward along the intestinal crypt wall; Paneth cells are the only cells that do not migrate. The cells are usually mature by the time they reach the upper third of the villus. Old and spent cells are extruded into the intestinal lumen at the tip of the villi, to face the same fate of digestion and absorption along with the ingesta. Overlying the Peyer's patches, epithelial cell differentiation includes the production of M cells.

The growth and integrity of the intestinal mucosa are maintained under the influence of the ingesta, several luminal factors as well as autocrine, endocrine and paracrine secretion from the surrounding cells. Thus, enteral nutrition is essential for the well-being of intestinal mucosa.

Furthermore, it is now clear that glucagon-like peptides secreted from enteroendocrine cells play a major cytoprotective and reparative role in the survival and proliferation of the intestinal mucosa.[18–21] The glucagon-like peptides, glucagon-like peptide (GLP) 1 and GLP-2, are released from enteroendocrine cells in response to nutrient ingestion. GLP-1 enhances glucose-stimulated insulin secretion and inhibits glucagon secretion, gastric emptying and feeding. It also has proliferative and antiapoptotic effects on pancreatic β cells. GLP-2 is a 33-amino-acid peptide, encoded carboxy-terminal to the sequence of GLP-1 in the proglucagon gene. It is an intestinal tropic peptide that stimulates cell proliferation and inhibits apoptosis in the intestinal crypts.[2] GLP-2 also regulates intestinal glucose transport and glucose transporter (GLUT) 2 expression, as well as food intake and gastric acid secretion, and gastric emptying and motility, and improves intestinal barrier function. GLP-2 reduces intestinal permeability and stimulates blood flow.[4] Additionally, GLP-2 reduces the death of enterocytes and decreases mucosal injury, cytokine expression and bacterial septicemia in the setting of small and large bowel inflammation. GLP-2 also enhances nutrient absorption and gut adaptation in rodents or humans with short bowel syndrome.

Absorptive cells

Lining both the villi and crypts is a layer of cells referred to as the enterocytes, or absorptive cells. These are tall columnar cells, each possessing a basally located, clear, oval-shaped nucleus and several nucleoli. The cells are tightly cemented to the basal lamina and are joined to the adjacent enterocytes at the apical pole by intracellular tight junctions. The luminal surface is studded with densely packed (1000–2000 per cell) finger-like, cylindrical projections termed microvilli. Each microvillus is about 1 μm long and 0.1 μm wide.[3] The microvilli are constantly bathed by luminal contents, and therefore contain the membrane-bound digestive proteins, transport proteins and other cellular elements necessary for nutrient absorption.

The intestinal microvillus is supported by a central core of cytoskeleton, which consists of highly concentrated microfilaments made up of five major proteins: actin, villin, fimbrin, brush border myosin I and spectrin.[22] Villin and fimbrin are bundling proteins that crosslink to support a central core of about 20 to 30 actin filaments (Fig. 29.4). The microfilaments are continuous and linked at the apical bases of the microvillus, forming a plexiform band called the terminal web, which consists mainly of spectrin. The terminal webs are also interconnected with the junctional complexes or tight junctions. The microvillus is rich in glycoprotein, cholesterol and glycolipids.

The apical surfaces of the intestinal epithelial cells carry multiple brush-border transporters that couple ion influxes to organic solute influxes, or exchange one ion for another. Three Na/H exchangers (NHEs) have since been localized to intestinal brush-border membranes and cloned. NHE2 and NHE3 are found in both small intestine and colon.[23] NHE1 is present only in the basolateral membrane of enterocytes and is thought to be involved with HCO_3 secretion. Two anion exchangers have also been localized to small-intestinal and colonic brush-border membranes and cloned. They are named 'downregulated in adenoma' (DRA) and putative anion transporter 1 (PAT1).

Contiguous enterocytes are tightly apposed at their apicolateral poles by the formation of junctional complexes. These consist of adherence membranes in three areas:

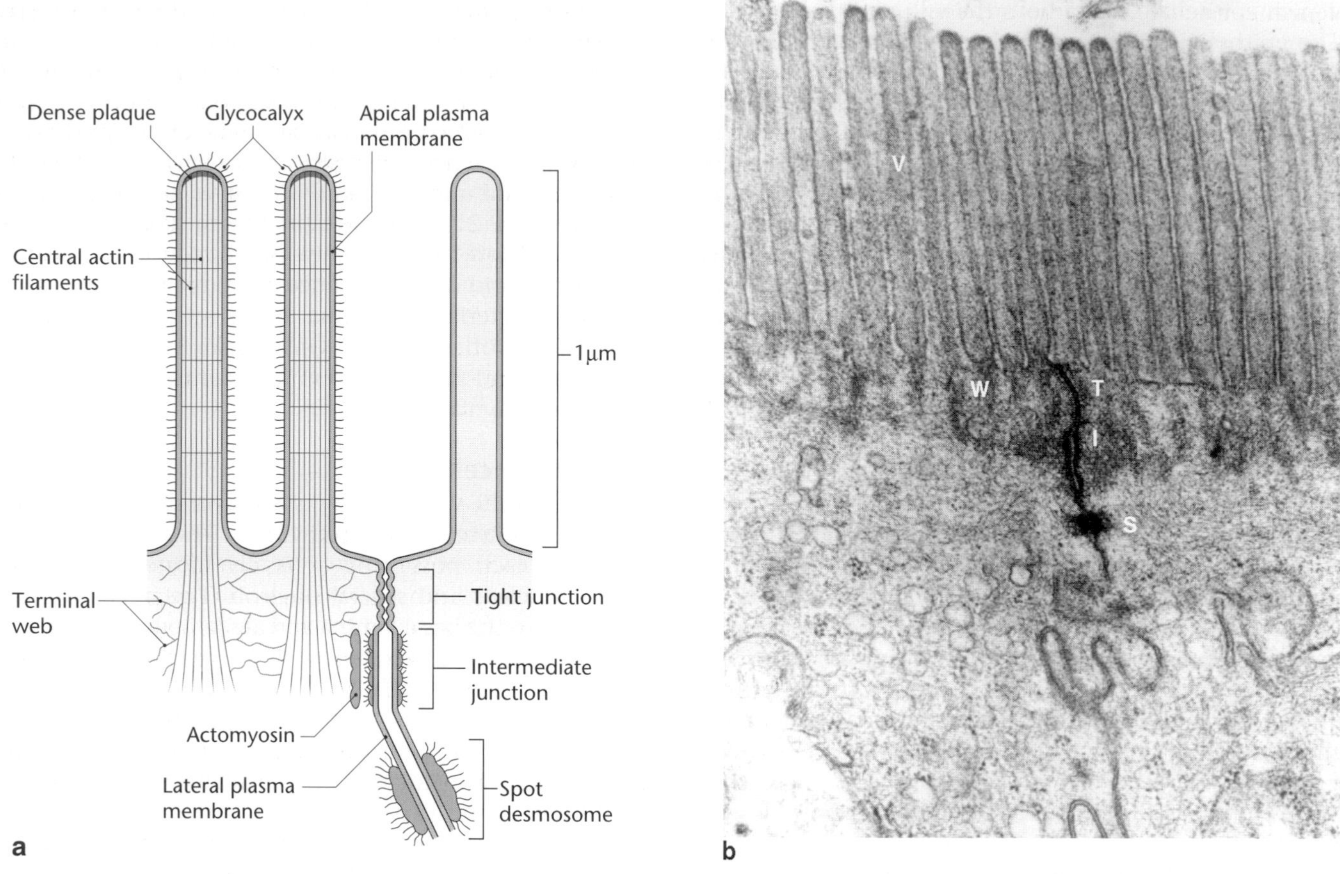

Figure 29.4: Microvillus membrane. **(a)** Schematic illustration of the microvillus membrane and specialized supporting structures of the apical cytoplasm of adjacent intestinal absorptive cells. **(b)** Electron micrograph of adjacent villous absorptive cells. The adjacent cells are tightly adherent through the formation of a junctional complex, containing a tight junction (T), intermediate junction (I) and spot desmosome (S). Thin supporting central filaments of actin are present within the microvillus (V) and terminate by embedding with filaments in the terminal web (W). Magnification ×15 000.

- The most proximal tight junction, or zonula occludens
- An intermediate junction, or zonula adherens
- A deeper junction, the spot desmosome or macular adherence zone.

Movements of fluid and ions through this intracelluar space from the apical to the basolateral compartment is termed *paracellular transport*, and is the dominant pathway for passive fluid and ion flow across the intestinal epithelial barrier into the endothelial cells. Permeability depends on the regulation of the tight junctions.[24]

Tight junctions consist of a family of transmembrane proteins – claudins, occludins and junctional adhesion molecules – which are anchored to the membranes of two adjacent cells and interact with one another to bind the cells together and prevent the passage of molecules between them. These membrane proteins are connected with the various signal transduction and transcriptional pathways involved in the regulation of tight junction function via interaction with scaffold proteins.[25,26]

Knowledge about the tight junction has evolved from a relatively simplistic view of it being a physical and permeability barrier in the paracellular space to one of a multicomponent, multifunctional complex that is involved in regulating numerous and diverse cell functions. The tight junction membrane proteins (occludins, claudins and junctional adhesion molecules) interact with an increasingly complex array of tight junction plaque proteins to regulate paracellular solute and water flux, as well as to integrate diverse processes such as gene transcription, tumor suppression, cell proliferation and cell polarity.

The tight junction, or zonula occludens, measures approximately 100–600 nm in depth,[27] serving as a regulatable, semipermeable diffusion barrier, and permitting the passage of ions while restricting the movement of large molecules. The tight junction is leakier and has a lower resistance in the proximal intestine, where absorption is most efficient, and tighter with a higher resistance in the ileum and large intestine. There is also strong evidence suggesting variations in the functional states of the junctional complexes, maintaining a relatively high resistance in the fasting state and a low resistance in the fed state.[28]

The zonula adherens, or intermediate junction, is located just below the zonula occludens on the lateral aspect of contiguous cells and is less adherent, with cells being separated by a 15–20-nm gap. Forming a belt-like region of cell-to-cell adhesion, the zonula adherens represents the clustering of cadherins, catenins and the actin cytoskeleton. The zonula adherens plays a dual role as a structural component of those junctions and as a signaling molecule in the Wnt signaling pathway. Adherens junctions have been implicated in signaling to the nucleus.[29]

Cadherins are a family of calcium-dependent cell–cell adhesion molecules that possess three major regions:[30]

- The extracellular region, critical for cell–cell binding
- A transmembrane domain, which spans the cell membrane
- A cytoplasmic domain, which protrudes into the cell.

The most distal portion of the junctional complex is a small circular junction located just below the zonula adherens, often referred to as the macula adherens or spot desmosome. The adjacent lateral membranes here are separated by a gap of about 30–50 nm.[29] Unlike the zonula occludens, spot desmosomes are not continuous around the circumference of the cell, but are rather scattered around the cell perimeter in an uneven row. The spot desmosomes are linked by tonofilaments (a type of intermediate filament), which are thought to represent transmembrane linkages extending across the intercellular gap. Cadherins are extremely important in establishing and maintaining cell–cell interactions between epithelial cells.[30] Three calcium-dependent adhesion molecules belonging to the cadherin family – desmoglein I and desmocollins I and II – mediate intercellular attachment. The overall function of this area appears to be primarily to support the overall continuity and integrity of the tight junction, as well as intercellular communication.

The remainder of the lateral wall of the enterocyte below the macula adherens is termed the basolateral membrane. This membrane has unique structural and biologic characteristics that differentiate it from the apical membrane. The basolateral membrane is often plicated and interdigitates with the adjacent lateral cellular membranes. Lacking the brush-border transporters, the Na/H exchangers and the digestive enzymes present on the apical membrane, it is embedded with basolateral membrane carriers that facilitate diffusion of organic solutes and are not coupled to ion movements. The basolateral membrane K^+ channels are responsible for K^+ extrusion from the cell and NaK_2Cl co-transporter which determines the maximal rate of chloride entry into the cell. Na/K-ATPase in the basolateral membrane uses energy from ATP hydrolysis to drive Na^+ extrusion and K^+ uptake.[23]

Gap junctions are essentially communication junctions; they consist of small, circular structures between contiguous cell membranes with a narrow gap in between. The gaps are traversed by tiny tubular channels, sometimes referred to as connexons, which allow the intercellular passage of ions and low-molecular-weight nutrients and intracellular messengers such as cyclic adenosine monophosphate (cAMP).

In addition to the basally located nuclei, other cellular organelles are present within the enterocyte in anticipated polarity. The Golgi apparatus, responsible for terminal glycosylation of synthesized proteins, lies in a supranuclear position, and just below the terminal web at the apical portion are numerous membrane-bound lysosomes.[3] Also scattered throughout the cytoplasm are free ribosomes, mitochondria, lysosomes, microtubules, and smooth and rough endoplasmic reticulum. The cellular structure and organelles are efficiently arranged and coordinated to work in concert for the absorption, packaging and subsequent extrusion of absorbed lipids, carbohydrate and peptides.

Goblet cells

Goblet cells are mucin-producing cells found scattered among other cells of the intestinal villi in lesser numbers than the absorptive cells. Overall, they are found in greater numbers in the large intestine and distal ileum than in the rest of the intestine. The term goblet cell derives from the characteristic wine-glass shape of these cells in conventionally fixed tissue: a narrow base and an oval-shaped apical portion (expanded with mucin-secreting granules) that sometimes extends into the intestinal lumen. If special precautions are taken during tissue fixation, goblet cells can be seen as cylindrically shaped.

Goblet cells usually assume a distinctly polarized morphology, with the nucleus and Golgi apparatus basally situated. The remaining cellular organelles are aligned along the lateral margins of the cell, being compressed to these regions by the abundant membrane-bound mucus-secreting granules within the cell interior.[31–33] Mucin secreted from the goblet cells is largely composed of highly glycosylated proteins suspended in an electrolyte solution. The mucin is secreted via two pathways: (1) a low-level, unregulated and essentially continuous secretion dependent on cytoskeletal movement of secretory granules; and (2) stimulated secretion via regulated exocytosis of granules in response to irritating extracellular stimuli. This second pathway ensures the capacity dramatically to increase mucin production and secretion. The goblet cell mucin provides a protective lubricant barrier against shear stress and shields the intestinal mucosa from peptic digestion and chemical damage. It is also thought to bind surface antigens and inhibit their attachment to the epithelial surfaces. Goblet cells retain the ability to differentiate, and do occasionally differentiate into epithelial cells as they migrate up the crypts onto the villus tips.

Gut endocrine cells

Enteroendocrine cells, or gut endocrine cells, are a highly specialized mucosal cell subpopulation, sparsely distributed throughout the entire length of the small intestine. The enteroendocrine lineage consists of at least 15 different cell types that are categorized based on their morphology, specific regional distribution and peptide

dominantly expressed in colon but scantily expressed in small intestine; with the duodenum being the site of greatest small intestinal expression.

The upper gastrointestinal tract, particularly the duodenum, is constantly exposed to an acidic chyme delivered from stomach, with the pH that sometimes reach as low as 1.5.[57,58] Mucin production from the goblet cells (as previously discussed) and secretion of bicarbonate to buffer the acid are the main defense mechanisms for protecting the duodenal mucosa against acid injury. DRA and PAT1 are abundant in the duodenum and present at higher density there than NHE2 and NHE3, suggesting a role in duodenal alkalinization.

To engage efficiently in the transcellular transport of ions, the enterocyte requires the simultaneous function and operation of more than two ion exchangers. In addition to the increased turnover of the Na^+/K^+ pump, the opening of basolateral membrane Cl^- and K^+ channels is essential to prevent swelling of the enterocyte by allowing serosal exit of the Cl^- taken up from the lumen and extrusion of the K^+ taken up by the Na^+/K^+ pump.

The third and final route of solute abruption is via the paracellular pathway. This is the dominant route for passive solute transport across the intestinal epithelial membrane.[59] The permeability of this pathway is modulated via the regulation of the intracellular tight junctions or zonula occludens, which function as a barrier between apical and basolateral compartments, restricting the flow of luminal contents into the blood and lymphatics, and vice versa. The tight junctions counter-regulate the gradient generated by the transcellular pathways by selectively allowing passive diffusion of small hydrophilic molecules and ions from the intestinal lumen into the bloodstream and the lymphatics. Tight junctions are dynamic structures constantly subjected to changes that dictate their functional status under a variety of physiologic and pathologic conditions.

The electrical resistance and permeability of these tight junctions are thought to be dependent upon a complex interaction of transmembrane protein microfilaments and discrete extracellular proteins, as described previously.

Secretion

Chloride secretion occurs in the intestinal crypt cells throughout the small intestine, whereas bicarbonate secretion is restricted solely to the ileum. Three specific cell membrane transporters, whose activity is mediated by cAMP via protein kinase signaling, are now functionally recognized to stimulate active intestinal chloride secretion. These are the apical anion channel, basolateral membrane K^+ channel and basolateral membrane NaK_2Cl co-transporters. The secretory cell is depolarized after chloride secretion has been initiated by the opening of the apical channels under the influence of cAMP, which is also said to recruit additional channels from the endoplasmic reticulum into the apical membrane. The basolateral membrane K^+ channel then opens to repolarize the cell, counteracting the depolarizing effect of the Cl^- channel. This sequence ensures the sustenance of the electrical driving force, namely chloride secretion into the intestinal lumen. Once the apical channels and the basolateral K^+ channels have been mobilized and activated, the basolateral membrane NaK_2Cl co-transporter is the rate-limiting factor for chloride entry into the cell from the serosa through the basolateral membrane.

Dysfunctional mutations of the apical anion channel result in cystic fibrosis, a recessively inherited disease.

Daily gastrointestinal tract fluid fluxes

On average, an adult secretes or ingests 7–8 liters of fluid into the gastrointestinal daily. (Table 29.1). Saliva and oral intake accounts for about 1.5 liters per day; 1.5 liters of gastric acid and digestive enzymes are sequestered daily, whereas bile and pancreatic secretion respectively contribute 1 liter each.

During the initial phase of intestinal digestion, a net flux of about 3 liters of fluid is secreted into the lumen following the osmotic gradient across the relatively loose 'tight' junction of the jejunal mucosa. However, 5 liters of secreted fluid and electrolytes are reabsorbed back within the jejunum and ileum, and only about 1.2 liters of fluid is released into the colon daily.

Endogenous neuroendocrine and paracrine regulation of absorption and secretion

Two distinct groups of regulatory compounds are known to mediate the intestinal epithelial function. One group inhibits active electrolyte absorption and stimulates active secretion (Table 29.2). The other group has the opposite effect, stimulating active absorption and inhibiting secretion (Table 29.3).[60]

The first group (pro-secretory and antiabsorptive) includes four classes of agents:

- Neurotransmitters, including acetylcholine, substance P, vasoactive intestinal peptide (VIP) and nucleotides (ATP and UDP)
- Paracrine agents, including serotonin and neurotensin
- Pro-inflammatory agents, including but not limited to histamine, serotonin, prostaglandins, leukotrienes and platelet-activating factor
- Guanylin.

The second group consists of compounds that promote active ion absorption and inhibit active bicarbonate and chloride secretion. These compounds include neuropeptide Y, norepinephrine, somatostatin and most neurotransmitters.

Ingestion	1–1.5
Saliva production	0.25–0.5
Gastric secretions	0.5–1
Bile production	0.5–1
Pancreatic secretion	0.5–5
Small bowel secretion	2–3

Table 29.1 Daily average influx of fluid into the gastrointestinal tract volume (liters)

Agent	Source	Target	Intracellular mediator(s)
Prostaglandin	Mesenchymal cells	Epithelial and neural cells	cAMP, Ca^{2+} and protein kinase C
Neurotensin	Epithelial endocrine cells	Enteric neurons	Protein kinase C and Ca^{2+}
Guanylin	Goblet cells	Epithelial cells	cGMP
Serotonin (5-hydroxytryptamine; 5-HT)	Mast and epithelial endocrine cells	Epithelial and neural cells	Protein kinase C and Ca^{2+}
Vasoactive intestinal peptide (VIP)	Enteric neural cells	Epithelial cells	Protein kinase C and Ca^{2+}
Acetylcholine (Ach)	Enteric neural cells	Epithelial, mesenchymal and neural cells	Ca^{2+} and protein kinase C
Substance P	Enteric neural cells	Mast, epithelial, neural cells	Ca^{2+} and protein kinase C
Histamine	Mast cells	Mesenchymal and neural cells	Ca^{2+}, cAMP and protein kinase C
Platelet-activating factors	Ca^{2+}, cAMP and protein kinase C	Mesenchymal cells	Ca^{2+}, cAMP and protein kinase C
Adenosine	Epithelial cells	Epithelial and mesenchymal cells	Ca^{2+}, cAMP and protein kinase C
Leukotrienes	Mesenchymal cells	Epithelial and neural cells	Ca^{2+}, cAMP and protein kinase C
Bradykinin	Vascular	Mesenchymal cells	Ca^{2+}, cAMP and protein kinase C
ATP/ADP	Enteric neurons	Epithelial and mesenchymal cells	Protein kinase C and Ca^{2+}

Table 29.2 Endogenous control of ion and water transport: secretory agents

Agent	Source	Target cell	Intracellular mediator(s)
12-Hydroxyeicosatetraenoic acid (12-HETE)	Mesenchymal cells	Epithelial and neural cells	Blockage of basolateral K^+ channel
Neuropeptide Y	Enteric neural and epithelial endocrine cells	Epithelial and neural cells	Unknown
Norepinephrine	Neural cells	Epithelial and neural cells	Activation of inhibitory G protein
Somatostatin	Enteric neural and epithelial endocrine cells	Epithelial and neural cells	Activation of somatostatin receptors

Table 29.3 Endogenous control of ion and water transport: antisecretory agents

Mast cells are the major effector cells for immediate hypersensitivity and chronic allergic reactions. Acting on the extensive interface between intestinal surface epithelium and the external environment, they elaborate a variety of autocrine/paracrine secretions including adenosine, leukotriene B_4, substance P, acetylcholine, histamine, serotonin and several chemokines. The presence of antigenic threats is detected by receptor-bound antigen-specific immunoglobulin E (IgE), priming the mast cells to recognize the sensitizing antigens and regulate the response to these threats. During future encounters the mast cells signal the presence of the inciting antigen to the enteric nervous system. The signal is interpreted as threat, and the enteric nervous system initiates a programmed secretory and propulsive motor behavior organized to eliminate the threat rapidly and effectively. This programmed alarm system protects the individual, but at the expense of often uncomfortable symptoms that include cramping abdominal pain, fecal urgency and diarrhea.

ANATOMY OF THE LARGE INTESTINE

The large intestine commences at the cecum as a blind pouch below the termination of the small intestine. It curves around, usually enclosing the convolutions of the small intestine, and terminates at the rectum. From cephalad to caudad, the large intestine consists of the following segments:

- Cecum and vermiform appendix
- Colon, which in turn is composed of four sections – ascending, transverse, descending and sigmoid colon
- Rectum
- Anal canal.

The colon is approximately 60 cm long in the newborn, increasing to approximately 150 cm in the adult. The caliber of the large intestine is greatest at the cecum and gradually diminishes as it approaches the rectum, where it balloons out considerably in size just above the anal canal.[3] The colonic wall remains fairly constant in thickness throughout its entire length. The colon functions as a receptacle and reservoir for fecal matter; periodic high-amplitude contractions propel the contents caudally. Absorption of fluids and electrolytes, which is its main function, takes place along the entire length. The colon is easily distinguished from the small intestine by several distinctive characteristic features:

- It is larger in caliber
- It is mostly fixed in position
- Its outer longitudinal muscular layer is congregated into three distinct longitudinal bands, or teniae coli, extending from the cecum to the rectum
- It has a characteristic sacculated and puckered appearance due to outpouchings (termed haustra) of its walls between the longitudinal bands

- Fatty projections of the mesentery and the serosa are found scattered over the free surface of the entire large intestine, with the exception of the cecum, vermiform appendix and rectum[3]
- The luminal surface is interrupted by intermittent irregular folds called plicae semilunares.

Extending as a reflection of the peritoneal lining, the mesentery envelopes the colon just as it does the small intestine. However, most of the large intestine is fixed in a retroperitoneal manner with only a small portion suspended by the mesentery. The transverse colon and sigmoid colon are fully suspended by the mesentery, whereas only a portion of the cecum is fully suspended. The prominent mesentery of the transverse colon is termed the transverse mesocolon, and the appendix is anchored by a short and well defined mesentery referred to as the mesoappendix. The proximal cecum, ascending colon, descending colon and rectum have only partial mesenteric covering on their anterior surfaces.

Originating from the midgut, the proximal colon, cecum, ascending colon and proximal two-thirds of the transverse colon all derive their blood supply from the superior mesenteric artery. The inferior mesenteric artery supplies the remaining one-third of the transverse colon, descending colon, sigmoid colon and rectum. In addition to the blood supply from the inferior mesenteric artery, the rectum and anal canal also receive blood from the internal iliac and median sacral arteries. The superior and inferior mesenteric veins drain the same regions of the large intestine supplied by the corresponding arteries.[3] With the exception of the lower half of the anal canal, the large intestine derives its nerve supply from the parasympathetic and sympathetic systems. The nerve distribution pattern closely mimics the arterial supply. The proximal colon receives its sympathetic neuronal innervation from the celiac and superior mesenteric ganglia, whereas the parasympathetic supply is from the vagus nerve. In each case the nerves are distributed to the proximal colon in plexuses around the branches of the superior mesenteric artery.[3] The distal colon receives its sympathetic nerve supply via branches from the lumbar segments of the sympathetic trunk, and the parasympathetic nerves originate from the pelvic splanchnic nerves.[61] The lymphatic drainage of the large intestine courses through the mesentery in close proximity to the arterial and venous supplies. First draining through groups of small pericolic nodes along the right and middle colic arteries and their branches, lymph flow from the colon drains into intermediate nodes located within the mesentery. The lymph ultimately terminates in the large colic pre-aortic nodes surrounding the superior and inferior mesenteric arteries. The rectum and anal canal drain into inferior mesenteric and iliac nodes via perirectal nodes, which lie in close apposition to the rectal walls.

As stated above, the primary function of the large intestine is water and electrolyte absorption; however, the large intestine is capable of absorbing small quantities of short-chain fatty acids (SCFAs), which are byproducts of the anaerobic bacterial fermentation of polysaccharides. The SCFAs absorbed by the colon contribute only about 7% of overall total body energy requirements,[62] with slightly higher amounts being contributed during infancy.[62,63] More importantly, the colonic epithelium depends on the luminal SCFAs for their energy supply,[64] as evidenced by the development of diversion colitis after surgical diversion of the fecal stream and resolution of the colitis with colonic instillation of *n*-butyric acid.[65]

Cecum

The cecum commences as a large pouch-like cul-de-sac in the right iliac fossa and continues superiorly with the ascending colon. Its diameter is greater than its length; the adult cecum measures approximately 6 cm in length and 7.5 cm in width.[3] The ileocecal valve, opening into the posteromedial wall of the cecum at its defined proximal end, passes through the wall in a perpendicular manner pointing slightly downwards. The superior and inferior folds of the ileocecal valve formed by the protrusion of the ileum are arranged in an elliptical manner, forming the orifice of the ileocecal valve. This arrangement allows the valve to function as a sphincter. The appendiceal orifice lies about 2.5 cm inferior to the ileocecal valve. Being supported by a distinct mesentery, the cecum, appendix and the last segment of the ileum are mobile. This mobility accounts for the observed positional variability of these structures within the right lower abdominal quadrant[3] and the rare predisposition for developing a cecal volvulus.[66,67]

Vermiform appendix

The adjective 'vermiform' literally means 'worm-like', and describes the narrow, elongated shape of the appendix. The appendix descends inferiorly as a small finger-sized tubular appendage of the cecum. It is typically anywhere between 2 and 20 cm long,[61] being longest in childhood. It generally shrinks during development and throughout adult life. The appendiceal wall is composed of all layers typical of the intestine. Its outer layer and that of the cecum are circumferential, and the teniae coli are not apparent until the level of the ileocecal valve. The appendix, once regarded as a vestigial organ, is now recognized as an important component of mammalian mucosal immune system, particularly B lymphocyte–mediated immune responses and extrathymically derived T lymphocytes.[68] It shares functional similarities with the pharyngeal tonsils and Peyer's patches. The vermiform appendix may vary greatly in location and be situated either dependently below the distal cecal pouch or behind the cecum, anteriorly or posteriorly to the ileum in a retroperitoneal manner.

Ascending colon

Originating at the level of the ileocecal valve, the ascending colon is narrower than the cecum.[3] It ascends in a cephalad manner to the inferior surface of the posterior lobe of the liver, where it angulates sharply to the left and slightly forward, forming the hepatic flexure. It measures about 20 cm in length in the adult,[69] and is situated retroperitoneally in about 75% of individuals.[61]

Transverse colon

The ascending colon merges from its retroperitoneal position, coursing anteriorly and medially to become the transverse colon. It becomes fully enveloped in mesentery (transverse mesocolon) and dips down to a variable extent toward the pelvis as it crosses the abdomen medially to the left upper abdominal quadrant. Here it curves acutely on itself, downward and then upward, forming the splenic flexure.[3] A thickened reflection of the peritoneum, termed the phrenicocolic ligament, anchors splenic flexure, suspending the splenic flexure higher than the hepatic flexure. The transverse colon lies anterior to the stomach and the small intestine throughout its course and measures approximately 40–50 cm in length.[61]

Descending colon

The descending colon emerges from the splenic flexure, continuing downward and posteriorly to take up a retroperitoneal position with only a partial peritoneal cover on its anterior surface in about 65% of individuals.[61] It measures approximately 25–45 cm in length, extending from the splenic flexure to the level of the left iliac crest.[3,61]

Sigmoid colon

The sigmoid colon begins at the pelvic brim where it is continuous with the descending colon as it emerges from a retroperitoneal position. The sigmoid colon forms a loop that varies greatly in length, averaging about 40 cm in an adult.[3] It is surrounded and supported by a mesentery termed the sigmoid mesocolon, longest at the center of the loop, then shortening and disappearing as it approaches the rectum. Thus, the sigmoid colon is somewhat fixed at its junctions with descending colon and rectum respectively. Enjoying a great range of mobility in its central region,[3] it is predisposed to volvulus depending upon the length of its mesocolon and/or the degree of distention. The sharpest angulations of the loop occur as the sigmoid turns downward to join the rectum.

Rectum

The rectum extends from the sigmoid colon at the level of the third sacral vertebra following the sacral curvature to the anal canal distally. It initially passes downward and posteriorly, and then directly downward before finally passing downward and anteriorly to join the anus.[3] It measures approximately 12–15 cm in length in the adult.[61] The peritoneum is reflected anteriorly at the rectosigmoid junction in most individuals; hence the entire rectum lies below the peritoneum in close relationship to structures within the pelvis. The anorectal junction usually lies 2–3 cm in front of and just below the tip of the coccyx.[3] The rectum is narrowest at its junction with the sigmoid, expanding out into the rectal ampulla at its lower end just before joining the anus. Unlike the sigmoid, the rectum lacks sacculations, appendices epiploicae and mesentery. The teniae coli converge and blend with the outer muscular layer about 5–6 cm above the rectosigmoid junction. The outer rectal wall becomes progressively thickened, forming prominent anterior and posterior muscular bands as it descends toward the anus. The luminal surface of the rectum has two longitudinal and transverse folds; the longitudinal folds are more apparent in the empty state, being easily effaced by rectal distention. The transverse folds or shelves are permanent and more prominent; commonly three folds are present, but this number may vary.[3]

Anal canal

The anal canal begins where the distal end of the rectal ampulla sharply narrows and passes inferiorly and outward to the anal opening. The anal canal is about 2 cm long in the infant, increasing to about 4.5 cm in the adult.[69] The canal occupies the ischiorectal fossa, where it is supported by a number of ligaments and muscular attachments as it pierces the pelvic diaphragm. The anorectal junction is situated within the pelvic diaphragm, which is made up of the levator ani and coccygeus muscles. The segment of the levator ani sling that encircles the anorectal junction is termed the puborectalis muscle. The contraction of this muscle pulls the rectum forward to retain stool, and the relaxation straightens the anal canal allowing defecation. The walls of the anal canal are surrounded by a complex of muscular fibers, arranged as the internal and external anal sphincters.[3] Commencing at the anorectal junction, the circular muscle layer of the large intestine thickens to become the internal anal sphincter. This sphincter, composed of smooth muscle fibers, surrounds the upper three-quarters of the anal canal.[3] The external sphincter is made up of striated muscle. Surrounding the entire length of the anal canal, the external anal sphincter consists of three parts, namely the subcutaneous, superficial and deep parts. Starting at about the middle of the anal canal, the luminal surface is thrown into a series of about six to ten longitudinal folds, termed the anal columns, which are more prominent in the child than the adult.[3] These columns converge distally to form small crescentic folds of tissue termed the anal valves. The level at which the anal columns converge to form the anal valves is termed the pectinate line; it is thought to represents the junction between the endodermal and ectodermal portions of the anal canal. Hence, beyond the pectinate line, the epithelial cell layer of the anal canal transitions from cuboidal to stratified squamous epithelium, which in turn continues and terminates in an irregular line or 'white' zone at the anal opening, termed the zona alba. Beyond the white zone, the epithelial layer changes to the typical squamous epithelium of the skin, with the full complement of sweat glands, sebaceous glands and hair follicles.[3]

Cellular morphology

Analogous to the walls of the small intestine, the walls of the large intestine are made up of four layers: the serosa or adventitia, the muscularis mucosa, the submucosa and the mucosa. The mucosa in turn can be further separated into three distinct layers: the epithelial cell layer, the lamina propria and the muscularis mucosae. On the outside, the large intestine is surrounded by a loose layer of connective tissue termed the adventitia, called the serosa when covered by the peritoneal reflection containing squamous mesothelial cells. Scattered macrophages, eosinophils, mast cells and fibroblasts are occasionally encountered within the serosa. The muscularis, just as observed in the small intestine, consists of two smooth muscle layers: an outer longitudinal and an inner circular layer. The outer longitudinal layer is thickened to form three prominent muscular bands, the teniae coli, which run in parallel to the long axis of colon throughout its entire length. The width of the teniae ranges from 6 to 12 mm in different individuals,[3] and their thickness increases caudally from the cecum to the sigmoid colon. The space between the longitudinal inner circular muscle layers houses a prominent nerve plexus, which runs in continuity with the myenteric (Auerbach's) plexus of the small intestine. The inner circular muscle layer is thin over the cecum and colon, running circumferentially, but maintaining a slightly oblique orientation to the long axis of the large intestine.[61] Its fibers are especially thickened in the rectum, and in the anal canal become numerous, forming the internal anal sphincter. Sandwiched between the muscularis and muscularis mucosae is the submucosa. It consists of a layer of loose connective tissue with a scattering of cellular elements, which include lymphocytes, macrophages, mast cells, plasma cells, eosinophils and fibroblasts. Present within the submucosa are also Meissner's nerve plexus and large blood vessels that supply the muscularis and the mucosa.

As stated above, the mucosa is composed of three layers: the epithelial cell layer, the lamina propria and the muscularis mucosae. The muscularis mucosae and lamina propria are similar to those of the small intestine, except that colonic muscularis mucosae is thicker and the thickness increases progressively from the cecum to the anal canal.[61]

Devoid of the villi that characterize the small intestine, the epithelial cell layer of the large intestine is smooth. Crescentic folds appear at intervals corresponding to the external sacculations.[3] The epithelial surface is also interrupted by numerous prominent crypts. Termed the crypts of Liberkuhn, they dip far down to reach just above the muscularis mucosae. Enteroendocrine cells and undifferentiated cells are restricted to the lower one-third of the crypts. The surface epithelium is of simple columnar type, interspaced with varying amounts of vacuolated cells, goblet cells and caveolated cells.

Surface epithelial cell

The epithelial surface and the upper one-third of the crypts are mostly lined with tall and slender absorptive columnar cells, also termed principal cells.[61] Constant supplies of these cells are provided by undifferentiated 'stem' cells at the bases and lower one-third of the crypts. Differentiation and maturation occur as they migrate upward along the lateral walls. Vacuolated cells are found lining the lateral walls of the crypts and are thought to be epithelial cells transitioning to mature surface epithelial cells. The luminal surfaces of the columnar cells are capped by apical membranes containing numerous microvilli supported by well developed terminal webs. The lateral borders of the luminal surfaces are bound by junctional complexes similar to those found in the small intestine. Their cytoplasm contains the usual cytoplasmic organelles. The nucleus is centrally located with a scattering of endoplasmic reticulum located both above and below it. The apical cytoplasm is particularly rich in secretory granules along with scant amounts of Golgi apparatus.

Goblet cell

Goblet cells are the second most abundant cells on the surface epithelium and the large intestinal crypts. They are similar in shape, configuration and morphology to that found in the small intestine. Copious amounts of mucin produced by the goblet cells is crucial in providing lubrication for the passage of feces.[3]

References

1. Reiquam CW, Allen RP, Akers DR, et al. Normal and abnormal small bowel lengths. Am J Dis Child 1965; 109:447–451.
2. Touloukian RJ, Walker-Smith GJ. Normal intestinal length in preterm infants. J Pediatr Surg 1983; 18:720–723.
3. Williams PL and Warwick R, eds. Gray's Anatomy, 36th British edn. Philadelphia, PA: WB Saunders.
4. Quigley EMM, Pfeiffer RF. Neuro-Gastroenterology. Philadelphia: Butterworth Heinemann; 0000:3–12.
5. Thuneberg L. Interstitial cells of Cajal. In: Shultz S, Wood JD, Rauner BB, eds. Handbook of Physiology, Vol. I. Motility and Circulation. Bethesda, MD: American Physiology Society; 1989:349–386.
6. Sanders KM. A case for interstitial cells of Cajal as the pacemakers and mediators of neuro-transmission in the gastrointestinal tract. Gastroenterology 1996; 111:492–515.
7. He CL, Burgart L, Wang L, et al. Decreased interstitial cells of Cajal volume in patients with slow-transit constipation. Gastroenterology 2000; 118:14–21.
8. Boeckxstaens GE, Rumessen JJ, de Wit L, et al Abnormal distribution of the interstitial cells of Cajal in an adult patient with pseudo-obstruction and megaduodenum. Am J Gastroenterol 2002; 97:2120–2126.
9. Cooke AR. The glands of Brunner. In: Code CF, ed. Hnadbook of Physiology: The Alimentary Canal, Vol. 2: Secretion. Baltimore, MD: Williams & Wilkins; 1967:1087–1095.
10. Nakajima K, Ota H, Zhang MX, et al. Expression of gastric gland mucous cell-type mucin in normal and neoplastic human tissues. J Histochem Cytochem 2003; 51: 1689–1698.

11. Wapnir RA, Fisher SE. Intestinal secretion and absorption. In: Silverberg M, Duam F, eds. Textbook of Pediatrics Gastroenterology, 2nd edn. Chicago, IL: Year Book Medical Publishers; 1988:40–71.
12. Madar JL. Functional morphology of the small intestine. In: Field M, ed. Handbook of Absorption and Secretion. New York: Oxford University Press; 1991:83–120.
13. Celemeti F Palade GE. Intestinal capillaries: 1. Permeability of peroxidase and ferritin. J Cell Biol 1969; 41:33–58.
14. Jepson MA, Clark MA, Foster N, et al. Targeting to intestinal M cells. J Anat 1996; 189:507–516.
15. Foster N, Hirst BH. Exploiting receptor biology for oral vaccination with biodegradable particulates. Adv Drug Deliv Rev 2005; 57:431–450.
16. Kraehenbuhl JP. Epithelial M cells: differentiation and function. Annu Rev Cell Dev Biol 2000; 16:301–332.
17. Madara JL, Bye WA, Trier JS. Structural features of the cholesterol distribution in the M-cell membranes in guinea pig, rat and mouse Peyer's patches. Gastroenterology 1984; 87:1091–1103.
18. Baggio LL, Drucker DJ. Clinical endocrinology and metabolism. Glucagon-like peptide-1 and glucagon-like peptide-2. Best Pract Res Clin Endocrinol Metab 2004; 18:531–554.
19. Burrin DG, Stoll B, Guan X, Cui L, Chang X, Holst JJ. Glucagon-like peptide 2 dose-dependently activates intestinal cell survival and proliferation in neonatal piglets. Endocrinology 2005; 146:22–32.
20. Jeppesen PB, Hartmann B, Thulesen J, et al. Treatment of short bowel patients with glucagon-like peptide-2 (GLP-2), a newly discovered intestinotrophic, anti-secretory, and transit-modulating peptide. Gastroenterology 2001; 120:806–815.
21. Drucker DJ. Glucagon-like peptide 2. J Clin Endocrinol Metab 2001; 86:1759–1764.
22. Bretscher A, Weber K.Villin: the major microfilament-associated protein of the intestinal microvillus. Proc Natl Acad Sci USA 1979; 76:2321–2325.
23. Field M. Intestinal ion transport and the pathophysiology of diarrhea. J Clin Invest 2003; 111:931–943.
24. Schneebergeer EE, Lynch RD. The tight junction: a multifunctional complex. Am J Physiol Cell Physiol 2004; 286:C1213–C1228.
25. Van Itallie CM, Anderson JM. The molecular physiology of tight junction pores. Physiology (Bethesda) 2004; 19:331–338.
26. Yin T, Green KJ. Regulation of desmosome assembly and adhesion. Semin Cell Dev Biol 2004; 15:665–677.
27. Fasano A. Intestinal zonulin: open sesame. Gut 2001; 49:159–162.
28. Wapnir RA, Fisher SE. Intestinal secretion and absorption. In: Silverberg M, Daum F, eds. Textbook of Pediatric Gastroenterology, 2nd edn. Chicago, IL: Year Book Medical Publishers; 1988:40–71.
29. Madara J. Functional morphology of the epithelium of the small intestines. In: Filed M, ed. Handbook of Physiology, Section 6: The Gastrointestinal System, Vol. 4: Intestinal Absorption and Secretion. New York: Oxford University Press; 1991:83–102.
30. Somoszy Z, Forgacs Z, Bognar G, Horvath K, Horvath G. Alteration of tight and adherens junctions on 50-Hz magnetic field exposure in Madin Darby canine kidney (MDCK) cells. Sci World J 2004; 4(Suppl 2):75–82.
31. Specian RD, Oliver MG. Functional biology of intestinal goblet cells. Am J Physiol 1991; 260:C183.
32. Verdugo P. Goblet cells secretion and mucogenesis. Annu Rev Physiol 1990; 52:157–176.
33. Merzel J. Leblond CP. Origin and renewal of goblet cells in the epithelium of the mouse small intestine. Am J Anat 1969; 124:281–306.
34. Lee CS, Kaestner KH. Clinical endocrinology and metabolism. Development of gut endocrine cells. Best Pract Res Clin Endocrinol Metab 2004; 18:453–462.
35. Rindi G, Leiter AB, Kopin AS, Bordi C, Solcia E. The 'normal' endocrine cell of the gut: changing concepts and new evidences. Ann N Y Acad Sci 2004; 1014:1–12.
36. Ouellette AJ. Defensin-mediated innate immunity in the small intestine. Best Pract Res Clin Gastroenterol 2004; 18:405–419.
37. Rumio C, Besusso D, Palazzo M, et al. Degranulation of paneth cells via toll-like receptor 9. Am J Pathol. 2004; 165:373–381.
38. Kelly P, Feakins R, Domizio P, et al. Paneth cell granule depletion in the human small intestine under infective and nutritional stress. Clin Exp Immunol 2004; 135:303–309.
39. Ayabe T, Satchell DP, Wilson CL, et al. Secretion of microbicidal alpha-defensins by intestinal Paneth cells in response to bacteria. Nat Immunol 2000; 1:113–118.
40. Ganz T. Defensins and host defense. Science 1999; 286:420–421.
41. Ganz T. Paneth cells – guardians of the gut cell. Nat Immunol 2000; 1:99–100.
42. Wilson CL, Ouellette AJ, Satchell DP, et al. Regulation of intestinal alpha-defensin activation by the metalloproteinase matrilysin in innate host defense. Science 1999; 286:113–117.
43. Madara JL, Carlson SL. Cup cells: further structural characterization of the brush border and the suggestion that they may serve as an attachment site for an unidentified bacillus in guinea pig ileum. Gastroenterology 1985; 89:1374–1386.
44. Fujimura Y, Iida M. A new marker for cup cells in the rabbit small intestine: expression of vimentin intermediate filament protein. Med Electron Microsc 2001; 34:223–229.
45. Barkla DH, Whitehead RH, Foster H, Tutton P. Tuft (caveolated) cells in two human colon carcinoma cell lines. Am J Pathol 1988; 132:521–525.
46. Camilleri M. Chronic diarrhea: a review on pathophysiology and management for the clinical gastroenterologist. Clin Gastroenterol Hepatol 2004; 2:198–206.
47. Schultz SG, Fuisz RE, Curran PF. Amino acid and sugar transport in rabbit ileum. J Gen Physiol 1966; 49:849–866.
48. Turnberg LA, Fordtran JS, Carter NW, Rector FC Jr. Mechanism of bicarbonate absorption and its relationship to sodium transport in the human jejunum. J Clin Invest1970; 49:548–556.
49. Turnberg LA, Bieberdorf FA, Morawski SG, Fordtran JS. Interrelationships of chloride, bicarbonate, sodium, and hydrogen transport in the human ileum. J Clin Invest1970; 49:557–567.
50. Hoogerwerf WA, Tsao SC, Devuyst O, et al. NHE2 and NHE3 are human and rabbit intestinal brush-border proteins. Am J Physiol 1996; 70:G29–G41.
51. Schultheis PJ, Clarke LL, Meneton P, et al. Renal and intestinal absorptive defects in mice lacking the NHE3 Na^+/H^+ exchanger. Nat Genet 1998; 19:282–285.
52. Melvin JE, Park K, Richardson L, Schultheis PJ, Shull GE. Mouse down-regulated in adenoma (DRA) is an intestinal Cl^-/HCO_3^- exchanger and is up-regulated in colon of mice lacking the NHE3 Na^+/H^+ exchanger. J Biol Chem 1999; 274:22855–22861.
53. Moseley RH, Hoglund P, Wu GD, et al. Downregulated in adenoma gene encodes a chloride transporter defective in congenital chloride diarrhea. Am J Physiol 1999; 276:G185–G192.

54. Kere J, Lohi H., Hoglund P. Genetic disorders of membrane transport. III. Congenital chloride diarrhea. Am J Physiol1999; 276:G7–G13.
55. Nozawa T, Sugiura S, Hashino Y, Tsuji A, Tamai I. Role of anion exchange transporter PAT1 (SLC26A6) in intestinal absorption of organic anions. J Drug Target 2004; 12:97–104.
56. Wang Z, Petrovic S, Mann E, Soleimani M. Identification of an apical Cl(+)/HCO_3(–) exchanger in the small intestine. Am J Physiol Gastrointest Liver Physiol 2002; 282:G573–G579.
57. Flemstrom G. Gastric and duodenal mucosal bicarbonate secretion. In: Johnson LR, Jacobson ED, Christensen J, Alpers D, Walsh JH, eds. Physiology of the Gastrointestinal Tract, 3rd edn. New York: Raven; 1994:1285–1309.
58. Hogan DL, Rapier RC, Dreilinger A, et al. Duodenal bicarbonate secretion eradication of *Helicobacter pylori* and duodenal structure and function in humans. Gastroenterology 1996; 110:705–716.
59. Diamond JM. The epithelia junction: bridge, gate and fence. Physiologist 1997; 20:10–18.
60. Wood JE. Enteric neuroimmunophysiology and pathophysiology. Gastroenterology 2004; 127:635–657.
61. Lacy ER. Functional morphology of the large intestines. In: Field M, ed. Handbook of Physiology, Section 6: The Gastroenterology System, Vol. 4. Intestinal Absorption and Secretion. New York: Oxford University Press; 1991:121–478.
62. Poster GD, Lester R. The developing colon and nutrition. J Pediatr Gastroenterol Nutr 1984; 3:485–487.
63. Bond JH, Levitt MD. Fate of soluble carbohydrate in the colon of rats and man. J Clin Invest 1976; 57:1158–1164.
64. Agarwal VP, Schimmel EM. Diversion colitis: a nutritional deficiency syndrome? Nutr Rev 1989; 47:257–261.
65. Harig JM, Soergel KH, Komorowski RA, Wood CA. Treatment of diversion colitis with short-chain-fatty acid irrigation. N Engl J Med 1989; 320:23–28.
66. Siveke JT, Braun GS. Small bowel and cecal volvulus due to mesenteric torsion. Emerg Med 2004; 26:237–239.
67. Shah SS, Louie JP, Fein JA. Cecal volvulus in childhood. Pediatr Emerg Care 2002; 18:300–302.
68. Judge T, Lichtenstein GR. Is the appendix a vestigial organ? Its role in ulcerative colitis. Gastroenterology 2001; 121:730–732.
69. Trier JS, Winter HS. Anatomy embryology, and developmental abnormalities of the small intestines and colon In: Sleisenger MH, Fordtran JS, eds. Gastrointestinal Disease, 4th edn. Philadelphia: WB Saunders; 1989:991–1021.
70. Bloom W-N, Fawcett DW. A Textbook of Histology. Philadelphia, PA: WB Saunders; 1968.
71. Sleisenger MH, Fordtran JS. Gastrointestinal Disease, 4th edn. Philadelphia, PA: WB Saunders; 1989.

Chapter 30
Maldigestion and malabsorption

Reinaldo Garcia-Naveiro and John N. Udall Jr

INTRODUCTION

Food assimilation is the major function of the gastrointestinal tract. Most nutrients cannot be absorbed in their natural form, for this reason they need to be digested. Food is chemically reduced to digestive end-products, small enough to participate in the absorption process across the intestinal epithelium. An understanding of the pathophysiology of maldigestion and malabsorption should be based on a knowledge of the normal steps of digestion and absorption. Normal intestinal assimilation can be divided into sequential physiologic stages: (1) hydrolysis and solubilization in the lumen and at the enterocyte membrane and (2) absorption across the intestinal mucosa and into systemic body fluids.

Hydrolysis is the basic process of digestion. Carbohydrates, fats and proteins undergo digestion by hydrolysis. The difference in the process for each nutrient lies in the enzymes required to promote the digestive reaction. Different physiologic processes, such as solubilization, intestinal motility and hormone secretion are also involved in normal digestion and absorption. Following digestion in the intestinal lumen and at the brush border, monosaccharides, monoglycerides, fatty acids, small peptides and amino acids are then absorbed and processed by the enterocyte. Vitamins, minerals and water also participate in the process. A nutrient must be transported into blood and lymph in order to be stored or metabolized in distant organs. Any disease that interrupts the delicate sequence of reactions important in digestion and absorption may lead to maldigestion, malabsorption and end in malassimilation.

These physiologic stages may be altered in intestinal disease (Table 30.1). For clinical purposes, maldigestion and malabsorption will be discussed by nutrient group, starting with carbohydrates, then lipids, proteins, vitamins, minerals and water.

CLASSES OF NUTRIENTS

Carbohydrates

The type of carbohydrates ingested varies with age. During infancy, lactose accounts for most of the dietary carbohydrate.[1] However, in older children and adults, starch makes up much of the ingested carbohydrates, with smaller amounts of lactose and sucrose.[2] Even when considered on a worldwide basis, carbohydrates constitute the major source of calories in the human diet. They are divided into four major groups: (1) monosaccharides or simple sugars, which cannot be hydrolyzed into a simpler form; (2) disaccharides, which yield two molecules when hydrolyzed; (3) oligosaccharides, which yield two to ten monosaccharides when hydrolyzed; and (4) polysaccharides, which yield more than ten molecules on hydrolysis. A schematic representation of digestion and absorption of dietary carbohydrates is shown in Figure 30.1.

People in the western world consume about 400 g of carbohydrates daily. Starches (glucose polymers), as noted above, represent the largest portion of ingested carbohydrates. Much of the starch in the diet is present in wheat, rice and corn as polysaccharides whose molecular weight ranges from 100 000 to greater than 1 000 000. The two chief constituents of starch are amylose, which is non-branching in structure, and amylopectin, which consists of highly branched chains.[2] Each is composed of a number of α-glucosidic chains having 24–30 glucose molecules a piece. The glucose residues are united by 1:4 or 1:6 linkages. Dietary fiber, which is non-starch polysaccharides and lignin from plants, is not subject to digestion in the intestine of humans but is an important source of 'bulk' in the diet.

Digestion of carbohydrates starts in the mouth. The carbohydrate comes in contact with saliva, produced by three pairs of salivary glands: the parotid, submandibular and sublingual. These three pairs of glands contribute 20%, 60% and 20%, respectively, to the total amount of saliva.[3] Numerous smaller glands are located in the lips, palate, tongue and cheeks; these glands also contribute to the exocrine fluid. Saliva contains mucin, a 'slimy' glycoprotein important for lubrication and a serous secretion rich in ptyalin, an α-amylase, which participates in the hydrolysis of starch.

Salivary and pancreatic α-amylases act on interior α1,4 glucose-glucose links of starch but cannot attack α1,4 linkages close to α1,6 branch point or the α1,6 branch point. Pancreatic α-amylase is normally secreted in excess. For this reason, carbohydrate hydrolysis is impaired in only severe forms of pancreatic insufficiency. Since α-amylase cannot hydrolyze the 1,6 branching links and has relatively little specificity for 1,4 links adjacent to these branch points, large oligosaccharides containing five to nine glucose units and consisting of one or more 1,6 branching links are produced by α-amylase action. The products of this digestion are the disaccharide maltose, the trisaccharide maltotriose and α-limit dextrins, branched polymers containing an average of about 8 glucose molecules.[2]

The final stages of carbohydrate digestion occur by enterocyte membrane-associated enzymes. Disaccharides are

Disease/condition	Pathophysiology
Intraluminal digestion	
Stomach	
Protein-calorie malnutrition	Decreased acid production, hypochlorhydria
Zollinger-Ellison syndrome	Inactivation of pancreatic enzymes at a low duodenal pH, and decreased ionization of conjugated bile salts
Pernicious anemia	Decreased intrinsic factor secretion, vitamin B_{12} malabsorption
Dumping syndrome	Rapid emptying of stomach contents into the small intestine, dilution of enzymes
Pancreas	
Cystic fibrosis	Impaired secretion of enzymes and bicarbonate
Shwachman–Diamond syndrome	Impaired secretion of enzymes
Acute/chronic pancreatitis	Impaired secretion of enzymes and bicarbonate
Protein-caloric malnutrition	Impaired secretion of enzymes
Trypsinogen deficiency	Impaired secretion of enzymes
Lipase deficiency	Impaired secretion of enzymes
Amylase deficiency	Impaired secretion of enzymes
Liver	
Cholestasis syndromes	Impaired secretion of bile salts with deficient micelle formation
surgery	Intestinal malabsorption of bile salts, deficient bile salt pool
Intestine	
Enterokinase deficiency	Impaired activation of luminal pancreatic enzymes
Protein-caloric malnutrition	Bacterial overgrowth with consumption of nutrients, toxin production, and deconjugation of bile acids
Anatomic duplication	Bacterial overgrowth with consumption of nutrients
Blind loop syndrome	Bacterial overgrowth with consumption of nutrients
Short bowel syndrome	Bacterial overgrowth with consumption of nutrients
Pseudo-obstruction	Bacterial overgrowth with consumption of nutrients
Digestion at the enterocyte membrane	
Congenital disaccharidase deficiency	Impaired digestion of a specific disaccharide leading to bacterial fermentation in the colon
Lactase	
Sucrase-isomaltase	
Trehalase	
Acquired/late-onset disaccharidase deficiency	Loss of enzyme activity due to mucosal injury or loss of activity with age
Lactase	
Sucrase-isomaltase	
Glucoamylase	
Enterocyte absorption	
Protein-calorie malnutrition	'Damage' *vs* 'adaptive regulation', altered mucosal architecture
Hartnup's disease	Transport defect of neutral amino acids
Lysinuric protein intolerance	Transport defect of dibasic amino acids in intestine and kidney
Blue diaper syndrome	Transport defect of tryptophan
Oasthouse syndrome	Transport defect of methionine in intestine and kidney
Lowe's syndrome	X-linked trait with defect in transport of lysine and arginine
Glucose-galactose malabsorption	Selective defect in glucose and galactose sodium cotransport system
Congenital chloride diarrhea	Selective defect in chloride transport by the intestine
A-β-lipoproteinemia	Absent production of apolipoprotein B, lipoproteins and chylomicrons
Hypobetalipoproteinemia	Impaired production of apolipoprotein B
Celiac disease	Damage to absorptive/digestive surface
Short bowel syndrome	Loss of absorptive/digestive surface, abnormal transit
Mucosal injury syndromes	Damage to digestive/absorptive surface
Milk/soy protein intolerance	
Post enteritis syndrome	
Tropical sprue	Damage to digestive/absorptive surface
Bacterial infection/inflammation	
Shigella	Damage to digestive/absorptive surface, abnormal motility
Salmonella	Damage to digestive/absorptive surface, abnormal motility
Campylobacter	Damage to digestive/absorptive surface, abnormal motility
Cholera	Secretory water and electrolyte loss
Giardiasis	Disruption of epithelial function secondary to adhesion or toxin(?)
Crohn's disease	Damage to digestive/absorptive surface, chronic gastrointestinal blood loss
Whipple's disease	Lymphatic obstruction, impaired lipid transport (?), patchy enteropathy
Viral infection	
Rotavirus	Damage to digestive/absorptive area
Human Immunodeficiency Virus	Damage to digestive/absorptive area, bacterial overgrowth, exocrine pancreatic and hepatic insufficiency

Table 30.1 Gastrointestinal diseases associated with maldigestion and malabsorption

(Continued)

Disease/condition	Pathophysiology
Acrodermatitis enteropathica	Impaired absorption of zinc
Uptake into blood and lymph	
Congestive heart failure	Venous distention, bowel wall edema
Intestinal lymphangiectasia	Obstructed lymphatic transport of lipid and fat-soluble vitamins, intestinal protein loss
Miscellaneous disorders	
Immune deficiency syndromes	Altered bacterial fora
Allergic gastroenteropathy	Unknown immune mechanism
Eosinophilic gastroenteropathy	Unknown immune mechanism
Drugs	
Methotrexate	Damage to mucosal surface by interference with enterocyte replication
Cholestyramine	Blocked reabsorption of bile salts in the ileum by drug; malabsorption of calcium, fat, bile acids, and fat-soluble vitamins
Phenytoin	Calcium, folic acid malabsorption
Sulfasalazine	Folic acid malabsorption
Histamine H_2 receptor antagonists	Impaired acid/proteolytic liberation of vitamin B_{12}

Table 30.1 Gastrointestinal diseases associated with maldigestion and malabsorption

hydrolyzed to monosaccharides by specific enzymes located in the brush border of intestinal epithelial cells. (Fig. 30.1) The disaccharidases are, in fact, mostly oligosaccharidases, which hydrolyze sugars containing three or more hexose units. They are present in highest concentration at the villous tips in the jejunum and persist throughout most of the ileum, but not in the colon.

Digestion and absorption of carbohydrates from the diet leads to the entry of three monosaccharides into the circulation; glucose, fructose and galactose. In normal subjects, the capacity of the small intestine is such that virtually all the free mono- and disaccharides present in the normal diet are completely absorbed. However, when there is malabsorption of disaccharides, monosaccharides or other carbohydrates, such as sorbitol or xylitol, these sugars are emptied into the colon. The unabsorbed carbohydrates may then be fermented by colonic bacteria, which leads to the production of carbon dioxide, hydrogen and methane. Propionic and butyric acids, both short chain fatty acids are also produced. Butyric acid can be utilized by colonic mucosal cells as an energy source and the bulk of the absorbed propionate is cleared by the liver.[4]

The most common type of carbohydrate maldigestion and malabsorption is caused by intestinal lactase deficiency. There are several types of lactase deficiency: congenital, adult-onset and secondary lactase deficiency. Congenital lactase deficiency is rare and is associated with symptoms occurring a short time after birth when lactose is present in the diet.[5] The largest group of patients with this disorder is from Finland, where at least 16 cases have been described.[6] Adult-onset lactase deficiency is extremely common and 'normal' for most humans, beginning as early as 2 years of age in some racial groups and as late as adolescence in others. Individuals with adult-onset lactase deficiency comprise the majority of the world's population. Individuals of northern European ancestry and certain groups in Africa and India, however, maintain lactase activity throughout adulthood. This ethnically-related lactase deficiency is the most common cause of lactose intolerance. On a global scale, it is obvious that persistence of the ability to digest lactose is the exception rather than the rule. Mutation of a regulatory gene for lactase has been postulated to explain the delayed onset of hypolactasia. There may be a genetically controlled 'switching off' of the lactase gene in susceptible individuals.[7–9] Continuing milk intake in populations known to become lactase deficient beyond the childhood years can affect the age of onset. Lactase does not behave as an inducible enzyme, but continued exposure to milk products can, to a certain degree, affect the regulatory gene.[10,11]

The prevalence of lactose intolerance in the Caucasian population of the USA is about 20%, while in American Indians, Eskimos, Japanese and Chinese, the prevalence is 80–100%. In the Scandinavian countries, lactose intolerance occurs in 2–15% of the population. As noted above, the age of onset of this ethnically associated lactase deficiency varies from early childhood to late teenage years. In African-Americans, symptomatic lactose intolerance increases after 10 years of age.

Secondary lactase deficiency occurs following infectious gastroenteritis or injury to the small intestinal mucosa caused by gluten or other sensitizing substances. Recovery of full function of this disaccharidase might take months, since lactase is the last disaccharidase to return to normal following injury. This secondary lactose intolerance has popularized the use of formulas containing sucrose or glucose polymers for children recovering from gastroenteritis. In addition, damage to the intestinal mucosa may increase the likelihood of not only lactose malabsorption, but also a cow's milk protein sensitivity. This has also encouraged the use of soy protein, protein hydrolyzates and amino acid-based formulas. There is evidence that implicates protein hypersensitivity in prolonged diarrhea seen in some children, with progression to a more chronic form of diarrhea. The damaged mucosa is thought to have decreased levels of disaccharidases. Continued ingestion of disaccharide when the enzyme important in hydrolysis is deficient may perpetuate the diarrhea.

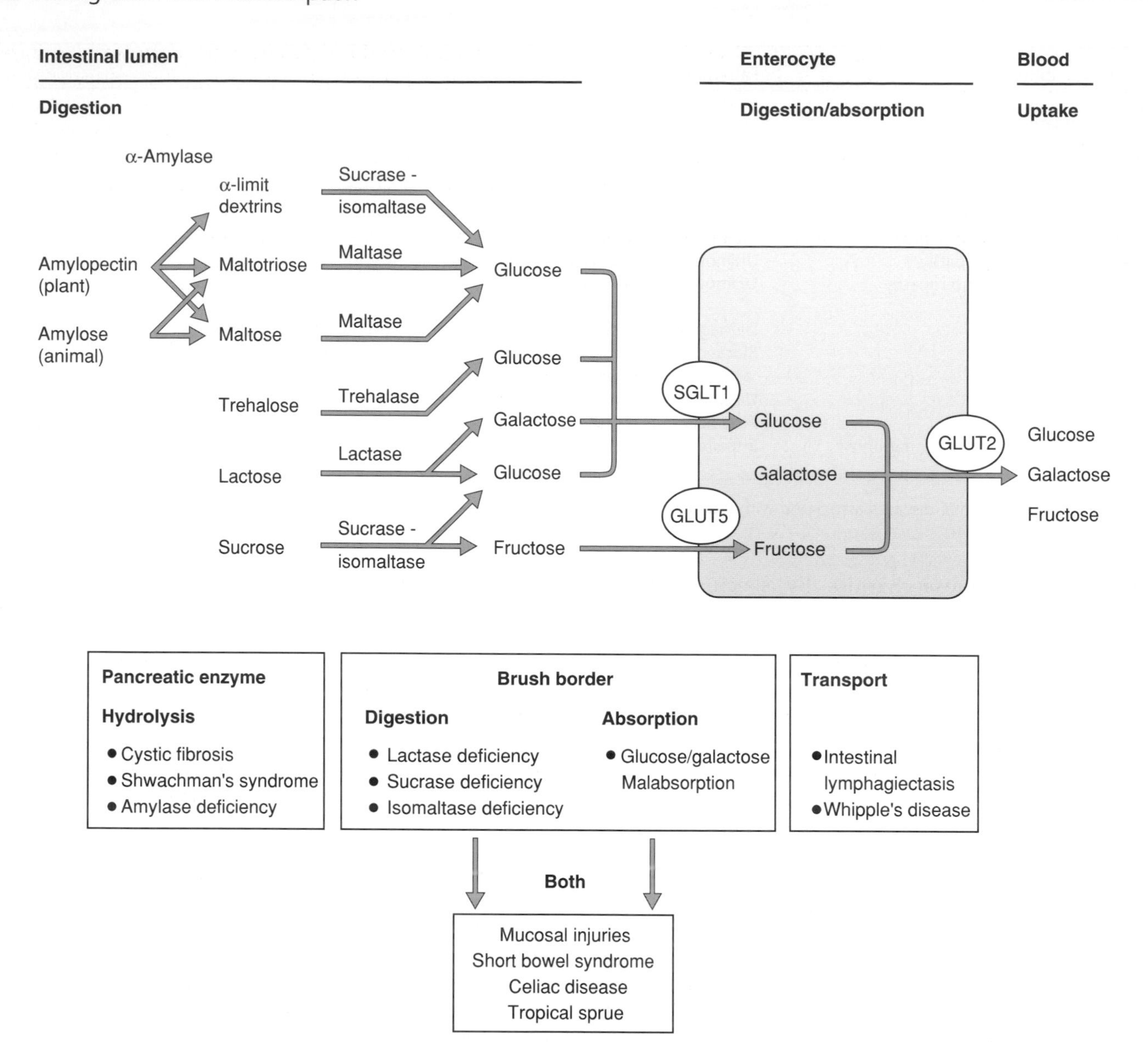

Figure 30.1: Digestion of carbohydrates is initiated by salivary and pancreatic α-amylase (endoenzymes). They digest the linear 'internal' α-1,4 linkages between glucose residues, but cannot break 'terminal' α-1,4 linkages. They also cannot split the α-1,6 linkages at the branch points of amylopectin or the adjacent α-1,6 linkages. The products of α-amylase action are linear glucose oligomers, maltotriose, maltose, trehalose, lactose and sucrose. Brush border oligosaccharidases, intrinsic membrane proteins with their catalytic domains facing the lumen, hydrolyze the products of α-amylase digestion. Absorption occurs by way of SGLT1, which is the sodium-coupled transporter that mediates the uptake of glucose and galactose from the lumen into the enterocyte and GLUT5, which mediates the facilitated diffusion of fructose into the enterocyte. Uptake of monosaccharides across the basolateral membrane and into the interstitial space occurs by GLUT2. GLUT, glucose transporter; SGLT, sodium/glucose co-transporter.

The presence of malabsorbed substrate in the intestinal lumen is responsible for the fluid shifts that occur in osmotic diarrhea. Fermentation by colonic bacteria contributes to cramps and bloating. It seems prudent to withhold lactose, or at least to decrease its total intake, in children with severe gastroenteritis for a period of 1–3 weeks if there is evidence of lactose intolerance. An exception to this guideline is the recommended practice of continuing breast feedings during acute gastroenteritis.[12,13]

Sucrase is a hybrid molecule consisting of two enzymes – one hydrolyzing sucrose into glucose and fructose and the other enzyme hydrolyzing the α1,6 branch points of α-limit dextrins. Therefore, sucrase-isomaltase and not 'sucrase' is the preferred term for this disaccharidase. The molecular relation and sharing of active sites between sucrase and isomaltase is still of great interest to geneticists and biochemists, since deficiency of one enzyme is accompanied by abnormal activity of the second. Congenital sucrase-isomaltase deficiency was first described in 1961 by Weijers and co-workers.[14] Although it is generally considered to be a rare condition, the heterozygote frequency in Caucasian subjects is 2%. The homozygote condition, rare in Caucasians, is as high as 5% in Greenlanders.[15] Symptoms vary from severe diarrhea in infancy to intermittent diarrhea, cramps and gas in the older child. The correct diagnosis may be missed for years with symptoms being attributed to 'toddler's diarrhea' or 'maternal anxiety'. When the diagnosis is suspected on clinical grounds, a breath hydrogen test after an oral sucrose load or an abnormal sucrose tolerance test will help identify sucrose as the offending carbohydrate. The diagnosis is established by the demonstration of deficient sucrase-isomaltase activity in a morphologically normal jejunal biopsy. Treatment of sucrase-isomaltase deficiency consists of strict avoidance of sucrose. A commercial preparation of sucrase is available and efficacious.[16] Starch can still be consumed in sucrase-isomaltase deficiency because most of its chemical make-up consists of amylose which is digested by pancreatic α-amylase or by brush border glucoamylase.

Several maltases (glucoamylases) have been identified. Maltases are responsible for the digestion of maltotriose. The enzyme differs from pancreatic α-amylase since maltase sequentially removes a single glucose from the non-reducing end of a linear α1,4 glucose chain, breaking down maltose into glucose. Theoretically, maltase deficiency may lead to carbohydrate maldigestion, although its clinical significance appears to be minimal.

Trehalose (α-D-glucopyranoside) is a non-reducing disaccharide that occurs in mushrooms, in some micro-organisms and in many insects. Trehalase deficiency can cause symptoms similar to those of lactase malabsorption.[17] An autosomal dominant type of inheritance has been suggested.

Brush border enzyme deficiencies are frequently acquired. The most common disaccharide deficiencies occur following infectious gastroenteritis or other damaging insults to the intestine including gluten-induced enteropathy, cow's protein sensitivity, giardiasis and rotavirus infection. A congenital defect involving the transport of glucose and galactose is extremely rare.

Once monosaccharides have been produced on the brush border, absorption depends on mechanisms coupled to energy-dependent, active sodium transport, requiring specific carrier proteins known as SGTL1. Glucose and galactose are two monosaccharides known to be absorbed through this pathway, while fructose and xylose appear to be absorbed by a process of facilitated diffusion where GLUT5 is the specific carrier for fructose.[18] Not all carbohydrate hydrolyzed at one site is absorbed at that site; rather, the sugar may be carried in intestinal juice to be absorbed further downstream. Glucose-galactose malabsorption was first described in 1962 by Lindquist and Meeuwisse.[19] *In vivo* and *in vitro* studies have shown markedly impaired or absent sodium-coupled mucosal uptake of glucose in this disease.[20] In many patients, clinical tolerance to the offending carbohydrates improves with age, despite the fact that the enzyme deficiency and transport defect persist.

Maldigestion and malabsorption can accompany severe disease of the pancreas. In addition, pancreatic amylase deficiency has been described. Lowe and May reported a 13-year-old boy whose duodenal juice showed a persistent absence of amylase with decreased levels of trypsin but a normal amount of lipase.[21] Another case of amylase deficiency was reported by Lilibridge and Townes.[22] They described a 2-year-old child who showed poor weight gain on a diet containing starch, despite a more than adequate caloric intake. Weight gain and growth improved when starch was eliminated from the diet and replaced by disaccharides.

Lipids

Greater than 90% of ingested lipid in the diet is in the form of neutral fats or triglycerides. The diet also contains small amounts of phospholipids, cholesterol and cholesterol esters. The schematic representation of the digestion and absorption of dietary lipids is shown in Figure 30.2.

Many of the steps in fat digestion, absorption and metabolism are not well-developed in the newborn human and even less so in the pre-term infant.[23] The full-term infant if fed with mother's milk receives nutrients that are well-adapted to the needs of the rapidly growing newborn. The fat in human milk is ideally suited to the requirements of full-term infants; however, in infants born extremely premature, the gastrointestinal tract is not always able to digest and absorb nutrients.[23]

As noted above, triglycerides are the main dietary fat throughout life and this applies to the infant as well. However, phospholipids and cholesterol also have important nutritional functions. It is open to question whether formulas that contain only trace amounts of cholesterol, compared with the cholesterol content of human milk (10–15 mg/dl) provide an adequate amount of this lipid. Cholesterol is not only a precursor for steroid hormones and bile acids, but it is also an essential component of cell membranes. At an average milk consumption of 750–850 ml/day, the rapidly growing infant absorbs 75–125 mg of cholesterol a day.

The newborn and especially the premature infant are deficient in pancreatic lipase and bile salts that are needed for digestion and solubilization of dietary fat. Pancreatic enzyme activity measured in the duodenum of full-term and preterm newborn infants under basal conditions shows considerable protease (trypsin and chymotrypsin) activity, but only trace amounts of lipase and no amylase.[23] During the first month of life, pancreatic lipase remains very low or absent not only under basal conditions, but also after cholecystokinin-pancreozymin stimulation.[23,24] At 2 years of age, basal activity and secretory response of pancreatic lipase are well-developed.[23,24]

Fat digestion in the newborn depends on the activities of the infant's lingual lipase, gastric lipase and the activity of a specific digestive lipase present in human milk. Gastric lipase is stable at a pH of 1.5–2.0 and has optimum activity at a pH of 3.0–6.5. This is different from pancreatic lipase, which requires a higher pH. Gastric lipase is also resistant to pepsin present in the stomach. In formula-fed premature infants, 30% of the fat is digested in the stomach. This compares with 40% of the ingested fat hydrolyzed in the

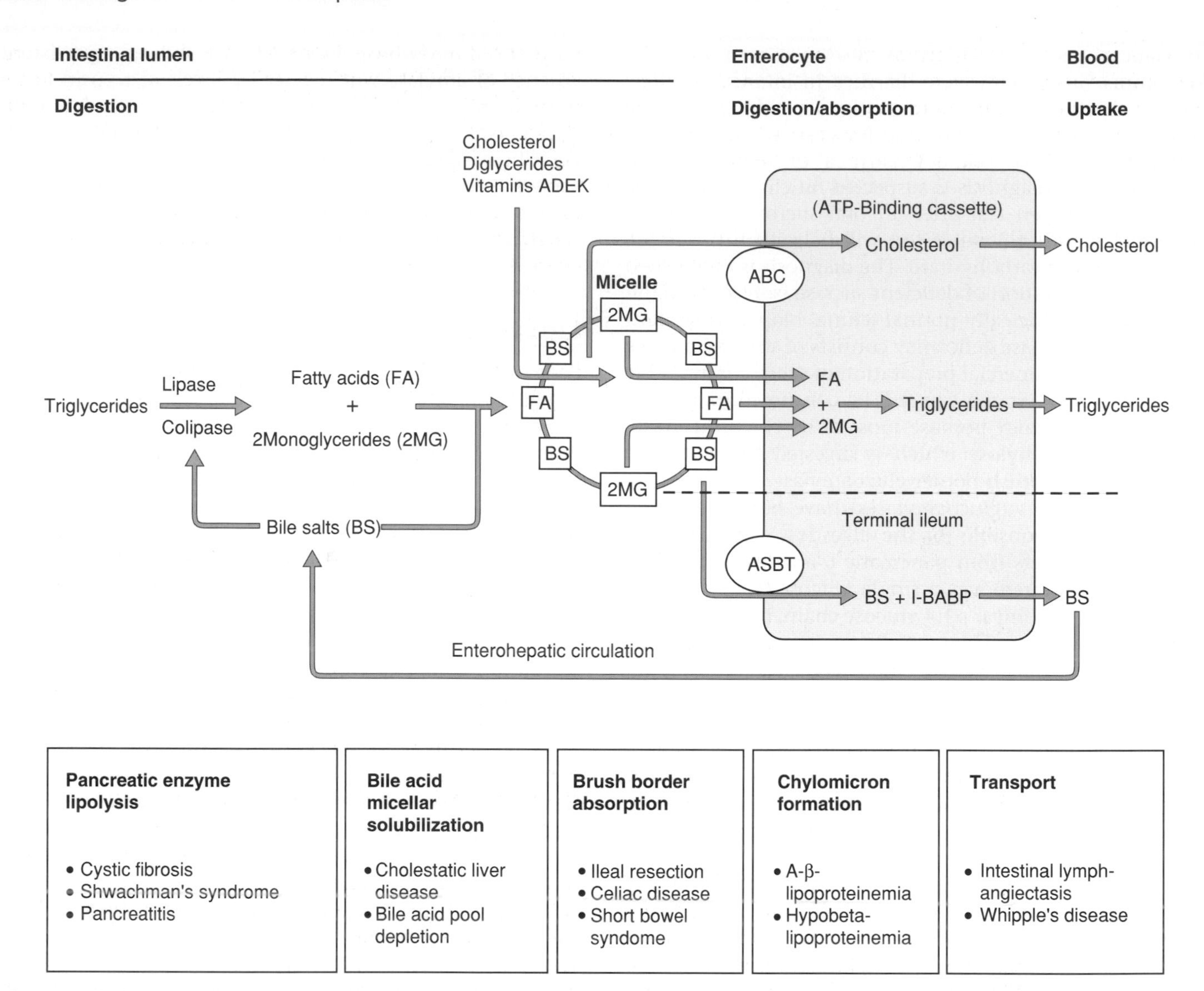

Figure 30.2: Digestion of triglycerides in the intestinal lumen occurs initially by lipase and colipase. Bile salts combine with the digestive products (fatty acids and monoglycerides). Mixed micelles of bile acids and lipid digestion products diffuse through the unstirred layer. Transport proteins such as ABC mediate the transport of cholesterol across the brush border membrane. Fatty acids and monoglycerides diffuse across the membrane. In the cytosol, fatty acids are bound to fatty acid-binding protein and cholesterol is bound to sterol carrier proteins. Uptake of cholesterol and triglycerides into the systemic circulation occurs at the basolateral membrane. In the terminal ileum, the uptake of bile salts occurs via ASBT. Intracellular I-BABP bind bile salts and transport them to the basolateral membrane where uptake occurs. ABC, ATP-Binding Cassette; BS, bile salts; FA, fatty acids; 2MG, 2 monoglyceride; ASBT, apical sodium-dependent bile transporter; I-BABP, ileal bile-acid binding protein

stomach of the breast-fed infant. Overall fat absorption attributable to lipolysis by non-pancreatic digestive lipase amounts to about 50–70% of ingested fat, suggesting that the excellent absorption of milk fat in the newborn depends on additional digestive enzymes, such as milk lipase.[23]

Little is known concerning the postnatal changes in pancreatic lipase activity from birth until adult levels are achieved.[23] However, with age, pancreatic lipase and colipase become more important in fat digestion. The products of pancreatic lipolysis, fatty acids and monoglycerides, must be solubilized. The mechanism to do this develops during maturation as bile salt production by the liver increases. The fatty acids and monoglycerides are solubilized in the intestinal lumen by bile salts to form micelles with the polar end facing the aqueous phase of intestinal fluid and non-polar hydrocarbon end inserted into the interior of the micelle. Bile salt micelles increase the capacity of water to carry fatty acids and allow for more efficient absorption.

In contrast to the immaturity of digestive function, fat uptake by the enterocyte from the intestine seems to be well-developed at birth. However, most of the studies on the mechanism of fat absorption have been carried out in suckling animals with only occasional observations in humans. Once inside the enterocyte, long-chain fatty acids are transported to the re-esterification site, the endoplasmic reticulum, by means of a cytosolic fatty-acid-binding protein.[25] Fatty-acid-binding proteins (FABP) are a family of cytosolic proteins that bind hydrophobic ligands and are thought to be important in the uptake and intracellular transport of fatty acids in the enterocyte. Much knowledge concerning these carrier proteins has accumulated since their initial description.[26–29] The fatty acids are activated to acyl CoA and their re-esterification to triglyceride then occurs. The newly synthesized triglyceride, together with phospholipids, cholesterol and protein is assembled into lipoproteins (chylomicrons and LDL). These large particles are released in the intercellular space by reverse pinocytosis and move across the basement membrane into lymphatics.[23,30] This complex sequence of events is necessary for the absorption of long-chain triglycerides. Short-chain and medium-chain triglycerides, because they are more water-soluble, may be absorbed directly into the portal blood system.

Failure to digest or absorb fats results in a variety of clinical symptoms and laboratory abnormalities. These manifestations are the result of both fat malassimilation *per se* and a deficiency of the fat-soluble vitamins. In general, malabsorption of fat deprives the body of calories and contributes to weight loss and malnutrition. Unabsorbed long-chain fatty acids interact with colonic mucosa to cause diarrhea by an irritant effect on the colon.[30] In addition, unabsorbed fatty acids bind calcium, a mineral normally present in the intestinal lumen. The calcium is then not available to bind oxalate. In fat malabsorption, oxalate not bound to calcium remains free and the oxalate is readily absorbed. This results in oxaluria and calcium oxalate kidney stones, which may occur in Crohn's disease.[31,32]

Recognition of fat malabsorption or steatorrhea is usually not difficult. The stools tend to be large and bulky. Because of their increased gas content, they tend to float in toilet water. In the infant, a film of oil can be seen or oiliness noticed when changing diapers. The smell is typically foul.

Fat malabsorption may occur in diseases that impair bile production or excretion or it may occur in pancreatic insufficiency. In certain conditions, bile acid excretion is impaired, but serum bilirubin concentration may be normal or near normal. This is seen in children with a paucity of intra-hepatic bile ducts. They may not be jaundiced, but have other biochemical signs of cholestasis such as pruritus, increased serum cholesterol, alkaline phosphatase or gamma glutamyl transpeptidase. Steatorrhea may be mild to severe in these children.

The most common cause of pancreatic insufficiency is cystic fibrosis. This disease affects not only enzymes important in fat digestion, but also those important in carbohydrate and protein digestion. Cystic fibrosis is a multi-organ disease that is characterized by the triad of malabsorption, failure to thrive and chronic sinopulmonary infections. The many potential features of cystic fibrosis include pancreatic insufficiency (approximately 85%), liver dysfunction (15–30%) and raised concentrations of sodium and chloride in the sweat, as well as obstructive azoospermia in postpubertal males.[33]

Some 15% of the patients have growth percentiles for height and weight exceeding the 75th percentile. Therefore, good stature does not exclude the diagnosis. The expression of the gene is highly variable, with hundreds of mutations: some patients are seriously handicapped physically, whereas others, who are experiencing minimal symptoms, are not identified until later in adulthood. Dr Harry Shwachman in Boston reported 70 patients that were not diagnosed until over 25 years of age.[34] Moreover, there are patients in whom a single clinical feature is the dominant finding, such as electrolyte abnormalities, pancreatitis, liver disease, sinusitis, or obstructive azoospermia and infertility.

Nutritional problems in cystic fibrosis are multifactorial, including not only maldigestion and malabsorption, but also increased energy expenditure, increased intestinal losses and increased caloric requirements.[35]

Pancreatic insufficiency is also part of Shwachman's syndrome, an inherited disease with abnormal bone marrow function, metaphyseal dysostosis, neutropenia, thrombocytopenia, anemia and eczema. Shwachman's syndrome may result in severe failure to thrive and the neutropenia is responsible for frequent and generalized infections, including chronic purulent otitis, mastoiditis and meningitis. The primary defect in this syndrome remains unknown.[36]

A-β-lipoproteinemia must be considered in the differential diagnosis of a child with steatorrhea, failure to thrive and anemia. A biochemical clue is the presence of very low serum cholesterol concentration generally less than 50 mg/dl. The presence of acanthocytes or spiculated red blood cells in a peripheral blood smear is also suggestive. The serum is not turbid after a fatty meal because of the basic inability to form chylomicrons and transport lipid from the enterocyte. The diagnosis is confirmed by serum lipoprotein electrophoresis along with a jejunal biopsy which shows fat-laden villi.[37,38] The progressive neurological deterioration, including retinitis pigmentosa, ataxia, ophthalmoplegia, was until recently considered an inseparable part of the disease; it has now been correlated with chronic vitamin E deficiency.[39] Early diagnosis and institution of adequate vitamin E replacement will prevent or modify the neurological deterioration.[40]

In congenital lipase deficiency, steatorrhea is present from birth.[41] Although pancreatic lipase, but not co-lipase, is deficient, a functioning gastric source of this lipolytic enzyme is present. There is also evidence of lingual/pharyngeal lipase activity. The diagnosis is confirmed by a secretin-pancreozymin test, which demonstrates normal proteolytic and amylolytic enzymes, but absent lipase activity in duodenal fluid.

Proteins

Infants fed 750–850 ml formula a day ingest approximately 12 g protein. Digestion of this protein begins in the stomach under the influence of pepsin. Although gastric proteolysis is extremely limited, intestinal protein digestion in the infant is probably adequate.[42] The efficiency with which proteins are digested and absorbed in the newborn relate more to the highly glycosylated form of some of the proteins in human milk than with the immaturity of neonatal digestive enzymes.

In the adult, the average protein intake varies considerably. The usual diet in a developed country provides 70–100 g protein/day.[43] Endogenous protein from secretions along the oro-gastro-intestinal tract contributes an additional 50–60 g/day. The bulk of dietary protein is hydrolyzed by pancreatic proteases secreted into the proximal duodenum in inactive form. Activation is catalyzed by the duodenal surface enzyme enterokinase, which converts trypsinogen to activated trypsin. Activation is virtually instantaneous. Intraluminal digestion of dietary protein occurs by sequential action of pancreatic endopeptidases and exopeptidases. The endopeptidases trypsin, chymotrypsin, elastase, DNAase and RNAase act on the peptide at the interior of the molecule. The peptides are then hydrolyzed by the exopeptidases carboxypeptidase A and B, which remove a single amino acid from the carboxyl terminal end of the peptide, yielding basic and neutral amino acids (AAs) as well as small peptides.[43] As shown in Figure 30.3, peptidases in the brush border then hydrolyze the residual di-, tri- and tetrapeptides.

The brush border proteases generate a large quantity and variety of short- and medium-sized peptides, as well as free amino acids. Most protein and oligopeptides are rapidly degraded. However, some structures are fairly resistant to hydrolysis and the rapidity of the digestive process is dependent on the protein's amino acid sequence and on post-translation modifications, such as glycosylation, which render peptides more resistant to hydrolysis.[42,43] Although oligopeptides of medium chain length are the primary products of the luminal phase of protein digestion, they are further cleaved by a spectra of membrane anchored peptidases at the brush border of intestinal epithelial cells. *In vitro* models used to study this have shown that when dipeptides are used as substrates, almost 90% of total mucosal hydrolysis is attributed to cytosolic enzymes, whereas with tripeptides, only around 50% of

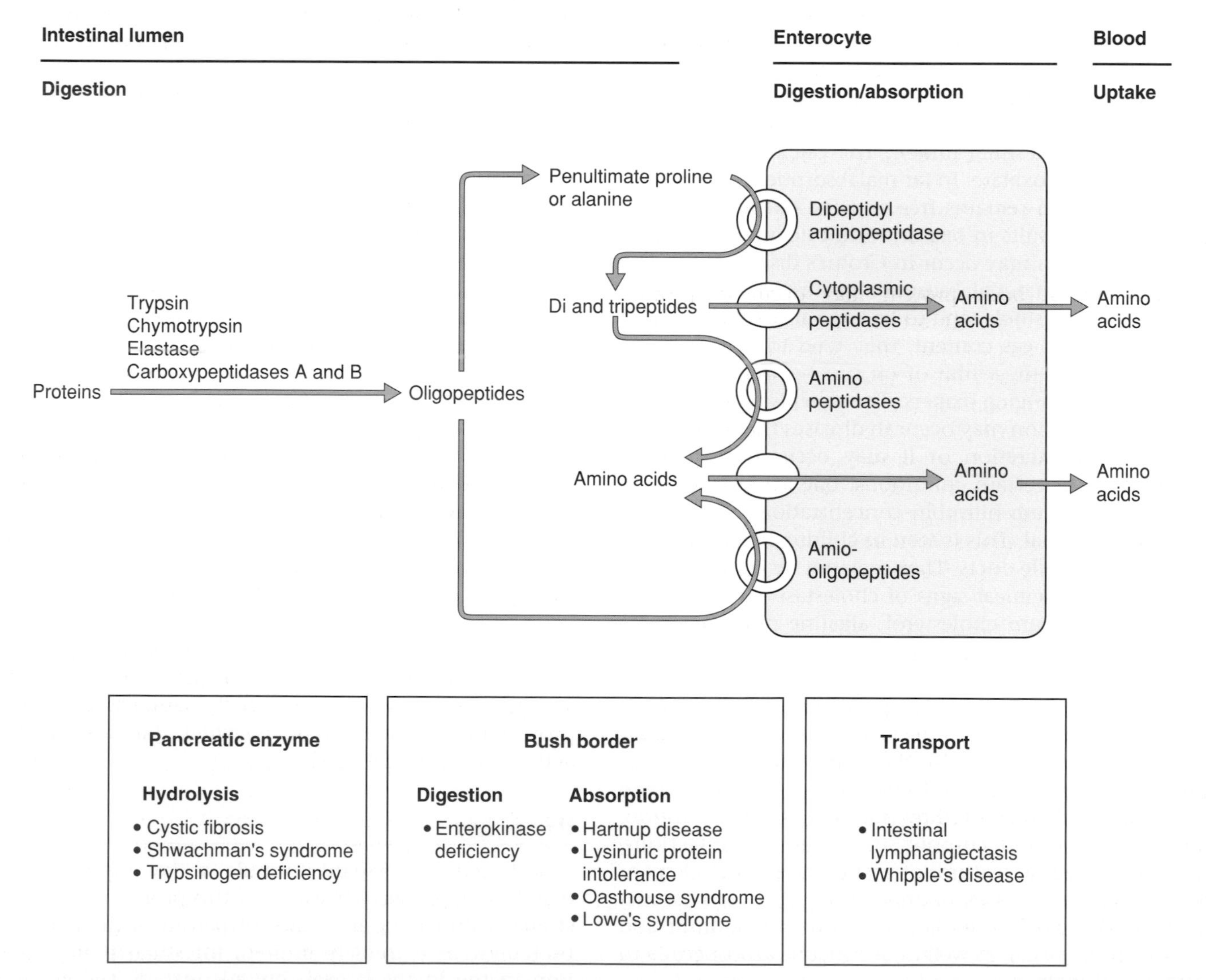

Figure 30.3: Digestion of proteins in the intestinal lumen is initiated by pancreatic trypsin, chymotrypsin, elastase and carboxypeptidases *A* and *B*. The pancreatic proteases convert dietary proteins to oligopeptides. Brush border peptidases (open circles) then hydrolyze the oligopeptides to amino acids, dipeptides, tripeptides and larger peptides. The amino acids are absorbed across the brush border membrane by amino acid transporters (closed circles) and the small peptides by a peptide transporter (closed circles). In the cytosol of the enterocyte, dipeptides, tripeptides and larger peptides are cleaved to single amino acids. Uptake of the single amino acids occurs across the basolateral membrane of the enterocyte.

the hydrolytic activity originates from the soluble cytosolic fraction. In the case of tripeptides and those peptides with more than four amino residues, essentially all hydrolytic activity is brush border membrane bound.[43] Luminal hydrolysis of normal di- and tripeptides occurs rapidly when the enzymes are not overloaded with substrates. When overloading does occur, some peptides then bypass hydrolysis and are taken up intact into the cell.

Multiple peptide transporters for the different substrate groups were initially postulated. Indeed, findings from experiments of intact tissue preparations have suggested, on the basis of cross-inhibition studies, that there could be more than one type of peptide carrier. However, cloning of the cDNA of the intestinal di-tripeptide carrier now designated as PEPT1, extensive analysis of mammalian genome databases, screening of intestinal tissue banks and immunohistology have not yet provided evidence for more than one peptide carrier in the brush border membrane of small intestinal epithelial cells.[43]

From these physiological considerations, protein malabsorption would be expected in diseases causing (1) pancreatic insufficiency; (2) loss of mucosal surface such as occurs in short bowel syndrome and celiac disease; (3) generalized impaired enterocyte function accompanying celiac disease; and (4) impaired dipeptide or amino acid transport by the enterocyte. The last possibility, impaired dipeptide or amino acid transport at the enterocyte membrane is extremely rare. Several of these diseases are noted in Table 30.1.

Severe loss of body protein may occur in protein maldigestion or malabsorption before there is evidence of laboratory abnormalities. This loss is more likely to occur when there is insufficient protein intake. Impaired protein synthesis from liver diseases and excessive protein loss in renal disease can further aggravate protein deficiencies. Clinically, protein deficiency results in edema and diminished muscle mass. Since the immune system is dependent upon adequate protein, protein deficiency can manifest as recurrent or severe infections. Alternatively, there may be growth retardation, mental apathy and irritability. Other features of protein deficiency include weakness, muscle atrophy, edema, hair loss, deformity of skeletal bone, anorexia, vomiting and diarrhea.

Vitamins

Fat-soluble vitamins

Diseases causing malabsorption of dietary fat commonly cause malabsorption of fat-soluble vitamins. This is especially important in diseases that also result in impaired micelle formation due to bile salt deficiency, such as biliary atresia. Failure to absorb the fat-soluble vitamins A, D, E and K results in a variety of symptoms. Vitamin A deficiency is associated with follicular hyperkeratosis. Vitamin E deficiency leads to a progressive demyelination of the central nervous system. Malabsorption of vitamin D causes osteopenia and rickets. Vitamin K deficiency may be associated with easy bruisability and/or bleeding into the nose, bladder, vagina, or gastrointestinal tract.

Water soluble vitamins

Folic acid The principal source of folic acid comes from dietary folates (folacins) that are widely distributed in foods; liver, yeast, leafy vegetables, legumes and some fruits. All folacins are hydrolyzed to folic acid, or pteroylglutamic acid, during digestion absorption. Pteroylglutamic acid is absorbed at a faster rate than larger polymers. Only 25–50% of dietary folacin is nutritionally available. Boiling destroys folate activity. The daily requirement for folate is approximately 100 μg. On the basis of a 50% food folate absorption, the recommended dietary allowance is 200 μg. Tissue stores of folate are only about 3 mg; therefore, malabsorption can deplete the body of folate within 1 month.

Polyglutamate forms of folate are hydrolyzed to the monoglutamate form. This hydrolysis takes place at the brush border by the enzyme folate conjugase. Folic acid is absorbed from the intestinal lumen by a sodium-dependent carrier. Once in the intestinal epithelial cell, folic acid is methylated and reduced to the tetrahydric form.

Interference with folic acid absorption at the brush-border carrier site occurs with drugs such as phenytoin and sulfasalazine. In addition, folic acid deficiency itself can impair folic acid absorption by producing 'megaloblastic' changes in columnar epithelial cells of the intestine creating an abnormal epithelium. Congenital isolated folate in malabsorption is rare, but has been described.[44]

Vitamin B_{12} Vitamin B_{12} is the generic term for compounds with bioactivity. Cobalamin refers to cobalt-containing compounds with a corrin ring. Cobalamin is the preferred term to distinguish those compounds that are active in humans from the many analogs produced by bacteria. Micro-organisms in the human colon synthesize cobalamin, which is absorbed in small amounts. However, strict vegetarians who do not eat cobalamin-containing meats may develop cobalamin deficiency. The average Western diet contains 10–20 μg/day. The daily requirement for cobalamin is 0.3 μg for infants and 2.0 μg for adult males. The human liver is the repository of approximately 5 mg of cobalamin. The large hepatic stores account for the delay of several years in the clinical appearance of vitamin B_{12} deficiency once cobalamin malabsorption begins.

When cobalamin is liberated from food, it is bound at acid pH to haptocorrin (R binder).[45] R binders or proteins are glycoproteins present in many body secretions, including serum, bile, saliva and gastric and pancreatic juices. Most of the gastric R protein is from swallowed saliva. The haptocorrin cannot mediate the absorption of cobalamin alone and its physiologic function is incompletely understood.

The cobalamin/haptocorrin complex, bound in the upper intestinal tract, leaves the stomach along with free intrinsic factor. In the duodenum, pancreatic proteases in the presence of bicarbonate hydrolyze the haptocorrin, thereby liberating free cobalamin. The cobalamin now combines with gastric intrinsic factor. A conformational change takes place, allowing the cobalamin/intrinsic-factor complex to be resistant to proteolytic digestion. This resistance allows the complex to safely traverse the small intestine and reach the ileum, its site of active absorption. In the ileum, the cobalamin/intrinsic-factor complex binds to a specific receptor located on the brush border. Free cobalamin without intrinsic factor does not bind to the ileal receptor. After passage across the enterocytes, cobalamin is transported in blood bound to circulating proteins known as transcobalamins.

Pancreatic insufficiency may lead to cobalamin deficiency, but lack of intrinsic factor or pernicious anemia is the most common cause of cobalamin deficiency. Bacterial overgrowth of the small intestine disrupts the cobalamin-intrinsic factor complex, decreasing cobalamin absorption. Giardia lamblia infestation is also associated with cobalamin malabsorption. Cobalamin absorption may be impaired after ileal resection or by diseases affecting more than 50 cm of the terminal ileum, such as Crohn's disease, celiac disease, tuberculosis and lymphoma. Finally, bariatric surgery is being performed on a limited number of morbidly obese teenagers. Vitamin B_{12} absorption has been shown to be compromised following gastric bypass surgery.[46] Clearly there is a wide diversity in the etiology of cobalamin deficiency and this requires a versatile diagnostic approach.

Other water soluble vitamins Most of the water-soluble vitamins, like the B vitamins and vitamin C (ascorbic acid) are absorbed in the small intestine by either carrier-mediated transport or by passive diffusion. Generalized malabsorption syndromes, such as occurs in Crohn's disease, impair the absorption of these vitamins and can lead to a deficiency state. However, water soluble vitamin malabsorption and deficiency is less frequent in the pediatric population than are malabsorption and deficiencies of fat-soluble vitamins.

Minerals

Iron

Iron is available for absorption from vegetables (non-heme iron) and from meats (heme iron). Heme iron is better absorbed (10–20%) than non-heme iron (1–6%). It is also less affected by intraluminal factors or dietary composition. The average dietary intake of iron is 10–20 mg/day. Men absorb 1–2 mg/day, while menstruating women and iron-deficient patients absorb 3–4 mg/day. In acute blood loss, increased absorption of iron does not occur for 3 days. Non-heme iron, in the ferric iron (Fe^{+++}) state, when ingested into a stomach unable to produce acid, forms insoluble iron complexes, which are not available for absorption. In the presence of gastric acid and ascorbic acid, ferrous iron (Fe^{++}) forms. The ferrous iron complexes to a mucopolysaccharide of about 200 000 MW and is transported as a complex into the duodenum and proximal jejunum. There in the presence of ascorbic acid, glucose and cysteine, the iron is absorbed. Dietary factors such as phosphate, phytate and phosphoproteins can render the iron insoluble and inhibit iron absorption.

Both heme and non-heme iron are absorbed most rapidly in the duodenum. Some of the iron absorbed is deposited as ferritin within the enterocyte and the remainder is transferred to plasma-bound transferrin. When the enterocyte defoliates, iron deposited as ferritin is lost into the intestinal lumen. This mechanism for loss is probably overwhelmed by the large amount of iron ingested. The amount of iron absorbed from the intestine depends largely upon two factors: (1) total body iron content and (2) rate of erythropoiesis.

Any disease that is associated with mucosal atrophy of the small intestine may be associated with iron malabsorption. Drugs that suppress gastric acid secretion can also contribute to the malabsorption of this mineral. Recent studies of *Helicobacter pylori* gastritis have shown that this infection raises gastric pH, depresses levels of gastric ascorbic acid and may contribute to the development of iron deficiency anemia.[47,48]

Calcium

Calcium absorption occurs in the proximal small intestine and is dependent on vitamin D intake. Calcium needs are greater during puberty than at any other time in life.[49] The efficiency of calcium absorption is increased during puberty as bone formation is optimized. Balance studies have indicated that for most healthy subjects, the maximal net calcium balance during puberty is achieved with intakes between 1200 and 1500 mg calcium/day. During puberty, the efficiency of conversion of 25-hydroxy-vitamin D to 1,25$(OH)_2$ vitamin D increases.

Calcium malabsorption is most frequently related to the direct damage of small intestine mucosa as occurs in celiac disease, with a significant reduction of the intestinal surface area. It also accompanies diseases causing fatty acid malabsorption. The malabsorbed fats complex with calcium forming insoluble calcium soaps. Deficiency of vitamin D and renal disease will contribute to calcium malabsorption, as will hypoparathyroidism and inborn defects in either 1, 25(OH)2 vitamin D formation or in defects in the intestinal vitamin D receptor.

Magnesium

In small intestine disorders, such as Crohn's disease, celiac disease and autoimmune-enteropathies, magnesium absorption may be affected by direct damage to the small intestine surface. In addition, the absorption of magnesium may be compromised by the luminal binding of the magnesium to the malabsorbed fat that occurs in these diseases. A congenital form of selective intestinal magnesium malabsorption has been reported.[50]

Zinc

Like other minerals, zinc is malabsorbed in mucosal disease of the small intestine. There is also zinc malabsorption in acrodermatitis enteropathica. Differentiating acrodermatitis from acquired zinc deficiencies can be difficult because both conditions present in the same manner. Some studies have shown that low zinc levels in the mother's milk may produce an acquired zinc deficiency in full-term, breast-fed infants. Acrodermatitis enteropathica tends to occur in the first few months of life shortly after discontinuation of breast-feeding. Two new proteins that are absent in the fibroblasts of patients with acrodermatitis enteropathica have recently been discovered.[51] These proteins may be responsible for the decreased zinc absorption and abnormal zinc metabolism that occurs in dermatitis enteropathica.

Water

Malabsorption of water can occur in diseases affecting the intestine. The epithelium of the small intestine exhibits passive permeability to salt and water. Osmotic equilibration between plasma and the intestinal lumen is fairly rapid; therefore, large differences in ion concentration do not develop. Intercellular junctions are more permeable to cations (positively charged ions) than anions (negatively charged ions). Therefore, intestinal lumen-to-blood concentration differences for Na^+ and K^+ are generally smaller than those for Cl^- and HCO_3^-. The colonic epithelium displays lower passive permeability to salt and water than the epithelium of the small intestine. One consequence of this lower passive ionic permeability (higher electrical resistance) is that electric potential differences across the colonic epithelium are an order of magnitude greater than those in the small intestine. Active Na^+ absorption, which is the main transport activity of the distal colon, generates a serosa-positive charge or potential difference (PD). Under the influence of aldosterone, this PD can be 60 mV or even higher. A 60 mV PD will sustain a 10-fold concentration difference for a monovalent ion such as K^+. Most of the high K^+ concentration in the rectum is accounted for by the PD. Despite the high fecal K^+ level, little K^+ is lost in the stool, since stool volume (about 200–300 ml/day) is normally so low. In contrast, during high-volume (>1000 ml/day) diarrhea of small bowel origin (rotavirus, cholera), the stool K^+ concentration is considerably lower, but stool K^+ loss is nonetheless great because of the large fluid volume that is malabsorbed. In such states, the stool K^+ concentration is low and the Na^+ concentration relatively high because diarrheal fluid passes through the colon too rapidly to equilibrate across the colonic epithelium.

In the small intestine, active electrolyte and fluid absorption can be conceived of as either nutrient-dependent or nutrient-independent. The absorptive processes for glucose and neutral amino acids are Na^+-dependent so that one Na^+ molecule is translocated across the brush border with each glucose or amino acid molecule. The sodium pump (Na^+/K^+-ATPase), which is located exclusively in the basolateral membrane of the enterocyte of the small intestine, extrudes Na^+ that has entered the cell from the lumen, thereby maintaining a low intracellular Na^+, a high intracellular K+ and a negative intracellular to extracellular electric potential. This Na^+/K^+ pump provides the potential energy for uphill sugar and amino acid absorption. Glucose is co-transported with sodium. Patients in intestinal secretory states such as cholera can absorb glucose normally. Sodium and water are also absorbed, accompanying the transport of glucose. As a consequence, the fluid losses of these patients can be replaced by oral glucose-electrolyte solutions.[52] These individuals generally do not require intravenous fluids unless they are comatose or too nauseated to drink the necessary large volumes of fluid to correct the dehydration. Application of this knowledge has had a major impact on the health of children worldwide. The oral rehydration therapy can be life-saving for children and adults with cholera-like diarrheas, which are so prevalent in developing countries, and state of the art facilities and hospitals are not required for this simple therapy.

In the distal colon, the luminal membrane contains Na^+ channels, which can be blocked by low concentrations of the diuretic amiloride. The Na^+ entering through these channels is then extruded across the basolateral membrane by the Na^+/K^+-ATPase pump discussed above. Aldosterone increases the number of these channels and also increases the number of Na^+/K^+-ATPase pumps. Aldosterone therefore enhances active Na^+ absorption in the distal colon. Chloride is absorbed along with Na^+ and traverses the epithelium by both cellular and paracellular routes. The transcellular route involves a Cl^-/HCO_3^- exchanger in the luminal membrane and Cl^- channels in the basolateral membrane. Intracellular mediators such as cyclic AMP (cAMP) do not appear to affect these Na^+ channels. Thus, patients with secretory diarrheas, especially those who are salt-depleted and therefore have elevated blood levels of aldosterone, are able to reabsorb some of the secreted fluid in their distal colon. Spironolactone, which inhibits the action of aldosterone, can increase the severity of diarrhea in such patients.

Water and electrolyte absorption and secretion in the small and large intestine can be adversely affected by a variety of hormones, bile salts, endotoxins, fatty acids and pathologic conditions. When this occurs and this finely tuned system of absorption and secretion is disrupted, water and electrolyte flux may be altered with significant or even massive losses of intestinal water and electrolytes.

DIAGNOSTIC APPROACH

History

A good history, a physical examination and judicious use of laboratory studies usually provide the information necessary to diagnose a maldigestion or malabsorption disorder.

The symptoms of diarrhea, weight loss and poor growth are not unique to malabsorption. Many disorders that do not directly affect the gastrointestinal tract may produce similar symptoms. Urinary tract infections and certain disease of the central nervous system may cause diarrhea and other signs or symptoms suggestive of malabsorption. However, with other clues from a complete and accurate clinical history, a cause can often be postulated. Important aspects of the history include the following:

1. A chronologic description of all symptoms (e.g. fever, diarrhea, abdominal pain), the relation of symptoms to changes in lifestyle or stress and information concerning the introduction of antibiotics or other medications should be obtained. Exacerbation of chronic medical problems should also be considered.
2. Assessment of appetite, activity and sleeping habits before the onset of the symptoms is important.
3. A dietary history is necessary to assess intake in terms of nutritional type and quantity. Note should be made of the dietary manipulations employed in an attempt to

controversial.[66,67] However, it does remain a relatively noninvasive screen for adequate proximal small intestinal surface area.

Third phase testing

Intestinal biopsy

The diagnostic value of small intestinal biopsy varies with the disease process. Capsule biopsy specimens are obtained from the area of the duodenojejunal junction and endoscopic biopsies are usually obtained from the proximal to middle duodenum. Serial biopsy specimens from other areas of the proximal small bowel can be considered when intermittent or patchy disease distribution is suspected. The careful mounting of the biopsy sample before fixation allows for proper orientation.

Pancreatic testing

Finally, there are a variety of specific tests for assessment of pancreatic secretory function. These include provocative pancreatic secretion testing. The bentiromide excretion test and, most recently, a noninvasive stable-isotope method to assess pancreatic exocrine function have also been used.[68]

MANAGEMENT

Only selected management principles are outlined here, because treatment principles have been noted elsewhere in this volume.

Therapy for malabsorptive disorders is based on first identifying the disease process and then applying specific treatment principles for the disease. Second, if protein-calorie malnutrition and/or any vitamin or trace mineral deficiency is present, it should be vigorously treated either enterally, parenterally, or by both approaches. The goal of nutritional support in pediatric practice is to provide adequate calories, lipids, protein, vitamins and trace minerals for catch-up growth and maintenance of normal growth.

Maldigestion

For altered luminal digestion, specific therapies can be initiated, depending on the cause of the maldigestion. Supplemental enzymes may be provided to augment depressed enzyme secretion by the pancreas, as in cystic fibrosis and Shwachman-Diamond syndrome. The enzymes can be given along with a histamine receptor antagonist or proton pump inhibitor to minimize acid-mediated degradation of the enzymes. However, with the high-potency pancreatic enzyme supplements used today, colonic strictures (fibrosing colonopathy) have been described and there are now specific recommendations for the use of these replacement enzymes.[69,70] Fat-soluble vitamin supplements can be provided in an attempt to overcome disorders of absorption. New pharmacologic strategies have been developed to enhance the absorption of vitamin E with the use of polyethylene glycol.[71,72] Dietary medium-chain triglycerides can improve fat absorption in patients with impaired triglyceride digestion and absorption. Liver disease and cholestasis can occur with cystic fibrosis. Some disorders of cholestasis can be improved by the use of ursodeoxycholic acid, which stimulates bile flow, resulting in improvement in fat digestion. Cotting and colleagues demonstrated improved liver function and nutritional status in eight cystic fibrosis patients treated with ursodeoxycholic acid.[73]

Dumping syndrome has been shown to be a complication of the Nissen fundoplication. Symptoms associated with dumping syndrome can be alleviated with the use of uncooked starch.[74]

Malabsorption

In patients with mild to moderate malabsorption, a slow continuous infusion of nutrients by way of a nasogastric tube or through a gastrostomy may increase absorption. The slow rate increases the contact time between nutrients and the absorptive surface. This form of therapy is ideal for nocturnal feedings, but an enteral infusion pump is necessary. Other methods, such as the use of taurine, may improve fat absorption in patients with cystic fibrosis.[75]

Patients with severe malabsorption that has resulted in significant protein-calorie malnutrition may require parenteral nutritional support, which can provide the necessary nutrients, including minerals, vitamins and iron.

In the future, new drugs as well as designer formulas and nutrients may allow healthcare professionals to optimize intestinal digestion and absorption in patients with diseases of the intestinal tract.

References

1. Ushijima K, Riby JE, Kretchmer N. Carbohydrate malabsorption. Pediatr Clin North Am 1995; 42(4):899–915.
2. Ganong WF. Gastrointestinal Function. Review of Medical Physiology. 14th edn. Los Altos, CA: Lange Medical Publications; 1989:398–407.
3. Granger DN, Barrowman JA, Kvietys PR. Eating: salivation, mastication and deglutition. Clinical Gastrointestinal Physiology: A Saunders Monograph in Physiology. Philadelphia, PA: WB Saunders; 1985:31–51.
4. Southgate DA. Digestion and metabolism of sugars. Am J Clin Nutr 1995; 62(1):203S–210S.
5. Vesa TH, Marteau P. Korpela R. Lactose Intolerance. J Am Coll Nutr 2000; 19(2):165S–175S.
6. Savilahti E, Launiala K, Kuitunen P. Congenital lactase deficiency. Arch Dis Child 1983; 58:246–252.
7. Sahi T, Launiala K. More evidence for the recessive inheritance of selective adult type lactose intolerance malabsorption. Gastroenterology 1977; 73:231–232.
8. Flatz G. The genetic polymorphism of intestinal lactase activity in adult humans. In: Scriver CR, Beaudet AL, Sly WS, Valle D, eds. The Metabolic and Molecular Bases of Inherited Disease, III, 7th ed. New York, NY: McGraw-Hill; 1995:4441–4450.
9. Järvellä I, Enattah NS, Kokkonen J, Varilo T, Savilahti E, Peltonen L. Assignment of the locus for congenital deficiency to 2q21, in the vicinity of but separate from the Lactase-Phlorizin Hydrolase Gene. Am J Hum Genet 1998; 63:1078–1085.

10. Reddy V, Pershad J. Lactase deficiency in Indians. Am J Clin Nutr 1972; 25:114–119.
11. Habte D, Sterky G, Hjalmarsson B. Lactose malabsorption in Ethiopian children. Acta Paediatr Scand 1973; 62(6):649–654.
12. Northrop-Clewes CA, Lunn PG, Downes RM. Lactose maldigestion in breast-feeding Gambian infants. J Pediatr Gastroenterol Nutr 1997; 24(3):257–263.
13. Vince JD. Diarrhoea in children in Papua New Guinea. Papua New Guinea Med J 1995; 38(4):262–271.
14. Weijers HA, va de Kamer JH, Dicke WK, Ijsseling J. Diarrhoea caused by deficiency of sugar splitting enzymes. I. Acta Paediatr 1961; 50:55–71.
15. Belmont JW, Reid B, Taylor W, et al. Congenital sucrase-isomaltase deficiency presenting with failure to thrive, hypercalcemia and nephrocalcinosis. BMC Pediatr 2002; 2(1):4.
16. Treem WR, McAdams L, Stanford L, Kastoff G, Justinich C, Hyams J. Sacrosidase therapy for congenital sucrase-isomaltase deficiency. J Pediatr Gastroenterol Nutr 1999; 28:137–142.
17. Arola H, Koivula T, Karvonen AL, Jokela H, Ahola T, Isokoski M. Low trehalase activity is associated with abdominal symptoms caused by edible mushrooms. Scand J Gastroenterol 2004; 34(9):898–903.
18. Wright EM, Martin MG, Turk E. Intestinal absorption in health and disease – sugars. Best Pr Res Clin Gastroenterol 2003; 17(6):943–956.
19. Linquist B, Meeuwisse G. Chronic diarrhoea caused by monosaccharide malabsorption. Acta Paediatr 1962; 51:674–685.
20. Wright EM. Genetic disorders of membrane transport. I. Glucose galactose malabsorption. Am J Physiol 1998; 275(38):G879–G882.
21. Lowe CV, May DC. Selective pancreatic deficiency: absent amylase, diminished trypsin and normal lipase. Am J Dis Child 1951; 82:459–464.
22. Lilibridge CB, Townes PL. Physiologic deficiency of pancreatic amylase in infancy: a factor in iatrogenic diarrhea. J Pediatr 1973; 82:279–282.
23. Hamosh M. Lipid metabolism in pediatric nutrition. Ped Clin North Am 1995; 42(4):839–862.
24. Lebenthal E, Lee PC. Development of functional response in human exocrine pancreas. Pediatrics 1980; 66:556–660.
25. Thomson ABR, Keelan M, Thiesen A, Clandinin MT, Ropeleski M, Wild GE. Small bowel review: Normal physiology Part 1. Dig Dis Sci 2001; 46(12):2567–2587.
26. Pelsers MM, Namiot Z, Kisielewski W, Namiot A, Januszkiewicz M, Hermens WT, Glatz JF. Intestinal-type and liver-type fatty acid-binding protein in the intestine. Tissue distribution and clinical utility. Clin Biochem 2003; 36(7):529–535.
27. Zimmerman AW, Veerkamp JH. New insights into the structure and function of fatty acid-binding proteins. Cell Mol Life Sci 2002; 59(7):1096–1116.
28. Stremmel W, Pohl L, Ring A, Herrmann T. A new concept of cellular uptake and intracellular trafficking of long-chain fatty acids. Lipids 2001; 36(9):981–989.
29. Clarke SD, Armstrong MK. Cellular lipid binding proteins: expression, function and nutritional regulation. FASEB J 1989; 3(13):2480–2487.
30. Tso P, Balint JA. Formation and transport of chylomicrons by enterocytes to the lymphatics. Am J Physiol 1986; 250(6):G715–G726.
31. Ben-Ami H, Ginesin Y, Behar DM, Fischer D, Edoute Y, Lavy A. Diagnosis and treatment of urinary tract complications in Crohn's disease: an experience over 15 years. Can J Gastroenterol 2002; 16(4):225–229.
32. Worchester EM. Stones from bowel disease. Endocrinol Metab Clin North Am 2002; 31(4):979–999.
33. Schwiebert EM, Benos DJ, Fuller C. Cystic fibrosis: A multiple exocrinopathy caused by dysfunctions in a multifunctional transport protein. Am J Med 1998; 104(6):576–590.
34. Shwachman H, Kowalski M, Khaw KT. Cystic fibrosis: a new outlook. 70 patients above 25 years of age. 1977. Medicine 1995; 74:48–58.
35. Pencharz PB, Durie PR. Pathogenesis of malnutrition in cystic fibrosis and its treatment. Clin Nutr 2000; 19(6):387–394.
36. Rothbaum R, Perrault J, Vlachos A, et al. Shwachman-Diamond syndrome: report from an international conference. J Pediatr 2002; 141(2):164–165.
37. Triantafillidids JK, Kottaras G, Sgourous S, et al. A-beta-lipoproteinemia: clinical and laboratory features, therapeutic manipulations and follow-up study of three members of a Greek family. J Clin Gastroenterol 1998; 26(3):207–211.
38. Berriot-Varoqueaux N, Aggerbeck LP, Samson-Bouma M, Wetterau JR. The role of the microsomal triglyceride transfer protein in abetalipoproteinemia. Annu Rev Nutr 2000; 20:663–697.
39. Stevenson VL, Hardie RJ. Acanthocytosis and neurological disorders. J Neurol 2001; 248(2):87–94.
40. Matthai J. Vitamin E updated. Indian J Pediatr 1996; 63(2):242–253.
41. Sheldon W. Congenital pancreatic lipase deficiency. Arch Dis Child 1964; 39:268–271.
42. Hamosh M. Digestion in the newborn. Clin Perinatol 1996;. 23(2):191–209.
43. Hannelore D. Molecular and integrative physiology of intestinal peptide transport. Ann Rev Physiol 2004; 66:361–384.
44. Malatack J, Moran MM, Moughan B. Isolated congenital malabsorption of folic acid in a male infant: Insights into treatment and mechanism of defect. Pediatrics 1999; 104(5):1133–1137.
45. Gueant JL, Champigneulle B, Gaucher P, Nicolas JP. Malabsorption of vitamin B12 in pancreatic insufficiency of the adult and of the child. Pancreas 1990; 5(5):559–567.
46. Smith CD, Herkes SB, Behrns KE, Fairbanks VF, Kelly KA, Sarr MG. Gastric acid secretion and vitamin B12 absorption after vertical Roux-en-Y gastric bypass for morbid obesity. Ann Surg 1993; 218(1):91–96.
47. Annibale B, Capurso G, Lahner E, et al. Concomitant alterations in intragastric pH and ascorbic acid concentration in patients with Helicobacter pylori gastritis and associated iron deficiency anaemia. Gut 2003; 52(4):496–501.
48. Hacihanefioglu A, Edebali F, Celebi A, et al. Improvement of complete blood count in patients with iron deficiency anemia and Helicobacter pylori infection after the eradication of Helicobacter pylori. Hepatogastroenterology 2004; 51(55):313–315.
49. Saggese G, Baroncelli GI, Bertelloni S. Puberty and bone development. Best Pr Res Clin Endocrinol 2002; 16(1):53–64.
50. Romero R, Meacham LR, Winn KT. Isolated magnesium malabsorption in a 10-year-old boy. Am J Gastroentol 1996; 91(3):611–613.
51. Grider A, Mouat MF. The acrodermatitis enteropathica mutation affects protein expression in human fibroblasts: analysis by two-dimensional gel electrophoresis. J Nutr 1998; 128(8):1311–1314.
52. Avery ME, Snyder JD. Oral therapy for acute diarrhea: The underused simple solution. N Engl J Med 1990; 323(13):891–894.

53. Silverman A, Roy CC. Physical signs. Pediatric Clinical Gastroenterology, 3rd edn. St Louis: Mosby; 1983:38–43.
54. Benson GD, Kowlessar OD, Sleisenger MH. Adult celiac disease with emphasis upon response to the gluten-free diet. Medicine (Baltimore) 1964; 43:1–10.
55. Fielding JF, Cooke WT. Finger clubbing and regional enteritis. Gut 1971; 12:412–444.
56. Hamilton JR, Bruce GA, Abdourhaman M, Gall DG. Inflammatory bowel disease in children and adolescents. Adv Pediatr 1979; 26:311–341.
57. Sondheimer JM. Office stool examination: A practical guide. Contemp Pediatr 1990; 7(2):63–82.
58. Hardt PD, Hauenschild A, Jaeger C, et al; S2453112/S2453113 Study Group. High prevalence of steatorrhea in 101 diabetic patients likely to suffer from exocrine pancreatic insufficiency according to low fecal elastase 1 concentrations: a prospective multicenter study. Dig Dis Sci 2003; 48(9):1688–1692.
59. Walkowiak J, Nousia-Arvanitakis S, Agguridaki C, et al. Longitudinal follow-up of exocrine pancreatic function in pancreatic sufficient cystic fibrosis patients using the fecal elastase-1 test. J Pediatr Gastroenterol Nutr 2003; 36(4):474–478.
60. Dormandy KM, Waters AH, Molin DL. Folic acid deficiency in celiac disease. Lancet 1963; 1:632–635.
61. Ater JL, Herbst J1, Landaw SA, O'Brien RT. Relative anemia and iron deficiency in cystic fibrosis. Pediatrics 1983; 71:810–814.
62. Lundh G. Pancreatic exocrine function in neoplastic and inflammatory disease: a simple and reliable new test. Gastroenterology 1962; 42:275–280.
63. Goldstein R, Blodheim O, Levy E, Stankiewicz H, Freier S. The fatty meal test: An alternative to stool fat analysis. Am J Clin Nutr 1983; 38:763–768.
64. Columbo C, Maiavacca R, Ronchi M, Consalvo E, Amoretti M, Giunta A. The steatocrit: a simple method for monitoring fat malabsorption in patients with cystic fibrosis. J Pediatr Gastroenterol Nutr 1987; 6:926–930.
65. Addison GM. Acid steatocrit. J Pediatr Gastroenterol Nutr 1996; 22:227.
66. Rolles CJ, Nutter S, Kendal MJ, Anderson CM. One-hour blood-xylose screening-test for coeliac disease in infants and young children. Lancet 1973; 2:1043–1045.
67. Lifschitz CH, Polanco I. The D-xylose test in pediatrics: Is it useful? Gastroenterology 1989; 97:246–247.
68. Deutsch JC, Santhosh-Kumar CR, Kolli VR. A noninvasive stableisotope method to simultaneously assess pancreatic exocrine function and small bowel absorption. Am J Gastroenterol 1995; 90:2182–2185.
69. Borowitz DS, Grand RJ, Durie PR. Use of pancreatic enzyme supplements for patients with cystic fibrosis in the context of fibrosing colonopathy. J Pediatr 1995; 127:681–684.
70. Littlewood JM. Management of malabsorption in cystic fibrosis: influence of recent developments on clinical practice. Postgrad Med J 1996; 72(suppl 2):S56–S62.
71. Sokol RJ, Henbi JE, Butler-Simon N. Treatment of vitamin E deficiency during chronic childhood cholestasis with oral D-alpha-tocopheryl polyethylene glycol-1000 succinate. Gastroenterology 1987; 93:975–985.
72. Sokol RJ. Vitamin E and neurologic deficits. Adv Pediatr 1990; 37:119–148.
73. Cotting J, Lentze MJ, Reichen J. Effects of ursodeoxycholic acid treatment on nutrition and liver function in patients with cystic fibrosis and longstanding cholestasis. Gut 1990(31):918–921.
74. Girtzelmann R, Hirsig J. Infant dumping syndrome: reversal of symptoms by feeding uncooked starch. Eur J Pediatr 1986; 145:504–506.
75. Belli DC, Levy E, Darling P, et al. Taurine improves the absorption of a fat meal in patients with cystic fibrosis. Pediatrics 1987; 80:517–523.

Chapter 31
Protracted diarrhea

Simon H. Murch

INTRODUCTION

Protracted diarrhea may occur in many conditions, including several congenital syndromes and a variety of infectious and immunologic states. There have been great advances recently in the understanding of disease mechanisms at the molecular level, which has altered some of the approaches to management of diseases characterized by chronic diarrhea.

Protracted diarrheal disease is one of the major causes of global childhood mortality. The burden of recurrent episodes of diarrheal and other infectious diseases upon infants and children growing in developing world countries is a major cause of nutritional failure. Tropical enteropathy, the enteric consequence of this continuing infectious challenge, may then cause chronic diarrheal disease even in the absence of pathogens, and contributes to malnutrition (Fig. 31.1). It is only within recent decades that mortality from acute diarrheal disease became uncommon in privileged countries of the developed world, and chronic diarrheal disease a relative rarity. Causes of chronic diarrheal disease in developed world countries are generally distinct from those found in the developing world, except in children with underlying immunodeficiency.

The rare syndromes of intractable diarrhea have conceptual importance because of the insights they provide into human physiology and immunology. Important findings have emerged recently from studies of these diseases that have much broader relevance than could have been forecast even a decade ago.

DIARRHEAL DISEASE

Diarrhea is defined on the basis of frequent passage of loose stools. This generally reflects an increased volume of stool water resulting from an increased secretion or decreased absorption. Diarrhea occurs when stool volume exceeds 200 ml per m^2 surface area per day, or loose stool weight of 150–200 g per m^2 surface area per day.[1] In practical terms, childhood diarrhea is usually defined on the basis of increased stool frequency together with a change in consistency towards loose or frankly watery stools. It is important to note the differences in stool frequency and consistency between breast-fed and formula-fed infants, as the stools of the former tend normally to be looser and more frequent than those of the latter.

Diarrheal disease is subdivided into acute diarrhea, of less than 2 weeks' duration, and chronic or persistent diarrhea, of more than 2 weeks' duration. The great majority of cases of acute diarrhea are due to infectious organisms, including bacteria (and their products), viruses and protozoa. There is geographic variability, largely due to the frequency of repeated episodes of bacterial gastroenteritis in developing world children. However, the breakdown of essential sanitation during warfare in countries previously viewed as developed shows that this infectious burden could return to any country. Analysis of infant mortality records from 100 years ago from the USA, UK and northern European countries confirms that chronic diarrheal disease was an important cause of death. In England and Wales in 1903, there were nearly 34 000 infant deaths

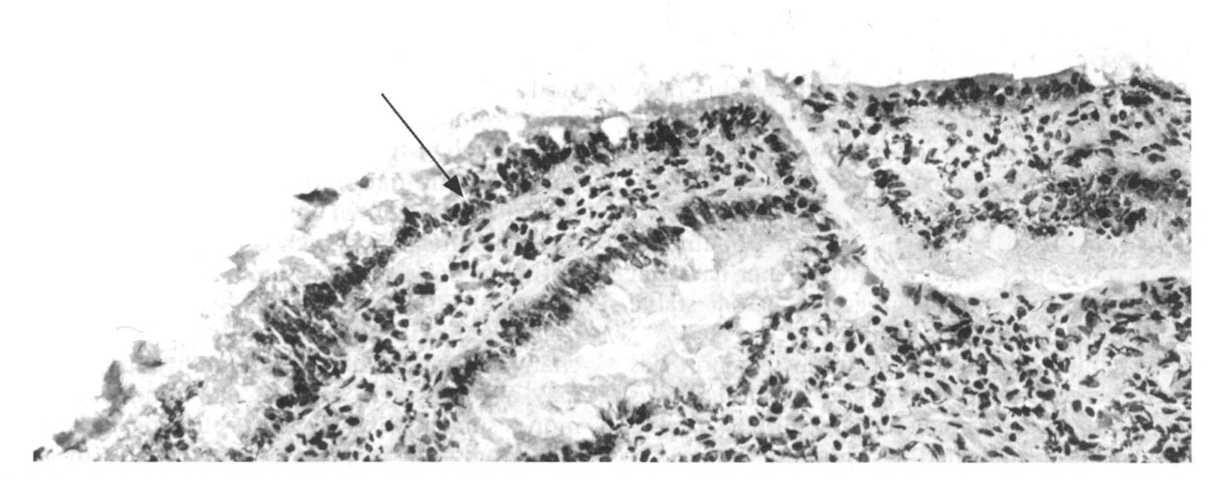

Figure 31.1: Tropical enteropathy in a Gambian infant with chronic diarrhea. Despite preservation of villous structure in this case, there is dense infiltration of γδ T cells (brown-staining; arrow) within the epithelial compartment. (Photomicrograph courtesy of Dr David Campbell.)(See plate section for color)

and either blockade of interleukin-5 or deviation towards Th1 inhibits clearance.[33]

It is uncommon for bacterial infections to persist as long as parasitic infections. Biopsy during the convalescent phase of acute infection may show enteropathy. Electron microscopy may demonstrate diagnostic features (i.e. enteropathogenic *E. coli* infection attaching–effacing lesion). In addition to infection with specific pathogens, malnourished children often suffer sequential infections with different pathogens. It is also important to recognize that persistent small intestinal mucosal inflammation may occur in congenital and acquired immunodeficiency syndromes. Some normally transient gastrointestinal infections, such as rotavirus, may become chronic in these conditions. As general physical health declines in malnourished developing world infants, a vicious circle may thus become established. Similar considerations apply to developed world infants with inborn primary immunodeficiencies. An important practical point is that carbohydrate malabsorption frequently supervenes, due to enteropathy and reduced disaccharidase expression. While lactose-free formulas may reduce the volume of diarrhea, they do not address the primary cause of the enteropathy. To view the complex pathophysiology of post-enteritis enteropathy as a straightforward situation of 'lactose intolerance' is a great oversimplification.[6]

Food-sensitive enteropathies

It has been recognized for many years that food antigens may induce chronic small intestinal enteropathy, and thus lead to persistent diarrhea if unrecognized or untreated. The most important specific enteropathy is celiac disease, which is covered elsewhere in this book. Testing of specific serology for celiac disease is thus important in the investigation of children with chronic diarrheal disease. While the specific HLA types predisposing to celiac disease (HLA-DQ2 and DQ8) are not found in children of ethnically sub-Saharan African origin, they do occur in other developing world populations. Thus celiac disease has been recognized as an important cause of chronic diarrhea in children from Saharan regions and the Indian subcontinent.[34,35]

There is additional evidence that some cases of post-enteritis enteropathy show a food-sensitive component, thought to be due to lost oral tolerance for these antigens after breach of the intestinal barrier.[36–38] Cow's milk enteropathy is the most frequent overlap condition, in which mucosal damage may be initiated by infection and perpetuated by continued antigen ingestion. Treatment with a lactose-free milk-derived formula minimizes symptoms while leaving the underlying pathology untreated. This was a relatively common cause of persistent diarrhea in developed world infants in the days when gastroenteritis was more common than it is now, as was bottle-feeding in the days when cow's milk-derived infant formulas were less well adapted to the human intestine than modern formulas.

Immunodeficiency and chronic diarrhea

Pediatric immunologists are familiar with the fact that many children with primary immunodeficiency have chronic diarrhea and failure to thrive.[20] Much has yet to be learned about specific patterns of enteropathy in different syndromes. Primary immunodeficiency syndromes can cause unexplained chronic diarrhea, presumably due to enteropathy, or may allow chronic pathogen infection. Although there have been significant advances in the recognition of the molecular basis of primary immunodeficiency,[21,39] there is still little knowledge about specific patterns of enteropathy in different syndromes. However, chronic diarrhea is particularly common in severe combined immune deficiency (SCID). Other primary immune deficiencies in which chronic diarrhea has been reported include thymic hypoplasia, class II major histocompatibililty complex (MHC) deficiency and CD40 ligand deficiency.[20] Evidence of severe immunodeficiency may not be apparent initially. The overall morphology of the small intestinal mucosa may be relatively normal or may show variable enteropathy. Secondary food sensitization is quite common, and many children benefit from exclusion diets.

Because lymphocyte function is important before birth, allowing negative selection (deletion by apoptosis) of potentially autoimmune T cells, there are specific links between some inborn immunodeficiencies and infant autoimmunity.[22,40] It is likely that many children with autoimmune gastrointestinal diseases will be found to have a specific abnormality in lymphocyte function. The indications for bone marrow transplantation as primary therapy may thus increase with time,[41] and gene transfer therapy may also become viable as the molecular basis of individual conditions is discovered.

It is not just major immunodeficiency that may be associated with gastrointestinal diseases causing chronic diarrhea. The association of minor immunodeficiency with dietary sensitization has been noted for many years, following the finding of low IgA in children with milk allergy by Soothill and colleagues.[42] This condition (transient IgA deficiency of infancy) occurs due to a developmental delay in maturation of IgA responses, possibly reflecting a relative lack of infectious exposures in early life, as it is not seen in developing world infants. Recent findings suggest that transient IgA deficiency is part of a broader pattern of delayed immune maturation that includes low circulating CD8 and natural killer cells, and IgG subclass deficiency.[43,44] In addition to chronic loose stools, children may present in early life with variable combinations of eczema, gut dysmotility and immediate hypersensitivity responses.

Inflammatory enteropathy

True Crohn's disease is uncommon in infants and young children, and many patients with inflammatory enteropathy have primary immunologic conditions, such as chronic granulomatous disease. Other conditions to exclude include Behçet's disease.[18,19] However, IBD is being recognized increasingly in young children, and full assessment may be required to exclude early-onset Crohn's disease or ulcerative colitis. The rare condition of intractable ulcerating enterocolitis of infancy shows predominantly colonic inflammation.[18]

Anatomic abnormalities

These may not present in early infancy, and presentation of malrotation is often much later in life. Secondary bacterial overgrowth may complicate anatomic abnormalities, and worsen malabsorption.

Lymphangiectasia is an important anatomic abnormality that causes protein-losing enteropathy, often also causing a low circulating lymphocyte count and visibly dilated lymphatics at endoscopy. This may also occur secondarily to cardiac lesions such as constrictive pericarditis or following a Fontan procedure.[45] The presentation may mimic celiac disease, with diarrhea and failure to thrive, and eventual hypoproteinemic edema. Small intestinal biopsy may show gross lymphatic dilation, but the lesion may be patchy and biopsies may be normal. Other overlap conditions include the rare enterocyte heparan sulfate deficiency and congenital disorders of glycosylation.[15]

Disorders of gut motility

The most common cause of chronic loose stools in an otherwise apparently healthy child is a benign motility disorder, variously called 'toddler's diarrhea', 'peas and carrots syndrome' (for reasons that are usually obvious on nappy changing) or 'chronic non-specific diarrhea of infancy'. Although 'benign', in the sense that it has no significant effects upon growth or development, its effects may be significant for social or educational reasons, and can sometimes lead to exclusion from nursery school or playgroup if the child remains dependent on nappies or is fecally incontinent.

This condition has been relatively under-researched, in terms of disease mechanism. Although there are frequently abnormal findings on formal study of gut motility, characterized by abnormal migrating eletromyogenic responses and fast small bowel transit, it has been uncertain whether this simply represented a transient stage of immaturity in neural development, or a specific change induced by a recognizable pathophysiologic mechanism.[46] Both viewpoints may be valid, and indeed there are frequently additional behavioral and psychologic issues.

There is now increasing recognition that gut motility may be disturbed by delayed antigen-specific hypersensitive responses, so-called allergic dysmotility due to non-IgE-mediated food allergy.[5] While in-depth discussion of specific mechanisms is beyond the scope of this chapter, it is noteworthy that antigen-induced degranulation of mast cells and eosinophils may play an important role in disturbance of motility and also intestinal secretion.[47] A review of a large British cohort of children with multiple food allergies identified several children with chronic loose stools induced by a variety of food antigens.[44] Thus a dietary history is a relevant undertaking in a child with troublesome 'toddler's diarrhea', and in selected cases a therapeutic trial of dietary exclusions can be helpful.

Pseudo-obstruction represents a much more malignant form of enteric dysmotility, and can be a cause of intestinal failure severe enough to warrant small intestinal transplantation.[48,49] Secretory and osmotic diarrhea may occur as a consequence of both neurogenic abnormalities and severe secondary bacterial overgrowth. This condition may occur due to failure of appropriate enteric neural migration *in utero*, failed development of intestinal pacemaker activity (dependent on the interstitial cells of Cajal), smooth muscle myopathy or acquired due to inflammatory destruction of enteric neural components.[48,50]

Enteropathy associated with primary metabolic diseases

Some metabolic diseases may cause protracted diarrhea, notably the mitochondrial cytopathies, and detection of a raised lactate concentration suggests the need for further assessment.[51] Children with a variety of other metabolic disorders, including mucopolysaccharidoses, have diarrhea, although this is understudied. The congenital disorders of glycosylation are particularly linked with protein-losing enteropathy.[15,52] These conditions are caused by defective synthesis of precursors in the *N*-glycosylation pathway, leading to underglycosylation of many proteins. Type 1 congenital disorders of glycosylation syndromes are particularly associated with enteropathy, and transferrin glycosylation screening should be considered in complex cases, particularly if there is hypoalbuminemia or prolonged clotting. Histologic findings include evidence of impaired localization of heparan sulfate within the enterocyte, potentially explaining protein-losing enteropathy.[15]

Enteropathy associated with malignancy

This is extremely rare in childhood, although small bowel lymphoma may present with chronic diarrhea, and may be missed on mucosal biopsy. Affected children are often systemically unwell, and imaging with CT or MRI, or sometimes even diagnostic laparotomy, may be needed.

Specific absorption failure

There are several syndromes of failed specific absorption mechanisms, including carbohydrates (glucose–galactose malabsorption, sucrase–isomaltase deficiency, congenital lactase deficiency), lipids and fat-soluble vitamins (abetalipoproteinemia, hypolipoproteinemia, Anderson's disease, ileal bile-salt receptor deficiency), zinc (acrodermatitis enteropathica) or electrolytes (congenital chloridorrhea, defective jejunal brush-border Na^+/H^+ exchange).[53] Apart from abetalipoproteinemia, in which vacuolated enterocytes are characteristic, there may be no specific histologic features.

Carbohydrate malabsorption syndromes

These autosomal recessive conditions vary from relatively common (sucrase–isomaltase deficiency) to the very rare

58. Hoglund P, Auranen M, Socha J, et al. Genetic background of congenital chloride diarrhea in high-incidence populations: Finland, Poland, and Saudi Arabia and Kuwait. Am J Hum Genet 1998; 63:760–768.
59. Yang H, Jiang W, Furth EE, et al. Intestinal inflammation reduces expression of DRA, a transporter responsible for congenital chloride diarrhea. Am J Physiol 1998; 275:G1445–1453.
60. Holmberg C, Perheentupa J. Congenital Na^+ diarrhea: a new type of secretory diarrhea. J Pediatr 1985; 106:56–61.
61. Booth IW, Stange G, Murer H, Fenton TR, Milla PJ. Defective jejunal brush-border Na^+/H^+ exchange: a cause of congenital secretory diarrhoea. Lancet 1985; i:1066–1069.
62. Schultheis PJ, Clarke LL, Meneton P, et al. Renal and intestinal absorptive defects in mice lacking the NHE3 Na+/H+ exchanger. Nat Genet 1998; 19:282–285.
63. Muller T, Wijmenga C, Phillips AD, et al. Congenital sodium diarrhea is an autosomal recessive disorder of sodium/proton exchange but unrelated to known candidate genes. Gastroenterology 2000; 119:1506–1513.
64. Sherman PM, Mitchell DJ, Cutz E. Neonatal enteropathies: defining the causes of protracted diarrhea of infancy. J Pediatr Gastroenterol Nutr 2004; 38:16–26.
65. Phillips AD, Schmitz J. Familial microvillous atrophy: a clinicopathological survey of 23 cases. J Pediatr Gastroenterol Nutr 1992; 14:380–396.
66. Olivia MM, Perman JA, Saavedra JM, et al. Successful intestinal transplantation for microvillous inclusion disease. Gastroenterology 1994; 106:771–774.
67. Herzog D, Atkinson P, Grant D, et al. Combined bowel–liver transplantation in an infant with microvillous inclusion disease. J Pediatr Gastroenterol Nutr 1996; 22:405–408.
68. Brown GR, Thiele DL, Silva M, Beutler B. Adenoviral vectors given intravenously to immunocompromised mice yield stable transduction of the colonic epithelium. Gastroenterology 1997; 112:1586–1594.
69. Pohl JF, Shub MD, Travelline EE, et al. A cluster of microvillous inclusion disease in the Navajo population. J Pediatr 1999; 134:103–106.
70. Reifen RM, Cutz E, Griffiths AM, Ngan BY, Sherman PM. Tufting enteropathy: a newly recognized clinicopathological entity associated with refractory diarrhea in infants. J Pediatr Gastroenterol Nutr 1994; 18:379–385.
71. Goulet O, Kedinger M, Brousse N, et al. Intractable diarrhoea of infancy with epithelial and basement membrane abnormalities. J Pediatr 1995; 127:212–219.
72. Patey N, Scoazec HY, Cuenod-Jabri B, et al. Distribution of cell adhesion molecules in infants with intestinal epithelial dysplasia (tufting enteropathy). Gastroenterology 1997; 113:833–843.
73. Pulkkinen L, Uitto J. Hemidesmosomal variants of epidermolysis bullosa. Mutations in the $\alpha_6\beta_4$ integrin and the 180-kD bullous pemphogoid antigen/type XV11 collagen genes. Exp Dermatol 1998; 7:46–64.
74. Lachaux A, Bouvier R, Loras-Duclaux I, et al. Isolated deficient $\alpha_6\beta_4$ integrin expression in the gut associated with intractable diarrhea. J Pediatr Gastroenterol Nutr 1999; 29:395–401.
75. Vernier RL, Klein DJ, Sisson SP, et al. Heparan sulfate-rich anionic sites in the human glomerular basement membrane: decreased concentration in congenital nephrotic syndrome. N Engl J Med 1983; 309:1001–1009.
76. Powers MR, Blumenstock FA, Cooper JA, MalikAB. Role of albumin arginyl sites in albumin-induced reduction of endothelial hydraulic conductivity. J Cell Physiol 1989; 141:558–564.
77. Kanwar YS, Linker A, Farquhar MG. Increased permeability of the glomerular basement membrane to ferritin after removal of glycosaminoglycans (heparan sulfate) by enzyme digestion. J Cell Biol 1980; 86:688–693.
78. Niehues R, Hasilik M, Alton G, et al. Carbohydrate-deficient glycoprotein syndrome type 1b – phosphomannose isomerase deficiency and mannose therapy. J Clin Invest 1998; 101:1414–1420.
79. Helenius A, Aebi M. Intracellular functions of *N*-linked glycans. Science 2001; 291:2364–2369.
80. Giraut D, Goulet O, Ledeist F, et al. Intractable diarrhea syndrome associated with phenotypic abnormalities and immune deficiency. J Pediatr 1994; 25:36–42.
81. Landers MC, Schroeder TL. Intractable diarrhea of infancy with facial dysmorphism, trichorrhexis nodosa, and cirrhosis. Pediatr Dermatol 2003; 20:432–435.
82. Powell BR, Buist NR, Stenzel P. An X-linked syndrome of diarrhea, polyendocrinopathy, and fatal infection in infancy. J Pediatr 1982; 100:731–737.
83. Walker-Smith JA, Unsworth DJ, Hutchins P, et al. Autoantibodies against gut epithelium in a child with small-intestinal enteropathy. Lancet 1982; i:566.
84. Mirakian R, Richardson A, Milla PJ, et al. Protracted diarrhoea of infancy: evidence of an autoimmune variant. BMJ 1986; 293:1132–1136.
85. Cuenod B, Brousse N, Goulet O, et al. Classification of intractable diarrhea in infancy using clinical and immunohistological criteria. Gastroenterology 1990; 99:1037–1043.
86. Kobayashi I, Imamura K, Kubota M, et al. Identification of an autoimmune enteropathy-related 75-kilodalton antigen. Gastroenterology 1999; 117:823–830.
87. Verpy E, Leibovici M, Zwaenepoel I, et al. A defect in harmonin, a PDZ domain-containing protein expressed in the inner ear sensory hair cells, underlies Usher syndrome type 1C. Nat Genet 2000; 26:51–55.
88. Bitner-Glindzicz M , Lindley KJ, Rutland P, et al. A recessive contiguous gene deletion causing infantile hyperinsulinism, enteropathy and deafness identifies the Usher type 1C gene. Nat Genet 2000; 26:56–60.
89. Hermiston ML, Gordon JI. Inflammatory bowel disease and adenomas in mice expressing a dominant negative N-cadherin. Science 1995; 270:1203–1207.
90. Cepek KL, Shaw SK, Parker CM, et al. Adhesion between epithelial cells and T lymphocytes mediated by E-cadherin and the $\alpha E\beta 7$ integrin. Nature 1994; 372:190–193.
91. Alarcón B, Regueiro JR, Arnaiz-Villena A, Terhorst C. Familial defect in the surface expression of the T-cell receptor–CD3 complex. N Engl J Med 1988; 319:1203–1208.
92. Arnaiz-Villena A, Timon M, Rodriguez-Gallego C, et al. T lymphocyte signalling defects and immunodeficiency due to the lack of CD3γ. Immunodeficiency 1993; 4:121–129.
93. Martín-Villa JM, Regueiro JR, de Juan D, et al. T-lymphocyte dysfunctions together with apical gut epithelial cell autoantibodies. Gastroenterology 1991; 101:390–397.
94. Moore L, Xu X, Davidson G, et al. Autoimmune enteropathy with anti-goblet cell antibodies. Hum Pathol 1995; 26:1162–1168.
95. Bennett CL, Yoshioka R, Kiyosawa H, et al. X-linked syndrome of polyendocrinopathy, immune dysfunction, and diarrhea maps to Xp11.23-Xq13.3. Am J Hum Genet 2000; 66:461–468.
96. Brunkow ME, Jeffery EW, Hjerrild KA, et al. Disruption of a new forkhead/winged-helix protein, scurfin, results in the fatal lymphoproliferative disorder of the scurfy mouse. Nat Genet 2001; 27:68–73.

97. Wildin RS, Ramsdell F, Peake J, et al. X-linked neonatal diabetes mellitus, enteropathy and endocrinopathy syndrome is the human equivalent of mouse scurfy. Nat Genet 2001; 27:18–20.
98. Bennett 1 CL, Christie J, Ramsdell F, et al. The immune dysregulation, polyendocrinopathy, enteropathy, X-linked syndrome (IPEX) is caused by mutations of *FOXP3*. Nat Genet 2001; 27:20–21.
99. Hori S, Nomura T, Sakaguchi S. Control of regulatory T cell development by the transcription factor Foxp3. Science 2003; 299:1057–1061.
100. Fontenot JD, Gavin MA, Rudensky AY. *Foxp3* programs the development and function of CD4+ CD25+ regulatory T cells. Nat Immunol 2003; 4:330–336.
101. Gambineri E, Torgerson TR, Ochs HD. Immune dysregulation, polyendocrinopathy, enteropathy, and X-linked inheritance (IPEX), a syndrome of systemic autoimmunity caused by mutations of *FOXP3*, a critical regulator of T-cell homeostasis. Curr Opin Rheumatol 2003; 15:430–435.
102. Wildin RS, Smyk-Pearson S, Filipovich AH. Clinical and molecular features of the immunodysregulation, polyendocrinopathy, enteropathy, X linked (IPEX) syndrome. J Med Genet 2002; 39:537–545.
103. Owen CJ, Jennings CE, Imrie H, et al. Mutational analysis of the *FOXP3* gene and evidence for genetic heterogeneity in the immunodysregulation, polyendocrinopathy, enteropathy syndrome. J Clin Endocrinol Metab 2003; 88:6034–6039.
104. Smyk-Pearson SK, Bakke AC, Held PK, Wildin RS. Rescue of the autoimmune *scurfy* mouse by partial bone marrow transplantation or by injection with T-enriched splenocytes. Clin Exp Immunol 2003; 133:193–199.
105. Padeh S, Theodor R, Jonas A, Passwell JH. Severe malabsorption in autoimmune polyendocrinopathy–candidosis–ectodermal dystrophy syndrome successfully treated with immunosuppression. Arch Dis Child 1997; 76:532–534.
106. Zuklys S, Balciunaite G, Agarwal A, et al. Normal thymic architecture and negative selection are associated with aire expression, the gene defective in the autoimmune–polyendocrinopathy–candidiasis –ectodermal dystrophy (APECED). J Immunol 2000; 165:1976–1983.
107. Chin RK, Lo JC, Kim O, et al. Lymphotoxin pathway directs thymic *Aire* expression. Nat Immunol 2003; 4:1121–1127.
108. Liston A, Lesage S, Wilson J, Peltonen L, Goodnow CC. *Aire* regulates negative selection of organ-specific T cells. Nat Immunol 2003; 4:350–354.
109. Anderson MS, Venanzi ES, Klein L, et al. Projection of an immunological self shadow within the thymus by the aire protein. Science 2002; 298:1395–1401.
110. Adamson KA, Pearce SH, Lamb JR, Seckl JR, Howie SE. A comparative study of mRNA and protein expression of the autoimmune regulator gene (*Aire*) in embryonic and adult murine tissues. J Pathol 2004; 202:180–187.
111. Chen W, Jin W, Hardegen N, et al. Conversion of peripheral CD4+ CD25− naive T cells to CD4+ CD25+ regulatory T cells by TGF-β induction of transcription factor Foxp3. J Exp Med 2003; 198:1875–1886.
112. Martin-Villa JM, Camblor S, Costa R, Arnaiz-Villena A. Gut epithelial cell autoantibodies in AIDS pathogenesis. Lancet 1993; 342:380.
113. Khattri R, Kasprowicz D, Cox T, et al. The amount of scurfin protein determines peripheral T cell number and responsiveness. J Immunol 2001; 167:6312–6320.
114. Goulet OJ, Brousse N, Canioni D, Walker-Smith JA, Schmitz J, Phillips AD. Syndrome of intractable diarrhoea with persistent villous atrophy in early childhood: a clinicopathological survey of 47 cases. J Pediatr Gastroenterol Nutr 1998; 26:151–161.

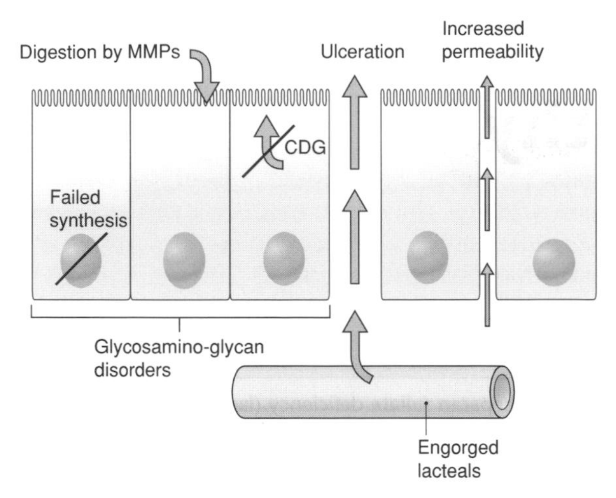

Figure 32.1: Mechanisms of protein-losing enteropathy. Protein can be lost through several mechanisms in the digestive tract, including increased permeability and discontinuity of the epithelial barrier (ulceration) as a result of inflammation, primary or secondary lymphangiectasia (due to engorged lacteals), or disorders of epithelial glycosaminoglycans. These can either be mislocalized (as in the case of congenital glycosylation disorders; CDGs), not synthesized (as in enterocyte heparan sulfate deficiency), or digested at the surface of the enterocyte by matrix metalloproteinases (MMPs). Any of these mechanisms will result in leakage of vascular proteins into the gut lumen.

CAUSES OF PLE

Abnormal enterocyte expression of heparan sulfate proteoglycan

Focal degradation of glycosaminoglycan during intestinal inflammation

Intestinal inflammation is characterized by a sustained inflammatory cascade that gives rise to the release of mediators capable of degrading and modifying bowel wall structure. An example of these mediators is matrix metalloproteinases (MMPs). These enzymes are capable of degrading extracellular matrix components and have been implicated in tissue remodeling and ulceration in inflammatory bowel disease, celiac disease and *Helicobacter pylori* infection.[2–5] Although normally there are mucosal inhibitors of these enzymes, their intestinal concentration can be decreased in patients with intestinal inflammation.[2] Therefore, during intestinal inflammation degradation of epithelial proteoglycans can go unopposed, with consequent protein leakage. In addition, increased epithelial permeability, local hyperemia and disruption of the integrity of the epithelial barrier (ulceration) can also contribute to the loss of intestinal protein (Fig. 32.1). Potentially, inflammation in any portion of the digestive tract can lead to PLE. These entities are discussed in detail elsewhere in this book, including esophagitis, gastritis, enteritis and colitis due to different etiologies. Therefore, the presence of PLE does not localize the pathologic process to any specific portion of the gastrointestinal tract.

Failed synthesis of enterocyte glycosaminoglycans

Murch et al.[6] described three young male infants who presented within the first weeks of life with massive enteric protein loss, secretory diarrhea and intolerance of enteral feeds in spite of normal intestinal biopsy findings. All required total parenteral nutrition and repeated albumin infusions. By specific histochemistry, a gross abnormality was detected in all three infants in the distribution of small intestinal glycosaminoglycans, with complete absence of enterocyte heparan sulfate. The distribution of vascular and lamina propria glycosaminoglycans was, however, normal. The authors suggested that these children had a congenital defect in the synthesis of enterocyte proteoglycans, and that these were important in normal intestinal function.

Congenital disorders of glycosylation

CGDs are multisystemic disorders characterized by defects in *N*-glycosylation of proteins. They can present with multisystemic involvement, including liver disease, PLE, cyclic vomiting and diarrhea.[7–9]

The pathophysiology of CDGs involves abnormalities in the intracellular processing of proteins. Most secreted, cell-surface and extracellular proteins are glycosylated. During normal *N*-glycosylation there are two distinct steps. The first phase involves the assembly and transfer of a 14-sugar-unit precursor from a lipid carrier to protein in the endoplasmic reticulum. This precursor is called the lipid-linked oligosaccharide. In the second step there is subsequent modification of the protein-bound sugar chains in the endoplasmic reticulum and Golgi apparatus to produce a properly folded protein. These proteins can then be directed to the cell membrane or exported by the cell.[9] When protein glycosylation is defective as a result of congenital causes, it can lead to disease in humans – the so-called CDGs. Defects in the steps up to and including the synthesis and transfer of the lipid-linked oligosaccharide to protein are called group I CDG. Group II consists of defects in subsequent oligosaccharide processing.

Perhaps the most interesting form of CDG for the pediatric gastroenterologist is CDG-Ib (OMIM 602579, 154550). This disorder is caused by phosphomannose isomerase (PMI) deficiency. Loss of PMI decreases the guanidine diphosphate (GDP)–mannose pools and limits the amount of available lipid-linked oligosaccharide that can bind to proteins. Although other forms of CDG are characterized by a wide variety of neurologic manifestations, patients with CDG-Ib have normal motor and mental development, and their clinical presentation is dominated by symptoms of gastrointestinal and liver disease.[8,9] These children may present with chronic diarrhea, cyclic vomiting, PLE, coagulopathy, hypoglycemia and hepatomegaly. Hypoalbuminemia, raised aminotransferase and low antithrombin III levels are characteristic. Partial villous atrophy from intestinal biopsies can falsely suggest celiac disease. Liver biopsy may reveal hepatic fibrosis with ductal plate malformations. Children with evidence of hepatomegaly, portal hypertension, hepatic fibrosis and/or steatosis, hypoglycemia, failure to thrive, coagulopathy or hypoglycemia should be tested for CDG-Ib by transferrin isoelectric focusing and enzymatic analysis. Other diagnostic modalities include transferrin mass spectrometry and molecular analysis of PMI mutations.[9]

PLE caused by lymphangiectasia

Intestinal lymphangiectasia is characterized histologically by dilation of the lacteals in the small intestine that distorts the villous architecture. Classically, there is absence of inflammation. Poor lymphatic drainage produces increased intestinal lymphatic pressure and leakage of lymph into the intestinal lumen, with consequent loss of protein and lymphocytes.[10] Intestinal lymphangiectasia can be congenital or secondary to a disease that interferes with intestinal lymphatic drainage.

Primary intestinal lymphangiectasia (OMIM 152800)

Waldmann and Schwab[11] reported that patients with edema of the legs and low serum protein levels had intestinal protein loss, presumably due to lymphangiectasia. Subsequently Murphy observed that these patients were lymphopenic and had double vortex pilorum ('hair whorl') and prominent 'floating ribs' (ribs 11 and 12).[11a] Strober et al.[10] then reported the presence of hypogammaglobulinemia, skin anergy and impaired allograft rejection (OMIM 4168730) in these patients. Later it was suggested that increased fibrinolysis in the gastrointestinal mucosa might play an important role in enhancing mucosal permeability to plasma proteins in intestinal lymphangiectasia.[12,13]

Patients with intestinal lymphangiectasia can present at any age during childhood, from premature infants[14] to adolescents.[15] Children typically complain of diarrhea as their first symptom, often before 3 years of age. Vomiting, growth retardation and peripheral lymphedema are also common. Children can present with seizures due to hypocalcemia. In some cases there is a family history of lymphedema. Lymphopenia may be present initially, but can appear years after the protein loss begins. Spontaneous remissions may occur.[16]

A number of distinct syndromes characterized by intestinal lymphangiectasia and a variety of congenital malformations have been described, including Hennekam lymphangiectasia–lymphedema syndrome (OMIM 235510), Urioste's syndrome (OMIM 235255) and a variant of macrocephaly – cutis marmorata telangiectatica congenita (OMIM 602501).[17] Intestinal lymphangiectasia has also been reported in some patients with autoimmune polyglandular disease type 1 (OMIM 240300),[18] aplasia cutis congenita[19] and Noonan's syndrome (OMIM 163950). Other organ systems can be affected in patients with intestinal lymphangiectasia, including the lung, uterus and conjunctiva.[20] Enamel changes and other dental problems have been described.[21] Rarely, a patient may present with gastrointestinal blood loss.[15,22,23]

Secondary lymphangiectasia

Cardiovascular causes Although structural heart defects,[24] constrictive pericarditis[25–27] and obstruction of the venous drainage can all engorge intestinal lymphatics and lead to PLE, the largest cardiac group with PLE comprises children with the cavopulmonary anastomosis for palliation of the univentricular heart, the so-called Fontan procedure. During the Fontan operation, the venous blood returning from the body is channeled to the lungs in a passive fashion without the use of a ventricular pumping chamber. For reasons that are not well understood, PLE develops in 4–11% of patients after Fontan palliation.[28] Chronically raised systemic venous pressure and increased thoracic duct pressure are thought to be responsible for the development of PLE in these patients, with immunologic or inflammatory factors perhaps superimposed.[28] Raised pulmonary resistance or obstruction to pulmonary blood flow can cause increased systemic venous pressure. However, it remains unclear what finally triggers the development of PLE and why it sometimes develops many years after surgery in children who are doing well from the hemodynamic point of view. Patient risk factors for the development of PLE post-Fontan include heterotaxia, polysplenia, anomalies of systemic venous return, ventricular anatomic variants (other than dominant left ventricle), increased pulmonary arteriolar resistance and increased left ventricular pressure. Interestingly, patients with tricuspid atresia are less likely to develop PLE than other groups.[28] Perioperative risk factors include longer cardiopulmonary bypass time, increased left atrial pressure after the operation, longer hospital stay and presence of postoperative renal failure.[29] Some laboratory findings have suggested an immune-mediated or autoimmune disorder with immune complex formation, complement activation and endothelial damage.[30] Coagulation disorders with low protein C levels correlate with the very early stage of PLE without clinical signs. PLE can start, as judged by increased fecal α1-antitrypsin concentration, before symptoms of diarrhea or hypoproteinemia appear.[31–33] Once the symptoms of PLE are established, there seems to be an ongoing progression, with intestinal lymphatic dysfunction and poor prognosis, with reported historical 5-year survival rates of 46–59%.

Systemic lupus erythematosus Hypoalbuminemia in systemic lupus erythematosus (SLE) is usually secondary to renal protein loss. The most common immune-mediated pathologic conditions involving the gastrointestinal tract during the course of SLE are represented by arterial vasculitis and abdominal vessel thrombosis. PLE is an uncommon cause of hypoalbuminemia in SLE, and may or may not be associated with lymphangiectasia.[34–44] Rarely it may present in association with chylothorax and chylous ascites.[45] PLE has been reported to respond to oral corticosteroids in adult patients, although in some patients more aggressive immunosuppression is needed to alleviate symptoms.[46] In addition, diet and octreotide have also been used in patients with SLE, with reported benefit.[46]

tify segmental intestinal involvement amenable to surgical resection, and computed tomography with intravenous and oral contrast.

TREATMENT

PLE associated with many forms of gastrointestinal inflammation improves by treating the underlying disease. The specific therapies for these disorders are reviewed elsewhere in this book.

CDG-Ib is a treatable disorder. Mannose supplementation circumvents the enzymatic defect and can correct defective glycosylation in patients. Doses of 0.1–0.15 g/kg four times daily are effective with no apparent side-effects. Free mannose does not occur in foods, and therefore it needs to be supplemented in these patients.

Intestinal lymphangiectasia can be treated with a high-protein, low-fat diet that is supplemented with medium-chain triglycerides (MCTs), which will be absorbed directly into the portal circulation. Octreotide has been helpful,[78–81] but should probably be reserved for patients who fail dietary therapy with MCT oil because of its cost and inconvenience. Antiplasmin therapy (*trans*-4-aminomethyl cyclohexane carboxylic acid) may have some role, based on the hypothesis that mucosal fibrinolysis increases mucosal permeability in patients with lymphangiectasia.[13,82] Surgery is reserved for palliation of large chylous ascites[83,84] or resection of isolated lesions.[85]

In PLE secondary to the Fontan procedure, the success rate of medical and surgical treatments aimed at treating PLE by reducing systemic venous pressure is very limited and ranges only from 19% to 40%. Medical treatments seem more promising than surgical revision. Some experts believe that therapeutic intervention may be most beneficial if started before the manifestation of symptoms of PLE, and advocate determination of serum albumin and serial fecal α1-antitrypsin levels after surgery. Surgical management options include the correction of small hemodynamic lesions and alteration of the primary hemodynamic derangement via fenestration of the systemic venous baffle. In refractory cases, resolution of PLE has been reported after heart transplant. Medical modalities include anticoagulation, medical treatment to improve hemodynamics, and intestinal cell membrane stabilization with high-dose steroids or subcutaneous high-molecular-weight heparin. It is not clear how parenteral heparin stops intestinal protein leakage. Low-molecular-weight heparin does not have the same effect. There is some evidence that performing the Fontan operation at an earlier age before ventricular dysfunction occurs may result in improved long-term results.

References

1. Murch SH. Toward a molecular understanding of complex childhood enteropathies. J Pediatr Gastroenterol Nutr 2002; 34(Suppl 1):S4–S10.
2. Louis E, Ribbens C, Godon A, et al. Increased production of matrix metalloproteinase-3 and tissue inhibitor of metalloproteinase-1 by inflamed mucosa in inflammatory bowel disease. Clin Exp Immunol 2000; 120:241–246.
3. Bebb JR, Letley DP, Thomas RJ, et al. *Helicobacter pylori* upregulates matrilysin (MMP-7) in epithelial cells *in vivo* and *in vitro* in a Cag dependent manner. Gut 2003; 52:1408–1413.
4. Daum S, Bauer U, Foss H-D, et al. Increased expression of mRNA for matrix metalloproteinases-1 and -3 and tissue inhibitor of metalloproteinases-1 in intestinal biopsy specimens from patients with coeliac disease. Gut 1999; 44:17–25.
5. Mori N, Sato H, Hayashibara T, et al. *Helicobacter pylori* induces matrix metalloproteinase-9 through activation of nuclear factor κB. Gastroenterology 2003; 124:983–992.
6. Murch SH, Winyard PJ, Koletzko S, et al. Congenital enterocyte heparan sulphate deficiency with massive albumin loss, secretory diarrhoea, and malnutrition. Lancet 1996; 347:1299–1301.
7. Westphal V, Murch S, Kim S, et al. Reduced heparan sulfate accumulation in enterocytes contributes to protein-losing enteropathy in a congenital disorder of glycosylation. Am J Pathol 2000; 157:1917–1925.
8. Kelly DF, Boneh A, Pitsch S, et al. Carbohydrate-deficient glycoprotein syndrome 1b: a new answer to an old diagnostic dilemma. J Paediatr Child Health 2001; 37:510–512.
9. Freeze HH. Congenital disorders of glycosylation and the pediatric liver. Semin Liver Dis 2001; 21:501–515.
10. Strober W, Wochner RD, Carbone PP, Waldmann TA. Intestinal lymphangiectasia: a protein-losing enteropathy with hypogammaglobulinemia, lymphocytopenia and impaired homograft rejection. J Clin Invest 1967; 46:1643–1656.
11. Waldmann TA, Schwab PJ. Igg (7 S gamma globulin) metabolism in hypogammaglobulinemia: studies in patients with defective gamma globulin synthesis, gastrointestinal protein loss, or both. J Clin Invest 1965; 44:1523–1533.

11a Murphy EA. Familial lymphatic dysplasia with intestinal lymphangiectasia. In: The Clinical Delineation of Birth Defects. GI Tract Including Liver and Pancreas. Part XIII. Baltimore, MD: Williams & Wilkins; 1972:180–181.

12. Kondo M, Nakanishi K, Bamba T, Hosokawa K, Masuda M. Experimental protein-losing gastroenteropathy: role of tissue plasminogen activator. Gastroenterology 1976; 71:631–634.
13. Kondo M, Bamba T, Hosokawa K, Hosoda S, Kawai K, Masuda M. Tissue plasminogen activator in the pathogenesis of protein-losing gastroenteropathy. Gastroenterology 1976; 70:1045–1047.
14. Salvia G, Cascioli CF, Ciccimarra F, Terrin G, Cucchiara S. A case of protein-losing enteropathy caused by intestinal lymphangiectasia in a preterm infant. Pediatrics 2001; 107:416–417.
15. MacLean JE, Cohen E, Weinstein M. Primary intestinal and thoracic lymphangiectasia: a response to antiplasmin therapy. Pediatrics 2002; 109:1177–1180.
16. Vardy PA, Lebenthal E, Shwachman H. Intestinal lymphagiectasia: a reappraisal. Pediatrics 1975; 55:842–851.
17. Megarbane A, Haddad J, Lyonnet S, Clayton-Smith J. Child with overgrowth, pigmentary streaks, polydactyly, and intestinal lymphangiectasia: macrocephaly-cutis marmorata telangiectatica congenita syndrome or new disorder? Am J Med Genet 2003; 116A:184–187.
18. Bereket A, Lowenheim M, Blethen SL, Kane P, Wilson TA. Intestinal lymphangiectasia in a patient with autoimmune polyglandular disease type I and steatorrhea. J Clin Endocrinol Metab 1995; 80:933–935.

19. Bronspiegel N, Zelnick N, Rabinowitz H, Iancu TC. Aplasia cutis congenita and intestinal lymphangiectasia. An unusual association. Am J Dis Child 1985; 139:509–513.
20. Mucke J, Hoepffner W, Scheerschmidt G, Gornig H, Beyreiss K. Early onset lymphoedema, recessive form – a new form of genetic lymphoedema syndrome. Eur J Pediatr 1986; 145:195–198.
21. Dummer PM, Cardiff BD. Severe enamel hypoplasia in a case of intestinal lymphangiectasia: a rare protein-losing enteropathy. Oral Surg Oral Med Oral Pathol 1977; 43:702–706.
22. Perisic VN, Kokai G. Bleeding from duodenal lymphangiectasia. Arch Dis Child 1991; 66:153–154.
23. Takami A, Nakao S, Sugimori N, et al. Management of disseminated intra-abdominal lymphangiomatosis with protein-losing enteropathy and intestinal bleeding. South Med J 1995; 88:1156–1158.
24. Gleason WA Jr, Roodman ST, Laks H. Protein-losing enteropathy and intestinal lymphangiectasia after superior vena cava–right pulmonary artery (Glenn) shunt. J Thorac Cardiovasc Surg 1979; 77:843–846.
25. Wilkinson P, Pinto B, Senior JR. Reversible protein-losing enteropathy with intestinal lymphangiectasia secondary to chronic constrictive pericarditis. N Engl J Med 1965; 273:1178–1181.
26. Nelson DL, Blaese RM, Strober W, Bruce R, Waldmann TA. Constrictive pericarditis, intestinal lymphangiectasia, and reversible immunologic deficiency. J Pediatr 1975; 86:548–554.
27. Kumpe DA, Jaffe RB, Waldmann TA, Weinstein MA. Constrictive pericarditis and protein losing enteropathy. An imitator of intestinal lymphangiectasis. Am J Roentgenol Radium Ther Nucl Med 1975; 124:365–373.
28. Mertens L, Hagler D, Sauer U, Somerville J, Gewillig M. Protein-losing enteropathy after the Fontan operation: an international multicenter study. J Thorac Cardiovasc Surg 1998; 115:1063–1073.
29. Powell AJ, Gauvreau K, Jenkins KJ, Blume ED, Mayer JE, Lock JE. Perioperative risk factors for development of protein-losing enteropathy following a Fontan procedure. Am J Cardiol 2001; 88:1206–1209.
30. Cheung YF, Tsang HY, Kwok JS. Immunologic profile of patients with protein-losing enteropathy complicating congenital heart disease. Pediatr Cardiol 2002; 23:587–593.
31. Fujii T, Shimizu T, Takahashi K, et al. Fecal alpha1-antitrypsin concentrations as a measure of enteric protein loss after modified fontan operations. J Pediatr Gastroenterol Nutr 2003; 37:577–580.
32. Rychik J. Management of protein-losing enteropathy after the Fontan procedure. Semin Thorac Cardiovasc Surg Pediatr Card Surg Annu 1998; 1:15–22.
33. Rychik J, Spray TL. Strategies to treat protein-losing enteropathy. Semin Thorac Cardiovasc Surg Pediatr Card Surg Annu 2002; 5:3–11.
34. Gattorno M, Buoncompagni A, Barabino A, et al. Severe hypoalbuminaemia in a systemic lupus erythematosus-like patient. Eur J Pediatr 2002; 161:84–86.
35. Gornisiewicz M, Rodriguez M, Smith JK, Saag K, Alarcon GS. Protein-losing enteropathy in a young African-American woman with abdominal pain, diarrhea and hydronephrosis. Lupus 2001; 10:835–840.
36. Northcott KA, Yoshida EM, Steinbrecher UP. Primary protein-losing enteropathy in anti-double-stranded DNA disease: the initial and sole clinical manifestation of occult systemic lupus erythematosus? J Clin Gastroenterol 2001; 33:340–341.
37. Yoshida M, Miyata M, Saka M, et al. Protein-losing enteropathy exacerbated with the appearance of symptoms of systemic lupus erythematosus. Intern Med 2001; 40:449–453.
38. Nakajima A, Ohnishi S, Mimura T, et al. Protein-losing enteropathy associated with hypocomplementemia and anti-nuclear antibodies. J Gastroenterol 2000; 35:627–630.
39. Molina JF, Brown RF, Gedalia A, Espinoza LR. Protein losing enteropathy as the initial manifestation of childhood systemic lupus erythematosus. J Rheumatol 1996; 23:1269–1271.
40. Sunheimer RL, Finck C, Mortazavi S, McMahon C, Pincus MR. Primary lupus-associated protein-losing enteropathy. Ann Clin Lab Sci 1994; 24:239–242.
41. Chung U, Oka M, Nakagawa Y, et al. A patient with protein-losing enteropathy associated with systemic lupus erythematosus. Intern Med 1992; 31:521–524.
42. Edworthy SM, Fritzler MJ, Kelly JK, McHattie JD, Shaffer EA. Protein-losing enteropathy in systemic lupus erythematosus associated with intestinal lymphangiectasia. Am J Gastroenterol 1990; 85:1398–1402.
43. Perednia DA, Curosh NA. Lupus-associated protein-losing enteropathy. Arch Intern Med 1990; 150:1806–1810.
44. Benner KG, Montanaro A. Protein-losing enteropathy in systemic lupus erythematosus. Diagnosis and monitoring immunosuppressive therapy by alpha-1-antitrypsin clearance in stool. Dig Dis Sci 1989; 34:132–135.
45. Lee CK, Han JM, Lee KN, et al. Concurrent occurrence of chylothorax, chylous ascites, and protein-losing enteropathy in systemic lupus erythematosus. J Rheumatol 2002; 29:1330–1333.
46. Yazici Y, Erkan D, Levine DM, Parker TS, Lockshin MD. Protein-losing enteropathy in systemic lupus erythematosus: report of a severe, persistent case and review of pathophysiology. Lupus 2002; 11:119–123.
47. Gerdes JS, Katz AJ. Neuroblastoma appearing as protein-losing enteropathy. Am J Dis Child 1982; 136:1024–1025.
48. D'Amico MA, Weiner M, Ruzal-Shapiro C, DeFelice AR, Brodlie S, Kazlow PG. Protein-losing enteropathy: an unusual presentation of neuroblastoma. Clin Pediatr (Phila) 2003; 42:371–373.
49. Coskun T, Ozen H, Buyukpamukcu M, Kale G. Neuroblastoma presenting as protein-losing enteropathy. Turk J Pediatr 1992; 34:107–109.
50. Sivaratnam DA, Pitman AG, Giles E, Lichtenstein M. The utility of Tc-99m dextran in the diagnosis and identification of melanoma metastases responsible for protein-losing enteropathy. Clin Nucl Med 2002; 27:243–245.
51. Case records of the Massachusetts General Hospital. Weekly clinicopathological exercises. Case 7-1999. A 50-year-old woman with severe diarrhea during radiation treatment for resected metastatic melanoma. N Engl J Med 1999; 340:789–796.
52. Chiu EK, Loke SL, Chan AC, Liang RH. T-lymphoblastic lymphoma arising in the small intestine. Pathology 1991; 23:356–359.
53. al-Izzi MS, Sidhu PS, Garside PJ, Menai-Williams R. Angiotropic large cell lymphoma (angioendotheliomatosis) presenting with protein-losing enteropathy. Postgrad Med J 1988; 64:313–314.
54. Konar A, Brown CB, Hancock BW, Moss S. Protein losing enteropathy as a sole manifestation of non-Hodgkin's lymphoma. Postgrad Med J 1986; 62:399–400.
55. Silbert AJ, Ireland JD, Uys PJ, Bowie MD. Hodgkin's lymphoma presenting as a protein-losing enteropathy: a case report. S Afr Med J 1980; 57:1009–1011.

56. Cockington RA. Leukaemic infiltration of the gastrointestinal tract. An unusual cause of protein-losing enteropathy. Med J Aust 1975; 1:103–105.
57. Thomas AG, Livingstone D, Miller V. Protein-losing enteropathy in an infant with a lymphangiomyoma. J Pediatr Gastroenterol Nutr 1989; 9:393–396.
58. Fishman SJ, Burrows PE, Leichtner AM, Mulliken JB. Gastrointestinal manifestations of vascular anomalies in childhood: varied etiologies require multiple therapeutic modalities. J Pediatr Surg 1998; 33:1163–1167.
59. Jackson AE Jr, Peterson C Jr. Hemangioma of the small intestine causing protein-losing enteropathy. Ann Intern Med 1967; 66:1190–1196.
60. Laine L, Garcia F, McGilligan K, Malinko A, Sinatra FR, Thomas DW. Protein-losing enteropathy and hypoalbuminemia in AIDS. Aids 1993; 7:837–840.
61. Novis BH, King H, Bank S. Kaposi's sarcoma presenting with diarrhea and protein-losing enteropathy. Gastroenterology 1974; 67:996–1000.
62. Raymond AR, Rorat E, Goldstein D, Lubat E, Strutynsky N, Gelb A. An unusual case of malignant melanoma of the small intestine. Am J Gastroenterol 1984; 79:689–692.
63. Arbeter AM, Courtney RA, Gaynor MF Jr. Diffuse gastrointestinal polyposis associated with chronic blood loss, hypoproteinemia, and anasarca in an infant. J Pediatr 1970; 76:609–611.
64. Muller AF, Pinder S, Toghill PJ. Juvenile gastric polyposis: reduction in blood- and protein-losing gastropathy with omeprazole. Am J Gastroenterol 1994; 89:444–446.
65. Gourley GR, Odell GB, Selkurt J, Morrissey J, Gilbert E. Juvenile polyps associated with protein-losing enteropathy. Dig Dis Sci 1982; 27:941–945.
66. Younes BS, Ament ME, McDiarmid SV, Martin MG, Vargas JH. The involvement of the gastrointestinal tract in posttransplant lymphoproliferative disease in pediatric liver transplantation. J Pediatr Gastroenterol Nutr 1999; 28:380–385.
67. Rao SS, Dundas S, Holdsworth CD. Intestinal lymphangiectasia secondary to radiotherapy and chemotherapy. Dig Dis Sci 1987; 32:939–942.
68. Thomas DW, Sinatra FR, Merritt RJ. Random fecal alpha-1-antitrypsin concentration in children with gastrointestinal disease. Gastroenterology 1981; 80:776–782.
69. Bunn SK, Bisset WM, Main MJ, Gray ES, Olson S, Golden BE. Fecal calprotectin: validation as a noninvasive measure of bowel inflammation in childhood inflammatory bowel disease. J Pediatr Gastroenterol Nutr 2001; 33:14–22.
70. Rugtveit J, Fagerhol MK. Age-dependent variations in fecal calprotectin concentrations in children. J Pediatr Gastroenterol Nutr 2002; 34:323–324; author reply 324–325.
71. Olafsdottir E, Aksnes L, Fluge G, Berstad A. Faecal calprotectin levels in infants with infantile colic, healthy infants, children with inflammatory bowel disease, children with recurrent abdominal pain and healthy children. Acta Paediatr 2002; 91:45–50.
72. Veldhuyzen van Zanten SJ, Bartelsman JF, Tytgat GN. Endoscopic diagnosis of primary intestinal lymphangiectasia using a high-fat meal. Endoscopy 1986; 18:108–110.
73. Connor FL, Angelides S, Gibson M, et al. Successful resection of localized intestinal lymphangiectasia post-Fontan: role of (99m)technetium-dextran scintigraphy. Pediatrics 2003; [illegible]
74. Yueh TC, Pui MH, Zeng SQ. Intestinal lymphangiectasia: value of Tc-99m dextran lymphoscintigraphy. Clin Nucl Med 1997; 22:695–696.
75. Maki M, Harmoinen A, Vesikari T, Visakorpi JK. Faecal excretion of alpha-1-antitrypsin in acute diarrhoea. Arch Dis Child 1982; 57:154–156.
76. Dossetor JF, Whittle HC. Protein-losing enteropathy and malabsorption in acute measles enteritis. BMJ 1975; 2:592–593.
77. Sarker SA, Wahed MA, Rahaman MM, Alam AN, Islam A, Jahan F. Persistent protein losing enteropathy in post measles diarrhoea. Arch Dis Child 1986; 61:739–743.
78. Weizman Z, Binsztok M, Fraser D, Deckelbaum RJ, Granot E. Intestinal protein loss in acute and persistent diarrhea of early childhood. J Clin Gastroenterol 2002; 34:427–429.
79. Bennish ML, Salam MA, Wahed MA. Enteric protein loss during shigellosis. Am J Gastroenterol 1993; 88:53–57.
80. Dansinger ML, Johnson S, Jansen PC, Opstad NL, Bettin KM, Gerding DN. Protein-losing enteropathy is associated with *Clostridium difficile* diarrhea but not with asymptomatic colonization: a prospective, case–control study. Clin Infect Dis 1996; 22:932–937.
81. Zwiener RJ, Belknap WM, Quan R. Severe pseudomembranous enterocolitis in a child: case report and literature review. Pediatr Infect Dis J 1989; 8:876–882.
82. Rybolt AH, Bennett RG, Laughon BE, Thomas DR, Greenough WB 3rd, Bartlett JG. Protein-losing enteropathy associated with *Clostridium difficile* infection. Lancet 1989; i:1353–1355.
83. Ehringhaus C, Dominick HC, Schuller M. Protein-losing enteropathy associated with *Clostridium perfringens* infection. Lancet 1989; ii:268–269.
84. Nakase T, Takaoka K, Masuhara K, Shimizu K, Yoshikawa H, Ochi T. Interleukin-1 beta enhances and tumor necrosis factor-alpha inhibits bone morphogenetic protein-2-induced alkaline phosphatase activity in MC3T3-E1 osteoblastic cells. Bone 1997; 21:17–21.
85. Lepinski SM, Hamilton JW. Isolated cytomegalovirus ileitis detected by colonoscopy. Gastroenterology 1990; 98:1704–1706.
86. Dubey R, Bavdekar SB, Muranjan M, Joshi A, Narayanan TS. Intestinal giardiasis: an unusual cause for hypoproteinemia. Indian J Gastroenterol 2000; 19:38–39.
87. Sherman P, Liebman WM. Apparent protein-losing enteropathy associated with giardiasis. Am J Dis Child 1980; 134:893–894.
88. Sutton DL, Kamath KR. Giardiasis with protein-losing enteropathy. J Pediatr Gastroenterol Nutr 1985; 4:56–59.
89. Korman SH, Bar-Oz B, Mandelberg A, Matoth I. Giardiasis with protein-losing enteropathy: diagnosis by fecal alpha 1-antitrypsin determination. J Pediatr Gastroenterol Nutr 1990; 10:249–252.
90. Sullivan PB, Lunn PG, Northrop-Clewes CA, Farthing MJ. Parasitic infection of the gut and protein-losing enteropathy. J Pediatr Gastroenterol Nutr 1992; 15:404–407.
91. Hill ID, Sinclair-Smith C, Lastovica AJ, Bowie MD, Emms M. Transient protein losing enteropathy associated with acute gastritis and *Campylobacter pylori*. Arch Dis Child 1987; 62:1215–1219.
92. Cohen HA, Shapiro RP, Frydman M, Varsano I. Childhood protein-losing enteropathy associated with *Helicobacter pylori* infection. J Pediatr Gastroenterol Nutr 1991; 13:201–203.
93. Badov D, Lambert JR, Finlay M, Balazs ND. *Helicobacter pylori* as a pathogenic factor in Menetrier's disease. Am J Gastroenterol 1998; 93:1976–1979.
94. Hochman JA, Witte DP, Cohen MB. Diagnosis of cytomegalovirus infection in pediatric Menetrier's disease by *in situ* hybridization. J Clin Microbiol 1996; 34:2588–2589.

95. Oderda G, Cinti S, Cangiotti AM, Forni M, Ansaldi N. Increased tight junction width in two children with Menetrier's disease. J Pediatr Gastroenterol Nutr 1990; 11:123–127.
96. Hardoff D, Attias D. Transient hypoproteinemia and hypoprothrombinemia in an infant. Eur J Pediatr 1981; 136:221–222.
97. Axton JH. Measles: a protein-losing enteropathy. BMJ 1975; 3:79–80.
98. Burke JA. Strongyloidiasis in childhood. Am J Dis Child 1978; 132:1130–1136.
99. Katz AJ, Twarog FJ, Zeiger RS, Falchuk ZM. Milk-sensitive and eosinophilic gastroenteropathy: similar clinical features with contrasting mechanisms and clinical course. J Allergy Clin Immunol 1984; 74:72–78.
100. Gregg JA, Luna L. Eosinophilic gastroenteritis. Report of a case with protein-losing enteropathy. Am J Gastroenterol 1973; 59:41–47.
101. Beishuizen A, van Bodegraven AA, Bronsveld W, Sindram JW. Eosinophilic gastroenteritis – a disease with a wide clinical spectrum. Neth J Med 1993; 42:212–217.
102. Kuri K, Lee M. Eosinophilic gastroenteritis manifesting with ascites. South Med J 1994; 87:956–957.
103. Moon A, Kleinman RE. Allergic gastroenteropathy in children. Ann Allergy Asthma Immunol 1995; 74:5–12.
104. Karademir S, Akcayoz A, Bek K, et al. Eosinophilic gastroenteritis presenting as protein-losing enteropathy (case report). Turk J Pediatr 1995; 37:45–50.
105. Wing-Harkins DL, Dellinger GW, Lynch C, Mihas AA. Eosinophilic gastro-enteritis associated with protein-losing enteropathy and protein C deficiency. J Int Med Res 1996; 24:155–163.
106. Couper RT, Durie PR, Stafford SE, Filler RM, Marcon MA, Forstner GG. Late gastrointestinal bleeding and protein loss after distal small-bowel resection in infancy. J Pediatr Gastroenterol Nutr 1989; 9:454–460.
107. Kano K, Ozawa T, Kuwashima S, Ito S. Uncommon multisystemic involvement in a case of Henoch–Schonlein purpura. Acta Paediatr Jpn 1998; 40:159–161.
108. Stanley AJ, Gilmour HM, Ghosh S, Ferguson A, McGilchrist AJ. Transjugular intrahepatic portosystemic shunt as a treatment for protein-losing enteropathy caused by portal hypertension. Gastroenterology 1996; 111:1679–1682.
109. Kobayashi A, Obe Y. Protein-losing enteropathy associated with arsenic poisoning. Am J Dis Child 1971; 121:515–517.
110. Plauth WH Jr, Waldmann TA, Wochner RD, Braunwald NS, Braunwald E. Protein-losing enteropathy secondary to constrictive pericarditis in childhood. Pediatrics 1964; 34:636–648.
111. Jaya Rao K, Jindal SK, Khattri HN, Bidwai PS, Sharma RR, Wahi PL. Protein losing enteropathy in constrictive pericarditis. Indian J Chest Dis Allied Sci 1977; 19:92–95.
112. Harada K, Seki I, Okuni M. Constrictive pericarditis with atrial septal defect in children. Jpn Heart J 1978; 19:531–543.
113. Muller C, Wolf H, Gottlicher J, Zielinski CC, Eibl MM. Cellular immunodeficiency in protein-losing enteropathy. Predominant reduction of CD3+ and CD4+ lymphocytes. Dig Dis Sci 1991; 36:116–122.
114. Liu DT, Sherman AM. Pregnancy and intestinal lymphangiectasis (familial neonatal hypoproteinaemia). Aust N Z J Obstet Gynaecol 1980; 20:58–59.
115. Smith S, Schulman A, Weir EK, Beatty DW, Joffe HS. Lymphatic abnormalities in Noonan syndrome: a case report. S Afr Med J 1979; 56:271–274.
116. Dousset B, Legmann P, Soubrane O, et al. Protein-losing enteropathy secondary to hepatic venous outflow obstruction after liver transplantation. J Hepatol 1997; 27:206–210.

Chapter 33
Celiac disease

Riccardo Troncone and Salvatore Auricchio

DEFINITION

Celiac disease (CD), also called gluten-sensitive enteropathy, is a permanent intestinal intolerance to dietary wheat gliadin and related proteins that produces mucosal lesions in genetically susceptible individuals.

HISTORICAL BACKGROUND

CD was first accurately described by Samuel Gee in 1888, but it was not until the early 1950s that Dicke in The Netherlands established the role of wheat and rye flour in the pathogenesis of the disease and identified the protein known as gluten as the harmful factor in those cereals.[1] A major contribution to the understanding of the disease came from the development of methods for peroral biopsy of the jejunal mucosa, which allowed definition of the mucosal lesion,[2] and from the definition of diagnostic criteria published in 1969 by the European Society of Paediatric Gastroenterology and Nutrition (ESPGAN).[3] In recent years a substantial amount of data have been produced that have profoundly changed our understanding of epidemiology, clinical aspects and pathogenesis of CD, opening new perspectives for treatment.

CEREAL PROTEINS AND OTHER ENVIRONMENTAL FACTORS

Cereal proteins

The cereals that are toxic for patients with CD are wheat, rye and barley; rice and maize are non-toxic and are usually used as wheat substitutes in the diet of patients with CD. The toxicity of oats has been reassessed in recent years. It has in fact been shown that the use of oats as part of a gluten-free diet has no unfavorable effects on adult patients in remission and does not prevent mucosal healing in patients with newly diagnosed disease.[4,5] Nonetheless, a few celiacs seem not to tolerate oats, showing raised levels of intestinal interferon gamma mRNA after challenge;[6] furthermore, the fear that small amounts of gliadin could contaminate oats, suggests caution before the inclusion of oats is advocated in the diet of celiac patients. Cereal grains belong to the grass family (*Gramineae*). Grains considered toxic for celiac patients (rye, barley and, to a lesser extent, oats) bear a close taxonomic relationship to wheat, whereas nontoxic grains (rice and maize) are taxonomically dissimilar (Fig. 33.1). Wheat seed endosperm contains heterogeneous protein classes differentiated, according to their extractability and solubility in different solvents, into albumins, globulins, gliadins and glutenins. Gliadins are monomers, whereas glutenins form large polymeric structures. Gliadins have been classified according to their N-terminal amino acid sequences into alpha, gamma and omega types; glutenins are subdivided into high molecular weight glutenins and low molecular weight glutenins. The wheat toxicity results from the gliadin protein fraction and the toxicity of cereals other than wheat is most likely associated with prolamin fractions equivalent to gliadins in the grain of these other species; on the other hand, glutenin peptides have been shown to be immunogenic for mucosal T cells from celiac patients.[7] The amino acid sequence(s) responsible for the disease have not been fully elucidated, also because different parts of the gliadin molecules show different biological properties, all potentially involved in the pathogenesis of the disease; several HLA-DQ2 restricted T-cell epitopes have been found clustering in regions of gliadin rich in proline residues,[8] target of the tissue transglutaminase (TG2) deamidating activity (see pathogenesis); other sequences have been shown to activate innate immunity mechanisms,[9] or interact with CD8+ cytotoxic T cells.[10] Organ culture systems have validated the biological activity of some of these sequences, but there is no doubt that *in vitro* methodology must be paralleled by *in vivo* challenge studies. In fact, histologic changes have been shown to occur in the celiac intestinal mucosa after challenge with synthetic peptides encompassing the 31–49,[11] 31–43 and 44–55,[12] and, more recently, the 56–75 sequence of A-gliadin.[13]

Other environmental factors

The high concordance rate for monozygotic twins and the similar risk shown by dizygotic twins and other siblings, suggest that a shared environment (gluten antigen aside) has little or no effect.[14] On the other hand, the relevance of environmental factors other than gluten in CD is suggested by the significant changes in the incidence of the disease by time and place. Feeding practices seem to be relevant. Recently, Sweden has experienced an epidemic of symptomatic celiac disease in children aged less than 2 years. The abrupt increase and decline in the incidence of the disease coincided with changes in the dietary pattern of infants.[15] The risk of celiac disease was found to be greater when gluten was introduced in the diet in large amounts;[16] on the contrary, it was reduced if children were still breast-fed when dietary gluten was introduced.[16] This finding add to previous case referent studies showing that breast-feeding is protective, while the age of introduction

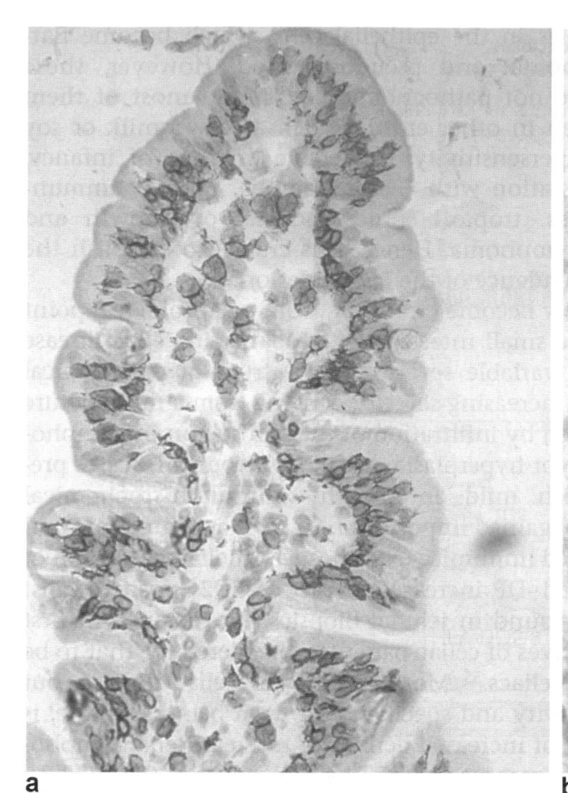

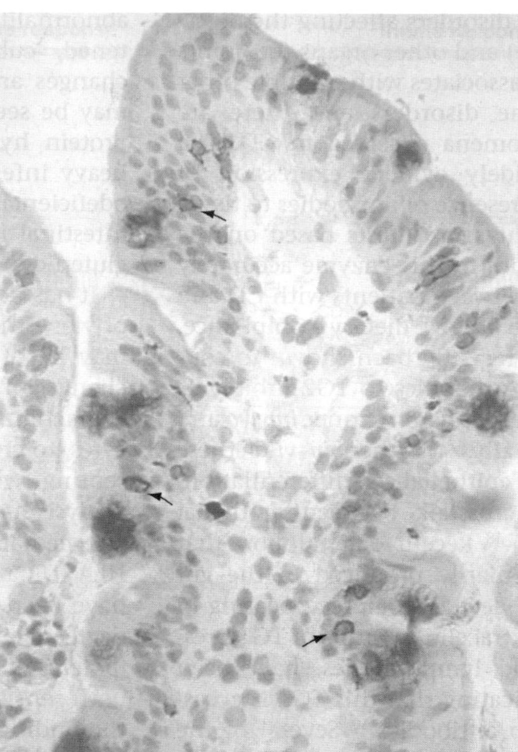

Figure 33.3: Increased density of (**a**) intraepithelial lymphocytes CD3+ and (**b**) intraepithelial lymphocytes expressing the gamma/delta T-cell receptor, in a celiac patient with serum positive antiendomysial antibodies, but normal jejunal architecture. (*See plate section for color*)

porosis has shown an incidence of CD ten-fold higher than in healthy people.[62] As a matter of fact the majority of adult celiac patients suffer from metabolic osteopathy; gluten free diet normalizes bone mass only in a proportion of subjects. Patients whose CD was diagnosed in childhood and who have since then been receiving gluten free diet have a bone mineral density similar to that of healthy controls.[63] The nervous system is also involved in CD. An Italian report has proposed an association between CD and epilepsy in patients with bilateral occipital calcifications[64] (Fig. 33.4); in such patients gluten-free diet beneficially affects the course of epilepsy only when started soon after epilepsy onset. Moreover, gluten sensitivity is proposed to be common in patients with neurological diseases of unknown etiology. One example is gluten ataxia,[65] a recently described condition, which seems to affect 60% of unclassified ataxia and which is identified on the basis of high serum titres of antigliadin antibody; up to 40% of them are celiacs. Peripheral neuropathies of axonal and demyelinating types have also been reported and may respond to elimination of gluten from the diet. There is no doubt that the liver is a target of gluten toxicity in CD. Isolated hypertransaminasemia has been recognized as a possible presentation of CD; it may be expression of chronic 'cryptogenic' hepatitis resolving on a gluten-free diet.[66] As 4% of patients with 'cryptogenic' hepatitis are affected by otherwise silent CD, serological screening for CD is mandatory in such patients.[67] Recently, patients with severe liver disease have been described in whom gluten-free diet prevented progression to hepatic failure, even in cases in which liver transplantation was considered.[68]

Patients having fertility problems may have subclinical CD: unexplained infertility may be the only sign of CD.[69] Similarly, unfavorable outcome of pregnancy such as recurrent abortions, or premature delivery, or low weight at birth, are more often observed in undiagnosed or untreated CD patients.[70] Different degrees of dental abnormalities have been described in children with CD; severe enamel hypoplasia is present in up to 30% of untreated CD children.[71] Alopecia areata has been reported to be the only clinical manifestation of CD.[72]

A special place in this list is taken by dermatitis herpetiformis (DH), a gluten dependent condition characterized by a symmetric pruritic skin rash with subepidermal blisters and granular subepidermal deposits of IgA in remote uninvolved skin. Most patients with DH have abnormal small intestinal biopsy pathology, histologically indistinguishable from that of CD, although usually less severe. Approximately 60% of children with DH have been reported to have subtotal villous atrophy and 30% have partial villous atrophy on jejunal biopsy.[73] The histologic changes return to normal after dietary exclusion of gluten. Therapy with dapsone usually leads to prompt clinical improvement; a strict gluten-free diet permits a reduction or discontinuation of dapsone over a period of months. Improvement of skin lesions on a gluten-free diet seems to occur also in patients with no evident mucosal abnormal-

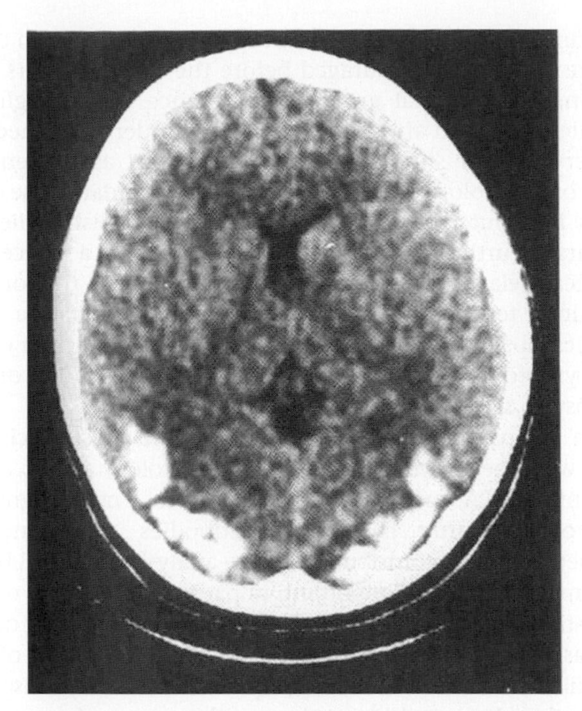

Figure 33.4: CT scan showing bilateral parieto-occipital calcifications in the cortico-subcortical layers in a patient with epilepsy and celiac disease.

ity; in the same patients the rash recurs with a gluten re-challenged.

The mechanisms operating in these different situations may be different. Such extradigestive manifestations may more likely result from the intestinal damage and consequent nutritional deficiencies (e.g. anemia, osteopenia) and/or due to the deranged (auto)immune response (e.g. skin, liver, joints, CNS involvement).

ASSOCIATED DISEASES

Some diseases, many with an autoimmune pathogenesis, are found with a higher than normal frequency in celiac patients; among these are thyroid diseases,[74] Addison's disease,[75] pernicious anemia,[76] autoimmune thrombocytopenia,[77] sarcoidosis,[78] insulin-dependent diabetes mellitus,[79] alopecia[80] and cardiomyopathies.[81] Such associations have been interpreted as a consequence of the sharing of identical HLA haplotypes (e.g. B8, DR3). Nevertheless, the relation between CD and autoimmunity is more complex. In CD patients there is evidence that the risk of developing autoimmune diseases seems to be directly correlated to the duration of gluten exposure.[82]

An increased incidence of CD has been found in Down syndrome patients compared with the general population.[83] Similarly in Turner's syndrome and Williams syndrome higher number of CD cases was also observed.[84,85] Selective IgA deficiency is also a condition associated with celiac disease.[86] Screening test alternatives to those based on the measurement of IgA isotype antibodies must be adopted in such patients.

LABORATORY FINDINGS

Tests for malabsorption and permeability

Tests for malabsorption may be of help in approaching the diagnosis of CD. Determination of hemoglobin, serum iron, calcium, phosphorus, alkaline phosphatase, magnesium and protein levels may be indicative of malabsorption. In particular, red blood cell folate levels have been found to be a sensitive index.[20] Prothrombin levels should be checked in any case before intestinal biopsy is performed.

Over the last few years, tests based on intestinal permeability to sugars have been found of value as a noninvasive screening tool. Most of them are based on the differential intestinal absorption of two non-metabolized sugars. In untreated CD the absorption of the smaller probe (mannitol, rhamnose) is reduced owing to the loss of intestinal surface area and that of the larger one (lactulose, cellobiose) is reported as increased, because paracellular pathways are 'leakier' and/or increased in number. Expression of the results as a ratio of disaccharide: monosaccharide recovery gives clear separation between normal cases and patients with CD.[87,88] Although this test has a sufficient sensitivity for abnormalities of jejunal mucosa, it is also characterized by a low specificity for CD and false-positive results occurring mainly in patients with mucosal abnormalities due to other causes (e.g. Crohn's disease, atopic eczema, food allergy and damage induced by non-steroidal anti-inflammatory agents).

Serological tests

Serological tests have also acquired a strong importance, in particular the search for antiendomysial antibodies; more recently, after the demonstration that tissue transglutaminase is the main autoantigen recognized by endomysial antibodies,[46] anti-tissue transglutaminase antibodies have shown a great sensitivity and specificity for the diagnosis of celiac disease[89] (Table 33.2). The specificity is almost absolute, also considering that subjects with positive serum endomysial antibodies and normal histology have a high chance to develop enteropathy in the following years.[90] On the other hand, a note of caution comes from studies in adult patients indicating a lower sensitivity, particularly in subjects with a milder form of enteropathy.[91] In the last years after first generation test based on the use of guinea pig antigen, the most recent assays, based on the use of recombinant human enzyme as coating antigen in ELISA, have further improved the diagnostic efficacy. We can expect further improvement by the definition of the epitopes of tissue transglutaminase recognized by celiac sera.[49] However, a series of technical problems common to other ELISA tests still are present, for example the correct definition of cut-off values. Furthermore, while it has now been clearly shown that the site of production of endomysial and tissue transglutaminase antibodies is the gut mucosa,[92] and that their presence in the serum is the result of their spillover, is more

Test	Sensitivity	Specificity	PPV	NPD
AGA IgG	57–100	42–98	20–95	41–88
AGA IgA	53–100	65–100	s28–100	65–100
AEA IgA	75–98	96–100	98–100	80–95
Guinea pig tTG	90.2	95		
Human tTg	98.5	98		

Table 33.2 Serological tests for celiac disease (Reproduced from Fasano A and Catassi C. Current approaches to diagnosis and treatment of celiac diseases: an evolving spectrum. Gastroenterology 2001; 121(6): 1527–1528, with permission from the American Gastroenterological Association.

than a working hypothesis the possibility that there are 'seronegative' subjects with presence of such antibodies only in their intestinal secretions.[93]

HLA

As already mentioned, celiac disease is strongly associated with some HLA allele specificities, namely those serologically recognized as HLA DQ2 (90–95% of cases) and HLA DQ8 (approximately 5% of cases); less than 2% of celiac patients lack both HLA specificities; at the same time approximately one-third of our 'normal' population has one or the other marker; that means that the demonstration of being DQ2 and/or DQ8 positive has a strong negative predictive value, but a very weak positive predictive value for the diagnosis of celiac disease. With these limitations, it may prove useful to exclude celiac disease in subjects on a gluten-free diet, or in subjects belonging to at risk groups (e.g. first degree relatives, insulin-dependent diabetics, patients with Down's syndrome) to avoid long term follow-up. Simplified methods based on molecular typing of only the alleles associated to celiac disease have been set up.[94]

DIAGNOSIS

The two requirements mandatory for the diagnosis of CD remain: (1) the finding of villous atrophy with hyperplasia of the crypts and abnormal surface epithelium, while the patient is eating adequate amounts of gluten; and (2) a full clinical remission after withdrawal of gluten from the diet. The finding of circulating IgA antibodies to gliadin, reticulin and endomysium at the time of diagnosis and their disappearance on a gluten-free diet, adds weight to the diagnosis. A control biopsy to verify the consequences on the mucosal architecture of the gluten-free diet is considered mandatory only in patients with equivocal clinical response to the diet and in patients asymptomatic at first presentation (as is often the case in patients diagnosed during screening programs, e.g. first-degree relatives of celiac patients).[95]

Gluten challenge is not considered mandatory, except under unusual circumstances. These include situations where there is doubt about the initial diagnosis, for example when no initial biopsy was done, or when the biopsy specimen was inadequate or not typical of CD. Gluten challenge should be discouraged before the age of 7 years and during the pubertal growth spurt. Once decided, gluten challenge should always be performed under strict medical supervision. It should be preceded by an assessment of mucosal histology and performed with a standard dose of at least 10 g gluten/day without disrupting established dietary habits. A further biopsy is taken when there is a noticeable clinical relapse or, in any event, after 3 to 6 months. Serologic tests (IgA gliadin, reticulin and endomysium antibodies, absorptive and permeability tests), more than clinical symptoms, can be of help in assessing the timing of the biopsy to shorten the duration of the challenge.[96]

In a situation where jejunal histology has lost specificity and with the growing contribution by serology and to a less extent by HLA, many propose to move to a new diagnostic approach mainly based on antibodies and genetics. Nonetheless, the contribution of the analysis of jejunal biopsies may still be very important; in particular the study of the intestinal mucosa could prove decisive in the definition of the disease state. In fact, considering that more than 30% of the population has the HLA alleles implicated in celiac disease and more than 1% a positive serology, with an increasing number of subjects showing signs of minor enteropathy, the same definition of disease and the consequent need of a gluten free diet still awaits a definitive response. It is quite clear that subjects with severe gluten dependent enteropathy face a series of health risks, mainly nutritional; they probably have also higher risk of developing autoimmunity and, although less than previously thought, of presenting neoplastic complications. On the contrary, little is known of those with minor enteropathy, maybe silent from a clinical point of view, for instance subjects belonging to groups such as first degree relatives or insulin-dependent diabetics. A recent report[57] showing nutritional deficiencies also in patients with minor enteropathy, positive serology and 'right' genetics, resolving on a gluten free diet, indicates, in all these subjects, the need for a gluten free diet. Prospective studies are necessary. Until serological methods are improved, the genetic make-up of celiac patients is better defined, it seems wise for a diagnosis of celiac disease still rely on a combined approach based of clinical criteria, histology, serology and genetics.

THERAPY

Gluten-free diet

Since the identification of gluten as etiologic factor in CD, a strict gluten-free diet has become the cornerstone of the management of such patients. Their diet should exclude wheat, rye and barley; the inclusion of oats is still debated, because the toxicity has not been definitively disproved and because of the fear that small amounts of gliadin could contaminate oats; rice and maize are non-toxic and are usually used as wheat substitutes.

The clinical response to withdrawal of gluten is often dramatic, but it must be stressed that the gluten-free diet is recommended for both symptomatic and asymptomatic patients with CD. Normalization of the jejunal histology occurs after about 6 months. The most likely cause of lack of response is failure to adhere strictly to the diet, but the possibility of sensitivity to other dietary proteins, lymphoma and immunodeficiency should also be considered.

All the present evidence strongly supports the view that restriction of gliadin and related prolamines should be complete and for life for all patients. A gluten-free diet is thought to be protective against the development of maligned disease. Patients with celiac disease have a risk of small bowel adenocarcinoma that is about 80-fold greater than that of the general population.[97] The predominant celiac-associated lymphoma is the enteropathy-associated T-cell lymphoma, which doses not respond well to chemotherapy and is rapidly fatal.[98] Malignancies are not the only risk that celiac patients not compliant with gluten-free diet are exposed to; nutritional deficiencies,[99] osteoporosis and more recent evidence that the risk of developing autoimmune diseases is related to the duration of exposure to gluten are additional concerns.[82]

Other therapeutic measures

Specific vitamin, mineral and trace element deficiencies should be corrected. Replacement therapy can generally be discontinued after clinical and histologic recovery on gluten-free diet has been documented.

Other dietary measures are rarely needed. The disaccharidase activity is greatly depressed in atrophic celiac mucosa, but it is advisable to remove milk and lactose-containing products only if intolerance is clinically manifest. Secondary lactase deficiency resolves rapidly after institution of a gluten-free diet and milk can usually be tolerated after 2 to 4 weeks of the diet.

When patients present in celiac crisis, rapid correction of volume depletion and fluid and electrolyte abnormalities is crucial; steroid therapy is helpful. Short-term administration of steroids (2 mg/kg per 24 h of prednisone for 1–2 weeks) may also be used in severely ill infants in whom anorexia and malabsorption do not rapidly respond to the gluten-free diet.

Therapeutic strategies for the future

Significant progress has been made in recent years in the understanding of the cellular and molecular basis of CD and in the consequent identification of possible targets for therapy. Recently it has been shown that, because of the high proline content, gliadin peptides are highly resistant to digestive processing by pancreatic and brush border proteases. Enzyme supplement therapy using bacterial endopeptidases has been proposed to promote complete digestion of cereal proteins and thus destroy T-cell multipotent epitopes. The identification of gliadin peptide sequences having biological effects, either through non immune-mediated mechanisms, or by activation of T cells, is important. Breeding programs and/or transgenic technology may lead to production of wheat that is devoid of biologically active peptide sequences. The identification of specific epitopes may also provide a target for immunomodulation of antigenic peptides. Engineered peptides may potentially bind to HLA molecules but not T-cell receptors (TCR), or bind TCR, but switch a proinflammatory Th1 to a Th2 or protective Th3 response. Other promising areas include inhibition of the innate immune response activated by gliadin peptides, preventing gliadin presentation to T cells by blocking HLA binding sites, use of TG2 inhibitors and assessing IL-10 as a tool to promote tolerance. An immunomodulatory approach will need to have a safety profile equivalent to that of the gluten-free diet, but with the advantage of increased compliance.

References

1. Dicke WM, Weijers HA, Kamer JK Van de. The presence in wheat of a factor having a deleterious effect in cases of coeliac disease. Acta Pediatr 1953; 42:34–42.
2. Shiner M, Doniach I. Histopathologic studies in steatorrhoea. Gastroenterology 1960; 38:419–440.
3. Meeuwisse G. Diagnostic criteria in coeliac disease. Acta Pediatr Scand 1970; 59:461–463.
4. Janatuinen EK, Pikkarainem PH, Kemppainen TA, et al. A comparison of diets with and without oats in adults with celiac disease. N Engl J Med 1995; 333:1033–1037.
5. Srinivasan U, Leonard N, Jones E, et al. Absence of oats toxicity in adult coeliac disease. BMJ 1996; 313:1330–1331.
6. Lundin KE, Nilsen EM, Scott HG, et al. Oats induced villous atrophy in coeliac disease. Gut 2003; 52:164–152.
7. Vader W, Kooy Y, Veelen P Van, et al. The gluten response in children with celiac disease is directed toward multiple gliadin and glutenin peptides. Gastroenterology 2002; 122:1729–1737.
8. Arentz-Hansen H, McAdam SN, Molberg O, et al. Celiac lesion T cells recognize epitopes that cluster in regions of gliadins rich in proline residues. Gastroenterology 2002; 123:803–809.
9. Maiuri L, Ciacci C, Ricciardelli I, et al. Association between innate response to gliadin and activation of pathogenic T cell in coeliac disease. Lancet 2003; 362:30–37.
10. Gianfrani C, Troncone R, Mugione P, et al. Celiac disease association with CD8+ T cell responses: identification of a novel gliadin-derived HLA-A2-restricted epitope. J Immunol 2003; 170:2719–2726.
11. Sturgess R, Day P, Ellis HJ, et al. Wheat peptide challenge in coeliac disease. Lancet 1994; 343:758–761.
12. Marsh MN, Morgan S, Ensari A, et al. In vivo activity of peptides 31–43,44–55, 55–68 of A-gliadin in gluten-sensitive enteropathy (GSE). 1995; 108:A871.
13. Fraser JS, Engel W, Ellisi HJ, et al. Celiac disease: in vivo toxicity of the putative immunodominant epitope. Gut 2003; 52:1698–1702.
14. Greco L, Romino R, Coto I, et al. The first large population based twin study of coeliac disease. Gut 2002; 50:624–628.
15. Ivarsson A, Persson LA, Nystrom L, et al. Epidemic of coeliac disease in Swedish children. Acta Paediat 2000; 89:165–171.
16. Ivarsson A, Hernell O, Stenlund H, et al. Breast-feeding protects against celiac disease. Am J Clin Nutr 2002; 75:914–921.
17. Auricchio S, Follo D, Ritis G de, et al. Working hypothesis: does breast feeding protect against the development of clinical symptoms of coeliac disease in children? J Pediatr Gastroenterol Nutr 1983; 2:428–433.

18. Monteleone G, Pender SL, Alstead E, et al. Role of interferon alpha in promoting T helper cell type 1 responses in the small intestine in coeliac disease. Gut 2001; 48:425–429.
19. Ivarsson A, Hernell O, Nystrom L, et al. Children born in the summer have increased risk for coeliac disease. J Epidemiol Community Health 2003; 57:36–39.
20. Auricchio S, Mazzacca G, Tosi R, et al. Coeliac disease as a familial condition: identification of asymptomatic coeliac patients within family groups. Gastroenterol Int 1988; 1:25–31.
21. Sollid ML, Markussen G, Ek J, et al. Evidence for a primary association of celiac disease to a particular HLA-DQ alpha/beta heterodimer. J Exp Med 1989; 169:345–350.
22. Karell K, Louka AS, Moodie SJ, et al. HLA types in celiac disease patients not carrying the DQA1*05-DQB1*02 (DQ2) heterodimer: results from the European Genetics Cluster on celiac disease. Hum Immunol 2003; 64:469–477.
23. Vader W, Stepniak D, Kooy Y, et al. The HLA-DQ2 gene dose effect in celiac disease is directly related to the magnitude and breadth of gluten-specific T cell responses. Proc Natl Acad Sci USA 2003; 100:12390–12395.
24. Djilali-Saiah I, Schmitz J, Harfouch-Hammoud E, et al. CTLA-4gene polymorphism is associated with predisposition to celiac disease. Gut 1998; 43:187–189.
25. Babron MC, Nilsson S, Adamovic S, et al. Meta and pooled analysis of European coeliac disease data. Eur J Hum Genet 2003; 11:828–834.
26. Greco L, Corazza G, Babron MC, et al. Genome search in celiac disease Am J Hum Genet 1998;. 62:669–675.
27. Belzen MJ Van, Meijer JW, Sandkuijl LA, et al. A major non-HLA locus in celiac disease maps to chromosome 19. Gastroenterology 2003; 125:1032–1041.
28. Greco L, Maki M, Di Donato F, Visakorpi IK. Epidemiology of coeliac disease in Europe and the Mediterranean area: a summary report on multicentre study by the European Society of Paediatric Gastroenterology and Nutrition. In: Auricchio S, Visakorpi JK, eds. Common Food Intolerances. Vol 1: Epidemiology of Coeliac Disease. Basel: Karger; 1992:25–44.
29. Maki M, Mustalahti K, Kokkonen J, et al. Prevalence of celiac disease among children in Finland. N Engl J Med 2003; 348:2517–2524.
30. Fasano A, Catassi C. Current approaches to diagnosis and treatment of celiac disease: an evolving spectrum. Gastroenterology 2001; 120:636–551.
31. Collin P, Rasmussen M, Kyronpalo S, et al. The hunt for coeliac disease in primary care. QJM 2002; 95:75–77.
32. Andria G, Cucchiara S, Vizia B De, et al. Brush border and cytosol peptidase activities of human small intestine in normal subjects and celiac disease. Pediatr Res 1980; 14:812–818.
33. Hausch F, Shan L, Santiago NA, et al. Intestinal digestive resistance of immunodominant gliadin peptides. Am J Physiol Gastrointest Liver Physiol 2002; 283:G996–G1003.
34. Shan L, Molberg O, Parrot I, et al. Structural basis for gluten intolerance in celiac sprue. Science 2002; 297:2275–2279.
35. Matysiak-Budnik T, Candalh C, Dugave C, et al. Alterations of the intestinal transport and processing of gliadin peptides in celiac disease. Gastroenterology 2003; 125:696–707.
36. Sollid L. Coeliac disease dissecting a complex inflammatory disorder. Nat Rev Immunol 2002; 9:647–655.
37. Salvati VM, MacDonald TT, Bajaj-Elliott M, et al. Interleukin 18 and associated markers of T Helper cell type 1 activity in coeliac disease. Gut 2002; 50:186–190.
38. Mazzarella G, MacDonald TT, Salvati VM, et al. Constitutive activation of the signal transducer and activator of transcription pathway in celiac disease lesions. Am J Pathol 2003; 162:1845–1855.
39. Salvati VM, MacDonald TT, Vecchio Blanco G Del, et al. Enhanced expression of interferon regulatory factor-1 in the mucosa of children with celiac disease. Pediatr Res 2003; 54:312–318.
40. Forsberg G, Hernell O, Melgar S, et al. Paradoxical coexpression of proinflammatory and Down-regulatory cytokines in intestinal T cells in childhood celiac disease. Gastroenterology 2002; 123:667–678.
41. Daum S, Bauer U, Foss HD, et al. Increased expression of mRNA for matrix metalloproteinases-1 and -3 and tissue inhibitor of metalloproteinases-1 in intestinal biopsy specimens from patients with coeliac disease. Gut 1999; 44:17–25.
42. Salvati VM, Bajaj-Elliott M, Poulsom R, et al. Keratinocyte growth factor and coeliac disease. Gut 2001; 49:176–181.
43. Jabri B, Serre NP De, Cellier C, et al. Selective expansion of intraepithelial lymphocytes expressing the HLA-E-specific natural killer receptor CD94 in celiac disease. Gastroenterology 2000; 118:867–879.
44. Maiuri L, Ciacci C, Raia V, et al. FAS engagement drives apoptosis of enterocytes of coeliac patients. Gut 2001; 48:418–424.
45. Ciccocioppo R, Di Sabatino A, Parroni R, et al. Cytolytic mechanisms of intraepithelial lymphocytes in coeliac disease. Clin Exp Immunol 2000; 120:235–240.
46. Dieterich W, Ehnis T, Bauer M, et al. Identification of tissue transglutaminase as the autoantigen of celiac disease. Mat Med 1997; 3:797–801.
47. Esposito C, Paparo F, Caputo I, et al. Anti-tissue transglutaminase antibodies from coeliac patients inhibit transglutaminase activity both in vitro and in situ. Anti-tissue transglutaminase antibodies from coeliac patients inhibit transglutaminase activity both in vitro and in situ. Gut 2002; 51:177–181.
48. Halttunen T, Maki M. Serum immunoglobulin A from patients with celiac disease inhibits human T84 intestinal crypt epithelial cell differentiation. Gastroenterology 1999; 116:566–572.
49. Marzari R, Sblattero D, Florian F, et al. Molecular dissection of the tissue transglutaminase autoantibody response in celiac disease. J Immunol 2001; 166:4170–4176.
50. Korponay-Szabo IR, Halttunen T, Szalai Z, et al. In vivo targeting of intestinal and extraintestinal transglutaminase 2 coeliac autoantibodies. Gut :in press.
51. Sollid LM, Molberg O, McAdam S, Lundin KE. Autoantibodies in coeliac disease: tissue transglutaminase-guilt by association? Gut 1997; 41:851–852.
52. Clemente MG, Musu MP, Frau F, et al. Immune reaction against the cytoskeleton in coeliac disease. Gut 2000; 47:520–526.
53. Sanchez D, Tuckova L, Mothes T, et al. Epitopes of calreticulin recognised by IgA autoantibodies from patients with hepatic and celiac disease. J Autoimmun 2003; 21:383–392.
54. Stulik J, Hernychova L, Porkertova S, et al. Identification of new celiac disease autoantigens using proteomic analysis. Proteomics 2003; 3:951–956.
55. Holm K, Savilahti E, Koskimies S, et al. Immunohistochemical changes in the jejunum in first degree relatives of patients with coeliac disease and the coeliac disease marker DQ genes. HLA class II antigen expression, interleukin-2 receptor positive cells and dividing crypt cells. Gut 1994; 35:55–60.
56. Spencer J, Isaacson PG, MacDonald TT, et al. Gamma/delta T cells and the diagnosis of coeliac disease. Clin Exp Immunol 1991; 85:109–113.

57. Kaukinen K, Maki M, Partanen J, et al. Celiac disease without atrophy. Dig Dis Sci 2001; 46:879–887.
58. Cacciari E, Volta U, Lazzari R, et al. Can antigliadin antibody defect symptomless coeliac disease in children with short stature? Lancet 1985; 1(8444):1469–1471.
59. Bottaro G, Cataldo F, Rotolo N, Spina M, Corazza GR. The clinical pattern of subclinical/silent celiac disease: an analysis on 1026 consecutive cases. Am J Gastroenterol 1999; 94:691–696.
60. Corazza GR, Valentini RA, Andreani ML, et al. Subclinical coeliac disease is a frequent cause of iron-deficiency anemia. Scand J Gastroenterol 1995; 30:153–156.
61. Maki M, Hallstrom O, Verronen P, et al. Reticulin antibody, arthritis and coeliac disease in children. Lancet 1988; 1(8583):479–480.
62. Lindh E, Ljungahall S, Larsson K, Lavo B. Screening for antibodies against gliadin in patients with osteoporosis. J Intern Med 1992; 231:403–406.
63. Molteni N, Caraceni MP, Bardella MT, et al. Bone mineral density in adult celiac patients and the effect of gluten-free diet from childhood. Am J Gastroenterol 1990; 85:51–53.
64. Gobbi G, Bouquet F, Greco L, et al. Coeliac disease, epilepsy and cerebral calcifications. Lancet 1992; 340:439–443.
65. Hadjivassiliou M, Gibson A, Davies-Jones GAB, et al. Does cryptic gluten sensitivity play a part in neurological illness? Lancet 1996; 347:369–371.
66. Vajro P, Fontanella A, Mayer M, et al. Elevated serum aminotransferase activity as a presentation of gluten-sensitive enteropathy. J Pediatr 1993; 122:416–419.
67. Volta U, Franceschi L De, Lari F, et al. Coeliac disease hidden by cryptogenic hypertransaminasemia. Lancet 1998; 352:26–29.
68. Kaukinen K, Halme L, Collin P, et al. Celiac disease in patients with severe liver disease: gluten-free diet may reverse hepatic failure. Gastroenterology 2002; 122:881–888.
69. Collin P, Vilska S, Heinonen PK, Hallstrom O, Pikkarainen P. Infertility and coeliac disease. Gut 1996; 39:382–384.
70. Martinelli P, Troncone R, Paparo F, et al. Coeliac disease and unfavourable outcome of pregnancy. Gut 2000; 46:332–335.
71. Aine L, Maki M, Collin P, Keyrilainen O. Dental enamel defects in celiac disease. J Oral Pathol 1990; 19:241–245.
72. Corazza GR, Andreani ML, Venturo N, et al. Celiac disease and alopecia areata: report of a new association. Gastroenterology 1995; 109:1333–1337.
73. Reunala T, Kosnai T, Karpati S, et al. Dermatitis herpetiformis: jejunal findings and skin response to gluten-free diet. Arch Dis Child 1984; 59:517–522.
74. Mulder CJJ. '1:Ytgat GNJ, Groenland F, Pena AS. Combined coeliac disease and thyroid disease: a study of 17 cases. J Clin Nutr Gastroenterol 1988; 3:89–92.
75. Reunala T, Salmi J, Karvonen J. Dermatitis herpetiformis and coeliac disease associated with Addison's disease. Arch Derm 1987; 123:930–932.
76. Stene-Larsen G, Mosvold J, Ly B. Selective vitamin B'2 malabsorption in adult coeliac disease: report on three cases with associated autoimmune diseases. Scand J Gastroenterol 1988; 23:1105–1108.
77. Stenhammar L, Ljunggren CG. Thrombocytopenic purpura and coeliac disease. Acta Paediatr Scand 1988; 77:764–766.
78. Douglas ID, Gillon J, Logan RFA, et al. Sarcoidosis and coeliac disease: an association. Lancet 1984; 2:13–14.
79. Savilahti E, Simell O, Koskimes S, et al. Coeliac disease in insulin-dependent diabetes mellitus. J Pediatr 1986; 108:690–693.
80. Corazza G, Andreani ML, Venturo N, et al. Coeliac disease and alopecia areata: report of a new association. Gastroenterology 1995; 109:1333–1337.
81. Not T, Faleschini E, Tommasini A, et al. Celiac disease in patients with sporadic and inherited cardiomyopathies and in their relatives. Eur Heart J 2003; 24:1455–1461.
82. Ventura A, Magazzu G, Greco L, et al. Autoimmune disorders, coeliac disease: relationship with duration of exposure to gluten. J Pediatr Gastroenterol Nutr 1997; 24:463.
83. Amil Dias J. Wa1ker-Smith J. Down's syndrome and coeliac disease. J Pediatr Gastroenterol Nutr 1990; 10:41–43.
84. Bonamico M, Pasquino AM, Mariani P, et al. Prevalence and clinical picture of celiac disease in Turner Syndrome. J Clin Endocrinol Metab 2002; 87:5495–5498.
85. Giannotti A, Tiberio G, Castro M, et al. Coeliac disease in Williams Syndrome. J Med Genet 2001; 38:767–768.
86. Savilahti E, Pelkonen P, Visakorpi JK. IgA deficiency in children: a clinical study with special reference to intestinal findings. Arch Dis Child 1971; 46:665–670.
87. Juby LD, Rothwell J, Axon ATR. Lactulose-mannitol test: an ideal screen for coeliac disease. Gastroenterology 1989; 96:79–85.
88. Juby LD, Rothwell J, Axon ATR. Cellobiose-mannitol sugar test-a sensitive tubeless test for coeliac disease: results on 1010 unselected patients. Gut 1989; 30:476–480.
89. Sulkanen S, Halttunen T, Laurila K, et al. Tissue transglutaminase autoantibody enzyme-linked immunosorbent assay in detecting celiac disease. Gastroenterology 1998; 115:1322–1328.
90. Collin P, Helin H, Maki M, Hallstrom O, Karvonen AL. Follow-up of patients positive in reticulin and gliadin antibody tests with normal small bowel biopsy findings. Scand J Gastroenterol 1993; 28:595–598.
91. Rostami K, Kerckhaert J, Tiemessen R, Blomberg ME von, Mejer JWR, Mulder CJJ. Sensitivity of anti-endomysium and anti-gliadin antibodies in untreated coeliac disease: disappointing in clinical practice. Am J Gastroenterol 1999; 94:888–894.
92. Picarelli A, Maiuri L, Frate A, Greco M, Auricchio S, Londei M. Production of antiendomysial antibodies after in vitro gliadin challenge of small intestinal biopsy samples from patients with coeliac disease. Lancet 1996; 348:1065–1067.
93. Wahnschaffe U, Urlich R, Riecken EO, Schulzke JD. Celiac disease-like abnormalities in a subgroup of patients with irritable bowel syndrome. Gastroenterology 2001; 121:1329–1338.
94. Sacchetti L, Calcagno G, Ferrajolo A, Sarrantonio C, Troncone R, Micillo M, et al. Discrimination between celiac and other gastrointestinal disorders in childhood by rapid HLA typing. Clin Chem 1998; 62:669–675.
95. Working Group of ESPGAN. Revised criteria for diagnosis of celiac disease. Arch Dis Child 1990; 65:909–911.
96. Mayer M, Greco L, Troncone R, et al. Early prediction of relapse during gluten challenge in childhood coeliac disease. J Pediatr Gastroenterol Nutr 1989; 8:474–479.
97. Swinson CM, Slavin G, Coles EC, et al. Coeliac disease and malignancy. Lancet 1983; 1:111–115.
99. Egan LJ, Walsh SV, Stevens FM, et al. Celiac-associated lymphoma. A single institution experience of 30 cases in the combination chemotherapy era. J Clin Gastroenterol 1995; 21:123–129.
99. Holmes GKT. Long-term health risks for unrecognized coeliac patients. In: Auricchio S, Visakorpi JK, eds. Common Food Intolerances. Vol I. Epidemiology of Coeliac Disease. Basel: Karger; 1992:105–118.

Chapter 34
Short bowel syndrome

Stuart S. Kaufman

DEFINITION

Short bowel syndrome (SBS) refers to the totality of functional impairments that result from a critical reduction in intestinal length. In the absence of therapy, features of SBS include diarrhea and chronic dehydration, malnutrition with weight loss and growth failure and numerous electrolyte and micronutrient deficiencies. Parenteral nutrition (PN) is the primary therapy that defines SBS. The term 'intestinal failure' has been used recently in reference to patients requiring PN because of severely compromised intestinal function of any etiology irrespective of bowel length, including mucosal disorders such as microvillus inclusion disease and tufting enteropathy, as well as severe intestinal pseudo-obstruction.[1] SBS is by far the most common cause of intestinal failure and continues to represent the model for management of these complex disorders.

ETIOLOGY

Frequency of pediatric SBS worldwide is unclear in the absence of a uniform reporting system. Sigalet has estimated an incidence in children of 4.8 per million, which is roughly two-fold greater than incidence in adults.[1,2] SBS most often originates in infancy as a result of congenital malformation of the gastrointestinal tract (Table 34.1). The single most common cause may be small intestinal atresia, particularly when multiple or 'apple-peel' in configuration.[3–7] Small intestinal volvulus secondary to intestinal malrotation is another common cause of SBS, about one-third of the total, as is gastroschisis. These etiologies are not mutually exclusive; malrotation and atresia commonly accompany severe gastroschisis. The other main etiology of SBS is necrotizing enterocolitis (NEC). Severity of NEC and resultant bowel loss is proportional to the degree of prematurity; most extensive gut necrosis requiring resection occurs in infants under 32 weeks gestation. However, NEC also occurs in full-term infants, often precipitated by pre-existing disorders that include severe congenital heart disease.[8] Severe expressions of omphalocele and aganglionosis involving the small bowel as well as colon contribute smaller numbers.

SBS beginning in later childhood and adolescence is caused by an amalgam of disorders that overlap the common etiologies in infancy and adulthood.[9] Rapidly developing, massive intestinal necrosis secondary to volvulus and previously non-symptomatic intestinal malrotation is a relatively common cause in this age group. Massive abdominal trauma and intra-abdominal neoplasia that requires abdominal and pelvic exenteration to complete tumor resection, particularly desmoid tumors in patients with familial adenomatous polyposis, are also observed.

- Neonates
  - Congenital malformation – 60%
    - Gastroschisis
    - Volvulus (secondary to malrotation, mainly; also Meckel's diverticulum, persistent omphalomesenteric duct)
    - Small intestinal atresia, especially multiple jejunal
    - Omphalocele
    - Congenital short bowel
  - Necrotizing enterocolitis – 40%
- Older children and adolescents
  - Volvulus secondary to malrotation
  - Trauma
  - Intra-abdominal neoplasia
  - Rare: Radiation enteropathy (associated with infantile abdominal/pelvic malignancy)

Table 34.1 Etiology of short bowel syndrome in children

INTESTINAL FUNCTION AND THE IMPACT OF INTESTINAL LOSS

Absorption and secretion in the gastrointestinal tract occur in steady state when the gastrointestinal tract is anatomically intact and functionally normal. The upper digestive tract, including stomach, duodenum and proximal jejunum, is principally secretory. In this area, water flows into the lumen passively in response to osmotic gradients originated by active particle transport at the epithelial basolateral plasma membrane. Approximately 8000 ml of fluid passes into the gut lumen daily in adults under the stimulus of food and dietary water.[10] Proximal gut secretion is essential, since dietary solids must first be liquefied before they can be absorbed. Net absorption occurs in all but the most proximal jejunoileum (6500 ml daily) and colon (1000–1500 ml daily) in adults, resulting in only about 200 ml of daily fecal water loss. Absorption, like secretion, of lumen water is passive in response to active and passive solute gradients that are inwardly directed in the distal bowel. Diarrhea in SBS results mainly when, following intestinal resection, aggregate secretion by remnant proximal bowel exceeds the absorptive capabilities of remnant distal bowel. Thus, the region(s) as well as the amount of intestine remaining after resection determine adequacy of assimilation.

Proximal intestinal loss

When mainly proximal intestine is lost, which is unusual in pediatric SBS, clinical impact on digestion is generally small. In some patients, increased gastric output of fluid offsets the usual contribution of the small bowel to the total volume secreted.[11] Gastric acid secretion increases in proportion to the magnitude of the resection, possibly because of a parallel reduction in release of enteric hormones such as somatostatin that inhibit acid production. In some patients, gastric hyperacidity may transiently cause malabsorption by inactivating pancreatic enzymes and precipitating bile acids. However, diarrhea is rarely substantial after proximal intestinal resection, because the more distal jejunum, ileum and colon have sufficient functional reserve to increase fluid uptake three- to five-fold.[10] Similarly, protein and carbohydrate absorption are minimally affected, because their complete assimilation requires only about one-third of normal small bowel length.[12] Rather, only lipids require the entire small bowel for normal uptake, so a substantial intestinal resection from any location may result in nutritionally significant lipid malabsorption.

Distal intestinal loss

Resection of more distal small intestine, particularly ileum, generally reduces nutrient, fluid and electrolyte absorption more than resection of an equivalent length of proximal jejunum.[10,13] The concept that loss of ileum should significantly impair nutrient assimilation is counterintuitive, since most macronutrients are assimilated in the upper small bowel. However, loss of all or most of this region of the small intestine has two consequences in addition to loss of length *per se*.

First, the ileum is *specialized* in comparison with the duodenum and jejunum in that it is the only intestinal segment that reabsorbs bile salts actively. If around one-third or more of the ileum is lost, about 100 cm in adults and 50 cm in children, the compensatory increase in hepatic bile salt synthesis will not keep pace with increased fecal bile salt loss.[1] In that case, the proximal intestinal lumen bile salt concentration will be inadequate for efficient lipid emulsification, contributing to fat malabsorption. Colon fluid losses are increased, both because the colon is impermeable to long chain fatty acids, resulting in an additional non-absorbable osmotic load and because long-chain fatty acids hydroxylated by colonic bacteria stimulate colonocyte electrolyte (and thereby water) secretion, particularly potassium and bicarbonate. A lesser amount of ileal loss may produce bile acid malabsorption without total body bile acid depletion or fat malabsorption. However, diarrhea may still result, since bile acids as well as long-chain fatty acids may stimulate colonic water secretion.[14]

Second, loss of ileum and probably also the ileocecal valve and colon, adversely affects motility of more proximal gut. Ileal loss, i.e. removal of the 'ileal brake', accelerates gastric emptying of liquids and increases proximal small bowel motility directly, thereby shortening total intestinal transit time independent of that resulting from reduction in intestinal length *per se*.[15] The result is a further reduction in contact between luminal contents and the mucosal surface, adding to the aggregate reduction in nutrient, fluid and electrolyte assimilation. Hormones normally secreted by the distal ileal and colonic mucosa, including peptide PYY and GLP-1, probably mediate the ileal brake.[16,17] The relative contributions of the distal ileum, ileocecal valve and proximal colon in slowing proximal motility remain incompletely defined.

Colon loss

The colon normally absorbs only a small fraction of total water reclaimed during digestion, only about 10–15% of the total. The colon also normally plays only a secondary role in digestion; at most, 20% of complex dietary starch and even less (<5%) dietary nitrogen and lipid escape small intestinal absorption.[10] Starches that escape absorption in the small intestine and also soluble fibers are salvaged to a considerable degree in the colon via fermentation to bioavailable short-chain fatty acids, primarily acetic, propionic and butyric acid, by resident anaerobic bacteria.[16,18] Reclamation by colonic fermentation of the increased load of carbohydrates (and proteins) not absorbed in the small intestine becomes a major source of nutrition following massive small intestinal resection. In adults, up to 1100 calories may be recovered daily in this fashion.[19–22] Uptake of short-chain fatty acid molecules in the colon also creates an osmotic gradient that enhances water absorption, thereby curtailing fecal water losses that accrue to malabsorption.

Patients who have lost most of their small bowel but retain continuity with all or some of the colon are at a distinct advantage compared to those with remnant small bowel of comparable length that terminates as an enterostomy, both in terms of nutrition and fluid balance. Conversely, the impact of losing all or most of the colon is determined by the magnitude of coincident small intestinal loss. Patients who have relatively preserved small bowel that ends in an enterostomy do not experience major nutrient impairments owing to the considerable digestive reserve of the small bowel and fluid and electrolyte depletion do not occur if modestly increased losses are compensated with additional intake.

FACTORS THAT DETERMINE PROGNOSIS OF SBS

Small intestinal length and absorptive function

The amount of small intestine remaining after a resection, not the amount removed, is the most import factor determining whether SBS shall develop and if so, whether PN dependence shall be permanent (Fig. 34.1).[3,5,23] It is useful to quantify anatomic intestinal deficiency in relation to

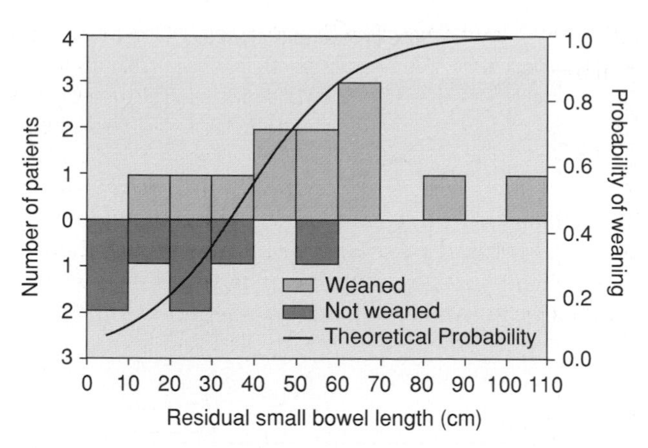

Figure 34.1: Theoretical relationship between probability from PN and residual measured small bowel length. (From Figure 2 in Andorsky DJ, Lund DP, Lillehei CW, et al. Nutritional and other postoperative management of neonates with short bowel syndrome correlates with clinical outcomes. J Pediatr 2001; 139:27–33.)[5]

normal small intestinal and colonic anatomy and function. In the full-term infant, small intestinal length ranges between 200 and 250 cm. Post-natal growth, which occurs predominantly in the first few years after birth,[23] is highly variable but on average, increases small intestinal length to between 400 and 700 cm, the average being approximately 550–600 cm, approximately one-third or 200–300 cm of which is functional jejunum. Children and adults who retain only about 30% of normal small intestinal length after resection, about 70 cm in infants and 150–200 cm in adults, are at risk to develop SBS.[24,25] In adults, PN is likely when total oral macronutrient absorption by the remnant gastrointestinal tract is less than one-third of that ingested or about 84% of the basal metabolic rate.[26] Medical and nutritional interventions short of PN are typical when oral nutrient assimilation ranges between one-third and two-thirds of that ingested. Similarly, parenteral fluid therapy can be expected when net assimilation falls below 1.4 kg (l) per day.[26] The implication is that adult patients with an extreme intestinal loss must become profoundly hyperphagic, increasing caloric intake up to three-fold, in order to avoid PN. Comparable data have not been definitively established in children. However, given the metabolic demands of growth and development, children probably need to tolerate an enteral intake two-fold greater than normal, i.e. assimilate at least 50% of calories consumed, to avoid PN.

Colon anatomy

Outcome of PN is influenced by coincident colon resection and, by implication, resection of the ileocecal valve (ICV). Because the ICV is rarely removed without some colon, prognostic significance of ICV loss independent of all other factors is very difficult to judge. Relative importance of these factors has been best established in adults with SBS and, by implication, patients with onset of SBS in later childhood or adolescence. In this group, resection of the entire colon and all but 100–115 cm of proximal small bowel, resulting in an end-jejunostomy, results in life-long PN dependence in the overwhelming majority of affected patients.[9,25] If at least 60 cm of proximal jejunum can be anastomosed to some length of colon, there is an 85–90% probability of ending PN, generally within 2 years. If the entire colon and ICV remain after resection, which implies preservation of some ileum, then PN can eventually be successfully discontinued in most patients with as little as 30–35 cm of jejunoileum. In contrast, no more than half of adults will end PN with 30–35 cm of small bowel, colon, but no ICV. Precisely comparable data are lacking in children, but termination of remnant small bowel as an enterostomy probably results in permanent intestinal failure if less than 70 cm of small bowel remains. In comparison, infants with as little as 20–25 cm of small bowel often recover from intestinal failure, i.e. wean from PN, if the remnant small bowel retains continuity with an intact colon including the ICV.[27–29] Overall, indefinite PN is a rarity when an intact colon and ICV are present with at least 40 cm of small bowel. In contrast, infants with a partial colon, i.e. no ICV, and 40 cm or less of small bowel are able to end PN in no more than half of all instances.[4,30]

Function of remnant gut

In addition to immediate post-resection anatomy of the gastrointestinal tract, several other factors determine whether PN shall be required indefinitely or, if not, then for how long. Among these is the efficiency of peristalsis and mucosal function of remnant bowel. Intestinal obstruction *in utero* secondary to gastroschisis or proximal jejunal atresia typically results in marked dilatation and atrophy of the muscularis propria. Persistently ischemic albeit viable segments of remnant bowel may also compromise motility, leading to a prolonged need for PN even if length of remnant small bowel is substantial. Studies of SBS in neonates generally fail to show that outcome is independently related to etiology, perhaps because the potential for permanent, sub-lethal injury to remnant bowel is high irrespective of the original cause of gut injury.[3] Gut function after resection is difficult to quantify directly, particularly in infants and early tolerance of enteral nutrition (EN) serves as a surrogate measure. Thus, in infants with 25 cm of small bowel remaining after neonatal resection, tolerance of 75% of calories via the gastrointestinal tract by age 3 months predicts a 90% probability of ending PN. Conversely, tolerance of only 25% of daily calories via the gastrointestinal tract with 25 cm of remnant small bowel at age 3 months predicts a 50% chance of ending PN (Fig. 34.2).[23]

Intestinal adaptation

Bowel function gradually improves following massive intestinal resection, thereby diminishing impact of gut loss to a variable degree through compensatory events collectively referred to as 'adaptation'. Central to the concept of adaptation is that global absorptive function of a segment of adapted remnant bowel is greater than that of an

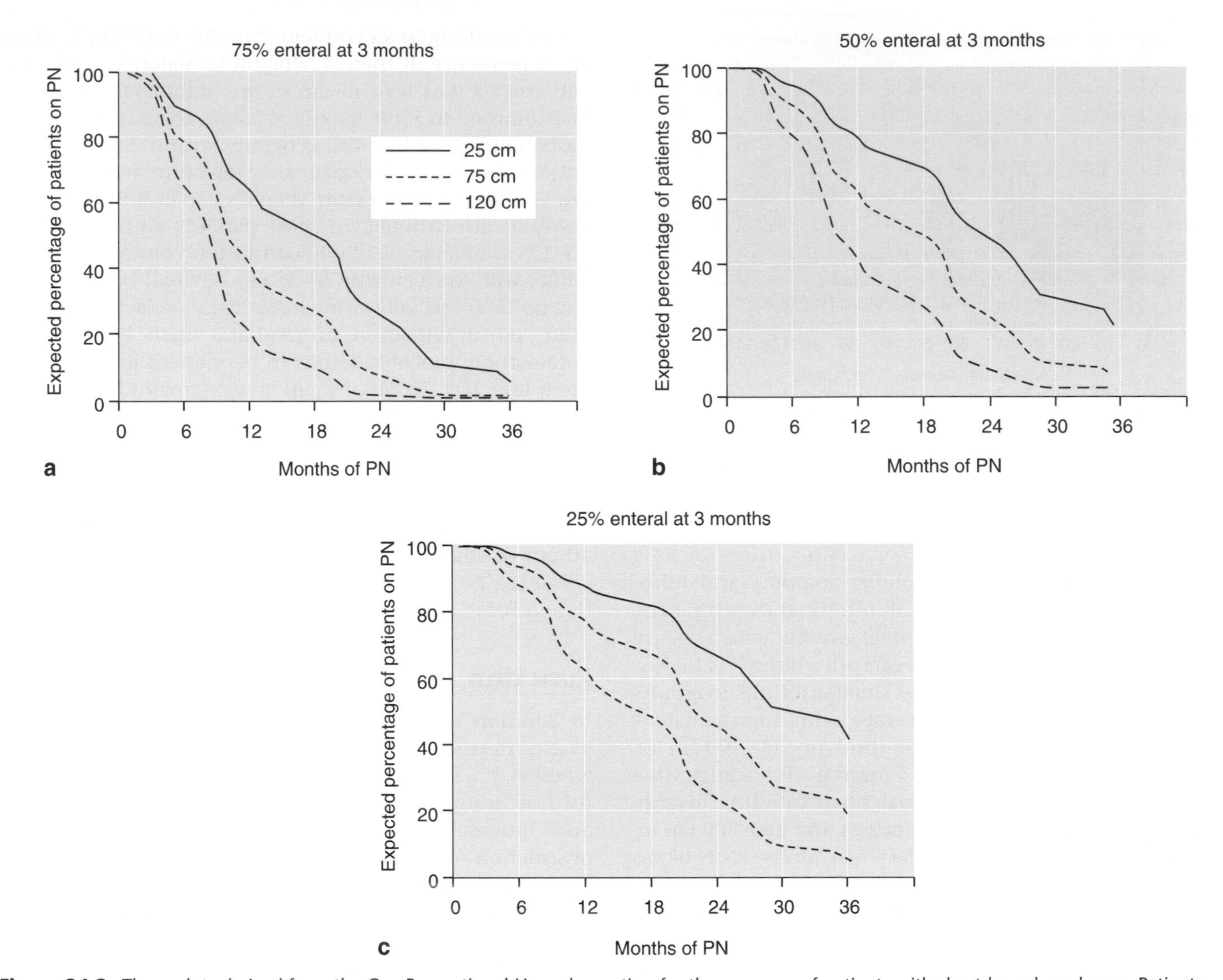

Figure 34.2: Three plots derived from the Cox Proportional Hazard equation for three groups of patients with short-bowel syndrome. Patients who receive (**a**) 75%; (**b**) 50% and (**c**) 25% of their daily calories by the enteral route at 3 months' adjusted age. The vertical axis shows expected percentage of patients who depend on PN at any age (months). Patients with three different residual intestinal lengths after initial surgery are shown (25 cm, 75 cm and 120 cm residual intestine, respectively). By using the Cox Proportional Hazard equations, survival curves such as these can be generated for any combination of the two variables. Care must be taken in applying these plots to patients whose medical management differs significantly from that described for subjects of this study. Variation of the model will require a prospective evaluation of its accuracy in more patients with neonatal intestinal resection. (From Figure 2 of Sondheimer JM, Cadnapaphornchai M, Sontag M, Zerbe GO. Predicting the duration of dependence of parenteral nutrition after neonatal intestinal resection. J Pediatr 1998;132:80–84.)[23]

equivalent segment of bowel immediately after resection. Most evidence for adaptation is derived from adult laboratory animal models of massive intestinal resection.[15] The applicability of this information to humans in general and to small infants in particular remains uncertain. Apart from species-specific differences in physiology, animal models usually do not account for congenital or acquired abnormalities of remnant bowel that might undermine subsequent reparative processes. Nonetheless, animal data constitute a useful working framework upon which SBS may be understood and physiological concepts of patient care developed. Following massive intestinal loss, generalized *cellular hyperplasia*, most notably affecting myocytes and enterocytes, ensues under the stimulus of enteral nutrients.[31,32] Mucosal hypoplasia occurs in the absence of enteral feeding, although this phenomenon may not be nearly as pronounced in humans as in experimental animals.[33,34] Complex nutrients are most effective in stimulating cellular hyperplasia, intact proteins more than free amino acids or peptides and long chain triglycerides more than medium chain triglycerides. Increased numbers of enterocytes lengthen the villus-crypt unit, increase the total surface area available for absorption and increase the total number of the various enzyme and transport molecules per crypt, although the absolute number of these molecules in individual enterocytes decreases. Expansion of the enterocyte and myocyte mass presumably contributes to expected *dilatation of remnant bowel*, further increasing total absorptive surface area. The time-frame over which hyperplasia occurs following resection is not precisely established in humans.[33] It is difficult to demonstrate adaptive hyperplasia months following resection, suggesting that adaptation occurs primarily if not exclusively within days to weeks following resection. EN appears to promote adaptation in humans as well as in animal models of SBS.

Although adaptation in humans at the molecular and cellular levels appears transient, clinical tolerance of enteral feeding improves for about 2 years after resection in adults[25] and up to 3–4 years thereafter in children.[3,23] Patients continuing to require PN after these intervals are very likely to need PN indefinitely. Thus, in the clinical setting, factors in addition to increased cellular mass per unit of small bowel length probably contribute to improved gut function over time. The obvious disparity in clinical adaptation between infants and adults is not surprising given the normal *linear growth of the intestinal tract* in childhood. The normally developing intestinal tract approximately doubles in length during the last trimester of pregnancy, which may explain the greater probability of premature infants obtaining complete adaptation, i.e. ending PN, compared with full-term infants with comparable amounts of gut loss. Most postnatal intestinal growth occurs within 3–4 years after birth, which corresponds to the peak window of opportunity for intestinal adaptation in this age group.[23] Whether intestinal lengthening greater than that associated with normal growth is stimulated by intestinal resection in either full-term or premature infants has not been established.

Aggregate digestive function may also improve over time without obvious changes in intestinal anatomy. Following massive intestinal resection, the quantity of carbohydrate and protein delivered to the colon potentially digestible by colonic flora, if in continuity with the small bowel, increases substantially. The time over which colonic bacterial fermentation increases has not been defined, but such increases may be gradual and clinically indistinguishable from increasing assimilation at the small intestinal level. Evidence concerning systemic metabolic adjustments to massive intestinal resection is scant. Limited data in children suggest that there is no significant alteration in total energy expenditure in SBS.[35] In contrast, adults may discontinue PN despite aggregate nutrient absorption well below the predicted basal metabolic rate, suggesting that metabolic compensation following massive intestinal resection and severe malabsorption can, in fact, occur. In infancy and childhood, energy expenditures, expressed per kg of total bodyweight or lean body mass, fall with advancing chronological age, which may also contribute to apparent adaptation, since the magnitude of increasing calories required to sustain growth gradually falls over time.

CLINICAL MANAGEMENT OF SBS

The early postoperative phase

The period of postoperative ileus ordinarily lasts less than one week if ongoing abdominal sepsis or other complications do not occur. At this time, fecal output is low as upper gastrointestinal secretions are drained, usually via a nasogastric or concurrently placed gastrostomy tube. Recovery of motility permits discontinuation of upper gastrointestinal tract decompression following which fecal output may variably increase. The clinical challenge at this time is to achieve continuous fluid and electrolyte balance based on the quantity and electrolyte content of ongoing fluid losses. Maintenance of appropriate fluid and electrolyte balance is most likely to be problematic when the small bowel terminates as an enterostomy, particularly if little or no distal jejunum and ileum remain. Given the fundamentally secretory character of proximal small bowel, a high enterostomy will be associated with outputs approximating 30–50 ml/kg per day even while the patient remains *nil per os*, in effect, a secretory diarrhea. Gastric hypersecretion may contribute to early, high fecal fluid loss. Histamine-2 receptor antagonists and proton pump inhibitors delivered intravenously have been advocated to reduce gastric hypersecretion during the first months after massive intestinal resection, although evidence that supports the efficacy of this practice in infants and children is lacking. Sodium and chloride concentrations in proximal jejunostomy effluent are relatively high, both up to 120 mEq/l and these electrolytes must be replaced intravenously in addition to fluid in order to prevent hyponatremia and hypochloremia as well as dehydration. In contrast, potassium and bicarbonate losses are low. The more distal the enterostomy, the lower fecal fluid loss as the fecal stream is exposed to more predominantly absorptive small bowel. Marked secretory diarrhea such as is common in patients with an enterostomy is generally absent in patients retaining a substantial length of colon. However, relatively more potassium and bicarbonate and relatively less sodium and chloride are likely to be needed, as these electrolytes are normally secreted in the colon.

PN is begun following establishment of stable fluid and electrolyte status. When remnant bowel anatomy predicts prolonged if not indefinite PN, a semi-permanent, cuffed catheter (Broviac®, Hickman®) can be placed at the time of original surgery or soon thereafter. Alternatively, parenteral feeding may be initiated via a peripherally inserted central catheter ('PICC line'). During the early period of PN in the hospital, it is usually useful to deliver stool replacement fluids separate from PN, since volume and composition of replacement fluid are likely to change much more frequently than PN, especially after EN is initiated.

Initiation of feeding

EN is begun when postoperative ileus has resolved, upper gastrointestinal tract decompression has ended and stable metabolic, fluid and electrolyte status has been achieved with PN and ancillary fluid and electrolyte support. In all ages, proprietary liquid diets are usually used. Most attention concerning EN in pediatric SBS has focused on young infants, the most common time that SBS is diagnosed in pediatrics. Optimal formula composition for infant SBS remains controversial. Controversies include nitrogen source, free amino acid, a mixture of amino acids and short peptides (protein hydrolysates), or intact protein and type and quantity of lipid, medium chain *vs* long chain

increasingly larger quantities of enteral feeding are tolerated, duration of the 'off' period can also be increased. Timing of the PN infusion is based largely on caretaker convenience. PN is customarily delivered to adults with SBS at night, because for continent adults, freedom from intravenous infusion during the daytime usually outweighs the inconvenience of frequent nocturnal urination. Nighttime infusion may be less advantageous to small children, since associated increases in urine production may further increase the risk of local skin breakdown.

Home PN in SBS

It is well established that pediatric as well as adult patients with SBS fare better when receiving PN in the home than in the institutional setting.[44] The benefit to patient life quality and family social structure is obvious. PN at home is relatively safe.[45] Although the annual cost of home PN remains substantial, around US$150 000–200 000, the expense is considerably less than the cost of continued confinement to a hospital or chronic care facility.[46]

Planning for discharge to home should begin soon after surgery, once patient survival appears to be a reasonable certainty. Assumption by parents and/or related family care providers of responsibility for all aspects of intravenous fluid delivery and routine central venous catheter care should be emphasized during teaching. After discharge, a multi-disciplinary team that includes physician, nursing, dietary and pharmaceutical components directs care. Professional nursing care should be provided in the home only as necessary to facilitate a smooth transition from the hospital. Formal mechanisms for regular communication between family care providers and the team, delivery of fluids, drugs and other supplies to the home and ambulatory laboratory support are established. This organization permits weaning of PN and advancement of EN as rapidly as possible, as caregivers assess response to dietary interventions, evaluate hydration and obtain scheduled and unscheduled laboratory testing, all in telephone, e-mail and office consultation with the team.

COMPLICATIONS OF SBS AND PN

Hepatobiliary disease

Patients with SBS who are receiving PN are more prone to develop *progressive liver disease* and liver failure than those receiving PN for other reasons. Incidence of progressive liver disease in infants with SBS is increased by sepsis developing within the first months following resection.[47] Liver failure associated with SBS also occurs in older children and adults in whom extreme small intestinal loss *per se* represents a statistical risk.[48] Inability to deliver enteral nutrition, loss of immunological protection associated with deficiency of gut-associated lymphoid tissue, lack of certain conditionally essential nutrients in PN such as choline and hepatotoxicity of some PN components including intravenous lipid emulsion, copper and manganese are postulated contributors.[49,50] The histological lesion is that of variable portal and lobular inflammation, cellular bilirubin and cholate stasis, macrophage hyperplasia and interlobular bile duct proliferation with varying degrees of portal and lobular fibrosis.[51] Progressive liver disease is suspected when hyperbilirubinemia fails to remit following several months of enteral feeding, particularly when greater than 3–6 mg/dl, in conjunction with indications of evolving portal hypertension, especially progressive splenomegaly and thrombocytopenia.[52] There is no proven therapy for PN-associated liver disease and ursodeoxycholic acid or related species have proven ineffective.[53] A platelet count of 100 000/μl is associated a 1-year survival of only about 30%,[54] while a total plasma bilirubin of about 10 mg/dl predicts death within 6 months.[55] Suspicion of progressive PN-associated liver disease in patients with SBS warrants early consideration of liver and intestinal transplantation.

Chronic *cholecystitis* with pigmented (calcium bilirubinate) stones is part of the spectrum of PN-associated liver disease in patients with SBS.[56] Loss of the ileum and enterohepatic circulation of bile acids and a lack of enteral nutrition contribute. Also important in the development of gallstones is absolute duration of PN, which has been reported to average about 30 months in affected patients.[57] The extent to which established parenchymal liver disease also contributes to formation of stones is unclear. Cholecystectomy is indicated for biliary tract obstruction and symptoms and signs of gallbladder inflammation.[58]

Small intestinal bacterial overgrowth (SIBO)

SIBO occurs in SBS when enteral nutrition is given in the setting of stasis of enteric succus in segments of bowel that are poorly peristaltic and/or excessively dilated as a result of *in utero* or post-natal obstruction. An ICV reduces occurrence but does not guarantee the absence of SIBO, which is present when $>10^5$ fecal bacteria/ml are present in duodenal-jejunal fluid.[3] Affected patients may also have elevated concentrations of breath hydrogen when fasting or following oral glucose challenge.[59] SIBO may undermine tolerance of enteral nutrition and thereby delay the ending of PN in patients with SBS by mechanisms that include direct injury to the enterocyte surface and inactivation of bile acids via deconjugation.[3] Symptoms of SIBO are similar to those of partial bowel obstruction and include abdominal distention, nausea and vomiting and increased stools with flatulence. Studies in adults demonstrate efficacy of amoxicillin-clavulanic acid and norfloxacin.[60] No comparable controlled studies have been performed in children, but trimethoprim-sulfamethoxazole and gentamicin (given by mouth) are often used for SIBO due to coliforms. Doses of gentamicin employed clinically usually range between 5 and 10 mg/kg per day, although markedly higher dosing has been utilized in clinical testing.[61] Verifying the absence of gentamicin absorption with blood levels is often recommended. Agents with efficacy against strict anaerobes such as metronidazole should be used with more caution, because they have the potential to suppress organisms largely responsible for converting complex carbohydrates to short-chain fatty acids and antibiotics may promote the formation of reservoirs of resistant organisms that may complicate treatment of future septic episodes. Since acid-suppressing agents promote SIBO,[62] their continuation beyond the initial postoperative period should be based on specific indications rather than empiric prophylaxis. Disadvantages of conventional antibiotic therapy of SIBO may be circumvented using probiotic bacteria, which are non-pathogenic organisms that can colonize the gastrointestinal tract and adhere to the surfaces of enterocytes and colonocytes.[63] These products competitively suppress replication of pathogens that probably contribute to SIBO and its complications and may promote adaptation by intensification of short-chain fatty acid production.[64] Most proprietary products (Culturelle®, VSL #3®) contain lactobacilli and bifidobacteria of various species. Although isolated case reports suggest a benefit in SBS, confirmation in controlled trials is lacking.

A special form of SIBO in patients with colon in continuity with the small bowel is overgrowth of lactobacilli strains that produce large quantities of d-lactic acid rather than hydrogen or other short-chain fatty acids.[65,66] *D-lactic acidosis* may be especially prone to develop when a high rate of gut lactic acid production and absorption is associated with impaired clearance, leading to encephalopathy characterized by lethargy and ataxia reminiscent of alcohol intoxication in association with metabolic acidosis and increased ion gap. Nystagmus may be present.[65] Diagnosis is suggested by the presence of large numbers of gram-positive rods in stools and confirmed by an elevated plasma concentration of d-lactic acid. Effective treatment of d-lactic acidosis includes suppression of production by reduced intake of mono- and disaccharides, the primary food substrates and antibiotics; oral gentamicin appears to be particularly effective.[61,67] The effect of vancomycin is inconsistent.[68] Probiotic therapy has also been successfully employed in isolated cases.[69]

Enterocolitis

The prevalence of enterocolitis in pediatric patients with SBS has not been precisely established but is probably more common than the few published reports would suggest.[3,70] Focal to variably diffuse aphthous ulceration is occasionally present and is distinct from peri-anastomotic ulceration that may develop following ileocolonic resection.[71,72] Symptoms are mainly due to chronic bleeding and secondary iron deficiency and generally do not include abdominal pain. Eosinophilia is often a prominent component of the inflammatory infiltrate. Enterocolitis associated with SBS may occur in infants early after resection, even when enteral nutrition consists of an amino acid-based formula. More commonly, enterocolitis is recognized when the remnant bowel is challenged with increasing quantities of EN in an attempt to end PN, implying that SIBO as well as occult food allergy may be responsible. Treatment remains largely empiric and has included mesalamine, corticosteroids and oral antibiotics in addition to iron replacement. Therapy is important, because inflammation may be severe enough to delay ending of PN.[3] Testing for food allergies may also be appropriate.

Structural and functional bowel obstruction

Viable bowel that is spared during a massive resection may not exhibit normal peristaltic function when challenged with enteral feeding, which is especially likely in the setting of chronic ischemia or obstruction pre-operatively, as in gastroschisis or proximal atresia. Furthermore, dilatation of remnant small bowel after resection, which is often marked, further contributes to inefficient peristalsis, SIBO, malabsorption and feeding intolerance. Compounding the deleterious effects of *dysmotility*, strictures may evolve in persistently ischemic regions, especially at anastomoses, leading to chronic, partial mechanical obstruction. When advancement of enteral nutrition is undermined by recurrent vomiting, abdominal distention and/or abdominal pain that suggest SIBO, either mechanical obstruction or dysmotility may be the culprit and should be evaluated with radiological imaging, endoscopy and biopsy. Management of these complications may be difficult, because *de facto* pseudo-obstruction may be hard to discriminate from mechanical obstruction in the setting of previous intestinal surgery. Medical therapy for symptomatic dysmotility may include antibiotics, anti-inflammatory drugs and prokinetic agents. These treatments may be of limited efficacy and when dysmotility is severe enough to interfere with advancement of enteral feeding and is unresponsive to medical management, surgical intervention is appropriate.

Numerous operations have been devised to improve bowel motility, most often by reducing bowel caliber. Simple anti-mesenteric longitudinal tapering efficiently reduces intestinal caliber, reduces stools and improves feeding tolerance in the short-term.[73] A potential long-term liability is the inherent reduction in an already diminished intestinal absorptive surface area. The longitudinal intestinal lengthening operation devised by Bianchi doubles the length of a dilated intestinal segment while reducing the diameter by one-half, effectively preserving surface area.[49] This is achieved by splitting the segment into two tubes in the mesenteric – anti-mesenteric plane with a stapler, which preserves perfusion to each, after which the two narrowed segments are anastomosed end to end. The operation appears to be most beneficial to patients beyond infancy who tolerate some EN and have not developed significant liver disease.[74] Conversely, results are disappointing when performed in younger infants who retain very little bowel, who tolerate minimal EN and have already developed significant liver disease.[75] Recently, Kim et al.[76] have devised a simplified but encouraging approach to intestinal lengthening, serial transverse enteroplasty or the 'STEP' procedure. In this operation, a series of staple lines, all perpendicular to the long axis of the bowel are placed, each staple line originating alternately from either side to create a maze-like tunnel within the dilated segment (Fig. 34.3).[77] No long-term experience is as yet reported.

spectrum of these disorders was defined solely by various case reports. As these reports became more frequent, various aspects of the disease became better described and stratified. Additional insight into the role of the eosinophil in health and disease has allowed further description of these disorders with respect to the underlying defect that drives the inflammatory response in those afflicted. Perhaps, most important to the definition of these disorders has been the understanding of the heterogeneity of the sites affected within the gastrointestinal tract (Table 35.1).

Eosinophilic gastroenteropathies are thought to arise from the interaction of genetic and environmental factors. Of note, approximately 10% of individuals with one of these disorders has a family history in an immediate family member.[8] In addition there is evidence for the role of allergy in the etiology of these conditions, including the observations that up to 75% of patients are atopic[9,10] and that an allergen-free diet can sometimes reverse disease activity.[9,10] Interestingly, only a minority of individuals with eosinophilic gastroenteropathies have food-induced anaphylaxis,[11] and therefore these disorders exhibit properties that are intermediate between pure IgE-mediated allergy and cellular mediated hypersensitivity disorders.

Gastric antrum	<10
Duodenum	<20
Colon	10–20
In infants	<10
Esophagus	0

Table 35.1 Typical number of gastrointestinal mucosal eosinophils in normal individuals

EOSINOPHILIC ESOPHAGITIS

Eosinophilic esophagitis (EoE) is characterized by an isolated, severe eosinophilic infiltration of the esophagus manifested by gastroesophageal reflux like symptoms, unresponsive to acid suppression therapy. This disorder has been given several names including eosinophilic esophagitis, allergic esophagitis, primary eosinophilic esophagitis and idiopathic eosinophilic esophagitis.

Etiology

EoE appears to be caused by an abnormal immunologic response to specific food antigens. While several studies have documented resolution of EoE with the strict avoidance of food antigens, in 1995, Kelly published the classic paper on EoE.[12] Because the suspected etiology was an abnormal immunologic response to specific unidentifiable food antigens, each patient was treated with a strict elimination diet which included an amino acid based formula (Neocate®). Patients were also allowed clear liquids, corn and apples. A total of 17 patients were initially offered a dietary elimination trial with 10 patients adhering to the protocol. The initial trial was determined by a history of anaphylaxis to specific foods and abnormal skin testing. These patients were subsequently placed on a strict diet consisting of an amino-acid-based formula for a median of 17 weeks. Symptomatic improvement was seen within an average of 3 weeks after the introduction of the elemental diet (resolution in eight patients; improvement in two). In addition, all 10 patients demonstrated a significant improvement in esophageal eosinophilia. Subsequently, all patients reverted to previous symptoms upon reintroduction of foods. Pre- and post-dietary trial evaluation demonstrated a significant improvement in clinical symptoms and almost complete resolution in esophageal eosinophilia, from a mean of 41 eosinophils per microscopic high power field (HPF) to <1 per HPF. Open food challenges were then conducted with a demonstration of a return of symptoms with challenges to milk (7 patients), soy (4), wheat (2), peanut (2) and egg (1).

While an exact etiology was not determined, Kelly suggested an immunologic basis, secondary to a delayed hypersensitivity or a cell-mediated hypersensitivity response, as the cause for EoE. A recent paper by Spergel demonstrated that foods which cause EoE are often not based on an immediate hypersensitivity reaction.[10] By using a combination of traditional skin testing and a newer technique of 'patch testing,' he established that a delayed cellular mediated allergic response may be responsible for many cases of EoE. Recently, CD8+ lymphocytes have been identified as the predominant T cell within the squamous epithelium of patients diagnosed with EoE.[13]

Previous studies have established the link between eosinophilic esophagitis and atopy over the last 8 years. It was these initial links between atopy and EoE that suggested food allergies may play a role in the pathogenesis of this disease. The role of food allergy was confirmed as patients improved on elemental diets. Elimination of the responsible food usually does not lead to rapid resolution of the symptoms. Rather, improvement of symptoms occurs approximately 1–2 weeks after the removal of the causative antigen. Also, in patients with EoE, symptoms do not typically occur immediately after reintroduction to the foods. It usually takes several days for symptoms to develop suggesting either a mixed IgE and T-cell mediated allergic response or strictly a T-cell delayed mechanism in the pathogenesis of this disease. While both IgE and T-cell mediated reactions have been identified as possible causative factors, T-cell mediated reactions seem to be the main mechanism of disease.

Several authors have suggested that aeroallergens may play a role in the development of EoE. Mishra et al. used a mouse model to show that the inhalation of Aspergillus caused EoE.[14] They found that the allergen-challenged mice developed elevated levels of esophageal eosinophils and features of epithelial cell hyperplasia that mimic EoE. In addition, Spergel reported a case of a 21-year-old female with asthma and allergic rhinoconjunctivitis who also had EoE.[15] The patient's EoE became symptomatic with exacerbations during pollen seasons, followed by resolution during the winter months.

Clinical manifestations

Patients, who are predominantly young males, typically present with one or more of the following symptoms: vomiting, regurgitation, nausea, epigastric or chest pain, water brash, globus, decreased appetite.[16] Less common symptoms include growth failure, hematemesis, esophageal dysmotility and dysphagia. Symptoms can be frequent and severe in some patients while extremely intermittent and mild in others. The majority of patients may experience daily dysphagia or chronic nausea or regurgitation while others may have infrequent or rare episodes of dysphagia. Up to 50% of patients manifest additional allergy related symptoms such as asthma, eczema, or rhinitis. Furthermore, more than 50% of patients have one or more parents with history of allergy (Table 35.2).

Walsh demonstrated comparable results.[9,10] He compared seven children with gastroesophageal reflux disease (GERD) with 21 children with EoE. Eleven of the EoE patients studied had normal pH probe results while all seven of the GERD patients had abnormal pH probes. Males outnumbered females in both groups. The symptoms of vomiting and abdominal pain occurred similarly in both groups. Dysphagia, diarrhea and growth failure were predominant in the EoE group. In addition, 80% of EoE patients had allergic symptoms compared with 29% of the GERD patients; 45% of EoE patients had another family member with an allergic history (0% GERD); and 50% of EoE patients had a peripheral eosinophilia (0% GERD). Patients with EoE had an average of 31 eosinophils per HPF compared with five eosinophils per HPF in the GERD group (Table 35.3).

Evaluation and diagnosis

Children with chronic refractory symptoms of gastroesophageal reflux disease or dysphagia should undergo evaluation for EoE. While laboratory and radiologic assessment is appropriate, the majority of these patients should undergo an upper endoscopy with biopsy. The diagnosis of EoE is made when an isolated severe histologic esophagitis unresponsive to aggressive acid blockade, associated with symptoms similar to those seen in gastroesophageal reflux disease, responds both clinically and histologically to the elimination of a specific food(s). In the past, a 24 h pH probe was required to demonstrate that the esophageal disease was not acid induced; however, over the past few years, the literature has shown that EoE is present when esophageal biopsy specimens reveal an isolated esophagitis of greater than 20 eosinophils per HPF, regardless of pH probe results. In contrast, individuals with reflux esophagitis typically show less than five eosinophils per HPF. Currently, upper endoscopy with biopsy is the only diagnostic test that can accurately determine if the esophageal inflammation of EoE is present.

Once EoE is suspected, patients should be encouraged to seek an allergy consultation. Skin prick testing and serum RAST tests may provide some clues to possible food allergens. Unfortunately, these tests are most useful in determining IgE-based allergic disorders. Since EoE is considered to be either a T-cell mediated disease or a mixed IgE and T-cell mediated disorder, the sensitivity and specificity of skin prick tests are low. Recently, investigators have demonstrated that patch testing (the placement of an antigen on the skin for several days) may be more useful in determining those antigens responsible for causing esophageal eosinophilia.[10] If no specific antigen(s) are found through allergy testing, a trial of an elimination diet, consisting of removal of the antigens that most commonly cause EoE, should be attempted. The most common foods identified as causing EoE are milk, soy, egg, wheat, nuts, fish and shellfish. If all of these measures fail, an elemental diet utilizing an amino acid based formula should be instituted. The assessment of success should be based on both the improvement of clinical symptoms and histologic improvement.

Once EoE has resolved, foods should be reintroduced individually every 5 to 6 days. This time period is usually sufficient to see a recurrence of symptoms; if symptoms persist the food should be discontinued. However, in some cases symptoms do not recur. A repeat endoscopy with

Clinical symptoms
- Similar to symptoms of GERD
  - Vomiting, regurgitation
  - Heartburn
  - Epigastric pain
  - Dysphagia
- Symptoms different in infants and adolescents
- Often intermittent symptoms
- Male > female

Associated signs and symptoms (>50% patients)
- Bronchospasm
- Eczema
- Allergic rhinitis

Family History (35–45% patients)
- Food allergy
- Asthma

Table 35.2 Characteristics of eosinophilic esophagitis

Eosinophilic esophagitis
- Intermittent symptoms
- pH probe
  - Normal
- Acid blockade
  - Unresponsive
- Number of esophageal eosinophils
  - >20 eosinophils/high-powered field (HPF)

Gastroesophageal reflux
- Persistent symptoms
- pH probe
  - Abnormal
- Acid blockade
  - Responsive
- Number of esophageal eosinophils
  - 1–5 eosinophils/HPF

Table 35.3 Contrasting characteristics of eosinophilic esophagitis and gastroesophageal reflux

biopsy is also required in order to evaluate for the presence of esophageal mucosal injury. Because clinical symptoms often occur sporadically, biopsy remains the most important way to accurately determine the presence or resolution of EoE.

While upper endoscopy with biopsy is the only test that can precisely determine the diagnosis, non-invasive diagnostic tests have proven to be less useful. These include the evaluation of serum IgE levels and quantitative peripheral eosinophils, radiographic upper gastrointestinal series (UGI), pH probe and manometry, RAST testing and skin prick and patch testing. When used alone, serum IgE levels and serum eosinophils have been found to be unreliable, as these tests usually respond to environmental allergens as well as ingested or inhaled allergens. While radiographs determine anatomic abnormalities, these tests cannot identify tissue eosinophilia. Patients with EoE usually have normal or borderline normal pH probes. These patients may have mild GERD secondary to abnormalities in esophageal motility due to tissue eosinophilic infiltration. Finally, while allergy testing, like serum RAST testing and skin prick testing are useful in diagnosing IgE mediated allergic disorders, these tests have been generally ineffective in diagnosing food allergy in EoE patients. Recently, Spergel has demonstrated that skin patch testing has increased the chance of finding possible food allergens.[10] The utilization of patch testing has improved the allergist's ability to identify potential food allergies in patients with EoE.

EoE is best defined as the presence of more than 20 eosinophils per high power field (HPF) isolated strictly to the esophageal mucosa. While some authors have suggested that the diagnosis can be made when 15–20 eosinophils are present, their results have been contradictory and confusing. In the past, early reports suggested that EoE patients developed an increased proximal or mid-esophageal tissue eosinophilia; however, recent information demonstrates that a severe mucosal eosinophilia can occur in either the distal or proximal esophagus.[17–19] To make an accurate diagnosis, the remainder of the gastrointestinal tract must be normal. EoE has been associated with visual findings on endoscopy: Concentric ring formation called 'trachealization' or a 'feline esophagus', longitudinal linear furrows and patches of small, white papules on the esophageal surface.[20] Most investigators believe that the esophageal rings and furrows are a response to full thickness esophageal tissue inflammation. The white papules appear to represent the formation of eosinophilic abscesses (Figs 35.1, 35.2).

In 1999, Ruchelli evaluated 102 patients presenting with GERD symptoms who also were found to have at least one esophageal eosinophil without any other gastrointestinal abnormalities.[21] Patients were subsequently treated with aggressive acid blockade. It was demonstrated that the treatment response could be classified into three categories. Patients who improved had on average 1.1 eosinophils per HPF, patients who relapsed upon completion of therapy had 6.4 eosinophils per HPF and patients who remained symptomatic had on average 24.5 eosinophils per HPF.

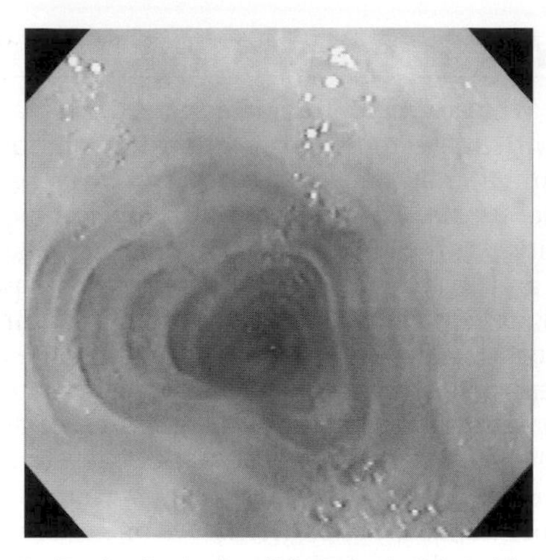

Figure 35.1: 'Trachealization' or 'felinization' of the mid-esophagus in a patient with eosinophilic esophagitis. The terms arise from the ringed appearance of the esophagus that cause it to resemble a human trachea or a cat esophagus (which has rings of cartilage).

In 2000, Fox utilized high resolution probe endosonography in patients with EoE in order to determine the extent of tissue involvement.[22] He compared eight patients identified with EoE to four control patients without esophagitis. He discovered that the layers of the esophageal wall were thicker in EoE patients than in control group (2.8–2.2 mm). Additionally, the mucosa to submucosa ratio was greater in EoE patients (1.6–1.1 mm) and the muscularis propria thickness was greater in EoE pts (1.3–1.0 mm). These findings suggested EoE patients had more than just surface involvement of eosinophils.

Management

The identification and removal of allergic dietary antigens is the mainstay of treatment for EoE. While removal of the offending food(s) reverses the disease process in patients with EoE, in many cases the isolation of these foods is

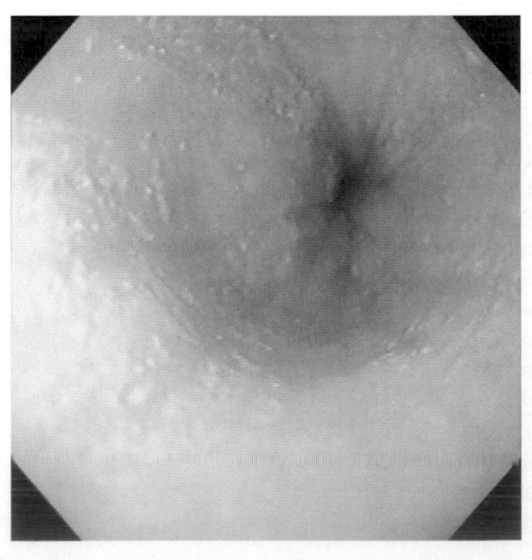

Figure 35.2: White plaques seen in the mid-esophagus in a patient with eosinophilic esophagitis.

extremely difficult. Often, patients with EoE cannot correlate their gastrointestinal symptoms with the ingestion of a specific food. This occurs due to the delayed hypersensitivity response. Several reports have demonstrated several days for symptoms to recur upon ingestion of antigens that cause EoE.[12,16] Even when a particular food causing EoE has been isolated, it may take days or weeks for the symptoms to resolve. In addition, although one food may be identified, there may be several other foods (not identified) that could also be contributing.

While attempts should be made to identify and eliminate potential food allergens through a careful history and the use of allergy testing, it may be difficult to determine the responsible allergic foods; the administration of a strict diet, utilizing an amino acid based formula, is often necessary. As established previously, the use of an elemental diet rapidly improves both clinical symptoms and histology in patients with EoE.[12,23] Because of poor palatability, the elemental formula is most often provided by continuous nasogastric feeding. The diet may be supplemented with water, one fruit (apples, grapes) and the corresponding pure fruit juice. Reversal of symptoms typically occurs within 10 days with histologic improvement in 4 weeks. Although the strict use of an amino acid based formula (typically provided by nasogastric tube feeding) may initially be difficult for patients (and parents) to accept, its benefits outweigh the risks of other treatments and the rapid improvement in symptoms proves very reinforcing to families. While the use of other medications, such as corticosteroids, may temporarily improve the disease and its symptoms, upon their discontinuation the disease recurs. In contrast, when foods that cause EoE are identified through a combination of allergy testing, endoscopy, elimination and selective reintroduction – then the disease for the individual patient is in effect cured and should not recur.

Treatment of EoE with aggressive acid blockade, including medical and surgical therapy, has not been proven effective. Several published reports have demonstrated the failure of H2 blocker and proton pump therapy in patients with EoE.[13,21,24] While acid blockade may improve clinical symptoms by improving acid reflux that occurs secondarily to the underlying inflamed esophageal mucosa, it does not reverse the esophageal histologic abnormality. Although some case reports suggested that fundoplication was beneficial for patients with EoE, in 1997, Liacouras reported on two cases of failed Nissen fundoplication in patients who were diagnosed with severe eosinophilic esophagitis.[25] Both patients underwent fundoplication for presumed acid reflux esophagitis unresponsive to medical therapy. However, post-surgical evaluation of both patients revealed ongoing clinical symptoms. Repeat EGD demonstrated persistent esophageal eosinophilia. Subsequently, both patients responded to oral corticosteroids with resolution of symptoms and histologic improvement.

Prior to 1997, reports suggested that systemic corticosteroids improved the symptoms of EoE in adults identified with a severe eosinophilic esophagitis.[26,27] In 1997, Liacouras was the first to publish the use of oral corticosteroids in 20 children diagnosed with EoE.[24] These patients were treated with oral methylprednisolone (average dose 1.5 mg/kg per day; maximum dose 48 mg/day) for 1 month. Symptoms were significantly improved in 19 of 20 patients by an average of 8 days. A repeat endoscopy with biopsy, 4 weeks after the initiation of therapy, demonstrated a significant reduction of esophageal eosinophils, from 34 to 1.5 eosinophils per HPF. However, upon discontinuation of corticosteroids, 90% had recurrence of symptoms.

In 1999, Faubion reported that swallowing a metered dose of inhaled corticosteroids was also effective in treating the symptoms of EoE in children.[28] Four patients diagnosed with EoE manifested by epigastric pain, dysphagia and a severe esophageal eosinophilia unresponsive to aggressive acid blockade were given fluticasone; four puffs twice a day. Patients were instructed to use an inhaler but to immediately swallow after inhalation in order to deliver the medication to the esophagus. Histologic improvement was not determined. Within 2 months, all four patients responded with an improvement in symptoms. Two patients required repeat use of inhalation therapy. Success with this therapy was recently confirmed.[13] While this therapy can improve EoE, the side-effects can include esophageal candidiasis and growth failure.[29,30] In addition, symptoms often recur in patients upon discontinuation of the therapy.[13]

The mast-cell-stabilizing agent cromolyn sodium has also been used to treat children with EoE.[31–33] In similar fashion to its use for children with EoG, oral cromolyn has been given to patients with a severe esophageal eosinophilia in conjunction with other systemic signs and symptoms of allergic disease. However, no controlled reports have been performed and efficacy for oral cromolyn in children with EoE has not been established.

Recently, leukotriene antagonists such as Montelukast, have been utilized in patients with EoE;[34] the rationale is that they selectively block the D4 receptor of cysteinyl leukotriene present in eosinophils. Leukotrienes have been implicated in causing eosinophil attraction and migration, powerful constriction of smooth muscle, airway edema, mucous hypersecretion and reduction of ciliary motility. Leukotrienes are predominately released by eosinophils, basophils and mast cells. By blocking these receptors, the inflammatory action of the eosinophil may be reduced. Thus, the eosinophils are not eliminated; instead, their actions are negated.

In a study in 2003, Attwood administered a leukotriene receptor antagonist to eight patients diagnosed with EoE.[35] Every patient underwent upper endoscopy with biopsies prior to beginning the medication. The mean age of these patients was 40 years of age and the average length of symptoms was 36 months. The primary symptom was dysphagia, although five patients reported regurgitation and six had heartburn. The median density of the eosinophils was 57 eosinophils per high-powered field. Seven of the eight patients demonstrated complete subjective improvement in dysphagia and were subsequently placed on a maintenance dose. Six of the eight patients had recurrence of symptoms within three weeks of cessation or reduction in medication. No biopsies were performed while patients were on medication.

EOSINOPHILIC GASTROENTERITIS

Eosinophilic gastroenteritis (EoG) is a general term that describes a constellation of symptoms attributable to the gastrointestinal tract, in combination with pathologic infiltration by eosinophils. This group includes eosinophilic gastritis, gastroenteritis and enteritis. There are no strict diagnostic criteria for this disorder and it has been largely shaped by multiple case reports and series. A combination of gastrointestinal complaints with supportive histologic findings is sufficient to make the diagnosis. These conditions are grouped together under the term EoG for the discussion here, though it is likely that they are distinct entities in most patients (Table 35.4).

EoG was originally described by Kaijser in 1937.[36] It is a disorder characterized by tissue eosinophilia that can affect different layers of the bowel wall, anywhere from mouth to anus. The gastric antrum and small bowel are frequently affected. In 1970, Klein classified EoG into three categories: a mucosal, muscular and serosal form.[37]

Etiology

EoG affects patients of all ages, with a slight male predominance. Most commonly, eosinophils infiltrate only the mucosa, leading to symptoms associated with malabsorption, such as growth failure, weight loss, diarrhea and hypoalbuminemia. Mucosal EoG may affect any portion of the gastrointestinal tract. A review of the biopsy findings in 38 children with EoG revealed that all patients examined had mucosal eosinophilia of the gastric antrum.[38] Some 79% of the patients also demonstrated eosinophilia of the proximal small intestine, with 60% having esophageal involvement and 52% having involvement of the gastric corpus. Those with colonic involvement tended to be under 6 months of age and were ultimately classified as having allergic colitis.

The exact etiology of EoG remains unknown, although it is now recognized as a result of both IgE and non-IgE mediated sensitivity.[39] The association between IgE-mediated inflammatory response (typical allergy) and EoG is supported by the increased likelihood of other allergic disorders such as atopic disease, food allergies and seasonal allergies.[40,41] Specific foods have been implicated in the cause of EoG.[42,43] In contrast the role of non-IgE mediated immune dysfunction, in particular the interplay between lymphocyte-produced cytokines and eosinophils, has also received attention. Interleukin (IL)-5 is a chemoattractant responsible for tissue eosinophilia.[44] Desreumaux et al. found that among patients with EoG, the levels of IL-3, IL-5 and granulocyte-macrophage colony stimulating factor (GM-CSF) were significantly increased as compared to control patients.[45] Once recruited to the tissue, eosinophils may further recruit similar cells through their own production of IL-3 and IL-5, as well as production of leukotrienes.[46] This mixed type of immune dysregulation in EoG has implications in the way this disorder is diagnosed, as well as the way it is treated.

Clinical characteristics
Nausea, vomiting, regurgitation
Severe abdominal pain
Diarrhea, protein losing enteropathy
Gastrointestinal bleeding
Ascites
Intestinal obstruction
>95%, gastric antrum involved
Peripheral eosinophilia (>50%)
Associated allergies, eczema, asthma, rhinitis, atopy

Table 35.4 Characteristics of eosinophilic gastroenteritis

Clinical manifestations

The most common symptoms of EoG include colicky abdominal pain, bloating, diarrhea, weight loss, dysphagia and vomiting.[32,47] In addition, up to 50% have a past or family history of atopy.[38] Other features of severe disease include gastrointestinal bleeding, iron deficiency anemia, protein losing enteropathy (hypoalbuminemia) and growth failure.[47] Approximately 75% of affected patients have an elevated blood eosinophilia.[48] Males are more commonly affected than females. Rarely, ascites can occur.[48,49]

In an infant, EoG may present in a manner similar to hypertrophic pyloric stenosis, with progressive vomiting, dehydration, electrolyte abnormalities and thickening of the gastric outlet.[50,51] When an infant presents with this constellation of symptoms, in addition to atopic symptoms such as eczema and reactive airway disease, an elevated eosinophil count, or a strong family history of atopic disease, then EoG should be considered in the diagnosis before surgical intervention if possible.

Uncommon presentations of EoG include acute abdomen (even mimicking acute appendicitis)[52] or colonic obstruction.[53] There have also been reports of serosal infiltration with eosinophils, with associated complaints of abdominal distention, eosinophilic ascites and bowel perforation.[49,54–58]

Evaluation and diagnosis

EoG should be considered in any patient with a history of chronic symptoms including vomiting, abdominal pain, diarrhea, anemia, hypoalbuminemia, or poor weight gain in combination with the presence of eosinophils in the gastrointestinal tract. Other causes of eosinophilic infiltration of the gastrointestinal tract include the other disorders of the eosinophilic gastroenteropathy spectrum, as well as parasitic infection, inflammatory bowel disease, neoplasm, chronic granulomatous disease, collagen vascular disease and the hypereosinophilic syndrome.[59–63]

A number of tests may aid in the diagnosis of EoG, however no single test is pathognomonic and there are no standards for diagnosis. Eosinophils in the gastrointestinal tract must be documented before EoG can be truly entertained as a diagnosis. This is most readily done with biopsies of either the upper gastrointestinal tract through esophagogastroduodenoscopy or the lower tract through flexible sigmoidoscopy or colonoscopy. A history of atopy supports the diagnosis, but is not a necessary feature. Peripheral eosinophilia or an elevated IgE level occurs in approximately 70% of affected individuals.[64] Measures of absorptive activity such as the *d-xylose* absorption test and lactose hydrogen breath testing may reveal evidence of malabsorption, reflecting small intestinal damage. Radiographic contrast studies may demonstrate mucosal irregularities or edema, wall thickening, ulceration, or lumenal narrowing. A lacy mucosal pattern of the gastric antrum known as *areae gastricae* is a unique finding that may be present in patients with EoG.[65]

Evaluation of other causes of eosinophilia should be undertaken, including stool analysis for ova and parasites. Signs of intestinal obstruction warrant abdominal imaging. RAST testing, as well as skin testing for environmental antigens are rarely useful. Skin testing using both traditional prick tests and patch tests may increase the sensitivity for identifying foods responsible for EoG by evaluating both IgE mediated and T-cell mediated sensitivities.[10]

Management

There is as much ambiguity in the treatment of EoG as there is in its diagnosis. This is in large part because the entity of EoG was defined mainly by case series, each of which employed their own mode of treatment. Because EoG is a difficult disease to diagnose, randomized trials for its treatment are uncommon, leading to considerable debate as to which treatment is best.

Food allergy is considered one of the underlying causes of EoG. The elimination of pathogenic foods, as identified by any form of allergy testing, or by random removal of the most likely antigens, should be a first line treatment. Unfortunately, this approach results in improvement in a limited number of patients. In severe cases, or when other treatment options have failed, the administration of a strict diet, utilizing an elemental formula, has been shown to be successful.[41,66] In these cases, formulas such as Neocate 1+™ or Elecare™ provided as the sole source of nutrition have been reported to be effective in the resolution of clinical symptoms and tissue eosinophilia.

When the use of a restricted diet fails, corticosteroids are often employed due to their high likelihood of success in attaining remission.[32] However, when weaned, the duration of remission is variable and can be short-lived, leading to the need for repeated courses or continuous low doses of steroids. In addition, the chronic use of corticosteroids carries an increased likelihood of undesirable side-effects, including cosmetic problems (cushingoid facies, hirsutism, acne), decreased bone density, impaired growth and personality changes. A response to these side-effects has been to look for substitutes that may act as steroid-sparing agents, while still allowing for control of symptoms.

Orally administered cromolyn sodium has been used with some success,[32,67–69] and recent reports have detailed the efficacy of other oral anti-inflammatory medications. Montelukast, a selective leukotriene receptor antagonist used to treat asthma, has been reported to successfully treat two patients with EoG.[34,70] Treatment of EoG with inhibition of leukotriene D4, a potent chemotactic factor for eosinophils, relies on the theory that the inflammatory response in EoG is perpetuated by the presence of the eosinophils already present in the mucosa causing an interruption in the chemotactic cascade breaking the inflammatory cycle. Suplatast tosilate, another suppressor of cytokine production has also been reported as a treatment for EoG.[71]

Given the possibilities for treatment of EoG, the combination of therapies incorporating the best chance of success with the smallest likelihood of side-effects should be employed. When particular food antigens that may be causing disease can be identified, elimination of those antigens should be employed as a first line therapy. When testing fails to identify potentially pathogenic foods, a systematic elimination of the most commonly involved foods[72] can be employed. If this approach fails, total elimination diet with an amino acid-based formula should be considered. Trials of non-steroid anti-inflammatory medications such as Cromolyn, montelukast and suplatast, are a reasonable option, although some might prefer to wait for more detailed studies.

When other treatments fail, corticosteroids remain a reliable treatment for EoG, with attempts at limiting the total dose, or the number of treatment courses where possible. Due to the diffuse and inconsistent nature of symptoms in this disease, serial endoscopy with biopsy is a useful and important modality for monitoring disease progression.

EOSINOPHILIC PROCTOCOLITIS

Eosinophilic proctocolitis (EoP), also known as allergic proctocolitis or milk-protein proctocolitis, has been recognized as one of the most common etiologies of rectal bleeding in infants.[38,73] This disorder is characterized by the onset of rectal bleeding, generally in children less than 2 months of age.

Etiology

The gastrointestinal tract plays a major role in the development of oral tolerance to foods. Through the process of endocytosis by the enterocyte, food antigens are generally degraded into non-antigenic proteins.[74,75] Although the gastrointestinal tract serves as an efficient barrier to ingested food antigens, this barrier may not be mature for the first few months of life.[76] As a result, ingested antigens may have an increased propensity for being presented intact to the immune system. These intact antigens have the potential for stimulating the immune system and driving an inappropriate response directed at the gastrointestinal tract. Because the major component of the young infant's diet is milk or formula, it stands to reason that the inciting antigens in EoP are derived from the proteins found in them. Cow's milk and soy proteins are the foods most frequently implicated in EoP.

Commercially available infant formulas most commonly utilize cow's milk as the protein source. There are at least 25 known immunogenic proteins within cow's milk, with beta-lactoglobulin and casein serving as the most antigenic.[77] It is felt that up to 7.5% of the population in developed countries exhibit cow's milk allergy, although there is wide variation in the reported data.[78–80] Soy protein allergy is felt to be less common than cow's milk allergy, with reported prevalence of approximately 0.5%.[77] However, soy protein intolerance becomes more prominent in individuals who have developed milk protein allergy, as there is significant cross-reactivity between these proteins, with prevalence from 15–50% or more in milk protein sensitized individuals.[81] For this reason, substitution of a soy protein-based formula for a milk protein-based formula in patients with suspected milk-protein proctocolitis is often unsuccessful.

Maternal breast milk represents a different challenge to the immune system. Up to 50% of the cases of EoP occur in breast-fed infants; but, rather than developing an allergy to human milk protein, it is felt that the infants are manifesting allergy to antigens ingested by the mother and transferred via the breast milk. The transfer of maternal dietary protein via breast milk was first demonstrated in 1921.[82] More recently, the presence of cow's milk antigens in breast milk has been established.[83–85]

When a problem with antigen handling occurs, whether secondary to increased absorption through an immature gastrointestinal tract or though a damaged epithelium secondary to gastroenteritis, sensitization of the immune system results. Once sensitized, the inflammatory response is perpetuated with continued exposure to the inciting antigen. This may explain the reported relationship between early exposures to cow's milk protein or viral gastroenteritis and the development of allergy.[86–88]

Clinical manifestations

Diarrhea, rectal bleeding and increased mucus production are the typical symptoms seen in patients who present with EoP.[38,89] There is a bimodal age distribution with the majority of patients presenting in infancy (mean age at diagnosis of 60 days)[90] and the other group presenting in adolescence and early adulthood.

The typical infant with EoP is well-appearing with no constitutional symptoms. Rectal bleeding begins gradually, initially appearing as small flecks of blood. Usually, increased stool frequency occurs accompanied by water-loss or mucus streaks. The development of irritability or straining with stools is also common and can falsely lead to the initial diagnosis of anal fissuring. Atopic symptoms, such as eczema and reactive airway disease may be associated. Continued exposure to the inciting antigen causes increased bleeding and may, on rare occasions, cause anemia, poor weight gain. Despite the progression of symptoms, the infants are generally well appearing and rarely appear ill. Other manifestations of gastrointestinal tract inflammation, such as vomiting, abdominal distention, or weight loss almost never occur (Table 35.5).

Evaluation and diagnosis

EoP is primarily a clinical diagnosis, although several laboratory parameters and diagnostic procedures may be useful. Initial assessment should be directed at the overall health of the child. A toxic appearing infant is not consistent with the diagnosis of EoP and should prompt evaluation for other causes of gastrointestinal bleeding. A complete blood count is useful, as the majority of infants with EoP have a normal or borderline low hemoglobin. An elevated serum eosinophil count may be present. Stool studies for bacterial pathogens, such as *Salmonella* and *Shigella*, should be performed in the setting of rectal bleeding. In particular, an assay for *Clostridium difficile* toxins A & B should also be considered. While *C. difficile* may cause colitis, infants may be asymptomatically colonized with this organism.[91,92] A stool specimen may be analyzed for the presence of white blood cells and specifically for eosinophils. The sensitivity of these tests is not well documented and the absence of a positive finding on these tests does not exclude the diagnosis.[93] Eosinophils can also accumulate in the colon in other conditions such as pin and hookworm infections, drug reactions, vasculitis and inflammatory bowel disease and it may be important to exclude these, especially in older children.

Although not always necessary, flexible sigmoidoscopy may be useful to demonstrate the presence of colitis. Visually, one may find erythema, friability, or frank ulceration of the colonic mucosa. Alternatively, the mucosa may appear normal, or show evidence of lymphoid hyperplasia.[94,95] Histologic findings typically include increased eosinophils in focal aggregates within the lamina propria, with generally preserved crypt architecture. Findings may be patchy, so that care should be taken to examine many levels of each specimen if necessary.[96,97]

Clinical symptoms
- Blood streaked stools
- Diarrhea
- Mild abdominal pain
- <3 months of age
- Usually normal weight gain
- Well-appearing
- Eczema, atopy – rare

Laboratory features
- Fecal leukocytes
- Mild peripheral eosinophilia
- Rarely
  - Hypoalbuminemia
  - Anemia
- Pin prick, RAST testing negative

Table 35.5 Characteristics of eosinophilic proctocolitis

Management

In a well appearing patient with a history consistent with EoP, it is acceptable to make an empiric change in the protein source of the formula. Because of the high degree of cross-reactivity between milk and soy protein in sensitized individuals, a protein-hydrolysate formula is often the best choice.[87] Resolution of symptoms begins almost immediately after the elimination of the problematic food. Although symptoms may linger for several days to weeks, continued improvement is the rule. If symptoms do not quickly improve or persist beyond 4–6 weeks, other antigens should be considered, as well as other potential causes of rectal bleeding. In breast-fed infants, dietary restriction of milk and soy containing products for the mother may result in improvement; however, care should be taken to ensure that the mother maintains adequate protein and calcium intake from other sources.

EoP in infancy is generally benign and withdrawing the milk protein trigger resolves the condition. Though gross blood in the stool usually disappears within 72 h, occult blood loss may persist for longer.[90] The prognosis is excellent and the majority of patients are able to tolerate the culprit milk protein by 1–3 years of age. In older individuals, it is more difficult to identify the food triggers and therefore patients usually require medical management. Though there is a paucity of clinical data regarding therapy for this condition, it appears that glucocorticoids and aminosalicylates are efficacious.[7] The prognosis for older onset EoP is less favorable than the infant presentation and is typically chronic and relapsing.

OTHER MANIFESTATIONS OF GASTROINTESTINAL ALLERGY IN INFANTS

Although we have described several specific manifestations of allergic bowel disease in the sections above, there remain numerous non-specific complaints that may occur in the infant that have also been linked to food allergy. These nonspecific complaints create an especially difficult situation for the practitioner, as only a proportion of infants with these complaints will have them as a result of allergy. Further, there are no specific findings that independently can confirm or exclude the diagnosis. Among these potential nonspecific manifestations are gastroesophageal reflux, colic and constipation.

Gastroesophageal reflux

Gastroesophageal reflux (GER) is a common complaint among infants, children and adults. Up to two-thirds of 4-month-old infants experience regurgitation on a daily basis,[98] with other complaints such as forceful vomiting, arching, irritability and feeding refusal occurring to varying degrees. Furthermore, many infants and children may experience GER without the presence of any overt signs or symptoms. Most cases of GER are not attributable to a specific underlying cause; however, one of the leading identifiable causes of GER in this population is food allergy.[99,100]

Relatively recently, the association between GER and cow's milk allergy (CMA) was prospectively investigated.[100] In a 3-year prospective study, infants with symptoms compatible with GER were given pH monitoring and endoscopy to confirm the presence of GER. Patients with a reflux index (percentage of time with acid reflux) of greater than 5% and the presence of esophagitis were considered as having GER. The presence of CMA in these patients was assessed using skin prick tests, the presence of eosinophils in fecal mucus, nasal mucus, or peripheral blood and by circulating levels of anti-betalactoglobulin IgG. Patients who had positive assays for CMA and GER were placed on a cow's milk restricted diet with a protein hydrolysate formula. After 3 months, a double-blind cow's milk challenge was performed to confirm the diagnosis of CMA.

This stringent method of diagnosing both GER and CMA revealed a surprisingly high prevalence (42%) of patients with GER who also had CMA. Further, this author group went on to show that 14 of 47 patients (30%) had GER that was attributable to the CMA itself, based on resolution of symptoms on restricted diet followed by return of symptoms when re-challenged.

Whether cow's milk or other food allergies are responsible for such a high proportion of GER in all populations remains to be seen; however these results imply that refractory cases of GER warrant consideration of food allergy as a contributing factor.

Infantile colic

Infantile colic is a term that is generally used to describe acute self-limited episodes of irritability (presumably due to abdominal pain) that occur in otherwise healthy infants in the first several months of life.[101] Although labeling an infant as having 'colic' implies there is no organic disease responsible, a subset of infants diagnosed with colic will have an underlying organic cause. Food allergies and specifically CMA, have been highly implicated in the organic etiologies of infantile colic.

In a trial of 70 formula-fed infants, 50 (71%) had resolution of colic symptoms when cow's milk protein was removed from the diet, with 100% relapse rate after two successive re-introductions of the protein.[102] Similarly, in a double-blind crossover study, cow's milk allergy was implicated in 24 of 27 infants with colic with significant reductions in daily crying when cow's milk protein was removed from the diet,[103] with worsening of symptoms when whey was reintroduced into the diet in a blinded fashion.

Traditionally, changing the infant's formula is a common way of dealing with colic; often several formula changes are made (e.g. from cow's milk based to soy based to hydrolyzed protein). It is often unclear, however, whether the formula change is responsible for the eventual resolution of symptoms as colic by definition begins to resolve by 4 to 5 months of age.

Diarrhea

The presence of diarrhea in the context of food allergies can be multifactorial. As discussed in previous sections,

EoG and EoP may both lead to intestinal mucosal damage and subsequent diarrhea. However, food allergy may also result in diarrhea in the absence of mucosal damage or eosinophilic infiltration.

Gastrointestinal symptoms, in particular diarrhea, are commonly seen among children with atopic eczema;[104,105] avoidance of particular foods in these patients will alleviate the symptoms.[105] In patients with GI symptoms related to milk ingestion (confirmed by double-blind challenge), the instillation of milk into the intestinal lumen resulted in increased production of histamine and eosinophil cationic protein within 20 min.[106] Albumin concentration in the intestine also increased, suggesting increased gut permeability and leakage; none of these findings were seen in normal controls.

Animal models suggest that food allergy may also increase intestinal motility, which in turn may lead to diarrhea.[107] Increased intestinal mast cell counts have been seen in subjects with increased intestinal motility.[108] However, diarrhea in relation to food allergy is almost certainly a multi-factorial event that may involve other processes such as secondary carbohydrate malabsorption or over ingestion of non-absorbable sugars.

Constipation

Constipation is a common problem among infants and children and although often short-lived or self-limited, a substantial proportion may have symptoms that persist for 6 months or more.[109] It has long been suggested that cow's milk plays a role in the development of chronic constipation,[110] but there is now growing evidence that CMA is a causative factor. One of the most compelling studies involved a blinded cross-over study of cow's milk restriction in children with chronic constipation.[111] In this trial, 65 children with chronic constipation (all of whom received cow's milk in their regular diet) were randomized to receive either cow's milk or soy milk for 15 days, followed by a washout period and reversal of the previous diet. A total of 68% of the children had improvement in their constipation while taking soy milk, while none had improvement on cow's milk. Re-challenging the responders with cow's milk resulted in return of constipation. Evidence of CMA was based upon higher frequencies of co-existent rhinitis, dermatitis and bronchospasm in responders, as well as increased likelihood of elevated IgE to cow's milk antigens and inflammatory cells on rectal biopsy. A subsequent study revealed further evidence of the causative nature of CMA in constipation.[112]

Approach to the potentially allergic infant with nonspecific GI symptoms

Because GI complaints such as those listed above are quite common in the infant population, the practitioner who cares for infants will commonly be faced with the issue of when to implicate food allergy. Further complicating the issue is that general allergic complaints such as atopic eczema and rhinitis are also quite common in this population. Optimally, the allergic contribution to any GI complaint would be investigated through double-blind food challenges. However, this is not practical for most practitioners.

Any infant with GI symptoms refractory to standard treatment may be manifesting signs of food allergy. Because CMA is implicated most commonly in this population, removal of this antigen from the diet is a reasonable approach. However, this change should be made in concert with appropriate investigations for other etiological factors (e.g. anatomic studies such as upper GI series in chronic reflux, stool cultures in chronic diarrhea). Soy formula may be substituted for cow's milk formula, with the understanding that there is a high cross-reactivity between cow's milk and soy protein in sensitized individuals. Protein-hydrolysate formulas represent a good option, more likely to result in improvement in a truly allergic infant. Breast-feeding mothers may need to restrict their intake of milk and soy for several weeks before the antigens no longer appear in breast milk. The use of amino-acid based elemental formulas should be reserved for those who have failed hydrolyzed protein formulas and preferably, in those who have some other objective positive findings of allergy. It should be remembered that the natural history of allergy in the infant is often self-limited and thus improvement with dietary elimination does not independently confirm food allergy. Formally re-challenging the infant with the suspected food antigen is a better way to confirm that allergy existed and was responsible for the symptoms in question. Formal consultation with an allergist in this context is highly advisable.

CONCLUSION

Eosinophilic disorders of the gastrointestinal tract are becoming increasingly recognized as distinct clinical entities with specific management strategies. While EoG is rare and difficult to diagnose, EoP and EoE are much more common and easily diagnosed by endoscopic biopsy. While EoP is a well-accepted entity, the diagnosis of EoE has recently been receiving a great deal of attention. Recent literature suggests a mini-epidemic of EoE in the pediatric population, though controversy still exists regarding the etiology and treatment. Further studies are needed to effectively differentiate patients with eosinophilic esophagitis from those with reflux esophagitis. It would appear that significant esophageal eosinophilia (>20 per HPF) suggests a diagnosis of eosinophilic esophagitis, while <5 per HPF and an improvement with acid blockade suggests GERD. The diagnosis is equivocal when an esophageal biopsy reveals 5–20 eosinophils per HPF.

Future research should focus on clarifying the prevalence and natural history (e.g. the potential development of strictures) and optimizing the diagnostic approach and treatment options of all gastrointestinal eosinophilic disorders. The particular management challenges posed by these conditions warrants close liaison between gastroenterologists, allergists and dietitians. In addition, patients and families require particular support, especially when trying to adopt restricted diets. Patient-founded, support advocacy groups have been established for this purpose (e.g. American Partnership for Eosinophilic Disorders, *www.APFED.org*).

Awareness of food-induced allergic and eosinophilic disease of the gastrointestinal tract has increased, but many unanswered questions remain. The variation in geographical distribution of EoG and EoE has yet to be explained. The pathogenesis of these conditions has to be fully elucidated, in particular the role of environmental and infectious agents. Advances need to be made in diagnosing these conditions, especially with the use of less invasive techniques than endoscopy with biopsy and also in better identifying offending food antigens and allergens. In addition, biochemical studies need to be pursued so that we can determine a cause of these disorders. Is the eosinophil dysregulation due to an immunologic defect or an allergy? These and other research questions reinforce the limitations of our current understanding of gastrointestinal eosinophilic disease.

References

1. Sampson HA. Differential diagnosis in adverse reactions to foods. J Allergy Clin Immunol 1986; 78:212–219.
2. Bock SA, Atkins FM. Patterns of food hypersensitivity during sixteen years of double-blind, placebo-controlled food challenges. J Pediatr 1990; 117:561–567.
3. Atkins FM, Steinberg SS, Metcalfe DD. Evaluation of immediate adverse reactions to foods in adult patients. II. A detailed analysis of reaction patterns during oral food challenge. J Allergy Clin Immunol 1985; 75:356–363.
4. Sampson HA. IgE-mediated food intolerance. J Allergy Clin Immunol 1988; 81:495–504.
5. Sampson HA, Albergo R. Comparison of results of skin tests, RAST and double-blind, placebo-controlled food challenges in children with atopic dermatitis. J Allergy Clin Immunol 1984; 74:26–33.
6. Heine RG. Pathophysiology, diagnosis and treatment of food protein-induced gastrointestinal diseases. Curr Opin Allergy Clin Immunol 2004; 4:221–229.
7. Rothenberg ME. Eosinophilic gastrointestinal disorders (EGID). J Allergy Clin Immunol 2004; 113:11–29.
8. Guajardo JR, Plotnick LM, Fende JM, Collins MH, Putnam PE, Rothenberg ME. Eosinophil-associated gastrointestinal disorders: a world-wide-web based registry. J Pediatr 2002; 141:576–581.
9. Walsh SV, Antonioli DA, Goldman H, et al. Allergic esophagitis in children: a clinicopathological entity. Am J Surg Pathol 1999; 23:390–396.
10. Spergel JM, Beausoleil JL, Mascarenhas M, Liacouras CA. The use of skin prick tests and patch tests to identify causative foods in eosinophilic esophagitis. J Allergy Clin Immunol 2002; 109:363–368.
11. Sampson HA. Food allergy. Part 1: immunopathogenesis and clinical disorders. J Allergy Clin Immunol 1999; 103:717–728.
12. Kelly KJ, Lazenby AJ, Rowe PC, Yardley JH, Perman JA, Sampson HA. Eosinophilic esophagitis attributed to gastroesophageal reflux: improvement with an amino acid-based formula. Gastroenterology 1995; 109:1503–1512.
13. Teitelbaum JE, Fox VL, Twarog FJ, et al. Eosinophilic esophagitis in children: immunopathological analysis and response to fluticasone propionate. Gastroenterology 2002; 122:1216–1225.
14. Mishra A, Hogan SP, Brandt EB, Rothenberg ME. An etiological role for aeroallergens and eosinophils in experimental esophagitis. J Clin Invest 2001; 107:83–90.
15. Fogg MI, Ruchelli E, Spergel JM. Pollen and eosinophilic esophagitis. J Allergy Clin Immunol 2003; 112:796–797.
16. Liacouras CA, Markowitz JE. Eosinophilic esophagitis: A subset of eosinophilic gastroenteritis. Curr Gastroenterol Rep 1999; 1:253–258.
17. Steiner SJ, Gupta SK, Croffie JM, Fitzgerald JF. Correlation between number of eosinophils and reflux index on same day esophageal biopsy and 24 hour esophageal pH monitoring. Am J Gastroenterol 2004; 99:801–805.
18. Straumann A, Spichtin HP, Grize L, Bucher KA, Beglinger C, Simon HU. Natural history of primary eosinophilic esophagitis: a follow-up of 30 adult patients for up to 11.5 years. Gastroenterology 2003; 125:1660–1669.
19. Katzka DA. Eosinophilic esophagitis. Curr Treat Options Gastroenterol 2003; 6:49–54.
20. Orenstein SR, Shalaby TM, Di Lorenzo C, et al. The spectrum of pediatric eosinophilic esophagitis beyond infancy: a clinical series of 30 children. Am J Gastroenterol 2000; 95:1422–1430.
21. Ruchelli E, Wenner W, Voytek T, Brown K, Liacouras C. Severity of esophageal eosinophilia predicts response to conventional gastroesophageal reflux therapy. Pediatr Dev Pathol 1999; 2:15–18.
22. Fox VL, Nurko S, Teitelbaum JE, Badizadegan K, Furuta GT. High-resolution EUS in children with eosinophilic 'allergic' esophagitis. Gastrointest Endosc 2003; 57:30–36.
23. Markowitz JE, Spergel JM, Ruchelli E, Liacouras CA. Elemental diet is an effective treatment for eosinophilic esophagitis in children and adolescents. Am J Gastroenterol 2003; 98:777–782.
24. Liacouras CA, Wenner WJ, Brown K, Ruchelli E. Primary eosinophilic esophagitis in children: successful treatment with oral corticosteroids. J Pediatr Gastroenterol Nutr 1998; 26:380–385.
25. Liacouras CA. Failed Nissen fundoplication in two patients who had persistent vomiting and eosinophilic esophagitis. J Pediatr Surg 1997; 32:1504–1506.
26. Vitellas KM, Bennett WF, Bova JG, Johnston JC, Caldwell JH, Mayle JE. Idiopathic eosinophilic esophagitis. Radiology 1993; 186:789–793.
27. Lee RG. Marked eosinophilia in esophageal mucosal biopsies. Am J Surg Pathol 1985; 9:475–479.
28. Faubion WA. Jr., Perrault J, Burgart LJ, Zein NN, Clawson M, Freese DK. Treatment of eosinophilic esophagitis with in haled corticosteroids. J Pediatr Gastroenterol Nutr 1998; 27:90–93.
29. Simon MR, Houser WL, Smith KA, Long PM. Esophageal candidiasis as a complication of inhaled corticosteroids. Ann Allergy Asthma Immunol 1997; 79:333–338.
30. Sharek PJ, Bergman DA. The effect of inhaled steroids on the linear growth of children with asthma: a meta-analysis. Pediatrics 2000; 106:E8.

31. Dahl R. Disodium cromoglycate and food allergy. The effect of oral and inhaled disodium cromoglycate in a food allergic patient. Allergy 1978; 33:120–124.
32. Whitington PF, Whitington GL. Eosinophilic gastroenteropathy in childhood. J Pediatr Gastroenterol Nutr 1988; 7:379–385.
33. Businco L, Cantani A. Food allergy in children: diagnosis and treatment with sodium cromoglycate. Allergol Immunopathol (Madr) 1990; 18:339–338.
34. Schwartz DA, Pardi DS, Murray JA. Use of montelukast as steroid-sparing agent for recurrent eosinophilic gastroenteritis. Dig Dis Sci 2001; 46:1787–1790.
35. Attwood SE, Lewis CJ, Bronder CS, Morris CD, Armstrong GR, Whittam J. Eosinophilic oesophagitis: a novel treatment using Montelukast. Gut 2003; 52:181–185.
36. Kaijser R. Zur Kenntnis der allergischen Affektioner desima Verdeanungaskanal von Standpunkt desmia Chirurgen aus. Arch Klin Chir 1937; 188:36–64.
37. Klein NC, Hargrove RL, Sleisenger MH, Jeffries GH. Eosinophilic gastroenteritis. Medicine (Baltimore) 1970; 49:299–319.
38. Goldman H, Proujansky R. Allergic proctitis and gastroenteritis in children. Clinical and mucosal biopsy features in 53 cases. Am J Surg Pathol 1986; 10:75–86.
39. Spergel JM, Pawlowski NA. Food allergy. Mechanisms, diagnosis and management in children. Pediatr Clin North Am 2002; 49:73–96.
40. Park HS, Kim HS, Jang HJ. Eosinophilic gastroenteritis associated with food allergy and bronchial asthma. J Korean Med Sci 1995; 10:216–219.
41. Justinich C, Katz A, Gurbindo C, et al. Elemental diet improves steroid-dependent eosinophilic gastroenteritis and reverses growth failure. J Pediatr Gastroenterol Nutr 1996; 23:81–85.
42. Leinbach GE, Rubin CE. Eosinophilic gastroenteritis: a simple reaction to food allergens? Gastroenterology 1970; 59:874–889.
43. Caldwell JH, Sharma HM, Hurtubise PE, Colwell DL. Eosinophilic gastroenteritis in extreme allergy. Immunopathological comparison with nonallergic gastrointestinal disease. Gastroenterology 1979; 77:560–564.
44. Cytokines KA. structure, function and synthesis. Curr Opin Immunol 1989; 2:215–225.
45. Desreumaux P, Bloget F, Seguy D, et al. Interleukin 3, granulocyte-macrophage colony-stimulating factor and interleukin 5 in eosinophilic gastroenteritis. Gastroenterology 1996; 110:768–774.
46. Takafuji S, Bischoff SC, Weck AL De, Dahinden CA. IL-3 and IL-5 prime normal human eosinophils to produce leukotriene C4 in response to soluble agonists. J Immunol 1991; 147:3855–3861.
47. Kelly KJ. Eosinophilic gastroenteritis. J Pediatr Gastroenterol Nutr 2000; 30(suppl):S28–S35.
48. Talley NJ, Shorter RG, Phillips SF, Zinsmeister AR. Eosinophilic gastroenteritis: a clinicopathological study of patients with disease of the mucosa, muscle layer and subserosal tissues. Gut 1990; 31:54–58.
49. Santos J, Junquera F, Torres I de, Molero X, Vilaseca J, Malagelada JR. Eosinophilic gastroenteritis presenting as ascites and splenomegaly. Eur J Gastroenterol Hepatol 1995; 7:675–678.
50. Aquino A, Domini M, Rossi C, D'Incecco C, Fakhro A, Lelli Chiesa P. Pyloric stenosis due to eosinophilic gastroenteritis: presentation of two cases in mono-ovular twins. Eur J Pediatr 1999; 158:172–173.
51. Khan S, Orenstein SR. Eosinophilic gastroenteritis masquerading as pyloric stenosis. Clin Pediatr (Phila) 2000; 39:55–57.
52. Redondo-Cerezo E, Cabello MJ, Gonzalez Y, Gomez M, Garcia-Montero M, Teresa J de. Eosinophilic gastroenteritis: our recent experience: one-year experience of atypical onset of an uncommon disease. Scand J Gastroenterol 2001; 36:1358–1360.
53. Shweiki E, West JC, Klena JW, et al. Eosinophilic gastroenteritis presenting as an obstructing cecal mass – a case report and review of the literature. Am J Gastroenterol 1999; 94:3644–3645.
54. Huang FC, Ko SF, Huang SC, Lee SY. Eosinophilic gastroenteritis with perforation mimicking intussusception. J Pediatr Gastroenterol Nutr 2001; 33:613–615.
55. Deslandres C, Russo P, Gould P, Hardy P. Perforated duodenal ulcer in a pediatric patient with eosinophilic gastroenteritis. Can J Gastroenterol 1997; 11:208–212.
56. Wang CS, Hsueh S, Shih LY, Chen MF. Repeated bowel resections for eosinophilic gastroenteritis with obstruction and perforation. Case report. Acta Chir Scand 1990; 156:333–336.
57. Hoefer RA, Ziegler MM, Koop CE, Schnaufer L. Surgical manifestations of eosinophilic gastroenteritis in the pediatric patient. J Pediatr Surg 1977; 12:955–962.
58. Lerza P. A further case of eosinophilic gastroenteritis with ascites. Eur J Gastroenterol Hepatol 1996; 8:407.
59. DeSchryver Kecskemeti K, Clouse RE. A previously unrecognized subgroup of 'eosinophilic gastroenteritis'. Association with connective tissue diseases. Am J Surg Pathol 1984; 8:171–180.
60. Dubucquoi S, Janin A, Klein O, et al. Activated eosinophils and interleukin 5 expression in early recurrence of Crohn's disease. Gut 1995; 37:242–246.
61. Levy AM, Yamazaki K, Keulen VP Van, et al. Increased eosinophil infiltration and degranulation in colonic tissue from patients with collagenous colitis. Am J Gastroenterol 2001; 96:1522–1528.
62. Griscom NT, Kirkpatrick JA Jr., Girdany BR, Berdon WE, Grand RJ, Mackie GG. Gastric antral narrowing in chronic granulomatous disease of childhood. Pediatrics 1974; 54:456–460.
63. Harris BH, Boles ET. Jr. Intestinal lesions in chronic granulomatous disease of childhood. J Pediatr Surg 1973; 8:955–956.
64. Caldwell JH, Tennenbaum JI, Bronstein HA. Serum IgE in eosinophilic gastroenteritis. Response to intestinal challenge in two cases. N Engl J Med 1975; 292:1388–1390.
65. Teele RL, Katz AJ, Goldman H, Kettell RM. Radiographic features of eosinophilic gastroenteritis (allergic gastroenteropathy) of childhood. AJR Am J Roentgenol 1979; 132:575–580.
66. Vandenplas Y, Quenon M, Renders F, Dab I, Loeb H. Milk-sensitive eosinophilic gastroenteritis in a 10-day-old boy. Eur J Pediatr 1990; 149:244–245.
67. Dellen RG Van, Lewis JC. Oral administration of cromolyn in a patient with protein-losing enteropathy, food allergy and eosinophilic gastroenteritis. Mayo Clin Proc 1994; 69:441–444.
68. Moots RJ, Prouse P, Gumpel JM. Near fatal eosinophilic gastroenteritis responding to oral sodium chromoglycate. Gut 1988; 29:1282–1285.
69. Di Gioacchino M, Pizzicannella G, Fini N, et al. Sodium cromoglycate in the treatment of eosinophilic gastroenteritis. Allergy 1990; 45:161–166.

70. Neustrom MR, Friesen C. Treatment of eosinophilic gastroenteritis with montelukast. J Allergy Clin Immunol 1999; 104:506.
71. Shirai T, Hashimoto D, Suzuki K, et al. Successful treatment of eosinophilic gastroenteritis with suplatast tosilate. J Allergy Clin Immunol 2001; 107:924–925.
72. Bengtsson U, Hanson LA, Ahlstedt S. Survey of gastrointestinal reactions to foods in adults in relation to atopy, presence of mucus in the stools, swelling of joints and arthralgia in patients with gastrointestinal reactions to foods. Clin Exp Allergy 1996; 26:1387–1394.
73. Jenkins HR, Pincott JR, Soothill JF, Milla PJ, Harries JT. Food allergy: the major cause of infantile colitis. Arch Dis Child 1984; 59:326–329.
74. Heyman M, Grasset E, Ducroc R, Desjeux JF. Antigen absorption by the jejunal epithelium of children with cow's milk allergy. Pediatr Res 1988; 24:197–202.
75. Husby S, Host A, Teisner B, Svehag SE. Infants and children with cow milk allergy/intolerance. Investigation of the uptake of cow milk protein and activation of the complement system. Allergy 1990; 45:547–551.
76. Kerner JA Jr. Formula allergy and intolerance. Gastroenterol Clin North Am 1995; 24:1–25.
77. Simpser E. Gastrointestinal allergy. In: Altschuler SM, Liacouras CA, eds. Clinical Pediatric Gastroenterology. Philadelphia, PA: Churchill Livingstone; 1998: 113–118.
78. Gerrard JW, MacKenzie JW, Goluboff N, Garson JZ, Maningas CS. Cow's milk allergy: prevalence and manifestations in an unselected series of newborns. Acta Paediatr Scand Suppl 1973; 234:1–21.
79. Host A, Halken S. A prospective study of cow milk allergy in Danish infants during the first 3 years of life. Clinical course in relation to clinical and immunological type of hypersensitivity reaction. Allergy 1990; 45:587–596.
80. Strobel S. Epidemiology of food sensitivity in childhood – with special reference to cow's milk allergy in infancy. Monogr Allergy 1993; 31:119–130.
81. Eastham EJ. Soy protein allergy. In: Hamburger, R. ed. Allergology, Immunology and Gastroenterology. New York, NY: Raven Press; 1989:223–236.
82. Shannon WR. Demonstration of food proteins in human breast milk by anaphylactic experiments in guinea pig. Am J Dis Child 1921; 22:223–225.
83. Makinen-Kiljunen S, Palosuo T. A sensitive enzyme-linked immunosorbent assay for determination of bovine beta-lactoglobulin in infant feeding formulas and in human milk. Allergy 1992; 47:347–352.
84. Axelsson I, Jakobsson I, Lindberg T, Benediktsson B. Bovine beta-lactoglobulin in the human milk. A longitudinal study during the whole lactation period. Acta Paediatr Scand 1986; 75:702–707.
85. Pittschieler K. Cow's milk protein-induced colitis in the breast-fed infant. J Pediatr Gastroenterol Nutr 1990; 10:548–549.
86. Vandenplas Y, Hauser B, Borre C Van den, Sacre L, Dab I. Effect of a whey hydrolysate prophylaxis of atopic disease. Ann Allergy 1992; 68:419–424.
87. Juvonen P, Mansson M, Jakobsson I. Does early diet have an effect on subsequent macromolecular absorption and serum IgE? J Pediatr Gastroenterol Nutr 1994; 18:344–349.
88. Kaczmarski M, Kurzatkowska B. The contribution of some environmental factors to the development of cow's milk and gluten intolerance in children. Rocz Akad Med Bialymst 1988; 33/34:151–165.
89. Katz AJ, Twarog FJ, Zeiger RS, Falchuk ZM. Milk-sensitive and eosinophilic gastroenteropathy: similar clinical features with contrasting mechanisms and clinical course. J Allergy Clin Immunol 1984; 74:72–78.
90. Hill SM, Milla PJ. Colitis caused by food allergy in infants. Arch Dis Child 1990; 65:132–133.
91. Donta ST, Myers MG. Clostridium difficile toxin in asymptomatic neonates. J Pediatr 1982; 100:431–434.
92. Cooperstock MS, Steffen E, Yolken R, Onderdonk A. Clostridium difficile in normal infants and sudden infant death syndrome: an association with infant formula feeding. Pediatrics 1982; 70:91–95.
93. Hirano K, Shimojo N, Katsuki T, Ishikawa N, Kohno Y, Niimi H. Eosinophils in stool smear in normal and milk-allergic infants. Arerugi 1997; 46:594–601.
94. Anveden-Hertzberg L, Finkel Y, Sandstedt B, Karpe B. Proctocolitis in exclusively breast-fed infants. Eur J Pediatr 1996; 155:464–467.
95. Odze RD, Bines J, Leichtner AM, Goldman H, Antonioli DA. Allergic proctocolitis in infants: a prospective clinicopathologic biopsy study. Hum Pathol 1993; 24:668–674.
96. Machida HM, Catto Smith AG, Gall DG, Trevenen C, Scott RB. Allergic colitis in infancy: clinical and pathologic aspects. J Pediatr Gastroenterol Nutr 1994; 19:22–26.
97. Goldman H. Allergic disorders. In: Ming S-C, Goldman H, ed. Pathology of the Gastrointestinal Tract. Philadelphia, PA: WB Saunders; 1992:171–187.
98. Nelson SP, Chen EH, Syniar GM, Christoffel KK. Prevalence of symptoms of gastroesophageal reflux during infancy. A pediatric practice-based survey. Pediatr Pract Res Group Arch Pediatr Adolesc Med 1997; 151:569–572.
99. Iacono G, Carroccio A, Cavataio F, et al. Gastroesophageal reflux and cow's milk allergy in infants: a prospective study. J Allergy Clin Immunol 1996; 97:822–827.
100. Cavataio F, Carroccio A, Iacono G. Milk-induced reflux in infants less than one year of age. J Pediatr Gastroenterol Nutr 2000; 30(suppl):S36–S44.
101. Wessel MA, Cobb JC, Jackson EB, Harris GS Jr, Detwiler AC. Paroxysmal fussing in infancy, sometimes called colic. Pediatrics 1954; 14:421–435.
102. Iacono G, Carroccio A, Montalto G, et al. Severe infantile colic and food intolerance: a long-term prospective study. J Pediatr Gastroenterol Nutr 1991; 12:332–335.
103. Lothe L, Lindberg T. Cow's milk whey protein elicits symptoms of infantile colic in colicky formula-fed infants: a double-blind crossover study. Pediatrics 1989; 83:262–266.
104. Ruuska T. Occurrence of acute diarrhea in atopic and nonatopic infants: the role of prolonged breast-feeding. J Pediatr Gastroenterol Nutr 1992; 14:27–33.
105. Caffarelli C, Cavagni G, Deriu FM, Zanotti P, Atherton DJ. Gastrointestinal symptoms in atopic eczema. Arch Dis Child 1998; 78:230–234.
106. Bengtsson U, Knutson TW, Knutson L, Dannaeus A, Hallgren R, Ahlstedt S. Eosinophil cationic protein and histamine after intestinal challenge in patients with cow's milk intolerance. J Allergy Clin Immunol 1997; 100:216–221.
107. Scott RB, Tan DT. Mediation of altered motility in food protein induced intestinal anaphylaxis in Hooded-Lister rat. Can J Physiol Pharm 1996; 74:320–330.

108. Gwee KA, Leong YL, Graham C, et al. The role of psychological and biological factors in postinfective gut dysfunction. Gut 1999; 44:400–406.
109. Loening-Baucke V. Constipation in children. N Engl J Med 1998; 339:1155–1156.
110. Clein NW. Cow's milk allergy in infants. Pediatr Clin North Am 1954; 25:949–962.
111. Iacono G, Cavataio F, Montalto G, et al. Intolerance of cow's milk and chronic constipation in children. N Engl J Med 1998; 339:1100–1104.
112. Daher S, Tahan S, Sole D, et al. Cow's milk protein intolerance and chronic constipation in children. Pediatr Allergy Immunol 2001; 12:339–342.

Chapter 36
Infectious diarrhea

Richard J. Noel and Mitchell B. Cohen

INTRODUCTION

In the USA, an estimated 21–37 million episodes of diarrhea occur annually in children younger than 5 years of age.[1] Some 10% of these children are seen by a physician, more than 200 000 are hospitalized and between 300 and 400 die from the illness. Worldwide, the number of childhood deaths from diarrhea is higher than 4 million per year.

Knowledge of diarrheal disease has increased remarkably during the past few decades.[2] Numerous bacterial pathogens and an increasing number of viral pathogens have been demonstrated to cause diarrhea. This increased understanding of pathogenic mechanisms has led to improvements in therapy. This chapter discusses the major viral and bacterial agents of infectious diarrhea, including their epidemiology, pathogenesis, clinical manifestations, diagnosis and therapy.

VIRAL GASTROENTERITIS

Diarrheal disease caused by viral agents occurs far more frequently than does similar disease of bacterial origin. In fact, viral gastroenteritis is the second most common illness in the USA, after the common cold.[3] Despite the frequent occurrence of viral enteritides, the identification of a specific virus as causative agent is a relatively recent development.[4] Rotavirus and a number of other small round structured viruses have been identified as a major cause of non-bacterial gastroenteritis in children and adults. This discussion focuses on these established pathogens, and then continues with a brief summary of several newer viral enteropathogens and the current status of several candidate pathogens.

Rotavirus

Rotavirus was first identified as a specific viral pathogen in duodenal cells of children with diarrhea by Bishop and associates in 1973.[5] Subsequent studies indicated that rotavirus is responsible not only for more cases of diarrheal disease in infants and children than any other single cause, but also for a significant portion of deaths caused by diarrhea in both developed and developing countries throughout the world.[6] Rotavirus is responsible for 20–70% of hospitalizations for diarrhea among children worldwide.[7]

Virology

The genus Rotavirus is classified as a member of the family Reoviridae of the RNA viruses. Rotaviruses are round particles 68 nm in diameter and are composed of two separate shells (capsids). The capsids surround a 38-nm icosahedral core structure, which in turn encloses the 11 double strands of RNA in the core. This structure gives the virus its characteristic appearance of a wide-rimmed wheel with spokes radiating from the hub, from which its name was derived (*rota* is Latin for 'wheel').[8]

Rotaviruses are classified based on antigenic properties of various proteins found in the capsid stricture. The VP6 protein on the inner capsid of the virus determines the rotavirus group.[4] Most viruses infecting humans are classified as group A, although rotaviruses from groups B and C have occasionally been associated with human diarrheal disease as well. The next level of classification is the subgroup, which is determined by other antigenic differences among the VP6 proteins. At least two subgroups are known to exist.[4] Subgroup typing has proved important in the study of patients who experience more than one episode of rotaviral infection. In these patients, recurrent infections usually but not necessarily involve agents of different subgroups, which suggests that subgroup antigens are not sufficient for inducing the production of protective antibodies.[9] Finally, the rotaviruses are classified into a variety of serotypes based on the antigenic differences of VP7 glycoprotein or the VP4 protease-sensitive hemagglutinin proteins that are found in the outer capsid.[10] VP7-based serotypes are now referred to as G types (for glycoprotein in VP7); G types 1 through 4 are responsible for most infections in children. VP4 serotypes are called P types (representing protease sensitivity of VP4). Reassortments of VP7 and VP4 have been used in candidate rotavirus vaccines.

Epidemiology

Rotavirus infection appears to occur throughout the world. In temperate climates, a sharp increase in incidence of cases occurs during the winter months.[6] In the USA, the peak rotavirus season begins in November in the Southwest and ends in the Northeast in April.[6] In the tropics, year-round transmission occurs, with seasonal variation in some areas.[11] Transmission is primarily from person to person, through contact with feces or contaminated fomites. Spread by water is likely. Respiratory transmission has been suggested but not proved.[12]

Although the virus may affect all age groups, it most commonly produces disease in children between 6 and 24 months of age. Most children have developed rotavirus antibodies by the age of 2 years, which helps to explain the observed decreased incidence of rotaviral infection in later childhood.[13] The disease does occur in the adult

some evidence that the norovirus is transmitted through a respiratory route in the form of aerosolized particles from vomitus.[62] Although previously referred to as 'winter vomiting disease',[48] norovirus produces outbreaks of disease that can occur throughout the year.

Pathophysiology The histologic changes induced by the norovirus in an infected host have been studied in small bowel biopsies from infected volunteers.[63] Those volunteers who remained free of clinical symptoms had normal biopsy specimens, whereas those with symptoms exhibited marked, but not specific, changes, including focal areas of villous flattening and disorganization of epithelial cells. On electron microscopy, microvilli were shortened and there was dilatation of the endoplasmic reticulum. These volunteers had repeat biopsies 2 weeks after the illness and normal histology was again present. Other investigators have demonstrated the presence of normal gastric and rectal histology in patients affected by norovirus as is typical of viral gastroenteritis.[55]

Clinical manifestations

The clinical manifestations of disease produced by the norovirus include nausea, vomiting and cramping abdominal pain (Table 36.1). Diarrhea is said to be a less consistent feature of this illness. In the original outbreak, only 44% of patients experienced diarrhea, whereas 84% had vomiting.[48] Other studies, however, have found that diarrhea occurs in most children and experimentally infected adult volunteers who become ill from this virus.[56,64,65] Fever occurs in approximately one-third of affected patients, but respiratory symptoms are not typically a part of this illness. An incubation period of approximately 24–48 h has been noted before the onset of symptoms,[48,56] and symptoms persist for 12–48 h.

Diagnosis and treatment

Development of techniques for diagnosis of norovirus has been difficult owing to the lack of methods for culturing the virus *in vitro* and the lack of an appropriate animal model. The use of molecular-based diagnostic assays is likely to improve our ability to recognize these infections and better understand their importance.[51,66,67]

The treatment for norovirus is supportive; oral rehydration solutions are used if necessary. Significant dehydration is uncommon and the need for hospitalization is rare.

Enteric adenovirus

The enteric adenoviruses are among the more recently recognized viral pathogens that cause acute gastroenteritis. Adenoviruses are a large group of viruses long recognized for their role in the pathogenesis of respiratory infections and keratoconjunctivitis. Most of the 47 serotypes are known to be shed in the feces of infected patients. In patients with predominantly gastrointestinal symptoms, the organisms are detectable by electron microscopy of stool samples; however, they fail to grow in standard tissue culture conditions.[23] Their unique cell culture requirements allow for the differentiation of nonenteric adenoviruses from the enteric serotypes (Ad40 and Ad41), which are recognized to be among the common causes of viral childhood gastroenteritis.[68,69]

Infection with enteric adenoviruses apparently occurs throughout the year, with only slight seasonal variation.[70,71] This disease tends to affect predominantly younger children, with most patients being younger than 2 years of age.[71,72] Enteric adenovirus is spread by the fecal-oral route. Transmission of the disease to family contacts is unusual.

Diarrhea is the most commonly reported symptom of enteric adenoviral infection. In contrast with diarrhea from other viral enteritides, diarrhea from enteric adenovirus typically persists for a prolonged period, sometimes as long as 14 days. Viruses may be excreted in the feces of infected patients for 1 to 2 weeks.[70] Vomiting frequently occurs but is usually mild and of a much shorter duration than is the diarrhea. Dehydration has been seen in approximately half of affected patients and hospitalization is sometimes necessary. The frequency of association of respiratory symptoms with enteric adenovirus infection is unclear.[72]

The diagnosis of enteric adenovirus is best made by electron microscopy or immunoelectron microscopy of stool samples or from intestinal biopsy specimens. ELISA[73] and PCR[74] techniques have also been used successfully in enteric adenovirus diagnosis. Treatment is mainly supportive and oral rehydration solutions are useful in cases of dehydration.

Astrovirus

Astrovirus, similar to HuCV, is a single-stranded RNA virus grouped with the small round structured viruses. However, the recently derived sequence of the astrovirus RNA genome reveals that this agent is sufficiently different to be classified in its own family as Astroviridae.[75] Astrovirus is worldwide in distribution and tends to infect mainly children in the 1 to 3-year age group. In controlled studies in Thailand, astrovirus infection was the second most common cause of enteritis, after rotavirus infection, in symptomatic children.[76] Astrovirus infection occurred in 9% of children with diarrhea, compared with 2% of controls. Comparable findings have been reported in daycare centers in North America and Japan.[77,78] Most children infected with astrovirus develop symptoms. Vomiting, diarrhea, abdominal pain and fever all are commonly seen with infection by this agent and symptoms typically last 1 to 4 days. Spread of the virus may occur via the fecal-oral route from person-to-person contact or through contaminated food or water. Asymptomatic shedding of astrovirus has also been reported.[79]

Other viruses

A variety of other viruses are being studied to determine what role, if any, they may play in the pathogenesis of human enteric infections. With the exception of those viruses previously discussed in detail, insufficient data are available to ascertain clinical and epidemiologic differences, if any, among the various small round viruses.

Pestivirus, a single-stranded RNA virus of the togavirus family, has been found in the feces of 24% of children living on an American Indian reservation who had diarrhea attributable to no other infectious agent.[80] These children experienced only mild diarrhea but had more severe respiratory complaints.

Coronavirus is known to cause an upper respiratory illness in humans and has been shown to cause diarrhea in some animals.[81] The role of this agent in human diarrheal disease is unclear and at least one study found coronavirus more commonly in children without diarrhea than in those who were ill.[82] Coronavirus was implicated in an outbreak of necrotizing enterocolitis.[83]

Toroviruses are pleomorphic viruses recognized to cause enteric illness in a variety of animals.[84] Members of this group, originally described in Berne, Switzerland and Breda, Iowa and named for those cities, have been seen in the feces of humans with diarrheal disease.[85] Because of the pleomorphic structure of toroviruses, electron microscopy was inadequate to prove an etiopathogenic role of these viruses in diarrheal disease. The more recent findings of torovirus-like particles by immunoassay, using validated anti-Breda virus antiserum, lends additional weight to the hypothesis that these are agents of human gastroenteritis.[86] Their causative role in human disease, however, remains unproven. Similarly, picobirnavirus is known to cause disease in animals and has been isolated from stools of humans with diarrheal illness.[87]

Cytomegalovirus has been associated with enteritis and colitis. Except for Ménétrier's disease, caused by gastric cytomegalovirus infection, enteritis and colitis seem to occur almost exclusively among immunocompromised patients. In this population, cytomegalovirus causes viremia and is carried by the blood stream to a variety of sites, including organs of the gastrointestinal tract. Diagnosis may be made by virus detection in feces, by demonstration of typical cytomegalic inclusion cells, or by *in situ* hybridization.[88]

BACTERIAL GASTROENTERITIS

Host-defense factors

For an infecting bacterial agent to cause diarrhea, it must first overcome the following gastrointestinal tract defenses: (1) gastric acidity, (2) intestinal motility, (3) mucus secretion, (4) normal intestinal microflora and (5) specific mucosal and systemic immune mechanisms. Gastric acidity is the first barrier encountered by infecting organisms.[89] Many studies have demonstrated the bactericidal properties of gastric juice at pH less than 4.[90] In patients with achlorhydria or decreased gastric acid secretion, the gastric pH is higher and this bactericidal effect is diminished. Gastric acidity serves to decrease the number of viable bacteria that proceed to the small intestine.

Organisms surviving the gastric acidity barrier are trapped within the mucus layer of the small intestine, facilitating their movement through the intestine by peristalsis. If motility in the intestine is abnormal or absent, organisms are more readily able to initiate the infectious process. Some organisms can elaborate toxic substances that impair intestinal motility. Increased intestinal peristalsis, which occurs during some enteric infections, may be an attempt by the host to rid itself of infective organisms.

In addition to its role in conjunction with intestinal motility, mucus also serves to provide a nonspecific barrier to bacterial proliferation and mucosal colonization. This barrier has been shown to be effective in preventing toxins from exerting their effects. Exfoliated mucosal cells trapped in the mucous layer may trap invading microorganisms. Mucus also contains carbohydrate analog of surface receptors, which may prevent invading organisms from binding to actual receptors.

The normal endogenous microflora of the gut serves as its next line of defense. Anaerobes, which are a large component of the normal flora, elaborate short-chain fatty acids and lactic acid, which are toxic to many potential pathogens. In breast-fed infants, this line of defense is enhanced by the presence of anaerobic lactobacilli, which produce fermentative products that act as toxins to foreign bacteria. Further evidence in support of the importance of endogenous microflora is the increase in susceptibility to infection after one's normal flora has been reduced by antibiotic administration, as is seen with *Clostridium difficile* infection.

The most complex element in the host-defense armamentarium involves the mucosal and systemic immune systems. Both serum and secretory antibodies may exert their protective effects at the intestinal level, even though the serum components are produced outside the gut. An immune response may be *specific* to a particular infective agent or *generalized* to a common group of bacterial antigens.

Mechanisms of bacterial disease production

Bacteria have developed a variety of virulence factors (Table 36.2) to overcome host defense mechanisms: (1) *invasion* of the mucosa, followed by intraepithelial cell multiplication or invasion of the lamina propria; (2) production of *cytotoxins*, which disrupt cell function via direct alteration of the mucosal surface; (3) production of *enterotoxins*, polypeptides that alter cellular salt and water balance yet leave cell morphology undisturbed; and (4) *adherence* to the mucosal surface with resultant flattening of the microvilli and disruption of normal cell functioning. Each of the bacterial virulence mechanisms acts on specific regions of the intestine. Enterotoxins are primarily effective in the small bowel but can affect the colon; the effects of cytotoxins and direct epithelial cell invasion occur predominantly in the colon. Enteroadhesive mechanisms appear to function in both the small intestine and colon.

Salmonella

Members of the species *Salmonella* are currently recognized as the most common cause of bacterial diarrhea among

severity from the typically mild gastroenteritis caused by other members of the genus; *S. typhi* infection also has a higher case-fatality rate.

Typhoid fever typically begins with a period of fever lasting approximately 1 week. Patients then complain of headache and abdominal pain. Diarrhea is not usually a manifestation of typhoid fever and many patients experience constipation. Hepatomegaly and splenomegaly have also been frequently noted.[97] The characteristic 'rose spots' (palpable, erythematous lesions), typical in adult cases of typhoid fever, occur with far less frequency in pediatric patients.[104] Patients may become chronic carriers.

Diagnosis of typhoid fever is made on the basis of positive blood cultures. *S. typhi* is usually sensitive to several antimicrobial agents, including ampicillin, chloramphenicol, trimethoprim-sulfamethoxazole, cefotaxime and ceftriaxone. Drug choice is based on site of infection and susceptibility of the organism.

A live oral vaccine from an attenuated strain of *S. typhi* (Ty21a) has been available in the USA since 1989; one recommended dosing schedule is four doses given every other day.[105] Current efforts are directed toward development of other attenuated strains, which may provide successful immunization in single-dose therapy.[105] Vaccine based on the Vi antigen from the *S. typhi* polysaccharide capsule produces seroconversion in 90% of subjects, lasting 3 years.[106,107] Newer oral vaccines based on either different attenuated strains of *S. typhi*[108] or *S. typhi* that constitutively express Vi antigen,[109] are currently under study.

Shigella

Bacillary dysentery, an illness caused by *Shigella*, was described in ancient Greece. Osler,[110] in 1892, referred to the disease as 'one of the four great epidemic diseases of the world'. He further stated: 'In the tropics it destroys more lives than cholera and it has been more fatal to armies than powder and shot'. Despite our increased knowledge of the pathogenesis and treatment of shigellosis, this organism continues to be a significant cause of diarrheal disease.

Microbiology

Shigella is a gram-negative, non-motile, non-lactose-fermenting aerobic bacillus, closely related to members of the genus *Escherichia*. The organisms are classified into four species or groups known as *Shigella dysenteriae, Shigella flexneri, Shigella boydii* and *Shigella sonnei* (groups A, B, C and D, respectively). Members of groups A, B and C exist in numerous serotypes, but only one serotype of group D is known.[101] *S. sonnei* is the most commonly recovered *Shigella* species in the developed world, accounting for 70% of isolates in the USA. *S. dysenteriae* and *S. flexneri* are the most commonly recovered species of *Shigella* in the developing world.[111]

Epidemiology

Shigella is worldwide in its distribution and the incidence and severity of shigellosis span an equally broad range. In Highland Mayan Indian children, the incidence of shigellosis is 1900 cases per 1000 children per year in the third year of life.[112] In the developed world, *Shigella* occurs much less frequently. However, in some studies *Shigella* is the second most common pathogen identified in cases of bacterial diarrhea in children aged 6 months to 10 years.[113] It may also be the most common bacterial cause of outbreaks of diarrhea in daycare settings. Outbreaks of shigellosis have also been described in residential institutions and on cruise ships. This disease is endemic on American Indian reservations in the Southwest.

Shigella is predominantly spread via the fecal-oral route, with person-to-person contact the most likely method. Secondary spread to household contacts may occur. The infection may be spread through contamination of food and water, as often occurs in areas of poor sanitation and inadequate personal hygiene.

Clinical manifestations

Patients infected with *Shigella* may experience a mild, self-limited, watery diarrhea that is clinically indistinguishable from gastroenteritis caused by a variety of other agents. The more classic form of shigellosis, however, is bacillary dysentery. This illness usually begins with fever and malaise, followed by watery diarrhea and cramping abdominal pain. By the second day of illness, blood and mucus are usually present in the stools and tenesmus has become a prominent symptom. At this point, in approximately 50% of affected patients, the stool volume decreases, with only scant amounts of blood and mucus being passed.[111] This pattern of bloody, mucus-containing stools is referred to as *dysentery*. Bacteremia is an uncommon feature of this illness, but several other complications have been reported, including seizures (in children), arthritis, purulent keratitis and the hemolytic-uremic syndrome (HUS). Non-suppurative arthritis is the most commonly occurring extraintestinal complication of shigellosis. Patients who carry the histocompatible locus antigen HLA-B27 may be predisposed to the development of this complication as well as to the development of Reiter's syndrome.[114] The association of seizures with shigellosis was earlier attributed to the neurotoxic effect of the *Shigella* toxin (Shiga toxin). It now seems likely, however, that the seizures may simply represent a subgroup of common febrile seizures and have no direct relation to the effects of Shiga toxin.

Pathogenesis

Shigella has been found to cause disease only in humans and in the higher apes.[111] The organisms are potent, with as few as 10 organisms being able to cause disease in a healthy adult.[111] Patients infected with *Shigella* may excrete 10^5 to 10^8 organisms/g of feces. This high rate of excretion and the relatively low number of organisms required to produce disease make possible the widespread distribution of disease.

For *Shigella* to exert its pathologic effect on a host, the bacteria must first come into contact with the surface of an intestinal epithelial cell and induce cytoskeletal rearrangements resulting in phagocytosis.[97,115,116] The bacteria then secrete enzymes that degrade the phagosomal membrane, releasing the bacteria into the host cytoplasm. Intracytoplasmic bacteria move rapidly, in association with a comet tail made up of host cell actin filaments. When moving bacteria reach the cell margin, they push out long protrusions with the bacteria at the tips that are then taken up by neighboring cells, allowing the infection to spread from cell to cell (Fig. 36.3).[97]

Shiga toxin is elaborated by all species, although in greater amounts by *S. dysenteriae* than by other species,[111] and may play a role in the pathogenesis of *Shigella* infection. The toxin has neurotoxic, enterotoxic and cytotoxic effects.[111] Structurally, it is composed of an active, or A, subunit (molecular weight 32 kD) surrounded by five binding, or B, subunits (77 kD).[111] The B subunits bind to cell-specific receptors and are taken up by endocytosis. Within the cells, the B subunits are cleaved away and the remaining A subunit is shortened by proteolysis. This molecule is thought then to bind to the 60S ribosome and inhibit protein synthesis, leading to cell death and sloughing.[117] This is the presumed mechanism for the cytotoxic effect. An enterotoxic effect of Shiga toxin in the ileum may account for the early watery diarrhea.

Diagnosis and treatment

In patients with signs and symptoms of colitis, the diagnosis of shigellosis should be considered. Stool culture provides the only definitive means to differentiate this organism from other invasive pathogens. *Shigella* may be cultured from stool specimens or rectal swabs, especially if mucopus is present, but there may be a delay of several days from the onset of symptoms to the recovery of organisms. Sigmoidoscopy or colonoscopy typically reveals a friable mucosa, possibly with discrete ulcers. Rectal biopsy may be useful to differentiate shigellosis from ulcerative colitis.[118]

In addition to rehydration, antimicrobial therapy has been recommended for *Shigella* (1) to shorten the course of the disease, (2) to decrease the period of excretion of the organisms[119] and (3) to decrease the secondary attack rate, since humans provide the only reservoir for the organism. However, handwashing, rather than use of antimicrobials, is the most effective method to prevent person-to-person spread. Those clinicians who advise against the routine treatment of shigellosis with antibiotics argue that (1) the disease is most often self-limited and (2) the use of antibiotics may facilitate the development of resistant strains[120] and may increase the likelihood developing HUS as a sequela.[112] We recommend antibiotic therapy only for patients who are severely ill at the time of diagnosis or who remain ill at the time of identification of *Shigella* in a stool culture.

A wide range of antibiotics has been used to treat *Shigella,* necessitated by the development of resistant strains. Currently, the agent of choice is trimethoprim-sulfamethoxazole (trimethoprim, 5 mg/kg, max. 160 mg, plus sulfamethoxazole, 25 mg/kg, max. 800 mg, per dose, given every 12 h, orally or intravenously, for 5 days). Ampicillin (25 mg/kg, max. 500 mg, per dose, given every 6 h, orally or i.v., for 5 days) may be used if local strains are typically susceptible.[102] Amoxicillin is ineffective against *Shigella.*[121] Nalidixic acid (55 mg/kg per day given every 6 h for 5 days) has also proved effective. Cefixime and ceftriaxone are alternative agents for resistant organisms.[111] Tetracycline, ciprofloxacin and norfloxacin have been used successfully for the treatment of *Shigella*, but these agents are approved for use only in adult patients. Multidrug-resistant strains have occurred in Latin America, Central Africa and Southeast Asia.[122]

Development of a vaccine for shigellosis is currently being pursued. These efforts include vaccines using a modified *Escherichia coli* strain; one using a mutant strain of *S. flexneri*, which lacks the ability to proliferate intracellularly; and one based on a strain with mutations in its virulence genes.[111]

Campylobacter

Campylobacter is a gram-negative, motile, curved or spiral-shaped rod, exhibiting a 'seagull' appearance when

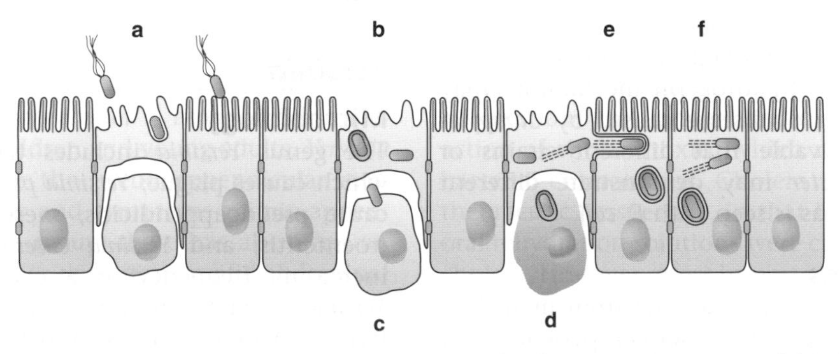

Figure 36.3: Interaction of *Shigella* species with the gut epithelium. Diagrammed is the putative interaction of shigellae with M cells overlying Peyer's patch follicles as well as absorptive epithelial cells. Invasion is diagrammed for an M cell. (**a,b**) Adherence to and intimate association of shigellae with an M cell followed by localization of the invading organism with an intracellular cytoplasmic vacuole. (**c,d,e**) Bacteria, having transcytosed the M cell, may interact with Peyer's patch macrophages and induce macrophage apoptosis. Bacteria free within the target cell cytoplasm also move within the host cell via an actin-associated tail. (**f**) Shigella intercellular invasion through a host cell membrane protrusion, followed by residence of the invading organism within a double-membraned intracellular cytoplasmic vacuole and escape from that vacuole. (From Hromockyj A, Falkow S. Interactions of bacteria with the gut epithelium. In: Blaser MJ, Smith PD, Ravdin JI, et al., eds. Infections of the Gastrointestinal Tract. New York: Raven Press; 1995,[97] with permission.)

Microbiology

Vibrio cholerae is a gram-negative, motile, curved bacillus that is free-living in bodies of salt water.[150] *V. cholerae* is classified on the basis of lipopolysaccharide antigens. Until recently, all epidemic strains of *V. cholerae* were of the O1 serotype. Group O1 is further subdivided into two biotypes: classic and El Tor. Other serotypes were thought to cause sporadic cases of diarrhea but not epidemic disease. This dictum was discarded by the development of an ongoing epidemic in Asia and South America caused by a new serotype, O139, synonym Bengal.[151,152] Although the pathogenesis and clinical features of O139 cholera are identical to those of O1 cholera, persons having immunity to serotype O1 are not immune to the Bengal serotype. This lack of immunity is primarily a result of the unique O139 cell surface antigen.

Epidemiology

V. cholerae is spread via contamination of food and water supplies. There is no evidence of an animal reservoir, but humans may serve as transient carriers.[153] On rare occasions, humans may chronically carry the organism.[154] Owing to the nature of its spread, persons living in areas with adequate sanitation are at minimal, if any, risk for encountering cholera. Cholera does occur in the USA, but usually as a result of imported food brought back by returning international travelers. Travelers from the USA to endemic areas are at low risk (about 1 per 30 000 travelers).[155] Cholera has also been isolated from oysters in the Gulf Coast.[156] However, owing to the frequency of international travel, it is important for the clinician who encounters a patient with severe cholera symptoms (dehydration and rice-water stools) to suspect this infection even in non-endemic areas.

Pathogenesis

V. cholerae enters its potential host through the oral route, usually in contaminated food or water. Volunteer studies have shown that a relatively large number of organisms (approximately 10^{11}) must be ingested to produce symptoms.[145] Similar to other ingested organisms, *V. cholerae* must survive the acidic gastric environment. The importance of gastric acidity as a host-protective factor is borne out by the increased occurrence of cholera in patients with absent or reduced gastric acidity.[89,157]

The organisms travel to the small intestine, where they adhere to the epithelium. This process may be aided by production of mucinase.[157] The intestinal epithelium remains intact with normal morphology.[158] *Vibrio* species produce a toxin that is composed of a central subunit (A) surrounded by five B subunits; the latter bind to a ganglioside, GM_1, which serves as the toxin receptor. This binding facilitates the transfer of the A subunit across the cell membrane, where it is cleaved into two components, denoted A_1 and A_2. The disulfide linkage between A_1 and A_2 is reduced to liberate an active A_1 peptide, which acts as a catalyst to facilitate the transfer of adenosine diphosphate-ribose from nicotinamide adenine dinucleotide to a guanyl nucleotide-binding regulatory protein (G_s). G_s then stimulates adenylate cyclase, located on the basolateral membrane, thereby increasing cyclic adenosine monophosphate. This result in turn leads to chloride secretion and a net flux of fluid into the intestinal lumen.[159]

Although this mechanism of toxin action adequately explains the clinical symptoms of cholera, similar symptoms have been noted in patients infected with strains that do *not* produce the classic cholera toxin. This has led to the recognition that *V. cholerae* harbors additional virulence factors in the bacterial genome that may contribute to diarrheal disease and must be considered in the design of a non-reactigenic vaccine. Newly recognized toxins produced by *V. cholerae* include zonula occludens toxin and the accessory cholera toxin.[160,161]

Clinical manifestations

After an incubation period, commonly 1–3 days, the symptoms of cholera usually begin abruptly with vomiting and profuse, watery diarrhea. The stool soon becomes clear, with bits of mucus giving it the so-called rice-water appearance. Patients do not experience tenesmus, but rather a sense of relief with defecation.[150] Typically there is no fever. The rate of fluid loss with cholera can be remarkable in severe disease, with purging rates in excess of 1 l/h reported in adult patients.[158] Despite the dramatic presentation and health risk of *'cholera gravis'*, most patients with cholera infection are asymptomatic or experience mild symptoms. In addition to people with reduced gastric acidity, people with blood group O are at increased risk for more severe disease. Other host factors that predispose to increased purging are less clear.

Diagnosis and treatment

V. cholerae is identified by colonial morphology and pigmentation on selective agar (e.g. thiosulfate citrate bile salt-sucrose agar). Further identification depends on biochemical markers (e.g. positive oxidase reaction) and motility of the organism. Specific serotyping is used to confirm the identification

The mainstay of cholera treatment is rehydration. In cases in which the disease is less severe and is recognized early, oral rehydration solutions are appropriate and effective. When purging is excessive (more than 10 ml/kg per h), intravenous rehydration is required.

Antibiotics have been shown to cause a decrease in duration of the diarrhea, total amount of fluid lost and length of time organisms are excreted.[150] Tetracycline (250–500 mg per dose, given every 6 h for 3 to 5 days) has been recommended as an appropriate antibiotic for adults,[158] and furazolidone (1.25 mg/kg, max. 100 mg, per dose, given every 6 h for 10 days) has been suggested for children and pregnant patients. Ampicillin, chloramphenicol, trimethoprim-sulfamethoxazole and doxycycline may also be used. Single-dose ciprofloxacin has also been shown to be effective in the treatment of *V. cholerae* O1 or O139,[162] although this drug is not approved for use in children.

Despite much progress, an ideal cholera vaccine is not yet available. An ideal vaccine would provide a high level of long-term protection even to those at high risk for severe illness (e.g. people with blood group type O) and this protection would commence shortly after administration of a single oral dose.[163] New oral vaccines have been developed for cholera, including both killed vaccines and live attenuated strains.[164,165] CVD 103-HgR, a vaccine strain with a 94% deletion of the *ctxA* proved efficacious against experimental challenge with *V. cholera* El Tor Inaba 3 months after inoculation, suggesting it may be useful for travelers to endemic areas.[166] Unfortunately, CVD 103-HgR was not effective in a field trial.[167] Peru-15, a non-motile strain that colonizes better than CVD 103-HgR, has been shown to be highly effective in volunteer studies.[168] Despite these successes, there remains a need to continue development of non-reactigenic O1 vaccines and vaccines against the new O139 epidemic strain. Neither the killed nor the live O1 vaccines protect against the new serotype O139, since most of the protection is lipopolysaccharide-mediated and the new serotype has a unique lipopolysaccharide. Therefore, the appearance of the new serotype reinforces the need for testing additional vaccine candidates.

Other vibrios

The non-cholera vibrios, *V. parahaemolyticus, V. fluvialis, V. mimicus, V. hollisae, V. furnissii* and *V. vulnificans*, have been shown to cause gastrointestinal illness, wound infections and septicemia.[169] Although each organism has its own characteristics, most non-cholera vibrios produce a protein toxin identical to the classic cholera toxin.[138] Some species also produce a heat-stable toxin similar to *E. coli* heat-stable toxin.[170] Although these organisms produce a cholera-like illness, the stool may sometimes contain blood and leukocytes and sepsis can occur. This has led to speculation that some members of this group, namely *V. parahaemolyticus*, may be capable of invasiveness as well as toxin production.[169] In the USA, gastroenteritis caused by these vibrios is most often associated with the ingestion of raw oysters.[171]

Gastroenteritis caused by non-O1 vibrios tends to be far milder than that caused by *V. cholerae*. In severe cases of diarrhea or septicemia, antibiotics may be helpful, with the agents used for *V. cholerae* recommended.

Escherichia coli

E. coli constitutes a diverse group of organisms, including nonpathogenic strains, which are among the most common bacteria in the normal flora of the human intestine and pathogenic strains. Pathogenic *E. coli* strains that cause diarrheal illness have been recognized since the 1940s.[172,173]

These diarrheagenic *E. coli* have been studied extensively and are currently classified, on the basis of serogrouping or pathogenic mechanisms, into six major groups: (1) enteropathogenic *E. coli* (EPEC), an important cause of diarrhea in infants in developing countries; (2) enterotoxigenic *E. coli* (ETEC), a cause of diarrhea in infants in developing areas of the world and a cause of traveler's diarrhea in adults; (3) enteroinvasive *E. coli* (EIEC), which cause either a watery ETEC-like illness or, less commonly, a dysentery-like illness; (4) Shiga toxin-producing *E. coli* (Stx-producing; formerly known as enterohemorrhagic *E. coli*), which cause hemorrhagic colitis and HUS; (5) enteroaggregative *E. coli* (EAggEC) and (6) diffusely-adherent *E. coli* (DAEC), which along with EPEC have been implicated as causes of persistent diarrhea. Each of these groups of *E. coli* has unique properties (Table 36.3).

Enteropathogenic *Escherichia coli*

EPEC is a major cause of diarrhea in developing countries. As many as 30–40% of cases of infant diarrhea, particularly in those infants less than 6-months of age, may be caused by EPEC and in some studies the frequency of EPEC infection exceeds that of rotavirus.[174–177] In North America and the UK, EPEC infections were common during the 1940s through the 1960s; now they are most commonly associated with sporadic cases and nosocomial or daycare outbreaks.[178,179] However, because of the general unavailability of serotyping, the true incidence of EPEC-associated diarrhea may be underestimated. A 1997 study in Seattle children with diarrhea, in which DNA probes were used to screen *E. coli* present in stool, found a high incidence of EPEC-like organisms (atypical EPEC) in this population.[180]

The hallmark of EPEC infection is the 'attaching and effacing' lesion seen in the intestine.[179,181] This lesion is characterized by destruction of microvilli and intimate

Name	Abbreviation	Pathogenic mechanisms	Illness
Enteropathogenic *E. coli*	EPEC	Adherence to enterocytes	Infantile diarrhea in developing countries
Enterotoxigenic *E. coli*	ETEC	Enterotoxin elaboration	Infantile diarrhea in developing countries; traveler's diarrhea
Enteroinvasive *E. coli*	EIEC	Invasion of epithelial cells; toxin elaboration	Watery diarrhea/dysentery
Stx-producing *E. coli*[a]	Stx-EC	Cytotoxin elaboration; Adherence	Hemorrhagic colitis; hemolytic-uremic syndrome
Enteroaggregative *E. coli*	EAggEC	?Adherence; Enterotoxin elaboration, IL 8 elaboration	Persistent diarrhea in developing countries, ?acute diarrhea in developed countries
Diffusely-adherent *E. coli*	DAEC	?Adherence	?Diarrhea

[a]Formerly enterohemorrhagic *E. coli* (EHEC).

Table 36.3 Diarrheagenic *Escherichia coli*

adherence between the bacterium and the epithelial cell membrane. Directly beneath the surface of the adherent organism, there are marked cytoskeletal changes in the enterocyte, including accumulation of actin polymers. Often, the bacteria are raised on a pedestal-like structure as a result of this actin accumulation. A number of steps are probably responsible for the development of this attaching and effacing lesion. As proposed by Donnenberg and Kaper,[182] EPEC pathogenesis consists of three phases: (1) localized adherence, which brings the bacteria in close contact with the enterocyte (e.g. docking); (2) signal transduction, including increases in intracellular calcium and protein phosphorylation; and (3) intimate adherence, a multigene process encoded in the bacterium by a locus of enterocyte effacement.[183,184] The dramatic loss of absorptive microvilli in the intestine presumably leads to diarrhea via malabsorption. Although this is probably the predominant mechanism, some evidence suggests that a separate secretory mechanism is also involved.

Patients with symptomatic EPEC infection typically experience diarrhea, vomiting, malaise and fever. The stool may contain mucus but does not usually contain blood. Symptoms with EPEC infection are more severe than with some other enteric infections and may persist for 2 weeks or longer.[172] In some patients, EPEC has caused protracted diarrhea with dehydration, malnutrition and zinc deficiency as complications; treatment with parenteral hyperalimentation has been required.[179] EPEC can be detected by serotyping of isolated *E. coli*,[178,185] by demonstration of the presence of the enterocyte adherence factor or other virulence genes using molecular probes,[186] or by identification of the attaching and effacing phenotype using tissue culture cells.[187] These assays are not commonly used in the clinical microbiology laboratory. Diagnosis of EPEC may be made by demonstrating the presence of adherent organisms on small intestinal or rectal biopsy.[178,179,185]

Although controlled studies of antibiotic therapy for EPEC have been few, the significant morbidity associated with this agent argues for treatment with antibiotics in most cases. Trimethoprim-sulfamethoxazole (trimethoprim, 5 mg/kg, max. 160 mg, plus sulfamethoxazole, 25 mg/kg, max. 800 mg, per dose, given every 12 h) has been used with some success, as have oral neomycin and gentamicin.

Enterotoxigenic *Escherichia coli*

ETEC are recognized as an important cause of diarrhea in infants in developing areas of the world. In endemic areas, children in the first few years of life may be infected several times each year.[188] In the USA, cases of ETEC among children are uncommon.[189] ETEC is also a major cause of traveler's diarrhea in adults. Fecal-oral transmission and consumption of heavily contaminated food or water are the most common vehicles for ETEC infection.

The production of disease by ETEC begins with colonization of the small intestine. There the bacteria depend on fimbriae (also called *pili*) to facilitate attachment to the mucosal surface and overcome the forward motion of peristalsis. This attachment process causes no detectable structural changes in the architecture of the brush border membrane but does allow the bacteria to release their enterotoxins, heat-labile toxin (LT) and heat-stable toxin (ST), in close proximity to the enterocyte brush border membrane where toxin receptors are present.[190] These toxins in turn stimulate adenylate cyclase (in the case of LT) or guanylate cyclase (in the case of ST) and both ultimately result in a net fluid secretion from the intestine (see the reviews by Cohen and Giannella[191] and by Sears and Kaper).[192] Two endogenous ligands for the ST receptor, guanylin and uroguanylin, have been identified.[193,194] This discovery is consistent with the hypothesis that ST is a superagonist and exerts its diarrheal action by means of usurping a normal secretory mechanisms in the intestine (e.g. by molecular mimicry of these less potent endogenous ligands). Uroguanylin may also act as a hormone regulating salt and water excretion in the kidney in response to an oral salt load.[195]

Clinically, ETEC infection causes nausea, abdominal pain and watery diarrhea. Stools typically contain neither mucus nor leukocytes. ETEC can be diagnosed with the use of bioassays such as the suckling mouse assay,[196] immunoassays, or gene probes specific for either ST[197] or LT.[198] PCR assays are also available. However, none of these assays is commonly used in the clinical microbiology laboratory. Supportive measures are sufficient therapy for most cases of ETEC diarrhea, with oral rehydration a mainstay of therapy. Antibiotics, including trimethoprim-sulfamethoxazole, have been shown to decrease the duration of fecal excretion of the organisms.[199] Quinolone antibiotics may be more effective,[200] but they are not recommended for use in children.

Enteroinvasive *Escherichia coli*

EIEC share many common features, including virulence mechanisms, with *Shigella*. These organisms preferentially colonize the colon and invade and replicate within epithelial cells, where they cause cell death.[172] In addition, both organisms elaborate one or more secretory enterotoxins. Clinically, both *Shigella* and EIEC infections are characterized by a period of watery diarrhea that precedes the onset of dysentery (scanty stools containing mucus, pus and blood). More commonly, in contrast to *Shigella*, only this first phase of watery diarrhea is seen in EIEC infection.[201] This illness is clinically indistinguishable from other causes of bacterial diarrhea (e.g. ETEC) or non-bacterial infectious diarrhea. In a minority of patients with EIEC infections, the dysentery syndrome of characteristic stools, tenesmus and fever is also seen. Bacteremia is not reported.

Infection due to EIEC is uncommon, but foodborne outbreaks of disease have occurred in the USA and aboard cruise ships. Diagnosis is dependent on bioassay (the Sereny test), serotyping, ELISA, or DNA probe techniques. None of these tests is commonly available in the clinical laboratory. Treatment is currently limited to supportive measures, although ampicillin given intramuscularly has been associated with bacteriologic cure and clinical improvement.[201]

Shiga toxin-producing *Escherichia coli*

Stx-producing *E. coli* are a distinct class of organisms that have been identified since 1983 as the cause of two recognizable syndromes: hemorrhagic colitis and HUS.[202,203] Hemorrhagic colitis is an illness characterized by crampy abdominal pain, initial watery diarrhea and subsequent development of grossly bloody diarrhea with little or no fever. Although there may be more than 100 serotypes in this class of diarrheagenic *E. coli*, in North America the *E. coli* serotype O157:H7 is the prototypic member of this family of organisms. *E. coli* O157:H7 is the most common cause of infectious bloody diarrhea in the USA.[204] Similarly, HUS, which is defined as the triad of acute renal failure, thrombocytopenia and microangiopathic hemolytic anemia, is also highly associated with antecedent *E. coli* O157:H7 infection.

Stx-producing *E. coli* infections may occur in sporadic cases, but they have also been associated with outbreaks of disease in nursing homes, daycare centers and other institutions; several reviews have been published.[205–208] It is estimated that *E. coli* O157:H7 causes approximately 10 000 to 20 000 infections per year in the USA alone and may be responsible for 250 deaths annually.[209] Inadequately cooked hamburgers were most likely the source of the first outbreak[186] and remain the most common vehicle of transmission. In 1993 there was a large epidemic in the western USA; inadequately cooked hamburgers were again implicated as the cause. Other, small epidemics have been attributed to apple juice or cider and large-scale outbreaks in Japan have been associated with bean sprouts. Contaminated water has also been a source of infection.[210,211] Common to all of these outbreaks is a reservoir of Stx-producing *E. coli* in the intestines of cattle and other animals who are asymptomatic. Infection is spread either by direct contact with intestinal contents or through droppings or water runoff from contaminated pastures. A low infectious dose for Stx-producing *E. coli* and the resistance of these organisms to gastric acid and to the food preserving process (high salt and drying) contribute to the high attack rate. The low infectious dose also contributes to frequent person-to-person transmission.[205–208]

Both the very old and the very young appear to be at increased risk for Stx-producing *E. coli* infection and its complications.[205–208] Clinical features and complications of *E. coli* O157:H7 infection include bloody diarrhea, nonbloody diarrhea, HUS, thrombotic thrombocytopenic purpura and, uncommonly, asymptomatic infection.[205] Symptoms may persist for several days or, less commonly, for several weeks. Early reports suggested that carriage of the organism was brief and that prompt culture was necessary to recover these organisms.[212,213] More recently, prolonged shedding has been observed.[214,215] This has led to the recommendation that two negative stool cultures be obtained before a child is allowed to return to daycare.[214]

The identification of Stx-producing *E. coli* is made difficult because it is not possible to differentiate disease-producing *E. coli* from normal enteric flora on the basis of standard microbiologic techniques. There are currently six techniques for identification of Stx-producing *E. coli*: biochemical markers with serotyping (most commonly used), serum antibody tests, cytotoxin bioassays, DNA hybridization, PCR-based tests and cytotoxin detection (including ELISAs). Some of these methods (e.g. toxin-based assays) detect the presence of cytotoxin-producing organisms, including non-O157 serotypes. It may be important to use both biochemical markers and toxin-based assays in clinical practice to identify these organisms.[216]

Prevention of disease transmission is made difficult by the fact that these organisms colonize the intestine of healthy cattle and other food animals, including beef, pork, lamb and poultry. Therefore, they can survive and multiply in the food chain. Proper cooking destroys these organisms; in hamburgers, an internal cooking temperature of 71°C (160°F) renders the meat safe. Practically, safe cooking most commonly results in a gray hamburger (not pink), with clear juices. Risk can be lowered by educating consumers about cross-contamination, use of warning labels now affixed to meat in the USA and improvements in meat processing and microbial contamination detection.

At present there is no effective therapy to treat Stx-producing *E. coli* disease, so prevention is the most important strategy. Hemorrhagic colitis has been confused with a number of other conditions, including ischemic colitis, appendicitis, Crohn's disease, ulcerative colitis, cecal polyp, pseudomembranous colitis and an acute abdomen (ileitis). Therefore, an important aspect of treatment of Stx-associated hemorrhagic colitis is making the correct diagnosis and avoiding unnecessary diagnostic studies such as angiography and laparotomy. The mainstay of therapy for hemorrhagic colitis is the management of dehydration, electrolyte abnormalities and gastrointestinal blood loss. Antimicrobial agents may help by killing the bacterial pathogens, but they may also cause harm by increasing the release and subsequent absorption of Shiga toxin.[217] Trials of antibiotic treatment of Stx-producing *E. coli* infection are inconclusive. Although these organisms are uniformly sensitive to antimicrobials *in vitro*, at present there is no convincing evidence that antimicrobial therapy is helpful in diminishing the severity of illness, shortening the duration of fecal excretion, or preventing HUS.[218,219] Of greater concern is a study suggesting an increased incidence of HUS in those treated with anti-microbials.[220] An attempt to assimilate findings of published series on the subject via a meta-analysis failed to identify an increased risk of HUS in those treated with antimicrobials.[221] Regardless, until more data is available on this topic, most experts would agree that treatment of Stx-producing *E. coli* with antimicrobials is not advisable.[222] A multi-center trial failed to demonstrate an improved clinical course in pediatric patients treated with Shiga toxin-binding resin.[223] Other toxin neutralizing therapies are currently under investigation.

Enteroaggregative and diffusely-adherent *Escherichia coli*

EAggEc and DAEC were initially categorized as part of a larger group of enteroadherent *E. coli*. These strains differed from classical EPEC strains in that they did not showlocalized adherence in the Hep-2 cell assay.[224] The aggregative or 'stacked brick' appearance of EAggEC in this bioassay permitted epidemiological investigation and EAggEc were found to be associated with persistent diarrhea in developing counties.[185,225] There was uncertainty about EAggEc pathogenicity because these organisms are found in apparently healthy individuals and because some epidemiologic studies failed to show an association with disease.[175,226,227] However, evidence from volunteer studies[228,229] and outbreaks[230] has confirmed the pathogenicity of some EAggEC strains. Recent studies at Cincinnati Children's Hospital Medical Center have shown that EAggEC are an important unrecognized cause of acute infant diarrhea.[231] The mechanisms by which these organisms cause disease is thought to involve adherence to the intestinal mucosa, possibly in both the small and large intestine, followed by secretion of one or more enterotoxins and/or stimulation of IL-8 release by a flagellar protein.[232–234] DAEC are less well characterized but have also been associated with diarrheal disease. Both the HEp-2 cell assay and DNA probes have been used to identify these organisms, but these are not routinely available in the clinical microbiology laboratory.

Clostridium difficile

C. difficile is a gram-positive anaerobic bacillus. Disease caused by this organism can manifest in a variety of ways, ranging from asymptomatic carriage to potentially life-threatening pseudomembranous colitis. This organism has been primarily, but not exclusively, associated with illness occurring after disruption of the normal intestinal flora by antibiotics.

Epidemiology

Of great interest in the study of *C. difficile* is the difference in the incidence of isolation of the organism and its toxin in various age groups. *C. difficile* toxin has been found in the feces of 10% of normal-term neonates and 55% of those in a neonatal intensive care unit.[235] Most infants found to have toxin in their stools are asymptomatic. A small group of toxin-positive infants have signs and symptoms of necrotizing enterocolitis, but no clear relation to *C. difficile* or its toxin has been demonstrated. The presence of *C. difficile* toxin in these asymptomatic infants may indicate the coexistence of some protective antitoxic substance[236] or may reflect a lack of appropriate toxin receptors in patients in this age group.[237]

The incidence of *C. difficile* toxin positivity decreases beyond the neonatal period. The incidence of asymptomatic carriage in children older than 2 years of age approaches that in healthy adults (about 3%). Furthermore, not all of these organisms are toxin producers. Adults who develop disease from *C. difficile* infection are also more likely than children to experience severe colitis symptoms.

Pathogenesis

C. difficile elaborates two important toxins. Toxin A probably mediates human disease; it is called an enterotoxin despite the fact that it causes cytotoxicity with hemorrhage and mucosal destruction in addition to having enterotoxic effects. Toxin A is a large protein (308 kD) that binds to an enterocyte surface receptor and activates an intracellular G protein-dependent signal transduction mechanism.[238] Bound toxin results in altered permeability, inhibition of protein synthesis and direct cytotoxicity. Toxin B is thought not to be an important mediator of human disease. However, this 'cytotoxin' is almost always found with toxin A and toxin B is the basis for the 'gold standard' cytotoxic tissue culture assay.

Clinical manifestations

C. difficile-related diarrhea almost always occurs in the setting of antimicrobial administration. Less commonly, the syndrome of pseudomembranous enterocolitis is seen after surgery (without antimicrobial agents) and after antineoplastic therapy. Any mucosal disease, including inflammatory bowel disease, is thought to be a risk factor, but only 1.7% of pediatric patients with inflammatory bowel disease were found to have *C. difficile* toxin in stool while in good control.[239] Hospitalization is a major risk factor for the acquisition of infection. Most patients experience mild, watery diarrhea that lasts only a few days and spontaneously resolves. In some patients, symptoms persist for weeks to months. Pseudomembranous colitis develops in a subset of patients. Patients with this disease are often extremely ill, with high fever, leukocytosis and hypoalbuminemia.

Diagnosis and treatment

C. difficile should be suspected in cases of colitis or mild diarrhea in which blood and leukocytes are noted in the stools. Concurrent or recent exposure (within several weeks) to antibiotics should increase the suspicion of *C. difficile* as the causative agent. The use of virtually any antibiotic may predispose to *C. difficile* disease.

Diagnosis of *C. difficile* can be made by culture of the organism or by examination for the presence of toxin in feces. The 'gold standard' for laboratory detection of *C. difficile* toxin requires the use of a tissue culture system, with demonstration of a cytopathic effect that can be neutralized by specific antitoxin. However, this is less commonly used and other assays, including a rapid toxin ELISA assay, have sensitivities and specificities approaching those of the tissue culture system and can be interpreted within hours. However, correct identification of *C. difficile* disease in children may require use of both toxin A and toxin B ELISA.[240] Sigmoidoscopy in cases of pseudomembranous colitis typically reveals friable white exudate overlying multiple ulcerated areas.[241] The histologic findings of such lesions are depicted in Figure 36.4. Less commonly, pseudomembranes may not be present in the rectosigmoid but may be present in the more proximal colon.

In cases of mild diarrheal illness caused by *C. difficile*, discontinuation of any antibiotics the patient is receiving may be sufficient therapy. In cases of severe illness and especially in cases of pseudomembranous colitis, treatment should also include oral vancomycin (5–10 mg/kg, max. 500 mg, per dose, given every 6 h for 7 days) or metron-

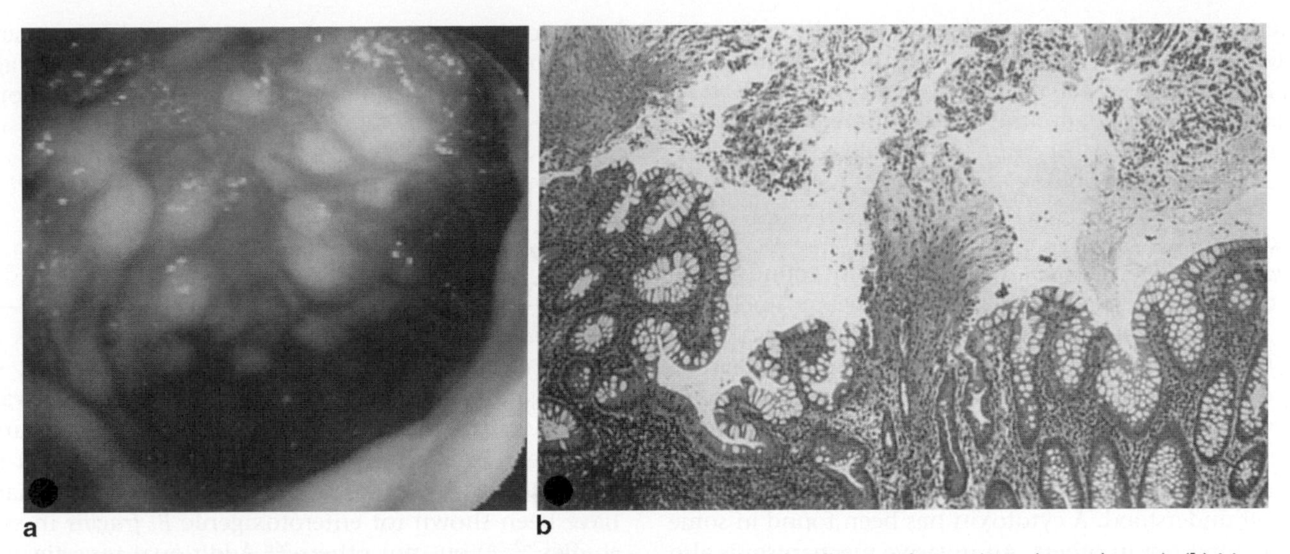

Figure 36.4: (**a**) The endoscopic appearance of the sigmoid colon with multiple densely adherent plaques (pseudomembranes). (**b**) Mucosal biopsy shows a focus of necrotizing enterocolitis with a typical volcano lesion (accumulated fibropurulent exudate intermixed with mucus). (From Bates M, Bove K, Cohen MB. Pseudomembranous colitis caused by *C. difficile*. J Pediatr 1997;130:146, with permission).[241]

idazole (5–10 mg/kg, max. 500 mg, per dose, given every 8 h for 7 days).[242] Compared with vancomycin, metronidazole is much less expensive, does not select for vancomycin-resistant organisms. and has similar efficacy.

There is a fairly high rate of relapse of illness, generally 15–20%, after treatment of *C. difficile*. These relapses usually occur within 1 month of completion of therapy and have been thought to result from the activation of *C. difficile* spores remaining from the primary infection.[243] Most of these cases of relapse are responsive to a second course of vancomycin or metronidazole or to repeated short courses of these drugs. There are reports of multiple relapses in which cholestyramine, given as a slurry (120 mg/kg per dose every 8 h) for 4 weeks and tapered over the following 3 weeks, was effective in eradication of the organism.[243] Intravenously administered gamma globulin is an alternative therapy for chronic *C. difficile* enterocolitis.[244] *Lactobacillus GG* has also been used successfully in a few pediatric patients with recurrent or persistent infection and Saccharomyces boulardii has been used effectively in adults.[245]

Aeromonas and *Plesiomonas*

Within the past decade, several organisms not previously recognized as enteric pathogens have been linked to diarrheal disease. This includes organisms of the genus *Aeromonas* and the closely related bacterium *Plesiomonas shigelloides* (previously classified as *Aeromonas shigelloides*). These organisms are gram-negative, facultatively anaerobic bacilli classified in the family Vibrionaceae. They are oxidase-positive, differentiating them from members of the Enterobacteriaceae.[246]

Aeromonas

Several members of the genus *Aeromonas*, including *Aeromonas hydrophila,* are common inhabitants of fresh and brackish water in the USA. These organisms were initially recognized as opportunistic pathogens in immunocompromised hosts, especially those with malignant hematologic diseases. The organisms also have been known to cause disease in patients with underlying hepatobiliary disease.[246] *Aeromonas* has been isolated from healthy persons as well and has therefore been thought to be part of the normal flora. Despite initial studies that yielded conflicting results,[247] it is now generally accepted that *A. hydrophila* is an enteric pathogen.

Studies in Australian children with diarrhea have found *Aeromonas* species present in 10% of patients.[248] Infection appears to occur most frequently in children younger than 2 years of age.[249] Of patients with *Aeromonas* isolated from stool cultures at Cincinnati Children's Hospital Medical Center approximately 50% were younger than 3 months. *Aeromonas* infection is also seasonal, occurring more often in the summer months.[246]

Not all *Aeromonas* species are pathogenic. The method of pathogenesis remains unclear. Both cytotoxic[249] and enterotoxic[246] properties have been observed, but neither these nor other pathogenic mechanisms are found consistently in strains isolated from patients with *Aeromonas*-associated disease.[247] *Aeromonas caviae*, a commonly isolated species, demonstrates both adherence and cytotoxin production.[250]

Clinical symptoms attributed to *Aeromonas* can be grouped into three categories: (1) acute watery diarrhea, the most common syndrome; (2) dysentery, which usually is self-limited; and (3) persistent watery diarrhea. Cramping abdominal pain and vomiting may also occur.[249] Symptoms may occasionally be severe and, especially when dysentery is present, have been incorrectly diagnosed as ulcerative colitis.[248]

In mild cases of *Aeromonas* infection, supportive treatment should suffice. In patients who are immunocompromised, are otherwise acutely ill, or have persistent illness, treatment with antibiotics is recommended.

Trimethoprim-sulfamethoxazole is usually effective (trimethoprim, 5 mg/kg, max. 160 mg, plus sulfamethoxazole, 25 mg/kg, max. 800 mg, per dose, given every 12 h for 14 days), as are tetracycline, chloramphenicol and the aminoglycosides.[246] Most strains of *Aeromonas* are resistant to the penicillins, including ampicillin.[246]

Plesiomonas

P. shigelloides, like *Aeromonas*, is commonly found in the environment,[251] especially in bodies of water, including water from a home aquarium.[252] Unlike *Aeromonas*, however, *Plesiomonas* has been reported to occur in epidemics, with contaminated water often found to be the cause.[251] *Plesiomonas* is also known to be spread through improperly cooked seafood.[253]

The pathogenesis of disease caused by *P. shigelloides* is not well understood. A cytotoxin has been found in some strains[251] but not in others. An invasive mechanism is also suspected, because of the colitis symptoms.[253] In addition to small-volume stools with leukocytes and possible blood, patients may also experience severe abdominal pain. Fever has been seen in approximately one-third of patients.[253] In one group of adult patients, symptoms persisted longer than 2 weeks in 75% and longer than 4 weeks in 32%.[253]

Diagnosis of *P. shigelloides* is made by stool culture. Although this illness is usually self-limited, treatment with antimicrobial agents has been shown to decrease the duration of symptoms,[253] with trimethoprim-sulfamethoxazole or aminoglycosides suggested as appropriate choices. There are no controlled trials of antimicrobial treatment of gastroenteritis caused by this organism.

Mycobacterium avium-intracellulare

Mycobacterium avium and *Mycobacterium intracellulare*, known collectively as *Mycobacterium avium-intracellulare* or *Mycobacterium avium* complex (MAC), are acid-fast bacilli that have been recognized primarily for their role in cases of atypical tuberculosis. These organisms are now recognized as causative agents of diarrheal symptoms as well. In a review of pediatric cases of atypical mycobacterial infections, Lincoln and Gilbert[254] described two immunocompetent patients whose clinical findings included diarrhea and colonic ulceration.

Of even greater significance than these sporadic cases of MAC infection in immunocompetent hosts is its occurrence among immunocompromised patients. In patients with the acquired immunodeficiency syndrome, MAC is among the most commonly isolated agents causing systemic bacterial infections.[255] These patients may also have chronic diarrhea and abdominal pain.[256,257] MAC has also been noted to cause diarrhea in patients undergoing bone marrow transplantation[258] and in a patient with cystic fibrosis.[259]

The MAC organisms may be cultured from gastric and duodenal aspirates obtained endoscopically and from the stool, the bone marrow and the blood.[255] Endoscopic examination in patients with MAC may reveal findings similar to those seen in Whipple's disease, with minute superficial ulcerations in the small bowel.[257] Treatment of MAC infections with conventional antituberculosis agents usually is unsuccessful in eradicating the organisms or alleviating symptoms.[255]

POTENTIAL DIARRHEAGENIC ORGANISMS

Enterotoxigenic *Bacteroides fragilis*

Bacteroides fragilis is an anaerobic organism that is commonly isolated from normal stool flora. However, some investigators have identified a toxin-producing variant that is enteropathogenic.[260] Enterotoxigenic organisms have been isolated from both healthy persons and those with diarrhea.[261] Epidemiologic associations with diarrhea have been shown for enterotoxigenic *B. fragilis* in several studies[262–265] but not others.[266] Additional investigation is required to fulfill Koch's postulates for this organism.

Brachyspira aalborgi

Intestinal spirochetosis, or the colonization of the large bowel by *Brachyspira aalborgi* and related spirochetes, has recently been implicated as a cause of diarrhea.[267] Some studies have shown an association between this organism and bloody diarrhea,[268] although asymptomatic colonization has also been reported.[269] The potential of this organism to cause diarrhea requires further evaluation.

Hafnia alvei

This organism has been associated with diarrhea in sporadic cases and in at least one hospital outbreak. Although a causal relation between *Hafnia alvei* and diarrhea has not been clearly established, a subset of this organism may be enteropathogenic. Organisms isolated from patients with diarrhea typically demonstrate the attaching and effacing lesion seen with EPEC, whereas non-pathogenic isolates do not show this characteristic.[270]

Listeria monocytogenes

Invasive illness caused by *Listeria* is well known. An outbreak of *Listeria* gastroenteritis and fever without invasive disease was reported in persons who had consumed contaminated chocolate milk.[271] The importance of *L. monocytogenes* in outbreaks of gastroenteritis caused by contaminated food has yet to be adequately determined.

CONCLUSION

Despite this chapter's extensive catalog of both bacterial and viral infectious agents, from 20–40% of cases of diarrhea are currently not attributable to any known cause. Undoubtedly, as techniques for identification and culture become more sophisticated, other causative agents will be identified and the percentage of diarrheal illnesses described as idiopathic or nonspecific will continue to decline. Advances in the widespread use of improved oral rehydration solutions have led to a decline in the morbidity and mortality associated with diarrhea. Future advances in preventive measures, including vaccines, may lead to a reduction of the incidence of diarrheal disease.

References

1. Glass RI, Lew JF, Gangarosa RE, LeBaron CW, Ho MS. Estimates of morbidity and mortality rates for diarrheal diseases in American children. J Pediatr 1991; 118:S27–S33.
2. Thielman NM, Guerrant RL. Clinical practice. Acute infectious diarrhea. N Engl J Med 2004; 350:38–47.
3. Blacklow NR, Cukor G. Viral gastroenteritis. N Engl J Med 1981; 304:397–406.
4. Kapikian AZ, Wyatt RG, Dolin R, Thornhill TS, Kalica AR, Chanock RM. Visualization by immune electron microscopy of a 27-nm particle associated with acute infectious nonbacterial gastroenteritis. J Virol 1972; 10:1075–1081.
5. Bishop RF, Davidson GP, Holmes IH, Ruck BJ. Virus particles in epithelial cells of duodenal mucosa from children with acute non-bacterial gastroenteritis. Lancet 1973; 2:1281–1283.
6. Ho MS, Glass RI, Pinsky PF, Anderson LJ. Rotavirus as a cause of diarrheal morbidity and mortality in the USA. J Infect Dis 1988; 158:1112–1116.
7. Kapikian AZ, Chanock RM. Rotaviruses. In: Fields BN, Knipe DM, Howley PM, eds. Fields Virology, Vol 2, 3rd edn. Philadelphia, PA: Lippincott-Raven Press; 1996:1657–1708.
8. Kapikian AZ, Hoshino Y, Chanock RM, Perez-Schael I. Efficacy of a quadrivalent rhesus rotavirus-based human rotavirus vaccine aimed at preventing severe rotavirus diarrhea in infants and young children. J Infect Dis 1996; 174(suppl 1):S65–S72.
9. Simhon A, Chrystie IL, Totterdell BM, Banatvala JE, Rice SJ, Walker-Smith JA. Sequential rotavirus diarrhoea caused by virus of same subgroup. Lancet 1981; 2:1174.
10. Blacklow NR, Greenberg HB. Viral gastroenteritis. N Engl J Med 1991; 325:252–264.
11. Rotavirus SMC. the first five years. J Pediatr 1980; 96:611–622.
12. Santosham M, Yolken RH, Wyatt RG, et al. Epidemiology of rotavirus diarrhea in a prospectively monitored American Indian population. J Infect Dis 1985; 152:778–783.
13. Yolken RH, Wyatt RG, Zissis G, et al. Epidemiology of human rotavirus Types 1 and 2 as studied by enzyme-linked immunosorbent assay. N Engl J Med 1978; 299:1156–1161.
14. Lycke E, Blomberg J, Berg G, Eriksson A, Madsen L. Epidemic acute diarrhoea in adults associated with infantile gastroenteritis virus. Lancet 1978; 2:1056–1057.
15. Meurman OH, Laine MJ. Rotavirus epidemic in adults. N Engl J Med 1977; 296:1298–1299.
16. Wenman WM, Hinde D, Feltham S, Gurwith M. Rotavirus infection in adults. Results of a prospective family study. N Engl J Med 1979; 301:303–306.
17. Totterdell BM, Chrystie IL, Banatvala JE. Rotavirus infections in a maternity unit. Arch Dis Child 1976; 51:924–928.
18. Bishop RF, Hewstone AS, Davidson GP, Townley RR, Holmes IH, Ruck BJ. An epidemic of diarrhoea in human neonates involving a reovirus-like agent and 'enteropathogenic' serotypes of *Escherichia coli*. J Clin Pathol 1976; 29:46–49.
19. Chrystie IL, Totterdell BM, Banatvala JE. Asymptomatic endemic rotavirus infections in the newborn. Lancet 1978; 1:1176–1178.
20. Ryder RW, McGowan JE, Hatch MH, Palmer EL. Reovirus-like agent as a cause of nosocomial diarrhea in infants. J Pediatr 1977; 90:698–702.
21. Delage G, McLaughlin B, Berthiaume L. A clinical study of rotavirus gastroenteritis. J Pediatr 1978; 93:455–457.
22. Bartlett ASI, Bednarz-Prashad AJ. DuPont HL. Rotavirus Gastroenteritis Annu Rev Med 1987; 38:399–415.
23. Morris CA, Flewett TH, Bryden AS, Davies H. Epidemic viral enteritis in a long-stay children's ward. Lancet 1975; 1:4–5.
24. Wilde J, Yolken R, Willoughby R, Eiden J. Improved detection of rotavirus shedding by polymerase chain reaction. Lancet 1991; 337:323–326.
25. Rodriguez WJ, Kim HW, Arrobio JO, et al. Clinical features of acute gastroenteritis associated with human reovirus-like agent in infants and young children. J Pediatr 1977; 91:188–193.
26. Riepenhoff-Talty M, Offor E, Klossner K, Kowalski E, Carmody PJ, Ogra PL. Effect of age and malnutrition on rotavirus infection in mice. Pediatr Res 1985; 19:1250–1253.
27. Gilger MA, Matson DO, Conner ME, Rosenblatt HM, Finegold MJ, Estes MK. Extraintestinal rotavirus infections in children with immunodeficiency. J Pediatr 1992; 120:912–917.
28. Davidson GP, Barnes GL. Structural and functional abnormalities of the small intestine in infants and young children with rotavirus enteritis. Acta Paediatr Scand 1979; 68:181–186.
29. Ball JM, Tian P, Zeng CQ, Morris AP, Estes MK. Age-dependent diarrhea induced by a rotaviral nonstructural glycoprotein. Science 1996; 272:101–104.
30. Christy C, Vosefski D, Madore HP. Comparison of three enzyme immunoassays to tissue culture for the diagnosis of rotavirus gastroenteritis in infants and young children. J Clin Microbiol 1990; 28:1428–1430.
31. Yolken RH, Miotti P, Viscidi R. Immunoassays for the diagnosis and study of viral gastroenteritis. Pediatr Infect Dis 1986; 5:S46–S52.
32. Nazarian LF, Berman JH, Brown G. Practice parameter: the management of acute gastroenteritis in young children. Pediatics 1996; 97:424–435.
33. Duggan C, Santosham M, Glass RI. The management of acute diarrhea in children: oral rehydration, maintenance and nutritional therapy. Centers for Disease Control and Prevention. MMWR Recomm Rep 1992; 41:1–20.
34. Cezard JP, Duhamel JF, Meyer M, et al. Efficacy and tolerability of racecadotril in acute diarrhea in children. Gastroenterology 2001; 120:799–805.
35. Salazar-Lindo E, Santisteban-Ponce J, Chea-Woo E, Gutierrez M. Racecadotril in the treatment of acute watery diarrhea in children. N Engl J Med 2000; 343:463–467.
36. Isolauri E, Juntunen M, Rautanen T, Sillanaukee P, Koivula T. A human Lactobacillus strain (Lactobacillus casei sp strain GG) promotes recovery from acute diarrhea in children. Pediatrics 1991; 88:90–97.
37. Kaila M, Isolauri E, Soppi E, Virtanen E, Laine S, Arvilommi H. Enhancement of the circulating antibody secreting cell response in human diarrhea by a human Lactobacillus strain. Pediatr Res 1992; 32:141–144.
38. Guandalini S, Pensabene L, Zikri MA, et al. Lactobacillus GG administered in oral rehydration solution to children with acute diarrhea: a multicenter European trial. J Pediatr Gastroenterol Nutr 2000; 30:54–60.
39. Saavedra JM, Bauman NA, Oung I, Perman JA, Yolken RH. Feeding of Bifidobacterium bifidum and Streptococcus thermophilus to infants in hospital for prevention of

diarrhoea and shedding of rotavirus. Lancet 1994; 344:1046–1049.

40. Guarino A, Canani RB, Russo S, et al. Oral immunoglobulins for treatment of acute rotaviral gastroenteritis. Pediatrics 1994; 93:12–16.
41. Velazquez FR, Matson DO, Calva JJ, et al. Rotavirus infections in infants as protection against subsequent infections. N Engl J Med 1996; 335:1022–1028.
42. Clark HF, Offit PA, Ellis RW, et al. The development of multivalent bovine rotavirus (strain WC3) reassortant vaccine for infants. J Infect Dis 1996; 174(suppl 1):S73–S80.
43. Treanor JJ, Clark HF, Pichichero M, et al. Evaluation of the protective efficacy of a serotype 1 bovine-human rotavirus reassortant vaccine in infants. Pediatr Infect Dis J 1995; 14:301–307.
44. Rennels MB, Glass RI, Dennehy PH, et al. Safety and efficacy of high-dose rhesus-human reassortant rotavirus vaccines – report of the National Multicenter Trial. US Rotavirus Vaccine Efficacy Group Pediatr 1996; 97:7–13.
45. Bernstein DI, Glass RI, Rodgers G, Davidson BL, Sack DA. Evaluation of rhesus rotavirus monovalent and tetravalent reassortant vaccines in US children. US Rotavirus Vaccine Efficacy Group JAMA 1995; 273:1191–1196.
46. Control CfD. Intussusception Among Recipients of Rotavirus Vaccine – USA, 1998–1999. MMWR 1999; 48:577–581.
47. Clark HF, Bernstein DI, Dennehy PH, et al. Safety, efficacy and immunogenicity of a live, quadrivalent human-bovine reassortant rotavirus vaccine in healthy infants. J Pediatr 2004; 144:184–190.
48. Adler JL, Zickl R. Winter vomiting disease. J Infect Dis 1969; 119:668–673.
49. Xi JN, Graham DY, Wang KN, Estes MK. Norwalk virus genome cloning and characterization. Science 1990; 250:1580–1583.
50. Jiang X, Wang M, Wang K, Estes MK. Sequence and genomic organization of Norwalk virus. Virology 1993; 195:51–61.
51. Jiang X, Wang J, Estes MK. Characterization of SRSVs using RT-PCR and a new antigen ELISA. Arch Virol 1995; 140:363–374.
52. Matson DO, Zhong WM, Nakata S, et al. Molecular characterization of a human calicivirus with sequence relationships closer to animal caliciviruses than other known human caliciviruses. J Med Virol 1995; 45:215–222.
53. Wang J, Jiang X, Madore HP, et al. Sequence diversity of small, round-structured viruses in the Norwalk virus group. J Virol 1994; 68:5982–5990.
54. Matson DO, Szucs G. Calicivirus infections in children. Curr Opin Infect Dis 2003; 16:241–246.
55. Cukor G, Blacklow NR. Human viral gastroenteritis. Microbiol Rev 1984; 48:157–179.
56. Graham DY, Jiang X, Tanaka T, Opekun AR, Madore HP, Estes MK. Norwalk virus infection of volunteers: new insights based on improved assays. J Infect Dis 1994; 170:34–43.
57. Lew JF, Valdesuso J, Vesikari T, et al. Detection of Norwalk virus or Norwalk-like virus infections in Finnish infants and young children. J Infect Dis 1994; 169:1364–1367.
58. Jenkins S, Horman JT, Israel E, Cukor G, Blacklow NR. An outbreak of Norwalk-related gastroenteritis at a boys' camp. Am J Dis Child 1985; 139:787–789.
59. Kuritsky JN, Osterholm MT, Greenberg HB, et al. Norwalk gastroenteritis: a community outbreak associated with bakery product consumption. Ann Intern Med 1984; 100:519–521.
60. Morse DL, Guzewich JJ, Hanrahan JP, et al. Widespread outbreaks of clam- and oyster-associated gastroenteritis. Role of Norwalk virus. N Engl J Med 1986; 314:678–681.
61. From the Centers for Disease Control and Prevention. Norovirus Activity–AcUSA, 2002. JAMA 2003; 289:693–696.
62. Greenberg HB, Wyatt RG, Kapikian AZ. Norwalk virus in vomitus. Lancet 1979; 1(55)
63. Agus SG, Dolin R, Wyatt RG, Tousimis AJ, Northrup RS. Acute infectious nonbacterial gastroenteritis: intestinal histopathology. Histologic and enzymatic alterations during illness produced by the Norwalk agent in man. Ann Intern Med 1973; 79:18–25.
64. Storr J, Rice S, Phillips AD, Price E, Walker-Smith JA. Clinical associations of Norwalk-like virus in the stools of children. J Pediatr Gastroenterol Nutr 1986; 5:576–580.
65. Kjeldsberg E, Anestad G, Greenberg H, Orstavik I, Pedersen R, Slettebo E. Norwalk virus in Norway: an outbreak of gastroenteritis studied by electron microscopy and radioimmunoassay. Scand J Infect Dis 1989; 21:521–526.
66. Tatsumi M, Nakata S, Sakai Y, Honma S, Numata-Kinoshita K, Chiba S. Detection and differentiation of Norwalk virus by reverse transcription-polymerase chain reaction and enzyme-linked immunosorbent assay. J Med Virol 2002; 68:285–290.
67. Honma S, Nakata S, Kinoshita-Numata K, Kogawa K, Chiba S. Evaluation of nine sets of PCR primers in the RNA dependent RNA polymerase region for detection and differentiation of members of the family Caliciviridae, Norwalk virus and Sapporo virus. Microbiol Immunol 2000; 44:411–419.
68. Wadell G, Allard A, Johansson M, Svensson L, Uhnoo I. Enteric adenoviruses. Ciba Found Symp 1987; 128:63–91.
69. Kotloff KL, Losonsky GA, Morris JG. Jr., Wasserman SS, Singh-Naz N, Levine MM. Enteric adenovirus infection and childhood diarrhea: an epidemiologic study in three clinical settings. Pediatrics 1989; 84:219–225.
70. Uhnoo I, Wadell G, Svensson L, Johansson ME. Importance of enteric adenoviruses 40 and 41 in acute gastroenteritis in infants and young children. J Clin Microbiol 1984; 20:365–372.
71. Grimwood K, Carzino R, Barnes GL, Bishop RF. Patients with enteric adenovirus gastroenteritis admitted to an Australian pediatric teaching hospital from 1981 to 1992. J Clin Microbiol 1995; 33:131–136.
72. Wood DJ. Adenovirus gastroenteritis. Br Med J (Clin Res Ed) 1988; 296:229–230.
73. Martin AL, Kudesia G. Enzyme linked immunosorbent assay for detecting adenoviruses in stool specimens: comparison with electron microscopy and isolation. J Clin Pathol 1990; 43:514–515.
74. Allard A, Girones R, Juto P, Wadell G. Polymerase chain reaction for detection of adenoviruses in stool samples. J Clin Microbiol 1990; 28:2659–2667.
75. Jiang B, Monroe SS, Koonin EV, Stine SE, Glass RI. RNA sequence of astrovirus: distinctive genomic organization and a putative retrovirus-like ribosomal frameshifting signal that directs the viral replicase synthesis. Proc Natl Acad Sci USA 1993; 90:10539–10543.
76. Herrmann JE, Taylor DN, Echeverria P, Blacklow NR. Astroviruses as a cause of gastroenteritis in children. N Engl J Med 1991; 324:1757–1760.
77. Lew JF, Moe CL, Monroe SS, et al. Astrovirus and adenovirus associated with diarrhea in children in day care settings. J Infect Dis 1991; 164:673–678.
78. Utagawa ET, Nishizawa S, Sekine S, et al. Astrovirus as a cause of gastroenteritis in Japan. J Clin Microbiol 1994; 32:1841–1845.
79. Ashley CR, Caul EO, Paver WK. Astrovirus-associated gastroenteritis in children. J Clin Pathol 1978; 31:939–943.

80. Yolken R, Dubovi E, Leister F, Reid R, Almeido-Hill J, Santosham M. Infantile gastroenteritis associated with excretion of pestivirus antigens. Lancet 1989; 1:517–520.

81. Prevention CfDCa. Viral agents of gastroenteritis: publich health importance and outbreak management. MMWR Morb Mortal Wkly Rep 1990; 39:1–3923.

82. Flewett TH, Beards GM, Brown DW, Sanders RC. The diagnostic gap in diarrhoeal aetiology. Ciba Found Symp 1987; 128:238–249.

83. Resta S, Luby JP, Rosenfeld CR, Siegel JD. Isolation and propagation of a human enteric coronavirus. Science 1985; 229:978–981.

84. Woode GN. Breda and Breda-like viruses: diagnosis, pathology and epidemiology. Ciba Found Symp 1987; 128:175–191.

85. Horzinek MC, Weiss M. Ederveen J. Toroviridae: a proposed new family of enveloped RNA viruses. Ciba Found Symp 1987; 128:162–174.

86. Koopmans M, Petric M, Glass RI, Monroe SS. Enzyme-linked immunosorbent assay reactivity of torovirus-like particles in fecal specimens from humans with diarrhea. J Clin Microbiol 1993; 31:2738–2744.

87. Pereira HG, Fialho AM, Flewett TH, Teixeira JM andrade ZP. Novel viruses in human faeces. Lancet 1988; 2:103–104.

88. Hochman JA, Witte DP, Cohen MB. Diagnosis of cytomegalovirus infection in pediatric Menetrier's disease by *in situ* hybridization. J Clin Microbiol 1996; 34:2588–2589.

89. Giannella RA, Broitman SA, Zamcheck N. Influence of gastric acidity on bacterial and parasitic enteric infections. A perspective. Ann Intern Med 1973; 78:271–276.

90. Giannella RA, Broitman SA, Zamcheck N. Gastric acid barrier to ingested microorganisms in man: studies *in vivo* and *in vitro*. Gut 1972; 13:251–256.

91. Hargrett-Bean NT, Pavia AT, Tauxe RV. Salmonella isolates from humans in the USA, 1984–1986. MMWR CDC Surveill Summ 1988; 37:25–31.

92. Bishop WP, Ulshen MH. Bacterial gastroenteritis. Pediatr Clin North Am 1988; 35:69–87.

93. Mahon BE, Ponka A, Hall WN, et al. An international outbreak of Salmonella infections caused by alfalfa sprouts grown from contaminated seeds. J Infect Dis 1997; 175:876–882.

94. Hennessy TW, Hedberg CW, Slutsker L, et al. A national outbreak of Salmonella enteritidis infections from ice cream. Invest Team N Engl J Med 1996; 334:1281–1286.

95. Duguid JP, North RA. Eggs and Salmonella food-poisoning: an evaluation. J Med Microbiol 1991; 34:65–72.

96. Blaser MJ, Newman LS. A review of human salmonellosis: I. Infective dose. Rev Infect Dis 1982; 4:1096–1106.

97. Hromockyj AE, Falkow S. Interactions of bacteria with the gut epithelium. In: Blaser MJ, Smith PD, Ravdin JI, eds. Infections of the Gastrointestinal Tract. New York, NY: Raven Press; 1995:603–616.

98. Torrey S, Fleisher G, Jaffe D. Incidence of Salmonella bacteremia in infants with Salmonella gastroenteritis. J Pediatr 1986; 108:718–721.

99. Buchwald DS, Blaser MJ. A review of human salmonellosis: II. Duration of excretion following infection with nontyphi Salmonella. Rev Infect Dis 1984; 6:345–356.

100. Aserkoff B, Bennett JV. Effect of antibiotic therapy in acute salmonellosis on the fecal excretion of salmonellae. N Engl J Med 1969; 281:636–640.

101. Geme JW. 3rd, Hodes HL, Marcy SM, Pickering LK, Rodriguez WJ, McCracken GH, Jr., Nelson JD. Consensus: management of Salmonella infection in the first year of life. Pediatr Infect Dis J 1988; 7:615–621.

102. Pickering LK. Therapy for acute infectious diarrhea in children. J Pediatr 1991; 118:S118–S128.

103. Lee LA, Puhr ND, Maloney EK, Bean NH, Tauxe RV. Increase in antimicrobial-resistant Salmonella infections in the USA, 1989–1990. J Infect Dis 1994; 170:128–134.

104. Colon AR, Gross DR, Tamer MA. Typhoid fever in children. Pediatrics 1975; 56:606–609.

105. Levine MM, Hone D, Stocker BAD. Vaccines to prevent typhoid. In: Woodrow G, Levine MM, eds. New-Generation Vaccines. New York, NY: Marcel Dekker; 1990:269–287.

106. Plotkin SA, Bouveret-Le Cam N. A new typhoid vaccine composed of the Vi capsular polysaccharide. Arch Intern Med 1995; 155:2293–2299.

107. Lin FY, Ho VA, Khiem HB, et al. The efficacy of a Salmonella typhi Vi conjugate vaccine in two-to-five-year-old children. N Engl J Med 2001; 344:1263–1269.

108. Tacket CO, Sztein MB, Wasserman SS, et al. Phase 2 clinical trial of attenuated Salmonella enterica serovar typhi oral live vector vaccine CVD 908-htrA in U.S. volunteers. Infect Immun 2000; 68:1196–1201.

109. Wang JY, Noriega FR, Galen JE, Barry E, Levine MM. Constitutive expression of the Vi polysaccharide capsular antigen in attenuated Salmonella enterica serovar typhi oral vaccine strain CVD 909. Infect Immun 2000; 68:4647–4652.

110. Olslcr W. Thc Principles and Practice of Medicine. D Appleton Co. 1892.

111. Acheson DWK, Keusch GT. Shigella and enteroinvasive Eschericha coli. In: Blaser MJ, Smith PD, Ravdin JI, eds. Infections of the Gastrointestinal Tract. New York, NY: Raven Press; 1995:763–784.

112. Mata LJ. The children of Santa Maria Caugue: a prospective field study of health and growth. Cambridge, Mass.: MIT Press; 1978:

113. Cohen MB. Etiology and mechanisms of acute infectious diarrhea in infants in the USA. J Pediatr 1991; 118:S34–S39.

114. Calin A. Fries JF. An experimental epidemic of Reiter's syndrome revisited. Follow-up evidence on genetic and environmental factors. Ann Intern Med 1976; 84:564–566.

115. Theriot JA. The cell biology of infection by intracellular bacterial pathogens. Annu Rev Cell Dev Biol 1995; 11:213–239.

116. Hale TL. Genetic basis of virulence in Shigella species. Microbiol Rev 1991; 55:206–224.

117. O'Brien AD, Holmes RK. Shiga and Shiga-like toxins. Microbiol Rev 1987; 51:206–220.

118. Surawicz CM, Belic L. Rectal biopsy helps to distinguish acute self-limited colitis from idiopathic inflammatory bowel disease. Gastroenterology 1984; 86:104–113.

119. Tong MJ, Martin DG, Cunningham JJ, Gunning JJ. Clinical and bacteriological evaluation of antibiotic treatment in shigellosis. JAMA 1970; 214:1841–1844.

120. Ross S, Controni G, Khan W. Resistance of shigellae to ampicillin and other antibiotics. Its clinical and epidemiological implications. JAMA 1972; 221:45–47.

121. Nelson JA, Haltalin KC. Amoxicillin less effective than ampicillin against Shigella in vitro and in vivo: relationship of efficacy to activity in serum. J Infect Dis 1974; 129(suppl):S222–S227.

122. Shears P. Shigella infections. Ann Trop Med Parasitol 1996; 90:105–114.

123. Williams EK, Lohr JA, Guerrant RL. Acute infectious diarrhea. II. Diagnosis, treatment and prevention. Pediatr Infect Dis 1986; 5:458–465.

124. Walker RI, Caldwell MB, Lee EC, Guerry P, Trust TJ, Ruiz-Palacios GM. Pathophysiology of Campylobacter enteritis. Microbiol Rev 1986; 50:81–94.

125. Goossens H, Vlaes L, De Boeck M, et al. Vandamme P. Is 'Campylobacter upsaliensis' an unrecognised cause of human diarrhoea? Lancet 1990; 335:584–586.

126. Sjogren E, Ruiz-Palacios G, Kaijser B. Campylobacter jejuni isolations from Mexican and Swedish patients, with repeated symptomatic and/or asymptomatic diarrhoea episodes. Epidemiol Infect 1989; 102:47–57.

127. Tauxe RV, Hargrett-Bean N, Patton CM, Wachsmuth IK. Campylobacter isolates in the USA, 1982–1986. MMWR CDC Surveill Summ 1988; 37:1–3713.

128. Blaser MJ, Reller LB. Campylobacter enteritis. N Engl J Med 1981; 305:1444–1452.

129. Spelman DW, Davidson N, Buckmaster ND, Spicer WJ, Ryan P. Campylobacter bacteraemia: a report of 10 cases. Med J Aust 1986; 145:503–505.

130. Rees JH, Soudain SE, Gregson NA, Hughes RA. Campylobacter jejuni infection and Guillain-Barre syndrome. N Engl J Med 1995; 333:1374–1379.

131. Salloway S, Mermel LA, Seamans M, et al. Miller-Fisher syndrome associated with Campylobacter jejuni bearing lipopolysaccharide molecules that mimic human ganglioside GD3. Infect Immun 1996; 64:2945–2949.

132. Karmali MA, Fleming PC. Campylobacter enteritis in children. J Pediatr 1979; 94:527–533.

133. Salazar-Lindo E, Sack RB, Chea-Woo E, et al. Early treatment with erythromycin of Campylobacter jejuni-associated dysentery in children. J Pediatr 1986; 109:355–360.

134. Cover TL, Aber RC. Yersinia enterocolitica. N Engl J Med 1989; 321:16–24.

135. Black RE, Jackson RJ, Tsai T, et al. Epidemic Yersinia enterocolitica infection due to contaminated chocolate milk. N Engl J Med 1978; 298:76–79.

136. Lee LA, Gerber AR, Lonsway DR, et al. Yersinia enterocolitica O:3 infections in infants and children, associated with the household preparation of chitterlings. N Engl J Med 1990; 322:984–987.

137. Lee LA, Taylor J, Carter GP, Quinn B, Farmer JJ. 3rd, Tauxe RV. Yersinia enterocolitica O:3: an emerging cause of pediatric gastroenteritis in the USA. The Yersinia enterocolitica Collaborative Study Group. J Infect Dis 1991; 163:660–663.

138. Marks MI, Pai CH, Lafleur L, Lackman L, Hammerberg O. Yersinia enterocolitica gastroenteritis: a prospective study of clinical, bacteriologic and epidemiologic features. J Pediatr 1980; 96:26–31.

139. Cover TL. Yersinia enterocolitica and Yersinia pseudotuberculosis. In: Blaser MJ, Smith PD, Ravdin JI, eds. Infections of the Gastrointestinal Tract. New York, NY: Raven Press; 1995:811–823.

140. Attwood SE, Mealy K, Cafferkey MT, et al. Yersinia infection and acute abdominal pain. Lancet 1987; 1:529–533.

141. Dequeker J, Jamar R, Walravens M. HLA-B27, arthritis and Yersinia enterocolitica infection. J Rheumatol 1980; 7:706–710.

142. Bottone EJ, Sheehan DJ. Yersinia enterocolitica: guidelines for serologic diagnosis of human infections. Rev Infect Dis 1983; 5:898–906.

143. Pai CH, Gillis F, Tuomanen E, Marks MI. Placebo-controlled double-blind evaluation of trimethoprim-sulfamethoxazole treatment of Yersinia enterocolitica gastroenteritis. J Pediatr 1984; 104:308–311.

144. Gayraud M, Scavizzi MR, Mollaret HH, Guillevin L, Hornstein MJ. Antibiotic treatment of Yersinia enterocolitica septicemia: a retrospective review of 43 cases. Clin Infect Dis 1993; 17:405–410.

145. Mofenson HC, Caraccio TR, Sharieff N. Iron sepsis: Yersinia enterocolitica septicemia possibly caused by an overdose of iron. N Engl J Med 1987; 316:1092–1093.

146. Sack DA, Sack RB, Nair GB. Siddique AK. Cholera Lancet 2004; 363:223–233.

147. Greenough WB. 3rd. The human, societal and scientific legacy of cholera. J Clin Invest 2004; 113:334–339.

148. Kaper JB, Morris JG. Jr., Levine MM. Cholera Clin Microbiol Rev 1995; 8:48–86.

149. Blake PA. Epidemiology of cholera in the Americas. Gastroenterol Clin North Am 1993; 22:639–660.

150. Morris JG. Jr, Black RE. Cholera and other vibrioses in the USA. N Engl J Med 1985; 312:343–350.

151. Ramamurthy T, Garg S, Sharma R, et al. Emergence of novel strain of Vibrio cholerae with epidemic potential in southern and eastern India. Lancet 1993; 341:703–704.

152. Albert MJ, Siddique AK, Islam MS, et al. Large outbreak of clinical cholera due to Vibrio cholerae non-O1 in Bangladesh. Lancet 1993; 341:704.

153. Cholera FRA. Critical Reviews in Microbiology 1973;. 2:553–623.

154. Azurin JC, Kobari K, Barua D, et al. A long-term carrier of cholera: cholera Dolores. Bull World Health Organ 1967; 37:745–749.

155. Weber JT, Levine WC, Hopkins DP, Tauxe RV. Cholera in the USA, 1965–1991. Risks at home and abroad. Arch Intern Med 1994; 154:551–556.

156. DePaola A, Capers GM, Motes ML, et al. Isolation of Latin American epidemic strain of Vibrio cholerae O1 from US Gulf Coast. Lancet 1992; 339:624.

157. Carpenter CC. Clinical and pathophysiologic features of diarrhea caused by Vibrio cholerae and *Escherichia coli*. In: Field M, Fordtran JS, Schutz SG, eds. Secretory Diarrhea. Bethesda, MD: American Physiological Society; 1980:66–73.

158. Carpenter CC. Cholera and other enterotoxin-related diarrheal diseases. J Infect Dis 1972; 126:551–564.

159. Moss J, Burns DL, Hsia JA, Hewlett EL, Guerrant RL, Vaughan M. NIH conference. Cyclic nucleotides: mediators of bacterial toxin action in disease. Ann Intern Med 1984; 101:653–666.

160. Fasano A, Baudry B, Pumplin DW, et al. Vibrio cholerae produces a second enterotoxin, which affects intestinal tight junctions. Proc Natl Acad Sci USA 1991; 88:5242–5246.

161. Trucksis M, Galen JE, Michalski J, Fasano A, Kaper JB. Accessory cholera enterotoxin (Ace), the third toxin of a Vibrio cholerae virulence cassette. Proc Natl Acad Sci USA 1993; 90:5267–5271.

162. Khan WA, Bennish ML, Seas C, et al. Randomised controlled comparison of single-dose ciprofloxacin and doxycycline for cholera caused by Vibrio cholerae 01 or 0139. Lancet 1996; 348:296–300.

163. Levine MM. Development of bacterial vaccines. In: Blaser MJ, Smith PD, Ravdin JI, eds. Infections of the Gastrointestinal Tract. New York, NY: Raven Press; 1995:1441–1470.

164. Levine MM, Kaper JB. Live oral vaccines against cholera: an update. Vaccine 1993; 11:207–212.

165. Trach DD, Clemens JD, Ke NT, et al. Field trial of a locally produced, killed, oral cholera vaccine in Vietnam. Lancet 1997; 349:231–235.

166. Tacket CO, Cohen MB, Wasserman SS, et al. Randomized, double-blind, placebo-controlled, multicentered trial of the efficacy of a single dose of live oral cholera vaccine CVD

103-HgR in preventing cholera following challenge with Vibrio cholerae O1 El tor inaba three months after vaccination. Infect Immun 1999; 67:6341–6345.

167. Richie EE, Punjabi NH, Sidharta YY, et al. Efficacy trial of single-dose live oral cholera vaccine CVD 103-HgR in North Jakarta, Indonesia, a cholera-endemic area. Vaccine 2000; 18:2399–2410.

168. Cohen MB, Giannella RA, Bean J, et al. Randomized, controlled human challenge study of the safety, immunogenicity and protective efficacy of a single dose of Peru-15, a live attenuated oral cholera vaccine. Infect Immun 2002; 70:1965–1970.

169. Morris JG Jr. Noncholera vibrio species. In: Blaser MJ, Smith PD, Ravdin JI, eds. Infections of the Gastrointestinal Tract. New York, NY: Raven Press; 1995:671–685.

170. Honda T, Arita M, Takeda T, Yoh M, Miwatani T. Non-O1 Vibrio cholerae produces two newly identified toxins related to Vibrio parahaemolyticus haemolysin and *Escherichia coli* heat-stable enterotoxin. Lancet 1985; 2:163–164.

171. Wilson R, Lieb S, Roberts A, et al. Non-O group 1 Vibrio cholerae gastroenteritis associated with eating raw oysters. Am J Epidemiol 1981; 114:293–298.

172. Levine MM. *Escherichia coli* that cause diarrhea: enterotoxigenic, enteropathogenic, enteroinvasive, enterohemorrhagic and enteroadherent. J Infect Dis 1987; 155:377–389.

173. Levine MM. *Escherichia coli* infections. N Engl J Med 1985; 313:445–447.

174. Cravioto A, Reyes RE, Ortega R, Fernandez G, Hernandez R, Lopez D. Prospective study of diarrhoeal disease in a cohort of rural Mexican children: incidence and isolated pathogens during the first two years of life. Epidemiol Infect 1988; 101:123–134.

175. Gomes TA, Blake PA, Trabulsi LR. Prevalence of *Escherichia coli* strains with localized, diffuse and aggregative adherence to HeLa cells in infants with diarrhea and matched controls. J Clin Microbiol 1989; 27:266–269.

176. Gomes TA, Rassi V, MacDonald KL, et al. Enteropathogens associated with acute diarrheal disease in urban infants in Sao Paulo, Brazil. J Infect Dis 1991; 164:331–337.

177. Robins-Browne RM, Still CS, Miliotis MD, et al. Summer diarrhoea in African infants and children. Arch Dis Child 1980; 55:923–928.

178. Sherman P, Drumm B, Karmali M, Cutz E. Adherence of bacteria to the intestine in sporadic cases of enteropathogenic *Escherichia coli*-associated diarrhea in infants and young children: a prospective study. Gastroenterology 1989; 96:86–94.

179. Rothbaum R, McAdams AJ, Giannella R, Partin JC. A clinicopathologic study of enterocyte-adherent *Escherichia coli*: a cause of protracted diarrhea in infants. Gastroenterology 1982; 83:441–454.

180. Bokete TN, Whittam TS, Wilson RA, et al. Genetic and phenotypic analysis of *Escherichia coli* with enteropathogenic characteristics isolated from Seattle children. J Infect Dis 1997; 175:1382–1389.

181. Moon HW, Whipp SC, Argenzio RA, Levine MM, Giannella RA. Attaching and effacing activities of rabbit and human enteropathogenic *Escherichia coli* in pig and rabbit intestines. Infect Immun 1983; 41:1340–1351.

182. Donnenberg MS, Kaper JB. Enteropathogenic *Escherichia coli*. Infect Immun 1992; 60:3953–3961.

183. McDaniel TK, Jarvis KG, Donnenberg MS, Kaper JB. A genetic locus of enterocyte effacement conserved among diverse enterobacterial pathogens. Proc Natl Acad Sci USA 1995; 92:1664–1668.

184. McDaniel TK, Kaper JB. A cloned pathogenicity island from enteropathogenic *Escherichia coli* confers the attaching and effacing phenotype on *E. coli* K-12. Mol Microbiol 1997; 23:399–407.

185. Bhan MK, Raj P, Levine MM, et al. Enteroaggregative *Escherichia coli* associated with persistent diarrhea in a cohort of rural children in India. J Infect Dis 1989; 159:1061–1064.

186. Gicquelais KG, Baldini MM, Martinez J, et al. Practical and economical method for using biotinylated DNA probes with bacterial colony blots to identify diarrhea-causing *Escherichia coli*. J Clin Microbiol 1990; 28:2485–2490.

187. Knutton S, Baldwin T, Williams PH, McNeish AS. Actin accumulation at sites of bacterial adhesion to tissue culture cells: basis of a new diagnostic test for enteropathogenic and enterohemorrhagic *Escherichia coli*. Infect Immun 1989; 57:1290–1298.

188. Black RE, Brown KH, Becker S, Yunus M. Longitudinal studies of infectious diseases and physical growth of children in rural Bangladesh. I. Patterns of morbidity. Am J Epidemiol 1982; 115:305–314.

189. Gorbach SL, Kean BH, Evans DG, Evans DJ Jr., Bessudo D. Travelers' diarrhea and toxigenic *Escherichia coli*. N Engl J Med 1975; 292:933–936.

190. Cohen MB, Guarino A, Shukla R, Giannella RA. Age-related differences in receptors for *Escherichia coli* heat-stable enterotoxin in the small and large intestine of children. Gastroenterology 1988; 94:367–373.

191. Cohen MB, Giannella R. Enterotoxigenic *E. coli*. In: Blaser MJ, Smith PD, Ravdin JI, Greenberg H, eds. Infections of the Gastrointestinal Tract. New York, NY: Raven Press; 2002:579–594.

192. Sears CL, Kaper JB. Enteric bacterial toxins: mechanisms of action and linkage to intestinal secretion. Microbiol Rev 1996; 60:167–215.

193. Currie MG, Fok KF, Kato J, Moore RJ, Hamra FK, Duffin KL, Smith CE. Guanylin: an endogenous activator of intestinal guanylate cyclase. Proc Natl Acad Sci USA 1992; 89:947–951.

194. Kita T, Smith CE, Fok KF, et al. Characterization of human uroguanylin: a member of the guanylin peptide family. Am J Physiol 1994; 266:F342–F348.

195. Lorenz JN, Nieman M, Sabo J, et al. Uroguanylin knockout mice have increased blood pressure and impaired natriuretic response to enteral NaCl load. J Clin Invest 2003; 112:1244–1254.

196. Giannella RA. Suckling mouse model for detection of heat-stable *Escherichia coli* enterotoxin: characteristics of the model. Infect Immun 1976; 14:95–99.

197. Moseley SL, Hardy JW, Hug MI, Echeverria P, Falkow S. Isolation and nucleotide sequence determination of a gene encoding a heat-stable enterotoxin of *Escherichia coli*. Infect Immun 1983; 39:1167–1174.

198. Moseley SL, Echeverria P, Seriwatana J, et al. Identification of enterotoxigenic *Escherichia coli* by colony hybridization using three enterotoxin gene probes. J Infect Dis 1982; 145:863–869.

199. Black RE, Levine MM, Clements ML, Cisneros L, Daya V. Treatment of experimentally induced enterotoxigenic *Escherichia coli* diarrhea with trimethoprim, trimethoprim-sulfamethoxazole, or placebo. Rev Infect Dis 1982; 4:540–545.

200. Heck JE, Staneck JL, Cohen MB, et al. Prevention of Travelers' Diarrhea: Ciprofloxacin versus Trimethoprim/Sulfamethoxazole in Adult Volunteers Working in Latin America and the Caribbean. J Travel Med 1994; 1:136–142.

201. DuPont HL, Formal SB, Hornick RB, et al. Pathogenesis of *Escherichia coli* diarrhea. N Engl J Med 1971; 285:1–9.

202. Riley LW, Remis RS, Helgerson SD, et al. Hemorrhagic colitis associated with a rare *Escherichia coli* serotype. N Engl J Med 1983; 308:681–685.
203. Karmali MA, Steele BT, Petric M, Lim C. Sporadic cases of haemolytic-uraemic syndrome associated with faecal cytotoxin and cytotoxin-producing *Escherichia coli* in stools. Lancet 1983; 1:619–620.
204. Slutsker L, Ries AA, Greene KD, Wells JG, Hutwagner L, Griffin PM. *Escherichia coli* O157:H7 diarrhea in the USA: clinical and epidemiologic features. Ann Intern Med 1997; 126:505–513.
205. Cohen MB. *Escherichia coli* O157:H7 infections: a frequent cause of bloody diarrhea and the hemolytic-uremic syndrome. Adv Pediatr 1996; 43:171–207.
206. Cohen MB, Giannella RA. Hemorrhagic colitis associated with *Escherichia coli* O157:H7. Adv Intern Med 1992; 37:173–195.
207. Griffin PM, Olmstead LC, Petras RE. *Escherichia coli* O157:H7-associated colitis. A clinical and histological study of 11 cases. Gastroenterology 1990; 99:142–149.
208. Tarr PI. *Escherichia coli* O157:H7: clinical, diagnostic and epidemiological aspects of human infection. Clin Infect Dis 1995; 20:1–2010.
209. Boyce TG, Swerdlow DL, Griffin PM. *Escherichia coli* O157:H7 and the hemolytic-uremic syndrome. N Engl J Med 1995; 333:364–368.
210. Swerdlow DL, Woodruff BA, Brady RC, et al. A waterborne outbreak in Missouri of *Escherichia coli* O157:H7 associated with bloody diarrhea and death. Ann Intern Med 1992; 117:812–819.
211. Keene WE, McAnulty JM, Hoesly FC, et al. A swimming-associated outbreak of hemorrhagic colitis caused by *Escherichia coli* O157:H7 and Shigella sonnei. N Engl J Med 1994; 331:579–584.
212. Milford DV, Taylor CM, Guttridge B, Hall SM, Rowe B, Kleanthous H. Haemolytic uraemic syndromes in the British Isles 1985–1988: association with verocytotoxin producing *Escherichia coli*. Part 1: Clinical and epidemiological aspects. Arch Dis Child 1990; 65:716–721.
213. Bitzan M, Ludwig K, Klemt M, Konig H, Buren J, Muller-Wiefel DE. The role of *Escherichia coli* O 157 infections in the classical (enteropathic) haemolytic uraemic syndrome: results of a Central European, multicentre study. Epidemiol Infect 1993; 110:183–196.
214. Belongia EA, Osterholm MT, Soler JT, Ammend DA, Braun JE, MacDonald KL. Transmission of *Escherichia coli* O157:H7 infection in Minnesota child day-care facilities. JAMA 1993; 269:883–888.
215. Karch H, Russmann H, Schmidt H, Schwarzkopf A, Heesemann J. Long-term shedding and clonal turnover of enterohemorrhagic *Escherichia coli* O157 in diarrheal diseases. J Clin Microbiol 1995; 33:1602–1605.
216. Klein EJ, Stapp JR, Clausen CR, et al. Shiga toxin-producing *Escherichia coli* in children with diarrhea: a prospective point-of-care study. J Pediatr 2002; 141:172–177.
217. Walterspiel JN, Ashkenazi S, Morrow AL, Cleary TG. Effect of subinhibitory concentrations of antibiotics on extracellular Shiga-like toxin I. Infection 1992; 20:25–29.
218. Griffin PM. *E. coli* 0157:H7 and other enterohemorrhagic *E. coli*. In: Blaser MJ, Smith PD, Ravdin JI, eds. Infections of the Gastrointestinal Tract. New York, NY: Raven Press; 1995:739–761.
219. Proulx F, Turgeon JP, Delage G, Lafleur L, Chicoine L. Randomized, controlled trial of antibiotic therapy for *Escherichia coli* O157:H7 enteritis. J Pediatr 1992; 121:299–303.
220. Wong CS, Jelacic S, Habeeb RL, Watkins SL, Tarr PI. The risk of the hemolytic-uremic syndrome after antibiotic treatment of *Escherichia coli* O157:H7 infections. N Engl J Med 2000; 342:1930–1936.
221. Safdar N, Said A, Gangnon RE, Maki DG. Risk of hemolytic uremic syndrome after antibiotic treatment of *Escherichia coli* O157:H7 enteritis: a meta-analysis. JAMA 2002; 288:996–1001.
222. Pediatrics Ao. Red Book: 2003 Report of the Committee on Infectious Diseases. Elk Grove Village, IL: American Academy of Pediatrics; 2003.
223. Trachtman H, Cnaan A, Christen E, et al. Effect of an oral Shiga toxin-binding agent on diarrhea-associated hemolytic uremic syndrome in children: a randomized controlled trial. JAMA 2003; 290:1337–1344.
224. Vial PA, Mathewson JJ, DuPont HL, Guers L, Levine MM. Comparison of two assay methods for patterns of adherence to HEp-2 cells of *Escherichia coli* from patients with diarrhea. J Clin Microbiol 1990; 28:882–885.
225. Nataro JP, Kaper JB, Robins-Browne R, Prado V, Vial P, Levine MM. Patterns of adherence of diarrheagenic *Escherichia coli* to HEp-2 cells. Pediatr Infect Dis J 1987; 6:829–831.
226. Cohen MB, Hawkins JA, Weckbach LS, Staneck JL, Levine MM, Heck JE. Colonization by enteroaggregative *Escherichia coli* in travelers with and without diarrhea. J Clin Microbiol 1993; 31:351–353.
227. Echeverria P, Serichantalerg O, Changchawalit S, et al. Tissue culture-adherent *Escherichia coli* in infantile diarrhea. J Infect Dis 1992; 165:141–143.
228. Mathewson JJ, Johnson PC, DuPont HL, Satterwhite TK, Winsor DK. Pathogenicity of enteroadherent *Escherichia coli* in adult volunteers. J Infect Dis 1986; 154:524–527.
229. Nataro JP, Deng Y, Cookson S, et al. Heterogeneity of enteroaggregative *Escherichia coli* virulence demonstrated in volunteers. J Infect Dis 1995; 171:465–468.
230. Okeke IN, Nataro JP. Enteroaggregative *Escherichia coli*. Lancet Infect Dis 2001; 1:304–313.
231. Cohen MB, Nataro JP, Bernstein DI, Hawkins J, Roberts N, Staat MA. Prevalence of diarrheagenic E. coli in acute childhood gastroenteritis: a prospective controlled surveillance study. J Pediatr 2005; 146:54–61.
232. Vial PA, Robins-Browne R, Lior H, et al. Characterization of enteroadherent-aggregative *Escherichia coli*, a putative agent of diarrheal disease. J Infect Dis 1988; 158:70–79.
233. Savarino SJ, Fasano A, Robertson DC, Levine MM. Enteroaggregative *Escherichia coli* elaborate a heat-stable enterotoxin demonstrable in an in vitro rabbit intestinal model. J Clin Invest 1991; 87:1450–1455.
234. Steiner TS, Nataro JP, Poteet-Smith CE, Smith JA, Guerrant RL. Enteroaggregative *Escherichia coli* expresses a novel flagellin that causes IL-8 release from intestinal epithelial cells. J Clin Invest 2000; 105:1769–1777.
235. Donta ST, Myers MG. Clostridium difficile toxin in asymptomatic neonates. J Pediatr 1982; 100:431–434.
236. Rolfe RD. Binding kinetics of Clostridium difficile toxins A and B to intestinal brush border membranes from infant and adult hamsters. Infect Immun 1991; 59:1223–1230.
237. Eglow R, Pothoulakis C, Itzkowitz S, et al. Diminished Clostridium difficile toxin A sensitivity in newborn rabbit ileum is associated with decreased toxin A receptor. J Clin Invest 1992; 90:822–829.
238. Pothoulakis C, LaMont JT, Eglow R, et al. Characterization of rabbit ileal receptors for Clostridium difficile toxin A. Evidence for a receptor-coupled G protein. J Clin Invest 1991; 88:119–125.

239. Hyams JS, McLaughlin JC. Lack of relationship between Clostridium difficile toxin and inflammatory bowel disease in children. J Clin Gastroenterol 1985; 7:387–390.
240. Kader HA, Piccoli DA, Jawad AF, McGowan KL, Maller ES. Single toxin detection is inadequate to diagnose Clostridium difficile diarrhea in pediatric patients. Gastroenterology 1998; 115:1329–1334.
241. Bates M, Bove K, Cohen MB. Pseudomembranous colitis caused by C. difficile. J Pediatr 1997; 130:146.
242. Teasley DG, Gerding DN, Olson MM, et al. Prospective randomised trial of metronidazole versus vancomycin for Clostridium-difficile-associated diarrhoea and colitis. Lancet 1983; 2:1043–1046.
243. Fekety R, Shah AB. Diagnosis and treatment of Clostridium difficile colitis. JAMA 1993; 269:71–75.
244. Leung DY, Kelly CP, Boguniewicz M, Pothoulakis C, LaMont JT, Flores A. Treatment with intravenously administered gamma globulin of chronic relapsing colitis induced by Clostridium difficile toxin. J Pediatr 1991; 118:633–637.
245. Biller JA, Katz AJ, Flores AF, Buie TM, Gorbach SL. Treatment of recurrent Clostridium difficile colitis with Lactobacillus GG. J Pediatr Gastroenterol Nutr 1995; 21:224–226.
246. Holmberg SD, Farmer JJ. 3rd. Aeromonas hydrophila and Plesiomonas shigelloides as causes of intestinal infections. Rev Infect Dis 1984; 6:633–639.
247. Challapalli M, Tess BR, Cunningham DG, Chopra AK, Houston CW. Aeromonas-associated diarrhea in children. Pediatr Infect Dis J 1988; 7:693–698.
248. Gracey M, Burke V, Robinson J. Aeromonas-associated gastroenteritis. Lancet 1982; 2:1304–1306.
249. Agger WA, McCormick JD, Gurwith MJ. Clinical and microbiological features of Aeromonas hydrophila-associated diarrhea. J Clin Microbiol 1985; 21:909–913.
250. Namdari H, Bottone EJ. Microbiologic and clinical evidence supporting the role of Aeromonas caviae as a pediatric enteric pathogen. J Clin Microbiol 1990; 28:837–840.
251. Olsvik O, Wachsmuth K, Kay B, Birkness KA, Yi A, Sack B. Laboratory observations on Plesiomonas shigelloides strains isolated from children with diarrhea in Peru. J Clin Microbiol 1990; 28:886–889.
252. Prevention CfDCa. Aquarium-associated Plesiomonas shigelloides infection -Missouri. MMWR Morb Mortal Wkly Rep 1989; 38:617–619.
253. Kain KC, Kelly MT. Clinical features, epidemiology and treatment of Plesiomonas shigelloides diarrhea. J Clin Microbiol 1989; 27:998–1001.
254. Lincoln EM, Gilbert LA. Disease in children due to mycobacteria other than Mycobacterium tuberculosis. Am Rev Respir Dis 1972; 105:683–714.
255. Young LS. Mycobacterium avium complex infection. J Infect Dis 1988; 157:863–867.
256. Hawkins CC, Gold JW, Whimbey E, et al. Mycobacterium avium complex infections in patients with the acquired immunodeficiency syndrome. Ann Intern Med 1986; 105:184–188.
257. Gillin JS, Urmacher C, West R, Shike M. Disseminated Mycobacterium avium-intracellulare infection in acquired immunodeficiency syndrome mimicking Whipple's disease. Gastroenterology 1983; 85:1187–1191.
258. Ozkaynak MF, Lenarsky C, Kohn D, Weinberg K, Parkman R. Mycobacterium avium-intracellulare infections after allogeneic bone marrow transplantation in children. Am J Pediatr Hematol Oncol 1990; 12:220–224.
259. Kinney JS, Little BJ, Yolken RH, Rosenstein BJ. Mycobacterium avium complex in a patient with cystic fibrosis: disease vs. colonization. Pediatr Infect Dis J 1989; 8:393–396.
260. Weikel CS, Grieco FD, Reuben J, Myers LL, Sack RB. Human colonic epithelial cells, HT29/C1, treated with crude Bacteroides fragilis enterotoxin dramatically alter their morphology. Infect Immun 1992; 60:321–327.
261. Myers LL, Shoop DS, Stackhouse LL, et al. Isolation of enterotoxigenic Bacteroides fragilis from humans with diarrhea. J Clin Microbiol 1987; 25:2330–2333.
262. Sack RB, Myers LL, Almeido-Hill J, et al. Enterotoxigenic Bacteroides fragilis: epidemiologic studies of its role as a human diarrhoeal pathogen. J Diarrhoeal Dis Res 1992; 10:4–9.
263. Sack RB, Albert MJ, Alam K, Neogi PK, Akbar MS. Isolation of enterotoxigenic Bacteroides fragilis from Bangladeshi children with diarrhea: a controlled study. J Clin Microbiol 1994; 32:960–963.
264. Sears CL, Myers LL, Lazenby A, Tassell RL Van. Enterotoxigenic Bacteroides fragilis. Clin Infect Dis 1995; 20(suppl 2):S142–S418.
265. San Joaquin VH, Griffis JC, Lee C, Sears CL. Association of Bacteroides fragilis with childhood diarrhea. Scand J Infect Dis 1995; 27:211–215.
266. Pantosti A, Menozzi MG, Frate A, Sanfilippo L, D'Ambrosio F, Malpeli M. Detection of enterotoxigenic Bacteroides fragilis and its toxin in stool samples from adults and children in Italy. Clin Infect Dis 1997; 24:12–16.
267. Lee JI, Hampson DJ. Genetic characterisation of intestinal spirochaetes and their association with disease. J Med Microbiol 1994; 40:365–371.
268. Cunha Ferreira RM da, Phillips AD, Stevens CR, Hudson MJ, Rees HC, Walker-Smith JA. Intestinal spirochaetosis in children. J Pediatr Gastroenterol Nutr 1993; 17:333–336.
269. Surawicz CM, Roberts PL, Rompalo A, Quinn TC, Holmes KK, Stamm WE. Intestinal spirochetosis in homosexual men. Am J Med 1987; 82:587–592.
270. Ismaili A, Bourke B, Azavedo JC de, Ratnam S, Karmali MA, Sherman PM. Heterogeneity in phenotypic and genotypic characteristics among strains of Hafnia alvei. J Clin Microbiol 1996; 34:2973–2979.
271. Dalton CB, Austin CC, Sobel J, et al. An outbreak of gastroenteritis and fever due to Listeria monocytogenes in milk. N Engl J Med 1997; 336:100–105.

Chapter 37
Enteric parasites

Jacqueline L. Fridge and Dorsey M. Bass

INTRODUCTION

Enteric parasites are important agents of disease throughout the world. Although the frequency and severity of parasitic diseases are most extreme in the developing world, changes in worldwide travel, immigration, commerce and daycare for young children and increasing numbers of patients with immune compromise have led to increased incidences of parasitic diseases in the developed world. Parasitic disease may mimic other gastrointestinal disorders, such as inflammatory bowel disease, hepatitis, sclerosing cholangitis, peptic ulcer disease and celiac disease. Parasitic infection can also trigger overt manifestations of quiescent chronic intestinal disorders.

EPIDEMIOLOGY

A variety of epidemiologic factors predispose patients to parasitic infestation worldwide, but the single most important factor is socioeconomic status. It has been shown repeatedly, in both the developed and developing world, that children of lower socioeconomic status have higher parasite loads and a greater prevalence of multiple infestations.[1,2] Travel to developing countries can expose an individual to parasites that may not cause symptoms until weeks, months, or years later. Immigrants from developing countries often harbor pathogens that are unfamiliar to physicians in their new homelands and may pass them on to their new countrymen. Less obvious sources of parasites include foodstuffs increasingly imported from all areas of the world. The United States has experienced outbreaks of intestinal cyclosporiasis from imported raspberries.[3]

Protozoan infections endemic to the developed world, such as *Giardia*sis, are transmitted with great efficiency in daycare centers, where fecal-oral contamination is quite common. Institutions for the mentally retarded are also common reservoirs for *Giardia, Entamoeba histolytica* and other protozoans. Pets and livestock are potential sources of *Cryptosporidium, Giardia* and *Toxocara* species, canine hookworm, *Balantidium coli* and other organisms.

Dietary habits can also be risk factors. Consumption of raw or undercooked fish can lead to *Diphyllobothrium latum, Capillaria philippinensis*, or *Anisakis* infection. Inadequate cooking of pork predisposes to *Taenia solium* and *Trichinella* infections. Beefsteak tartare and other raw or rare bovine delicacies can harbor *Taenia saginata*. Furthermore, a variety of protozoan organisms can be transmitted via produce that has been exposed to human or animal waste. Unpasteurized apple juice has been reported as a cause of *Cryptosporidium* outbreaks.[4]

HOST FACTORS

Children, particularly toddlers, are more susceptible to these infestations, owing to their habits of 'mouthing' all sorts of environmental objects, their propensity to go barefoot and their immunologic 'naiveté'. Patients with compromised immune systems, whether due to congenital defects, infections such as human immunodeficiency virus (HIV), or medical ministrations (transplant and oncology patients) may have severe, protracted, or unusual manifestations of parasitic disease. Patients with hypogammaglobulinemia and immunoglobulin A (IgA) deficiency may suffer severe protozoan infections such as *Giardia*sis. Patients with acquired immunodeficiency syndrome (AIDS) infected with *Cryptosporidium* organisms may have severe, prolonged diarrhea as well as unusual manifestations in the biliary tree and lungs, despite high levels of luminal IgA antibody directed against *Cryptosporidium*.[5] Sexual practices, particularly those that involve anal penetration, are also associated with transmission of parasitic diseases.[6,7]

CLINICAL PRESENTATIONS

Enteric parasites most often produce gastrointestinal symptoms-abdominal pain, diarrhea, flatulence and distention.[8] In a children's hospital laboratory survey of stool ova and parasite tests, it was found that stools sent from the gastroenterology clinic were most likely to be positive, as compared with stools submitted from other outpatient clinics, the emergency room, or inpatient settings.[9] Heavy infestations of large worms such as *Ascaris* can lead to intestinal obstruction or, if they migrate into the biliary system, biliary obstruction with cholangitis or pancreatitis. *Amoeba* and *Trichuris* organisms can cause enterocolitis with tenesmus and mucoid, bloody stool.

Liver disease from enteric parasites can be due to bile duct obstruction by organisms such as *Ascaris* worms or liver flukes or from portal hypertension due to inflammatory reactions to ova, as in schistosomiasis. Some protozoans such as *Cryptosporidium* can infect biliary epithelium and produce syndromes such as cholangitis and cholecystitis. Other protozoans such as *E. histolytica* can cause hepatic parenchymal necrosis resulting in liver abscesses.

Systemic manifestations of parasitic infestation are also common. Intestinal luminal blood and protein loss can lead to anemia and edema. Fever is often the most prominent feature of amebic liver abscess. Malabsorption is common in *Giardiasis* and cryptosporidiosis and can lead to wasting, fat soluble-vitamin deficiency and failure to thrive.

DIAGNOSIS

Stool examination

The mainstay of diagnosing enteric parasites is a skilled microscopist in the parasitology laboratory. At least 35 species of enteric parasites may be identified by stool examination.[10] Furthermore, the observation of fecal leukocytes, eosinophils and macrophages in preserved specimens may provide clues to nonparasitic gastrointestinal diseases. Because microscopists' skills vary, clinicians are advised to select reference laboratories with care. Careful attention to the appropriate collection, preservation and examination of samples is critical to successful diagnosis of enteric parasites.

Appropriate sample collection begins with ascertaining that no interfering substances are present in the stool that will invalidate the results. Common interfering substances include barium (from contrast radiography), bismuth preparations, antacids and mineral oil. Antibiotics can also make detection of protozoans difficult. It is preferable to wait 2 weeks after the ingestion of any of these substances before obtaining a specimen. Clinicians evaluating gastrointestinal symptoms should obtain stool specimens before initiating gastrointestinal radiology studies and certain forms of empiric therapy. Water and urine contamination of stool lead to rapid lysis of trophozoites and should be avoided.

Although examination of a fresh stool specimen is useful for identification of motile trophozoites, it is rarely performed in laboratories in the USA. Most stools are collected in preservatives, which allows for convenience in both collection and examination. The commonly used preservatives, such as formalin and polyvinyl alcohol, are quite toxic if ingested.

The appropriate number and frequency of stool examinations are matters of some controversy. It is clear that repeated samples obtained on separate days enhance sensitivity by at least 20%, owing to variable shedding of eggs, cysts and trophozoites.[11] For patients with very low clinical-epidemiologic risk factors, one sample may be adequate, but for those with a high index of suspicion, more than three samples may be needed, particularly for *E. histolytica* and *Dientamoeba fragilis*.

Some enteric parasites, most notably *Cryptosporidium* and *Cyclospora* species, are not detected on routine ova and parasite examinations. These organisms require either acid-fast staining or special immunofluorescence techniques.

Immunoassay

Enzyme-linked immunoassay (ELISA) tests for antigen in stool samples are widely available for *Giardia* and *Cryptosporidium* species. These sensitive and specific assays can be useful adjuncts to standard stool examinations. Because several common organisms can cause the clinical picture of *Giardia*sis, ELISA is not recommended as the sole means of evaluating patients, except in the context of a known outbreak.

Macroscopic examination

Ascaris lumbricoides worms can be passed intact in the stool or vomited, particularly during febrile illness. They are easily recognized because of their size (15–40 cm) and resemblance to earthworms. Cestodes, or more commonly, segments of cestodes, can also be passed per rectum. Species identification is possible by microscopic examination. *Enterobius* organisms venture nocturnally onto the perianal area to lay eggs. The small thread-like worms may be visualized or the 'Scotch tape' test may be employed to identify the eggs of this common parasite.

Serology

Serologic detection of antibodies to *E. histolytica* is possible in 85% of patients with dysentery and 95% of infected patients who have liver abscesses in non endemic areas. Specific IgM serology for *Giardia* and *Strongyloides* may be useful in obscure cases.

Eosinophilia

Eosinophils are granulocytes with cytoplasm that stains strongly with acid dyes such as eosin. They normally make up less than 5% of circulating granulocytes, or an absolute count of less than 500/mm^3. Elevation of eosinophils in the peripheral blood is associated with allergy, connective tissue disease, infections and malignancy.[12] Only invasive parasitic infections are associated with a peripheral eosinophilia and the degree of elevation is proportional to the degree of invasion.[13] Protozoal infections rarely cause eosinophilia. Circulating eosinophils are a marker of much higher tissue aggregations of eosinophils, usually in the skin and epithelial tissues. Eosinophil production is stimulated by cytokines released by Th2 cells. The Th2 immune response is triggered by allergens and helminths and differs from the Th1 response involved in bacterial and viral infections. Eosinophilia is not a sensitive screening tool for parasitic infection. However, if eosinophilia is present, infection with *Ascaris*, hookworm, visceral or cutaneous larva migrans, *Strongyloides*, *Trichinella*, *Trichuris* or tapeworm must be considered.

Intestinal fluid and biopsy

Duodenal fluid may be useful in diagnosis of *Giardiasis* or strongyloidiasis when stool specimens are negative. Fluid may be obtained by duodenal intubation or during endoscopy. It should be examined immediately. The Entero-Test is a gelatin capsule that contains a string that adsorbs duodenal fluid. It is swallowed and then retrieved by a string taped to the patient's cheek. This technique may be difficult to perform in young children.

In selected patients, duodenal biopsy may reveal *Giardia, Cryptosporidium*, Microsporidia, or *Strongyloides* organisms. Biopsy of the edges of colon ulcers may reveal trophozoites of *E. histolytica*. The sensitivity of intestinal biopsy for diagnosis of parasitic disease depends to a large degree on the interest and experience of the pathologist.

BENEFITS OF PARASITES

Interest is growing in a hypothesized link between lack of exposure to helminth infection and the development of allergy. Several studies have shown that children with chronic parasitic infections have reduced skin reactivity to common environmental allergens such as the house dust mite, as compared to non-infected children with otherwise similar exposures.[14] There seems to be benefit both from current parasite infection and from repetitive infection in infancy.[15] Inflammation triggers CD4+ T cell production of either a Th1 or Th2 predominant response. Th1 cytokines stimulated by bacterial and viral infections are the cytokines which mediate a normal inflammatory response. Th2 cytokines are stimulated by parasites and allergens and cause an allergic response, but in the case of parasitic infections the response is modified and IgE degranulation is inhibited. Recurrent exposure to parasites in infancy is thought to downregulate the Th2 response and lessen the likelihood of induction of allergy. Current parasite infection also downregulates the inflammatory response, possibly to allow the parasite to mature and reproduce. The role of the anti-inflammatory cytokines such as interleukin 10 (IL-10) are important as repetitive parasitic and other infections upregulate IL-10 and ensure a normal termination of inflammation.[16]

As with allergy, the incidence of inflammatory bowel disease is said to be inversely related to the prevalence of parasitic infection. Immune tolerance and autoimmunity, mediated by Th3/Tr1 cells also depends on the balance of anti-inflammatory cytokines IL-10 and transforming growth factor beta (TGF-beta) with pro-inflammatory cytokines from the Th1 pathway. Parasitic infections downregulate Th1 responses which are implicated in the mucosal inflammation seen in inflammatory bowel disease.[17] After promising experiments on mice, humans with inflammatory bowel disease have been dosed with *Trichuris suis* (pig whipworm). The results suggest efficacy, but repeated dosing is needed to sustain remission.[18]

PATHOGENIC ORGANISMS

Protozoa

Giardia lamblia

Giardiasis is the most common pathogenic intestinal protozoan infection in the world. It has been estimated that some 2–5% of the population of the industrialized world and 20% of those in the developing world are infected at any time.[19–23] The majority of these infections are asymptomatic. Prevalence of infection increases through infancy and early childhood, not decreasing until early adolescence. A major pediatric health concern is that this protozoan may be contributing to failure of growth and cognitive development in the developing world.[24] However *Giardia* was only recognized as a major pathogen in the 1970s and was listed as a parasitic pathogen by the World Health Organization in 1981.[25] *Giardia* was also the first described human protozoan agent of intestinal disease. Von Leeuwenhoek observed them in 1681 in his own diarrheal stool and described them as 'animalcules'. *Giardia* is an ancient organism and was recently demonstrated in the stools of prehistoric Peruvian human populations.[26] It is a primitive eukaryocyte and relies on anaerobic metabolism as it lacks mitochondria. They share many properties with bacteria and hence are susceptible to antibiotics. *Giardia* are also of interest because of their relationship to archeobacteria by comparison of ribosomal RNA sequence.[27] This relationship suggests that organisms such as *Giardia* may have been among the first eukaryotic life forms. The *Giardia* Genome Project has successfully sequenced 90% the genetic material of *Giardia* and is a valuable resource for further study of this organism (*www.mbl.edu/Giardia*).[28]

G. lamblia exists in two forms: the encysted, environmentally stable form that is responsible for transmission and the small intestine-dwelling trophozoite, which is the motile form observed by von Leeuwenhoek. The process of excystation is thought to be pH dependent and follows the transition of the cyst from acid stomach to alkaline duodenum causing the characteristic heavy infestation in the proximal small bowel.[29] In the small intestine, the trophozoites adhere to enterocytes by a ventral disc, causing local effacement of the microvilli. *Giardia* is a water-borne pathogen that can be transmitted via the feco-oral route. The study of *Giardia* species has been hampered by multiple naming systems. The *Giardia* pathogenic to mammals is known as *Giardia lamblia* and also as *G. intestinalis* and *G. duodenalis*.[30] Several different assemblage types identified within *G. lamblia* have relevance for host specificity, but evidence is lacking for effect on clinical disease severity.[31] A variety of domestic mammals including dogs and cats, wild mammals such as beavers, raccoons and rodents and domestic livestock such as cattle and sheep can harbor the organism.[32–35] The role of animals in the transmission of *Giardia* to humans remains controversial, partly because of emerging data about the relevance of assemblage types within the *G. lamblia* species which may determine host specificity.[36]

The pathophysiology of *Giardiasis* is unclear. Pathologic changes in the small intestine are quite variable. Although most symptomatic patients have normal or nearly normal villi,[37] 5–10% or more have subtotal villus atrophy. Patients with immunoglobulin deficiency are particularly prone to histological abnormality, but AIDS patients do not seem to be at increased risk of severe or persistent *Giardiasis*.[25] There are no reported cases of *Giardiasis* associated with commonly used immunosuppressive agents such as steroids or ciclosporin. Secretory IgA is thought to have an important role in host defenses to *Giardia*, but the deficiency must be severe to be clinically relevant.[38,39] Invasive disease may rarely occur with spread to the gallbladder and urinary system. Most symptomatic patients have lactose intolerance, both clinically and as measured by the hydrogen breath test.

Symptoms of *Giardiasis* can include diarrhea, flatulence, malabsorption with weight loss, constipation and abdominal pain. The 2–3 week incubation period may be followed by a phase of acute illness, but more than half of infected children will be asymptomatic. Symptoms can be intermittent or continuous. Stools may be watery, malabsorptive, or formed, but are not bloody and do not contain leukocytes. Urticaria may occur and may be prolonged.[40]

Laboratory findings are generally nonspecific. Fat may be found in the stool. Rarely, serum albumin is decreased and fecal alpha$_1$-antitrypsin is increased. Eosinophilia does not occur. Radiological findings are generally nonspecific. *Giardiasis* localized to the terminal ileum may radiologically mimic Crohn's disease.[41] Ophthalmoscopy may demonstrate salt and pepper retinal degeneration in preschool children, but progressive retinal disease does not occur.[42]

Diagnosis is based on demonstration of *Giardia* trophozoites, cysts, or antigen in stool, duodenal fluid, or intestinal biopsy specimens (Fig. 37.1). Microscopic examination of a single stool specimen is approximately 70% sensitive for detection. Sensitivity increases to approximately 85% with three samples. Examination of duodenal fluid has been reported to be 40–90% sensitive. Antigen detection assays by direct fluorescence antibody (DFA) or enzyme immunoassays (EIA) on stool offer 89–100% sensitivity and 99.3–100% specificity on a single specimen, but do not identify other protozoans that can cause similar symptoms.[43–45]

Treatment options for *Giardiasis* include metronidazole (and its derivatives), quinacrine and furazolidone (Table 37.1). Immunocompromised patients may require prolonged therapy to clear the organism. Some apparent clinical treatment failures are due to lactose intolerance, which can persist for weeks after successful treatment. There is no clear role for the use of probiotics in the treatment or prevention of *Giardia* infection.[46]

Prevention of infection is a major public health concern. An inoculum of only 10–100 cysts can cause infection in humans. *Giardia* is more resistant than bacteria and the cyst can survive 3 months in water at 4°C. Water-borne infections account for 60% of cases in the USA.[47] Standard iodine water purification tablets will not reliably kill *Giardia* in infected water and it is relatively resistant to chlorination and ozonolysis.[31,48] Swimming pools and even tap water are common sources of infection. Filtration of water and ultraviolet light treatment are most effective at eradicating *Giardia* from the water supply.[49] Food-borne infection outbreaks are usually secondary to infected or excreting food handlers, but viable *Giardia* have been found on fruits and vegetables such as lettuce and strawberries.[47] Outbreaks in daycare centers are also common. Thorough handwashing is essential to disease prevention. Antigenic variation in the *Giardia* surface antigens has slowed development of a vaccine for humans, but a veterinary vaccine for cats and dogs is commercially available.[50] Breast-feeding is protective for preventing infection and symptomatic infection.[51]

Entamoeba histolytica

Although a variety of species of amoebae inhabit the human intestine only *E. histolytica* is clearly pathogenic.

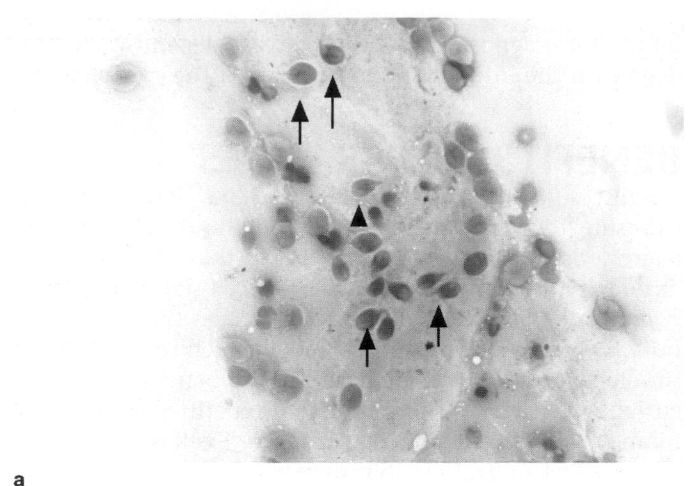

a

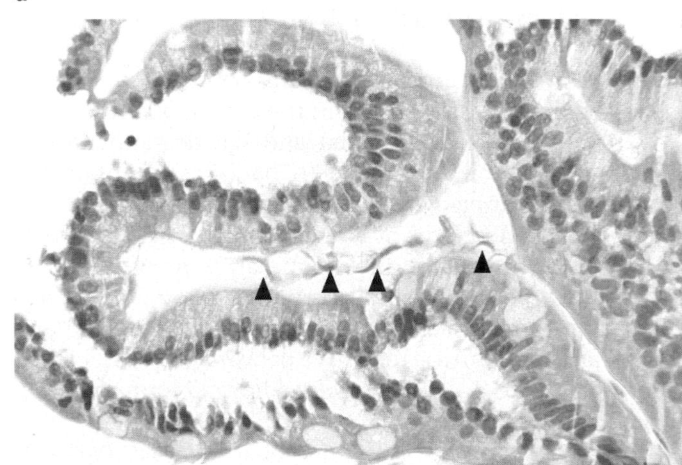

b

Figure 37.1: Trophozoites (arrows) of *Giardia lamblia* from small bowel biopsy. (**a**) Giemsa stain of touch prep. (**b**) Routine section (H&E). (Courtesy of Drs Gerald Berry and Terry Longacre). (See plate section for color)

Although identical on light microscopy, newer biochemical, immunologic and DNA analyses exist that distinguish between pathogenic and non-pathogenic strains.[56–59] Nonpathogenic strains are now named *Entamoeba dispar*.[60,61] In addition, only certain strains of *E. histolytica* are capable of invading the mucosa and causing disease. Even within an endemic area there are genetically distinct strains of *E. histolytica* that cause intestinal *vs* hepatic disease.[62] Virulence factors are related to a number of proteins produced by the parasite including a lectin that mediates adherence to epithelial cells, a peptide that lyses cells by creating a pore and matrix digesting proteases.[63] Indeed, the name *histolytica* refers to the amoeba's ability to breakdown extracellular matrix proteins and cause necrosis of host cells.[64]

The life cycle of these unicellular eukaryocytes is quite similar to that of *Giardia*. Ingested cysts are stimulated by gastric acid to excystate in the small intestine. The resulting trophozoites colonize the large intestine, where they multiply in the mucin layer. The trophozoites then either invade the mucosa, or encystate, depending on local

Disease	Drug	Dosage	Comments
Amebiasis (*E. histolytica*)			
Asymptomatic and luminal clearance	Iodoquinol or	30–40 mg/kg per day in 3 doses × 20 days (max. 2 g/day)	Currently suggested that asymptomatic cyst passers in non-endemic areas be treated
	Paromomycin or	25–35 mg/kg per day in 3 doses × 7 days (max. 1.5 g/day)	
	Diloxanide furoate or	20 mg/kg per day in 3 doses × 10 days (max. 1.5 g/day)	Not commercially available in USA
Colitis, liver abscess	Metronidazole or	35–50 mg/kg per day in 3 doses × 7–10 days (max. 2.25 g/day)	Metronidazole absorbed very well orally. Follow with luminal clearance
	Nitazoxanide	500 mg b.i.d. × 3 days (adult dose)	
Liver abscess	Tinidazole or	50 mg/kg per day in 3 doses × 5 days (max. 2 g/day)	May be less effective but better tolerated. Follow with luminal clearance as above
	Ornidazole	25 mg/kg per day × 5–10 days	Alternates include dehydroemetine or combination therapy with chloroquine phosphate
Ancylostoma caninum (dog hookworm, eosinophilic enterocolitis)	Albendazole or	400 mg once (10 mg/kg once, may repeat in 3 weeks)	Serologic/clinical diagnosis; no ova or parasites are found in stool
	Pyrantel pamoate or	11 mg/kg per day × 3 days (max. 1 g/day)	
	Mebendazole or Endoscopic removal	100 mg b.i.d. × 3 days	
Anisakiasis (fish worm)	Surgical or endoscopic removal		
Ascariasis	Albendazole or	400 mg once	For symptoms of obstruction use nasogastric infusion of piperazine citrate 75 mg/kg per day (max. 3.5 g).
	Mebendazole or	100 mg b.i.d. × 3 days or 500 mg once	
	Pyrantel pamoate or	11 mg/kg once (max. 1 g)	
	Ivermectin	150–200 μg/kg once	
Balantidium coli	Tetracycline or	40 mg/kg per day in 4 doses × 10 days (max. 2 g/day)	Contraindicated in pregnant women and children less than 8 years old. Paromomycin is alternate for pregnant women.
	Iodoquinol or	40 mg/kg per day in 3 doses × 20 days (max. 2 g/day)	
	Metronidazole	35–50 mg/kg per day in 3 doses × 5 days (max. 2.25 g/day)	
Blastocystis hominis	Metronidazole or	35–50 mg/kg per day in 3 doses × 5–10 days (max. 2.25 g/day)	Clinical importance of infection is debatable.
	Iodoquinol	40 mg/kg per day in 3 doses × 20 days (max. 2 g/day)	Alternate trimethoprim-sulfamethoxazole and nitazoxanide.
Capillaria philippinensis	Mebendazole or	200 mg b.i.d. × 20 days	Non-compliance with prolonged course leads to frequent relapse
	Albendazole or	400 mg daily × 10 days	
	Thiabendazole	25 mg/kg per day in 2 doses × 30 days	
Cryptosporidiosis	Nitazoxanide or	200 mg b.i.d. × 3 days (children 4–11 years old) 100 mg b.i.d. × 3 days (children 1–3 years old)	Consider oral human immune globulin or bovine colostrum in immunocompromised patients. Improved immune function is best prognosis.[52]
	Azithromycin dihydrate alone or with Paromomycin (minimally effective)	25 mg/kg per day b.i.d. × 14 days 30 mg/kg per day in 3 doses (max. 4 g/day)	
Cyclospora	Trimethoprim-sulfamethoxazole (TMP-SMZ)	TMP 5 mg/kg per day, SMZ 25 mg/kg per day b.i.d. × 7–10 days (max. 1 DS tablet b.i.d.)	HIV infected patients may need higher dose and longer treatment. Ciprofloxacin is an alternate for sulfa allergic patients.
Dientamoeba fragilis	Iodoquinol or	30–40 mg/kg per day in 3 doses × 20 days (max. 2 g/day)	Contraindicated in pregnant women and children less than 8 years old.
	Tetracycline or	40 mg/kg per day in 4 doses × 10 days (max. 2 g/day)	

Table 37.1 Treatment of enteric parasites

(*Continued*)

Disease	Drug	Dosage	Comments
	Metronidazole or	20–40 mg/kg per day in 3 doses × 10 days (max. 2.25 g/day)	
	Paromomycin	25–35 mg/kg per day in 3 doses × 7 days	
Enterobius vermicularis (pinworm)	Pyrantel pamoate or	11 mg/kg (max. 1 g) once; repeat in 2 weeks	Treatment of household contacts is often advised
	Mebendazole or	100 mg once; repeat in 2 weeks	
	Albendazole	400 mg × once; repeat in 2 weeks	
Giardiasis	Metronidazole or	15 mg/kg per day in 3 doses × 5 days (max. 750 mg/day)	Other alternates include bacitracin.
	Tinidazole or Ornidazole or Nitroimidazole	50 mg/kg once (max. 2 g)	
	Furazolidone or	6 mg/kg per day in 4 doses × 7–10 days (max. 400 mg/day)	For resistant *Giardia*[52]
	Albendazole or	400 mg once × 5 days	
	Nitazoxanide or	200 mg b.i.d. × 3 days children 4–11 years old, 100 mg b.i.d. × 3 days children 1–3 years old	With metronidazole for resistant strains.[53]
	Paromomycin or	25–35 mg/kg per day in 3 doses × 7 days (max. 1.5 g/day)	Least efficacious, but recommended for pregnant women.
	Quinacrine or	2 mg/kg t.i.d. × 5 days (max. 300 mg/day)	Colors skin yellow.
Hookworm	Albendazole or	400 mg once	
(*Ancylostoma duodenale,*	Pyrantel pamoate or	11 mg/kg per day × 3 days (max. 1 g)	
Necator americanus)	Mebendazole	100 mg b.i.d. × 3 days or 500 mg once	
Isospora belli	TMP-SMZ	TMP 5 mg/kg per day, SMZ 25 mg/kg per day b.i.d. × 10 days (max. 1 DS tab b.i.d.)	Pyrimethamine and ciprofloxacin are alternates for sulfa allergic patients.
Microsporidiosis (Intestinal)	Fumagillin or	60 mg/d × 14 days (adult dose)	*S. Intestinalis responds* much better to treatment.
(*Enterocytozoon bieneusi, Septata intestinalis*)	Albendazole	400 mg b.i.d. × 21 days(adult dose)	Alternatives include metronidazole, atovaquone, and nitazoxanide.
Schistosomiasis			
S. japonicum	Praziquantel	60 mg/kg in 3 doses × 1 day	Treatment does not reverse established portal hypertension.
S. mansoni	Praziquantel or	40 mg/kg in 2 doses × 1 day	
	Oxamniquine	20 mg/kg in 2 doses × 1 day	Contraindicated in pregnancy.
S. haematobium	Praziquantel	40 mg/kg in 2 doses × 1 day	
S. mekongi	Praziquantel	60 mg/kg in 3 doses × 1 day	
Strongyloidiasis (*Stongaloides stercoralis*)	Ivermectin or	200 µg/kg per day × 2 days	Discontinuing large doses of steroids is important in fulminant, disseminated disease.
	Thiabendazole or	50 mg/kg per day in 2 doses × 2 days (max. 3 g/day)	
	Albendazole	400 mg b.i.d. × 7 days	
Tapeworm (adult worm)	Praziquantel or	5–10 mg/kg once	
(*D. latum, T. solium, T. saginata, D. canium*)	Niclosamide	50 mg/kg once	
Tapeworm		25 mg/kg once	
(*Hymenolepis nana*)	Praziquantel or Nitazoxanide	200 mg b.i.d. × 3 days (children 4–11 years old), 100 mg b.i.d. × 3 days (children 1–3 years old)	
Trichuris trichiura	Mebendazole or	100 mg b.i.d. × 3 days or 500 mg once	
(whipworm)	Albendazole or	400 mg × 3 days	
	Ivermectin	200 µg/kg per day × 3 days	

Table 37.1 Treatment of enteric parasites

conditions and the nature of the particular strain. The interaction of the genetic capabilities of the strain and host factors such as the bacterial flora of the gut determine virulence.[65] Invading trophozoites destroy epithelial target cells by releasing substances such as hemolysins, which disrupt cell membranes by creating an amoebapore. A variety of excreted cysteine proteases disrupt the extra cellular matrix. Injury to epithelial cells triggers release of cytokines leading to chemotaxis of leukocytes, which also contribute to the local inflammatory response. Eventually, ulceration of the mucosa occurs and invading amoebae may enter the portal circulation and eventually the liver. *In vitro*, the trophozoites have a powerful ability to kill T lymphocytes, neutrophils and macrophages. Virulence may also be related to the trophozoites ability to cause apoptosis in these inflammatory cells and then phagocytose them, thus limiting further inflammatory response.[63] Unlike intestinal lesions, hepatic abscesses contain few inflammatory cells, consisting almost entirely of necrotic liver cells. In patients treated with large doses of steroids, amoebae may spread to a variety of organs, including lungs, brain and eyes. For reasons unknown, such systemic dissemination is not common in AIDS patients, who are often infected with *Entamoeba* species.[66]

The WHO estimates there are 100 000 deaths per year due to *E. histolytica*, second only to malaria for parasitic related death.[61] Risk factors for amoebiasis include poverty, crowding, poor hygiene, travel in endemic areas and male homosexual promiscuity. Risk factors for severe disease include young age (particularly infants), malnutrition and corticosteroid use. Although physicians in the USA think of amebic disease as exotic, prevalence of infection here has been estimated as high as 5% among the general population and 30% among homosexual men. However, most prevalence data predates the ability to distinguish *histolytica* from *dispar*.[7,67] Even in patients with symptomatic AIDS, *E. dispar* is not pathogenic. *E. histolytica* accounts for about 10% of diarrheal illnesses in children in endemic areas.[68] Asymptomatic infections commonly last more than a year and latency periods as long as several years are possible.[69] Clinicians need to take a detailed and distant travel history and maintain a high index of suspicion for late development of liver abscesses.

Symptoms of intestinal amoebiasis vary with the location and extent of the infection. *E. histolytica* may invade any portion of the colon, though the cecum and ascending colon are most commonly affected. Patients often complain of abdominal pain, anorexia, malaise and intermittent diarrhea. Patients with rectosigmoid involvement suffer from tenesmus and more frequent diarrhea. Patients with extensive involvement have symptoms similar to those of ulcerative colitis, with frequent mucous, bloody stools. In non-fulminant cases, fever is uncommon, but with fulminant colitis or hepatic abscess, fever can be prominent. Toxic megacolon or perforation can occur and are leading causes of mortality in untreated patients. In some cases, a localized granulomatous reaction to *E. histolytica* known as an *ameboma* occurs. Amebomas are difficult to distinguish from colon carcinoma. Amebic dysentery may mimic inflammatory bowel disease leading to institution of high-dose steroid therapy, which can be lethal in persons with amoebiasis. Painful cutaneous ulcers may complicate colitis. Salpingitis and lymphadenitis due to *E. histolytica* have also been reported.[70,71] Cases of post-infectious glomerulonephritis have been reported following amebic liver abscess.[72]

Amebic liver abscess is manifested by right upper quadrant pain, leukocytosis, fever and hepatomegaly. Liver abscess usually occurs in the absence of current or recent overt intestinal disease. Liver function tests, including bilirubin and transaminases, are often normal. Ultrasonography shows one or more cystic masses in the hepatic parenchyma. Complications of abscesses include rupture, with possible pericardial or pleural spread.

Diagnosis of colonic amebiasis is best made by microscopic examination of fresh stool. Three to six samples should be adequate to identify 90% of cases. Biopsies taken from the edge of colon ulcers may also be useful in identifying trophozoites, particularly with periodic acid-Schiff (PAS) stain (Fig. 37.2). Stool enzyme immunoassay (EIA) panels are available to detect *E. histolytica/E. dispar* with 96% sensitivity and 99% specificity[73,74] ELISA (enzyme-linked immunosorbent assay) tests are available to distinguish *histolytica* from *dispar*. Polymerase chain reaction (PCR) tests are slightly more reliable, although costly, time consuming and not yet commercially available.[75] PCR and ELISA cannot be performed on fixed stool, the stool must be fresh or frozen.[76]

Serologic testing is particularly useful for suspected amebic liver abscess. Most patients have neither overt intestinal symptoms nor detectable cysts or trophozoites in their stool. Unfortunately, standard serology is difficult to interpret in endemic areas. Newer serum antigen tests are being developed that can distinguish *E. histolytica* from *dispar* and become negative with successful treatment. The antigen test can also be performed on material aspirated from a liver abscess.[77] In non-endemic areas, suspected liver abscesses may require aspiration to exclude bacterial causes.

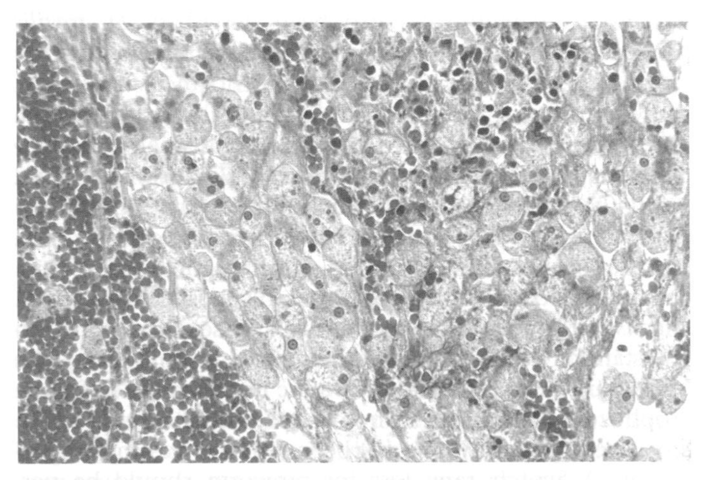

Figure 37.2: *Entamoeba histolytica* trophozoites in a colonic biopsy. (Courtesy of Drs Gerald Berry and Terry Longacre.) (*See plate section for color*).

tries where asymptomatic carriage may be relatively common among local children and may increase in the rainy season.[147] There is no clear animal host. Infection is water-borne and not person to person because oocysts excreted in stool are not immediately infectious. Several large food-borne outbreaks have been documented. For example in the USA, a multistate outbreak due to *C. cayetanensis* was traced to raspberries imported from Guatemala.[148] Treatment is trimethoprim-sulfamethoxazole; ciprofloxacin is a less effective alternate for sulfa allergic patients.[149] Prophylaxis against relapses may be needed for immunocompromised patients.

Isospora belli is a cause of traveler's diarrhea in normal hosts and of protracted diarrhea in immunocompromised hosts.[150] Although infection is much more common in the tropics, daycare outbreaks have been reported in the USA. Unlike *Cryptosporidia*, scant numbers of the large 30 μm oocysts are excreted in the stool, making diagnosis difficult. However, excreted oocyst may by infectious and person-to-person transmission is possible.[145] Small intestine biopsy may be helpful in establishing the diagnosis. Accurate diagnosis is important because the organism is sensitive to trimethoprim-sulfamethoxazole. As with *Cylospora*, ciprofloxacin is a less effective alternate. Maintenance therapy to prevent relapses may be necessary for immunocompromised patients.

Microsporidia is a unique group of unicellular protozoa of the microspora phylum with 1000 separate species.[145] Human pathogens include *Enterocytozoon bieneusi, Septata (Encephalitozoon) intestinalis, Trachipleistophora hominis and Vittaforma corneae*. They are all intracellular parasites that have been reported principally in patients with AIDS and more recently in recipients of solid organ transplants.[151–154] However, cases in apparently normal patients have been described. Animal reservoirs such as pigs, domestic pets and rodents exist and zoonotic infection is possible, but water-borne or sexual spread is probably the more common mode of infection.[155,156] The illness is similar to that found with *Cryptosporidium* infection: prolonged watery diarrhea with weight loss. Microsporidia can also cause cholangiopathy, keratoconjunctivitis and respiratory tract infections in patients with AIDS.[127,157–160] Although special techniques for visualizing spores are reported, diagnosis often requires intestinal biopsy, preferably jejunal.[161] Experienced, or reference laboratories should be used when possible.[162] The more common *E. bieneusi* is difficult to recognize in standard paraffin hematoxylin and eosin sections and may require embedding in plastic resin, special stains, or electron microscopy. *S. intestinalis* is larger and more easily seen on routine sections. Albendazole has been reported helpful for these infections, particularly for *S. intestinalis*, with fumagillin and nitazoxanide as alternatives.[163,164] The combination of albendazole and furazolidone has been proposed for *E. bieneusi* infections in AIDS patients.[165] The organisms are very resistant to environmental conditions and immunocompromised patients may reduce risk of infection by avoidance of swimming, drinking unfiltered tap water and contact with pets such as rabbits, birds and dogs.[166]

Nematodes (roundworms)

Ascaris lumbricoides

A. lumbricoides is the largest and most common helminthic infection worldwide.[167] Adult worms live in the jejunum, where the 20–49 cm long females may produce 200 000 eggs per day. The fertilized eggs are excreted in the feces and must mature in the soil for 10–14 days before the first-stage larvae, which are infectious, develop. When such embryonated eggs are ingested and reach the intestine, second-stage larvae develop that penetrate the intestinal mucosa to migrate via the liver to the lungs. The tiny larvae then pass through the alveolar wall, to the respiratory tract and back to the gut after being swallowed. Then mature worms develop that may live 12–18 months. The respiratory phase may induce an eosinophilic pneumonitis, Loeffler's syndrome, which may clinically resemble seasonal asthma.

Under normal circumstances, the intestinal phase of infection is asymptomatic. Serious complications arise either during heavy infestations, which may produce intestinal obstruction, or during migration of worms, which is frequently precipitated by an unrelated febrile illness. Infected patients may vomit or cough up the large earthworm-like ascarids during such illnesses. Alternatively, the worms can obstruct the biliary or pancreatic ducts, producing cholangitis or pancreatitis.[168–170] Ascaris obstruction of the bowel lumen may lead to volvulus or perforation.[171]

The role of *Ascaris* worms in chronic malnutrition of children in the tropics is unclear. Heavy infestation is probably one of many factors affecting such children. Some studies have shown improvement in nutritional status after ascaris eradication.[172]

Diagnosis of ascariasis can be made by finding the eggs in stools. Adult worms may be expelled from the mouth or anus, observed during endoscopy, or outlined by barium during radiologic studies. Eosinophilia is prominent only during larval migrations through tissues.

Treatments include pyrantel pamoate, which paralyzes *Ascaris worms* and can be given by nasogastric tube for cases of intestinal obstruction. Mebendazole and albendazole are also effective in uncomplicated cases. Endoscopic or surgical therapy is necessary for some complications although most cases of biliary ascariasis and intestinal obstruction respond to conservative medical management. Mass treatment programs are useful in communities with high prevalences of infection.

Trichuris trichiura

T. trichiura (whipworm) is named for the morphology of adult worms. *Trichuris* worms differ from other human nematodes in two ways. First, there is no tissue migration during its life cycle. Second, adult *Trichuris* worms reside in the colon rather than the small intestine (Fig. 37.4). Like *Ascaris* eggs, those of *Trichuris* must mature in the soil before being ingested, making direct person-to-person transmission impossible. The larvae hatch and mature in the distal small bowel before migrating to the cecum,

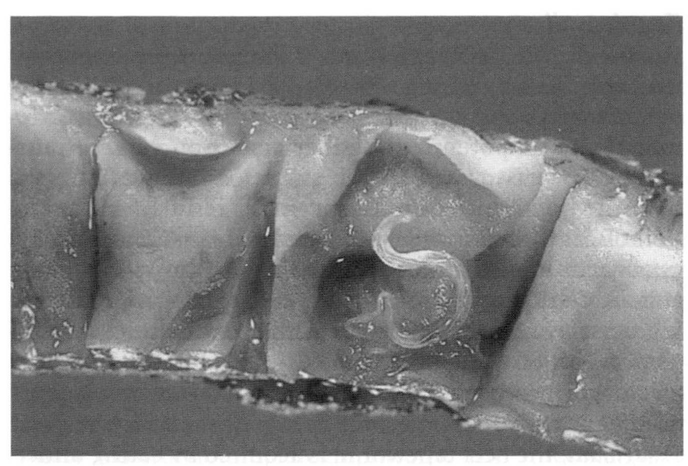

Figure 37.4: *Trichuris trichiura* in a resected colon. (Courtesy of Drs Gerald Berry and Terry Longacre.) (*See plate section for color*).

where they attach to the bowel wall via their narrow anterior ('whip') end. They may reside in the colon for as long as 8 years.

Trichuris has a worldwide distribution similar to that of *Ascaris*. The infection is most common in the tropics, especially Asia, but an estimated 2 million people are infected in the USA. Toddlers and young children tend to have the heaviest worm burdens.

Most light infections are asymptomatic. Moderate infections produce a picture of chronic colitis with diarrhea, abdominal pain and weight loss.[173] Heavy infections can produce a dysentery-like picture that may feature rectal prolapse.[174] Chronic infections in children are associated with stunted growth, anemia and delayed cognitive development.[175]

Necator americanus and *Ancylostoma duodenale* (hookworms)

Hookworm infestation affects approximately 1 billion people.[174,176] There are two species of human hookworms, *N. americanus* and *A. duodenale*. Transmission of hookworm requires contamination of soil with human fecal material and an unshod population (usually young children). Filiform infective larvae in the contaminated soil invade the host via the skin (usually the bare foot) and are carried by the circulation to the lungs, where they penetrate the alveoli. They then proceed up the airway until they are swallowed into the gut. Hookworms reside in the small intestine, where they attach to the mucosa with their specialized mouthparts. Each worm is capable of ingesting up to 250 μl of blood per day. Symptoms of hookworm are the sequelae of this blood loss – mainly anemia and hypoproteinemia.[177] Patients may also report intense pruritic rashes on the feet during the initial larval penetration. Some patients with heavy worm burdens also report epigastric distress. Diagnosis of significant hookworm infection is made by finding the characteristic ova in fresh or preserved stool specimens. Treatment of choice is mebendazole or albendazole (Table 37.1).

Strongyloides stercoralis

Strongyloides is a small (1–10 mm long) nematode that is capable of replicating completely within the host.[178] Because of this capability, patients with suppressed immune systems can acquire an enormous worm burden, with potentially fatal dissemination. Infection begins when filiform larvae in contaminated soil penetrate the skin. The larvae then migrate via blood or lymph to the lungs, where they penetrate the alveoli and proceed up the airway to the pharynx and are swallowed. The larvae mature in the proximal small intestine and females burrow into the lamina propria to lay eggs (Fig. 37.5). The eggs hatch locally and the resulting rhabditiform larvae migrate into the intestinal lumen. Most of the rhabditiform larvae are passed with stool into the environment, where they mature into infectious filiform larvae. A variable number are able to differentiate into filiform larvae in the host colon. These infectious progeny are capable of re-infecting the host and maintaining a state of chronic infection.

In most hosts an equilibrium state seems to be reached in which a small number of adult worms are maintained. In severely malnourished or steroid-treated hosts the equilibrium becomes impaired and huge worm burdens can develop. In such circumstances larvae may disseminate to all organs, carrying with them associated enteric bacteria. This syndrome, known as *disseminated strongyloidiasis*, is usually fatal.[179] *Strongyloides* organisms are present in virtually all tropical and subtropical regions. They are also found in the southern USA and in small pockets of industrialized nations. Institutionalized patients are often infected.

Whereas most normal patients with chronic low-grade infections are asymptomatic, *Strongyloides* can cause significant gastrointestinal illness. Most common is a syndrome similar to *Giardiasis*, with bloating, heartburn and malabsorptive stools. Intractable diarrhea has been described in infants. Rarely, an ulcerative colitis-like picture may be seen with prominent pseudopolyp formation.[180]

The disseminated strongyloidiasis syndrome most often follows high-dose corticosteroid therapy.[181] Interestingly, the hyperinfection syndrome does not appear to be very

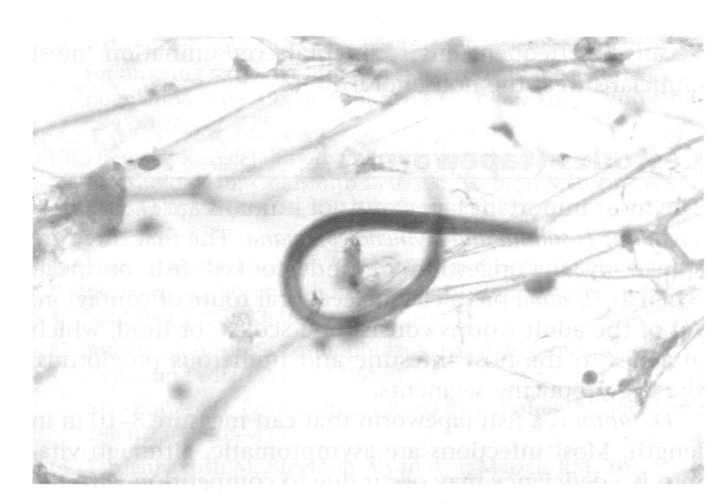

Figure 37.5: *Strongyloides stercoralis* (adult form). (Courtesy of Drs Gerald Berry and Terry Longacre.) (*See plate section for color*).

15. Kim DS, Drake-Lee AB. Infection, allergy and the hygiene hypothesis: historical perspective. J Laryngol Otol 2003; 117(12):946–950.
16. Yazdanbakhsh M, Matricardi PM. Parasites and the hygiene hypothesis: regulating the immune system? Clin Rev Allergy Immunol 2004; 26(1):15–24.
17. Elliott D, Urban JJ, Argo C, Weinstock J. Does the failure to acquire helminthic parasites predispose to Crohn's disease? FASEB J 2000; 14(12):1848–1855.
18. Summers RW, Elliott DE, Qadir K, Urban JF. Jr., Thompson R, Weinstock JV. Trichuris suis seems to be safe and possibly effective in the treatment of inflammatory bowel disease. Am J Gastroenterol 2003; 98(9):2034–2041.
19. Grimmond T, Radford A, Brownridge T, et al. *Giardia* carriage in aboriginal and non-aboriginal children attending urban day-care centers in South Australia. Aust Paediatr J 1988; 24:304–305.
20. Pickering L, Engelkirk P. *Giardia lamblia*. Pediatr Clin North Am 1988; 35:565–577.
21. Mason P, Patterson B. Epidemiology of *Giardia lamblia* infection in children: cross-sectional and longitudinal studies in urban and rural communities in Zimbabwe. Am J Trop Med Hyg 1987; 37:277–282.
22. Woo P, Paterson W. *Giardia lamblia* in children in day-care centres in southern Ontario, Canada and susceptibility of animals to G. *lamblia*. Trans R Soc Trop Med Hyg 1986; 80:56–59.
23. Newman RD, Moore SR, Lima AA, et al. A longitudinal study of *Giardia lamblia* infection in north-east Brazilian children. Trop Med Int HealTh2001; 6(8):624–634.
24. Berkman DS, Lescano AG, Gilman RH, Lopez SL, Black MM. Effects of stunting, diarrhoeal disease and parasitic infection during infancy on cognition in late childhood: a follow-up study. Lancet 2002; 359(9306):564–571.
25. Faubert G. Immune response to *Giardia* duodenalis. Clin Microbiol Rev 2000; 13(1):35–54.
26. Ortega YR, Bonavia D. Cryptosporidium, *Giardia* and Cyclospora in ancient Peruvians. J Parasitol 2003; 89(3):635–636.
27. Kabnick K, Peattie D. *Giardia*: a missing link between prokaryotes and eukaryotes. Am Sci 1991; 79:34–43.
28. McArthur AG, Morrison HG, Nixon JE, et al. The *Giardia* genome project database. FEMS Microbiol Lett 2000; 189(2):271–273.
29. Hetsko ML, McCaffery JM, Svard SG, et al. Cellular and transcriptional changes during excystation of *Giardia lamblia* in vitro. Exp Parasitol 1998; 88(3):172–183.
30. Thompson RC, Hopkins RM, Homan WL. Nomenclature and genetic groupings of *Giardia* infecting mammals. Parasitol Today 2000; 16(5):210–213.
31. Ali SA, Hill DR. *Giardia* intestinalis. Curr Opin Infect Dis 2003; 16(5):453–460.
32. Ruest N, Faubert GM, Couture Y. Prevalence and geographical distribution of *Giardia* spp. and Cryptosporidium spp. in dairy farms in Quebec. Can Vet J 1998; 39(11):697–700.
33. Collins G, Pope S, Griffin D, et al. Diagnosis and prevalence of *Giardia* spp in dogs and cats. Aust Vet J 1987; 64:89–90.
34. Kiorpes A, Kirkpatrick C, Bowman D. Isolation of *Giardia* from a llama and from sheep. Can J Vet Res 1987; 51:277–280.
35. Pacha R, Clark G, Williams E, et al. Small rodents and other mammals associated with mountain meadows as reservoirs of *Giardia* spp. and *Campylobacter* spp. Appl Environ Microbiol 1987; 53:1574–1579.
36. Monis PT, Thompson RC. Cryptosporidium and *Giardia*-zoonoses: fact or fiction? Infect Genet Evol 2003; 3(4):233–244.
37. Oberhuber G, Kastner N. Stolte M. *Giardia*sis: a histologic analysis of 567 cases. Scand J Gastroenterol 1997; 32:48–51.
38. Eckmann L. Mucosal defences against *Giardia*. Parasite Immunol 2003; 25(5):259–270.
39. Langford TD, Housley MP, Boes M, et al. Central importance of immunoglobulin A in host defense against *Giardia* spp. Infect Immun 2002; 70(1):11–18.
40. Blaser MJ, Smith PD, Ravdin JI, Greenberg HB, Guerrant RL (eds). Infections of the Gastrointestinal Tract, 2nd edn. Philadelphia, PA: Lippincott Williams & Wilkins; 2002.
41. Gunasekaran T, Hassall E. *Giardiasis* mimicking inflammatory bowel disease. J Pediatr 1992; 120:424–426.
42. Corsi A, Nucci C, Knafelz D, et al. Ocular changes associated with *Giardia lamblia* infection in children. Br J Ophthalmol 1998; 82(1):59–62.
43. Aldeen WE, Carroll K, Robison A, Morrison M, Hale D. Comparison of nine commercially available enzyme-linked immunosorbent assays for detection of *Giardia lamblia* in fecal specimens. J Clin Microbiol 1998; 36(5):1338–1340.
44. Aziz H, Beck CE, Lux MF, Hudson MJ. A comparison study of different methods used in the detection of *Giardia lamblia*. Clin Lab Sci 2001; 14(3):150–154.
45. Maraha B, Buiting AG. Evaluation of four enzyme immunoassays for the detection of *Giardia lamblia* antigen in stool specimens. Eur J Clin Microbiol Infect Dis 2000; 19(6):485–487.
46. Perez PF, Minnaard J, Rouvet M, et al. Inhibition of *Giardia* intestinalis by extracellular factors from Lactobacilli: an in vitro study. Appl Environ Microbiol 2001; 67(11):5037–5042.
47. Rose JB. Slifko TR. *Giardia*, Cryptosporidium and Cyclospora and their impact on foods: a review. J Food Prot 1999; 62(9):1059–1070.
48. Lane S, Lloyd D. Current trends in research into the water-borne parasite *Giardia*. Crit Rev Microbiol 2002; 28(2):123–147.
49. Linden KG, Shin GA, Faubert G, Cairns W, Sobsey MD. UV disinfection of *Giardia lamblia* cysts in water. Environ Sci Technol 2002; 36(11):2519–2522.
50. Olson ME, Ceri H, Morck DW. *Giardia* vaccination. Parasitol Today 2000; 16(5):213–217.
51. Mahmud MA, Chappell CL, Hossain MM, et al. Impact of breast-feeding on *Giardia lamblia* infections in Bilbeis, Egypt. Am J Trop Med Hyg 2001; 65(3):257–260.
52. No authors listed. Nitazoxanide (Alinia) – a new anti-protozoal agent. Med Lett Drugs Ther 2003; 45(1154):29–31.
53. Nash TE. Surface antigenic variation in *Giardia lamblia*. Mol Microbiol 2002; 45(3):585–590.
54. Med Lett. Drugs for Parasitic Infections. Med Lett Drugs Ther 16 August 2004; Issue 1189: http://medletbest.securesites.com/freedocs/parasitic.pdf
55. American Academy of Pediatrics. Red Book: 2003 Report of the Committee on Infectious Diseases. Elk Grove Village, IL: American Academy of Pediatrics; 2003.
56. Cevallos M, Porta H, Alagon A, Lizardi P. Sequence of the 5.8S ribosomal gene of pathogenic and non-pathogenic isolates of Entamoeba histolytica. Nucl Acids Res 1993; 21:355.
57. Carrero J, Laclette J. Molecular biology of Entamoeba histolytica: a review. Arch Med Res 1996; 27:403–412.
58. Mann BJ. Entamoeba histolytica Genome Project: an update. Trends Parasitol 2002; 18(4):147–148.

59. Tannich E. Royal Society of Tropical Medicine and Hygiene Meeting at Manson House, London, 19 February 1998. Amoebic disease. Entamoeba histolytica and E. dispar: comparison of molecules considered important for host tissue destruction. Trans R Soc Trop Med Hyg 1998; 92(6):593–596.
60. Jackson TF. Entamoeba histolytica and Entamoeba dispar are distinct species; clinical, epidemiological and serological evidence. Int J Parasitol 1998; 28(1):181–186.
61. WHO. WHO/Pan American Health Organization/UNESCO Expert Consultation on Amoebiasis; 4 April: WHO, Weekly Epidemiological Record. Mexico City, Mexico: WHO; 1997:97–100.
62. Ayeh-Kumi PF, Ali IM, Lockhart LA, Gilchrist CA, Petri WA. Jr, Haque R. Entamoeba histolytica: genetic diversity of clinical isolates from Bangladesh as demonstrated by polymorphisms in the serine-rich gene. Exp Parasitol 2001; 99(2):80–88.
63. Stauffer W, Ravdin JI. Entamoeba histolytica: an update. Curr Opin Infect Dis 2003; 16(5):479–485.
64. Berninghausen O, Leippe M. Necrosis versus apoptosis as the mechanism of target cell death induced by Entamoeba histolytica. Infect Immun 1997; 65(9):3615–3621.
65. Bhattacharya A, Anand MT, Paul J, Yadav N, Bhattacharya S. Molecular changes in Entamoeba histolytica in response to bacteria. J Eukaryot Microbiol 1998; 45(2):28S–33S.
66. Allason-Jones E, Mindel A, Sargeaunt P, Katz D. Outcome of untreated infection with Entamoeba histolytica in homosexual men with and without HIV antibody. Br Med J 1988; 297:654–657.
67. Tachibana H, Kobayashi S, Nagakura K, Kaneda Y, Takeuchi T. Asymptomatic cyst passers of Entamoeba histolytica but not Entamoeba dispar in institutions for the mentally retarded in Japan. Parasitol Int 2000; 49(1):31–35.
68. Haque R, Mondal D, Kirkpatrick BD, et al. Epidemiologic and clinical characteristics of acute diarrhea with emphasis on Entamoeba histolytica infections in preschool children in an urban slum of Dhaka, Bangladesh. Am J Trop Med Hyg 2003; 69(4):398–405.
69. Blessmann J, Ali IK, Nu PA, Dinh BT, Viet TQ. Van AL, et al. Longitudinal study of intestinal Entamoeba histolytica infections in asymptomatic adult carriers. J Clin Microbiol 2003; 41(10):4745–4750.
70. Calore EE, Calore NM, Cavaliere MJ. Salpingitis due to Entamoeba histolytica. Braz J Infect Dis 2002; 6(2):97–99.
71. Mayhew KM, Dundoo M, Dunne EF, Dwinnell BG, Stephens JK. Inguinal lymphadenitis caused by Entamoeba histolytica: case report and literature review. Mayo Clin Proc 2000; 75(5):513–516.
72. Lecuit M, Martinez F, Deray G, et al. Clinical and pathophysiological aspects of immune complex glomerulonephritis associated with Entamoeba histolytica abscess of the liver. Clin Infect Dis 1997; 25(2):335–336.
73. Pillai DR, Keystone JS, Sheppard DC, et al. Entamoeba histolytica and Entamoeba dispar: epidemiology and comparison of diagnostic methods in a setting of nonendemicity. Clin Infect Dis 1999; 29(5):1315–1318.
74. Schunk M, Jelinek T, Wetzel K, Nothdurft HD. Detection of *Giardia lamblia* and Entamoeba histolytica in stool samples by two enzyme immunoassays. Eur J Clin Microbiol Infect Dis 2001; 20(6):389–391.
75. Mirelman D, Nuchamowitz Y, Stolarsky T. Comparison of use of enzyme-linked immunosorbent assay-based kits and PCR amplification of rRNA genes for simultaneous detection of Entamoeba histolytica and E. dispar. J Clin Microbiol 1997; 35(9):2405–2407.
76. Gonin P, Trudel L. Detection and differentiation of Entamoeba histolytica and Entamoeba dispar isolates in clinical samples by PCR and enzyme-linked immunosorbent assay. J Clin Microbiol 2003; 41(1):237–241.
77. Haque R, Mollah NU, Ali IK, et al. Diagnosis of amebic liver abscess and intestinal infection with the TechLab Entamoeba histolytica II antigen detection and antibody tests. J Clin Microbiol 2000; 38(9):3235–3239.
78. Orozco E, Lopez C, Gomez C, et al. Multidrug resistance in the protozoan parasite Entamoeba histolytica. Parasitol Int 2002; 51(4):353–359.
79. Rossignol JF, Ayoub A, Ayers MS. Treatment of diarrhea caused by *Giardia* intestinalis and Entamoeba histolytica or E. dispar: a randomized, double-blind, placebo-controlled study of nitazoxanide. J Infect Dis 2001; 184(3):381–384.
80. Chen KT, Chen CJ, Chiu JP. A school water-borne outbreak involving both Shigella sonnei and Entamoeba histolytica. J Environ Health 2001; 64(4):9–13.
81. Braga LL, Gomes ML, Silva MW Da, Facanha FE. Jr., Fiuza L, Mann BJ. Household epidemiology of Entamoeba histolytica infection in an urban community in northeastern Brazil. Am J Trop Med Hyg 2001; 65(4):268–271.
82. Pai HH, Ko YC, Chen ER. Cockroaches (*Periplaneta americana and Blattella germanica*) as potential mechanical disseminators of *Entamoeba histolytica*. Acta Trop 2003; 87(3):355–359.
83. Mann BJ, Burkholder BV, Lockhart LA. Protection in a gerbil model of amebiasis by oral immunization with Salmonella expressing the galactose/N-acetyl D-galactosamine inhibitable lectin of Entamoeba histolytica. Vaccine 1997; 15(6/7):659–663.
84. Petri WA. Entamoeba histolytica: Clinical update and vaccine prospects. Curr Infect Dis Rep 2002; 4(2):124–129.
85. Miller-Sims VC, Petri WA. Jr. Opportunities and obstacles in developing a vaccine for Entamoeba histolytica. Curr Opin Immunol 2002; 14(5):549–552.
86. Butler W. Dientamoeba fragilis. An unusual intestinal pathogen. Dig Dis Sci 1996; 41:1811–1813.
87. Chan F, Stewart N, Guan M, et al. Prevalence of Dientamoeba fragilis antibodies in children and recognition of a 39 kDa immunodominant protein antigen of the organism. Eur J Clin Microbiol Infect Dis 1996; 15:950–954.
88. Chang S. Parasitization of the parasite. JAMA 1973; 223:1510–1513.
89. Grendon J, DiGiacomo R, Frost F. Descriptive features of Dientamoeba fragilis infections. J Trop Med Hyg 1995; 98:309–315.
90. Norberg A, Nord CE, Evengard B. Dientamoeba fragilis–fragilia protozoal infection which may cause severe bowel distress. Clin Microbiol Infect 2003; 9(1):65–68.
91. Cuffari C, Oligny L, Seidman EG. Dientamoeba fragilis masquerading as allergic colitis. J Pediatr Gastroenterol Nutr 1998; 26(1):16–20.
92. Girginkardesler N, Coskun S, Cuneyt Balcioglu I, Ertan P, Ok UZ. Dientamoeba fragilis, a neglected cause of diarrhea, successfully treated with secnidazole. Clin Microbiol Infect 2003; 9(2):110–113.
93. Windsor JJ, Johnson EH. Dientamoeba fragilis: the unflagellated human flagellate. Br J Biomed Sci 1999; 56(4):293–306.
94. Shlim D, Hoge C, Rajah R, et al. Is Blastocystis hominis a cause of diarrhea in travelers? A prospective controlled study in Nepal. Clin Infect Dis 1995; 21:97–101.
95. Markell E. Is there any reason to continue treating Blastocystis infections? (Editorial comment). Clin Infect Dis 1995; 21:104–105.

96. Sinniah B, Rajeswari B. Blastocystis hominis infection, a cause of human diarrhea. Southeast Asian J Trop Med Public HealTh1994; 25:490–493.
97. Jelinek T, Peyerl G, Loscher T, Sonnenburg F von, Nothdurft HD. The role of Blastocystis hominis as a possible intestinal pathogen in travellers. J Infect 1997; 35(1):63–66.
98. Brites C, Barberino MG, Bastos MA, Sampaio Sa M, Silva N. Blastocystis hominis as a Potential Cause of Diarrhea in AIDS Patients: a Report of Six Cases in Bahia, Brazil. Braz J Infect Dis 1997; 1(2):91–94.
99. Cirioni O, Giacometti A, Drenaggi D, Ancarani F, Scalise G. Prevalence and clinical relevance of Blastocystis hominis in diverse patient cohorts. Eur J Epidemiol 1999; 15(4):389–393.
100. Rao K, Sekar U, Iraivan KT, Abraham G, Soundararajan P. Blastocystis hominis–hominan emerging cause of diarrhoea in renal transplant recipients. J Assoc Physicians India 2003; 51:719–721.
101. Abe N, Wu Z, Yoshikawa H. Zoonotic genotypes of Blastocystis hominis detected in cattle and pigs by PCR with diagnostic primers and restriction fragment length polymorphism analysis of the small subunit ribosomal RNA gene. Parasitol Res 2003; 90(2):124–128.
102. O'Gorman M, Orenstein S, Proujansky R, et al. Prevalence and characteristics of Blastocystis hominis infection in children. Clin Pediatr 1993; 32:91–96.
103. Hussain R, Jaferi W, Zuberi S, et al. Significantly increased IgG2 subclass antibody levels to Blastocystis hominis in patients with irritable bowel syndrome. Am J Trop Med Hyg 1997; 56(3):301–306.
104. Leelayoova S, Taamasri P, Rangsin R, et al. In-vitro cultivation: a sensitive method for detecting Blastocystis hominis. Ann Trop Med Parasitol 2002; 96(8):803–807.
105. Ok UZ, Girginkardesler N, Balcioglu C, et al. Effect of trimethoprim-sulfamethaxazole in Blastocystis hominis infection. Am J Gastroenterol 1999; 94(11):3245–3247.
106. Anargyrou K, Petrikkos GL, Suller MT, et al. Pulmonary Balantidium coli infection in a leukemic patient. Am J Hematol 2003; 73(3):180–183.
107. Cermeno JR, Hernandez Cuesta I De, Uzcategui O, et al. Balantidium coli in an HIV-infected patient with chronic diarrhoea. Aids 2003; 17(6):941–942.
108. Nine F, Burek J, Page D, et al. Acute enterocolitis in a human being infected with the protozoan Cryptosporidium. Gastroenterology 1976; 70:592–598.
109. Izumiyama S, Furukawa I, Kuroki T, et al. Prevalence of Cryptosporidium parvum infections in weaned piglets and fattening porkers in Kanagawa Prefecture, Japan. Jpn J Infect Dis 2001; 54(1):23–26.
110. McReynolds CA, Lappin MR, Ungar B, et al. Regional seroprevalence of Cryptosporidium parvum-specific IgG of cats in the United States. Vet Parasitol 1999; 80(3):187–195.
111. Chalmers RM, Sturdee AP, Bull SA, Miller A, Wright SE. The prevalence of Cryptosporidium parvum and C. muris in Mus domesticus, Apodemus sylvaticus and Clethrionomys glareolus in an agricultural system. Parasitol Res 1997; 83(5):478–482.
112. Fayer R, Lewis EJ, Trout JM, et al. Cryptosporidium parvum in oysters from commercial harvesting sites in the Chesapeake Bay. Emerg Infect Dis 1999; 5(5):706–710.
113. Graczyk TK, Fayer R, Trout JM, et al. *Giardia* sp. cysts and infectious Cryptosporidium parvum oocysts in the feces of migratory Canada geese (Branta canadensis). Appl Environ Microbiol 1998; 64(7):2736–2738.
114. Graczyk TK, Fayer R, Knight R, et al. Mechanical transport and transmission of Cryptosporidium parvum oocysts by wild filth flies. Am J Trop Med Hyg 2000; 62(3/4):178–183
115. Morgan-Ryan UM, Fall A, Ward LA, et al. Cryptosporidium hominis n. sp. (Apicomplexa: Cryptosporidiidae) from Homo sapiens. J Eukaryot Microbiol 2002; 49(6):433–440.
116. Widmer G. Population genetics of Cryptosporidium parvum. Trends Parasitol 2004; 20(1):3–6.
117. Peng MM, Xiao L, Freeman AR, et al. Genetic polymorphism among Cryptosporidium parvum isolates: evidence of two distinct human transmission cycles. Emerg Infect Dis 1997; 3(4):567–573.
118. Chacin-Bonilla L, Bonilla MC, Soto-Torres L, et al. Cryptosporidium parvum in children with diarrhea in Zulia State, Venezuela. Am J Trop Med Hyg 1997; 56(4):365–369.
119. Dietz V, Vugia D, Nelson R, et al. Active, multisite, laboratory-based surveillance for Cryptosporidium parvum. Am J Trop Med Hyg 2000; 62(3):368–372.
120. Dietz VJ, Roberts JM. National surveillance for infection with Cryptosporidium parvum, 1995-1998: what have we learned? Public Health Rep 2000; 115(4):358–363.
121. Egorov A, Paulauskis J, Petrova L, et al. Contamination of water supplies with Cryptosporidium parvum and *Giardia lamblia* and diarrheal illness in selected Russian cities. Int J Hyg Environ Health 2002; 205(4):281–289.
122. Tumwine JK, Kekitiinwa A, Nabukeera N, et al. Cryptosporidium parvum in children with diarrhea in Mulago Hospital, Kampala, Uganda. Am J Trop Med Hyg 2003; 68(6):710–715.
123. Checkley W, Epstein LD, Gilman RH, et al. Effects of Cryptosporidium parvum infection in Peruvian children: growth faltering and subsequent catch-up growth. Am J Epidemiol 1998; 148(5):497–506.
124. Leach CT, Koo FC, Kuhls TL, Hilsenbeck SG, Jenson HB. Prevalence of Cryptosporidium parvum infection in children along the Texas-Mexico border and associated risk factors. Am J Trop Med Hyg 2000; 62(5):656–661.
125. Pereira MD, Atwill ER, Barbosa AP, Silva SA, Garcia-Zapata MT. Intra-familial and extra-familial risk factors associated with Cryptosporidium parvum infection among children hospitalized for diarrhea in Goiania, Goias, Brazil. Am J Trop Med Hyg 2002; 66(6):787–793.
126. Chappell CL, Okhuysen PC, Sterling CR, et al. Infectivity of Cryptosporidium parvum in healthy adults with pre-existing anti-C parvum serum immunoglobulin G. Am J Trop Med Hyg 1999; 60(1):157–164.
127. Bouche H, Housset C, Dumont J, et al. AIDS-related cholangitis: diagnostic features and course in 15 patients. J Hepatol 1993; 17:34–39.
128. Goddard EA, Mouton SC, Westwood AT, Ireland JD, Durra G. Cryptosporidiosis of the gastrointestinal tract associated with sclerosing cholangitis in the absence of documented immunodeficiency: Cryptosporidium parvum and sclerosing cholangitis in an immunocompetent child. J Pediatr Gastroenterol Nutr 2000; 31(3):317–320.
129. Norby SM, Bharucha AE, Larson MV, Temesgen Z. Acute pancreatitis associated with Cryptosporidium parvum enteritis in an immunocompetent man. Clin Infect Dis 1998; 27(1):223–224.
130. Garcia LS, Shimizu RY. Evaluation of nine immunoassay kits (enzyme immunoassay and direct fluorescence) for detection of *Giardia lamblia* and *Cryptosporidium parvum* in human fecal specimens. J Clin Microbiol 1997; 35(6):1526–1529.
131. Amenta M, Dalle Nogare ER, Colomba C, et al. Intestinal protozoa in HIV-infected patients: effect of rifaximin in Cryptosporidium parvum and Blastocystis hominis infections. J Chemother 1999; 11(5):391–395.
132. Rossignol JF, Ayoub A, Ayers MS. Treatment of diarrhea caused by Cryptosporidium parvum: a prospective

randomized, double-blind, placebo-controlled study of Nitazoxanide. J Infect Dis 2001; 184(1):103–106.

133. Hicks P, Zwiener R, Squires J, Savell V. Azithromycin therapy for Cryptosporidium parvum infection in four children infected with human immunodeficiency virus. J Pediatr 1996; 129:297–300.

134. Trad O, Jumaa P, Uduman S, Nawaz A. Eradication of Cryptosporidium in four children with acute lymphoblastic leukemia. J Trop Pediatr 2003; 49(2):128–130.

135. Greenberg P, Cello J. Treatment of severe diarrhea caused by Cryptosporidium parvum with oral bovine immunoglobulin concentrate in patients with AIDS. J Acquir Immune Defic Syndr Hum Retrovirol 1996; 13:348–354.

136. Kuhls T, Orlicek S, Mosier D, et al. Enteral human serum immunoglobulin treatment of cryptosporidiosis in mice with severe combined immunodeficiency. Infect Immun 1995; 63:3582–3586.

137. Brantley RK, Williams KR, Silva TM, et al. AIDS-associated diarrhea and wasting in Northeast Brazil is associated with subtherapeutic plasma levels of antiretroviral medications and with both bovine and human subtypes of Cryptosporidium parvum. Braz J Infect Dis 2003; 7(1):16–22.

138. Alak JI, Wolf BW, Mdurvwa EG, et al. Supplementation with Lactobacillus reuteri or L. acidophilus reduced intestinal shedding of cryptosporidium parvum oocysts in immunodeficient C57BL/6 mice. Cell Mol Biol 1999; 45(6):855–863.

139. MacKenzie W. A massive outbreak in Milwaukee of Cryptosporidium infection transmitted through the public water supply. N Engl J Med 1994; 331:161–168.

140. Patel S, Pedraza-Diaz S, McLauchlin J, Casemore DP. Molecular characterisation of Cryptosporidium parvum from two large suspected water-borne outbreaks. Outbreak Control Team South and West Devon 1995, Incident Management Team and Further Epidemiological and Microbiological Studies Subgroup North Thames 1997. Commun Dis Public Health 1998; 1(4):231–233.

141. Ackers J. Gut coccidia-Isospora, Cryptosporidium, Cyclospora and Sarcocystis. Semin Gastrointest Dis 1997; 8:33–44.

142. Arness MK, Brown JD, Dubey JP, Neafie RC, Granstrom DE. An outbreak of acute eosinophilic myositis attributed to human Sarcocystis parasitism. Am J Trop Med Hyg 1999; 61(4):548–553.

143. Brennan M, MacPherson D, Palmer J. Keystone J. Cyclosporiasis: a new cause of diarrhea. Can Med Assoc J 1996; 155:1293–1296.

144. PHLS. Diagnosis of Cyclospora cayetanensis infections. Commun Dis Rep CDR Wkly 1997; 7(37):329, 332.

145. Curry A, Smith HV. Emerging pathogens: Isospora, Cyclospora and microsporidia. Parasitology 1998; 117(suppl):S143–S159.

146. Zar FA, El-Bayoumi E, Yungbluth MM. Histologic proof of acalculous cholecystitis due to Cyclospora cayetanensis. Clin Infect Dis 2001; 33(12):E140–E141.

147. Chacin-Bonilla L, Mejia Young M de, Estevez J. Prevalence and pathogenic role of Cyclospora cayetanensis in a Venezuelan community. Am J Trop Med Hyg 2003; 68(3):304–306.

148. Herwaldt BL. Cyclospora cayetanensis: a review, focusing on the outbreaks of cyclosporiasis in the 1990s. Clin Infect Dis 2000; 31(4):1040–1057.

149. Verdier RI, Fitzgerald DW, Johnson WD Jr, Pape JW. Trimethoprim-sulfamethoxazole compared with ciprofloxacin for treatment and prophylaxis of Isospora belli and Cyclospora cayetanensis infection in HIV-infected patients. A randomized, controlled trial. Ann Intern Med 2000; 132(11):885–888.

150. Marshall M, Naumovitz D, Ortega Y, Sterling C. Water-borne protozoan pathogens. Clin Microbiol Rev 1997; 10:67–85.

151. Schwartz D, Sobottka I, Leitch G, et al. Pathology of microsporidiosis: emerging parasitic infections in patients with acquired immunodeficiency syndrome. Arch Pathol Lab Med 1996; 120:173–188.

152. Croft S, Williams J, McGowan I. Intestinal microsporidiosis. Semin Gastrointest Dis 1997; 8:45–55.

153. Asmuth D, DeGirolami P, Federman M, et al. Clinical features of microsporidiosis in patients with AIDS. Clin Infect Dis 1994; 18:819–825.

154. Gumbo T, Hobbs RE, Carlyn C, Hall G, Isada CM. Microsporidia infection in transplant patients. Transplantation 1999; 67(3):482–484.

155. Franzen C, Muller A. Cryptosporidia and microsporidia–micwater-borne diseases in the immunocompromised host. Diagn Microbiol Infect Dis 1999; 34(3):245–262.

156. Dengjel B, Zahler M, Hermanns W, et al. Zoonotic potential of Enterocytozoon bieneusi. J Clin Microbiol 2001; 39(12):4495–4499.

157. Didier E, Rogers L, Brush A, et al. Diagnosis of disseminated microsporidian Encephalitozoon hellem infection by PCR-Southern analysis and successful treatment with albendazole and fumagillin. J Clin Microbiol 1996; 34:947–952.

158. Garvey M, Ambrose P, Ulmer J. Topical fumagillin in the treatment of microsporidial keratoconjunctivitis in AIDS. Ann Pharmacother 1995; 29:872–874.

159. Rossi R, Wanke C, Federman M. Microsporidian sinusitis in patients with the acquired immunodeficiency syndrome. Laryngoscope 1996; 106:966–971.

160. Botterel F, Minozzi C, Vittecoq D, Bouree P. Pulmonary localization of Enterocytozoon bieneusi in an AIDS patient: case report and review. J Clin Microbiol 2002; 40(12):4800–4801.

161. Svedhem V, Lebbad M, Struve J, et al. Microsporidia in duodenal biopsies from 72 HIV-infected patients with abdominal complaints. Apmis 1998; 106(5):535–538.

162. Rinder H, Janitschke K, Aspock H, et al. Blinded, externally controlled multicenter evaluation of light microscopy and PCR for detection of microsporidia in stool specimens. The Diagnostic Multicenter Study Group on Microsporidia. J Clin Microbiol 1998; 36(6):1814–1818.

163. Bicart-See A, Massip P, Linas MD, Datry A. Successful treatment with nitazoxanide of Enterocytozoon bieneusi microsporidiosis in a patient with AIDS. Antimicrob Agents Chemother 2000; 44(1):167–168.

164. Molina JM, Goguel J, Sarfati C, et al. Potential efficacy of fumagillin in intestinal microsporidiosis due to Enterocytozoon bieneusi in patients with HIV infection: results of a drug screening study. Fr Microsporidiosis Study Group Aids 1997; 11(13):1603–1610.

165. Dionisio D, Manneschi LI, Di Lollo S, et al. Persistent damage to Enterocytozoon bieneusi, with persistent symptomatic relief, after combined furazolidone and albendazole in AIDS patients. J Clin Pathol 1998; 51(10):731–736.

166. Deplazes P, Mathis A, Weber R. Epidemiology and zoonotic aspects of microsporidia of mammals and birds. Contrib Microbiol 2000; 6:236–260.

167. Ascariasis KM. Gastroenterol Clin North Am 1996; 25:553–577.

168. Asrat T, Rogers N. Acute pancreatitis caused by biliary ascaris in pregnancy. J Perinatol 1995; 15:330–332.

Chapter 38
Gastrointestinal manifestations of primary immunodeficiency

Qian Yuan and Athos Bousvaros

INTRODUCTION

In 1995 and 1999, an expert panel of the World Health Organization identified more than 80 primary and secondary immunodeficiency syndromes.[1,2] If selective immunoglobulin A (IgA) deficiency is excluded, approximately 400 children with primary immunodeficiency syndromes are born in the USA each year,[3] whereas human immunodeficiency virus (HIV) infects 1000–2000 American children born each year.[4] This chapter reviews the gastrointestinal manifestations and complications of the more common primary immunodeficiency syndromes (Table 38.1). A more detailed discussion of the systemic complications of each syndrome can be found elsewhere.[3]

INNATE *VS* ADAPTIVE IMMUNITY

The immune response is a complex process, and can be divided into innate and adaptive responses. The differences between these two arms of the immune system are summarized in Table 38.2. The *innate immune system* is the first line of defense against invading micro-organisms. The innate system serves a prominent protective function in all tissues and organs, especially the intestinal tract, genitourinary tract, respiratory tract and the skin, where there is greater exposure to the external environment and foreign antigens. The cellular components of the innate immune system include cells residing in host tissues and cells that may migrate to areas of inflammation. The principal cells of the innate immune system are Langerhans cells of the skin, tissue dendritic cells and macrophages, natural killer (NK) cells and γδ T-cell intraepithelial lymphocytes of the gut.[5] Cells involved in innate immunity (e.g. dendritic cells and macrophages) utilize Toll-like receptors (TLRs) present on the cell surface to recognize certain specific molecules, such as lipopolysaccharide (LPS) and heat shock proteins (HSPs). As the protein structure of molecules such as LPS and HSPs is similar between bacterial species, the term pathogen-associated molecular pattern (PAMP) is utilized to describe microbial products that are conserved throughout evolution and are structurally similar in different organisms. The interaction of an organism's PAMP product with a cell's Toll-like receptor triggers a signaling cascade, which can in turn produce an immediate immune response, for example the production of cytokines by dendritic cells, or activation and phagocytosis by a macrophage[5,6] (Fig. 38.1).

In contrast, the *adaptive immune system* utilizes T and B lymphocytes to mediate and amplify antigen-specific humoral and cellular responses. Given that a human is exposed to a wide variety of different infections, and that many viruses and bacteria can modify their cellular and protein structures to escape detection, the immune system must adapt to recognize new pathogens and proteins. In the adaptive immune system, macrophages and dendritic cells take up and digest antigens, process and present the antigen to T cells, which can in turn stimulate the production of antibody-producing B cells and cytotoxic cells.

Thus, the human immune system can generate new antibodies and new cellular receptors to allow it to recognize pathogens and fight infections more efficiently. However, these responses often take days to weeks to achieve maximal activity and require a somatic gene rearrangement, which results in immunologic memory. The majority of immunodeficiency syndromes described in this chapter represent defects in adaptive immunity.

COMPONENTS OF THE ADAPTIVE IMMUNE RESPONSE

To trigger the cascade of immunologic events summarized in Table 38.3, an exogenous antigen must penetrate the physical barriers at epithelial surfaces. In certain specialized regions of gut epithelium termed *follicle-associated epithelium* (dome epithelium), modified epithelial cells (M cells) preferentially bind bacteria and viruses. These M cells are located over lymphoid nodules and Peyer's patches in the gut. They provide a portal of entry that directly exposes potential pathogens to the systemic and mucosal immune systems.[7,8]

On exposure to cells of the immune system, antigen is endocytosed and processed by antigen-presenting cells (APCs). Although many different types of cell can present antigen to T cells, the two principal APCs in the body are monocyte–macrophages and dendritic cells. APCs are characterized by their ability to phagocytose proteins or peptides, degrade them intracellularly, complex these peptides with proteins of the major histocompatibility complex (MHC) and transport the peptide–MHC protein to the APC cell surface.[9] Antigen presentation to a CD4 (helper) T lymphocyte occurs when a peptide complexed to an MHC class II protein on the surface of an APC comes in contact with the T-cell receptor complex on the surface of the

Disease	Proposed cause
Predominantly antibody deficiencies	
X-linked agammaglobulinemia	Mutations in *BtK* in B cells
Hyper-IgM syndrome	Mutations of gp39 (CD40 ligand) on T cells
Selective IgA deficiency	Failure of terminal differentiation in IgA+ B cells
Transient hypogammaglobulinemia of infancy	Delayed maturation of helper T-cell function
Combined cellular–hymoral defects	
Common variable immunodeficiency	Impaired B-cell differentiation; molecular defect unknown
Severe combined immunodeficiency	Multiple causes, including adenosine deaminase deficiency, purine nucleotidyl phosphorylase deficiency, absence of IL-2 receptor γ chain (in X-linked SCID), mutations in Rag1/2, T-cell maturation defects (e.g. ZAP-70 kinase mutation)
Bare lymphocyte syndrome	MHC class I and/or class II deficiency caused by mutations in transcription factors (such as *CIITA* or *RFX5*, *RFXAP*, *RFXANK* genes for MHC class II molecules)
Immunodeficiency with other systemic disease	
Ataxia telangiectasia (AT)	Mutation in AT gene (*ATM*) causes disorder of cell cycle checkpoint pathway leading to chromosomal instability
Wiskott–Aldrich syndrome	Mutations in *WASp* gene cause cytoskeletal defect affecting hematopoietic stem cell derivatives
DiGeorge syndrome	Contiguous gene defect causes thymic hypoplasia
X-linked proliferative syndrome	Defect in SAP
Other primary immunodeficiency diseases **Defects of phagocytic function**	
Chronic granulomatous disease	Deficiency of 91-kDa chain of cytochrome *b* in X-linked CGD; deficiencies of 22-kDa chain of cytochrome *b* or p47 or p67 cytosol factors in autosomal recessive CGD
Leukocyte adhesion deficiency	Deficiency of β chain (CD18) of LFA-1, Mac-1 and p150,95 in LAD type 1; failure to convert GDP mannose to fucose in LAD type 2
Shwachman syndrome	Defect in neutrophil chemotaxis; molecular defect unknown
Complement deficiencies	
Immunodeficiency associated with other diseases	
Chromosomal defects (e.g. Down syndrome, Fanconi's anemia, xeroderma)	
Generalized growth retardation (e.g. Dubowitz syndrome, Hutchinson–Gildord syndrome)	
Hereditary metabolic defects (e.g. glycogen storage disease 1B)	
Hypercatabolism of immunoglobulin (e.g. intestinal lymphangiectasia)	
Malnutrition	
Malignancy	
Drug-induced (sulfasalazine, gold, chloroquine, penicillamine, captopril, hydantoin, carbamazepine, valproate, etc.)	
Acquired immune deficiency syndrome	

Adapted from Rosen et al.,[1] International Union of Immunological Societies[2] and Hammarstrom et al.[199]

Table 38.1 Classification and etiology of primary immunodeficiency diseases with prominent gastrointestinal manifestations

	Innate immunity	Adaptive immunity
Response	Immediate	Delayed (days to weeks)
Stimuli	Limited (bacterial LPS, HSP, etc.)	Variable
Receptors	Toll-like receptors	MHC–TCR
Cells	Dendritic cells, macrophages, NK cells, intraepithelial lymphocytes of the gut	T and B lymphocytes
Mechanisms	Variety Mechanical barriers – epithelial cells, cytotoxic (defensins and other secretory enzymes), gastric acid, mucins, commensal intestinal flora, intestinal motility	Cellular and humoral immune responses

LPS, lipopolysaccharide; HSP, heat shock protein; NK, natural killer T cells; MHC, major histocompatibility complex; TCR, T-cell receptor.

Table 38.2 Innate *vs* adaptive immunity

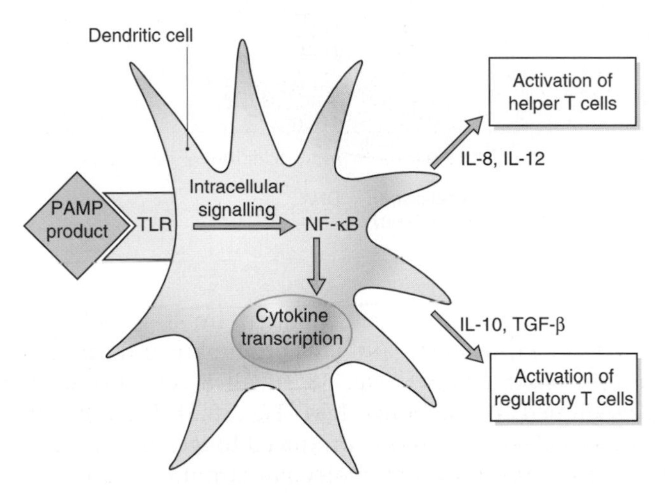

Figure 38.1: Mechanisms of innate immune response. Binding of bacterial proteins with pathogen-associated molecular patterns (PAMP products, e.g. lipopolysaccharide) to Toll-like receptors (TLR) on dentritic cells results in signal transduction. The signal generated at the cell membrane results in the activation of a complex signaling pathway involving the proteins MyD88, TNF receptor-associated factor 6 (TRAF-6), NIK and IKK. As a result, the protein NF-κB enters the nucleus and stimulates cytokine transcription. Depending on the cytokines released, different T-cell populations may be activated.

lymphocyte. Stimulation of the T-cell receptor alone is not sufficient to promote T-lymphocyte activation, and a second signal (either through another cell surface molecule such as CD28, through surface cell adhesion molecules such as leukocyte functional antigen 1 (LFA-1), or through cytokine signaling) is necessary to activate a T cell.[10–12]

- Antigen uptake by antigen presenting cells (dendritic cells, macrophages)
- Antigen processing
- Antigen presentation to T cells
- T-lymphocyte activation
- B-cell activation, switching and immunoglobulin production
- Leukocyte homing and adhesion to tissues
- Effector cell recruitment
- Release of inflammatory mediators (e.g. prostaglandin, leukotriene, complement, etc.)

Adapted from Rhee and Bousvaros, 2004, with permission.[201]

Table 38.3 Components of the adaptive immune response

If antigenic stimulation and co-stimulation occur, a signal is transduced through the CD3 complex, characterized by phosphorylation of tyrosine molecules in the CD3 and zeta chains[13] (Fig. 38.2). Subsequently, tyrosine kinases, including Lck and zeta-associated protein 70 (ZAP-70), are activated and induce phosphorylation of phospholipase Cγ1, which in turn converts inositol 4,5-biphosphate to inositol 1,4,5-triphosphate (IP_3).[14] IP_3 formation results in increased cytosolic free calcium from intracellular stores and activation of the molecule calcineurin. A second intracellular signal transduction pathway initiated by phospholipase Cγ1 involves the molecules diacylglycerol and protein kinase C[14,15] (Fig. 38.2). These pathways are separate but synergistic, and inhibition of one or the other may abrogate T-cell activation.

Calcineurin and protein kinase C enzymes in turn promote increased transcription of cytokine gene products mediated by nuclear binding factors, including NF-AT and NF-κB. NF-κB essential modifier (NEMO), also known as inhibitor of NF-κB kinase γ (IKK-γ), is required for the activation and subsequent translocation to the nucleus of the transcription factor NF-κB, where NF-κB activates multiple target genes.[16,17] A third T-cell activation pathway triggered by antigen recognition involves a group of kinases termed mitogen-activated protein (MAP) kinases, which in turn activate the transcription factor AP-1 (18).

Based on studies performed with murine T-lymphocyte clones, helper (CD4) T lymphocytes have been categorized into two broad types. Type 1 helper T cells (Th1) promote cellular immune responses and delayed-type hypersensitivity by secreting interleukin (IL) 2, interferon γ (INF-γ) and tumor necrosis factor β (TNF-β). In contrast, type 2 helper T cells (Th2) promote humoral responses by secreting IL-4, IL-5, IL-10 and IL-13.[19] IL-4, IL-5 and IL-13 in turn promote B-lymphocyte differentiation into plasma cells and antibody synthesis. Both Th1 and Th2 cell subsets develop from naive CD4 cells, depending on the types of antigen processed by dendritic cells or macrophages. A Th1 cytokine response promotes macrophage activation with the aim of eliminating intracellular microbes, whereas a Th2 response results in mast cell activation, clearing of

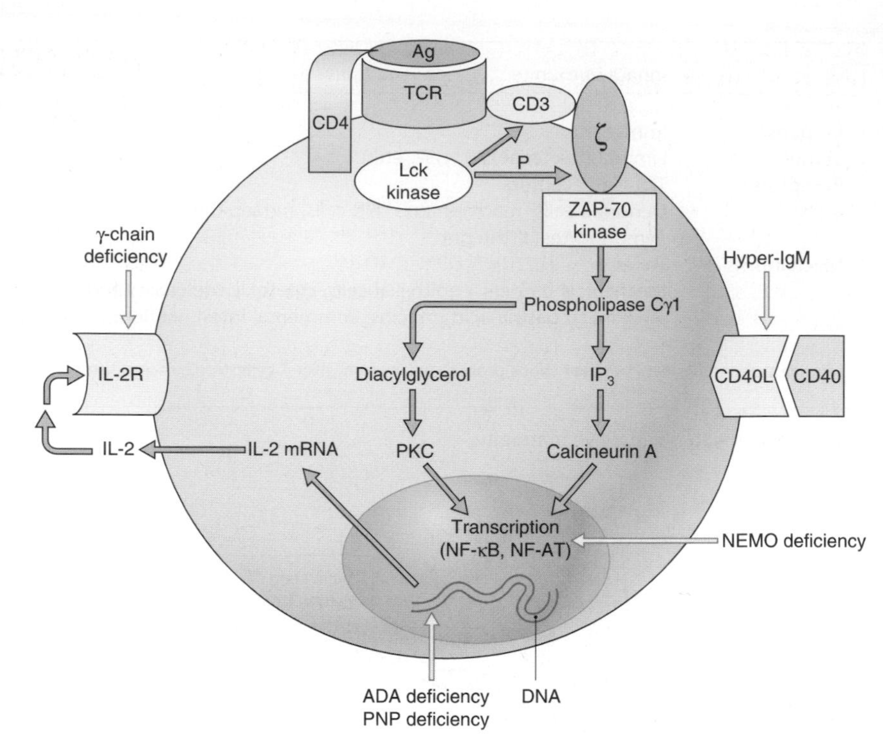

Figure 38.2: Signaling effects in T-lymphocyte activation and sites of effects of immunodeficiency syndromes. Binding of antigen (Ag), in association with MHC proteins, to the T-cell receptor (TCR)–CD3 complex activates two intracellular pathways of signaling. The first pathway involves diacylglycerol (DAG) and protein kinase C (PKC); the second involves inositol triphosphate (IP_3) and calcineurin. The end-result of this intracellular signaling is increased DNA synthesis by T cells and increased synthesis of cytokine (e.g. IL-2) messenger RNA as mediated by the nuclear factor of activated T cells (NF-AT). The activated T-cell expresses CD40 ligand (CD40L). Patients with adenosine deaminase (ADA) deficiency and purine nucleotidyl phosphorylase (PNP) deficiency have impaired synthesis of DNA; patients with X-linked severe combined immunodeficiency have defective IL-2 receptor γ-chain expression. Patients with hyper-IgM syndrome have defective expression of CD40L. (Adapted from Rhee and Bousvaros, 2004, with permission.)[201]

parasites and allergic reactions.[20] Th1 cells are implicated in the pathogenesis of Crohn's disease, whereas Th2 cells have been implicated in the pathogenesis of ulcerative colitis and allergic disorders.

Two other groups of regulatory T-cell subsets, Th3 and CD4+ CD25+ cells, decrease inflammation and promote tolerance by secreting anti-inflammatory cytokines, such as IL-10 and transforming growth factor β (TGF-β).[20] IL-10 inhibits microphage activation and antagonizes the pro-inflammatory cytokine INF-γ, whereas TGF-β inhibits B- and T-cell proliferation.[21]

Humoral immunity is generated by B lymphocytes, which, on exposure to antigen, proliferate and differentiate into plasma cells[22] (Fig. 38.3). All B cells are initially programmed to synthesize IgM (Fig. 38.3). For a B cell to switch its class of antibody produced to IgG or IgA (isotype switching), several other molecular stimuli need to occur (Fig. 38.3). The CD40 ligand (gp39, CD154) is a molecule on the surface of the T cell that binds to CD40 on B cells. This interaction promotes B-cell activation and differentiation, and isotype switching from IgM to IgG, IgA or IgE. Conversely, the CD40–CD154 interaction also promotes

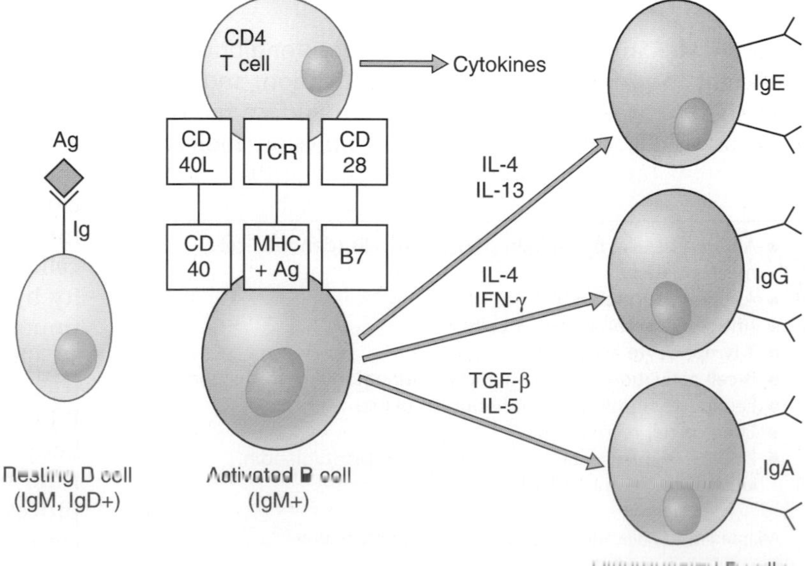

Figure 38.3: B-cell differentiation and the role of helper T cells. For a resting B cell to differentiate into an antibody-producing plasma cell, three steps are necessary. The first step involves binding of antigen (Ag) on to immunoglobulin molecules (Ig) on the surface of the B cell, which provides an initial signal for B-cell activation. The second step involves physical contact with a helper T lymphocyte, which further activates both the B cell and the T cell. The three major molecular interactions mediating the B- and T-cell contact involve CD40–CD40 ligand, MHC+ antigen with the T-cell receptor (TCR), and B7–CD28. This physical contact promotes B-cell proliferation and differentiation. The third step in B-cell differentiation involves cytokine stimulation. The activated T cell may produce different cytokines that promote immunoglobulin class switching (isotype switching). Differentiation into IgE-producing B cells and plasma cells is promoted by IL-4 and IL-5; IgG-producing B cells are promoted by IL-4 and INF-γ; and IgA-producing B cells are promoted by TGF-β and IL-5.

activation of CD4+ T cells. Deficiency of this molecule results in an unusual form of immunodeficiency termed the hyper-IgM syndrome.[23] Cytokines, such as IL-4, are responsible in switching B cells from IgM to IgE production, and TGF-β has been shown to play a role in B-cell switching to IgA production.[24] Immunodeficiencies that inhibit T-cell differentiation and proliferation commonly impair B-cell function and humoral immunity.

Activated cells of the immune system, including macrophages, monocytes, and B and T lymphocytes, produce a large number of multifunctional cytokines and chemokines. These can be categorized functionally into Th1-type cytokines, which stimulate cell-mediated immunity and cytotoxicity, and Th2-type cytokines, which stimulate humoral immunity and allergic responses.[25,26] These molecules promote activation of cells of the immune system, recruitment of effector cells such as neutrophils and eosinophils, and the production of acute-phase reactants by the liver. Many cytokines have both pro-inflammatory and anti-inflammatory effects. For example, IL-2 promotes differentiation of Th1 cells, which in turn mediate macrophage activation. However, IL-2 can also have anti-inflammatory effects, such as promoting lymphocyte apoptosis and increasing the population of CD4+CD25+ regulatory T cells.[27] Cytokines, such as IL-1 and tumor necrosis factor α (TNF-α), mediate clinical effects (including fever, diarrhea and hypotension) seen in rejection, shock and sepsis. IL-5 recruits eosinophils, whereas INF-γ activates macrophages to phagocytose and kill microbes.

The end-result of the immune response is the recruitment of activated effector cells (cytotoxic lymphocytes, macrophages, neutrophils, eosinophils and mast cells) to an infected or inflamed tissue.[3] In bacterial infections, neutrophils can phagocytose and degrade micro-organisms; this process is facilitated by opsonization of bacteria by immunoglobulin and complement.[3] In viral infections, infected cells are typically lysed by CD8 (cytotoxic) T cells, which have two distinct mechanisms of cytotoxicity: perforin and Fas ligand.[28] Perforin is a membrane pore-forming molecule, which allows release of granular enzymes (e.g. granzymes) directly into the cytosol of the target cells. Granzyme B induces rapid apoptosis of the target cell in caspase-dependent and caspase-independent manners.

The immune system also has ways of suppressing and downregulating immune responses. Regulatory T lymphocytes (CD4+ CD25+) release molecules that inhibit inflammation, including IL-10 and TGF-β. Oral tolerance to an antigen develops when dendritic cells exposed to dietary antigens produce IL-10 and TGF-β.[29]

Derangements at any point in this complex pathway may result in three principal types of clinical disorder in immunodeficient patients:

- Susceptibility to infection may be increased
- Autoimmune disease, including enteropathy, colitis and hepatitis, may occur, because dysfunctional mononuclear cells may be unable to suppress unwanted immune responses properly
- Increased risk of malignancy.

HUMORAL IMMUNODEFICIENCIES

Selective IgA deficiency

Selective IgA deficiency is the most common primary immunodeficiency, with a prevalence of approximately 1 in 500.[30] It has a male predominance, and in patients with IgA deficiency the serum IgA levels are significantly higher in winter than in other seasons.[31] The decreased IgA production probably results from a wide variety of potential immunologic derangements.[32–35] Individuals with this disorder have extremely low levels (less than 5 mg/dl) of serum and mucosal IgA; in addition, 15–20% of patients with selective IgA deficiency also have low levels of IgG subclasses IgG_2 and IgG_4. A compensatory increase in biologically active secretory IgM frequently protects against infection.[36,37] The pathogenesis of IgA deficiency is not known, although abnormalities in immunoglobulin class switching and the cytokines involved in isotype switching have been implicated. Studies of T-cell function have been normal in most patients with selective IgA deficiency. In a recent fine-scale genetic mapping at the *IGAD1* locus, a susceptibility locus for selective IgA deficiency/common variable immunodeficiency (CVI), the HLA-DQ/DR was found to be the major hereditary determinant of susceptibility to IgA deficiency/CVI.[38]

Most persons with selective IgA deficiency are asymptomatic. The precise mechanism of this lack of disease in IgA deficiency is unclear and is thought in part to be due to a compensatory increase in secretory IgM, and possibly in IgG as well.[39] However, patients with IgA deficiency are at increased risk for infections, gastrointestinal disease and autoimmune disease[39,40] (Table 38.4). Recurrent giardiasis refractory to antibiotic therapy may result in partial villus atrophy and secondary malabsorption.[30] Chronic

- Upper respiratory infections
- Otitis media
- Sinusitis
- Bronchiectasis
- Allergic disorders (including food allergies, asthma, eczema)
- Anaphylaxis to intravenous immunoglobulin
- Giardiasis
- Strongyloidiasis
- Nodular lymphoid hyperplasia
- Celiac disease (with false-negative antiendomysial antibody)
- Achlorhydria
- Malabsorption villus atrophy
- Cholelithiasis
- Inflammatory bowel disease
- Primary biliary cirrhosis
- Gastrointestinal carcinoma and lymphoma
- Henoch–Schönlein purpura
- Hepatitis C

Data from Cunningham-Rundles,[30,39] Leung et al.[41] and Meini et al.[44]

Table 38.4 Disorders associated with selective immunoglobulin A deficiency

Strongyloides infection, poorly responsive to antihelminthic therapy, has also been reported.[41]

The most common non-infectious complication of selective IgA deficiency is celiac disease. Antigliadin IgA, antiendomysial IgA and anti-tissue transglutaminase IgA antibodies commonly yield false-negative results and are unreliable screening tools in this population.[42] Heneghan et al.[43] found that, of 604 subjects with celiac sprue, 14 (2.3%) had IgA deficiency. In a prospective study in which jejunal biopsy was performed in 65 consecutive children with selective IgA deficiency, 7.7% showed diagnostic features of celiac disease.[44] In a separate study with pediatric population, Cataldo et al.[45] found that 12 (1.7%) of 688 patients with untreated celiac disease had selective IgA deficiency and did not produce endomysial antibody and IgA antigliadin antibody. In addition, there is an increased incidence of nodular lymphoid hyperplasia, food allergy, pernicious anemia and idiopathic villus atrophy in IgA-deficient patients.[30] There have been reported cases of a patient with selective IgA deficiency, celiac disease and ulcerative colitis,[46] a girl with selective IgA deficiency, celiac disease and atypical Turner syndrome,[47] and a patient with selective IgA deficiency and Crohn's disease.[48]

Antibiotic therapy with metronidazole or nitazoxanide should be administered to patients with selective IgA deficiency and giardiasis.[49] If diarrhea persists and biopsy demonstrates villus atrophy, a gluten-free diet may be therapeutic. Intravenous immunoglobulin (IVIG) should be avoided in patients with selective IgA deficiency, because it does not cross mucosal surfaces and may result in systemic anaphylaxis.[50] Finally, a small number of patients with selective IgA deficiency may develop common variable immunodeficiency (CVI), which has a much higher prevalence of gastrointestinal complications[51] (see below).

X-linked agammaglobulinemia

X-linked (Bruton's) agammaglobulinemia (XLA) manifests with recurrent infections after 9 months of age. In a study by Conley and Howard,[52] the mean age at diagnosis in the 60 patients with sporadic XLA was 35 (median 26, range 2–11) months. Affected boys have a paucity of peripheral lymphoid tissue and low serum levels of all classes of immunoglobulin. Humoral responses to specific antigens are markedly depressed or absent. The gene for XLA has been localized to chromosome Xq21.3-q22. B cells from affected persons have a defect in a B cell-specific tyrosine kinase gene (*BtK*).[53–55] Defects in the *Btk* gene affect the early stages of B-cell differentiation.[56]

The onset of recurrent bacterial infections is typically during the latter part of the first year of life, when the levels of maternal antibodies acquired passively through the placenta are no longer protective. Recurrent sinusitis, otitis media, pneumonia and bronchitis are the most common reported illnesses in persons with XLA. Autoimmune disease (including arthritis and dermatomyosis) may also develop.[57] Patients with XLA are at risk for disseminated echovirus infection with central nervous system involvement.[58] Chronic enteritis develops in 10%; identifiable causes of the enteritis include *Giardia*, *Salmonella*, *Campylobacter*, *Cryptosporidium*, rotavirus, coxsackievirus and poliovirus. In a multicenter survey, gastrointestinal infections with recurrent diarrhea were seen in 13% of patients with XLA.[59] Associations with sclerosing cholangitis and a sprue-like illness have also been noted.[60–63] Patients with XLA, small bowel strictures and transmural intestinal fissures resembling Crohn's disease have been seen. In contrast to Crohn's disease, however, no granulomas or plasma cells are identified when strictures are resected.[57,64] In a reported case, the regional enteritis of the terminal ileum in a patient with XLA was thought to be due to enterovirus infection.[65] Patients with XLA may also be at increased risk for small and large bowel cancers.[61,66]

Hyper-IgM syndrome

This syndrome is a rare humoral immune disorder that affects mainly boys (55–65%) and is characterized by severe recurrent bacterial infections with decreased serum levels of IgG, IgA and IgE but raised IgM levels.[67] The molecular basis for the X-linked form of immunodeficiency with hyper-IgM (HIGM) has been identified as a T-cell defect, in which mutations in the gene that encodes the CD40 ligand molecule are present. The T cell's CD40 ligand cannot interact with the CD40 molecule on the B-cell surface, resulting in impaired isotype switching from IgM to IgG or IgA, and reduced functional antibody.[53,68,69]

An autosomal recessive form of hyper-IgM syndrome has also been reported.[70,71] Family consanguinity is frequent. These patients express CD40 ligand normally, and the surface expression of CD40 on B cells is also normal.[72] Molecular studies have shown that the defect in the autosomal variant of HIGM syndrome (HIGM2) is a mutation in the gene that encodes activation-induced cytidine deaminase (AID).[71]

Boys with hyper-IgM syndrome present at between 1 month and 10 years of life with opportunistic infections. Chronic encephalitis and idiopathic neurologic deterioration may occur.[73] Gastrointestinal complications reported include histoplasmosis of the esophagus, cryptosporidiosis, giardiasis, hepatosplenomegaly, intestinal lymphoid hyperplasia and recurrent large painful oral ulcerations[63,73–76] (Figs 38.4 and 38.5). Protracted or recurrent diarrhea is common, occurring in about one-third of the patients, and *Cryptosporidium* is the most frequently isolated pathogen.[77] Patients with hyper-IgM syndrome are also at increased risk for intestinal lymphoma.

Abnormal transaminase and alkaline phosphatase levels are seen in 50% of patients. Two separate series have suggested that sclerosing cholangitis and cirrhosis occur in up to 35% of patients older than 10 years of age.[73,78] Pancreatic and hepatobiliary malignancies have been reported in patients as young as 7 years of age.[78] In a recent case report, a child with CHARGE association was found to have hyper-IgM syndrome, but it is unclear whether these conditions are related.[79]

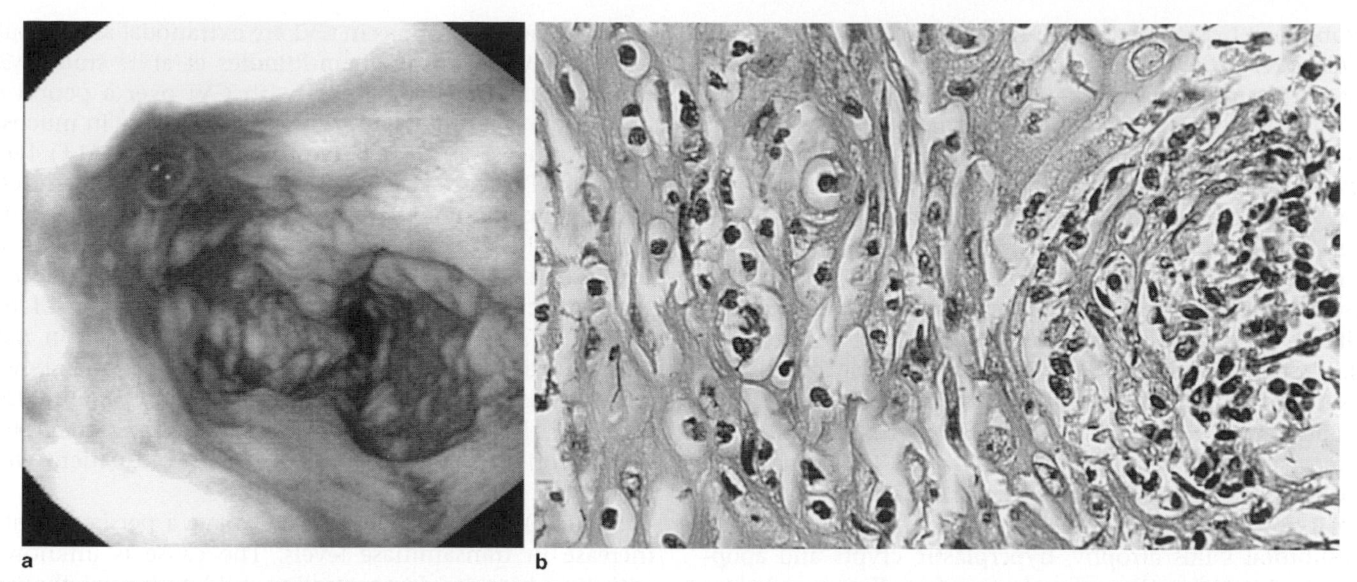

Figure 38.4: Esophageal candidiasis in a patient with the hyper-IgM syndrome. (**a**) Endoscopic view of the esophagus demonstrates near-complete coating of the esophageal mucosa with a creamy white exudate. (Courtesy of Drs Carine Lenders and Samuel Nurko.) (**b**) Esophageal histology demonstrates inflammatory cells and pseudohyphae. (Courtesy of Dr. Kameran Badizadegan, Children's Hospital, Boston, MA.)

Transient hypogammaglobulinemia of infancy

Transient hypogammaglobulinemia of infancy (THI) is a poorly defined condition characterized by low serum immunoglobulin levels in infancy, with attainment of normal levels at a later time. Serum IgG is typically low, without any subclass specificity; IgA or IgM levels may also be decreased. Kilic et al.[80] found that 33 of 40 children with THI recovered before 36 months of age. The prevalence of this condition in infants with recurrent infections ranges from 0.1% to 5% in different studies.[81,82] Children with THI typically present with recurrent respiratory infections at 6–12 months of age. Although the immunoglobulin deficiency usually resolves in later childhood, a subset of children has persistent hypogammaglobulinemia, which may evolve into CVI.[3]

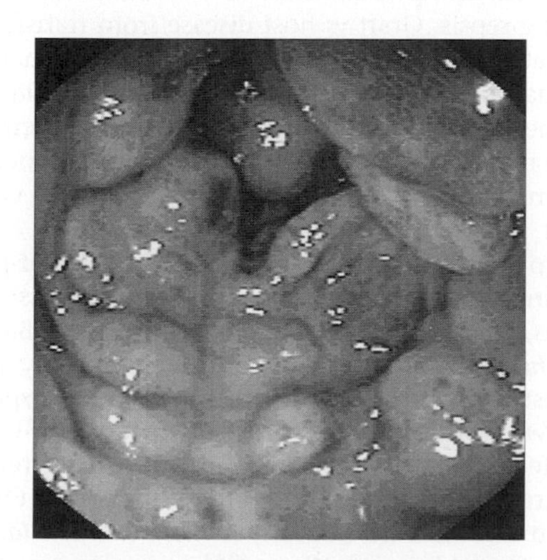

Figure 38.5: Massive lymphoid nodular hyperplasia seen in the colon of a patient with hyper-IgM syndrome. (Courtesy of Dr. Victor Fox, Children's Hospital, Boston, MA.)

Chronic diarrhea is the second most common complication in these patients after respiratory illness. Lactose intolerance, *Giardia lamblia* infestation or *Clostridium difficile* infection were found in one-third of 55 children with low serum immunoglobulin levels and chronic diarrhea. Small bowel histology demonstrated enteritis or villus atrophy in up to 50% of these patients. It is unclear whether these patients had THI or enteric protein loss from the intestinal illness.[84] In children with recurrent *C. difficile* infection unresponsive to antibiotics and low antibody titers to *C. difficile*, IVIG has resulted in clearance of the infection.[85]

COMBINED CELLULAR–HUMORAL IMMUNODEFICIENCIES

Common variable immunodeficiency

CVI, also called acquired hypogammaglobulinemia, adult-onset hypogammaglobulinemia or dysgammaglobulinemia, is a rare heterogeneous group of disorders affecting between 1 in 50 000 and 1 in 200 000 persons. It is characterized by hypogammaglobulinemia, recurrent infections, enteropathy, autoimmune disease and malignancy. Up to 45% of cases are diagnosed in childhood.[86] The cause of CVI is unknown, but B-lymphocyte differentiation into plasma cells is impaired.[87–90] The different abnormalities reflect the variability of CVI, and support the concept that more than one gene is probably responsible for the immune abnormalities in CVI.

Patients typically present in late childhood and young adulthood with recurrent sinusitis, bronchitis and pneumonia. Common causes of the respiratory illness include *Streptococcus pneumoniae*, *Haemophilus influenzae* and *Mycoplasma pneumoniae*; mycobacteria, *Pneumocystis* and fungi are less frequent pathogens. Diagnosis of CVI is established by demonstration of persistently low antibody levels over time and impaired responses to standard pediatric immunizations; in a male, XLA must be excluded.[87,91]

Gastrointestinal disease occurs in up to 70% of patients and accounts for much of the morbidity (Table 38.5). Infectious diarrhea caused by a wide variety of pathogens may occur. Nodular lymphoid hyperplasia is detected radiographically or endoscopically in up to 20% of patients, and may predispose to either malabsorption or gastrointestinal bleeding.[92,93] In one case report, a 40-year-old patient with CVI developed cytomegalovirus infection of the stomach and small bowel with multiple ulcers and strictures, resulting in intestinal obstruction.[94]

Between 10% and 20% of patients with CVI have an enteropathy characterized by weight loss, abdominal pain and severe diarrhea in the absence of enteric infection. Small bowel biopsy in these patients demonstrates partial or subtotal villus atrophy, hyperplastic crypts and apoptotic bodies.[64,95,96] Gluten- or lactose-free diets may help a subset of patients, but most improve when treated with an elemental diet, although parenteral nutrition may also be required.[95,97–99] The severe malabsorption may result in vitamin B_{12} deficiency and/or zinc deficiency.[97,100]

An inflammatory bowel disease-like syndrome, characterized by small intestinal strictures and microscopic colitis, may occur.[57,95] Unlike Crohn's disease, there is generally no granulomatous inflammation in this enteropathy. A necrotizing variant of this enteropathy requiring colectomy at 10 months of age was reported in an infant with CVI.[101] Another condition that may be confused with inflammatory bowel disease is a non-infectious granulomatous illness resembling sarcoidosis, which also involves the skin and lung.[102,103]

Patients with CVI are at a 30-fold increased risk for the development of gastric carcinoma or malignant lymphoma. The lymphomas in CVI are extranodal and usually B cell in type. Cunningham-Rundles et al.[104] studied 22 B-cell lymphomas in patients with CVI over a period of 25 years, and found that five lymphomas arose in mucosal sites – mucosa-associated lymphoid tissue (MALT) lymphomas. These MALT lymphomas are low-grade B-cell lymphomas and tend to occur in organs that have acquired lymphoid tissue as a result of long-term infectious or autoimmune stimulation (e.g. chronic gastric *Helicobacter pylori* infection and chronic hepatitis C infection of the liver).[104] *H. pylori* infection and *p53* gene mutation may play a role in the gastric carcinogenesis.[105] The small bowel lymphomas reported may manifest with intestinal malabsorption.[64,87] In addition, a cecal carcinoma of neuroendocrine origin was reported in a 16-year-old patient with CVI.[106]

Some 20% of patients with CVI have a persistent mild increase in transaminase levels. The cause is unknown, with liver biopsies demonstrating mild periportal changes or granulomas.[57] Hepatitis C is now reported as a complication of IVIG infusion in patients with CVI,[107,108] and it may progress rapidly to cirrhosis with a poor outcome.[109–111]

Therapy for CVI consists of monthly IVIG infusions and symptomatic treatment of infections and malabsorption.[112] Epstein–Barr virus infections in patients with CVI may respond to IFN-α.[113]

- Enteric infections (including *Shigella, Salmonella* and dysgonic fermenter 3)
- Giardiasis
- Cryptosporidiosis
- Nodular lymphoid hyperplasia
- Enterocolitis
- Enteropathy, malabsorption, wasting syndrome
- Perirectal abscess
- Short stature
- Zinc deficiency
- Inflammatory bowel disease
- Ménétrier's disease
- Atrophic gastritis or pernicious anemia
- Gastric adenocarcinoma
- Intestinal lymphoma
- Cecal carcinoma (undifferentiated)
- Hepatitis C with cirrhosis

Data from Sneller et al.,[87] Cunningham-Rundles,[91] Sperber and Mayer,[97] de Bruin et al.,[106] Quinti et al.,[107] Eisenstein and Sneller,[112] and Cunningham-Rundles and Bodian.[200]

Table 38.5 Gastrointestinal complications of common variable immunodeficiency

Severe combined immunodeficiency

The term severe combined immunodeficiency (SCID) refers to a group of diseases characterized by molecular defects interfering with T-and/or B-cell differentiation and resulting in an infant with failure to thrive and extreme susceptibility to infections.[114–116] Approximately 20 defective genes have been associated with SCID; patients are classified according to the specific mutation present, the associated lymphocyte phenotype and mode of inheritance[2,53,114,117–120] (see Table 38.1). Presenting features include growth impairment, chronic diarrhea, persistent thrush or candidiasis, and overwhelming sepsis. Graft *vs* host disease from transfusions of unirradiated blood, or disseminated illness from live vaccines, may occur if the diagnosis is delayed. Diagnosis is established by the demonstration of low or absent T-lymphocyte numbers in peripheral blood; B-cell and neutrophil counts may also be depressed, depending on the variant of SCID.[115]

Gastrointestinal illness occurs in up to 90% of patients. Organisms frequently associated with illness include rotavirus, *Candida*, cytomegalovirus, Epstein–Barr virus and *Escherichia coli*. Although candidiasis rarely involves the intestine, candidal esophagitis should be suspected in infants with SCID and decreased oral intake.[63,121] Chronic viral infection is the most frequent cause of enteritis and may be responsible for death in 80% of cases.[122] Other less common causes of enteropathy include *Salmonella, Shigella* and *Cryptosporidium* infections.[60,63]

Autoimmune enteropathy has been described in at least one patient with defective T-lymphocyte function;[123] in addition, patients with SCID are prone to various autoimmune complications (including hemolytic anemia and glomerulonephritis).[121] Boeck et al.[124] found clinically significant gastroesophageal reflux in 20.5% of patients with SCID, much higher than that reported for the normal population (0.1–0.3%), but the mechanism is unknown.

Hepatic abnormalities are also common in patients with SCID, and include graft *vs* host disease of the liver, adenovirus and cytomegalovirus hepatitis, rotavirus hepatitis, parenteral nutrition-associated liver disease, and lymphoproliferative disorder.[125,126] Pancreatic infection by viruses has also been described.[127]

One variant of SCID that seems to render a patient particularly prone to gastrointestinal complications is *bare lymphocyte syndrome*. Gastrointestinal candidiasis is common in addition to giardiasis, cryptosporidiosis and other bacterial enteritides. A high incidence of hepatobiliary abnormalities is noted, including sclerosing cholangitis associated with biliary cryptosporidiosis. Bacterial cholangitis secondary to *Pseudomonas, Enterococcus* and *Streptococcus* infections has been described.[128]

The principal therapy for patients with SCID is bone marrow transplantation, ideally from a matched sibling. In patients with SCID with adenosine deaminase deficiency, infusions of a long-acting form of adenosine deaminase correct metabolic abnormalities and provide some restoration of immune function.[129] In addition, gene replacement therapy has also been used in these patients, with some success.[130]

OTHER PRIMARY IMMUNODEFICIENCIES

Wiskott–Aldrich syndrome

Wiskott–Aldrich syndrome (WAS) is an X-linked immunodeficiency characterized by the classic triad of severe eczema, thrombocytopenia with small platelets, and recurrent opportunistic and pyogenic infections. The gene for this syndrome has been identified on the short arm of the X chromosome at Xp11.22-p11.23.[131] The gene product, WAS protein (WASp), is expressed only in hematopoietic cells, and belongs to a unique family of proteins that are responsible for transduction of signals from the cell membrane to the actin cytoskeleton. The interaction between WASp, the Rho family GTPase CDC42, and the cytoskeletal organizing complex Arp2/3 is critical to many of these functions, which, when disturbed as a result of WASp mutations, translate into measurable defects of cell signaling, polarization, motility and phagocytosis.[132–134] Children are usually diagnosed before 2 years of age, after presenting with epistaxis, purpura, recurrent otitis, sinusitis, pneumonia, opportunistic infections or diarrhea.[135]

Gastrointestinal complications occur in 10–30% of patients. Gastrointestinal bleeding from thrombocytopenia can antedate the diagnosis. Infectious diarrhea occurs in up to 25% of cases, although opportunistic pathogens are unusual. Henoch–Schönlein purpura may occur in up to 5% of patients, and necrotizing enterocolitis has been reported in one patient.[135] A steroid-responsive inflammatory bowel disease characterized by bloody diarrhea and colonic pseudo-polyps has been seen.[136] Finally, patients with Wiskott–Aldrich syndrome are at a 100-fold increased risk of developing lymphoma, which may originate in the gut.[135]

Chronic granulomatous disease

Chronic granulomatous disease (CGD) refers to a group of immunodeficiencies characterized by the inability of an affected patient's neutrophils to generate superoxide and hydrogen peroxide, leaving the patient susceptible to infections with catalase-positive organisms.[137] The disease has an estimated incidence of 1 in 250 000 persons, with an X-linked inheritance pattern seen in two-thirds of patients and autosomal recessive inheritance in the remainder.[138,139] The X-linked form is due to a mutation in the gene for the phagocytic oxidase cytochrome glycoprotein of 91 kDa (gp91^{phox}), and the autosomal recessive form is due to a mutation in the gene for a cytosolic component of 47-kDa (p47^{phox}) protein.[140] The most common presenting features involve suppurative infections by catalase-positive organisms, such as *Staphylococcus aureus, Serratia, Aspergillus, Candida* and *Nocardia*.[141,142]

Gastrointestinal involvement is often pronounced. Many patients with CGD present with gastric outlet obstruction secondary to pronounced antral narrowing[141,143] (Fig. 38.6). The antral narrowing is usually caused by a combination of infection and granulomatous inflammation. It may resolve with a combination of antibiotics and corticosteroid therapy, but may also require surgical intervention.[143,144] Similar obstructive lesions of the esophagus occur less frequently.[141] Small bowel involvement may mimic Crohn's disease, with multifocal abscesses, fistulae and granulomatous colitis. The presence of lipid-containing histiocytes in the mucosa and submucosa of colonic biopsies strongly suggests CGD colitis.[145,146] Such colitis may respond to therapy with corticosteroids, IFN-γ or ciclosporin, but surgical resection may be necessary for intractable colitis or acute obstruction.[145–147] Pyogenic or fungal liver abscess is also a common complication of CGD; it is treated with appropriate antimicrobial agents, surgical drainage and possibly IFN-γ.[148] Prophylactic IFN-γ may reduce the frequency of opportunistic infections.[142,149]

Chronic mucocutaneous candidiasis

Chronic mucocutaneous candidiasis is characterized by a diminished T-cell response to candidal antigens. Infants with this disorder present with persistent thrush or candidal dermatitis, failure to thrive and dystrophic nails. Candidal esophagitis may result in refusal of foods. A polyglandular endocrinopathy syndrome characterized by hypoparathyroidism, hypothyroidism, adrenal insufficiency and pernicious anemia develops in up to 70% of older children. Malabsorption secondary to pancreatic insufficiency contributes to the poor weight gain in 10% of patients. Therapy includes eradication of *Candida* with topical antibiotics plus

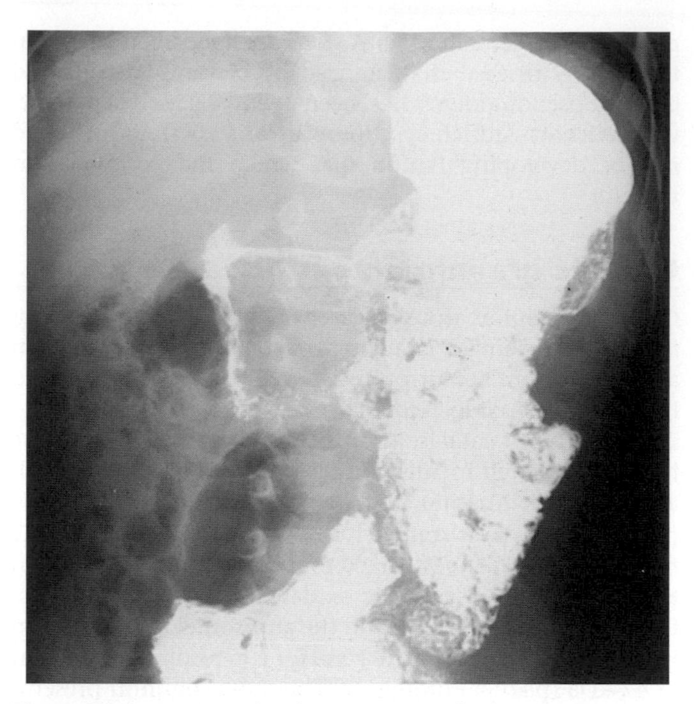

Figure 38.6: Gastric outlet obstruction secondary to antral narrowing in a patient with chronic granulomatous disease. The patient underwent partial gastrectomy, with inflammatory cells and granulomas identified in the hypertrophied antral tissue. (Courtesy of Dr. Thorne Griscom and Children's Hospital, Boston, Radiology Teaching File.)

ketoconazole or fluconazole, as well as hormone or pancreatic enzyme replacement when appropriate.[150,151]

Leukocyte-adhesion deficiency

Leukocyte-adhesion deficiency type I is characterized by impaired phagocytic function secondary to deficiencies of adhesion molecules (CD18/β2 integrin) necessary for cell migration and interactions, and is an autosomal recessive disorder.[152] The second type of leukocyte adhesion deficiency is a defect of carbohydrate fucosylation and is associated with growth retardation, dysmorphic features and neurologic deficits.[153–155] The genetic defect of the second type has not been determined. Necrotic infections of the skin (including pyoderma gangrenosum) and mucous membranes, otitis media and episodes of microbial sepsis are the principal features.[156,157] Gastrointestinal complications include intraoral infections and periodontitis, candidal esophagitis, gastritis, appendicitis, necrotizing enterocolitis and perirectal abscess.[156,158,159] Fatal enterocolitis similar to that of necrotizing enterocolitis or Hirschsprung's disease has been described in an infant with leukocyte adhesion deficiency.[160,161]

Intestinal lymphangiectasia

Primary lymphangiectasia is a congenital disorder of the lymphatic system characterized by marked ectasia of the lymphatic vessels resulting in obstruction and leakage of lymph fluid.[162] Intestinal lymphangiectasia is characterized by a protein-losing enteropathy resulting in hypoproteinemia and lymphocytopenia due to blocked intestinal lymphatics and loss of lymph fluid into the gastrointestinal tract. Intestinal lymphangiectasia is diagnosed definitively by small bowel biopsy demonstrating dilated lymphatics in the mucosa, submucosa and serosa in the absence of coexisting inflammation.[163–165] Clinical symptoms include diarrhea, vomiting, peripheral edema, lymphedematous limbs, generalized malaise and weight loss.[163–167] Bacterial and viral infections have been reported in patients with primary intestinal lymphangiectasia.[168,169] Intestinal lymphangiectasia may occur in isolation or simultaneously in the same patient as part of a generalized lymphatic dysplasia. It primarily affects children and young adults, but has also been described prenatally, in full-term infants and in premature infants.[170,171] Treatment includes corticosteroids,[172] dietary modifications,[173] surgery,[174] octreotide[175,176] and antiplasmin therapy.[177,178]

NF-κB essential modifier mutations

NF-κB essential modifier (NEMO) mutations have been identified in patients with X-linked hyper-IgM and hypohidrotic ectodermal dysplasia (HED).[179] B-cell switching and antigen-presenting cell activation are impaired with NEMO mutations. Certain mutations of NEMO are associated with deficient natural killer (NK) cell cytotoxicity,[180] and dysgammaglobulinemia with very poor specific antibody production.[181] Patients display features of HED with conical teeth and absence (or hypoplasia) of hair, teeth and sweat glands.[181] Recurrent bacterial and viral infections often occur in infancy.

Gastrointestinal symptoms include persistent vomiting, chronic diarrhea, recurrent cytomegalovirus colitis and giardiasis.[180–182] Growth delay is common as a result of infection and poor nutrition due to gastrointestinal symptoms. Parenteral nutrition is often used to provide adequate nutritional support.

X-linked lymphoproliferative disease

X-linked lymphoproliferative disease (XLP) is characterized by three major clinical phenotypes: fulminant infectious mononucleosis (50%), B-cell lymphomas (20%) and dysgammaglobulinemia (20%).[183,184] An XLP registry was established in 1978 and has approximately 300 patients registered from over 80 families.[183] The mutated gene in XLP has been identified on the long arm of the X chromosome at Xq24-25, encoding for the protein SH2D1A, also known as SAP for SLAM (signaling lymphocytic activation molecule)-associated protein.[185,186] This protein plays an important role in intracellular signaling by associating with the surface activating receptors SLAM (CD105) and 2B4 (CD244) that are present on T and NK cells.[187]

Hepatosplenomegaly, fulminant hepatitis and hepatic necrosis are the common gastrointestinal manifestations in patients with XLP with fulminant infectious mononucleosis. Uncontrolled lymphocyte proliferation, organ infiltration and T-cell cytotoxic activity lead to multiorgan failure; hepatic necrosis and bone marrow failure constitute the most common events that determine death in these patients.[188] Intestinal lymphoma involving the ileum and cecum is well described, and the malignant lymphomas are usually non-Hodgkin's lymphoma of the Burkitt type.[189] Chemotherapy is often used for treatment, but outcome is generally poor. The mortality rate of XLP is 100% by the age of 40 years, and XLP is generally fatal in the first decade of life in patients with XLP with either fulminant infectious mononucleosis or B-cell lymphoma.

Glycogen storage disease

Patients with glycogen storage disease type 1B (GSD-1B) present with severe hypoglycemia, failure to thrive and hepatomegaly. In contrast to von Gierke's disease (GSD-1A), these patients have severe neutropenia and phagocytic dysfunction.[190] GSD-1B is characterized by absence of the hepatic glucose 6-phosphate transport protein.[191]

Patients with GSD-1B may develop an idiopathic colitis clinically similar to Crohn's disease.[192,193] Granulocyte–macrophage colony-stimulating factor was used in the treatment of two patients with GSD-1B, and increased neutrophil counts with concurrent improvement in the bowel inflammation were noted.[194]

Ataxia telangiectasia

Ataxia telangiectasia is a recessive disorder characterized by progressive neurologic degeneration, ocular and skin telangiectasias, and immunodeficiency predisposing to infections and malignancies.[195] Chronic diarrhea and gastrointestinal cancers have both been reported as complications of ataxia telangiectasia.[196,197]

Novel immunodeficiency

Bernard et al.[198] have recently described a novel syndrome characterized by severe prenatal and postnatal growth failure, mild skeletal and facial abnormalities, and primary immunodeficiency including mild neutropenia, low peripheral CD8+ αβ T cells and lack of NK cells. One of the two patients died when aged 18 months from cytomegalovirus disease, and the younger sibling is now well at 5 years of age without significant infection. The molecular basis has not yet been identified.

Shwachman's syndrome

Shwachman's syndrome, characterized by pancreatic insufficiency, neutropenia and metaphyseal dysostosis, is reviewed elsewhere in the book.

References

1. Rosen F, Wedgwood R, Eibl M, et al. Primary immunodeficiency disease: report of a WHO scientific group. Clin Exp Immunol 1995; 1(Suppl 99):1-24.
2. International Union of Immunological Societies. Primary immunodeficiency. Report of an IUIS Scientific Committee. Clin Exp Immunol 1999; 118(Suppl 1):1–28.
3. Stiehm ER, Ochs HD, Winkelstein JA. Immunologic Disorders in Infants and Children. Philadelphia, PA: Elsevier Saunders; 2004.
4. Centers for Disease Control and Prevention. AIDS among children – United States, 1996. MMWR Morbid Mortal Wkly Rep 1996; 45:1005–1010.
5. Yuan Q, Walker WA. Innate immunity of the gut: mucosal defense in health and disease. J Pediatr Gastroenterol Nutr 2004; 38:463–473.
6. Medzhitov R. Toll-like receptors and innate immunity. Nat Rev Immunol 2001; 1:135–145.
7. Sanderson I, Walker W. Uptake and transport of macromolecules by the intestine: possible role in clinical disorders. Gastroenterology 1993; 104:622–639.
8. Pabst E. The anatomical basis for the immune function of the gut. Anat Embryol (Berl) 1987; 176:135–143.
9. Grey H, Sette A, Buus S. How T cells see antigen. Sci Am 1989; 261:56–64.
10. Abbas A, Lichtman A. Antigen processing and presentation to T lymphocytes. In: Cellular and Molecular Immunology, 5th edn. Philadelphia, PA: WB Saunders; 2003:81–104.
11. Shimizu Y, van Seventer GA, Ennis E, et al. Crosslinking of the T cell-specific accessory molecules CD7 and CD28 modulates T cell adhesion. J Exp Med 1992; 175:577–582.
12. van der Merwe P, Davis S. Molecular interactions mediating T cell antigen recognition. Annu Rev Immunol 2003; 21:659–684.
13. Wecker H, Auchinchloss H. Cellular mechanisms of rejection. Curr Opin Immunol 1992; 4:561–566.
14. Abbas A, Lichtman A. Activation ofT lymphocytes. In: Cellular and Molecular Immunology, 5th edn. Philadelphia, PA: WB Saunders; 2003:163–188.
15. Sigal N, Dumont F. Cyclosporin A, FK-506, and rapamycin: pharmacologic probes of lymphocyte signal transduction. Annu Rev Immunol 1992; 10:519–560.
16. Rothwarf DM, Zandi E, Natoli G, et al. IKK-gamma is an essential regulatory subunitofthe IkappaB kinase complex. Nature 1998; 395:297–300.
17. Yamaoka S, Courtois G, Bessia C, et al. Complementation cloning of the NEMO, a compent of the IkappaB kinase complex essential for NF-kappaB activation. Cell 1998; 93:1231–1240.
18. Dong C, Davis R, Flavell R. MAP kinases in the immune response. Annu Rev Immunol 2002; 20:55–72.
19. Mosmann T, Coffman R. TH1 and TH2 cells: different patterns of lymphokine secretion lead to different functional properties. Annu Rev Immunol 1989; 7:145–173.
20. Neurath MS, Finotto S, Glimcher L. The role of Th1/Th2 polarization in mucosal immunity. Nat Med 2002; 8:567–573.
21. Abbas A, Lichtman A. Immunological tolerance. In: Cellular and Molecular Immunology. Philadelphia, PA: Saunders; 2003:216–239.
22. Rudin C, Thompson C. B cell development and maturation. Semin Oncol 1998; 25:435–446.
23. Alien RC, Armitage RJ, Conley ME, et al. CD40 ligand gene defects responsible forX-linked hyper-IgM syndrome. Science 1993; 259:990–993.
24. Abbas A, Lichtman A. B cell activation and antibody production. In: Cellular and Molecular Immunology, 5th edn. Philadelphia, PA: WB Saunders; 2003:189–205.

25. Yoshie 0, Imai T, Nomiyama H. Chemokines in immunity. Adv Immunol 2001; 78:57–110.
26. Hill N, Sarvetnick N. Cytokines: promoters and dampeners of autoimmunity. Curr Opin Immunol 2002; 14:791–797.
27. O'Shea J, Ma A, Lipsky P. Cytokines and autoimmunity. Nat Immunol 2002; 2:37–45.
28. Russell JH, Ley TJ. Lymphocyte-mediated cytotoxicity. Annu Rev Immunol 2002; 20:323–370.
29. Mowat A. Anatomical basis of tolerance and immunity to intestinal antigens. Nat Immunol 2003; 3:331–341.
30. Cunningham-Rundles C. Selective IgA deficiency and the gastrointestinal tract. Immunol Allergy Clin North Am 1988; 8:435–449.
31. Weber-Mzell D, Kotanko P, Hauer AC, et al. Gender, age and seasonal effects on IgA deficiency: a study of 7293 Caucasians. Eur J Clin Invest 2004; 34:224–228.
32. StroberW, Harriman G. The regulation of IgA B cell differentiation. Gastroenterol Clin North Am 1991; 20:473–494.
33. Strober W, Krakauer R, Klaeveman H, et al. Secretory component deficiency: a disorder of the IgA immune system. N Engl J Med 1976; 294:351–356.
34. Conley M, Cooper M. Immature IgA B cell in IgA deficient patients. N Engl J Med 1981; 305:475–479.
35. Briere F, Bridon J, Chevet D, et al. Interleukin 10 induces B lymphocytes from IgA deficient patients to secrete IgA. J Clin Invest 1994; 94:94–104.
36. Morgan G, Levinsky R. Clinical significance of IgA deficiency. Arch Dis Child 1988; 63:579–581.
37. Oxelius V, Laurell A, Lindquist B, et al. IgG subclasses in selective IgA deficiency: common occurrence of lgG2a deficiency. N Engl J Med 1981; 304:1476–1477.
38. Kralovicova J, Hammarstrom L, Plebani A, et al. Fine-scale mapping at IGAD1 and genome-wide genetic linkage analysis implicate HLA-DQ/DR as a major susceptibility locus in selective IgA deficiency and common variable immunodeficiency. J Immunol 2003; 170:2765–2775.
39. Cunningham-Rundles C. Physiology of IgA and IgA deficiency. J Clin Immunol 2001; 21:303–309.
40. Zinneman H, Kaplan A. The association of giardiasis with reduced secretory immunoglobulin A. Am J Dig Dis 1972; 17:793–797.
41. Leung V, Liew C, Sung J. Strongyloidiasis in patient with IgA deficiency. Trop Gastroenterol 1995; 16:27–30.
42. Rittmeyer C, Rhoads J. IgA deficiency causes false-negative endomysial antibody results in celiac disease. J Pediatr Gastroenterol Nutr 1996; 23:504–506.
43. Heneghan MA, Stevens FM, Cryan EM, et al. Celiac sprue and immunodeficiency states: a 25-year review. J Clin Gastroenterol 1997; 25:421–425.
44. Meini A, Pillan N, Villanacci V, et al. Prevalence and diagnosis of celiac disease in IgA deficient children. Ann Allergy Asthma Immunol 1996; 77:333–336.
45. Cataldo F, Marino V, Bottaro G, et al. Celiac disease and selective immunoglobulin A deficiency. J Pediatr 1997; 131:306–308.
46. Falchuk K, Falchuk Z. Selective immunoglobulin A deficiency, ulcerative colitis, and gluten-sensitive enteropathy: a unique association. Gastroenterology 1975; 69:503–506.
47. Schewior S, Brand M, Santer R. Celiac disease and selective IgA deficiency in a girl with atypical Turner syndrome. J Pedia Gastroenterol Nutr 1999; 28:353–354.
48. Lizuka M, Itou H, Sato M, et al. Crohn's disease associated with selective immunoglobulin A deficiency. J Gastroenterol Hepatol 2001; 16:951.
49. Shepherd R, Boreham P. Recent advances in the diagnosis and management of giardiasis. Scand J Gastroenterol 1989; 24(Suppl 169):60–64.
50. Burks A, Sampson H, Buckley R. Anaphylactic reactions following gammaglobulin administration in patients with hypogammaglobulinemia: detection of IgE antibodies to IgA. N Engl J Med 1986; 314:560–564.
51. Espanol T, Catala M, Hernendez M, et al. Development of a common variable immunodeficiency in IgA deficient patients. Clin Immunol Immunopathol 1996; 80:333–335.
52. Conley ME, Howard V. Clinical findings leading to the diagnosis of X-linked agammaglobulinemia. J Pediatr 2002; 141:566–571.
53. Ochs H, Aruffo A. Advances in X-linked immunodeficiency diseases. Curr Opin Pediatr 1993; 5:684–691.
54. Tsukada S, Saffran D, Rawlings D, et al. Deficient expression of a B cell cytoplasmic tyrosine kinase in human X-linked agammaglobulinemia. Cell 1993; 72:279–290.
55. Holinski-Feder E, Weiss M, Brandau O, et al. Mutation screening of the BTK gene in 56 families with X-linked agammaglobulinemia (XLA): 47 unique mutations without correlation to clinical course. Pediatrics 1998; 101: 276–284.
56. Conley ME. B cells in patients with X-linked agammaglobulinemia. J Immunol 1985; 134:3070–3074.
57. Hermaszewski R, Webster A. Primary hypogammaglobulinemia: a survey of clinical manifestations and complications. Q J Med 1993; 86:31–42.
58. Ochs HD, Smith CI. X-linked agammaglobulinemia. A clinical and molecular analysis. Medicine (Baltimore) 1996; 75:287–299.
59. Plebani A, Soresina A, Rondelli R, et al. Clinical, immunological, and molecular analysis in a large cohort of patients with X-linked agammaglobulinemia: an Italian multicenter study. Clin Immunol 2002; 104:221–230.
60. Arbo A, Santos J. Diarrheal diseases in the immunocompromised host. Pediatr Infect Dis 1987; 6:894–906.
61. Lederman H, Winkelstein J. X-linked agammaglobulinemia: an analysis of 96 patients. Medicine (Baltimore) 1985; 64:145–156.
62. Sisto A, Feldman P, Garel L, et al. Primary sclerosing cholangitis in children: study of 5 cases and review of the literature. Pediatrics 1987; 80:918–923.
63. Stiehm E, Chin T, Haas A, et al. Infectious complications of the primary immunodeficiencies. Clin Immunol Immunopathol 1986; 40:69–86.
64. Washington K. Gastrointestinal pathology in patients with common variable immunodeficiency and X-linked agammaglobulinemia. Am J Surg Pathol 1996; 20: 1240–1252.
65. Collier C, Foray S, Hermine O. Regional enteritis associated with enterovirus in a patient with X-linked agammaglobulinemia. N Engl J Med 2000; 342:1611–1612.
66. van der Meer J, Weening R, Schellekens P, et al. Colorectal cancer in patients with X-linked agammaglobulinemia. Lancet 1993; 341:1439–1440.
67. Notarangelo LD, Duse M, Ugazio AG. Immunodeficiency with hyper-IgM (HIM). Immunodefic Rev 1992; 3:101–122.
68. Fuleihan R, Ramesh N, Loh R, et al. Defective expression of the CD40 ligand in X chromosome linked immunoglobulin deficiency with normal or elevated IgM. Proc Natl Acad Sci USA 1993; 90:2170–2173.
69. Alien R, Armitage R, Conley M, et al. CD40 ligand defects responsible for X-linked hyper-IgM syndrome. Science 1993; 259:990–993.

70. Minegishi Y, Lavoie A, Cunningham-Rundles C, et al. Mutations in activation induced cytidine deaminase in patients with hyper IgM syndrome. Clin Immunol 2000; 97:203–210.

71. Revy P, Muto T, Levy Y, et al. Activation-induced cytidine deaminase (AID) deficiency causes the autosomal recessivce form of the hyper-IgM syndrome (HIGM2). Cell 2000; 102:565–575.

72. Oliva A, Quinti I, Scala E, et al. Immunodeficiency with hyperimmunoglobulinemia M in two female patients is not associated with abnormalities of CD40 or CD40 ligand expression. J Allergy Clin Immunol 1995; 96:403–410.

73. Banatvala N, Davies J, Kanariou M, et al. Hypogammaglobulinemia associated with normal or increased IgM (the hyper IgM syndrome): a case series review. Arch Dis Child 1994; 71:150–152.

74. Hostohoffer R, Berger M, Clark H, et al. Disseminated *Histoplasma capsulatum* infection in a patient with hyper IgM immunodeficiency. Pediatrics 1994; 94:234–236.

75. Quartier P, Bustamante J, Sanal O, et al. Clinical, immunologic and genetic analysis of 29 patients with autosomal recessive hyper-IgM syndrome due to activation-induced cytidine deaminase deficiency. Clin Immunol 2004; 110:22–29.

76. Chang MW, Romero R, Scholl PR, et al. Mucocutaneous manifestations of the hyper-IgM immunodeficiency syndrome. J Am Acad Dermatol 1998; 38:191–196.

77. Winkelstein JA, Marino MC, Ochs H, et al. The X-linked hyper-IgM syndrome: clinical and immunologic features of 79 patients. Medicine (Baltimore) 2003; 82:373–384.

78. Hayward A, Levy J, Facchetti F, et al. Cholangiopathy and tumors of the pancreas, liver and biliary tree in boys with X-linked immunodeficiency and hyper-IgM. J Immunol 1997; 158:977–983.

79. Bahillo P, Cantero T, Solis P, et al. Hyper-IgM syndrome with CHARGE association. Pediatr Allergy Immunol 2003; 14:487–489.

80. Kilic SS, Tezcan I, Sanal O, et al. Transient hypogammaglobulinemia of infancy: clinical and immunologic features of 40 new cases. Pediatr Int 2000; 42:647–650.

81. Cano F, Mayo D, Ballow M. Absent viral antibodies in patients with transient hypogammaglonulinemia of infancy. J Allergy Clin Immunol 1990; 85:510–513.

82. Dressier F, Peter H, Muller W, et al. Transient hypogammaglobulinemia of infancy: five new cases, review of the literature, and redefinition. Acta Paediatr Scand 1989; 78:767–774.

83. McGeady S. Transient hypogammaglobulinemia of infancy: need to reconsider name and definition. J Pediatr 1987; 110:47–50.

84. Perlmutter D, Leichtner A, Goldman H, et al. Chronic diarrhea associated with hypogammaglobulinemia and enteropathy in infants and children. Dig Dis Sci 1985; 30:1149–1155.

85. Leung D, Kelly C, Boguniewicz M, et al. Treatment with intravenously administed gamma globulin of chronic relapsing colitis induced by *Clostridium difficile* toxin. J Pediatr 1991; 118:633–637.

86. Cunningham-Rundles C. Clinical and immunologic studies of common variable immunodeficiency. Curr Opin Pediatr 1994; 6:676–681.

87. Sneller M, Strober W, Eisenstein E, et al. New insights into common variable immunodeficiency. Ann Intern Med 1993; 118:720–730.

88. Farrington M, Grosmaire L, Nonoyama S, et al. CD40 ligand expression is defective in a subset of patients with common variable immunodeficiency. Proc Natl Acad Sci USA 1994; 91:1099–1103.

89. Nonoyama S, Farrington M, Ishida H, et al. Activated B cells from patients with common variable immunodeficiency proliferate and synthesize immunoglobulin. J Clin Invest 1993; 92:1282–1287.

90. Punnonen J, Kainulainen L, Ruuskanen O, et al. IL-4 synergizes with IL-10 and anti-CD40 MoAbs to induce B-cell differentiation in patients with common variable immunodeficiency. Scand J Immunol 1997; 45:203–212.

91. Cunningham-Rundles C. Clinical and immunologic analysis of 103 patients with common variable immunodeficiency. J Clin Immunol 1989; 9:22–33.

92. Bastlein C, Burlefinger R, Holzberg E. Common variable immunodeficiency syndrome and nodular lymphoid hyperplasia in the small intestine. Endoscopy 1988; 20:272–75.

93. Bennett W, Watson R, Heard J, et al. Home hyperalimentation for common variable hypogammaglobulinemia with malabsorption secondary to intestinal nodular lymphoid hyperplasia. Am J Gastroenterol 1987; 82:1019–1095.

94. Tahan V, Dobrucali A, Canbakan B, et al. Cytomegalovirus infection of gastrointestinal tract with multiple ulcers and strictures, causing obstruction in a patient with common variable immunodeficiency syndrome. Dig Dis Sci 2000; 45:1781–1785.

95. Teahon K, Webster A, Price A, et al. Studies on the enteropathy associated with primary hypogammaglobulinemia. Gut 1994; 35:1244–1249.

96. Luzi G, Zullo A, Iebba F, et al. Duodenal pathology and clinical–immunological implications in common variable immunodeficiency patients. Am J Gastroenterol 2003; 98:118–121.

97. Sperber K, Mayer L. Gastrointestinal manifestations of common variable immunodeficiency. Immunol Allergy Clin North Am 1988; 8:423–434.

98. Conley M, Park C, Douglas S. Childhood common variable immunodeficiency with autoimmune disease. J Pediatr 1986; 108:915–922.

99. Catassi C, Mirakian R, Natalini G, et al. Unresponsive enteropathy associated with circulating antienterocyte antibodies in a boy with common variable hypogammaglobulinemia and type I diabetes. J Pediatr Gastroenterol Nutr 1988; 7:608–613.

100. Litzman J, Dastych M, Hegar P. Analysis of zinc, iron, and copper serum levels in patients with common variable immunodeficiency. Allergol Immunopathol (Madr) 1995; 23:117–120.

101. John H, Sullivan K, Smith C, et al. Enterocolitis in common variable immunodeficiency. Dig Dis Sci 1996; 41:621–623.

102. Pierson J, Camisa C, Lawlor K, et al. Cutaneous and visceral granulomas in common variable immunodeficiency. Cutis 1993; 52:221–222.

103. Spickett G, Zhang J, Green T, et al. Granulomatous disease in common variable immunodeficiency: effect on immunoglobulin replacement therapy and response to steroids and splenectomy. J Clin Pathol 1996; 49:431–434.

104. Cunningham-Rundles C, Cooper DL, Duffy TP, et al. Lymphomas of mucosal-associated lymphoid tissue in common variable immunodeficiency. Am J Hematol 2002; 69:171–178.

105. Zullo A, Romiti A, Rinaldi V, et al. Gastric pathology in patients with common variable immunodeficiency. Gut 1999; 45:77–81.

106. de Bruin NC, de Groot R, den Hollander JC, et al. Small-cell undifferentiated (neuroendocrine) carcinoma of the cecum in a child with common variable immunodeficiency. Am J Pediatr Hematol Oncol 1993; 15:258–261.
107. Quinti I, Pandoiti F, Paganelli R, et al. HCV infection in patients with primary defects of Ig production. Clin Exp Immunol 1995; 102:11–16.
108. Webster A, Brown D, Franz A, et al. Prevalence of hepatitis C in patients with primary antibody deficiency. Clin Exp Immunol 1996; 103:5–7.
109. Smith M, Webster D, Dhillon A, et al. Orthotopic liver transplantation for chronic hepatitis in two patients with common variable immunodeficiency. Gastroenterology 1995; 108:879–884.
110. Sumazaki R, Matsubara T, Moki T, et al. Rapidly progressive hepatitis C in a patient with common variable immunodeficiency. Eur J Pediatr 1996; 155:532–534.
111. Bjoro K, Skaug K, Haaland T, et al. Long-term outcome of chronic hepatitis C virus infection in primary hypogammaglobulinaemia. Q J Med 1999; 92:433–441.
112. Eisenstein E, Sneller M. Common variable immunodeficiency: diagnosis and management. Ann Allergy 1994; 73:285–294.
113. Toraldo R, D'Avanzo M, Tolone C, et al. Effect of interferon-gamma in a patient with common variable immunodeficiency and chronic Epstein–Barr virus infection. Pediatr Hematol Oncol 1995; 12:489–493.
114. Buckley RH. Primary cellular immunodeficiencies. J Allergy Clin Immunol 2002; 109:747–757.
115. Stephan J, Vlekova V, LeDiest F, et al. Severe combined immunodeficiency: a retrospective single-center study of clinical presentation and outcome in 117 patients. J Pediatr 1993; 123:564–572.
116. Buckley RH, Schiff Rl, Schiff SE, et al. Human severe combined immunodeficiency: genetic, phenotypic, and functional diversity in one hundred eight infants. J Pediatr 1997; 130:378–387.
117. Leonard W. The molecular basis of X-linked severe combined immunodeficiency: the role of the interleukin-2 receptor gamma chain as a common gamma chain. Immunol Rev 1994; 138:61–86.
118. Leonard W. The molecular basis of X-linked severe combined immunodeficiency: defective cytokine receptor signalling. Annu Rev Med 1996; 47:229–239.
119. Fischer A. Severe combined immunodeficiency (SCID). Clin Exp Immunol 2000; 122:143–149.
120. Fischer A. Primary immunodeficiency disease: an experimental model for molecular medicine. Lancet 2001; 357:1863–1869.
121. Berthet F, LeDiest F, Dulliege A, et al. Clinical consequences and treatment of primary immunodeficiency syndromes characterized by functional T and B lymphocytes anomalies (combined immune deficiency). Pediatrics 1994; 93:265–270.
122. Jarvis W, Middleton P, Gelfand E. Significance of viral infections in severe combined immunodeficiency disease. Pediatr Infect Dis 1983; 2:187–192.
123. Murch S, Meadows N, Morgan G, et al. Severe enteropathy and immunodeficiency in interleukin-2 deficiency (abstract). J Pediatr Gastroenterol Nutr 1994; 19:A335.
124. Boeck A, Buckley RH, Schiff RI. Gastroesophageal reflux and severe combined immunodeficiency. J Allergy Clin Immunol 1997; 99:420–424.
125. Washington K, Gossage D, Gottfried M: Pathology of the liver in severe combined immunodeficiency and DiGeorge syndrome. Pediatr Pathol 1993; 13:485–504.
126. Gilger M, Matson D, Conner M, et al. Extraintestinal rotavirus infections in children with immunodeficiency. J Pediatr 1992; 120:912–917.
127. Washington K, Gossage D, Gottfried M. Pathology of the pancreas in severe combined immunodeficiency and DiGeorge syndrome. Hum Pathol 1994; 25:908–914.
128. Klein C, Lisowska-Grospierre B, LeDiest F, et al. Major histocompatibility complex class II deficiency: clinical manifestations, immunologic features, and outcome. J Pediatr 1993; 123:921–928.
129. Hershfield M. PEG-ADA: an alternative to haploidentical bone marrow transplantation and an adjunct to gene therapy for adenosine deaminase deficiency. Hum Mutat 1995; 5:107–112.
130. Blaese R, Culver K, Miller A, et al. T lymphocyte directed gene therapy for ADA-SCID: initial trial results after 4 years. Science 1995; 270:475–480.
131. Derry JM, Ochs HD, Francke U. Isolation of a novel gene mutated in Wiskott–Aldrich syndrome. Cell 1994; 78:635–644.
132. Thrasher AJ, Kinnon C. The Wiskott–Aldrich syndrome. Clin Exp Immunol 2000; 120:2–9.
133. Thrasher AJ. WASp in immune-system organization and function. Nat Rev Immunol 2002; 2:635–646.
134. Snapper SB, Rosen FS. A family of WASPs. N Engl J Med 2003 ;348:350–351.
135. Sullivan K, Mullen C, Blaese R, et al. A multiinstitutional survey of the Wiskott–Aldrich syndrome. J Pediatr 1994; 125:876–885.
136. Hsieh K, Chang M, Lee C, et al. Wiskott–Aldrich syndrome and inflammatory bowel disease. Ann Allergy 1988; 60:429–431.
137. Roos D, deBoer M, Kuribayashi F, et al. Mutations in the X-linked and autosomal recessive forms of chronic granulomatous disease. Blood 1996; 87:1663–1681.
138. Liese J, Jendrossek V, Jansson A, et al. Chronic granulomatous disease in adults. Lancet 1995; 346:220–223.
139. Hadzic N, Heaton N, Baker A, et al. Successful orthotopic liver transplantation for fulminant liver failure in a child with autosomal recessive chronic granulomatous disease. Transplantation 1995; 60:1185–1186.
140. Winkelstein JA, Marino MC, Johnston RB Jr, et al. Chronic granulomatous disease: report on a national registry of 368 patients. Medicine (Baltimore) 2000; 79:155–169.
141. Eckert J, Abramson S, Starke J, et al. The surgical implications of chronic granulomatous disease. Am J Surg 1995; 169:320–323.
142. Fischer A, Segal A, Seger R, et al. The management of chronic granulomatous disease. Eur J Pediatr 1993; 152:896–899.
143. Griscom N, Kirkpatrick J, Girdany B, et al. Gastric antral narrowing in chronic granulomatous disease of childhood. Pediatrics 1974; 54:456–460.
144. Danziger R, Goreb A, Becker J, et al. Outpatient management with oral corticosteroid therapy for obstructive conditions in chronic granulomatous disease. J Pediatr 1993; 122:303–305.
145. Werlin S, Chusid M, Caya J, et al. Colitis in chronic granulomatous disease. Gastroenterology 1982; 82:328–331.
146. Sloan J, Cameron C, Maxwell R, et al. Colitis complicating chronic granulomatous disease: a clinicopathological case report. Gut 1996; 38:619–622.
147. Rosh J, Tang H, Mayer L, et al. Trearment of intractable gastrointestinal manifestations of chronic granulomatous disease with cyclosporine. J Pediatr 1995; 126:143–145.

148. Hague R, Eastham E, Lee R, et al. Resolution of hepatic abscess after interferon gamma in chronic granulomatous disease. Arch Dis Child 1993; 69:443–445.

149. International Chronic Granulomatous Disease Study Group. A controlled trial of interferon gamma to prevent infection in chronic granulomatous disease. N Engl J Med 1991; 324:509–516.

150. Herrod H. Chronic mucocutaneous candidiasis in childhood and complications of non-*Candida* infection. J Pediatr 1990; 116:377–382.

151. Kirkpatrick C. Chronic mucocutaneous candidiasis. Eur J Clin Microbiol Infect Dis 1989; 8:448–456.

152. Etzioni A, Doerschuk CM, Harland JM. Of man and mouse: leukocyte and endothelial adhesion molecule deficiencies. Blood 1999; 94:3281–3288.

153. Etzioni A, Frydman M, Pollack S, et al. Recurrent severe infections caused by a novel leukocyte adhesion deficiency. N Engl J Med 1992; 327:1789–1792.

154. Phillips ML, Schwartz BR, Etzioni A, et al. Neutrophil adhesion in leukocyte adhesion deficiency syndrome type 2. J Clin Invest 1995; 96:2898–2906.

155. Marquardt T, Brune T, Luhn K, et al. Leukocyte adhesion deficiency II syndrome, a generalized defect in fucose metabolism. J Pediatr 1999; 134:681–688.

156. Anderson D, Springer T. Leukocyte-adhesion deficiency: an inherited defect in the Mac-1, LFA-1, and p150,95 glycoproteins. Annu Rev Immunol 1987; 38:175–194.

157. Voss L, Rhodes K. Leukocyte adhesion deficiency presenting with recurrent otitis media and persistent leukocytosis. Clin Pediatr 1992; 31:442–445.

158. Todd R, Freyer D. The CD11/CD18 leukocyte glycoprotein deficiency. Hematol Oncol Clin North Am 1988; 2:13–31.

159. Roberts M, Atkinson J. Oral manifestations associated with leukocyte adhesion deficiency: a five year case study. Pediatr Dent 1990; 12:107–111.

160. Hawkins H, Heffelfinger S, Anderson D. Leukocyte adhesion deficiency: clinical and postmortem observations. Pediatr Pathol 1992; 12:119–130.

161. Rivera-Matos I, Rakita R, Marisaico M, et al. Leukocyte-adhesion deficiency mimicking Hirschsprung disease. J Pediatr 1995; 127:755–757.

162. Faul JL, Berry GJ, Colby TV, et al. Thoracic lymphangiomas, lymphangiectasis, lymphangiomatosis, and lymphatic dysplasia syndrome. Am J Respir Crit Care Med 2000; 161:1037–1046.

163. Roberts SH, Douglas AP. Intestinal lymphangiectasia: the variability of presentation. A study of five cases. Q J Med 1976; 45:39–48.

164. Levine C. Primary disorders of the lymphatic vessels – a unified concept. J Pediatr Surg 1989; 24:233–240.

165. Hilliard RI, McKendry JB, Phillips MJ. Congenital abnormalities of the lymphatic system: a new clinical classification. Pediatrics 1990; 86:988–994.

166. Abramowsky C, Hupertz V, Kilbridge P, et al. Intestinal lymphangiectasia in children: a study of upper gastrointestinal endoscopic biopsies. Pediatr Pathol 1989; 9:289–297.

167. Berezin S, Newman L, Russe J. Hemorrhage and shock due to intestinal malabsorption. Pediatr Emerg Care 1986; 2:91–92.

168. Hallevy C, Sperber AD, Almog Y. Group G streptococcal empyema complicating primary intestinal lymphangiectasia. J Clin Gastroenterol 2003; 37:270.

169. Ross IN, Chesner I, Thompson RA, et al. Cutaneous viral infection as a presentation of intestinal lymphangiectasia. Br J Dermatol 1982; 107:357–363.

170. Hardikar W, Smith AL, Chow CW. Neonatal protein-losing enteropathy caused by intestinal lymphatic hypoplasia in siblings. J Pediatr Gastroenterol Nutr 1997; 25:217–221.

171. Salvia G, Cascioli CF, Ciccimarra F, et al. A case of protein-losing enteropathy caused by intestinal lymphangiectasia in a preterm infant. Pediatrics 2001; 107:416–417.

172. Fleisher TA, Strober W, Muchmore AV, et al. Corticosteroid-responsive intestinal lymphangiectasia secondary to an inflammatory process. N Engl J Med 1979; 300:605–606.

173. Tift WL, Lloyd JK. Intestinal lymphangiectasia. Long-term results with MCT diet. Arch Dis Child 1975; 50:269–276.

174. Persic M, Browse NL, Prpic I. Intestinal lymphangiectasia and protein losing enteropathy responding to small bowel restriction. Arch Dis Child 1998; 78:194.

175. Ballinger AB, Farthing MJ. Octreotide in the treatment of intestinal lymphangiectasia. Eur J Gastroenterol Hepatol 1998; 10:699–702.

176. Bac DJ, Van Hagen PM, Postema PT, et al. Octreotide for protein-losing enteropathy with intestinal lymphangiectasia. Lancet 1995; 345:1639.

177. Mine K, Matsubayashi S, Nakai Y, et al. Intestinal lymphangiectasia markedly improved with antiplasmin therapy. Gastroenterology 1989; 96:1596–1599.

178. MacLean JE, Cohen E, Weinstein M. Primary intestinal and thoracic lymphangiectasia: a response to antiplasmin therapy. Pediatrics 2002; 109:1177–1180.

179. Jain A, Ma CA, Liu S, et al. Specific missense mutations in NEMO result in hyper-IgM syndrome with hypohydrotic ectodermal dysplasia. Nat Immunol 2001; 2:223–228.

180. Orange JS, Brodeur SR, Jain A, et al. Deficient natural killer cell cytotoxicity in patients with IKK-gamma/NEMO mutations. J Clin Invest 2002; 109:1501–1509.

181. ZonanaJ, Elder ME, Schneider LC, et al. A novel X-linked disorder of immune deficiency and hypohidrotic ectodermal dysplasia is allelic to incontinetia pigmenti and due to mutations in IKK-gamma (NEMO). Am J Hum Genet 2000; 67:1555–1562.

182. Dupuis-Girod S, Corradini N, Hadj-Rabia S, et al. Osteopetrosis, lymphedema, anhidrotic ectodermal dysplasia, and immunodeficiency in a boy and incontinentia pigmenti in his mother. Pediatrics 2002; 109:e97.

183. Hamilton JK, Paquin LA, Sullivan JL, et al. X-linked lymphoproliferative syndrome registry report. J Pediatr 1980; 96:669–673.

184. Howie D, Sayos J, Terhorst C, et al. The gene defective in X-linked lymphoproliferative disease controls T cell dependent immune surveillance against Epstein–Barr virus. Curr Opin Immunol 2000; 12:474–478.

185. Coffey AJ, Brooksbank RA, Brandau O, et al. Host response to EBV infection in X-linked lymphoproliferative disease results from mutation in an SH2-domain encoding gene. Nat Genet 1998; 20:129–135.

186. Sayos J, Wu C, Morra M, et al. The X-linked lymphoproliferative-disease gene product SAP regulates signals induced through teh co-receptor SLAM. Nature 1998; 395:462–469.

187. Tangye SG, Phillips JH, Lanier LL, et al. Functional requirement for SAP in 2B4-mediated activation of human natural killer cells as revealed by the X-linked lymphoproliferative syndrome. J Immunol 2000; 165:2932–2936.

188. Morra M, Howie D, Grande MS, et al. X-linked lymphoproliferative disease: a progressive immunodeficiency. Annu Rev Immunol 2001; 19:657–682.

189. Harrington DS, Weisenburger DD, Purtilo DT. Malignant lymphoma in the X-linked lymphoproliferative syndrome. Cancer 1987; 59:1419–1429.
190. Gitzelmann R, Bosshard N. Defective neutrophil and monocyte functions in glycogen storage disease Ib: a literature review. Eur J Pediatr 1993; 152(Suppl 1): S33–S38.
191. Nordlie RC, Sukalski KA, Johnson WT. Human microsomal glucose-6-phosphatase system. EurJ Pediatr 1993; 152(Suppl 1):S2–S6.
192. Couper R, Kapelushnik J, Griffiths A. Neutrophil dysfunction in glycogen storage disease Ib: association with Crohn's like colitis. Gastroenterology 1991; 100:549–554.
193. Roe T, Thomas D, Gilsanz V, et al. Inflammatory bowel disease in glycogen storage disease Ib. J Pediatr 1986; 109:55–59.
194. Roe T, Coates T, Thomas D, et al. Treatment of chronic inflammatory bowel disease in glycogen storage disease Ib with colony stimulating factors. N Engl J Med 1992; 326:1666–1669.
195. Lavin M, Shiloh Y. Ataxia telangiectasia: a multifaceted genetic disorder associated with defective signal transduction. Curr Opin Immunol 1996; 8:459–464.
196. Abdullah A. Aetiology of chronic diarrhea in children: experience at King Khalid University Hospital, Riyadh, Saudi Arabia. Ann Trop Pediatr 1994; 14:111–117.
197. Ceroni M, Karau J, Pergami P, et al. High incidence of gastrointestinal cancer in a family with ataxia telangiectasia. Acta Neurol 1994; 16:33–37.
198. Bernard F, Picard C, Cormier-Daire V, et al. A novel developmental and immunodeficiency syndrome associated with intrauterine growth retardation and a lack of natural killer cells. Pediatrics 2004; 113:136–141.
199. Hammarstrom L, Vorechovsky I, Webster D. Selective IgA deficiency (SIgAD) and common variable immunodeficency (CVID). Clin Exp Immunol 2000; 120:225–231.
200. Cunningham-Rundles C, Bodian C. Common variable immunodeficiency: clinical and immunological features of 248 patients. Clin Immunol 1999; 92:34–48.
201. Rhee SJ, Bousvaros A. Immunosuppressive therapies. In: Walker WA, Goulet O, Kleinman RE, et al., eds. Pediatric Gastrointestinal Disease, 4th edn. Lewiston, NY: BC Decker; 2004:

Chapter 39
Gastrointestinal complications of secondary immunodeficiency syndromes

Tracie L. Miller

Secondary immunodeficiency syndromes constitute a wide array of non-gastrointestinal disorders. The gastrointestinal complications of these disorders often follow a common theme, with patients being at significant risk for infections of the gastrointestinal tract. In addition, cellular changes in the gastrointestinal tract (the largest immune organ in the body), malabsorption, peptic disorders and dysmotility are other problems faced by these children. Worldwide, human immunodeficiency virus (HIV-1) infection and malnutrition are by far the most common secondary immunodeficiency states. However, in the USA and other developed countries, HIV-1 disease has come under excellent control with the advent of highly active antiretroviral therapy (HAART), resulting in a decreased incidence of gastrointestinal complications. Nevertheless, review of the gastrointestinal complications of HIV-1 disease in children is important, as HIV-1 is prevalent worldwide and serves as a model for complications of other secondary immunodeficiency states.

PEDIATRIC HIV INFECTION

The first cases of the acquired immune deficiency syndrome (AIDS) were described in the early 1980s. Later in 1984,[1] HIV-1 was determined to be the causative agent, and HIV-1 infection was recognized as a spectrum of disease, ranging from asymptomatic infection to full-blown AIDS. The AIDS epidemic claimed an estimated 3 million lives in 2004, and an estimated 5 million people acquired HIV-1 in 2004, bringing to 40 million the estimated number of people globally living with the virus.[1a] With the successful preventive strategies of elective cesarian section delivery and chemoprophylaxis of pregnant HIV-1-infected women, the transmission rates plummeted from 15–30% to less than 2% of all HIV-1-infected women delivering infants.[2] Furthermore, with the advent of HAART in 1996, the natural history of HIV-1 in children in developed countries has altered markedly.[3] However, the successes of prevention and prophylaxis have not been realized in developing countries, where HIV infection continues to increase. Thus there are grave implications for children, especially in some developing nations, where more than 25% of the women are infected with HIV-1 and therapeutic options for pregnant women at this time are limited.[4]

HIV-1 is an RNA virus that belongs to the lentivirus family. It has a particular tropism for the CD4 surface antigen of cells, and the binding of HIV-1 to the CD4 receptor initiates the viral cycle. The virus may subsequently replicate within the host cell or, alternatively, the proviral DNA within the host cells may remain latent until cellular activation occurs. Human T lymphocytes and monocytes–macrophages are the primary cells that are infected with HIV-1, although other cell lines may be infected as well. The net effect is suppression of the immune system and a progressive decline in CD4+ T lymphocytes, which leaves patients susceptible to opportunistic and recurrent bacterial infections.

HIV AND THE CELLULAR COMPONENTS OF GASTROINTESTINAL TRACT

The gastrointestinal tract is the main source of HIV-1 infection when parenteral transmission is excluded. In vertical transmission, HIV-1 is found in the gastrointestinal tract after the fetus swallows infected amniotic fluid, blood, cervical secretions or breast milk. Virus, inoculated in the gastrointestinal tract, infects the fetus as it enters into the gut-associated lymphoid tissue (GALT) through the tonsil or upper intestinal tract. The rates of acquisition of HIV-1 through the gastrointestinal tract are likely related to the quantity of virus in the person transmitting it[5–7] and the immunologic function and maturity of the patient being infected. Mucosal infections with opportunistic infections may increase HIV-1 transmission. Mycobacterial infections upregulate CC chemokine recptor 5 (CCR5) expression in monocytes, which facilitates the entry of CCR5-tropic HIV-1. Other factors, such as tumor necrosis factor-α (TNF-α), which is induced by nuclear factor (NF)-κB (which itself is pathogen induced), are potent inducers of HIV-1.[8,9]

Cellular routes that potentially can transmit HIV-1 across the gastrointestinal tract include M cells, dendritic cells and epithelial cells. M cells are specialized epithelial cells that overlay the Peyer's patches and transport large macromolecules and micro-organisms from the apical surface to the basolateral surface. Human transport of HIV-1 by M cells *in vivo* has not been reported. Dendritic cells bind HIV-1 through a specific dendritic cell-specific adhension molecule. *In vitro* studies support the role of dendritic cells in transmitting HIV-1;[10–13] however, the role of the dendritic cell in *in vivo* transmission of HIV-1 has yet to be determined. Epithelial cells express CCR5 and can selectively transfer CCR5-tropic HIV-1. The epithelial cell can transport HIV-1 *in vitro* from the apical to the basolateral surface.[14,15] The R5-tropic viruses are transferred *in vitro* through epithelial cell lines.[16]

Once transmitted, the lamina propria lymphocytes express CCR5 and CXC4 chemokine receptor 4 (CXCR4), which support HIV-1 replication.[17,18] Early after infection there is a greater proportion of infected lymphocytes in the lamina propria than in peripheral blood.[19,20] The lymphocytes are able to disseminate the virus to distant sites, with depletion of CD4 cells in the lamina propria[19,21] and then in the blood. As mucosal and peripheral T cells are depleted, monocytes and macrophages become important reservoirs for the virus. The intestinal macrophages do not promote inflammation and do not carry the receptor for CCR5 or CXCR4; however, the blood monocytes are different in their profile and are infected by HIV-1. They are found infected in the blood and thereafter take up residence in the gut.[22] They are stimulated by opportunistic agents and proinflammatory cytokines.[23]

Villous atrophy and gastrointestinal tract dysfunction are coincident with high levels of HIV-1 viral load in the gut.[24] A dysfunctional gastrointestinal tract can produce significant clinical symptoms that contribute to both morbidity and mortality in children with HIV-1 infection. These symptoms include weight loss, vomiting, diarrhea and malabsorption (Table 39.1).

Cause	
Anorexia, nausea, weight loss, vomiting	
Peptic disease	Idiopathic, gastroesophageal reflux, medications, *H. pylori*
Opportunistic infections of upper gastrointestinal tract	*Candida*, CMV, HSV
Pancreatic or hepatobiliary disease	Pancreatitis, cholangitis, infectious
Encephalopathy/CNS disorders	HIV
Idiopathic aphthous ulcers	HIV, cytokines
Primary anorexia	HIV, cytokines
Gastrointestinal dysmotility	HIV, autonomic, infectious, inflammatory
Medication toxicity	Specified in Table 39.3
Gastrointestinal malabsorption, diarrhea Mucosal disease	
Infectious	Bacterial, parasitic, viral
Inflammatory	HIV enteropathy, IBD
Disaccharidase deficiency	Infectious, inflammatory
Protein-losing enteropathy	Infectious, inflammatory
Fat malabsorption	Infectious, inflammatory
Hepatobiliary disease	
Sclerosing cholangitis	Infectious
Chronic pancreatitis	Infectious, drug-induced
Cirrhosis	Hepatitis B and C infection

IBD, inflammatory bowel disease.

Table 39.1 Gastrointestinal symptoms and causes in HIV-1-infected children

STRUCTURE AND FUNCTION OF THE INTESTINAL TRACT IN HIV INFECTION

As reviewed above, there are distinct changes in the cellular milieu of the gastrointestinal tract in HIV-1-infected patients. Previous studies have shown that activated mucosal T cells play a role in the pathogenesis of enteropathy in the human small intestine[25] and can affect the morphology of the villi and crypts in a manner similar to that seen in patients with HIV-1 infection. Recently the magnitude of viral burden in the gastrointestinal tract has been associated with villous blunting and other abnormal morphology.[24] A number of studies in the 1980s associated a distinct enteropathy with HIV-1. This was first described by Kotler et al.,[26] who studied 12 homosexual men with HIV-1 and controls. Seven of the patients had diarrhea, weight loss, an abnormally low D-xylose absorption and steatorrhea, without evidence of intestinal infection. Jejunal and rectal biopsies were obtained in all patients with diarrhea. Jejunal biopsies showed partial villous atrophy with crypt hyperplasia and increased numbers of intraepithelial lymphocytes. This was the first histologic description of a specific pathologic process that occurred in the lamina propria of the small intestine in some patients with HIV-1. Ullrich et al.[27] also defined small intestinal structure in adult patients with HIV-1. Microscopically, he found low-grade small bowel atrophy and maturational defects of enterocytes in 45 HIV-1-infected patients. These findings also support an HIV-1 enteropathy, characterized by mucosal atrophy with hyporegeneration. However, some investigators have challenged this concept, suggesting the findings could be attributed to an undiagnosed enteric infection.

Miller et al.[28] published histologic findings in 43 children with HIV-1 infection. The majority of patients had normal villous architecture and many of the children with villous blunting had an associated intercurrent enteric infection. Distinct features of hyperplasia of the lamina propria and increased intraepithelial lymphocytes were not apparent.

In order to link the altered morphology with abnormal intestinal function, Bjarnason et al.[29] studied intestinal inflammation and ileal structure and function in patients with a wide spectrum of HIV-1 disease states. HIV-1-infected patients who were minimally symptomatic had normal intestinal absorption and permeability, yet had increasing gastrointestinal dysfunction as they progressed to AIDS. Malabsorption of bile acids and vitamin B_{12} did not correlate with morphometric analysis of ileal biopsies and were unremarkable in these patients. Thus, there was significant mucosal dysfunction with only minor ileal morphologic changes. Malabsorption of bile acids may play a pathologic role in patients with AIDS diarrhea. The absorptive defect of AIDS enteropathy using a D-xylose kinetic model of proximal absorption was studied,[30] and correlated with the results of a Schilling test for cobalamin absorption, which measures distal intestinal function. There were minimal histologic abnormalities in both the proximal and distal biopsy sites in patients with diarrhea and no enteric infection. D-Xylose absorption was low, and the absorptive defect was more severe and greater than would be expected from the histologic abnormalities found. Thus, these findings support other studies that showed little association between histologic characteristics of the small bowel and its absorptive function in patients with HIV-1 infection.

Most studies do not support a direct role for gastrointestinal malabsorption on growth failure or weight loss. Ullrich et al.[27] described gastrointestinal malabsorption in HIV-1-infected patients who had low levels of lactase enzyme in the brush border, crypt death, decreased villous surface area and decreased mitotic figures per crypt when compared with control patients. In addition, Keating et al.[31] described absorptive capacity and intestinal permeability in HIV-1-infected patients. Malabsorption was prevalent in all groups of patients with AIDS, but was not as common in the asymptomatic HIV-1-infected patients. Malabsorption correlated significantly with the degree of immune suppression and with body mass index. There were mild decreases in the jejunal villous height to crypt depth ratio, yet not as severe as the subtotal villous atrophy found in celiac disease. Lim et al.[32] found disaccharidase activity to decrease proportionately with increasing HIV-1 disease severity, although there was no association between disaccharidase levels and weight loss. In addition, Mosavi et al.[33] found no correlation between diarrhea and weight loss in HIV-1-positive patients. More recently, Taylor et al.[34] found mild histologic changes accompanied by severe disaccharidase abnormalities; however, symptoms were severe enough to withdraw lactose in only 25% of the patients. Collectively these studies suggest that gastrointestinal malabsorption may be present, but is not always associated with weight loss and diarrhea.

Formal studies of intestinal absorption in children with HIV-1 are more limited. Malabsorption occurs frequently in HIV-1-infected children and may progress with the disease. In one study, 40% of children had non-physiologic lactose malabsorption and 61% had generalized carbohydrate malabsorption that was not associated with gastrointestinal symptoms or nutritional status.[35] These findings have been confirmed by others.[36] Another study in children revealed an association between diarrhea and nutrition.[37] Abnormal D-xylose absorption has also been associated with enteric infections in children.[35] Fat and protein loss or malabsorption have also been described. Sentongo et al.[38] evaluated fat malabsorption and pancreatic exocrine insufficiency using fecal elastase-1 enzyme assay in 44 HIV-1-infected children. Hormone-stimulated pancreatic function testing and 72-h stool and dietary fat sample collection were performed in children with abnormal fecal elastase levels. The prevalence of steatorrhea was 39% and that of pancreatic insufficiency was 0% (95% confidence interval 0–9%). There were no associations between steatorrhea and pancreatic insufficiency, growth, HIV-1 RNA viral load, CD4 status or type of antiretroviral therapy. Others studies support the absence of association.[39] Thus, the clinical significance of steatorrhea in pediatric HIV-1, similar to absorption of other nutrients, is unclear.

The etiology of malabsorption in HIV-1 infection is probably multifactorial. The cellular milieu of the lamina propria is altered significantly with HIV-1 infection.[24,40] The depletion of the CD4 T lymphocytes in the intestinal tract may cause change in the cytokine environment and alter intestinal function. Viral load in the intestinal tract may be considerably higher than that measured peripherally, and this can also affect mucosal gastrointestinal structure and function. Studies suggesting these hypotheses include that of Kotler et al.[41] which looked at intestinal mucosal inflammation in 74 HIV-1-infected individuals. These authors found abnormal histopathology in 69% of the patients, and this finding was associated with altered bowel habits. High tissue P24 antigen levels were observed, and these correlated with more advanced HIV-1 disease. Tissue P24 detection was associated with both abnormal bowel habits and mucosal histology. The tissue content of cytokines, including TNF, α-interferon and interleukin-1β, were higher in HIV-1-infected individuals than in controls, and these increases were independent of intestinal infection. Thus, HIV-1 reactivation in the intestinal mucosa could be associated with an inflammatory bowel-like syndrome in the absence of other enteric pathogens.

Small bowel bacterial overgrowth can be another source of gastrointestinal dysfunction leading to malabsorption. Bacterial overgrowth may be due to AIDS gastropathy[42,43] in which the stomach produces only small amounts of hydrogen chloride, allowing bacterial pathogens to escape the acid barrier of the stomach and colonize the duodenum. Additionally, iatrogenic hypochlorhidria may be due to the use of acid-blocking agents as treatment for ongoing peptic disease. Interestingly, some authors have found no relationship between gastric pH, small bowel bacterial colonization and diarrhea in HIV-1-infected patients.[44] Enteric pathogens[45] have been associated with enteric dysfunction, as discussed below.

With the advent of HAART, gastrointestinal symptoms, especially those associated with opportunistic infections, are less common. As viral burden decreases, immunosuppression has less effect on gastrointestinal function. Ritonavir, a protease inhibitor, in combination therapy resulted in restoration of gastrointestinal function in 10 children with carbohydrate malabsorption, steatorrhea, protein loss and iron deficiency.[46] However, one study in adults found similar rates of fat malabsorption in patients taking HAART and in those not taking HAART.[47]

INFECTIONS OF THE GASTROINTESTINAL TRACT

The gastrointestinal tract is a major target for opportunistic infections in immunocompromised HIV-1-infected children. The spectrum of these infections is dependent on

HIV-1 disease progression. In developed countries, with improved viral suppression associated with HAART, opportunistic infections of the gut and elsewhere are less common.[48] However, immunocompromised children continue to be at risk for infections with cytomegalovirus (CMV), herpes simplex virus (HSV), *Cryptosporidium* and microsporidia. Previous dogma that much of the diarrhea found in children with HIV-1 infection is not associated with enteric pathogens has been challenged. Unusual viral and parasitic infections can be diagnosed as a result of better diagnostic techniques. However, the cause of diarrhea in a significant number of patients with HIV-1 remains undiagnosed.[49]

Viral infections

The detection of viral gastrointestinal infections in HIV-1-infected children can sometimes be difficult owing to the limitations of diagnostic techniques. The most common gastrointestinal viral pathogen in HIV-1-infected children is CMV. Other pathogens, such as HSV, adenovirus, Epstein–Barr virus and a variety of other unusual viruses, can also contribute to intestinal dysfunction and diarrhea.

Herpes simplex virus

HSV infection in an immunocompromised child usually represents reactivation of a latent virus that had been acquired earlier in life. Gastrointestinal infection with HSV most commonly involves the esophagus and causes multiple small discrete ulcers. HSV can also involve other areas of the intestinal tract, including the colon and small bowel. The diagnosis of HSV relies on recognizing the multinucleated intranuclear inclusion bodies (Cowdry type A) with a ground-glass appearance and molding of the nuclei. The squamous epithelium is usually infected, although there may also be involvement of intestinal glandular epithelium in the mesenchymal cells. HSV monoclonal antibody staining is confirmatory for the diagnosis. In extensive involvement, there may be transmural necrosis and development of tracheo-esophageal fistulae. Treatment of HSV and other common gastrointestinal pathogens and their primary site of involvement are outlined in Table 39.2.

Other herpesviruses have also been detected in the gut of HIV-1-infected individuals. A case report of one 34-year-old HIV-1-infected man with intestinal pseudo-obstruction and disseminated cutaneous herpes zoster revealed positive immunohistochemistry against herpes zoster in a resected portion of the terminal ileum. This area had focal ulceration. The virus was localized to the muscularis propria and myenteric plexi throughout the entire length of the specimen. The authors postulated that the location of the virus in the gut may have been the etiologic factor for the pseudo-obstruction.[50]

Cytomegalovirus

CMV in the immunocompromised child, like HSV, represents reactivation of a latent virus that was acquired in earlier life. CMV is one of the more common viral pathogens of HIV-1-infected children. The reported incidence of gastrointestinal involvement in the pre-HAART era varied from 4.4% to 52% of patients studied. The incidence rates may have varied based on the techniques of diagnosis.[43] CMV infection is rare in patients with CD4 T-lymphocyte counts greater than 50 cells/mm^3.[51] Thus, in the HAART era, morbidity and mortality rates from CMV-associated gastrointestinal disease have diminished.[52] CMV may involve any part of the gastrointestinal tract, with an increased incidence in the esophagus or colon. CMV infection usually results in one or two discrete single and large ulcers of the esophagus and colon. Lesions may lead to severe gastrointestinal bleeding and hemodynamic instability. CMV inclusion bodies can be discovered incidentally in an asymptomatic patient, and this does not necessarily reflect disease.

In patients with upper intestinal CMV disease, there can be dysphagia and upper abdominal symptoms; whereas diarrhea is more common with colitis. The diarrhea can be watery or bloody in nature. Children may be systemically ill.[53] The colitis from CMV infection is patchy in nature and can be associated with severe necrotizing colitis and hemorrhage.[54] CMV usually affects the cecum and the right colon. Diagnosis is confirmed by endoscopy and biopsy. The histologic appearance of CMV-infected cells is quite unique (Fig. 39.1). These cells are enlarged and contain intranuclear and cytoplasmic inclusion bodies. The nuclear inclusion bodies are acidophilic and are often surrounded by a halo. Cytoplasm inclusion bodies are multiple, granular and often basophilic. Cells that are dying may appear smaller and smudged, with poorly defined inclusion bodies. Staining for CMV antigen shows that many of the infected cells are endothelial cells with others being perivascular mesenchymal cells. CMV can cause vasculitis because of its target cell population. Thus, the spread of CMV occurs with circulating infected endothelial cells. Treatment options are outlined in Table 39.2. Once HAART is established, with decreased viral burden (both HIV-1 and CMV) and improved CD4 counts, CMV treatment may be discontinued without concern of reactivation.[52]

Other viral infections

Infections with other unusual viral pathogens have been described. These include the human papilloma virus and Epstein–Barr virus, which have been identified in esophageal ulcers of patients with HIV-1. Adenovirus of the stomach and colon have also been reported and are often difficult to identify.[55] In the pre-HAART era, patients who excreted adenovirus from their gastrointestinal tract had a shorter survival.[56] There are unusual enteric viruses that have been associated with diarrhea in HIV-1-infected children.[57] These viruses, among others, include astrovirus and picobirnavirus.[58] Cegielski et al.[59] studied 59 children with HIV-1 infection in Tanzania. They looked for enteric viruses identified by electron microscopy of fecal specimens. Small round structured viruses (SRSVs) were found more frequently in HIV-1-infected children than in uninfected children with chronic diarrhea. Rotavirus and coronavirus-like particles were not associated with HIV-1

Pathogen	Drug treatment
Bacteria (*)	
Salmonella (SI, C)	Ampicillin; TMP–SMZ; cefotaxime sodium, ceftriaxone sodium; fluoroquinolones (>18 years)
Shigella (SI, C)	Ampicillin, TMP–SMZ; ceftriaxone sodium; azithromycin; fluoroquinolones (>18 years)
Campylobacter (SI)	Erythromycin; azithromycin dihydrate; doxycycline (>8 years); fluoroquinolones (>18 years)
Yersina (SI, C)	TMP–SMZ; tetracycline (>8 years); cefotaxime sodium; chloramphenicol; fluoroquinolones (>18 years)
Clostridium difficile (C)	Discontinue antibiotics, if possible; metronidazole; vancomycin; bacitracin; cholestyramine (may bind toxin and relieve symptoms); lactobacillus GG
Mycobacteria (*)	
Mycobacterium tuberculosis (SI)	Isoniazid; rifampin; pyrazinamide; ethambutol; aminoglycoside
MAC (SI)	(1) Clarithromycin or azithromycin combined with (2) ethambutol with adding (3) rifabutin (not in combination with PIs) or rifampin, plus (4) amikacin or streptomycin
Viruses (*)	
Cytomegalovirus (SI, C)	Ganciclovir; foscarnet; CMV–IVIG; valganciclovir hydrochloride
Herpes simplex virus (O/P, E)	Aciclovir; foscarnet; famciclovir; penciclovir
Fungi (*)	
Candida albicans (O/P, E)	Fluconazole, itraconazole, ketoconazole, amphotericin B
Histoplasma (SI)	Amphotericin B; fluconazole; itraconazole
Cryptococcus (SI)	Amphotericin B with oral flucytosine (serious systemic infections); fluconazole; itraconazole
Pneumocystis jiroveci (SI)	TMP–SMZ; pentamidine; atovaquone; dapsone
Parasites (*)	
Cryptosporidia (SI)	Nitazoxanide; azithromycin; paromomycin, octreotide; human immune globulin; bovine hyperimmune colostrum
Microsporidia (SI)	Albendazole; metronidazole; atovaquone; nitazoxanide; fumagillin
Isospora belli (SI)	TMP–SMZ; pyrimethamine; fluoroquinolones (>18 years)
Giardia lamblia (SI)	Metronidazole; furazolidone; nitazoxanide

*O/P, oropharynx; E, esophagus; S, stomach; SI, small intestine; C, colon; MAC, *Mycobacterium avium intracellulare* complex; PI, protease inhibitor; TMP–SMZ, trimethoprim–sulfamethoxazole.

Table 39.2 Primary location and drug therapy for common enteric pathogens infecting immunocompromised children

infection. These authors considered that these SRSVs may be associated with HIV-1 infection and could lead to chronic diarrhea in Tanzanian children.

Bacterial infections

Bacterial infections that involve the gastrointestinal tract of children with HIV-1 infection may be divided into three groups: bacterial overgrowth of normal gut flora; pathogens that can affect immunocompromised children as well as immunocompetent children (*Salmonella, Shigella, Campylobacter, Clostridium difficile* and *Aeromonas*); and bacterial infections that are more unique to immunocompromised children (*Mycobacterium avium intracellulare* complex; MAC).

Few studies have evaluated bacterial overgrowth in HIV-1-infected children, although gastric hypoacidity has been associated with opportunistic enteric infections and bacterial overgrowth in adult patients with HIV-1.[60] Other studies have not found this association. Small bowel bacterial overgrowth was not a common finding in a group of 32 HIV-1-infected patients, regardless of the presence of diarrhea, and it was not associated with hypochlorhydria.[44] Lactose hydrogen breath testing has shown high baseline readings in children that may indirectly suggest bacterial overgrowth of the small intestinal tract.[35] Detection of bacterial overgrowth in the small bowel is usually performed by quantitative duodenal aspirate for bacterial culture, with therapy directed at treating the organisms, which are often anaerobic.

Common bacterial infections

Common bacterial pathogens include *Salmonella, Shigella, Campylobacter, C. difficile* and *Aeromonas*. Infection with

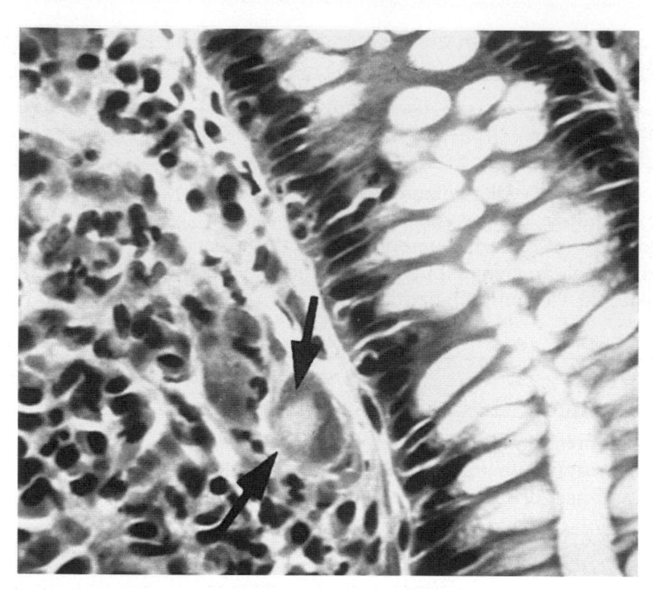

Figure 39.1: Small bowel biopsy of a child with HIV infection showing cytomegalovirus inclusion (arrows) within the lamina propria.

these organisms occurs more frequently in immunocompromised patients. The decline in the incidence of infections with these bacterial pathogens in developed countries has been linked to the improved immunity associated with HAART. However, combined morbidity and mortality rates associated with HIV-1 and these bacterial pathogens in developing countries approach 50% in some studies.[61] HIV-1-infected patients with *Campylobacter* infection have higher rates of bacteremia than the general population. Deaths from sepsis due to this organism have been reported in severely immunodeficient patients with AIDS, despite HAART.[62]

Colitis from *C. difficile* is also more common in the immunosuppressed population owing to chronic antibiotic use and impaired immune system.[63] Pulvirenti et al.[64] studied 161 HIV-1-infected patients with *C. difficile* and found that they had longer hospital stays and more admissions than patients without *C. difficile* infection, as well as other opportunistic infections such as herpes virus. They found *C. difficile*-associated diarrhea in 32% of all study patients with diarrhea. However, infection with *C. difficile* appeared to have little impact on morbidity or mortality. In a 1998, New York state screening study[65] of hospitalized HIV-1-infected patients in the HAART era, 2.8% were admitted with a diarrheal diagnosis, with 51.3% of these having a *C. difficile* infection. Thus, even with HAART, diarrhea is prevalent and is often associated with identifiable pathogens. Because of the serious complications that are associated with active bacterial enteric infections in immunodeficient children, treatment options are outlined in Table 39.2.

Mycobacteria

Intestinal infections with mycobacteria, including *Mycobacterium tuberculosis*, MAC and other atypical mycobacteria, were the most frequently encountered bacterial infections in HIV-1-infected patients in the pre-HAART era,[66] and became more prevalent in the pre-HAART era as patients were living longer with CD4 counts below 200 cells/mm^3.[67,68] In the HAART era, disseminated MAC in colonized patients can be successfully prevented; however, the effects of HAART on restoration of CD4 counts does not prevent MAC colonization.[69]

Infection with MAC usually occurs in the very late stages of AIDS in children, when CD4 counts are lower than 200 cells/mm^3. The most common clinical manifestations of gastrointestinal infections with MAC include fever, weight loss, malabsorption and diarrhea. Intestinal obstruction, resulting from lymph node involvement and intussusception, terminal ileitis, which resembles Crohn's disease, and refractory gastric ulcers are often found. Severe gastrointestinal hemorrhage has also been described.[70] Endoscopically, fine white nodules may be seen in the duodenum, or the duodenal mucosa may look velvety and grayish in appearance. Segments of the gastrointestinal tract can become infected with MAC. Histologically, there is a diffuse histiocytic infiltrate in the lamina propria with blunting of the small intestinal villi. These histiocytic infiltrates can be recognized on hematoxylin and eosin staining and on acid-fast stains, and are pathognomonic for infection (Fig. 39.2). With the advent of HAART, immune reconstitution disease has been described.[71,72] This is likely an immune reaction in which previously quiescent organisms become active because of the improved immune function associated with HAART. This can occur in as many as 25% of patients who respond to HAART.[73] Lymphadenitis is the most common condition, although abscesses can appear anywhere. Severe abdominal complaints may result.

Appropriate therapies are outlined in Table 39.2, yet this organism is often frustrating to treat. Azithromycin 600 mg, when given in combination with ethambutol, is an effective agent for the treatment of disseminated *M. avium* disease in patients infected with HIV-1.[74] Caution must be exercised in administering these multidrug regimens for

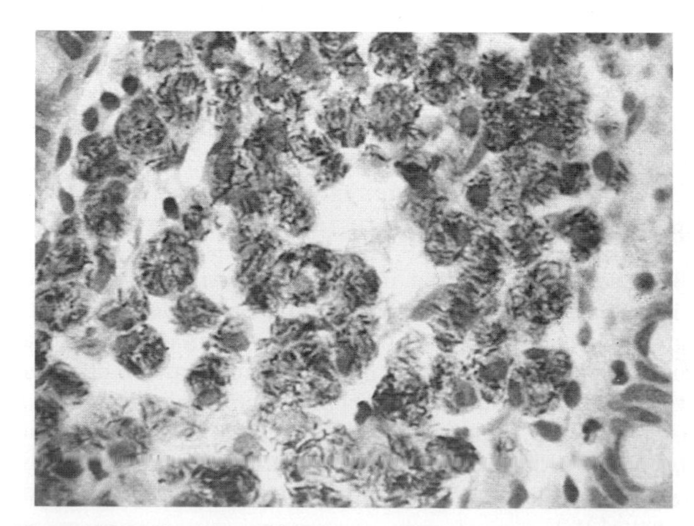

Figure 39.2: Small bowel biopsy of a child with HIV infection showing histiocytes infiltrated with *Mycobacterium avium intracellulare* within the lamina propria.

MAC in patients receiving concurrent HAART. Rifamycins induce cytochrome P450 enzymes and accelerate the metabolism of clarithromycin and HIV-1 protease inhibitors. Conversely, clarithromycin inhibits these enzymes, resulting in increased rifabutin toxicity. The net result is treatment regimens that can be extremely difficult to tolerate and manage, especially for the sicker patients. Clarithromycin and azithromycin must be administered in combination with other agents, such as ethambutol, to prevent the emergence of macrolide resistance.[75]

Escherichia coli

Other entities, such as bacterial enteritis, have been described in adults with HIV-1. A study by Orenstein and Kotler[76] evaluated ileal and colonic biopsies in patients with AIDS and diarrhea, and found bacteria similar to adherent *E. coli* along the intestinal epithelial border. Similar findings were documented by Kotler et al.,[77] who showed adherent bacteria in 17% of all adult patients with AIDS. The infection was localized primarily to the cecum and right colon, and three distinct histopathologic patterns of adherence observed: attachment on effacing lesions, bacteria intercalated between microvilli, and aggregates of bacteria more loosely attached to the damaged epithelium. The bacterial cultures of frozen rectal biopsies yielded *E. coli* in 12 of the 18 patients. These findings suggest that chronic infection with adherent bacteria can also produce the syndrome of AIDS-associated diarrhea. In a 'look back' evaluation, Orenstein and Dieterich[55] found that enteropathogenic bacterial infections were overlooked on initial examination and concluded that, for accurate diagnoses, specimens should be evaluated by laboratories with expertise in HIV.

Helicobacter pylori

H. pylori prevalence is not significantly different between HIV-1-infected patients and HIV-1-negative patients.[78,79] Some investigators have found the seroprevalence of *H pylori* to be lower in HIV-1-infected patients,[80] especially as CD4 counts decline with advancing disease.[78] The protection from *H. pylori* may be a result of frequent antibiotic use or correlated with a more advanced, dysfunctional immune state that results in a decreased inflammatory response to the organism.[81] Remission of a high-grade gastric mucosa-associated lymphoid tissue (MALT) lymphoma followed *H. pylori* eradication and HAART in a patient with AIDS.[82] Treatment of *H. pylori* in HIV-1-infected children is similar to non-infected children, with special attention to drug interactions.

Parasitic infections

Cryptosporidium parvum

In the early 1980s, cryptosporidiosis was regarded as an AIDS-defining disease and an opportunistic intestinal pathogen. It became an important cause of chronic diarrhea, leading to high morbidity and mortality rates in immunocompromised patients. To date, no effective chemotherapy is available. With the introduction of protease inhibitors in HAART regimens, the incidence of cryptosporidiosis in patients with AIDS has declined substantially in developed countries.[83] However, in developing nations, gastrointestinal infection with *C. parvum* is prevalent, and carries high morbidity and mortality rates.[84,85]

Although *Cryptosporidium* was initially described in animals, it was first noted to cause an enterocolitis in both immunocompromised and immunocompetent humans in 1976.[86,87] An intact T-cell response is the primary mechanism that confers protection against this organism; thus patients with abnormal T-cell function or number are at risk. The spectrum and severity of disease in immunocompromised individuals with cryptosporidiosis correlates with most severe disease found in individuals with defects in the T-cell response.[83] The overall frequency of infection seems to be related to the severity of immunodeficiency and not the specific disorder.[88]

Cryptosporidium usually affects the gastrointestinal tract, although it has been found in other organs including the biliary tract,[89] pancreas[90] and respiratory tract.[91] In immunocompetent individuals, the diarrhea is self-limiting, whereas in immunocompromised patients it may be protracted and associated with significant malabsorption and nutritional compromise. The small intestine is the primary target, although it can occur in any part of the intestinal tract. Esophageal cryptosporidiosis has also been described in one child[92] and in adults. Clayton et al.[93] described two patterns of enteric cryptosporidiosis. One was accompanied by severe clinical disease with significant malabsorption, with the majority of the organisms found in the proximal small bowel, whereas less severe clinical disease was seen in patients with colonic disease or with infection only noted in the stool. Patients with proximal small bowel infection with *Cryptosporidium* showed crypt hyperplasia, villous atrophy, lamina propria inflammatory infiltrates, abnormal D-xylose absorption, greater weight loss, and shorter survival, with greater need for intravenous hydration and hyperalimentation than patients with colonic disease. In other studies, absorption of nutrients showed an inverse correlation with active infection,[94] as shown by altered vitamin B_{12} and D-xylose absorption, and lactulose and mannitol urinary excretion ratios. Intestinal function improved in patients whose oocyte counts were reduced by treatment with paromomycin.

Symptomatic cryptosporidiosis has been documented in as many as 6.4% of immunocompetent children and 22% of immunodeficient children, whereas in an asymptomatic population, *Cryptosporidium* was found in 4.4% of immunocompetent and 4.8% of immunodeficient children.[94a] Spiramycin at 100 mg per kg daily for 14 days caused a significant reduction in the shedding of infectious oocysts, and no gastrointestinal symptoms developed in children treated for asymptomatic infection, whereas children who were not treated developed gastrointestinal symptoms.[94a]

The diagnosis of cryptosporidiosis is made by identifying the organisms in a duodenal aspirate, stool or tissue sample (biopsies). On hematoxylinand eosin-stained sections, these organisms can be found as rows or clusters of basophilic spherical structures 2–4 μm in diameter, attached to the microvillous border of the epithelial cells (Fig. 39.3). The tips in the lateral aspect of the villi show the greatest number of organisms in the small intestine. In the colonic epithelium, the crypt and surface epithelial involvement appear equal. *Cryptosporidium* also stain positively with Giemsa, and negatively with mucous stains. The acid-fast stain on a stool sample is one of the most widely used methods of determining whether a patient has cryptosporidiosis. More recent sensitive and specific methods for diagnosing cryptosporidiosis include fluorescein-labeled IgG monoclonal antibodies.[95,96]

Treatment of cryptosporidiosis in children with HIV-1 infection is often difficult. The disease can be chronic and protracted with diffuse watery diarrhea and dehydration. Several different agents are used to eradicate the organism, with varying success rates. The most effective treatment is to improve immunologic function and nutritional status. With the advent of HAART, many children's immune function has been restored with a lower incidence and prevalence of *Cryptosporidium* infection.[97] The introduction of HAART in a patient with severe debilitating *Cryptosporidium* infection not only resulted in an increased CD4 count in the peripheral blood and clearance of the organism, but also produced a marked increase in CD4 count in the rectal mucosa on biopsy, suggesting this may have been the main mechanism of clearing the parasite.[98] Octreotide therapy of acute and chronic diarrhea, with coincident improvement in nutritional status, eradicated *Cryptosporidium* in one patient.[96,99] Other investigators have used bovine hyperimmune colostrum with benefit.[100,101] The macrolides, such as azithromycin, have shown some promise in the treatment of *Cryptosporidium* infection.[102,103] The effect of protease inhibitors as therapy against *Cryptosporidium* has been tested in a cell culture system.[104] Nelfinavir moderately inhibited the host cell invasion over a period of 2 h. Indinavir, nelfinavir and ritonavir inhibited parasite development significantly. The inhibitory effect was increased when the aminoglycoside paromomycin was combined with the protease inhibitors indinavir, ritonavir and, to a lesser extent, saquinavir, compared with the protease inhibitor alone. Thus protease inhibitor therapy may directly (rather than indirectly, through its effects on the immune system) inhibit growth of *Cryptosporidium*. Amadi et al.[84] found that a 3-day course of nitazoxanide improved diarrhea, helped eradicate the parasite and improved mortality in HIV-1-seronegative, but not HIV-1-seropositive, children in Zambia.

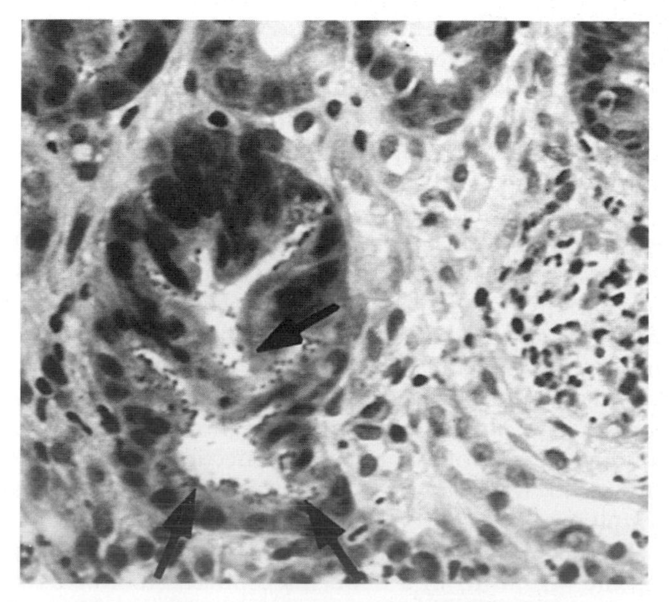

Figure 39.3 Small bowel biopsy of a child with HIV infection showing *Cryptosporidium* attached to the villus (arrows).

Microsporidia

Microsporidia are obligate intracellular protozoal parasites that infect a variety of cell types in many different species of animals. These organisms were first described in 1857, when recognized as a cause of disease in non-human hosts.[105] The first description of microsporidia (*Enterocytozoon bieneusi*) as a human pathogen was in 1985, and microsporidia have since been described as more common human pathogens.[106] Infection with microsporidia typically occurs in patients with severely depressed CD4 T-lymphocyte counts. One of the largest case studies of intestinal microsporidiosis in patients with HIV-1 infection was described by Orenstein et al.[107] in 67 adult patients with AIDS and AIDS-related complex and chronic non-pathogenic diarrhea. *E. bieneusi* was diagnosed by electromicroscopy in 20 of the patients. Jejunal biopsies were more positive than duodenal biopsies. The parasites and spores were clearly visible by light microscopy in 17 of the 21 biopsies. Infection was confined to enterocytes located at the tip of the intestinal villus, and the histologic findings included villous atrophy, cell degeneration, necrosis and sloughing. Other investigators[108–110] found microsporidia in as many as 50% of HIV-1-infected patients with chronic and unexplained diarrhea evaluated in the pre-HAART era. *E. bieneusi* has been documented in 15–25% of children with[111] or without[112] diarrhea in developing countries, making it fairly ubiquitous in these regions of the world. Other species of microsporidia, including *Encephalitozoon (septata) intestinalis*, can cause significant enteric disease with diarrhea, wasting and malabsorption. *Septata intestinalis* differs from *E. bieneusi* in its tendency to disseminate, and can infect enterocytes, as well as macrophages, fibroblasts and endothelial cells.

Microsporidia are found with increasing frequency in HIV-1-negative patients.[113] Infection has been documented in almost every tissue and organ in the body, and in epithelial, mesenchymal and neural cells. Microsporidia can cause inflammation and cell death, and a variety of symptoms including shortness of breath, sinusitis and diarrhea with wasting. If left untreated, microsporidiosis can be a significant cause of mortality.

Treatments for microsporidia include albendazole, which can relieve clinical symptoms and eliminate microsporidial spores in the feces, especially of the less common pathogen, *E. intestinalis*. *E. bieneusi* is more challenging to treat, although therapy with fumagillin or its analog, TNP-470 (antiangiogenesis agents) have shown promising results.[114–116] Other studies show atovaquone as an effective treatment as well.[117] Indirect treatment by improving the immune system with HAART has also effectively cleared these organisms.[97,118,119]

Isospora belli

Isospora belli is recognized as an opportunistic small bowel pathogen in patients with HIV-1 infection. This organism is most common in tropical and subtropical climates. Isosporiasis can be diagnosed by identification of the oocyte in the stool or by biopsy. The diagnosis is critical because, unlike cryptosporidiosis or microsporidiosis, the therapy is very effective. *I. belli* is found within the enterocyte and within the cytoplasm. The organism stains poorly, although the central nucleus, large nucleolus and perinuclear halo give it a characteristic appearance. The infection produces mucosal atrophy and tissue eosinophilia. A 10-day course of trimethoprim–sulfamethoxazole is effective therapy, and recurrent disease can be prevented by ongoing prophylaxis with this combination drug.[120] Ciprofloxacin, although not as effective, is an acceptable alternative for those with sulfa allergies.[120] Other therapies for *Isospora* include pyrimethamine, also indicated for patients with sulfa allergies.[121]

Other parasites

Blastocystis hominis is usually considered a non-pathologic parasite, but has been described in patients with chronic diarrhea and HIV-1 infection.[122] This organism is more pathogenic in immunocompromised patients and can cause mild, prolonged or recurrent diarrhea. Effective therapy includes di-iodohydroxyquinoline 650 mg orally three times daily for 21 days. Other protozoan infections that can be found in HIV-1-infected patients are *Entameba histolytica, Entameba coli, Entameba hartmanni, Endolimax nana* and *Giardia lamblia* in 4% of cases.

Fungal infections

Candida albicans

Candidiasis of the gastrointestinal tract is the most common fungal infection in HIV-1-infected children. The esophagus is the primary target of *Candida* and this infection occurred in the majority of patients during the course of their illness in the pre-HAART era. It was also the second most frequent AIDS-defining disease, second in prevalence only to *Pneumocystis carinii*. Currently, with successful viral suppression, invasive *Candida* is rare with children on HAART. Patients with *Candida* esophagitis complain of odynophagia or dysphagia, and may often have vomiting and recurrent abdominal pain. Children often have oral thrush, coincident with more disseminated and invasive *Candida* esophagitis, although the absence of oral thrush does not preclude the diagnosis of *Candida* esophagitis.[28] In one study, oral candidiasis preceded the diagnosis of *Candida* esophagitis in 94% of children.[123] Other risk factors include low CD4 count and prior antibiotic use.[123] Histopathologically, yeast forms within an intact mucosa confirm invasive disease. This is in contrast to colonization, where the yeast is found overlying intact mucosal surfaces or necrotic tissue. These organisms are best seen with Grocott's methenamine silver method or periodic acid–Schiff stain. Upper gastrointestinal studies are suggestive of *Candida* esophagitis with diffuse mucosal irregularities (Fig. 39.4). Upper gastrointestinal endoscopy with biopsy and appropriate staining is the most sensitive test for determining invasive candidiasis of the esophagus. Candidiasis can also occur in the stomach, as well as the small bowel if the acid barrier has been suppressed either through an intrinsic decrease in gastric acid production or iatrogenically with the use of potent acid blockers. Numerous effective therapies have been described to treat *Candida* of the upper gastrointestinal tract, including fluconazole, ketoconazole and itraconazole.[124,125] Ketoconazole has more hepatic side-effects than fluconazole. Itraconazole is usually well tolerated and is effective. In severe and invasive disease, either topical or intravenous amphotericin can be used. Agents such as oral miconazole and nystatin are not indicated for invasive *Candida*.

Other fungal infections

Disseminated histoplasmosis develops in 5% of adult patients with AIDS in the mid-western region of the United States, and elsewhere. The clinical signs and symptoms related to this infection may be indolent, but left untreated can carry significant morbidity and mortality.[126] The likelihood of disease is higher in patients with CD4 counts under 200 cells/mm^3.[127] There is enterocolitis associated

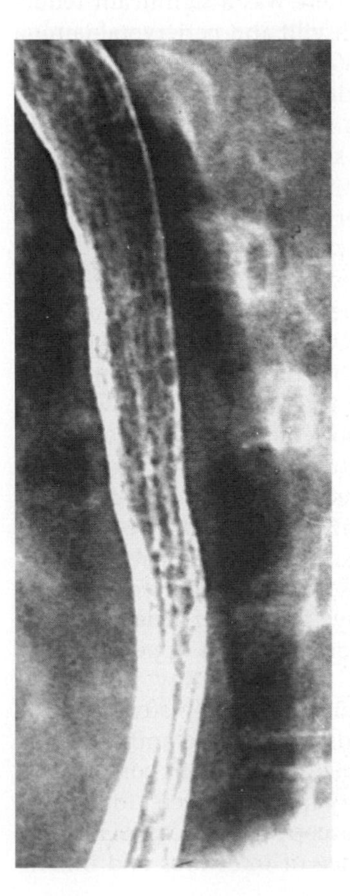

Figure 39.4: Radiographic contrast study showing mucosal irregularities seen with *Candida* esophagitis.

with infection, and at colonoscopy, plaques, ulcers, pseudopolyps and skip areas are frequently seen. Cryptococcal gastrointestinal disease has been identified in patients with disseminated *Cryptococcus* infection. The esophagus and colon are involved most frequently. *P. carinii* infection of the gastrointestinal tract has also been described.[45] Gastrointestinal pneumocystosis develops after hematogenous or lymphatic dissemination from the lungs, or reactivation of latent gastrointestinal infection. The administration of aerosolized pentamidine has increased the risk of developing extrapulmonary spread of PCP. PCP infection can occur throughout the gastrointestinal tract. In the lamina propria there are foamy exudates with *P. carinii* organisms found within them. Although more rare, infection of the colon can also cause diarrhea.

MOTILITY OF THE GASTROINTESTINAL TRACT IN HIV INFECTION

In up to 15–25% of HIV-1-infected children, the etiology of the diarrhea is unclear. Autonomic dysfunction is another potential mechanism of non-infectious diarrhea not previously described. Clinically, children with autonomic neuropathy have sweating, urinary retention and abnormal cardiovascular hemodynamics. It is possible that this autonomic denervation may contribute to the diarrhea in patients with HIV-1 infection, as suggested by Griffin et al.[128] when neuron-specific polyclonal antibodies were applied to jejunal biopsies. There was a significant reduction in axonal density in both villi and pericryptal lamina propria in patients with HIV-1 infection compared with controls, with the greatest reduction in patients with diarrhea. Octreotide therapy has shown promising results in some patients.[129] Lastly, drug side-effects should be considered, with many of the antiretroviral therapies causing chronic diarrhea and other gastrointestinal toxicities (Table 39.3).

Motility problems of the esophagus and stomach have been reported[130–132]and can be a source of upper gastrointestinal complaints including vomiting, dysphagia, nausea and dyspepsia. The motility abnormalities may be primary, or secondary to infectious or inflammatory disease of the respective organ. Hypertension of the lower esophageal sphincter with incomplete relaxation, esophageal hypocontraction and non-specific motility disorders have been described in patients with normal intact esophageal mucosa.[131] Gastric emptying, especially in patients with infections or advanced disease, may be delayed, as documented by gastric scintigraphy.[130] However, delayed gastric emptying does not always correlate with upper gastrointestinal symptoms or small bowel motility studies. In adults with HIV-1 infection and minimally advanced disease, gastric emptying of solids was delayed and emptying of liquids accelerated compared with that in controls. No abnormal esophageal motility patterns were found. All patients had a normal endoscopy prior to the motility studies.[132] Thus, in the absence of infectious and inflammatory disease in patients with appropriate symptoms, motility studies or empiric trials of prokinetic agents should be considered, with careful consideration of drug interactions.

IDIOPATHIC ESOPHAGEAL ULCERATION

Esophageal ulceration can be a result of an intercurrent opportunistic infection. Idiopathic oral and esophageal ulcers have been described in both children and adults with HIV-1.[133] These ulcers are characteristically large and may be single or multiple in nature (Fig. 39.5). The ulcers are located in the mid to distal esophagus. Controversy exists regarding the pathogenesis of these ulcers, with some investigators identifying HIV-1 at the ulcer base,[134] whereas others have not.[135] Treatment options for these ulcers are limited, but include steroid therapy, with encouraging results,[134] and thalidomide.[136,137] However, chronic low-dose thalidomide does not prevent recurrence of the oral or esophageal aphthous ulcers.[138] In addition to the potentially teratogenic effects, a significant portion of children receiving thalidomide develop a rash, which precludes use of the drug. Significant caution should be exercised when using thalidomide. Overall, HAART has had a positive impact on esophageal disease occurrence and relapse.[139]

CLINICAL MANAGEMENT OF GASTROINTESTINAL DISORDERS IN HIV INFECTION

The diagnostic approach to the child with HIV-1 and gastrointestinal symptoms is outlined in Table 39.4. A comprehensive clinical history should be taken with a focus on estimating caloric intake and evaluating abdominal symptoms, such as diarrhea, vomiting and abdominal pain. Growth history should also be reviewed. The physical examination should focus on an assessment of nutritional state and the possibility of intestinal or hepatobiliary disease. With diarrheal symptoms, every HIV-1-infected child should have a complete evaluation for bowel pathogens. This should precede all other diagnostic studies, as treatment of the pathogen may result in resolution of the symptoms. Investigation for enteric infections should include studies for the organisms outlined in the preceding section on infectious diarrhea. The child's antiretroviral regimen and initiation of new medications should be noted as many of these medications produce significant gastrointestinal side-effects (see Table 39.2). Every effort should be made to correlate timing of the initiation of a drug with onset of symptoms. The clinician should keep in mind that children with active enteric infections may also have secondary problems with malabsorption.

If the clinical history and physical examination are suspicious for malabsorption without enteric infection, the next step should include an evaluation of specific nutrient

Medication	Action	Side-effects
Abacavir	NRTI	Nausea, vomiting, abdominal pain, pancreatitis, abnormal liver function
Aciclovir	Antiviral	Nausea, abdominal pain, diarrhea, abnormal liver function
Amprenavir	PI	Abdominal pain, diarrhea
Atazanavir	PI	Nausea, diarrhea, abdominal pain, hyperbilirubinemia
Azithromycin	Antibacterial	Nausea, vomiting, melena, jaundice
Ciprofloxacin	Antibacterial	Ileus, jaundice, bleeding, diarrhea, anorexia, oral ulcers, hepatitis, pancreatitis, vomiting, abdominal pain
Clarithromycin	Antibacterial	Nausea, diarrhea, abdominal pain, abnormal taste
Combivir (zidovudine–lamivudine)	Combination	Nausea, vomiting, abdominal pain, abnormal liver function, pancreatitis
Delavirdine	NNRTI	Pancreatitis; hepatitis; nausea, vomiting, diarrhea, abdominal pain
Dideoxycytidine (ddC)	NRTI	Nausea, vomiting, abdominal pain
Dideoxyinosine (ddI)	NRTI	Nausea, vomiting, abdominal pain, pancreatitis, abnormal liver function
Efavirenz	NNRTI	Nausea, vomiting, abnormal liver function
Emtricitabine	NRTI	Lactic acidosis, hepatomegaly
Erythromycin	Antibacterial	Nausea, vomiting, abdominal pain
Fosamprenavir	PI	Nausea, diarrhea, vomiting, abdominal pain
Ganciclovir	Antiviral	Nausea, vomiting, diarrhea, anorexia, abnormal liver function
Indinavir	PI	Nausea, vomiting, abdominal pain, diarrhea, changes in taste, jaundice, abnormal liver function
Ketoconazole	Antifungal	Hepatotoxicity
Lamivudine (3TC)	NRTI	Nausea, diarrhea, vomiting, abdominal pain, pancreatitis, abnormal liver function
Lopinavir	PI	Diarrhea, nausea, abdominal pain
Nelfinavir	PI	Nausea, diarrhea, fatigue, abnormal liver function
Nevirapine	NNRTI	Stomatitis, nausea, abdominal pain, raised gamma-glutamyl transpeptidase level, hepatotoxicity
Pentamidine	Antiparasitic	Abdominal pain, bleeding, hepatitis, pancreatitis, nausea, vomiting
Rifampin	Antibacterial	Abdominal pain, nausea, vomiting, diarrhea, jaundice
Ritonavir	PI	Nausea, vomiting, diarrhea, abdominal pain, pancreatitis, abnormal liver function
Saquinavir	PI	Mouth ulcers, nausea, abdominal pain, diarrhea, pancreatitis, abnormal liver function
Stavudine (d4T)	NRTI	Nausea, vomiting, abdominal pain, diarrhea, pancreatitis, abnormal liver function, hepatic failure
Sulfonamides	Antibacterial	Hepatitis, pancreatitis, stomatitis, nausea, vomiting, abdominal pain
Trizivir (abacavir–lamivudine–zidovudine)	Combination	Nausea, vomiting, abdominal pain, pancreatitis, abnormal liver function
Zalcitabine	NRTI	Pancreatitis, hepatic failure (with HBV), steatosis, lactic acidosis
Zidovudine (ZDV)	NRTI	Nausea, vomiting, abdominal pain, abnormal liver function

HBV, hepatitis B virus; NRTI, nucleoside analog–reverse transcriptase inhibitor; NNRTI, non-nucleoside–reverse transcriptase inhibitor; PI, protease inhibitor.

Table 39.3 Medications and common gastrointestinal side-effects

absorption. Carbohydrate malabsorption can be detected through lactose breath hydrogen testing, which measures hydrogen production as a response to an oral lactose load. A raised baseline breath hydrogen or early peak of hydrogen production suggests bacterial overgrowth, and appropriate treatment can be initiated. Lactose malabsorption results in a level of hydrogen production more than 10–15 parts per million over baseline, 60 min after ingestion. Dietary changes can then be made.

D-Xylose absorption testing also helps to determine the absorptive capacity of the gastrointestinal tract. D-Xylose is an absorbable sugar that does not require active transport for uptake by enterocytes. Thus, the D-xylose serum level, after administration of a test dose, reflects the absorptive ability of the gastrointestinal tract and the integrity of the mucosal surface. In younger children, the administered dose is 0.5 g per kg bodyweight, given orally after an overnight fast. In older children and adolescents, the maximum dose is 25 g. A serum level is obtained 1 h after ingestion. Urine samples may be obtained for 5 h after ingestion as well.

Fat malabsorption is determined by a 72-h fecal fat collection. A high-fat diet is administered several days before the collection is initiated and throughout the collection

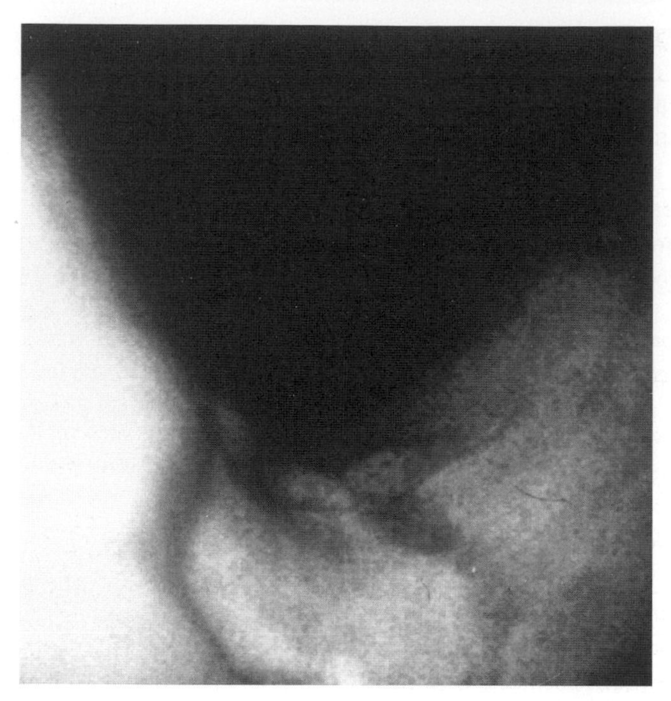

Figure 39.5: Endoscopic view of the esophagus in an HIV-infected child with a large idiopathic esophageal ulcer.

period. An alternative method is to keep a dietary fat intake record during the period of fecal fat collection.The stool is analyzed for total fat content and the fecal fat is compared with the amount ingested; a coefficient of fat absorption is then calculated. Ten percent or more of ingested fat in the stool is considered abnormal. Alternatively, a Sudan stain may be performed on a random stool sample. This may be helpful as a quick test for fat malabsorption, although it is not so reliable. Quantification of fecal elastase may help to determine whether the fat malabsorption is pancreatic in origin. Lastly, raised fecal alpha$_1$-antitrypsin levels suggest protein loss from the gut.

If noninvasive studies, such as those described above, are not helpful in documenting and determining the etiology of the malabsorption, diarrhea or vomiting, endoscopy (either upper or lower) with biopsy and appropriate culture of fluid may be useful. Miller et al.[28] confirmed histologic abnormalities in 72% of children undergoing upper endoscopy. In 70% of patients in this series the clinical management of the child was changed because of the endoscopic evaluation. A high diagnostic yield has been supported by other investigators.[140] Specific gastrointestinal symptoms are not predictive of abnormal findings at endoscopy; advanced HIV-1 disease stage and an increased number of symptoms seem to be more predictive.[28] Histologic studies of the small bowel may aid in determining the degree of the villous blunting, and electron microscopy and special staining for opportunistic pathogens can be performed. Quantitative bacterial cultures and parasite evaluation of the duodenal fluid should be obtained when an endoscopy is performed. Characteristically, the detection of more than 10^5 organisms per ml of duodenal fluid confirms bacterial overgrowth. It is important to obtain both anaerobic and quantitative cultures. However, other studies have shown that endoscopy does not improve the diagnostic yield compared with stool examination in patients with intestinal infection. The only exception is the diagnosis of CMV.[141] An additional study found that flexible sigmoidoscopy was as useful as a full colonoscopy for diagnosing infection.[142] Special histologic stains for fungal, mycobacterial or viral infections did not increase the diagnostic yield over routine hematoxyline and eosin staining.[143]

Treatment of intestinal infections has been outlined in Table 39.2 and previous sections. Therapy for gastrointestinal malabsorption should be directed toward the underlying diagnosis. If clinically symptomatic lactose malabsorption is found, a lactose-free diet should be initiated. Compliance may be difficult, because many foods contain lactose. Children can limit the effects of dietary lactose by taking exogenous lactase or using lactase-treated milk. There should be careful consideration of calcium and vitamin D intake, as children with HIV-1 infection are susceptible to low bone mineral density.[144] If there is malabsorption of protein and fat, a protein hydrolysate diet

Preliminary evaluation

1. **Complete history and physical examination**
   - Caloric intake, anthropometrics, gastrointestinal symptoms
   - Drug interactions
   - Oropharyngeal, abdominal and rectal examinations
2. **Laboratory**
   - Complete blood count, viral load, immune function (CD4 T-lymphocyte count), chemistries (liver function studies, lactate dehydrogenase, pancreatic studies)
3. **Evaluation for enteric pathogens**
   - Bacterial, viral, parasite cultures, examination of stool

Secondary evaluation

1. **Malabsorption studies**
   - Hydrogen breath test analysis
   - Fecal fat determination
   - Fecal elastase
   - D-Xylose absorption
   - Stool alpha$_1$-antitrypsin
2. **Radiographic studies (contrast, computed tomography, ultrasonography)**

Tertiary evaluation

1. **Diagnostic endoscopy**
   - Biopsies, routine stains
   - Brushings, cytology
   - Duodenal aspirate (quantitative bacterial culture, ova and parasite)
   - MAC culture, AFB stains (CD4 count < 200 cells/mm^3)
   - Electron microscopy
2. **Motility studies (in the appropriate clinical setting)**

MAC, *Mycobacterium avium intracellulare* complex.

Table 39.4 Approach to diagnosis of gastrointestinal tract disease in HIV-1-infected children

should be tried. Many of these supplements are poorly tolerated because they are unpalatable. In some circumstances, specialized supplements may need to be administered through a supplemental feeding tube.[145,146] Peptic and motility disorders can be treated as in other non-HIV-1-infected children, paying careful attention to potential drug interactions with antiretroviral regimens.

OTHER SECONDARY IMMUNODEFICIENCIES

A variety of other disorders (Table 39.5) can cause secondary immunodeficiencies with effects on the gastrointestinal tract. Overall, these disorders are more prevalent than either primary or HIV-1-associated immunodeficiencies. Premature infants, children with cancer and associated exposure to immunosuppressant and cytotoxic medications (including children with graft *vs* host disease), and children with protein-losing enteropathy with associated loss of immunoglobulins from the gastrointestinal tract, can all be immunodeficient because of the underlying disorder. In general, children with these immunodeficiencies are at risk for many of the same complications that are experienced by children with HIV-1 infection. Gastrointestinal tract infections are among the most common problems facing children with other secondary immunodeficiencies.

Prematurity
Metabolic disorders
- Down syndrome
- Malnutrition
- Micronutrient deficiency
- Uremia, nephrotic syndrome
- Sickle cell disease
- Diabetes mellitus
- Protein-losing enteropathy

Immunosuppression
- Drug
- Radiation

Infectious diseases
- HIV
- Congenital rubella
- Cytomegalovirus
- Epstein–Barr virus
- Acute bacterial disease
- Disseminated fungal disease

Hematologic or malignancy
- Leukemia, lymphoma
- Graft *vs* host disease
- Aplastic anemia, agranulocytosis

Surgery or trauma
- Splenectomy
- Burns

Inflammatory bowel disease
Systemic lupus erythematosus
Cirrhosis

Table 39.5 Causes of secondary immunodeficiencies

Malnutrition and micronutrient deficiencies

Malnutrition is the most common cause of immunodeficiency worldwide. Nutritional status and immunity have long been linked in many disease states. Before HIV-1 was described, *P. carinii* pneumonia and Kaposi's sarcoma, known opportunistic diseases, were first described in otherwise healthy, but malnourished, children and adults in developing nations.[147,148] This association led investigators to conclude that nutrition alone can affect the immunologic response of an individual. In malnourished children there is a profound involution of lymphoid tissues, including thymic atrophy and diminished paracortical regions of lymph nodes.[149] In young infants and children, protein-calorie malnutrition increases the risk of death by severalfold by increasing the susceptibility to infection.[150] In many countries, the mortality rate increases from 0.5% in children whose weight-for-height percentage of standard is greater than 80%, to 18% in children whose weight-for-height percentage of standard is less than 60%.[151] In other diseases such as cystic fibrosis and cancer, nutritional status has been linked closely to survival rates and morbidity. With leukemia and lymphoma, the incidence of infection with *P. carinii* is higher in patients with protein-calorie malnutrition.[147]

Biochemically, protein-calorie malnutrition leads to changes in several aspects of the immune system. Cell-mediated immunity, microbial function of phagocytes, complement systems, secretory antibodies and antibody affinity, are consistently impaired in patients with significant malnutrition. Additionally, deficiencies of micronutrients, especially zinc and iron, as well as many others, may also have deleterious effects on the immune system. Other aspects of immunity that are altered by protein-calorie malnutrition include impaired chemotaxis of neutrophils, decreased lysozyme levels in serum and secretions, and interferon production in antibody response to T cell-dependent antigens. A child with protein-calorie malnutrition may also have impaired mucosal immunity with lowered concentrations of secretory IgA in saliva, nasopharynx, tears and the gastrointestinal tract compared with well-nourished control children.

Similar to children and adults with HIV-1 infection, in patients with malabsorption T-cell function is depressed not only in the peripheral circulation but also in the intestinal tract. Subsequently, plasma cell function and macrophage activity may be impaired, leading to more frequent intestinal infections in children with severe protein-calorie malnutrition. Not only does nutrition improve the immunologic functioning of the intestinal tract, but nutrients themselves are trophic and essential for the maintenance of the absorptive capacity of the intestines. In some studies, weight loss greater than 30%, due to other disorders, was associated with a reduction in pancreatic enzyme secretion of over 80%, villous atrophy, and impaired carbohydrate and fat absorption.[152] These disorders are promptly reversed with appropriate nutritional rehabilitation. In addition, with villous blunting, increased antigen uptake may also occur, leaving the child at higher risk of enteric infection. The pathogenesis of villous blunting is currently unclear, but may be due to crypt hyperplasia as the primary event with premature sloughing at the villus tip[153] *vs* loss of enterocytes at the villus tip with resultant proliferation at the crypts.[154]

Immunosuppressive therapy

Immunosuppressant medications are the mainstay of therapy for many diseases in children with autoimmune disorders, inflammatory bowel disease, chronic pulmonary disease, cancer and organ transplantation. The best known immunosuppressants include corticosteroids, azathioprine, ciclosporin, tacrolimus and antithymocyte globulin. Unfortunately, the effects of these medications are not targeted toward specific organs, but rather indiscriminately suppress immune function throughout the child. Thus, several immunologic functions including a decrease in monocyte adherence, neutrophil chemotaxis and overall suppression of the inflammatory response are found. Children are at risk of enteric infections, similar to those described in children with HIV-1 infection.

SUMMARY

Gastrointestinal problems are common, with significant accompanying morbidity for HIV-1-infected children. Primary problems of the gastrointestinal tract are associated with gastrointestinal malabsorption and infections. Scientific progress has been made regarding the detection of novel pathogens that can contribute to the gastrointestinal dysfunction, yet there continues to be a subset of children with persistent diarrhea and abdominal pain that is of indeterminate etiology, despite extensive evaluations. Future efforts should focus on improved therapeutic options for treatment of unusual infections as well as further delineation of the etiology of chronic non-pathogenic diarrhea. Although the etiology of immunodeficiencies in disorders such as cancer and malnutrition is different than that associated with HIV 1, many of the same diagnostic and management principles apply. Clinicians should be aggressive in the evaluation of diarrhea and gastrointestinal tract dysfunction in children with ongoing secondary immunodeficiencies.

References

1. Gallo RC, Salahuddin SZ, Popovic M, et al. Frequent detection and isolation of cytopathic retroviruses (HTLV-III) from patients with AIDS and at risk for AIDS. Science 1984; 224:500–503.

1a. UNAIDS. AIDS epidemic update. Online. Available: http://www.unaids.org/en/resources/epidemiology.asp. 22 December 2004.

2. Kourtis AP, Duerr A. Prevention of perinatal HIV transmission: a review of novel strategies. Expert Opin Investig Drugs 2003; 12:1535–1544.

3. van Rossum AM, Fraaij PL, de Groot R. Efficacy of highly active antiretroviral therapy in HIV-1 infected children. Lancet Infect Dis 2002; 2:93–102.

4. Stringer EM, Sinkala M, Kumwenda R, et al. Personal risk perception, HIV knowledge and risk avoidance behavior, and their relationships to actual HIV serostatus in an urban African obstetric population. J Acquir Immune Defic Syndr 2004; 35:60–66.

5. Daar ES, Moudgil T, Meyer RD, Ho DD. Transient high levels of viremia in patients with primary human immunodeficiency virus type 1 infection. N Engl J Med 1991; 324:961–964.

6. Kinloch-De Loes S, Hirschel BJ, Hoen B, et al. A controlled trial of zidovudine in primary human immunodeficiency virus infection. N Engl J Med 1995; 333:408–413.

7. Mellors JW, Rinaldo CRJ, Gupta P, White RM, Todd JA, Kingsley LA. Prognosis in HIV-1 infection predicted by the quantity of virus in plasma. Science 1996; 272:1167–1170.

8. Wahl SM, Greenwell-Wild T, Peng G, et al. *Mycobacterium avium* complex augments macrophage HIV-1 production and increases CCR5 expression. Proc Natl Acad Sci 1998; 95:12574–12579.

9. Smith PD, Saini SS, Raffeld M, Manischewitz JF, Wahl SM. Cytomegalovirus induction of tumor necrosis factor-alpha by human monocytes and mucosal macrophages. J Clin Invest 1992; 90:1642–1648.

10. McDonald D, Wu L, Bohks SM, Kewal Ramani VN, Unutmaz D, Hope TJ. Recruitment of HIV and its receptors to dendritic cell–T cell junctions. Science 2003; 300:1295–1298.

11. Frankel SS, Wenig BM, Burke AP, et al. Replication of HIV-1 in dendritic cell-derived syncytia at the mucosal surface of the adenoid. Science 1996; 272:115–117.

12. Geijtenbeek TB, Kwon DS, Torensman R, et al. DC-SIGN, a dendritic cell-specific HIV-1-binding protein that enhances trans-infection of T cells. Cell 2000; 100:587–597.

13. Cameron PU, Freudenthal PS, Barker JM, Gezelter S, Inaba K, Steinman RM. Dendritic cells exposed to human immunodeficiency cirus type-1 transmit a vigorous cytopathic infection to CD4+ T cells. Science 1992; 257:383–387.

14. Fantini J, Cook DG, Nathanson N, Spitalnik SL, Gonzalez-Scarano F. Infection of colonic epithelial cell lines by type 1 human immunodeficiency virus is associated with cell surface expression of galactosylceramide, a potential alternative gp120 receptor. Proc Natl Acad Sci 1993; 90:2700–2704.

15. Bomsel M. Transcytosis of infectious human immunodeficiency virus across a tight human epithelial cell line barrier. Nat Med 1997; 3:42–47.

16. Meng G, Wei X, Wu X, et al. Primary intestinal epithelial cells selectively transfer R5 HIV-1 to CCR5+ cells. Nat Med 2002; 8:150–156.

17. Meng G, Sellers M, Mosteller Barnum M, Rogers T, Shaw G, Smith P. Lamina propria lymphocytes, not macrophages, express CCR5 and CXCR4 and are likely target cell for HIV-1 in the intestinal mucosa. J Infect Dis 2000; 182:785–791.

18. Smith PD, Meng G, Sellers MT, Rogers TS, Shaw GM. Biological parameters of HIV-1 infection in primary intestinal lymphocytes and macrophages. J Leukoc Biol 2000; 68:360–365.

19. Veazey RS, DeMaria M, Chalifoux LV, et al. Gastrointestinal tract as a major site of CD4+ T cell depletion and viral replication in SIV infection. Science 1998; 280:427–431.

20. Burgio VT, Fais S, Boirivant M, Perrone A, Pallone F. Peripheral monocyte and naive T-cell recruitment and activation in Crohn's disease. Gastroenterology 1995; 109:1029–1038.

21. Kewenig S, Schneider T, Hohloch K, et al. Rapid mucosal CD4(+) T-cell delpetion and enteropathy in simian

immunodeficiency virus-infected rhesus macaques. Gastroenterology 1999; 116:1115–1123.

22. Smythies LE, Sellers M, Clements RH, et al. Human intestinal macrophages display profound inflammatory anergy despite avid phagocytic and bacteriocidal activity. J Clin Invest 2005; 115:66–75.
23. Wahl SM, Orenstein JM, Smith PD. Macrophage functions in HIV-1 infection. In: Gupta SD, ed. Immunology of Human Immunodeficiency Virus Type 1 Infection. New York: Plenum; 1996:303–336.
24. Smith PD, Meng G, Salazar-Gonzalez JF, Shaw GM. Macrophage HIV-1 infection and the gastrointestinal tract reservoir. J Leukoc Biol 2003; 74:642–649.
25. MacDonald T, Spencer J. Evidence that activated mucosal T cells play a role in the pathogenesis of enteropathy in human small intestine. J Exp Med 1988; 167:1341–1349.
26. Kotler DP, Gaetz HP, Lange M, Klein EB, Holt PR. Enteropathy associated with the acquired immunodeficiency syndrome. Ann Intern Med 1984; 104:421–428.
27. Ullrich R, Zeitz M, Heise W, L'age M, Hoffken G, Riecken EO. Small intestinal structure and function in patients infected with human immunodeficiency virus (HIV): evidence for HIV-induced enteropathy. Ann Intern Med 1989; 111:15–21.
28. Miller TL, McQuinn LB, Orav EJ. Endoscopy of the upper gastrointestinal tract as a diagnostic tool for children with human immunodeficiency infection. J Pediatr 1997; 130:766–773.
29. Bjarnason I, Sharpstone DR, Frances DR, et al. Intestinal inflammation, ileal structure and function in HIV. AIDS 1996; 10:1385–1391.
30. Carlson S, Yokoo H, Craig RM. Small intestinal human immunodeficiency virus-associated enteropathy: evidence for panintestinal enterocyte dysfunction. Lab Clin Med 1994; 124:652–659.
31. Keating J, Bjarnason I, Somasundaram S, et al. Intestinal absorptive capacity, intestinal permeability and jejunal histology in human immundeficiency virus and their relation to diarrhea. Gut 1995; 37:623–629.
32. Lim SG, Menzies IS, Nukajam WS, Lee CA, Johnson MA, Pounder RE. Intestinal disaccharidase activity in human immunodeficiency disease. Scand J Gastroenterol 1995; 30:235–241.
33. Mosavi AJ, Hussain MF, DuPont HL, Mathewson JJ, White AC. Lack of correlation between diarrhea and weight loss in HIV-positive outpatients in Houston, Tx. J Clin Gastroenterol 1995; 21:61–64.
34. Taylor C, Hodgson K, Sharpstone D, et al. The prevalence and severity of intestinal disaccharidase deficiency in human immunodeficiency virus-infected subjects. Scand J Gastroenterol 2000; 35:599–606.
35. Miller TL, Orav EJ, Martin SR, Cooper ER, McIntosh K, Winter HS. Malnutrition and carbohydrate malabsorption in children with vertically-transmitted human immunodeficiency virus-1 infection. Gastroenterology 1991; 100:1296–1302.
36. Italian Paediatric Intestinal/HIV Study Group. Intestinal malabsorption of HIV-infected children: relationship to diarrhoea, failure to thrive, enteric microorgansims and immune impairment. AIDS 1993; 7:1435–1440.
37. Yolken RH, Hart W, Oung I, Schiff C, Greenson J, Perman JA. Gastrointestinal-dysfunction and disaccharide intolerance in children infected with human immunodeficiency virus. J Pediatr 1991; 118:359–363.
38. Sentongo TA, Rutstein RM, Stettler N, Stallings VA, Rudy B, Mulberg AE. Association between steatorrhea, growth, and immunologic status in children with perinatally acquired HIV infection. Arch Pediatr Adolesc Med 2001; 155:149–153.
39. Carroccio A, Fontana M, Spagnuolo MI, et al. Pancreatic dysfunction and its association with fat malabsorption in HIV infected children. Gut 1998; 43:558–563.
40. Schneider T, Jahn HV, Schmidt W, et al. Loss of CD4 T lymphocytes in patients infected with human immunodeficiency virus type 1 is more pronounced in the duodenal mucosa than in the peripheral blood. Gut 1995; 37:524–529.
41. Kotler DP, Reka S, Clayton F. Intestinal mucosal inflammation associated with human immunodeficiency virus infection. Dig Dis Sci 1993; 38:1119–1127.
42. Lake-Bakaar G, Tom W, Lake-Bakaar D, et al. Gastropathy and ketoconazole malabsorption in the acquired immuno-deficiency syndrome (AIDS). Ann Intern Med 1988; 109:471–473.
43. Smith PD, Lane HC, Gill VJ, et al. Intestinal infections in patients with the acquired immunodeficiency syndrome (AIDS): etiology and response to therapy. Ann Intern Med 1988; 108:328–333.
44. Wilcox CM, Waites KB, Smith PD. No relationship between gastric pH, small bowel bacterial colonisation, and diarrhoea in HIV-1 infected patients. Gut 1999; 44:101–105.
45. Ramos-Soriano AG, Saavedra JM, Wu TC, et al. Enteric pathogens associated with gastrointestinal dysfunction in children with HIV infection. Mol Cell Probes 1996; 10:67–73.
46. Canani RB, Spagnuolo MI, Cirillo P, Guarino A. Ritonavir combination therapy restores intestinal function in children with advanced HIV disease. J Acquir Immune Defic Syndr 1999; 21:307–312.
47. Poles MA, Fuerst M, McGowan I, et al. HIV-related diarrhea is multifactorial and fat malabsorption in commonly present, independent of HAART. Am J Gastroenterol 2001; 96:1831–1837.
48. Monkemuller KE, Call SA, Lazenby AJ, WIlcox CM. Declining prevalence of opportunistic gastrointestinal disease in the era of combination antiretroviral therapy. Am J Gastroenterol 2000; 95:457–462.
49. Brink AK, Mahe C, Watera C, et al. Diarrhea, CD4 counts and enteric infections in a community-based cohort of HIV-infected adults in Uganda. J Infect 2002; 45:99–106.
50. Pui JC, Furth EE, Minda J, Montone KT. Demonstation of varicella-zoster virus infection in the muscularis propria and myenteric plexi of the colon in an HIV-positive patient with herpes zoster and small bowel pseudo-obstruction (Ogilvie's syndrome). Am J Gastroenterol 2001; 96:1627–1629.
51. Tendero DT. Laboratory diagnosis of cytomegalovirus (CMV) infections in immunodepressed patients, mainly in patients with AIDS. Clin Lab 2001; 47:169–183.
52. Pollok RC. Viruses causing diarrhoea in AIDS. Novartis Found Symp 2001; 238:276–283.
53. Ukarapol N, Chartapisak W, Lertprasertsuk N, et al. Cytomegalovirus-associated manifestations involving the digestive tract in children with human immunodeficiency virus infection. J Pediatr Gastroenterol Nutr 2002; 35:669–673.
54. Zanolla G, Resener T, Knebel R, Verney Y. Massive lower gastrointestinal hemorrhage caused by CMV disease as a presentation of HIV in an infant. Pediatr Surg Int 2001; 17:65–67.
55. Orenstein JM, Dieterich DT. The histopathology of 103 consecutive colonoscopy biopsies from 82 symptomatic patients with acquired immunodeficiency syndrome: original and look-back diagnoses. Arch Pathol Lab Med 2001; 125:1042–1046.

56. Sabin CA, Clewley GS, Deayton JR, et al. Shorter survival in HIV-positive patients with diarrhoea who excrete adenovirus from the GI tract. J Med Virol 1999; 58:280–285.
57. Grohmann GS, Glass RI, Monroe SS, Hightower AW, Weber R, Bryan RT. Enteric viruses and diarrhea in HIV-infected patients. N Engl J Med 1993; 329:14–20.
58. Giordano MO, Martinez LC, Rinaldi D, et al. Detection of picobirnavirus in HIV-infected patients with diarrhea in Argentina. J Acquir Immune Defic Syndr Hum Retrovirol 1998; 18:380–380.
59. Cegielski JP, Msengi AE, Miller SE. Enteric viruses associated with HIV infection in Tanzanian children with chronic diarrhea. Pediatric AIDS HIV Infect 1994; 5:296–299.
60. Belitsos PC, Greenson JK, Yardley JH, Sisler JR, Bartlett JG. Association of gastric hypoacidity with opportunistic enteric infections in 12 patients with AIDS. J Infect Dis 1992; 166:277–284.
61. Gordon MA, Banda HT, Gondwe M, et al. Non-typhoidal salmonella bacteraemia among HIV-infected Malawian adults: high mortality and frequent recrudenscence. AIDS 2002; 16:1633–1641.
62. Manfredi R, Calza L, Chiodo F. Enteric and disseminated *Campylobacter* species infection during HIV disease: a persisting but significantly modified association in the HAART era. Am J Gastroenterol 2002; 97:510–511.
63. Buchner AM, Sonnenberg A. Medical diagnoses and procedures associated with *Clostridium difficile* colitis. Am J Gastroenterol 2001; 96:766–772.
64. Pulvirenti JJ, Mehra T, Hafiz I, et al. Epidemiology and outcome of *Clostridium difficile* infection and diarrhea in HIV infected inpatients. Diagn Microbiol Infect Dis 2002; 44:325–330.
65. Anastasi JK, Capili B. HIV and diarrhea in the era of HAART: 1998 New York State hospitalizations. Am J Infect Control 2000; 28:262–266.
66. Nightingale SD, Byrd LT, Southern PM, et al. Incidence of *Mycobacterim avium-intracellulare* complex bacteremia in human immunodeficiency virus-positive patients. J Infect Dis 1992; 165:1082–1085.
67. Chaisson RE, Gallant JE, Keruly JC, Moore RD. Impact of opportunistic disease on survival in patients with HIV infection. AIDS 1998; 12:29–33.
68. Rolla VC, Gadelha AJ, Accacio N, et al. Opportunistic diseases incidence and survival in AIDS patients who experienced very low CD4+ cell counts in the protease inhibitors era (TuPe 3341). Ninth International Conference on AIDS, 2000, Durban, South Africa.
69. Gadelha A, Accacio N, Grinzstejn B, et al. Low incidence of colonization and no cases of disseminated *Mycobacterium avium* complex infection (DMAC) in Brazilian AIDS patients in the HAART era. Brazil J Infect Dis 2002; 6:252–257.
70. Nguyen HN, Frank D, Handt S, et al. Severe gastrointestinal hemorrhage due to *Mycobacterium avium* complex in a patient receiving immunosuppressive therapy. Am J Gastroenterol 1999; 94:232–235.
71. Race EM, Adelson Mitty J, Kriegel GR, et al. Focal mycobacterial lymphadenitis following initiation of protease-inhibitor therapy in patients with advanced HIV-1 disease. Lancet 1998; 351:252–255.
72. Desimone JA, Babinchak TJ, Kaulback KR, Pomerantz RJ. Treatment of *Mycobacterium avium* complex immune reconstitution disease in HIV-1-infected individuals. AIDS Patient Care STDs 2003; 17:617–622.
73. French MA, Lenzo N, John M, et al. Immune restoration disease after the treatment of immunodeficient HIV-infected patients with highly active antiretroviral therapy. HIV Med 2000; 1:107–115.
74. Dunne M, Fessel J, Kumar P, et al. A randomized, double-blind trial comparing azithromycin and clarithromycin in the treatment of disseminated *Mycobacterium avium* infection in patients with human immunodeficiency virus. Clin Infect Dis 2000; 31:1245–1252.
75. Griffith DE. Risk–benefit assessment of therapies for *Mycobacterium avium* complex infections. Drug Saf 1999; 21:137–152.
76. Orenstein JM, Kotler DP. Diarrheogenic bacterial enteritis in acquired immunodeficiency syndrome: a light and electron microscopy study of 52 cases. Hum Pathol 1995; 26:481–492.
77. Kotler DP, Giang TT, Thim M, Nataro JP, Sordillo EM, Orenstein JM. Chronic bacterial enteropathy in patients with AIDS. J Infect Dis 1995; 171:552–558.
78. AliMohamed F, Lule GN, Nyong'o A, Bwayo J, Rana FS. Prevalence of *Helicobacter pylori* and endoscopic findings in HIV seropositive patients with upper gastrointestinal tract symptoms at Kenyatta National Hospital, Nairobi. East Afr Med J 2002; 79:226–231.
79. Sud A, Ray P, Bhasin DK, Wanchu A, Bambery P, Singh S. *Helicobacter pylori* in Indian HIV infected patients. Trop Gastroenterol 2002; 23:79–81.
80. Fernando N, Holton J, Zulu I, Vaira D, Mwaba P, Kelly P. *Helicobacter pylori* infection in an urban African population. J Clin Microbiol 2001; 39:1323–1327.
81. Lichterfeld M, Lorenz C, Nischalke HD, Scheurlen C, Sauerbruch T, Rockstroh JK. Decreased prevalence of *Helicobacter pylori* infection in HIV patients with AIDS defining diseases. Z Gastroenterol 2002; 40:11–14.
82. Ribeiro JM, Lucas M, Palhano MJ, Victorino RM. Remission of a high-grade gastric mucosa associated lymphoid tissue (MALT) lymphoma following *Helicobacter pylori* eradication and highly active antiretroviral therapy in a patient with AIDS. Am J Med 2001; 111:328–329.
83. Hunter PR, Nichols G. Epidemiology and clinical features of *Cryptosporidium* infection in immunocompromised patients. Clin Microbiol Rev 2002; 15:145–154.
84. Amadi B, Kelly P, Mwiya M, et al. Intestinal and systemic infection, HIV, and mortality in Zambian children with persistent diarrhea and malnutrition. J Pediatr Gastroenterol Nutr 2001; 32:550–554.
85. Cegielski JP, Ortega YR, McKee S, et al. *Cryptosporidium*, enterocytozoon, and *Cyclospora* infections in pediatric and adult patients with diarrhea in Tanzania. Clin Infect Dis 1999; 28:314–321.
86. Nime FA, Burek JB, Page DL, Holscher MA, Yardley JH. Acute enterocolitis in a human being infected with the protozoon *Cryptosporidium*. Gastroenterology 1976; 70:592–598.
87. Mersel JL, Perera DR, Meligro C, Rubin CE. Overwhelming watery diarrhea associated with a cryptosporidium in an immunosuppressed patient. Gastroenterology 1976; 70:1156–1160.
88. Botero JH, Castano A, Montoya MN, Ocampo NE, Hurtado MI, Lopera MM. A preliminary study of the prevalence of intestinal parasites in immunocompromised patients with and without gastrointestinal manifestations. Rev Inst Med Trop S Paulo 2003; 45:197–200.
89. Westrope C, Acharya A. Diarrhea and gallbladder hydrops in an immunocompetent child with cryptosporidium infection. Pediatr Infect Dis J 2001; 20:1179–1181.
90. Calzetti C, Magnani G, Confalonieri D, et al. Pancreatitis caused by *Cryptosporidium parvum* in patients with severe immunodeficiency related to HIV infection. Ann Ital Med Int 1997; 12:63–66.

91. MacKenzie WR, Hoxie NJ, Proctor ME, et al. A massive outbreak in Milwaulkee of *Cryptosporidium* infection transmitted through the public water supply. N Engl J Med 1994; 331:161–167.

92. Kazlow PG, Shah K, Benkov KJ, Dische R, LeLeiko NS. Esophageal cryptosporidiosis in a child with acquired immune deficiency syndrome. Gastroenterology 1986; 91:1301–1303.

93. Clayton F, Heller T, Kotler DP. Variation in the enteric distribution of cryptosporidia in acquired immunodeficiency syndrome. Am J Clin Pathol 1994; 102:420–425.

94. Goodgame RW, Kimball K, Ou CN, et al. Intestinal function and injury in acquired immunodeficiency-related cryptosporidiosis. Gastroenterology 1995; 108:1075–1082.

94a Pettoello-Mantovani M, Di Martino L, Dettori G et al. Asymptomatic carriage of intestinal *Cryptosporidium* in immunocompetent and immunodeficient children: a prospective study. Pediatr Infect Dis J 1995; 14:1042–1047.

95. Soave R, Johnson WD. *Cryptosporidium* and *Isospora belli* infection. J Infect Dis 1988; 157:225–229.

96. Kreinik G, Burstein O, Landor M, Bernstein C, Weiss LM, Wittner M. Successful management of intractable cryptosporidial disease with intravenous octreotide, a somatostatin analogue. AIDS 1991; 5:765–767.

97. Miao YM, Awad El Kariem FM, Franzen C, et al. Eradication of cryptosporidia and microsporidia following successful antiretroviral therapy. J Acquir Immune Defic Syndr 2000; 25:124–129.

98. Schmidt W, Wahnschaffe U, Schafer M, et al. Rapid increase of mucosal CD4 T cells followed by clearance of intestinal cryptosporidiosis in an AIDS patient receiving highly active antiretroviral therapy. Gastroenterology 2001; 120:984–987.

99. Simon D, Weiss L, Tanowitz HB, Wittner M. Resolution of *Cryptosporidium* infection in an AIDS patient after improvement of nutritional and immune status with octreotide. Am J Gastrenterol 1991; 86:615–618.

100. Nord J, Pearl M, DiJohn D, Tzipori S, Tacket CO. Treatment with hyperimmune colostrum of cryptosporidial diarrhea in AIDS patients. AIDS 1990; 4:581–584.

101. Ungar BL, Ward DJ, Fayer R, Quinn CA. Cessation of *Cryptosporidium*-associated diarrhea in an acquired immunodeficiency patient after treatment with hyperimmune bovine colostrum. Gastroenterology 1990; 98:486–489.

102. Hicks P, Zwiener J, Squires J, Savell V. Azithromycin therapy for *Cryptosporidium parvum* infection in 4 children infected with HIV. J Pediatr 1996; 129:297–300.

103. Kadappu KK, Nagaraja MV, Rao PV, Shastry BA. Azithromycin as treatment for cryptosporidiosis in human immunodeficienccy virus disease. J Postgrad Med 2002; 48:179–181.

104. Hommer V, Eichholz J, Pertry F. Effect of antiretroviral protease inhibitors alone, and in combination with paromomycin, on the excystation, invasion and *in vitro* development of *Cryptosporidium parvum*. J Antimicrob Chemother 2003; 52:359–364.

105. Bryan RT, Cali A, Owen RL, Spencer HC. Microsporidia: opportunistic pathogens in patients with AIDS. Prog Clin Parasitol 1991; 2:1–26.

106. Desportes I, Le Charpentier Y, Galian A, et al. Occurrence of a new microsporidian: *Enterocytozoon bieneusi* n.g., n. sp., in the enterocytes of a human patient with AIDS. J Protozool 1985; 32:250–254.

107. Orenstein JM, Chiang J, Steinberg W, Smith PD, Rotterdam H, Kotler DP. Intestinal microsporidiosis as a cause of diarrhea in human immunodeficiency virus infected patients: a report of 20 cases. Hum Pathol 1990; 21:475–481.

108. Molina JM, Sarfati C, Beauvais B, et al. Intestinal microsporidiosis in human immunodeficiency virus-infected patients with chronic unexplained diarrhea: prevalence and clinical and biologic features. J Infect Dis 1993; 167:217–221.

109. Coyle CM, Wittner M, Kotler DP, et al. Prevalence of microsporidiosis due to *Enterocytozoon bieneusi* and *Enterocytozoon (Spetata) intestinalis* among patients with AIDS-related diarrhea: determination of polymerase chain reaction to the micrsporidian small-subunit rRNA gene. Clin Infect Dis 1996; 23:1002–1006.

110. Kotler DP, Orenstein JM. Prevalence of intestinal microsporidia in HIV-infected individual referred for gastroenterolgical evaluation. Am J Gastroenterol 1994; 89:1998–2002.

111. Wanachiwanawin D, Chokephaibulkit K, Lertlaituan P, Ongratchanakun J, Chinabut P, Thakerngpol K. Intestinal microsoporidiosis in HIV-infected children with diarrhea. SE Asian J Trop Med Public Health 2002; 33:241–245.

112. Tumwine JK, Kekitiinwa A, Nabukeera N, Akiyoshi DE, Buckholt MA, Tzipori S. *Enterocytozoon bieneusi* among children with diarrhea attending Mulago Hospital in Uganda. Am J Trop Med Hyg 2002; 67:299–303.

113. Orenstein JM. Diagnostic pathology of microsporidiosis. Ultrastruct Pathol 2003; 27:141–149.

114. Molina JM, Goguel J, Sarfati C, et al. Potential efficiency of funagillin in intestinal microspordiosis due to *Enterocytozoon bieneusi* in patients with HIV infection: results of a drug screening study. AIDS 1997; 11:1603–1610.

115. Coyle CM, Kent M, Tanowitz HB, Wittner M, Weiss LM. NP 470 is an effective antimicrosporidial agent. J Infect Dis 1998; 177:515–518.

116. Didier ES. Effects of albendazole, fumagillin and TNP-470 on microsporidial replication *in vitro*. Antimicrob Agents Chemother 1997; 41:1541–1546.

117. Anwar-Bruni DM, Hogan SE, Schwartz DA, Wilcox CM, Bryan RT, Lennox JL. Atovaquone is effective treatment for the symptoms of gastrointestinal microsporidiosis in human immundeficiency virus-1 infected patients. AIDS 1996; 10:619–623.

118. Conteas CN, Berlin OGW, Ash LR, Pruthi JS. Therapy for human gastrointestinal microsporidiosis. Am J Trop Med Hyg 2000; 63:121–127.

119. Maggi P, Larocca AM, Quarto M, et al. Effect of antiretroviral therapy on cryptosporidiosis and microsporidiosis in patients infected with human immunodeficiency virus type 1. Eur J Clin Microbiol Infect Dis 2000; 19:213–217.

120. Verdier RI, Fitzgerald DW, Johnson WD, Pape JW. Trimethoprim–sulfamethoxazole compared with ciprofloxacin for treatment and prophylaxis of *Isospora belli* and *Cyclospora cayetanensis* infection in HIV-infected patients. A randomized, controlled trial. Ann Intern Med 2000; 132:885–888.

121. Weiss LM, Perlman DC, Sherman J, Tanowitz H, Wittner M. *Isospora belli* infection: treatment with pyrimethamine. Ann Intern Med 1988; 109:474–475.

122. Germani Y, Minssart P, Vohito M, et al. Etiologies of acute, persistent, and dysenteric diarrheas in adults in Bangui, Central African Republic, in relation to human immunodeficiency virus serostatus. Am J Trop Med Hyg 1998; 59:1008–1014.

123. Chiou CC, Groll AH, Gonzalez CE, et al. Esophageal candidiasis in pediatric acquired immunodeficiency syndrome: clinical manifestations and risk factors. Pediatr Infect Dis 2000; 19:729–734.

124. Saag MS, Fessel WJ, Kaufman CA, et al. Treatment of fluconazol-refractory oropharyngeal candidiasis with itraconazole oral solution in HIV-positive patients. AIDS Res Hum Retroviruses 1999; 15:1413–1417.
125. Groll AH, Wood L, Roden M, et al. Safety, pharmacokinetics, and pharmacodynamics of cyclodextrin itraconazole in pediatric patients with oropharyngeal candidiasis. Antimicrob Agents Chemother 2002; 46:2554–2563.
126. Suh KN, Anekthananon T, Mariuz PR. Gastrointestinal histoplasmosis in patients with AIDS: case report and review. Clin Infect Dis 2001; 32:483–491.
127. Wheat LJ, Connolly Stringfield PA, Baker RL, et al. Disseminated histoplasmosis in the acquired immune deficiency syndrome: clinical findings, diagnosis and treatment, and review of the literature. Medicine 1990; 69:361–374.
128. Griffin GE, Miller A, Batman P, et al. Damage to jejunal intrinsic autonomic nerves in HIV infection. AIDS 1988; 2:379–382.
129. Neild PJ, Evans DF, Castilla FD, et al. Effect of octreotide on small intestinal motility in HIV-infected patients with chronic refractory diarrhea. Dig Dis Sci 2001; 46:2636–2642.
130. Neild P, Nijran KS, Yazaki E, et al. Delayed gastric emptying in human immunodeficiency virus infection: correlation with symptoms, autonomic function, and intestinal motility. Dig Dis Sci 2000; 45:1491–1499.
131. Zalar AE, Olmos MA, Piskorz EL, Magnanini FL. Esophageal motility disorders in HIV patients. Dig Dis Sci 2003; 48:962–967.
132. Konturek JW, Fischer H, van der Voort IR, Domschke W. Disturbed gastric motor activity in patients with human immunodeficiency virus infection. Scand J Gastroenterol 1997; 32:221–225.
133. Blitman NM, Ali M. Idiopathic giant esophageal ulcer in an HIV-positive child. Pediatr Radiol 2002; 32:907–909.
134. Kotler DP, Reka S, Orenstein JM, Fox CH. Chronic idiopathic esophageal ulceration in the acquired immunodeficiency syndrome, characterization and treatment with corticosteroids. J Clin Gastroenterol 1992; 15:284–290.
135. Wilcox CM, Schwartz DA, Clark WS. Esophageal ulceration in human immunodeficiency virus infection. Ann Intern Med 1995; 122:143–149.
136. Naum SM, Molloy PJ, Kania RJ, McGarr J, Van Thiel DH. Use of thalidomide in treatment and maintenance of idiopathic esophageal ulcers in HIV+ individuals. Dig Dis Sci 1995; 40:1147–1148.
137. Jacobson JM, Spritzler J, Fox L, et al. Thalidomide for the treatment of esophageal aphthous ulcers in patients with human immunodeficiency virus infection. National Institute of Allergy and Infectious Disease AIDS Clinical Trials Group. J Infect Dis 1999; 180:61–67.
138. Jacobson JM, Greenspan JS, Spritzler J, et al. Thalidomide in low intermittent doses does not prevent recurrence of human immunodeficiency virus-associated apthous ulcers. J Infect Dis 2001; 183:343–346.
139. Bini EJ, Micale PL, Weinshel EH. Natural history of HIV-associated esophageal disease in the era of protease inhibitor therapy. Dig Dis Sci 2000; 45:1301–1307.
140. Bashir RM, Wilcox CM. Symptom-specific use of upper gastrointestinal endoscopy in human immunodeficiency virus-infected patients yields high dividends. J Clin Gastroenterol 1996; 23:292–298.
141. Weber R, Ledergerber B, Zbinden R, et al. Enteric infections and diarrhea in human immunodeficiency virus-infected persons: prospective community-based cohort study. Swiss HIV cohort study. Arch Intern Med 1999; 159:1473–1480.
142. Kearney DJ, Steuerwald MS, Koch J, Cello JP. A prospective study of endoscopy in HIV-associated diarrhea. Am J Gastroenterol 1999; 94:596–602.
143. Monkemuller KE, Bussian AH, Lazenby AJ, Wilcox CM. Special histologic stains are rarely beneficial for the evaluation of HIV-related gastrointestinal infections. Am J Clin Pathol 2000; 114:387–394.
144. Jacobson D, Spiegelman D, Duggan C et al. (2005) Predictors of bone mineral density in human immunodeficiency virus-1 infected children. J Pediatr Gastroenterol and Nutr (in press)
145. Miller TL, Awnetwant EL, Evans S, Morris VM, Vazquez IM. Gastrostomy tube supplementation for HIV-infected children. Pediatrics 1995; 96:696–702.
146. Henderson RA, Saavedra JM, Perman JA, Hutton N, Livingston RA, Yolken RH. Effect of enteral tube feeding on growth of children with symptomatic human immunodeficiency virus infection. J Pediatr Gastroenterol Nutr 1994; 18:429–434.
147. Chandra RK, ed. Immunocompetence of Nutritional Disorders. London: Arnold; 1980.
148. Centers for Disease Control, Task Force on Kaposi's Sarcoma and Opportunistic Infections. Epidemiologic aspects of the current outbreak of Kaposi's sarcoma and opportunistic infection. N Engl J Med 1982; 306:248–252.
149. Chandra, RK and Newbuerne, PM, Nutrition, immunity and infection: mechanisms of interactions, ed. Chandra RK, NP. 1977, New York: Plenum.
150. Scrimshaw NS, Taylor CE, Gordon JE. Interactions of nutrition and infection. WHO Monograph Series World Health Organ 1968; 57.
151. Hughes WT, Price RA, Sisko F, et al. Protein-calorie malnutrition: a host determinant for *Pneumocystis carinii* infection. Am J Dis Child 1974; 128:44–52.
152. O'Keefe SJ. Nutrition and gastrointestinal disease. Scand J Gastroenterol 1996; 220S:52–59.
153. Bhan MK. The gut in malnutrition. In: Walker WA, ed. Pediatric Gastrointestinal Disease: Pathophysiology, Diagnosis, and Management, 3rd edn. Philadelphia, PA: BC Decker; 1991:603–612.
154. Booth CC. The enterocyte in celiac disease. BMJ 1970; 3:725–731.

Chapter 40
Crohn's disease

Jeffrey S. Hyams

INTRODUCTION

Crohn's disease continues to challenge basic scientists, to vex skilled clinicians and to impair the quality of life for hundreds of thousands of children and adults. Despite decades of intense research, we have a limited understanding of the basic pathophysiologic events that start and continue the often panenteric inflammatory process; this information gap restricts our therapies to those that mitigate inflammation rather than prevent it. Nonetheless, there have been many seminal advances in the treatment of this disorder and a better appreciation of how genotype–phenotype interactions affect natural history and influence therapeutic choices.

EPIDEMIOLOGY

Defining the exact epidemiology of Crohn's disease has been made difficult by the insidious onset of disease, frequent marked delay in diagnosis, occasional presentation with extraintestinal manifestations, and occasional misclassification of patients. Despite these limitations, recent data suggest that the incidence of Crohn's disease has increased dramatically.[1] In Sweden, the incidence is 4.9 per 100 000 children, more than twice that of ulcerative colitis, with a marked increase noted between 1990 and 2001.[2] A statewide population-based study of children in Wisconsin revealed an overall inflammatory bowel disease (IBD) incidence of 7.05 per 100 000, with that for Crohn's disease of 4.56 – more than twice that of ulcerative colitis.[3] There is generally a slight female preponderance and a bimodal distribution of age at diagnosis, with a peak in the second to third decades of life, followed by a smaller peak in the sixth and seventh decades. Although Crohn's disease can be found in infancy, most pediatric cases occur in the mid-adolescent years, with a peak incidence at 14–15 years of age.

Recent observations have challenged many of the old tenets of IBD epidemiology. The emerging pattern suggests similar patterns of disease incidence in whites and nonwhites, those who live in urban and those who live in rural areas, and those in more northern and southern latitudes.[3,4] The large discrepancy between disease incidence in Jews and non-Jews has greatly decreased.[5]

The most important risk factor for developing Crohn's disease is a family history of IBD (see below), but several other risk factors have emerged. Improved living conditions early in life increase the likelihood of developing the condition.[6,7] Other factors that appear to increase risk include previous appendectomy,[8] older maternal age during pregnancy for females developing Crohn's disease[9] and possibly maternal smoking. Data concerning the permissive or protective role of breast-feeding and the development of IBD are conflicting.[10] There are conflicting reports as to whether measles vaccination or exposure in early life is associated with a greater risk of Crohn's disease, but the bulk of evidence argues against an association.[11] Conditions associated with a higher frequency of Crohn's disease include Turner's syndrome,[12] Hermansky–Pudlak syndrome[13] and glycogen storage disease type Ib.[14]

ETIOLOGY

It is likely that a complex interaction of genetic and environmental factors results in the development of Crohn's disease. Animal models have provided important insight into this relationship.[15]

Genetics

The single greatest risk factor for the development of IBD is having a first-degree relative with the condition, with the estimated risk 30–100 times greater than in the general population.[16] The age-adjusted risk for a first-degree relative of a proband with Crohn's disease developing the condition during their lifetime is about 4%, with a slightly greater risk for females than for males.[17] Daughters of an individual with Crohn's disease have a 12.6% lifetime risk of developing IBD, compared with a 7.9% risk for male offspring.[17] If both parents have Crohn's disease, offspring have a 33% risk of developing the condition by the age of 28 years.[18] At the time of diagnosis of Crohn's disease, the likelihood of finding IBD in a first-degree relative of the proband is 10–25%.[17,19] Concordance in monozygotic twins is greater for Crohn's disease (50%)[20] than for insulin-dependent diabetes, asthma or schizophrenia. Although early observations of families with multiple affected members suggested genetic anticipation (earlier onset of disease, increased severity, or both, in succeeding generations of affected families), more recent evidence has not supported this finding.[21] Subclinical intestinal inflammation has been demonstrated in healthy relatives of patients with Crohn's disease, suggesting a possible inherited defect with less destructive expression in some individuals than in others.[22] This subclinical inflammation may also be associated with increased gut permeability,[23] another phenomenon demonstrated in the relatives of patients with Crohn's disease.[24] A similar phenomenon

Neuroendocrine

Inflammatory mediators may alter the structure and function of enteric nerves, and enteric neurotransmitters (e.g. substance P) may have a pro-inflammatory effect.[60] Calcitonin gene-related peptide (CGRP)-containing nerves are prominent in Crohn's disease tissue;[61] in experimental models of colitis, CGRP appears to have an anti-inflammatory effect.[62]

Pathway for tissue injury

The signature feature of Crohn's disease is the intense bowel infiltration with inflammatory cells. Levels of vascular adhesion molecules are greatly increased, resulting in exaggerated migration of circulating inflammatory cells into the mucosa.[63] Tissue concentrations of prostaglandins, leukotrienes, free radicals, nitric oxide, pro-inflammatory cytokines and various chemokines are increased. These substances induce various proteases that result in degradation of extracellular matrix and ulceration. The matrix metalloproteinases (MMPs) are divided into four groups (collagenases, gelatinases, stromelysins and membrane type) and are produced by mesechymal cells, mononuclear inflammatory cells and neutrophils. MMPs are overexpressed in IBD tissue.[64] They are inhibited by several molecules, the most important of which is α_2-microglobulin.[65] In addition, lipoxins, lipoxygenase-derived eicosanoids produced during cell–cell interactions, serve to mitigate inflammation by inhibiting neutrophil chemotaxis and adhesion to epithelium, epithelial chemokine release, TNF-α-stimulated inflammatory responses, cyclo-oxygenase product generation and epithelial cell apoptosis.[66]

Bowel wall thickening and fibrosis is common in Crohn's disease. Mucosal thickening comes from both the epithelium and the lamina propria. Keratinocyte growth factors are overexpressed in the mucosa in IBD.[67] Lamina propria expansion appears to be mediated by multiple cytokines including TNF-α and IL-1β, which are mitogens for subepithelial colonic myofibroblasts,[68] and connective tissue growth factor (CTGF), which promotes extracellular matrix formation and proliferation.[69]

The balance between ongoing inflammatory tissue injury, healing and remodeling appears to dictate the degree to which there is growth of the intestinal muscularis and eventually fibrosis and stenosis. Microvessels from chronically inflamed Crohn's disease tissue demonstrate microvascular endothelial cell dysfunction, characterized by loss of nitric oxide-mediated vasodilation which may lead to reduced perfusion, impaired healing and maintenance of inflammation.[70] Fibrosis results from the deposition of excessive fibrillar collagen and other extracellular matrix materials, and by the overgrowth of smooth muscle. Upregulation of fibrogenic activity by subepithelial myofibroblasts,[71] increased type III collagen production by fibroblasts in response to TGF-β[72] and possible mediation of fibrogenic activity by mast cells[73] occurs.

A schematic representation of the theoretical pathogenesis of Crohn's disease is shown in Figure 40.3.

PATHOLOGY

Macroscopic pathology

Gross inspection of the bowel in well established Crohn's disease reveals marked wall thickening as a result of transmural edema and chronic inflammation. Mural thickening is accompanied by narrowing of the bowel lumen, and may be severe enough to cause clinical obstruction. The mesentery is thickened with edematous, indurated fat that migrates over the serosal surface of the bowel (Fig. 40.4). Mesenteric lymph nodes are frequently enlarged. The bowel mucosa may reveal small aphthous lesions, which may coalesce into larger irregular and deeper ulcers (Fig. 40.5). Bowel inflammation and ulceration may be confluent, but more characteristically is punctuated by 'skip areas' of grossly and even microscopically normal mucosa. Cobblestoning of the surface lining may occur as a result of extensive linear and serpiginous mucosal ulceration with associated regeneration and hyperplasia, in addition to marked submucosal thickening (Fig. 40.6). Stricture formation may occur in the setting of chronic inflammation as a result of fibrous tissue proliferation involving first the submucosa and then the deeper layers of the bowel wall.

Loops of adjacent bowel may become matted together because of serosal and mesenteric inflammation. Fistulae are thought to arise when transmural bowel inflammation extends through the serosa into adjacent structures, such as bowel, abdominal wall, bladder, vagina or perineum. Frequently, a fistulous tract may end blindly in an inflammatory mass (phlegmon) adjacent to the bowel and involves the bowel itself as well as the mesentery, lymph nodes and, occasionally, a chronic active abscess cavity.

Microscopic appearance

The findings on histologic examination of the bowel in Crohn's disease are highly dependent on the duration of disease involvement. Early disease may manifest as superficial aphthoid lesions of the mucosa, usually overlying a lymphoid follicle (Fig. 40.7). Mucosal ulcers may become confluent, producing broad, depressed ulcer beds. There is sequential progression from mucosal disease to profound transmural infiltration of the bowel with lymphocytes, histiocytes and plasma cells. The inflammation is characteristically extensive in the submucosa and is characterized by edema, lymphatic dilation and collagen deposition. The latter is responsible for obliteration of the submucosa, resulting in stricture, obstruction or both. Deep fissuring ulceration into the muscularis propria frequently occurs and, when prominent, is highly characteristic of Crohn's disease even in the absence of granulomas. Crypt abscesses and goblet cell depletion are common but may not be as marked as in ulcerative colitis (Fig. 40.8). Mucosa that is

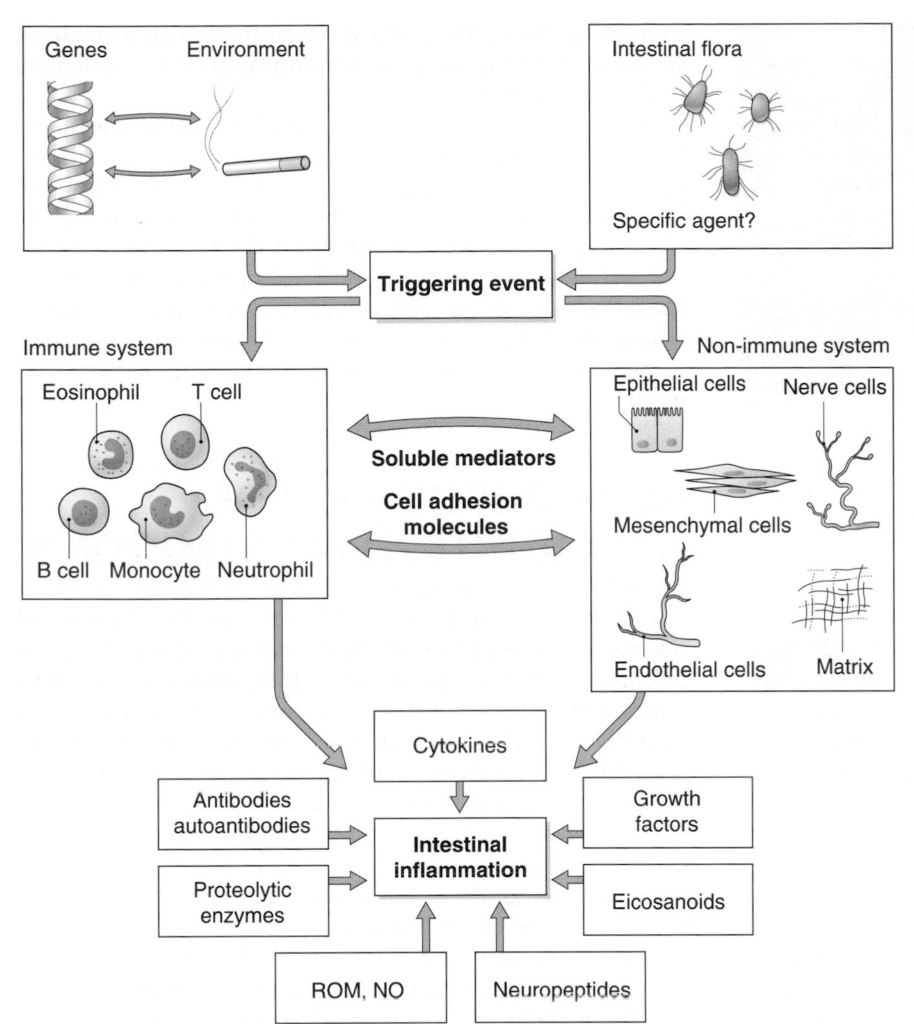

Figure 40.3: Schematic representation of possible contributing factors to the development of Crohn's disease. NO, nitric oxide; ROM, reactive oxygen metabolites. (Courtesy of Claudio Fiocchi MD.)

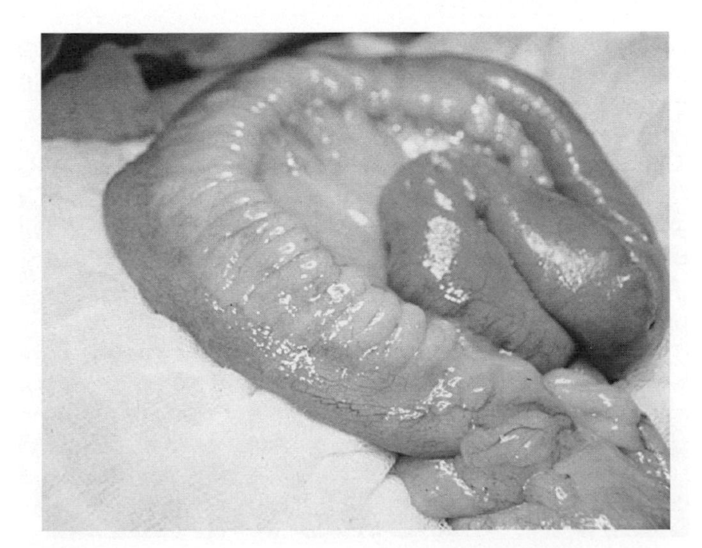

Figure 40.4: Mesenteric fat creeping over inflamed bowel.

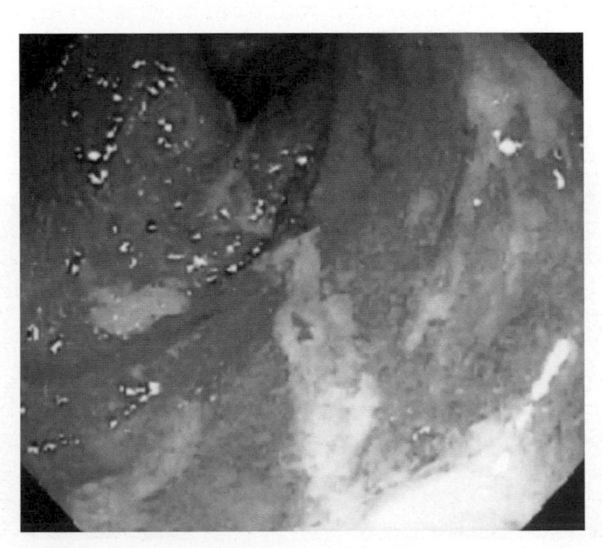

Figure 40.5: Cecal ulceration in Crohn's disease.

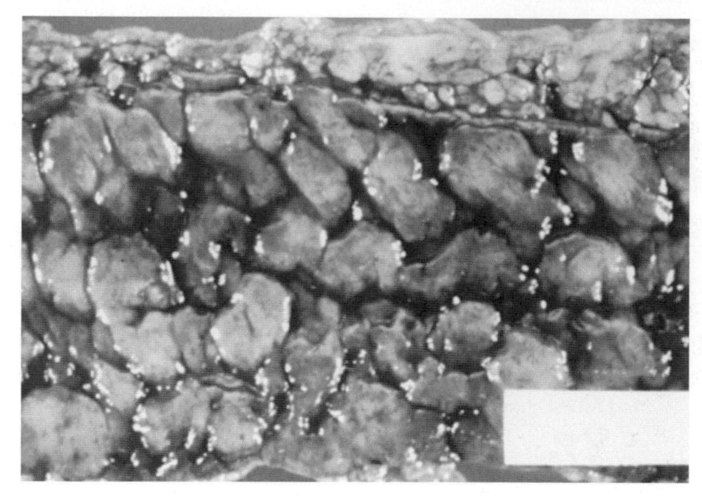

Figure 40.6: Colonic resection specimen showing marked bowel wall thickening with cobblestoning.

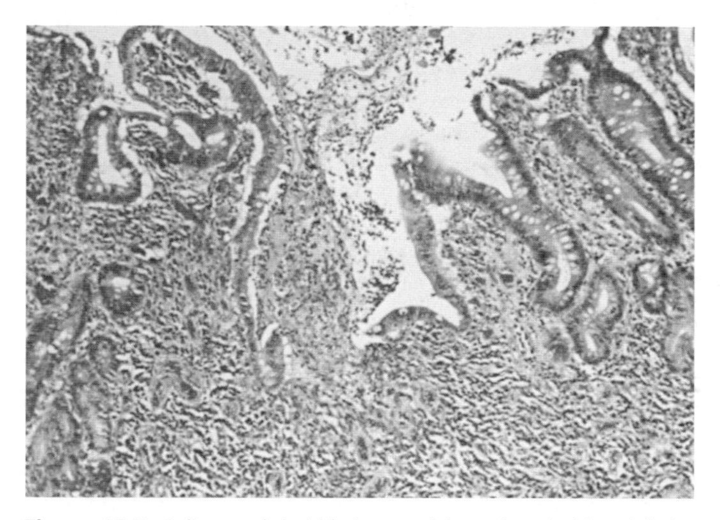

Figure 40.7: Solitary aphthoid lesion overlying a lymphoid nodule in early Crohn's disease.

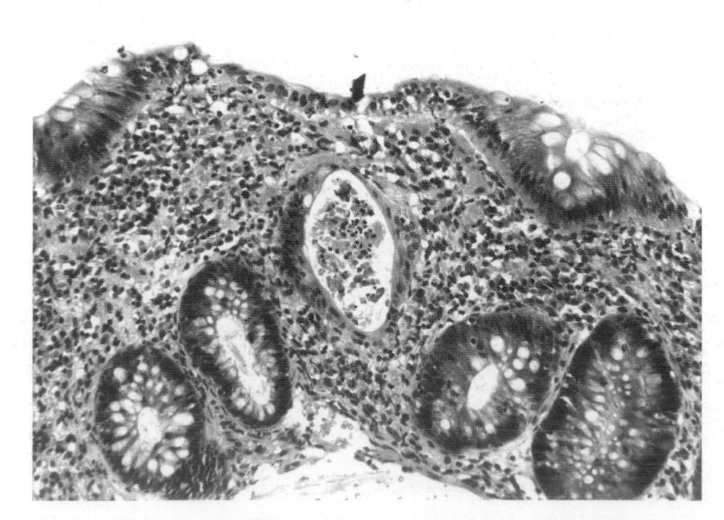

Figure 40.8: Neutrophilic crypt abscess and crypt architectural distortion. (*See plate section for color*).

thought to be normal grossly often reveals abnormalities such as edema and an increase in mononuclear cell density in the lamina propria.

Granulomas are not always found in pathologic specimens from individuals with Crohn's disease, being absent in up to 40% of surgically resected specimens and 60–80% of mucosal biopsies.[74] Granulomas may be found in any layer of the bowel wall, although most commonly in the superficial submucosa (Fig. 40.9). Biopsies from ulcers or the edge of aphthoid lesions may have the highest yield of granuloma. Granulomas may also be present in extraintestinal structures such as lymph nodes, mesentery and peritoneum.

PATHOPHYSIOLOGY OF GASTROINTESTINAL SYMPTOMS

The presence of inflammation in the small and large intestine, bowel wall thickening, or both, leads to a number of derangements that culminate in diarrhea, gastrointestinal bleeding and abdominal pain. Inflammatory mediators released by activated immune cells lead to increased mucosal electrolyte secretion. Extensive jejunal and ileal disease may result in malabsorption. Malabsorbed fatty acids entering the colon impair electrolyte and water absorption. Abnormal terminal ileal function may result in bile acid loss, with an eventual decrease in the luminal bile acid concentration, worsening steatorrhea. Bile salts may significantly impair colonic absorption of electrolytes. Bacterial overgrowth in the small intestine associated with obstruction, stasis or enteroenteric fistula may lead to mucosal damage and bile salt deconjugation, further worsening symptoms. Diffuse mucosal disease leads to exudation of serum proteins and bleeding. Cramping abdominal pain may result from gut distention, usually associated with obstruction or abnormalities in intestinal motility. The pain of Crohn's disease may also result from the inflammation-mediated recruitment of silent nociceptors in the ileocecal region.

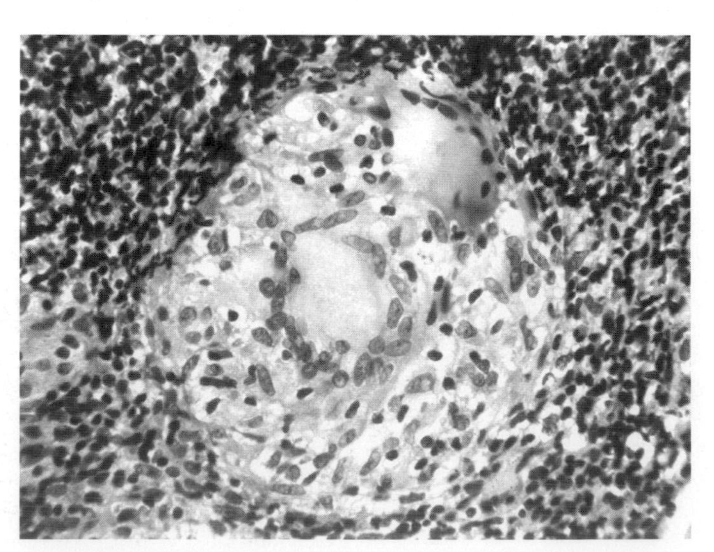

Figure 40.9: Epitheliod granuloma with multinucleated giant cells (*See plate section for color*).

CLASSIFICATION OF SUBGROUPS IN CROHN'S DISEASE

The complex interaction of an individual's genetic composition, immunologic status and environment as described above lead to the heterogeneous manifestations of Crohn's disease. Attempts to categorize patients with Crohn's disease by their variable clinical and laboratory manifestations is called 'phenomics' (Table 40.1).

The Vienna classification was published by an international panel of experts to define subgroups of patients with Crohn's disease.[75] Disease location was classified as terminal ileum only, colon only, ileocolon, or upper gastrointestinal, which reflected any involvement proximal to the terminal ileum. Biologic behavior was classified as non-stricturing non-perforating (inflammatory), stricturing, or penetrating:

- Stricturing disease was defined as the occurrence of persistent luminal narrowing with prestenotic dilation or obstructive signs and symptoms without evidence of penetrating disease.
- Penetrating disease was defined as the occurrence of intra-abdominal or perianal fistulae, inflammatory masses and/or abscess at any time in the course of the disease.

Longitudinal observation of patients shows considerable evolution of biologic behavior, with many patients presenting with inflammatory disease and then manifesting stricturing or penetrating disease over time. A high degree of concordance for anatomic site and biologic behavior is often noted in families with more than one affected member.

Anatomic location
Gastroduodenal (30–40% of subjects)
Jejunoileal (15–20%)
Ileal (30–35%)
Ileocolonic (50–60%)
Colonic (15–20%)
Perirectal (20–30%)
Biologic behavior
Inflammatory
Stricturing (fibrostenosing)
Penetrating
Laboratory markers
ANCA
ASCA
Anti-OmpC
Anti I2
Genetic markers
NOD2/CARD15 (multiple polymorphisms)

Table 40.1 Clinical and laboratory subgroups of patients with Crohn's disease

The presence or absence of immunologic markers has been used to categorize patients with IBD. Antineutrophil cytoplasmic antibody (ANCA), anti-*Saccharomyces cerevisiae* antibody (ASCA) and an antibody to the *Escherichia coli*-related outer membrane porin C (anti-OmpC) have been examined most closely. Perinuclear (p)ANCA associated with IBD is produced by mucosal B cells responding to various antigens.[76] Although present in the serum of 60–70% of patients with ulcerative colitis, pANCA is also detected in 15% of patients with Crohn's disease.[77,78] Patients with Crohn's disease who are pANCA positive exhibit an ulcerative colitis-like picture with left-sided colonic disease and histopathologic expression similar to that of ulcerative colitis.[79] Levels of ASCA (IgG or IgA) are detected in about 50–60% of patients with Crohn's disease.[78] The presence of high-titer ASCA in the absence of ANCA is highly predictive of Crohn's disease.[78,80] Higher levels of IgG and IgA ASCA correlate with the presence of small bowel involvement, as well as with fibrostenosing or perforating disease.[81] Antibodies to I2 (Crohn's disease-associated bacterial sequence) and OmpC are associated with a greater number of strictures and internal perforations.[82] pANCA-positive patients with Crohn's disease are less likely to respond to infliximab than those who are ASCA positive or totally seronegative for these markers.[83] Antibodies to OmpC are present in 38% of patients with Crohn's disease, particularly in those who are ASCA negative.[84]

CLINICAL FEATURES

The presenting clinical features of Crohn's disease are depicted in Table 40.2. Minor discrepancies are seen in different case series, but the most common geographic distribution of disease is ileocolitis (40–60%), followed by small bowel alone (20–30%) and colon alone (20%). Children under 5 years of age have a higher likelihood of colonic involvement.[85] Gastroduodenal involvement is found in up to 30% of children with Crohn's disease.[86]

Terminal ileal and cecal disease is associated with right lower quadrant discomfort; examination often reveals tenderness on palpation and a fullness or distinct mass in this area. Periumbilical pain is common with colonic disease or more diffuse small bowel disease. Gastroduodenal inflammation is common and may be associated with epigastric pain. Odynophagia and dysphagia are observed in most patients with Crohn's disease of the esophagus. The

Feature	Proportion affected (%)
Abdominal pain	75
Diarrhea	65
Weight loss	65
Growth retardation	25
Nausea/vomiting	25
Perirectal disease	25
Rectal bleeding	20
Extraintestinal manifestations	25

Table 40.2 Clinical features of Crohn's disease

abdominal pain associated with Crohn's disease tends to be persistent and severe, and frequently awakens the child from sleep. At times, the acute development of right lower quadrant pain without a well established previous history of illness suggests a diagnosis of appendicitis, but laparotomy findings are consistent with Crohn's disease.

Diarrhea is seen in two-thirds of children, and may be severe and nocturnal. Gross blood in the stool is unusual with isolated small bowel disease, and more common when the colon is involved. Severe hemorrhage, however, may be seen in the setting of small bowel disease when bowel ulceration extends deeply into the bowel wall and involves a larger blood vessel.

Fever can be low grade or spiking, and may persist for extended periods before a diagnosis is made. Nausea and vomiting are frequent and may be seen with involvement of any part of the bowel; they are particularly common in the setting of severe colitis. Fatigue is a common complaint. Anorexia, weight loss and diminution in growth velocity may be seen in 20–60% of children.

About 20–30% of affected children develop perirectal inflammation with fissures, fistulae or tags, and may be misdiagnosed as having hemorrhoids or perianal condyloma. The perirectal disease may prompt a suspicion of abuse. Drainage from these fistulae may be impressive, but perirectal pain is unusual unless there is actual abscess formation.

Gastrointestinal complications

Hemorrhage

Massive acute gastrointestinal hemorrhage is seen in less than 1% of patients with Crohn's disease, but may be severe enough to cause exsanguination. Mesenteric angiography is used to guide surgical resection.

Obstruction

Intestinal obstruction may occur secondary to severe bowel wall inflammation with or without localized phlegmon or abscess formation, stricture formation associated with chronic inflammation, undigested food occluding the lumen of a strictured bowel, carcinoma or adhesions associated with previous surgery. Chronic low-grade obstruction may lead to proximal small bowel bacterial overgrowth.

Perforation

Free perforation (i.e. that not accompanying an abscess or chronic fistula) is unusual in Crohn's disease. It is most common in the ileum. Rarely it can be the initial presentation of the disease. No relationship to perforation has been established between corticosteroid therapy, duration of disease, toxic dilation or obstruction.[87] Classic signs of peritonitis may be masked in the presence of corticosteroid therapy.

Abscess

Transmural bowel inflammation with fistulization and perforation may lead to the formation of abscesses. Fever and abdominal pain are usually present, although it may be difficult to differentiate clinically between an abscess and an exacerbation of the underlying disease with phlegmon formation. Fecal flora is found when these abscesses are cultured. Hip pain may indicate the presence of an ileopsoas abscess.

Fistula formation

Although perianal and perirectal fistulization are most common, other types of fistula include enteroenteric, enterovesical, enterovaginal and enterocutaneous ones. A small proportion of children have highly destructive perianal disease, which often does not respond well to medical therapy. The most common enteroenteric fistula is between the ileum and the sigmoid colon. Enterocolic fistulae may lead to bacterial overgrowth of the proximal bowel.

Toxic megacolon

Toxic megacolon is rare in Crohn's disease.

Carcinoma

Subjects with Crohn's colitis may be at similar risk of developing carcinoma of the colon as those with ulcerative colitis. Carcinoma of the small bowel has also been described.

Extraintestinal manifestations

Extraintestinal manifestations are seen in 25–35% of patients with IBD and can be classified in four groups:[88]

- Those related directly to intestinal disease activity; these usually respond to therapy directed against bowel disease
- Those whose course appears to be unrelated to bowel disease activity
- Those that are a direct result of the presence of disease bowel, such as ureteral obstruction or nephrolithiasis
- Complications arising from therapy.

Joints

Arthralgia (30–40% of patients) and frank arthritis (10%) may be seen.[89] Either the axial skeleton or peripheral joints may be involved. A recent schema has been proposed to classify peripheral joint problems in patients with Crohn's disease.[90] Type 1 arthropathy involves fewer than five joints (pauciarticular), usually involves large joints, is brief in duration, and temporally is related to flares of intestinal inflammation. It is clinically and genetically similar to the reactive arthritis that is associated with human leukocyte antigen (HLA) class I genes. Type 2 arthritis involves multiple small joints and has a course independent of intestinal inflammation; it is not associated with HLA class I genes. In children, arthritis may precede clinical evidence of gastrointestinal inflammation and occasionally children are diagnosed as having juvenile rheumatoid arthritis only to have the diagnosis change once diarrhea and rectal bleeding have begun.

Ankylosing spondylitis is a seronegative arthropathy affecting the vertebral column and is characterized by sacroiliitis and progressive ankylosis or fusion of the vertebral column. It is strongly associated with HLA-B27: up to 50% of patients with IBD who are positive for HLA-B27 develop ankylosing spondylitis. Ileocolonoscopy in individuals with idiopathic ankylosing spondylitis demonstrates gut inflammation resembling early IBD.[91] Clubbing, a form of hypertrophic osteoarthropathy, is common in children with Crohn's disease, particularly when the small bowel is affected.

Musculoskeletal

Muscle diseases described include vasculitic myositis, granulomatous myositis, pyomyositis and dermatomyositis. Proximal muscle weakness is rarely associated with high-dose daily corticosteroid therapy.

Cutaneous

The most common cutaneous manifestation is perianal disease. Erythema nodosum occurs in up to 10% of patients with Crohn's disease, usually during a period of increased intestinal inflammatory activity; recurrence is common. Pyoderma gangrenosum is reported in up to 1–2% of patients with Crohn's disease; its course is not necessarily related to bowel disease activity. Metastatic Crohn's disease is characterized by granulomatous skin lesions distant from the perineum (often the lower extremities), and its course is independent of bowel activity.[92] Epidermolysis bullosa acquisita, a blistering condition of the skin and mucous membranes, is rarely seen. Trace metal deficiency (zinc) and vitamin deficiency (pyridoxine) may be complicated by rashes. Acne is often worsened by corticosteroid therapy, which can also produce striae.

Oral

Oral ulceration (canker sores) range in severity from painless to severe. Biopsy may contain granuloma. Orofacial granulomatosis is a rare condition associated with inflammation and cobblestone ulceration of the oral cavity, and may precede overt intestinal inflammation. Pyostomatitis vegetans is characterized by friable erythematous plaques and is considered the mucosal equivalent of pyoderma gangrenosum.

Ocular

Ocular problems such as uveitis, episcleritis and iritis are often seen in the setting of other extraintestinal manifestations, such as arthritis and erythema nodosum.[93] Slit-lamp examination reveals uveitis in about 6% of children with Crohn's disease; most are asymptomatic.[94] Increased intraocular pressure and posterior subcapsular cataracts may be seen with prolonged corticosteroid therapy.

Vascular

Hypercoagulability from thrombocytosis, hyperfibrinogenemia, rasied levels of factor V and factor VIII, and depression in free protein S concentration is seen in some patients with IBD.[95] Vascular complications have included deep vein thrombosis, pulmonary emboli and neurovascular disease. Vasculitis is a rare complication of Crohn's disease.

Renal

Urinary tract abnormalities may include ureteral obstruction and hydronephrosis secondary to an ileocecal phlegmon encasing the right ureter, enterovesical fistula, perinephric abscess and nephrolithiasis. Oxalate, urate and phosphate stones may be found. The development of proteinuria or raised creatinine levels in a patient with long-standing Crohn's disease suggests amyloidosis. Drug-related interstitial nephritis has been described following 5-aminosalicylic acid (5-ASA) therapy;[96] however, some patients develop chronic interstitial nephritis before taking any medication.[97]

Hepatobiliary

Abnormal serum levels of aminotransferases are seen during the course of disease in approximately 14% of children with IBD.[98] When increased enzyme levels are prolonged (for more than 6 months), the patient usually has either sclerosing cholangitis or chronic hepatitis.[98] A brief increase in serum aminotransferase levels may be associated with increased bowel disease activity, medications (e.g. 6-mercaptopurine), parenteral nutrition and massive weight gain. Other hepatobiliary disorders include hepatic granuloma, hepatic abscess, cholelithiasis and acalculous cholecystitis. Terminal ileal resection or significant ileal disease is associated with increased enteric bile acid loss and an interruption of the enterohepatic circulation of bile acids. Bile may then become supersaturated with cholesterol, leading to gallstone formation.

Autoimmune hepatitis or primary sclerosing cholangitis (PSC) occurs in less than 1% of children with Crohn's disease. Of children with IBD who develop sclerosing cholangitis, about 10% have Crohn's disease.[99] In contrast to adults, there may be significant overlap in the clinical and histologic expression of autoimmune hepatitis and PSC in children with IBD.[100] Serum γ-glutamyl transferase (GGT) appears to be a better screen for PSC than serum alkaline phosphatase.[100]

Pancreas

Pancreatitis may develop as a reaction to drug therapy (6-mercaptopurine, sulfasalazine), from periampullary duodenal disease, associated with sclerosing cholangitis, and in an idiopathic form.[101,102]

Bone

Osteopenia may result from malnutrition, inadequate calcium intake or malabsorption, vitamin D deficiency, excessive pro-inflammatory cytokine production by diseased bowel, prolonged inactivity and corticosteroid therapy.[103] Reduced bone mineral density can occur prior to diagnosis or during the course of illness.[104,105] It has been proposed that bone formation may be inhibited in the presence of bowel inflammation.[106] Both cortical and trabecular bone loss may occur, with resultant fractures, loss of height, severe pain and disability. Although the absolute risk of fracture development in children and adolescents is unknown, data in adults suggest an increase compared with a control population.[107] Risk likely relates to disease severity and duration and the total amount of corticosteroids taken. Aseptic necrosis (osteonecrosis) is very rare in the pediatric population with IBD.

Hematologic

Anemia may be secondary to iron deficiency, folic acid deficiency, vitamin B_{12} deficiency, hemolysis (drug induced or autoimmune) and bone marrow suppression (6-mercaptopurine). Immune activation with the elaboration of pro-inflammatory cytokines may suppress erythrocyte production. It may also be the operative mechanism for thrombocytosis seen in many patients. Neutropenia is a rare accompanying condition.

Malnutrition

Weight loss is seen in most children with Crohn's disease at the time of presentation, and anthropometric observations during the course of disease commonly show abnormalities compared with age-matched control children.[108] Causes of malnutrition in these patients include suboptimal dietary intake, increased gastrointestinal losses, malabsorption and possibly increased requirements associated with marked inflammatory activity (Fig. 40.10). Anorexia may be severe enough to mimic anorexia nervosa. Children who fear exacerbation of gastrointestinal symptoms as a result of eating decrease their intake. Delayed gastric emptying may be associated with early satiety. Marked mucosal inflammation leads to the loss of cellular constituents and hematochezia, with the development of protein-losing enteropathy and iron deficiency anemia. Fecal calcium and magnesium losses may be increased.[109] Deficiency states for iron, folic acid, vitamin B_{12}, nicotinic acid, vitamin D, vitamin K, calcium, magnesium and zinc have been noted.[110] Abnormalities in lipoprotein composition and oxidant antioxidant status have been demonstrated, along with essential fatty acid deficiency.[111]

Limited studies have suggested increased resting energy expenditure,[112,113] together with decreased diet-induced thermogenesis. Corticosteroid therapy affects both energy expenditure and lipid oxidation.[114]

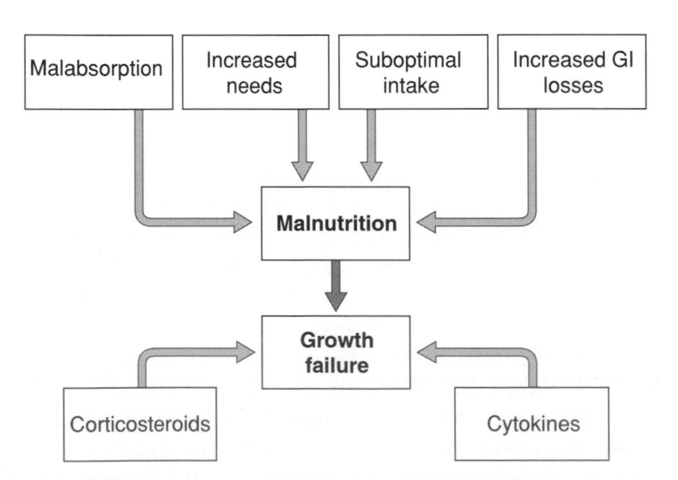

Figure 40.10: Factors contributing to the development of malnutrition and growth failure in children and adolescents with Crohn's disease.

Growth failure

A decrease in growth velocity may precede overt gastrointestinal symptoms in up to 40% of children with Crohn's disease,[115] and evidence of impaired linear growth at the time of diagnosis may be present in 30%.[115,116] There is evidence that some patients with disease onset early in life fail to reach predicted adult height.[117]

There are likely several pathogenetic mechanisms that lead to growth failure (Fig. 40.10), including chronic undernutrition secondary to inadequate intake, excessive losses and increased energy requirement, as well as the effect of bowel inflammation on the growth process.[118,119] The anorexia present in some patients with Crohn's disease is striking and out of proportion to the severity of abdominal pain or diarrhea. In most patients, both basal and stimulated growth hormone levels are normal, but the concentration of insulin-like growth factor (IGF) 1 is reduced, suggesting a degree of hepatic growth hormone insensitivity. In an animal model of colitis, data suggest that part of the diminution in IGF-1 levels is from malnutrition and the remainder secondary to the effects of inflammation.[120] In this same animal model, appetite suppression appeared to be linked to increased serotonin release from the paraventricular nucleus of the hypothalamus, possibly induced by circulating pro-inflammatory cytokines.[121]

Chronic administration of high-dose daily corticosteroid therapy may be an iatrogenic cause of growth failure. Daily corticosteroid therapy for a period as short as 7–14 days is associated with decreased type I collagen production, a prerequisite for linear growth.[122] Alternate-day therapy appears to have little impact on growth velocity[122] or on type I or III collagen production.[123] It is often difficult to separate the growth-retarding effects of increased disease severity from those of the concomitant use of high doses of corticosteroids.

Psychologic disturbances

Depression and anxiety may be present at diagnosis or during the course of the disease. Neither disease activity nor the use of corticosteroids is correlated with the development of depression.

DIAGNOSIS

A combination of clinical and laboratory observations suggests a diagnosis of Crohn's disease, which is then confirmed with radiologic, endoscopic and histologic findings (Table 40.3). Delayed diagnosis is common because the clinical findings may involve systems outside the gastrointestinal tract.

History and physical examination

A complete clinical history is mandatory and will elicit both gastrointestinal and extraintestinal manifestations detailed above. Physical examination should include careful abdominal palpation with particular attention to

History
Abdominal pain Diarrhea Rectal bleeding Fever Arthritis Rash Family history of IBD
Physical examination
Abdominal tenderness Abdominal mass Perirectal disease Clubbing Stomatitis Erythema nodosum Pyoderma gangrenosum
Growth data
Height and weight velocity Decreased for age Delayed puberty
Laboratory tests
Anemia Increased erythrocyte sedimentation rate Increased C-reactive protein level Hypoalbuminemia Thrombocytosis Positive stool occult blood Serology (ANCA, ASCA)
Imaging
Nodularity Skip areas Luminal narrowing (string sign) Fistula Ulceration Bowel wall thickening, abscess (computed tomography) Abnormal isotope scan Abnormal finding on magnetic resonance imaging
Endoscopy
Ulcers Inflammation Cobblestoning Rectal sparing

Table 40.3 Clinical and laboratory findings used to establish a diagnosis of Crohn's disease

tenderness, fullness or mass. Careful inspection of the perirectal area and perineum is mandatory. Rectal examination and stool guaiac should be part of the routine physical examination in a child suspected of having IBD. The presence of stomatitis, clubbing, arthritis, erythema nodosum or pyoderma gangrenosum is suggestive of IBD. Height and weight should be measured and compared with previous values to calculate the rate of change and to compare with expected values from standard growth curves.

Laboratory evaluation

Appropriate stool cultures and examination should be made to exclude enteric bacterial pathogens and parasites including *Salmonella, Shigella, Campylobacter, E. coli* 0157:H7, *Yersinia, Aeromonas, Clostridium difficile, Cryptosporidium* and *Giardia*. Acute onset of bloody diarrhea with fever and vomiting is more suggestive of a bacterial pathogen than Crohn's disease.

Laboratory abnormalities frequently found include anemia (70% of patients), raised erythrocyte sedimentation rate (80%), hypoalbuminemia (60%) and guaiac-positive stools (35%).[124] Although thrombocytosis is common (60%), total leukocyte count is often normal. There may be bandemia. In the nutritionally depleted patient, serum zinc, magnesium, calcium and phosphorus levels may be low. Serum aminotransferase levels are raised at the time of diagnosis in approximately 10% of patients.[98] Testing for ASCA and ANCA may be performed as described previously, and usually serves as adjunctive evidence in the diagnosis.

Breath hydrogen testing for lactose malabsorption may be helpful in subsequent dietary management. Urinalysis should be performed to exclude pyuria or infection associated with enterovesical fistula.

Radiographic evaluation

Contrast imaging

Upper gastrointestinal series with small bowel follow-through is required in all patients with Crohn's disease. Careful fluoroscopy with abdominal palpation is used to identify irregular, nodular (cobblestoned) and thickened bowel loops, as well as stenotic areas (string sign), ulcers and fistulae (Fig. 40.11). Pathologic terminal ileal nodularity is common in Crohn's disease and must be distinguished from non-pathologic nodular lymphoid hyperplasia. In the latter the nodules are usually 3 mm or less in diameter.

Ultrasonography

The presence of a tender mass in the right lower quadrant in a patient with Crohn's disease suggests the presence of an inflammatory phlegmon or abscess. Ultrasonographic examination may help reveal bowel wall thickening as well as extraluminal fluid suggesting abscess. Color Doppler ultrasonography has been used to evaluate vascular changes in bowel loops as a means of assessing disease activity.[125]

Computed tomography

Computed tomography (CT) may be useful in delineating extramural extension of inflammation by fistulization to adjacent structures and in diagnosing abscesses (Fig. 40.12). The clinician must be aware of the significant radiation exposure associated with abdominal CT, especially in the situation of repeated imaging.

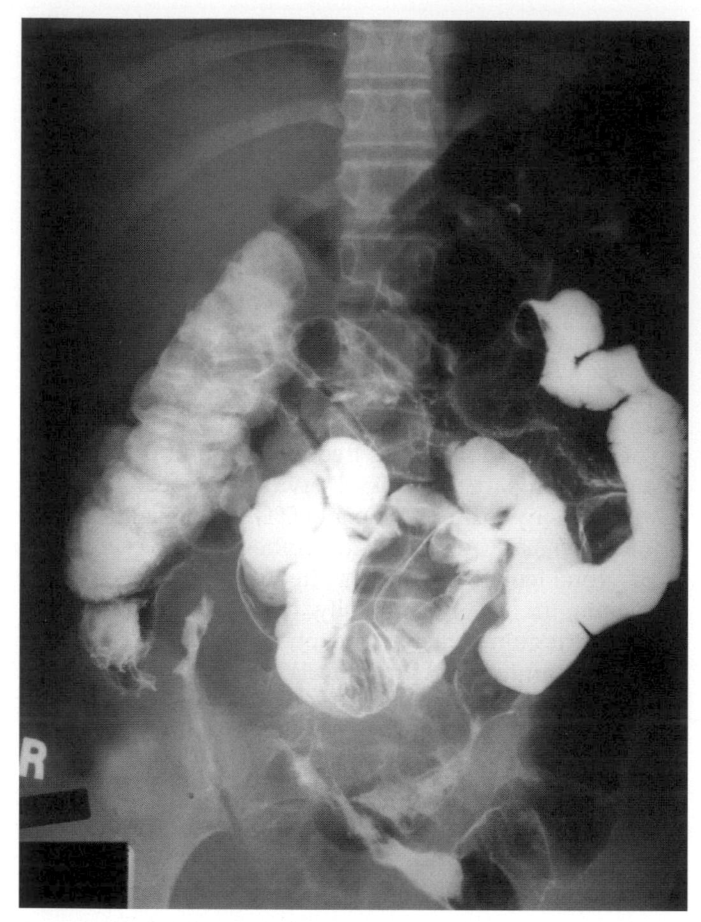

Figure 40.11: Distal ileal narrowing and distortion in an adolescent with newly diagnosed Crohn's disease.

Magnetic resonance imaging

Although more costly than CT, magnetic resonance imaging involves no radiation exposure and appears to have similar sensitivity to contrast imaging.[126,127] It also has the advantage of revealing extraintestinal pathology.

Nuclear scans

Radio-isotope studies are expensive, time consuming, and generally use either ^{111}indium[128] or ^{99m}technetium[129] for *in vitro* leukocyte labeling of a phlebotomized blood sample, which is then returned to the patient. Antigranulocyte monoclonal antibody scinitigraphy using ^{99m}technetium-labeled antibody has been used in children with Crohn's disease, but has poor specificity.[130]

Endoscopic and histologic evaluation

Examination of the colon is often performed early in the evaluation of a child with chronic bloody diarrhea with the aim of distinguishing ulcerative colitis from Crohn's disease. The finding of aphthous lesions (small ulcers on an erythematous base) in the setting of an otherwise normal-looking colon is highly suggestive of Crohn's disease (Fig. 40.13). Rectal sparing is unusual in ulcerative colitis and common in Crohn's disease. Patchiness of inflammation with abnormal areas interspersed with grossly normal-appearing areas is characteristic of Crohn's disease. Deep fissuring ulcers and heaped-up edematous mucosa (pseudopolyps) may be present. The ileocecal valve may appear granular, friable and edematous. Intubation of the terminal ileum may reveal marked nodularity and inflammation (Fig. 40.14).

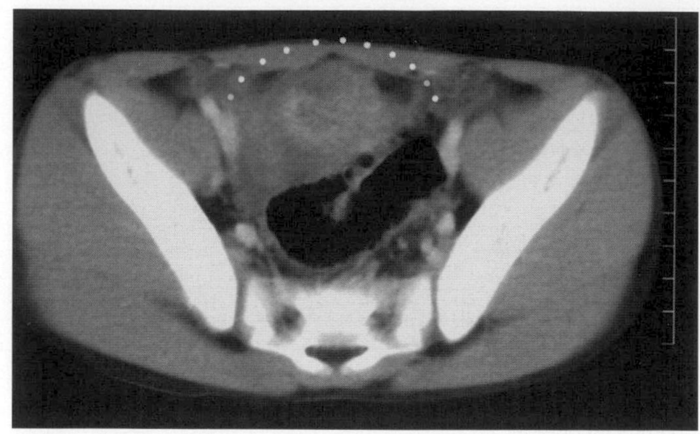

Figure 40.12: Marked distal small bowel wall thickening in an 8-year-old with Crohn's disease.

Mucosal biopsies should be taken from normal- and abnormal-appearing areas. Biopsies of normal-appearing areas may reveal inflammation and, rarely, granuloma, diagnostic of Crohn's disease. Although focally enhanced gastritis is common in Crohn's disease, it can also be present in patients with ulcerative colitis and so its presence does not reliably differentiate between the two disorders.[131]

Wireless capsule endoscopy is now being used with increasing frequency in adults, and occasionally in children capable of swallowing the capsule in whom conventional evaluative techniques have been unrevealing but in whom a high suspicion for Crohn's disease of the small bowel still exists.[132] Prior to capsule endoscopy it is important that any bowel stenosis or stricture that might impair passage of the capsule has been evaluated.

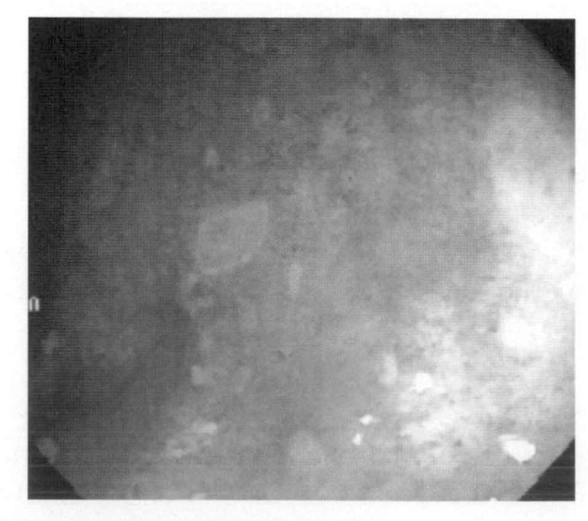

Figure 40.13: Colonic aphthous lesions in an adolescent with newly diagnosed Crohn's disease.

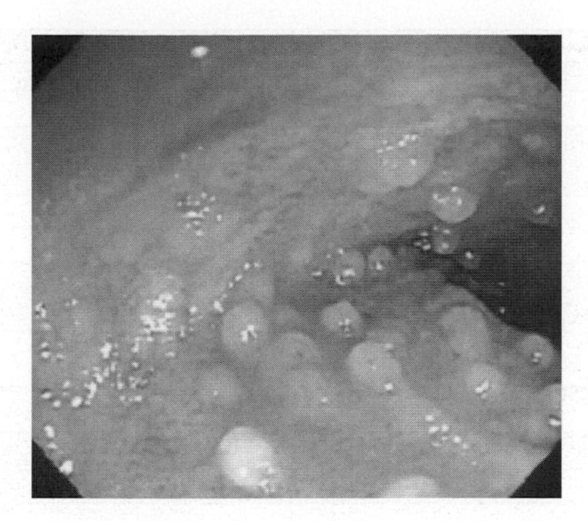

Figure 40.14: Marked lymphoid hyperplasia in Crohn's disease. (*See plate section for color*).

DIFFERENTIAL DIAGNOSIS

The protean manifestations of Crohn's disease create a long differential diagnosis. Disease entities to be considered are reviewed in Table 40.4.

THERAPY

Emerging therapies have made bowel healing and long-lasting remission the therapeutic goal. Nonetheless, care must be taken to use common sense, and treatment should be directed toward symptoms and quality of life, not necessarily abnormal laboratory tests, biopsies or radiographs. Assessment of disease activity in any patient is problematic as there is no 'gold standard'. Inflammation may be present without symptoms,[133] and symptoms may be present without inflammation (e.g. stricture, irritable bowel syndrome). There may be a considerable dissociation between abnormal test results and clinical activity.[133,134] The clinician must decide whether the target of therapy is to reduce inflammation (medical therapy), alleviate a surgical condition (stenosis, abscess), promote growth (nutritional intervention), improve quality of life (treating anxiety, depression), or a combination of these. Successful therapy for one indication may lead to problems in other areas (e.g. corticosteroid therapy leading to depression). Instruments have been devised to give an overall assessment of disease activity (Pediatric Crohn's Disease Activity Index (PCDAI),[135] Crohn's Disease Activity Index (CDAI)).[136]

Pharmacologic therapy

Multiple medications have proven efficacy in reducing symptoms, inducing remission and maintaining remission. Traditionally, a stepwise approach has been used with less 'powerful' and presumably safer agents tried first, and more powerful agents used subsequently if good results are not realized. Increased experience with immunomodulators and biologic therapy has challenged this approach. Pharmacologic agents used to treat Crohn's disease can be divided into the following categories: aminosalicylates, corticosteroids, immunomodulators, antibiotics and biologics[137,138] (Table 40.5).

Aminosalicylates

Aminosalicylates act at multiple levels in the inflammatory response. Actions include inhibition of leukotriene and thromboxane synthesis, scavenging of reactive oxygen metabolites, inhibition of platelet-activating factor synthesis and formation of nitric oxide, and alteration of mucosal prostaglandin profiles.[139]

Sulfasalazine (Azulfidine™) and mesalamine (Asacol™, Pentasa™, Claversal™, Salofalk™) are the two aminosalicylates used to treat mild to moderate Crohn's disease. The vehicle for Pentasa™ is ethylcellulose microgranules, which facilitates release from the jejunum to colon, whereas Asacol™ is released primarily in the terminal ileum and colon.

Active disease Sulfasalazine is usually effective for mild to moderate Crohn's colitis but has no documented efficacy in small bowel disease.[140] The efficacy of mesalamine in the treatment of active Crohn's disease of the distal small bowel or large bowel is largely dose related. In adults, 3.2 g daily of Asacol™'[141] or 4 g per day Pentasa™'[142] have been shown to be more effective than placebo in inducing remission. Mesalamine was equally as efficacious as 6-methylprednisolone (6-MP) in one study of adults with mild to moderate ileitis.[143] A recent meta-analysis of several large 5-ASA trials showed this drug to be superior to placebo in decreasing the score on

Primary presenting symptom	Diagnostic considerations
Right lower quadrant abdominal pain, with or without mass	Appendicitis, infection (e.g. *Campylobacter*, *Yersinia*), lymphoma, intussusception, mesenteric adenitis, Meckel's diverticulum, ovarian cyst
Chronic periumbilical or epigastric abdominal pain	Irritable bowel, constipation, lactose intolerance, peptic disease
Rectal bleeding, no diarrhea	Fissure, polyp, Meckel's diverticulum, rectal ulcer syndrome
Bloody diarrhea	Infection, hemolytic–uremic syndrome, Henoch–Schönlein purpura, ischemic bowel, radiation colitis
Watery diarrhea	Irritable bowel, lactose intolerance, giardiasis, cryptosporidium, sorbitol, laxatives
Perirectal disease	Fissure, hemorrhoid (rare), streptococcal infection, condyloma (rare)
Growth delay	Endocrinopathy
Anorexia, weight loss	Anorexia nervosa
Arthritis	Collagen vascular disease, infection
Liver abnormalities	Chronic hepatitis

Table 40.4 Differential diagnosis of presenting symptoms of Crohn's disease

Drug category	Indications	Daily dose (mg/kg)	Maximum dose
Aminosalicylates			
Sulfasalazine	Mild colonic disease	40–50	3–4 g
Mesalamine			
Pentasa™	Mild small bowel or colonic disease	50–80	4 g
Asacol™	Mild distal small bowel or colonic disease	50–80	4.8 g
Corticosteroids			
Prednisone	Moderate to severe small bowel or colonic disease	1–2	40–80 mg
Budesonide	Distal small bowel or ascending colon disease	?	9 mg
Immunomodulators			
Azathioprine	Steroid dependent or refractory disease; minimize	2–3	150–200 mg[a]
6-Mercaptopurine	steroid use prospectively; perirectal disease	1–2	100–150 mg
Methotrexate	Steroid dependent or refractory disease	15 mg/m^2 (weekly, i.m.)	25 mg (weekly, i.m.)
Antibiotics			
Metronidazole	Perirectal disease; colonic disease	10–20	1.5 g
Ciprofloxacin	Perirectal disease	?	1 g
Ciprofloxacom			
Infliximab	Steroid dependent or refractory disease; steroid sparing; perirectal disease; maintenance of remission; refractory extraintestinal disease	5–10 mg/kg[b] (i.v.)	1 g[b] (i.v.)

[a] Maximum doses of azathioprine or 6-mercaptopurine are relative values and will be determined by clinical response, laboratory tolerance as reflected by complete blood count and serum aminotransferase levels, and 6-thioguanine levels.
[b] Infliximab is generally initially administered as a three-infusion series at 0, 2 and 6 weeks. Maintenance therapy is initially given every 8 weeks, and then every 4–12 weeks as determined by clinical course.

Table 40.5 Pharmacologic therapy for Crohn's disease

the CDAI, but speculated whether the numeric difference observed was clinically significant.[144] One very small study showed efficacy of Pentasa™ in children with active small bowel disease when used in a dose of 50 mg/kg daily.[145] Mesalamine enemas may be used for distal colonic disease.

Maintenance and postoperative therapy There is considerable controversy as to the role of 5-ASA in maintaining remission.[146] A large meta-analysis of 2097 patients showed that mesalamine significantly reduced the relapse rate following surgical induction of remission, but not medically induced remission.[147] Another study failed to show postsurgical benefit.[148] Several other studies have shown benefit in both medically induced[149–151] and surgically induced[152, 153] remission. When used in an attempt to maintain remission, the drug should be used at full induction dosage.

Toxicity 5-ASA is usually well tolerated, but dose-related and idiosyncratic reactions can occur. Worsening disease can be seen with any of these agents. Nausea and vomiting are more common with sulfasalazine. Less common but important complications include pancreatitis, blood dyscrasias, hair loss, hepatitis, nephritis and pericarditis.[154,155]

Corticosteroids

The effects of corticosteroids in mitigating the inflammation has been reviewed in detail elsewhere.[156] Corticosteroids bind to corticosteroid receptors on target cells, regulating the expression of certain genes. An interaction between NF-κB and activated corticosteroid receptors may be crucial in the downregulation of pro-inflammatory mediators[157,158] such as IL-1, IL-6, IL-8, IFN-γ, TNF-α, adhesion molecules and leukotrienes. The two corticosteroids used in clinical practice are prednisone (and its equivalents) and budesonide.

Active disease Systemic corticosteroids are effective in the treatment of active disease in virtually all distributions of Crohn's disease.[140,159] Response rates of up to 90% have been demonstrated.[133,159] Oral therapy is usually initiated with prednisone at a dose of 1–2 mg/kg daily, with a maximum of 40–80 mg/day. Intravenous therapy is occasionally used for particularly severe disease. The dose is tapered over several weeks to months to an alternate-day schedule, and then discontinued depending on the patient's response. Corticosteroid dependence demonstrated by recurrent symptoms upon tapering or shortly after withdrawal is common[160] and often necessitates the use of additional therapy (see below). Resistance to corticosteroids can develop over time and appears to result from several mechanisms, including decreased cytoplasmic glucocorticoid concentration associated with overexpression of the multidrug resistance gene (*MDR1*), impaired glucocorticoid signaling because of dysfunction at the level of the glucocorticoid receptor, and proinflammatory mediator-induced inhibition of glucocorticoid receptor transcriptional activity.[161]

Budesonide, a synthetic steroid with high affinity for the glucocorticoid receptor (15 times that of prednisone), potent anti-inflammatory activity and low systemic bioavailability (85% first-pass metabolism), is being used in the treatment of Crohn's disease.[156] Studies have shown that budesonide is superior to placebo[162] and mesalamine[163] in the treatment of ileal or ileocolonic disease, and similar but not quite as good as prednisolone.[164,165] Efficacy in adults is greatest at a dose of 9 mg/day. A nonblinded pediatric report showed similar findings.[166] Compared with prednisone, budesonide generally has fewer corticosteroid side-effects and a diminished effect on the pituitary–adrenal axis, but these problems may still be found.[164,165,167] Some data suggest a switch from prednisone to budesonide in patients with prednisone-dependent remission to decrease corticosteroid-associated side-effects.[168] Corticosteroid enemas may be used for relief of symptoms caused by inflammation of the sigmoid and rectum.

Maintenance and postoperative therapy Prednisone does not decrease the risk of relapse in patients with medically induced remission.[159] In comparison with placebo, budesonide has no beneficial effect in decreasing relapse rates at 1 year following medically or surgically induced remission.[169–171] In a small study of corticosteroid-dependent patients in remission, those switched to budesonide had a lower relapse rate at 1 year than patients tapered off prednisone and switched to mesalamine (55% *vs* 82%).[172]

Toxicity The toxicity of corticosteroid therapy relates to the size and duration of the dose administered. Growth inhibition is a major problem with daily therapy, but normal growth rates may be preserved with alternate-day therapy.[122] In one small study budesonide did not appear to improve growth in children who had decreased gastrointestinal symptoms.[173] Compliance with prednisone therapy may be problematic in children and adolescents who suffer mood swings and develop cosmetic problems associated with corticosteroid therapy. Adequate calcium intake and maintaining physical activity are important in preventing corticosteroid-induced bone disease.

Immunomodulators

Immunomodulator therapy is commonly used in the treatment of Crohn's disease refractory to corticosteroids or when patients cannot be weaned from corticosteroids, and increasingly as primary therapy. The potential mechanisms of action and pharmacology of these medications have been reviewed previously.[174] Azathioprine and 6-MP remain the most commonly used immunomodulators. The metabolism of 6-MP and its pro-drug azathioprine are shown in Figure 40.15. Deficiency of the enzyme thiopurine methyltranferase (TPMT) (severe in 0.3% of the population and mild in 11%) can lead to high 6-thioguanine levels, which may exert severe bone marrow toxicity.[175]

Active disease 6-MP (1–1.5 mg/kg daily) and azathioprine (2–3 mg/kg daily) are effective in patients with active disease when added to corticosteroid therapy. They facilitate the development of remission and promote tapering of corticosteroids.[176,177] Either medication usually requires 3–6 months to show efficacy, and neither is effective as primary therapy as a single agent. A double-blind placebo-controlled trial showed that the addition of 6-MP to corticosteroids at initiation of therapy in children was associated with lower cumulative corticosteroid

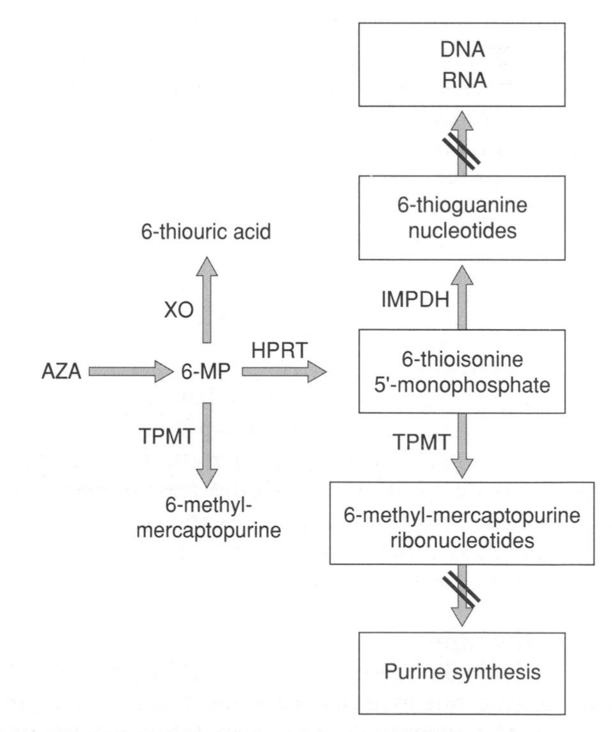

Figure 40.15: Metabolism of azathioprine (AZA) and 6-mercaptopurine (6-MP). HPRT, hypoxanthine phosphoribosyl transferase; IMPDH, inosine 5′-monophosphate dehydrogenase; TPMT, thiopurine methyltranferase; XO, xanthine oxidase.

requirements and prolonged remission.[176] It has been suggested that therapeutic effect and toxicity correlate with 6-MP metabolite levels.[178–180] If TPMT phenotype is measured before initiating therapy and is normal, full-dose therapy can be started. If TPMT is not measured, it is preferable to start at a lower dose and to monitor blood counts frequently (at 1–2 weeks, 2–4 weeks, 1 month, and then every 2–3 months). 6-Thioguanine therapy should not used because of the risk of serious liver injury.[179]

Methotrexate (25 mg intramuscularly, once weekly) was more effective than placebo in facilitating remission in adult patients receiving prednisone for chronically active disease.[181] Published data in children are limited, but one small non-blinded study suggested efficacy in children refractory to or intolerant of 6-MP.[182] The co-administration of folic acid may minimize side-effects.

The utility of cyclosporin to treat active inflammatory disease is uncertain, with conflicting studies on efficacy.[183,184] It may be helpful in the treatment of severe perirectal fistula.[185] Oral tacrolimus is associated with fistula improvement but not resolution.[186]

Maintenance therapy 6-MP and azathioprine have been shown to decrease significantly the likelihood of recurrent disease in patients in remission.[187,188] Once remission has been maintained for 4 years without steroids, the risk of relapse is the same whether either medication is stopped or continued.[189] Neither methotrexate nor cyclosporin has been shown to maintain remission. Immunomodulator therapy was shown to lessen intra-abdominal septic complications in adults with Crohn's disease undergoing bowel reanastomosis or strictureplasty.[190]

Toxicity All immunomodulators predispose patients to an increased risk of infection. Myelosuppression is a potentially serious side-effect of azathioprine/6-MP, particularly in those with TPMT deficiency; however, leukopenia can be seen with 6-MP therapy in the absence of TPMT deficiency at any time during administration, and blood counts should be monitored periodically (every 2–3 months).[191] TPMT activity may be inhibited by aminosalicylates or infliximab, and leukopenia may be more common with the co-administration of these drugs.[192,193] Other side-effects associated with azathioprine/6-mercaptopurine include pancreatitis, hepatitis, fever, rash and arthralgia. A theoretical risk for the development of malignancy has been suggested for long-term therapy, but is thought to be quite low.[174] Methotrexate therapy has been associated with hepatitis, nausea and rash. The risk of hepatic fibrosis is thought to be low in patients with IBD treated with methotrexate.

Biologic therapy

Numerous biologic agents have been developed to treat Crohn's disease but extensive experience is available only for the anti-TNF-α antibody infliximab. Infliximab has been used for moderate to severe luminal disease, corticosteroid-dependent or -refractory disease and fistulous disease, and to address a variety of extraintestinal manifestations.

Infliximab is a chimeric (70% human, 30% mouse) IgG_1 monoclonal antibody that binds to soluble and membrane-bound TNF-α. It induces apoptosis of lamina propria and peripheral blood T lymphocytes using a caspase-dependent pathway;[194] this action, rather than neutralizing soluble TNF-α, is thought to underlie its therapeutic effect.

Active disease

Anti-TNF therapy. Controlled data in adults have shown efficacy in treating moderate to severe luminal[195] and fistulous[196] disease. Large, uncontrolled patient series have confirmed these observations in adults,[197] and smaller series have shown similar results in children.[198,199] The ability of anti-TNF therapy to allow a decrease in dosage or elimination of corticosteroid therapy in some patients has proven very beneficial.[200] In luminal inflammatory disease, short-term response rates range from 50% to 80%, and endoscopic healing of diseased bowel has been demonstrated in some patients. Relapse of active disease is common, especially in the absence of concomitant immunomodulator therapy. Healing of perirectal fistula occurs in some patients, but recurrence is common. The drug is given initially as three infusions of 5 mg per kg per dose at 0, 2 and 6 weeks. Higher dosing (up to 10 mg per kg per dose) can be given if necessary. Single-episode dosing appears to be associated with a higher risk of subsequent allergic reactions (see below).

Improved response rates are seen in patients on concomitant immunomodulatory therapy.[201] Extraintestinal complications of Crohn's disease such as pyoderma gangrenosum have been treated successfully with infliximab. Limited data are available on several other agents. CDP571 is a humanized moclonal antibody to TNF that has shown marginal efficacy compared with placebo.[202] The MAPK inhibitor CNI-1493, a guanylhydrazone, was associated with clinical improvement and endoscopic healing in a small study of 12 patients with severe disease.[203] Thalidomide, which increases the degradation of messenger RNA for TNF, has been used in an open-label fashion in a small number of patients.[204]

Anti-adhesion molecule therapy. Natalizumab is a monoclonal antibody directed against α_4-integrin that is expressed on lymphocytes, monocytes and eosinophils. α_4-Integrin mediates attachment to vascular endothelium adhesion molecules (vascular cell adhesion molecule (VCAM) 1, mucosal adressin cell adhesion molecule (MAdCAM) 1) and facilitates their migration into tissue.[205] Mild improvement compared with placebo was noted for patients with moderate to severely active luminal Crohn's disease who received two infusions of 3 mg/kg 4 weeks apart.[206] ISIS 2302 is an antisense oligodeoxynucleotide that reduces *in vitro* ICAM activity in inflamed tissue. Potential efficacy was suggested in one study in adults.[207]

Other. Other agents that have shown potential value include growth hormone[208] and GM-CSF.[59]

Maintenance therapy Infliximab is more effective than placebo in maintaining remission in adults with luminal Crohn's disease.[209] Regularly scheduled maintenance treatment regimens (every 8–12 weeks) improve outcomes compared with that in patients receiving maintenance therapy in an episodic fashion.[210] Remission of active fistula is also improved with maintenance infliximab, but recurrence is common once therapy is stopped.[211] Anecdotal experience in children and adults is the same. Data on other agents are sparse.

Toxicity Numerous minor and significant acute and late complications have been seen with infliximab therapy. Infusion reactions are most common (5–10% of patients) and are generally associated with the presence of higher-titer antibody to infliximab (ATI).[212–214] High-titer ATI may also be associated with shorter duration of action of the drug.[212,215] Concomitant immunodulator therapy as well as regular dosing of infliximab (every 8 weeks) reduces ATI formation.[212,216] Intravenous hydrocortisone premedication prior to infliximab infusion reduces ATI levels but does not eliminate formation or infusion reactions.[216] Single-dose infliximab, especially in the absence of immunomodulator therapy, should be avoided as it fosters an immunogenic reaction. Maintenance scheduled infusions also appear to be associated with a lower likelihood of antibody development.[210] A delayed serum sickness-like reaction has been described in 1–3% of patients.[213,217] A high percentage of treated adult patients develop antinuclear antibodies (>50%), but clinical autoimmunity is rare.[218] Fatal tuberculosis as well as other opportunistic infections such as cytomegalovirus, histoplasmosis, aspergillosis, listeria, pneumocystis and varicella infection among others have been seen. Purified protein derivative (PPD) testing should always precede infliximab therapy. Intra-abdominal infection is an absolute contraindication to infliximab therapy, and any abscess should be drained and treated prior to therapy. Lymphoproliferative disease has been described in adults[219] and a pediatric patient (personal communication) in the setting of infliximab therapy. Cause and effect of this serious latter problem is not established, but great care is required in selecting patients for this therapy and in monitoring their course. Any patient with a previous history of lymphoma should not receive infliximab. Further contraindications to infliximab therapy include multiple sclerosis or optic neuritis, and congestive heart failure. The occurrence of progressive multifocal leukoencephalopathy has been described in several patients receiving natalizumab, including one with Crohn's disease.[219a]

Antibiotics

These medications have long been used as both primary treatment and to address the complications of Crohn's disease. The precise mechanisms of their action in this disorder are not clear.

Active disease Metronidazole has similar efficacy to sulfasalazine in the treatment of Crohn's disease of the colon.[220] It has been used as the drug of choice for perirectal fistula, although the problem usually flares upon discontinuation of therapy. Metronidazole plus ciprofloxacin had a similar efficacy to methylpredisolone in a small group of adults with active disease.[221] Ciprofloxacin is commonly used to treat perirectal disease, although controlled data are lacking.

Maintenance therapy Metronidazole (20 mg/kg daily) decreases the likelihood of endoscopic recurrence at 3 months and clinical recurrence by 1 year following ileal resection.[222]

Toxicity Peripheral neuropathy is the most serious side-effect of metronidazole therapy. Rarely, paresthesias may persist despite discontinuing the medication. Nausea and a metallic taste are common. *Candida* esophagitis has been seen in adolescents treated with broad-spectrum antibiotics who are also receiving immunosuppressive therapy (personal observation).

Adjunctive therapy At present there are no controlled data suggesting efficacy of prebiotics or probiotics in the acute or chronic management of Crohn's disease.[223] A study in adults showed no efficacy of *Lactobacillus GG* in preventing recurrent disease after definitive resection.[224] An enteric-coated fish oil preparation has been used to maintain remission.[225] Loperamide may help control diarrhea. Anticholinergics such as dicycloverine may be helpful in subjects with Crohn's disease who also have irritable bowel syndrome-like symptoms. Low-dose tricyclic antidepressant therapy (e.g. amitriptyline 10–20 mg/day) may also be helpful in this situation. Colestyramine, a bile acid-binding resin, may decrease diarrhea in patients who have had terminal ileal resection or extensive ileal disease with the attendant loss of bile acids into the colon stimulating colonic secretion. Individuals with extensive resection of the terminal ileum are at risk for developing vitamin B_{12} deficiency and should receive parenteral supplementation. Calcium supplementation should be provided to at least meet the recommended daily requiremnt if not met by dietary intake. Non-steroidal anti-inflammatory drugs (NSAIDs) may exacerbate Crohn's disease and should be avoided if possible.

Nutritional therapy

Nutritional therapy can be used as primary therapy without accompanying pharmacologic intervention or as adjunctive therapy with medications. It should always be used in patients suffering malnutrition.

Active disease Total parenteral nutrition and bowel rest may be effective in inducing remission in up to 60–80% of subjects.[226] A large meta-analysis of exclusive enteral nutrition therapy, with either elemental or polymeric diets, showed a large range (20–80%) of remission.[227] In general, enteral therapy was less effective than corticosteroids in effecting remission in studies where a comparison was made. No differences have been demonstrated between elemental and non-elemental diets. Relapse rate after enteral nutrition-induced remission is greater than that following remission achieved with prednisolone.[228] In selected children with growth failure, particularly those with predominantly small bowel disease, enteral nutritional therapy may be preferable to corticosteroids as initial therapy. Most children require nasogastric tube administration of these formulas as oral acceptance is low. It has been suggested and disputed that the fat content of these enteral formulas might affect the success rate, with fat blends that promote pro-inflammatory mediator production (n6 polyunsaturated fatty acids) being inferior to those containing monounsaturated fatty acids.[229,230] Glutamine supplementation of the enteral formula appears to offer no advantage.

Maintenance therapy Data are limited. One study showed that after successful treatment of active Crohn's disease in children and adolescents by exclusive enteral nutritional therapy, supplementary enteral nutrition prolonged remission and was associated with improved growth.[231] Gastrostomy placement is safe and well tolerated in children being treated with long-term enteral therapy who do not want to use a nasogastric tube.

Other indications Intensive nutritional support, primarily through enteral supplementation via tube feedings, has been shown to be effective in reversing growth retardation in most patients.[116] It is *imperative* that nutritional support be started well before physiologic bone maturation and fusion of epiphyses if catch-up growth is to be expected, and that non-corticosteroid regimens be used to suppressive bowel inflammation.

Surgery

Following terminal ileal resection, endoscopic evidence of recurrent disease is present at the neoterminal ileum in more than 70% of adults at 1 year after surgery, although only 35% are symptomatic.[234] In one pediatric series, clinical recurrence rates were 17%, 38% and 60% at 1, 3 and 5 years respectively.[235] Higher PCDAI scores, the preoperative use of 6-MP and colonic disease were associated with higher recurrence rates, perhaps reflecting more aggressive disease at the time of surgery. Segmental colonic resection with reanastomosis is associated with a higher risk of recurrence than ileal or ileocecal resection.[235,236] The recurrence rate at the neoterminal ileum 5–10 years after panproctocolectomy and ileostomy is 70% when ileal disease was present at the time of surgery *vs* only 10% when disease was limited to the colon.[237]

Strictureplasty is a well accepted method in the surgical management of adult and pediatric patients with Crohn's disease.[238,239] In this procedure, a longitudinal incision is made through the stenotic bowel and the opening is then closed transversely. The risk of reoperation following strictureplasty is no greater than when resection is performed. Strictureplasty is generally performed on small intestinal strictures or at an ileocolonic anastomosis in the presence of mostly fibrotic disease. Mild inflammation does not preclude strictureplasty.

Unless perianal hygiene is severely compromised, perianal skin tags are generally not excised. A variety of surgical techniques has been developed to help address severe perirectal disease refractory to medical management. Anal fissures generally heal and should not be treated surgically. Superficial perianal abscesses can be treated with incision and drainage. Deep abscesses are frequently associated with high perianal fistula and are treated with incision and drainage followed by placement of a non-cutting seton. While the seton facilitates drainage of the abscess, it also perpetuates the fistula. Complex fistulae may require long-term drainage and staged fistulotomy. Control of symptoms is the realistic goal of such therapy. Proctectomy and diversion of the fecal stream may be required for particularly severe perirectal disease. Marked rectal disease, with or without complex fistula formation, may eventually lead to rectal stenosis requiring dilation.

Despite intensive medical and nutritional therapy, growth failure still persists in some children with Crohn's disease. Provided the subject is prepubertal or in early puberty, surgery may significantly improve growth in most of these children if good nutrition can be maintained, and corticosteroid therapy can be discontinued or weaned to an alternate-day schedule.[240]

Homeopathy

Homeopathic remedies are frequently used by patients and families in the management of Crohn's disease. To date, no controlled data have shown efficacy. These remedies are often used without the knowledge of the attending physician as families may want to avoid confrontation.

Psychologic therapy

Education of both patient and family is essential in the management of Crohn's disease. Demystification of the disease course and thorough explanation of the rationale for and complications of therapy often relieve unjustified fears. Counseling and attendance at age- and sex-matched peer groups may be helpful. Antidepressant and antianxiety therapy can be offered, and are quite helpful when indicated.

NATURAL HISTORY

Disease course

Crohn's disease is marked by periods of exacerbation and remission. Historically, only 1% of adult patients with well-documented Crohn's disease do not suffer at least one relapse following diagnosis and initial therapy;[241] of a cohort of 480 adults, only 10% maintained long-term remission free of corticosteroids following their initial presentation.[242] Children with ileocolitis generally have a poorer response to medications and a greater need for surgery than those with small bowel disease alone. Yet to be determined in either of these populations is whether current immunomodulatory therapy and emerging biologic therapy will affect the likelihood of disease exacerbation and need for surgery. Data have suggested that markers of inflammation such as C-reactive protein, orosomucoid and erythrocyte sedimentation rate identify patients at higher risk for recurrence.[243] Younger age (<25 years) appears to be associated with a greater risk of relapse. A history of multiple previous relapses is probably the greatest predictor of subsequent relapses. Smoking is a significant risk factor for recurrence.

Malignancy

There have been concerns raised regarding three types of malignancy and Crohn's disease: colorectal cancer, small bowel cancer and lymphoma.

The risk of colorectal cancer appears to be similar in ulcerative colitis and Crohn's colitis, and is affected by disease duration and severity,[244] occurring a median of 18 years after the onset of Crohn's disease.[245] Chronic 5-ASA administration may decrease the risk.[244] Yearly screening colonoscopy for patients with colonic inflammation of greater than 8–10 years' duration appears warranted. Adenocarcinoma of the small bowel is rare, but occurs more frequently than in the general population; the rare affected patients often have disease for more than 20 years at the time of cancer development, tend to be male, have fistulizing disease, and often have surgically excluded loops.[244,246]

Most current evidence does not support a primary relationship between Crohn's disease and an increased risk of non-Hodgkin's lymphoma.[247,248] A slightly increased risk may be observed with the administration of azathioprine or 6-MP,[247,248] but improved quality-adjusted life expectancy because of therapeutic effect on the disease course may outweigh this incremental risk. Lymphoproliferative disease has been described in recipients of anti-TNF-α therapy;[219] after discontinuation of this therapy, outcome has ranged from lymphoma regression to death.

Mortality

Death from Crohn's disease in the pediatric population is extremely rare. Adults with Crohn's disease appear to have a slight increased mortality risk compared with age-matched controls.[249]

Acknowledgement

The author is indebted to Andrew Ricci, Jr, MD and Fabiola Balerezo, MD for their contribution to the pathology section of this chapter.

References

1. Loftus EV Jr, Schoenfeld P, Sandborn WJ. The epidemiology and natural history of Crohn's disease in population-based patient cohorts from North America: a systematic review. Aliment Pharmacol Ther 2002; 16:51–60.
2. Hildebrand H, Finkel Y, Grahnquist L, et al. Changing pattern of paediatric inflammatory bowel disease in northern Stockholm 1990–2001. Gut 2003; 52:1432–1434.
3. Kugathasan S, Judd RH, Hoffmann RG, et al. Epidemiologic and clinical characteristics of children with newly diagnosed inflammatory bowel disease in Wisconsin: a statewide population-based study. J Pediatr 2003; 143:525–531.
4. Shivananda S, Lennard-Jones J, Logan R, et al. Incidence of inflammatory bowel disease across Europe: is there a difference between north and south? Results of the European Collaborative Study on Inflammatory Bowel Disease (EC IBD). Gut 1996; 39:690–697.
5. Alic M. Crohn's disease epidemiology at the turn of the century – solving the puzzle. Am J Gastroenterol 2000; 95:321–323.
6. Feeney MA, Murphy F, Clegg AJ, et al. A case–control study of childhood environmental risk factors for the development of inflammatory bowel disease. Eur J Gastroenterol Hepatol 2002; 14:529–534.
7. Blanchard JF, Bernstein CN, Wajda A, et al. Small-area variations and sociodemographic correlates for the incidence of Crohn's disease and ulcerative colitis. Am J Epidemiol 2001; 154:328–335.
8. Andersson RE, Olaison G, Tysk C, et al. Appendectomy is followed by increased risk of Crohn's disease. Gastroenterology 2003; 124:40–46.
9. Montgomery SM, Wakefield AJ, Ekbom A. Sex-specific risks for pediatric onset among patients with Crohn's disease. Clin Gastroenterol Hepatol 2003; 1:303–309.
10. Corrao G, Tragnone A, Caprilli R, et al. Risk of inflammatory bowel disease attributable to smoking, oral contraception and breastfeeding in Italy: a nationwide case–control study. Cooperative Investigators of the Italian Group for the Study of the Colon and the Rectum (GISC). Int J Epidemiol 1998; 27:397–404.
11. Robertson DJ, Sandler RS. Measles virus and Crohn's disease: a critical appraisal of the current literature. Inflamm Bowel Dis 2001; 7:51–57.
12. Hayward PA, Satsangi J, Jewell DP. Inflammatory bowel disease and the X chromosome.Qart J Med 1996; 89:713–718.
13. Anderson PD, Huizing M, Claassen DA, et al. Hermansky–Pudlak syndrome type 4 (HPS-4): clinical and molecular characteristics. Hum Genet 2003; 113:10–17.
14. Dieckgraefe BK, Korzenik JR, Husain A, et al. Association of glycogen storage disease 1b and Crohn disease: results of a North American survey. Eur J Pediatr 2002; 16(Suppl 1): S88–S92.
15. Bouma G, Strober W. The immunological and genetic basis of inflammatory bowel disease. Nat Rev Immunol 2003; 3:521–533.
16. Ahmad T, Satsangi J, McGovern D, et al. The genetics of inflammatory bowel disease. Aliment Pharmacol Ther 2001; 15:731–748.
17. Peeters M, Nevens H, Baert F, et al. Familial aggregation in Crohn's disease: increased age-adjusted risk and concordance in clinical characteristics. Gastroenterology 1996; 111:597–603.
18. Laharie D, Debeugny S, Peeters M, et al. Inflammatory bowel disease in spouses and their offspring. Gastroenterology 2001; 120:816–819.
19. Meucci G, Vecchi M, Torgano G, et al. Familial aggregation of inflammatory bowel disease in northern Italy: a multicenter study. The Gruppo di Studio per le Malattie Infiammatorie Intestinali (IBD Study Group). Gastroenterology 1992; 103:514–519.
20. Halfvarson J, Bodin L, Tysk C, et al. Inflammatory bowel disease in a Swedish twin cohort: a long-term follow-up of concordance and clinical characteristics. Gastroenterology 2003; 124:1767–1773.

97. Izzedine H, Simon J, Piette AM, et al. Primary chronic interstitial nephritis in Crohn's disease. Gastroenterology 2002; 123:1436–1440.
98. Hyams J, Markowitz J, Treem W, et al. Characterization of hepatic abnormalities in children with inflammatory bowel disease. Inflamm Bowel Dis 1995; 1:27–33.
99. Faubion WA Jr, Loftus EV, Sandborn WJ, et al. Pediatric 'PSC-IBD': a descriptive report of associated inflammatory bowel disease among pediatric patients with PSC. J Pediatr Gastroenterol Nutr 2001; 33:296–300.
100. Feldstein A, Angula P, El-Youssef M, et al. Overlap with autoimmune hepatitis in pediatric patients with primary sclerosing cholangitis. Gastroenterology 2002; 122:202–209.
101. Keljo DJ, Sugerman KS. Pancreatitis in patients with inflammatory bowel disease. J Pediatr Gastroenterol Nutr 1997; 25:108–112.
102. Barthet M, Hastier P, Bernard JP, et al. Chronic pancreatitis and inflammatory bowel disease: true or coincidental association? Am J Gastroenterol 1999; 94:2141–2148.
103. Sentongo TA, Semaeo EJ, Stettler N, et al. Vitamin D status in children, adolescents, and young adults with Crohn disease. Am J Clin Nutr 2002; 76:1077–1081.
104. Semeao EJ, Jawad AF, Zemel BS, et al. Bone mineral density in children and young adults with Crohn's disease. Inflamm Bowel Dis 1999; 5:161–166.
105. Ghosh S, Cowen S, Hannan WJ, et al. Low bone mineral density in Crohn's disease, but not in ulcerative colitis, at diagnosis. Gastroenterology 1994; 107:1031–1039.
106. Sylvester FA, Wyzga N, Hyams JS, et al. Effect of Crohn's disease on bone metabolism *in vitro*: a role for interleukin-6. J Bone Miner Res 2002; 17:695–702.
107. van Staa TP, Cooper C, Brusse LS, et al. Inflammatory bowel disease and the risk of fracture. Gastroenterology 2003; 125:1591–1597.
108. Sentongo TA, Semeao EJ, Piccoli DA, et al. Growth, body composition, and nutritional status in children and adolescents with Crohn's disease. J Pediatr Gastroenterol Nutr 2000; 31:33–40.
109. Motil KJ, Altchuler SI, Grand RJ. Mineral balance during nutritional supplementation in adolescents with Crohn disease and growth failure. J Pediatr 1985; 107:473–479.
110. Motil KJ, Grand RJ. Nutritional management of inflammatory bowel disease. Pediatr Clin North Am 1985; 32:447–469.
111. Levy E, Rizwan Y, Thibault L, et al. Altered lipid profile, lipoprotein composition, and oxidant and antioxidant status in pediatric Crohn disease. Am J Clin Nutr 2000; 71:807–815.
112. Azcue M, Rashid M, Griffiths A, et al. Energy expenditure and body composition in children with Crohn's disease: effect of enteral nutrition and treatment with prednisolone. Gut 1997; 41:203–208.
113. Rigaud D, Cerf M, Alberto L, et al. Increased resting energy expenditure in acute attacks of Crohn's disease. Gastroenterol Clin Biol 1993; 17:932–937.
114. Al-Jaouni R, Schneider SM, Piche T, et al. Effect of steroids on energy expenditure and substrate oxidation in women with Crohn's disease. Am J Gastroenterol 2002; 97:2843–2849.
115. Kanof ME, Lake AM, Bayless TM. Decreased height velocity in children and adolescents before the diagnosis of Crohn's disease. Gastroenterology 1988; 95:1523–1527.
116. Ferry G, Buller H. Mechanisms of growth retardation, drug therapy, and nutritional support in pediatric inflammatory bowel disease. Inflamm Bowel Dis 1995; 1:313–330.
117. Sawczenko A, Ballinger AB, Croft NM, et al. Adult height in patients with early onset of Crohn's disease. Gut 2003; 52:454–455.
118. Savage MO, Beattie RM, Camacho-Hubner C, et al. Growth in Crohn's disease. Acta Paediatr Suppl 1999; 88:89–92.
119. Ballinger A. Fundamental mechanisms of growth failure in inflammatory bowel disease. Horm Res 2002; 58(Suppl 1):7–10.
120. Ballinger AB, Azooz O, El-Haj T, et al. Growth failure occurs through a decrease in insulin-like growth factor 1 which is independent of undernutrition in a rat model of colitis. Gut 2000; 46:694–700.
121. Ballinger A, El-Haj T, Perrett D, et al. The role of medial hypothalamic serotonin in the suppression of feeding in a rat model of colitis. Gastroenterology 2000; 118:544–553.
122. Hyams JS, Moore RE, Leichtner AM, et al. Relationship of type I procollagen to corticosteroid therapy in children with inflammatory bowel disease. J Pediatr 1988; 112:893–898.
123. Hyams JS, Treem WR, Carey DE, et al. Comparison of collagen propeptides as growth markers in children with inflammatory bowel disease. Gastroenterology 1991; 100:971–975.
124. Thomas DW, Sinatra FR. Screening laboratory tests for Crohn's disease. West J Med 1989; 150:163–164.
125. Esteban JM, Maldonado L, Sanchiz V, et al. Activity of Crohn's disease assessed by colour Doppler ultrasound analysis of the affected loops. Eur Radiol 2001; 11:1423–1428.
126. Schreyer AG, Golder S, Seitz J, et al. New diagnostic avenues in inflammatory bowel diseases. Capsule endoscopy, magnetic resonance imaging and virtual enteroscopy. Dig Dis 2003; 21:129–137.
127. Rieber A, Wruk D, Potthast S, et al. Diagnostic imaging in Crohn's disease: comparison of magnetic resonance imaging and conventional imaging methods. Int J Colorectal Dis 2000; 15:176–181.
128. Saverymuttu SH, Camilleri M, Rees H, et al. Indium 111-granulocyte scanning in the assessment of disease extent and disease activity in inflammatory bowel disease. A comparison with colonoscopy, histology, and fecal indium 111-granulocyte excretion. Gastroenterology 1986; 90:1121–1128.
129. Charron M. Inflammatory bowel disease activity assessment with biologic markers and ^{99m}Tc-WBC scintigraphy: are there different trends in ileitis versus colitis? J Nucl Med 2003; 44:1586–1591.
130. Bruno I, Martelossi S, Geatti O, et al. Antigranulocyte monoclonal antibody immunoscintigraphy in inflammatory bowel disease in children and young adolescents. Acta Paediatr 2002; 91:1050–1055.
131. Sharif F, McDermott M, Dillon M, et al. Focally enhanced gastritis in children with Crohn's disease and ulcerative colitis. Am J Gastroenterol 2002; 97:1415–1420.
132. Mow WS, Lo SK, Targan SR, et al. Initial experience with wireless capsule enteroscopy in the diagnosis and management of inflammatory bowel disease. Clin Gastroenterol Hepatol 2004; 2:31–40.
133. Modigliani R, Mary JY, Simon JF, et al. Clinical, biological, and endoscopic picture of attacks of Crohn's disease. Evolution on prednisolone. Groupe d'Etude Therapeutique des Affections Inflammatoires Digestives. Gastroenterology 1990; 98:811–818.
134. Hyams JS, Mandel F, Ferry GD, et al. Relationship of common laboratory parameters to the activity of Crohn's disease in children. J Pediatr Gastroenterol Nutr 1992; 14:216–222.
135. Hyams JS, Ferry GD, Mandel FS, et al. Development and validation of a pediatric Crohn's disease activity index. J Pediatr Gastroenterol Nutr 1991; 12:439–447.

136. Best WR, Becktel JM, Singleton JW, et al. Development of a Crohn's disease activity index. National Cooperative Crohn's Disease Study. Gastroenterology 1976; 70:439–444.

137. Escher JC, Taminiau JA, Nieuwenhuis EE, et al. Treatment of inflammatory bowel disease in childhood: best available evidence. Inflamm Bowel Dis 2003; 9:34–58.

138. Hanauer SB, Present DH. The state of the art in the management of inflammatory bowel disease. Rev Gastroenterol Disord 2003; 3:81–92.

139. Zimmerman MJ, Jewell DP. Cytokines and mechanisms of action of glucocorticoids and aminosalicylates in the treatment of ulcerative colitis and Crohn's disease. Aliment Pharmacol Ther 1996; 10(Suppl 2):93–98; discussion 99.

140. Malchow H, Ewe K, Brandes JW, et al. European Cooperative Crohn's Disease Study (ECCDS): results of drug treatment. Gastroenterology 1984; 86:249–266.

141. Tremaine WJ, Schroeder KW, Harrison JM, et al. A randomized, double-blind, placebo-controlled trial of the oral mesalamine (5-ASA) preparation, Asacol, in the treatment of symptomatic Crohn's colitis and ileocolitis. J Clin Gastroenterol 1994; 19:278–282.

142. Singleton JW, Hanauer SB, Gitnick GL, et al. Mesalamine capsules for the treatment of active Crohn's disease: results of a 16-week trial. Pentasa Crohn's Disease Study Group. Gastroenterology 1993; 104:1293–1301.

143. Prantera C, Cottone M, Pallone F, et al. Mesalamine in the treatment of mild to moderate active Crohn's ileitis: results of a randomized, multicenter trial. Gastroenterology 1999; 116:521–526.

144. Hanauer SB, Stromberg U. Oral Pentasa in the treatment of active Crohn's disease: a meta-analysis of double-blind, placebo-controlled trials. Clin Gastroenterol Hepatol 2004; 2:379–388.

145. Griffiths A, Koletzko S, Sylvester F, et al. Slow-release 5 aminosalicylic acid therapy in children with small intestinal Crohn's disease. J Pediatr Gastroenterol Nutr 1993; 17:186–192.

146. Feagan BG. Maintenance therapy for inflammatory bowel disease. Am J Gastroenterol 2003; 98(Suppl):S6–S17.

147. Camma C, Giunta M, Rosselli M, et al. Mesalamine in the maintenance treatment of Crohn's disease: a meta-analysis adjusted for confounding variables. Gastroenterology 1997; 113:1465–1473.

148. Lochs H, Mayer M, Fleig WE, et al. Prophylaxis of postoperative relapse in Crohn's disease with mesalamine: European Cooperative Crohn's Disease Study VI. Gastroenterology 2000; 118:264–273.

149. Modigliani R, Colombel JF, Dupas JL, et al. Mesalamine in Crohn's disease with steroid-induced remission: effect on steroid withdrawal and remission maintenance, Groupe d'Etudes Therapeutiques des Affections Inflammatoires Digestives. Gastroenterology 1996; 110:688–693.

150. Messori A, Brignola C, Trallori G, et al. Effectiveness of 5 aminosalicylic acid for maintaining remission in patients with Crohn's disease: a meta-analysis. Am J Gastroenterol 1994; 89:692–698.

151. Steinhart AH, Hemphill D, Greenberg GR. Sulfasalazine and mesalazine for the maintenance therapy of Crohn's disease: a meta-analysis. Am J Gastroenterol 1994; 89:2116–2124.

152. Sutherland LR, Martin F, Bailey RJ, et al. A randomized, placebo-controlled, double-blind trial of mesalamine in the maintenance of remission of Crohn's disease. The Canadian Mesalamine for Remission of Crohn's Disease Study Group. Gastroenterology 1997; 112:1069–1077.

153. Brignola C, Cottone M, Pera A, et al. Mesalamine in the prevention of endoscopic recurrence after intestinal resection for Crohn's disease. Italian Cooperative Study Group. Gastroenterology 1995; 108:345–349.

154. Marteau P, Nelet F, Le Lu M, et al. Adverse events in patients treated with 5-aminosalicyclic acid: 1993–1994 pharmacovigilance report for Pentasa in France. Aliment Pharmacol Ther 1996; 10:949–956.

155. Ransford RA, Langman MJ. Sulphasalazine and mesalazine: serious adverse reactions re-evaluated on the basis of suspected adverse reaction reports to the Committee on Safety of Medicines. Gut 2002; 51:536–539.

156. Yang YX, Lichtenstein GR. Corticosteroids in Crohn's disease. Am J Gastroenterol 2002; 97:803–823.

157. Barnes PJ, Karin M. Nuclear factor-kappaB: a pivotal transcription factor in chronic inflammatory diseases. N Engl J Med 1997; 336:1066–1071.

158. Auphan N, DiDonato JA, Rosette C, et al. Immunosuppression by glucocorticoids: inhibition of NF-kappa B activity through induction of I kappa B synthesis. Science 1995; 270:286–290.

159. Summers RW, Switz DM, Sessions JT Jr, et al. National Cooperative Crohn's Disease Study: results of drug treatment. Gastroenterology 1979; 77:847–869.

160. Faubion WA Jr, Loftus EV Jr, Harmsen WS, et al. The natural history of corticosteroid therapy for inflammatory bowel disease: a population-based study. Gastroenterology 2001; 121:255–260.

161. Farrell RJ, Kelleher D. Glucocorticoid resistance in inflammatory bowel disease. J Endocrinol 2003; 178:339–346.

162. Greenberg GR, Feagan BG, Martin F, et al. Oral budesonide for active Crohn's disease. Canadian Inflammatory Bowel Disease Study Group. N Engl J Med 1994; 331:836–841.

163. Thomsen OO, Cortot A, Jewell D, et al. A comparison of budesonide and mesalamine for active Crohn's disease. International Budesonide–Mesalamine Study Group. N Engl J Med 1998; 339:370–374.

164. Rutgeerts P, Lofberg R, Malchow H, et al. A comparison of budesonide with prednisolone for active Crohn's disease. N Engl J Med 1994; 331:842–845.

165. Gross V, Andus T, Caesar I, et al. Oral pH-modified release budesonide versus 6-methylprednisolone in active Crohn's disease. German/Austrian Budesonide Study Group. Eur J Gastroenterol Hepatol 1996; 8:905–909.

166. Levine A, Broide E, Stein M, et al. Evaluation of oral budesonide for treatment of mild and moderate exacerbations of Crohn's disease in children. J Pediatr 2002; 140:75–80.

167. Campieri M, Ferguson A, Doe W, et al. Oral budesonide is as effective as oral prednisolone in active Crohn's disease. The Global Budesonide Study Group. Gut 1997; 41:209–214.

168. Andus T, Gross V, Caesar I, et al. Replacement of conventional glucocorticoids by oral pH-modified release budesonide in active and inactive Crohn's disease: results of an open, prospective, multicenter trial. Dig Dis Sci 2003; 48:373–378.

169. Ferguson A, Campieri M, Doe W, et al. Oral budesonide as maintenance therapy in Crohn's disease – results of a 12 month study. Global Budesonide Study Group. Aliment Pharmacol Ther 1998; 12:175–183.

170. Hellers G, Cortot A, Jewell D, et al. Oral budesonide for prevention of postsurgical recurrence in Crohn's disease. The IOIBD Budesonide Study Group. Gastroenterology 1999; 116:294–300.

171. Ewe K, Bottger T, Buhr HJ, et al. Low-dose budesonide treatment for prevention of postoperative recurrence of Crohn's disease: a multicentre randomized placebo-controlled

trial. German Budesonide Study Group. Eur J Gastroenterol Hepatol 1999; 11:277–282.

172. Mantzaris GJ, Petraki K, Sfakianakis M, et al. Budesonide versus mesalamine for maintaining remission in patients refusing other immunomodulators for steroid-dependent Crohn's disease. Clin Gastroenterol Hepatol 2003; 1:122–128.
173. Kundhal P, Zachos M, Holmes JL, et al. Controlled ileal release budesonide in pediatric Crohn disease: efficacy and effect on growth. J Pediatr Gastroenterol Nutr 2001; 33:75–80.
174. Sandborn WJ. A review of immune modifier therapy for inflammatory bowel disease: azathioprine, 6-mercaptopurine, cyclosporine, and methotrexate. Am J Gastroenterol 1996; 91:423–433.
175. Givens RC, Watkins PB. Pharmacogenetics and clinical gastroenterology. Gastroenterology 2003; 125:240–248.
176. Markowitz J, Grancher K, Kohn N, et al. A multicenter trial of 6-mercaptopurine and prednisone in children with newly diagnosed Crohn's disease. Gastroenterology 2000; 119:895–902.
177. Verhave M, Winter HS, Grand RJ. Azathioprine in the treatment of children with inflammatory bowel disease. J Pediatr 1990; 117:809–814.
178. Dubinsky MC, Lamothe S, Yang HY, et al. Pharmacogenomics and metabolite measurement for 6-mercaptopurine therapy in inflammatory bowel disease. Gastroenterology 2000; 118:705–713.
179. Dubinsky MC, Vasiliauskas EA, Singh H, et al. 6-Thioguanine can cause serious liver injury in inflammatory bowel disease patients. Gastroenterology 2003; 125:298–303.
180. Cuffari C, Hunt S, Bayless T. Utilisation of erythrocyte 6 thioguanine metabolite levels to optimise azathioprine therapy in patients with inflammatory bowel disease. Gut 2001; 48:642–646.
181. Feagan BG, Rochon J, Fedorak RN, et al. Methotrexate for the treatment of Crohn's disease. The North American Crohn's Study Group Investigators. N Engl J Med 1995; 332:292–297.
182. Mack DR, Young R, Kaufman SS, et al. Methotrexate in patients with Crohn's disease after 6-mercaptopurine. J Pediatr 1998; 132:830–835.
183. Brynskov J, Freund L, Norby Rasmussen S, et al. Final report on a placebo-controlled, double-blind, randomized, multicentre trial of cyclosporin treatment in active chronic Crohn's disease. Scand J Gastroenterol 1991; 26:689–695.
184. Jewell D, Lennard-Jones J. Oral cyclosporine for chronic active Crohn's disease: a multicentre controlled trial. The Cyclosporin Study Group of Great Britain and Ireland. Eur Hepatol Gastroenterol 1994; 6:499–505.
185. Present DH, Lichtiger S. Efficacy of cyclosporine in treatment of fistula of Crohn's disease. Dig Dis Sci 1994; 39:374–380.
186. Sandborn WJ, Present DH, Isaacs KL, et al. Tacrolimus for the treatment of fistulas in patients with Crohn's disease: a randomized, placebo-controlled trial. Gastroenterology 2003; 125:380–388.
187. Candy S, Wright J, Gerber M, et al. A controlled double blind study of azathioprine in the management of Crohn's disease. Gut 1995; 37:674–678.
188. O'Donoghue DP, Dawson AM, Powell-Tuck J, et al. Double-blind withdrawal trial of azathioprine as maintenance treatment for Crohn's disease. Lancet 1978; ii:955–957.
189. Bouhnik Y, Lemann M, Mary JY, et al. Long-term follow-up of patients with Crohn's disease treated with azathioprine or 6 mercaptopurine. Lancet 1996; 347:215–219.
190. Tay GS, Binion DG, Eastwood D, et al. Multivariate analysis suggests improved perioperative outcome in Crohn's disease patients receiving immunomodulator therapy after segmental resection and/or strictureplasty. Surgery 2003; 134:565–572; discussion 572–573.
191. Connell WR, Kamm MA, Ritchie JK, et al. Bone marrow toxicity caused by azathioprine in inflammatory bowel disease: 27 years of experience. Gut 1993; 34:1081–1085.
192. Lowry PW, Franklin CL, Weaver AL, et al. Leucopenia resulting from a drug interaction between azathioprine or 6 mercaptopurine and mesalamine, sulphasalazine, or balsalazide. Gut 2001; 49:656–664.
193. Roblin X, Serre-Debeauvais F, Phelip JM, et al. Drug interaction between infliximab and azathioprine in patients with Crohn's disease. Aliment Pharmacol Ther 2003; 18:917–925.
194. Van den Brande JM, Braat H, van den Brink GR, et al. Infliximab but not etanercept induces apoptosis in lamina propria T-lymphocytes from patients with Crohn's disease. Gastroenterology 2003; 124:1774–1785.
195. Targan SR, Hanauer SB, van Deventer SJ, et al. A short-term study of chimeric monoclonal antibody cA2 to tumor necrosis factor alpha for Crohn's disease. Crohn's Disease cA2 Study Group. N Engl J Med 1997; 337:1029–1035.
196. Present DH, Rutgeerts P, Targan S, et al. Infliximab for the treatment of fistulas in patients with Crohn's disease. N Engl J Med 1999; 340:1398–1405.
197. Farrell RJ, Shah SA, Lodhavia PJ, et al. Clinical experience with infliximab therapy in 100 patients with Crohn's disease. Am J Gastroenterol 2000; 95:3490–3497.
198. Stephens MC, Shepanski MA, Mamula P, et al. Safety and steroid-sparing experience using infliximab for Crohn's disease at a pediatric inflammatory bowel disease center. Am J Gastroenterol 2003; 98:104–111.
199. Hyams JS, Markowitz J, Wyllie R. Use of infliximab in the treatment of Crohn's disease in children and adolescents. J Pediatr 2000; 137:192–196.
200. Sandborn WJ, Loftus EV. Balancing the risks and benefits of infliximab in the treatment of inflammatory bowel disease. Gut 2004; 53:780–782.
201. Parsi MA, Achkar JP, Richardson S, et al. Predictors of response to infliximab in patients with Crohn's disease. Gastroenterology 2002; 123:707–713.
202. Sandborn WJ, Feagan BG, Hanauer SB, et al. An engineered human antibody to TNF (CDP571) for active Crohn's disease: a randomized double-blind placebo-controlled trial. Gastroenterology 2001; 120:1330–1338.
203. Hommes D, van den Blink B, Plasse T, et al. Inhibition of stress-activated MAP kinases induces clinical improvement in moderate to severe Crohn's disease. Gastroenterology 2002; 122:7–14.
204. Vasiliauskas EA, Kam LY, Abreu-Martin MT, et al. An open-label pilot study of low-dose thalidomide in chronically active, steroid-dependent Crohn's disease. Gastroenterology 1999; 117:1278–1287.
205. Sandborn WJ, Yednock TA. Novel approaches to treating inflammatory bowel disease: targeting alpha-4 integrin. Am J Gastroenterol 2003; 98:2372–2382.
206. Ghosh S, Goldin E, Gordon FH, et al. Natalizumab for active Crohn's disease. N Engl J Med 2003; 348:24–32.
207. Yacyshyn BR, Chey WY, Goff J, et al. Double blind, placebo controlled trial of the remission inducing and steroid sparing properties of an ICAM-1 antisense oligodeoxynucleotide,

alicaforsen (ISIS 2302), in active steroid dependent Crohn's disease. Gut 2002; 51:30–36.

208. Slonim AE, Bulone L, Damore MB, et al. A preliminary study of growth hormone therapy for Crohn's disease. N Engl J Med 2000; 342:1633–1637.
209. Hanauer SB, Feagan BG, Lichtenstein GR, et al. Maintenance infliximab for Crohn's disease: the ACCENT I randomised trial. Lancet 2002; 359:1541–1549.
210. Rutgeerts P, Feagan BG, Lichtenstein GR, et al. Comparison of scheduled and episodic treatment strategies of infliximab in Crohn's disease. Gastroenterology 2004; 126:402–413.
211. Sands BE, Anderson FH, Bernstein CN, et al. Infliximab maintenance therapy for fistulizing Crohn's disease. N Engl J Med 2004; 350:876–885.
212. Baert F, Noman M, Vermeire S, et al. Influence of immunogenicity on the long-term efficacy of infliximab in Crohn's disease. N Engl J Med 2003; 348:601–608.
213. Cheifetz A, Smedley M, Martin S, et al. The incidence and management of infusion reactions to infliximab: a large center experience. Am J Gastroenterol 2003; 98:1315–1324.
214. Crandall WV, Mackner LM. Infusion reactions to infliximab in children and adolescents: frequency, outcome and a predictive model. Aliment Pharmacol Ther 2003; 17:75–84.
215. Miele E, Markowitz JE, Mamula P, et al. Human antichimeric antibody in children and young adults with inflammatory bowel disease receiving infliximab. J Pediatr Gastroenterol Nutr 2004; 38:502–508.
216. Farrell RJ, Alsahli M, Jeen YT, et al. Intravenous hydrocortisone premedication reduces antibodies to infliximab in Crohn's disease: a randomized controlled trial. Gastroenterology 2003; 124:917–924.
217. Colombel JF, Loftus EV Jr, Tremaine WJ, et al. The safety profile of infliximab in patients with Crohn's disease: the Mayo Clinic experience in 500 patients. Gastroenterology 2004; 126:19–31.
218. Vermeire S, Noman M, Van Assche G, et al. Autoimmunity associated with anti-tumor necrosis factor alpha treatment in Crohn's disease: a prospective cohort study. Gastroenterology 2003; 125:32–39.
219. Brown SL, Greene MH, Gershon SK, et al. Tumor necrosis factor antagonist therapy and lymphoma development: twenty-six cases reported to the Food and Drug Administration. Arthritis Rheum 2002; 46:3151–3158.

219a. Van Assche G, Van Ranst M, Sciot R et al. Progressive multifocal leukoencephalopathy after natalizumab therapy for Crohn's disease. N Engl J Med 2005; 353(4):362–368.

220. Sutherland L, Singleton J, Sessions J, et al. Double blind, placebo controlled trial of metronidazole in Crohn's disease. Gut 1991; 32:1071–1075.
221. Prantera C, Zannoni F, Scribano ML, et al. An antibiotic regimen for the treatment of active Crohn's disease: a randomized, controlled clinical trial of metronidazole plus ciprofloxacin. Am J Gastroenterol 1996; 91:328–332.
222. Rutgeerts P, Hiele M, Geboes K, et al. Controlled trial of metronidazole treatment for prevention of Crohn's recurrence after ileal resection. Gastroenterology 1995; 108:1617–1621.
223. Famularo G, Mosca L, Minisola G, et al. Probiotic lactobacilli: a new perspective for the treatment of inflammatory bowel disease. Curr Pharm Des 2003; 9:1973–1980.
224. Prantera C, Scribano ML, Falasco G, et al. Ineffectiveness of probiotics in preventing recurrence after curative resection for Crohn's disease: a randomised controlled trial with Lactobacillus GG. Gut 2002; 51:405–409.
225. Belluzzi A, Brignola C, Campieri M, et al. Effect of an enteric-coated fish-oil preparation on relapses in Crohn's disease. N Engl J Med 1996; 334:1557–1560.
226. Ostro MJ, Greenberg GR, Jeejeebhoy KN. Total parenteral nutrition and complete bowel rest in the management of Crohn's disease. JPEN J Parenter Enteral Nutr 1985; 9:280–287.
227. Griffiths AM, Ohlsson A, Sherman PM, et al. Meta-analysis of enteral nutrition as a primary treatment of active Crohn's disease. Gastroenterology 1995; 108:1056–1067.
228. Gorard DA, Hunt JB, Payne-James JJ, et al. Initial response and subsequent course of Crohn's disease treated with elemental diet or prednisolone. Gut 1993; 34:1198–1202.
229. Gassull MA, Cabre E. Nutrition in inflammatory bowel disease. Curr Opin Clin Nutr Metab Care 2001; 4:561–569.
230. Gassull MA, Fernandez-Banares F, Cabre E, et al. Fat composition may be a clue to explain the primary therapeutic effect of enteral nutrition in Crohn's disease: results of a double blind randomised multicentre European trial. Gut 2002; 51:164–168.
231. Wilschanski M, Sherman P, Pencharz P, et al. Supplementary enteral nutrition maintains remission in paediatric Crohn's disease. Gut 1996; 38:543–548.
232. Davies G, Evans CM, Shand WS, et al. Surgery for Crohn's disease in childhood: influence of site of disease and operative procedure on outcome. Br J Surg 1990; 77:891–894.
233. Farmer RG, Michener WM. Prognosis of Crohn's disease with onset in childhood or adolescence. Dig Dis Sci 1979; 24:752–757.
234. Rutgeerts P, Geboes K, Vantrappen G, et al. Predictability of the postoperative course of Crohn's disease. Gastroenterology 1990; 99:956–963.
235. Baldassano RN, Han PD, Jeshion WC, et al. Pediatric Crohn's disease: risk factors for postoperative recurrence. Am J Gastroenterol 2001; 96:2169–2176.
236. Griffiths AM, Wesson DE, Shandling B, et al. Factors influencing postoperative recurrence of Crohn's disease in childhood. Gut 1991; 32:491–495.
237. Hyams JS, Grand RJ, Colodny AH, et al. Course and prognosis after colectomy and ileostomy for inflammatory bowel disease in childhood and adolescence. J Pediatr Surg 1982; 17:400–405.
238. Dietz DW, Laureti S, Strong SA, et al. Safety and longterm efficacy of strictureplasty in 314 patients with obstructing small bowel Crohn's disease. J Am Coll Surg 2001; 192:330–337; discussion 337–338.
239. Di Abriola GF, De Angelis P, Dall'oglio L, et al. Strictureplasty: an alternative approach in long segment bowel stenosis Crohn's disease. J Pediatr Surg 2003; 38:814–818.
240. Hyams JS, Moore RE, Leichtner AM, et al. Longitudinal assessment of type I procollagen in children with inflammatory bowel disease subjected to surgery. J Pediatr Gastroenterol Nutr 1989; 8:68–74.
241. Binder V, Hendriksen C, Kreiner S. Prognosis in Crohn's disease – based on results from a regional patient group from the county of Copenhagen. Gut 1985; 26:146–150.
242. Veloso FT, Ferreira JT, Barros L, et al. Clinical outcome of Crohn's disease: analysis according to the Vienna classification and clinical activity. Inflamm Bowel Dis 2001; 7:306–313.
243. Sahmoud T, Hoctin-Boes G, Modigliani R, et al. Identifying patients with a high risk of relapse in quiescent Crohn's disease. The GETAID Group. The Groupe d'Etudes Therapeutiques des Affections Inflammatoires Digestives. Gut 1995; 37:811–818.

244. Munkholm P. The incidence and prevalence of colorectal cancer in inflammatory bowel disease. Aliment Pharmacol Ther 2003; 18(Suppl 2):1–5.
245. Choi PM, Zelig MP. Similarity of colorectal cancer in Crohn's disease and ulcerative colitis: implications for carcinogenesis and prevention. Gut 1994; 35:950–954.
246. van Hogezand RA, Eichhorn RF, Choudry A, et al. Malignancies in inflammatory bowel disease: fact or fiction? Scand J Gastroenterol Suppl 2002; 236:48–53.
247. Loftus EV Jr, Tremaine WJ, Habermann TM, et al. Risk of lymphoma in inflammatory bowel disease. Am J Gastroenterol 2000; 95:2308–2312.
248. Lewis JD, Bilker WB, Brensinger C, et al. Inflammatory bowel disease is not associated with an increased risk of lymphoma. Gastroenterology 2001; 121:1080–1087.
249. Card T, Hubbard R, Logan RF. Mortality in inflammatory bowel disease: a population-based cohort study. Gastroenterology 2003; 125:1583–1590.
250. Neurath MF. T-lymphocyte dysregulation. In: Sartor R, Sandborn W, eds. Kirsner's Inflammatory Bowel Diseases, 6th edn. Edinburgh: Saunders; 2004:199–211.

Chapter 41
Ulcerative colitis in children and adolescents

James F. Markowitz

INTRODUCTION

Ulcerative colitis (UC) is an important pediatric gastrointestinal disease, given its potential for significant morbidity and even mortality during childhood, its chronicity and its premalignant nature. Although significant advances in our understanding of its immunologic basis have led to novel approaches to its therapy, UC remains medically incurable. Nevertheless, current medical and surgical therapeutic options have improved the overall outlook for children with this condition.

EPIDEMIOLOGY

As opposed to the documented rise in incidence of pediatric Crohn's disease over the last 30 years, incidence rates of UC in children appear to have remained fairly stable or to have decreased slightly. Recent population-based studies from Wisconsin[1] and northern Stockholm[2] identified incidence rates of 2.1 and 2.2 per 100 000 population respectively, rates that fall in the middle of the range of estimates of 0.5–4.3 per 100 000 population reported in earlier studies.[3] The incidence rates for UC appear to be about half of that seen for Crohn's disease in the same population.[1,2] Estimated prevalence rates in children are 18–30 per 100 000. Males and females are equally affected. While the majority of pediatric patients with UC present as adolescents (87% of subjects in a review from the Cleveland Clinic)[4], very young children with UC are not unusual[5,6] and about 40% of children with UC present by the age of 10 years.[7] Overall, 10–15% of children with UC have first-degree relatives with inflammatory bowel disease (IBD).[7,8] However, 22.6% of Jewish children with UC have affected relatives, compared with only 13.7% of non-Jewish children.[8] Children with UC are more likely than their unaffected siblings to have had diarrhea during infancy.[9] However, children who received formula feedings as infants appear to be at no greater risk of developing UC than those who were breast-fed.[10] Appendectomy for acute appendicitis before 20 years of age clearly protects against the development of UC in adults,[11] but it is not clear to what degree this factor protects against the development of UC during childhood. The effect of either active or passive cigarette smoking on the risk of developing UC during childhood is also not clear. Epidemiologic studies have documented that passive smoking during childhood protects against developing UC as an adult.[12] However, although passive smoking may increase the risk of developing Crohn's disease as a child, a protective effect against the development of UC during childhood has not been clearly demonstrated.[9,13] In fact, a recent case–control study questions whether cigarette smoking is protective against UC in adults at all, as adults who had never smoked could not be shown to have an increased risk of UC compared with active smokers.[14] In this study, the risk of UC appeared to be increased only in smokers who had stopped smoking, suggesting the possibility that the disease was either triggered or unmasked by the removal of an immunosuppressive effect exerted by cigarette smoke.

GENETICS

Genetic factors are important in UC, although to a lesser degree than in Crohn's disease. Studies consistently demonstrate a lower rate of IBD in relatives of probands with UC than in those with Crohn's disease.[8,15,16] Similarly, the rate of concordant disease is much less for monozygotic twin pairs with UC than it is for those with Crohn's disease.[17]

Despite this, a number of genetic breakthroughs in UC have been made. Among the first was the recognition of an association between HLA class II alleles and UC. HLA-DR2 has been found in 40% of a US population with UC, confirming previous studies in which 70% of a Japanese population with UC was found to have the same association.[18,19] A specific allele of another HLA-associated gene, major histocompatibility complex (MHC) class I chain-related gene A, has been shown to be associated with UC in a Japanese population, and homozygosity for the allele is associated with earlier age of disease onset.[20]

A number of other genes have been identified as potentially important in the susceptibility to or development of UC. Polymorphisms in the tumor necrosis factor α (TNF-α) gene are found more commonly in patients with UC than in those with Crohn's disease or in normal controls.[21] An association with polymorphisms of the intracellular adhesion molecule 1 gene,[22] the interleukin 11 gene[23] and the interleukin 1 receptor antagonist gene[24] have also been described.

Another gene of interest is the multidrug resistance 1 (*MDR1*) gene, located on chromosome 7 in a region identified by genome-wide scans as a potential site of an IBD susceptibility gene. Abnormal gene expression is characterized

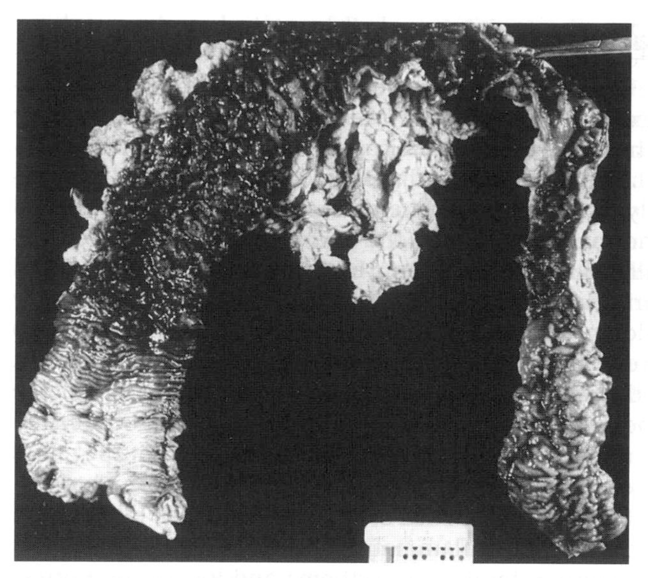

Figure 41.2: Macroscopic appearance of the colon of a 16-year-old patient with ulcerative colitis at the time of subtotal colectomy. Note the mucosa characterized by diffuse ulceration and multiple pseudo-polyps. (Courtesy of Ellen Kahn MD).

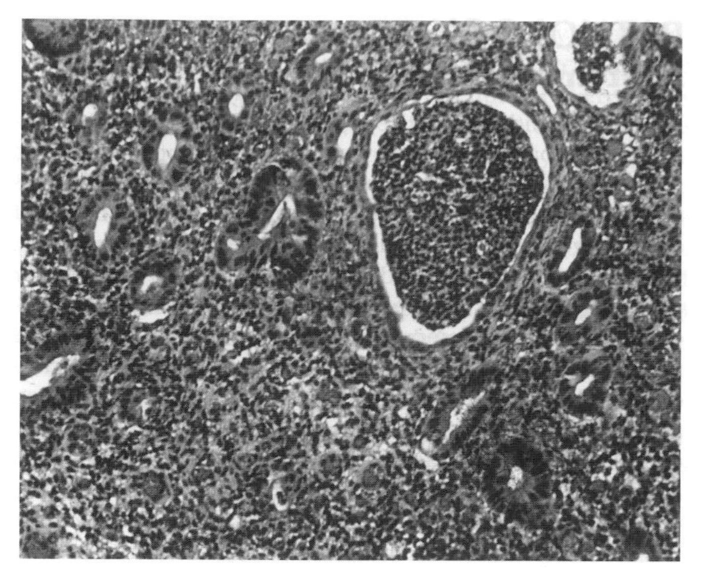

Figure 41.3: Colonic biopsy. Active ulcerative colitis, characterized by neutrophilic infiltration of the crypts, crypt abscesses and crypt distortion. Hematoxylin–eosin stain, × 125. (Courtesy of Ellen Kahn MD).

to the surface epithelium and Paneth cell metaplasia. None of these findings is pathognemonic for UC, as similar changes can be seen in severe Crohn's colitis. Infectious colitis may also have a similar appearance, although histologic differentiation of UC from acute self-limiting colitis is generally possible.[60] Although diffuse histologic involvement of the affected bowel is typical in the untreated patient, a few children have manifested patchy inflammation and rectal sparing.[57–59] In surgical specimens obtained from patients with severe or fulminant disease, ulceration can, at times, extend into the submucosa or rarely the deeper layers of the bowel wall.

CLINICAL FEATURES

Symptoms and signs

Children with UC most commonly present with diarrhea, rectal bleeding and abdominal pain (Table 41.1). Frequent watery stools can contain either streaks of blood or clots, and are most common on arising in the morning, after eating and during the night. Children often describe both tenesmus and urgency, although the former symptom is at times misinterpreted as constipation by the child or parent. Acute weight loss is common, but abnormalities of linear growth are unusual (see below).

The severity of symptoms at presentation is variable. Some 40–50% of children and adolescents present with mild symptoms, characterized by fewer than four stools per day, only intermittent hematochezia and minimal (if any) systemic symptoms or weight loss.[7] These children generally have normal findings on physical examination, or only minimal tenderness on palpation of the lower abdomen. Stools may have streaks of blood or may be positive only for occult blood. Laboratory studies can reveal mild anemia and raised acute-phase reactants such as the erythrocyte sedimentation rate. However, some children have entirely normal laboratory findings.

Another third of children are moderately ill, often displaying weight loss, more frequent diarrhea and systemic

	Toronto[a] (diagnosed 1970–1978)		Cleveland[b] (diagnosed before 1967)	
	No. of patients (n = 87)	% of population	No. of patients (n = 125)	% of population
Hematochezia	84	96	107	86
Diarrhea	82	94	116	93
Abdominal pain	77	88	107	86
Anorexia	44	50	–	–
Nocturnal diarrhea	43	49	–	–
Weight loss	37	42	64	51
Fever	12	13	46	37
Vomiting	10	11	53	42

Data from [a]Hamilton et al.[48] and [b]Michener.[188]

Table 41.1 Symptoms at diagnosis of ulcerative colitis

symptoms. Physical examination demonstrates abdominal tenderness, whereas laboratory studies often are characterized by moderate leukocytosis, mild anemia and raised acute-phase reactants.

The final 10–15% of the pediatric UC population has an acute fulminant disease presentation. These patients appear moderately to severely toxic and have severe crampy abdominal pain, fever, more than six diarrheal stools per day and, at times, copious rectal bleeding. They frequently manifest tachycardia, orthostatic hypotension, diffuse abdominal tenderness without peritoneal signs, and distension. Laboratory studies reveal leukocytosis, often with numerous band forms, anemia, thrombocytosis and hypoproteinemia. Toxic megacolon represents the most dangerous extreme of acute fulminant colitis, and is quite rare in the pediatric age group.

EXTRAINTESTINAL MANIFESTATIONS

Extraintestinal manifestations are common in children with UC, and can affect almost every organ system of the body. The more common sites of involvement are the skin, eye, biliary tree and joints. Although the etiology for these extraintestinal manifestations remains unknown, it has been shown that an anticolonocyte antibody detectable in the serum of patients with UC cross-reacts with antigens present in the skin, ciliary body of the eye, bile duct and joints.[34,35,61] Many of the extraintestinal manifestations tend to occur at times of increased colitis activity. It is therefore tempting to speculate that extraintestinal symptoms develop when autoantibodies capable of recognizing these non-intestinal tissues are produced as part of the humoral response characteristic of UC.

Hepatobiliary

The most serious hepatobiliary diseases associated with UC are primary sclerosing cholangitis (PSC) and autoimmune hepatitis. The presentation and severity of these manifestations are generally independent of the activity of colitis, and often do not appear to be affected by medical management of UC or by colectomy. PSC occurs in 3.5% of children and adolescents with UC, whereas autoimmune hepatitis is seen in less than 1%.[62] Either may be present at the time of, or even precede, the initial diagnosis of UC, or may develop during the course of the illness.

Both illnesses cause variable degrees of chronic liver disease, ranging from mild to end-stage liver disease requiring transplantation, or death.[62–64] PSC also is a risk factor for the development of cholangiocarcinoma.

PSC does not appear to affect the severity of UC. However, the presence of PSC enhances the risk of colorectal aneuploidy, dysplasia and cancer in patients with UC.[65] The absolute cumulative risk for colorectal cancer in patients with UC with PSC is 9%, 31% and 50% after 10, 20 and 25 years of disease respectively, compared with 2%, 5% and 10% in patients with UC without PSC.[66] In patients with UC and PSC who have a colectomy and ileal pouch, the risk of severe mucosal atrophy, aneuploidy and dysplasia in the pouch also appears to be increased.[67] In addition, those with PSC and UC complicated by colorectal cancer are at increased risk of cholangiocarcinoma, compared with patients with PSC and UC but no colorectal malignancy.[66] Although treatment with ursodeoxycholic acid has shown some potential benefit in decreasing the risk of colonic cancer in adult patients with UC and PSC,[68] earlier initiation and increased frequency of colonic surveillance is indicated.

In addition, liver function abnormalities can be seen in a variety of other clinical circumstances, for instance during periods of increased colitis activity, as well as in association with specific therapies used for colitis including corticosteroids, sulfasalazine, parenteral hyperalimentation, azathioprine and 6-mercaptopurine (6-MP), or with fatty changes associated with massive acute weight gain.[62]

Joints

Arthralgia has been described in up to 32% of children with UC at some time during their course.[69] Arthritis, either a peripheral migratory type affecting the large joints or a monoarticular non-deforming arthritis primarily affecting the knees or ankles, has been reported in 10–20% of children.[69,70] The presence and activity of arthritis and arthralgia generally, but not invariably, correlate with the activity of the bowel disease. Ankylosing spondylitis occurs in up to 6% of adults with UC, but is rare during childhood.

Skin

Cutaneous manifestations occur during periods of enhanced colitis activity, with erythema nodosum occurring more commonly than pyoderma gangrenosum.[71] Erythema nodosum lesions appear as raised, erythematous, painful circular nodules that usually occur over the tibia, but may also be present on the lower leg, ankle or extensor surface of the arm. Lesions persist for several days to a few weeks, and generally remit with treatments directed at the enhanced colitis activity.[71] Pyoderma gangrenosum usually appears as small, painful, sterile pustules that coalesce into a larger sterile abscess (Fig. 41.4). This ultimately drains, forming a deep necrotic ulcer. Lesions usually occur on the lower extremities, although the upper extremities, trunk and head are not spared. A variety of possibly beneficial therapies have been reported, although at present systemic or local ciclosporin, tacrolimus and intravenous infliximab appear to be the treatments of choice.[72–76]

Thromboembolic disorders

Case reports document the occurrence of thromboembolic complications in children with UC. Sites of venous or arterial thrombosis include the extremities, portal or hepatic vein, lung and central nervous system. While thromobophilia,[77] hyperhomocysteinemia possibly due to

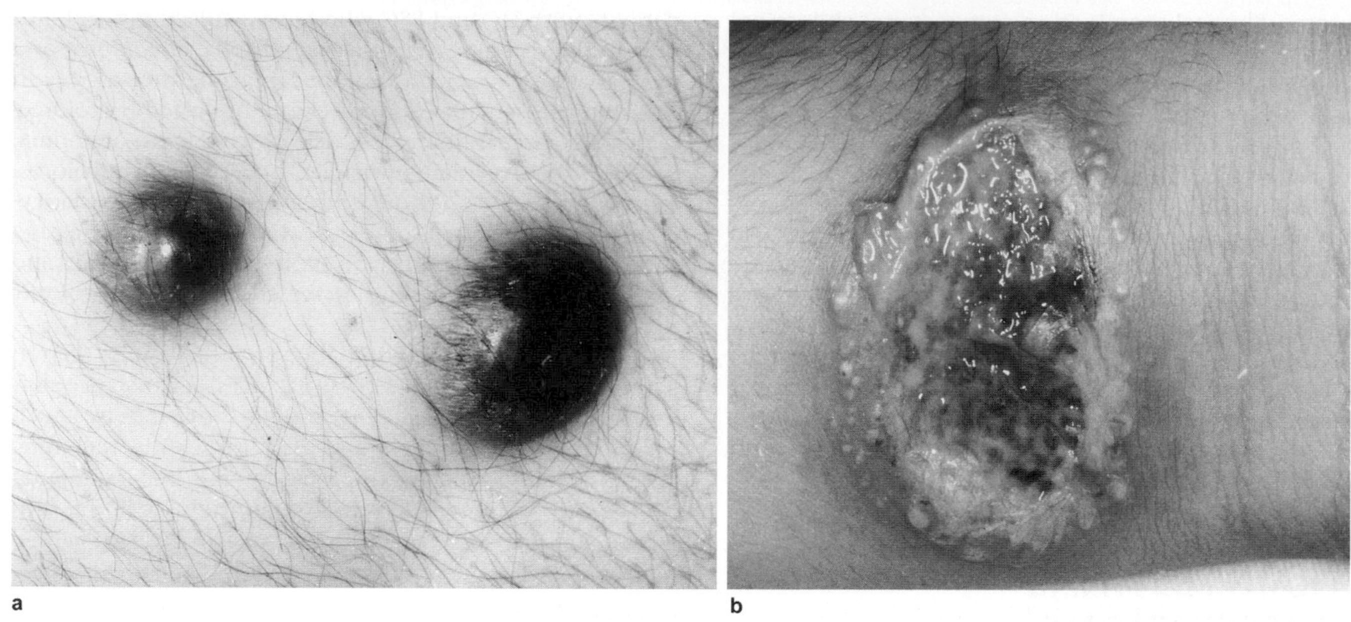

Figure 41.4: (a) Pustular phase of pyoderma gangrenosum in a 15-year-old boy with ulcerative colitis. Cutaneous lesions began to appear 2 weeks after initial gastrointestinal symptoms. (b) Typical chronic ulcer of pyoderma gangrenosum from the same patient, located on the dorsal surface of the forearm.

folate deficiency[78] or vitamin B_6 deficiency[79] and specific mutations of coagulation factors such as factor V Leiden[80] have been described in individual patients with UC and a history of thrombosis, no consistent abnormality has been identified to explain why only a subset of patients develops thrombotic complications.

Ocular disorders

Eye involvement in UC is rare in children, although episcleritis and asymptomatic uveitis have been described.[81] Other ocular disorders such as posterior subcapsular cataracts or increased ocular pressure may be the result of corticosteroid therapy.[82,83]

COMPLICATIONS

Bleeding

Hematochezia is nearly universal in UC, but severe hemorrhage requiring urgent or multiple transfusions occurs in less than 5% of cases. When present, severe hemorrhage is usually the result of diffuse, active, mucosal ulceration. Children who continue to require blood transfusions after 7–14 days of intensive medical therapy have been shown to be at risk for significant complications and colectomy.[84]

Perforation

Free perforation of the colon is an emergent complication of UC that occurs rarely. Circumstances that predispose to perforation include acute fulminant colitis, toxic megacolon and diagnostic interventions such as barium enema or colonoscopy. In these settings, gaseous distension or direct pressure from an endoscope can generate sufficient force to perforate the inflamed colon. Peritonitis and septic shock can result. These potentially life-threatening complications require appropriate fluid resuscitation, broad-spectrum antibiotics and emergent surgery. Plain radiographs of the abdomen may be required to identify a possible free perforation in children with UC who develop worsening symptoms or shoulder pain, as concomitant corticosteroid therapy may mask physical findings such as board-like rigidity or diffuse rebound tenderness.

Toxic megacolon

This complication has been described in up to 5% of children and adolescents with UC, and represents a medical and potentially surgical emergency.[47,84] Improper diagnosis or treatment can lead to a rapidly progressive deterioration complicated by severe electrolyte disturbances, hypoalbuminemia, hemorrhage, perforation, sepsis and/or shock. Precipitating factors include the use of antidiarrheal agents such as anticholinergics or opiates, and excessive colonic distension during barium enema or colonoscopy. Possibly as the result of recognizing and minimizing these factors, the frequency of toxic megacolon in the pediatric population appears to be decreasing. In fact, in a review of the clinical outcome of children with UC treated at Hartford Hospital and North Shore University Hospital between 1975–1994, only one patient with toxic megacolon was seen in 171 children followed for a total of 823 patient-years.[7]

Carcinoma

The colorectal tumors that develop in the setting of chronic ulcerative colitis are adenocarcinomas. In contrast to sporadic adenocarcinomas, tumors that arise in UC do not begin as adenomatous polyps, but rather as flat lesions characterized by the presence of dysplasia.[85] The genetic alterations that precede the development of dysplasia occur multifocally in the colon, so that the resulting adenocarcinomas are evenly distributed about the colon.[86] Multifocal or synchronous tumors are present in 10–20% of patients.[87]

Individuals who develop UC during childhood have a particularly high lifetime risk of colorectal cancer because duration (>10 years) and extent (pancolitis > left-sided colitis > proctitis) of colitis are the two most critical risk factors for cancer in these conditions.[88–90] Other less well characterized risk factors include concomitant sclerosing cholangitis,[65,66] an excluded, defunctionalized or bypassed segment,[76,91] and depressed red blood cell folate levels.[92] Patients as young as 16 years of age have been demonstrated to have colonic aneuploidy, dysplasia or cancer, although as in adults the risk for these changes does not appear to be significant in the first decade of illness.[47,88,93]

Population-based studies support the observation that children with UC have an increased lifetime risk of colorectal cancer.[94–97] A large Swedish study revealed that children with onset of UC before the age of 15 years have a standardized incidence ratio (SIR – the ratio of observed to expected cases) of colorectal cancer of 118 (162 for those with pancolitis), compared with a SIR ranging from 2.2 to 16.5 in individuals older than 15 years at diagnosis.[94] These values translate into cumulative colorectal cancer incidence rates of 5% at 20 years and 40% at 35 years for patients with colitis onset at ages 0–14 years, and 5% and 30% respectively for those whose colitis began between the ages of 15 and 39 years.[94] These values are strikingly similar to those originally reported by Devroede from the Mayo Clinic in children with onset of colitis at less than 14 years of age (3% in the first 10 years, 43% at 35 years).[88] In addition, 52–68% of patients with colitis-associated cancers detected because of symptoms have regional node involvement or distant metastasis, resulting in an overall 5-year survival rate of 31–55%.[98–100] Therefore, it is estimated that there is an 8% risk of dying from colonic cancer 10–25 years after diagnosis of colitis if colectomy is not performed for control of disease symptoms.[101]

Given the high risk of colorectal cancer, surveillance colonoscopy has been advocated as an approach that might lessen the need for prophylactic proctocolectomy. Surveillance programs as currently practised suffer from lack of objective premalignant markers and the problems associated with invasive testing. A standardized definition of dysplasia (negative, indefinite, low grade, high grade)[85] is in widespread use, but interobserver variability using these definitions results in major discrepancy rates of 4–7.5% between expert pathologists reviewing the same slides.[102,103] In addition, evaluations must be made, but have not always been reported, based on an 'intent to treat' model, as non-compliance with the surveillance protocol (refusal to enroll or maintain regular examination schedule) and inability to evaluate the entire colon adequately due to stricture, poor bowel preparation or active disease constitute realities of surveillance that have a direct bearing on the efficacy of the surveillance strategy.

The literature generally reflects the practice of performing colectomy only when high-grade dysplasia or cancer is detected. With this approach, a review of recent prospective cohort studies has revealed that surveillance detects cancer at an early and potentially curable stage 65% of the time, thereby reducing the frequency of detecting advanced lesions from 60% to 35%.[101] However, the data suggest that 33 patients would have to be under regular surveillance for 15 years to prevent one incurable cancer. With biannual examinations resulting in seven to eight colonoscopies per patient, a total of about 250 procedures would be performed to prevent one incurable cancer.[101] Analyses such as these have led to a vigorous discussion regarding the cost-effectiveness of surveillance as currently practised.[104,105]

These data have led to a search for better markers to enhance the predictive accuracy of surveillance. Expanding indications for surgery to include the identification of low-grade dysplasia might enhance the effectiveness of surveillance, as low-grade dysplasia has been shown to advance to high-grade dysplasia or cancer in 54% of cases within 5 years.[106] Other markers, including aneuploidy,[93,107–109] loss of tumor suppressor gene (e.g. *p53*)[110] function, expression of proto-oncogenes (e.g. K-*ras*)[111] and expression of abnormal mucin-associated antigens (e.g. sialosyl-Tn)[112], have also been investigated as adjuncts to surveillance for dysplasia.

No prospective studies have assessed the optimal schedule of surveillance, although a cost–benefit analysis has suggested colonoscopies every 3 years for the first 10 years of surveillance, with more frequent investigations as the duration of colitis increases.[113] Current practice generally begins with bi-yearly colonoscopies 7–10 years after diagnosis. Although many advocate initiating surveillance only after 15–20 years of disease in adults with left-sided colitis or proctosigmoiditis, the frequent proximal extension of these disease distributions in patients with onset of disease during childhood suggests that all patients with childhood-onset UC of any extent be enrolled in a surveillance program within 10 years of initial diagnosis. Procedures require panendoscopy to the cecum, with two to four biopsies every 10 cm from the cecum to the sigmoid, and every 5 cm in the sigmoid and rectum. Additional biopsies must be performed if a mass or other suspicious lesion is identified. Current recommendations for colectomy include any identification of dysplasia (low or high grade) confirmed by two independent experienced pathologists. Repeat colonoscopy for confirmation of dysplasia on new biopsies is not recommended, as there is no way to guarantee that the identical site can be biopsied on a subsequent procedure. If indefinite dysplasia is identified, aggressive medical management to reduce active inflammation followed by repeat surveillance colonoscopy within 3–6 months is indicated.

Growth and development

As opposed to Crohn's disease, only about 10% of children with UC demonstrate significantly impaired linear growth,[114] even though, for many patients, periods of poor caloric intake associated with episodes of active disease can result in acute weight loss. Why linear growth impairment is so unusual in UC, compared with Crohn's disease, remains to be explained, although the different cytokine profiles seen in the two diseases may be important. Although serum from children with Crohn's disease produced marked impairment in bone growth in an *in vitro* animal model, serum from children with UC and from normal controls does not.[115] Further study is necessary before it can be determined whether this effect is mediated by circulating proinflammatory cytokines or some other serum factor.

- Complete blood count, differential, reticulocyte count
- Erythrocyte sedimentation rate, C-reactive protein
- Electrolytes, serum chemistries (including total protein, albumin, liver function)
- Serum iron, total iron binding capacity, ferritin
- Stools for enteric pathogens (including Salmonella, Shigella, Campylobacter, Yersinia, Aeromonas, Escherichia coli)
- Stool for *Clostridium difficile* toxins
- Direct microscopic examination of the stool for ova and parasites, Charcot–Leyden crystals, leukocytes
- Perinuclear antineutrophilic cytoplasmic antibody, anti-*Saccharomyces cerevisiae* antibody, anti-ompC (anti-outer membrane porin of *E. coli*) antibody
- Fecal calprotectin

Table 41.2 Laboratory studies in suspected ulcerative colitis

DIAGNOSIS

History

Many children present with obvious symptoms of diarrhea and rectal bleeding. However, in others symptoms are less obvious and more difficult to elicit, especially in children or adolescents who are unwilling or too embarrassed to discuss the frequency and consistency of their bowel movements. Awakening with pain or the need to defecate is an especially important symptom to elicit, as it often helps to differentiate the child with organic illness from one with a functional condition. The history should seek to identify evidence of recent weight loss, poor growth, arrested sexual development or, in the postmenarchal adolescent, secondary amenorrhea. When family history reveals other relatives with IBD, the possibility that UC is present is increased.

Physical examination

A careful physical examination may demonstrate a number of findings that help suggest the appropriate diagnosis. Children with active colitis often have mild to moderate abdominal tenderness, especially in the left lower quadrant or mid-epigastric area. Tender bowel loops may be palpable, although inflammatory masses are lacking. With fulminant disease, marked tenderness can be present. Perianal inspection is generally normal, and the presence of perianal tags or fistulae suggests Crohn's disease. The presence of skin lesions, such as erythema nodosum, pyoderma gangrenosum or cutaneous vasculitis, or arthritis is an important clue to the autoimmune nature of the child's illness.

Laboratory studies

Once UC is suspected, the laboratory studies outlined in Table 41.2 help to exclude other illnesses and provide evidence to support proceeding to more invasive radiologic and endoscopic diagnostic procedures. Microcytic anemia, mild to moderate thrombocytosis, raised erythrocyte sedimentation rate and hypoalbuminemia are present in 40–80% of patients. Total white blood cell count is normal to only mildly increased, unless the illness is complicated by acute fulminant colitis. Abnormal liver function is found in 3% of children at the time of initial diagnosis, and reflect signs of potentially serious concomitant liver disease (chronic active hepatitis or sclerosing cholangitis) in about half of them.[62] In a number of children, however, all laboratory studies can be normal. Fecal levels of calprotectin, a neutrophil-associated protein present in the stools in conditions associated with intestinal inflammation, are higher in patients with active UC than in healthy controls.[116] Although calprotectin levels can also be raised in patients with enteric infection or Crohn's disease, an increased fecal calprotectin assay can help determine which children with abdominal pain or diarrhea should undergo more invasive testing for UC or Crohn's disease.[116]

Enteric pathogens must be excluded in all patients. Particular attention should be given to the possibility of *Clostridium difficile*-mediated colitis, given the frequency with which children are often exposed to antibiotics. If a pathogen is identified, it must be treated and the patient followed, as it is not unusual for children with UC to present initially with superimposed infection. If symptoms persist despite eradication of the identified pathogen, workup should continue.

Serologic tests for the detection of circulating perinuclear antineutrophil cytoplasmic antibody (pANCA) can be useful in differentiating UC from other colitides, including Crohn's disease.[29,117] pANCA can be detected in about 70% of patients with UC, but is present in only 6% of Crohn's patients and 3% of controls. The other serologic markers commonly identified in patients with IBD – anti-*Saccharomyces cerevisae* antibody (ASCA) and anti-outer membrane porin of *Escherichia coli* (ompC) – are found only rarely in children with UC. Utilizing an assay for both pANCA and ASCA, a recent pediatric study revealed that a positive pANCA coupled with a negative ASCA titer had a sensitivity of 69.2%, specificity of 95.1%, positive predictive value of 90.0% and negative predictive value of 87.1% for the diagnosis of UC.[118] Although children with indeterminate colitis may be negative for all serologic markers, at times the markers can be helpful in determining whether the child actually has Crohn's disease or UC. In adults with indeterminate colitis, a finding of pANCA+/ASCA– predicts UC in 64%, whereas pANCA–/ASCA+ findings predict Crohn's disease in 80%.[119]

Radiography

Traditionally, when UC was suspected, a barium enema was performed to identify radiographic signs of inflammation. Barium enema can, at times, differentiate between Crohn's and UC, but the classic radiographic findings attributed to one form of colitis can be mimicked by the other. Currently, barium enema is performed only rarely, having been replaced by colonoscopy. In most circumstances, however, the child with suspected UC should still undergo upper gastrointestinal series with small bowel follow-through to help exclude the possibility of Crohn's disease.

Abdominal ultrasonography, computed tomography and various scintigraphic techniques including technetium-99m–HMPAO-labelled white cell scan can be used to assess the presence and extent of intestinal inflammation, although these studies are not used widely to establish the initial diagnosis. Overall, these modalities are more useful in identifying complications associated with Crohn's disease than for UC.

Endoscopy

Colonoscopy allows accurate determination of the extent and distribution of colitis through direct visualization and biopsy of the affected segments. UC is characterized by diffuse inflammation, which begins at the anal verge and progresses proximally to a variable degree. Although rectal sparing is generally associated with Crohn's disease, untreated children can have rectal sparing at initial colonoscopy yet subsequently evidence typical UC.[57,120,121] In mild UC, the rectal and colonic mucosa appears erythematous, the normal vascular markings are lost, and there is increased friability evidenced by petechiae or contact hemorrhage (see Fig. 41.1a). With more active disease, exudate, ulcerations and marked hemorrhage are evident (see Fig. 41.1b,c). Skip lesions, aphthous ulcerations and significant ileal inflammation are indicative of Crohn's disease. All children who undergo endoscopy should be biopsied, as the histologic appearance can often help differentiate between acute self-limiting colitis, Crohn's disease and UC.[60]

Although UC is described as an inflammatory disease confined to the colon, endoscopic studies can reveal inflammation of the proximal gastrointestinal tract. A pattern of focally enhanced gastritis is seen in 21% of children with UC, and 50% can have features of chronic gastritis.[122] These observations require that clinicians do not automatically exclude the possible diagnosis of UC in a child with colitis who is shown to have endoscopic or histologic gastritis.

DIFFERENTIAL DIAGNOSIS

The differential diagnosis is summarized in Table 41.3. Most can easily be excluded by history, physical examination, laboratory evaluation, or endoscopy and biopsy. In contrast to adults, neoplastic disease, ischemia and radiation-induced injury are rarely significant diagnostic concerns in the child or adolescent.

Enteric infection
- Salmonella
- *Shigella*
- Campylobacter
- Aeromonas
- *Yersinia*
- Enterohemorrhagic *E. coli*
- Entameba histolytica
- *Giardia lamblia*[a]

Pseudomembranous (post-antibiotic) enterocolitis
- *Clostridium difficile*

Carbohydrate intolerance[a]
- Lactose
- Sucrose
- Non-digestible carbohydrates (sorbitol, xylitol, mannitol, maltitol, sucralose)

Vasculitis
- Henoch–Schönlein purpura
- Hemolytic–uremic syndrome

Allergic enterocolitis[b]
Hirschsprung's enterocolitis[b]
Eosinophilic gastroenteritis
Celiac disease[a]
Laxative abuse[a]
Neoplasms
- Juvenile polyp[b]
- Adenocarcinoma
- Intestinal polyposis

[a] Watery, non-bloody diarrhea.
[b] Pimarily in the young child.
(Modified from Park S-D, Markowitz JF. Ulcerative colitis (pediatric). In: Johnson L, ed. Encyclopedia of Gastroenterology. USA: Academic Press; 2004: 400–408, with permission).

Table 41.3 Differential diagnosis of ulcerative colitis in children

MEDICAL THERAPIES

As curative medical therapy does not exist, current treatment remains symptomatic and supportive. Treatment aims include the suppression of symptoms and the control of unavoidable complications. In many cases, UC and Crohn's disease respond to the same therapeutic modalities, and the reader may wish to review Chapter 40 for additional details of the various pharmacologic agents discussed below.

The treatment of children and adolescents presents the challenge of promoting normal growth and sexual development while controlling disease symptoms. Current treatment options at times promote one goal while hindering another. Therapy, therefore, may require striking a balance between potentially conflicting effects. Therapeutic options are listed in Table 41.4. Many of the data supporting the use of these medications have been extrapolated from adult studies. The following discussion focuses on aspects of treatment that have been shown to be particularly effective in the pediatric population.

Nutritional therapy

Although nutritional therapies have a role as primary treatment in Crohn's disease, UC is less amenable to nutritional interventions. Elimination diets rarely result in significant

Nutritionals
Appropriate dietary intake (with or without food supplements) Short-chain fatty acids n-3 fatty acids (fish oils)
Anti-inflammatories
Corticosteroids • Prednisone, prednisolone, hydrocortisone • Budesonide 5-Aminosalicylates • Sulfasalazine • Olsalazine • Mesalamine • Balsalazide
Immunomodulators
6-Mercaptopurine Azathioprine Ciclosporin Tacrolimus Methotrexate
Biologics
Infliximab

Table 41.4 Medical therapeutic options in ulcerative colitis

improvement in symptoms, and can promote inadequate nutritional intake in the child who finds the elimination diet prescribed unpalatable or too restrictive. Similarly, although 'bowel rest' can ameliorate symptoms in Crohn's disease of the small bowel, it is often ineffective in UC, possibly because the colonocyte derives energy from the fecal stream in the form of short-chain fatty acids. In addition, as growth failure is a much more frequent and dramatic problem in Crohn's disease than in UC, the nutritional therapy of growth failure becomes more central to the treatment of the former illness. Therefore, nutritional interventions in UC are generally adjunctive to other treatments. In UC, an adequate dietary intake promotes normal growth and prevents catabolism, thereby enhancing the effect of other treatment modalities.[123] Nutritional support can successfully be accomplished by a number of approaches, including dietary supplementation, enteral or parenteral nutrition.

The therapeutic use of short-chain fatty acids may represent one area where a 'nutritional' intervention can offer benefit as primary therapy in UC. Adults with UC have been shown to have impaired butyrate metabolism. Similarly, fecal concentrations of *n*-butyrate are raised in children with inactive or mild UC, suggesting impaired utilization of this metabolic fuel.[46] A number of placebo-controlled trials of short-chain fatty acid or butyrate enemas have demonstrated limited improvement in symptom score and endoscopic appearance in actively treated adult subjects. The combination of 5-aminosalicylate (5-ASA) treatment and butyrate enemas has also been shown to be beneficial.[124] An additional study in adults has reported decreased mucosal hyperproliferation after short-chain fatty acid or butyrate enemas, suggesting that such treatment might have a role in decreasing the risk of colonic cancer in patients with UC.[125] More recent studies have explored the possibility that fecal butyrate concentrations can be effectively increased in patients with UC by adding specific dietary fibers such as oat bran[126] or a prebiotic such as germinated barley foodstuff[127] in an attempt to enhance the growth and metabolism of enteric butyrate-producing bacteria.

The oral supplementation of *n*-3 fatty acids derived from fish oil has also received some attention. Initial studies suggested that early relapse of UC could be delayed by supplementing the diet with 5.1 g/day of *n*-3 fatty acids, although relapse rates after 3 months were comparable to those in placebo-treated controls.[128] Similarly, *n*-3 fatty acids provided no, or only modest, steroid-sparing effect compared with placebo in the treatment of acute UC.[129] Only a single small pediatric trial has been reported. Compared with pretreatment values, children with UC in remission who were supplemented orally with purified eicosapentaenoic acid for 2 months had decreased leukocyte and rectal production of leukotriene B_4.[130] Whether this was clinically important could not be determined. Although no child relapsed during the study, there was no control group with whom clinical response could be compared. Clearly, further studies are necessary before the usefulness of this therapy in UC can be fully assessed.

Corticosteroids

Corticosteroids appear to downregulate multiple steps in the inflammatory cascade that results in UC.[131,132] The initial use of corticosteroids as treatment for children with UC was largely extrapolated from studies in adults. Pediatric treatment regimens have evolved through empiric use and clinical experience, rather than controlled clinical trial. Prednisone, methylprednisolone and hydrocortisone are the agents most frequently employed. Commonly prescribed dosages are comparable to those prescribed for children with Crohn's disease. Oral corticosteroids are well absorbed, although occasional children with poor absorption or corticosteroid resistance may benefit from intravenous bolus or continuous infusion dosing. Rectal corticosteroids are particularly beneficial in children with severe tenesmus and urgency, but many children have difficulty retaining enema formulations, so that foam-based treatments or suppositories may be preferable in selected individuals. One adult study has demonstrated better efficacy for systemically administered corticotropin (adrenocorticotropic hormone; ACTH) as compared to intravenous hydrocortisone,[133] although pediatric experience with this therapy is lacking.

The decision to use corticosteroids must be balanced by their potential adverse effects. A wide spectrum of complications occasionally occurs (Table 41.5). Importantly, systemically active corticosteroids can interfere with linear

Cosmetic
Moon facies
Acne
Hirsutism
Striae
Central obesity
Metabolic
Hypokalemia
Hyperglycemia
Hyperlipidemia
Systemic hypertension
Endocrinologic
Growth suppression
Delayed puberty
Adrenal suppression
Musculoskeletal
Osteopenia
Aseptic necrosis of bone
Vertebral collapse
Myopathy
Ocular
Cataracts
Increased intraocular pressure

Table 41.5 Side-effects of corticosteroid therapy

bone growth, even in the face of adequate dietary intake.[134] Alternate-day dosing minimizes these effects while maintaining reduced disease activity,[135–137] and appears to have no deleterious effect upon bone mineralization in children.[138] However, in patients who have not completed their linear growth and whose disease activity cannot be controlled by alternate-day dosing regimens, the anti-inflammatory effects of daily corticosteroids must be weighed against the coincident suppression of linear growth.

Topically active corticosteroids such as budesonide have the potential to provide anti-inflammatory activity to the gut without systemic toxicity because of their high first-pass metabolism.[139] These agents may offer particular advantages for the treatment of children if they prove to be minimally growth suppressive, but pediatric studies in UC have yet to be reported. In adults, the enema formulation of budesonide is as effective as rectal mesalamine[140] and rectal prednisolone or hydrocortisone[141,142] in the treatment of left-sided and distal colitis. A budesonide rectal foam is also as effective as a hydrocortisone foam in adults with proctosigmoiditis, and 52% of previous rectal mesalamine failures responded to the budesonide foam.[143] In adults, budesonide enemas (2 mg) are associated with fewer abnormal ACTH stimulation test results than rectal hydrocortisone (100 mg).[142] Multiple courses of rectal budesonide are safe and effective for recurrent flares of UC.[142] Data on the effect of oral budesonide in UC are limited. A single study in adults with active extensive and distal UC demonstrated that oral budesonide (10 mg) delivered as a controlled-release preparation was as effective as oral prednisolone (40 mg), but did not suppress plasma cortisol levels.[144] Additional studies are required to determine whether the current oral formulation, which is designed to deliver active budesonide to the ileum and right colon, will be an effective therapy in children with UC.

Corticosteroid resistance remains a difficult problem for many patients. A number of different mechanisms appear to result in corticosteroid resistance, including IL-2-induced inhibition of glucocorticoid receptor activity and decreased intracellular glucocorticoid levels due to overexpression of the multidrug resistance gene 1.[145] Therapeutic strategies designed to overcome these factors are under investigation. In two different preliminary trials, adults with corticosteroid-resistant UC responded dramatically to treatment with either daclizumab or basiliximab, anti-IL-2 receptor monoclonal antibodies that block the lymphocyte IL-2 receptor and prevent IL-2-induced inhibition of the glucocorticoid receptor.[146,147] Whether these agents will ultimately be shown to be useful in the management of children with active or fulminant UC remains to be determined.

5-Aminosalicylates

It is postulated that the 5-ASA drugs (sulfasalazine, mesalamine, olsalazine, balsalazide) exert local anti-inflammatory effects through a number of different mechanisms. These include inhibition of 5-lipoxygenase with resulting decreased production of leukotriene B_4, scavenging of reactive oxygen metabolites, prevention of the upregulation of leukocyte adhesion molecules and inhibition of IL-1 synthesis.[132,148] As 5-ASA is rapidly absorbed from the upper intestinal tract upon oral ingestion, different delivery systems have been employed to prevent absorption until the active drug can be delivered to the distal small bowel and colon. Sulfasalazine (Azulfidine®) links 5-ASA via an azo bond to sulfapyridine. Bacterial enzymes in the colon break the azo linkage, releasing 5-ASA to exert its anti-inflammatory effect in the colon. Because the sulfapyridine moiety causes most of the untoward reactions to sulfasalazine and is thought to have no therapeutic activity, newer agents have been designed to deliver 5-ASA without sulfapyridine. Olsalazine (Dipentum®) links two molecules of 5-ASA via an azo bond, and balsalazide (Colazal®, Colazide®) links 5-ASA via an azo bond to an inert, non-absorbed carrier. A number of other delayed release preparations (Asacol®, Claversal®, Mesasal®, Salofalk®) prevent rapid absorption of 5-ASA (also known generically as mesalamine) by coating it with Eudragit®, a pH-sensitive acrylic resin. Another preparation (Pentasa®) coats microgranules of mesalamine with ethylcellulose, releasing it in a time-dependent fashion. Uncoated mesalamine is also available as a rectal suppository (Canasa®, Salofalk®) or enema formulation (Rowasa®).

Overall, the 5-ASA drugs have been shown to be effective in controlling mild to moderate UC in adults in 50–90% of cases, and effective in maintaining remission in 70–90%.[149,150] Despite extensive studies in adults, few pediatric studies exist. Clinical experience with sulfasalazine in children with UC has generally mirrored the adult experience.[151] One pediatric study made a direct comparison of the efficacy of sulfasalazine and olsalazine.[152] In this study, 79% of children with mildly to moderately active UC treated with sulfasalazine (60 mg/kg daily) improved clinically, compared with only 39% of those treated with olsalazine (30 mg/kg daily). Several smaller open-label or double-blind pediatric trials, and one larger retrospective analysis of 10 years' clinical experience with Eudragit®-coated 5-ASA preparations in children, have reported therapeutic benefits in active UC as well as in active Crohn's colitis and active small-bowel Crohn's disease.[153–156] Adverse reactions to all of the 5-ASA preparations have been described, requiring discontinuation of treatment in 5–15% of cases. The more serious complications reported in children have included pancreatitis, nephritis, exacerbation of disease, and sulfa- or salicylate-induced allergic reactions. Although some toxicities (e.g. headache) to sulfasalazine have been attributed to slow acetylation of the drug, a recent study has demonstrated no association between *N*-acetyltransferase 1 or 2 genotype and efficacy or toxicity from either mesalamine or sulfasalazine.[157]

Antibiotics

There is little role for antibiotics in the primary therapy of active UC. Based on experience in adults, metronidazole is occasionally used for the treatment of mild to moderate UC or the maintenance of remission in the 5-ASA-intolerant or -allergic patient.[158] A controlled trial of ciprofloxacin as an adjunct to corticosteroids in adults with active UC demonstrated no benefit compared with placebo.[159] No pediatric studies exist.

Immunomodulators

6-Mercaptopurine and azathioprine

Despite the surgically curable nature of UC (see below), many parents and physicians are reluctant to perform colectomies in children, even those with severely active UC. As a consequence, immunomodulators are increasingly being used therapeutically. The most commonly prescribed agents are 6-mercaptopurine (6-MP) and azathioprine.[160] These purine analogs inhibit RNA and DNA synthesis, thereby downregulating cytotoxic T-cell activity and delayed hypersensitivity reactions.

Clinical experience in children with UC has mirrored adult studies, demonstrating that 6-MP and azathioprine can act as steroid-sparing agents and induce and maintain remission in 60–75% of patients.[160,161] Onset of action is delayed, with a mean time to response of 4.5 ± 3.0 months.[162] In adults with UC achieving complete remission with 6-MP, 65% maintain continuous remission for 5 years if they remain on the medication, compared with only 13% of those who electively discontinue 6-MP after induction of remission.[163] These data are comparable to those from an earlier study using azathioprine in which 64% of adults maintained on azathioprine after induction of remission remained well at 1 year, compared with only 41% of those switched to placebo after remission induction.[164] No comparable pediatric data have been published. Finally, studies have shown that azathioprine and 6-MP are effective agents for maintaining long-term remission induced by intravenous ciclosporin in both children and adults with severe UC.[165,166]

As maintenance drugs, the long-term safety profile of these therapies is especially important. At a 6-MP dose of 1.0–1.5 mg/kg daily, adverse reactions requiring discontinuation of treatment such as allergic reactions, pancreatitis or severe leukopenia occur in less than 5% of pediatric patients.[167] The recognition of patients with subnormal or absent thiopurine methyltransferase (TPMT) activity (the major inactivating enzyme for both azathioprine and 6 MP), by screening for TPMT genotype before initiation of therapy, can reduce but not eliminate the potential for severe leukopenia.[168] Ongoing assessment of 6-MP and azathioprine metabolites can also identify subjects at risk for either leukopenia or hepatotoxicity.[169]

Ciclosporin and tacrolimus

Ciclosporin and tacrolimus (FK506) are potent inhibitors of cell-mediated immunity. Both agents bind to their respective intracellular receptors (immunophilins). The resulting drug–immunophilin complex inhibits the action of another intracellular mediator, calcineurin, which in turn inactivates the genes responsible for the production of IL-2 and IL-4.[170] As a consequence, T cell, and to a lesser extent B cell, function is impaired.

The use of these agents for the treatment of severe UC in children has had mixed results. Initial response rates, defined as avoidance of imminent surgery and discharge from the hospital, of 20–80% have been reported with either oral or intravenous ciclosporin.[171,172] Responses generally occur within 7–14 days of initiating treatment, but relapses requiring colectomy occur within 1 year in 70–100% of initial responders during or after discontinuation of ciclosporin.[171,172] Addition of 6-MP or azathioprine to the therapeutic regimen once ciclosporin has induced remission results in long-term remission in 60–90% of patients.[166]

Oral tacrolimus can also be used to treat children with fulminant colitis. An open-label pediatric experience demonstrated that 69% of treated subjects initially avoided surgery and were discharged from hospital after tacrolimus was initiated. Despite addition of 6-MP or azathioprine, however, only 38% of the initial cohort avoided colectomy after 1 year.[173]

Tremors, hirsutism and systemic hypertension are the most common toxic effects of ciclosporin and tacrolimus that have been described in children with IBD. However, isolated reports of *Pneumocystis carinii* pneumonia, lymphoproliferative disease, and serious bacterial and fungal infection merit careful monitoring in all children treated with ciclosporin, especially those treated in combination with corticosteroids and 6-MP or azathioprine. Prophylaxis against *Pneumocystis* is necessary during the phase when ciclosporin or tacrolimus is used in conjunction with corticosteroids and 6-MP.

Other immunomodulators

Methotrexate has been used with beneficial effects in a few children with severe Crohn's disease, but published pediatric experience in UC is lacking. Although studies in adult patients with UC suggest that methotrexate can provide benefit in the induction and maintenance of remission, a double-blind trial demonstrated no benefit compared with placebo for either indication.[174]

Infliximab

The chimeric anti-TNF-α monoclonal antibody infliximab dramatically improves disease activity in patients with Crohn's disease. Much less experience is available with this agent as a treatment for UC. Open-label clinical experience in adults suggests that 50–75% of patients with chronic or fulminant UC respond to an initial infusion of infliximab, but that repeat infusions are necessary to maintain response and, despite therapy, about 33% require colectomy within 1 year.[175,176] However, a small placebo-controlled trial has not supported these data.[177] Open-label pediatric experience from a single US center identified a short-term response in 82% of children and sustained improvement in 62%, with most requiring repeated infliximab infusions.[178] Adverse reactions are usually minor infusion reactions, although more severe delayed infusion reactions, anaphylaxis, reactivation of latent tuberculosis and possibly lymphoma development have all been described.

SURGERY

UC is a surgically curable condition, and within 5 years of diagnosis intractable or fulminant symptoms result in 19% of children and adolescents undergoing colectomy (see section on Prognosis).[7] Indications for surgery in UC are summarized in Table 41.6. Curative surgery requires total mucosal proctocolectomy. Although proctocolectomy and ileostomy result in a healthy patient with no risk of future recurrence, few children or parents readily accept the option of a permanent ileostomy. Most instead opt for restorative surgery, which allows the child to continue to defecate by the normal route.

As it is often difficult to distinguish definitively between fulminant UC and Crohn's colitis before the operation, many centers perform a staged procedure in the child with active colitis who requires surgery. Initially subtotal colectomy and ileostomy are performed, followed at a later date by restorative surgery if the colectomy specimen confirms a diagnosis of UC. The most commonly performed restorative surgery is currently the ileal pouch–anal anastomosis (IPAA) (Fig. 41.5). The continent ileostomy (Kock pouch) is rarely, if ever, performed in children, given the success of IPAA. Summaries of pediatric surgical experience document that IPAA utilizing an ileal J-pouch (or less commonly a W- or S-pouch) results in fewer daytime and nocturnal bowel movements, and less fecal soiling, than an ileoanal anastomosis without a pouch.[179–182] Anorectal function is well preserved in children, and postoperative fecal soiling is unusual.[181] When growth retardation is evident before surgery, significant increases in height velocity can be expected after surgery.[183]

Small bowel obstruction is the most common early postoperative complication of IPAA.[184] Pouchitis is the most common late complication, occurring in a mild form in 48% of cases, and in a severe chronic form in a further 7%.[184] Pouchitis generally responds to treatment with metronidazole, ciprofloxacin, 5-ASA or corticosteroids.[181,182,184] Chronic and at times intractable complications do occur, with pouch failure requiring resection of the pouch occurring in 8.6 % of cases.[184]

Indications for surgery
Failure of medical therapy
• Intractable symptoms
• Drug toxicity
Persistent hemorrhage requiring transfusion
Perforation
Toxic megacolon
Low- or high-grade dysplasia
Carcinoma

Table 41.6 Indications for surgery in ulcerative colitis

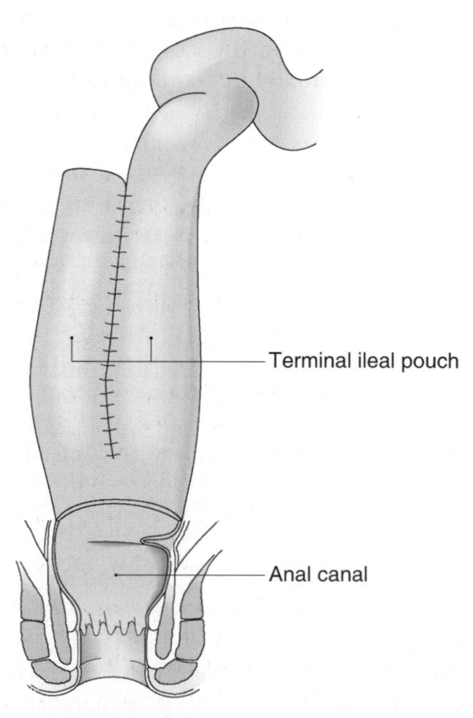

Figure 41.5: Ileal J-pouch–anal anastomosis (IPAA) – restorative surgery for ulcerative colitis.

COURSE AND PROGNOSIS

The course and prognosis of UC in children based on clinical experience derived after 1975 has been reported.[7] Seventy percent of children can be expected to enter remission within 3 months of initial diagnosis, irrespective of whether their initial attack is characterized as mild, moderate or severe, and 45–58% remain inactive over the first year after diagnosis.[7] However, 10% of those whose symptoms are characterized as moderate or severe can be expected to remain continuously symptomatic. Over the ensuing 7–10-year intervals, approximately 55% of all patients have inactive disease, 40% have chronic intermittent symptoms and 5–10% have continuous symptoms. These data are similar to those reported for adult populations.[185–187]Colectomy is required in 5% of all children within the first year after diagnosis, and in 19–23% by 5 years after diagnosis.[7,49] However, these rates rise to 9% and 26% respectively in the subgroup of children initially presenting with moderate or severe symptoms.[7] Overall these rates appear comparable to those recently reported in a Swedish pediatric population treated between 1961 and 1990,[187] and lower than those from older US data that revealed colectomy rates of nearly 50% by 5 years after diagnosis in children presenting between 1955 and 1964, and 26% in those presenting between 1965 and 1974.[47]

Children with proctitis or proctosigmoiditis appear to follow a somewhat more benign course. More than 90% are asymptomatic within 6 months of diagnosis. In any given year of follow-up, 55% remain asymptomatic and less than 5% have continuously active disease.[51] In contrast to adults, however, proximal extension of disease occurs frequently, so that within 3 years of initial diagnosis as many as 25% of children may demonstrate signs of proximal extension. This rate of proximal extension may increase up to 70% over the course of follow-up.[49,51,52] Colectomy may eventually be required in 5% of patients.

References

1. Kugathasan S, Judd RH, Hoffmann RG, et al. Wisconsin Pediatric Inflammatory Bowel Disease Alliance. Epidemiologic and clinical characteristics of children with newly diagnosed inflammatory bowel disease in Wisconsin: a statewide population-based study. J Pediatr 2003; 143:525–531.
2. Hildebrand H, Finkel Y, Grahnquist L, Lindholm J, Ekbom A, Askling J. Changing pattern of paediatric inflammatory bowel disease in northern Stockholm 1990–2001. Gut 2003; 52:1432–1434.
3. van der Zaag-Loonen HJ, Casparie M, Taminiau JAJM, Escher JC, Rodrigues Pereira R, Derkx HHF. The incidence of pediatric inflammatory bowel disease in the Netherlands: 1999–2001. J Pediatr Gastroenterol Nutr 2004; 38:302–307.
4. Michener WM, Caulfield ME, Wyllie RW, Farmer RG. Management of inflammatory bowel disease: 30 years of observation. Cleve Clin J Med 1990; 58:685–691.
5. Gryboski JD. Ulcerative colitis in children 10 years old or younger. J Pediatr Gastroenterol Nutr 1993; 17:24–31.
6. Mamula P, Telega GW, Markowitz JE, et al. Inflammatory bowel disease in children 5 years of age and younger. Am J Gastroenterol 2002; 97:2005–2010.
7. Hyams JS, Davis P, Grancher K, Lerer T, Justinich CJ, Markowitz J. Clinical outcome of ulcerative colitis in children. J Pediatr 1996; 129:81–88.
8. Griffiths A, Harris K, Smith C, Ray P, Corey M, Sherman P. Prevalence of inflammatory bowel disease in first-degree relatives of children with IBD. Gastroenterology 1997; 112:A985.
9. Gilat T, Hacohen D, Lilos P, Langman MJS. Childhood factors in ulcerative colitis and Crohn's disease: an international cooperative study. Scand J Gastroenterol 1987; 22:1009–1024.
10. Koletzko S, Griffiths A, Corey M, Smith C, Sherman P. Infant feeding practices and ulcerative colitis in children. BMJ 1991; 302:1580–1581.
11. Andersson RE, Olaison G, Tysk C, Ekbom A. Appendectomy and protection against ulcerative colitis. N Engl J Med 2001; 344:808–814.
12. Sandler RS, Sandler DP, McDonnell CW, Wurzelman JI. Childhood exposure to environmental tobacco smoke and the risk of ulcerative colitis. Am J Epidemiol 1992; 135:603–608.
13. Lashner BA, Shaheen NJ, Hanauer SB, Kirschner BS. Passive smoking is associated with an increased risk of developing inflammatory bowel disease in children. Am J Gastroenterol 1993; 88:356–359.
14. Abraham N, Selby W, Lazarus R, Solomon M. Is smoking an indirect risk factor for the development of ulcerative colitis? An age- and sex-matched case–control study. J Gastroenterol Hepatol 2003; 18:139–146.
15. Roth M-R, Petersen GM, McElree C, Vadheim CM, Panish JF, Rotter JI. Familial empiric risk estimates of inflammatory bowel disease in Ashkenazi Jews. Gastroenterology 1989; 96:1016–1020.
16. Yang H, McElree C, Roth M-P, Shanahan F, Targan SR, Rotter JI. Familial empiric risks for inflammatory bowel disease: differences between Jews and non-Jews. Gut 1993; 34:517–524.
17. Tysk C, Lindberg E, Jarenot G, Floderus-Myrhed B. Ulcerative colitis and Crohn's disease in an unselected population of monozygotic and dizygotic twins. A study of heredibility and the influence of smoking. Gut 1988; 29:990–996.
18. Toyoda H, Wang SJ, Yang HY, et al. Distinct associations of HLA class II genes with IBD. Gastroenterology 1993; 104:741–748.
19. Asakura H, Tsuchiya M, Aiso S, et al. Association of human lymphocyte-DR2 antigen with Japanese ulcerative colitis. Gastroenterology 1982; 82:413–418.
20. Sugimura K, Ota M, Matsuzawa J, et al. A close relationship of triplet repeat polymorphism in MHC class I chain-related gene A (*MICA*) to the disease susceptibility and behavior in ulcerative colitis. Tissue Antigens 2001; 57:9–14.
21. Sashio H, Tamura K, Ito R, et al. Polymorphisms of the TNF gene and the TNF receptor superfamily member 1B gene are associated with susceptibility to ulcerative colitis and Crohn's disease, respectively. Immunogenetics 2002; 53:1020–1027.
22. Braun C, Zahn R, Martin K, Albert E, Folwaczny C. Polymorphisms of the ICAM-1 gene are associated with inflammatory bowel disease, regardless of the p-ANCA status. Clin Immunol. 2001; 101:357–360.
23. Klein W, Tromm A, Griga T, et al. A polymorphism in the IL11 gene is associated with ulcerative colitis. Genes Immun 2002; 3:494–496.
24. Carter MJ, di Giovine FS, Jones S, et al. Association of the interleukin 1 receptor antagonist gene with ulcerative colitis in Northern European Caucasians. Gut 2001; 48:461–467.

25. Schwab M, Schaeffeler E, Marx C, et al. Association between the C3435T *MDR1* gene polymorphism and susceptibility for ulcerative colitis. Gastroenterology 2003; 124:26–33.
26. Panwala CM, Jones JC, Viney JL. A novel model of inflammatory bowel disease: mice deficient for the multiple drug resistance gene, *mdr1a*, spontaneously develop colitis. J Immunol 1998; 161:5733–5744.
27. Ogura Y, Bonen DK, Inohara N, et al. A frameshift mutation in NOD2 associated with susceptibility to Crohn's disease. Nature 2001; 411:603–606.
28. Armuzzi A, Ahmad T, Ling KL, et al. Genotype–phenotype analysis of the Crohn's disease susceptibility haplotype on chromosome 5q31. Gut 2003; 52:1133–1139.
29. Duerr RH, Targan SR, Landers CJ, Sutherland LR, Shanahan F. Anti-neutrophil cytoplasmic antibodies in ulcerative colitis: comparison with other colitides/diarrheal illnesses. Gastroenterology 1991; 100:1590–1596.
30. Shanahan F, Duerr RH, Rotter JI, et al. Neutrophil autoantibodies in ulcerative colitis: familial aggregation and genetic heterogeneity. Gastroenterology 1992; 103:456–461.
31. Achkar JP, Barmada MM, Duerr RH. Perinuclear neutrophil antibodies are not markers for genetic susceptibility or indicators of genetic heterogeneity in familial ulcerative colitis. Am J Gastroenterol 2002; 97:2343–2349.
32. Sartor RB. Cytokines in intestinal inflammation: pathophysiological and clinical considerations. Gastroenterology 1994; 106:533–539.
33. MacDermott RP, Nash GS, Auer IO, et al. Alterations in serum immunoglobulin G subclasses in patients with ulcerative colitis and Crohn's disease. Gastroenterology 1989; 96:764–768.
34. Das KM, Dasgupta A, Mandal A. Autoimmunity to cytoskeletal protein tropomyosin(s): a new to the pathogenetic mechanism for ulcerative colitis. J Immunol 1993; 150:2487–2493.
35. Bhagat S, Das KM. A shared unique peptide in human colon, eye, and joint detected by a novel monoclonal antibody. Gastroenterology 1994; 107:103–108.
36. Kambham N, Vij R, Cartwright CA, Longacre T. Cytomegalovirus infection in steroid-refractory ulcerative colitis: a case–control study. Am J Surg Pathol 2004; 28:365–373.
37. Jewell DP, Truelove SC. Circulating antibodies to cow's milk proteins in ulcerative colitis. Gut 1972; 13:796–801.
38. Candy S, Borok G, Wright JP, Boniface V, Goodman R. The value of an elimination diet in the management of patients with ulcerative colitis. S Afr Med J 1995; 85:1176–1179.
39. Bruce T. Emotional sequelae of chronic inflammatory bowel disease in children and adolescents. Clin Gastroenterol 1986; 15:89–104.
40. Burke P, Meyer V, Kocoshis S, et al. Depression and anxiety in pediatric inflammatory bowel disease and cystic fibrosis. J Am Acad Child Adolesc Psychiatry 1989; 28:948–951.
41. Wood B, Watkins JB, Boyle JT, Nogueira J, Zimand E, Carroll L. Psychological functioning in children with Crohn's disease and ulcerative colitis: implications for models of psychobiological interaction. J Am Acad Child Adolesc Psychiatry 1987; 26:774–781.
42. Burke P, Meyer V, Kocoshis S, Orenstein D, Chandra R, Sauer J. Obsessive-compulsive symptoms in childhood inflammatory bowel disease and cystic fibrosis. J Am Acad Child Adolesc Psychiatry 1989; 28:525–527.
43. Krall V, Szajnberg NM, Hyams JS, Treem WP, Davis P. Projective personality tests of children with inflammatory bowel disease. Percept Mot Skills 1995; 80:1341–1342.
44. North CS, Clouse RE, Spitznagel EL, Alpers DH. The relation of ulcerative colitis to psychiatric factors: a review of findings and methods. Am J Psychiatry 1990; 147:974–981.
45. Roediger WE. The colonic epithelium in ulcerative colitis: an energy-deficiency disease? Lancet 1980; ii:712–715.
46. Treem WR, Ahsan N, Shoup M, Hyams JS. Fecal short-chain fatty acids in children with inflammatory bowel disease. J Pediatr Gastroenterol Nutr 1994; 18:159–164.
47. Michener WM, Farmer RG, Mortimer EA. Long-term prognosis of ulcerative colitis with onset in childhood or adolescence. J Clin Gastroenterol 1979; 1:301–305.
48. Hamilton JR, Bruce GA, Abdourhaman M, Gall DG. Inflammatory bowel disease in children and adolescents. In: Barness LA, ed. Advances in Pediatrics, vol. 26. Chicago, IL: Year Book Medical; 1979:311–341.
49. Langholz E, Munkholm P, Krasilnikoff PA, Binder V. Inflammatory bowel diseases with onset in childhood: clinical features, morbidity, and mortality in a regional cohort. Scand J Gastroenterol 1997; 32:139–147.
50. Mamula P, Telega GW, Markowitz JE, et al. Inflammatory bowel disease in children 5 years of age and younger. Am J Gastroenterol 2002; 97:2005–2010.
51. Hyams J, Davis P, Lerer T, et al. Clinical outcome of ulcerative proctitis in children. J Pediatr Gastroenterol Nutr 1997; 25:149–152.
52. Mir-Madjlessi SH, Michener WM, Farmer RG. Course and prognosis of idiopathic ulcerative proctosigmoiditis in young patients. J Pediatr Gastroenterol Nutr 1986; 5:571–575.
53. Abdullah BA, Gupta SK, Croffie JM, et al. The role of esophagogastroduodenoscopy in the initial evaluation of childhood inflammatory bowel disease: a 7-year study. J Pediatr Gastroenterol Nutr 2002; 35:636–640.
54. Sharif F, McDermott M, Dillon M, et al. Focally enhanced gastritis in children with Crohn's disease and ulcerative colitis. Am J Gastroenterol 2002; 97:1415–1420.
55. Berrebi D, Languepin J, Ferkdadji L, et al. Cytokines, chemokine receptors, and homing molecule distribution in the rectum and stomach of pediatric patients with ulcerative colitis. J Pediatr Gastroenterol Nutr 2003; 37:300–308.
56. Groisman GM, George J, Harpaz N. Ulcerative appendicitis in universal and nonuniversal ulcerative colitis. Mod Pathol 1994; 7:322–325.
57. Markowitz J, Kahn E, Grancher K, Hyams J, Treem W, Daum F. Atypical rectosigmoid histology in children with newly diagnosed ulcerative colitis. Am J Gastroenterol 1993; 88:2034–2037.
58. Glickman JN, Bousvaros A, Farraye FA, et al. Pediatric patients with untreated ulcerative colitis may present initially with unusual morphologic findings. Am J Surg Pathol 2004; 28:190–197.
59. Rajwal SR, Puntis JW, McClean P, et al. Endoscopic rectal sparing in children with untreated ulcerative colitis. J Pediatr Gastroenterol Nutr 2004; 38:66–69.
60. Surawicz CM, Haggitt RC, Husseman M, McFarland LV. Mucosal biopsy diagnosis of colitis: acute self-limited colitis and inflammatory bowel disease. Gastroenterology 1994; 107:755–763.
61. Das KM, Squillante L, Chitayet D, Kalousek DK. Simultaneous appearance of a unique common epitope in fetal colon, skin and biliary epithelial cells: a possible link for extracolonic manifestations in ulcerative colitis. J Clin Gastroenterol 1992; 15:311–316.
62. Hyams J, Markowitz J, Treem W, Davis P, Grancher K, Daum F. Characterization of hepatic abnormalities in children with

inflammatory bowel disease. Inflamm Bowel Dis 1995; 1:27–33.

63. Quigley EMM, LaRusso NF, Ludwig J, MacSween RNM, Birnie GG, Watkinson G. Familial occurrence of primary sclerosing cholangitis and ulcerative colitis. Gastroenterology 1983; 85:1160–1165.
64. Wilschanski M, Chait P, Wade JA, et al. Primary sclerosing cholangitis in 32 children: clinical, laboratory, and radiographic features, with survival analysis. Hepatology 1995; 22:1415–1422.
65. Soetikno RM, Lin OS, Heidenreich PA, Young HS, Blackstone MO. Increased risk of colorectal neoplasia in patients with primary sclerosing cholangitis and ulcerative colitis: a meta-analysis. Gastrointest Endosc 2002; 56:48–54.
66. Broome U, Lofberg R, Veress B, Eriksson LS. Primary sclerosing cholangitis and ulcerative colitis: evidence for increased neoplastic potential. Hepatology 1995; 22:1404–1408.
67. Stahlberg D, Veress B, Tribukait B, Broome U. Atrophy and neoplastic transformation of the ileal pouch mucosa in patients with ulcerative colitis and primary sclerosing cholangitis: a case control study. Dis Colon Rectum 2003; 46:770–778.
68. Pardi DS, Loftus EV Jr, Kremers WK, Keach J, Lindor KD. Ursodeoxycholic acid as a chemopreventive agent in patients with ulcerative colitis and primary sclerosing cholangitis. Gastroenterology 2003; 124:889–893.
69. Passo MH, Fitzgerald JF, Brandt KD. Arthritis associated with inflammatory bowel disease in children: relationship of joint disease to activity and severity of bowel lesion. Dig Dis Sci 1986; 31:492–497.
70. Lindsey CB, Schaller JG. Arthritis associated with inflammatory bowel disease in children. J Pediatr 1974; 84:16–20.
71. Mir-Madjlessi SH, Taylor JS, Farmer RG. Clinical course and evolution of erythema nodosum and pyoderma gangrenosum in chronic ulcerative colitis: a study of 42 patients. Am J Gastroenterol 1985; 80:615–620.
72. Matis, WL, Ellis CN, Griffiths CEM, Lazarus GS. Treatment of pyoderma gangrenosum with cyclosporine. Arch Dermatol 1992; 128:1060–1064.
73. Friedman S, Marion JF, Scherl E, Rubin PH, Present DH. Intravenous cyclosporine in refractory pyoderma gangrenosum complicating inflammatory bowel disease. Inflamm Bowel Dis 2001; 7:1–7.
74. Kimble RM, Tickler AK, Nicholls VS, Cleghorn G. Successful topical tacrolimus (FK506) therapy in a child with pyoderma gangrenosum. J Pediatr Gastroenterol Nutr 2002; 34:555–557.
75. Kugathasan S, Miranda A, Nocton J, Drolet BA, Raasch C, Binion DG. Dermatologic manifestations of Crohn disease in children: response to infliximab. J Pediatr Gastroenterol Nutr 2003; 37:150–154.
76. Regueiro M, Valentine J, Plevy S, Fleisher MR, Lichtenstein GR. Infliximab for treatment of pyoderma gangrenosum associated with inflammatory bowel disease. Am J Gastroenterol 2003; 98:1821–1826.
77. Magro F, Dinis-Ribeiro M, Araujo FM, et al. High prevalence of combined thrombophilic abnormalities in patients with inflammatory bowel disease. Eur J Gastroenterol Hepatol 2003; 15:1157–1163.
78. Nakano E, Taylor CJ, Chada L, McGaw J, Powers HJ. Hyperhomocystinemia in children with inflammatory bowel disease. J Pediatr Gastroenterol Nutr 2003; 37:586–590.
79. Saibeni S, Cattaneo M, Vecchi M, et al. Low vitamin B(6) plasma levels, a risk factor for thrombosis, in inflammatory bowel disease: role of inflammation and correlation with acute phase reactants. Am J Gastroenterol 2003; 98:112–117.
80. Kader HA, Berman WF, Al-Seraihy AS, Ware RE, Ulshen MH, Treem WR. Prevalence of factor V G1691A (Leiden), prothrombin G20210A, and methylene tetrahydrofolate reductase C677T thrombophilic mutations in children with inflammatory bowel disease. J Pediatr Gastroenterol Nutr 2002; 35:629–635.
81. Hofley P, Roarty J, McGinnity G, et al. Asymptomatic uveitis in children with chronic inflammatory bowel diseases. J Pediatr Gastroenterol Nutr 1993; 17:397–400.
82. Tripathi RC, Kipp MA, Tripathi BJ, et al. Ocular toxicity of prednisone in pediatric patients with inflammatory bowel disease. Lens Eye Toxic Res 1992; 9:469–482.
83. Tripathi RC, Kirschner BS, Kipp M, et al. Corticosteroid treatment for inflammatory bowel disease in pediatric patients increases intraocular pressure. Gastroenterology 1992; 102:1957–1961.
84. Werlin SL, Grand RJ. Severe colitis in children and adolescents: diagnosis, course, and treatment. Gastroenterology 1977; 73:828–832.
85. Riddell RH, Goldman H, Ranshohoff DF, et al. Dysplasia in inflammatory bowel disease: standardized classification with provisional clinical applications. Hum Pathol 1983; 14:931–968.
86. Itzkowitz S. Colorectal cancer in inflammatory bowel disease. Prog Inflamm Bowel Dis 1993; 14:1–5.
87. Ransohoff DF. Colon cancer in ulcerative colitis. Gastroenterology 1988; 94:1089–1091.
88. Devroede GJ, Taylor WF, Sauer WG, Jackman RJ, Stickler GB. Cancer risk and life expectancy of children with ulcerative colitis. N Engl J Med 1971; 285:17–21.
89. Sugita A, Sachar DB, Bodian C, Ribiero MB, Aufses AH Jr, Greenstein AJ. Colorectal cancer in ulcerative colitis. Influence of anatomical extent and age at onset on colitis–cancer interval. Gut 1991; 32:167–169.
90. Gillen CD, Walmsley RS, Prior P, Andrews HA, Allen RN. Ulcerative colitis and Crohn's disease: a comparison of the colorectal cancer risk in extensive colitis. Gut 1994; 35:1590–1592.
91. Lavery IC, Jagelman DG. Cancer in the excluded rectum following surgery for inflammatory bowel disease. Dis Colon Rectum 1982; 25:522–524.
92. Lashner BA. Red blood cell folate is associated with the development of dysplasia and cancer in ulcerative colitis. J Cancer Res Clin Oncol 1993; 119:549–554.
93. Markowitz J, McKinley M, Kahn E, et al. Endoscopic screening for dysplasia and mucosal aneuploidy in adolescents and young adults with childhood onset colitis. Am J Gastroenterol 1997; 92:2001–2006.
94. Ekbom A, Helmick C, Zack M, Adami H-O. Ulcerative colitis and colorectal cancer: a population-based study. N Engl J Med 1990; 323:1228–1233.
95. Ekbom A, Helmick C, Zack M, Adami H-O. Increased risk of large-bowel cancer in Crohn's disease with colonic involvement. Lancet 1990; 336:357–359.
96. Brostrom O, Lofberg R, Nordenvall B, Ost A, Hellers G. The risk of colorectal cancer in ulcerative colitis: an epidemiologic study. Scand J Gastroenterol 1987; 22:1193–1199.
97. Langholz E, Munkholm P, Davidsen M, Binder V. Colorectal cancer risk and mortality in patients with ulcerative colitis. Gastroenterology 1992; 103:1444–1451.
98. Lavery IC, Chiulli RA, Jagelman DG, Fazio VW, Weakley FL. Survival with carcinoma arising in mucosal ulcerative colitis. Ann Surg 1982; 195:508–512.
99. Gyde SN, Prior P, Thompson H, Waterhouse JA, Allan RN. Survival of patients with colorectal cancer complicating ulcerative colitis. Gut 1984; 25:228–231.

100. Choi PM, Nugent FW, Schoetz DJ Jr, Silverman ML, Haggitt RC. Colonoscopic surveillance reduces mortality from colorectal cancer in ulcerative colitis. Gastroenterology 1993; 105:418–424.

101. Griffiths AM, Sherman PM. Colonoscopic surveillance for cancer in ulcerative colitis: a critical review. J Pediatr Gastroenterol Nutr 1997; 24:202–210.

102. Dixon MF, Brown LJ, Gilmour HM, et al. Observer variation in the assessment of dysplasia in ulcerative colitis. Histopathology 1988; 13:385–397.

103. Melville DM, Jass JR, Shepherd NA, et al. Dysplasia and deoxyribonucleic acid aneuploidy in the assessment of precancerous changes in chronic ulcerative colitis: observer variation and correlations. Gastroenterology 1988; 95:668–675.

104. Jonsson B, Ahsgren L, Andersson LO, Stenling R, Rutegard J. Colorectal cancer surveillance in patients with ulcerative colitis. Br J Surg 1994; 81:689–691.

105. Axon AT. Colonic cancer surveillance in ulcerative colitis is not essential for every patient. Eur J Cancer 1995; 31A:1183–1186.

106. Lennard-Jones JE, Melville DM, Morson BC, Ritchie JK, Williams CB. Precancer and cancer in extensive ulcerative colitis: findings among 401 patients over 22 years. Gut 1990; 31:800–806.

107. Lofberg R, Brostrom O, Karlen P, Ost A, Tribukait B. DNA aneuploidy in ulcerative colitis: reproducibility, topographic distribution and relation to dysplasia. Gastroenterology 1992; 102:1149–1154.

108. Rubin CE, Haggitt RC, Burmer GC, et al. DNA aneuploidy in colonic biopsies predicts future development of dysplasia in ulcerative colitis. Gastroenterology 1992; 103:1611–1620.

109. Befrits R, Hammarberg C, Rubio C, Jaramillo E, Tribukait B. DNA aneuploidy and histologic dysplasia in long-standing ulcerative colitis. A 10-year follow-up study. Dis Colon Rectum 1994; 37:313–319.

110. Yin J, Harpaz N, Tong Y, et al. *P53* point mutations in dysplastic and cancerous ulcerative colitis lesions. Gastroenterology 1993; 104:1633–1639.

111. Burmer GC, Levine DS, Kulander BG, Haggitt RC, Rubin CE, Rabinovitch PS. C-Ki-*ras* mutations in ulcerative colitis and sporadic colon carcinoma. Gastroenterology 1990; 99:416–420.

112. Itzkowitz SH, Young E, Dubois D, et al. Sialosyl-Tn antigen is prevalent and precedes dysplasia in ulcerative colitis: a retrospective case–control study. Gastroenterology 1996; 110:694–704.

113. Lashner BA. Recommendations for colorectal cancer screening in ulcerative colitis: a review of research from a single university-based surveillance program. Am J Gastroenterol 1992; 87:168–175.

114. Markowitz J, Grancher K, Rosa J, Aiges H, Daum F. Growth failure in pediatric inflammatory bowel disease. J Pediatr Gastroenterol Nutr 1993; 16:373–380.

115. Hyams JS, Wyzga N, Kreutzer DL, Justinich CJ, Gronowicz GA. Alterations in bone metabolism in children with inflammatory bowel disease: an in vitro study. J Pediatr Gastroenterol Nutr 1997; 24:289–295.

116. Olafsdottir E, Aksnes L, Fluge G, Berstad A. Faecal calprotectin levels in infants with infantile colic, healthy infants, children with inflammatory bowel disease, children with recurrent abdominal pain and healthy children. Acta Paediatr. 2002; 91:45–50.

117. Ruemmele FM, Targan SR, Levy G, Dubinsky M, Braun J, Seidman EG. Diagnostic accuracy of serological assays in pediatric inflammatory bowel disease. Gastroenterology 1998; 115:822–829.

118. Gupta SK, Fitzgerald JF, Croffie JM, Pfefferkorn MD, Molleston JP, Corkins MR. Comparison of serological markers of inflammatory bowel disease with clinical diagnosis in children. Inflamm Bowel Dis 2004; 10:240–244.

119. Joossens S, Reinisch W, Vermeire S, et al. The value of serologic markers in indeterminate colitis: a prospective follow-up study. Gastroenterology 2002; 122:1242–1247.

120. Rajwal SR, Puntis JW, McClean P, et al. Endoscopic rectal sparing in children with untreated ulcerative colitis. J Pediatr Gastroenterol Nutr 2004; 38:66–69.

121. Glickman JN, Bousvaros A, Farraye FA, et al. Pediatric patients with untreated ulcerative colitis may present initially with unusual morphologic findings. Am J Surg Pathol 2004; 28:190–197.

122. Sharif F, McDermott M, Dillon M, et al. Focally enhanced gastritis in children with Crohn's disease and ulcerative colitis. Am J Gastroenterol 2002; 97:1415–1420.

123. Kleinman RE, Balistreri WF, Heyman MD, et al. Nutritional support for pediatric patients with inflammatory bowel disease. J Pediatr Gastroenterol Nutr 1989; 8:8–12.

124. Vernia P, Annese V, Bresci G, et al. Gruppo Italiano per lo Studio del Colon and del Retto. Topical butyrate improves efficacy of 5-ASA in refractory distal ulcerative colitis: results of a multicentre trial. Eur J Clin Invest 2003; 33:244–248.

125. Scheppach W, Muller JG, Boxberger F, et al. Histological changes in the colonic mucosa following irrigation with short-chain fatty acids. Eur J Gastroenterol Hepatol 1997; 9:163–168.

126. Hallert C, Bjorck I, Nyman M, Pousette A, Granno C, Svensson H. Increasing fecal butyrate in ulcerative colitis patients by diet: controlled pilot study. Inflamm Bowel Dis 2003; 9:116–121.

127. Kanauchi O, Serizawa I, Araki Y, et al. Germinated barley foodstuff, a prebiotic product, ameliorates inflammation of colitis through modulation of the enteric environment. J Gastroenterol 2003; 38:134–141.

128. Loeschke K, Ueberschaer B, Pietsch A, et al. *n*-3 Fatty acids only delay early relapse of ulcerative colitis in remission. Dig Dis Sci 1996; 41:2087–2094.

129. Hawthorne AB, Daneshmend TK, Hawkey CJ, et al. Treatment of ulcerative colitis with fish oil supplementation: a prospective 12 month randomised controlled trial. Gut 1992; 33:922–928.

130. Shimizu T, Fujii T, Suzuki R, et al. Effects of highly purified eicosapentaenoic acid on erythrocyte fatty acid composition and leukocyte and colonic mucosa leukotriene B_4 production in children with ulcerative colitis. J Pediatr Gastroenterol Nutr 2003; 37:581–585.

131. Thiesen A, Thomson ABR. Older systemic and newer topical glucocorticosteroids and the gastrointestinal tract. Aliment Pharmacol Ther 1996; 10:487–496.

132. Zimmerman MJ, Jewell DP. Cytokines and mechanisms of action of glucocorticoids and aminosalicylates in the treatment of ulcerative colitis and Crohn's disease. Aliment Pharmacol Ther 1996; 10(Suppl 2):93–98.

133. Meyers S, Sachar DB, Goldberg JD, Janowitz HD. Corticotropin versus hydrocortisone in the intravenous treatment of ulcerative colitis: a prospective, randomized, double-blind clinical trial. Gastroenterology 1983; 85:351–357.

134. Hyams JS, Moore RE, Leichtner AM, Carey DE, Goldberg BD. Relationship of type I procollagen to corticosteroid therapy in children with inflammatory bowel disease. J Pediatr 1988; 112:893–898.

135. Hyams JS, Carey DE, Leichtner AM, Goldberg BD. Type I procollagen as a biochemical marker of growth in children with inflammatory bowel disease. J Pediatr 1986; 109:619–624.

136. Hyams JS, Treem WR, Carey DE, et al. Comparison of collagen propeptides as growth markers in children with inflammatory bowel disease. Gastroenterology 1991; 100:971–975.

137. Whittington PF, Barnes V, Bayless TM. Medical management of Crohn's disease in adolescence. Gastroenterology 1977; 72:1338–1344.

138. Issenman RM, Atkinson SA, Radoja C, Fraher L. Longitudinal assessment of growth, mineral metabolism and bone mass in pediatric Crohn's disease. J Pediatr Gastroenterol Nutr 1993; 17:401–406.

139. Lofberg R. New steroids for inflammatory bowel disease. Inflamm Bowel Dis 1995; 1:135–141.

140. Lemann M, Galian A, Rutgeerts P, et al. Comparison of budesonide and 5-aminosalicylic acid enemas in active distal ulcerative colitis. Aliment Pharmacol Ther 1995; 9:557–562.

141. Lofberg R, Ostergaard Thomsen O, et la. Budesonide versus prednisolone retention enemas in active distal ulcerative colitis. Aliment Pharmacol Ther 1994; 8:623–629.

142. Hanauer SB, Robinson M, Pruitt R, et al. Budesonide enema for the treatment of active, distal ulcerative colitis and proctitis: a dose-ranging study. US Budesonide Enema Study Group. Gastroenterology 1998; 115:525–532.

143. Bar-Meir S, Fidder HH, Faszczyk M, et al. International Budesonide Study Group. Budesonide foam *vs.* hydrocortisone acetate foam in the treatment of active ulcerative proctosigmoiditis. Dis Colon Rectum 2003; 46:929–936.

144. Lofberg R, Danielsson A, Suhr O, et al. Oral budesonide versus prednisolone in patients with active extensive and left-sided ulcerative colitis. Gastroenterology 1996; 110:1713–1718.

145. Farrell RJ, Kelleher D. Glucocorticoid resistance in inflammatory bowel disease. J Endocrinol 2003; 178:339–346.

146. Van Assche G, Dalle I, Noman M, et al. A pilot study on the use of the humanized anti-interleukin-2 receptor antibody daclizumab in active ulcerative colitis. Am J Gastroenterol 2003; 98:369–376.

147. Creed TJ, Norman MR, Probert CS, et al. Basiliximab (anti-CD25) in combination with steroids may be an effective new treatment for steroid-resistant ulcerative colitis. Aliment Pharmacol Ther 2003; 18:65–75.

148. Greenfield SM, Punchard NA, Teare JP, Thompson RPH. Review article: the mode of action of the aminosalicylates in inflammatory bowel disease. Aliment Pharmacol Ther 1993; 7:369–383.

149. Sutherland L, MacDonald JK. Oral 5-aminosalicylic acid for induction of remission in ulcerative colitis (Cochrane Review). In: The Cochrane Library, Issue 2. Chichester, UK: John Wiley; 2004.

150. Sutherland L, Roth D, Beck P, May G, Makiyama K. Oral 5 aminosalicylic acid for maintenance of remission in ulcerative colitis (Cochrane Review). In: The Cochrane Library, Issue 2. Chichester, UK: John Wiley; 2004.

151. Leichtner AM: Aminosalicylates for the treatment of inflammatory bowel disease. J Pediatr Gastroenterol Nutr 1995; 21:245–252.

152. Ferry GD, Kirschner BS, Grand RJ, et al. Olsalazine versus sulfasalazine in mild to moderate childhood ulcerative colitis: results of the Pediatric Gastroenterology Collaborative Research Group Clinical Trial. J Pediatr Gastroenterol Nutr 1993; 17:32–38.

153. Tolia V, Massoud N, Klotz U. Oral 5-aminosalicylic acid in children with colonic inflammatory bowel disease: clinical and pharmacokinetic experience. J Pediatr Gastroenterol Nutr 1989; 8:333–338.

154. Barden L, Lipson A, Pert P, Walker-Smith JA. Mesalazine in childhood inflammatory bowel disease. Aliment Pharmacol Ther 1989; 3:597–603.

155. Griffiths A, Koletzko S, Sylvester F, Marcon M, Sherman P. Slow-release 5-aminosalicylic acid therapy in children with small intestinal Crohn's disease. J Pediatr Gastroenterol Nutr 1993; 17:186–192.

156. D'Agata ID, Vanounou T, Seidman E. Mesalamine in pediatric inflammatory bowel disease: a 10 year experience. Inflamm Bowel Dis 1996; 2:229–235.

157. Ricart E, Taylor WR, Loftus EV, et al. *N*-acetyltransferase 1 and 2 genotypes do not predict response or toxicity to treatment with mesalamine and sulfasalazine in patients with ulcerative colitis. Am J Gastroenterol 2002; 97:1763–1768.

158. Gilat T, Leichtman G, Delpre G, Eshchar J, Bar Meir S, Fireman Z. A comparison of metronidazole and sulfasalazine in the maintenance of remission in patients with ulcerative colitis. J Clin Gastroenterol 1989; 11:392–395.

159. Mantzaris GJ, Archavlis E, Christoforidis P, et al. A prospective randomized controlled trial of oral ciprofloxacin in acute ulcerative colitis. Am J Gastroenterol 1997; 92:454–456.

160. Markowitz J, Grancher K, Kohn N, Daum F. Immunomodulatory therapy for pediatric inflammatory bowel disease: changing patterns of use, 1990–2000. Am J Gastroenterol 2002; 97:928–932.

161. Verhave M, Winter HS, Grand RJ. Azathioprine in the treatment of children with inflammatory bowel disease. J Pediatr 1990; 117:809–814.

162. Markowitz J, Grancher K, Mandel F, Daum F. Immunosuppressive therapy in pediatric inflammatory bowel disease: results of a survey of the North American Society for Gastroenterology and Nutrition. Am J Gastroenterol 1993; 88:44–48.

163. George J, Present DH, Pou R, Bodian C, Rubin PH. The long-term outcome of ulcerative colitis treated with 6 mercaptopurine. Am J Gastroenterol 1996; 91:1711–1714.

164. Hawthorne AB, Logan RFA, Hawkey CJ, et al. Randomised controlled trial of azathioprine withdrawal in ulcerative colitis. BMJ 1992; 305:20–222.

165. Fernandez-Banares F, Bertran X, Esteve-Comas M, et al. Azathioprine is useful in maintaining long-term remission induced by intravenous cyclosporine in steroid-refractory severe ulcerative colitis. Am J Gastroenterol 1996; 91:2498–2499.

166. Ramakrishna J, Langhans N, Calenda K, Grand RJ, Verhave M. Combined use of cyclosporine and azathioprine or 6 mercaptopurine in pediatric inflammatory bowel disease. J Pediatr Gastroenterol Nutr 1996; 32:296–302.

167. Kirschner BS. Safety of azathioprine and 6-mercaptopurine in pediatric patients with inflammatory bowel disease. Gastroenterology 1998; 115:813–821.

168. Colombel JF, Ferrari N, Debuysere H, et al. Genotypic analysis of thiopurine *S*-methyltransferase in patients with Crohn's disease and severe myelosuppression during azathioprine therapy. Gastroenterology 2000; 118:1025–1030.

169. Seidman EG. Clinical use and practical application of TPMT enzyme and 6-mercaptopurine metabolite monitoring in IBD. Rev Gastroenterol Disord 2003; 3(Suppl 1):S30–S38.

170. Ho S, Clipstone N, Timmermann L, et al. The mechanism of action of cyclosporin A and FK506. Clin Immunol Immunopathol 1996; 80:S40–S45.

171. Benkov KJ, Rosh JR, Schwerenz AH, Janowitz HD, LeLeiko NS. Cyclosporine as an alternative to surgery in children with inflammatory bowel disease. J Pediatr Gastroenterol Nutr 1994; 19:290–294.

172. Treem WR, Cohen J, Davis P, Justinich CJ, Hyams JS. Cyclosporine for the treatment of fulminant ulcerative colitis in children. Dis Colon Rectum 1995; 38:474–479.

173. Bousvaros A, Kirschner BS, Werlin SL, et al. Oral tacrolimus treatment of severe colitis in children. J Pediatr 2000; 137:794–799.

174. Oren R, Arber N, Odes S, et al. Methotrexate in chronic active ulcerative colitis: a double-blind, randomized, Israeli multicenter trial. Gastroenterology 1996; 110:1416–1421.

175. Gornet JM, Couve S, Hassani Z, et al. Infliximab for refractory ulcerative colitis or indeterminate colitis: an open-label multicentre study. Aliment Pharmacol Ther. 2003; 18:175–181.

176. Sands BE, Tremaine WJ, Sandborn WJ, et al. Infliximab in the treatment of severe, steroid-refractory ulcerative colitis: a pilot study. Inflamm Bowel Disord 2001; 7:83–88.

177. Probert CS, Hearing SD, Schreiber S, et al. Infliximab in moderately severe glucocorticoid resistant ulcerative colitis: a randomised controlled trial. Gut 2003; 52:998–1002.

178. Mamula P, Markowitz JE, Cohen LJ, von Allmen D, Baldassano RN. Infliximab in pediatric ulcerative colitis: two year follow-up. J Pediatr Gastroenterol Nutr 2004; 38:298–301.

179. Rintala RJ, Lindahl H. Restorative proctocolectomy for ulcerative colitis in children – is the J-pouch better than the straight pull-through? J Pediatr Surg 1996; 31:530–533.

180. Fonkalsrud EW. Long-term results after colectomy and ileoanal pull-through procedure in children. Arch Surg 1996; 131:881–885.

181. Shamberger RC, Lillehei CW, Nurko S, Winter HS. Anorectal function in children after ileoanal pull-through. J Pediatr Surg 1994; 29:329–332.

182. Sarigol S, Caulfield M, Wyllie R, et al. Ileal pouch–anal anastomosis in children with ulcerative colitis. Inflamm Bowel Disord 1996; 2:82–87.

183. Nicholls S, Vieira MC, Majrowski WH, Shand WS, Savage MO, Walker-Smith JA. Linear growth after colectomy for ulcerative colitis in childhood. J Pediatr Gastroenterol Nutr 1995; 21:82–86.

184. Alexander F, Sarigol S, DiFiore J, et al. Fate of the pouch in 151 pediatric patients after ileal pouch anal anastomosis. J Pediatr Surg 2003; 38:78–82.

185. Langholz E, Munkholm P Davidsen M, Binder V. Course of ulcerative colitis: analysis of changes in disease activity over years. Gastroenterology 1994; 107:3–11.

186. Hendriksen C, Kreiner S, Binder V. Long term prognosis in ulcerative colitis – based on results from a regional patient group from the county of Copenhagen. Gut 1985; 26:158–163.

187. Ahsgren L, Jonsson B, Stenling R, Rutegard J. Prognosis after early onset of ulcerative colitis. A study from an unselected patient population. Hepatogastroenterology 1993; 40:467–470.

188. Michener WM. Ulcerative colitis in children. Problems in management. Pediatr Clin North Am 1967; 14:159–173.

189. Park S-D, Markowitz JF. Ulcerative colitis (pediatric). In: Johnson L, cd. Encyclopedia of Gastroenterology. USA: Academic Press; 2004:400–408.

Chapter 42
Chronic intestinal pseudo-obstruction

Paul E. Hyman

INTRODUCTION

Chronic intestinal pseudo-obstruction is a rare, severe, disabling disorder characterized by repetitive episodes or continuous symptoms and signs of bowel obstruction, including radiographic documentation of dilated bowel with air-fluid levels, in the absence of a fixed, lumen-occluding lesion.[1] Chronic intestinal pseudo-obstruction is a clinical diagnosis based on phenotype, not pathology or manometry. The most common signs are abdominal distention and failure to thrive. The most common symptoms are abdominal pain, vomiting and constipation or diarrhea. Chronic intestinal pseudo-obstruction represents a number of different conditions that vary in cause, severity, course and response to therapy (Table 42.1). Examples of genetic heterogeneity in pseudo-obstruction include, but are not limited to, a wide spectrum of abnormal gastric, small intestinal and colonic myoelectrical activity and contractions as well as histologic abnormalities in nerve and muscle. Although these diseases have distinctive pathophysiologic characteristics, they are considered together because of their clinical and therapeutic similarities.

ETIOLOGY

Pseudo-obstruction may occur as a primary disease or as a secondary manifestation of a large number of other conditions that transiently (e.g. hypothyroidism, phenothiazine overdose), or permanently (e.g. scleroderma, amyloidosis) alter bowel motility (Table 42.2).

Most congenital forms of neuropathic and myopathic pseudo-obstruction are both rare and sporadic, possibly representing new mutations. That is, there is no family history of pseudo-obstruction, no associated syndrome and no evidence of other predisposing factors such as toxins, infections, ischemia, or autoimmune disease. In some cases, chronic intestinal pseudo-obstruction results from a familial inherited disease. There are reports of autosomal-dominant[2,3] and -recessive[4–6] neuropathic and dominant[7–9] and recessive[10,11] myopathic, patterns of inheritance. In the autosomal-dominant diseases, expressivity and penetrance are variable; some of those affected die in childhood, but those less handicapped are able to reproduce. An X-linked recessive form of neuropathic pseudo-obstruction has been mapped to its locus, Xq28.[12] When counseling families, a thorough family history is essential and screening tests of relatives should be considered to seek milder phenotypic expression.

Pseudo-obstruction may result from exposure to toxins during critical developmental periods in utero. A few children with fetal alcohol syndrome[13] and a few exposed to narcotics *in utero* have neuropathic forms of pseudo-obstruction. Presumably, any substance that alters neuronal migration or maturation might affect the development of the myenteric plexus and cause pseudo-obstruction.

Children with chromosomal abnormalities or syndromes may suffer from pseudo-obstruction. Children with Down syndrome have a higher incidence of Hirschsprung's disease than the general population and may have abnormal esophageal motility[14] and neuronal dysplasia in the myenteric plexus. Rare children with Down syndrome have a myenteric plexus neuropathy so generalized and so severe that they present with pseudo-obstruction. Children with neurofibromatosis, multiple endocrine neoplasia type IIB (MEN IIB) and other

Onset
Congenital
Acquired
Acute
Gradual
Presentation
Megacystis-microcolon intestinal hypoperistalsis syndrome
Acute neonatal bowel obstruction, with or without megacystis
Chronic vomiting and failure to thrive
Chronic abdominal distention and failure to thrive
Cause
Sporadic
Familial
Toxic
Ischemic
Viral
Inflammatory
Autoimmune
Area of Involvement
Entire gastrointestinal tract
Segment of gastrointestinal tract
Megaduodenum
Small bowel
Colon
Pathology
Myopathy
Neuropathy
Absent neurons
Immature neurons
Degenerating neurons
Intestinal neuronal dysplasia
No microscopic abnormality

Table 42.1 Features of chronic intestinal pseudo-obstruction in pediatric patients

Causes
Primary pseudo-obstruction
Visceral myopathy: sporadic or familial
Visceral neuropathy: sporadic or familial
Secondary pseudo-obstruction: related or associated recognized causes
Muscular dystrophies
Scleroderma and other connective tissue diseases
Postischemic neuropathy
Postviral neuropathy
Generalized dysautonomia
Hypothyroidism
Diabetic autonomic neuropathy
Drugs: anticholinergics, opiates, calcium channel blockers, many others
Severe inflammatory bowel disease
Organ transplantation
Amyloidosis
Chagas' disease
Fetal alcohol syndrome
Chromosome abnormalities
Multiple endocrine neoplasia IIB
Radiation enteritis

Table 42.2 Causes of chronic pseudo-obstruction in children

chromosome aberrations and autonomic neuropathies may suffer from neuropathic constipation. Children with Duchenne's muscular dystrophy sometimes develop pseudo-obstruction, especially in the terminal stages of life. Esophageal manometry and gastric emptying are abnormal in Duchenne's dystrophy, suggesting that the myopathy includes gastrointestinal smooth muscle even in asymptomatic children.[15]

Acquired pseudo-obstruction may be a rare complication of infection from cytomegalovirus[16] or Epstein-Barr virus.[17] Immunocompromised children and immunosuppressed transplant recipients seem at higher risk than the general population. Many of the acquired cases of pseudo-obstruction might be a result of myenteric plexus neuritis from persistent viral infection or an autoimmune inflammatory response. Mucosal inflammation causes abnormal motility. With celiac disease,[18] Crohn's disease and the chronic enterocolitis associated with Hirschsprung's disease some patients develop dilated bowel and symptoms due, not to anatomic obstruction, but to a neuromuscular disorder presumably related to the effects of inflammatory mediators on mucosal afferent sensory nerves or motor nerves in the enteric plexuses. Other rare causes of pseudo-obstruction associated with inflammation include myenteric neuritis associated with antineuronal antibodies[19] and intestinal myositis.[20]

PATHOLOGY

There may be histologic abnormalities in the muscle or nerve or, rarely, both.[21] Histology is normal in about 10% of cases that are studied appropriately. In such cases there may be an abnormality in some biochemical aspect of stimulus-contraction coupling.

When laparotomy is imminent for a child with pseudo-obstruction, there must be timely communication between the surgeon and the pathologist. A laparotomy is not indicated for biopsy alone,[22] perhaps because a pathologic diagnosis usually does not alter the clinical management or the clinical course. When surgery is indicated (e.g. for colectomy, cholecystectomy or creation of an ileostomy) a plan should be made to obtain a full-thickness bowel biopsy specimen at least 2 cm in diameter. The tissues should be processed for studies: histology, histochemistry for selected neurotransmitters and receptors, electron microscopy and silver stains.

Muscle disease may be inflammatory but more often is not. In light microscopy of both familial and sporadic forms of hollow visceral myopathy, the muscularis appears thin. The external longitudinal muscle layer is more involved than the internal circular muscle and there may be extensive fibrosis in the muscle tissue. By electron microscopy there are vacuolar degeneration and disordered myofilaments (Fig. 42.1).

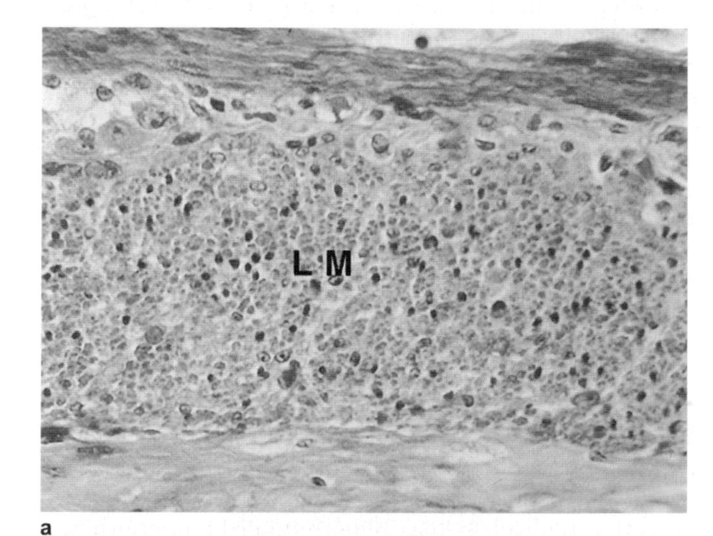

a

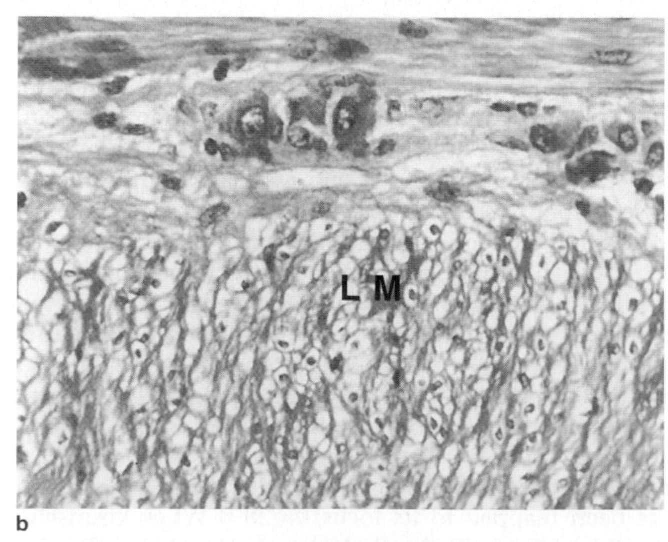

b

Figure 42.1: Visceral myopathy. **(a)** Longitudinal muscle cut in cross section from the small intestine of a control infant. **(b)** Longitudinal muscle from an infant with visceral myopathy shows classic vacuolar degeneration. Note the normal neurons in the myenteric plexus above the longitudinal muscle. ×136. (Courtesy of Michael D. Schuffler.)

Neuropathic disease is best examined with silver stains of the myenteric plexus[23,24] and routine histologic techniques. The presence of neurons in the submucous plexus of a suction biopsy specimen eliminates Hirschsprung's disease as a diagnostic possibility but is inadequate for the evaluation of other neuropathies. There may be maturational arrest of the myenteric plexus (Fig. 42.2). This hypoganglionosis is characterized by fewer neurons, which may be smaller than normal. Maturational arrest can be a primary congenital disorder or can occur secondary to ischemia or infection. Changes can be patchy or generalized.

Intestinal neuronal dysplasia,[25] or hyperganglionosis, is a histologic diagnosis defined by these findings: (1) hyperplasia of the parasympathetic neurons and fibers of the myenteric (and sometimes submucous) plexus, characterized by increases in the number and size of ganglia, thickened nerves and increases in neuron cell bodies; (2) increased acetyl cholinesterase-positive nerve fibers in the lamina propria; (3) increased acetylcholine esterase-positive nerve fibers around submucosal blood vessels; (4) heterotopic neuron cell bodies in the lamina propria, muscle and serosal layers. The first two criteria are obligatory.

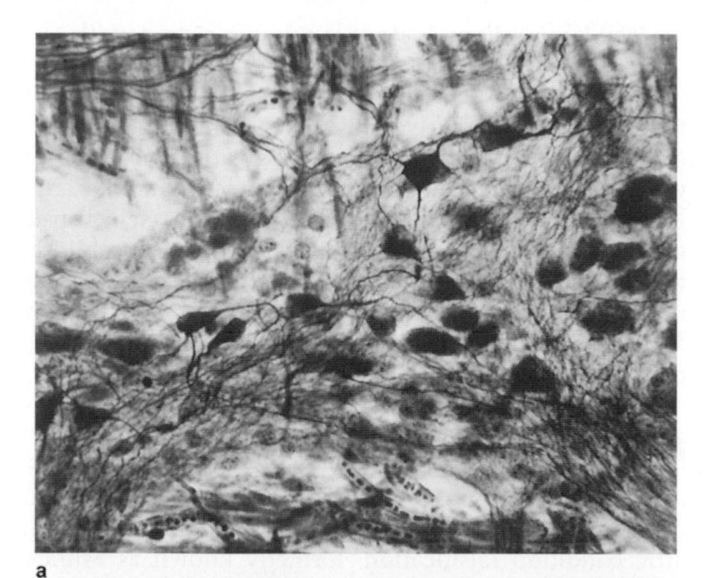

a

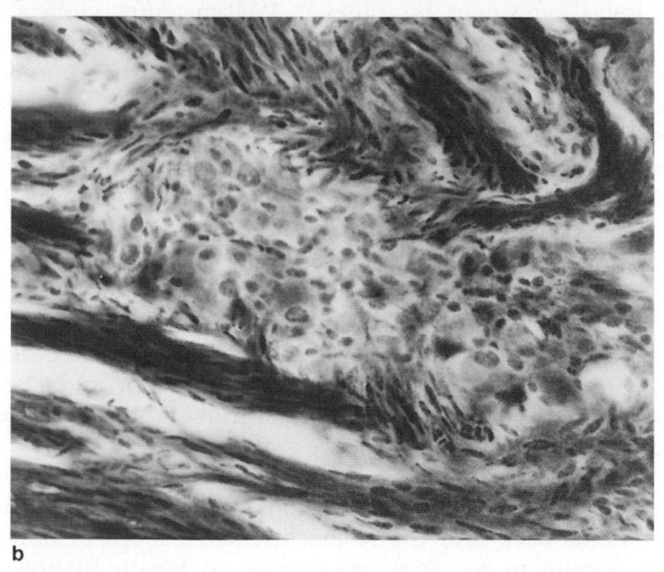

b

Figure 42.2: Maturational arrest of myenteric plexus. (**a**) Ganglionic area of myenteric plexus from the small intestine of a control infant. Note the numerous argyrophilic neurons and axons. (**b**) Ganglionic area of myenteric plexus from the small intestine of an infant with chronic intestinal pseudo-obstruction caused by maturational arrest. Note the absence of argyrophilic neurons and axons. The ganglion is filled with numerous cells, which are probably glial cells and immature neurons. ×544. (Courtesy of Michael D. Schuffler.)

Children with intestinal neuronal dysplasia are a heterogeneous group. Children with primary pseudo-obstruction due to neuronal dysplasia may have disease that is limited to the colon or disseminated. Other children may have neuronal dysplasia associated with prematurity, protein allergy, chromosome abnormalities, MEN IIB and neurofibromatosis; however, intestinal neuronal dysplasia is an occasional incidental finding in bowel specimens examined for reasons unrelated to motility. Intestinal neuronal dysplasia correlates poorly with motility-related symptoms.[26] Thus, a pathologic diagnosis of intestinal neuronal dysplasia neither predicts clinical outcome nor influences management.

CLINICAL FEATURES

Presentation

More than half of the affected children develop symptoms at or shortly after birth. A few cases are diagnosed *in utero*, by ultrasound findings of polyhydramnios and megacystis and marked abdominal distention (Fig. 42.3). Intestinal malrotation is found in both neuropathic and myopathic congenital forms of pseudo-obstruction. Of children who present at birth, about 40% have an intestinal malrotation. In the most severely affected infants, symptoms of acute bowel obstruction appear within the first hours of life. Less severely affected infants present months later with symptoms of vomiting, diarrhea and failure to thrive. A few patients have megacystis at birth and insidious onset of gastrointestinal symptoms over the first few years. More than three-quarters of the children develop symptoms by the end of the first year of life and the remainder present sporadically through the first two decades.

Although there is individual variation in the number and intensity of signs and symptoms, it may be useful to note the relative frequencies in this population. Abdominal distention and vomiting are the most common features (75%). Constipation, episodic or intermittent abdominal pain and poor weight gain are features in about 60% of cases. Diarrhea is a complaint in one-third. Urinary tract smooth muscle is affected in those with both hollow visceral neuropathy and hollow visceral myopathy, about one-fifth of all pseudo-obstruction patients. Often these children are severely affected at birth and are described by the phenotype *megacystis-microcolon intestinal hypoperistalsis syndrome*.[27]

The majority of children's clinical course is characterized by relative remissions and exacerbations. Many are able to identify factors that precipitate deteriorations, including intercurrent infections, general anesthesia, psychological stress and poor nutritional status.

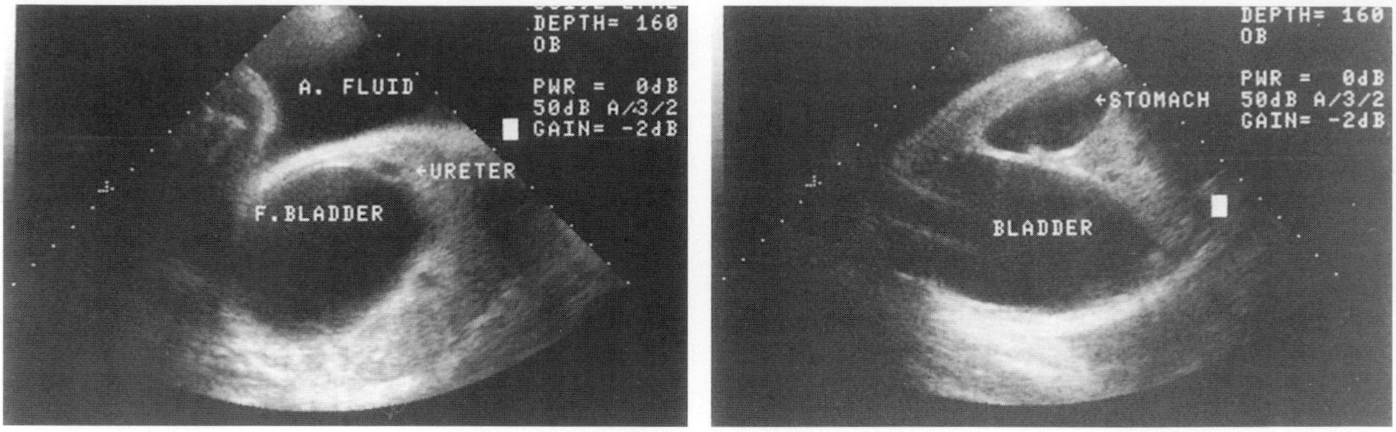

a

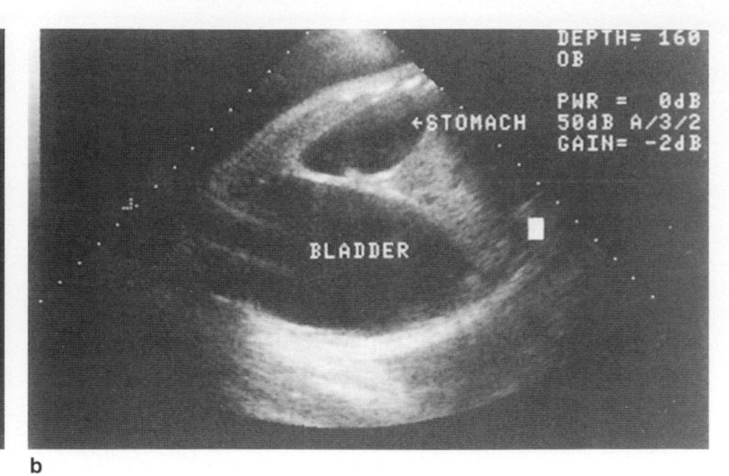

b

Figure 42.3: Ultrasound of infant with pseudo-obstruction diagnosed *in utero*. There is polyhydramnios as well as distention of the stomach and urinary bladder. (Courtesy of Radha Cherukuri.)

The radiographic signs are those of intestinal obstruction, with air-fluid levels (Fig. 42.4), dilated stomach, small intestine and colon, or microcolon in those studied because of obstruction at birth.[28] There may be prolonged stasis of contrast material placed into the affected bowel, so it is prudent to plan how to evacuate the contrast fluid or to use a nontoxic, isotonic, water-soluble medium to prevent barium from solidifying into a true anatomic obstruction. Children who feel well can still show radiographic evidence of bowel obstruction. The greater problem arises when children develop an acute deterioration. Radiographs demonstrate the same patterns of bowel obstruction that are seen when the child feels well. In children who previously had surgery, it can be difficult to discriminate between physical obstruction related to adhesions and an episodic increase in the symptoms of pseudo-obstruction.

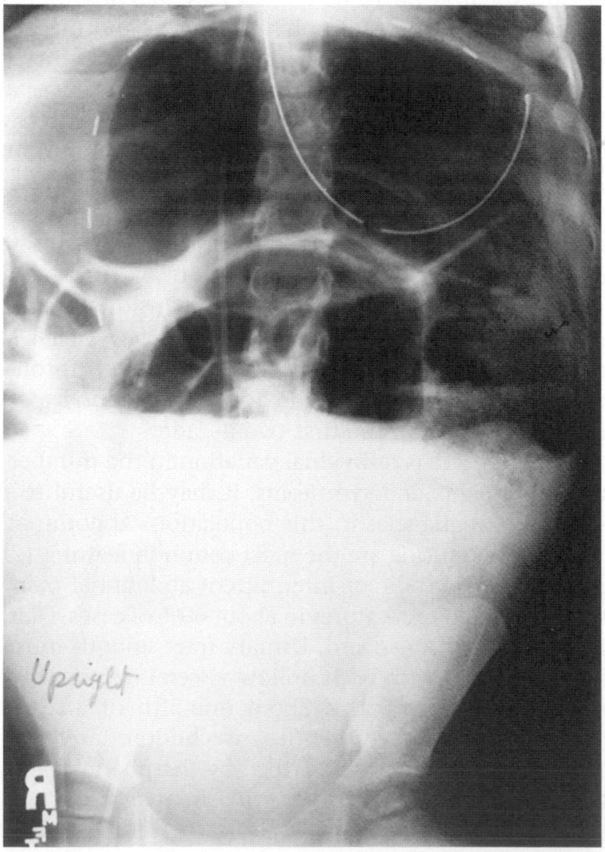

Figure 42.4: Upright abdominal radiograph in a 4-year-old boy with hollow visceral myopathy. Note bowel dilatation and air-fluid levels, central venous catheter in the inferior vena cava and antroduodenal manometry catheter in the stomach and duodenum.

Diagnosis

An incorrect diagnosis of pseudo-obstruction can result from misdiagnosis of infant and toddler victims of pediatric condition falsification, formerly known as Münchausen's syndrome by proxy.[29] Well-meaning clinicians inadvertently co-create disease as they respond to a parent's symptom fabrications by performing tests and procedures, including parenteral nutrition support, repeated surgery and even small bowel transplantation.[30] Adolescents with disabling abdominal pain arising from psychiatric diseases such as visceral pain disorder, post-traumatic stress disorder and Asperger's syndrome may also confuse gastroenterologists.[31,32]

Diagnostic testing provides information about the nature and severity of the pathophysiology. Manometric studies are more sensitive than radiographic tests to evaluate the strength and coordination of contraction and relaxation in the esophagus, gastric antrum, small intestine, colon and anorectal area.

In affected children scintigraphy demonstrates delayed gastric emptying of solids or liquids and reflux of intestinal contents back into the stomach. Dilated loops of bowel predispose to bacterial overgrowth, so breath hydrogen testing may reveal elevations in fasting breath hydrogen and a rapid increase in breath hydrogen with a carbohydrate meal.

Esophageal manometry is abnormal in about half those affected by pseudo-obstruction. In children with myopathy, contractions are low amplitude but coordinated in the distal two-thirds of the esophagus. Lower esophageal sphincter pressure is low and sphincter relaxation is complete. When the esophagus is affected by neuropathy, contraction amplitude in the esophageal body may be high, normal, low, or absent. There may be simultaneous, spontaneous, or repetitive contractions. Relaxation of the lower esophageal sphincter may be incomplete or absent.

Antroduodenal manometry findings are always abnormal with intestinal pseudo-obstruction involving the upper gastrointestinal tract; however, manometry is often abnormal in partial or complete small bowel obstruction. Although the manometric patterns of true obstruction differ from those of pseudo-obstruction in adults,[33,34] such a distinction was not possible in children we have studied. Antroduodenal manometry should not be used as a test to differentiate true bowel obstruction from pseudo-obstruction. Manometry should be done after a diagnosis of pseudo-obstruction is established, to determine the physiologic correlates for the symptoms, to assess drug responses and for prognosis.[35–37] Contrast radiography and, as a last resort, exploratory laparotomy are best for differentiating true obstruction from pseudo-obstruction.

As in the esophagus, intestinal myopathy causes low-amplitude coordinated contractions and neuropathy causes uncoordinated contractions. Interpretation of antroduodenal manometry requires recognition of normal and abnormal features (Table 42.3). The abnormalities in pseudo-obstruction are commonly discrete and easily interpreted by eye (Fig. 42.5). They contrast markedly with normal features of antroduodenal manometry (Fig. 42.6).

In most cases the manometric abnormality correlates with clinical severity of the disease. For example, children with total aganglionosis have contractions of normal amplitude that are never organized into migrating motor complexes (MMCs), fed patterns, or even bursts or clusters of contractions but are simply a monotonous pattern of random events. Children with such a pattern are dependent on total parenteral nutrition (TPN). More than 80% of children with MMCs are nourished enterally, but more than 80% of children without MMCs require partial or total parenteral nutrition. Discrete abnormalities in the organization of intestinal contractions are listed in Table 48.3.

Normal antroduodenal manometry and absence of dilated bowel in a patient with symptoms of chronic

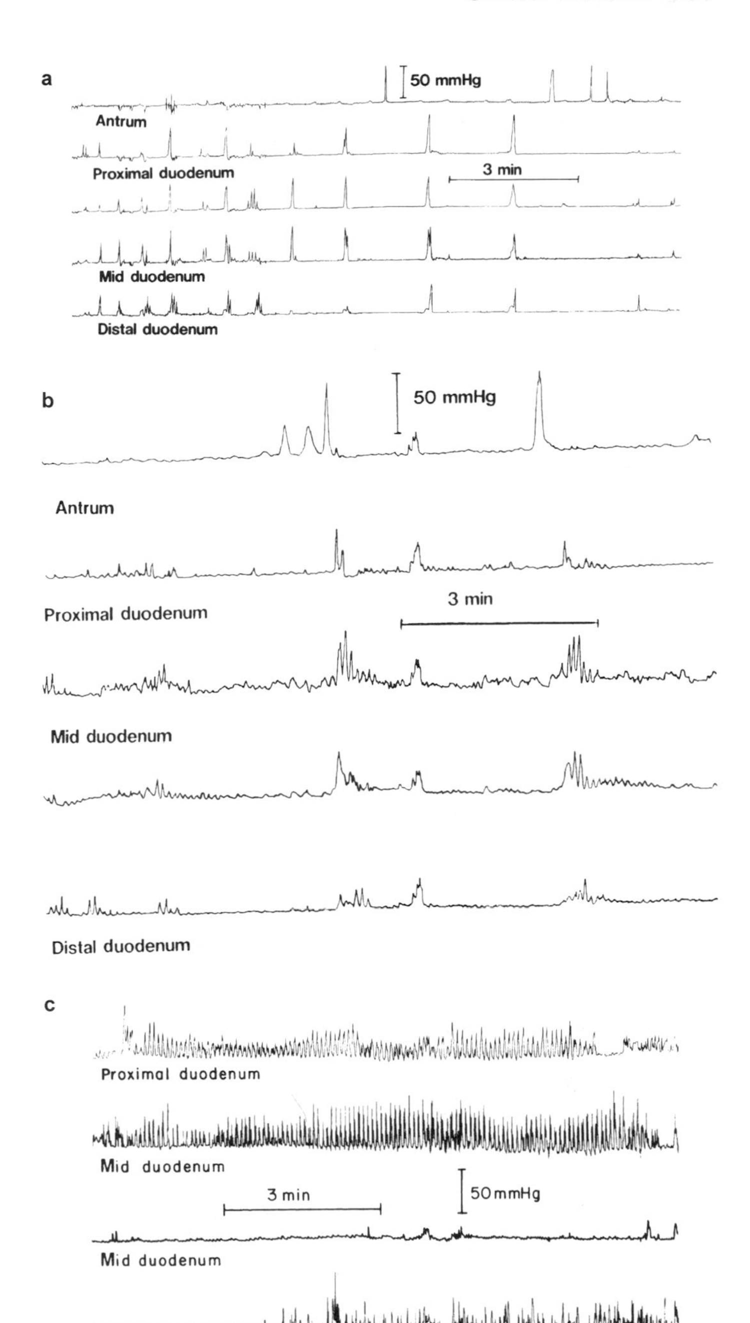

Figure 42.5: Discrete abnormalities in antroduodenal manometry. (**a**) Single propagating high-amplitude duodenal contractions. These 'single ring' contractions are associated with irritable bowel disorders when the migrating motor complex is present. (**b**) Non-propagating, simultaneous, short clusters in monotonous pattern continuing uninterrupted for a 6-h study. (**c**) Long burst of non-propagating duodenal contractions.

Table 42.3 Antroduodenal manometric features from studies of 300 children[a]

- Normal features
  - Migrating motor complex (MMC) (fasting)
  - Postprandial (phase 2-like) pattern
- Abnormal features in duodenum
  - Absent MMC phase 3
  - Sustained tonic contractions
  - Retrograde propagation of phase 3
  - Giant single-propagating contractions
  - Absent phase 2 with increased phase 3 frequency
  - Persistently low-amplitude or absent contractions
  - Prolonged non-propagating clusters
- Postprandial abnormalities
  - Antral hypomotility after a solid nutrient meal
  - Absent or decreased motility
  - Failure to induce a fed pattern (MMC persists)

[a] Each of these features is easily recognized by visual inspection of the recording. (Reproduced from Tomomasa T, DiLorenzo C, Morikawa A, et al. Analysis of fasting antroduodenal manometry in children. Dig Dis Sci 1996; 41:195–203, with permission of Springer Science and Business Media.)[35]

mucosal injury.[1] Nonetheless there is a paucity of evidence to suggest that episodes of identifiable hypoxic–ischemic events contribute to the pathogenesis of NEC in most infants.[1] Of all the suggested ischemic risk factors for NEC, only polycythemia, exchange transfusion, severe cyanotic congenital heart disease and, possibly, *in utero* exposure to cocaine are thought to be associated with the development of NEC.[1]

Enteral alimentation

Because 95% of infants with NEC have been fed enterally before its onset, enteral alimentation has been proposed as a contributing factor in NEC.[12,14] Various hypotheses propose that it is the composition of the milk, the rate of milk volume increments, the immaturity of gastrointestinal motility, absorptive or host defense processes, or other variables (high luminal osmolality) that contribute to the pathogenesis of NEC.[1,12,14]

Human milk reduces the risk for NEC.[24] Animal models support a role for the breast milk macrophage, but human data suggest that anti-inflammatory cytokines and enzymes as well as immunoglobulins, specifically IgA, may have a protective advantage. Indeed, both enterally administered serum-derived IgA and human milk may reduce the incidence of NEC.[25] Human milk may also reduce allergic reactions and facilitate the development of a favorable intestinal bacterial flora, while enhancing digestion and absorption of normal nutrients.

The volume of milk fed to infants may also predispose the patient to NEC.[14,15,26–28] Excessively rapid increments of milk feeding may overcome the infant's intestinal absorptive capability, especially in the presence of altered motility, resulting in malabsorption. Malabsorbed carbohydrates contribute to enhanced intestinal bacterial gas production, resulting in abdominal distention.[1,12,14] High intraluminal pressure from gaseous distention may reduce mucosal blood flow, producing secondary intestinal ischemia. In addition, dissection of bacterial gas products from the intestinal lumen may produce pneumatosis intestinalis or, if gas enters the portal venous system, hepatic venous gas may be evident. Analysis of gas from the intestinal lumen and cysts of pneumatosis intestinalis reveals a profile typical of intestinal bacterial fermentation of malabsorbed carbohydrates (e.g. hydrogen, methane, carbon dioxide).[1]

Earlier hypotheses had suggested that giving patients at risk nothing by mouth might reduce the incidence of NEC. Delayed feeding for asphyxiated infants or those with umbilical arterial or venous catheters and respiratory distress syndrome has not reduced the incidence of NEC.[1,12,14] In fact, delayed feeding may do more harm than good by increasing the risk of intestinal mucosal atrophy, cholestatic jaundice, osteopenia of prematurity and hyperalimentation-related complications.[14]

Large-volume milk feedings, increased too rapidly during the feeding schedule, may place undue stress on a previously injured or immature intestine. Feeding increments in excess of 20–30 ml/kg per 24 h were associated with an increased risk of NEC in at least two studies.[12,14] Two other studies have demonstrated the safety of 30–35 ml/kg per 24 h feeding increments.[26,29] Such information should temper enthusiasm for excessively rapid feeding protocols for low-birthweight infants. It suggests that daily increments should be based on the clinical examination, evidence of feeding intolerance and a recommended volume increment of 20–35 ml/kg per 24 h.

Hypertonic formula and enteric medications may have direct adverse effects on mucosal blood flow and intestinal motility. Subsequent injury may predispose to NEC.[1,12,14] Alternatively, direct pharmacologic effects of an agent on systemic host defense (vitamin E), motility (morphine) or regional blood flow (indomethacin) may result in mucosal injury, increasing the risks for NEC in susceptible neonates. H_2-blocking agents may decrease the risk of NEC.

Infectious–inflammatory agents

There are multiple epidemiologic investigations that have provided circumstantial or direct evidence to suggest that NEC is associated with one or more microbiologic agents.[1,30] NEC has been reported to occur in epidemics or clustered episodes due to an identifiable enteric pathogen; more often no identifiable agent is discovered.[1,30] When no agent is identifiable, this may be due to the unculturable nature of the pathogen. The suspicion of a transmissible agent is corroborated by the observation that epidemics abate following the institution or reinforcement of specific infectious disease-control measures (gowning, gloving, nurse cohorts and, especially, careful hand-washing).[1,30] Epidemics have been associated with the recovery of no specific agent, or with the recovery of a single pathogen such as *Escherichia coli*, *Klebsiella*, *Salmonella*, *Staphylococcus epidermidis*, *Clostridium butyricum*, coronavirus, rotavirus and enteroviruses.[1,31] An outbreak of NEC has been associated with *Enterobacter sakazakii*-contaminated powdered milk formula.[31]

Additional evidence suggesting that NEC is due to an infectious agent includes the observation of related infantile diarrheal illnesses within a community or among personnel in the neonatal intensive care unit.[1] Furthermore, there are similarities between NEC (pathology, symptoms, immature susceptibility) and many enterotoxemias of young animals and humans. Such enteric toxin-mediated illnesses may be due to *Clostridium*, *S. epidermidis* or other toxin-producing enteric pathogens.[32–34] Alternatively, endotoxin production by the 'normal' Gram-negative enteric flora during enteral alimentation may predispose the immature intestine to mucosal injury if endotoxin production exceeds elimination.[35] In addition transcytosis (crossing of epithelial cells by *E. coli*, etc.) could initiate this process; *E. coli* from patients with NEC has this capacity in animal models.[36] Endotoxin stimulates host inflammatory cells to produce various mediators such as tumor necrosis factor and platelet-activating factor.[35] Both of these and other inflammatory cytokines can initiate or propagate the pathologic process characterized by coagulation necrosis, inflammation, increased vascular permeability, edema, hemorrhage, local thrombosis and platelet consumption. Indeed, the immature enterocyte (epithelial cell) tends to react with excessive local production of pro-inflammatory cytokines when stimulated with endotoxin or interleukin 1β. The resulting cytokine mediator-induced thrombocytopenia, neutropenia, hypotensive–hypovolemic shock (third-space fluid losses), metabolic acidosis and hemorrhagic diarrhea are quite similar to the clinical manifestations of NEC in human neonates.[37]

The blood culture is positive in 20–30% of patients with NEC.[1,4] Reports of the responsible bacteremic pathogens before 1980 demonstrated a predominance of *E. coli* and *Klebsiella*.[1] Current reports of agents producing bacteremia in patients with NEC suggest that *S. epidermidis* is another common blood isolate.[4] It remains to be determined whether the organisms recovered in blood or peritoneal cultures are the primary pathogens or secondary invading organisms that gain access to the circulation or peritoneum through a compromised intestinal mucosa.

Unifying hypothesis of pathophysiology

The predominant risk factor for NEC is prematurity, *not* the associated diseases of premature infants. Nonetheless, multiple potentially adverse events may produce mucosal injury, the net result being manifest as NEC. Figure 43.2 provides potential initiating events, and Figure 43.3 identifies additional pathologic factors that may propagate NEC once mucosal injury exceeds the immature host's ability to repair the process. Although it is hoped that one microbiologic agent or other process will be found to be responsible for NEC, it is more probable that NEC is a final common pathway for an immature intestinal response to injury. Indeed, NEC is a common cause of the systemic inflammatory response syndrome (SIRS) in neonates.

CLINICAL MANIFESTATIONS

Early signs and symptoms of NEC are often non-specific; they include subtle signs of the 'sepsis syndrome' and more specific but equally subtle signs of gastrointestinal disease.[1] Non-specific extra-gastrointestinal manifestations include apnea, bradycardia, lethargy, temperature instability (hypothermia or the need to increase the Isolette temperature to maintain normal body temperature), cyanosis, mottling, cool extremities and acidosis.[1] More specific but not diagnostic gastrointestinal manifestations are related to ileus, third-space fluid losses, local coagulopathy and intestinal hemorrhage. Gastrointestinal signs and symptoms include abdominal distention, abdominal tenderness, emesis, sudden increased gastric residual volume, hematemesis, bright red blood from the rectum, absent bowel sounds, abdominal guarding and diarrhea. The latter is an uncommon isolated manifestation of NEC.

Monitoring pre-feed gastric residuals (gastric aspirates) is not helpful in predicting NEC as many unaffected neonates have gastric residuals.[38] A sudden change in the volume of gastric residuals plus abdominal distention is more ominous for NEC. Monitoring for subtle signs of gastrointestinal bleeding with stool guaiac testing is also not helpful as many unaffected premature infants have stools with occult blood, and patients with NEC may have stools negative for occult blood. Gross blood in the stool is more suggestive of NEC but is not diagnostic.

As the disease progresses in severity, there is disseminated intravascular coagulation, hypotensive (septic and hypovolemic) shock, ascites, peritonitis and intestinal perforation. Focal findings may include erythematous streaking of the anterior abdominal wall around the umbilicus and the course of the subcutaneous umbilical vein, and erythema with a mass in the right lower quadrant, representing a local perforation, with matted bowel forming a local abscess.

Disease stage should be classified as noted in Table 43.1 (modified Bell's criteria).[1,38–40] Stage I represents subclinical (no diagnostic radiographic or ultrasonographic signs) NEC or another gastrointestinal or systemic disturbance. Stage II and III NEC are documented disease and often present with a sudden onset. Progression from one stage to another usually occurs within 24 h after onset of symptoms. Once stabilized, patients with NEC rarely progress to another stage; most episodes of perforation occur at presentation (stage IIIB) or among patients with stage IIIA that progresses to stage IIIB. Perforation usually occurs within 48–72 h of the onset of disease manifestations in patients with stage IIIA NEC. The modified Bell's staging criteria are also useful in comparing cases of NEC in the literature.

DIAGNOSIS

The diagnosis of NEC is confirmed by the radiographic presence of pneumatosis intestinalis or hepatic venous gas (Figs 43.4 and 43.5). Gastrointestinal perforation (pneumoperitoneum; Figs 43.6 and 43.7) is strong evidence for NEC, but the diagnosis must then be confirmed by histopathologic evidence.

Hepatic venous gas and ascites may also be demonstrated by abdominal ultrasonography or magnetic resonance imaging, and inapparent pneumatosis intestinalis may become more evident by performing a contrast enema.[1,41,42] Nonetheless, except under unusual circumstances (to rule out volvulus), contrast studies are not needed to determine the diagnosis of NEC. Ancillary laboratory evaluations may reveal thrombocytopenia with or without evidence of disseminated intravascular coagulation, anemia, neutropenia, metabolic acidosis from septic or hypovolemic shock, respiratory acidosis from increased intra-abdominal pressure and poor diaphragm excursion, increased breath hydrogen excretion, raised fecal calprotectin levels and radiographic signs of ileus, an isolated dilated intestinal loop or ascites.[1,43] The differential diagnosis of NEC is outlined in Table 43.2. Idiopathic, focal, spontaneous, isolated intestinal perforation is also a common cause of pneumoperitoneum in the pre-term and, less often, full-term neonate. The onset is usually sudden and occurs earlier in life than that of NEC. Prior feeding may not be present and pneumatosis intestinalis is absent. Affected patients usually have respiratory distress

THERAPY

NEC has a wide spectrum of severity. The mildest form manifests as hemorrhagic colitis with or without pneumatosis coli; the more fulminant state is similar to that noted in patients with Gram-negative septic shock, commonly referred to as SIRS.

Abdominal distention is a universal feature of NEC. Significant abdominal distention may reduce the mesenteric arterial perfusion pressure, thus exacerbating a previously compromised intestinal blood flow. Models of the effects of increased intra-abdominal pressure have reported such adverse consequences as increased systemic vascular resistance, decreased cardiac output, decreased urine output and 'apparent' hypovolemia.[53,54] Surgical decompression of increased intra-abdominal pressure in human adults restores systemic arterial oxygenation, cardiac output and urine production within 15 min of the procedure.[53]

Increased intra-abdominal pressure in patients with NEC is due to the development of tense ascites, marked intestinal gas production, stasis (ileus) and inflammatory fluid exudation with hemorrhage into the lumen of the small and large intestines. It is imperative to reduce abdominal distention with nasogastric tube placement and no further formula feeding (NPO – nil *per os*). The decompression tube should be the largest that the patient can tolerate. Paracentesis with placement of an intra-abdominal drain under local anesthesia has been helpful in stage II or III disease. Finally, if the patient fails to respond to medical management or abdominal drain placement within 24–48 h of the onset of illness, exploratory laparotomy can result in abdominal decompression by removal of necrotic tissue and inflammatory exudate (Table 43.3).

The associated bacteremia in approximately 20–30% of patients with NEC is probably not the primary cause of the disease. Nonetheless, appropriate antimicrobial therapy must be directed against these bacteria, even when the bacteremia is due to bowel injury and secondary bacterial invasion. Patients with both NEC and bacteremia usually have more severe disease and a higher mortality rate.[1] Although the precise antibiotic regimen for the treatment of NEC has not been determined, the clinician must remain flexible, as there are changes in the pathogens recovered in patients with NEC, and each neonatal intensive care unit has different bacteria with different antimicrobial resistent patterns.[1,4,30,50] This may reflect a bacterial shift in the fecal colonization of premature infants. Nonetheless, the changing pattern of the agents recovered during bacteremia requires close scrutiny and appropriate modification of antimicrobial therapy. Traditional antimicrobial treatment of NEC employs systemic administration of a semisynthetic penicillin (ampicillin, ticarcillin) and an aminoglycoside (gentamicin, kanamycin). Evidence suggests a beneficial response with the use of vancomycin and cefotaxime.[55] Many recommend anaerobic coverage with clindamycin or metronidazole. Vigilant attention to the microbiology of blood, fecal and peritoneal cultures in patients with NEC is needed for appropriate modification of antibiotic therapy (see Table 43.1 for duration of antimicrobial therapy)[56,57].

Abnormality	Interventions	Goals
Presumed infection	Broad-spectrum antibiotics	Eradicate infection
Peritonitis or intestinal perforation	Antibiotics plus surgery or paracentesis with abdominal drain	Eradicate nidus of infection; remove necrotic bowel, ascites; decrease distention
Intestinal distention or ileus	NPO; nasogastric tube drainage, paracentesis with abdominal drain	Decrease intestinal gas production; remove intestinal secretions; decompress abdomen
Hypotension	Volume expansion, vasopressor agents	Restore gestational and postnatal age-appropriate blood pressure
Hypoperfusion/oxygen delivery	Volume expansion, vasopressor and inotropic agents; mechanical ventilation, oxygen, packed red blood cell transfusions	Hemoglobin 12–14 g/dl Oxygen saturation >95% Normal blood lactate level (pH) Normal cardiac index
Organ system dysfunction	Volume expansion, vasopressor and inotropic agents; mechanical ventilation, oxygen; packed red blood cells, platelet, fresh frozen plasma transfusions; diuretics, dialysis–hemofiltration	Normalize or reverse abnormalities: *Renal*: urine output, BUN, creatinine *Hepatic*: bilirubin, coagulopathy, albumin *Pulmonary*: alveolar–arterial gradient, hypercapnia *Cardiac*: pulse, blood pressure, cardiac index *CNS*: level of consciousness *Hematologic*: correct anemia, DIC (if active bleeding)
Poor nutritional intake	Parenteral alimentation (central or peripheral); enteral feedings during recovery	Reverse catabolism; improve nitrogen balance and healing; prevent hypoglycemia

BUN, blood urea nitrogen; DIC, disseminated intravascular coagulopathy.
Modified from Kliegman, 1996.[68]

Table 43.3 Approach to management of patients with necrotizing enterocolitis

Perforation with subsequent bacterial peritonitis is managed with abdominal drain placement or surgery.

The treatment of severe NEC manifested as SIRS is not unlike that of other causes of bacteremia-associated hypotension. Endotoxin-stimulated production of inflammatory mediators such as bradykinin, tumor necrosis factor or platelet-activating factor results in increased vascular permeability, large transcapillary fluid loss, increased pulmonary artery pressure with hypoxia, lactic acidosis and hypotension. Hypermetabolism increases oxygen requirements. Once stabilized from the septic shock state, all patients require parenteral nutrition while NPO. Fluid losses plus the initial vasodilation increase water and electrolyte requirements. Despite rapid killing of bacteria by antibiotics, the diverse effects of bacterial products (endotoxin, etc.) are still evident. The net result is a markedly reduced cardiopulmonary ability to meet the oxygen requirements of the peripheral tissues.[58–60]

The decreased cardiac output in septic shock (and NEC) may be due to pooling of blood and fluid in the capacitance peripheral vessels and loss of fluid in third spaces as well as a specific myocardial dysfunction characteristic of severe bacteremic states. The myocardial depression is not due to ischemia but rather to various mediators released as a response to inflammation and hypotension. Circulatory failure results in a flow-limited ability to provide the oxygen necessary to support energy metabolism (local tissue oxygen consumption). Circulatory failure causes tissue hypoxia and metabolic (lactic) acidosis. Some of the cellular defects of oxygen utilization may not be due to hypoxia–ischemia alone. Tumor necrosis factor produced during endotoxemia has various metabolic consequences that may interfere with mitochondrial oxygen utilization.[58]

Methods used to treat septic shock must take into consideration the linear relationship between oxygen delivery and local tissue oxygen consumption.[58] This flow-dependent relationship can be improved by restoring the circulating blood volume (preload) with fluid resuscitation and by improving myocardial contractility with inotropic sympathomimetic agents.

An acute 'adult' respiratory distress-like syndrome (ARDS) may be observed in patients with NEC. This is due in part to inflammatory or vasoactive mediators producing non-cardiogenic pulmonary edema. Hypoxia is exacerbated by increased pulmonary artery pressure, abdominal distention with reduced diaphragmatic excursion, and myocardial contractile failure. Adequate oxygen delivery is closely dependent on appropriate ventilator management of patients with NEC. Methods that improve oxygen delivery also reduce local lactate production and improve metabolic acidosis. A successful outcome in patients with septic shock is related to the ability of the therapeutic measures to improve cardiac output. In addition to support for the failing circulation, careful attention must be given to the pulmonary problems associated with NEC.

The application of these principles to the therapy of NEC must emphasize aggressive use of fluid resuscitation. If fluid administration is unsuccessful in restoring perfusion and urine production, or in correcting the metabolic acidosis, inotropic drugs (dopamine, dobutamine) can be used to improve oxygen delivery by improving myocardial contractility and occasionally by vasodilation. The administration of inotropic, vasodilator or vasopressor agents must be carefully titrated against peripheral perfusion, blood pressure, urine production, metabolic acidosis and central venous pressure if available. The therapeutic balance between vasopressor (myocardial contractility) agents and vasodilation (afterload reduction) is often difficult to achieve but may benefit from additional fluid therapy.

Abdominal drainage by percutaneous drain placement may acutely decompress the abdomen and improve many of the adverse cardiopulmonary complications of NEC due to a tense abdomen and compromised diaphragms. It may be particularly helpful in improving oxygenation and ventilation.[61]

Intestinal perforation is a traditional indication for exploratory laparotomy. In certain high-risk, unstable patients (often weighing less than 1000 g with stage IIb or III NEC), percutaneous placement of an abdominal drain under local anesthesia has been performed.[61–64] In many but not all patients with NEC managed with paracentesis and a drain, exploratory laparotomy is necessary 24–72 h later. Drain placement is even more beneficial for patients with isolated idiopathic intestinal perforations. Fewer patients with isolated perforations may require immediate exploratory laparotomy in 24–48 h. Additional indications for surgery include progressive clinical deterioration despite aggressive medical management (see Table 43.3), and in the convalescent stages for the resection of strictures and enteric fistulae. All patients treated with abdominal drain placement must be considered at risk for stricture formation. If percutaneous drainage is used as the first surgical treatment, exploratory laparatomy is then indicated for deterioration, signs of intestinal obstruction or failure of a second drain to relieve pneumoperitoneum.

Surgical management should attempt to preserve as much viable bowel as possible, resecting only the most obviously necrotic and gangrenous tissue. In circumstances of NEC totalis, a high diverting jejunostomy is recommended.[65] A second laparotomy is performed within 48–72 h if the patient remains critically ill to determine whether what previously looked like non-viable tissue was actually viable.[65] This approach may avoid massive resection and subsequent development of the short gut syndrome.[66]

For patients with minimal and well defined disease, some surgeons recommend that primary anastomosis be performed after resection of dead bowel, at the time of the initial laparotomy. Such patients should be observed carefully for development of strictures (at the anastomosis and other sites) or recurrent NEC. Strictures may present with signs of obstruction (emesis, obstipation, abdominal distention), sepsis or gastrointestinal bleeding.

References

1. Kliegman RM, Walsh MC. Neonatal necrotizing enterocolitis: pathogenesis, classification and spectrum of disease. Curr Prob Pediatr 1987; 17:213–288.

2. Bolisetty S, Lui K, Oei J, et al. A regional study of underlying congenital diseases in term neonates with necrotizing enterocolitis. Acta Paediatr 2000; 89:1226–1230.
3. Holman RC, Stehr-Green JK, Zelasky MT. Necrotizing enterocolitis mortality in the United States, 1979–85. Am J Publ Health 1989; 79:987–989.
4. Palmer SR, Biffin A, Gamsu HR. Outcome of neonatal necrotising enterocolitis: results of the BAPM/CDSC surveillance study, 1981–1984. Arch Dis Child 1989; 64:388–394.
5. Bisquera JA, Cooper TR, Berseth CL. Impact of necrotizing enterocolitis on length of stay and hospital charges in very low birth weight infants. Pediatrics 2002; 109:423–428.
6. Gaynes R, Edwards J, Jarvis W, et al. National Nosocomial Infections Surveillance System. Nosocomial infections among neonates in high-risk nurseries in the United States. Pediatrics 1996; 98:357–361.
7. Andorsky DJ, Lund DP, Lillebei CW, et al. Nutritional and other postoperative management of neonates with short bowel syndrome correlates with clinical outcomes. J Pediatr 2001; 139:27–33.
8. Grosfeld J, Molinari F, Chaet M, et al. Gastrointestinal perforation and peritonitis in infants and children: experience with 179 cases over ten years. Surgery 1996; 120:650–656.
9. Noerr B. Part 1: Current controversies in the understanding of necrotizing enterocolitis. Adv Neonatal Care 2003; 3:107–120.
10. Llanos AR, Moss ME, Pinzon MC, et al. Epidemiology of neonatal necrotizing enterocolitis: a population-based study. Paediatr Perinat Epidemiol 2002; 16:342–349.
11. Hällström M, Koivisto AM, Janas M. Frequency of and risk factors for necrotizing enterocolitis in infants born before 33 weeks of gestation. Acta Paediatr 2003; 92:111–113.
12. Kliegman RM. Neonatal necrotizing enterocolitis: bridging the basic science with the clinical disease. J Pediatr 1990; 117:833–835.
13. McElhinney DB, Hedrick HL, Bush DM, et al. Necrotizing enterocolitis in neonates with congenital heart disease: risk factors and outcomes. Pediatrics 2000; 106:1080–1087.
14. Kliegman RM. The relationship of neonatal feeding practices and the pathogenesis and prevention of necrotizing enterocolitis. Pediatrics 2003; 111:671–672.
15. Kennedy KA, Tyson JE, Chamnanvanakij S. Rapid *versus* slow rate of advancement of feedings for promoting growth and preventing necrotizing enterocolitis in parenerally fed low-birth-weight infants. Cochrane Database of Systematic Reviews 2002; 3.
16. Ballance WA, Dahms BB, Shenker N, et al. Pathology of neonatal necrotizing enterocolitis: a ten-year experience. J Pediatr 1990; 117:S6–S13.
17. Ewer AK. Role of platelet-activating factor in the pathophysiology of necrotizing enterocolitis. Acta Paediatr Suppl 2002; 437:2–5.
18. Nadler EP, Stanford A, Zhang XR, et al. Intestinal cytokine gene expression in infants with acute necrotizing enterocolitis: interleukin-11 mRNA expression inversely correlates with extent of disease. J Pediatr Surg 2001; 36:1122–1129.
19. Pender SLF, Braegger C, Gunther U, et al. Matrix metalloproteinases in necrotizing enterocolitis. Pediatr Res 2003; 54:160–164.
20. Nowicki P. Intestinal ischemia and necrotizing enterocolitis. J Pediatr 1990; 117:S14–S19.
21. Coombs RC, Morgan MEI, Durbin GM, et al. Gut blood flow velocities in the newborn: effects of patent ductus arteriosus and parenteral indomethacin. Arch Dis Child 1990; 65:1067–1071.
22. Lopez SL, Taeusch HW, Findlay RD, Walther FJ. Time of onset of necrotizing enterocolitis in newborn infants with known prenatal cocaine exposure. Clin Pediatr 1995; 34:424–429.
23. Craigo S, Beach M, Harvey-Wilkes K, D'Alton M. Ultrasound predictors of neonatal outcome in intrauterine growth restriction. Am J Perinatol 1996; 13:465–471.
24. McGuire W, Anthony MY. Donor human milk *versus* formula for preventing necrotizing enterocolitis in preterm infants: systematic review. Arch Dis Child Fetal Neonatal Ed 2003; 88:F11–F14.
25. Eibl MM, Wolf HM, Furnkranz H, et al. Prevention of necrotizing enterocolitis in low-birth-weight infants by IgA – IgG feeding. N Engl J Med 1988; 319:1–7.
26. Rayyis SF, Ambalavanan N, Wright L, et al. Randomized trial of 'slow' *versus* 'fast' feed advancements on the incidence of necrotizing enterocolitis in very low birth weight infants. J Pediatr 1999; 134:293–297.
27. Berseth CL, Bisquera JA, Paje V. Prolonging small feeding volumes early in life decreases the incidence of necrotizing enterocolitis in very low birth weight infants. Pediatrics 2003; 111:529–534.
28. Kamitsuka MD, Horton MK, Williams MA. The incidence of necrotizing enterocolitis after introducing standardized feeding schedules for infants between 1250 and 2500 grams and less than 35 weeks of gestation. Pediatrics 2000; 105:379–384.
29. Caple JI, Armentrout DC, Huseby VD, et al. The effect of feeding volume on the clinical outcome in premature infants. Pediatr Res 1997; 41:229A.
30. Boccia D, Stolfi I, Lana S, et al. Nosocomial necrotizing enterocolitis outbreaks: epidemiology and control measures. Eur J Pediatr 2001; 160:385–391.
31. Van Acker J, De Smet F, Muyldermans G, et al. Outbreak of necrotizing enterocolitis associated with *Enterobacter sakazakii* in powdered milk formula. J Clin Microbiol 2001; 39:293–297.
32. Scheifele DW. Role of bacterial toxins in neonatal necrotizing enterocolitis. J Pediatr 1990; 117:S44–S46.
33. Rotbart HA, Johnson ZT, Reller LB. Analysis of enteric coagulase-negative staphylococci from neonates with necrotizing enterocolitis. Pediatr Infect Dis J 1989; 8:140–142.
34. Fink MP, Cohn SM, Lee PC, et al. Effect of lipopolysaccharide on intestinal intramucosal hydrogen ion concentration in pigs: evidence of gut ischemia in a normodynamic model of septic shock. Crit Care Med 1989; 17:641–646.
35. Duffy LC, Zielezny MA, Carrion V, et al. Bacterial toxins and enteral feeding of premature infants at risk for necrotizing enterocolitis. In: Newberg DS, ed. Bioactive Components of Human Milk. New York: Kluwer Academic/Plenum; 2001:519–527.
36. Panigrahi P, Bamford P, Horvath K, et al. *Escherichia coli* transcytosis in a caco-2 cell model: implications in neonatal necrotizing enterocolitis. Pediatr Res 1996; 40:415–421.
37. Nanthakumar NN, Fusunyan RD, Sanderson I, et al. Inflammation in the developing human intestine: a possible pathophysiologic contribution to necrotizing enterocolitis. PRoc Natl Acad Sci 2000; 97:6043–6048.
38. Pinheiro JMB, Clark DA, Benjamin KG. A critical analysis of the routine testing of newborn stools for occult blood and reducing substances. Adv Neonatal Care 2003: 3:133–138.
39. Hoehn T, Stover B, Buhrer C. Colonic pneumatosis intestinalis in preterm infants: different to necrotizing enterocolitis with a more benign course? Eur J Pediatr 2001; 160:369–371.
40. Travadi JN, Patole SK, Gardiner K. Pneumatosis coli – a benign form of necrotizing enterocolitis. Indian Pediatr 2003; 40:349–351.

41. Buras R, Guzzetta P, Avery G, et al. Acidosis and hepatic portal venous gas: indications for surgery in necrotizing enterocolitis. Pediatrics 1986; 78:273–277.

42. Weinberg B, Peralta VE, Diakoumakis EE, et al. Sonographic findings in necrotizing enterocolitis with paucity of abdominal gas as the initial symptom. Mt Sinai J Med 1989; 56:330–333.

43. Carroll D, Corfield A, Spicer R, et al. Faecal calprotectin concentrations and diagnosis of necrotizing entercolitis. Lancet 2003; 361:310–311.

44. Okuyama H, Kubota A, Oue T, et al. A comparison of the clinical presentation and outcome of focal intestinal perforation and necrotizing entercolitis in very-low-birth-weight neonates. Pediatr Surg Int 2002; 18:704–706.

45. Pumberger W, Mayr M, Kohlhauser C, et al. Spontaneous localized intestinal perforation in very-low-birth-weight infants: a distinct clinical entity different from necrotizing enterocolitis. J Am Coll Surg 2002; 195:796–803.

46. Foster J, Cole M. Oral immunoglobulin for preventing necrotizing enterocolitis in preterm and low birth-weight neonates. Cochrane Database of Systematic Reviews 2003; 3.

47. Dugdale AE. Breast milk and necrotising enterocolitis. Lancet 1991; 337:435.

48. Halac E, Halac J, Begue EF, et al. Prenatal and postnatal corticosteroid therapy to prevent neonatal necrotizing enterocolitis: a controlled trial. J Pediatr 1990; 117:132–138.

49. Amin HJ, Zamora SA, McMillan DD, et al. Arginine supplementation prevents necrotizing enterocolitis in the premature infant. J Pediatr 2002; 140:425–431.

50. Siu YK, Fung SCK, Lee CH, et al. Double blind, randomized, placebo controlled study of oral vancomycin in prevention of necrotizing enterocolitis in preterm, very low birthweight infants. Arch Dis Child Fetal Neonatal Ed 1998; 79:F105–F109.

51. Bury RG, Tudehopr D. Enteral antibiotics for preventing necrotizing enterocolitis in low birthweight or preterm infants. Cochrane Database of Systematic Reviews 2003; 3.

52. Meis PJ, Klebanoff M, Thom E, et al. Prevention of recurrent preterm delivery by 17alpha-hydroxyprogesterone caproate. N Engl J Med 2003; 348:2379–2385.

53. Cullen DJ, Coyle JP, Teplick R, et al. Cardiovascular, pulmonary, and renal effects of massively increased intra-abdominal pressure in critically ill patients. Crit Care Med 1989; 17:118–121.

54. Richards WO, Scovill W, Baekhyo S, et al. Acute renal failure associated with increased intra-abdominal pressure. Ann Surg 1983; 197:183–187.

55. Scheifele DW, Ginter GL, Olsen E, et al. Comparison of two antibiotic regimens for neonatal necrotizing enterocolitis. J Antimicrob Chemother 1987; 20:421–429.

56. Gorbach SL. Intraabdominal infections. Clin Infect Dis 1993; 17:961–967.

57. Montravers P, Gauzit R, Muller C, et al. Emergence of antibiotic-resistant bacteria in cases of peritonitis after intraabdominal surgery affects the efficacy of empirical antimicrobial therapy. Clin Infect Dis 1996; 23:486–494.

58. Rackow EC, Astiz ME, Weil MH. Cellular oxygen metabolism during sepsis and shock: the relationship of oxygen consumption to oxygen delivery. JAMA 1988; 259:1989–1993.

59. Natanson C, Danner RL, Elin RJ, et al. Role of endotoxemia in cardiovascular dysfunction and mortality: *Escherichia coli* and *Staphylococcus aureus* challenges in a canine model of human septic shock. J Clin Invest 1989; 83:243–251.

60. Carcillo JA, Pollack MM, Ruttimann UE, et al. Sequential physiologic interactions in pediatric cardiogenic and septic shock. Crit Care Med 1989; 17:12–16.

61. Dzakovic A, Notrica DM, O'Brian Smith E. Primary peritoneal drainage for increasing ventilatory requirements in critically ill neonates with necrotizing enterocolitis. J Pediatr Surg 2001; 36:730–732.

62. Nadler EP, Upperman JS, Ford HR. Controversies in the management of necrotizing enterocolitis. Surg Infect 2001; 2:113–120.

63. Demestre X, Ginovart G, Figueras-Aloy J, et al. Peritoneal drainage as primary management in necrotizing enterocolitis: a prospective study. J Pediatr Surg 2002; 37:1534–1539.

64. Moss RL, Dimmitt RA, Henry MCW, et al. A meta-analysis of peritoneal drainage *versus* laparotomy for perforated necrotizing enterocolitis. J Pediatr Surg 2001; 36:1210–1213.

65. Sugarman ID, Kiely EM. Is there a role for high jejunostomy in the management of severe necrotizing enterocolitis? Pediatr Surg Int 2001; 17:122–124.

66. Horwitz JR, Lally KP, Cheu HW, et al. Complications after surgical intervention for necrotizing enterocolitis: a multicenter review. J Pediatr Surg 1995; 30:994–999.

67. Polin R, Fox W. Neonatal and Fetal Medicine: Physiology and Pathophysiology. Philadelphia, PA: WB Saunders; 1992.

68. Kliegman R. Necrotizing enterocolitis. In: Burg FD, Ingelfinger JR, Wald ER, Polin RA, eds. Gellis & Kagan's Current Pediatric Therapy, 15th edn. Philadelphia, PA: WB Saunders; 1996: 217–220.

Chapter 44
Appendicitis

S.T. Lau and Michael G. Caty

INTRODUCTION

Acute appendicitis is one of the most common surgical conditions occurring in children and adults. Approximately 250 000 cases of acute appendicitis occur annually in the USA, with the highest incidence occurring between the ages of 10 to 19 years, at about 23 per 10 000 population per year. The lifetime risk of developing appendicitis has been estimated at 8.6% for males and 6.7% for females, with a lifetime incidence of an appendectomy estimated at 12% for males and 23% for females.[1] In the pediatric population, the usual age of presentation is 11–12 years. Between 30 and 50% of children will present with a perforated appendix. In children younger than 5 years old, the perforation rate is 60–65%. In those less than 2 years of age, the perforation rate approaches 95%.[2] In today's medical community, a non-surgical physician is usually the first to evaluate a patient with appendicitis. Therefore, a thorough understanding of this common disease is essential for all physicians.

Leonardo da Vinci was the first to describe and illustrate the appendix in 1492, however his work remained unpublished. In 1543, Andreas Vesalius was credited with the first published illustration of a normal appendix. Claudius Amyand, one of the surgeons and founders of St George's Hospital in London, performed the first reported appendectomy in 1735. In 1886, Reginald Fitz, professor of pathological anatomy at Harvard Medical School, proposed surgical intervention as the proper treatment for this disease. That same year, Richard Hall reported the first case of an appendectomy in North America in a patient who survived an operation for perforated appendicitis. Thomas Morton, in 1887, performed an appendectomy for a non-perforated appendicitis with a correct preoperative diagnosis. In 1889, Charles McBurney presented his description of the point of maximal tenderness known as McBurney's point. Five years later he published his paper advocating the gridiron 'McBurney' incision.[3–5]

More recently, the emergence of new technology has allowed several advances in the treatment of appendicitis. As both laparoscopic skills and laparoscopic technology have continued to improve, there has been an increasing trend towards performing laparoscopic appendectomies. Advances in interventional radiology have given the surgeon more options in the treatment of perforated appendicitis. Many surgeons are initially treating patients with antibiotics and percutaneous drainage followed by an interval appendectomy.

EMBRYOLOGY

The development of the appendix begins during the eighth week of gestation. The appendix initially projects from the apex of the cecum, but as the right terminal haustrum develops, the appendix is displaced medially towards the ileocecal valve.[6] The colonic teniae arise from the base of the appendix and is also displaced by the growth of the right haustrum. By the 7th month of gestation, a few lymph nodules are present and the lymphoid tissue continues to develop until puberty and then diminishes.[7]

In 1827, Melier first discussed the variations in the shape and location of the appendix.[8] Its position within the abdomen is quite variable.[6] In 1885, Treves further described the position of the appendix with respect to the ileum and cecum. He examined 100 autopsies and reported the most frequent position to be post-ileal, pointing towards the spleen.[9] In 1933, Wakeley reviewed 10 000 post mortem cases looking for the position of the appendix (Table 44.1).[10] Maisel reviewed autopsies of 100 fetuses of 30–40 weeks gestation and 300 adult autopsies. He found the most common position of the appendix to be pelvic (53% in the fetal group and 58% in the adult group). The second most common position was retrocecal (26% in the fetal group and 26.7% in the adult group).[11]

In the adult, the appendix is variable in length, but averages about 8 cm; it is relatively longer and narrower in children. The appendix has its own mesentery, called the mesoappendix, which contains the appendicular artery, a branch of the ileocolic artery, which is a branch of the superior mesenteric artery. The ileocolic vein drains blood from the cecum and appendix and enters the superior mesenteric vein to drain into the portal vein.

PATHOPHYSIOLOGY

The etiology of appendicitis was outlined in 1939 by Wangensteen and Dennis in their paper 'Experimental Proof of the Obstructive Origin of Appendicitis in Man'[12]

Position	(%)
Retrocecal	65.28
Pelvic	31.01
Subcecal	2.26
Preileal	1.00
Right pericolic and postileal	0.40

From Wakeley, 1933.[10]

Table 44.1 Positions of the vermiform appendix

and in previous work by Wangensteen and Bowers.[13] Appendicitis is initiated by obstruction of the appendiceal lumen. When the lumen of the appendix becomes obstructed, the flow of normal mucosal secretions is inhibited. This leads to increased intraluminal pressure and compromised venous drainage, which leads to ischemic breakdown of the mucosa. Simultaneously, luminal bacteria proliferate and invade the appendiceal wall. This combination results in acute appendicitis, gangrene and ultimately perforation.

The bacteria involved in acute appendicitis are the normal colonic flora. It is usually a polymicrobial process, involving both aerobes and anaerobes. The typical species are *Escherichia coli, Bacteroides fragilis* and *Clostridial* species, although *Streptococcus, Pseudomonas* and *Enterobacter* can also be found.[14,15]

It is also possible for the luminal obstruction (such as a fecalith) to pass from the lumen into the cecum, allowing decompression and relief of symptoms. The appendix could potentially heal at this point. Even if there were a perforation, it is possible that the inflammatory process could be isolated by the omentum and loops of small bowel, allowing healing without any intervention. These processes would be associated with an element of fibrosis, which could lead to narrowing of the lumen and a predisposition to formation of another fecalith and another episode of acute appendicitis or appendiceal colic, which will be discussed later in the chapter.

PATHOLOGY

The appendix is comprised of the same four layers as the rest of the intestine (the mucosa, submucosa, muscularis propria and serosa). The mucosa is made of a surface layer of epithelial cells, a loose connective tissue layer known as the lamina propria, as well as the muscularis mucosa that is the boundary between the mucosa and the submucosa. The epithelial surface contains a combination of columnar cells with basally located nuclei, goblet cells with apical mucin and absorptive cells. Scattered Paneth cells containing secretory granules and neuroendocrine cells are present in this layer as well. These neuroendocrine cells are the origin of the carcinoid tumor, which is the most common appendiceal neoplasm. The lamina propria, just underneath the surface epithelial layer, contains the crypts of Lieberkühn as well as lymphoid follicles with germinal centers. As previously mentioned, the muscularis mucosa lies between the mucosa and submucosa, but this layer is less developed in the appendix compared with other areas of the intestine.

The submucosa contains a rich network of blood vessels, lymphatics and nerves. The network of ganglion cells and Schwann cells found within this layer is known as Meissner's plexus. The next level of the appendiceal wall is the muscularis propria, which consists of two layers of smooth muscle. The muscle fibers of the inner layer are arranged in a circular fashion, while the fibers of the outer layer are arranged longitudinally. Another neural network, known as Auerbach's plexus, lies between these muscle layers. The outermost level of the appendiceal wall, the serosa, is made up of a band of fibrous tissue with an overlying layer of cuboidal mesothelial cells.

In acute appendicitis, the appendix becomes swollen, with subserosal vascular congestion. With transmural inflammation, a serosal exudate and perforation may be found. The mucosa is often hyperemic and ulcerated. As the inflammatory process progresses, there are an increased number of neutrophils associated with cryptitis and crypt abscesses. The submucosa and muscularis propria become inflamed and may result in perforation.[16]

When compared with appendicitis specimens from patients who undergo immediate appendectomy, interval appendectomy specimens commonly have granulomatous and xanthogranulomatous inflammation. Most have mural fibrosis and thickening as well as transmural chronic inflammation with lymphoid aggregates. The mucosa is also often distorted with abnormally shaped crypts or crypt loss and, like acute appendicitis specimens, there may be focal cryptitis and crypt abscesses.[17]

CLINICAL PRESENTATION

Early diagnosis is vital to providing optimal management. While laboratory and radiologic studies are often useful aids in making the diagnosis, the key components are the history and physical exam.

The initial symptom is usually periumbilical abdominal pain. This initial vague pain is due to distension of the appendix, transmitted by visceral afferent fibers entering the spine at T10, causing referred pain in the associated dermatome. As the inflammation develops, the somatic afferent pain fibers of the parietal peritoneum become involved, causing localized pain in the right lower quadrant, usually at McBurney's point, which is located two-thirds of the distance along a line extending from the umbilicus to the anterior superior iliac spine. Localized pain may also occur in the right upper quadrant, the right flank, or the suprapubic area if the appendix is high and retrocolic or retrocecal or located in the pelvis. If the patient is malrotated or has situs inversus, pain may occur in the epigastrium or left lower quadrant. Urinary symptoms may also be precipitated by a close proximity of the appendix to the bladder or right ureter.

Nausea and vomiting are common symptoms that follow the onset of pain. Vomiting that occurs before the onset of pain is almost never due to appendicitis. Anorexia is also very common, although somewhat less frequent in the pediatric population. Diarrhea can also occur with appendicitis, especially in younger children. If perforation occurs, the resulting decompression of the appendiceal lumen may transiently relieve the symptoms.

It is extremely important to pay attention to the time course of the onset and transition of the site of pain. The clinician should attempt to define the onset of the pain. Inquiring when a child ate their last full meal, or whether they slept well, can provide clues as to the timing of the onset of pain. Children may have the onset of pain during sleep and then give the misleading history that the pain began when 'they woke up', when in fact it may have started 6–8 h earlier. Diagnostic confusion may occur during the onset of the pain resulting from visceral distension of the appendix. This occurs because the pain is often poorly located and mimics other more common sources of abdominal pain. The transition of pain which is diffuse to a localized pain raises the concern for appendicitis. The source of confusion in the diagnosis of appendicitis when the pain is localized results from the variability of the location of the appendix. A pelvic or retrocecal appendix may not manifest the same degree of 'anterior' peritoneal signs and mislead the clinician. These are the situations where CT scanning and ultrasound provide the greatest importance in distinguishing the pain from nonoperative conditions such as gastroenteritis and ovarian cysts. While it is often difficult to make the diagnosis within the first 12 h, it is also unlikely that perforation will occur within this time period. Most perforations will occur greater than 24 h after the onset of symptoms.[2,18,19] Symptoms that last >40 h are suggestive of complicated appendicitis.

Appendicitis in infants presents its own set of unique difficulties. There is often a delay in diagnosis and a resultant increase in the incidence of perforation and morbidity and mortality. While it is often difficult for parents to appreciate pain in an infant, most babies will present with vomiting and a fever. Irritability, lethargy and anorexia are also common symptoms noted by parents. A physical exam will usually reveal abdominal tenderness, either diffuse or localized to the right lower quadrant. Since there is usually a prolonged time interval between the onset of symptoms and the time of diagnosis, most infants will have a perforated appendicitis. In addition, they have a diminished ability to contain the infection once perforation has occurred and will more frequently develop generalized peritonitis.[18–22]

PHYSICAL EXAM

A low-grade fever is often present early in the process and worsens as the illness progresses. The most consistent physical finding with acute appendicitis is abdominal tenderness. The child will usually lie still on the table, resist examination and guard their abdomen. As mentioned, the usual point of maximal tenderness is McBurney's point in the right lower quadrant. Muscle spasm and involuntary guarding is common. Pain that occurs with specific maneuvers has been described. Rovsing's sign is positive when palpation of the left lower quadrant causes pain in the right lower quadrant. The psoas sign is positive when extension of the right hip causes pain. The obturator sign is pain with internal rotation of the flexed right thigh.

A rectal examination can be an important component of the physical exam in a patient with acute appendicitis. If the appendix is located in the pelvis, the abdominal exam may lack the symptoms mentioned above and transrectal palpation of the right pelvic sidewall may elicit focal pain.

As mentioned, a variation of the location of the appendix can lead to localized pain in the right upper quadrant, the right flank, or the suprapubic area. Pain may even occur in the epigastrium or the left lower quadrant in a child with malrotation or situs inversus.

DIAGNOSTIC TESTS

The most reliable test for acute appendicitis is the history and physical exam. However, laboratory studies and diagnostic imaging can clarify or confirm the diagnosis. A number of serum studies have been analyzed for their utility in diagnosing acute appendicitis; however most have been found to have a limited role in clinical practice. The C-reactive protein (CRP) is an acute phase protein synthesized in the liver in response to inflammation. While some studies have concluded that CRP has some diagnostic value, it is typically in conjunction with a white blood cell count. In fact, other studies have shown no benefit compared with using the leukocyte count alone.[23,24] Usually, the white blood count (WBC) is slightly elevated with a left shift.[25] The sensitivity is only about 80%, however, as up to 20% of patients with acute appendicitis may have a normal WBC as well as a normal CRP.[26,27] Similar to the CRP, the erythrocyte sedimentation rate has been examined and found to have limited clinical utility.[27,28]

The urinalysis may be helpful to clarify cases where a urinary tract infection may be suspected; although if the appendix is close to the ureter or bladder, the inflammation can cause elevation of the RBC and WBC in the urine. Bacteriuria will not be present in acute appendicitis and its presence should suggest a urinary tract infection. A urine pregnancy test should be done in all adolescent females.

Imaging studies can be especially useful in equivocal cases of abdominal pain. Abdominal radiographs may identify a calcified fecalith in the appendiceal lumen, corresponding to the area of maximal tenderness. Other abdominal X-ray findings suggestive of appendicitis correspond to a right lower quadrant ileus, such as dilated loops of bowel with air fluid levels or a paucity of gas in the right lower quadrant. One might also see a scoliosis of the spine with the concavity towards the right. It is unusual to see intraperitoneal free air even in the case of appendiceal rupture.

Computerized tomography (CT) is a highly accurate and effective imaging technique for diagnosing acute appendicitis. The sensitivity of helical CT has been reported to be 90–100%, with a specificity of 91–99%, a positive predictive value of 92–98% and a negative predictive value of 95–100%.[29] Typical appendiceal CT protocols include 5-mm sectioning with both intravenous and oral contrast agents, particularly in children.[30] Intravenous contrast material helps to identify the inflamed appendix, which is especially helpful in those patients with mild appendicitis and a paucity of mesenteric fat. Oral contrast material opacifying the terminal ileum and cecum helps to avoid mistaking fluid-filled terminal ileal loops for the appendix. Furthermore, opacification of a normal appendix helps to exclude a diagnosis of appendicitis.

A CT diagnosis of acute appendicitis is clear in those cases where an abnormal appendix can be identified or if a calcified appendicolith is found in the setting of pericecal inflammation. (Fig. 44.1) In cases of mild appendicitis where a CT is obtained early in the disease process, the findings can be more subtle. The appendix may be minimally distended and seen as a fluid-filled tubular structure surrounded by homogeneous-appearing mesenteric fat. Most patients will have more distension of the appendiceal lumen with circumferential and symmetric appendiceal wall thickening. Most patients will also have periappendiceal inflammation with linear fat stranding and a clouding appearance to the mesentery. Often, focal cecal apical thickening can also be found as well as the 'arrowhead sign' of cecal contrast material funneling symmetrically to the cecal apex at the point of appendiceal occlusion. Perforated appendicitis can be associated with a pericecal phlegmon or abscess, easily seen on CT. Other findings seen with a perforated appendix are extraluminal free air, significant ileocecal thickening and localized lymphadenopathy.[29,31]

As technology has improved, along with radiologic experience, ultrasound has become a useful diagnostic tool that is both quick and inexpensive. Although the success of this modality is operator-dependent, the sensitivity has been reported to be 75–90%, with a specificity of 86–100%, a positive predictive value of 91–94% and a negative predictive value of 89–97%.[29] The inflamed appendix can often be visualized as an immobile, blind-ending tubular structure that is dilated with a thickened wall. There is loss of wall compressibility as well as increased echogenicity of the surrounding fat. (Fig. 44.2) Circumferential color in the appendiceal wall on Doppler images is strongly indicative of active inflammation. Appendicoliths are seen as bright, echogenic foci with acoustic shadowing. If the appendix has ruptured, it will be decompressed and may not be visualized[31]; however periappendiceal signs can still be seen. Inflamed fat can appear as an echogenic mass, with the hyperemia seen on color Doppler. A periappendiceal fluid collection may be found. Gas bubbles within the fluid collection suggest perforation or gas-forming organisms.

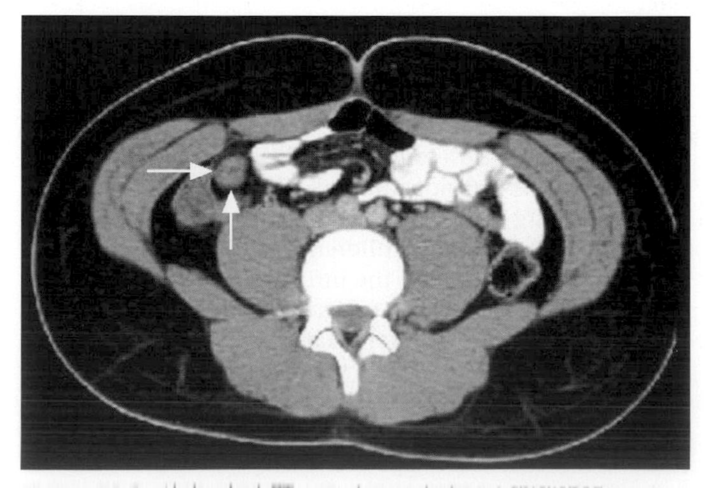

Figure 44.1: Abdominal CT scan demonstrating a thickened appendix (arrow) adjacent to the cecum.

The role of a radiolabeled white blood cell scan is perhaps less clear than that of CT and ultrasound. The literature reports a sensitivity of 79–97%, a specificity of 80–94%, a positive predictive value of 88–93% and a negative predictive value of 71–98%.[32–34]

This imaging test requires an intravenous injection of technetium-labeled white blood cells and serial abdominal scans with a gamma camera. The availability and logistical difficulty of this test limit its utility, leaving ultrasound and CT as the preferred diagnostic imaging modalities.

The choice of ultrasound or CT is often institutionally dependent, as the accuracy of ultrasound is somewhat operator-dependent unlike CT.[29,31,35] Ultrasound offers the advantage of being fast, noninvasive, inexpensive and uses no ionizing radiation. It also has the advantage of not requiring any patient preparation or use of intravenous or oral contrast. For these reasons, ultrasound is often the first choice in children.

DIFFERENTIAL DIAGNOSIS

The clinical presentation of appendicitis can mimic many different conditions (Table 44.2); conversely, many different conditions can present like appendicitis. Laboratory studies and radiologic imaging can aid in making the diagnosis.

Acute gastroenteritis is a frequent cause of abdominal pain. Typically, the child will have vomiting and diarrhea, fever and generalized abdominal pain. These symptoms are usually self-limited and resolve within 48 h. The pattern of diarrhea helps distinguish gastroenteritis from appendicitis. Children with gastroenteritis have watery diarrhea early in their illness. Diarrhea associated with perforated appendicitis presents at least 3–4 days after the onset of illness and is attributed to the effects of pelvic inflammation on the sigmoid colon.

Mesenteric adenitis is often indistinguishable from acute appendicitis. This enlargement of the terminal ileal mesenteric nodes usually occurs with an upper respiratory infection, causing pain and often fever and nausea. This diagnosis may only be made after other conditions are excluded and may require a negative appendectomy. A CT scan may show significant adenopathy in the absence of appendiceal inflammation.

Gynecologic conditions must be included in the differential diagnosis of appendicitis. The typical female patient with a tubo-ovarian abscess has had multiple sex partners and often has a history of recurrent episodes of pelvic pain. She will have cervical tenderness on pelvic examination, often with vaginal discharge and adnexal enlargement. Lower abdominal pain may also occur with an ovarian cyst that is either ruptured or hemorrhagic. Torsion of an ovary, ovarian cyst, or ovarian tumor will also cause acute intense pain. An ectopic pregnancy must be considered in any female after menarche. The classic presentation is abdominal pain, vaginal bleeding and amenorrhea and the diagnosis can be made with a pregnancy test and ultrasound.

Meckel's diverticulitis may be impossible to differentiate from acute appendicitis. Operative exploration is usually

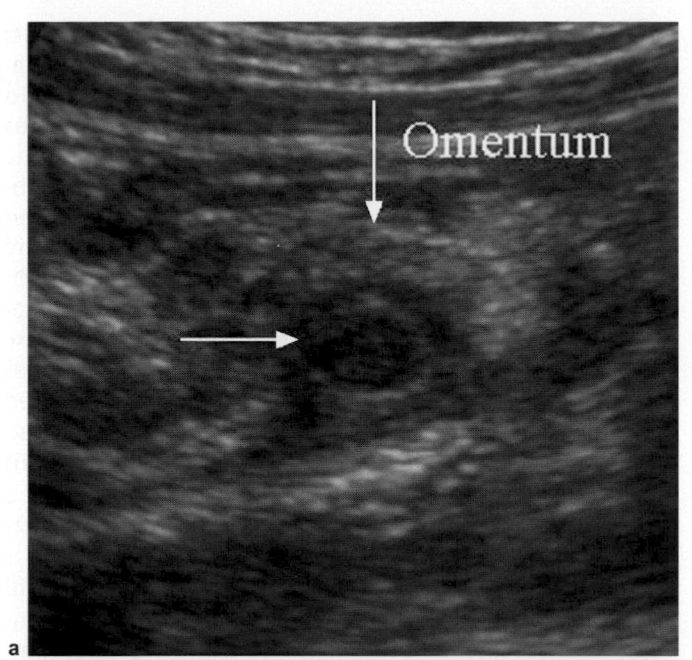

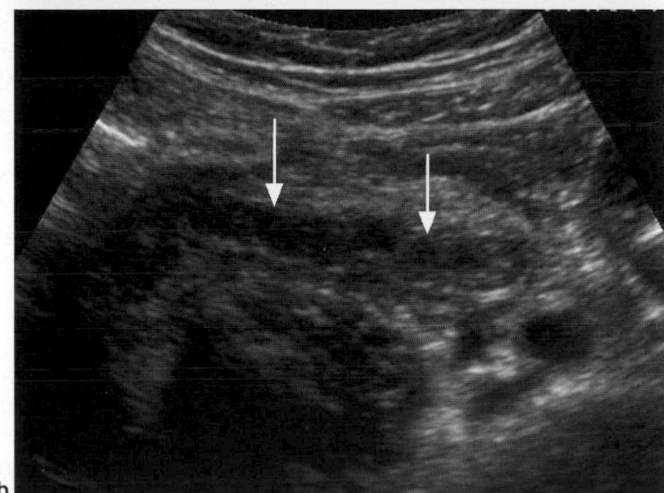

Figure 44.2: (a) Abdominal sonogram demonstrating a thickened appendix (arrows) surrounded by omentum. (b) Abdominal sonogram demonstrating a non-compressible appendix.

Infant
Abdominal trauma – child abuse
Gastroenteritis
Intussusception
Pneumonia
Urinary tract infection
Meckel's diverticulitis
Child
Constipation
Gastroenteritis
Henoch Schönlein purpura
Hemolytic uremic syndrome
Meckel's diverticulitis
Mesenteric adenitis
Omental torsion
Ovarian torsion
Pneumonia
Urinary tract infection
Crohn's disease
Adolescent
Constipation
Crohn's disease
Gastroenteritis
Meckel's diverticulitis
Mesenteric adenitis
Mittelschmerz
Omental torsion
Ovarian cyst rupture
Urinary tract infection

Table 44.2 Differential diagnosis of appendicitis

indicated in either condition and preoperative distinction is unnecessary.

Idiopathic intussusception (no pathologic lead point) typically occurs in children under 2 years old and often follows a viral illness that causes enlargement of the lymphoid tissue in the distal ileum (Peyer's patches). The majority of patients over 5 years old with intussusception have a pathologic lead point. This condition typically presents in a healthy-appearing infant with attacks of sudden abdominal pain. The child appears normal between these attacks but will usually pass a bloody stool. Physical examination may reveal a sausage-shaped mass in the right lower quadrant of the abdomen. The diagnosis and often successful treatment, can be accomplished with a radiologic reduction (hydrostatic or pneumatic enema).

Several common medical conditions may also present in a fashion similar to acute appendicitis. Constipation can present with abdominal pain, vomiting and fever. Abdominal plain films can suggest this diagnosis. A right lower lobe pneumonia may also cause right lower quadrant abdominal pain. The typical patient would also have symptoms of coughing, tachypnea and pleuritic chest pain, as well as a fever and leukocytosis. A chest radiograph would confirm this diagnosis. A urinary tract infection can cause lower abdominal pain, fever and dysuria. Laboratory studies may reveal a leukocytosis and a urinalysis is key to making this diagnosis.

Henoch-Schönlein purpura may also cause severe abdominal pain. This syndrome typically occurs several weeks after a streptococcal or viral infection. Usually the child will also have joint pains, purpura and occasionally, nephritis.

Crohn's disease can present in children and adolescents and mimic appendicitis. The most common location of disease involves the terminal ileum. There is usually a history of weight loss, fever and possibly vomiting and diarrhea. Abdominal pain may occur in the right lower quadrant or periumbilical location. While careful history usually reveals more chronic symptoms, occasional patients present with an acute picture.

TREATMENT

The treatment of choice for uncomplicated acute appendicitis is an appendectomy, either open or laparoscopic.[36,37] If an open approach is chosen, a right lower quadrant incision is typically used with specific placement adjusted to the point of maximal tenderness. A muscle-splitting technique usually allows adequate exposure for removal of the appendix. A digital exploration is used to palpate and locate the appendix, which is then delivered through the wound and removed. If a normal-appearing appendix is found, an appendectomy should still be performed. A search should then be made for a Meckel's diverticulum or terminal ileitis, as well as for any gynecologic pathology. This effort may require extending the incision to allow adequate visualization or palpation.

Kurt Semm, a gynecologist from Switzerland, described the first laparoscopic appendectomy in 1980. Since that time, improvements in technology have increased the popularity of this approach, but some debate still exists over the benefits of the laparoscopic approach *vs* the standard open technique. Proponents of the laparoscopic technique report a decreased incidence of wound infection, less postoperative pain, a faster recovery time and an improved cosmetic result. Another benefit, perhaps even more convincing, is the greater visualization of the abdominal cavity. This can be particularly helpful in those patients in whom the diagnosis is uncertain. In this situation, laparoscopy offers an advantage both diagnostically and therapeutically, as other surgical conditions may be addressed at the time of operation. Those who favor the open approach argue that laparoscopy results in longer operative times and more expensive operative equipment with minimal difference in outcomes. A recent review of randomized trials comparing the open and laparoscopic techniques in the adult population addressed many of these issues.[37] While there were studies demonstrating a longer operative time with the laparoscopic approach, there were also studies showing no difference. There seemed to be a trend towards no difference in operative time in the later studies, perhaps reflecting the learning curve of laparoscopy. Using narcotic use as a measurement of postoperative pain, the laparoscopic approach was superior to the open technique; however the length of hospital stay did not appear to be significantly different between the two groups and the hospital cost of laparoscopy was significantly higher compared with the open approach. While the incidence of local wound infections was lower in the laparoscopic groups, there were studies that showed an increased risk of intra-abdominal abscess formation with laparoscopy as well as studies that demonstrated no difference in the rate of intra-abdominal complications. In summary, there is no clearly superior method of approaching the appendectomy and the choice of performing a laparoscopic appendectomy *vs* an open appendectomy should be based upon the surgeon's experience and preference.

In patients who present with perforated appendicitis, the appropriate management is more controversial. There has been a growing trend of treating nontoxic patients with antibiotics, intravenous fluids and possible percutaneous drainage followed by an interval appendectomy in an elective setting.[38–43] The option of percutaneous drainage of an abscess is relatively new and has become feasible with the evolution of ultrasonographic or computed tomographic guidance. There is even controversy in the literature about whether an interval appendectomy after initial nonoperative management is necessary.[38,44–46]

All patients with acute appendicitis should receive preoperative antibiotics. This has been shown to decrease both the complication rate as well as mortality.[18] The two organisms most commonly isolated from perforated appendicitis are *Esherichia coli* and *Bacteroides fragilis*, so both aerobic and anaerobic coverage must be used. In uncomplicated appendicitis, single-drug therapy with a second-generation cephalosporin that has anaerobic coverage (e.g. cefotetan) or with piperacillin tazobactam is appropriate. In complicated cases, most institutions will use a combination of ampicillin, gentamicin and clindamycin in order to provide coverage of enterococcus, Gram-negative rods and anaerobic organisms.

Many institutions use treatment algorithms to determine length of antibiotic treatment as well as hospital stay in the postoperative management of appendicitis, particularly complicated appendicitis. These algorithms can be adjusted based on the patient's clinical response (i.e. physical exam, fever curve and white blood cell count). Such treatment courses have helped to shorten hospital stay while maintaining good clinical outcomes.[47]

COMPLICATIONS

The most common postoperative complication after an appendectomy is a wound infection. This typically presents with pain, erythema and fluctuance or drainage from the wound and usually requires opening the wound to allow adequate drainage. In cases of simple appendicitis, the wound infection rate is approximately 3%. This incidence is higher with complicated appendicitis (6–8%).

An intra-abdominal abscess typically occurs in the setting of complicated appendicitis, with an incidence of up to 20% reported in the literature. The use of antibiotics has dramatically reduced the incidence of this complication. The abscesses usually occur in the pelvis, but can occur anywhere within the abdomen. This complication must be considered with a persistent fever and/or leukocytosis. A rectal examination may reveal a fluctuant mass. A CT scan of the abdomen and pelvis should be obtained to confirm the diagnosis. Treatment consists of drainage, most often performed percutaneously by the interventional radiologist, as well as intravenous antibiotics.

A small bowel obstruction may also occur due to adhesion formation, with a higher incidence in patients with complicated appendicitis. While this complication can sometimes be managed non-operatively with nasogastric suction, bowel rest and fluid replacement, operative intervention may be necessary.

CHRONIC APPENDICEAL PAIN

Chronic appendiceal pain may be due to one of three different etiologies. Long-term appendiceal pain is referred to as chronic appendicitis. The histologic implication of this term, however, includes an infiltration of the appendix with chronic inflammatory cells.[48] Recurrent appendicitis occurs after an episode of low-grade appendicitis that spontaneously resolves, leaving an area of fibrosis and narrowing of the appendiceal lumen, which predisposes the patient to another episode. Appendiceal colic is due to a partial or intermittent obstruction of the appendiceal lumen. This obstruction is typically associated with an underlying pathology causing narrowing of the lumen. This pathology is usually fibrosis, but may include lymphoid hyperplasia or carcinoid tumors. The spasm of the obstructed appendix produces the symptoms, which are relieved with extrusion of the obstructing material until the next episode. The frequency, severity and duration of these episodes are quite variable. A physical exam performed during an episode of appendiceal colic will help to confirm the diagnosis, as the patient will be reproducibly tender over the location of the appendix. If the patient is examined between episodes, the physical exam may be unremarkable and should be re-examined during a symptomatic episode.

Imaging and laboratory studies are helpful to rule out other causes for pain, but are often normal in the setting of appendiceal colic. This entity remains a clinical diagnosis and often the best course of action is to proceed with a diagnostic laparoscopy or laparotomy and appendectomy.[49,50]

References

1. Addiss DG, Shaffer N, Fowler BS, Tauxe RV. The epidemiology of appendicitis and appendectomy in the United States. Am J Epidemiol 1990; 132(5):910–925.
2. Stevenson RJ. Appendicitis. In: Ziegler MM, Azizkhan RG, Weber TR, eds. Operative Pediatric Surgery. New York, NY: McGraw-Hill; 2003:671–689.
3. Corman ML. Classic articles in colonic and rectal surgery, Charles Heber McBurney. Dis Colon Rectum 26(4):291–303.
4. Rutkow IM. American Surgery: An Illustrated History. Philadelphia, PA: Lippincott-Raven; 1998:236–237, 402–403.
5. Appendicitis SA. A Historical Review. Can J Surg 1981; 24(4):427–433.
6. Garis CF De. Topography and development of the cecum-appendix. Ann Surg 1939; 113(4):540–548.
7. Skandalakis LJ, Gray SW, Ricketts R, Skandalakis JE. The colon and rectum. In: Skandalakis JE, Gray SW, eds. Embryology for Surgeons. Baltimore, MD: Williams & Wilkins; 1994:244–245, 274–277.
8. Melier F. Memoire et observations sur quelques maladies de l'appenice caecale. J Gen Med Chir Pharm Paris 100(1827):317–345.
9. Treves F. The anatomy of the intestinal canal and peritoneum in man. Br Med J 1885; 1:415–419, 470–474, 527–530, 580–583.
10. Wakeley CPG. The position of the vermiform appendix as ascertained by an analysis of 10,000 cases. J Anat 1933; 67:277–283.
11. Maisel H. The position of the human vermiform appendix in fetal and adult age groups. Anat Rec 1960; 1960(136):385–389.
12. Wangensteen OH, Dennis C. Experimental proof of the origin of appendicitis in man. Ann Surg 1939; 110:629–647.
13. Wangensteen OH, Bowers WF. Significance of the obstructive factor in the genesis of acute appendicitis: An experimental study. Arch Surg 1935; 34:496–526.
14. Marchildon MB, Dudgeon DL. Perforated appendicitis: Current experience in a children's hospital. Ann Surg 1977; 186(1):84–87.
15. Roberts JP. Quantitative bacterial flora of acute appendicitis. Arch Dis Child 1988; 63(5):536–540.
16. Petras RE, Goldblum JR. Appendix. In: Damjanov I, Linder J, eds. Anderson's Pathology, 10th edn. St Louis, MO: Mosby; 1996:1728–1740.
17. Guo G, Greenson JK. Histopathology of interval (delayed) appendectomy specimens: strong association with granulomatous and xanthogranulomatous appendicitis. Am J Surg Pathol 2003; 27(8):1147–1151.
18. Foster JH, Edwards WH. Acute appendicitis in infancy and childhood: A twenty-year study in a general hospital. Ann Surg 1957; 146(1):70–77.
19. Graham JM, Pokorny WJ, Harberg FJ. Acute appendicitis in preschool age children. Am J Surg 1980; 139(2):247–250.
20. Bartlett RH, Eraklis AJ, Wilkinson RH. Appendicitis in infancy. Surgery. Gynecol Obstet 1970; 130(1):99–104.
21. Grosfeld JL, Weinberger M, Clatworthy HW Jr. Acute appendicitis in the first two years of life. J Pediatr Surg 1973; 8(2):285–293.
22. Janik JS, Firor HV. Pediatric appendicitis: A 20-year study of 1,640 children at Cook County (Illinois) Hospital. Arch Surg 1979; 114(6):717–719.
23. Kessler N, Cyteval C, Gallix B, et al. Appendicitis: evaluation of sensitivity, specificity and predictive values of US, Doppler US and laboratory findings. Radiology 2004; 230(2):472–478.
24. Rodríguez-Sanjuán JC, Martín-Parra JI, Seco I, et al. C-reactive protein and leukocyte count in the diagnosis of acute appendicitis in children. Dis Colon Rectum 1999; 42(10):1325–1329.
25. Bower RJ, Bell MJ, Ternberg JL. Diagnostic value of the white blood count and neutrophil percentage in the evaluation of abdominal pain in children. Surgery. Gynecol Obstet 1981; 152(4):424–426.
26. Gronroos JM. Do normal leucocyte count and C-reactive protein value exclude acute appendicitis in children? Acta Paediatr 2001; 90(6):649–651.
27. Amland PF, Skaane P, Ronningen H, et al. Ultrasonography and parameters of inflammation in acute appendicitis. A comparison with clinical findings. Acta Chir Scand 1989; 155(3):185–189.
28. Dieijen-Visser MP van, Go PM, Brombacher PJ. The value of laboratory tests in patients suspected of acute appendicitis. Eur J Clin Chem Clin Biochem 1991; 29(11):749–752.
29. Birnbaum BA, Wilson SR. Appendicitis at the millennium. Radiology 2000; 215(2):337–348.
30. Friedland JA, Siegel MJ. CT appearance of acute appendicitis in childhood. Am J Roentgenol 1997; 168:439–442.
31. Teo ELHJ, Tan KPAA, Lam SL, et al. Ultrasonography and computed tomography in a clinical algorithm for the evaluation of suspected acute appendicitis in children. Singapore Med J 2000; 41(8):387–392.
32. Chang CC, Tsai CY, Lin CC, et al. Comparison between technetium-99m hexamethylpropylenamineoxide labeled white blood cell abdomen scan and abdominal sonography to

detect appendicitis in children with an atypical clinical presentation. Hepatogastroenterology 2003; 50(50):426–429.
33. Turan C, Tutus A, Ozokutan BH, et al. The evaluation of technetium 99m-citrate scintigraphy in children with suspected appendicitis. J Pediatr Surg 1999; 34(8):1272–1275.
34. Yan DC, Shiau YC, Wang JJ, et al. Improving the diagnosis of acute appendicitis in children with atypical clinical findings using the technetium-99m hexamethylpropylene amine oxime-labelled white-blood-cell abdomen scan. Pediatr Radiol 2002; 32(9):663–666.
35. Zielke A, Hasse C, Sitter H, Rothmund M. Influence of ultrasound on clinical decision making in acute appendicitis: A prospective study. Eur J Surg 1998; 164(3):201–209.
36. Blakely ML, Spurbeck WW, Lobe TE. Current status of laparoscopic appendectomy in children. Semin Pediatr Surg 1998; 7(4):225–227.
37. Fischer CP, Castaneda A, Moore F. Laparoscopic appendectomy: Indications and controversies. Semin laparoscopic Surg 2002; 9(1):32–39.
38. Brown CVR, Abrishami M, Muller M, Velmahos GC. Appendiceal abscess: Immediate operation or percutaneous drainage? Am Surg 2003; 69(10):829–832.
39. Bufo AJ, Shah RS, Li MH, et al. Interval appendectomy for perforated appendicitis in children. Journal Laparoendoscopic Adv Surg Tech 1998; 8(4):209–213.
40. Mazziotti MV, Marley EF, Winthrop AL, et al. Histopathologic analysis of interval appendectomy specimens: Support for the role of interval appendectomy. J Pediatr Surg 1997; 32(6):806–809.
41. Powers RJ, Andrassy RJ, Brennan LP, Weitzman JJ. Alternate approach to the management of acute perforating appendicitis in children. Surg Gynecol Obstet 1981; 152(4):473–475.
42. Samuel M, Hosie G, Holmes K. Prospective evaluation of nonsurgical versus surgical management of appendiceal mass. J Pediatr Surg 2002; 37(6):882–886.
43. Yamini D, Vargas H, Bongard F, et al. Perforated appendicitis: Is it truly a surgical urgency? Am Surg 1998; 64(10):970–975.
44. Ein SH, Shandling B. Is interval appendectomy necessary after rupture of an appendiceal mass? J Pediatr Surg 1996; 31(6):849–850.
45. Friedell ML, Perez-Izquierdo M. Is there a role for interval appendectomy in the management of acute appendicitis? Am Surg 2000; 66(12):1158–1162.
46. Willemsen PJ, Hoorntje LE, Eddes EH, Ploeg RJ. The need for interval appendectomy after resolution of an appendiceal mass questioned. Dig Surg 2002; 19:216–222.
47. Keller MS, McBride WJ, Vane DW. Management of complicated appendicitis: A rational approach based on a clinical course. Arch Surg 1996; 131(3):261–264.
48. Falk S, Schutze U, Guth H, Stutte HJ. Chronic recurrent appendicitis. A clinicopathologic study of 47 cases. Eur J Pediatr Surg 1991; 1(5):277–281.
49. Gorenstein A, Serour F, Katz R, Usviatsov I. Appendiceal colic in children: A true clinical entity? J Am Coll Surg 1996; 182(3):246–250.
50. Stevenson RJ. Chronic right-lower-quadrant abdominal pain: Is there a role for elective appendectomy? J Pediatr Surg 1999; 34(6):950–954.

Chapter 45
Intussusception in infants and children

David K. Magnuson

INTRODUCTION

Intussusception is a curious anatomic condition characterized by the invagination of one segment of the gastrointestinal tract into the lumen of an adjacent segment. Once initiated, additional intestine telescopes into the distal segment, causing the invaginated intestine to propagate distally within the bowel lumen. This advancing tube of proximal intestine is referred to as the *intussusceptum*, and the distal recipient intestine is referred to as the *intussuscipiens*.

Although any segment of the infradiaphragmatic gastrointestinal tract may be involved, more than 80% of cases in infants and children involve invagination of the ileocecal valve or terminal ileum into the right colon – an *ileocolic* intussusception. The intussusceptum usually extends no further than the hepatic flexure or proximal transverse colon, although rarely it may advance to the rectum and even extrude through the anus. Isolated small intestinal (enteroenteric, jejunoileal and ileoileal) and colocolonic intussusceptions also occur, although much less commonly. Gastroduodenal intussusceptions have been reported, usually in association with placement of a gastrostomy tube or duodenal polyps, but are exceedingly rare.[1]

Whatever the location and extent, the great majority of intussusceptions result in two distinct but related clinical problems: complete obstruction of the intestinal tract proximal to the intussusception, and the progressive vascular compromise and eventual infarction of the intussusceptum. These two factors are largely responsible for the morbidity, and occasional mortality, associated with intussusception. Diagnostic and therapeutic measures must be approached with a sense of urgency as the pathophysiologic consequences of intestinal obstruction and ischemia may progress rapidly in infants and children.

PATHOPHYSIOLOGY

The pathogenesis of intussusception is not precisely known, but is believed to be related to unbalanced forces created when a normal wave of peristaltic contraction encounters a focal structural abnormality in the intestinal wall. In some cases, the structural abnormality is clearly definable and is referred to as a `lead point'. When present, this lead point is always found at the apex of the intussusceptum and is therefore presumed to have had a causative role in the initiation of the process. Early theories proposed that the lead point projected into the peristaltic stream and was simply pulled downstream, dragging the intestinal wall along with it. However, this hypothesis did little to explain the vast majority of cases in which no pathologic lead point could be identified. In these instances of 'idiopathic' intussusception, lymphoid hyperplasia within the intestinal wall is thought to produce the functional equivalent of a pathologic lead point. This hypothesis is supported by the observation that the vast majority of idiopathic intussusceptions are ileocolic in distribution and that the terminal ileum is the richest repository of gut-associated lymphoid tissue (GALT) within the gastrointestinal tract. When a peristaltic wave encounters an area of intestinal wall with different mechanical properties due to lymphoid hyperplasia (or a pathologic lead point), the imbalance of contractile forces causes the wall to kink or buckle, creating an infolding of the wall that extends radially around the bowel wall until the entire circumference is involved. This invaginated rim of intestinal wall initiates the intussusception and becomes its apex, and distal propagation requires elongation of the intussusceptum by the infolding of additional bowel both proximal and distal to the point of origination.[2]

One advantage of this model is that the proposed mechanism satisfactorily explains the occurrence of intussusception in certain disease states that are not associated with definable lead points or lymphoid hyperplasia. Among these are postoperative intussusception and intusussception occurring in patients with cystic fibrosis. In postoperative intussusception, the resumption of peristaltic activity after a period of paralytic ileus results in the juxtaposition of contracting and non-contracting regions of the intestine where peristaltic waves meet flaccid, unresponsive bowel. In cystic fibrosis with mucoviscidosis, inspissated putty-like secretions adhere to the intestinal wall and alter its mechanical properties, resulting in a focal area of altered compliance and elasticity. Intussusception has also been reported in other conditions characterized by purely functional disturbances in intestinal muscular contraction. An association between neonatal intussusception and severe cerebral hypoxia suggests that altered gut peristalsis resulting from altered central nervous system function may be sufficient to produce intussusception in some patients.[3] Enteroenteric intussusception has also been documented surgically in a child with major burn injury and no pathologic lead point or identifiable lymphoid hyperplasia, suggesting that extreme physiologic stress alone may be a risk factor for intussusception in certain patients.[4]

Once the intussusceptum begins to advance distally, its mesentery is pulled along as well. The mesenteric vascular supply to the intussusceptum is acutely angulated and compressed at the point where it enters the intussuscipiens. Initially, this results in venous outflow obstruction and leads to venous congestion and edema of the intussusceptum, exacerbating the compressive pressures and generating a vicious cycle of venous hypertension, swelling and ischemia. Progressive injury to the bowel results in loss of barrier function, leading to endotoxemia and the development of a systemic inflammatory state characterized by increased levels of circulating cytokines.[5] Eventually, arterial inflow is also compromised, and infarction of the apex of the intussusceptum supervenes. The ischemic mucosa sloughs, leading to the passage of blood, desquamated epithelium and mucus, often described as `currant jelly stools'. If uncorrected, ischemic necrosis extends to the entire intussusceptum and intussuscipiens, culminating in perforation and peritonitis. Furthermore, the pathologic events taking place in the intussusception are superimposed on the effects of a complete bowel obstruction, including fluid sequestration, dehydration and electrolyte disturbances.

Although this sequence of events consistently applies to the common ileocolic intussusceptions, other types of intussusception may have a different natural history. Isolated small-intestinal intussusceptions may indeed progress to infarction, perforation and peritonitis. However, the increased use of ultrasonography and computed tomography (CT) has led to the recognition that many small intestinal intussusceptions are asymptomatic and reduce spontaneously.[6] Fetal intussusception can now be detected on prenatal ultrasonography, and has recently been proposed to explain some cases of jejunoileal atresia in neonates.[7,8] The infarction of the intussusception in the sterile *in utero* environment is thought to result in the resorption of the involved intestine instead of necrosis and perforation, leaving an atretic segment and mesenteric defect. In spite of the sterile environment, perforation and meconium peritonitis can also accompany intussusception in the fetus.[9]

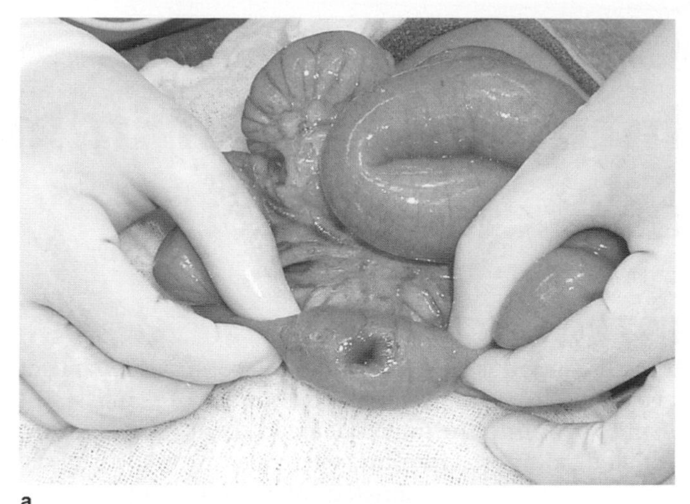

a

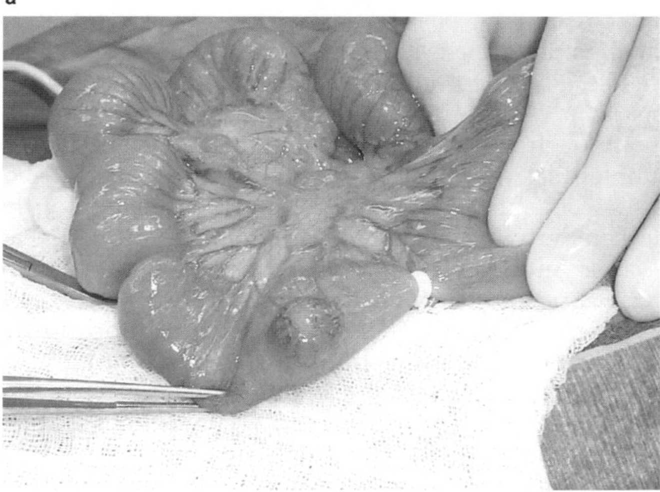

b

Figure 45.1: Surgically reduced ileocolic intussusception secondary to Meckel's diverticulum as lead point. (**a**) Inverted diverticulum as lead point. (**b**) Everted diverticulum in normal orientation (See plate section for color).

ETIOLOGY

Overall, only 10% of intussusceptions in children are associated with a pathologic lead point.[10,11] The actual incidence of lead points varies with age. In infants and toddlers below the age of 2 years, lead points can be identified in fewer than 4% of cases.[12] Above the age of 2 years, lead points are found in as many as one-third of patients; above 4 years, the reported incidence is as high as 57%.[13] The likelihood of finding a causative lead point continues to increase with age, exceeding 90% in adults.[14] In 90% of children, however, no structural abnormality can be found and the etiology has long been presumed to be related to lymphoid hyperplasia.[15,16] No bacterial or viral agent has been implicated consistently as a causative factor in this disease, although multiple reports of intussusception in infants following administration of tetravalent rhesus-human rotavirus vaccine ultimately forced its withdrawal from the market.[17]

The most common pathologic lead point in children of all ages is a Meckel's diverticulum (Fig. 45.1).[12,18,19] Almost any process that results in a structural abnormality of the bowel wall has been described as a pathologic lead point (Table 45.1)[19–23] Intestinal duplication cysts, ectopic pancreatic and gastric rests, vascular anomalies, inverted postappendectomy stumps, and anastomotic suture lines have all been implicated as lead points in intussusception. Neoplastic lead points include intestinal polyps, Peutz–Jeghers' hamartomas, carcinoids, leiomyomas and leiomyosarcomas, and lymphomas (particularly Burkitt's lymphoma). Other causes include Crohn's pseudopolyps, post-transplant lymphoproliferative disease, submucosal hemorrhage and foreign bodies.

Two medical conditions commonly associated with intussusception are cystic fibrosis and Henoch–Schönlein purpura (HSP). Approximately 1% of patients with gastrointestinal manifestations of cystic fibrosis will experience at least one episode of intussusception owing to the thick, tenacious secretions that adhere to the intestinal wall. HSP is an autoimmune vasculitis of uncertain etiology that is associated with multifocal hemorrhage due to the loss of vascular endothelial integrity. Among other bleeding sites, HSP results in multiple areas of submucosal hemorrhage within the wall of the small intestine.[24] These

	No. of cases						
Type of lead point	Ref 12	Ref 19	Ref 21	Ref 22	Ref 23	Ref 25	Total (*n* = 179)
Meckel's diverticulum	27	6	14	7	12	7	73 (40.8)
Intestinal polyps	12	2	8	1	8	3	34 (19.0)
Duplication cyst	4	4	5	2	3	1	19 (10.6)
Lymphoma	5	1	1	6	3	1	17 (9.5)
Henoch–Schönlein purpura		2	1		6		9 (5.0)
Massive lymphoid hyperplasia				5	1		6 (3.4)
Cystic fibrosis		2			4		6 (3.4)
Appendiceal disease/mucocele			1	2	2	1	6 (3.4)
Carcinoid	2						2 (1.1)
Ectopic pancreatic tissue				2			2 (1.1)
Neutropenic colitis					2		2 (1.1)
Celiac disease		1					1 (0.6)
Leiomyoma				1			1 (0.6)
Leukemia		1					1 (0.6)

Values in parentheses are percentages.

Table 45.1 Relative incidence of pathologic lead points in childhood intussusception (Reproduced from Navarro O, Daneman A. Intussusception, Part 3: Diagnosis and Management of those with an identifiable predisposing cause and those that reproduce spontaneouly. Pediatr. Radiol 2004; 34(4):305–312 with permission of Springer Science and Media).

areas of intramural hemorrhage may act as lead points for intussusception. Other conditions predisposing to intramural hemorrhage may behave similarly, including idiopathic thrombocytopenic purpura, hemophilia, leukemia and anticoagulation therapy.

CLINICAL PRESENTATION

Intussusception can present at any age, but is typically segregated into three general age ranges: infants and toddlers, older children, and adults. Within the pediatric age group, the vast majority of cases occur in within the first 2 years of life, with a peak incidence between 6 months and 1 year of age.[10] The remainder of cases in the pediatric population are distributed more evenly throughout childhood and adolescence. As described above, the majority of cases within the first 2 years of life are idiopathic and related to lymphoid hyperplasia. Conversely, the majority of cases in patients older than 2 years are associated with a pathologic lead point.[25] There is a slight male predominance. Institutions from different geographic regions report inconsistent seasonal variations, and no pattern emerges when data from these institutions are grouped together.

Children with intussusception present with an acute bowel obstruction. In fact, intussusception ranks as one of the leading causes of mechanical bowel obstruction in younger patients, accounting for more than 50% of cases in some series.[26] Infants with intussusception are usually previously healthy and present with an acute onset of abdominal pain. The pain is typically severe, crampy or colicky, and intermittent. The infant draws up its knees and flexes at the waist during the paroxysms of pain. Pallor and diaphoresis are commonly described. These episodes may last for several minutes, and are separated by variable periods of relief lasting from 30 minutes to several hours. During these quiescent periods, the infant may behave normally, but more often exhibits a significant degree of lethargy and somnolence. This classic pattern of violent, colicky pain alternating with periods of profound lethargy should alert the examiner to the likelihood of intussusception.

Other findings at presentation may include a history of vomiting, the passage of grossly bloody stools with mucus (currant jelly stools), the presence of occult blood on digital rectal examination, and the presence of a palpable abdominal mass. Initially the vomiting is reflexive and non-bilious, but eventually becomes bilious as the mechanical obstruction becomes clinically manifest. The abdominal mass is usually felt in the right upper quadrant and is associated with an `emptiness' in the right lower quadrant. In rare cases, the intussusceptum can be felt on digital rectal examination or may even be seen extruding from the anus, in which case it must be distinguished from a simple rectal prolapse. In prolapse, the dentate line is everted and visible, and there is no groove or sulcus between the anus proper and the intussusceptum. Non-bloody diarrhea, resulting from evacuation of the distal gastrointestinal tract following intussusception but prior to mucosal slough, occurs in 10% of patients.[27] Interpreting the presence of diarrhea as conclusive evidence excluding the possibility of a proximal obstruction (and, therefore, intussusception) is a frequent diagnostic error.

The presence of these various signs and symptoms has been reported to have well defined predictive power.[10] Pain and vomiting each occur in over 80% of cases, a palpable abdominal mass in 55–65%, and occult or gross rectal bleeding in 50–60%. The classic triad of paroxysmal pain, vomiting and passage of currant jelly stools, however, occurs in less than one-third of patients. Some investigators have found that certain combinations of these findings can increase diagnostic accuracy significantly.[28] The combination of pain, vomiting and a palpable right upper quadrant mass has a positive predictive value (PPV) of 93%. The addition of rectal bleeding to this triad increases the PPV to virtually 100%. Some retrospective studies, however, have failed to identify patterns of clinical predictors that have sufficient accuracy to allow for the exclusion of the diagnosis on clinical grounds alone.[29] This apparent discrepancy may be related to the level of examiner expertise and the degree of precision in identifying diagnostic criteria.

The infant with advanced intussusception may present with a more dramatic clinical picture. Obtundation, abdominal distention, peritonitis, dehydration, metabolic acidosis and hypotension may all be present when ischemic infarction of the involved bowel has occurred. Clearly, these patients require nasogastric decompression, systemic antibiotics, aggressive resuscitation, correction of electrolyte and acid–base abnormalities, and possibly airway control and ventilatory support concurrent with an expeditious diagnostic evaluation. The rare occurrence of intussusception in the premature neonate is usually misdiagnosed as complicated necrotizing enterocolitis, the correct diagnosis usually being made only at laparotomy. Most of these patients do not have pathologic lead points yet require resection for advanced disease.[30]

DIAGNOSTIC WORK-UP

Most infants and children presenting with acute abdominal complaints undergo plain abdominal radiography, which may demonstrate several helpful findings in the child with intussusception. The presence of a soft-tissue mass in the right upper quadrant or epigastrum is essentially pathognomonic for intussusception in an infant with clinical features suggesting the diagnosis, and is present in 25–60% of cases (Fig. 45.2).[31] This is particularly true if the soft tissue mass exhibits the characteristic appearance of two concentric circles of soft tissue density representing the intussusceptum and intussuscipiens respectively. Other indirect signs such as a paucity of gas in the right iliac fossa are not sufficiently reliable to be of much help in further directing the work-up (Fig. 45.3). Occasionally, the only plain radiographic finding is a bowel gas pattern suggesting a small bowel obstruction. In all infants and children with radiographic evidence of a mechanical small bowel obstruction, the differential diagnosis must include intussusception.

Usually, physical examination and plain radiography alone are insufficient to establish the diagnosis of intussusception with sufficient precision to proceed with a specific management plan. Definitive diagnostic studies include non-invasive modalities such as ultrasonography and CT; invasive studies such as contrast enema are highly accurate and may also be therapeutic. The decision to evaluate a child by non-invasive means prior to contrast enema must be based on certain considerations. If the diagnosis of intussusception is strongly suspected on the basis of rigorous diagnostic criteria and the child is an acceptable candidate for non-operative treatment, proceeding directly to contrast enema without prior ultrasonography or CT is a

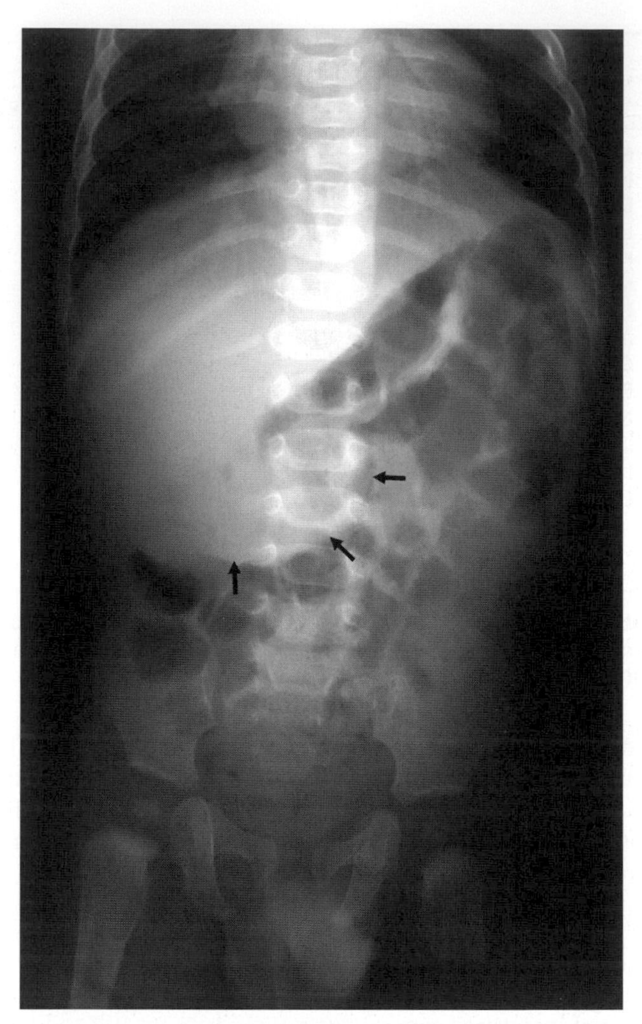

Figure 45.2: Plain abdominal radiograph demonstrating a soft tissue mass in the right upper quadrant. (From Vasavada P, 2004, with permission.)[79]

reasonable approach and eliminates the delay caused by multiple imaging studies. Alternatively, if the diagnosis is less certain, or if certain features of the presentation make surgical intervention preferable in the event that the diagnosis of intussusception is confirmed, non-invasive screening can decrease the expense, discomfort and exposure to radiation associated with unnecessary contrast enemas in a large number of children.[32] Retrospective studies document that more than 60% of children suspected of having intussusception and subjected to barium enema on the basis of non-rigorous clinical criteria have normal study findings.[33]

Since the 1980s, ultrasonography has emerged as the 'gold standard' for non-invasive imaging of intussusception. The characteristic cross-sectional appearance of the intussusception is that of a 'target' or 'doughnut' (Fig. 45.4), and when viewed along the longitudinal axis a 'pseudo-kidney sign' is appreciated (Fig. 45.5). These findings are extremely reliable and reproducible, allowing the accurate diagnosis of intussusception even in less experienced hands.[34] In multiple reports, the positive and negative predictive values of ultrasonography approach 100%.[35,36] Ultrasonography also has the advantages of

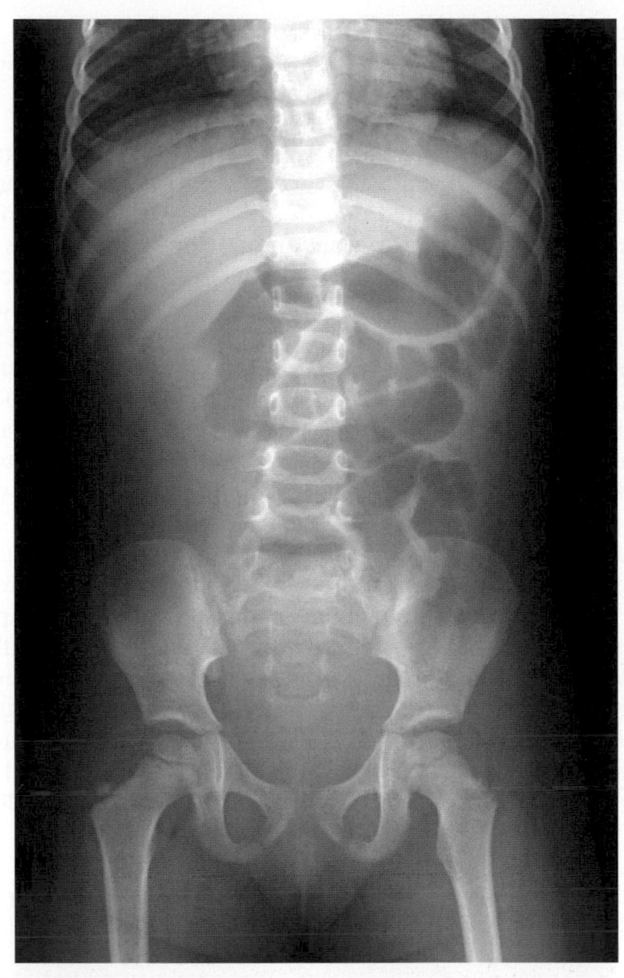

Figure 45.3: Plain abdominal radiograph exhibiting indirect signs of intussusception, including paucity of gas in the right lower quadrant, displacement of the small intestine and abrupt cut-off of gas in the transverse colon.

detecting isolated small bowel intussusceptions, identifying lead points, avoiding ionizing radiation, and maintaining superior patient comfort and compliance. Reduced blood flow in the intussusceptum assessed by color Doppler sonography has been shown to be highly predictive of irreducibility or irreversible ischemia (Fig. 45.6).[37]

CT can be highly accurate in the diagnosis of intussusception, although it offers little advantage over ultrasonography to justify the additional expense and exposure to radiation. Although CT is not commonly used as a primary diagnostic modality for intussusception, unsuspected intussusceptions are occasionally demonstrated on abdominal CT performed for other indications. The diagnostic accuracy of CT in this setting is quite high.[38] One potential advantage of CT over ultrasonography in the diagnosis of intussusception is its uniform availability – it may be difficult or cost-prohibitive for some institutions to make ultrasonographic expertise immediately available around the clock. The actual performance of CT imaging is not operator-dependent, requires only a technician, and the images can be digitally transferred to an available radiologist. As CT protocols become better defined, faster, more focused and less expensive, this technology may replace ultrasonography for the imaging of intussusception, much as it has done for acute appendicitis.

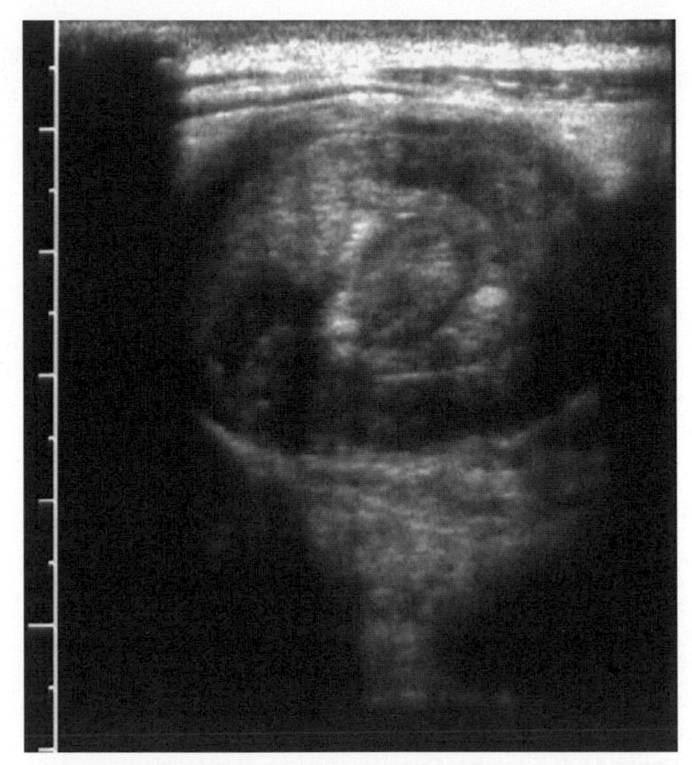

Figure 45.4: Sonographic image of intussusception in the transverse section demonstrating the echodense intussusceptum within the echolucent intussuscipiens. Note the bright mesenteric vessels on end, running along the intestinal wall.

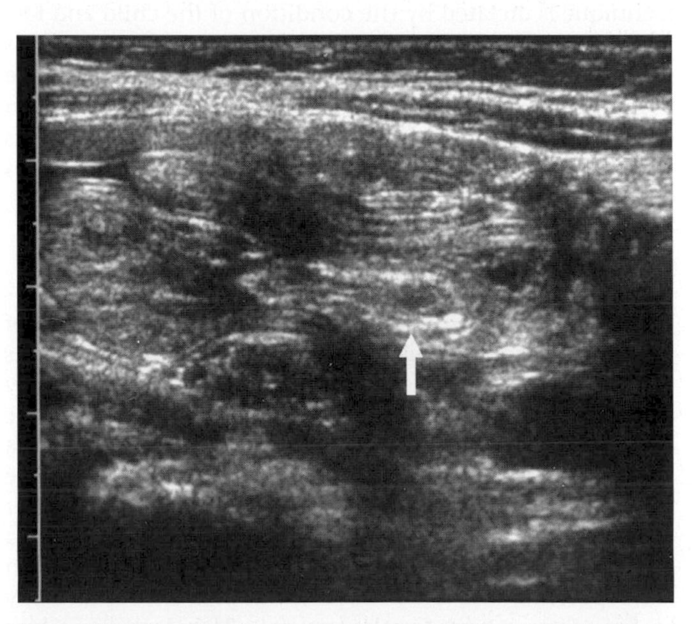

Figure 45.5: Sonographic image of intussusception in longitudinal section demonstrating the 'pseudo-kidney' sign. (From Vasavada P, 2004, with permission.)[79]

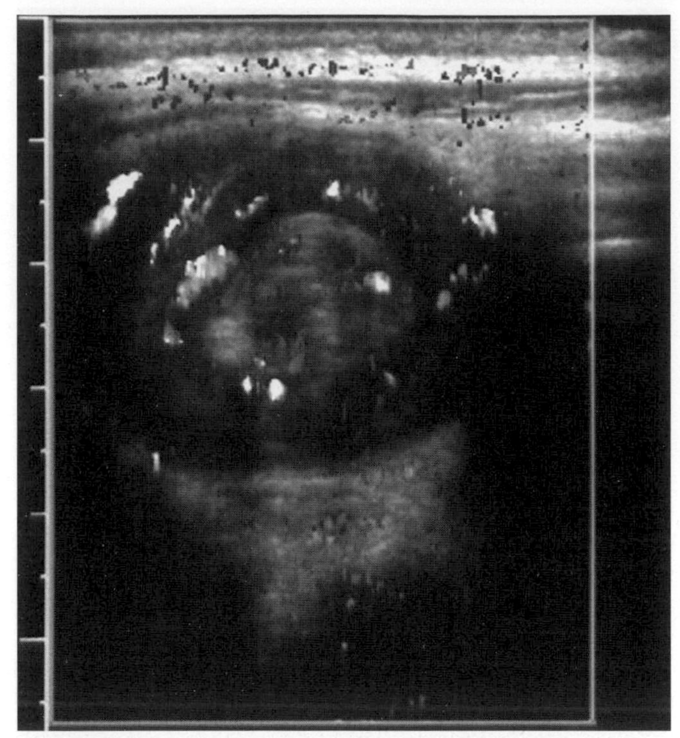

Figure 45.6: Transverse Doppler sonogram of reducible intussusception demonstrating intact blood flow. (From Vasavada P, 2004, with permission.)[79]

THERAPEUTIC OPTIONS

Once the diagnosis has been established, attention is immediately focused on reducing the intussusception in the safest and most expeditious manner. The likelihood of successful reduction and avoidance of complications decreases rapidly with the passage of time. Strategies for reduction include both non-operative and surgical techniques. The choice of technique is dictated by the condition of the child and factors that predict the probability of complications such as perforation and presence of pathologic lead points. The presence of clinical peritonitis, pneumoperitoneum on plain abdominal films and shock are absolute contraindications to non-operative reduction, and patients with these features should be resuscitated and undergo surgical exploration.

Hydrostatic reduction

The reduction of intussusception by the application of pressure to the intussusceptum via a column of liquid is the most common method of reduction currently employed. Hirschprung advocated the use of a therapeutic enema to reduce intussusception in 1876, and presented a large series of successful attempts in 1905. Following the introduction of diagnostic barium enema techniques after the turn of the twentieth century, the use barium enema for the controlled, monitored reduction of intussusception was reported in the late 1920s and adopted enthusiastically in Scandinavia and South America. This technique was introduced in the USA in 1939, and became the preferred management strategy following the standardization of techniques by Ravitch, who published his findings in 1948.[39] Subsequently, the use of barium enema reduction became universal in its application, and is reported to be successful in 50–85% of cases (Fig. 45.7).[10,11,18]

All children subjected to hydrostatic reduction should have adequate intravenous access established and fluid resuscitation completed prior to the attempt. Patients with more significant vomiting, abdominal distention or signs of systemic toxicity should also have a nasogastric tube placed and receive broad-spectrum antibiotics. Hydrostatic reduction by gravity feed with 60% barium suspension should be limited to a column height of 100 cm, generating a retrograde pressure of 100–120 mmHg. Pressures greater than this were found by Ravitch to be capable of reducing a gangrenous intussusceptum, resulting in perforation.[39] Water-soluble agents may also be used, although their lower specific gravity dictates a higher fluid column in order to generate comparable pressures. The intussusception is subjected to the enema pressure for 3–5 min and the progress of reduction monitored fluoroscopically. Several attempts may be required to reduce the intussusception fully. Complete reduction is established when contrast flows freely past the ileocecal valve and fills the terminal ileum. After successful reduction, fluid resuscitation is continued and feedings are withheld for 12–24 h while the child is observed for complications of reduction or early recurrence.

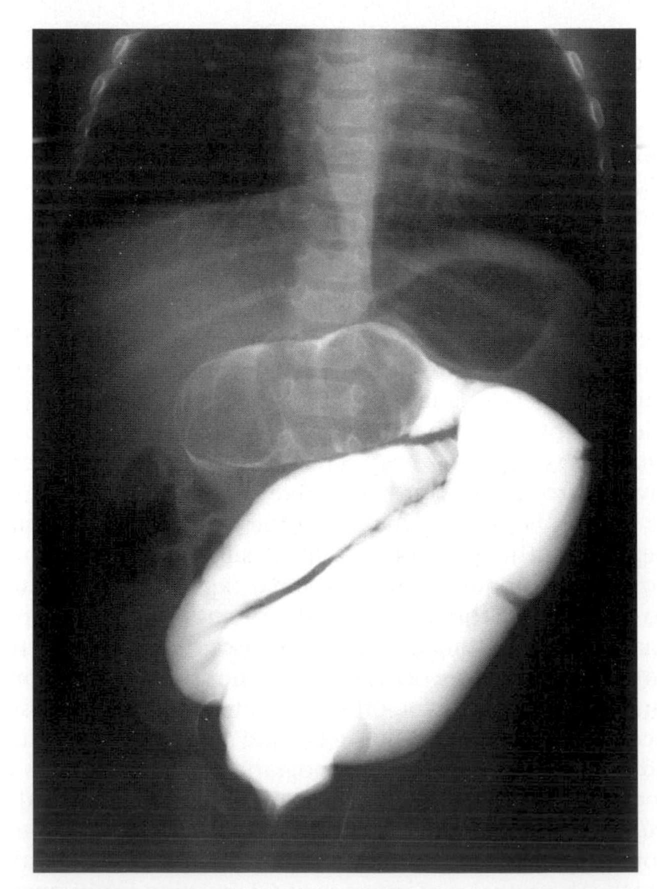

Figure 45.7: Hydrostatic reduction of ileocolic intussusception by barium enema. This intussusceptum was encountered in the transverse colon.

Although barium reduction under fluoroscopic guidance is a technique favored by most radiologists utilizing hydrostatic reduction, recent experience with saline reduction has yielded excellent results.[40] Saline reduction can be performed under ultrasonographic guidance, and is therefore incorporated easily and efficiently into the diagnostic imaging sequence while avoiding ionizing radiation. Some radiologists use a very dilute solution of water-soluble contrast agent so that complete reduction can be documented by plain radiography, demonstrating contrast in the terminal ileum. Although perforation rates with any form of pressure enema reduction are 1% or less, perforation with barium leads to complicated peritonitis, which can be avoided with saline. Furthermore, published success rates for saline enema range from 70% to 90%, exceeding those for barium enema reduction.[41,42]

Pneumatic reduction with air under fluoroscopic guidance is another variation on the theme of pressure enema reduction, and is replacing hydrostatic reduction as the preferred non-operative strategy in many institutions. With pneumatic reduction, air is introduced at a constant pressure of 120 torr, which is more easily and precisely controlled than barium. Success rates of 75–95% have been reported, exceeding those for both barium and saline reduction.[43–45] It is likely that the enhanced success rates for saline and air enema reduction compared with barium are related to the perception that perforation, although undesirable, is less catastrophic when barium is not present. This perception may result in more aggressive and repeated attempts at reduction with air or saline. Unlike ultrasonographically guided saline enema, however, standard air contrast enema reduction still requires exposure to radiation. A recent large series of more than 6000 consecutive cases of intussusception from China documented the efficacy of pneumatic reduction without fluoroscopic guidance.[46] As with hydrostatic reduction, ultrasonography may be used to monitor reduction without radiation. Initial reports of ultrasonographically guided pneumatic reduction have documented its feasibility and a successful reduction rate of 92–95%.[47,48]

Failure to achieve complete reduction after three or four attempts usually mandates surgical exploration. In a stable patient with incomplete reduction, however, some surgeons and radiologists advocate repeated attempts at hydrostatic or pneumatic reduction after a rest period of 2–3 h.[49] If the radiologist feels the reduction was complete but reflux of contrast into the terminal ileum was prevented by edema at the ileocecal valve, close observation may be undertaken if the child is stable. Follow-up imaging by ultrasonography to confirm reduction may be possible if saline has been used or the majority of the barium has been evacuated.

Certain features identifiable at presentation may serve as relative contraindications to non-surgical reduction, as they predict a low probability of successful reduction, a high probability of perforation or the presence of a pathologic lead point requiring surgical resection.[43] These factors include premature or neonatal status, age greater than 2 years, duration of symptoms greater than 48 h, radiographic evidence of a small bowel obstruction, isolated small intestinal (e.g. jejunoileal) intussusception defined by non-invasive imaging, and multiple recurrences. In these patients, a decision to proceed initially with non-operative reduction must take into consideration these negative prognostic factors.

Surgical management

Despite the wide variety of effective non-operative options for infants and children with intussusception, surgery remains a common therapeutic mainstay for the 10–50% of infants in whom pressure enema reduction fails, and for other children with pathologic lead points or ischemic complications. The traditional open operation is usually performed through a transverse incision in the right lower abdomen, although small-intestinal intussusceptions can be managed through a limited midline incision. Once the peritoneal cavity has been entered and explored, the involved intestine is externalized and inspected (Fig. 45.8). Obvious perforation or infarction of the intussuscipiens mandates resection without an attempt at manual reduction.

If no absolute indications for resection are encountered, reduction is attempted by carefully and gradually compressing the bowel just distal to the apex of the intussusceptum and gently pushing it retrograde until reduction is accomplished. The intussusceptum is never pulled out of the intussuscipiens as traction injuries are common in the compromised bowel. Irreversible ischemic injury may be apparent only after successful manual reduction. Failure of manual reduction usually indicates a gangrenous intussusceptum, and resection is indicated. Resection of any pathologic lead point is also mandatory. Regardless of the reason for resection, primary anastomosis is usually recommended over the creation of an enterostomy unless the resection involves unprepared colon in a compromised patient. Laparoscopy may be beneficial in the occasional infant with idiopathic intussusception who fails pressure enema reduction, and in cases where complete reduction by non-operative means is uncertain (Fig. 45.9).

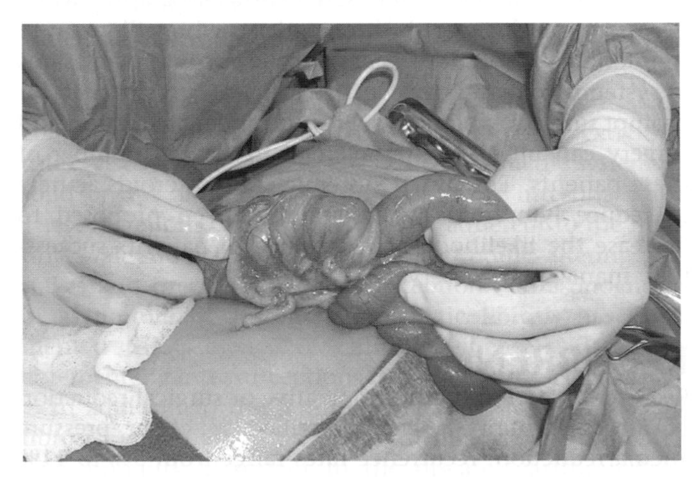

Figure 45.8: Intraoperative photograph of an ileocolic intussusception through the ileocecal valve. The absence of ischemic changes predicts successful manual reduction (See plate section for color).

obstruction syndrome (DIOS) in which thick, inspissated secretions aggregate and block the terminal ileum, producing a mechanical bowel obstruction. This syndrome is analogous to meconium ileus in the neonate with cystic fibrosis, and has therefore also been termed meconium ileus equivalent (MIE). These patients present with acute, colicky abdominal pain, abdominal distention, vomiting and the radiographic appearance of an acute small bowel obstruction. On examination, many of these patients have a palpable right lower quadrant mass. The diagnostic overlap between DIOS and intussusception is obvious.

Distinguishing DIOS from intussusception at the outset is crucial, as the treatment for DIOS frequently involves antegrade administration of a large volume of a hyperosmotic solution such as polyethylene glycol in order to flush the meconium-like plug out of the ileum and into the colon. Such treatment might easily precipitate an abdominal crisis in a patient with intussusception. As there is no reliable clinical feature that can differentiate intussusception from DIOS, sonographic examination of the abdomen should be performed promptly in patients with severe pain, systemic toxicity or bloody stools. If ultrasonography documents intussusception, the treatment options are essentially the same as for other varieties of intussusception: hydrostatic, pneumatic or surgical reduction. The success rate for hydrostatic reduction is sufficiently high to recommend it for most patients with cystic fibrosis and ileocolic intussusception.[74] The safety and efficacy of a conservative strategy involving careful observation and supportive measures in patients with cystic fibrosis and enteroenteric intussusceptions have not been studied by any prospective trial, and surgical exploration and reduction should still be considered the current standard of care in these patients.

References

1. Fisher D, Hadas-Halpern I. Jejunoduodenogastric intussusception – a rare complication of gastrostomy tube migration. Pediatr Radiol 2001; 31:455.
2. Reymond RD. The mechanism of intussusception: a theoretical analysis of the phenomenon. Br J Radiol 1972; 45:1–11.
3. Ueki I, Nakashima E, Kumagai M, et al. Intussusception in neonates: analysis of 14 Japanese patients. J Paediatr Child Health 2004; 40:388–391.
4. Kincaid MS, Vavilala MS, Faucher L, et al. Feeding intolerance as a result of small-intestinal intussusception in a child with major burns. J Burn Care Rehabil 2004; 25:212–214.
5. Willetts IE, Kite P, Barclay GR, et al. Endotoxin, cytokines and lipid peroxides in children with intussusception. Br J Surg 2001; 88:878–883.
6. Doi O, Aoyama K, Hutson JM. Twenty-one cases of small bowel intussusception: the pathophysiology of idiopathic intussusception and the concept of benign small bowel intussusception. Pediatr Surg Int 2004; 20:140–143.
7. Yang JI, Kim HS, Chang KH, et al. Intrauterine intussusception presenting as fetal ascites at prenatal ultrasonography. Am J Perinatol 2004; 21:241–246.
8. Rattan KN, Singh Y, Sharma A, et al. Intrauterine intussusception – a cause for ileal atresia. Indian J Pediatr 2000; 67:851–852.
9. Shimotake T, Go S, Tsuda T, Iwai N. Ultrasonographic detection of intrauterine intussusception resulting in ileal atresia complicated by meconium peritonitis. Pediatr Surg Int 2000; 16:43–44.
10. Stringer MD, Pablot SM, Brereton FJ. Pediatric intussusception. Br J Surg 1992; 79:867–876.
11. Bruce J, Huhy S, Coney DR, et al. Intussusception: evolution of current management. J Pediatr Gastr Nutr 1987; 6:663–674.
12. Ong NT, Beasley SW. The lead point in intussusception. J Pediatr Surg 1990; 25:640–643.
13. Turner D, Rickwood AMK, Brereton RJ. Intussusception in older children. Arch Dis Child 1980; 55:544–546.
14. Azar T, Berger DL. Adult intussusception. Ann Surg 1997; 226:134–138.
15. O'Sullivan WD, Child CG. Ileocecal intussusception caused by lymphoid hyperplasia. J Pediatr 1951; 38:320–324.
16. Cornes JS, Dawson IM. Papillary lymphoid hyperplasia at the ileocaecal valve as a cause of acute intussuception in infancy. Arch Dis Child 1963; 38:89–91.
17. Centers for Disease Control and Prevention. Suspension of rotavirus vaccine after reports of intussusception – United States, 1999. MMWR Morb Mortal Wkly Rep 2004; 53:786–789.
18. Chung JL, Kong MS, Lin JN, et al. Intussusception in infants and children: risk factors leading to surgical reduction. J Formos Med Assoc 1994; 93:481–485.
19. Navarro O, Daneman A. Intussusception. Part 3: Diagnosis and management of those with an identifiable or predisposing cause and those that reduce spontaneously. Pediatr Radiol 2004; 34:305–312.
20. DiFiore JW. Intussusception. Semin Pediatr Surg 1999; 8:214–220.
21. Ein SH. Leading points in childhood intussusception. J Pediatr Surg 1976; 11:209–211.
22. Pang LC. Intussusception revisited: clinicopathologic analysis of 261 cases, with emphasis on pathogenesis. South Med J 1989; 82:215–228.
23. Navarro O, Dugougeat F, Kornecki A, et al. The impact of imaging in the management of intussusception owing to pathologic lead points in children. A review of 43 cases. Pediatr Radiol 2000; 30:594–603.
24. Nistala K, Hyer W, Halligan S. Jejunal hemorrhage in Henoch–Schönlein syndrome. Arch Dis Child 2003; 88:434.
25. Eklof OA, Johanson L, Kohr G. Childhood intussusception: hydrostatic reducibility and incidence of leading points in different age groups. Pediatr Radiol 1980; 10:83–86.
26. Ikeda H, Matsuyama S, Suzuki N, et al. Small bowel obstruction in children: review of 10 years experience. Acta Paediatr Jpn 1993; 35:504–507.
27. Ein SH, Stephens CA. Intussusception: 354 cases in 10 years. J Pediatr Surg 1971; 6:16–21.
28. Harrington L, Connolly B, Hu X, et al. Ultrasonographic and clinical predictors of intussusception. J Pediatr 1998; 131:836–839.
29. Klein EJ, Kapoor D, Shugerman EP. The diagnosis of intussusception. Clin Pediatr 2004; 43:343–347.
30. Avansino JR, Bjerke S, Hendrickson M, et al. Clinical features and treatment outcome of intussusception in premature neonates. J Pediatr Surg 2003; 38:1818–1821.
31. Meradji M, Hussain SM, Robben SGF, et al. Plain film diagnosis in intussusception. Br J Radiol 1994; 67:147.
32. Henrikson S, Blane CE, Koujok K, et al. The effect of screening sonography on the positive rate of enemas for intussusception. Pediatr Radiol 2003; 33:190–193.

33. Eklof O, Thonell S. Conventional abdominal radiography as a means to rule out ileo-caecal intussusception. Acta Radiol (Diagn) 1984; 25:265–268.
34. Eshed I, Gorenstein A, Serour F, Witzling M. Intussusception in children: can we rely on screening sonography performed by junior residents? Pediatr Radiol 2004; 34:134–137.
35. Verschelden P, Filiatrault D, Garel L, et al. Intussusception in children: reliability of US in diagnosis – a prospective study. Radiology 1992; 184:741–744.
36. Stanley A, Logan H, Bate TW, et al. Ultrasound in the diagnosis and exclusion of intussusception. Irish Med J 1997; 90:64–65.
37. Lim HK, Bae SH, Lee KH, et al. Assessment of reducibility of ileocolic intussusception in children: usefulness of color Doppler sonography. Radiology 1994; 191:781–785.
38. Strouse PJ, DiPietro MA, Saez F. Transient small bowel intussusception in children on CT. Pediatr Radiol 2003; 33:316–320.
39. Ravitch MM, McCune RM. Reduction of intussusception by hydrostatic pressure: an experimental study. Bull Johns Hopkins Hosp 1948; 82:550–568.
40. Crystal P, Hertzanu Y, Farber B, et al. Sonographically guided hydrostatic reduction of intussusception in children. J Clin Ultrasound 2002; 30:343–348.
41. Chan KL, Saing H, Peh WC. Childhood intussusception: ultrasound-guided Hartmann's solution hydrostatic reduction or barium enema reduction? J Pediatr Surg 1997; 32:3–6.
42. Rohrschneider WK, Troger J. Hydrostatic reduction of intussusception under US guidance. Pediatr Radiol 1995; 25:530–540.
43. Daneman A, Alton DJ. Intussusception: issues and controversies related to diagnosis and reduction. Radiol Clin North Am 1996; 34:743–756.
44. Miles SG, Cumming WA, Williams JL. Pneumatic reduction of ileocolic intussusception in children. Pediatr Radiol 1988; 18:3–5.
45. Stein M, Alton DJ, Daneman A. Pneumatic reduction of intussusception: clinical experience and pressure correlates. Radiology 1991; 181:169–172.
46. Guo J, Ma X, Zhou A. Results of air pressure enema reduction of intussusception: 6396 cases in 13 years. J Pediatr Surg 1986; 21:1201–1203.
47. Yoon CH, Kim KJ, Goo HW. Intussusception in children: US-guided pneumatic reduction – initial experience. Radiology 2001; 218:85–88.
48. Gu L, Zhu H, Wang S, et al. Sonographic guidance of air enema for intussusception reduction in children. Pediatr Radiol 2000; 30:339–342.
49. Navarro OM, Daneman A, Chae A. Intussusception: the use of delayed, repeated attempts and the management of intussusceptions due to pathological lead points in pediatric patients. AJR Am J Roentgenol 2004; 182:1169–1176.
50. Kornecki A, Daneman A, Navarro O, et al. Spontaneous reduction of intussusception: clinical spectrum, management and outcome. Pediatr Radiol 2000; 30:58–63.
51. Sonmez K, Turkyilmaz Z, Demirogullari B, et al. Conservative treatment for small intestinal intussusception associated with Henoch–Schönlein's purpura. Surg Today 2002; 32:1031–1034.
52. Ein SH. Recurrent intussusception in children. J Pediatr Surg 1975; 10:751–754.
53. Olcay I, Zorludemir U. Idiopathic postoperative intussusception. Z Kinderchir 1989; 44:86–87.
54. Kidd J, Jackson R, Wagner CW, Smith SD. Intussusception following the Ladd procedure. Arch Surg 2000; 135:713–715.
55. West KW, Stephens B, Rescorla FJ, Vane DW, Grosfeld JL. Postoperative intussusception: experience with 36 cases in children. Surgery 1988; 104:781–787.
56. Linke F, Eble F, Berger S. Postoperative intussusception in childhood. Pediatr Surg Int 1998; 14:175–177.
57. Tatekawa Y, Muraji T, Nishijima E, et al. Postoperative intussusception after surgery for malrotation and appendectomy in a newborn. Pediatr Surg Int 1998; 14:171–172.
58. Holcomb GW 3rd, Ross AJ 3rd, O'Neill JA Jr. Postoperative intussusception: increasing frequency or increasing awareness? South Med J 1991; 84:1334–1339.
59. Hulbert WC Jr, Valvo JR, Caldamone AA, et al. Intussusception following resection of Wilm's tumor. Urology 1983; 21:578–580.
60. Kaste SC, Wilimas J, Rao BN. Postoperative small-bowel intussusception in children with cancer. Pediatr Radiol 1995; 25:21–23.
61. Pumberger W, Pomberger G, Wiesbauer P. Postoperative intussusception: an overlooked complication in pediatric surgical oncology. Med Pediatr Oncol 2002; 38:208–210.
62. de Vries S, Sleeboom C, Aronson DC. Postoperative intussusception in children. Br J Surg 1999; 86:81–83.
63. Chen SY, Kong MS. Gastrointestinal manifestations and complications of Henoch–Schönlein purpura. Chang Gung Med J 2004; 27:175–181.
64. Choong CK, Beasley SW. Intra-abdominal manifestations of Henoch–Schönlein purpura. J Paediatr Child Health 1998; 34:405–409.
65. Hu SC, Feeney MS, McNicholas M, et al. Ultrasonography to diagnose and exclude intussusception in Henoch–Schönlein purpura. Arch Dis Child 1991; 66:1065–1067.
66. Katz S, Borst M, Seekri I, Grosfeld JL. Surgical evaluation of Henoch–Schönlein purpura. Experience with 110 children. Arch Surg 1991; 126:849–853.
67. Cull DL, Rosario V, Lally KP, et al. Surgical implications of Henoch–Schönlein purpura. J Pediatr Surg 1990; 25:741–743.
68. Mir E. Surgical complications in Henoch–Schönlein purpura in childhood. Z Kinderchir 1988; 43:391–393.
69. Connolly B, O'Halpin D. Sonographic evaluation of the abdomen in Henoch–Schönlein purpura. Clin Radiol 1994; 49:320–323.
70. Couture A, Veyrac C, Baud C, et al. Evaluation of abdominal pain in Henoch–Schönlein syndrome by high frequency ultrasound. Pediatr Radiol 1992; 22:12–17.
71. Sonmez K, Turkyilmaz Z, Demirogullari B, et al. Conservative treatment for small intestinal intussusception associated with Henoch–Schönlein's purpura. Surg Today 2002; 32:1031–1034.
72. Kornecki A, Daneman A, Navarro O, et al. Spontaneous reduction of intussusception: clinical spectrum, management and outcome. Pediatr Radiol 2000; 30:58–63.
73. Holsclaw DS, Rocmans C, Schwachman H. Intussusception in patients with cystic fibrosis. Pediatrics 1971; 48:51–56.
74. Gross K, Desanto A, Grosfeld JL, et al. Intra-abdominal complications of cystic fibrosis. J Pediatr Surg 1985; 20:431–435.
75. Wilschanski M, Fisher D, Hadas-Halperin I, et al. Findings on routine ultrasonography in cystic fibrosis patients. J Pediatr Gastroenterol Nutr 1999; 28:182–185.
76. Vasavada P. Ultrasound evaluation of acute abdominal emergencies in infants and children. Radiol Clin North Am 2004; 42:445–456.

Chapter 46
Inguinal hernia and hydrocele

Frederick Alexander

INTRODUCTION

Inguinal hernia is one of the more common surgical problems of infancy and childhood. It occurs in 0.8–4.4% of children;[1] however, in premature infants, the incidence may increase to 30%, depending on the age of gestation.[2] The peak incidence occurs in the neonatal period, when the defect is also most likely to cause symptoms usually related to incarceration and strangulation. The incidence subsequently declines with age, but remains approximately six times more common in boys than in girls.[3]

Inguinal hernia usually presents as an intermittent bulge in the groin that may extend into the scrotum or labia majora with crying or straining. These findings contrast with the fluctuant scrotal swelling that is characteristic of a hydrocele. On the other hand, because congenital inguinal hernias and hydroceles share a common origin, the patent processus vaginalis, they may be difficult to distinguish clinically or may occur in conjunction with one another. Their management relative to the timing of surgery and contralateral exploration remains controversial.

HISTORY

Hernias were described in ancient times, but not until the early nineteenth century was the anatomy of the inguinal canal accurately described. Bassini[4] in 1887 was the first author to describe the successful use of high ligation of the hernia sac in combination with anatomic repair. This concept was modified in 1899 by Ferguson,[5] who advocated incision of the external oblique fascia to improve surgical exposure. In 1950, Potts and co-workers[6] recommended simple high ligation and removal of the hernia sac for routine hernia repair in children that has become the standard of care.

EMBRYOLOGY AND PATHOGENESIS

The processus vaginalis is a tubular extension of the peritoneal membrane that passes through the internal ring and into the scrotum during the third month of gestation. This membrane surrounds the testis and gubernaculum and probably contributes to testicular descent in the seventh month of gestation by downward transmission of intra-abdominal pressure.[7] The processus vaginalis usually obliterates some time after testicular descent is complete, although the timing and mechanism of closure are unknown. Failure of the processus vaginalis to obliterate is the most common cause of inguinal hernia and hydrocele in infants and children. However, autopsy studies have shown that the processus vaginalis may remain patent in a larger number of asymptomatic children and adults,[8,9] suggesting that other factors also may be involved. For example, an increase in abdominal pressure or fluid may play an important role in the clinical development of a hernia or a hydrocele. Ascites from any cause, or placement of a ventriculoperitoneal shunt or a peritoneal dialysis catheter in a formerly asymptomatic patient frequently lead to the development of a clinical hernia or hydrocele.

CLINICAL PRESENTATION

Incomplete obliteration of the processus vaginalis may lead to a variety of clinical presentations (Fig. 46.1). For example, closure of the processus may occur at any point between the internal ring and the scrotum, leading to various degrees of herniation into the inguinal canal. The processus vaginalis may remain open into the scrotum forming a complete inguinal hernia. On the other hand, the processus vaginalis may close incompletely along its longitudinal axis, leading to fluid accumulation in the scrotum defined as a hydrocele. If the processus remains open sufficiently to allow bidirectional movement of fluid, a *communicating hydrocele* may result that usually fluctuates in size. Late obliteration of the processus may entrap fluid within the tunica vaginalis surrounding the testis, resulting in a *non-communicating hydrocele*.

Usually the child with a hernia presents with a history of intermittent pain or swelling of the groin. Incarceration occurs when a segment of intestine becomes entrapped within the hernia sac. Incarceration often produces bilious vomiting and obstipation and is a common cause of small bowel obstruction in infants and children who have not had prior surgery. Therefore, an incarcerated inguinal hernia should be greatly suspected in any child with signs of intestinal obstruction. When incarceration leads to diminished circulation within the herniated viscus, strangulation with ischemic necrosis may result. In its late stages, strangulation may result in erythema and edema overlying a tender groin mass. In contrast, children with hydroceles usually present with asymptomatic scrotal swelling.

Examination of a child for inguinal hernia or hydrocele may be facilitated by placing the child in an upright position or by encouraging straining or coughing. The scrotum may be inverted into the distal inguinal canal over the thumb or forefinger in order to detect a groin mass. Manual palpation of the groin and scrotum often reveals the

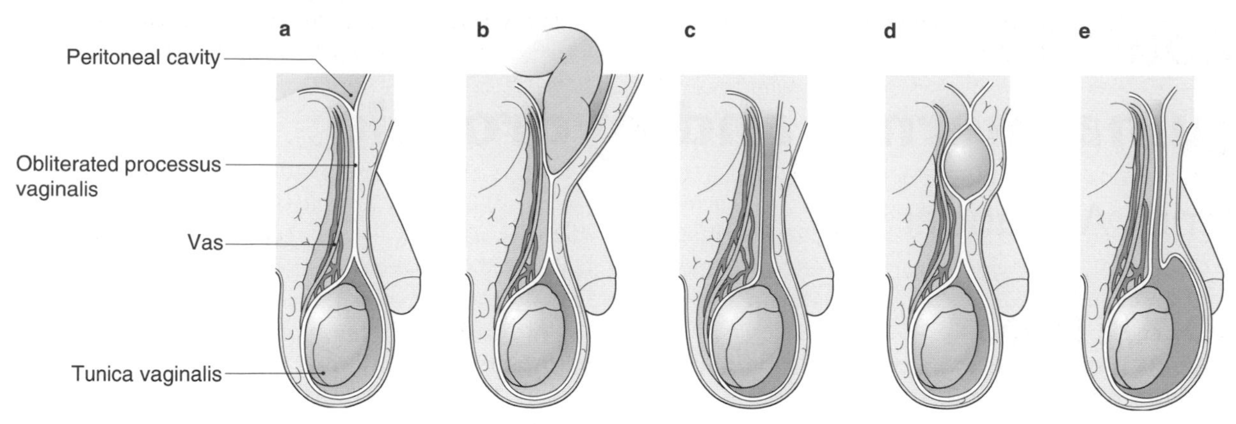

Figure 46.1: Spectrum of anatomic abnormalities of the processus vaginalis. (**a**) Normal anatomy. (**b**) Inguinal hernia. (**c**) Complete hernia. (**d**) Hydrocele of the cord. (**e**) Communicating hydrocele.

significant findings described previously. It is important to palpate both testicles within the scrotum, since an undescended or retractile testis may often pose as a groin mass. Usually, gentle pressure applied bimanually in a cephalad and posterior direction will result in a sudden reduction of an inguinal hernia. Reduction of the hernia may be confirmed by simultaneous palpation of the contralateral groin, which should feel absolutely symmetric following reduction of the hernia. Transillumination is the hallmark of a hydrocele and hydroceles frequently fluctuate in size, becoming less prominent at night when the child is sleeping. If scrotal swelling is reduced by gentle caudal pressure leaving the scrotum decompressed and symmetric with the contralateral side, then the presence of a hydrocele has been confirmed. Occasionally it may be difficult to distinguish between an incarcerated hernia and a loculated hydrocele of the cord, particularly in premature or neonatal infants. Both conditions may transilluminate and may be irreducible; however, a hydrocele of the cord is otherwise asymptomatic as opposed to an incarcerated hernia, which is generally tender and associated with intestinal symptoms. Failure to reduce a hernia after administration of intramuscular morphine sulfate or meperidine, or a plain radiographic film of the abdomen that reveals signs of small bowel obstruction or a gas bubble below the inguinal ligament, indicate an incarcerated hernia. If the clinician is unable to distinguish an incarcerated hernia (Fig. 46.2) from a loculated hydrocele, surgical exploration is recommended.

In some instances, a bulge in the groin may be seen by the parents or pediatrician but may not be apparent on examination. In this situation, several findings including thickening of the cord at the ring or an associated hydrocele may suggest the presence of a hernia. Otherwise, the surgeon may accept the diagnosis based on the description or may re-evaluate the child during a second visit.

MANAGEMENT

Inguinal hernias should be repaired promptly after the diagnosis is made in order to prevent incarceration. Although the overall risk of incarceration is unknown, this

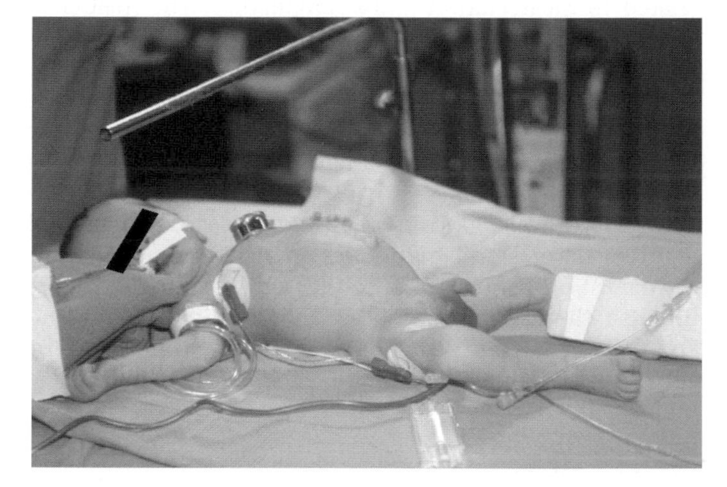

Figure 46.2: Typical appearance of an incarcerated hernia in a premature infant prior to surgical reduction and repair.

risk is much higher during the first year of life. Rowe and Clatworthy[10] found that two-thirds of incarcerated hernias occur in children younger than 1 year of age and that two-thirds of these children required surgical reduction. Given proper technique and adequate sedation, most children may now undergo manual reduction and thus avoid the anesthetic hazards of emergent surgical reduction. If manual reduction is easily and promptly accomplished, the child may be discharged and scheduled for elective outpatient surgery. In the more difficult cases, successful manual reduction should be followed by admission and subsequent elective hernia repair prior to discharge from the hospital. In those infants and children with hernias who are hospitalized for unrelated severe or life-threatening problems hernia repair is best deferred until the primary problem is resolved. In premature infants, repair is often deferred until just prior to discharge from the neonatal intensive care unit, so that they may be closely observed postoperatively for apnea and bradycardia.

In contrast to inguinal hernia, hydroceles frequently resolve spontaneously during the first 2 years of life. Both non-communicating and communicating hydroceles in infancy often resolve spontaneously during the first 12–18 months of life (Fig. 46.3). Thus, in the absence of a hernia, it is prudent to observe a hydrocele for at least 18 months before recommending surgical repair. If the hydrocele shows no signs of resolution between 18 and 24 months of life, then surgical repair should be recommended. Because a persistent hydrocele in this setting is most likely to be communicating repair should be performed through the groin and should include high ligation of the processus vaginalis. The distal portion of the hydrocele sac should be trimmed with care so as not to injure the testis or structures of the cord.

Surgical repair of hernias and hydroceles in children is usually performed under general anesthesia as an outpatient procedure. A transverse skin incision is made within the skin crease midway between the symphysis pubis and anterior iliac crest. This incision is carried down through Scarpa's fascia, exposing the external oblique fascia. The external oblique is then opened, exposing the inguinal canal and the structures of the cord. At this point, the cremasteric muscle is gently separated exposing the hernia sac, which always lies anterior to the structures of the cord. The hernia sac is gently dissected away from the structures of the cord and is then divided and traced to its origin at the internal ring, where it is ligated and amputated. The distal sac may be trimmed but not completely removed, since this is unnecessary and even hazardous. In a premature infant or in any child with an associated undescended testicle, orchiopexy must be performed in conjection with the hernia repair. Sliding hernias are rare in children and may include the appendix, salpinx, or Meckel's diverticulum (Littre's hernia) as part of the hernia sac. In this situation, the structure must be carefully dissected away from the wall of the sac prior to high ligation. When exploration is carried out for incarceration, the incarcerated viscera should be carefully inspected for signs of ischemic necrosis and, if none are found, subsequently reduced. As a general rule, if an incarcerated hernia may be successfully reduced manually prior to surgery, it is unnecessary to inspect the intestine at the time of the subsequent hernia repair.

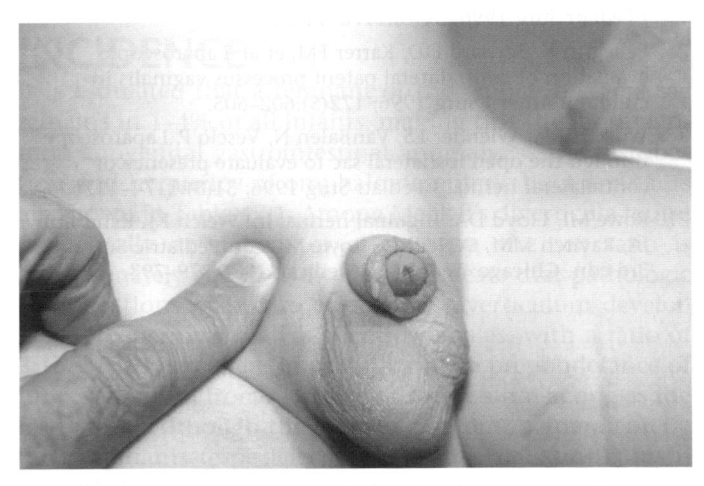

Figure 46.3: Typical appearance of a hydrocele, which frequently regresses by 2 years of age.

There has been considerable controversy over the issue of contralateral exploration. Many surgeons[11–13] have reported a high incidence of contralateral inguinal hernia or patent processus vaginalis when routine contralateral groin exploration is carried out in children with a unilateral, clinically apparent inguinal hernia. Thus, Gilbert and Clatworthy[14] concluded that it was justifiable to perform a bilateral inguinal hernia repair in any healthy infant or child with a unilaterally apparent hernia, irrespective of age, sex, or side involved.

On the other hand, Sparkman,[15] in a large review found that although a contralateral patent processus vaginalis may be found in 50–60% of all infants and children, unilateral hernia repair was followed by the subsequent development of a contralateral hernia in only 15–20% of the operated group. Bock and Sobye[16] reported only a 15% incidence of contralateral hernia in a group of 174 children who underwent unilateral hernia repair and were followed for 27 to 36 years. More recently, Muraje et al. reported a 6% occurrence of contralateral hernia following unilateral hernia repair in 206 patients aged 11 days to 13 years.[17] Puri[18] found that 10% of 165 infants (aged 1 week to 6 months) developed a contralateral hernia an average of 6 months after unilateral hernia repair. Finally, in a review of 2764 infants and children, Rowe and colleagues[19] found a contralateral patent processus vaginalis in 63% within 2 months which declined to 41% at 2 years of age. From these reports, it would appear that the contralateral processus vaginalis obliterates near birth in approximately 40% of cases, with obliteration of another 20% during the first 2 years of life. After 2 years of age, nearly 40% of children still have a contralateral patent processus vaginalis, but fewer than half of these children develop a clinically apparent hernia.

The major advantage of routine contralateral exploration is the avoidance of a second operation with its cost and risk of anesthesia. The major disadvantages of routine contralateral exploration include the possibility of a technical mishap leading to infertility, (a minimal risk in experienced hands) as well as increased cost and postoperative pain.

A number of studies[16,20–23] have examined whether age, sex, or the side of the hernia may be used to predict the need for contralateral exploration. Of these factors, only age has any relationship to the risk of development of a contralateral hernia. Bock and Sobye[16] found that 47% of children whose primary hernia was repaired before the age of 1 year developed a contralateral hernia, compared with only 11% of those whose primary hernia was repaired after the first year of life. These data suggest that routine contralateral exploration may be justified during the first year of life, but not in older children. Several studies[16,20] have shown a slightly increased risk of contralateral hernia when the clinically apparent hernia appears on the left side as compared with the right; however, these findings are disputed by other studies in which little or no difference was found.[21,22] Finally, Bock and Sobye[16] found that the occurrence of contralateral hernia in girls who underwent unilateral hernia repair was only 8%. Thus, sex and the

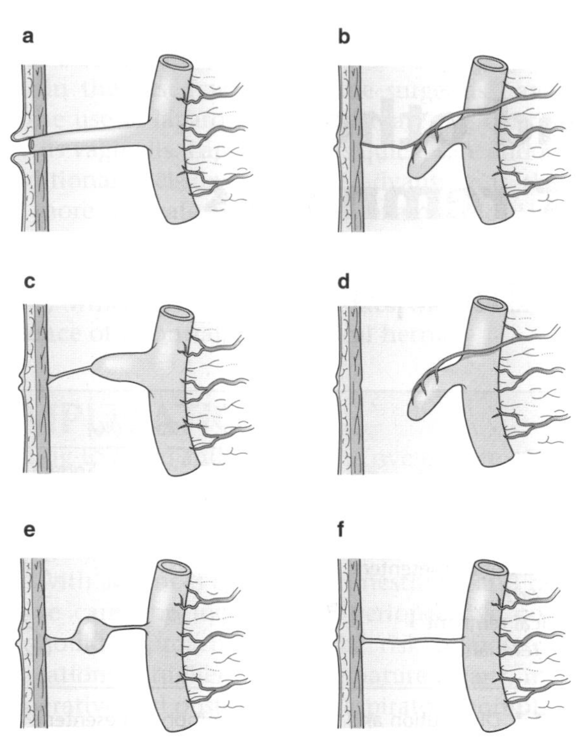

Figure 47.1: Illustrated are some of the more common residual congenital abnormalities that result from the embryonic yolk sac, as follows: (**a**) Patent omphalomesenteric duct representing a communication from the terminal ileum to the umbilicus; (**b**) Meckel's diverticulum with a patent right vitelline artery as blood supply to the Meckel's diverticulum and a residual of the vitelline artery illustrated as a cord to the undersurface to the umbilicus; (**c**) Meckel's diverticulum with a cord connecting the tip of the Meckel's diverticulum to the undersurface of the umbilicus. The cord (band) represents the distal residual of the omphalomesenteric duct; (**d**) Typical appearance of a Meckel's diverticulum with persistence of the vitelline artery; (**e**) Involution of the proximal and distal ends of the omphalomesenteric duct with residual cord or band and central preservation of the omphalomesenteric duct resulting in a mucosa-lined cyst; (**f**) Intraperitoneal band from the ileum to the undersurface of the umbilicus representing involution without resolution of the omphalomesenteric duct.

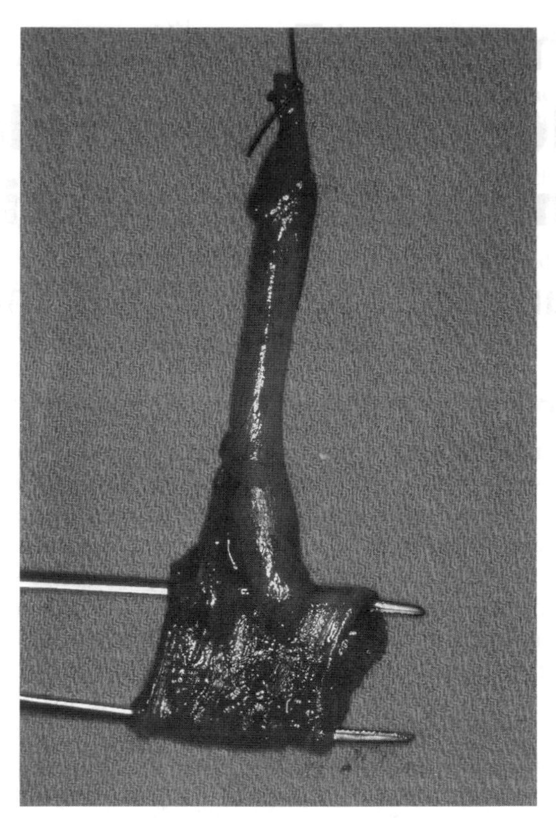

Figure 47.2: Operative specimen showing a segment of the terminal ileum (with forceps through the lumen) and a patent omphalomesenteric duct with a tie around the distal portion that extended through the umbilicus.

undersurface of the umbilicus by a solid cord, either as a residual from the yolk sac (Fig. 47.1c) or the vitelline vessels (Fig. 47.1b). Persistence of the vitelline artery can be the source of subsequent bleeding.

There are many abnormalities that result from remnants of the embryonic yolk sac. The numerous variations can be generally categorized in the following sections.

Patent omphalomesenteric (vitelline) duct

A patent omphalomesenteric (vitelline) duct is the result of the persistence of the normal *in utero* connection between the distal ileum and umbilicus (Fig. 47.2). This anomaly accounts for 2.5–6% of the spectrum of omphalomesenteric duct remnants.[6,9] Males predominate by a ratio of 5:1.[6] Ectopic gastric mucosa is identified in approximately one-third of the patients with a complete fistula.[6] Clinical presentation of this anomaly usually occurs in the first 1 to 2 weeks of life. After the natural atrophy and separation of the umbilical cord stump, drainage from the umbilicus occurs that has the appearance of intestinal contents. Inspection of the umbilicus reveals either an opening or a polypoid mass, which represents a limited prolapse of the patent omphalomesenteric duct (Fig. 47.3). Confirmation of the diagnosis can be made by injection of contrast material into the opening of the sinus tract with resultant drainage of the contrast agent into the distal small intestine. Complications of a patent omphalomesenteric duct include prolapse through the umbilicus of the patent duct only or the duct and the attached ileum. This can lead to increased intestinal drainage through the opening or to a partial intestinal obstruction. Partial prolapse of the duct or ileum has been mistaken for an umbilical polyp and amputated, with significant adverse sequelae.

Meckel's diverticulum

The most common of the embryonic yolk sac remnants which represents at least 80% of all these anomalies is a Meckel's diverticulum.[6,9] The diverticulum contains all three layers of the intestinal wall and is typically located within 40–50 cm of the ileocecal valve.[13] However, considerable variation in this distance is related to the age of the patient at the time of diagnosis. A Meckel's diverticulum can develop in a variety of shapes and lengths. The diverticulum

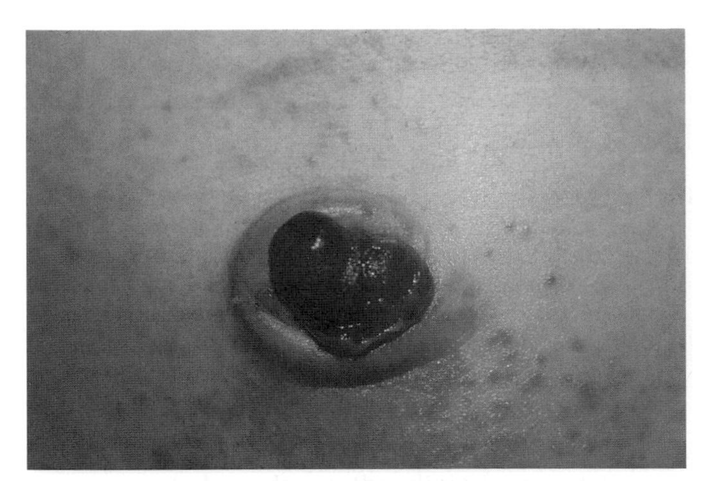

Figure 47.3: Distal end of an omphalomesenteric duct with the appearance of a stoma at the umbilicus.

originates from the antimesenteric border of the bowel and is typically 3–6 cm in length and slightly smaller than the diameter of the small intestine (Fig. 47.4). However, it can have a wide base, and the length can range from only 1 or 2 cm to more than 6 cm. Occasionally, a Meckel's diverticulum is attached to the undersurface of the umbilicus, to another portion of the abdominal wall, or to another segment of bowel or its mesentery by a fibrous cord. Of considerable significance is the presence of ectopic tissue within a Meckel's diverticulum. Meckel's diverticula are usually lined with ileal mucosa. However, gastric, duodenal, and colonic mucosa have been described.[13] In addition, bile duct mucosa and ectopic pancreatic tissue have also been demonstrated in Meckel's diverticula.[13] Numerous studies have indicated that, in symptomatic patients, 40–80% of Meckel's diverticula contain ectopic tissue.[14–17] In most of these cases the ectopic tissue is gastric mucosa, with pancreatic tissue being the second most common finding.

Omphalomesenteric duct cyst

Involution of the omphalomesenteric duct at the umbilicus and at the ileum can result in a mucosa-lined, cystic mass in either the intraperitoneal (Fig. 47.1e) or the preperitoneal space. These cysts contain all three layers of the small intestine and can present as either abdominal wall infections (particularly with preperitoneal cysts) or intestinal obstruction (with intraperitoneal cysts).

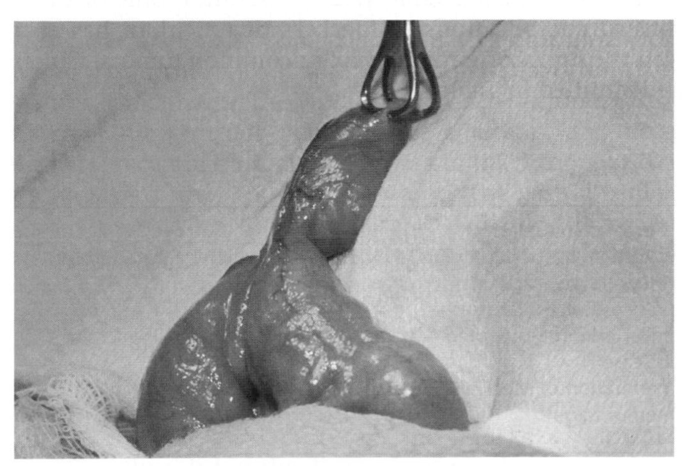

Figure 47.4: Typical appearance of a Meckel's diverticulum.

Omphalomesenteric duct remnants at the umbilicus

Although the omphalomesenteric duct is present at the umbilicus *in utero*, remnants at the umbilicus are uncommon. When present, these remnants usually are identifiable after the first 1–2 weeks of life following separation of the umbilical stalk. What remains is a polypoid mass covered by mucosa at the umbilicus or a limited sinus that ends blindly. Omphalomesenteric duct remnants at the umbilicus are frequently confused with umbilical granulomas. Umbilical sinuses usually become evident because of persistent drainage at the umbilicus. The drainage is small in amount and does not have the typical appearance of intestinal contents. Treatment for both lesions is excision.

Omphalomesenteric band

An omphalomesenteric band results from involution of the omphalomesenteric duct mucosa and muscle, producing a solid cord connecting the ileum to the undersurface of the umbilicus (see Fig. 47.1f). This abnormality clinically becomes evident at abdominal exploration (laparotomy or laparoscopy) as the cause of an intestinal obstruction. These remnants may also be diagnosed as an incidental finding at the time of surgical exploration.

Vitelline blood vessel remnants

Occlusion, but failure of involution of vitelline blood vessel remnants also results in a fibrous cord within the peritoneal cavity. It may extend from the ileum or a Meckel's diverticulum to the undersurface of the umbilicus (Fig. 47.1b, f). This remnant becomes clinically evident when it produces intestinal obstruction as a result of the twisting of a segment of small intestine around the band.

CLINICAL PRESENTATION

Hemorrhage

Intermittent and painless bleeding per rectum is the most common presentation of a Meckel's diverticulum and therefore, the most common presentation of all the variations of yolk sac remnants. The cause of the bleeding is peptic ulceration at the junction of the ectopic gastric mucosa and normal ileal mucosa. Acid production by the gastric mucosal parietal cells is not neutralized because of the absence of duodenal bicarbonate. Thus, a 'marginal' ulcer develops at the junction of the gastric and ileal mucosa. *Helicobacter pylori*, an organism known to be associated with gastritis and peptic ulcer disease, has been

magnetic resonance (MR) angiography are less invasive and may be useful diagnostic tools. However, there is little clinical experience with these techniques in determining the presence of a vitelline artery or Meckel's diverticulum.

^{99m}Tc-labeled red blood cells

An additional study that has been helpful in certain cases uses ^{99m}Tc-labeled red blood cells. This nuclear medicine technique is not specific for a Meckel's diverticulum, but it can be used for localizing the site of bleeding in patients with intermittent and relatively low rates of bleeding.[41] Successful use of an *in vitro*, commercially available labeling kit has been reported.[42]

Ultrasonography

As visualization using ultrasonography has improved, the ability to diagnose intestinal abnormalities such as appendicitis and intussusception has been increasingly reported. Similarly, a study by Daneman and colleagues reported that, in a group of 31 children that had a false negative Meckel's scan, ultrasonography was successful in visualizing the Meckel's diverticulum in 14 patients (44%).[43]

Laparoscopy

Laparoscopy has not only gained wide acceptance in adult patients but also in the pediatric age group. As a diagnostic tool in children, laparoscopy has been very helpful in evaluating unusual abdominal symptoms or other diagnostic dilemmas. It is also a mechanism for treatment which will be discussed in the next section. However, it is important to note a word of caution that, because it is routine to place the initial access port through the umbilicus, there have been reports of injury to the bowel as a result of an omphalomesenteric duct remnant attached to the umbilicus.[44]

TREATMENT

In patients who present with intestinal obstruction from an omphalomesenteric duct remnant, the cause of the obstruction is rarely determined preoperatively. Intussusception of a Meckel's diverticulum can produce symptoms and signs of intestinal obstruction or more vague symptoms. Thus, diagnosis of this event can be difficult. As noted above, ultrasonography and CT can be successful in visualizing an inverted Meckel's diverticulum.[43,45] Patients with obstruction from a Meckel's diverticulum require prompt surgical exploration to relieve the obstruction. Patients with inflammation of a Meckel's diverticulum also require prompt surgical exploration. Most often these patients undergo abdominal exploration with the preoperative diagnosis of appendicitis. However, one differentiating factor may be the presence of significant free intraperitoneal air. This radiographic finding is exceptionally rare in patients with perforated appendicitis, but it is not unusual in those patients with perforation of a Meckel's diverticulum.

Although the approach and procedures may vary, the management of omphalomesenteric duct remnants is surgical resection. The one significant exception is the asymptomatic Meckel's diverticulum that does not contain ectopic tissue.

Meckel's diverticulum

Symptomatic Meckel's diverticula should always be surgically removed. Adequate preoperative resuscitation with intravenous fluid and (if indicated) packed red blood cell transfusion is necessary. If the presenting problem is hemorrhage, the extent of the resection will depend on the extent of ectopic gastric mucosa within the Meckel's diverticulum. In general, the ectopic gastric mucosa is limited to the distal portion of the Meckel's diverticulum. However, in some circumstances the ectopic mucosa extends to the junction of the ileum or even into the ileum (Fig. 47.7). When the gastric mucosa involves only the distal portion of the diverticulum, a stapling device can be used to excise only the diverticulum at the antimesenteric border of the bowel. If the ectopic mucosa extends into the ileum, a very limited ileal resection, including the diverticulum, with end-to-end anastomosis is appropriate. The surgical approach has generally been through a right lower quadrant transverse incision (Fig. 47.8). However, laparoscopy has been reported to be successful for both the diagnosis and surgical excision of a Meckel's diverticulum.[46,47] An alternative to either the open or the laparoscopic approach is to make the diagnosis laparoscopically and then slightly enlarge the umbilical port site and deliver the Meckel's diverticulum through this site. This allows the surgeon to palpate the diverticulum to define the extent of the gastric

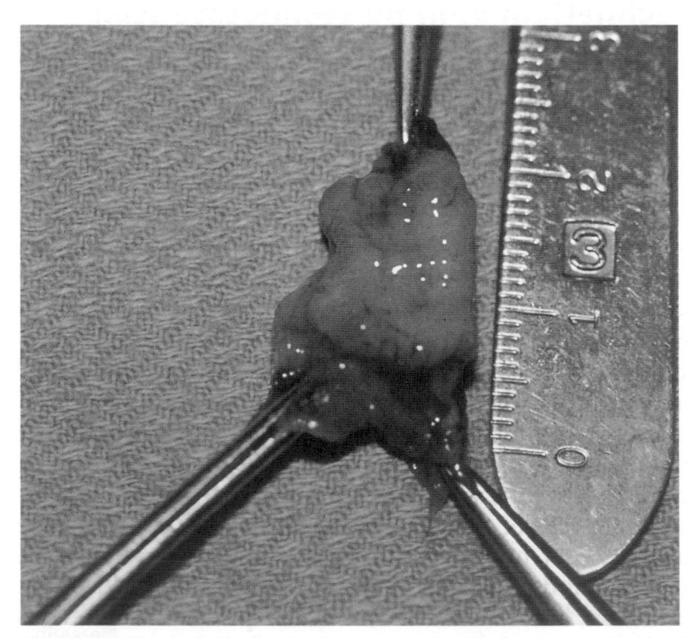

Figure 47.7: Meckel's diverticulum opened with the upper two-thirds containing ectopic gastric mucosa and the lower one-third containing normal ileal mucosa. An area of ulceration at the junction of the gastric mucosa and ileal mucosa could be seen at the time of surgery, but is difficult to see in the operative photograph.

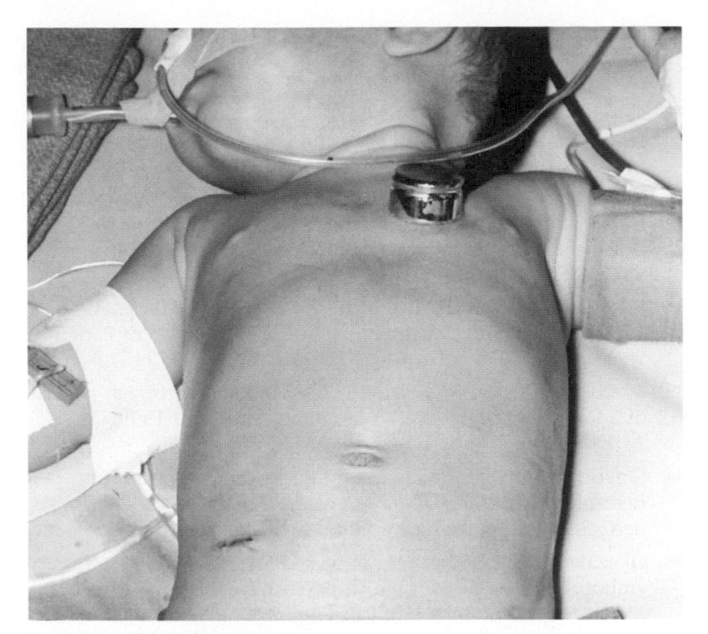

Figure 47.8: Typical short right lower quadrant transverse incision used for resection of a Meckel's diverticulum.

mucosa (which feels thicker) to determine the degree of resection. It also allows the surgeon to do an 'open' bowel anastomosis if indicated which can be easier and faster.

The surgical approach for intussusception induced by a Meckel's diverticulum is similar to that for the idiopathic variety. However, it is unusual for the cause of the intussusception to be known before laparotomy. The index of suspicion that a lead point is present should increase in children older than 2 to 3 years of age. If at exploration a Meckel's diverticulum is identified as the lead point, it should be excised.

Complications are uncommon after excision of a Meckel's diverticulum. The most common postoperative complications are infection (either intraperitoneal or wound) and a leak at the site of ileal closure or from the anastomosis after a limited bowel resection. However, these complications should not occur in more than 2% of cases.

There is little controversy that symptomatic Meckel's diverticula should be removed. However, an area of ongoing controversy is the approach to a Meckel's diverticulum found incidentally at the time of laparotomy being performed for another reason. Some authors believe that a Meckel's diverticulum should always be removed when found.[5,19,48,49] This is based on the potential risks of bleeding, perforation, obstruction, and the development of neoplasms. Those authors opposed to incidental diverticulectomy point to the low lifetime risk of development of symptoms related to the presence of a Meckel's diverticulum[11] and the potential risk of postoperative complications.[7,50,51] If, at surgical exploration, palpation of the Meckel's diverticulum reveals ectopic gastric mucosa or if its base is narrow (which increases the risk of obstruction) then most pediatric surgeons would proceed with resection. If none of the above findings are present, the unresolved question of elective resection remains.

Patent omphalomesenteric duct

A patent omphalomesenteric duct should always be surgically excised from the junction of the umbilicus to its junction with the ileum. Care should be taken to remove all portions of the communication at the umbilicus to avoid subsequent complications. Laparoscopy would not be advantageous in this situation because the diagnosis is known and it would not be feasible to place the umbilical port.

Omphalomesenteric duct cyst

Frequently, omphalomesenteric duct cysts manifest as an infected mass around or inferior to the umbilicus. As previously noted, they are either preperitoneal or intraperitoneal. These cystic remnants can become very large during the course of an infection, and an effort at excision at that time may be inappropriate. Incision and drainage followed, several weeks later, by cyst excision after the infection has resolved would diminish the risk for complications.

SUMMARY

Omphalomesenteric duct remnants are common and can result in a variety of presentations and complications, some of which are life threatening. Symptomatic lesions should always be surgically removed. Asymptomatic lesions, such as intraperitoneal bands or cysts, discovered at the time of surgical exploration for other reasons should also be removed to avoid a future bowel obstruction or other complications. Remnants at the umbilicus should be resected as they are likely to cause symptoms (especially infection) at some point in time. The ongoing controversy of what to do about asymptomatic, non-ectopic tissue containing Meckel's diverticula remains. It has been our bias to not resect them.

References

1. Fabricius Hildanus W. Opera observationum et curationum medicochirurgicarum, quae extant omina. Francof J Beveri, 1646.
2. Lavater JH. Dissertatio medico-chirurgica, de 'enteroperistole' seu intestinorum compressione, Basilae, 1672.
3. Ruysch F. Opera Omnia. Amsterdam, Jansson-Waesberg, 1757.
4. Meckel JF. Ueber die Divertikel am Darmkanal. Arch Physiol 1809(9):421–453.
5. Gray SW, Skanddalakis JE. Embryology for Surgeons. Philadelphia, PA: WB Saunders; 1972:156–167.
6. Soderlund S. Meckel's diverticulum, a clinical and histologic study. Acta Chir Scand Suppl 1959; 118:1–233.
7. Soltero MJ, Bill AH. The natural history of Meckel's diverticulum and its relations to incidental removal. Am J Surg 1976; 132:168–173.
8. Collins DC. A study of 50,000 specimens of the human vermiform appendix. Surg Gynecol Obstet 1955; 101:137–145.
9. Moses WR. Meckel's diverticulum. N Engl J Med 1947; 237:118–122.
10. Androulakis JA, Gray SW, Lionakis B, et al. The sex ratio of Meckel's diverticulum. Am Surg 1969; 35:455–460.

11. Amory RA. Meckel's diverticulum. In: Welch KJ, Randolph JG, Ravitch MM, et al., eds. Pediatric Surgery, 4th edn. Chicago, IL: Year Book Medical Publishers; 1986:859–867.
12. Gross RE. The Surgery of Infancy and Childhood. Philadelphia, PA: WB Saunders; 1953:212–220.
13. Yamaguchi M, Takeuchi S, Awazu S. Meckel's diverticulum: investigation of 600 patients in Japanese literature. Am J Surg 1978; 136:247–249.
14. Jewett TC Jr, Duszynski DO, Allen JE. The visualization of Meckel's diverticulum with ^{99m}Tc-pertechnetate. Surgery 1970; 68:567–570.
15. Wansbrough RM, Thompson S, Leckey RG. Meckel's diverticulum: a 42-year review of 273 cases at the Hospital for Sick Children, Toronto. Can J Surg 1957; 1:15–20.
16. Kiesewetter WB. Meckel's diverticulum in children. Arch Surg 1957; 75:914–919.
17. Ludtke FE, Mende V, Kohler H, et al. Incidence and frequency of complications and management of Meckel's diverticulum. Surg Gynecol Obstet 1989; 169:537–542.
18. Bemelman WA, Bosma A, Wiersman PH, et al. Role of Helicobacter pylori in the pathogenesis of complications of Meckel's diverticula. Eur J Surg 1993; 159:171–175.
19. Oguzkurt P, Talim B, Tanyel FC, et al. The Role of Heterotopic Gastric Mucosa With or Without Colonization of Helicobacter pylori upon the Diverse Symptomatology of Meckel's Diverticulum in Children. Turk J Pediatr 2001; 43:312–316.
20. Rutherford RB, Akers DR. Meckel's diverticulum: a review of 148 pediatric patients, with special reference to the pattern of bleeding and to mesodiverticular vascular bands. Surgery 1966; 59:618–626.
21. Seagram CGF, Louche RE, Stephens CA, et al. Meckel's diverticulum: a 10-year review of 218 cases. Can J Surg 1968; 11:369–373.
22. Andreyev HJ, Owen RA, Thompson I, et al. Association between Meckel's diverticulum and Crohn's disease: a retrospective review. Gut 1994; 35:788–790.
23. Neidlinger NA, Madan AK, Wright MJ. Meckel's Diverticulum Causing Cecal Volvulus. Am Surg 2001; 67:41–43.
24. Tosato F, Corsini F, Marano S, et al. Ileal Occlusion caused by enterolith migrated from Meckel's diverticulum. Ann Ital Chir 71:393–396.
25. Hudson HM, Millham FH, Dennis R. Vesico-diverticular fistula: a rare complication of Meckel's diverticulum. Am Surg 1992; 58:784–786.
26. Henneberg HC, Thorlacius-Ussing O, Teglbjaerg PS, et al. Inverted Meckel's diverticulum masquerading Crohn's disease in the small intestine. Scand J Gastroenterol 2003; 38:225–227.
27. Jelenc F, Strlic M, Gvardijancic D. Meckel's Diverticulum Perforation with Intraabdominal Hemorrhage. J Pediatr Surg 2002; 37:E18.
28. Stolk MF. deJong AE, van Ramshorst B, et al: Intestinal Bleeding Due to a Stromal Tumor in a Meckel's Diverticulum. Gastrointest Endosc 2002; 56:147–149.
29. Harden RMcG. Alexander WD, Kennedy I: Isotope uptake and scanning of stomach in man with ^{99m}Tc-pertechnetate. Lancet 1967; 1:1305–1307.
30. Anderson GF, Sfakianakis G, King DR, et al. Hormonal enhancement of technetium-99m pertechnetate uptake in experimental Meckel's diverticulum. J Pediatr Surg 1980; 15:900–905.
31. Khettery J, Effmann E, Grand RJ, et al. Effect of pentagastrin, histamine, glucagon, secretin, and perchlorate on the gastric hoarding of ^{99m}Tc pertechnetate in mice. Radiology 1976; 120:629–631.
32. Treves S, Grand RJ, Eraklis AJ. Pentagastrin stimulation of technetium 99m uptake by ectopic gastric mucosa in a Meckel's diverticulum. Radiology 1978; 128:711–712.
33. Cooney DR, Duszynski DO, Camboa E, et al. The abdominal technetium scan (a decade of experience). J Pediatr Surg 1982; 17:611–619.
34. Keramidas DC, Coran AG, Zaleska RW. An experimental model for assessing the radiopertechnetate diagnosis of gastric mucosa in Meckel's diverticulum. J Pediatr Surg 1974; 9:879–883.
35. Swaniker F, Soldes O, Hirschl RB. The Utility of Technetium 99m Pertechnetate Scintigraphy in the Evaluation of Patients with Meckel's Diverticulum. J Pediatr Surg 1999; 34:760–764.
36. McKevitt EC, Baerg JE, Nadel HR, et al. Laparoscopy as a cause of a false-positive Meckel's scan. Clin Nucl Med 1999; 24:102–104.
37. Emamian SA, Shalaby-Rana E, Majd M. The spectrum of heterotopic gastric mucosa in children detected by Tc-99m pertechnetate scintigraphy. Clin Nucl Med 2001; 26:529–535.
38. Okazaki M, Higashihara H, Yamasaki S, et al. Arterial embolization to control life-threatening hemorrhage from a Meckel's diverticulum. Am J Roentgenol 1990; 154:1257–1258.
39. Routh WD, Lawdahl RB, Lund E, et al. Meckel's diverticula: angiographic diagnosis in patients with no acute hemorrhage and negative scintigraphy. Pediatr Radiol 1990; 20:152–156.
40. Okazaki M, Higashihara H, Saida Y, et al. Angiographic findings of Meckel's diverticulum: the characteristic appearance of the vitelline artery. Abdom Imaging 1993; 18:15–19.
41. Winzelberg GG, McKusick KA, Strauss HW, et al. Evaluation of gastrointestinal bleeding by red blood cells labeled in vivo with technetium 99m. J Nucl Med 1979; 20:1080–1086.
42. Kwok CG, Lull RJ, Yen CK, et al. Feasibility of Meckel's scan after RBC gastrointestinal bleeding study using in vitro labeling technique. Clin Nucl Med 1995; 20:959–961.
43. Daneman A, Lobo E, Alton DJ, et al. The value of sonography, CT, and air enema for detection of complicated Meckel diverticulum in children with nonspecific clinical presentation. Pediatr Radiol 1998; 28:928–932.
44. Westcott CJ, Westcott RJ, Kerstein MD. Perforation of a Meckel's diverticulum during laparoscopic cholecystectomy. South Med J 1995; 88:661.
45. Pantongrag-Brown L, Levine MS, Elsayed AM, et al. Inverted Meckel's diverticulum: clinical radiologic and pathologic findings. Radiology 1996; 199:693–696.
46. Schier F, Hoffman K, Waldschmidt J. Laparoscopic removal of Meckel's diverticula in children. Eur J Pediatr Surg 1996; 6:38–39.
47. Sanders LE. Laparoscopic treatment of Meckel's diverticulum. Surg Endosc 1995; 9:724–727.
48. Arnold JF, Pellicane JV. Meckel's diverticulum: a ten-year experience. Am Surg 1997; 63:354–355.
49. Cullen JJ, Kelly KA, Moir CR, et al. Surgical management of Meckel's diverticulum: an epidemiologic, population-based study. Ann Surg 1994; 220:564–568.
50. Kashi SH, Lodge JP. Meckel's diverticulum: a continuing dilemma? J R Col Surg Edin 1995; 40:392–394.
51. Mackey WC, Dinen P. A fifty-year experience with Meckel's diverticulum. Surg Gynecol Obstet 1983; 156:56–64.

Chapter 48
Hirschsprung's disease

Anthony Stallion and Tzuyung Doug Kou

HISTORY

In 1886 Harald Hirschsprung gave the first comprehensive account of the condition that now bears his name. It was in 1888 that he summarized his findings in a publication entitled 'Constipation in newborns as a consequence of dilatation and hypertrophy of the colon', in which he gave a typical clinical presentation of the infants he had encountered. Hirschsprung suggested that the condition was congenital, but did not offer any specific etiology or therapeutic option.[1] He had noted a somewhat narrow rectum in one of his early cases, but did not fully understand that the cause of the megacolon was the non-dilated distal bowel. The recognition of distal intestinal obstruction as the pathologic basis of Hirschsprung's disease (HD) was not discovered until the early twentieth century. It was not until 1945 that a group of physicians led by Orvar Swenson at the Boston Children's Hospital was able to determine that the disease process of HD was secondary to functional distal obstruction. The functional obstruction results from chronic contraction of the distal rectum with secondary proximal bowel dilation.[2] Swenson's group was able to document that the internal pressure of the distal segment of bowel was higher than that in the normal colon, which also had no peristalsis. Eventually it was recognized that there is an absence of ganglion cells in HD, specifically of Auerbach's plexus in the distal segment of bowel. In addition, it was subsequently demonstrated that removal of this abnormal segment of bowel with anastomosis of the proximal bowel to the anus resulted in resolution of the problem.

Swenson and Bill in 1948 were the first to advocate full-thickness rectal biopsy to make the diagnosis of HD. They subsequently developed a life-saving surgical procedure that spared patients an invariably premature death secondary to toxic megacolon and enterocolitis. This procedure involved resecting the aganglionic bowel and replacing it with normal innervated proximal intestine.[3] The resulting improved patient survival and subsequent reproduction revealed a previously unsuspected familial transmission of HD.

EPIDEMIOLOGY

HD is a rare disorder affecting approximately 1 in 5000 live births, showing a male : female predominance of approximately 4:1. In long-segment disease, the ratio approaches 1 : 1. The rates of distribution are equal between Caucasians and African-Americans. Most cases of HD occur in full-term infants. Less than 10% of cases occur in infants with a birthweight of less than 3 kg.

HD (non-syndromic) occurs as an isolated trait in 70% of patients. Syndromic HD occurs in 30% of cases, and 40% of these are associated with a chromosomal abnormality, representing 12% of total cases; trisomy 21 is by far the most frequent chromosomal abnormality, found in more than 90% of instances.[3] Children with Down's syndrome have an increased incidence of HD (3–10% of patients with HD) compared with the general population. In the remaining 60% of syndromic HD cases (18% of the total), there are multiple congenital anomalies or recognized genetic syndromes such as multiple endocrine neoplasia (MEN) IIA, congenital deafness, Waardenberg's syndrome and Von Recklinghausen's disease. Syndromic HD can be classified as a pleiotrophic syndrome with colonic aganglionosis as a mandatory feature accompanied by recognizable syndromes.[3]

HD is usually subdivided into short- and long-segment disease. The internal anal sphincter is the lowermost limit in both types. Some 80% of patients have short-segment HD involving the colon distal to the splenic flexure; 20% have long-segment disease involving the colon proximal to the splenic flexure. In rare cases, approximately 3–5%, there is total colonic aganglionosis, and even less common is total intestinal HD. There is also a very rare form of HD in which there is an ultra-short segment involving only the very distal 2–5 cm of rectum.

GENETICS

A large number of chromosomal abnormalities have been described in association with HD. The most common associated syndromic abnormality (3–10% of all ascertained cases; 90% of all chromosomal cases) is trisomy 21 (Down's syndrome).[4,5] Genetic inheritance has long been appreciated in that HD may affect more than one family member in 37% of cases, and some familial forms of HD have a 50% inheritance rate. Studies have demonstrated that the longer the segment of aganglionosis, the higher rate of familial incidence. HD is a complex multigenetic disorder in which there is significant interplay between different genes potentially resulting in multiple abnormalities. The products of different associated genes are important in the determination of the HD phenotype. Thus, there is a complex proteinomic network involved in the pathogenesis of HD.

In 1967, Passarge reported 60 families with HD with autosomal recessive and autosomal dominant inheritance. It became clear that HD did not strictly follow the rules of mendelian inheritance. In syndromic forms of HD, the genes encoding for the proteins of the *RET* signalling pathway (*RET*, *GDNF* and *NTN*), as well as those in the endothelium (*EDN*) type B receptor pathway (*EDNRB*, *EDN-3*) are found in more than 50% of affected individuals (Table 48.1).[4,6–12] The majority of these mutations are incompletely penetrant, so that many family members carrying them are completely asymptomatic. The interplay between the actual ligands and receptors accounting for these genetic mutations are not completely understood. Most likely, there needs to be overlapping of multiple genetic mutations, rather than a single mutation, for HD to occur.[13]

By the mid-1980s it was apparent that non-syndromic HD was a multifactorial disorder. Segregation studies in non-syndromic HD have shown that the recurrent risk in siblings varies from 1% to 33% depending on the sex and the length of the aganglionic segment in the affected child, as well as the sex of the sibling. The first association of a specific genetic defect in HD was reported in 1992 as a deletion in the short arm of chromosome 10.[14] Further investigation revealed the location of the mutation between 10-Q 11.2 and Q-21.2. This overlapped the region of the *RET* proto-oncogene. Mutations of the *RET* gene are responsible for approximately half of familial cases, and 10% of cases of sporadic HD. In non-syndromic HD, abnormalities have been described in three loci of the *RET* locus, which encodes for the RET receptor. It has been postulated that different mutations in the *RET* proto-oncogene predispose to either HD or MENII syndrome. There is evidence that the degree of mutation in the *RET* proto-oncogene is associated with the severity of presentation of HD. Approximately 15% of all HD cases are accounted for by mutations in the two genes *RET* and *EDNRB*. The *RET* polymorphic variance may contribute to the occurrence of total intestinal aganglionosis (TIA).[15] HD is one of the first polymorphic multifactorial human diseases with a defined multigenic etiology to have been identified.

The authors have obtained microarray data to evaluate human colonic biopsy specimens from patients with HD and those with chronic constipation. A significant downregulation of the genes that encode molecules responsible for regulating leukocyte, epithelial, nerve and muscle cells was found in aganglionic compared with ganglionic tissue from patients with HD. In addition, a significant upregulation of genes coding for similar molecules was observed when aganglionic and ganglionic tissue from a patient with HD was compared with tissue from a control patient with constipation (Fig. 48.1a–c; Table 48.2). In the future, having a better understanding of the actual genetic mutations involved may lead to gene therapy for fetuses suspected of having HD based on a strong family history confirmed by the presence of one or more genetic mutations.

Gene	Location	Main effect	Penetrance (%)
PMX2B	4p13	Recessive	50–60
RET	10q11.2	Dominant, loss of function	50–72
GDNF	5p13.1	Dominant or recessive	Unknown
EDNRB	13q22	Recessive	30–85
EDN3	20q13	Recessive	Unknown
SOX10	22q13	Dominant or recessive	>80
NTN	19p13	Unknown	Unknown
SIP1	2q22	Sporadic	Unknown

Table 48.1 Genes associated with Hirschsprung's disease

EMBRYOLOGY

Normal ganglion cells are recognized in the esophagus at 6 weeks of gestation, in the transverse colon by 8 weeks and in the rectum by 12 weeks. The initial caudal migration of intramuscular neuroblasts is followed by intramural dispersal of neuroblasts to the superficial and deep submucosal nerve plexus. There is then concurrent and subsequent maturation of neuroblasts into ganglion cells well into infancy. Congenital intestinal aganglionosis or HD is the result of arrested fetal development of the myenteric nervous system; however, the precise pathologic mechanisms involved are not completely understood.

ETIOLOGY

Classic theory regarding the embryologic development of HD is that there is failure of migration of ganglion cells along the gastrointestinal tract during the 5th through 12th weeks of embryologic development. Ganglion cells that form as the intrinsic nerves of the colon migrate caudally along the embryonic gut, originating from the vagal neural crest.[16] Another theory is that there is a hostile micro-environment owing to decreased neural crest adhesion molecule (NCAM) reactivity in the aganglionic colon compared with that in normal age- and sex-matched controls. NCAM is believed to be important in neuron-site migration and localization to specific sites during embryogenesis.[17,18] Although there are experimental data to support individual theories, it is likely that the cause of HD is multifactorial.

PATHOPHYSIOLOGY

Aganglionosis is confined to the sigmoid colon or rectum in 75–80% of affected infants. Classically, the proximal bowel is distended with histologic evidence of muscular hypertrophy. The characteristic lesion in the distal bowel is the absence of ganglion cells in the intermuscular and submucosal plexus (Fig. 48.2). In addition, many large,

	No. of genes upregulated	No. of genes downregulated
HD aganglionic tissue *vs* normal tissue	274	82
HD ganglionic tissue *vs* normal tissue	110	22
HD aganglionic tissue *vs* HD ganglionic tissue	81	127

Table 48.2 Genes upregulated or downregulated in patients with HD and controls

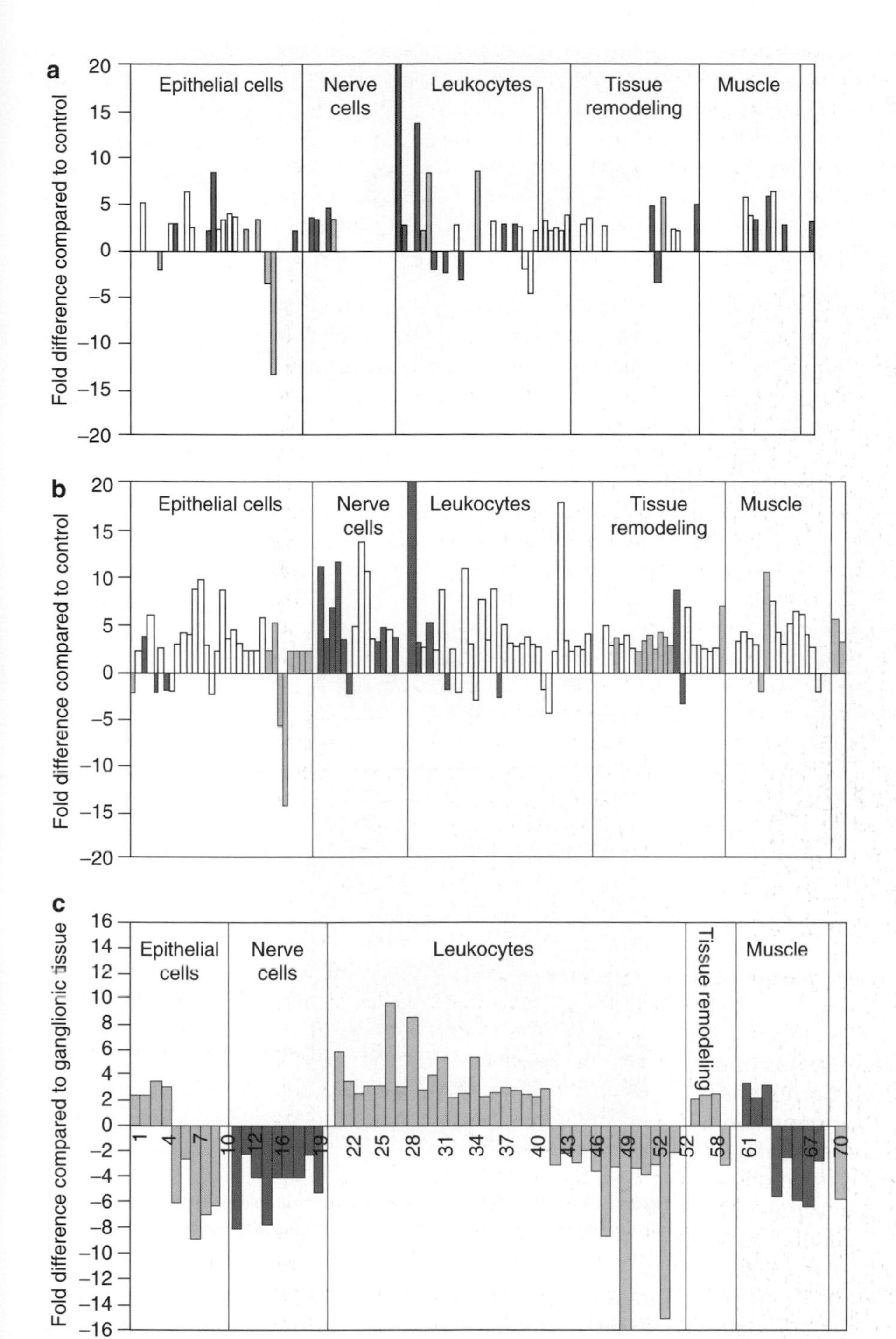

Figure 48.1: Microarray data on biopsy specimens from patients with HD and constipation as control. (**a**) Aganglionic tissue from patients with HD *vs* controls. (**b**) Ganglionic tissue from patients with HD *vs* controls. (**c**) Aganglionic and ganglionic tissue from patients with HD.

thickened, non-myelinated nerve fibers are found within the muscularis mucosa, lamina propria, submucosa and Auerbach's intramuscular plexus. Most of these fibers are cholinergic. Thus, an important diagnostic test involves histochemical staining for acetylcholinesterase (Fig. 48.3).

HD is a form of intestinal pseudo-obstruction or functional bowel obstruction with the absence of mechanical blockage of the lumen. It is the most common form of pseudo-obstruction. Normal intestinal motility depends on a coordinated segmental contraction wave immediately preceded by smooth muscle relaxation as it propagates caudally. In HD there is a lack of a functional myenteric nervous system in the affected distal intestine, and thus ineffective distal peristalsis secondary to an inability to have smooth muscle relaxation. There are also other potential abnormalities within the more proximal transition and ganglionic bowel.[19] The clinical outcome is incomplete distal bowel obstruction in neonates or chronic constipation in older children. Patients with HD do not have the normal internal sphincter relaxation that should follow rectal dilation, and thus diagnosis may be made by manometric studies.

Interposed between normal ganglionic proximal bowel and the abnormal distal bowel is a transition zone characterized by hypoganglionosis and a progressive increase in

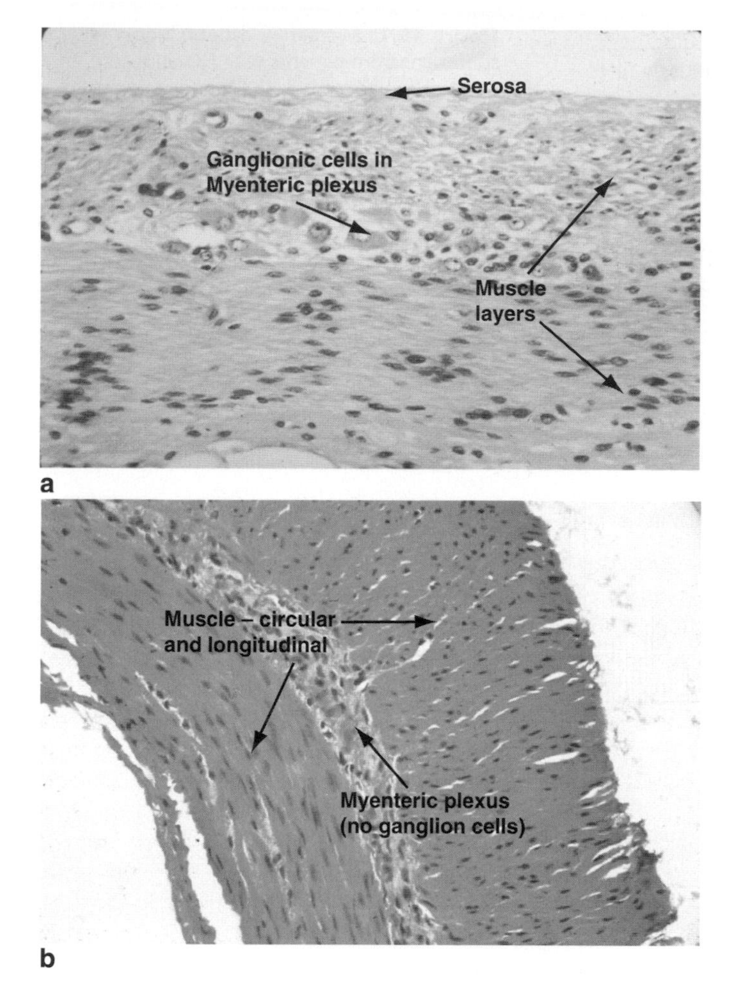

Figure 48.2: Hematoxylin and eosin stain of colonic biopsy showing myenteric plexus from (**a**) a normal subject and (**b**) a patient with HD (*See plate section for color*).

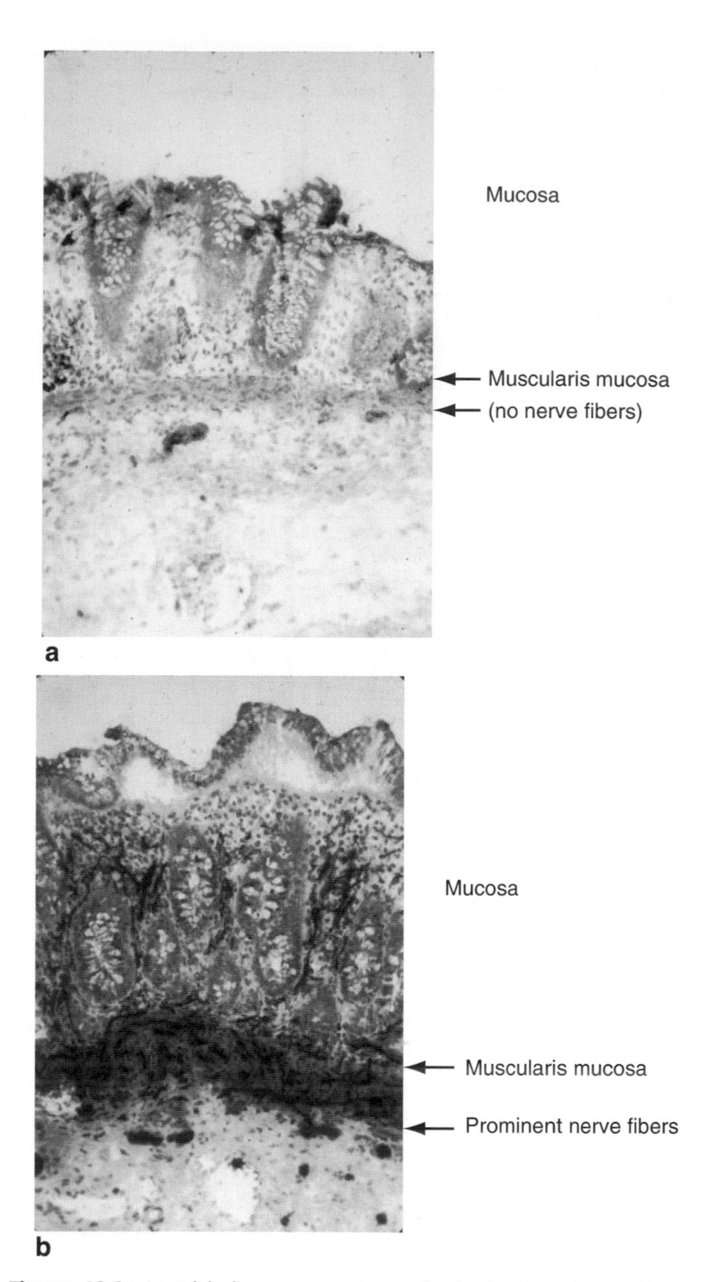

Figure 48.3: Acetylcholinesterase staining of colonic biopsy from (**a**) a normal subject and (**b**) a patient with HD (*See plate section for color*).

the number of thickened, non-myelinated neurons as one moves distally toward the aganglionic bowel. Correlation between the gross and microscopic anatomy is not precise, so histologic confirmation is always necessary for intraoperative decision-making. The transition zone is often obvious grossly or radiographically by a few weeks of age, as the obstruction leads to progressive proximal dilation and eventually to 'congenital megacolon'. A normal barium enema study can never rule out the diagnosis of HD. Most evidence supports the concept that HD is a continuous disorder starting in the distal rectum and moving proximally. Although the length of involved rectal segment may be short, a correctly obtained rectal biopsy specimen showing ganglion cells precludes the existence of HD. Intestinal atresia is occasionally found in association with HD.

Neural crest cells play an important role throughout the body, particularly in the gastrointestinal tract in the formation of the enteric nervous system (ENS). The complexity of the ENS rivals that of the brain, and it shares many of the neurotransmitters found in the central nervous system (CNS). The ENS also has a reflex arc that acts independently of the CNS. The ENS communicates with the CNS via the parasympathetic and sympathetic ganglia, but is capable of independently controlling the functions of the gastrointestinal tract. The ENS is derived from the neural crest cells that give rise to the vagal crest and subsequently the submucosal ganglia. At the completion of migration, neural crest cells differentiate into diverse cell types including neurons and glia of the sensory, sympathetic and parasympathetic ganglia, neuroendocrine cells adrenal medulla, pigmented cells and facial cartilage. Failure of the vagally derived neural crest cells to colonize the hindgut results in failure of ENS development. The earlier the migration arrest, the longer is the portion of distal aganglionic intestine. It has been demonstrated experimentally that ablation of the vagal neural crest can result in total intestinal aganglionosis. Iwashita et al.[20]demonstrated, by gene expression profiling combined with reversed genetic analysis of stem cell function, that HD may be caused by defects in neural crest stem cell function.

In summary, HD is a developmental disorder of the ENS characterized by absence of ganglion cells in the myenteric and submucosal plexuses along a variable portion of the distal intestine. The most widely accepted etiopathogenic hypothesis involves a defect of the craniocaudal migration of neuroblasts originating from the neural crest.

NEUROCRISTOPATHIES

This encompasses an array of syndromes that arise from abnormalities in the development of the pluripotential neural crest cells. The diseases arising from neural crest are diverse in clinical presentation, including endocrine, cutaneous, neurologic, digestive and/or associated with syndromes. With its constellation of symptoms, in 1974, Bolande suggested the term 'neurocristopathies'.[21] The neural crest cells are important in the development of the neural and endocrine systems; thus there is a link that associates HD with abnormalities in other neural crest-derived systems. HD is classified as a simple neurocristopathy.

Syndromes associated with HD include the Shah–Waardenburg syndrome, congenital central hypoventilation syndrome (CCHS), MENII and Haddad syndrome, which is short-segment HD associated with a congenital central hypoventilation syndrome. Therefore, awareness of a possible neurocristopathy associated with neurologic abnormalities should be taken into account in any patient newly diagnosed with HD. In a small study, a number of patients with HD demonstrated measurable autonomic dysfunction on pupillary and cardiovascular testing of sympathetic, parasympathetic and cardiovagal cholinergic function.[22]

Cheng et al.[23] demonstrated moderate to severe sensory neural hearing loss, abnormal otoacoustic transmission and marked abnormalities in tests of peripheral nerve function in patients with HD compared with controls. Thus, HD may be a more generalized neuropathy than simply involving the affected bowel.

There are also multiple non-neurocristopathies that are associated with HD, including the Smith–Lemli–Opitz syndrome, and distal limb anomalies that are all quite rare. Goldberg–Shprintzen syndrome, with its distinct dysmorphic facial features, microcephaly and intellectual impairment, along with agenesis of the corpus callosum and cortical malformations associated with intractable seizures, has also been associated with HD. There is a rare combination of congenital aganglionosis of the intestine and CCHS (Ondine's curse).[21,23,24] Currarino's triad is a form of caudal regression syndrome that is a rare complex of congenital caudal anomalies that include anorectal malformations, sacral bone deformity and presacral tumor. This has been described in association with HD by Baltogiannis et al.[25]

INTESTINAL AGANGLIONOSIS

Absence of ganglion cells in the small intestine is a rare form of HD. It is a condition found in the newborn and is associated with increased morbidity and mortality compared with the more common rectosigmoid disease. There may be histopathologic differences between total colonic aganglionosis and rectosigmoid HD. Total colonic HD demonstrates a lack of neuronal nitric oxide synthesis and peripherin immunoreactivity. In addition, in total colonic HD there is a lack of interstitial cells of Cajal (ICCs), which act as pacemakers within the myenteric plexus, thus playing a role in bowel motility.[26] Puri[27] demonstrated that ICCs, which also play a role in development of the gastrointestinal tract, have an altered distribution in the entire resected bowel of patients with HD. This may suggest that the persistent dysmotility problems after pull-through operations in patients with HD may be due to altered distribution and impaired function of these ICCs.[26,28]

Puri also described carbon monoxide as a proposed endogenous messenger molecule for ICCs and smooth muscle cells in the gastrointestinal tract that may be altered along with heme oxygenase 2 (HO2), which is the main physiologic mechanism for generating carbon monoxide in human cells. He further demonstrated the presence of HO2 immunoreactivity in the ICCs of normal human colon and the absence of HO2 immunoreactivity in sparsely appearing ICCs in the bowel of patients with HD.[27] This lack of HO2 in the ICCs may result in impaired intracellular communication between the ICCs and smooth muscle cells, causing motility dysfunction. Wedel et al.[18] demonstrated structural abnormalities in the basal lamina of patients with HD. The observed ultrastructural alterations in the basal lamina of both neural and non-neural cells, as well as the increased amount of perineural and endoneural collagen, provided further evidence that the extracellular matrix components are abnormally distributed and overproduced within the bowel wall of patients affected by HD.[18]

CLINICAL PRESENTATION

HD often presents in newborns as distal intestinal obstruction with or without sepsis. The incidence of enterocolitis is variable and always a concern. Thus, the diagnosis must be undertaken with some degree of urgency. The newborn may present as acutely ill secondary to the distal bowel obstruction. Other findings may include abdominal distention and bilious or feculent vomiting associated with failure to pass meconium. In the most severe cases, the patient may present with overwhelming sepsis and/or peritonitis secondary to intestinal perforation. At times, the delayed passage of meconium more than 48h after delivery is the mode of presentation. Between 40% and 95% of patients have been reported to have failure of passage of meconium by 48 h. However, it must be understood that the passage of meconium within 48 h does not exclude the diagnosis of HD. A high index of suspicion must be maintained for the neonate with an abnormal presentation.

Age at diagnosis can vary widely, with approximately 50% of patients being diagnosed in the neonatal period and the vast majority of the remainder before the age of 2 years. Occasionally a patient will make it to later childhood or as a young adult before diagnosis. Usually they are

Calibration and subsequent dilation starting in the early postoperative period will usually prevent these complications. If the patient is having difficulties and there is no stricture present, repeat biopsy is warranted to rule out a retained segment of aganglionic bowel. Other diagnoses such as neuronal dysplasia or hypoganglionosis should also be ruled out.

Myectomy may be useful in patients who have persistent enterocolitis or constipation with failed medical treatment, and who have been shown by biopsy not to have an aganglionic segment. In addition, myectomy may be helpful in the patient who has been demonstrated to have a retained length of aganglionic bowel of less than 5 cm. Its success has been attributed to the use of a lateral sphincter myotomy including the external sphincter in patients with severe outlet obstruction and constipation.[70] This has resulted in significant symptomatic relief in two-thirds of patients. The use of botulism toxin (botox) injections into the internal anal sphincter in patients with severe constipation or recurrent enterocolitis has demonstrated good results. Patients with a good response are those who may benefit most from a myectomy. There may also be lasting effects of the botox injection, so that the patient may not need any further intervention.

Indications for repeat pull-through may be retained aganglionosis, severe stricturing, dysfunctional bowel or neuronal dysplasia, severe enterocolitis, anastomotic stricture, leaking anastomosis and persistent rectal septum.[66,71] Additionally, there are patients with marked dilation of the rectosigmoid secondary to years of constipation and loss of muscular tone of the bowel. In patients who have had an endorectal pull-through, either transabdominal or laparoscopic, an attempt at a repeat endorectal pull-through may be possible. If not, a decision should be made whether to perform a Duhamel- or Swenson-type procedure. Patients with a failed pull-through procedure may do best with a Duhamel pull-through performed as a secondary procedure, owing to its lower risk for injury to pelvic structures and preservation of a previously dissected sphincter complex. Patients who have a Swenson or Duhamel procedure will require a transabdominal repeat of either of those procedures. An endorectal pull-through gives similar results to Duhamel and Swenson procedures for repeat pull-through operations, as long as there is an adequate rectal cuff for repeat anastomosis.[72] The posterior sagittal approach is a useful alternative in difficult repeat pull-through surgery with maintenance of continence and minimal complications.[73]

INTESTINAL DYSMOTILITY SYNDROMES

As demonstrated by Miele et al.[74] in a subset of patients with HD, gastrointestinal dysmotility persists long after surgical correction. The basic defects of HD could provide further motor abnormalities that are responsible for the continuation of symptoms after surgical correction. Baillie et al.[75] demonstrated that there is persistence of gastrointestinal motor dysfunction in the majority of children with HD long after surgical treatment of the aganglionic segment. The objective abnormalities include abnormal colonic transit, delayed total gut transit and previously unrecognized delays in gastric emptying. Transit abnormalities are also found in more than half of asymptomatic children, suggesting that additional factors are required to induce the symptomatic state. Thus, those caring for patients with HD must be aware that the manifestations of the disease are not localized only to the aganglionic colonic segment, and that once the disease has been treated surgically there may be postoperative symptoms.

Intestinal neuronal dysplasia (IND) associated with HD may also result in persistence of symptoms. IND was initially described by Meier-Ruge in 1971 and was classified as a colonic dysplasia. IND has a varied histologic appearance with hyperplasia of the enteric ganglia; increased acetylcholinesterase staining is characteristic. The typical presentation of IND is variable. Most children complain of abdominal distention; some have constipation and develop enterocolitis. The extent of IND may range from a short colonic segment to the entire length of the gastrointestinal tract. In contrast to HD, the internal sphincteric relaxation reflex is absent or atypical in only 75% of patients. HD-associated IND was found in 40% of cases.[27,57] There are two types of IND: A and B. Type B is seen much more commonly, yet type A presents at a younger age. Initial symptoms are related to the length of the aganglionic segment, but not to the presence of HD-associated IND. After surgery, the presence of long-segment aganglionosis or associated IND implies a delay in the restoration of normal defecation.[76] Persistent constipation is found in 40% of patients with associated disseminated IND at 6-month follow-up, compared with 20% in patients with isolated HD. These children need secondary intervention more often than those with associated localized IND or isolated HD. Thus, HD-associated IND has clinical implications for the postoperative period if IND is disseminated. Intraoperative histochemical examination could be of importance in looking for dysganglionic and hypoganglionic segments that may be responsible for postoperative bowel dysfunction.

References

1. Jay V. Legacy of Harald Hirschsprung. Pediatr Dev Pathol 2001; 4:203–204.
2. Swenson O. How the cause and cure of Hirschsprung's disease were discovered. J Pediatr Surg 1999; 34:1580–1581.
3. Amiel J, Lyonnet S. Hirschsprung disease, associated syndromes, and genetics: a review. J Med Genet 2001; 38:729–739.
4. Parisi MA, Kapur RP. Genetics of Hirschsprung disease. Curr Opin Pediatr 2000; 12:610–617.
5. Stewart DR, von Allmen D. The genetics of Hirschsprung disease. Gastroenterol Clin North Am 2003; 32:819–837, vi.
6. Sancandi M, Ceccherini I, Costa M, et al. Incidence of *RET* mutations in patients with Hirschsprung's disease. J Pediatr Surg 2000; 35:139–142, discussion 142–143.

7. Benailly HK, Lapierre JM, Laudier B, et al. *PMX2B*, a new candidate gene for Hirschsprung's disease. Clin Genet 2003; 64:204–209.
8. Garavelli L, Donadio A, Zanacca C, et al. Hirschsprung disease, mental retardation, characteristic facial features, and mutation in the gene *ZFHX1B* (*SIP1*): confirmation of the Mowat–Wilson syndrome. Am J Med Genet 2003; 116A:385–388.
9. Garcia-Barcelo M, Sham MH, Lui VC, Chen BL, Ott J, Tam PK. Association study of *PHOX2B* as a candidate gene for Hirschsprung's disease. Gut 2003; 52:563–567.
10. Eketjall S, Ibanez CF. Functional characterization of mutations in the *GDNF* gene of patients with Hirschsprung disease. Hum Mol Genet 2002; 11:325–329.
11. Duan XL, Zhang XS, Li GW. Clinical relationship between *EDN-3* gene, *EDNRB* gene and Hirschsprung's disease. World J Gastroenterol 2003; 9:2839–2842.
12. Kruger GM, Mosher JT, Tsai YH, et al. Temporally distinct requirements for endothelin receptor B in the generation and migration of gut neural crest stem cells. Neuron 2003; 40:917–929.
13. McCabe ER. Hirschsprung's disease: dissecting complexity in a pathogenetic network. Lancet 2002; 359:1169–1170.
14. Borrego S, Wright FA, Fernandez RM, et al. A founding locus within the *RET* proto-oncogene may account for a large proportion of apparently sporadic Hirschsprung disease and a subset of cases of sporadic medullary thyroid carcinoma. Am J Hum Genet 2003; 72:88–100.
15. Gath R, Goessling A, Keller KM, et al. Analysis of the *RET*, *GDNF*, *EDN3*, and *EDNRB* genes in patients with intestinal neuronal dysplasia and Hirschsprung disease. Gut 2001; 48:671–675.
16. Rayhorn NJ, Ingebo KR. Aganglionosis of the small intestine: a rare form of Hirschsprung's disease. Gastroenterol Nurs 1999; 22:164–166.
17. Puri P, Ohshiro K, Wester T. Hirschsprung's disease: a search for etiology. Semin Pediatr Surg 1998; 7:140–147.
18. Wedel T, Holschneider AM, Krammer HJ. Ultrastructural features of nerve fascicles and basal lamina abnormalities in Hirschsprung's disease. Eur J Pediatr Surg 1999; 9:75–82.
19. Kubota M, et al. Electrophysiological properties of the aganglionic segment in Hirschsprung's disease. Surgery 2002; 131(Suppl):S288–S293.
20. Iwashita T, et al. Hirschsprung disease is linked to defects in neural crest stem cell function. Science 2003; 301: 972–976.
21. Bolande RP. The neurocristopathies: a unifying concept of disease arising in neural crest maldevelopment. *Hum Path* 1974; 5:409–429.
22. Staiano A, Santoro L, De Marco R, et al. Autonomic dysfunction in children with Hirschsprung's disease. Dig Dis Sci 1999; 44:960–965.
23. Cheng W, Au DK, Knowles CH, Anand P, Tam PK. Hirschsprung's disease: a more generalised neuropathy? J Pediatr Surg 2001; 36:296–300.
24. Shahar E, Shinawi M. Neurocristopathies presenting with neurologic abnormalities associated with Hirschsprung's disease. Pediatr Neurol 2003; 28:385–391.
25. Baltogiannis N, Mavridis G, Soutis M, Keramidas D. Currarino triad associated with Hirschsprung's disease. J Pediatr Surg 2003; 38:1086–1089.
26. Piotrowska AP, Solari V, de Caluwe D, Puri P. Immunocolocalization of the heme oxygenase-2 and interstitial cells of Cajal in normal and aganglionic colon. J Pediatr Surg 2003; 38:73–77.
27. Puri P. Intestinal neuronal dysplasia. Semin Pediatr Surg 2003; 12:259–264.
28. Rolle U, Piotrowska AP, Nemeth L, Puri P. Altered distribution of interstitial cells of Cajal in Hirschsprung disease. Arch Pathol Lab Med 2002; 126:928–933.
29. Meyrat BJ, Lesbros Y, Laurini RN. Assessment of the colon innervation with serial biopsies above the aganglionic zone before the pull-through procedure in Hirschsprung's disease. Pediatr Surg Int 2001; 17:129–135.
30. Lewis NA, Levitt MA, Zallen GS, et al. Diagnosing Hirschsprung's disease: increasing the odds of a positive rectal biopsy result. J Pediatr Surg 2003; 38:412–416.
31. Proctor ML, Traubici J, Langer JC, et al. Correlation between radiographic transition zone and level of aganglionosis in Hirschsprung's disease: implications for surgical approach. J Pediatr Surg 2003; 38:775–778.
32. Mazziotti MV, Langer JC. Laparoscopic full-thickness intestinal biopsies in children. J Pediatr Gastroenterol Nutr 2001; 33:54–57.
33. Maia DM. The reliability of frozen-section diagnosis in the pathologic evaluation of Hirschsprung's disease. Am J Surg Pathol 2000; 24:1675–1677.
34. Petchasuwan C, Pintong J. Immunohistochemistry for intestinal ganglion cells and nerve fibers: aid in the diagnosis of Hirschsprung's disease. J Med Assoc Thai 2000; 83:1402–1409.
35. Chentanez V, Chittmittrapap S, Cheepsoonthorn P, Agthong S. New classification of histochemical staining patterns of acetylcholinesterase activity in rectal suction biopsy in Hirschsprung's disease. J Med Assoc Thai 2000; 83:1196–1201.
36. Chentanez V, Chittmittrapap S, Kasantikul V. Modification of the acetylcholinesterase (AchE) staining method in Hirschsprung's disease. J Med Assoc Thai 2000; 83:1101–1104.
37. Nakao M, Suita S, Taguchi T, Hirose R, Shima Y. Fourteen-year experience of acetylcholinesterase staining for rectal mucosal biopsy in neonatal Hirschsprung's disease. J Pediatr Surg 2001; 36:1357–1363.
38. Huang SF, Chen CC, Lai HS. Prediction of the outcome of pull-through surgery for Hirschsprung's disease using acetylcholinesterase activity. J Formos Med Assoc 2001; 100:798–804.
39. Yang S, Donner LR. Detection of ganglion cells in the colonic plexuses by immunostaining for neuron-specific marker NeuN: an aid for the diagnosis of Hirschsprung disease. Appl Immunohistochem Mol Morphol 2002; 10:218–220.
40. Osatakul S, Patrapinyokul S, Osatakul N. The diagnostic value of anorectal manometry as a screening test for Hirschsprung's disease. J Med Assoc Thai 1999; 82:1100–1105.
41. Reid JR, Buonomo C, Moreira C, Kozakevich H, Nurko SJ. The barium enema in constipation: comparison with rectal manometry and biopsy to exclude Hirschsprung's disease after the neonatal period. Pediatr Radiol 2000; 30:681–684.
42. Georgeson KE, Cohen RD, Hebra A, et al. Primary laparoscopic-assisted endorectal colon pull-through for Hirschsprung's disease: a new gold standard. Ann Surg 1999; 229:678–682, discussion 682–683.
43. Georgeson KE. Laparoscopic-assisted pull-through for Hirschsprung's disease. Semin Pediatr Surg 2002; 11:205–210.
44. Langer JC, Durrant AC, de la Torre L, et al. One-stage transanal Soave pullthrough for Hirschsprung disease: a multicenter experience with 141 children. Ann Surg 2003; 238:569–583, discussion 583–585.
45. Langer JC, Seifert M, Minkes RK. One-stage Soave pull-through for Hirschsprung's disease: a comparison of the transanal and open approaches. J Pediatr Surg 2000; 35:820–822.

Imperforate anus without fistula

In these patients the rectum ends blindly, without a fistula, approximately 1–2 cm above the perineum. The sacrum and sphincter mechanism are usually good, and about 80% of these patients achieve bowel control after the main repair.[1,2,9] Approximately 50% of patients with this defect have Down's syndrome. Conversely, 95% of patients with Down's syndrome who have anorectal malformations have this specific type.[9] Interestingly, babies with Down's syndrome babies also have a good functional prognosis. This malformation can be repaired primarily at birth, without a colostomy, provided the surgeon has enough experience and the baby is in good condition.

Vestibular fistula

This is the most common defect in females. The rectum opens into the vestibule of the female genitalia, which is the wet area located outside the hymen (Fig. 49.2). The rectum and vagina share a very thin common wall. The sacrum and sphincters are usually of good quality. Approximately 93% of these patients achieve bowel control after surgery,[1,2] and 30% have associated urologic defects.[10]

This malformation can also be repaired primarily, without a colostomy, provided the patient is in good health and the surgeon has experience in the management of newborn babies with these defects.

Rectourethral fistula

This is by far the most common defect in males (Fig. 49.3). The rectum communicates with the posterior urethra through a narrow orifice (fistula). This fistula may be located in the lower posterior urethra (bulbar fistula) or in the upper posterior urethra (prostatic fistula). Some 85% of patients with rectourethral bulbar fistula achieve fecal continence after the main repair, but only 60% of those with rectoprostatic fistula do so.[1,2] About 30% of patients with bulbar urethral fistula have associated urologic defects,[10] as do 60% of patients with rectoprostatic fistula.[10] The quality of the sacrum usually is good in the former case, but is frequently abnormal in the latter. Most of these patients must have a colostomy at birth, particularly those who were born with a prostatic fistula. Patients with rectourethral bulbar fistula can be repaired at birth without a previous protective colostomy, provided the baby is in good condition and the surgeon has enough experience.

Recto-bladderneck fistula

This is the highest defect seen in males. The rectum opens into the bladder neck. Some 90% of these patients have significant associated urologic defects.[10] Only 15% achieve bowel control after the main repair.[1,2] The sacrum usually has poor quality. In these patients, the repair includes a posterior sagittal approach plus a laparotomy or laparoscopy to reach a very high rectum. The perineum in these patients is usually flat: they do not have the normal midline groove and an anal dimple cannot be seen (Fig. 49.4).

Cloaca

This is by far the most complex problem seen in females. This defect is defined as a malformation in which rectum, vagina and urethra are fused together into a single common channel that opens into a single orifice in the perineum[11] (Fig. 49.5). The prognosis varies depending on the quality of the sacrum and the length of the common channel. Most patients with a common channel longer than 3 cm require intermittent catheterization after the main repair in order to empty the bladder. About 50% of these patients have voluntary bowel movements.[12]

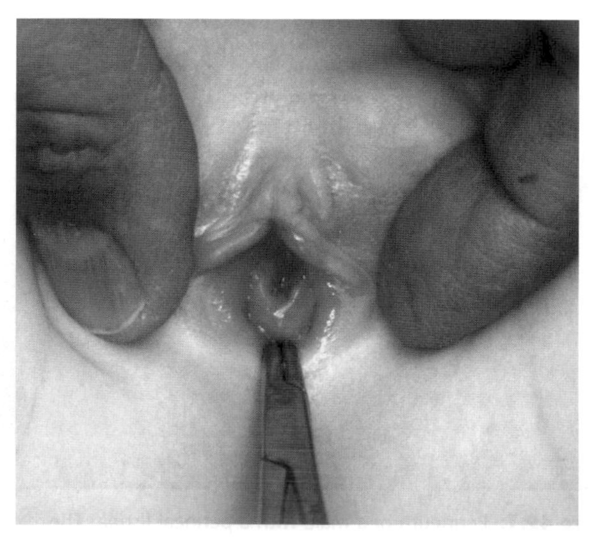

Figure 49.2: External appearance of a girl with a rectovestibular fistula.

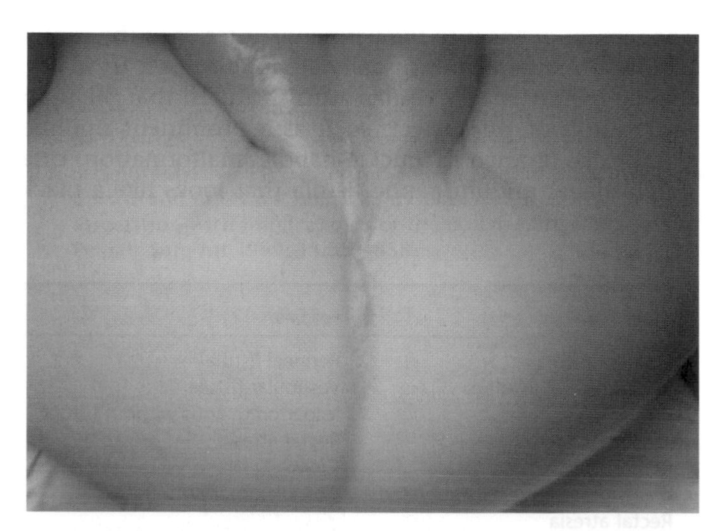

Figure 49.3: Perineum of a patient with a rectourethral fistula. The patient has a good perineal groove, well formed buttocks and an anal dimple.

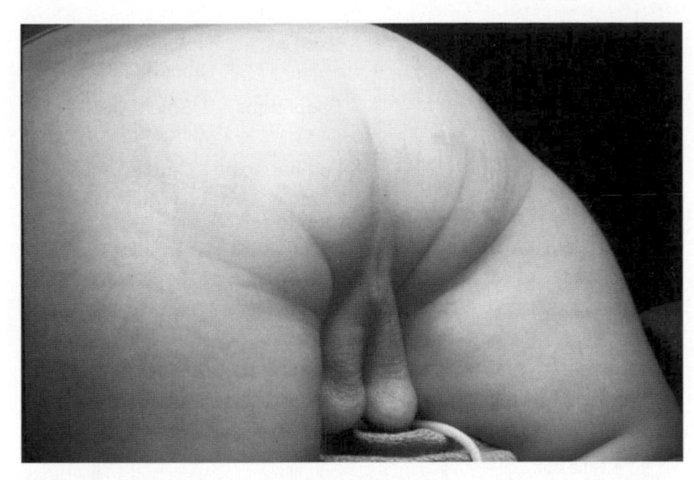

Figure 49.4: Perineum of a patient with a recto-bladder neck fistula. These patients with very high defects have a flat bottom, no perineal groove and frequently have a bifid scrotum.

However, if the common channel is shorter than 3 cm, 20% of the patients require intermittent catheterization to empty the bladder and about 70% have voluntary bowel movements.[11,12]

Ninety percent of patients with cloaca have an important associated urologic problem.[10] This may represent a serious urologic emergency that the clinician should recognize early in life, in order to detect and treat an obstructive uropathy.

More than 40% of these patients also have hydrocolpos, which is a very distended, tense, giant vagina that may compress the opening of the ureters, provoking bilateral megaureters.[11,12] A significant number also have massive vesicoureteral reflux. At birth, these patients require the opening of a colostomy, drainage of the hydrocolpos when present, and sometimes some sort of urinary diversion to take care of the obstructive uropathy. After 1 month of life they undergo an extensive operation during which the three main structures (rectum, vagina and urethra) are separated and placed in their normal location. Patients suffering from cloacas with a common channel shorter than 3 cm require an operation posterior sagittally; usually it is not necessary to open the abdomen. In doing this procedure, a maneuver called total urogenital mobilization is performed,[13] which facilitates the procedure. This type of malformation can therefore be repaired by most general pediatric surgeons.

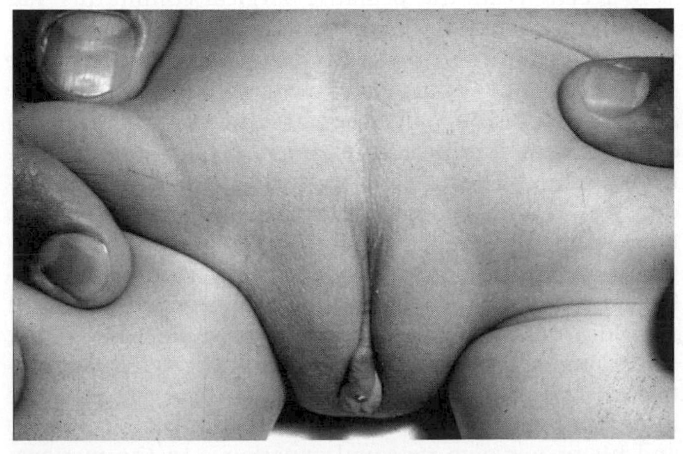

Figure 49.5: Perineum of a patient with a cloaca. The patient has a single perineal orifice.

Patients suffering from a cloaca with a common channel longer than 3 cm require not only the posterior sagittal approach but also a laparotomy and a series of decision-making steps that require a significant amount of experience. These malformations should be repaired by specialized surgeons in specialized centers with wide experience in this area.[12]

ASSOCIATED DEFECTS

The most common defects associated with anorectal malformations are urologic. The frequency of these associations has already been described.[1,2] The next most common associated defects are those of the spine and sacrum. The quality of the sacrum has a direct relation to the prognosis for bowel and urinary control. A very hypoplastic or absent sacrum correlates directly with fecal and urinary incontinence.

Another significant group of patients have gastrointestinal defects, including esophageal atresia, duodenal atresia and other kinds of atresia in the intestinal tract. Approximately 30% of all patients suffer from some sort of cardiovascular defect, but only 10% are hemodynamically unstable and require an operation. The other 20% usually have patent ductus arteriosus, atrial septal defects or ventricular septal defects with no hemodynamic implications.

EARLY MANAGEMENT AND DIAGNOSIS

When a child is born with an anorectal malformation two main questions must be answered within the first 24 h of life:

1 Does the infant have an associated defect (most likely urologic or cardiac) that endangers his or her life and requires immediate treatment?
2 Does the infant need a colostomy or can the malformation be repaired in a primary way without a colostomy?

These two questions must be answered in this order. The higher and more complex the anorectal defect, the greater the chance of a dangerous associated defect. Figures 49.6 and 49.7 show decision-making algorithms used in the early management of these newborns.

All infants with anorectal malformations should have an abdominal and pelvic ultrasonographic examination during the first hours of life. This simple test can exclude hydronephrosis, megaureters and hydrocolpos. If the study results are normal, no further urologic evaluations are required. If the patient has any of these conditions, further urologic evaluation may be needed. Echocardiography can

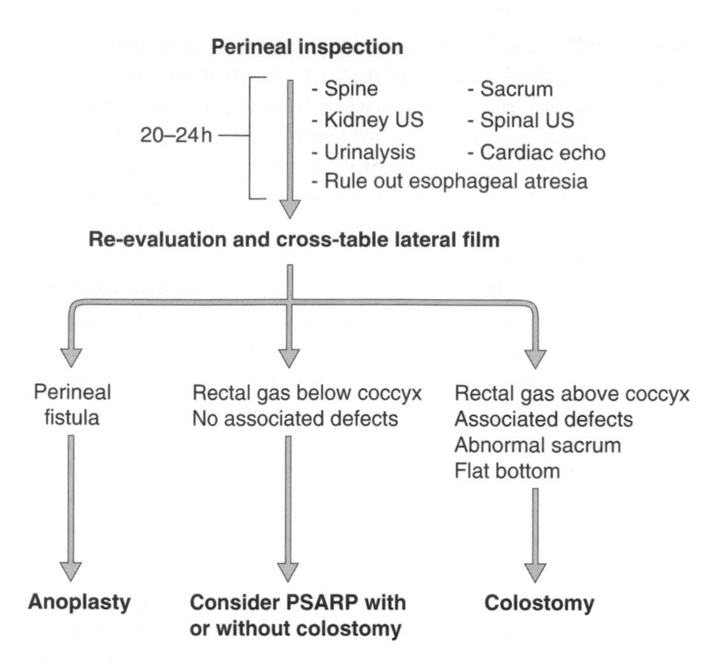

Figure 49.6: Decision-making algorithm for male newborn babies with anorectal malformations. PSARP, posterior sagittal anorectoplasty.

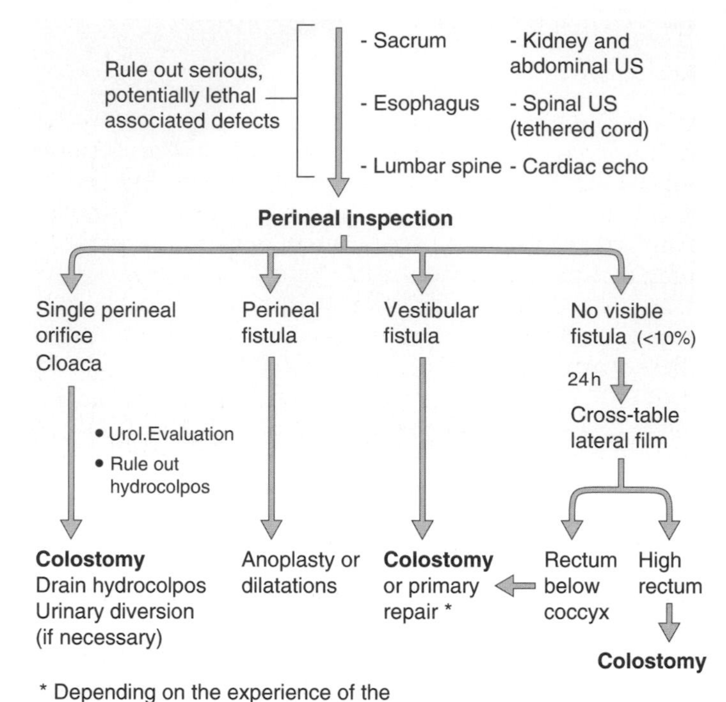

Figure 49.7: Decision-making algorithm for female newborn babies. *Depending on the experience of the surgeon and general condition of the patient.

also be performed during the first hours of life. The perineum must be evaluated meticulously, because it provides a series of clues that help to answer the second question. The presence of a midline groove with two well-formed buttocks and a conspicuous anal dimple (see Fig. 49.3) is a good prognostic sign indicating that the patient probably has a rather low type of malformation. One should always look for the presence of a perineal fistula, which is sometimes extremely small. However, a flat bottom (no midline groove and absence of an anal dimple) occurs in infants with very high defects (see Fig. 49.4). Ultrasonography of the lower spine should also be performed in the first few days of life to rule out the presence of tethered cord, which is associated with a very high type of anorectal malformation with poor prognosis.[14]

When a child is born with an anorectal malformation, the abdomen is not distended. During the following 18–24 h, the abdomen becomes distended and the intraluminal pressure of the bowel increases significantly, forcing the meconium through the lowest part of the rectum, which is surrounded by the sphincter mechanism. One can expect that the meconium will pass through a fistula, usually after 18–24 h. The golden rule in the early diagnosis of these children is to wait at least 18–24 h before making a decision. Male infants need a urinalysis to look for traces of meconium. A piece of gauze placed on the tip of the penis may filter the meconium when the infant voids, leading to the diagnosis of a rectourinary fistula, which is an indication to open a colostomy in most cases. A tiny perineal fistula may remain unnoticed and after 20–24 h a drop of meconium may become evident. The presence of meconium in the perineum or an obvious perineal fistula establishes the diagnosis of perineal fistula, which can be treated with an anoplasty and without a colostomy.

In about 5% of all patients a perineal fistula cannot be found. There is no evidence of a cloaca, there is no evidence of vestibular fistula, and no meconium is found in the urine. Such patients may have an imperforate anus without fistula. To confirm this, a cross-table lateral film with the child prone and the pelvis elevated is taken with a radio-opaque marker placed on the anal dimple. The location of the rectum full of gas can be demonstrated radiologically, and the distance between the rectum and the perineum measured. A primary approach without a colostomy can be considered when the image of the rectum full with gas is seen below the coccyx.

In recent years the pediatric surgical community has shown a tendency to operate on more and more anorectal malformations primarily, without a protective colostomy. The rationale is to try to avoid the three-stage approach (colostomy, main repair and colostomy closure) of traditional routine, decreasing the number of operations to one. The present authors agree with this tendency with the specific purpose to decrease the trauma to the patient. However, the colostomy is still the safest way to avoid complications during the repair of anorectal malformations. The authors believe that every surgeon should make an individual decision concerning colostomy or primary repair, based on the general condition of the patient, the surrounding circumstances, the infrastructure of the hospital where the surgeon works and his or her own personal experience in the management of these babies.

MAIN REPAIR

Anoplasty

An anoplasty is a small operation performed with the patient in prone position and the pelvis elevated. A newborn does not require bowel preparation. The operation takes about 30–45 min but requires many meticulous and delicate maneuvers to avoid damage to important continence structures, as well as injury to the urethra in male patients.

An older child with an untreated perineal fistula usually presents with severe fecal impaction and megasigmoid. These patients require a full bowel preparation before the operation, and after the procedure they also need parenteral nutrition and fasting for several days to avoid potential infection.

Posterior sagittal anorectoplasty

Most anorectal malformations can be repaired by using a posterior sagittal approach between the buttocks. The rationale behind this operation is that the entire sphincter mechanism can be divided in the midline to avoid nerve damage. An electric stimulator is used to determine the precise limits of the sphincter. The goal of the operation is to separate the rectum from the genitourinary tract, to dissect it sufficiently to reach the perineum, and to place it within the limits of the sphincter mechanism. Sometimes the rectum is so dilated that some degree of tapering is needed to achieve this goal. In 10% of males it is necessary to open the abdomen or to perform a laparoscopic procedure in addition to the posterior sagittal approach in order to reach a rectum that is located extremely high in the abdomen (recto-bladder neck fistula).[1,2] In such cases, the posterior sagittal procedure is started and the surgeon creates a path immediately behind the urinary tract, through which the rectum is to be pulled down. A rubber tube is placed in the desired tract, the patient is turned to the supine position, the abdomen is opened or approached laparoscopically, the rectum is separated from the bladder neck, and the rectum is then anchored to the rubber tube, which is found in the retroperitoneal space. The rubber tube is pulled down, bringing with it the rectum, which is then placed within the limits of the sphincter mechanism and anastomosed to the perineum.

About 40% of females born with a cloaca also need a laparotomy to reach a very high rectum, a very high vagina, or both. In these cases, the operation is called posterior sagittal anorectovaginourethroplasty.

These are very specialized, delicate, demanding operations that have as a goal the anatomic reconstruction of the rectum, urethra and vagina.[12]

FUNCTIONAL SEQUELAE

Elements required for bowel control

Three main elements are necessary for bowel continence: sensation, sphincters and normal rectosigmoid motility.

Sensation

The most important sensation that is useful for bowel control resides in the anal canal, from a few millimeters above the pectinate line to the anal verge. In that area, it is possible for the patient to discriminate between gas, liquid and solid contents, and even to discern changes in temperature.[15] There is another type of sensation that resides in the rectum and is elicited when the rectum is distended, and supposedly stretches the voluntary muscles that surround the rectum. This type of sensation is vague and is called proprioception. The rectal mucosa has no sensation; the proprioception receptors reside in the voluntary muscle that surrounds the rectum.[16,17]

Sphincters

There are two types of sphincter. The first is the voluntary external sphincter mechanism, represented by a funnel-like voluntary muscle structure that inserts in the middle portion of the pelvic rim and extends all the way down to the skin surrounding the rectum and anus. The internal sphincter is a more controversial structure, defined as a thickening of the circular layer of the smooth muscle in the lowest part of the intestine. This is an involuntary sphincter.

Rectosigmoid motility

Normal rectosigmoid colonic motility is extremely important for bowel control. Under normal circumstances, the rectosigmoid acts like a reservoir: it catches all the solid stool that comes from the rest of the colon. Once a day, or every other day depending on the person's habit, the rectosigmoid gives signs of trying to empty by pushing the fecal contents toward the anal canal. The contact of the rectal contents with the anal canal gives the person the necessary information to note the nature of the rectal contents.

Depending on the surrounding social circumstances, the person may elect to relax the voluntary sphincter or to contract it. Once the decision is made to empty the rectosigmoid, the voluntary sphincter is relaxed and the next wave of peristaltic contraction empties the rectosigmoid. Children with anorectal malformations have deficiencies in all three of these main elements of bowel control. The sensation that resides in the anal canal exists only in those with anorectal malformations in which an anal canal is present. There is only one specific defect with that characteristic; it is called rectal atresia and occurs in only 1% of all cases.[1,2] These patients have a normal-looking anus with an atresia located 1–2 cm above the anal verge. All other patients with anorectal malformations are born with no anal canal or with a very abnormal one. Therefore, very precise discrimination cannot be expected in these children. However, all of them have different degrees of proprioception, usually good enough to be toilet trained provided the prognosis for their type of defect is good. The presence of a solid piece of stool moving in the rectum is perceived by the patient in a rather vague manner but strongly enough to give the signal to defecate. Liquid stool is more difficult to sense.

more often in infants with more proximal obstructions. Jaundice is seen in over 30% of babies with jejunal atresia and 20% with ileal atresia. This is believed to result from delay in the maturation of the glucuronyl transferase enzyme in the absence of normal enteral feedings.

In abdominal radiographs of infants with proximal intestinal atresia, there are few dilated bowel loops and air-fluid levels (Fig. 51.3). The more distal atresias tend to have more dilated intestine on radiograph. A dominant dilated loop of intestine may be present. A contrast enema usually shows a microcolon in patients with small intestinal atresia although this is nonspecific. This study may also aid in establishing the diagnosis of meconium plug or Hirschsprung's disease.

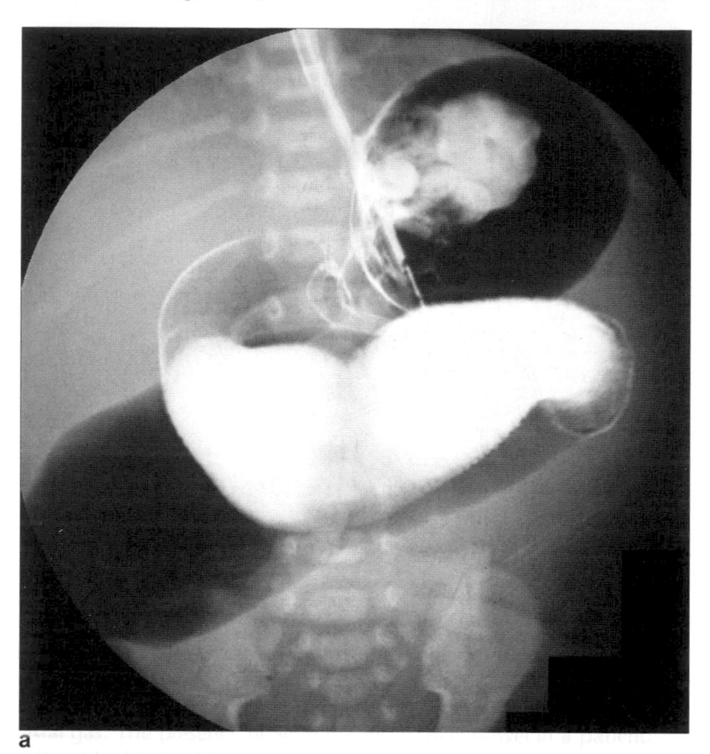

a

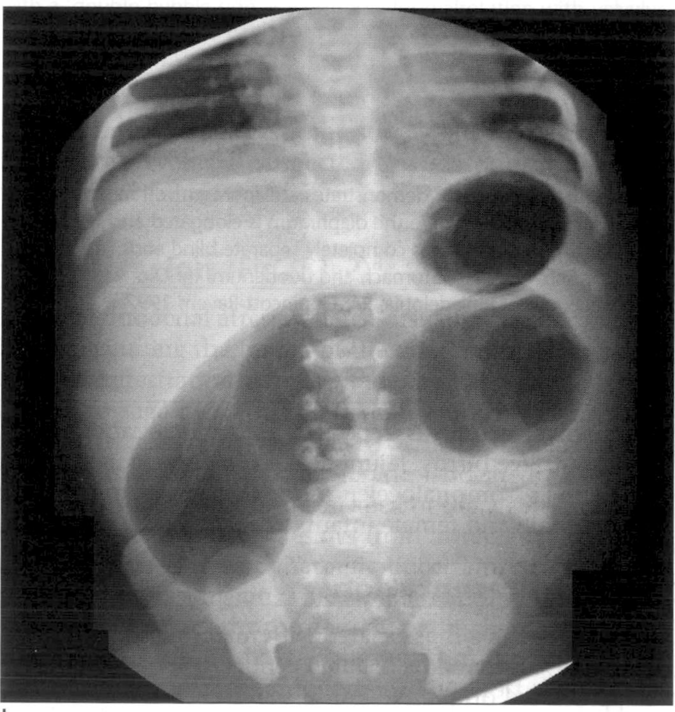

b

Figure 51.3: (a) Plain abdominal radiograph in a baby with jejunal atresia. (b) A contrast study demonstrates the blind end in the same baby.

Classification (Fig. 51.4)[12]

Grosfeld[13] and Touloukian[14] have modified an intestinal atresia classification proposed by Martin[15] to yield an anatomic system in use today. Type I intestinal atresia has an intraluminal diaphragm in continuity with the muscular layers of the proximal and distal segments. In type II atresias, fibrous bands separate the ends of the two relevant segments. Type IIIa atresias are characterized by a V-shaped mesenteric defect and intestinal discontinuity. Type IIIb atresias have an extensive mesenteric defect, with the distal ileum receiving its entire blood supply retrograde via the ileocolic or right colic artery. In this circumstance, the distal intestine coils itself around the artery, giving rise to descriptive terms such as 'apple-peel' or 'Christmas tree' deformity. This type of anomaly is often associated with particularly small distal bowel and a significant loss in overall bowel length.[16] Type IV atresias are composed of multiple atresias within the length of the small bowel, and sometimes these require multiple anastomoses to preserve bowel length.

Treatment

Preoperative care is similar for that of duodenal atresia. Gastric decompression, intravenous fluid resuscitation and antibiotic administration are required. It is important to remember that the dilated proximal segment can serve as a fixed point, around which the bowel can volvulize. Prompt abdominal exploration is required and is generally performed through a transverse supraumbilical incision. The entire bowel is eviscerated and the point(s) of obstruction identified. It is imperative to explore the distal intestine for the presence of other atresias. A small caliber rubber catheter may be introduced into the distal segment and the remaining intestine flushed with saline for this purpose. Colonic patency is confirmed either by inserting a rectal tube and filling the colon intraoperatively or a preoperative contrast enema.

The surgeon must determine the length of the functional intestine. If the baby has adequate length of bowel, then the bulbous proximal intestine may be resected to perform an end-to-end anastomosis between two ends of bowel with relatively equal sizes. However, if the bowel length is limited, a tapering enteroplasty should be considered to preserve as much bowel length as possible.

Reported operative mortality rates are about 1%.[7] Long-term survival is 84%[7] in our report, usually related to other medical problems or from short bowel syndrome. The prognosis for patients with small intestinal atresia is dependent on the length of residual functional small bowel.[17] At least 40 cm of small intestine without an ileocecal valve or 20 cm

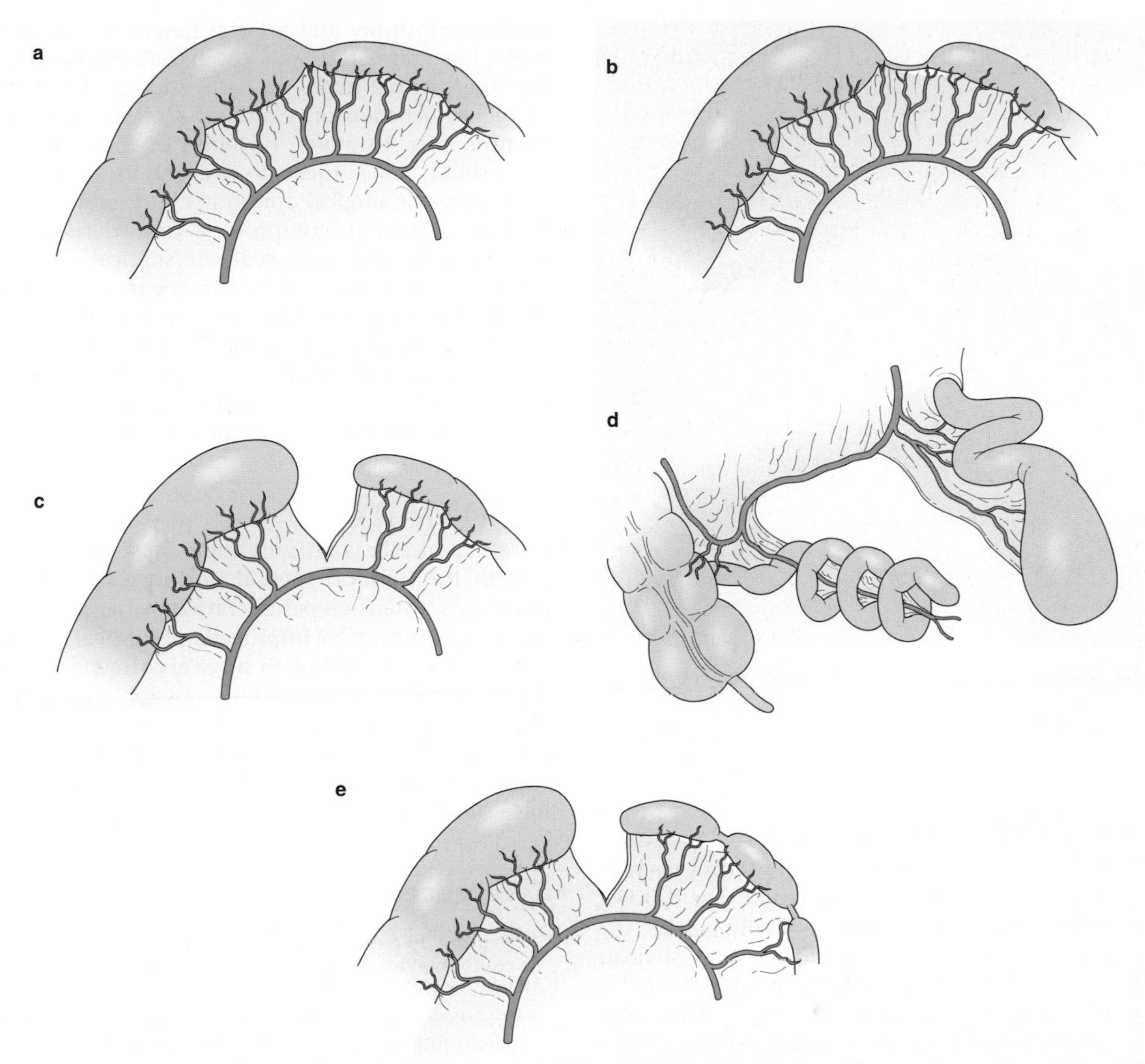

Figure 51.4: Classification of small intestinal atresia. (**a**) Type I atresia has an obstructing membrane with musculoserosal continuity. (**b**) Type II atresia has a fibrous band between the two atretic ends. (**c**) Type IIIA is characterized by two blind intestinal ends with no intervening mesentery. (**d**) Type IIIB (apple peel atresia) is characterized by a bulbous proximal small intestine, which is usually foreshortened. The distal, small-caliber intestine is wrapped around the ileo-colic artery. (**e**) Type IV atresia has multiple segments of atretic bowel. (Adapted from Grosfeld JL. Jejunoileal atresia and stenosis. In: Welch KJ, Randolph JG, Ravitch MM, et al., eds. Pediatric Surgery. Chicago: Year Book Medical Publisher; 1986:843.)[12]

with an ileocecal valve is considered necessary for adequate long intestinal adaptation, although these must be considered generalizations only.[18] Postoperatively, an orogastric tube is left in place until intestinal motility resumes. The infant's diet is then slowly advanced to goal volume. A child with short bowel syndrome requires complex post-surgical care and this is discussed elsewhere in this text.

COLONIC ATRESIA

Embryology

Similar to jejunoileal atresia, colonic atresia is thought to occur due to vascular compromise of a colon segment in utero. This happens after the midgut has returned into the celomic cavity between the 10th and 12th week of gestation.[19] Although atresias may occur anywhere along the length of the colon, some evidence suggests that they are more likely to occur in the 'vascular watershed areas' of the hepatic flexure.[20]

Incidence

The incidence of colon atresia is approximately 1 in 20 000 live births and it is the least common of all intestinal atresias.[21] There is a 2% incidence of Hirschsprung's disease in patients with colon atresia,[22] therefore this possibility should be ruled out with a rectal suction biopsy prior to re-establishing intestinal continuity in patients with colon atresia. Jejunal-ileal atresia, cardiac anomalies and abnormalities of the musculoskeletal system have been reported to coexist with this entity.

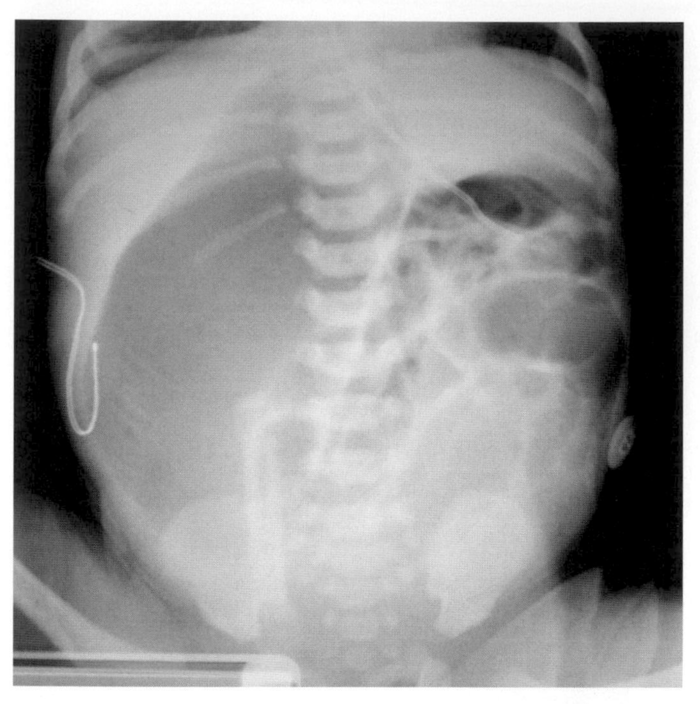

Figure 51.5: Plain abdominal radiograph in a baby with colonic atresia.

Clinical presentation

Prenatal ultrasound of a fetus with colonic atresia may show an enlarged loop of intestine or colon that is larger for gestational age 20, but one cannot reliably localize the site of obstruction. Infants with colonic atresia or stenosis usually have no acute problems at birth but develop a distended abdomen within 24–48 h (Fig. 51.5). They may require mechanical ventilation secondary to the distention. Failure to pass meconium is typical, but some infants do pass a small amount of mucous per rectum. Plain abdominal radiographs show multiple distended small intestinal loops. In infants, it is difficult to differentiate between small and large intestine on abdominal X-rays, therefore, making the distinction between distal ileal obstruction and colonic obstruction is difficult.

Contrast radiography with isotonic contrast agent may establish the diagnosis of colon atresia or stenosis. This study is important in evaluating patients for other causes of distal obstruction such as meconium plug syndrome, Hirschsprung's disease or small left colon syndrome. Therefore, it is routinely recommended in the clinical setting of neonatal distal bowel obstruction.

Treatment

After resuscitation, gastric decompression and administration of intravenous antibiotics, exploratory laparotomy is done. The most common finding in colon atresia is two blind ending segments of colon with no intervening mesentery. Historically, surgical correction often involved staged procedures, initially with the creation of a functioning colostomy and a distal mucus fistula. In this scenario, the dilated proximal colon is allowed to decompress and the luminal diameter reduce to roughly normal size before an ileocolostomy or a colocolostomy is performed months later. However, resection of the dilated segment and primary anastomosis to establish intestinal continuity is a reasonable surgical option in children without perforation, hemodynamic compromise, or medical contraindications. In contemporary pediatric surgical practice this is now often done. Regardless, patency of the distal segment should be evaluated either preoperatively or intraoperatively. If a primary anastomosis is performed, it is imperative to make sure that the distal segment has normal ganglion cells using either suction or open rectal biopsy.

Operative mortality for colon atresia is low.[7]

SUMMARY

Intestinal atresia is an important cause of bowel obstruction in the newborn period. Advancements in neonatal anesthesia, intensive perioperative management, and parenteral nutrition have improved the survival and outcomes of these patients. Although surgical correction can be technically complex, it is generally possible today, but higher rates of morbidity and mortality are still observed in patients with concurrent anatomic anomalies of other systems, especially congenital heart disease and those who have short gut syndrome.

References

1. Calder J. Two examples of children born with preternatural conformation of the guts. Medical Essays and Observations, Edinburgh 1733; 1:203–206
2. Ernst NP. A case of congenital atresia of the duodenum treated successfully by operation. BMJ 1916; 1:1644.
3. Webb CJ, Wangensteen OH. Congenital intestinal atresia. Am J Child 1931; 41:262.
4. Grosfeld JL, Rescorla FJ. Duodenal atresia and stenosis: reassessment of treatment and outcome based on antenatal diagnosis, pathologic variance, and long-term follow-up. World J Surg 1993; 17(3):301–309
5. Tandler J. Entwicklunggeschichte des menschlichen Duodenum. Morhol Jahrb 1902; 29:187.
6. Mandell G. Duodenal atresia. www.emedicine.com, 2002.
7. Dalla Vecchia LK, Grosfeld JL, West KW, Rescorla FJ, Scherer LR, Engum SA. Intestinal atresia and stenosis: a 25-year experience with 277 cases. Arch Surg 1998; 133(5):490–497.
8. Magnuson D, Schwartz MZ, Stomach and duodenum. In: Oldham KT, Colombani PM, Foglia RP, eds. Surgery of Infants and Children. Scientific Principles and Practice. Philadelphia, PA: Lippincott-Raven; 1997
9. Kimura K, Mukohara N, Nishijima E, Muraji T, Tsugawa C, Matsumoto Y. Diamond-shaped anastomosis for duodenal atresia: an experience with 44 patients over 15 years. J Pediatr Surg 1990; 25(9):977–979.
10. Louw JH, Barnard CN. Congenital intestinal atresia; observations on its origin. Lancet 1955; 269(6899):1065–1067.
11. Louw, JH. Congenital intestinal atresia and stenosis in the newborn: observations on its pathogenesis and treatment. Ann R Coll Surg (Eng) 1959;25:209–234.

12. Grosfeld JL. Jejunoileal atresia and stenosis. In: Welch KJ, Randolph JG, Ravitch MM, et al., eds. Pediatric Surgery. Chicago: Year Book Medical Publisher; 1986:843.
13. Grosfeld JL, Ballantine TVN, and Shoemaker R. Operative management of intestinal atresia and stenosis based on pathologic findings. J Pediatr Surg 1979; 14:368.
14. Touloukian RJ. Intestinal atresia. Clin Perinatol 1978; 5:3.
15. Martin LW, Zerella JT. Jejuno-ileal atresia: a proposed classification. J Pediatr Surg 1976; 11:399.
16. Dickson JAS. Apple peel small bowel. An uncommon variant of duodenal and jejunal atresia. J Pediatr Surg 1970; 5:575.
17. Weber TR, Vane DW, Grosfeld JL. Tapering enteroplasty in infants with bowel atresia and short gut. Arch Surg 1982; 117:684.
18. Rescorla FJ, Grosfeld JL. Intestinal atresia and stenosis: analysis of survival in 120 cases. Surgery 1985; 98:668.
19. Garza JJ. Intestinal atresia, stenosis, and webs. www.emedicine.com, 2004.
20. Boles ET Jr, Vassy Le, Ralston M. Atresia of the colon. J Pediatr Surg 1976; 11:69.
21. Oldham K. Atresia, stenosis and other obstructions of the colon. In: O' Neill JA Jr, Rowe MI, Grosfeld JL, Fonkalsrud EW, Coran AG, eds. Pediatric Surgery, 5th edn, St Louis, MO: Mosby; 1998.
22. Anderson N, Malpas T, Robertson R. Prenatal diagnosis of colon atresia. Pediatr Radiol 1993; 23(1):63–64.

Chapter 52
Newborn abdominal wall defects

Donald R. Cooney and Danny C. Little

HISTORICAL BACKGROUND AND TERMINOLOGY

Ambrose Pare[1] recorded the first description of omphalocele during the sixteenth century emphasizing the serious nature of the condition and poor prognosis. The first description of gastroschisis is attributed to Calder in 1733.[1] Nomenclature included many confusing terms such as epiomphaschisis and hologastroestroschisis. In 1953, Moore and Stokes[1] established the present day classification, distinguishing omphalocele from gastroschisis on the basis of the site of the umbilical cord, the presence or absence of a covering sac and the appearance of eviscerated bowel (Table 52.1).

The first child to survive with an omphalocele was treated non-operatively in 1751. In 1899, Ahlfeld[1] described treatment with alcohol dressings. In 1957, Grob[1] described the use of 2% aqueous solution of merbromin as a topical agent, producing a dry crust on the sac with a granulating surface beneath. Gradual epithelialization occurred over many weeks.

The first surgical cures of omphalocele were reported in 1803 and 1806.[1] Except for small defects, most of the early surgical attempts were unsuccessful. In 1887, Olshausen[1] described mobilization of abdominal skin flaps to cover the sac. This method was not adopted until 1948 when Gross[1] reported this technique to close three giant omphaloceles.

Factor	Omphalocele	Gastroschisis
Location	Umbilical ring	Lateral to cord
Size of defect	2.0–10.0 cm	Small (4.0 cm)
Umbilical cord	Inserts in sac	Normal insertion
Sac	Present (amnion and peritoneum)	None
Contents	Liver, bowel, etc.	Bowel, stomach
B = bowel appearance	Normal	Matted, foreshortened exudate
Malrotation	Present	Present
Small abdominal cavity	Present	Present
Postoperative alimentary function	Normal	Prolonged ileus
Associated anomalies	Common (50–67%)	Unusual (15% atresia of gut)

Table 52.1 Clinical findings in infants with abdominal wall defects

Skin flap closure necessitated future repair of the resultant ventral hernia. Adoption of this technique was a major advance in the survival of infants with omphaloceles.

Watkins[1] performed the first successful surgical repair of gastroschisis in 1943. During the 1940s and 1950s, drastic measures to close the defect utilizing partial hepatectomy, splenectomy and bowel resection[1] usually led to the death of the baby. Izant[1] in 1966, recommended manual stretching of the abdominal wall to enlarge the cavity. In 1967, Schuster[1] reported a new technique that revolutionized surgical management. He drew attention to the fact that in omphaloceles the rectus muscles approximate each other behind the eviscerated mass and skin flap closure did little to alter intraabdominal forces which provided little stimulus for growth of the abdominal cavity. The resulting huge ventral hernias were just as difficult to repair as the original omphalocele. By attaching sheets of prosthetic material to the abdominal fascia, the intraabdominal forces could be altered favoring enlargement of the abdominal cavity. Schuster used sheets of mesh that were sewn to lateral margins of the defect, the mesh was sutured together under tension and the skin closed. Subsequent stages involved reopening the skin and excising redundant mesh as the abdominal cavity grew until the mesh could be removed.

In 1968 Gilbert[1] reported a modification of Schuster's technique utilizing reinforced sheets of silicone that were sutured to the abdominal fascia and left to protrude from the wound. To improve on this technique, Allen and Wrenn[1] in 1969 used silicone sheets to construct a silo around the eviscerated mass. Gradually, the silo was reduced until closure of the fascia was achieved. This technique continues to play a prominent role in the management of abdominal wall defects.

Despite successful surgical treatment prior to the 1970s, many infants died from starvation as a result of prolonged ileus. In 1971 Filler[1] first reported using parenteral nutrition to provide nutrition for five infants with ruptured omphalocele and gastroschisis. Today, TPN remains part of the standard management of infants with abdominal wall defects.

EMBRYOGENESIS DICTATES THE TYPE OF DEFECT

Closure of the body wall begins at 2 weeks gestation and results from growth and longitudinal infolding of the embryonic disk. The cephalic fold forms the thoracic and epigastric wall. The caudal fold contributes the hindgut, bladder and hypogastric wall. The lateral folds form the lateral abdominal walls. The four folds meet in the center to form the umbilical ring, which is usually fully developed by the fourth week. During the 6th week, growth of the midgut causes a physiologic herniation of the gut out through the umbilical ring. The midgut then rotates as it reenters the abdominal cavity so that the small intestine and colon come to lie in their correct anatomical positions. The intestine migrates to its normal intraperitoneal location by the end of the 10th week of development. Since this process does not occur in cases of omphalocele and gastroschisis these patients always have malrotation.

The embryogenesis of omphalocele remains controversial. Duhamel[1] suggested that failure of body wall morphogenesis of the cephalic fold would result in an 'epigastric omphalocele'. These infants have an omphalocele associated with cleft sternum, anterior diaphragmatic hernia, possible ectopia cordis, congenital heart defects and absence of a portion of the pericardium. This group of anomalies, first described in 1958, is now recognized as the pentalogy of Cantrell. With small omphalocele or hernia into the umbilical cord, the umbilical ring is only slightly widened. These defects probably represent failure of the intestine to return completely after its normal period of extracolonic development. Failure to form the caudal fold results in hypogastric omphalocele. Both the somatic and splanchnic layers of the fold are affected so that there may be agenesis of the hindgut, exstrophy of the bladder or cloaca and a fistula between the intestine and bladder. If only the lateral folds fail to develop, the umbilical orifice remains widely open resulting in a centrally located omphalocele allowing for prolapse of the liver, stomach, spleen and ovaries, small intestine and colon.

The embryogenesis of gastroschisis is more controversial. Duhamel[1] proposed that gastroschisis was caused by failure of differentiation of embryonic mesenchyme of the lateral folds which is supported by de Vries study[1] of serial sections of human fetuses in the Carnegie collection. Involution of the right umbilical vein results in the mesenchymal defect at the junction of the body stalk with the body wall.

FACTORS THAT MAY CAUSE THE DEFECT

Etiologic factors causing omphalocele or gastroschisis have not been identified in humans. These anomalies may be induced in rats by folic acid deficiency,[1] administration of salicylates,[1] hypoxia,[1] carbon monoxide and protein-zinc deficiencies.[2] In addition, vasoconstricting medications such as pseudoephedrine, phenylpropanolamine and ephedrine and nicotine increase the risk of gastroschisis and intestinal atresia.[3] Familial cases of both defects have been reported and major chromosomal anomalies are associated with 10–38% of cases of omphalocele.[4,5] Some cases of omphalocele and gastroschisis may be genetically determined. Obtaining an accurate family history enables the physician to provide recurrence risk counseling in rare cases of familial or syndromic cases. However, providing specific information to families regarding the risk to future pregnancies must be done cautiously until additional studies clarify the genetic and environmental roles.

A CHANGING EPIDEMIOLOGY

The Center of Disease Control estimates the combined incidence of omphalocele and gastroschisis is approximately 1 in 2000 live births in the USA. In the past, omphalocele was clearly the most common condition; however, the global incidence of gastroschisis appears to be increasing as noted from reports from Utah,[6] California,[1] Sweden,[1] Finland,[1] and Spain.[7] The incidence of omphalocele has remained unchanged.

The incidence of gastroschisis is inversely related to maternal age[8] and is most common in young mothers with low gravidity.[8–10]Although both conditions are associated with lower gestational age, prematurity is more common in gastroschisis.[7] Infants have lower birth weight than normal babies of the same gestational age. Gastroschisis infants are often smaller than omphalocele newborns. These observations suggest that abdominal wall defects may be related to prenatal care of the mother. This supposition is reinforced by a recent study indicating that periconceptional use of multivitamins is associated with a 68% reduction in nonsyndromic omphalocele.[11]

No racial or geographic associations have been observed for either condition. A slight male predominance (1.5:1) is reported for omphalocele but not for gastroschisis.[9] Omphaloceles have occurred in consecutive children, twins and in different generations of the same family.

A SPECTRUM OF DEFECTS

Congenital hernia of the cord (the very small omphalocele)

Congenital hernias of the umbilical cord should be no larger than 4 cm in diameter and the sac contain only a few bowel loops. Careless cord clamping can cause injury to the intestine. Hernias of the cord should be differentiated from larger omphaloceles since the intestine is easily reduced, surgical closure is simple and excellent results are expected (Fig. 52.1a). If left untreated, these small hernias of the cord may gradually re-epithelialize (cutis navel).

Omphaloceles

An omphalocele is an umbilical ring defect, varying in size from a small, easily treated, condition to a 'giant' omphalocele requiring special care (Fig. 52.1a, b). The eviscerated contents are contained within a sac consisting of a translucent avascular membrane composed of peritoneum, Wharton's jelly and amnion. The umbilical cord is inserted directly onto the sac. The abdominal wall defect varies from 4 to 12 cm and usually contains stomach and loops of large and small intestine. The liver remains extraperitoneal in

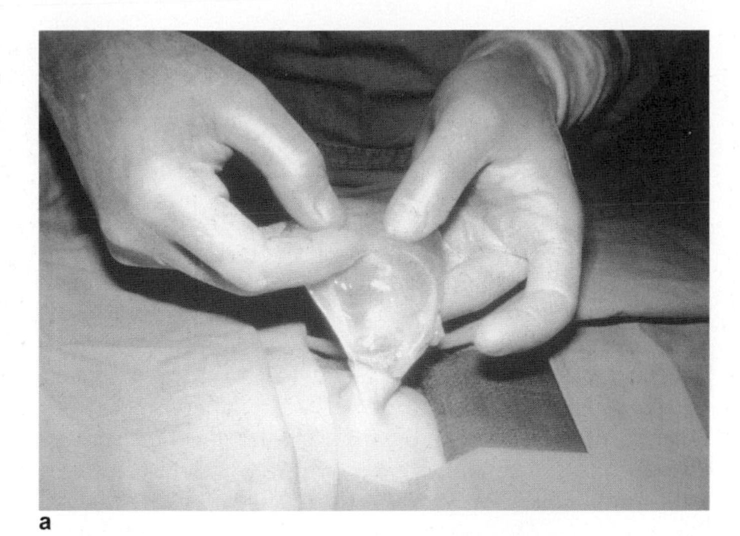

a

b

Figure 52.1: (**a**) Congenital hernia of the cord; a very small omphalocele that is easily reduced and repaired by primary closure of the fascia. (**b**) A giant omphalocele, difficult to close, place in a silo, or cover with skin flaps; associated with much higher morbidity and mortality.

48% of cases.[12] Giant omphaloceles have a massive sac that contains most of the abdominal viscera, including the liver, spleen, bladder, gonads, entire intestinal tract as well as a small underdeveloped peritoneal cavity. Successful management in these cases is challenging and associated with higher morbidity (Fig. 52.1b).

The omphalocele sac may rupture *in utero*, during labor (4% of cases),[4] or after birth (Fig. 52.2a). Prenatal rupture of the sac has been reported to occur in 10–18% of cases.[13,14] With early disruption, the eviscerated intestine may be covered by thick matted exudate. Gastroschisis may have a similar appearance, but a prenatally ruptured omphalocele can be differentiated by its midline position, abnormal insertion of the umbilical cord and presence of sac remnants (Fig. 52.2a).

Gastroschisis

In gastroschisis, the small smooth-edged opening is located to the right of the umbilical cord (Fig. 52.2b). Rare cases of left-sided gastroschisis have been reported.[15] The size of the defect may be dangerously small, varying from 2 to 5 cm. The stomach as well as the small and large intestine are herniated, but the liver is rarely involved. Evisceration of the gallbladder, uterus, fallopian tubes, urinary bladder, testes and ovaries have been reported.[16] The extruded intestine has an abnormal appearance and may be at risk for vascular compromise (Fig. 52.2b). The abdominal musculature is normally developed and the underdeveloped abdominal cavity is usually larger than that seen is cases of omphalocele. Associated anomalies are rare. Clinical differences between omphalocele and gastroschisis are summarized in Table 52.1.

ASSOCIATED ANOMALIES (THE MAJOR DETERMINANT OF MORBIDITY AND MORTALITY)

Congenital anomalies are frequently associated with omphalocele. Cardiovascular anomalies may be encountered in 20% of patients.[17] Tetralogy of Fallot (33%) and atrial defects (25%) are most common. Congenital heart disease is more common with epigastric omphaloceles and may be associated with a diaphragmatic hernia and sternal defect. More than half of patients with omphalocele and congenital heart disease have multiple congenital anomalies or a specific syndrome.[17]

Omphalocele may be associated with trisomies 13, 14, 15, 18, or 21. Beckwith Wiedemann syndrome is found in approximately 12% of patients. These infants have enlarged tongues, large, rounded craniofacial features, visceromegaly and are prone to develop hypoglycemia, presumably caused by hyperplasia of the pancreatic islet cells.

Genitourinary anomalies may be associated with omphalocele as part of the syndrome of bladder exstrophy or hindgut agenesis in cases of hypogastric omphalocele. Renal malrotation has been documented in cases of omphalocele.[18] Cryptorchidism is associated with both omphalocele and gastroschisis.

Lower midline syndrome consists of hypogastric omphalocele, cloacal exstrophy; possible duplication of the colon and/or appendix, imperforate anus, colonic atresia, sacral anomalies; myelomeningocele, hydro- or diastematomyelia and skeletal or limb deformities. This syndrome is very rare and requires sophisticated multidisciplinary management to avoid excessive morbidity. Pentalogy of Cantrell consists of an epigastric omphalocele, diastasis recti, central midline diaphragmatic hernia, distal sternal cleft, pericardial defect, anterior displacement of the heart and congenital heart disease. Again, individualized management is required.

Other associated anomalies include musculoskeletal abnormalities, cleft palate, Rieger's syndrome, hydrocephalus, pulmonary hypoplasia and respiratory distress. Prune-belly syndrome is associated with omphaloceles. Abnormalities of the intestinal tract occur with both omphalocele and gastroschisis. Malrotation occurs in all cases of omphalocele and gastroschisis. Lack of intestinal

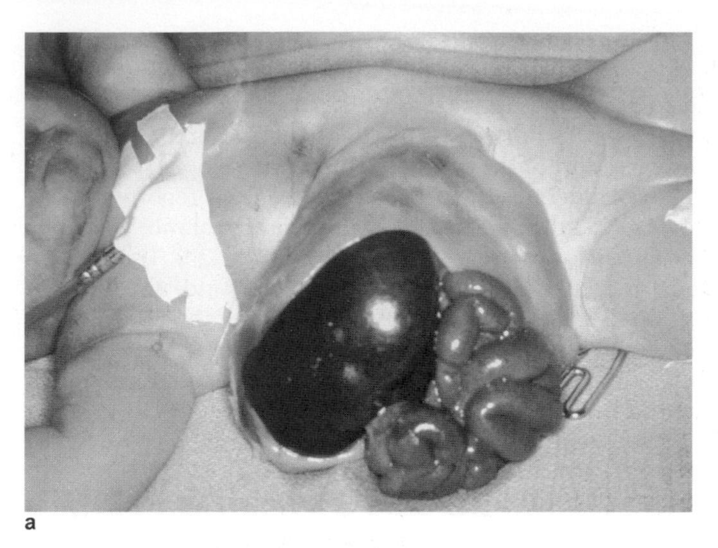

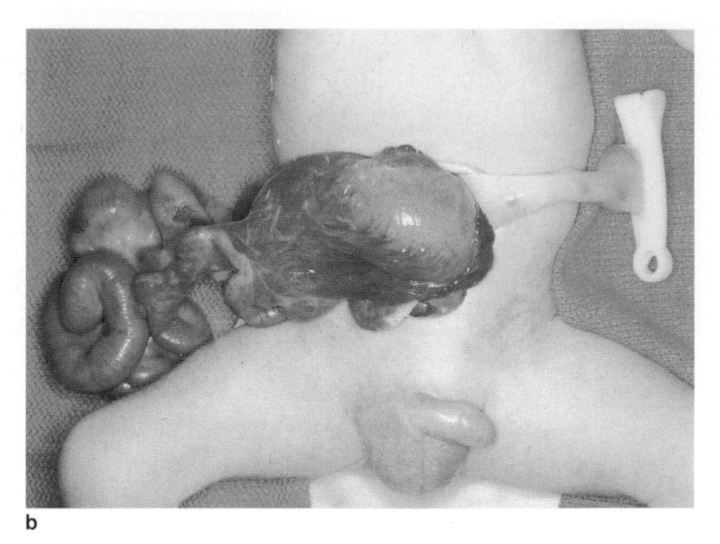

Figure 52.2: (**a**) Depicts an infant with a ruptured omphalocele with a large defect; liver is present; the umbilical cord is distorted and remnants of the sac remain. (**b**) A gastroschisis presenting to the right of a normal appearing umbilical cord; the bowel is covered with exudate and a portion appears to be experiencing vascular compromise.

fixation and a narrow mesentery leads to an increased risk of midgut volvulus. Intestinal atresia, Meckel's diverticulum and intestinal duplication may be encountered and are especially common in cases of gastroschisis (10–15%).[16] The eviscerated intestine is thickened, inflamed, edematous and matted together, often appearing congested and ischemic. The mesentery is also thickened and short. The length of intestine in most cases of gastroschisis is foreshortened (mean = 70 cm) but this is not necessarily of clinical importance since it seems to reverse spontaneously as the inflammation and edema resolves.[19] Irving's[1] postoperative radiographic studies have confirmed the early return to near normal length. Prolonged ileus with delayed transit has been demonstrated in both omphalocele and gastroschisis and particularly when exudates are present.[19] The period of dysfunction usually lasts 20–30 days.[19] Studies have documented decreased carbohydrate, fat and protein absorption. Transit and absorption patterns usually return to normal within 6 months (Fig. 52.3).[19]

The severity of intestinal macroscopic damages may be related to the duration the intestine is exposed to amniotic fluid. Gastrointestinal function returns sooner in patients with fewer exudative changes. Intestinal wall inflammation is usually less severe in ruptured omphalocele than in gastroschisis. Alteration in amniotic fluid composition with the onset of fetal renal function may contribute to the deleterious effect on the exposed intestine.[19] In fetal lambs with gastroschisis, atrophy of myenteric ganglion cells can be observed, resulting in disordered peristalsis.[20] Moreover, decreased blood flow may be responsible for the changes in 'motility' and absorption. Intestinal compression at the neck of the defect results in edema and ischemic damage. In an *in utero* fetal model, a ligature placed around the herniated bowel causing constriction resulted in bowel dysmotility.[21] It appears that both constriction and ischemia of the intestine as well as exposure to amniotic fluid contribute to the intestinal changes.

PRENATAL MANAGEMENT

Prenatal diagnosis allows for rational decisions regarding such issues as timing, location and method of delivery as well as risk to the mother, termination of the pregnancy and parental counseling. If the defect is associated with other severe anomalies, moral, religious and ethical questions may arise, including discussion regarding termination of the pregnancy.

Unborn infants with abdominal wall defects should be monitored by serial ultrasonography to detect intrauterine growth retardation. Prenatal diagnosis allows for appropriate referral to a tertiary care center to plan for the delivery and the surgical care of the newborn.

Gastroschisis and omphalocele may be detected by an elevated maternal serum alpha-fetoprotein (MSAFP) but must be differentiated from other fetal abnormalities, especially spina bifida, which may result in an elevation of the MSAFP. Omphalocele may be distinguished from gastroschisis by determining the ratio of acetylcholinesterase to pseudocholineseterase in the amniotic fluid.[22]

Ultrasound has become part of good prenatal care. Ultrasonography allows for detection of abdominal wall defects after the bowel returns to the peritoneal cavity at the 10th week of gestation. Infants with omphalocele are distinguished from those with gastroschisis by a membranous sac and liver protruding from the abdomen. Children with gastroschisis are characterized by the presence of loops of intestine floating freely in the amniotic fluid. Fetal echocardiography should be performed to detect cardiac defects. In a recent study, 15% of gastroschisis babies and 45% of omphalocele infants had congenital heart disease.[23] This information is critical to advise the parents and prepare the medical team for delivery.

Doppler ultrasonography can be used to evaluate visceral blood flow to the bowel. In cases of gastroschisis, the ultra-

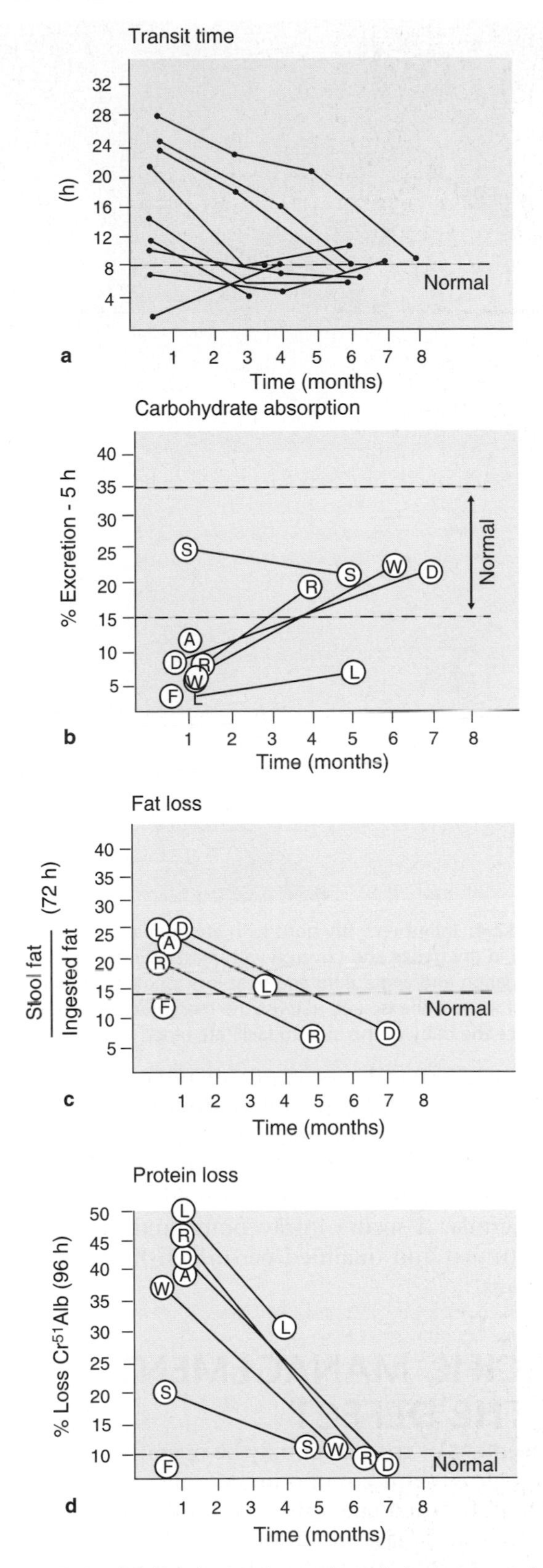

Figure 52.3: (a–d) Initial changes in transit, carbohydrate, protein and fat absorption as a relationship to time in abdominal wall defect patients.

sonographic appearance of the intestine may be related to the clinical outcome. In addition, polyhydramnios may be a predictor of bowel complications such as atresia or obstruction.[24] In one series, small intestinal dilatation and wall thickening were associated with intestinal atresia or stenosis as well as a poor outcome.[25] The appearance of the intestine on ultrasonography is not, however, an indication for early delivery of the child.

Amniocentesis

Amniocentesis and chromosomal analysis should be considered in all cases to detect abnormalities that commonly occur. Amnio-exchange may reduce inflammation in the exposed gastroschisis by reducing gastrointestinal waste in the amniotic fluid.[26] Luton's recent publication described transabdominal amniotic fluid drainage. Beginning at 30 weeks gestation, approximately 900 cc amniotic fluid would be removed and replaced with an equal amount of warm normal saline. This procedure was repeated every 2–3 weeks. No adverse incidents were identified and significant improvement was noted in degree of intestinal exudate, duration of ventilation and length of stay in the NICU.

Caesarean section *vs* vaginal delivery

Large omphaloceles may cause obstructed labor or liver injury necessitating C-section. Several years ago these anecdotal reports led to proposals that caesarean section was the preferred method of delivery. Cameron set the precedence in 1978 describing elective caesarean section for a prenatally diagnosed omphalocele.[27] Lenke and Hatch[1] claimed that babies with gastroschisis delivered by caesarean section have less intestinal edema, were easier to repair and had shorter hospital stays with lower mortality.

However, numerous recent studies have concluded that caesarean section is unwarranted. Bethel, Carpenter, Davidson and Kirk[1] have concluded that caesarean section does not confer any advantage with regard to survival or other neonatal postoperative parameters. Although medical and legal issues may influence maternal obstetric care, there are currently no prospective, well-controlled studies that support the contention that Caesarean section provides an additional measure of safety for babies with abdominal wall defects.[28]

INITIAL MANAGEMENT FOLLOWING DELIVERY

Resuscitation should begin immediately. An orogastric tube is inserted to prevent vomiting and aspiration, to improve ventilation, to decrease intestinal distention and to facilitate visceral reduction. Patients with signs of respiratory distress should undergo immediate endotracheal intubation. Fluid resuscitation must be initiated promptly to avoid hypothermia. An intravenous canula should be placed preferably in an upper limb since inferior vena caval compression may occur during reduction. However, catheters inserted into the lower limbs and advanced into the inferior vena cava may be useful in determining the intraabdominal pressure. A 6-French Foley catheter should be inserted into the bladder to monitor urine output and intravesicular pressure. Hematocrit, serum electrolytes, blood glucose and arterial blood gas values should be obtained soon after birth to guide resuscitation.

Although normal neonates require limited maintenance volumes for the first few days of life (60–80 ml/kg per day of bodyweight), infants with abdominal wall defects experience abnormal fluid losses particularly with gastroschisis and ruptured omphalocele. The previously described intestinal changes result in substantial water, electrolyte and protein losses. Atmospheric exposure of the intestine results in increased insensible fluid and heat losses. Initial fluid resuscitation should consist of rapid bolus infusion of 20 ml/kg of crystalloid solution. Tradition has maintained that solutions low in electrolytes are most appropriate for infants; however, this is not true for infants with omphalocele or gastroschisis. The rate of infusion should be guided by the clinical condition of the baby as determined by pulse rate, mean arterial blood pressure and urine output. Infusion of D_5 0.5NS at two to three times maintenance requirements is usually necessary. Babies with eviscerated intestines have abnormally low levels of immunoglobulin and are probably at greater risk for developing infection. Contamination of the intestine is inevitable and broad-spectrum antibiotics should be administered as well as Vitamin K in anticipation of the surgical procedure.

Once fluid resuscitation has begun, attention should be directed to the herniated intestine and avoidance of hypothermia. If the intestine is contained within a sac, it should be left intact. In some cases of gastroschisis, it may be apparent that the defect is so small that it is causing vascular compromise of the intestine. In these cases, the physician should immediately enlarge the defect. Occasionally, loops of intestine will require untwisting to restore circulation. The eviscerated bowel or the omphalocele sac should be carefully wrapped and supported with sterile dry gauze dressing. The eviscerated mass should be positioned to avoid vascular obstruction during wrapping with sterile gauze. The infant should be placed on their side with the organs arranged to avoid injury or vascular compromise. Gauze should be covered by enclosing the torso of the infant in a sterile transparent bowel bag or clear plastic wrap to reduce the evaporative loss of heat and fluid and to allow for frequent examination (Fig. 52.4). Hypothermia is a frequent and serious problem that can be avoided by placing the infant under a radiant heater immediately after birth and maintaining the infant in a heated incubator or infant care island.

After initial resuscitation, the infant should undergo careful evaluation for associated anomalies. Episodes of cyanosis, absence of the xiphoid, or cleft sternum should alert the clinician to the possibility of a cardiac or diaphragmatic defect. Chest radiographs may be helpful in identifying associated cardiac anomalies, diaphragmatic defects, or aspiration. If trisomy 13 or 18 is confirmed, the prognosis is poor and consultation with the parents is advisable before further treatment is undertaken. Discussions with the family and ethics committee may be helpful in defining the most appropriate course.

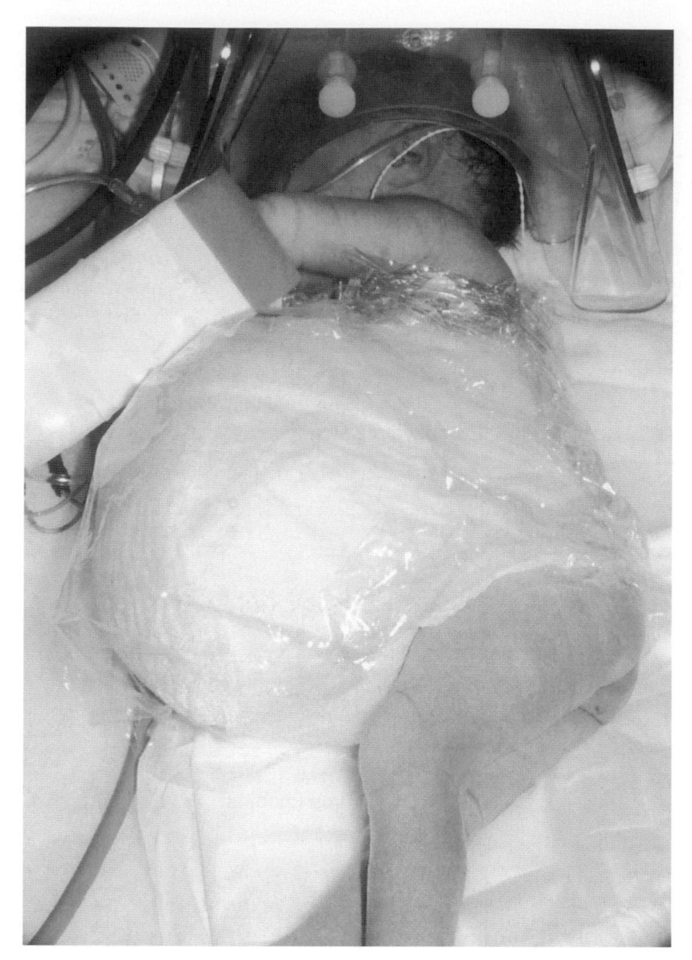

Figure 52.4: Infant recently born with abdominal wall defect wrapped in dry gauze and covered with plastic wrap to protect from contamination and avoid fluid and heat loss; prior to wrapping bowel, one must inspect the bowel, untwist the mesentery, if necessary and then place the baby on his side to facilitate blood flow return.

Although surgical procedures are not especially difficult, intraoperative judgment and postoperative expertise are major determinants of good outcome. Transfer of these infants to an appropriate tertiary care center is always recommended. Heated incubators should be used to prevent hypothermia. A secure intravenous fluid infusion should be continued and qualified personnel should accompany the infant.

SPECIFIC MANAGEMENT OF THE DEFECT

Management of the defect may be operative or non-operative. Surgical treatment of omphalocele and gastroschisis is similar and should take into account the size of the defect, the eviscerated mass, gestational age, birthweight and the presence of other anomalies. The goal is to achieve closure of the defect as soon as possible, avoid complications and shorten hospital stay. Non-operative topical treatment is rarely indicated but may be helpful when transportation to a tertiary care facility is impossible or when ethical issues are encountered.

Non-operative treatment

Non-operative treatment is associated with a significant risk for infection, sac rupture during the gradual epithelialization phase and prolonged hospitalization. In addition, the infant is left with a large ventral hernia that must be repaired later (Fig. 52.5a,b). However, non-operative management may be indicated in infants who have other life-threatening conditions, severe cardiac lesions, or chromosomal syndromes. Two percent Mercurochrome solution for topical application to the omphalocele sac[29] can result in toxic mercury levels necessitating monitoring of serum mercury levels. Alternative topical agents include silver sulfadiazine, 0.5% silver nitrate solution, 70% alcohol, or biologic dressings. Improved surgical therapy and NICU care have relegated topical therapy to a secondary role.

General principles of surgical management

Before proceeding with operative care, it is imperative to ensure that the infant has received adequate fluid resuscitation and is not hypothermic or acidotic. A planned delay prior to surgery, during which time these factors are corrected, will outweigh any potential advantage of 'rushing' into the operating theater. Heat loss during the procedure should be prevented by placing the patient on a neonatal warming unit, wrapping the head and limbs, increasing the ambient temperature of the room and using conduction or radiant heat warmers.

Surgery is performed under general anesthesia with muscle relaxation. Bacterial contamination can be reduced by thorough cleansing of the exposed intestine with povidone-iodine solution, which is washed off with warm sterile saline solution. Rectal irrigation with warm saline helps to evacuate meconium from the intestine, reduce the intestinal mass and aids in achieving primary closure. Once the intestine has been washed and the meconium evacuated, the skin is prepared and the infant is draped for the surgical procedure. A Foley catheter is inserted once the sterile field has been established.

An intact omphalocele sac should be excised while avoiding injury to adherent liver. The hepatic veins may be elongated and can kink with excessive torsion. Usually, the defect will be enlarged to allow adequate inspection and reduction of the intestine. Ladd's bands may be present in association with malrotation and should be divided to preclude duodenal obstruction. In gastroschisis, inspection of the intestine may be difficult because of the covering inflammatory peel, which should not be removed because considerable blood loss or inadvertent intestinal perforation may occur. The volume of viscera may be reduced by manually milking intestinal contents out of the rectum. Atretic areas may be detected during the irrigation and milking procedure. If primary closure is feasible and areas of intestinal atresia are encountered, the bowel can be resected and primary anastomosis accomplished without undue risk.[10] If a prosthetic silo is to be applied and inflammation of the intestine is severe, it may be prudent to leave the segment of atresia *in situ* and plan for delayed repair when the inflammation has resolved. Some authors have advocated the use of temporary exteriorizing ostomies for atresias while others have suggested that an intestinal anastomosis in these babies may be complicated by an increased risk of a postoperative stricture.[30,31] However, we believe that, because of the risk of infection, exteriorization of the intestine is

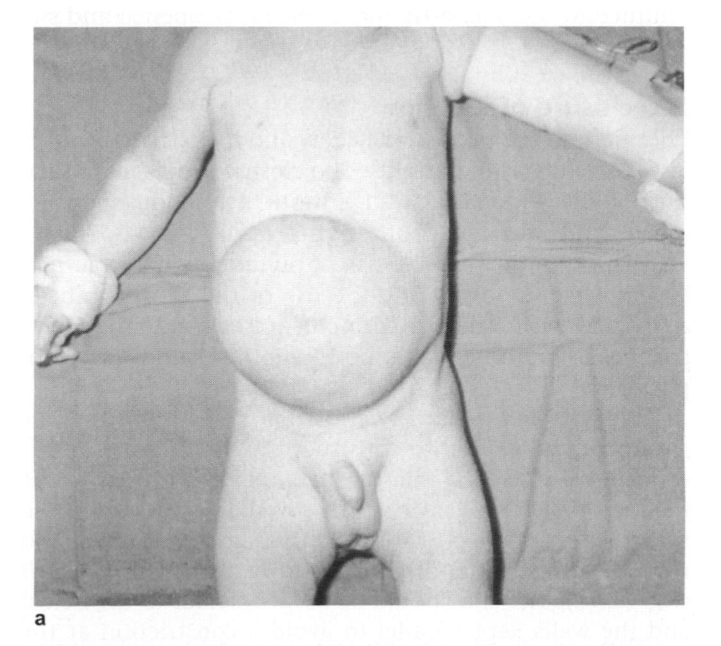

a

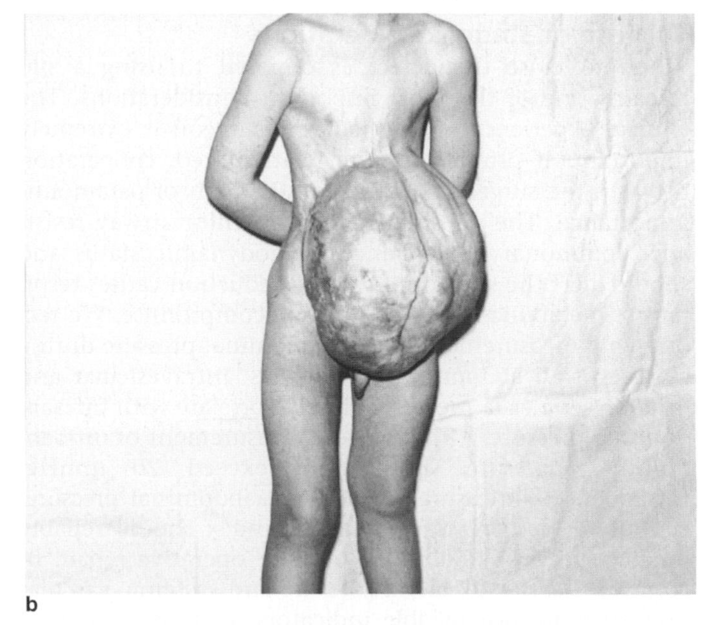

b

Figure 52.5: (**a**) Infant treated by skin flap closure with resultant large ventral hernia. (**b**) Child with same treatment in which hernia has enlarged and peritoneal cavity has become relatively smaller.

unnecessary and unwise. When a silo is used, the atresia may be excised when the edema has partially resolved. A primary anastomosis can be safely performed at the time of final fascial closure.[32]

After the intestine has been inspected, the diaphragm must be examined since a diaphragmatic hernia may not become apparent until the intestine is returned. If the liver is herniated, careful division of the diaphragmatic attachments allows for easier reduction. The liver has an abnormal globular shape and it may be difficult to reduce the organ to the normal anatomical position. Care must be taken not to injure elongated hepatic veins, obstruct the stomach, or compress the inferior vena cava during reduction of the liver.

The decision whether to repair the abdominal wall defect by primary fascial closure or to utilize a staged repair is a critical one. No consensus exists regarding the optimal approach. In fact, the best approach should be determined by the clinical situation. For hernias of the cord or small omphaloceles, primary closure is clearly preferred and is associated with the fewest complications. For larger defects, the degree of viscero-abdominal disproportion often makes it difficult to reduce the viscera in one stage without causing hemodynamic or respiratory compromise. A few years ago, one of the immediate problems facing the surgical team at the conclusion of the operation was achieving safe extubation of the patient. For this reason, infants were allowed to breathe spontaneously during surgery. Muscle relaxants were not used. This concern dictated the use of the staged silo approach and during the late 1960s and 1970s, staged closure using the silastic silo gained widespread acceptance. With improved postoperative ventilator care, primary closure has been accepted as the most appropriate management for babies born with abdominal wall defects.

To close or stage considerations

When to close the defect as opposed to using a silo remains one of the most important considerations. The clinical experience of the pediatric surgeon is extremely important. If primary closure is attempted, cooperation between the surgeon and the anesthetist is of paramount importance. The anesthetist must monitor airway resistance, pulmonary compliance, hemodynamic status and should alert the surgeon if visceral reduction causes respiratory, metabolic, or hemodynamic compromise. We recommend measurement of intraabdominal pressure during closure of all abdominal wall defects. Intravesicular and inferior vena cava pressures closely correlate with intraabdominal pressure.[33] The indirect measurement of intraabdominal pressure should not exceed 20 mmHg. Intraoperative measurement of intraabdominal pressure, central venous pressure or cardiac index should reliably predict success or failure of primary operative repair. In contrast, heart rate, blood pressure and systemic vascular resistance are not reliable indicators. In most instances, the surgeon will also have to rely on his or her clinical experience.

Primary closure guidelines

Primary closure is always the goal since it is associated with an excellent outcome.[34] Muscle relaxants during the operation are necessary to achieve safe primary closure. Respiratory assistance will usually be required during the initial postoperative period. Patients treated by primary closure have a shorter hospital stay compared to staged silo closure as well as improved survival, reduced risk of sepsis and less intestinal dysfunction.[35] Transient edema of the lower limbs is common and is not usually associated with any morbidity. With primary closure, the loops of intestine are carefully returned to the abdominal cavity with care taken to orient the mesentery correctly and to avoid vascular compromise. The fascia is approximated with interrupted suture and the skin is closed with absorbable subcuticular suture. By stretching the abdominal wall an incision may be unnecessary. A portion of the umbilical cord is preserved, sutured to the inferior margin of the defect and allowed to heal by secondary intention. The cosmetic results as depicted in (Fig. 52.6a) have been excellent. Years later, the uninformed clinician may not recognize that the patient has had an operation (Fig. 52.6b).

Respiratory compromise can be avoided by monitoring the intraoperative airway pressure. As a guide, airway pressure should not exceed 25 mmHg. Although it is possible to overcome respiratory problems encountered during the primary closure, other consequences of a 'tight' closure may occur. Cardiac output may be reduced and corrected by intravascular volume expansion, ionotropic agents, or both. Renal blood flow and glomerular filtration rate can be dramatically reduced and may not be restored by fluid volume replacement. Intraabdominal pressures that exceed 20 mmHg may cause renal vein thrombosis and renal failure. If the pressure exceeds this level, the baby should be returned to the operating room, the fascia opened and silo applied.

Silo closure guidelines

This method has been used widely and is associated with,[36] low morbidity and mortality. Silo closure avoids manipulation of the abdominal wall, intestinal milking of meconium and the use of high-pressure postoperative ventilation mitigating the risk of pulmonary barotraumas. Recent reviews advocating the use of the silo have been associated with a decreased incidence of abdominal compartment syndrome, better bowel motility and fewer complications.[37,38]

If staged silo closure is chosen for treatment, silastic sheeting may be used to construct the silo or a preformed silo can be utilized. A silastic sheet may be sutured to the margin of the defect. All skin is saved and not sutured to silastic sheeting. A closed silo is then constructed around the intestine by stapling or suturing the sheet to itself (Fig. 52.7a). The silo should be perpendicular to the defect and the walls kept parallel to avoid a constriction at the base of the silo where the prosthesis joins the abdominal wall (Fig. 52.8a). Pre-fashioned silos have been improved in

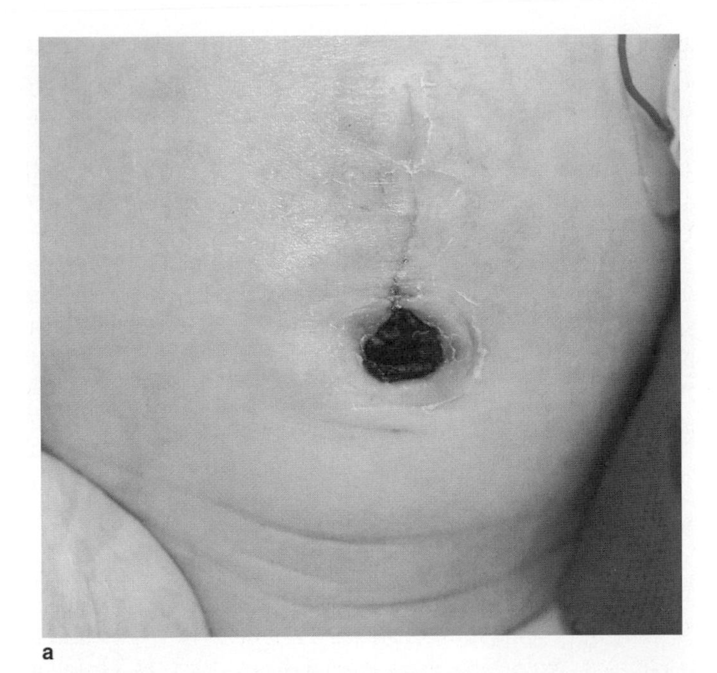

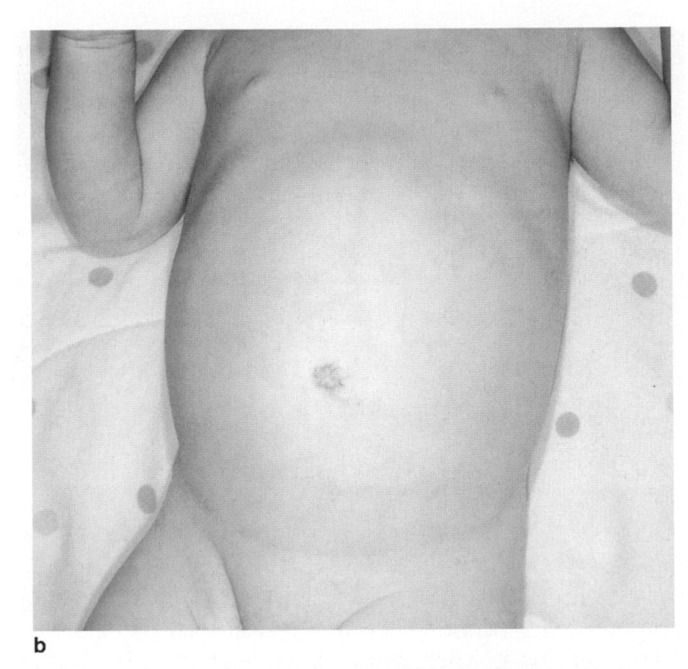

a b

Figure 52.6: (**a**) Shows immediate postoperative appearance of a baby with upper midline incision and use of umbilical cord umbilicoplasty, forming a near normal appearance of the abdominal wall. (**b**) Older child following primary closure of gastroschisis; note that there is no incision and the neo-umbilicus appears relatively normal with an excellent cosmetic appearance.

the last few years. They have become the preferred method since they are applied quickly and avoid suturing to the abdominal wall. After the silo is applied, it should be wrapped in sterile, thick gauze bandages to protect the silo and prevent evaporation and contamination. When the infant is returned to an open incubator, the apex of the silo should be suspended from the overhead warming lights to prevent it from tilting over and to allow gravity to encourage reduction (Fig. 52.7b).

POSTOPERATIVE MANAGEMENT

Infants with large defects require postoperative ventilation until the abdominal wall relaxes and edema resolves sufficiently to allow for adequate spontaneous respiration. Arterial blood gas values should be carefully monitored and the respiratory rate, inspired oxygen, peak airway pressure and tidal volume should be adjusted as necessary to maintain optimal ventilation and oxygenation. A decrease in urine output may represent decreased preload from vena cava compression or increased intraabdominal pressure. Fluid resuscitation should be aggressive. If a fluid challenge fails to improve renal function, re-operation to relieve intraabdominal pressure and application of a silo may be required to avert serious renal damage.

Fluid management

Even if preoperative and intraoperative fluid resuscitation has been vigorous, postoperative fluid requirements are much higher for babies with abdominal wall defects. Abdominal wall defect infants require as much as 312 ml/kg or as little as 83 ml/kg in the first 24 h of life to support tissue perfusion as determined by muscle pH studies. A mean fluid volume of 146 ± 35 mg/kg may be required for the first day.[39] The requirements for the first, second and third days after surgical repair, respectively, may vary as follows: 160.7 ml/kg on the first day, 125.4 ml/kg on the second day and 141.5 ml/kg on the third day. Urinary output should be used to adjust the actual volumes administered. Postoperative fluid requirements for infants with gastroschisis and babies with silos may be higher compared with patients with omphalocele and primary closure patients throughout the first postoperative week.

Delay in the return of intestinal functions must be anticipated. Prokinetic agents such as erythromycin have not proven effective in randomized trials at speeding return of intestinal function.[40] The orogastric tube should be left in position and frequently aspirated to keep the intestine decompressed. Parenteral nutrition will be necessary for all infants. During the period of prolonged ileus, trophic feedings to facilitate intestinal recovery have been well established as safe and effective.[41] Total parenteral nutrition (TPN) is best started early in anticipation that intestinal motility will not return immediately. Patients with ruptured omphalocele or gastroschisis are most likely to require prolonged TPN. Insertion of a central venous catheter or PIC line is beneficial. Catheter-related sepsis and liver disease are significant complications of TPN therapy. Blood cultures should be obtained if fever is detected and the central catheter should be removed if there are laboratory or clinical signs of infection. Some surgeons defer insertion of TPN catheters for several days to minimize the chance of contamination induced by the initial operative

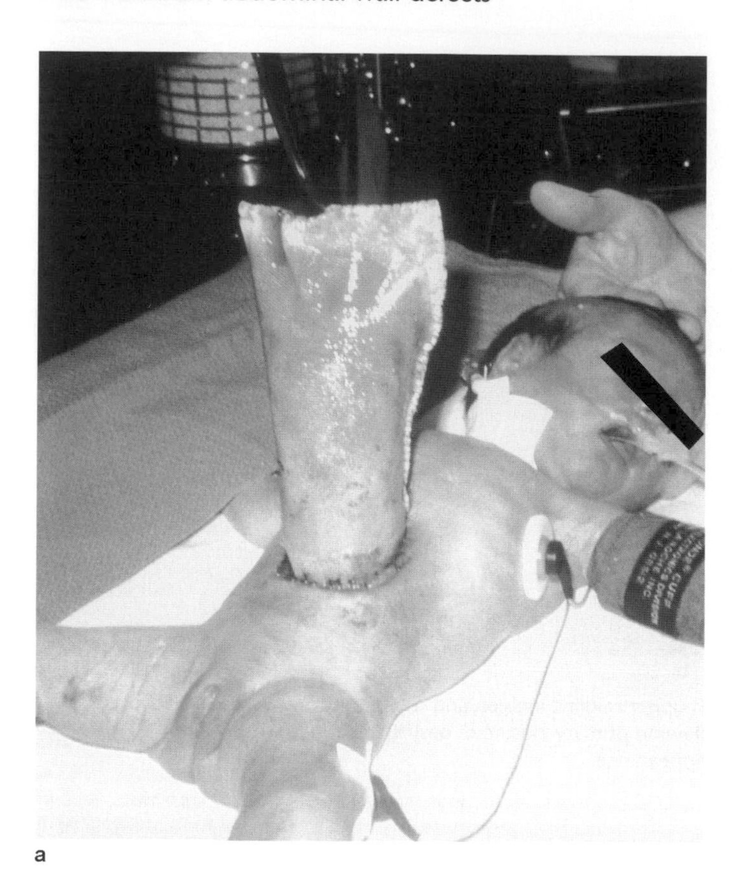
a

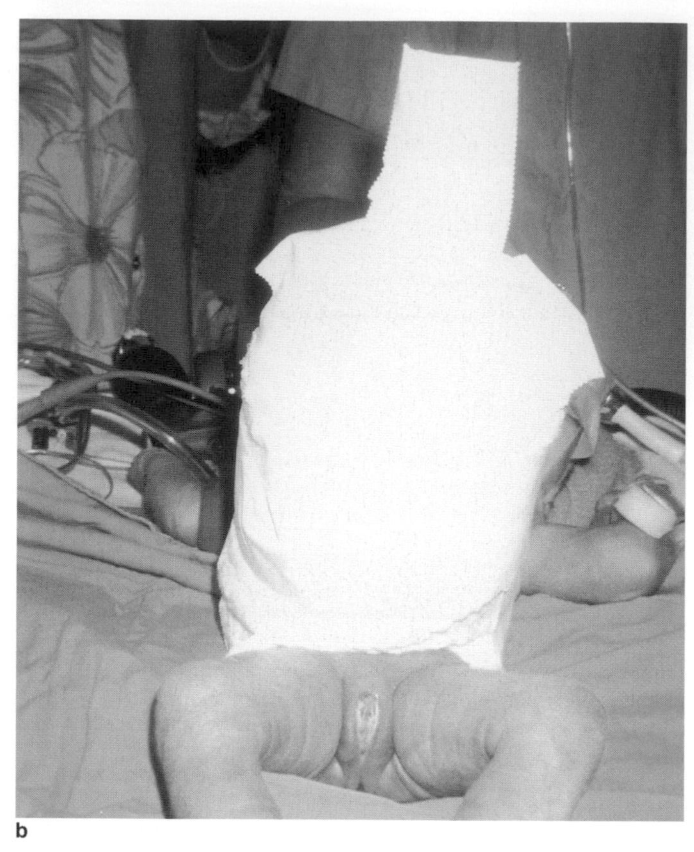
b

Figure 52.7: (a) Newborn requiring placement of bowel within a 'constructed' silo; bowel loops and exudative fluid are visible. (b) Silo covered with thick dry gauze dressings; suspension avoids kinking of the silo and facilitates effects of gravity.

procedure. Liver enzyme values should be monitored to evaluate liver function. Oral feeding should not be started until orogastric aspirates are negligible and stools are passed. Because infants with these disorders often have some degree of malabsorption, it is advisable to begin feeding with semi-elemental or predigested formulas.

Infants with silo closure are at risk for dehydration and septicemia as long as the prosthetic material is in place. As the abdominal wall relaxes and the edema resolves, the contents of the silo should be reduced every 12–24 h, with care being taken not to cause excessive elevation of intraabdominal pressure. Manipulation of the silo must be done under strict aseptic conditions. Each time the viscera are reduced, the silo volume must be adjusted accordingly. This can be done by suturing the sac, or more easily, with a stapling device (Fig. 52.8b). Once complete reduction is achieved, the infant may be returned to the operating theater for removal of the prosthesis and closure of the defect.

ALTERNATIVE METHODS OF CLOSURE

Gross's skin flap closure techniques have assumed a secondary role. This technique may still be useful when a prosthesis is not available, premature separation of the silo occurs, or when the surgeon determines that fascial closure is dangerous. Although Gross originally advised leaving the omphalocele sac intact, most surgeons today advise removing the sac to inspect the viscera. Barlow[1] recommended the application of an external bandage silo to reduce the giant omphalocele for several days before operation is undertaken. Jona suggested that the effects of gravity and time may be sufficient to reduce the bowel within a silo while avoiding the potential complications of abdominal compartment syndrome or respiratory compromise.[42] Hendrickson recommended sequential bedside clamping without a prosthesis as a useful alternative to silo or skin flap closure for omphalocele.[43] In 1990, Klein[1] reported the treatment of infants with abdominal wall defects utilizing dura to close the abdominal wall. Saxena recommended this method for cases of giant omphalocele when a silo is not available or skin flaps would not cover the defect.[44] Meddings[1] recently reported the use of polyglactin mesh to achieve closure of the abdominal wall. Yazbeck[1] reported use of a polyamide mesh that was glued to the abdominal wall and reduced by segmental infolding of the mesh. Hong[1] suggested sequential reduction of the intact sac to reduce giant omphaloceles. Bax[1] and DeUgarte[45] reported a new concept using tissue expanders that are placed into the peritoneal cavity for several days. After the expander is progressively enlarged and sufficient volume is achieved, the expander is removed and the abdomen is closed.

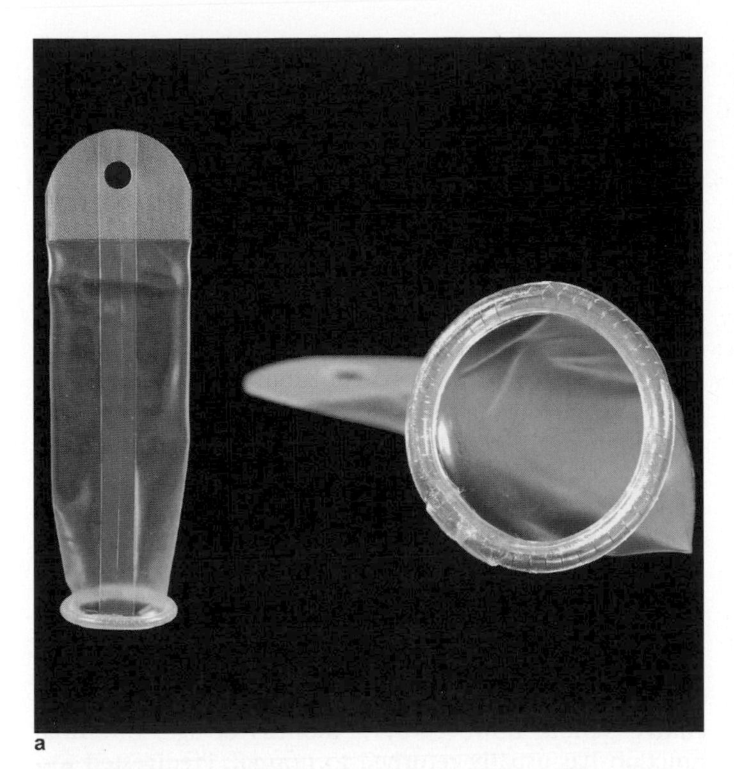

a

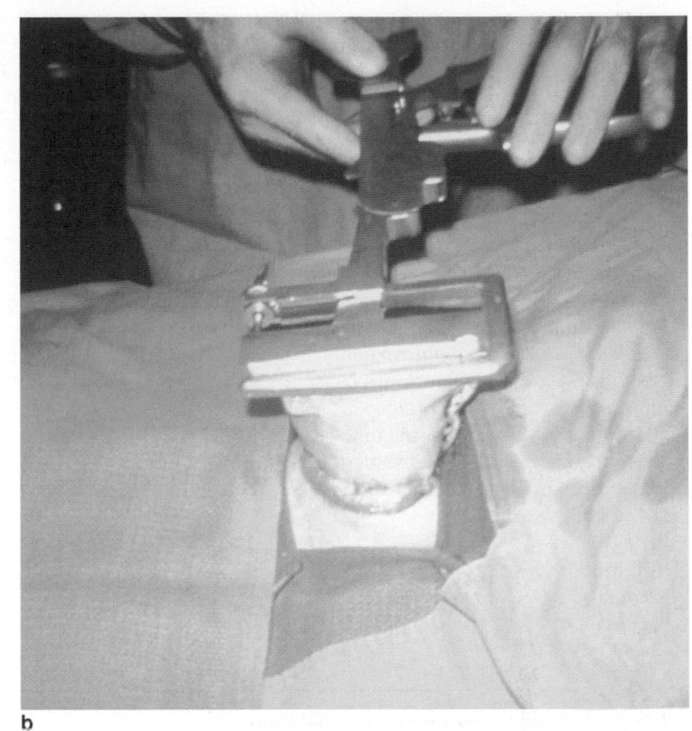

b

Figure 52.8: (**a**) Shows preformed silo with spring coil at base opening; easy to place bowel in silo and quick to insert beneath the fascia; avoids time consuming attachment to the abdominal wall. (**b**) Depicts the use of the stabling device to sequentially and safely reduce the size of the silo.

EXPECTED MORTALITY

Until the 1960s and 1970s, omphalocele and gastroschisis were associated with a very high mortality rate. The advent of parenteral nutrition and staged methods of closure in the late 1970s contributed to improved survival. The size of the defect and the presence of herniated liver appear to have no influence on mortality. In cases of omphalocele, babies weighing less than 2500 g have a higher rate of mortality. In cases of gastroschisis, the mortality rate is not related to birthweight. Multiple congenital anomalies continue to be the major cause of death in omphalocele patients and mortality rates have not improved over the last several years. In contrast, the overall survival rate for patients with gastroschisis markedly improved to 90% during the last several decades. Prematurity, intestinal complications and sepsis associated with parenteral nutrition have been the major contributors to mortality.[1]

In general there is a gratifying trend toward improved survival and simpler procedures. In the future, morbidity and mortality will most likely be determined by associated anomalies, prematurity and unexpected post-surgical complications.

INCREASING HOSPITAL COSTS

Patient care continues to be the paramount concern. however, the cost of hospital care is becoming an increasing concern. The average cost of hospitalization has been reported as US$123 000.[46] Room charges contributed to 43% of total costs. Additional costs included physician fees collected (15%), respiratory care (10%), supplies (10%), pharmacy (6%), lab (4%), operating room charges (4%) and other (8%). Cost per day was nearly US$2700. Significant cost differences between staged repair (US$154 000) and primary repair (US$93 800) were noted. Cost for babies with gastrointestinal complications averaged US$219 200 *vs* US$83 800 for those without such complications. There was strong correlation between hospital costs, the use of the NICU and overall length of stay.[46] Clearly every effort should be made to use methods that minimize the risk of complications and at the same time avoid over use of the neonatal intensive care unit.

POSTOPERATIVE COMPLICATIONS

Postoperative complications can be divided into early, intermediate and late (Table 52.2). Whichever method of closure has been used, high-volume bilious aspirates and failure to defecate may suggest obstruction. The radiographic appearance of dilated intestine may mimic intestinal obstruction. However, mechanical obstruction is relatively uncommon and these signs usually indicate prolonged postoperative ileus. If there is clinical suspicion of obstruction, upper gastrointestinal radiographic contrast studies may be helpful. Moreover, water-soluble contrast examination of the colon may actually help to evacuate meconium, provide information regarding the distal small intestine, demonstrate sites of obstruction and stimulate peristalsis. Occasionally, sites of

Early	Intermediate	Late
Respiratory distress	Inguinal hernia	Growth delay
Sepsis	Gastroesophageal reflux	Low IQ
Wound infection	Cryptorchidism	Malpositioned viscera
Postsurgical ileus	Ventral hernia	Atypical appendicitis
Dehydration	Small intestinal obstruction	Intestinal obstruction
Enteric fistula	Malrotation with obstruction	
Necrotizing enterocolitis	Necrotizing enterocolitis	
Gastric outlet obstruction	Gastric outlet obstruction	
Malabsorption	Malabsorption	
Lower limb swelling		
Renal vein thrombosis		
Premature separation of silo		

Table 52.2 Possible postsurgical complications

atresia or obstruction due to Ladd's bands will be missed at the time of the initial operation. However, the abdomen should only be re-explored if there is definite radiographic evidence of mechanical obstruction. Intestinal obstruction may occur months or years after the original operation and can be related to intraperitoneal adhesions or malrotation. However, such adhesions do not seem to be a common long-term problem. If not corrected at the time of original surgery, malrotation may lead to duodenal obstruction and volvulus.

One of the most problematic complications has been the development of postoperative necrotizing enterocolitis.[47] During the past few years, this complication has contributed to approximately 20% of the deaths at one institution. Management consists of orogastric tube decompression, antibiotics and physiologic support. Operative intervention is reserved for patients with physiologic deterioration or perforation.

Enteric fistulae may develop at the site of inadvertent intestinal injury, unrecognized areas of ischemia, or atresia. Compression of intestinal loops by tight closure or erosion due to contact with suture may cause intestinal injury and lead to fistula formation. Perforation of intestine in a silo is possible. Moreover, a fistula may develop if a primary anastomosis fails. Fistulae without distal obstruction often close spontaneously. If further complications develop, re-operation and exterioration may be desirable.

Development of inguinal hernia after closure of the defect has been reported and is presumably caused by increased intraabdominal pressure. In one series, inguinal hernias occurred in 14% of patients with omphalocele and 2% of patients with gastroschisis.[13] Ventral hernias occasionally occur in infants who are treated by skin flap closure or by nonoperative measures. Similarly, failure of prosthetic silo method to achieve fascial closure necessitates skin flap closure, resulting in a ventral hernia. In addition, because the fascial closure is sometimes done under considerable tension, hernias may occur along the closure line and necessitate repair. Small hernias may heal spontaneously. Late secondary hernia repairs in older children may require staged closure or the use of prosthetic materials.

Increased intraabdominal pressure may also lead to gastroesophageal reflux.[10,12] Nissen fundoplication should be considered. Conversely, low intraabdominal pressure during fetal development may contribute to the increased incidence of cryptorchidism, which is seen frequently in male infants with abdominal wall defects.[18]

LATE MORBIDITY AND QUALITY OF LIFE

Long-term problems related to intestinal function are uncommon. As noted, absorption of carbohydrate, protein and fat may be abnormal at birth and in the early postoperative period, however by 7 months of age, intestinal function has usually returned to normal. Predigested formulas should be used initially. Similarly, Berseth[1] studied 22 survivors of omphalocele and gastroschisis. Fecal fat excretion and serum chemistry were normal in all patients at 3 years of age. However, at 1 year of age, these patients were between the 3rd and 15th percentile for weight and height and by 10 years of age, no child demonstrated a height or weight above the 50th percentile.

The cause of poor growth is unclear, although it must be remembered that many patients with gastroschisis have low birthweight and failure to attain normal growth may be caused by underlying prenatal factors or associated anomalies. Berseth[1] found that one-third of their patients had IQs of less than 90. Intellectual impairment seemed to be related to the length of hospital stay. The authors concluded that this complication might be related to prematurity, low birthweight and other non-gastrointestinal neonatal complications.

Koivusalo[48] reviewed 57 patients, 17 years or older with congenital abdominal wall defects. With the exception of rheumatoid arthritis, the prevalence of acquired disease in abdominal wall defect patients was comparable to the general population. A number of patients had concerns related to the abdominal scar (37%), while 51% appeared to have disturbances best characterized as functional gastrointestinal disorders. Most importantly, overall quality of life and education levels of these patients were similar to the general population.[48]

In his review, Zaccara[49] focused on possible long-term physiologic limitations of children with abdominal wall defects. Following the Bruce protocol for children, 18 children ranging in age from 7 to 18 years with previous abdominal wall defects, underwent stress treadmill testing with a stepwise workload increase until exhaustion. Ergometric data were compared with the normal pediatric population. Parameters included exercise time, maximal oxygen consumption, heart rate, systolic blood pressure and forced vital capacity. These patients exhibited normal cardiopulmonary function with no abnormalities detected at rest or exertion.[49] No limitation to motor performances should exist for these patients.

Finally, malposition of the abdominal viscera may cause problems. Gastric outlet obstruction caused by displacement of the spleen or other organs has been documented.[50] The previously eviscerated globular liver may be misdiagnosed as an epigastric abdominal mass is more susceptible to traumatic injury.[50] Finally, the associated malrotation may create a diagnostic dilemma if the child develops appendicitis later in life since the cecum may not reside in the right lower quadrant. For this reason, removal of the appendix through an inversion appendectomy should be considered if it can be safely done during the original operation and if no associated genitourinary anomalies requiring bladder augmentation are present.

References

1. Cooney DR. Defects of the abdominal wall. In: O'Neill JA, Rowe MI, Grosfeld JL, Fonkalsrud EW, Coran AG, eds. Pediatric Surgery. St Louis, MO: Mosby; 1998:1045–1069.
2. Singh J. Gastroschisis is caused by the combination of carbon monoxide and protein-zinc deficiencies in mice. Birth Defects Research (Part B) 2003; 68(4):355–362.
3. Werler MM, Sheehan JE, Mitchell AA. Association of vasoconstrictive exposures with risks of gastroschisis and small intestinal atresia. Epidemiology 2003; 14:349–354.
4. Irving IM, Rickham PP. Umbilical abnormalities. In: Rickham PP, Lister J, Irving M, eds. Neonatal Surgery, 2nd edn. London: Butterworths; 1978.
5. Izant RJ, Brown F, Rothmann BF. Current embryology and treatment of gastroschisis and omphalocele. Arch Surg 1966; 93(1):49–53.
6. Houghland KT, Hanna AM, Meyers R, et al. Increasing prevalence of gastroschisis in Utah: a thirty-one year review. J Pediatr Surg 2004; in press.
7. Martinez-Frias ML, Salvador J, Prieto L, et al. Epidemiological study of gastroschisis and omphalocele in Spain. Teratology 1984; 29(3):377–382.
8. Roeper PJ, Harris J, Lee G. Secular rates and correlates for gastroschisis in California (1968–1977). Teratology 1987; 35(2):203–210.
9. Colombani PM, Cunningham MD. Perinatal aspects of omphalocele and gastroschisis. Am J Dis Child 1977; 131(12):1386–1388.
10. Grosfeld JL, Dawes L, Weber TR. Congenital abdominal wall defects: current management and survival. Surg Clin North Am 1981; 61(5):1037–1049.
11. Botto LD, Mulinare J, Erickson JD. Occurrence of omphalocele in relation to maternal multivitamin use: a population-based study. Pediatrics 2002; 109(5):904–908.
12. Stringel G, Filler RM. Prognostic factors in omphalocele and gastroschisis. J Pediatr Surg 1979; 14(5):515–519.
13. Knight PJ, Sommer A, Clatworthy HW. Omphalocele: a prognostic classification. J Pediatr Surg 1981; 16:599–604.
14. Mahour GH, Weitzmann JJ, Rosenkrantz JG. Omphalocele and gastroschisis. Annals of Surgery 1973; 177(4):478–482.
15. Caniano DA, Brokaw B, Ginn-Pease ME. An individualized approach to the management of gastroschisis. J Pediatr Surg 1990; 25(3):297–300.
16. Grosfeld JL, Weber TR. Congenital abdominal wall defects: gastroschisis and omphalocele. Curr Probl Surg 1982; 19(4):157–213.
17. Greenwood RG, Rosenthal A, Nadas AS. Cardiovascular malformations associated with omphalocele. J Pediatr 1974; 85(6):818–821.
18. Aliotta PJ, Piedmonte M, Karp M, et al. Cryptorchidism in newborns with gastroschisis and omphalocele. Urology 1992; 40(1):84–86.
19. O'Neill JA, Grosfeld JL. Intestinal malfunction after antenatal exposure of viscera. Am J Surg 1974; 127(2):129–132.
20. Haller JA Jr, Kehrer BH, Shaker IJ, et al. Studies of the pathophysiology of gastroschisis in fetal sheep. J Pediatr Surg 1974; 9(5):627–632.
21. Langer JC, Longaker MT, Crombleholme TM, et al. Etiology of intestinal damage in gastroschisis: effects of amniotic fluid exposure and bowel constriction in a fetal lamb model. J Pediatr Surg 1989; 24(10):992–997.
22. Burton BK. Positive amniotic fluid acetylcholinesterase: distinguishing between open spina bifida and ventral wall defects. Am J Obstet Gynecol 1986; 155(5):984–986.
23. Gibbin C, Touch S, Broth RE, et al. Abdominal wall defects and congenital heart disease. Ultrasound Obstet Gynecol 2003; 21(4):334–337.
24. Japaraj RP, Hockey R, Chan FY. Gastroschisis: can prenatal sonography predict neonatal outcome? Ultrasound Obstetrics Gynecol 2003; 21(4):329–333.
25. Bond SJ, Harrison MR, Filly RA, et al. Severity of intestinal damage in gastroschisis correlation with prenatal sonographic findings. J Pediatr Surg 1988; 23(6):520–525.
26. Luton D, Guibourdenche J, Vuillard E, et al. Prenatal management of gastroschisis: the place of the amnioexchange procedure. Clin Perinatology 2003; 30:551–572.
27. Cameron GM, McQuown DS, Modanlou HD, et al. Intrauterine diagnosis of an omphalocele by diagnostic ultrasonography. Am J Obstet Gynecol 1978; 131(7):821–822.
28. Heider AL, Strauss RA, Kuller JA. Omphalocele: clinical outcomes in cases with normal karyotypes. Am J Obstet Gynecol 2004; 190:135–141.
29. Dudrick SJ, Wilmore DW, Vars HM, et al. Long-term total parenteral nutrition with growth, development and positive nitrogen balance. Surgery 1968; 64(1):134–142.
30. Hollabaugh RS, Boles ET. The management of gastroschisis. J Pediatr Surg 1973; 8(2):263–270.
31. Hrabovsky EE, Boyd JB, Savrin RA, et al. Advances in the management of gastroschisis. Ann Surg 1980; 192(2):244–248.
32. Snyder CL, Miller KA, Sharp RJ, et al. Management of intestinal atresia in patients with gastroschisis. J Pediatr Surg 2001; 36(10):1542–1545.
33. Lacey SR, Bruce J, Brooks SP, et al. The relative merits of various methods of indirect measurement of intraabdominal pressure as a guide to closure of abdominal wall defects. J Pediatr Surg 1987; 22(12):1207–1211.
34. Reynolds M. Abdominal wall defects in infants with very low birth weight. Seminars in Pediatric Surgery 2000; 9(2):88–90.
35. Ein SM, Rubin SZ. Gastroschisis: primary closure of silon pouch. J Pediatr Surg 1980; 15(4):549–552.
36. Schwartz MZ, Tyson KR, Milliorn K, et al. Staged reduction using a silastic sac is the treatment of choice for large congenital abdominal wall defects. J Pediatr Surg 1983; 18(6):713–719.

37. Kidd RN Jr, Jackson RJ, Smith SD, et al. Evolution of staged versus primary closure of gastroschisis. Ann Surg 2003; 237(6):759–764.
38. Schlatter M, Norris K, Uitvlugt N, et al. Improved outcomes in the treatment of gastroschisis using a preformed silo and delayed repair approach. J Pediatr Surg 2003; 38(3):459–464.
39. Mollitt DL, Ballantine TV, Grosfeld JL, et al. A critical assessment of fluid requirements in gastroschisis. J Pediatr Surg 1978; 13(3):217–219.
40. Curry JI, Lander AD, Stringer MD, et al. A multicenter, randomized, double-blind, placebo-controlled trial of the prokinetic agent erythromycin in the postoperative recovery of infants with gastroschisis. J Pediatr Surg 2004; 39(4):565–569.
41. Singh SG, Fraser A, Leditschke JF, et al. Gastroschisis: determinants of neonatal outcome. Pediatr Surg Int 2003; 19(4):260–265.
42. Jona JZ. The 'Gentle Touch' technique in the treatment of gastroschisis. J Pediatr Surg 2003; 38(7):1036–1038.
43. Hendrickson RJ, Partrick DA, Janik JS. Management of giant omphalocele in a premature low-birth-weight neonate utilizing a bedside sequential clamping technique without prosthesis. J Pediatr Surg 2003; 38(10):14–16.
44. Saxena AK, Hulskamp G, Schleef J, et al. Gastroschisis: a 15 year, single center experience. Pediatr Surg Int 2002; 18(5/6):420–424.
45. Ugarte DA De, Asch MJ, Hedrick MH, et al. The use of tissue expanders in the closure of a giant omphalocele. J Pediatr Surg 2004; 39(4):613–615.
46. Sydorak RM, Nijagal A, Sbragia L, et al. Gastroschisis: small hole, big cost. J Pediatr Surg 2002; 37(12):1669–1672.
47. Oldham KT, Coran AG, Drongowski RA, et al. The development of necrotizing enterocolitis following repair of gastroschisis: a surprisingly high incidence. J Pediatr Surg 1988; 23(10):945–949.
48. Koivusalo A, Lindahl H, Rintala RJ. Morbidity and quality of life in adult patients with a congenital abdominal wall defect: a questionnaire survey. J Pediatr Surg 2002; 37(11):1594–1601.
49. Zaccara A, Iacobelli BD, Calzolari A, et al. Cardiopulmonary performances in young children and adolescents born with large abdominal wall defects. J Pediatr Surg 2003; 38(3):478–481.
50. Schuster SR. Omphalocele and gastroschisis. In: Welch KJ, Randolph JG, Ravitch MM, et al. eds. Pediatric Surgery, 4th edn. Chicago: Year Book; 1986:

Chapter 53
Stomas of the small and large intestine

Michael W. L. Gauderer

INTRODUCTION

Enterostomies play an important role in the management of numerous gastrointestinal conditions in the pediatric age group. Indications for such stomas comprise a broad spectrum ranging from decompression for congenital to acquired bowel obstructions, from diversion for neonatal intestinal perforations to abdominoperineal trauma, from foregut access for long-term enteral feedings to hindgut access for antegrade enemas.

Although often considered fairly basic, enterostomies actually encompass a wide variety of types, techniques and methods of care. Pediatric stomas differ from those in adult patients in many aspects, including the criteria for the selection of the most appropriate type, the importance of technical precision in the placement, the specialized age-related care, growth and the consideration of the psychologic needs of the child.

HISTORICAL NOTE

The word stoma comes from the Greek *stomoun* (to provide with an opening or mouth). The history of intestinal stomas is long and colorful.[1] Indeed, the concept of treating intestinal obstruction with exteriorization of the colon dates back to the eighteenth century, and among the first survivors were children with imperforate anus.[2] However, despite a few early successes, the use of stomas in the large intestine and later in the small intestine in children evolved slowly. There was, understandably, a reluctance to use such drastic interventions, which were associated with major complications. Gradually, as surgeon's experience increased toward the end of the nineteenth century and beginning of the twentieth century, colostomies and occasionally jejunostomies were employed to manage a handful of pediatric pathologies. With the advent of modern pediatric surgical practice and survival of children with conditions that were formally likely to be fatal, the need for stomas increased. Enterostomal construction techniques, initially developed for adults,[1,3] were modified and adapted for pediatric patients. Early approaches focused on newborns with congenital intestinal obstruction.[4–7] These were followed by new techniques combining proximal decompression with distal feeding for neonates with high intestinal atresia.[8–10] A number of other special, child-oriented stomas of the small and large intestine were introduced next.[11–19] In the last couple of decades, in great part because of the increased incidence of foregut dysmotility, new procedures aimed at providing postpyloric feeding access continue to be developed and evaluated.[11,14,16,20] Additionally, the advent of minimally invasive techniques provides new and exciting opportunities for the creation of feeding as well as venting, decompressing and irrigating stomas.[21–23]

Several factors have contributed to the safety, effectiveness and ease of care of pediatric stomas. Paramount among these is the advent of enterostomal therapy, which has evolved into a specialty in its own right.[24–26] The knowledge and experience derived from enterostomal care has led to the creation of child-specific appliances in a wide variety of types and sizes, as well as better tolerated biomaterials and sophisticated management techniques. Another important development has been the creation of non-medical support systems and organizations for ostomates.[27] Along with this is the availability of a significant number of publications for parents, caregivers and teenage patients.[28] Greater awareness and acceptance of ostomates, as well as the recognition of their needs and rights among the lay population, has also helped to improve their quality of life.[29] On the physician's side, understanding of stomal physiology and of specialized enteral and parenteral nutrition, as well as the diagnosis and management of stoma-related complications, has further improved care and outcome.[21,30] Although surgeons and gastroenterologists caring for children are continuously developing and evaluating alternatives to stomas,[31] the creation, management and closure of these accesses to the intestinal tract continue to occupy a substantial portion of their practice.[32]

THE CHILD WITH A STOMA

An enterostomy in a child is a major disruption of normality and frequently leads to significant psychologic trauma for the child and parents.[33] Fortunately, however, most intestinal stomas in the pediatric age group are temporary, and correction of the underlying problem often leads to closure of the diverting opening. On the other hand, in several instances of non-correctable and crippling pathologic conditions of the intestines, a permanent well-functioning stoma contributes to an improved quality of life.[29]

Despite many advances related to enterostomies, their placement, care and closure are associated with a surprisingly high rate of both early and late complications.[34–42] These facts present the surgeon, the gastroenterologist, the enterostomal therapist, the nurses, the parents and the child with major challenges. Therefore, when the need for a stoma arises, the best results are achieved by carefully evaluating the child's pathologic condition and health-status, weighing the pros and cons of diversion, planning ahead (for closure) whenever possible, and considering both construction and takedowns as major interventions. In addition to the well-defined guidelines for stomal placement established for adult patients, such factors as anatomic and physiologic differences, delicate structures, growth, and physical and emotional maturity need to be considered. It must always be kept in mind that the quality of life of a patient with a stoma is largely related to the quality of that stoma.

TYPES OF INTESTINAL STOMA AND THEIR APPLICATIONS

Depending on their *primary purpose*, enterostomas can be divided into four basic types.

1 Administration of feeding, medication or both (Fig. 53.1)

The access can be done indirectly, *without entering the small bowel wall*, employing nasojejunal or gastrostomy–jejunostomy tubes.[43] This approach works well if used for a limited number of days or a few of weeks. However, catheter plugging as well as dislodgement through accidental removal or displacement back into the stomach is common, restricting this modality largely to short-term use.

For long-term use, *direct access through the small bowel wall* is preferred. The options are needle–catheter jejunostomy,[11] tunneled catheter jejunostomy,[16] placement of a T tube[13] or a button.[14] Additionally, in selected patients, a direct percutaneous endoscopic jejunostomy or a laparoscopically assisted jejunostomy[21] may be employed, obviating the need for a laparotomy. Because of mechanical problems, particularly leakage, some surgeons use an isolated jejunal loop brought directly to the abdominal wall in the Roux-en-Y manner.[20] In this latter modality, the distal (feeding) limb can be made to exit through the abdominal wall and be catheterized intermittently, or the limb can remain under the abdominal wall and be accessed by means of a skin-level device such as a button.

2 Proximal decompression and distal feeding (Fig. 53.2)

Here, too, the access can be done *without entering the smal bowel wall*, as with a gastrostomy–jejunostomy

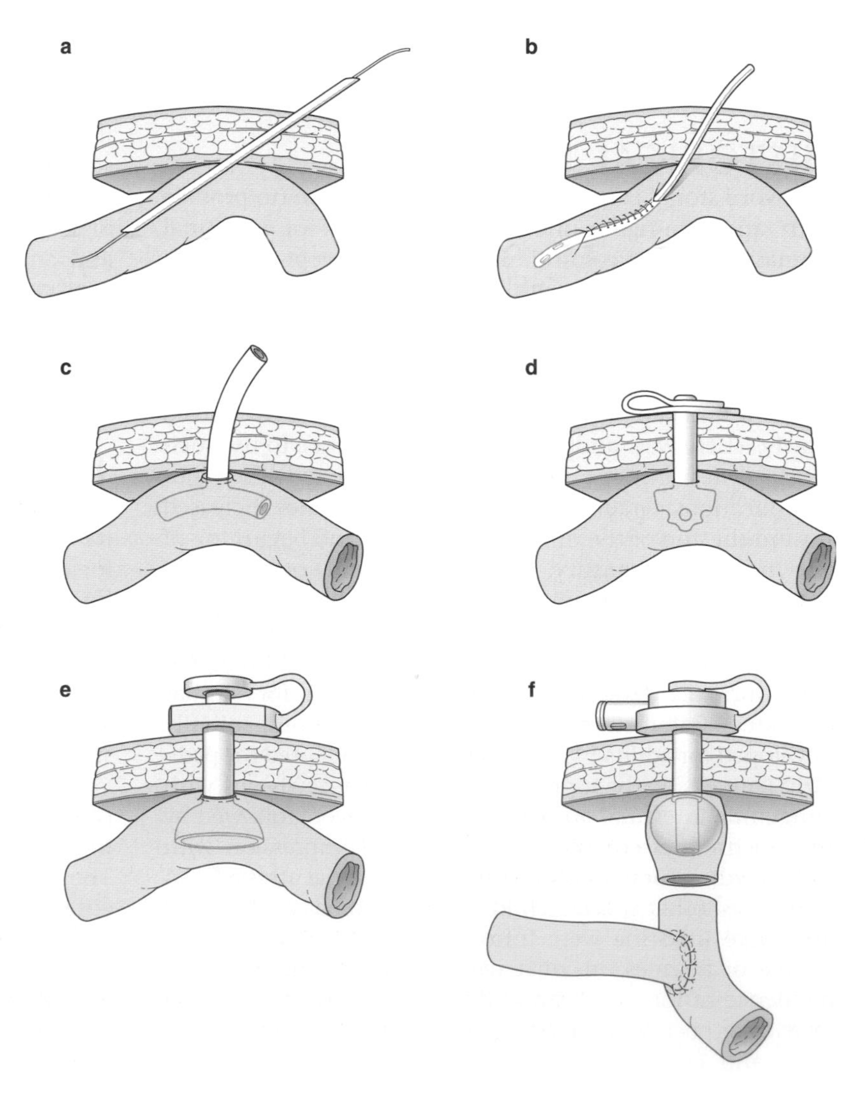

Figure 53.1: Diagram of select feeding jejunostomies. (**a**) Needle catheter.[11] (**b**) Tunneled catheter.[16] (**c**) T tube.[13] (**d**) Button.[14] (**e**) Direct percutaneous endoscopic jejunostomy converted to a skin-level device.[52] (**f**) Roux-en-Y feeding jejunostomy with a balloon-type skin-level device.[20] (Adapted from Gauderer, 1998.)[63]

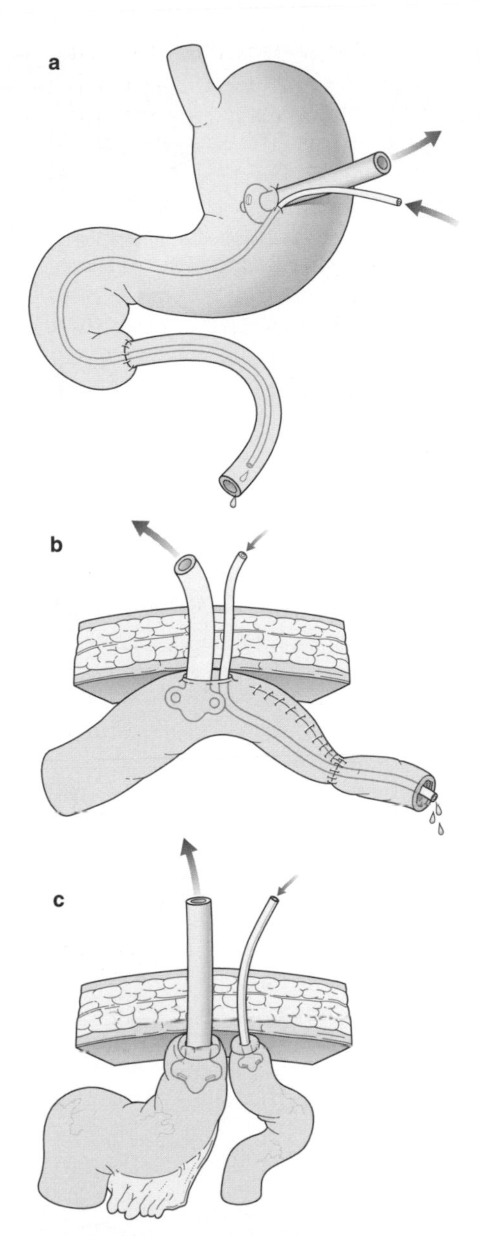

Figure 53.2: Diagram of selected feeding–decompressing jejunostomies. (**a**) Classic gastrostomy–jejunostomy arrangement for children with duodenal atresia.[9] (**b**) Similar arrangement for high jejunal atresia.[8] (**c**) Temporary decompression–feeding using catheters when primary anastomosis is unsafe and intestinal exteriorization is undesirable.[10] (Adapted from Gauderer, 1998.)[63]

combination.[43] An early classic example of this arrangement is the use of a gastrostomy along with a transpyloric, transanastomotic feeding tube in newborns with duodenal atresia.[9] A variant of this setup, but *entering the bowel wall*, can be employed in children with jejunal atresia and very dilated proximal bowel. The decompressing catheter is placed in the dilated, commonly tapered (and often hypoperistaltic), segment and a second, smaller tube advanced either transanastomotically or directly into the narrower distal bowel.[8] A third option is the placement of a large decompressing tube in the proximal bowel and a smaller feeding tube into the distal bowel's proximal end when a primary anastomosis is unsafe and intestinal exteriorization is undesirable or impossible following an intra-abdominal catastrophe leading to bowel resection.[10]

3 Access for antegrade irrigation

The appendix or other specially modified colonic conduit can be brought *through the abdominal wall* for intermittent catheterization.[19] Long-term access can also be established by means of a device such as a catheter, a T tube or a skin-level button-type device implanted in a *non-exteriorized segment* of colon.[13,14,17,22]

4 Decompression, diversion or evacuation (Fig. 53.3)

This is the largest group and comprises the most commonly employed types of stoma.[1,2] The bowel can be exteriorized as an *end-stoma* with a single opening,[3] a *double-barrel* opening[6] or a *loop-stoma*.[7] Variations include end-to-side anastomosis with a distal vent for irrigation, or the reverse type, side-to-end with a proximal vent.[5] Additional types include open or closed loops accessed with large catheters or occluding valve-type devices allowing controlled egress of liquid or semi-liquid stools.[3,30] Further variants comprise special stomas, such as a catheterizable pouch.[44]

The *exit* of an enterostomy through the abdominal wall can be handled in several ways (Figs 53.4 & 53.12).

Proximal stoma

The bowel segment may be brought out *through the laparotomy incision, through a separate incision, with proximal and distal limbs close to each other* or with *both openings* apart. The patient may require multiple stomas and, at times, variations of the above.

Distal stoma

The intestine may be exteriorized as a *mucus fistula adjacent to*, or *separate from*, the proximal stoma. It may also be *closed and replaced into the abdominal cavity*. As a variant to this approach, a catheter may be placed into the closed distal segment for subsequent access for irrigation or contrast studies.

INDICATIONS FOR ENTEROSTOMIES IN CHILDREN

Stomas of the small and large intestine, whether temporary or permanent, are employed in the management of a wide variety of surgical and non-surgical conditions in neonates, infants and children. Their primary uses are described below.

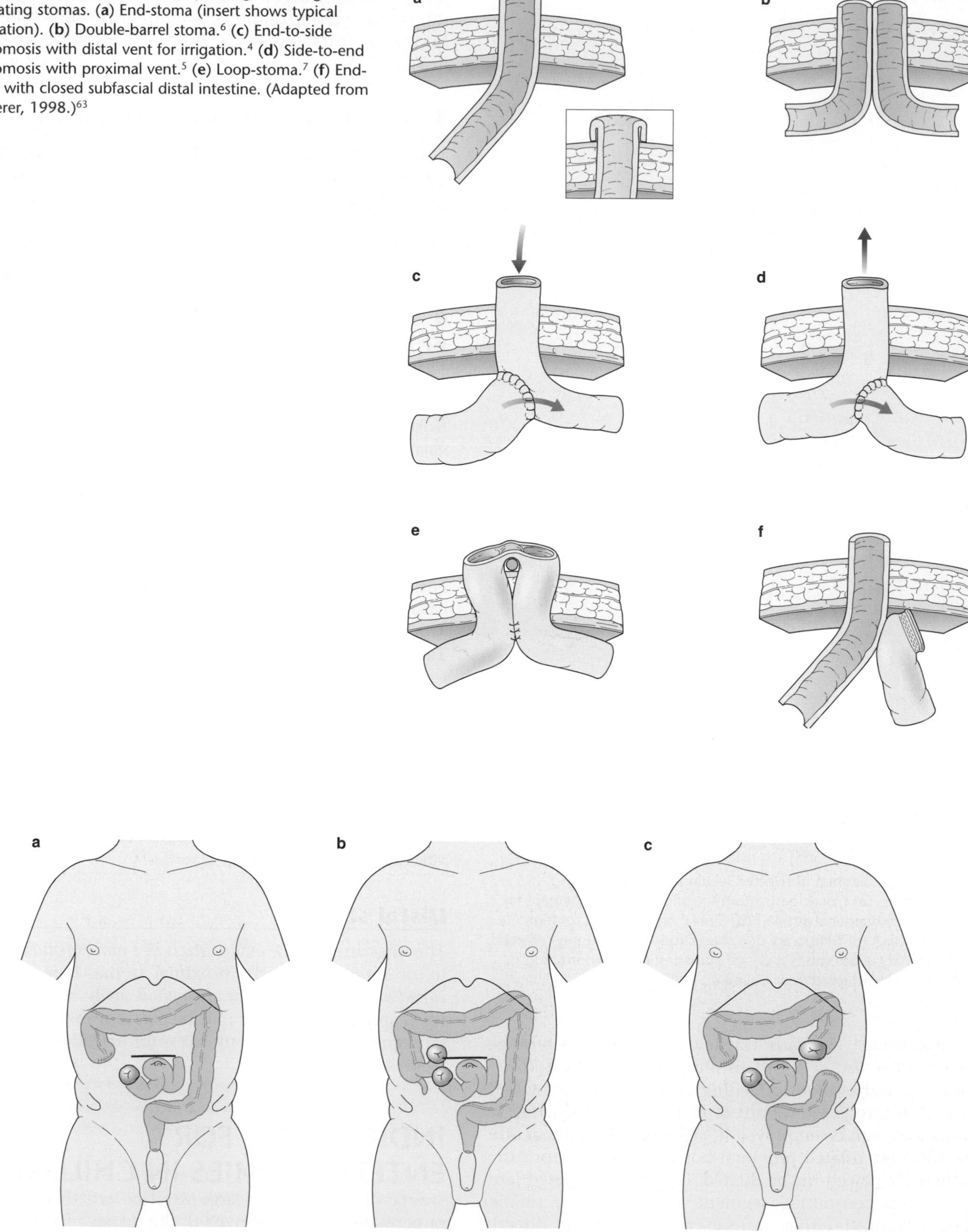

Figure 53.3: Examples of decompressing, diverting and evacuating stomas. (**a**) End-stoma (insert shows typical maturation). (**b**) Double-barrel stoma.[6] (**c**) End-to-side anastomosis with distal vent for irrigation.[4] (**d**) Side-to-end anastomosis with proximal vent.[5] (**e**) Loop-stoma.[7] (**f**) End-stoma with closed subfascial distal intestine. (Adapted from Gauderer, 1998.)[63]

Figure 53.4: Example of options for the management of infants after intestinal resection. (**a**) Exteriorization of proximal intestine through a counter-incision and closure of distal intestine beneath the abdominal wall. (This is our preferred arrangement.) (**b**) Same procedure as in (**a**), with exteriorization of proximal end of distal intestine through the wound edge. (**c**) Arrangement after resection of two intestinal segments. (Adapted from Gauderer, 1998.)[63]

Jejunostomies

Direct access to the proximal small bowel is primarily an alternative to a gastrostomy, the preferred route for long-term enteral alimentation.[43] The majority of patients requiring a feeding jejunostomy are neurologically impaired children, usually with complex medical problems associated with foregut dysmotility. At times, both a gastrostomy and a jejunostomy are required (Fig. 53.5). Additionally, jejunostomies can be useful in the care of patients with acute surgical problems benefiting from early enteral nutrition, such as major trauma or burns, and in children needing long-term supplemental feedings (e.g. cystic fibrosis). Various types of exteriorized jejunal segments were once employed in the management of children with biliary atresia, primarily in an attempt to reduce ascending cholangitis. However, this approach is no longer used, in part because of secondary problems such as bleeding from stomal varices associated with portal hypertension,[45] and because the stomas can add possible problems at the time of a future liver transplantation. On the other hand, the use of a segment of intestine interposed between the gallbladder and the abdominal wall for partial drainage of bile has been helpful in the management of children with certain cholestatic syndromes (Fig. 53.6).[18,46] Stomas are also employed in the monitoring of the intestinal graft in patients with small bowel transplantation. As with other segments of the intestine, exteriorization or tube decompression is clearly indicated after jejunal resection when peritonitis or severe ischemia is present.

Ileostomies

These more distal small bowel stomas are widely used when primary anastomosis is impossible or unsafe.

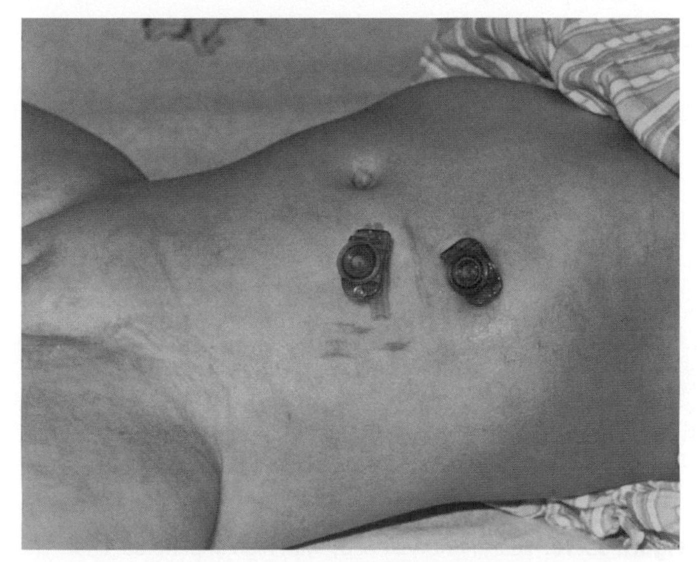

Figure 53.5: Neurologically impaired child with both a gastrostomy and feeding jejunostomy. The jejunostomy was placed using a small laparotomy. The gastrostomy was placed previously using the percutaneous endoscopic technique.[43] The small cross-bar under the jejunostomy was placed for temporary immobilization and removed. Both skin-level devices are of the changeable external-valve type.[52]

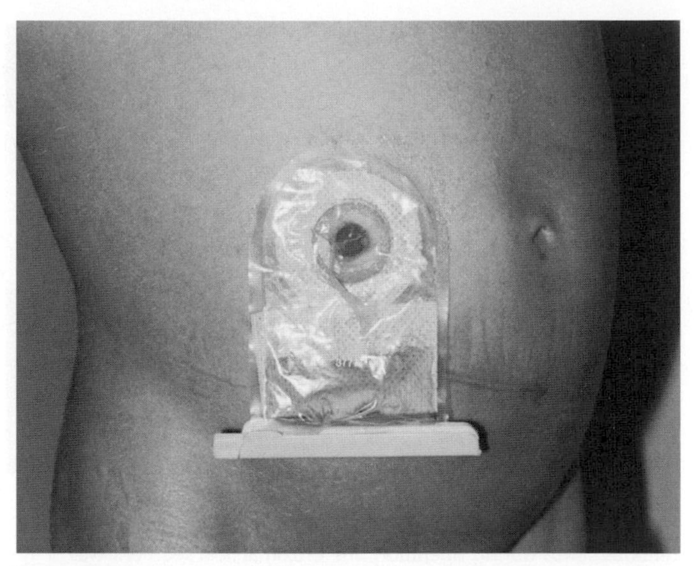

Figure 53.6: An 11-year-old child with Alagille syndrome, 2 months after cholecystoappendicostomy.[18] Note the bile-filled one-piece infant-type pouch.

Typical indications include neonatal necrotizing enterocolitis[32,47] or other adverse intra-abdominal events (Fig. 53.7). Ileostomies are essential in the management of neonates with certain types of distal intestinal obstruction, such as long-segment Hirschsprung's disease, complex meconium ileus, and gastroschisis with atresia (Fig. 53.8). Ileostomies are employed extensively in the management of ulcerative colitis and familial polyposis as temporary, protective or, at times, permanent stomas[3,24,48] (see Figs 53.13, 53.14 & 53.16). Less common indications include other forms of inflammatory bowel disease and rare manifestations of colonic dysmotility.[24]

Appendicostomies, tube cecostomies and tube sigmoidostomies

The main indication for these interventions is to provide access sites for antegrade intestinal irrigation in children with complex anal sphincter and hindgut problems (Fig. 53.9), as well as those with myelodysplasia.[1,17,19,22]

Colostomies

Stomas of the large bowel have the longest history, and extensive experience with these enterostomies has accrued.[1,2,24] Although modern pediatric surgical practice has led to a decrease in the use of preliminary colostomies in selected children with conditions such as Hirschsprung's disease,[31] diversion of the fecal stream is essential in the management of several congenital and acquired pathologies such as high forms of imperforate anus[32,49] (Fig. 53.10), complex pelvic malformations and colonic atresia. Additionally, colostomies have a place in the care of patients with colonic, anorectal and anoperineal trauma[50] (Fig. 53.11), and malignant conditions.[41]

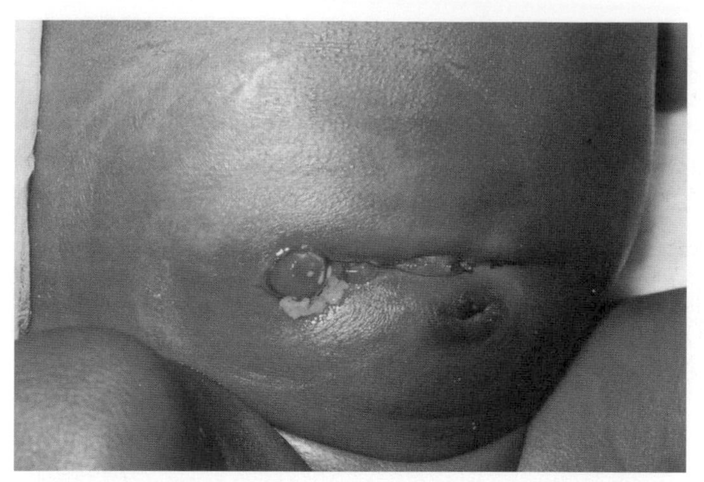

Figure 53.7: Two-month-old premature baby, 6 weeks after bowel resection for severe neonatal necrotizing enterocolitis. Because of the tenuous status during operation, the proximal ileal segment was brought out through the lateral portion of the incision rather than through a counter-incision, which is our preferred approach (see Fig. 53.4a). Notice the slight retraction of the stoma, the undesirable crease formed by the incision following weight gain (rendering pouch application more difficult) and the presence of granulation tissue around absorbable sutures at the fascial level. To control leakage, a paste was placed in the 'groove' adjacent to the stoma to allow for proper fit of the pouch.

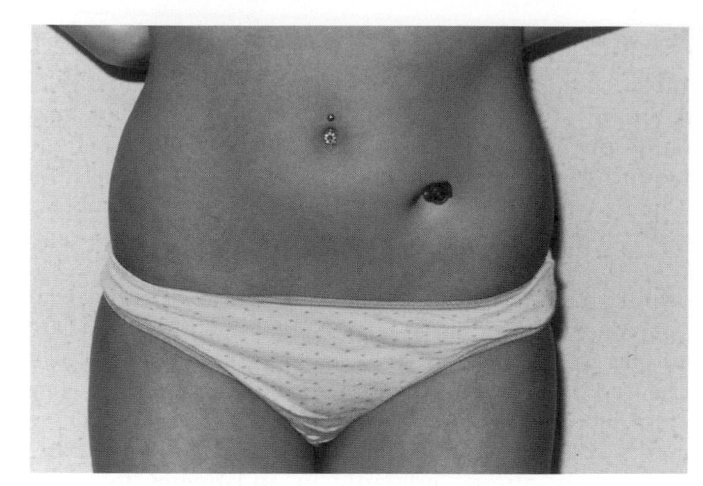

Figure 53.9: A 16-year-old girl 7 years after placement of a sigmoid irrigation tube.[22] She had been unable to evacuate without enemas since early infancy. Rectal biopsies were normal. Colonic transit of radio-opaque markers and anal manometry confirmed the diagnosis of pelvic floor dysfunction with complications of acquired megarectum and increased rectal sensitivity threshold. The patient had failed to respond to laxative, prokinetic and biofeedback therapy. She irrigates herself every 2–3 days with 600–900 ml of tap water and has no stooling-related difficulties. The skin-level device[52] was changed twice.

Urostomies

Exteriorized segments of ileum or colon have been utilized as conduits in the management of urinary tract pathologies, although these external diversions are seldom employed today. However, the mobilized appendix, interposed between the bladder and the abdomen, is still used in children with various urinary dysfunctions to provide a catheterizable conduit to the urinary bladder.[12,51]

CHOICE OF ENTEROSTOMY

Feeding jejunostomy

Of the various options available to provide long-term jejunal access in children, we prefer the 'open' placement through a small, left upper quadrant incision[14] (see Fig. 53.5). This approach permits unequivocal identification of the stoma site in the proximal jejunum with minimal manipulation, as well as a secure attachment of the

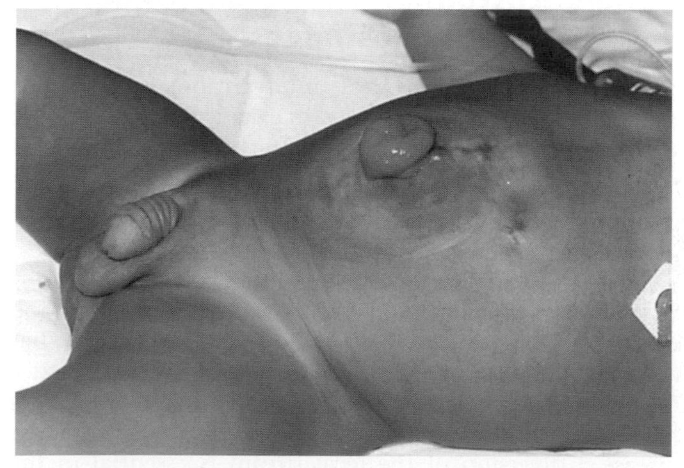

Figure 53.8: Two-month-old baby with gastroschisis and bowel atresia, prior to stoma closure with re-establishment of bowel continuity. Because of the large size of the exposed bowel, a silo pouch was needed for its reduction. At the time of the abdominal wall closure, at 1 week of age, the end of the distended atretic bowel was brought out through the incision, at the umbilical level. Because short gut syndrome was suspected, a gastrostomy (since removed) was added.

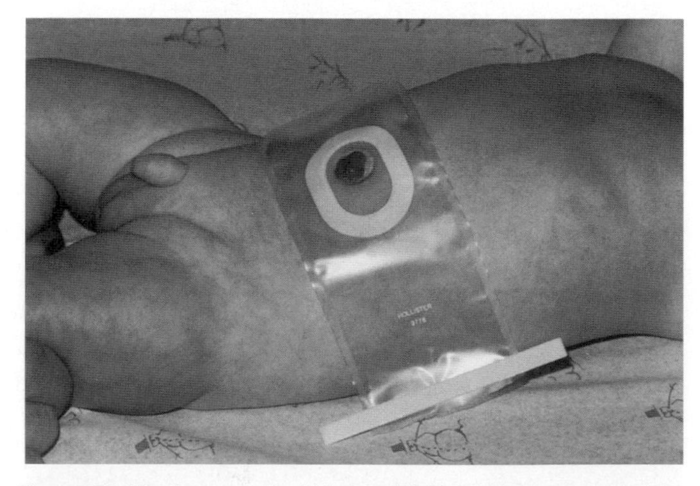

Figure 53.10: Four-month-old baby with high imperforate anus. The high sigmoid loop colostomy is in a position that allows for maximum mobility of the child without the separation of the one-piece pouch. The stoma was taken down after posterior sagittal anorectoplasty.

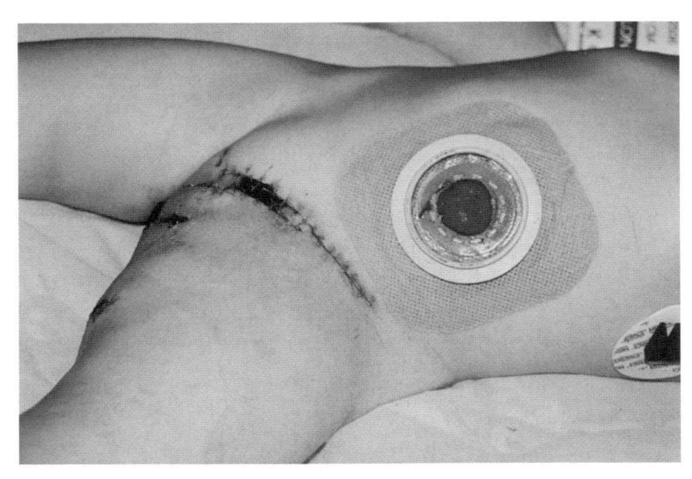

Figure 53.11: Three-year-old child who sustained severe anorectoperineal and limb injuries after falling from a riding lawn mower. A temporary diverting sigmoid loop colostomy was placed at the time of the initial repair. A two-piece pouching system was selected. The skin barrier with its flange is in a good anatomic position.

bowel to the abdominal wall with sutures. The laparoscopic approach is a good alternative.[21] Direct percutaneous jejunostomies are difficult in small children because of limitations imposed by the endoscopic equipment. The technique is, however, applicable to older patients.[21] Because conventional tunneled straight catheters can be difficult to immobilize or replace, our preference is for a T tube for infants and small children (because these do not obstruct the narrow lumen) (see Fig. 53.5), and a button[14] or a non-balloon skin-level device[52] for older pediatric patients. These devices are replaceable as an office procedure. An alternative for long-term jejunal access, purported to have fewer problems with peristomal leakage, is the more complex approach constructing a Roux-en-Y.[20]

Ileostomy

The child's underlying condition, age and the estimated length of use of the stoma help determine the choice of ileostomy. In neonatal necrotizing enterocolitis or other major intra-abdominal events requiring intestinal resection, we prefer to bring a single end-stoma out through a counter incision (see Fig. 53.4a). A more expedient alternative is to bring the proximal intestine through the end of the incision (see Figs 53.4b,c & 53.7). However, with this approach, wound complications tend to be more common and, if the stoma must remain for a prolonged period of time and the child gains weight, the fold created by the laparotomy incision may interfere with fitting of the stoma appliance (see Fig. 53.7). With a healthy distal intestine and anticipated downstream patency, we close the distal limb and place it intra-abdominally adjacent to the proximal stoma. Otherwise, exteriorization as a mucous fistula is prudent. The use of a loop-stoma rather than an end-stoma is an alternative in which the intact mesentery provides maximal perfusion.[53] A double-barrel stoma is another option.[6,47] To save as much intestine as possible, the placement of multiple stomas may be necessary (see Fig. 53.4c).

In children with ulcerative colitis or familial polyposis, the enterostomal principles are similar to those established for adult patients. Choices for a temporary protective diverting ileostomy include a simple loop, an end-loop and an end-stoma, with the closed end under the fascia[48] (see Figs 53.14 & 53.16).

Appendicostomy, tube cecostomy or tube sigmoidostomy

The choice of antegrade enema depends on the type of colonic pathology being managed. With normal peristalsis, either the right[17,19] or the left[22] colon may be chosen for the access. However, if dysmotility is a concern, access to the right colon is indicated. If the appendix is present, it is exteriorized with or without interposition of a valve by either an 'open' or a laparoscopic approach. If the appendix is not available, the wall of the cecum may be fashioned into a conduit that is then brought to the skin level. Either the appendix or the conduit so constructed is then catheterized to instill the enema fluid. A simpler technique, when there is no appendix, is the placement of a skin-level device.[17] For patients with normal colonic motility, our preference is for access to the left colon by means of a sigmoid irrigation tube[22] (see Fig. 53.9).

Colostomy

Most colostomies fall into three categories: right transverse, left transverse and sigmoid.[1,2,7,24] The significant physiologic and anatomic differences between these three segments must be taken into consideration when choosing the site for the stoma.

For infants with high imperforate anus, the high sigmoid is the preferred site for exteriorization.[49] The main advantages are firmer stools with less tendency for skin excoriation, less tendency for prolapse, less surface for urine absorption in male children with rectovesical fistula, and the possibility of evacuation of distal sigmoid meconium during the initial procedure. Additionally the surgeon is better able to identify the correct site, using the pelvic peritoneal reflection as a guide. A further advantage is that there are no scars in the epigastrium. However, if the low- or mid-sigmoid is exteriorized, there may be interference with the blood supply as well as insufficient bowel length for the future pull-through.[49] If the transverse colon is exteriorized, there is always adequate bowel length for a pull-through; the intestine is easy to mobilize and has a smaller diameter and no meconium. However, the disadvantages of the transverse colon colostomy are far greater: the stools are looser and skin maceration and dehydration more common, there is a higher prolapse rate, and a greater absorptive surface for urine in the distal limb.[34] Additionally adequate evacuation of meconium is nearly impossible. Our preference is for a high sigmoid loop colostomy (see Fig. 53.10). However, many surgeons

procedure is usually possible by incising all layers around the strictured stoma and bringing out healthy, at times dilated, bowel. The opening should not be excessive, though, because this might lead to prolapse. If the problem is more complex or a parastomal hernia is present, the pathology is best addressed through a separate incision. Retraction of an end-stoma may lead to skin-level stricture and obstruction. It also results in poor fitting of the appliance. Retraction of a loop-stoma interferes with proper evacuation and leads to filling of the distal intestinal loop with stool.

Stoma takedown and bowel reanastomosis is also associated with a high rate of complications, most notably wound infection, dehiscence, fistula formation and intestinal obstruction.[42,47,57,59] Among the various factors contributing to this morbidity are poor timing, inadequate bowel preparation, technical errors and shortcuts. As expected, malnourished, debilitated, anemic patients and those on steroids are at greatest risk for complications. These contributing factors should be corrected before re-establishment of intestinal continuity is planned.

Placement and takedown of any stoma should be planned carefully and considered a major procedure. Likewise, monitoring of the stoma and early recognition and correction of problems is essential. Pediatric stomas are quite different from adult stomas, and the importance of meticulous attention to detail cannot be overemphasized.

References

1. Cataldo PA. History of stomas. In: MacKeigan JM, Cataldo PA, eds. Intestinal Stomas: Principles, Techniques, and Management. St. Louis. MO: Quality Medical Publishers; 1993:3–37.
2. Schärli WF. The history of colostomy in childhood. Prog Pediatr Surg 1986; 20:188–198.
3. Brooke BN. Historical perspectives. In: Dozois RR, ed. Alternatives to Conventional Ileostomy. Chicago, IL: Year Book Medical; 1985:19–28.
4. Bishop HC, Koop CE. Management of meconium ileus: resection, Roux-en-Y anastomosis and ileostomy irrigation with pancreatic enzymes. Ann Surg 1957; 145:410–414.
5. Santulli TV, Blanc WA. Congenital atresia of the intestine, pathogenesis and treatment. Ann Surg 1961; 154:939–948.
6. Randolph JG, Zolinger RM Jr, Gross RE. Mikulicz resection in infants and children: a 20 year survey of 196 patients. Ann Surg 1963; 158:481–485.
7. Nixon HH. Colostomy: a simple technique, and observations on indications. Z Kinderchir 1966; 3:98–103.
8. Rehbein F, Halsband M. A double-tube technique for the treatment of meconium ileus and small bowel atresia. J Pediatr Surg 1968; 3:723–726.
9. Coln D, Cywes S. Simultaneous drainage gastrostomy and feeding jejunostomy in the newborn. Surg Gynecol Obstet 1977; 145:594–595.
10. Gauderer MWL. Double-tube enterostomy for temporary small bowel decompression. Pediatr Surg Int 1986; 1:60–62.
11. Andrassy RJ, Page CP, Feldtman RW, et al. Continual catheter administration of an elemental diet in infants and children. Surgery 1977; 82:205–210.
12. Mitrofanoff P. Cystostomie continente trans-appendiculaire dans le traitement des vessies neurologiques. Chir Pediatr 1980; 21:297–305.
13. Harberg FJ, Senekjian EK, Pokorny WJ. Treatment of uncomplicated meconium ileus via T-tube ileostomy. J Pediatr Surg 1981; 16:61–63.
14. Stellato TA, Gauderer MWL. Jejunostomy button as a new method for long-term jejunostomy feedings. Surg Gynecol Obstet 1989; 168:552–554.
15. Fitzgerald PG, Lau GY, Cameron GJ. Use of the umbilical site for temporary ostomy: review of 47 cases. J Pediatr Surg 1989; 24:973.
16. Schimpl G, Mayr J, Gauderer MWL. Jejunostomy with replaceable feeding tube: a new technique. J Am Coll Surg 1997; 184:652–654.
17. Shandling B, Chait PG, Richards HF. Percutaneous cecostomy: a new technique in the management of fecal incontinence. J Pediatr Surg 1996; 31:534–537.
18. Gauderer MWL, Boyle JT. Cholecystoappendicostomy in a child with Alagille syndrome. J Pediatr Surg 1997; 32:166–167.
19. Driver CP, Barrow C, Fishwick J, et al. The Malone antegrade colonic enema procedure: outcome and lessons of six years' experience. Pediatr Surg Int 1998; 13:370–372.
20. DeCou JM, Shorter NA, Karl SR. Feeding Roux-en-Y jejunostomy in the management of severely neurologically impaired children. J Pediatr Surg 1993; 28:1276–1279.
21. Nagle AP, Murayama KM. Laparoscopic gastrostomy and jejunostomy. J Long Term Eff Med Implants 2004; 14:1–11.
22. Gauderer MWL, DeCou JM, Boyle JT. Sigmoid irrigation tube for the management of chronic evacuation disorders. J Pediatr Surg 2002; 37:348–351.
23. Koga H, Yamataka A, Yoshida R, et al. Laparoscopic-assisted repair for prolapsed colostomy in an infant. Pediatr Endosurg Innov Tech 2004; 8:275–278.
24. Winkler R. Stoma Therapy: An Atlas and Guide for Intestinal Stomas. New York: Thieme; 1986.
25. Turnbull RW, Turnbull GB. The history and current status of paramedical support for the ostomy patient. J ET Nurs 1993; 20:102–104.
26. Borkowski S. Pediatric stomas, tubes and appliances. Pediatr Clin North Am 1998; 101:642–648.
27 Davies A. Children with ostomies: parents helping parents. J ET Nurs 1992; 19:207–212.
28. Mullen BD, McGinn KA. The Ostomy Book: Living Comfortably with Colostomies, Ileostomies and Urostomies. Palo Alto: Bull Publishing; 1992.
29. Branagan G, Tromans A, Finnis D. Effect of stoma formation on bowel care and quality of life in patients with spinal cord injury. Spinal Cord 2003; 41:680–683.
30. Hill GL. Physiology of conventional ileostomy. In: Dozois RR, ed: Alternatives to Conventional Ileostomy. Chicago, ,IL: Year Book Medical; 1985:129–139.
31. Teitelbaum DH, Cilley RE, Sherman NJ, et al. A decade of experience with the primary pull-through for Hirschsprung's disease in the newborn period: a multicenter analysis of outcomes. Ann Surg 2000; 232:372–380.
32. Millar AJ, Lakhoo K, Rode M, et al. Bowel stomas in infants and children: a five-year audit of 203 patients. S Afr J Surg 1993; 31:110–113.
33. Phillips RM. Coping with an ostomy. Wayne, NJ: Avery Publishing; 1986.
34. Caldamone AA, Emmens RW, Rabinowitz R. Hyperchloremic acidosis and imperforate anus. J Urol 1979; 122:817–818.

35. Mollitt DL, Malangoni MA, Ballantine TV, et al. Colostomy complications in children: an analysis of 146 cases. Arch Surg 1980; 115:455–458.

36. Festen C, Severijnen RS, vd Staak FH. Early closure of enterostomy after exteriorization of the small intestine for abdominal catastrophies. J Pediatr Surg 1987; 22:144–145.

37. Bower TR, Pringle KC, Soper RT. Sodium deficit causing decreased weight gain and metabolic acidosis in infants with ileostomy. J Pediatr Surg 1988; 23:567–572.

38. Al-Salem AH, Grant C, Khawaja S. Colostomy complications in infants and children. Int Surg 1992; 77:164–166.

39. Nour S, Beck J, Stringer MD. Colostomy complications in infants and children. Ann R Coll Surg Engl 1996; 78:526–530.

40. Smith D, Soucy P. Complications of long-term jejunostomy in children. J Pediatr Surg 1996; 31:787–790.

41. Rokhsar S, Harrison EA, Shaul DB, et al. Intestinal stoma complications in immunocompromised children.. J Pediatr Surg 1999; 34:1757–1761.

42. Chandramouli B, Srinivasan K, Jagdish S, et al. Morbidity and mortality of colostomy and its closure in children. J Pediatr Surg 2004; 39:596–599.

43. Gauderer MWL, Stellato TA. Gastrostomies: evolution, techniques, indications and complications. Curr Probl Surg 1986; 23:657–719.

44. Ein SH. A ten-year experience with the pediatric Kock pouch. J Pediatr Surg 1987; 22:764–766.

45. Smith S, Wiener ES, Starzl TE, et al. Stoma-related variceal bleeding: an under-recognized complication of biliary atresia. J Pediatr Surg 1988; 23:243–245.

46. Emond JC, Whitington PF. Selective surgical management of progressive familial intrahepatic cholestasis (Byler's disease). J Pediatr Surg 1995; 30:1635–1641.

47. Musemeche CA, Kosloske AM, Ricketts RR. Enterostomy in necrotizing enterocolitis: an analysis of techniques and timing of closure. J Pediatr Surg 1987; 22:479–483.

48. Fonkalsrud EW, Thakur A, Roof L. Comparison of loop versus end ileostomy for fecal diversion after restorative proctocolectomy for ulcerative colitis. J Am Coll Surg 2000; 190:418–422.

49. Wilkins S, Pena A. The role of colostomy in the management of anorectal malformations. Pediatr Surg Int 1988; 3:105–109.

50. Quarmby CJ, Millar AJ, Rode H. The use of diverting colostomies in paediatric peri-anal burns. Burns 1999; 25:645–650.

51. Stein JP, Daneshmand S, Dunn M, et al. Continent right colon reservoir using a cutaneous appendicostomy. Urology 2004; 63:577–580.

52. Gauderer MWL, Abrams RS, Hammond JH. Initial experience with the changeable skin-level port-valve: a new concept for long-term gastrointestinal access. J Pediatr Surg 1998; 33:73–75.

53. Alaish SM, Krummel TM, Bagwell CE, et al. Loop enterostomy in newborns with necrotizing enterocolitis. J Am Coll Surg 1996; 182:457–458.

54. Morris DM, Rayburn D. Loop colostomies are totally diverting in adults. Am J Surg 1991; 161:668–671.

55. Kirkland S. Ostomy dolls for pediatric patients. J Enterostomal Ther 1985; 12:104–105.

56. Gertler JP, Seashore JH, Touloukian RJ. Early ileostomy closure in necrotizing enterocolitis. J Pediatr Surg 1987; 22:140–143.

57. Kiely EM, Sparnon AL. Stoma closure in infants and children, Pediatr Surg Int 1987; 2:95–97.

58. Haberlik A, Höllwarth ME, Windhager U, et al. Problems of ileostomy in necrotizing enterocolitis. Acta Paediatr Suppl 1994; 396:74–76.

59. Weber TR, Tracy TF Jr, Silen ML, et al. Enterostomy and its closure in newborns. Arch Surg 1995; 130:534–537.

60. Sangkhathat S, Patrapinyokul S, Tadyathikom K. Early enteral feeding after closure of colostomy in pediatric patients. J Pediatr Surg 2003; 38:1516–1519.

61. Krasna IH. A simple pursestring suture technique for treatment of colostomy prolapse and intussusception. J Pediatr Surg 1979; 14:801–802.

62. Gauderer MWL, Izant RJ Jr. A technique for temporary control of colostomy prolapse in children. J Pediatr Surg 1985; 20:653–655.

63. Gauderer MWL. Stomas of the small and large intestine. In: O'Neill JA, Rowe MI, Grosfeld JL, et al., eds. Pediatric Surgery, 5th edn. St Louis, MO: Mosby; 1998:1349–1359.

Chapter 54
Disorders of the anorectum: fissures, fistulae, prolapse, hemorrhoids, tags

Marian D. Pfefferkorn and Joseph F. Fitzgerald

The anal sphincter consists of an inner ring of smooth muscle, the internal anal sphincter, the intersphincteric space and an outer ring of skeletal muscle, the external anal sphincter. The internal sphincter is an involuntary muscle that maintains anal tone. It is in a continuous state of partial contraction and relaxes in response to rectal distension. The external sphincter is a voluntary muscle extending from the puborectalis and levator ani muscles that provides short-term augmentation of anal pressure to postpone defecation. The transitional and columnar epithelium of the rectum is separated from the squamous epithelium of the anus by the dentate line, which is located in the mid-portion of the anal canal (Fig. 54.1). Anal crypts are located at the dentate line, and anal glands are found at the base of these crypts.

ANAL FISSURE

Anal fissure is a split in the skin of the anus. The passage of a hard stool commonly causes anal fissures; however, a history of constipation preceding the onset of an anal fissure is obtained in only one of four cases, and diarrhea is a predisposing factor in 4–7% of patients.[1] Fissures are usually located in the anterior or posterior midline. Other processes, for example infectious or inflammatory, should be entertained when the fissure is positioned laterally.[2] Blood is often seen on the surface of the stool, on the toilet tissue, or even dripping from the anus. There may be severe anal pain associated with the fissure, especially during defecation.

Physical examination of the patient in a lateral decubitus position involves gently parting the buttocks and stretching the anal skin laterally. An acute fissure is a superficial split in the anoderm with sharply demarcated edges. Induration at the edges of the fissure may be seen when the fissure is chronic (Fig. 54.2). A skin tag may be present. Rectal examination using the fifth finger in an infant younger than 3 years, or the index finger in an older child, should then be performed.

Most acute anal fissures heal with conservative therapy. The inciting factor, whether constipation or diarrhea, should be corrected. The presence of fecal material within the fissure inhibits healing; hence, it is ideal to instruct the caregivers to clean the child's anus after every stool. The application of a local anesthetic is unnecessary. Dietary bran supplements and warm Sitz baths have been shown to be superior to topically applied local anesthetic or hydrocortisone cream in the treatment of acute anal fissure, with healing in 87% after 3 weeks.[3]

Chronic fissures are unusual in children who have no underlying predisposing factors, such as inflammatory bowel disease or immunodeficiency (Fig. 54.3). In adults, chronic fissures may not respond to conservative treatment and may require lateral internal sphincterotomy. Local injection of botulinum toxin and topical application of nitrates or calcium channel blockers are therapies under investigation.[4–8]

RECTAL PROLAPSE

Rectal prolapse is the abnormal protrusion of one or more layers of the rectum through the anus. Mucosal or partial prolapse is less serious and less pronounced[9] (Fig. 54.4). A complete rectal prolapse (procidentia), consisting of all

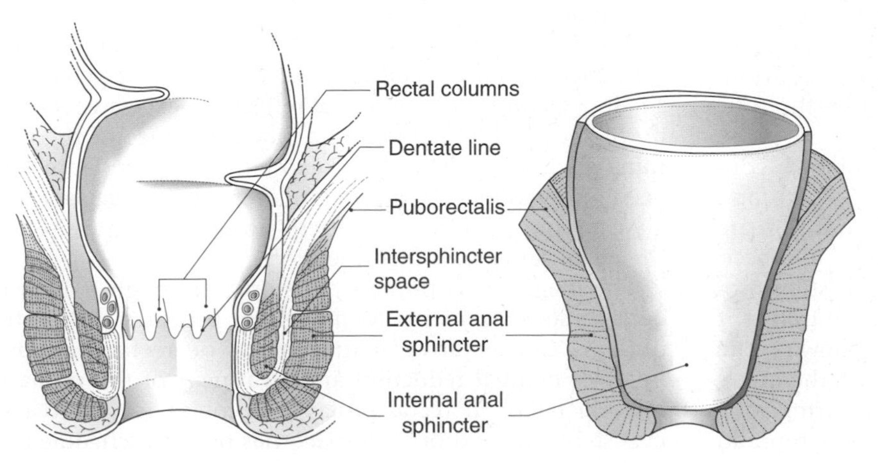

Figure 54.1: Schematic diagram of the perianal region. (Reproduced from Sandborn et al., AGA technical review on perianal Crohn's disease. Gastroenterology 2003; 125:1508–1530, with permission)[27]

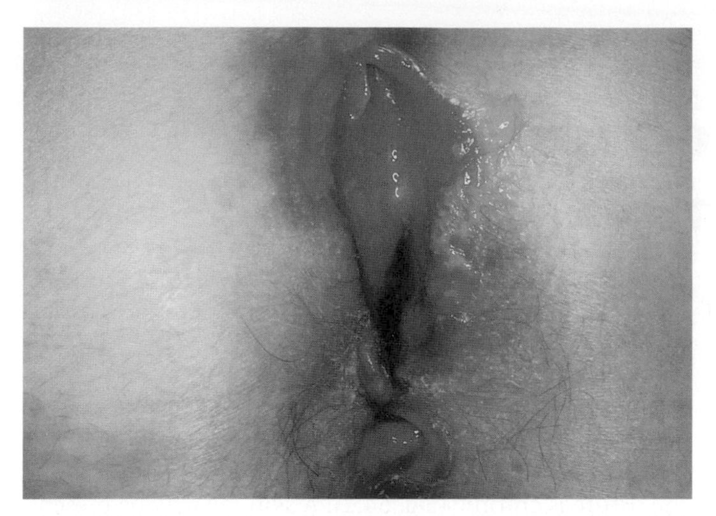

Figure 54.2: Large, indurated, chronic fissure associated with Crohn's disease.

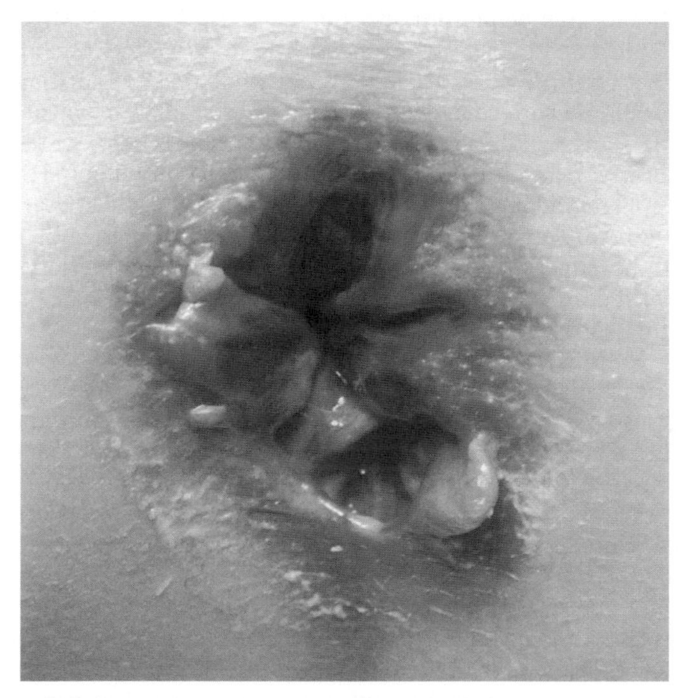

Figure 54.3: Crohn's disease associated anal fissures with undermining of the edges.

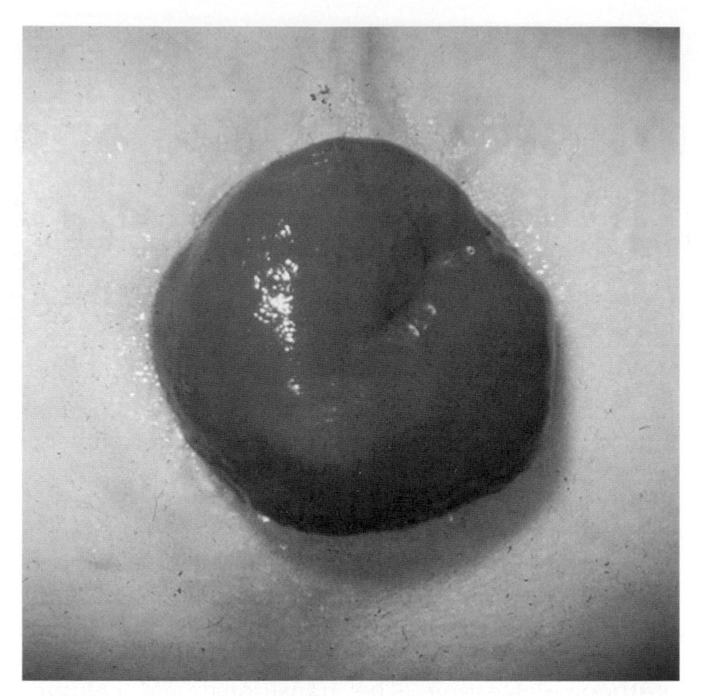

Figure 54.4: Mucosal prolapse. (Photo courtesy of Frederick Rescorla MD.)

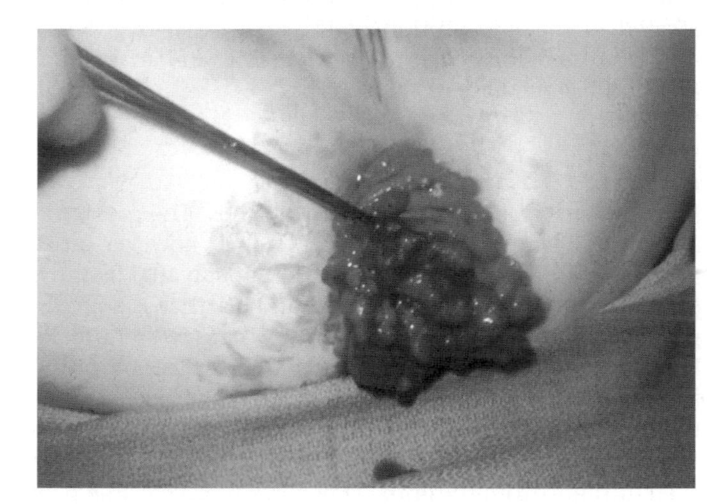

Figure 54.5: Prolapsed rectal juvenile polyps. (Photo courtesy of Frederick Rescorla MD.)

layers of the rectal wall, frequently requires manual reduction.[10] Rectal prolapse is usually detected by the child's parents and is urgently brought to medical attention; however, it has often spontaneously reduced by the time the child is examined by medical personnel.

Prolonged straining during toilet training or with constipation is a frequent cause in children.[11,12] Acute and chronic diarrhea, intestinal parasites and malnutrition are other common etiologies.[12–14] Rectal prolapse has been reported in up to 19% of 605 patients with cystic fibrosis.[15,6] Rectal prolapse in these patients was often transient and usually resolved at 3–5 years of age, or following the institution of pancreatic enzyme replacement therapy.[15] There have been reports of rectal prolapse occurring with juvenile polyps (Fig. 54.5), inflammatory polyps, lymphoid hyperplasia, solitary rectal ulcer, meningocele, pertussis and Ehlers–Danlos syndrome.[17–21] Certain anatomic factors, such as loose rectal mucosa, deficiency of pelvic fat, shallow sacrum, low peritoneal reflection, excessive mobility of the sigmoid colon and a straight course of the rectum, predispose to rectal prolapse.[12] Rectal prolapse has been reported in a 6-year-old girl after she was sucked onto a swimming pool drain.[22] Often, no underlying cause for the rectal prolapse is identified.[12,14]

The diagnosis is primarily historic, although it is prudent to screen patients for intestinal parasites and cystic fibrosis. Conservative management of rectal prolapse involves manual reduction and treatment of the primary inciting factor. If rectal prolapse becomes recurrent and persistent, the authors' approach has been to schedule the

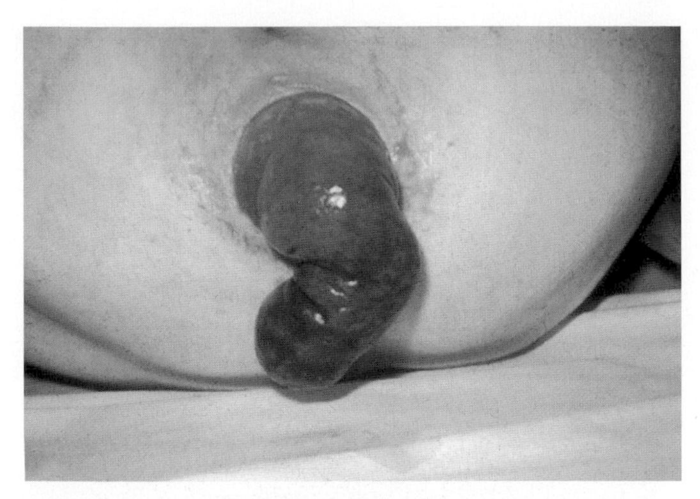

Figure 54.6: Necrotic rectal prolapse. (Photo courtesy of Frederick Rescorla MD.)

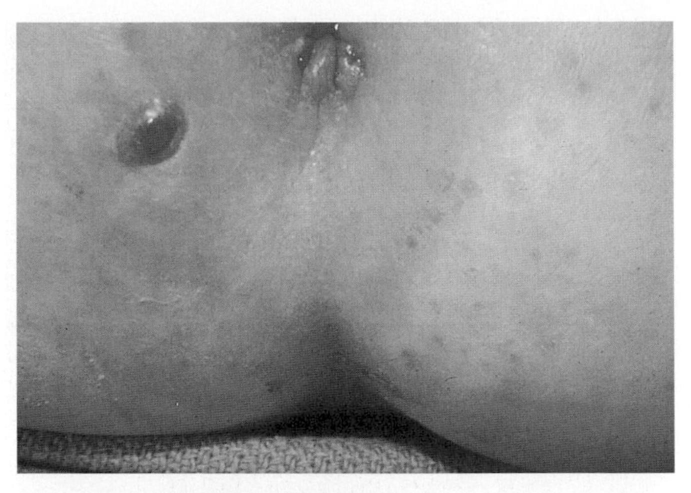

Figure 54.7: Fistula-*in-ano*. (Photo courtesy of Frederick Rescorla MD.)

patient for examination under anesthesia to exclude an anatomic lead point for the prolapse, such as a polyp. If none is found, a surgeon then treats the patient with submucosal injection of a sclerosant, such as 5% phenol in almond oil, 50% dextrose, 25% saline or 1% sodium morrhuate.[11,13,23,24] Resolution of rectal prolapse was reported in 91 of 100 children who were treated with rectal submucosal injection of 5% phenol in oil.[25] Indications for surgical management are rare in children, but may include the development of mucosal ulceration with bleeding, irreducible prolapse, no improvement with conservative treatment and rectal prolapse longer than 3 cm[26] (Fig. 54.6).

FISTULAE

A perianal fistula is a chronic track of granulation tissue connecting two epithelial-lined surfaces, whereas a sinus track is a track of granulation tissue that is open only at one end.[27] In infants and young children who develop a diaper rash, a small perianal pustule or infected anal gland may spread to the intersphincteric space and result in a fistulous abscess.[28] A fistulous abscess becomes a fistula when it ruptures. At least 50% of perianal abscesses recur as fistulae.[28]

Most fistulas-*in-ano* originate below the dentate line[29] (Fig. 54.7). The internal opening in infants is radially opposite the external opening, unlike in adults where it is often in the posterior midline (Goodsall's rule). The earliest sign of a perianal abscess is an indurated tender area, which may occur at any site around the anus. When the abscess ruptures, it discharges pus and/or blood. It may heal temporarily, only to recur with the next episode of inflammation. Once detected, management should include immediate drainage except in patients with known or suspected Crohn's disease in whom management may be more complex, as outlined below.[30] Abscesses do not generally need to be cultured unless they persist or recur within days of drainage. The abscess cavity can be loosely packed to encourage hemostasis, or a catheter may be placed within the abscess cavity. Sitz or tub baths are initiated, along with analgesics, stool softeners and dietary fiber supplementation. Antibiotics may be used as an adjunctive therapy to incision and drainage when there is extensive cellulitis, or in the presence of immunosuppression, valvular heart disease and diabetes.[30]

When a fistula is present, a surgeon inserts a probe into the external opening (Fig. 54.8). The internal opening of the fistula in children is on the pectinate line radially opposite the external orifice. The probe is passed out of the internal opening and the fistula is then unroofed by incising down onto the probe. After surgery the area needs to be kept clean with soap and water until it heals.[28]

The more complex forms of abscess and fistula are rarely encountered in children, but may be a complication of inflammatory bowel disease (IBD), especially Crohn's disease (Figs 54.9a,b). The frequency of perianal fistulae in Crohn's disease in referral populations varies from 17% to 43%.[31] In a review of 141 children and adolescents with Crohn's disease, 13% had significant perianal disease.[32] The American Gastroenterological Association Clinical Practice Committee published a technical review on perianal Crohn's disease in 2003.[27] It recommends physical examination of the perianal area to identify any perianal

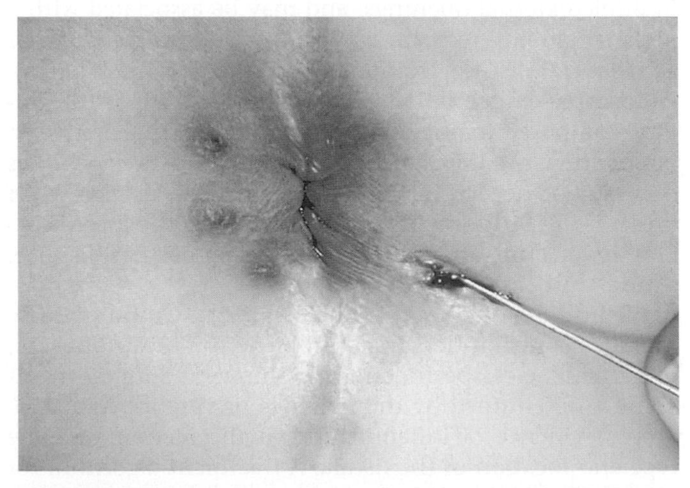

Figure 54.8: Multiple fistulae-*in-ano*. A probe is inserted in the external opening of one fistula. (Photo courtesy of Frederick Rescorla MD.)

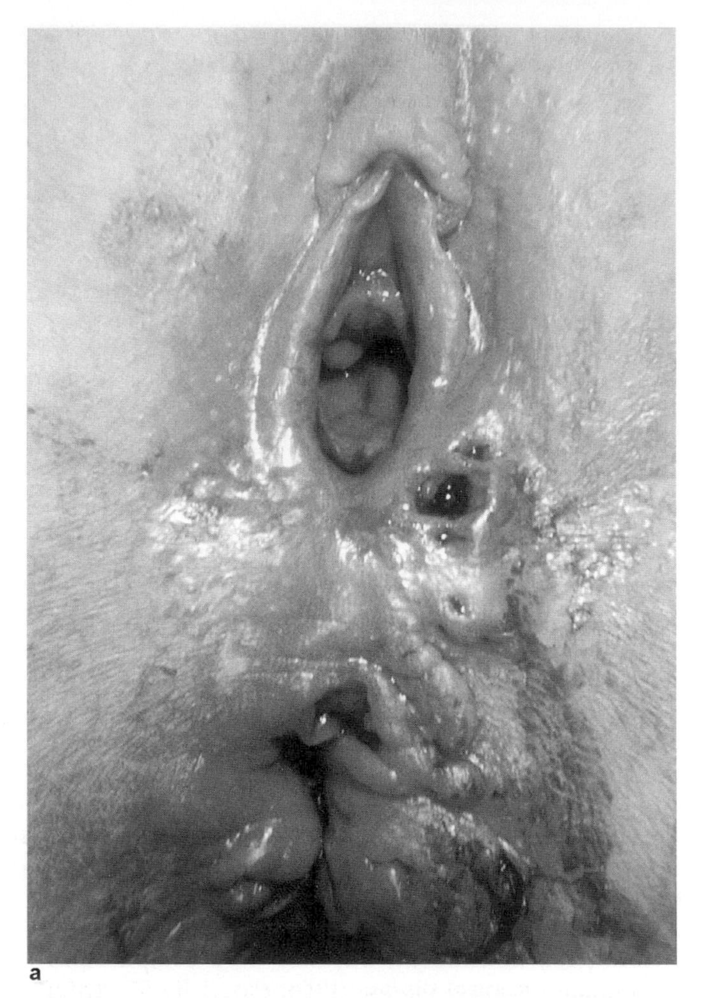

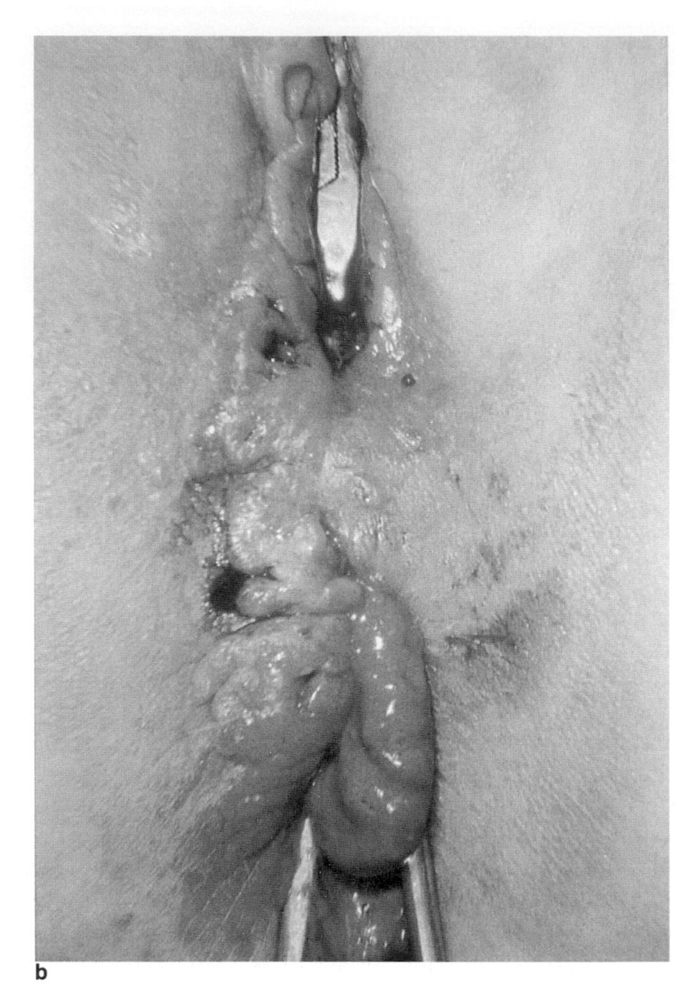

Figure 54.9: (**a**) Perineal fistula associated with Crohn's disease. (**b**) Rectovaginal fistula.

disease, and endoscopic examination to determine any rectal inflammation. Fistulae are then classified as either simple or complex. A simple fistula is low, has a single external opening, has no pain or fluctuation to suggest a perianal abscess and there is no evidence of rectovaginal fistula or anorectal stricture. A complex fistula is high, may have multiple external openings, and may be associated with a perianal abscess, rectovaginal fistula, anorectal stricture or active rectal disease. Examination under anesthesia (EUA), endoscopic endoanal ultrasonography (EUS), fistulography, computed tomography (CT) and pelvic magnetic resonance imaging (MRI) are additional diagnostic modalities that may be needed to classify some fistulae accurately. Of these, EUA, with or without EUS, has been the most accurate in detecting and correctly classifying perianal fistulae, sinuses and abscesses.

Medical treatment of perianal fistulae in Crohn's disease includes antibiotics, azathioprine/6-mercaptopurine, infliximab, ciclosporin and tacrolimus.[27] Surgical treatment is determined by the presence or absence of macroscopic evidence of inflammation in the rectum, and the type and location of the fistula. A treatment algorithm for managing patients with Crohn's perianal fistulae has been proposed (Fig. 54.10).[27]

HEMORRHOIDS

Small asymptomatic hemorrhoids found incidentally on perianal examination are not uncommon in children. Symptomatic hemorrhoids are unusual in the pediatric age group, but may occur with chronic straining associated with constipation, as a result of an anal infection spreading to the hemorrhoidal veins, or with underlying Crohn's disease or portal hypertension. Symptoms include bleeding, prolapse, discomfort/pain, fecal soiling and pruritus (Fig. 54.11).

The anal canal is lined by three fibrovascular cushions of submucosal tissue, suspended by a connective tissue framework.[33] A venous plexus fed by arteriovenous communications is present within each cushion. Loss of connective tissue supporting the cushions leads to their descent. Straining with the passage of hard stools produces an increase in venous pressure and engorgement, and hard stools alone produce a mechanical insult to the cushions. Hemorrhoids are classified as external, internal or mixed. External hemorrhoids originate from the external hemorrhoidal venous plexus below the dentate line; internal hemorrhoids originate from the internal hemorrhoidal venous plexus above the dentate line. Hemorrhoids are

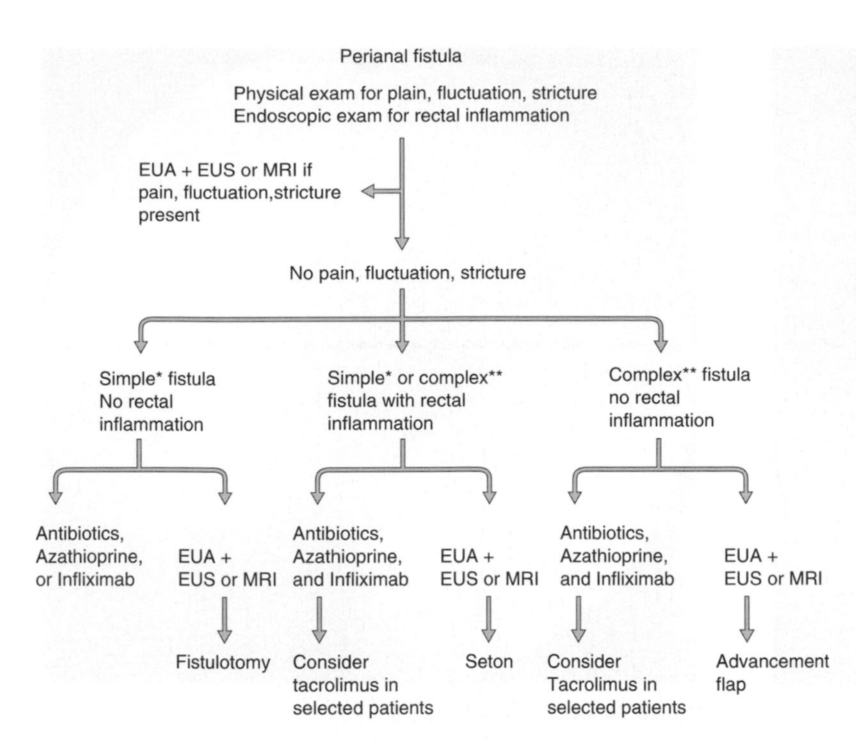

Figure 54.10: Treatment algorithm for patients with Crohn's disease with a perianal fistula. *A simple fistula is low, has a single external opening, and is not associated with perianal abscess, rectovaginal fistula, anorectal stricture or macroscopically evident rectal inflammation. **A complex fistula is high and/or has multiple external openings, perianal abscess, rectovaginal fistula, anorectal stricture or macroscopic evidence of rectal inflammation. EUA, examination under anesthesia; EUS, endoscopic anorectal ultrasonsography; MRI, pelvic magnetic resonance imaging. (Reproduced from Sandborn et al., AGA technical review on perianal Crohn's disease. Gastroentrology 2003; 125:1508–1530, with permission).[27]

also classified according to the degree of prolapse.[34] The prolapsed cushion has an impaired venous return resulting in dilation of the plexus and venous stasis. Inflammation occurs with erosion of the cushion's epithelium, resulting in bleeding. First-degree hemorrhoids protrude into the anal canal but do not prolapse. Second-degree hemorrhoids prolapse on straining and reduce spontaneously. Third-degree hemorrhoids prolapse on straining and require manual reduction. Fourth-degree hemorrhoids are prolapsed and irreducible.

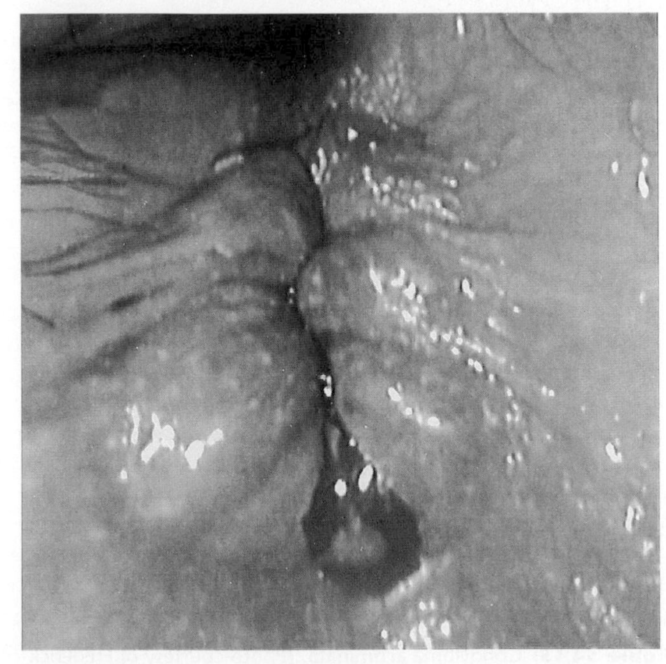

Figure 54.11: Bleeding external hemorrhoids.

Asymptomatic hemorrhoids require no treatment. Conservative management of symptomatic hemorrhoids includes avoidance of straining with defecation, and providing relief of constipation by increasing fluid and fiber intake and/or prescribing a stool softener. Topical ointments or enemas containing local anesthetics and mild astringents or steroids may provide short-term symptomatic relief, but there is no evidence to support their long-term use.[33,34] Prolonged use may cause skin sensitization, and rectal absorption may lead to systemic side-effects. Non-surgical interventional procedures are reserved for recalcitrant hemorrhoids and include rubber band ligation, infrared coagulation, bipolar electrocoagulation, low-voltage direct current, injection sclerotherapy, laser therapy and cryosurgery. Two meta-analyses compared these non-operative methods and found that rubber band ligation and infrared coagulation were the most effective.[35,36] Surgical hemorrhoidectomy is the definitive treatment for symptomatic hemorrhoids.

TAGS AND MISCELLANEOUS CONDITIONS

An anal skin tag is usually asymptomatic and may be a remnant of a healed anal fissure or previously thrombosed external hemorrhoid (Fig. 54.12). Anal tags that cause chronic pruritus or problems with hygiene can be excised when they are not associated with IBD.[2] Excision should be avoided for tags associated with Crohn's disease.

Hypertrophied anodermal papillae can evert during (and after) defecation; this is an annoyance, but rarely requires surgical management (Fig. 54.13).

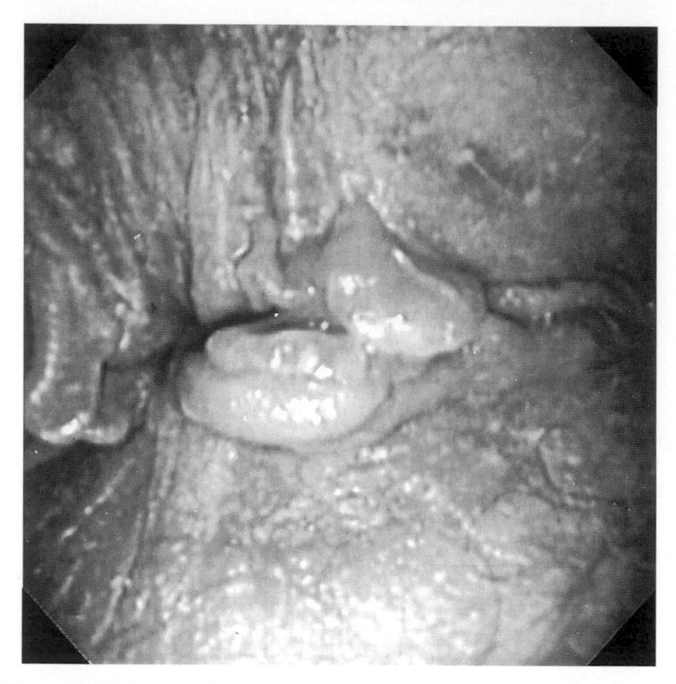

Figure 54.12: Anal skin tags.

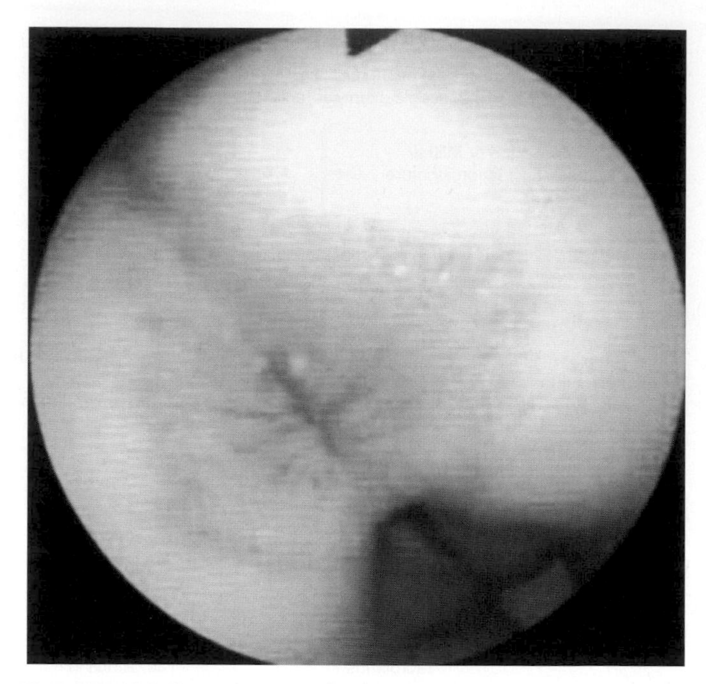

Figure 54.14: β-Streptococcal anusitis.

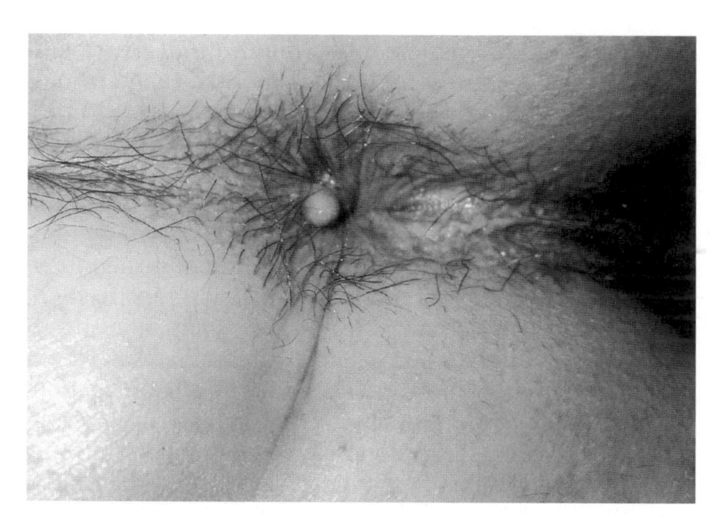

Figure 54.13: Hypertrophied anodermal papilla. (Photo courtesy of Frederick Rescorla MD.)

Perianal cellulitis due to group A β-hemolytic streptococcal infection occurs more frequently in children than in adults.[37] Examination of the perianal area reveals a well demarcated erythematous rash surrounding the anal opening (Fig. 54.14). It is often associated with pain, pruritus and bleeding, without fever and other systemic symptoms. Treatment with an oral antibiotic against streptococcus is effective.[38]

Enterobius vermicularis (pinworm) infestation affects pediatric patients prevalently, and commonly presents with anal pruritus. The most common physical finding of enterobiasis is excoriated perianal skin, which may be complicated by a secondary bacterial infection. Dead parasites or eggs deposited in the perianal area and other ectopic sites may also cause abscesses and granulomas.[39]

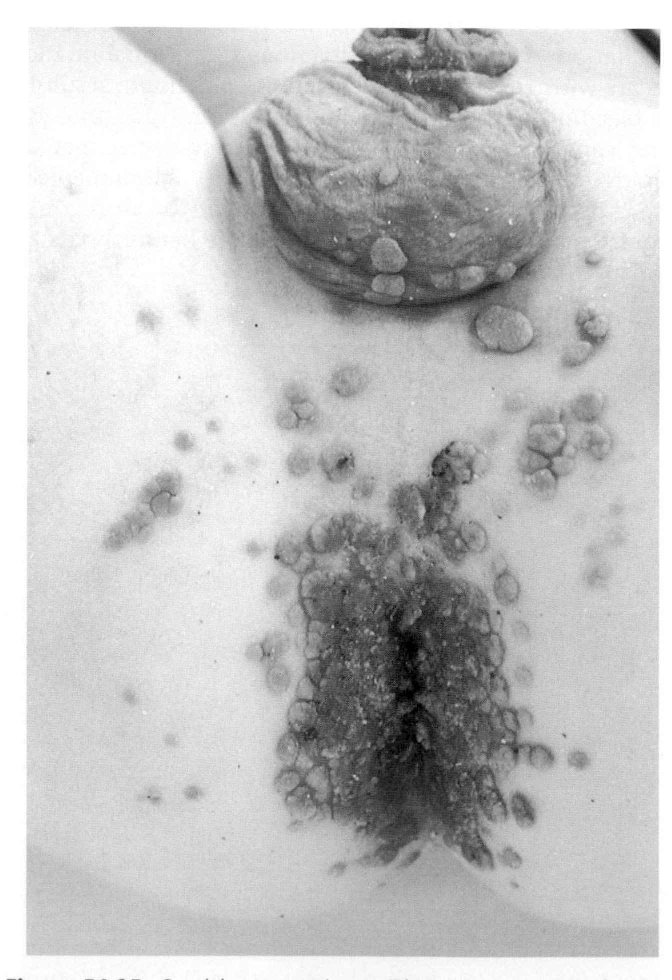

Figure 54.15: Condyloma acuminata. (Photo courtesy of Frederick Rescorla MD.)

A human papillomavirus (HPV) causes anogenital warts called condyloma acuminata (Fig. 54.15). There has been an increase in the number of reported cases of anogenital warts in children since the 1980s.[40] Most HPV infections are subclinical and asymptomatic, and benign skin lesions are the most common manifestations.[41] They can, however, cause other problems including functional impairment, discomfort and psychologic distress; malignant transformation is a concern.[42] Transmission of HPV occurs by direct sexual contact and raises the concern of sexual abuse in children. HPV may also be passed transplacentally to the fetus or during the passage of an infant through an infected birth canal. Non-sexual transmission may result from autoinoculation of HPV lesions on the hands. Fomites have also been implicated.[43] The usual therapeutic options include cryotherapy, podophyllin, curettage and electrocautery.

References

1. Lund JN, Scholefield JH. Aetiology and treatment of anal fissure. Br J Surg 1996; 83:1335–1344.
2. Pfenninger JL, Zainea GG. Common anorectal conditions. Obstet Gynecol 2001; 98:1130–1139.
3. Jensen SL. Treatment of first episodes of acute anal fissure: prospective randomized study of lignocaine ointment versus hydrocortisone ointment or warm sitz baths plus bran. BMJ 1986; 292:1167–1169.
4. Jost WH, Schimrigk K. Therapy of anal fissure using botulinum toxin. Dis Colon Rectum 1994; 45:719–722.
5. Altomare DF, Rinaldi M, Milito G, et al. Glyceryl trinitrate for chronic anal fissure – healing or headache? Results of a multicenter, randomized, placebo-controlled, double-blind trial. Dis Colon Rectum 2000; 43:174–181.
6. Richard CS, Gregoire R, Plewes EA, et al. Internal sphincterotomy is superior to topical nitroglycerine in the treatment of chronic anal fissure: results of a randomized, controlled trial by the Canadian Colorectal Surgical Trials Group. Dis Colon Rectum 2000; 43:1048–1058.
7. Antropoli C, Perrotti P, Rubino M, et al. Nifedipine for local use in conservative treatment of anal fissures: preliminary results of a multicenter study. Dis Colon Rectum 1999; 42:1011–1015.
8. Carapeti EA, Kamm MA, Evans BK, Phillips RK. Topical diltiazem and bethanecol decrease anal sphincter pressure without side effects. Gut 1999; 45:719–722.
9. Qvist N, Rasmussen L, Klaaborg K, Hansen L, Pederson S. Rectal prolapse in infancy: conservative *vs* operative treatment. J Pediatr Surg 1986; 21:887–888.
10. Freeman NV. Rectal prolapse in children. J R Soc Med 1984; 77(Suppl 3):9–12.
11. Severijnen R, Festen C, Van der Staak F, Rieu P. Rectal prolapse in children. Neth J Surg 1989; 41:149–151.
12. Zemspky W, Rosenstein B. The cause of rectal prolapse in children. Am J Dis Child 1988; 142:338–339.
13. Fehri M, Harouchi A, Reffas, el Andaloussi M, Benbachir M, Guessous N. Rectal prolapse in children. Review of 260 cases. Chir Pediatr 1988; 29:313–317.
14. Eriksen C, Hadley G. Rectal prolapse in childhood – the role of infections and infestations. S Afr Med J 1985; 68:790–791.
15. Stern R, Izant RJ Jr, Boat T, Wood R, Matthews L, Doershuk C. Treatment and prognosis of rectal prolapse in cystic fibrosis. Gastroenterology 1982; 82:707–710.
16. Gross K, Desanto A, Grosfeld J, West K, Eigen H. Intra-abdominal complications of cystic fibrosis. J Pediatr Surg 1985; 20:431–435.
17. Colorectal prolapse in a child with severe form of juvenile polyposis. Acta Med Port 1995; 8:369–372.
18. Rittmeyer C, Nakayama D, Ulshen M. Lymphoid hyperplasia causing recurrent rectal prolapse. J Pediatr 1997; 131:487–488.
19. Pena A. Rectal prolapse. In: Behrman R, Kliegman R, Arvin A, Nelson W, eds. Nelson Textbook of Pediatrics. Philadelphia, PA: WB Saunders; 1996:1113.
20. Chetty R, Bhatahl P, Slavin J. Prolapse-induced inflammatory polyps of the colorectum and anal transition zone. Histopathology 1993; 23:63–67.
21. Godbole P, Botterill I, Newell S, Sagar P, Stringer M. Solitary rectal ulcer syndrome in children. J R Coll Surg Edinb 2000; 45:411–414.
22. Davison A, Puntis J. Awareness of swimming pool suction injury among tour operators. Arch Dis Child 2003; 88:584–586.
23. Lukram AS. Management of complete rectal prolapse. J Indian Med Assoc 1989; 87:284–285.
24. Chan W, Kay S, Laberge J, Gallucci J, Bensoussan A, Yazbeck S. Injection of sclerotherapy in the treatment of rectal prolapse in infants and children. J Pediatr Surg 1998; 33:255–258.
25. Wyllie GG. The injection treatment of rectal prolapse. J Pediatr Surg 1979; 14:62–64.
26. Sander S, Vural O, Unal M. Management of rectal prolapse in children: Ekehorn's rectosacropexy. Pediatr Surg Int 1999; 15:111–114.
27. Sandborn W, Fazio V, Feagan B, Hanauer S. AGA technical review on perianal Crohn's disease. Gastroenterology 2003; 125:1508–1530.
28. Shandling B. Perianal lesions. In: Walker WA, Durie PR, Hamilton JR, Walker-Smith JA, Watkins JB, eds. Pediatric Gastrointestinal Disease, 3rd edn. Hamilton, Ontario: BC Decker; 2000:580–584.
29. Goligher J. Fistula-*in-ano*. In: Goligher J, ed. Surgery of the Anus, Rectum, and Colon, 5th edn. London: Baillière Tindall; 1984:178–220.
30. Wexner S, Roberts P, Lowry A, et al. Practice parameters for treatment of fistula-*in-ano* – supporting documentation. Dis Colon Rectum 1996; 39:1363–1372.
31. Schwartz D, Pemberton J, Sandborn W. Diagnosis and treatment of perianal fistulas in Crohn disease. Ann Intern Med 2001; 135:906–918.
32. Tolia V. Perianal Crohn's disease in children and adolescents. Am J Gastroenterol 1996; 91:922–926.
33. Nisar P, Scholefield J. Managing haemorrhoids. BMJ 2003; 327:847–851.
34. Alonso-Coello P, Castillejo M. Office evaluation and treatment of hemorrhoids. J Fam Pract 2003; 52:366–374.
35. Johanson J, Rimm A. Optimal nonsurgical treatment of hemorrhoids: a comparative analysis of infrared coagulation, rubber band ligation, and injection sclerotherapy. Am J Gastroenterol 1992; 87:1600–1606.
36. MacRae H, McLeod R. Comparison of hemorrhoidal treatment modalities: a meta-analysis. Dis Colon Rectum 1995; 38:687–694.
37. Barzilai A, Choen H. Isolation of group A streptococci from children with perianal cellulitis and from their siblings. Pediatr Infect Dis J 1998; 17:358–360.
38. Krol A. Perianal streptococcal cellulitis. Pediatr Dermatol 1990; 7:97–100.

39. Avolio L, Avolyini V, Ceffa F, Bragheri R. Perianal granuloma caused by *Enterobius vermicularis*: report of a new observation and review of the literature. J Pediatr 1998; 132:1055–1056.
40. Favre M, Ramoz N, Orth G. Human papillomaviruses: general features. Clin Dermatol 1997; 15:181–198.
41. Gibbs N. Anogenital papillomavirus infections in children. Curr Opin Pediatr 1998; 10:393–397.
42. Tyring S. Introduction: perspectives on human papillomavirus infection. Am J Med 1997; 102:1–2.
43. Pacheco B, Di Paola G, Ribas J, Vighi S, Rueda N. Vulvar infections caused by human papillomavirus in children and adolescents without sexual contact. Adolesc Pediatr Gynecol 1991; 4:136–142.

Chapter 55
Neoplasms of the gastrointestinal tract and liver

Karen F. Murray and Laura S. Finn

INTRODUCTION

In contrast to the adult population, neoplasms of the gastrointestinal (GI) tract are uncommon in children. Furthermore, the symptoms leading to their diagnosis are usually nonspecific and may be erroneously attributed to a chronic underlying GI condition. Having an understanding of chronic conditions from which neoplasms can arise is important, however, most encountered neoplasms will be unanticipated and the ability to arrive at a prompt and correct diagnosis can be crucial to the survival of the patient. Consequently, this chapter will review the most common GI neoplasms encountered in childhood.

NEOPLASMS OF THE LUMINAL GASTROINTESTINAL TRACT

The GI tract is a relatively common site for involvement by childhood cancers, with approximately 5% of childhood cancers presenting in this organ system. Primary GI cancer in the pediatric population is rare, however. When neoplasms do arise from the GI tract, the presenting symptoms are variable and relatively nonspecific. The symptoms or signs may include abdominal pain, abdominal distention, vomiting, a palpable mass, anemia, GI bleeding, or weight loss. The finding of a neoplasm at surgery for intussusception, bowel obstruction, or perforation as well as the incidental finding during a surgical or radiological procedure for other reasons, also occurs. Definitive diagnosis usually requires a biopsy for histopathological examination and possibly immunotyping and cytogenetics, depending on the tumor.

Neoplasms of the GI tract can be divided into categories based on their tissue of origin (Table 55.1). The most commonly encountered tumors in children arise from the lymphoid or epithelial tissues. Mesenchymal tumors are less frequent. Both benign and malignant tumors can be found within all of these categories. In the following sections we will discuss the most commonly encountered neoplasms within these categories, their epidemiology, pathology, molecular biology, prognosis and treatment.

Tissue of origin	Tumor	Most common GI sites
Lymphoid	Lymphonodular hyperplasia	Ileum, colon
	Lymphoma	Ileum, appendix, colon
Epithelial	Carcinoid	Appendix
	Adenocarcinoma	Colon
Mesenchymal	Leiomyoma/ leiomyosarcoma	Colon
	Gastrointestinal stromal tumor	Stomach, small intestine
	Primitive neuroectodermal tumor	Small intestine
	Schwannoma/ malignant nerve sheath tumor/ neurofibroma	Small intestine
	Hemangioma	All levels
	Lipoma	Colon

Table 55.1 Pediatric gastrointestinal tumors

NEOPLASMS OF LYMPHOID ORIGIN

The gastrointestinal tract is a lymphoid tissue-rich organ system, beautifully adapted to respond in a stimulatory or repressive fashion to recognized luminal antigens. Although there is lymphoid tissue throughout the GI tract, in the form of lymphoid follicles or scattered T and B lymphocytes in the lamina propria, they are particularly prominent in the ileum where they aggregate into Peyer's patches, well-organized germinal follicles of B lymphocytes with T lymphocytes in the interfollicular zones.

Lymphonodular hyperplasia

Lymphonodular hyperplasia (LNH) is a common condition that can affect children of all ages. Its peak ages of occurrence are in early childhood and adolescents as these are times of developmental lymphoid proliferation. Males more commonly than females usually present with right lower quadrant abdominal pain, diarrhea, intussusception, or gastrointestinal bleeding. Endoscopically seen is patchy exaggeration of lymphoid nodules in the large and small bowel, at times distorting the overlying mucosa into prominent folds. Histologically there is reactive hyperplasia with prominent germinal center formation, but no disruption in the normal lymphoid architecture or cellular pleomorphism (Fig. 55.1). Assuming acute management of symptoms is unnecessary, this condition is usually benign with no specific therapy required and an excellent prognosis.

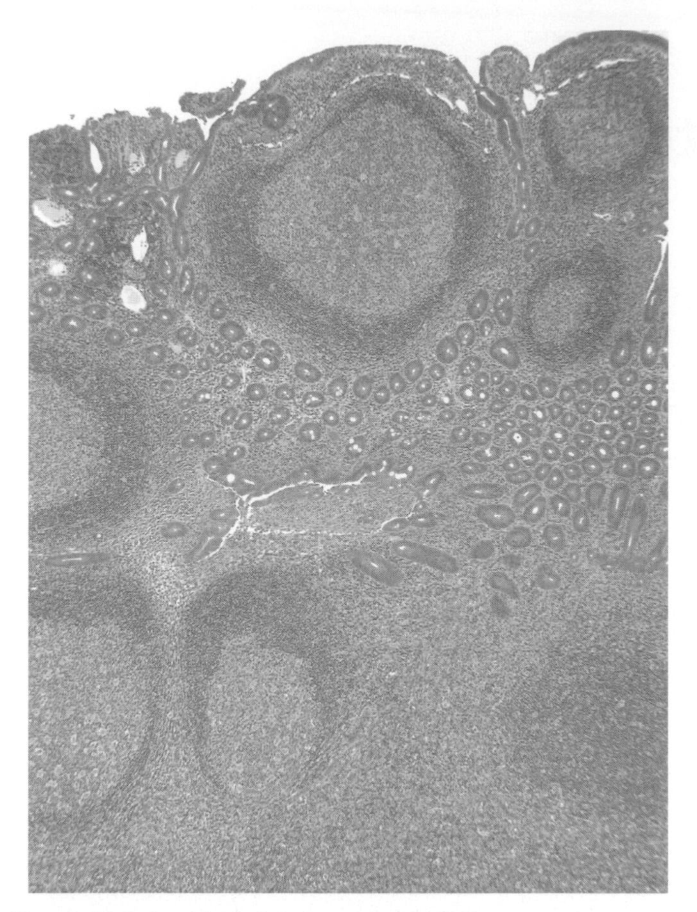

Figure 55.1: Lymphonodular hyperplasia. Numerous reactive germinal centers distort the normal villous architecture of the small bowel. (*See plate section for color*).

In the setting of primary immunodeficiencies (hypogammaglobulinemias), however, LNH may occur with associated diarrhea, malabsorption and chronic intestinal infections such as giardiasis. In adults, this lesion complicates primary hypogammaglobulinemia in approximately 20% of patients.[1] The presence of intestinal lymphomas of either B or T cell type is now well described adjacent to hyperplastic nodules in some of these patients.[2,3]

Lymphoma

The gastrointestinal tract is the most common site of primary extranodal lymphomas. Primary gastrointestinal lymphomas are defined as tumors originating from the mucosal associated lymphoid tissue and contiguous lymph nodes, where the main bulk of the disease is located in that particular region of the gastrointestinal tract (i.e. stomach, ileum, etc.). Lymphoma accounts for approximately 15% of all small bowel malignancies in individuals from North America and Western Europe. In young people under the age of 20 years, lymphoma, the most common malignant neoplasm of the GI tract, is almost universally non-Hodgkin's lymphoma.[4–6] In children under 15 years of age, however, lymphoma is the third most common malignant neoplasm, where it accounts for 10% of all neplasms.[7,8] The gastrointestinal distribution differs between adults and children. Whereas 40–50% of primary GI lymphomas occur in the stomach of adults, the most common sites in children are the terminal ileum, appendix and cecum with the frequency decreasing distally such that 10–20% occur in the colon.

Some 80% of primary intestinal non-Hodgkins lymphomas are of B-cell origin,[4] collectively classified by the World Health Organization (WHO) as precursor or mature B-cell lymphomas, or proliferations of uncertain malignant potential, as are seen in secondary immunodeficiency states.[9] In this same population, or in those individuals immunosuppressed by medications, Epstein–Barr virus (EBV) associated B-cell lymphoma can be a complicating development in their care.[10,11] EBV is also tightly linked to Burkitt's lymphoma in equatorial Africa, but there is a much weaker association in patients from North America. Celiac disease is associated with a variety of small bowel neoplasms but the most common is T-cell lymphoma (70%). The mean age of presentation in the setting of Celiac disease is in the 5th decade, with the jejunum being the most common location.[12] No pediatric cases have been reported.

Diagnosis usually requires surgical biopsy of a mass lesion, however, many lymphomas of the GI tract can be diagnosed through endoscopic biopsies if the lesion involves mucosa or submucosa. Rapid ascertainment of tumor distribution with abdominal computed tomography (CT), bone scan, lumbar puncture and bone marrow aspirate is required and consultation with an oncologist mandatory.

The most common lymphoma arising in the pediatric gastrointestinal tract is Burkitt lymphoma, which most frequently involves the ileocecal region where it presents as an abdominal mass or as the lead-point for intussusception. Burkitt lymphoma is a highly aggressive tumor, comprised of sheets of mitotically active monomorphic medium sized cells with scanty cytoplasm and round to oval nuclei containing small nucleoli. Within the sheets there is apoptotic debris and numerous macrophages, producing a 'starry-sky' appearance (Fig. 55.2). The lymphoma invades through all layers of the bowel, eroding surface mucosa and infiltrating mesenteric lymph nodes (Fig. 55.3). Genetic abnormalities, typically translocations involving the C-MYC gene at chromosome 8q24 leading to deregulation of the oncogene, are crucial in lymphomagenesis. The tumor cells have clonal immunoglobin heavy and light chain rearrangements and *TP53* inactivating mutations in up to 25%.[13]

The gastrointestinal tract is the most common extranodal site for diffuse large B-cell lymphoma (DLBCL), which develops in the pediatric ileocecal region, like Burkitt's, or commonly the stomach in adults, where it may result from secondary transformation of a less aggressive lymphoma. This latter phenomenon is virtually unheard of in children, given the exceedingly low incidence of extranodal marginal zone B-cell lymphoma of mucosa-associated lymphoid tissue ('MALT' lymphoma) that is associated with *H. pylori* infection. DLBCL in the gastrointestinal tract is

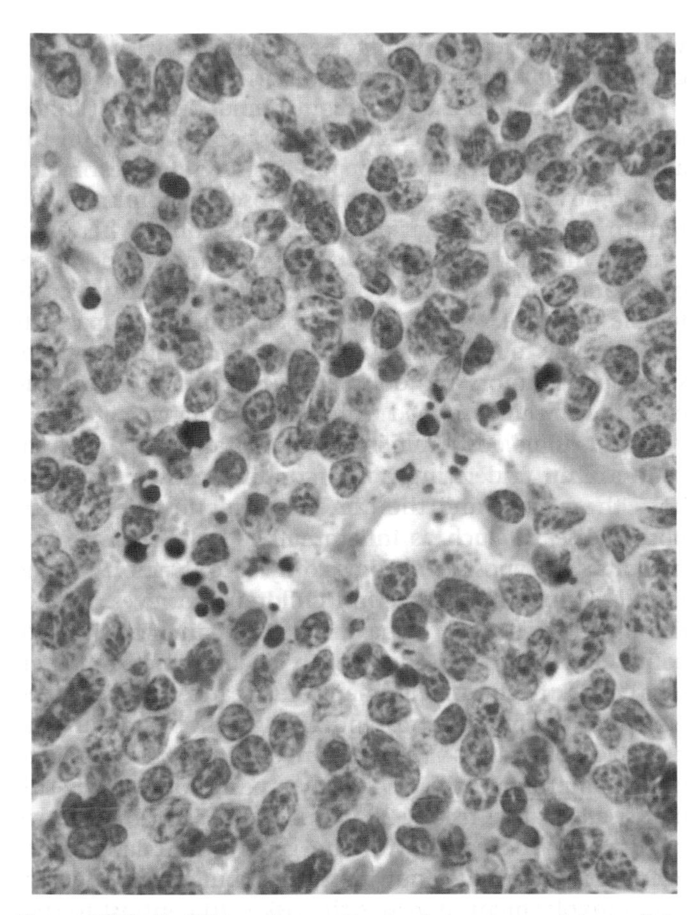

Figure 55.2: Burkitt lymphoma. Sheets of monotonous intermediate sized lymphoid cells have indiscreet nucleoli. Abundant apoptotic nuclear debris is present centrally. (*See plate section for color*)

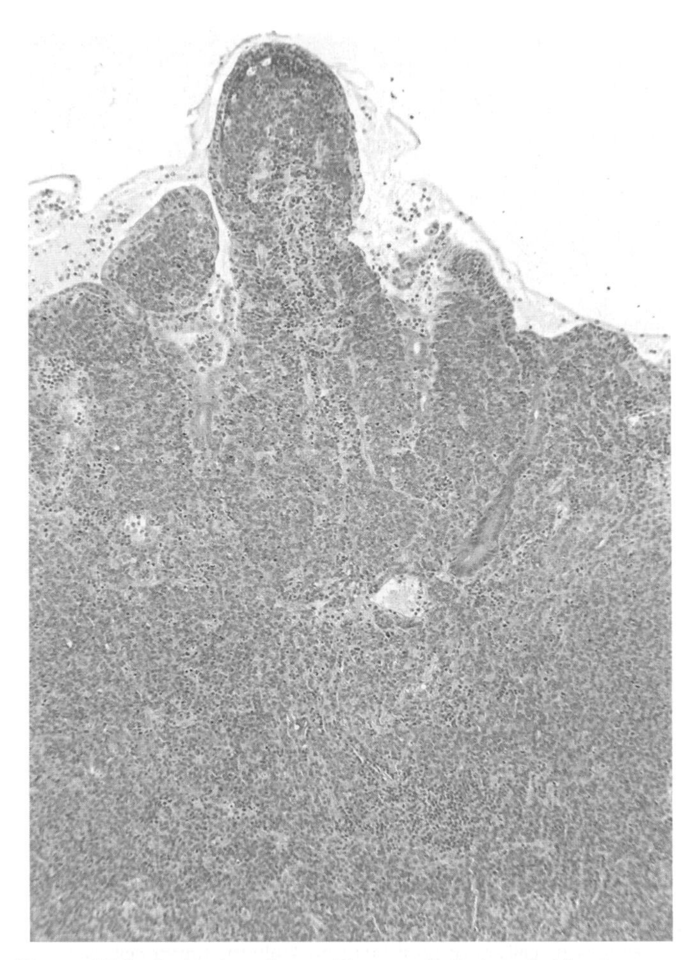

Figure 55.3: Burkitt lymphoma. The neoplastic lymphoid cells diffusely infiltrate the mucosa, overrunning the epithelium. Contrast with the benign lymphoid reaction in Figure 55.1. (*See plate section for color*)

indistinguishable from those arising within lymph nodes. The intestinal architecture is often destroyed by medium to large cells with vesicular nuclei and typically prominent nucleoli (Fig. 55.4). Most cases have clonal rearrangement of the immunoglobulin heavy and light chain genes and display often complex but not specific cytogenetic abnormalities. *BLC2* gene translocation (t(14;18)) occurs in 20–30% of adult cases but has not been described in pediatric DLBCL.[14] Abnormalities involving the *BCL6* protooncogene localized to 3q27 region are identified in over 30% of adult DLBCL but extensive investigations have not been carried out in childhood DLBCL.[15]

Treatment of GI lymphoma is largely chemotherapy based, augmented with radiation therapy. Surgical resection is limited only to the rare circumstance of focal disease. The length and type of chemotherapeutic intervention depends on the extent of disease (Table 55.2) but generally requires both systemic therapy as well as intrathecal delivery of agents to prevent or treat involvement in the cerebral spinal fluid. The most commonly employed chemotherapeutic agents include cyclophosphamide, doxorubicin, vincristine, prednisone and intrathecal methotrexate. The best prognosis is with stage A and B lymphoma (greater that 90% long-term survival),[16,17] with stage AR having an equally favorable prognosis. Involvement with unresectable abdominal tumor carries a less favorable prognosis. With large tumor burden the potential for tumor-lysis syndrome due to rapid cell turnover and consequent release of uric acid, potassium and phosphorus into the blood stream must be anticipated with the initiation of therapy.

NEOPLASMS OF EPITHELIAL ORIGIN

Neoplasms of epithelial origin include carcinomas as well as tumors derived from neuroendocrine elements. This group of tumors includes adenocarcinomas and carcinoids, which are uncommon in childhood but cause significant morbidity and mortality when they occur.

Carcinoma of the colon

Colorectal cancer is the second leading cause of death in the USA,[18] with an average lifetime risk equal in men and women of 6%. Most colon cancer occurs in older adults, with only 1–4% occurring in individuals under 30 years of age.[19] Despite this infrequency, however, carcinoma of the colon is the most common primary solid malignancy of

Smooth muscle tumors in the gastrointestinal tract are identical to those that occur in more common locations. Typically beginning as intramural lesions, they expand as well circumscribed spherical or sausage-shaped masses toward the lumen or mediastinal or peritoneal cavities. Benign smooth muscle tumors, leiomyomas, consist of interlacing bundles of bland spindled cells with cigar-shaped nuclei and a moderate amount of eosinophilic cytoplasm. Their smooth muscle origin is confirmed by demonstrating smooth muscle actin and desmin expression; these tumors are negative for CD34 and CD117 (C Kit). Malignant tumors, leiomyosarcomas, have increased cellularity and mitotic activity compared to their benign counterparts.[63,64] Epstein–Barr virus associated smooth muscle tumors in children infected with the human immunodeficiency virus (HIV) not infrequently involve the gastrointestinal tract.[65]

Diagnosis is usually made incidentally during radiographic, endoscopic, or surgical evaluation of unrelated symptoms. The mainstay of therapy is surgical resection, however, extensive local spread is possible with both benign and metastatic tumors, making complete resection difficult and leading to a high incidence of local recurrence. Survival is variable and both local and distant metastases have occurred years after the primary resection.[66–68]

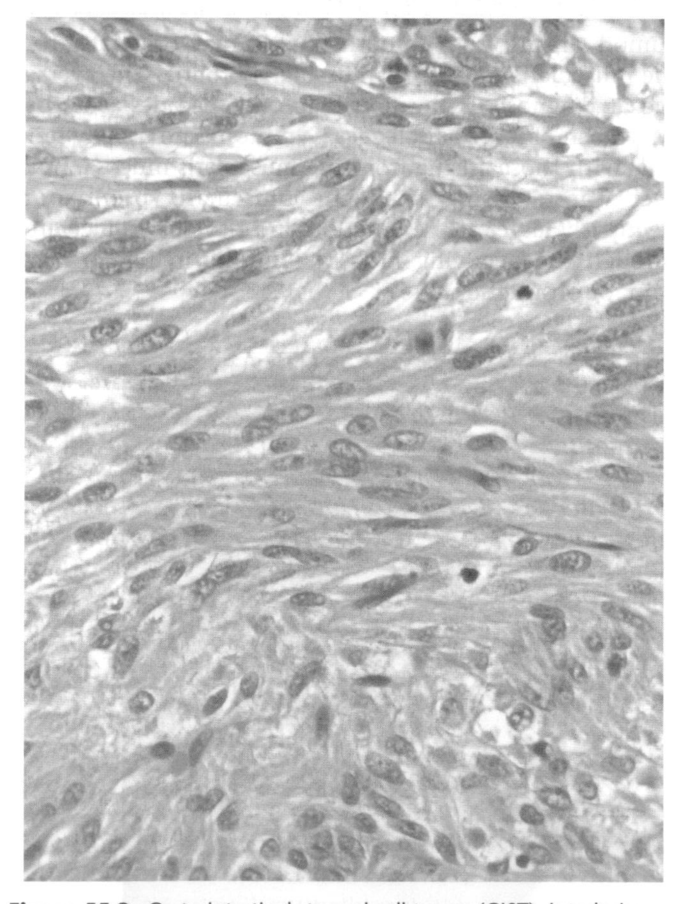

Figure 55.9: Gastrointestinal stromal cell tumor (GIST). Interlacing fascicles of plump cigar-shaped cells with tapered ends, comprise the spindle cell GIST. (*See plate section for color*).

Stromal cell origin

GI stromal tumors arise from the intestinal wall, mesentery, omentum, or retroperitoneum.[69] The Finnish Cancer Registry estimates the incidence of these tumors to be roughly 4 per million although the true incidence is not known. Rare in childhood, the peak prevalence is in the fifth and sixth decades, although pediatric cases have been described. Some 60–70% of the tumors arise in the stomach, 20–30% in the small intestine and less than 10% from the remainder of the GI tract, omentum, mesentery and retroperitoneum.

Stromal cell tumors may be derived from the interstitial cells of Cajal of the autonomic nervous system, as they usually express the transmembrane tyrosine kinase receptor CD 117(c-kit proto-oncogene protein), in contrast to leiomyomas and leiomyosarcomas.[70] Staining for CD 117 is frequently necessary as these tumors can have deceptively heterogeneous morphology. Most of the tumors also show immunopositivity for CD34.[71] These unique features have revolutionized the diagnosis of GIST. What in the mid-1990s became known as GISTs were generically classified as 'stromal tumors' after the advent of immunohistochemistry in the 1980s demonstrated a lack of smooth muscle differentiation; prior to that they had been erroneously regarded as smooth muscle tumors, earning appellations such as 'cellular leiomyomas' or 'leiomyoblastomas'. Constitutive overexpression of KIT oncoproteins in GISTs is critical to its pathogenesis and most commonly results from oncogenic mutations in the KIT gene on the long arm of chromosome 4. Both benign and malignant GISTs frequently show losses in chromosomes 14 and 22 by karyotypic analysis.[72]

The histopathology of GISTs typically falls into one of three categories: spindle cell type (70%); epithelioid type (20%) or mixed.[71] The spindle cell type is comprised of uniform plump eosinophilic cells arranged in short fascicles and whorls while nests of moderately sized round cells with clear to eosinophilic cytoplasm constitute the epithelioid type (Figs 55.9, 55.10). Criteria for malignancy is disputed, but larger, mitotically active tumors carry a higher risk of aggressive behavior including peritoneal cavity or hepatic metastases.

Primary treatment is surgical with chemotherapy reserved for metastatic or unresectable tumors. Although standard chemotherapeutic agents are ineffective, imatinib mesylate, a selective inhibitor of tyrosine kinase, has been shown to reduce tumor size in 54.7% and 69.4% of cases.[73,74]

As imatinib mesylate has only been used in the treatment of stromal cell tumors in recent years, the long-term survival with this therapy has not yet been realized. The 5 year survival with surgical resection alone is 20–78%.

NEOPLASMS OF THE LIVER

Hepatic tumors make up only 1–4% of pediatric solid tumors and most of these are metastatic lesions from an extrahepatic site. Five primary hepatobiliary tumors occur

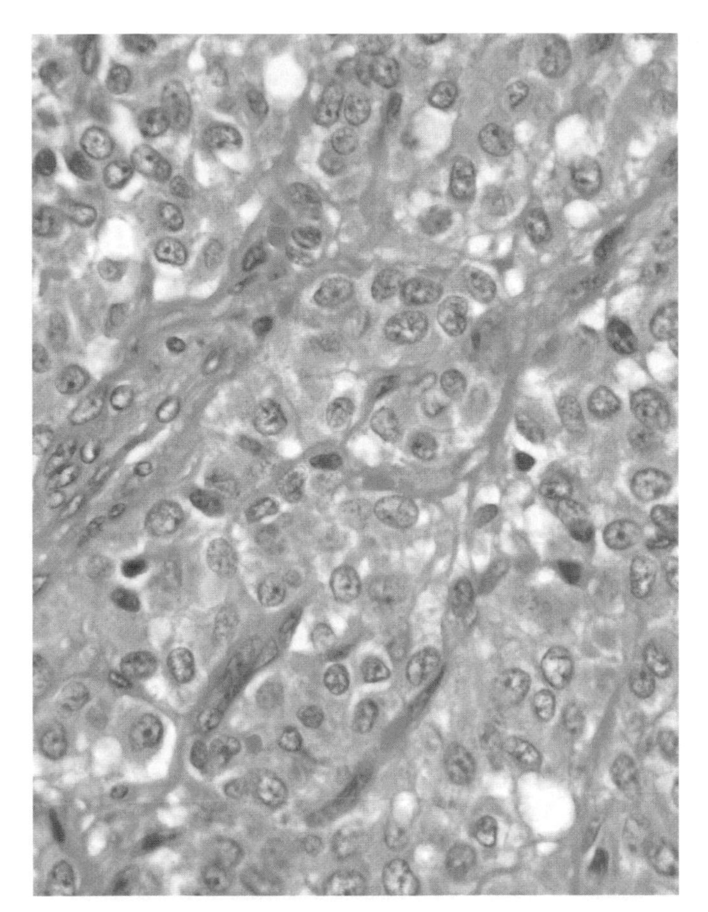

Figure 55.10: Gastrointestinal stromal cell tumor (GIST). Nests of medium-sized epithelioid cells with a moderate amount of eosinophilic cytoplasm comprise the epithelioid GIST. (*See plate section for color*).

uniquely in childhood, however, including hepatoblastoma, infantile hemangioendothelioma, mesenchymal hamartoma, undifferentiated embryonal sarcoma and embryonal rhabdomyosarcoma of the biliary system. Of these tumors infantile hemangioendotheliomas usually occur in the first 6 months of life and 90% of hepatoblastomas in the first 5 years of life (68% in the first 2 years) with these two tumors representing roughly 80% of liver tumors in children under the age of 2 years. In contrast, undifferentiated embryonal sarcomas are most commonly encountered in school aged children.[75] In this section, we will review the most common pediatric primary liver tumors with a complete list found in Table 55.4.

Hepatoblastoma

The first case of hepatoblastoma was described in 1898[76] and this tumor is now known to be the most common pediatric liver malignancy, accounting for 1% of all pediatric malignancies with an incidence of 0.5 to 1.5 cases per million children under the age of 15 years in Western countries.[77]

Patients usually present when family members notice an enlarging abdomen or an irregular mass in the right upper quadrant is palpated on a routine physical examination. The mass is usually non-tender. Accompanying anorexia,

Tumor	Most common age at presentation
Hepatoblastoma	Under 5 years, most under 2 years
Infantile hemangioendothelioma	Under 6 months
Hepatocellular carcinoma	>5 years
Fibrolamellar variant of hepatocellular carcinoma	2nd decade
Focal nodular hyperplasia	2nd decade
Mesenchymal hamartoma	Most under 2 years
Undifferentiated embryonal sarcoma	5 to 10 years
Nodular regenerative hyperplasia	All ages
Hepatocellular adenoma	All ages
Angiosarcoma	All ages
Embryonal rhabdomyosarcoma	3–15 years
Teratoma	Under 1 year

Table 55.4 Pediatric primary liver neoplasms

weight loss, nausea, vomiting, or abdominal pain is less commonly observed and jaundice is uncommon (5%).[75]

Diagnosis is made with a combination of radiographic and laboratory tests. CT or MRI can be helpful in defining the size and distribution of the mass and can identify features that distinguish it from other liver tumors. The finding of speckled calcifications is well described and found in roughly 50% of cases.[78] At diagnosis, approximately 20% of tumors have metastasized, most commonly to the lungs.[79] The most diagnostically useful laboratory finding seen with hepatoblastomas is a significant elevation in serum α-fetoprotein (AFP), which is present in approximately 90% of the cases. The extent of AFP elevation correlates with tumor size or presence of metastases and its decrease, with tumor clearance after therapy. AFP levels are helpful in monitoring recurrence. The 10% of hepatoblastomas that do not have elevated AFP levels tend to be of small-cell undifferentiated histology and carry a poor prognosis.[75,80] Confirmation of the diagnosis and documentation of the histological features require a biopsy.

Multiple scoring systems, preoperative and postoperative, have been developed over the years to predict prognosis. The simplest of these, the Children's Cancer Study Group/Pediatric Oncology Group staging system has a highly significant predictive value for survival ($p = 0.0009$) (Table 55.5).

Hepatoblastomas are derived from undifferentiated embryonal tissue and do not have a characteristic chromosomal anomaly though trisomies of chromosomes 20, 2 and 8 are frequent.[81] These tumors are associated with some familial conditions such as Beckwith Wiedemann syndrome and Familial Adenomatous Polyposis and with Trisomy 18. Hepatoblastomas are typically a single mass and involve the right lobe in slightly more than half of the cases. Their gross appearance varies tremendously and is dependent on the proportion of mesenchymal elements. Most commonly, hepatoblastomas contain purely 'fetal' epithelial cells, which are uniform, small to medium

very primitive mesenchymal cells and account for 9–13% of childhood hepatic tumors.[102–104]

As with the other hepatic tumors developing in this age group, the most common presenting sign is abdominal enlargement or a mass, but fever, vomiting and weight loss may also occur.[105] Diagnosis requires a biopsy to differentiate this tumor from other malignant tumors of the liver. By US these tumors are solid, however, CT and MRI sometimes suggests a cystic quality.

The majority of tumors are in the right lobe and typically measure 10–20 cm.[82] Tumor cells are stellate to spindled and often have markedly pleomorphic or bizarre giant nuclei. They are loosely or compactly arranged within abundant myxoid stroma that may focally become more fibrous. A characteristic and helpful diagnostic feature is the presence of numerous eosinophilic globules in tumor cells and extracellularly (Fig. 55.14). Immunohistochemical and ultrastructural analyses have demonstrated limited differentiation along various lines including fibroblastic, rhabdomyoblastic and leiomyoblastic.[106]

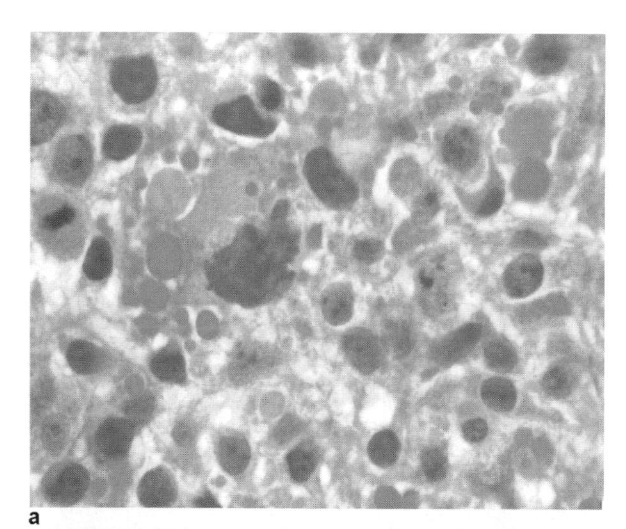
a

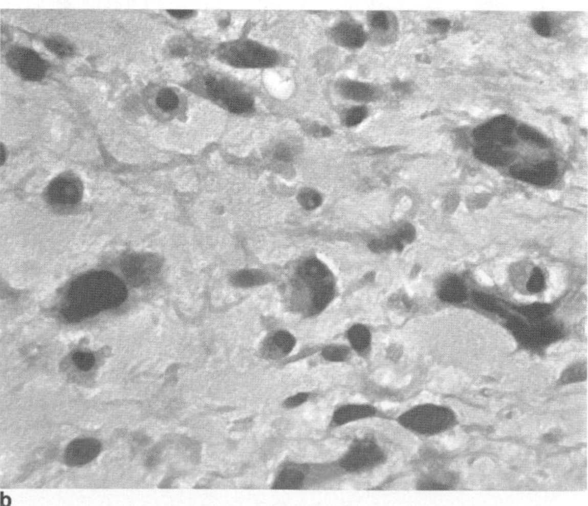
b

Figure 55.14 Undifferentiated embryonal sarcoma. Marked pleomorphism is characteristic and cellular density is variable. Scattered atypical hyperchromatic multinucleated cells are sporadically distributed within abundant myxoid stroma **(b)**. Another more cellular tumor has abundant eosinophilic hyaline globules **(a)**.

The prognosis of children with undifferentiated embryonal sarcomas is poor, however, recent advances in preoperative chemotherapy followed by surgical resection has improved the long-term survival to as high as 70%.[105,107,108]

Embryonal rhabdomyosarcoma of the biliary tree

Rhabdomyosarcomas are the most common sarcomas in children, but those involving the biliary system are rare, accounting for only 1% of liver tumors. They typically occur between 5 and 15 years of age and present with jaundice in as many as 80% of cases.[109,110]

Although laboratory values are non-specific and simply reflective of biliary ductal obstruction, CT, MRI, or US can localize the mass lesion to the intrahepatic or more commonly the extrahepatic ductal system.

Primary therapy is surgical resection although this is successful in fewer than 50% of cases due to local extension of the tumor into the liver, other intra-abdominal organs, or lymphatic metastasis. Chemotherapy with subsequent second surgical exploration has raised the long-term survival to above 20%.[75,111]

References

1. Webster ADB, Kenwright S, Ballard J, et al. Nodular lymphoid hyperplasia of the small bowel in primary hypogammaglobulinaemia: a study of in vivo and in vitro lymphocyte function. Gut 1997; 18(5):364–372.
2. Freiman JS, Gallagher ND. Mesenteric lymph node enlargement as a cause of intestinal variceal hemorrhage in nodular lymphoid hyperplasia. J Clin Gastroenterol 1985; 7:422–424.
3. Matuchanksky C, Morichau-Beauchant M, Touchard G, et al. Nodular lymphoid hyperplasia of the small bowel associated with primary jejunal malignant lymphoma; evidence favoring a cytogenetic relationship. Gastroenterology 1980; 78:1587–1592.
4. Guillerman RP. Primary intestinal non-Hodgkin lymphoma. J Pediatr Hematol Oncol 2000; 22(5):476–478.
5. North JH, Pack MS. Malignant tumors of the small intestine: a review of 144 cases. Am Surg 2000; 66(1):46–51.
6. Rambaud J-C. Small intestinal lymphomas and alpha-chain disease. Clin Gastroenterol 1983; 12:743–766.
7. Young JL, Miller RW. Incidence of malignant tumors in US children. J Pediatr 1975; 86:254–258.
8. Leichtner AM, Hoppin AG. Intestinal neoplasms. In: Walker WA, Durie PR, Hamilton JR, Walker-Smith JA, Watkins JB, eds. Pediatric Gastrointestinal Disease, Pathophysiology, Diagnosis, Management, 2nd edn. St Louis, MO: Mosby; 1996:922–936.
9. Jaffe ES, Harris NL, Stein H, Vardiman JW, eds. World Health Organization Classification of Tumours. Pathology and Genetics. Tumours of haematopoietic and lymphoid tissues. Lyon: IARCPress; 2001.
10. Smets F, Sokal EM. Lymphoproliferation in children after liver transplantation. J Pediatr Gastroenterol Nutr 2002; 34:499–505.
11. Purtillo DT, DeFlorio D, Hutt LM Jr, et al. Variable phenotype expression of an X-linked lymphoproliferative syndrome. N Engl J Med 1977; 297:1077–1080.

12. Pricolol VE, Mangi AA, Aswad B, Bland KI. Gastrointestinal malignancies in patients with celiac sprue. Am J Surg 1998; 176(4):344–347.
13. Sanchez-Beato M, Sanchez-Aguilera A, Piris MA. Cell cycle deregulation in B-cell lymphomas. Blood 2003; 101(4):1220–1235.
14. Weiss LM, Warnke RA, Sklar J, Cleary ML. Molecular analysis of the chromosomal translocation in malignant lymphomas. N Engl J Med 1987; 317:1185–1189.
15. Vitolo U, Botto B, Capello D, et al. Point mutations of the BCL-6 gene: clinical and prognostic correlation in B-diffuse large cell lymphoma. Leukemia 2002; 16(2):268–275.
16. Patte C, Gerrard M, Auperin A, et al. Results of the randomised international trial FAB LMB 96 for the 'intermediate risk' childhood and adolescent B-cell lymphoma: reduced therapy is efficacious. Pediatr Cancer 2003; 22:796.
17. Patte C, Auperin A, Michon J, et al. The Societe Francaise d'Oncologie Pediatrique LMB89 protocol: highly effective multiagent chemotherapy tailored to the tumor burden and initial response in 561 unselected children with B-cell lymphomas and L3 leukemia. Blood 2001; 97(11):3370–3379.
18. Jemal A, Murray T, Samuels A, et al. Cancer statistics. CA Cancer J Clin 2003; 2003; 53(1):5–26.
19. Hoerner MT. Carcinoma of the colon and rectum in persons under 20 years of age. Am J Surg 1958; 96:47–53.
20. Griffin PM, Liff JM, Greenberg RS, Clark WS. Adenocarcinoma of the colon and rectum on persons under 40 years old. Gastroenterology 1991; 100:1033–1040.
21. Kern WH, William CW. Adenocarcinoma of the colon in a nine-month old infant. Report of a case. Cancer 1958; 11:855–857.
22. Fitzgibbons RJ, Lynch HT Jr, Stanislav GV, et al. Recognition and treatment of patients with hereditary nonpolyposis colon cancer (lynch syndromes I and II). Ann Surg 1987; 206:289–295.
23. Aiges HW, Kahn E, Silverberg M, Daum F. Adenocarcinoma of the colon in an adolescent with the family cancer syndrome. J Pediatr 1979; 94:632–633.
24. Winawer S, Fletcher R, Rex D, et al. Colorectal cancer screening and surveillance: clinical guidelines and rationale-update based on new evidence. Gastroenterology 2003; 124:544–560.
25. Greenstein AJ, Sachar DB, Smith H, et al. Cancer in universal and left-sided ulcerative colitis: factors determining risk. Gastroenterology 1979; 77:290–294.
26. Greenstein AJ, Sachar DB, Smith H, Janowitz HD, Aufses AH Jr. Patterns of neoplasia in Crohn's disease and ulcerative colitis. Cancer 1980; 46:403–407.
27. Sigel JE, Petras RE, Lashner BA, Fazio VW, Goldblum JR. Intestinal adenocarcinoma in Crohn's disease: a report of 30 cases with a focus on coexisting dysplasia. Am J Surg Path 1999; 23(6):651–655.
28. Sessions RT, Riddell DH, Kaplan HJ, Foster JH. Carcinoma of the colon in the first two decades of life. Ann Surg 1965; 162:279–284.
29. Middelkamp JN, Haffner H. Carcinoma of the colon in children. Pediatrics 1963; 32:558–571.
30. Falterman KW, Hill CB, Markey JC, Fox JW, Cohn I Jr. Cancer of the colon, rectum and anus: a review of 2313 cases. Cancer 1974; 34:951–959.
31. Brown RA, Rode H, Millar AJW, Sinclair-Smith C, Cywes S. Colorectal carcinoma in children. J Pediatr Surg 1992; 27(7):919–921.
32. Needle MN. Cancer of the gastrointestinal tract. In: Altschuler SM, Liacouras CA, eds. Clinical pediatric Gastroenterology, 1st edn. Philadelphia, PA: Churchill Livingstone; 1998:243–246.
33. Riddell RH, Petras RE, Williams GT, Sobin LH, eds. Atlas of Tumor Pathology. Tumors of the Intestine. Bethesda: Armed Forces Institute of Pathology; 2003.
34. Hamilton SR, Aaltonen LA. World Health Organization Classification of Tumours. Pathology and Genetics. Tumours of the digestive system. Lyon: IARC Press; 2000.
35. Kinzler KW, Vogelstein B. Lessons from hereditary colorectal cancer. Cell 1996; 87(2):159–170.
36. Datta RV, LaQuaglia MP, Paty PB. Genetic and phenotypic correlates of colorectal cancer in young patients. N Engl J Med 2000; 342:137–138.
37. Gryfe R, Kim H, Hsieh ETK, et al. Tumor microsatellite instability and clinical outcome in young patients with colorectal cancer. N Engl J Med 2000; 342:69–77.
38. Andersson A, Bergdahl L. Carcinoma of the colon in children: a report of six new cases and review of the literature. J Pediatr Surg 1976; 11:967–971.
39. Rao BN, Pratt CB, Fleming ID, et al. Colon carcinoma in children and adolescents, a review of 30 cases. Cancer 1985; 55:1322–1326.
40. Odone V, Chang L, Caces J, George SL, Pratt CB. The natural history of colorectal carcinoma in adolescents. Cancer 1982; 49:1716–1720.
41. Munck A, Bellaiche M, Ferkadji L, et al. Carcinoma of the stomach in a child. J Pediatr Gastroenterol Nutr 1993; 16:334–336.
42. McGill TW, Downey EC, Westbrook J, Wade D, de la Garza J. Gastric carcinoma in children. J Pediatr Surg 1993; 28:1620–1621.
43. Murphy S, Shaw K, Blanchard H. Report of three gastric tumors in children. J Pediatr Surg 1994; 29:1202–1204.
44. Berge T, Linell F. Carcinoid tumors. Acta Pathol Microbiol Scand 1976; 84:322–330.
45. Horie H, Iwasaki I, Takahashi H. Carcinoid in a gastrointestinal duplication. J Pediatr Surg 1986; 21:902–904.
46. Hecks B, Kadinski S. Carcinoid tumor of a Meckel's diverticulum. Lancet 1992; ii:70.
47. Chow CW, Sane S, Campbell PE, Carter RF. Malignant carcinoid tumors in children. Cancer 1982; 49:802–811.
48. Andersson A, Bergdahl L. Carcinoid tumors of the appendix in children: a report of 25 cases. Acta Chir Scand 1977; 143(3):173–175.
49. Ryden SE, Drake RM, Franciosi RA. Carcinoid tumors of the appendix in children. Cancer 1975; 36(4):1538–1542.
50. Soga J. Carcinoids of the colon and ileocecal region: a statistical evaluation of 363 cases collected from the literature. J Exp Clin Cancer Res 1998; 17(2):139–148.
51. Biorck G, Axen O, Thorson A. Unusual cyanosis in a boy with congenital pulmonary stenosis and tricuspid insufficiency: fatal outcome after angiocardiography. Am Heart J 1952; 44(1):143–148.
52. Godshall D. The carcinoid syndrome: an unusual cause of valvular heart disease. J Emerg Med 2001; 21(1):21–25.
53. Attanoos R, Williams GT. Epithelial and neuroendocrine tumors of the duodenum. Semin Diagn Pathol 1991; 8(3):149–162.
54. Dayal Y, Tallberg KA, Nunnemacher G, DeLellis RA, Wolfe HJ. Duodenal carcinoids in patients with and without neurofibromatosis: A comparative study. Am J Surg Pathol 1986; 10:348–357.
55. McCormick D. Carcinoid tumors and syndrome. Gastroenterol Nurs 2002; 25(3):105–111.

56. Moertel CG, Weiland LH, Nagorney DM, Dockerty MB. Carcinoid tumor of the appendix: treatment and prognosis. N Engl J Med 1987; 317(27):1699–1701.
57. Moertel CG. Treatment of the carcinoid tumor and the malignant carcinoid syndrome. J Clin Oncol 1983; 1(11):727–740.
58. Boushey RP, Dackiw AP. Carcinoid tumors. Curr Treat Options Oncol 2002; 3(4):319–326.
59. Arnold R. Medical treatment of metastasizing carcinoid tumors. World J Surg 1996; 20(2):203–207.
60. Shapiro RS, Shafir M, Sung M, Warner R, Glajchen N. Cryotherapy of metastatic carcinoid tumors. Abdom Imaging 1998; 23(3):314–317.
61. Roche A, Girish BV, Baere T de, et al. Trans-catheter arterial chemoembolization as first-line treatment for hepatic metastases from endocrine tumors. Eur Rad 2003; 13(1):136–140.
62. Shebani KO, Souba WW, Finkelstein DM, et al. Prognosis and survival in patients with gastrointestinal tract carcinoid tumors. Ann Surg 1999; 229(6):815–824.
63. Miettinen M, Kopczynski J, Makhlouf HR, et al. Gastrointestinal stromal tumors, intramural leiomyomas and leiomyosarcomas in the duodenum. A clinicopathologic, immunohistochemical and molecular genetic study of 167 cases. Am J Surg Pathol 2003; 27:625–641.
64. Miettinen M, Sarlomo-Rikala M, Sobin LH, Lasota J. Esophageal stromal tumors: A clinicopathologic, immunohistochemical and molecular genetic study of 17 cases and comparison with esophageal leiomyomas and leiomyosarcomas. Am J Surg Pathol 2000; 24:211–222.
65. Jenson HB, Leach CT, McClain KL, et al. Benign and malignant smooth muscle tumors containing Epstein-Barr virus in children with AIDS. Leuk Lymphoma 1997; 27(3/4):303–314.
66. Evans HL. Smooth muscle tumors of the gastrointestinal tract. A study of 56 cases followed for a minimum of 10 years. Cancer 1985; 56:2242–2250.
67. Nemer FD, Stoeckinger JM, Evans OT. Smooth muscle rectal tumours: A therapeutic dilemma. Dis Colon Rectum 1977; 20:405–13.
68. Walsh TH, Mann CV. Smooth muscle neoplasms of the rectum and anal canal. Br J Surg 1984; 71:597–599.
69. Davila RE, Faigel DO. GI stromal tumors. Gastrointest Endosc 2003; 58:80–88.
70. Tornoczky T, Kover E, Pajor L. Frequent occurrence of low grade cases among metastatic gastrointestinal stromal tumours. J Clin Pathol 2003; 56(6):363–367.
71. Fletcher CDM, Berman JJ, Corless C, et al. Diagnosis of gastrointestinal stromal tumors: a consensus approach. Hum Pathol 2002; 33:459–465.
72. Heinrich MC, Rubin BP, Longley BJ, Fletcher JA. Biology and genetic aspects of gastrointestinal stromal tumors: KIT activation and cytogenetic alterations. Hum Pathol 2002; 33:484–495.
73. Demetri GD, Mehren M von, Blanke CD, et al. Efficacy and safety of imatinib mesylate in advanced gastrointestinal stromal tumors. N Engl J Med 2002; 347:472–480.
74. van Oosterom AT, Judson I, Verweik J, et al. Safety and efficacy of imatinib (ST1571) in metastatic gastrointestinal stromal tumours: a phase I study. Lancet 2001; 358(9291):1421–1423.
75. Stocker JT. Hepatic tumors in children. Clin liver Dis 2001; 5(1):259–281.
76. Misick OS. A case of teratoma hepatis. J Pathol Bacteriol 1898(5):128–137.
77. Schnater JM, Kohler SE, Lamers WH, Schweinitz D von, Aronson DC. Where do we stand with hepatoblastoma? Cancer 2003; 98:668–678.
78. Miller J, Greenspan B. Integrated imaging of hepatic tumors in children: I. Malignant lesions (primary and metastatic). Radiology 1985; 145:83–90.
79. Perilongo G, Brown J, Shafford E, et al. Hepatoblastoma presenting with lung metastases. Cancer 2000; 89:1845–1853.
80. Schweinitz D von, Hecker H. Schmidt-von-Arndt G, Harms D. Prognostic factors and staging systems in childhood hepatoblastoma (abstract). Int J Cancer 1997; 74:593–599.
81. Surace C, Leszl A, Perilongo G, et al. Fluorescent in situ hybridization (FISH) reveals frequent and recurrent numerical and structural abnormalities in hepatoblastoma with no informative karyotype. Med Pediatr Oncol 2002; 39(5):536–539.
82. Ishak KG, Goodman ZD, Stocker JT. Atlas of Tumor Pathology. Tumors of the liver and intrahepatic bile ducts. Bethesda: Armed Forces Institute of Pathology; 2001.
83. Kasai M, Watanabe I. Histologic classification of liver-cell carcinoma in infancy and childhood and its clinical evaluation: A study of 70 cases collected in Japan. Cancer 1970; 25(3):551–563.
84. Schnater JM, Aronson DC, Plaschkes J, et al. Surgical view of the treatment of patients with hepatoblastoma. Results from the first prospective trial of the international Society of Pediatric Oncology Liver Tumor Study Group (SIIOPEL-1). Cancer 2002; 94:1111–1120.
85. Pritchard J, Brown J, Shafford E, et al. Cisplatin, doxorubicin and delayed surgery for childhood hepatoblastoma: a successful approach. Results of the first prospective study of the International Society of Pediatric Oncology (SIOP)-SIOPEL 1. J Clin Oncol 2000; 18:3819–3828.
86. Daller JA, Bueno J, Gutierrez J, et al. Hepatic hemangioendothelioma: clinical experience and management strategy. J Pediatr Surg 1999; 34:98–105.
87. Hase T, Kodama M, Kishida A, et al. Successful management of infantile hepatic hilar hemangioendothelioma with obstructive jaundice and consumption coagulopathy. J Pediatr Surg 1995; 30:1485–1487.
88. Selby DM, Stocker JT, Waclawiw MA, Hitchcock CL, Ishak KG. Infantile hemangioendothelioma of the liver. Hepatology 1994; 20:39–45.
89. Horton KM, Bluemke DA, Hurban RH, Soyer P, Fishman EK. CT and MR imaging of benign hepatic and biliary tumors. Radiographics 1999; 19:431–451.
90. Helmberger TK, Ros PR, Mergo PJ, Tomczak R, Reiser MF. Pediatric liver neoplasms: a radiologic-pathologic correlation. Eur Radiol 1999; 9:1339–1347.
91. North PE, Waner M, Mizeracki A, Mihm MC. GLUT1: a newly discovered immunohistochemical marker for juvenile hemangiomas. Hum Pathol 2000; 31(1):11–22.
92. Mo JQ, Dimashkieh HH, Bove KE. GLUT1 endothelial reactivity distinguishes hepatic infantile hemangioma from congenital hepatic vascular malformation with associated capillary proliferation. Hum Pathol 2004; 35:200–209.
93. Berenguer B, Mulliken JB, Enjolras O, et al. Rapidly involuting congenital hemangioma: clinical and histopathologic features. Pediatr Dev Pathol 2003; 6(6):495–510.
94. Becker JM, Heitler MS. Hepatic hemangioendotheliomas in infancy. Surg Gynecol Obstet 1989; 168:189–200.
95. McHugh K, Burrows PE. Infantile hepatic hemangioendothelioma: significance of portal venous and

systemic collateral arterial supply. J Vasc Interv Radiol 1992; 3:337–344.

96. Rosch J, Petersen BD, Hall LD, Ivancev K. Interventional treatment of hepatic arterial and venous pathology: a commentary. Cardiovasc Intervent Radiol 1990; 13:183–188.
97. Achilleos OA, Buis LJ, Kelly DA, et al. Unresectable hepatic tumors in childhood and the role of liver transplantation. J Pediatr Surg 1996; 31:1563–1567.
98. Calder CI, Raafat F, Buckels JA, Kelly DA. Orthotopic liver transplantation for type 2 hepatic infantile hemangioendothelioma. Histopathology 1996; 28:271–273.
99. George J, Cohen M, Tarver R, Rosales RN. Ruptured cystic mesenchymal hamartoma: an unusual cause of neonatal ascites. Pediatr Radiol 1994; 24:304–305.
100. Bessho T, Kubota K, Komori S, et al. Prenatally detected hepatic hamartoma: another cause of non-immune hydrops. Prenat Diagn 1996; 16:337–341.
101. Balmer B, Le Coultre C, Feldges A, Hanimann B. Mesenchymal liver hamartoma in a newborn; case report. Eur J Pediatr Surg 1996; 6:303–305.
102. Weinberg AJ, Finegold MJ. Primary hepatic tumors in childhood. In: Feingold MJ, ed. Pathology of neoplasia in children and adolescents. Philadelphia, PA: WB Saunders; 1986:333–372.
103. Stocker JT. Hepatic tumors in children. In: Suchy FJ, ed. Liver Disease in Children. Philadelphia, PA: Lippincott; 1994:901–929.
104. Stocker JT. Ishak KG. Undifferentiated (embryonal) sarcoma of the liver. Cancer 1978; 42:336–348.
105. Bisogno G, Pilz T, Perilongo G, et al. Undifferentiated sarcoma of the liver in childhood: a curable disease. Cancer 2002; 94(1):252–257.
106. Parham DM, Kelly DR, Donnelly WH, Douglass EC. Immunohistochemical and ultrastructural spectrum of hepatic sarcomas of childhood: evidence for a common histogenesis. Mod Pathol 1991; 4(5):648–653.
107. Babin-Boilletot A, Flamant F, Terrier-Lacombe MJ, Marsden B, van Unnik, Demeocq F, et al. Primitive malignant nonepithelial hepatic tumors in children. Med Pediatr Oncol 1993; 21:634–639.
108. Urban CE, Mache CJ, Schwinger W, et al. Undifferentiated (embryonal) sarcoma of the liver in childhood. Successful combined-modality therapy in four patients. Cancer 1993; 72:2511–2516.
109. Lack EE, Perez-Atayde AR, Schuster SR. Botryoid rhabdomyosarcoma of the biliary tract. Am J Surg Pathol 1981; 5:643–652.
110. Sanz N, Florez ML, Rollan V. Rhabdomyosarcoma of the biliary tree. Pediatr Surg Int 1997; 12:200–201.
111. Pollono DG, Tomarchio S, Berghoff R, et al. Rhabdomyosarcoma of extrahepatic biliary tree: Initial treatment with chemotherapy and conservative surgery. Med Pediatr Oncol 1998; 30:290–293.

Chapter 56
Other diseases of the small intestine and colon

Elizabeth Gleghorn

HENOCH–SCHÖNLEIN PURPURA

Henoch–Schönlein purpura (HSP) shows an acute leukocytoclastic vasculitis that affects mostly children. Some 75–90% of affected children are less than 10 years of age,[1,2] although the reported age range is from 6 months to 86 years.[1] Heberden described the palpable purpuric lesions in 1801. The combination of purpura and arthritis was described by Schönlein in 1899, and Henoch added the descriptions of gastrointestinal disease and kidney lesions in 1874 and 1899.[3] The American College of Rheumatology established diagnostic criteria in 1990. Two of the following four criteria must be present:

1 Age less than 20 years at onset
2 Palpable purpura
3 Bowel angina (pain, ischemia or bloody diarrhea
4 Histologic evidence of leukocytes in the walls of arterioles or venules.

The presence of two or more criteria gives 87.1 % sensitivity and 87.7% specificity for HSP.[4] If the rash is absent or atypical, sepsis, polyarteritis nodosa, systemic lupus erythematosus and Wegener's granulomatosis could be considered.[1]

Clinical presentation

The rash – purpuric or urticarial – is the hallmark of the disease. It usually occurs on the extensor and dependent areas of the body (Fig. 56.1). The rash can also manifest as edema or hemorrhagic edema, especially in the youngest children.[5] Other manifestations may precede the rash. Arthritis occurs in 60–84% of patients. It involves noticeable swelling, usually in the knees and ankles.[6] The pain may be debilitating but the arthritis does not cause articular damage. Renal disease occurs in 20–100% of children,[1,6] and ranges from hematuria with or without proteinuria, to nephritis/nephrosis, to rapidly progressive crescentic glomerulonephritis. Renal disease presents the greatest risk of long-term health problems. The vasculitis may present with cerebral symptoms, commonly headache but also coma, seizures, paresis,[1] blindness[6] or cerebral hemorrhage.[3,6] Guillain–Barré syndrome, parotitis and carditis have also been reported.[1,6] Pulmonary findings include interstitial edema and loss of diffusing capacity as well as pulmonary hemorrhage. Scrotal edema and pain can imitate testicular torsion.[1] Priapism and other penile lesions have been reported.[3]

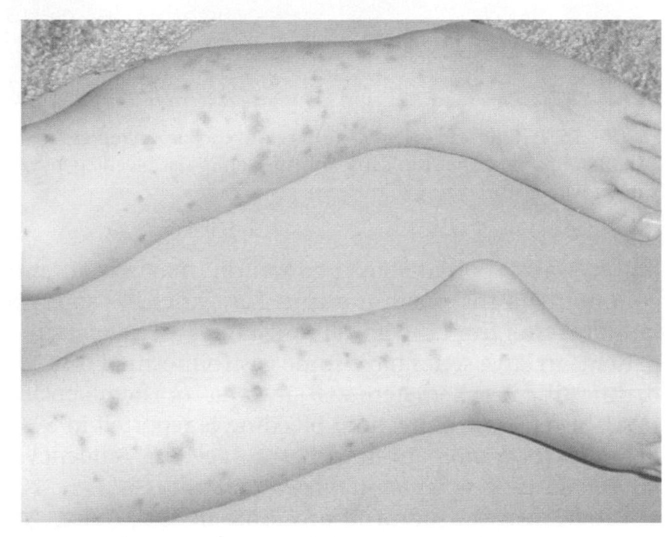

Figure 56.1: Palpable purpura on the back and legs of a four year old with abdominal pain from Henoch–Schönlein purpura. (See plate section for color)

Gastrointestinal disease occurs in 65–76% of patients.[1,6] Edema and hemorrhage of the bowel wall lead to severe colicky abdominal pain. The ultrasonographic correlation of uncomplicated pain shows mural thickening and hemorrhage. Plain films may show dilated, thickened bowel loops.[7] Contrast radiology, when employed, shows thickened mucosal folds and small barium flecks, presumably in small ulcers. Radiographic evidence of intramural hemorrhage may be present (Fig. 56.2). Endoscopic findings include ulceration, erythema, edema, hematoma-like protrusions and petechiae.[8,9] In 14–36% of patients, the rash may occur later in the course than the gastrointestinal manifestations, leading to diagnostic difficulties. Pain consistent with appendicitis can occur prior to the rash and lead to 'unnecessary' appendectomy. Vasculitis and hemorrhage of the abdominal wall musculature can occur, leading to severe pain that may be difficult to diagnose.[7]

Intussusception, with areas of hemorrhage and edema acting as the lead point, develops in 4–5% of cases. Intussusception associated with HSP, in contrast to the usual early childhood presentation, occurs in the small bowel in 58% of cases and at an average age of 6 years.[7] Paralytic ileus or pseudo-obstruction may occur,[7] most likely secondary to ischemia. On occasion this has necessitated parenteral nutrition support, but is usually transient.[7] Ischemia can clearly lead to infarction and necrosis of the

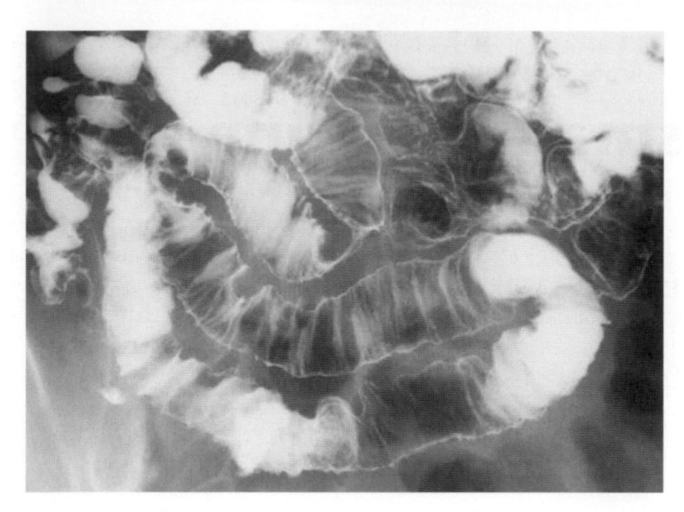

Figure 56.2: Characteristic protrusions into the lumen represent intramural purpura that can cause intussusception or bleeding in a patient with HSP.

bowel wall. Spontaneous perforation may occur, most commonly in the small intestine. Late strictures and fistulae may result from the bowel wall damage. Fifty percent of patients in large series have some gastrointestinal bleeding, manifesting as hematemesis, melena or heme-positive stool. Severe gastrointestinal bleeding is reported in 5% of patients. In combination with the bleeding tendency of renal failure, this can be life-threatening.[7]

Pancreatitis can occur at any time in the course, with vasculitis and hemorrhage.[7,10] Symptoms and laboratory findings are typical for pancreatitis of any cause and may mimic an acute abdomen. Gallbladder involvement, with hydrops or necrosis, has been reported, but is rare.[7]

Epidemiology

Estimates for the incidence of HSP range from 13.8 to 22.1 per 100 000.[1,3] Boys are affected more often than girls. Most patients are aged between 4 and 7 years, with a peak at 5 years.[9] HSP is more frequent from late fall through spring. It is often reported after viral or bacterial infections, but no one pathogen can be identified.[2,3] Medications have also been associated with HSP, probably from non-specific stimulation of the immune cascade.[9] Recurrent disease, often with abdominal pain, may occur in 3–40%, usually within the first year.[6] Renal disease is usually detected within the first 3–6 months.[11] Of all children with HSP, 1–5% progress to end-stage renal disease over time,[1,3,11] and to 18% may have mild renal impairment. Patients without early renal disease usually remain well, whereas those with severe renal disease at onset, severe abdominal pain or extended persistence of rash seem more likely to have kidney damage.[1,3,11–13] Women who have had HSP are especially likely to display renal symptoms when pregnant. Thus, all girls who have had HSP should be monitored carefully during pregnancy.[3,12]

The disease does occur in adults but more rarely, with an incidence of about 2 in 1 000 000. The male:female ratio is equal and there is no obvious seasonality in adult cases. Nephritis occurs in 20–40% and end-stage renal disease in 10–20%.[2] HSP may account for 5–15% of all cases of end-stage renal failure.[1]

Etiopathogenesis

HSP is a disorder of the inflammatory cascade leading to pathologic inflammation of blood vessels. There is probably an inciting immune stimulus, perhaps infectious. It most commonly involves abnormalities in IgA, with raised serum IgA levels, circulating IgA-containing immune complexes, and usually IgA deposition in blood vessel walls and in the kidney mesangium.[1,2,14] Factors that increase pathologic immune activation increase patient susceptibility to HSP.

Increased incidence has been described with mutations of the familial Mediterranean fever gene,[15] HLA-B35,[2] certain polymorphisms of interleukin-1 receptor antagonists,[16] and impaired regulation of pro- and anti-inflammatory cytokines.[17] Overall, aberrant glycosylation of IgA1 subclasses seems to lead to increased formation of immune complexes that are more likely to deposit in the kidney.[2] Understanding this phenomenon and its genetic substrate may ultimately help to identify individuals who are likely to develop renal disease. Abnormal nailfold capillaroscopy persisted for 16 months after diagnosis in one study, a finding that implies ongoing autoimmune activation in all patients.[18] Clearer understanding of the prognosis and need for therapy in HSP depends on further elucidation of the immune mechanisms.

Management

Management depends on recognition of the characteristic features of HSP and then monitoring for complications. If the rash and other extraintestinal features are absent, ultrasonography and occasionally contrast radiography can be helpful, although the findings may simply be edema. Biopsy of the endoscopic lesions may show characteristic leukocytoclastic vasculitis.[8] It is accepted that glucocorticoids will lessen the severity or duration of abdominal pain as well as the rash and the arthritis,[19,20] although this has not been subjected to prospective trial. Steroids are usually begun at 1 mg/kg daily and continued for a week, then tapered slowly. Most immunoactive medications have been used, from prednisone through cyclosporin, methotrexate, thalidomide[21] and plasmapheresis;[2] treatment is escalated when simple steroid therapy seems insufficient or the disease is prolonged. It is important to remember that steroids can mask catastrophic intra-abdominal events. Some authorities recommend ongoing ultrasonographic surveillance.[19,20] However, as significant surgical lesions occur in only 2–6% of patients,[22] it would seem more rational to follow patients clinically and perform imaging, either abdominal plain radiography or ultrasonography, for only the most worrisome patients. A combination of anti-inflammatory therapy to decrease the vasculitis and direct endoscopic or surgical intervention may be necessary to treat intussusception, perforation and massive gastrointestinal bleeding.[6] Repeat courses of steroids, other immunomodulators and intravenous immunoglobulin therapy[23] have been used for refractory recurrent illness.

The most vexing question of HSP is whether therapy can prevent or modify the long-term renal consequences. The issue is clouded by lack of controls and the fact that those with abdominal pain are both more likely to be treated with steroids and more likely to suffer renal disease.[11] Overall, it does seem that steroid therapy may ameliorate renal disease. More aggressive therapy with cyclophosphamide, dipyridamole, warfarin, or combinations, may have greater effect. The use of fish oil supplements, tonsilectomy, or angiotensin-converting enzyme (ACE) inhibitors is not supported by the literature.[11]

ACRODERMATITIS ENTEROPATHICA

This autosomal recessive disorder was recognized as a zinc deficiency in the mid-1970s by Moynahan, Barnes, Michaelsson and Thyresson.[24] Investigation of the inherited disease and its clinical imitators has helped to illuminate the complicated biologic role of zinc. Primary acrodermatitis enteropathica occurs mostly in formula-fed infants or in children weaned from the breast. The full-fledged disease includes a characteristic acro-orificial rash, alopecia and diarrhea. Lesions at the corners of the eyes and mouth and in the perineum can spread rapidly to a weeping desquamation. Poor weight gain, stunting, susceptibility to infection, sepsis, and even death can occur. Response to large (5–10 mg/kg daily) oral doses of zinc is immediate. The need for zinc supplementation is lifelong because the underlying defect is profoundly depressed zinc absorption. Zinc in breast milk has a much greater bioavailability than zinc in formula or cow's milk,[25] which leads to the typical weanling onset of the disease. Zinc deficiency can also occur because of a zinc-deficient diet or the ingestion of large amounts of phytates and other compounds that interfere with zinc absorption.[25] Abnormal zinc losses can occur in diarrhea with Crohn's disease, celiac disease and cystic fibrosis, and in urine in some liver diseases, diabetes mellitus, sickle cell disease, nephritic syndrome and any disease with high metabolic stress. The requirement for zinc in severe illness or tissue repair, such as premature infants, postsurgical patients or those with multiple episodes of infection, may outstrip the dietary supply and lead to acquired symptoms of acrodermatitis enteropathica, which may be subtle.[25] Conditions due to mild to moderate zinc deficiency include short stature, poor appetite, abnormalities of the immune system (especially T-cell function),[26] a variety of skin and nail conditions, behavioral problems including irritability and withdrawal, delayed sexual maturation or impaired reproductive performance, eye lesions and delayed wound healing.

The originally reported patients with inherited acrodermatitis enteropathica had low plasma zinc levels. However, because of the volatile nature of zinc homeostasis, this is not a universal finding. Plasma zinc concentrations below 60 μg/dl may occur in moderate to severe zinc deficiency, but can also occur as a result of stress, infection or pregnancy.[25] Alternatively, symptoms of zinc deficiency, and response to zinc therapy, may occur in children with normal serum or plasma zinc levels. Alkaline phosphatase levels may be depressed in zinc deficiency and are often used as a surrogate test. However, this is not at all specific or sensitive because there are other conditions that involve altered alkaline phosphatase levels. Determination of hair zinc concentration has been suggested as a diagnostic tool, but is unreliable in young children and in those with severe disease with arrest of hair growth. Measurement of urine zinc levels is insensitive. Response to therapy remains the best diagnostic tool.[25]

Pathobiology

There are more than 100 zinc metalloenzymes, involved in every major enzyme classification.[25] These include alkaline phosphatase, alcohol dehydrogenase, carbonic anhydrase and DNA polymerase. 'Zinc fingers', which are zinc-complexed conformations of nuclear DNA-binding proteins, are the most frequent binding motif for transcription factor proteins[25] and are essential to all gene expression. Zinc stabilizes polysomes during protein synthesis and stabilizes the biomembranes of circulating cellular elements.[27] The essential involvement of zinc in these basic processes of life offers a rationale for the long list of disorders associated with zinc deficiency.

The defect in primary acrodermatitis enteropathica has been localized to 8q24.3 by homozygosity mapping.[28,29] This gene encodes a protein that is a member of the ZIP family of metallotransporters.[29] ZIP4 appears to be abnormal in congenital acrodermatitis enteropathica.[29] Several different mutations in SLC39A4 have been found in different acrodermatitis enteropathica families.[30] Normal ZIP4 appears to be upregulated in conditions of low zinc availability, either by increased transcription or increased expression on the cell membrane.[29] ZIP4 appears to function in the upper small intestine, where zinc absorption occurs. Some breast milk is actually deficient in zinc, implying the occasional occurrence of an abnormal ZIP protein in breast tissue.[25]

HEMOLYTIC UREMIC SYNDROME

Hemolytic uremic syndrome (HUS) consists of a microangiopathic hemolytic anemia with some degree of thrombocytopenia and uremia. Some 90% of cases of this syndrome in children follow a diarrheal illness, often with blood in the stool. Most of these cases occur in children under the age of 5 years. This type (called D^+ HUS by most writers) is, of course, more interesting to gastroenterologists. The cause of this syndrome is usually a Shiga-like toxin. In the USA, most of the cases are due to enterotoxigenic *Escherichia coli* type O157:H7(31). Other *E. coli* strains have been identified, more frequently in other countries, but probably accounting for 25% of cases in the USA.[32]

Other bacteria and viruses have also been linked to this disorder. Non-diarrheal HUS may be caused by bacterial infections in other locations or by other causes of increased thrombotic tendency, such as pregnancy, certain drugs and inherited susceptibility. These 'endemic' cases tend to have more severe consequences than the 'epidemic' postdiarrheal form. Between 276 and 736 new cases of HUS occur in the USA each year, leading to 24–63 patients needing chronic dialysis or a transplant.

Pathogenesis

Causal bacteria for D+ HUS attach to enterocytes via the intestinal adherence factor intimin. This causes effacement of villi and induces water and electrolyte efflux, producing the early watery diarrhea. A Shiga-like toxin, also called verocytotoxin, causes the major symptoms of this illness. The toxin binds via its B subunits to galactose disaccharides in globotriasylceramide (GB3) receptors in the membranes of glomerular, colonic and cerebral epithelial or microvascular endothelial cells, renal mesangial and tubular cells, platelets and monocytes. Subjects vary in the amount of GB3 receptor that is present in different tissues. This may account for some of the variability in susceptibility to gastrointestinal, kidney and nervous system disease.[33] Binding stimulates secretion of cytokines and chemoattractants, and also activates platelets. The toxin is internalized into the cell. The A subunit binds enzymatically to ribosomes, ending protein synthesis and eventually causing cell death. Damage to vascular endothelial cells in the susceptible tissues leads to localized clotting, intravascular hemolysis and platelet trapping. Microangiopathic damage is seen first in the intestine and later in the kidney. There is direct cellular damage as well.

Clinical presentation

The usual clinical prodrome for D+ HUS is an acute gastroenteritis with vomiting, abdominal pain, fever and watery diarrhea. In about 70%, bloody diarrhea follows. Diarrhea can last for weeks. The hemolysis and uremia occur within 5–14 days of the initial illness.[34] The child is pale, lethargic, sometimes jaundiced, and oliguric. In 10%, a seizure will herald the uremia.[34] There is intravascular hemolysis, burr cells, raised plasma hemoglobin levels and hyperbilirubinemia, and a negative Coombs' test. Platelets usually fall to 20 000–100 000 per μl, and the white count may be increased. HUS occurs in 8–31% of patients infected with *E. coli* 0157:H7.[31] Some 10–30% of these develop chronic renal disease and 5% die from the acute illness.[32] HUS is the most common cause of acute renal failure in children in many countries. Not surprisingly, the severity of disease at presentation predicts the seriousness of sequelae.

Imaging studies and gross pathology demonstrate mucosal and submucosal hemorrhage and edema in the intestine (Fig. 56.3). Barium enema may show spasm and ulceration. Both small and large intestine may be involved, although the colon suffers the majority of the significant damage. Some 10% of patients have rectal prolapse. There

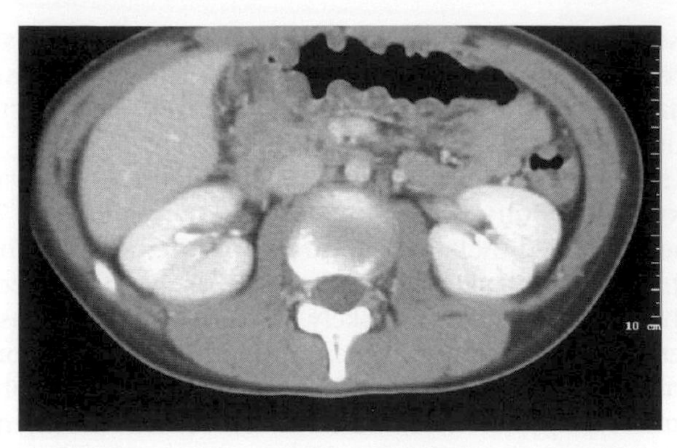

Figure 56.3: Edema of the bowel wall produces the characteristic thumbprinting in hemolytic uremic syndrome.

may be jaundice, petechiae, purpura and lethargy. Ulcerative colitis, Crohn's disease, intussusception and appendicitis may be considered early in the course of the illness. The acute nature of the illness and the usually young age of the patients make inflammatory bowel disease less likely. There are surgical complications in 2–7%, including intussusception, severe colitis, sigmoid volvulus, rectal prolapse and intestinal perforation. The surgical literature points out that, if there is perforation, it usually occurs 10 days or more after the onset of illness.[35] Colitis usually resolves, but colectomy or colostomy has been required in up to 2% of cases. There have been reports of late stricture formation in 3%.[34] Other gastrointestinal complications include raised levels of transaminases in 40% and increased lipase or amylase levels in 20%.[34] Ongoing diabetes mellitus occurs in 8%.[34]

Cultures should be performed in cases of serious bloody diarrhea and D+ HUS. *E. coli* strains, such as O111:H− in Australia and O26:H11 in Germany, have caused the syndrome. The verocytotoxin for HUS is plasmid encoded, allowing for transfer to other *E. coli* or even other species. In Germany, a *Citrobacter freundii* making this toxin caused a kindergarten outbreak of HUS. The major reservoir for *E. coli* 0157:H7 is cattle, for which it is normal flora, colonizing up to 44% of beef cattle awaiting slaughter. A single meatpacking plant can send food all over the USA, so outbreaks can be widespread. Ground meat, in which the pathogen can be mixed throughout the entire lot, is most likely to spread infection. Larger solid cuts of meat are more easily sterilized in the usual cooking process. An interesting approach to reducing the burden of colonization is to alter feeding practices for beef cattle. Changing to hay rather than grain for 5 days prior to slaughter decreases fecal *E. coli* markedly. Healthcare professionals are increasingly aware of unusual sources of *E. coli* transmission, such as raw vegetables and juices, as well as lakes and pools. The incidence of the illness is higher in the summer months, corresponding to higher colonization in cattle and presumably higher exposure to environmental water sources and raw vegetables.

It is generally accepted that antibiotic treatment of the diarrhea should be withheld because it may increase the likelihood of uremia. Fosfomycin has been shown to increase release of verocytotoxin from *E. coli in vitro*.[36] However, it is not clear whether this occurs in a clinically meaningful way. Antibiotic treatment did not seem to increase the risk of HUS in the 1993 Jack-in-the-Box outbreak, and actually seemed protective in an outbreak in Japan in 1996.[32] It is not obvious that antibiotics would be helpful in treating the colitis, in which the damage may have already occurred. It has been shown that antibiotic therapy does not shorten the diarrheal illness. Thus, except for rare cases of sepsis, it seems safer to not treat.[31,34,37] Physicians considering antibiotics for non-bloody diarrhea in children should bear in mind the possible prodrome relationship before treating. A randomized prospective study addressing this question is unlikely to occur because of the numbers needed and the ethical dilemmas involved.

RADIATION ENTERITIS

Radiation therapy is an effective agent for the treatment of malignancy. In pediatric oncology, it is used for leukemia, intracranial malignancy, Wilm's tumor, sarcoma and preparation for bone marrow transplant, among other indications.[38] Children may be more susceptible to the acute effects of radiation therapy, most likely because more of their tissues are actively growing. The intestine is quite sensitive to radiation, also because of rapid cell turnover. Radiation injury occurs through free radical formation from water in the irradiated tissue.[39] The free radicals disrupt DNA, leading to cell death as replication proceeds. The therapeutic goal is to cause more damage to tumor tissue than to healthy tissue. However, the therapeutic dose range, which maximizes tumor cell death, is often close to the toxic dose range for the tissue.[39] Sequelae of radiation to the intestine occur acutely, and in a more chronic phase within the next year or even delayed for a decade or more.[39–42]

The acute consequences of radiation to the abdomen are visible as a sequence of histologic changes.[41] Damage to the small intestine is obvious in the first 12 h. Over the first week, cell loss exceeds the mitotic ability of the crypt cells to regenerate new cells. The villi of the small intestine shorten and disaccharidases are lost. Edema and inflammation follow, leading to loss of absorptive capacity.[41] Bile salt malabsorption leads to cholerectic diarrhea. Damage to the rectum is similar. Crypt abscesses in the rectum may contain a high proportion of eosinophils, suggesting a localized allergic-type response, although the target is unclear.[41]

Intravenous nutrition is now used routinely to support the child through mucositis, diarrhea and anorexia. Some 70% of children subjected to radiotherapy in one early study exhibited diarrhea and vomiting during the course of radiation; 30% of these were severe enough to require intervention to maintain fluid and electrolyte balance. Fifty percent of children had weight loss.[40] There is abdominal pain, bloating and tenesmus. Radiographic studies may show dilation of bowel loops, wall edema and loss of normal motility. Patients are treated empirically with lactose restriction or hypoallergenic diet, proton pump inhibitors, bile acid-binding resins, loperamide and probiotics. Hydrophilic stool softeners, steroid enemas and Sitz baths are used for proctitis. Kinsella and Bloomer[41] showed normalization of tests of malabsorption after 1 year, whereas others found that most patients had permanent late alterations in bowel habit even though they did not voice any complaints.[43,44] Some authors feel that patients who had more severe symptoms early on are more likely to have late complications.

Donaldson et al.[40] described subacute damage in 11% of radiated children in the 2–12 months after therapy. These children presented with obstructive symptoms of vomiting and diarrhea as well as radiographic evidence of obstruction. There was an inflammatory infiltrate in the intestine with lymphangiectasia and villous atrophy. Exuberant fibrosis and adhesions caused the obstruction; vascular damage was not mentioned.

Later complications of radiation therapy are a consequence of ischemia. There is an obliterative endarteritis and fibrosis leading to ulceration, necrosis, perforation and stricture.[41] Some 85% of patients with these problems present within 2 years, although the remainder may exhibit symptoms 15 or more years later.[42] Proctitis with tenesmus and bleeding is the major symptom in 75% of patients. The diagnosis is made on endoscopy, which shows erythema, edema, friability and often numerous telangiectasiae.[39] There may be deep ulceration. Alternatively, the mucosa may be thin, translucent and clearly extremely fragile.[41] Bleeding tends to be difficult to treat, but is self-limiting in about 80% of adults. In adults, a transfusion requirement predicts a low rate of remission and substantial mortality. Treatment for proctitis includes enemas of 2 g sucralfate suspended in 4% methylcellulose, hyperbaric oxygen and the use of an argon laser for coagulation of the telangiectasiae.[45] In adult patients, ulcers are also treated with instilation of a 4% solution of formaldehyde directly into the rectum or applied with gauze sponges. Studies show no evidence that mesalamine or steroids are helpful either orally or rectally.[45] Surgical resection of the rectum for severe bleeding is more effective than diversion, but all surgical procedures are subject to high complication rates. Better results are obtained when it is possible to use non-irradiated bowel for any anastomosis or stoma formation.[39]

Other late consequences of radiation stem from bowel fibrosis, which causes stricture formation. Fistulization and perforation are less common. Bacterial overgrowth may occur in the relatively stagnant loop, leading to irritant diarrhea, vitamin B_{12} loss, and destruction to villi with accompanying disaccharidase deficiency and loss of intraluminal bile salts due to deconjugation and early reabsorption. Malabsorption of sugars and fat leads to diarrhea and fat-soluble vitamin deficiency. The scarred intestine may have abnormal motility, leading to rapid intestinal transit, or perhaps to ileus or a functional motility disorder.[44] Therapy should be directed at the most likely cause of the symptoms and carried out systematically. Empiric medication and diet change are the same as for acute radiation reaction, but may need to be continued indefinitely.[45] Nutritional supplementation may be crucial. If strictures cause only low-grade symptoms, surgery should be avoided if possible. The same problems with anastomosing radiated bowel occur in these situations.

Damage to the bowel and later consequences are increased by several different factors, some of which can be modified.[38] Normally the intestine, except for the rectum, is constantly moving during the application of radiation. This diminishes the point exposure time of any one segment and decreases damage. Bowel that is fixed by previous inflammation or surgery is less mobile and therefore more vulnerable. It is possible to place a polyglycolic acid mesh sling to raise the small bowel out of the range of pelvic irradiation, thus preventing much of the damage.[46] Certain chemotherapeutic drugs, such as 5-fluorouracil, doxorubicin, actinomycin D and methotrexate, increase the risk of enteritis.[41] Newer treatment protocols may avoid using these agents or may time the dosing to allow maximal recovery of normal tissue while causing maximal damage to tumor cells.[38] Advances in radiation therapy technique permit targeting of therapy directly to small areas and scaling doses to the size of individual children. There is new research into medications that protect normal tissues from radiation (amifostine or ethylol, amongst others) and into techniques that preferentially sensitize tumor cells to the radiation.[38] Once fully developed and implemented, these techniques will help to prevent a large proportion of radiation damage to the intestine.

MALAKOPLAKIA

Malakoplakia is a rare and poorly understood chronic inflammatory process that seems to occur mostly in the setting of some type of immunodeficiency.[47] Michaelis and Gutmann, and their mentor Von Hansemann, described it almost simultaneously in the early 1900s.[48,49] About 75% of cases involve the genitourinary tract, with about 200 described in the intestine.[50] The disorder presents as friable yellow plaques or polypoid lesions on the mucosa of the gastrointestinal tract, sometimes with narrowing or stricturing of the colon. Fistulae can occur. There may be bleeding, pain or obstructive symptoms. The plaques can grow very large and may present as an abdominal or rectal mass (Fig. 56.4). Anemia, raised erythrocyte sedimentation rate, leukocytosis, night sweats and fatigue may be present.[50] Large masses concentrate gallium in nuclear medicine scanning.[47] The most common site of involvement in the gastrointestinal tract is the rectum, with the sigmoid and right colon being less common. Most examples of malakoplakia occur in middle age, but there is a small peak in childhood.[50]

The diagnosis of malakoplakia is made by the characteristic pathology. Abnormal phagocytic macrophages (von Hansemann cells) can be shown on electron microscopy to contain lysosomes swollen with partially degraded bacteria. Michaelis–Gutmann bodies, lamelated basophilic collections of calcified mucopolysaccharides and lipids that are similar to bacterial cell walls, must be evident in the lysosomes to substantiate the diagnosis (Fig. 56.5).[47]

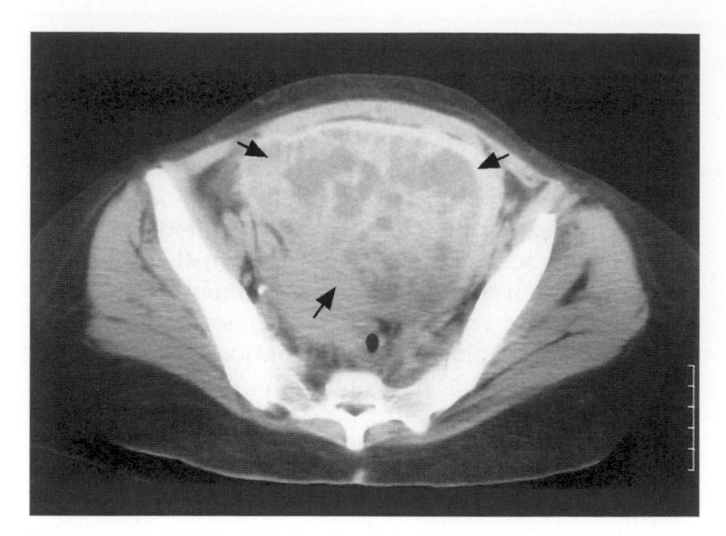

Figure 56.4: Malakoplakia – a large non-homogeneous mass with internal septa and peripheral enhancement seen on CT with intravenous contrast.

The ultramicroscopic appearance of the lesion gives a clue as to the pathogenesis of the problem, which is still poorly understood. There seems to be defective bacterial killing, as a result of a primary disease state or immunosuppressive medication. In many of the cases, *E. coli* has been cultured. *Mycobacterium tuberculosis*, *Proteus* and *Klebsiella* have also been cultured, but many lesions do not yield any organisms despite the fragments of bacteria therein.[47] The disease has been reported in patients taking prednisone or azathioprine. In these cases, withdrawal of the medications led to resolution. Other patients have had hypogammaglobulinemia, IgA deficiency, acquired immune deficiency syndrome (AIDS) or neoplasm.[50] One patient was found to have a selective defect in killing *Proteus* and *Salmonella*.[48] It has been theorized that deficient cyclic guanosine monophosphate (cGMP) in the macrophage could lead to deficient fusion of lysosomes with phagosomes containing bacterial products.[47,50] Overall, this could lead to incomplete bacterial killing and ongoing inflammation. There is a substantial mortality

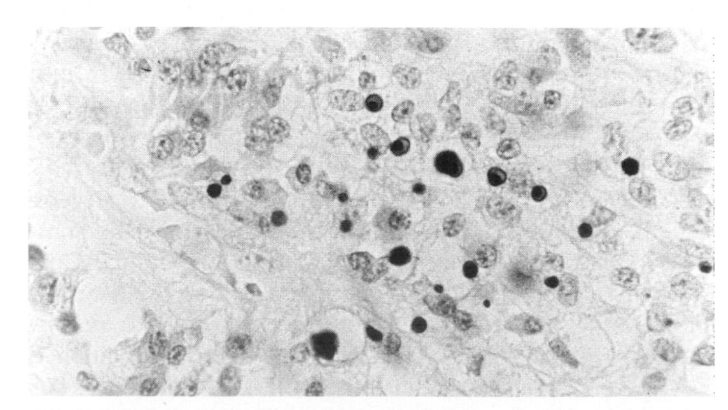

Figure 56.5: Light microscopy of malakoplakia. Xanthogranulomatous inflammation in an area of malakoplakia, showing clear phagocytic cells (von Hansemann cells) surrounding dense black dots (Michaelis–Gutmann bodies).

rate in adult series: up to 80% of untreated patients and 15% for all cases.[47] Therapy with a cholinergic agent, bethanechol, to increase cGMP levels, has occasionally been helpful. Ascorbic acid is thought to be synergistic with this therapy, by increasing cGMP levels. More frequently, therapy with trimethoprim–sulfamethoxazole or quinolones, antibiotics that are internally concentrated by macrophages, results in cure of the lesion. Surgical removal of large mass lesions may aid cure.[47]

BEHÇET'S SYNDROME

Behçet's disease is a chronically recurring inflammatory disorder of unknown cause. It occurs most frequently along the ancient Silk Route, which extends from the Far East through the Middle East to the Mediterranean, the trade route taken by Marco Polo on his voyage to Cathay. The prevalence of Behçet's syndrome in Western countries is low: 0.64 per 100 000 population in the UK and 0.12–0.33 per 100 000 in the USA. The disease is more common in Japan, Korea, China, Saudi Arabia and Iran (13.5–20 cases per 100 000), but is rare in Japanese immigrants to the USA.[51] It has been reported to occur in clusters in families, up to 15% in the Middle East but only 2–5% elsewhere. It is more common in females in the Far East and in males in the Middle East. Monozygotic twin pairs have been reported, both concordant and discordant. Both environment and genetics are important in the epidemiology of the condition.[52]

Behçet's syndrome is a vasculitis that causes lesions in many different organ systems. There are no pathognomonic findings, so the diagnosis depends on the presence of major and minor manifestations as defined by the International Study Group for Behçet's Disease. In some patients, the interesting phenomenon of pathergy can help make the diagnosis. Pathergy is a characteristic reaction to sterile needle disturbance of the skin, joint or eye. Pathergy is a characteristic reaction to sterile needle disturbance of the skin, joint or eye. Pathergy is a characteristic reaction to sterile needle disturbance of the skin, joint or eye. The manifestations may occur over the course of years. The condition is quite rare in children, in part because the diagnostic symptoms may not appear rapidly enough to meet the definition until the child is older. Gastrointestinal disease is more common in children than in adults, whereas ocular disease is much less common.[51]

Oral ulcers, occurring in 70–90% of subjects with Behçet's disease, are painful round lesions with a sharp erythematous border, covered by a yellow pseudomembrane. These occur on the buccal and labial mucosa, the tongue and the gingiva. The ulcers heal in 7–14 days without scarring; recurrence of lesions is the norm. Oral ulcers may be the first symptom of Behçet's disease, but can occur in up to 10% of normal persons. *Genital ulcers,* of similar frequency, occur on the vulva, scrotum and penis. They are painful, deeper and more serpiginous than the oral lesions. They heal within 2 weeks with scarring, and may also recur periodically.[51]

Ocular lesions are usually the most serious problem in Behçet's disease in adults, occurring in 80%. Only 20% of children develop this manifestation of the disease. Symptoms include pain, blurring, photophobia, floaters, tearing and redness. Uveitis may be recurrent, and eventually leads to scarring of the iris and glaucoma. Occlusive vascular disease results in a painless decrease in visual acuity. Hypopyon, inflammatory cells layering out in the anterior chamber, is a visible characteristic, but can also occur in spondyloarthropathy.[51] A number of different *skin lesions* are associated with Behçet's syndrome. Erythema nodosum, pseudofolliculitis, acneiform nodules and migratory thrombophlebitis occur.[51]

Minor criteria include gastrointestinal disease, arthritis and neurologic disease. *Intestinal symptoms* include nonspecific pain, vomiting, diarrhea, flatulence and constipation. There can be more serious disease, with bloody diarrhea, perforation and fistulae. The radiographic signs are thickened folds, mucosal ulcerations, deformation of bowel loops and fistulae. The gut disease resembles ulcerative colitis histologically, but can occur in the ileum (25%) and esophagus (12%). Granulomas are absent, but differentiation from the classic inflammatory bowel diseases can be difficult. The bowel lesions are deeper than in ulcerative colitis and the ulcers seem more isolated than in Crohn's disease. Gastrointestinal involvement varies in different geographic populations, being rare in patients in Turkey and in Caucasian patients in the West, but occurring in up to 15% of patients in Japan.[51] *Arthritis* in Behçet's disease is usually non-destructive, involving the large joints. Acneiform lesions and arthritis seem to occur together in the same patient, with the same severity and timing.

Neurologic disease, occurring in up to 20% of Behçet's patients, can be useful in differentiating this from other inflammatory bowel diseases. Acute aseptic meningitis or meningoencephalitis may occur early on, but is more frequent 5 years or more into the illness. There are brainstem symptoms and motor problems as well as personality changes. Cranial nerve palsies, pseudotumor cerebri, thromboses and seizures can occur. Irreversible damage and dementia may evolve in 30% of affected patients. Magnetic resonance imaging shows typical multiple high-intensity focal lesions in the brainstem, white matter and basal ganglia.[51]

Diffuse vascular disease can cause serious problems in Behçet's disease, including thrombophlebitis, large vessel aneurysms, infarction and organ failure. Coronary vasculitis and valvular disease may occur. Dyspnea, cough, chest pain and hemoptysis can result from pulmonary vasculitis.[51] A hypersensitivity reaction occurs at the needle track, causing a papule or pustule, synovitis or panophthalmitis, lesions filled with activated neutrophils.[51,52]

Etiopathogenesis

Behçet's disease may more accurately be described as a syndrome[52] because of the lack of homogeneity in its manifestations and even in its treatments. The disease is frequently associated with HLA-B51 in the Silk Route countries: up to 80% in Asian patients and 55% in Japan. Japanese carriers of HLA-B51 have a relative risk of 6.7 for Behçet's disease, but only a 1.3 risk in the USA. HLA-B51 seems to be associated with a high prevalence and severity of eye and neurologic disease in Asia, but severe disease does occur without it. Other manifestations vary with geography. Intestinal involvement is common in the Far East but not the Middle East. Pathergy is frequent in the Mediterranean but not in Europe. Some treatments are effective for female but not male patients, whereas other treatments help some symptoms and exacerbate others.[52]

Behçet's disease seems to be a disease of cells rather than of circulating factors.[52] Neutrophils and lymphocytes function abnormally in Behçet's syndrome. Neutrophils are excessively active, leading to tissue injury through the release of tumor necrosis factor, interleukin 1β and interleukin 8. Lymphocytes home specifically to abnormal self-proteins derived from heat shock proteins. These self-proteins are present in the affected tissues of Behçet's patients, but not in unaffected persons. They seem to resemble bacterial heat shock proteins but are different from the abnormal heat shock proteins of rheumatoid arthritis.[51] Vasculitis is found near all of the characteristic lesions. Endothelial cells and platelets are activated. Despite the tendency to thrombosis, circulating levels of thrombophilic factors are normal.[53] Behçet's disease has also been associated with microbial infections, but no one organism is found in all subjects. Instead, it seems that cross-reactivity to self may be an important mechanism in this, as in many similar diseases. However, some syndromes that commonly accompany other autoimmune diseases, such as Raynaud's phenomenon and autoantibodies, are absent in Behçet's syndrome.[52]

Therapy

Treatment depends on the type of involvement. Medications are usually those directed against autoimmune reactions. Treatment of the most serious lesions in the eyes, gut and nervous system, and those causing large vessel disease, takes precedence.[51]

Colchicine, steroids, azathioprine, chlorambucil and cyclophosphamide are used for ocular lesions. Unfortunately, 10–25% of patients still progress to blindness. Cyclosporin is also used, but has a declining response over time. Interferon α2a has been used with greater success, but data are limited. Gastrointestinal disease can be treated like Crohn's disease, with salicylates and steroids. Disease can be recurrent. Acute neurologic disease responds to corticosteroids, whereas chronic disease may be refractory. Large-vessel pulmonary disease can be fatal if hemoptysis begins; steroids, antiplatelet drugs and (sometimes and with caution) anticoagulants are used.[51,52] Because of the involvement of tumor necrosis factor, thalidomide and infliximab have been used in a few cases, with success.[54]

TYPHLITIS

Also known as neutropenic enterocolitis and ileocecal syndrome, this ulcerating disease of the intestine occurs in patients who are profoundly neutropenic from chemotherapy for malignancy or from other drug therapy. It has also occurred in AIDS, aplastic anemia or from leukemia itself.[55,56] Typhlitis has been described most often in children, perhaps because their chemotherapeutic regimens have traditionally been very intense. Some authors suggest that adults are experiencing an increasing incidence as their therapeutic regimens are made more toxic. Postmortem series from large pediatric oncology services collecting cases up to the 1990s documented typhlitis in 10–24% of autopsied children.[57] Early series allow a crude estimate of overall incidence to be 5% of all pediatric patients treated for leukemia.[57,58] Case fatality rates for this problem seemed high in the beginning; cases were often recognized clinically because of complications that necessitated surgery. Operation was attempted but was often unsuccessful because the children were already moribund. Since then, greater awareness of the symptom complex has enabled clinicians to suspect the illness in its early presentations. More accurate imaging has most likely expanded the discovery and allowed earlier, more effective therapy.[58–60]

Symptoms of typhlitis include abdominal pain, which may be diffuse and localized to the right lower quadrant, or may be absent, most likely due to concomitant corticosteroid therapy. There is usually fever, abdominal distention, nausea and vomiting. Constipation may occur, but diarrhea is more common. There may be gross blood in the stool. In most cases, chemotherapy was given 2–4 weeks prior to the onset of typhlitis.[58,60,61] The absolute neutrophil count is usually less than 5000 per μl. Plain films may show thumbprinting of the colon, a dilated fluid-filled cecum, a soft tissue mass in the right lower quadrant, pneumatosis or absence of air in most of the colonic lumen. Barium enema is now felt to be contraindicated, but would show ileus, small bowel obstruction and 'non-filling' of the colon. Ultrasonography has given way to routine abdominal computed tomography (CT), which may demonstrate edema of the colon, inflammation surrounding the colon and in the mesenteric fat, and sometimes pneumatosis.[55,57,59,62] The differential diagnosis includes appendicitis, perforation from other cause, and volvulus or intussusception. It is not clear that any particular chemotherapeutic regimen is more likely to give rise to this complication.[59,62]

Autopsy and surgical findings show dilation, edema and hemorrhage of the bowel, with frank necrosis sometimes evident. The cecum alone may be involved, but other portions of the bowel, including appendix, ileum and ascending colon, or sporadic involvement of any portion of the intestine, can be seen in varied combinations.[58] Ulceration and diffuse necrotizing loss of the mucosa are seen. There is little inflammatory infiltrate, and leukemic infiltrate is not usually seen. Fungal or bacterial forms are frequently found in the necrotic tissue. Blood cultures are positive for bacteria in 70–80% of patients and for fungus in about 30%. Bacteria include *Pseudomonas, Staphylococcus aureus, E. coli* and *α-Streptococcus*.[55,57,58,61]

The pathogenesis of typhlitis is unclear. Many of the chemotherapeutic regimens cause ileus as well as damage to the gastrointestinal mucosa. In combination with leukopenia or the immunoincompetence of leukemic cells, bacterial invasion of the bowel wall can occur. Subsequent toxin production could lead to further bowel wall damage and vascular compromise.[57,62] The cecum may be more vulnerable because of its watershed location, as in neonatal necrotizing enterocolitis – in some ways a similar situation.

Therapy of typhlitis begins prospectively with vigilance for the symptoms of fever and pain. Prompt CT may reveal suspicious findings. The patient is placed on bowel rest, often with nasogastric suction. Parenteral nutrition is usually started and antibiotics are begun, if not already used. Immunosuppressants should be weaned if possible. Antifungal therapy is often started if fever does not decrease within 2–3 days. Filgrastim (granulocyte colony-stimulating factor) is given, based on the observation that regaining a leukocyte count to greater than 1000 dl correlates with survival.[55,57,60,61] Laparoscopy should be performed when there is clinical suspicion of necrosis or CT evidence of perforation. The mortality rate in early series was 50% or greater,[55,60] but with earlier recognition and more effective therapy is now falling below 10%.[55] Because repeated courses of chemotherapy often bring on repeated bouts of typhlitis, prophylactic colectomy has been recommended for children who have suffered this once and need further cytotoxic therapy.[57]

LYMPHOCYTIC AND COLLAGENOUS COLITIS

These disorders present mostly in middle-aged women who are symptomatic with copious watery, non-bloody diarrhea and cramping abdominal pain. Biopsies show an inflammatory infiltrate in the lamina propria. Lymphocytes predominate over plasma cells, mast cells and eosinophils. Lymphocytes also infiltrate the crypts and the surface epithelium, and should account for more than 10–25% of surface epithelial cells.[63] Subepithelial type I or III collagen layers vary in thickness in both of these conditions. There may be marked variation in an individual patient. Biopsy findings of these diseases are sparse and discontinuous, adding to the difficulty of characterizing the findings in individual patients as well as in compiling meaningful case series.[64] Thus, there is controversy as to whether these are truly distinct diseases. The etiology is also unclear. Various medications, including non-steroidal anti-inflammatory medications, and autoimmune conditions are associated with the biopsy findings in adults.

Lymphocytic colitis (LC) and collagenous colitis (CC) are uncommon in children. There are case series showing LC in children with regressive autism, although the characteristic symptom of profuse diarrhea was not always reported.[65,66] A child with neurologic disease developed LC after carbamazepine.[63] Classic LC/CC was seen in a small case series in which recovery occurred over the course of a year.[67] A third series showed patients with a similar presentation evolving into more classic inflammatory bowel disease.[68] Up to 30% of children with celiac disease also have LC/CC.[69] All series emphasize the dictum that tends to distinguish pediatric from adult endoscopists: systematic biopsies throughout the entire colon are indicated in children when non-specific symptoms of diarrhea prompt endoscopy, even if the mucosa is grossly normal.[70]

In childhood, as in adulthood, therapy for these diseases is unclear. Celiac disease should be excluded and possible causal medications stopped. Cholestyramine, bismuth subsalicylate and sulfasalazine are safe medications that have helped some patients. Prednisone and budesonide have been useful in adults[71] and could be tried in children.

EHLERS–DANLOS SYNDROME

This is a group of heritable diseases of collagen formation. The vascular type of Ehlers–Danlos syndrome (EDS) is characterized by mutations in the *COL3A1* gene on chromosome 2q31, which leads to synthesis of abnormal type III procollagen molecules that are not secreted normally out of the cell. This type of collagen is widespread in the body, present in skin, blood vessels, bowel and solid organs. Lack of this collagen leads to thin, tight skin, easy scarring, excessive mobility of joints, frequent breakage of blood vessels and easy bruising. Rupture of large blood vessels is common. Patients frequently die from vascular complications before the end of their fifth decade. Further symptoms outside the gastrointestinal tract include aneurysm and fistula formation, diaphragmatic hernia, joint dislocation, cardiac abnormalities and hypospadias. Pregnancy can end in uterine rupture. Fetuses with the syndrome may be premature and of low birthweight.[72]

EDS is inherited in an autosomal dominant fashion, but almost half of cases appear to be new mutations.[72,73] Characteristic features of this type are a thin face, narrow pinched nose, thin lips, prominent eyes, asthenic habitus, easily visible vessels, and hands that appear elderly in childhood. The symptoms may be subtle in early childhood and a dangerous complication may be the first sign.[74] Diagnosis depends on awareness of the physical findings, a possible family history of vascular rupture, and the culture of skin fibroblasts. These cultured cells secrete reduced quantities or abnormal variants of type III collagen. Messenger RNA sequencing shows an abnormal gene.[72] Ultrastructural examination of involved tissues shows reduced amounts of type III collagen, and broken and fragmented elastic fibers.[73]

The major intestinal complication of this disorder is spontaneous perforation of the bowel. The most common location of perforation is the colon, especially the sigmoid. Multiple perforations are not uncommon. Sutures easily rip out of repaired tissues; wound infection and poor healing is common.[72,73] It is recommended that emergency surgery for perforation should consist of exteriorization of the perforation, or resection and end-colostomy with closure or mucous colostomy of the distal portion.[72] Many children who had closure of the bowel have had recurrent perforation.[72,75] Therefore, a permanent colostomy is recommended.[72,75,76] Other gastrointestinal symptoms include constipation, diverticulosis, gastrointestinal bleeding and perhaps dysmotility.[76]

PNEUMATOSIS INTESTINALIS

This interesting condition was first described in 1730 by DuVernoi and documented in humans by Bang in 1730.[77] This radiographic finding has an ominous meaning to most pediatricians, based on its frequent occurrence in moribund premature infants with necrotizing enterocolitis. However, the condition is much more widespread and less dangerous overall than is commonly appreciated.[78–82]

Intraluminal gas in the intestine may be detected on plain abdominal radiography, by ultrasonography, endoscopically and even found incidentally on histologic examination,[83,84] but is best visualized by CT[80] (Fig. 56.6). It may be associated with a wide variety of non-intestinal conditions, as well as intra-abdominal illnesses and even in healthy children (Table 56.1). Not all instances of pneumatosis intestinalis are dangerous, and most do not require operation.[80,85,86] The underlying illness, if any, the precipitating event and the clinical course dictate the management.

Conditions
Healthy child
Asthma
Pulmonary fibrosis
Cystic fibrosis
Chronic obstructive pulmonary disease
Pyloric stenosis
Peptic ulcer
Intestinal obstruction
Intestinal pseudo-obstruction and other motility disorders
Inflammatory bowel disease
Celiac disease
Hirschsprung's disease
Jejunoileal bypass
Endoscopy (with or without biopsy)
Enteric tube placement (needle catheter jejunostomy)
Collagen vascular disease
Organ and bone marrow transplant
Graft *vs* host disease
Acquired immune deficiency syndrome
Medications –: prednisone, lactulose, cancer chemotherapy
Iron overdose
Decompensated heart disease
Gastroschisis
Short bowel syndrome
Closed abdominal trauma
Intestinal surgery

Table 56.1 Conditions associated with pneumatosis intestinalis[77,78,80,82,86]

There are several different possible theoretical mechanisms to explain gas entry into the abdominal wall.[78,80,83,84,86] The mechanical theory suggests that gas dissects into the bowel wall under pressure. This could occur with pulmonary obstructive disease, violent coughing, trauma[86] or vomiting. In these situations, air could travel through lymphatics or vessels to the abdomen. This theory is supported by analysis of intramural gas showing composition consistent with alveolar air in some patients.[77] Not all cysts contain this composition, however. Gas could also be forced from the bowel lumen into the walls if there is intestinal obstruction from any cause, or if there is an increase in intraluminal pressure from endoscopy or trauma. Another possibility suggests intraluminal bacterial action to produce a great increase in the partial pressure of hydrogen or methane. The excess gas may diffuse passively into the bowel wall. This could occur as a result of carbohydrate malabsorption of any cause. In some cases, such as short bowel syndrome, the gas in the wall is indeed high in hydrogen content.[77] Children with short bowel syndrome may have pneumatosis that fluctuates with the level of carbohydrate in their diet.[78] A bacterial invasion theory suggests that gas-forming bacteria enter the bowel wall under conditions of infection or inflammation, such as necrotizing enterocolitis or graft *vs* host disease colitis. The finding of high levels of breath hydrogen in some of these patients supports this theory as well. However, the cysts are usually sterile and bacteria are not usually found on histologic examination. The intramural gas may again represent increased intraluminal gas forcing its way through microscopic vents in the tissue.[77] Most cases of pneumatosis can theoretically fit into one or a combination of these mechanisms.

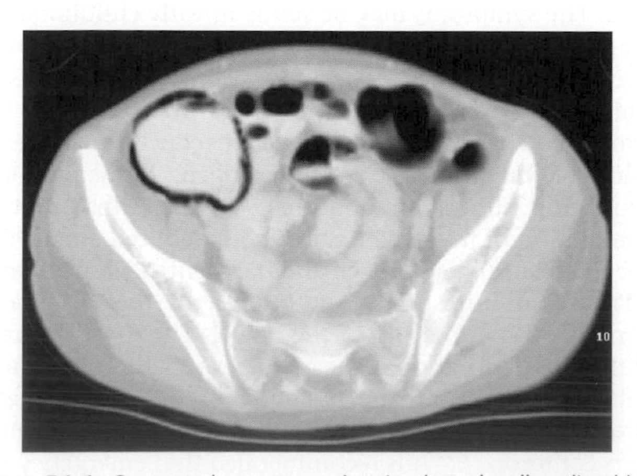

Figure 56.6: Computed tomogram showing bowel wall outlined by a black rim of air in pneumatosis intestinalis.

There are several reviews of pneumatosis in children.[78,81,82] Short bowel syndrome, organ and bone marrow transplant, intestinal dysmotility, congenital heart disease, and toxicity from iron ingestion were common associated illnesses, perhaps reflecting in part the specialties of the reporting institutions. Healthy children also made up a considerable proportion of reported cases.[78] The inciting events were frequently infectious enteritis, non-infectious colitis or ischemia.[78] Symptoms most commonly noted were abdominal distention, bloody diarrhea, vomiting and lethargy.[77,78,82] Poor outcome and the need for surgical intervention were associated with more serious underlying disorders which increased the risk of multisystem disease and bowel necrosis. These disorders included decompensated heart disease and transplant status, as well as iron toxicity.[78,82] Poor outcome was also associated with acidosis, hypotension and portal venous gas.[78,82] Some children with pneumoperitoneum or portal venous gas did not require surgery and recovered with supportive care.[79,81] Surgery, most often resection of an infarcted or perforated section of bowel, was indicated because of steady deterioration, increased abdominal pain and rebound, and as well as the presence of free air.[28,77,78,82]

Pneumatosis intestinalis may be an incidental finding. Rarely, crepitation may be felt in the abdomen or on rectal examination; air blebs may simulate polyps on rectal examination or endoscopy.[83,84] There may be abdominal distention or pain. Symptoms usually relate to the underlying disease. On rare occasions, the air blebs may cause pain or obstruction.[83,84] Treatment for pneumatosis itself may be indicated for mechanical problems. Treatment for the underlying disease may help to decrease pneumatosis and prevent its recurrence. Conservative therapy includes placing the bowel at rest, using suction and giving antibiotics (metronidazole, ampicillin or ciprofloxacin).[83,84] Oxygen may be administered at moderate to high concentrations (40–100%) to achieve a moderate to high partial pressure of oxygen (200–300 mmHg).[77,83,84] Hyperbaric oxygen has been used. Some children receive no treatment and recover rapidly.[78]

SOLITARY RECTAL ULCER SYNDROME AND COLITIS CYSTICA PROFUNDA

Solitary rectal ulcer syndrome (SRS) is probably underdiagnosed in both children and adults because it is not always recognized as a distinct entity. This syndrome seems to result from disordered defecation.[71,83,84,87] There is a high incidence of rectal prolapse, either obvious or occult. Prolapse may result from persistent contraction of the puborectalis muscle, keeping the anal canal closed with very high intrarectal pressure. The external anal sphincter may fail to relax, again leading to high pressure. Another mechanism is excessive perineal descent, so that the anterior rectal wall protrudes into the anal canal. Each of these mechanisms has been observed in some adult patients on defecography or manometry.[71] The dysfunction leads to straining to stool, pressure necrosis of the anal mucosa, or congestion and traction of the submucosal vessels.[84] Self-induced trauma due to digital removal of stool has also been described with this syndrome.[71,84]

The end result of this process is pressure necrosis of the bowel wall. The endoscopic appearance of SRS often belies the singularity implied by its name.[84] There frequently may be several shallow round or serpiginous ulcers with a thin erythematous rim. They range from 0.5 to 5 cm in diameter. The lesions are seen most often on the anterior wall but may be circumferential.[88] They are located 5–15 cm from the anal verge.[71] Early in the evolution of the lesion, or in a healing phase, there may be only erythema and edema. Less commonly, polypoid lesions may be found, and may themselves prolapse.[88]

Madison and Morson described the characteristic histologic picture of SRS in 1969.[71] The features include obliteration of the lamina propria by fibromuscular proliferation of the muscularis mucosa, streaming of muscle fibers and fibroblasts between contorted branching crypts, thickening of the muscularis mucosa, and diffuse collagen infiltration of the lamina propria.[84] Orientation of the muscle fibers perpendicular to the lamina propria is pathognomonic.[88] The diffuse fibrosis in these cases differs from the focal fibrosis of inflammatory bowel disease or ischemia.[69] Some patients also have colitis cystica profunda (CCP), with submucosal cysts in the muscularis propria or even the serosa.[71,84] The cysts may have benign colonic epithelium lining, or may have no lining. It is postulated that these cysts result from translocation of surface epithelium into the deeper mucosal layers under pressure.[71] Up to 54% of patients with CCP have rectal prolapse, further strengthening the association of these two entities.[84]

Patients with these two syndromes have variable symptoms; probably 25% are asymptomatic. Up to 89% have rectal bleeding, which rarely is profuse enough to require transfusion.[84] There may be muccorhea, diarrhea, constipation, incontinence, proctalgia, abdominal pain and tenesmus.[71,84] There may be actual obstruction of defecation by the prolapse.[71,84]

Therapy for solitary rectal ulcer is poorly defined. Conservative therapy may be more effective in children, especially those in whom the lesion is polypoid rather than ulcerative.[71] This medical therapy includes stool softening, bowel retraining in positions to decrease straining, and reassurance. Corticosteroids, salicylates and sucralfate have been tried; probably each is useful for some patients. Local electrocautery, caustics and antibiotics have been used.[84] Rectopexy tends to be the most successful procedure. Simple excision of the lesion is not successful.[84,89] Success with surgery ranges from 65% to 94%, with most series in the lower range. Thus surgery should be reserved for those with intractable and disabling symptoms. Total diversion of the fecal stream can be used for the most symptomatic cases.[84,89]

AMYLOIDOSIS

Deposition of amyloid is an infrequent consequence of a variety of inflammatory diseases (Table 56.2). Exactly how inflammation causes this deposition is not completely clear, but the molecular nature of amyloid has been thoroughly explored. Amyloid exists as a β-pleated sheet of long non-branching fibrils 7.5–10 nm in diameter. The pleating accounts for its pathognomonic birefringence when stained with Congo Red. Most of the fibrils in gastrointestinal disease are of two types:

- AL (amyloid light chains, derived from immunoglobulin light chains) are found in monoclonal B-cell proliferation.
- AA (amyloid associated protein made by the liver) deposits in tissues of persons affected with infectious

Diseases associated with amyloid deposition
Tuberculosis
Bronchiectasis
Chronic osteomyelitis
Rheumatoid arthritis (3%)
Cystic fibrosis
Glycogenosis
Ankylosing spondylitis
Inflammatory bowel disease
'Skin popping' narcotics (chronic infection)
Familial Mediterranean fever
Hemodialysis (β_2-microglobulin not removed by dialysis membrane)
Diabetes mellitus type II

Table 56.2 Diseases associated with amyloid deposition[50,71]

and non-infectious inflammation. AA amyloid is also called secondary amyloidosis.

Amyloid deposits first around the blood vessels of the intestine but later infiltrates the submucosa, muscularis and subserosa. The consequences of this are changes in motility and possibly ischemia. Clinically amyloidosis of the intestine may be silent or may manifest as irregular contours of the bowel, which does not change function. Other radiographic signs include dilation,[71] granularity, 3–4-mm nodules and polypoid lesions measuring up to 10 mm. Endoscopically visible lesions occur in the duodenum in 75% and in the colon of 54% of patients. Deep biopsies containing submucosa demonstrate a higher percentage of involvement.[50]

Poor motility, obstruction and pseudo-obstruction, abdominal pain, nausea and vomiting may occur. There may be malabsorption, diarrhea and weight loss. Occasionally there is bleeding, even massive hemorrhage, due to ischemia. Ischemic perforation may occur.[71] Therapy for the underlying disease may decrease the deposition of amyloid, and rarely the deposits themselves may shrink. If therapy is not successful, nutritional support and even parenteral nutrition may be necessary. Severe ischemic disease may necessitate resection.[50]

References

1. Tizard EJ. Henoch–Schönlein purpura. Arch Dis Child 1999; 80:380–383.
2. Saulsbury FT. Epidemiology of Henoch–Schönlein purpura. Cleve Clin Med J 2002; 69(Suppl 2):SII87–SII89.
3. Ballinger S. Henoch–Schönlein purpura. Curr Opin Rheumatol 2003; 15:591–594.
4. Mills JA, Michel BA, Bloch DA, et al. The American College of Rheumatology 1990 criteria for the classification of Henoch–Schönlein purpura. Arthritis Rheum 1990; 33:1114–1121.
5. Caksen H, Odabas D, Kosem M, et al. Report of eight infants with acute infantile hemorrhagic edema and review of the literature. J Dermatol 2002; 29:290–295.
6. Dillon M. Henoch–Schönlein purpura (treatment and outcome). Clev Clin J Med 2002; 69(Suppl 2):SII121–SII123.
7. Choong CK, Beasley SW. Intra-abdominal manifestations of Henoch–Schönlein purpura. J Paediatr Child Health 1998; 34:405–409.
8. Esaki M, Matsumoto T, Nakamura S, et al. GI involvement in Henoch–Schönlein purpura. Gastrointest Endosc 2002; 56:920–923.
9. Pore G. GI lesions in Henoch–Schönlein purpura. Gastrointest Endosc 2002; 55:283–286.
10. Sharief N, Ward HC, Wood CB. Functional intestinal obstruction in Henoch–Schönlein purpura. J Pediatr Gastroenterol Nutr 1991; 12:272–275.
11. Wyatt RJ, Hogg RJ. Evidence-based assessment of treatment options for children with IgA nephropathies. Pediatr Nephrol 2001; 16:156–167.
12. Rigante D, Candelli M, Federico G, Bartolozzi F, Porri MG, Stabile A. Predictive factors of renal involvement or relapsing disease in children with Henoch–Schönlein purpura. Rheumatol Int 2005; 25:45–48.
13. Ronkainen J, Nuutinen M, Koskimies O. The adult kidney 24 years after childhood Henoch–Schönlein purpura: a retrospective cohort study. Lancet 2002; 360:666–670.
14. Gibson LE. Cutaneous vasculitis update. Dermatol Clin 2001; 19:603–615, vii.
15. Gershoni-Baruch R, Broza Y, Brik R. Prevalence and significance of mutations in the familial Mediterranean fever gene in Henoch–Schönlein purpura. J Pediatr 2003; 143:658–661.
16. Amoli MM, Calvino MC, Garcia-Porrua C, Llorca J, Ollier WE, Gonzalez-Gay MA. Interleukin 1beta gene polymorphism association with severe renal manifestations and renal sequelae in Henoch–Schönlein purpura. J Rheumatol 2004; 31:295–298.
17. Rostoker G, Rymer JC, Bagnard G, Petit-Phar M, Griuncelli M, Pilatte Y. Imbalances in serum proinflammatory cytokines and their soluble receptors: a putative role in the progression of idiopathic IgA nephropathy (IgAN) and Henoch–Schönlein purpura nephritis, and a potential target of immunoglobulin therapy? Clin Exp Immunol 1998; 114:468–476.
18. Martino F, Agolini D, Tsalikova E, et al. Nailfold capillaroscopy in Henoch–Schönlein purpura: a follow-up study of 31 cases. J Pediatr 2002; 141:145.
19. Hyams JS. Corticosteroids in the treatment of gastrointestinal disease. Curr Opin Pediatr 2000; 12:451–455.
20. Rosenblum ND, Winter HS. Steroid effects on the course of abdominal pain in children with Henoch–Schönlein purpura. Pediatrics 1987; 79:1018–1021.
21. Choi SJ, Park SK, Uhm WS, et al. A case of refractory Henoch–Schönlein purpura treated with thalidomide. Korean J Intern Med 2002; 17:270–273.
22. Martinez-Frontanilla LA, Haase GM, Ernster JA, Bailey WC. Surgical complications in Henoch–Schönlein purpura. J Pediatr Surg 1984; 19:434–436.
23. Lamireau T, Rebouissoux L, Hehunstre JP. Intravenous immunoglobulin therapy for severe digestive manifestations of Henoch–Schönlein purpura. Acta Paediatr 2001; 90:1081–1082.
24. Perafan-Riveros C, Franca LF, Alves AC, Sanches JA Jr. Acrodermatitis enteropathica: case report and review of the literature. Pediatr Dermatol 2002; 19:426–431.
25. Krebs N, Hambidge N. Trace elements in human nutrition. In: Walker W, Watkins J, eds. Nutrition in Pediatrics. Hamilton: BC Decker; 1997:94–100.
26. Fraker PJ, King LE, Laakko T, Vollmer TL. The dynamic link between the integrity of the immune system and zinc status. J Nutr 2000; 130(Suppl):1399S–1406S.
27. Solomon N. Zinc. In: Baumgartner T, ed. Clinical Guide to Parenteral Micronutrition, 2nd edn. USA: Fujisawa; 1991:217–229.
28. Wang K, Pugh EW, Griffen S, et al. Homozygosity mapping places the acrodermatitis enteropathica gene on chromosomal region 8q24.3. Am J Hum Genet 2001; 68:1055–1060.

29. Dufner-Beattie J, Wang F, Kuo YM, Gitschier J, Eide D, Andrews GK. The acrodermatitis enteropathica gene *ZIP4* encodes a tissue-specific, zinc-regulated zinc transporter in mice. J Biol Chem 2003; 278:33474–3381.
30. Kury S, Kharfi M, Kamoun R, et al. Mutation spectrum of human SLC39A4 in a panel of patients with acrodermatitis enteropathica. Hum Mutat 2003; 22:337–338.
31. Trachtman H, Christen E. Pathogenesis, treatment, and therapeutic trials in hemolytic uremic syndrome. Curr Opin Pediatr 1999; 11:162–168.
32. Bower JR. Foodborne diseases: Shiga toxin producing *E. coli* (STEC). Pediatr Infect Dis J 1999; 18:909–910.
33. Proulx F, Seidman EG, Karpman D. Pathogenesis of Shiga toxin-associated hemolytic uremic syndrome. Pediatr Res 2001; 50:163–171.
34. Siegler RL. The hemolytic uremic syndrome. Pediatr Clin North Am 1995; 42:1505–1529.
35. Saltzman DA, Chavers B, Brennom W, Vernier R, Telander RL. Timing of colonic necrosis in hemolytic uremic syndrome. Pediatr Surg Int 1998; 13:268–270.
36. Yoh M, Honda T. The stimulating effect of fosfomycin, an antibiotic in common use in Japan, on the production/release of verotoxin-1 from enterohaemorrhagic *Escherichia coli* O157:H7 *in vitro*. Epidemiol Infect 1997; 119:101–103.
37. Taylor CM, Monnens LA. Advances in haemolytic uraemic syndrome. Arch Dis Child 1998; 78:190–193.
38. Swift P. Novel techniques in the delivery of radiation in pediatric oncology. Pediatr Clin North Am 2002; 49:1107–1129.
39. Otchy DP, Nelson H. Radiation injuries of the colon and rectum. Surg Clin North Am 1993; 73:1017–1035.
40. Donaldson SS, Jundt S, Ricour C, Sarrazin D, Lemerle J, Schweisguth O. Radiation enteritis in children. A retrospective review, clinicopathologic correlation, and dietary management. Cancer 1975; 35:1167–1178.
41. Kinsella TJ, Bloomer WD. Tolerance of the intestine to radiation therapy. Surg Gynecol Obstet 1980; 151:273–284.
42. Rao SP, Anderson V, Shlasko E, Miller ST, Choi K, Rabinowitz S. Intestinal perforation 14 years after abdominal irradiation and chemotherapy for Wilms tumor. J Pediatr Hematol Oncol 1996; 18:187–190.
43. Galland RB, Spencer J. The natural history of clinically established radiation enteritis. Lancet 1985; i:1257–1258.
44. Yeoh E, Horowitz M, Russo A, et al. Effect of pelvic irradiation on gastrointestinal function: a prospective longitudinal study. Am J Med 1993; 95:397–406.
45. McGarrity T. Nonoperative management of radiation enteritis and colitis. In: Digestive Disease Week, New Orleans, LA, 2004:124–127.
46. Meric F, Hirschl RB, Mahboubi S, et al. Prevention of radiation enteritis in children, using a pelvic mesh sling. J Pediatr Surg 1994; 29:917–921.
47. van der Voort P tVJ, Wassenaar R, Silberbusch J. Malacoplakia: two case reports and a comparison of treatment modalities based on a literature review. Arch Intern Med 1996; 156:577–583.
48. van Crevel R, Curfs J, van der Ven AJ, Assmann K, Meis JF, van der Meer JW. Functional and morphological monocyte abnormalities in a patient with malakoplakia. Am J Med 1998; 105:74–77.
49. Hartman G, Yong SL, Chejfec G. Malakoplakia of liver diagnosed by a needle core biopsy: a case report and review of the literature. Arch Pathol Lab Med 2002; 126:372–374.
50. Blumberg D, Wald A. Other diseases of the small intestine and colon. In: Feldman M, Scharscmidt B, Sleisenger M, eds. Schlesinger and Fordtran's Gastrointestinal and Liver Disease: Pathophysiology, Diagnosis, Management, 7th edn. Philadelphia, PA: WB Saunders; 2002:1982–1984.
51. Sakane T, Takeno M, Suzuki N, Inaba G. Behçet's disease. N Engl J Med 1999; 341:1284–1291.
52. Yazici H. Behçet's syndrome: where do we stand? Am J Med 2002; 112:75–76.
53. Espinosa G, Font J, Tassies D, et al. Vascular involvement in Behçet's disease: relation with thrombophilic factors, coagulation activation, and thrombomodulin. Am J Med 2002; 112:37–43.
54. Brik R, Shamali H, Bergman R. Successful thalidomide treatment of severe infantile Behçet disease. Pediatr Dermatol 2001; 18:143–145.
55. Schlatter M, Snyder K, Freyer D. Successful nonoperative management of typhlitis in pediatric oncology patients. J Pediatr Surg 2002; 37:1151–1155.
56. Paulino AF, Kenney R, Forman EN, Medeiros LJ. Typhlitis in a patient with acute lymphoblastic leukemia prior to the administration of chemotherapy. Am J Pediatr Hematol Oncol 1994; 16:348–351.
57. Safdar A, Armstrong D. Infectious morbidity in critically ill patients with cancer. Crit Care Clin 2001; 17:531–570, vii–viii.
58. Katz JA, Wagner ML, Gresik MV, Mahoney DH Jr, Fernbach DJ. Typhlitis. An 18-year experience and postmortem review. Cancer 1990; 65:1041–1047.
59. Otaibi AA, Barker C, Anderson R, Sigalet DL. Neutropenic enterocolitis (typhlitis) after pediatric bone marrow transplant. J Pediatr Surg 2002; 37:770–772.
60. Wade DS, Nava HR, Douglass HO Jr. Neutropenic enterocolitis. Clinical diagnosis and treatment. Cancer 1992; 69:17–23.
61. Sloas MM, Flynn PM, Kaste SC, Patrick CC. Typhlitis in children with cancer: a 30-year experience. Clin Infect Dis 1993; 17:484–490.
62. Blair SL, Schwarz RE. Critical care of patients with cancer. Surgical considerations. Crit Care Clin 2001; 17:721–742, ix.
63. Mahajan L, Wyllie R, Goldblum J. Lymphocytic colitis in a pediatric patient: a possible adverse reaction to carbamazepine. Am J Gastroenterol 1997; 92:2126–2127.
64. Bonner GF, Petras RE, Cheong DM, Grewal ID, Breno S, Ruderman WB. Short- and long-term follow-up of treatment for lymphocytic and collagenous colitis. Inflamm Bowel Dis 2000; 6:85–91.
65. Furlano RI, Anthony A, Day R, et al. Colonic CD8 and gamma delta T-cell infiltration with epithelial damage in children with autism. J Pediatr 2001; 138:366–372.
66. Torrente F, Ashwood P, Day R, et al. Small intestinal enteropathy with epithelial IgG and complement deposition in children with regressive autism. Mol Psychiatry 2002; 7:375–382.
67. Mashako MN, Sonsino E, Navarro J, et al. Microscopic colitis: a new cause of chronic diarrhea in children? J Pediatr Gastroenterol Nutr 1990; 10:21–26.
68. Heyman MB, Perman JA, Ferrell LD, Thaler MM. Chronic nonspecific inflammatory bowel disease of the cecum and proximal colon in children with grossly normal-appearing colonic mucosa: diagnosis by colonoscopic biopsies. Pediatrics 1987; 80:255–261.
69. Kocoshis SA. Other diseases of the small intestine and colon. In: Wyllie R, Hyams J, eds. Pediatric Gastrointestinal and Liver Disease. London: Elsevier; 0000:532–550.

70. Sanderson IR, Boyle S, Williams CB, Walker-Smith JA. Histological abnormalities in biopsies from macroscopically normal colonoscopies. Arch Dis Child 1986; 61:274–277.
71. Sartor RB, Murphy ME, Rydzak E. Miscellaneous inflammatory and structural disorders of the colon. In: Yamada T, ed. Textbook of Gastroenterology. Philadelphia, PA: Lippincott Williams & Wilkins; 1999:1857–1883.
72. Pepin M, Schwarze U, Superti-Furga A, Byers PH. Clinical and genetic features of Ehlers–Danlos syndrome type IV, the vascular type. N Engl J Med 2000; 342:673–680.
73. Collins MH, Schwarze U, Carpentieri DF, et al. Multiple vascular and bowel ruptures in an adolescent male with sporadic Ehlers–Danlos syndrome type IV. Pediatr Dev Pathol 1999; 2:86–93.
74. Soucy P, Eidus L, Keeley F. Perforation of the colon in a 15-year-old girl with Ehlers–Danlos syndrome type IV. J Pediatr Surg 1990; 25:1180–1182.
75. Sykes EM Jr. Colon perforation in Ehlers–Danlos syndrome. Report of two cases and review of the literature. Am J Surg 1984; 147:410–413.
76. Sigurdson E, Stern HS, Houpt J, el-Sharkawy TY, Huizinga JD. The Ehlers–Danlos syndrome and colonic perforation. Report of a case and physiologic assessment of underlying motility disorder. Dis Colon Rectum 1985; 28:962–966.
77. Heng Y, Schuffler MD, Haggitt RC, Rohrmann CA. Pneumatosis intestinalis: a review. Am J Gastroenterol 1995; 90:1747–1758.
78. Kurbegov AC, Sondheimer JM. Pneumatosis intestinalis in non-neonatal pediatric patients. Pediatrics 2001; 108:402–406.
79. Luks FI, Chung MA, Brandt ML, et al. Pneumatosis and pneumoperitoneum in chronic idiopathic intestinal pseudoobstruction. J Pediatr Surg 1991; 26:1384–1386.
80. Pear BL. Pneumatosis intestinalis: a review. Radiology 1998; 207:13–19.
81. Reynolds HL Jr, Gauderer MW, Hrabovsky EE, Shurin SB. Pneumatosis cystoides intestinalis in children beyond the first year of life: manifestations and management. J Pediatr Surg 1991; 26:1376–1380.
82. West KW, Rescorla FJ, Grosfeld JL, Vane DW. Pneumatosis intestinalis in children beyond the neonatal period. J Pediatr Surg 1989; 24:818–822.
83. Davila AD, Willenbucher RF. Other diseases of the colon and rectum. In: Feldman M, Scharschmidt B, Sleisinger M, eds. Gastrointestinal and Liver Disease. Philadelphia, PA: WB Saunders; 1998:1979–1982.
84. Davila AD, Willenbucher RF. Other disease of the colon and rectum. In: Feldman M, Scharschmidt B, Sleisinger M, eds. Gastrointestinal and Liver Disease. Philadelphia, PA: WB Saunders; 1998:1977–2001.
85. Rescorla FJ, Grosfeld JL, West KJ, Vane DW. Changing patterns of treatment and survival in neonates with meconium ileus. Arch Surg 1989; 124:837–840.
86. St Peter SD, Abbas MA, Kelly KA. The spectrum of pneumatosis intestinalis. Arch Surg 2003; 138:68–75.
87. Gopal DV. Diseases of the rectum and anus: a clinical approach to common disorders. Clin Cornerstone 2002; 4:34–48.
88. Ertem D, Acar Y, Karaa EK, Pehlivanoglu E. A rare and often unrecognized cause of hematochezia and tenesmus in childhood: solitary rectal ulcer syndrome. Pediatrics 2002; 110:e79.
89. Marchal F, Bresler L, Brunaud L, et al. Solitary rectal ulcer syndrome: a series of 13 patients operated with a mean follow-up of 4.5 years. Int J Colorectal Dis 2001; 16:228–233.

SECTION SIX
THE LIVER AND BILE DUCTS

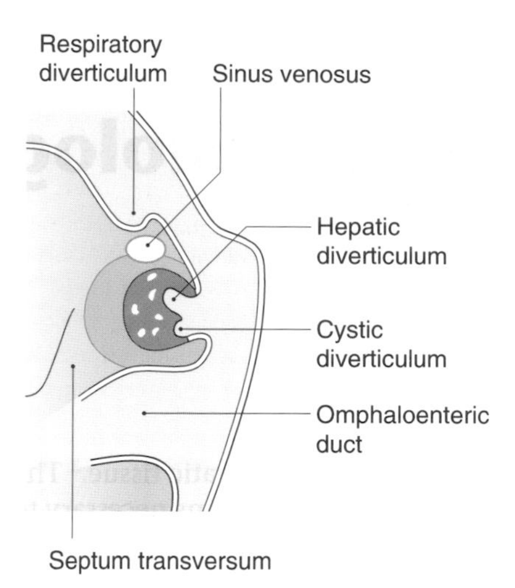

Figure 57.2: Midline section of the developing vertebrate embryo at the level of the anterior endoderm. Cranial (hepatic) diverticulum and caudal (cystic) diverticulum. Both are adjacent to the developing lung diverticula, consistent with a common anterior endodermal lineage. (Modified from O'Rahilly, R, Muller F. The digestive system-the liver. In: O'Rahilly, R, Muller F (1992) Human Embryology and Teratology 2nd edn, with permission of John Wiley & Sons, Inc)

results in both migration and proliferation of the hepatoblasts. In addition, as the hepatoblasts invade the ST mesenchyme, so do other cell types, including hematopoietic and endothelial precursors. There is a significant amount of cross-talk between these different cell types. This interaction has been illustrated recently in the mouse knockout of hepatocyte nuclear factor 6 (HNF-6). In the absence of this important transcription factor, the mouse liver displays both liver and vascular anomalies.[5]

As the organ structure matures, so do its individual cells. Hepatoblasts become hepatocytes and biliary epithelial cells (as discussed in the section on biliary development). This transition is not quite complete at birth and goes on into the first 2 months of life. Importantly, a small proportion of hepatoblasts do not differentiate, but retain their bipotentiality and may participate in the ability of the adult liver to respond to injury (see section on liver regeneration).

Overall, once the bud has emerged, the immature organ undergoes intense growth until it reaches its encapsulated and lobulated structure by the end of the sixth week of human gestation. Thereafter, the rate of cell replication is low, but sufficient to maintain an organ mass proportionate to the size of the child.

DEVELOPMENT OF THE BILIARY TREE

Biliary tree development begins at the end of the second month of gestation. It occurs simultaneously in two neighboring areas of the liver bud (Fig. 57.2):

- The hepatic (cranial) diverticulum, which gives rise to the hepatic parenchyma
- The cystic (caudal) diverticulum, which gives rise to the gallbladder and cystic duct.

As development proceeds, and the intrahepatic biliary tree develops, the common bile duct, derived from the cranial bud, merges with the cystic duct derived from the caudal bud. Anomalies in this crucial step, although not well understood, may lead to some of the congenital hepatobiliary disorders, such as choledochal cyst and biliary atresia, and to the pathogenesis of some rare conditions including spontaneous perforation of the common bile duct.

Understanding the development of the intrahepatic bile ducts has particular clinical relevance. The most commonly accepted theory,[6–8] known as the *ductal plate theory*, proposed by Desmet, suggests that the early hepatic epithelial cells, or hepatoblasts, are bipotential precursors giving rise to both hepatocytes and biliary epithelial cells (BECs). The hepatocytes also participate in the formation of the smallest unit of the intrahepatic biliary system by forming intercellular bile canaliculi (canals of Hering) with their apical membrane. These small canaliculi, in turn, drain into the lobular and interlobular bile ducts lined by the BECs (Fig. 57.3).

According to Desmet, hepatoblasts acquire characteristics similar to those of the cholangiocytes of the extrahepatic biliary tree when they come in contact with the mesenchyme surrounding the larger branches of the portal vein. This is the *formation of the ductal plate*. As the hepatoblast changes fate, morphologic changes are subtle, but cell identity can be traced by means of immunocytochemistry: hepatoblasts fated to become BECs express cytokeratins, and hepatoblasts fated to become hepatocytes begin to express α-fetoprotein and albumin, as well as staining for glycogen.[9] Development proceeds, and this continuous monolayer around the portal vein branches stratifies into a bilayer and then becomes fenestrated; this is known as *remodeling of the ductal plate* (Fig. 57.4). Finally, only a few segments of the stratified biliary epithelial cells become bile ducts as they in turn *invade* the mesenchyme and become part of the functional unit called the portal triad. Both ductal plate formation and remodeling, and migration of the bile ducts into the mesenchyme, occur in a centrifugal fashion, starting at the hilum. Importantly, this process continues postnatally at the periphery of the organ; this should be considered when obtaining and interpreting the biopsies of very young infants.

In addition, this theory offers insight into the pathogenesis of an array of conditions known as 'ductal plate malformations', which include congenital hepatic fibrosis, Caroli's disease, Meckel's syndrome, and the recessive and dominant forms of polycystic kidney disease.[7,11] The development of the biliary tree is a strong example of the developmentally conserved principle of interactions between epithelium and mesenchyme in the determination of cellular identity and position.

Development of the biliary tree is intimately linked to that of the hepatic vasculature. Indeed, ductal plates form only where there is a branch of the portal vein. Knockout

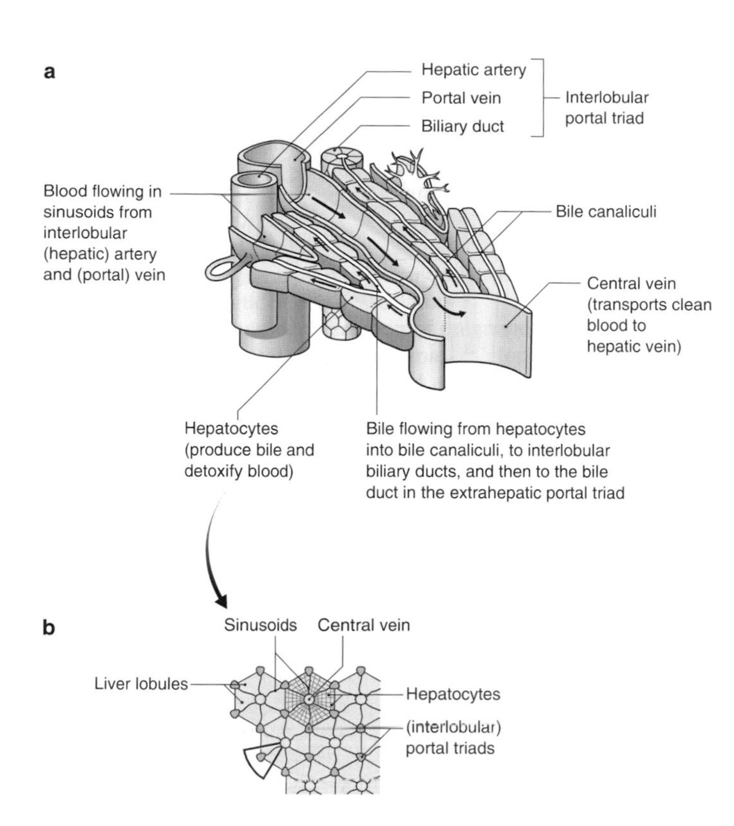

Figure 57.3: (**a**) Three-dimensional section across a liver lobule. The hepatocytes form rows, separated by the sinusoids which flow from the portal trial to the centrilobular vein. The biliary pole of the hepatocyte drains into the canaliculi, which are oriented perpendicular to sinusoidal flow. (**b**) Cross-section across a vertebrate liver lobule, as seen in histologic sections. (From Moore and Dalley, 1999, with permission.)[10]

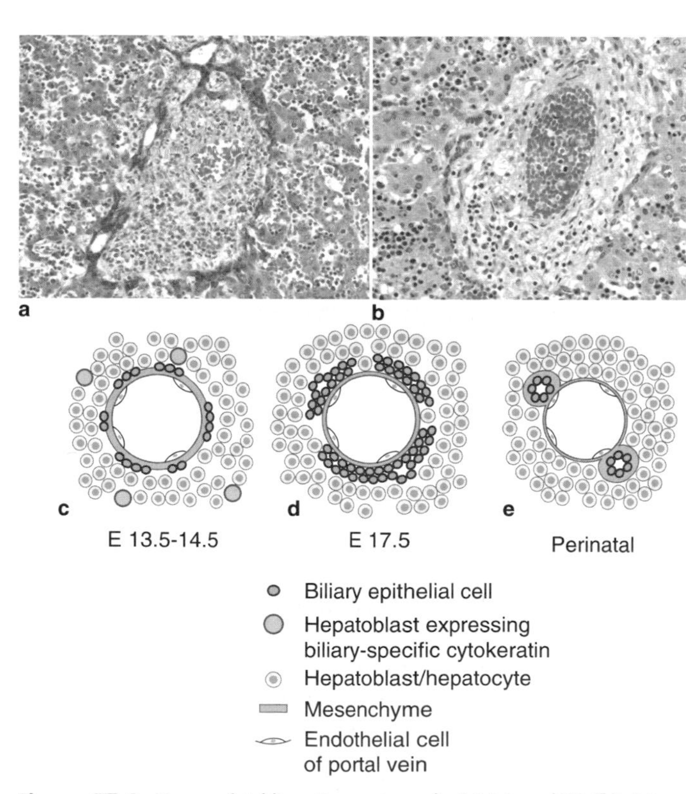

Figure 57.4: Human fetal liver tissue at weeks 16 (**a**) and 20 (**b**). (**a**) Remodeling of the ductal plate. (**b**) Remodeling is almost complete. (**c–e**) Illustrate schematically the remodeling of the ductal plate in the mouse embryo. (From Lemaigre, 2003, with permission.)[11] Pictures courtesy of Gail Deutsch, MD (*See plate section for color*).

studies in mice have shown that when genes affecting biliary development (*HNF6*, *HNF1β*, *Notch2* and *Jagged1* in varying combinations) are absent, the resulting phenotype includes vascular defects affecting branches of the portal vein, or of the hepatic artery and its peribiliary capillaries.[11] It is not excluded that the *primum movens* in ductal plate malformations could be a defect in a mesenchymal protein, or in a vascular gene, which would lead to secondary biliary defects.

In summary, understanding the cross-regulation involved in the development of the liver and biliary tree not only aids our understanding of liver histopathology, but also, on a broader level, our comprehension of syndromic associations.

DEVELOPMENT OF THE HEPATIC VASCULATURE

Development of the hepatic vasculature mimics that of the bile ducts.

At the *intrahepatic* level, there is evidence in vertebrate models that endothelial cells are required for liver induction and migration of the early hepatic epithelium into the ST mesenchyme.[12] These early endothelial cells go on to form the fenestrated lining of the hepatic sinusoids.[13] They participate in the early organization of the liver into its structural unit, the lobule, by directing the migration of the hepatoblasts into cords[8] (Fig. 57.5).

an infected maternal genital tract, postnatally via maternal breast milk or saliva, or iatrogenically from transfusion of blood products.

From 90–95% of neonates with congenital CMV infection are asymptomatic in the neonatal period. Typical clinical features in those with overt disease in the neonatal period include hepatomegaly, splenomegaly, jaundice, petechiae or purpura, pneumonia, microcephaly, chorioretinitis and cerebral calcifications. Hepatosplenomegaly is caused by mild hepatitis, a reticuloendothelial response to chronic infection and extramedullary hematopoiesis.[41] CMV hepatitis is associated with conjugated and unconjugated hyperbilirubinemia and mild elevation of liver transaminases. Although CMV hepatitis is usually mild, recurrent ascites, bleeding diathesis, disseminated intravascular coagulopathy, secondary bacterial infections and ensuing death have been reported.[42–44] CMV infection also has been associated with obliteration of bile ducts and paucity of intrahepatic bile ducts.[45] Hepatic histopathology includes multi-nucleated giant cell transformation, large inclusions-bearing cells, cholestasis, cholangitis and extramedullary hematopoiesis. The characteristic finding is an enlarged (endothelial, hepatocyte, or bile duct epithelial) cell containing basophilic granules in the cytoplasm and a swollen nucleus. An amphophilic intranuclear inclusion is surrounded by a clear halo, resembling an owl's eye (Fig. 58.2). Both nuclear and cytoplasmic inclusions represent closely packed virions.[46] Liver calcifications are found on imaging.[47]

CMV infection should be excluded in all neonates with prolonged cholestasis. Isolation of the virus from tissue cultures or detection in urine, saliva, blood, cerebrospinal fluid and tissue biopsies by culture or polymerase chain reaction (PCR) all can be used to diagnose CMV infection. Assessment of extra-hepatic involvement should be part of the routine work up including fundoscopy, brain ultrasound and CT scan and assessment of hearing by brain stem evoked potentials.

Potential options for the treatment for congenital CMV-infected neonates include the use of intravenous ganciclovir and CMV immunoglobulin.[48] A recent randomized controlled study of ganciclovir therapy for congenitally infected newborns with central nervous system disease suggests that treatment decreases the risk of hearing impairment.[49] Although hepatomegaly and mild alteration in liver function test results may persist for several months after birth, severe chronic liver disease rarely occurs.

Herpes simplex virus

In newborns, herpes simplex virus (HSV) infection manifests as a disseminated disease involving multiple organs, most prominently liver and lungs; localized central nervous system (CNS) disease; or disease localized to the skin, eye and mouth. Asymptomatic HSV infection of the neonate rarely occurs. HSV type 2 strains cause disease in neonates more commonly than HSV type 1 strains. The incidence of neonatal HSV infection is estimated to range from 1:3000 to 1:20 000 live births.[22] Prematurity is a risk factor with premature infants accounting for 40–50% of cases of neonatal herpes and having a greater likelihood of having a fatal outcome. Whether the increased frequency of prematurity among neonates with herpes indicates a greater propensity of mothers with genital herpes to deliver prematurely or a greater susceptibility of premature infants to HSV infection remains unknown. Transmission occurs during delivery via exposure to an infected maternal genital tract or ascending infection (even through apparently intact membranes); or postpartum from a parent or other caregiver (most often from a non-genital infection such as the mouth or hands), or from another infected infant or caregiver in the nursery (probably via the hands of a health care professional attending the infant).

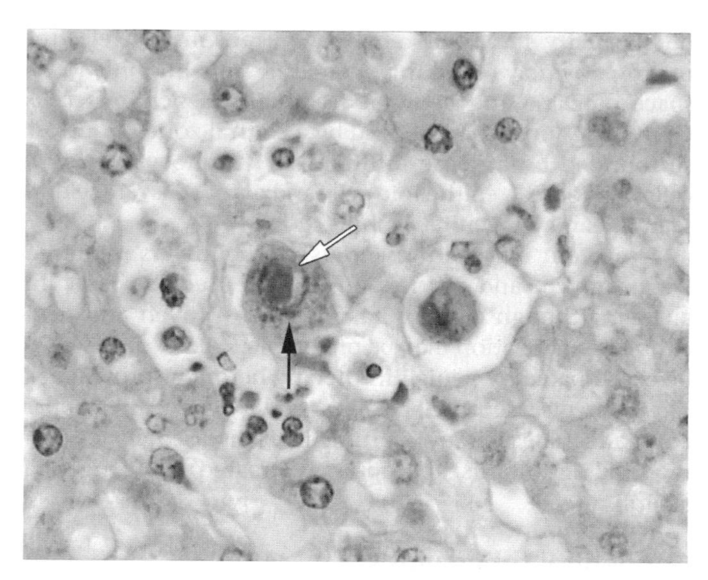

Figure 58.2: Cytomegalovirus infection. Enlarged hepatocyte contains basophilic granules in the cytoplasm (→). Intranuclear inclusions are surrounded by a clear halo (→). Both the nuclear and cytoplasmic inclusions represent closely packed virions. (H&E, original magnification ×600).

HSV hepatitis presents as part of a generalized herpetic disease in the newborn infant. Hepatic manifestations may be mild, but most commonly are severe with jaundice, hepatomegaly, conjugated hyperbilirubinemia and elevated transaminases, major abnormalities of blood clotting factors and bleeding complications. Disseminated HSV infection can present as neonatal liver failure with an accompanying dismal prognosis.[50] Liver histopathology reveals generalized or multifocal hepatocyte necrosis and cholestasis with characteristic intra-nuclear acidophilic inclusion bodies representing the herpes simplex virions (Fig. 58.3, inset).[17,51]

Diagnosis of neonatal HSV infection is confirmed by isolation of virus from the skin or body secretions, detection of viral DNA by PCR, or rapid diagnosis from skin lesion by direct immunofluorescence or enzyme immunoassay. Serology testing is of little value due to lack of or delayed production of IgM in the neonatal period and the inability to differentiate between HSV 1 and 2. Immunohistochemistry has been used to confirm the diagnosis in liver tissue specimens.

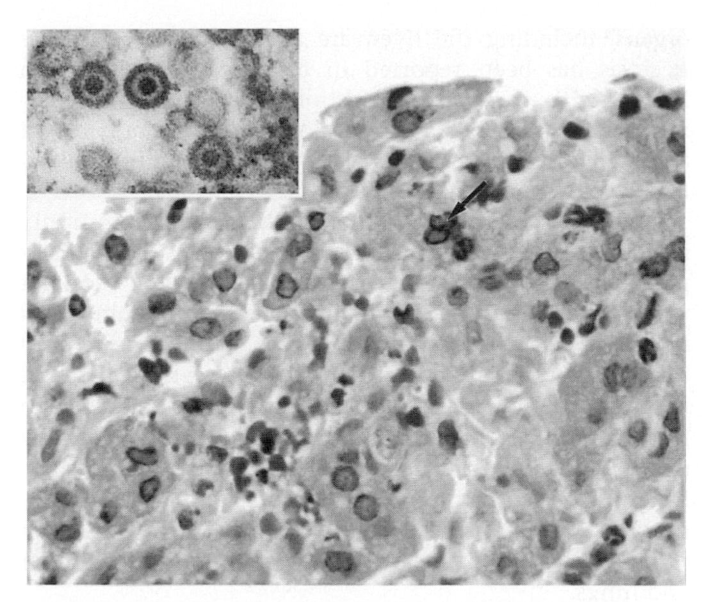

Figure 58.3: Herpes simplex infection. Generalized necrosis with characteristic pale intranuclear inclusions surrounded by rim of chromatin (arrow) in hepatocytes are noted. Significant giant cell transformation present. (Hematoxylin and eosin, original magnification ×600.) Inset: Electron microscopy shows herpes simplex virons. (Original magnification ×10 0000.)

Parenteral acyclovir is the treatment of choice for neonatal HSV infections, with the results of a vidarabine-acyclovir comparison trial in the treatment of neonatal herpes not showing any difference in efficacy and safety between the two drugs.[52] Acyclovir should be administered to all neonates with confirmed HSV infection, regardless of clinical manifestations. Intravenous immunoglobulin has no role in the treatment of neonatal HSV infection. Adequate hydration during treatment is important to prevent acyclovir-induced renal toxicity. Successful liver transplantation for fulminant hepatitis secondary to HSV 2 has been reported.[53,54]

Congenital rubella

Rubella virus is an enveloped RNA virus in the family *Togaviridae*. Although rubella usually is a mild, often subclinical disease affecting school-age children and young adults, congenital rubella syndrome is associated with multiple anomalies. These congenital malformations include ophthalmologic (cataracts, retinopathy and congenital glaucoma), cardiac (patent ductus arteriosus and peripheral pulmonary artery stenosis), auditory (sensorineural hearing impairment) and neurologic (behavioral disorders, meningoencephalitis and mental retardation). Additional features include growth retardation, radiolucent bone disease, hepatosplenomegaly, thrombocytopenia and purpuric skin lesions of the 'blueberry muffin' appearance.

Congenital rubella is associated with giant-cell transformation in neonatal hepatitis. Clinical manifestations include jaundice, hepatosplenomegaly and transient cholestasis to a late anicteric hepatitis.[55] Hepatosplenomegaly persists for longer periods of time and resolves after 12 months or even longer.[17] Diagnosis of congenital rubella is made by the detection of rubella-specific immunoglobulin (Ig) M antibody at birth, stable or increasing serum rubella-specific IgG over several months and isolation of rubella virus from nasopharyngeal or other body fluid specimens. Liver histology typically demonstrates giant-cell hepatitis.[56] Infants with congenital rubella usually recover from the hepatitis and progression to cirrhosis is rare. Treatment for congenital rubella is supportive. Mass immunization of prepubertal females offers the best hope for prevention of this disease.

Enteroviruses

The non-polio enteroviruses are single-stranded RNA viruses belonging to the family *Picornaviridae*, which include coxsackieviruses, echoviruses and enteroviruses.[57] Neonatal infection with coxsackieviruses and echoviruses can result from transplacental viral transmission, contact infection during birth and human-to-human contact after birth. Coxsackieviral and echoviral infections in neonates result in a wide variety of clinical manifestations ranging from asymptomatic infection to fetal encephalitis and myocarditis. The most common manifestation is a non-specific febrile illness, which leads to an evaluation for bacterial sepsis. Important factors in the clinical diagnosis of enteroviral infection include the seasonal (summer and fall) prevalence, exposure (positive maternal history in the summer and fall), incubation period and clinical symptoms.[57]

Hepatitis is an important neonatal non-polio enteroviral illness, with 2% of neonates with clinically severe enteroviral disease having hepatitis.[57] Severe hepatitis, frequently with hepatic necrosis, has been noted with echoviruses 6, 9, 11, 14, 19 and 21. Liver involvement with fatal massive hepatic necrosis has also been noted with coxsackie group B virus and enterovirus 71, manifest by rapidly progressive hepatic failure, jaundice and disseminated intravascular coagulation.[58–60] Mortality rates range between 31% and 83% in case series of neonates with hepatitis.[61] Liver calcifications may complicate survivors of coxsackievirus B1 hepatitis.

Specimens providing the highest rate of virus isolation are those obtained from the throat, stool and rectum. Diagnosis is made using PCR or direct viral detection in cell cultures. Serology testing is of limited value due to low sensitivity resulting from a lack of a common antigen in so many antigenically different enteroviruses.[61]

Treatment is primarily supportive. No specific therapy is currently available, although the antiviral agent, pleconaril, is undergoing clinical evaluation.[59,60] Intravenous immune globulin (IVIG) containing high antibody titers to the infecting virus may be beneficial for selected patients, including those with life-threatening neonatal infections.

Hepatotrophic viruses

The five hepatotrophic viruses, hepatitis A (HAV), hepatitis B (HBV), C (HCV), D (HDV) and E (HEV) cause hepatitis as their primary disease manifestation, but likely play a limited role in neonatal hepatitis. The known hepatitis viruses are not responsible for a large number of cases of neonatal hepatitis syndrome. In infants, HAV and HBV infections are generally asymptomatic.[62] Neonatal cholestasis resulting from vertical transmission of HAV infection was recently reported.[63] HBV is vertically transmitted during pregnancy or delivery. The transmission rate is approximately 70% in mothers who are both hepatitis B surface antigen and hepatitis B e antigen positive.[64] Most infected infants will become asymptomatic carriers. In contrast, infants born to mothers who are hepatitis B e antigen negative, have a higher risk of developing fulminant hepatitis.[64] HCV can be transmitted perinatally, with some infected infants having mild to moderate elevation of aminotransferase levels.[65] Perinatal transmission of HDV is uncommon.[66] Vertical transmission of HEV has been described, with rare instances of acute icteric hepatitis possible.[67] Hence, screening for the hepatotropic viruses in infants presenting with prolonged cholestasis remains in diagnostic algorithms. Further discussion of these viruses in older children and adolescents is discussed in Chapter 63.

Human immunodeficiency virus (HIV)

HIV infection in children causes a broad spectrum of disease and a varied clinical course. Acquired immunodeficiency syndrome (AIDS) represents the most severe end of the clinical spectrum. The established modes of HIV transmission include sexual contact; percutaneous or mucous membrane exposure to contaminated blood or other body fluids with high titers of HIV; mother-to-infant transmission before or around the time of birth; and breastfeeding. Pediatric HIV often involves the intestinal tract and liver. Clinical manifestations include failure to thrive, recurrent diarrhea, oral candidiasis, hepatitis, hepatomegaly and splenomegaly as well as generalized lymphadenopathy, parotitis, cardiomyopathy, nephropathy, central nervous system disease (including developmental delay), lymphoid interstitial pneumonia, recurrent invasive bacterial infections, opportunistic infections and specific malignant neoplasms.[68] Giant cell hepatitis has been reported in an infant born to HIV positive parents.[69] Ultrastructural evidence of tubuloreticular inclusions in endothelial cells and non-hepatocyte cylindrical confronting cisternae were noted and attributed directly to HIV infection.[69]

Other viruses

Human herpes virus (HHV)-6, the cause of childhood roseola infantum with fever and exanthem subitum, has been associated with cholestasis, neonatal hepatitis, giant cell transformation[70] and fatal fulminant hepatitis.[71] The histopathology is of a non-specific lobular hepatitis. Diagnosis is confirmed by serology or PCR on body fluids and infected tissues.

Human parvovirus (B19 virus), the cause of erythema infectiosum in childhood, is thought to principally attack pronormoblastic erythroid cells, resulting in severe hemolytic anemia in the fetus with hydrops.[72] Many fetal organs, including the liver, are affected and hepatocyte necrosis has been reported in fetuses and in newborn infants with parvovirus infection.[72,73] Diagnosis of parvovirus B19 is confirmed by serology with detection of IgM and IgG in blood samples or by the detection of virus by PCR in blood or tissue samples.

Adenoviruses are DNA viruses, which most commonly infect the upper respiratory tract. Transmission is either perinatal during delivery or postnatal through contact with infected caregivers. Life-threatening disseminated infection occasionally occurs among young infants and immunocompromised hosts, with severe hepatitis and liver failure.[74,75] The pathology is similar to that seen in Herpes simplex infection, with widespread liver cell necrosis and intranuclear viral inclusion bodies. Diagnosis is confirmed by isolation of the virus from nasopharyngeal or pulmonary secretions or by detection of viral DNA by PCR in infected tissues, such as the liver and lungs.

Congenital varicella syndrome refers to the onset of chickenpox within the first 10 days of life. The incubation period, defined as the interval between the onset of rash in the mother and onset in the fetus or neonate, usually is 9–15 days, with a range of between 1 and 16 days. Infants at risk are those whose mother suffers from chickenpox during the last 1–2 weeks of pregnancy or within the first few days post partum. Severe hepatitis may occur as a feature of multi-system involvement that may include extensive skin lesions, pneumonitis and meningoencephalitis.[57]

Transfusion-Transmitted Virus (TTV) is a newly discovered unenveloped single-stranded DNA virus initially implicated as a cause of posttransfusion hepatitis. Maternal-neonatal transmission has been reported.[76] The detection of the TTV genome in the liver of 3 infants with idiopathic neonatal hepatitis and favorable response to gammaglobulin therapy suggest a potential cause-and-effect relationship.[77,78]

Reovirus-3 has been proposed as a candidate virus serving as an etiologic agent for neonatal hepatitis as well as biliary atresia. Infection of weanling mice results in hepatic lesions similar to those observed in neonates with neonatal hepatitis. However, studies in humans using molecular techniques have yielded mixed results.[79,80]

Paramyxovirus infection has been attributed as the etiologic agent in a rare form of neonatal hepatitis called syncytial giant-cell hepatitis affecting both children and adults.[81] The clinical liver disease varies with the age of the patient. In neonates, syncytial giant-cell hepatitis is associated with a severe hepatitis, with progression to chronic cholestasis and decompensated cirrhosis over the first year of life. Liver histology and electron microscopy reveal both the hallmark syncytial-type giant cells replacing hepatocyte cords most prominently in the centrilobular region, as well as severe acute and chronic hepatitis with bridging necrosis of hepatocytes, ballooning and drop-out of hepatocytes, cholestasis and small round cell inflammation within the lobule. Ultrastructural studies revealed the presence of virus-like structures within giant cells resembling the nucleocapsids of paramyxovirus. These giant cells are larger and of different morphology than the giant cells typically encountered in neonatal liver disease.[82] The putative virus from the paramyxoviruses family has not been subsequently identified since this entity was first described. Treatment with the anti-viral drug ribavirin was beneficial in one infant with syncytial giant cell hepatitis.[83] Liver transplantation is life-saving. Recurrence of the disease after liver transplantation has been reported and supports the hypothesis of a transmissible viral agent as the etiological agent.

Parasitic infections

Toxoplasmosis

Toxoplasma gondii is an obligate intracellular protozoan parasite that can cross the placenta and infect the fetus. Congenital infection occurs primarily as a result of maternal infection during pregnancy acquired by consumption of undercooked meat or direct contact with the feces of infected animals, such as cats or kittens. IgM screening has documented the prevalence of congenital infection to range from 0.08 per 1000 live births to 3 to 10 per 1000 live births.[57,84]

Most infants born with congenital *Toxoplasma* infection are asymptomatic in the neonatal period, with clinical signs and symptoms being present in only approximately 25% of infants.[57] The clinical manifestations of congenital toxoplasmosis in the newborn generally are indistinguishable from those associated with other agents of congenital infection such as CMV or *Treponema pallidum*. The most characteristic clinical findings, frequently referred to as the classic triad of congenital toxoplasmosis, are chorioretinitis, intracranial calcifications and hydrocephalus. They are often accompanied by a combination of other signs and symptoms, including hepatosplenomegaly and jaundice.[57] Serum aminotransferase levels are elevated and progressive liver dysfunction with ascites may occur. Liver histopathology features include a non-specific giant-cell hepatitis with focal necroses associated with parasitized sinusoidal cells. The commonest clinical association is now with accompanying HIV infection.[57]

The diagnosis of congenital toxoplasmosis is made prenatally by the detection of *T. gondii* in fetal blood or amniotic fluid, or from the placenta, umbilical cord, or infant peripheral blood via polymerase chain reaction (PCR). Serologic diagnosis can be made by immunoglobulin M (IgM) or IgA or persistent (over 12 months) IgG anti-*Toxoplasma* antibody tests determined in the infant's blood. A case of congenital toxoplasmosis diagnosed by the use of exfoliative cytology of neonatal ascites has been reported.[85] Treatment may prevent further progression of tissue damage. Pyrimethamine and sulfadiazine are synergistic and are the most commonly used drugs in the treatment of infants with documented infection. The focus of prevention should be on education of women of childbearing age to avoid ingestion of infective cysts and contact with sporulated oocysts.

SYSTEMIC CONDITIONS ASSOCIATED WITH NEONATAL HEPATITIS

Endocrinopathies

Conjugated hyperbilirubinemia has been associated with disturbance of the pituitary-adrenal axis. The initial manifestations of congenital anterior hypopituitarism may be hypoglycemia with prolonged neonatal cholestasis.[86] In male infants, micropenis and undescended testes can be associated features. Hypoglycemia typically occurs after fasting, due to deficiencies of the hormones that antagonize insulin.[87] The resultant cholestasis is probably a secondary feature of an inadequate development of the hepatobiliary secretory apparatus from the absence of the trophic hormones modulating or stimulating bile canalicular development and bile acid synthesis, conjugation and secretion. The presence of 'wandering' nystagmus on physical examination diagnoses septooptic dysplasia as seen with the de Morsier's syndrome, also known as optic nerve hypoplasia.[88] In the absence of physical findings suggestive of hypopituitarism, the diagnosis is less apparent. In these babies, clinical suspicion can be confirmed by assay of cortisol, growth hormone and insulin levels. A liver biopsy is typically not helpful, with nonspecific features of neonatal hepatitis.

Infants with isolated thyroid hormone deficiency also may develop cholestasis. There has been no clearly documented case of cholestasis and hypoglycemia secondary to isolated GH deficiency, although animal studies support growth hormone deficiency as a factor responsible for hepatic dysfunction. Cortisol deficiency as the primary cause of altered liver function in infants with hypopituitarism and adrenal insufficiency[89] and neonatal cholestasis has been seen in infants with congenital insensitivity of adrenocorticotropin (ACTH).[90,91] Clinical suspicion and early diagnosis with appropriate treatment of the underlying endocrinopathy results in rapid resolution of the hepatic dysfunction.

Chromosomal disorders

Neonatal hepatitis syndrome is reported in association with trisomy 17, trisomy 18 and trisomy 21 (Down syndrome).[92] Paucity of the intrahepatic bile duct in infants and children has been reported in trisomy 21.[92] The mechanisms underlying these associations remain unknown.

Autoimmune conditions

Neonatal lupus erythematosus (NLE) is an uncommon autoimmune disease caused by the passage of maternal anti-Ro (SS-A) or anti-La (SS-B) antibodies across the placenta. Affected organs include the heart, skin and liver, because these are the fetal tissues which express the Ro and La antigens. Disease presentation occurs during gestation or immediately after birth. A maternal history of systemic lupus erythematosus is common. The most striking manifestations are congenital complete heart block and a discoid lupus erythematosus rash, appearing either in the newborn period or weeks later.

A retrospective analysis of a United States NLE research registry revealed that 9% of newborns with NLE have some degree of hepatic involvement.[93] Three clinical variants of hepatobiliary disease are observed: (1) severe liver failure present during gestation or in the neonatal period, often with a phenotype mimicking neonatal iron storage disease; (2) conjugated hyperbilirubinemia with mild or no elevations of aminotransferases, occurring in the first few weeks of life; and (3) mild elevations of aminotransferases occurring at approximately 2–3 months of life. The prognosis for children in the last two categories is excellent.

Hepatobiliary disease is a relatively common finding in NLE and can be the sole clinical manifestation of NLE. Liver manifestations include hepatomegaly, jaundice, hepatosplenomegaly, mild-moderate increase in transaminases, conjugated hyperbilirubinemia and, in severe cases, fulminant hepatic failure.[93,94] Liver histology resembles giant cell hepatitis with giant cell transformation, ductal or ductular obstruction and extramedullary hematopoiesis. In fatal cases, liver pathology was consistent with the typical findings of neonatal hemochromatosis.[93]

Diagnosis is based on a maternal history of SLE, typical clinical findings and the presence of anti-Ro or anti-La antibodies in serum. Anti nuclear antibody can be detected in some of the cases with hepatic involvement and might have a role in the pathogenesis of liver disease.[95] Immunosuppressive treatment with prednisone in selected cases in the first few months of life led to improvement in the liver function tests.

Ischemic hepatitis

Ischemic hepatitis refers to diffuse hepatic injury resulting from acute hypoperfusion. Hepatic ischemia, like ischemia involving other organs, results from an imbalance between oxygen supply and tissue demands. As the metabolic rate of the liver is relatively constant, oxygen supply, not demand, is the principal determinant of hepatic ischemia.

Hepatic dysfunction occurs frequently in children with disorders that compromise blood flow, despite the unique dual circulation of the liver conferring relative protection against ischemic injury. With 25% of cardiac output directed to the liver, two thirds of the hepatic blood flow arrives through the portal vein and the remainder through the hepatic artery. In the periportal zone of the hepatic lobule, the highly oxygenated blood from the hepatic artery mixes with less well oxygenated portal blood rich in nutrients and hormones from the gastrointestinal tract. Under normal conditions, oxygen and nutrients in the blood decrease from periportal (zone 1) to pericentral (zone 3) areas. The low oxygen tension in the sinusoidal blood in zone 3 of the hepatic acinus makes pericentral hepatocytes in this zone relatively vulnerable to ischemic injury and necrosis.[96]

Hence, ischemic hepatitis, which clinically may mimic toxic or infectious hepatitis, occurs in association with congenital heart disease (such as hypoplastic left heart syndrome and coarctation of the aorta), shock, cardiorespiratory arrest, asphyxia, prolonged seizures, severe dehydration or pericardial tamponade.[97] Ischemic hepatitis is associated with a decrease in cardiac output, although the hypotension frequently has not been documented. Left-hearted heart failure tends not to cause hepatic symptoms until hypotension or reduced cardiac output is present.[98] Ischemic hepatitis is also seen in neonates following cardiopulmonary bypass.[99]

Ischemic hepatitis is characterized by a marked and rapid elevation of serum transaminases within 24–48 h after the initial insult, with a rapid decline by 3–11 days if perfusion and oxygenation are restored.[100] Serum aminotransferase concentrations peak to 5000–10 000 IU/l; alkaline phosphatase is usually normal. Hepatomegaly, jaundice and coagulopathy are detected in up to 50% of affected patients. Elevations of serum creatinine phosphokinase (CPK) and serum creatinine reflect hypotensive injury to other organs and are helpful indicators of global hypoperfusion. As the diagnosis may be made on clinical and biochemical review, liver biopsy is usually not necessary. The prognosis for children with ischemic hepatitis depends primarily on the response of the underlying disorder to therapy.[101]

Parenteral nutrition

Total parenteral nutrition (TPN) has been associated with a wide spectrum of adverse hepatobiliary consequences. In infants, cholestasis is the primary form of TPN-associated liver disease. The severity of cholestasis spans the spectrum in individual patients from mild increases in serum aminotransferase and bilirubin levels that may remit despite continued TPN to progressive disease that results in liver failure. TPN-induced liver disease develops in 40–60% of infants who require long-term TPN for intestinal failure.[102] The rate of progression of TPN-associated liver disease may vary from months to several years.

Infants particularly susceptible are those born prematurely and of low birthweight. In most affected infants, cholestasis occurs in a complex clinical context, making it difficult to ascribe the liver injury to a single insult. For example, the small, critically ill neonate has a clinical picture dominated by hypotension and multiple episodes of sepsis with accompanying multi-organ system failure or dysfunction. Another high-risk group includes infants with intestinal disease such as necrotizing enterocolitis and the short gut syndrome. Although the high prevalence of TPN-associated cholestasis in premature infants suggests that immaturity of hepatic excretory function is an etiologic factor, it is this group of patients who usually require prolonged TPN. The infant liver may well be more vulnerable to cholestatic stresses, as bile acid processing is relatively inefficient in this age group.

The pathogenesis of TPN-associated liver cholestasis in infants remains ill defined. The severity of cholestasis appears to be associated with insults of hypoxemia (shock/reperfusion) and hypotension. The degree and severity of the liver disease also is related to recurrent sepsis including catheter sepsis, bacterial translocation and cholangitis. Lack of enteral feeding leading to reduced gut hormone secretion, reduction of bile flow and biliary stasis also likely are important factors in the development of cholestasis, biliary sludge and cholelithiasis. TPN contributes to the cholestatic effect of sepsis by promoting bacterial translocation from the gut via impairment of intestinal defense mechanisms and induction of small bowel bacterial overgrowth. The administration of a nutrient solution in TPN can be directly damaging to the hepatocyte. The common denominator in these situations is oxidant stress. It is proposed that oxidant stress and stimulation of hepatic Kupffer cells by bacterial cell wall products absorbed from the injured intestine are major factors leading to cholestasis and liver injury during prolonged parenteral nutrition.[103,104]

The morphological changes of TPN-associated cholestasis in infants are non-specific and variable. As the diagnosis is one of exclusion, liver biopsy is not commonly performed, particularly in the setting of the critically ill infant with coagulopathy and multisystem involvement. Bilirubinostasis affecting hepatocytes and canaliculi is consistently present and may develop in a matter of days; cholestatic rosettes are frequently observed; bile plugs also may be present in interlobular bile ducts. Steatosis may be present. Portal tracts show a variable mixed inflammatory cell infiltrate and, with prolonged therapy, a periportal ductular reaction with progressive hepatic fibrosis ultimately leading to biliary cirrhosis.[51]

TPN-associated cholestasis remains a diagnosis of exclusion since specific clinical, biochemical and histologic criteria are lacking. Consideration must be given to alternative causes of conjugated hyperbilirubinemia; otherwise, reversible disorders may be overlooked or the parenteral nutrition inappropriately discontinued. The risk:benefit ratio of parenteral nutrition must be individualized for each neonate. The dilemma is based on weighing the risk of progressive cholestasis and its attendant complications against the risk of starvation, malnutrition and their consequences.

Management strategies for the prevention of TPN-induced liver disease include early enteral feeding and aseptic catheter techniques to reduce episodes of sepsis. The administration of ursodeoxycholic acid may improve bile flow and reduce gallbladder and intestinal stasis.[104] Avoiding excessive nutrient infusion and providing even minimal enteral calories has been touted to mitigate cholestasis. Routine monitoring of hepatic transaminases and synthetic function in all neonates receiving parenteral nutrition allows early detection and potential interventions. As survival from isolated intestinal transplantation improves, this therapeutic option should be considered before TPN liver disease becomes irreversible and combined liver and small bowel transplantation is required.[103]

IDIOPATHIC NEONATAL HEPATITIS

Idiopathic neonatal hepatitis continues to be a descriptive term and 'default' diagnosis applied to infants with prolonged cholestasis in whom extrahepatic obstruction has been ruled out and known infectious and metabolic diseases have been excluded. The liver injury is highlighted by the presence of variable numbers of multi-nuclear 'giant' cells.[105] Neonatal hepatitis may be familial or non-familial. The familial form can be progressive, with or without the development of cirrhosis, or the course may be characterized by recurrent cholestasis.[106,107] The pattern of inheritance is considered to be autosomal recessive. Idiopathic neonatal hepatitis represents a common diagnosis for infants presenting with clinical or biochemical evidence of cholestasis, with incidence rates ranging from 1:4800 to 1:9000 live births.[108] However, reliable figures do not exist regarding the current incidence, as specific entities continue to be discovered and described, allowing re-categorization and re-definition of patients previously labeled as idiopathic neonatal hepatitis.

Clinical features

Affected infants usually present with jaundice in the first week of life. While idiopathic neonatal hepatitis may be associated with low birthweight, a cause-and-effect relationship is not evident. The clinical course is highly variable. Most infants appear well; however, poor feeding and vomiting with failure to thrive, which should be suggestive of metabolic disease, complicates the clinical course in a small percentage of affected infants. Hepatomegaly is present in almost all patients and splenomegaly occasionally may be present. Serum bile acid levels are markedly increased. A bleeding diathesis, resulting from vitamin K deficiency and or decreased synthesis of clotting factors, may be present in those with a more fulminant course. The presence of associated abnormalities such as microcephaly, ophthalmologic, vascular or skeletal anomalies should suggest alternative diagnoses.

Treatment and prognosis

The major issue in the management of infants with idiopathic neonatal hepatitis is to carry out an exhaustive search for recognizable and treatable causes for the common phenotype presentation. Idiopathic neonatal hepatitis represents a heterogeneous disorder without a unitary etiology. By definition, there are no specifically delineated causative or perpetuating factors; hence, therapy is not specific. Management is directed toward the consequences of cholestasis, including nutritional support and vitamin supplementation.

The overall prognosis in idiopathic neonatal hepatitis is difficult to estimate, particularly because of the variability of the clinical course and the generally ill-defined pathogenesis. Furthermore, it is not well understood what factors allow the perpetuation of the cholestatic process and hepatocyte injury. There are no specific biochemical or histologic correlates with clinical outcome. Cumulative data indicate that 60% of patients with sporadic (non-familial) neonatal hepatitis will recover; 10% will have persisting fibrosis or inflammation; 2% will develop cirrhosis and 30% will die. This outcome differs from that of familial cases, or cases in which consanguinity was present in whom 30% recover, 10% develop chronic liver disease and cirrhosis and 60% die.[109–112] Some investigators identify a group of babies with a good clinical outcome; this group is referred to as transient neonatal cholestasis.[113]

COMPLICATIONS AND MANAGEMENT OF NEONATAL HEPATITIS SYNDROME

A summary of medical treatment options for cholestasis is provided in Table 58.3.

The ultimate prognosis for affected infants is related to the severity of the complications resulting from chronic and persisting cholestasis. These complications are attributed to decreased delivery of bile acids to the proximal intestine with decreased intraluminal bile acid concentrations (resulting in malnutrition and malabsorption of fat and fat-soluble vitamins); regurgitation of bile constituents (both known and unknown) into the systemic circulation leading to pruritus, xanthoma/xanthelasma production and fatigue; and retention by the liver of substances causing ensuing hepatotoxicity progressing to portal hypertension, cirrhosis and chronic liver failure (Fig. 58.4). Such departures from normal physiology lead to discomfort, failure to thrive, specific nutrient deficiencies and psychological or behavioral problems in the developing child. Currently, no specific therapy either reverses existing cholestasis or prevents ongoing damage. Therefore, although therapy is empiric, meticulous attention is aimed at improving nutritional status, maximizing growth potential and minimizing discomfort.[114] Success of therapeutic interventions is further limited by the residual capacity of the damaged liver and by the rate of progression of the underlying disorder.

- Malabsorption/Undernutrition
  - Optimize caloric intake – via enteral nutrition if possible
  - Administer medium-chain triglycerides (MCT)
  - Decrease the percentage of dietary long-chain triglycerides (LCT)
  - Ensure adequate essential fatty acid intake
  - Ensure adequate protein intake
  - Consider branched chain amino acids supplements
- Vitamin and micronutrient deficiency
  - Careful and serial monitoring of levels in serum
  - Supplement fat-soluble vitamins (A, D, E and K) as necessary
  - Supply water-soluble vitamins
  - Correct and prevent mineral and trace element deficiencies
- Pruritus/xanthomata
  - Ursodeoxycholic acid
  - Hydroxyzine
  - Rifampicin
  - Cholestyramine
  - Phenobarbital
  - Opioid antagonists
  - Others with potential benefit
    - Chlorpromazine
    - Carbamazepine
  - Partial external biliary diversion
- Progression of liver disease
  - Ascites
    - Restrict sodium intake
    - Diuretics
      - Spironolactone
      - Furosemide
    - Therapeutic paracentesis
  - Portal hypertension and variceal hemorrhage
    - Medication
    - Endoscopy (banding, sclerotherapy)
    - Surgery (shunts)
  - Liver transplantation

Table 58.3 Medical management of neonatal cholestasis

Malabsorption and undernutrition

Malnutrition, growth failure and debilitation seen in the child with chronic cholestasis are attributed to multiple factors.[115] The decreased delivery of bile acids to the duodenum during cholestasis leads to intraluminal bile acid concentrations that are inadequate for the formation of micelles, resulting in the malabsorption of dietary lipids and the fat-soluble vitamins. Other contributing factors include abnormalities in amino acid and glucose metabolism, increased resting energy expenditure, recurrent infections, anorexia and early satiety and gastroesophageal reflux or vomiting secondary to compression of abdominal viscera by an enlarged liver or spleen and ascites.[116–119] Cholestasis, hepatocyte injury and undernutrition interact to impair adequate growth.[120] The impact of malnutrition on brain growth, mental development and immune function further support prioritizing an early and aggressive approach to the nutritional status of the child with chronic cholestasis.[121]

Adequate protein intake is paramount (2.0–3.0 mg protein/kg ideal bodyweight/day in small infants), while delivering optimal energy intake. The goal for caloric intake should be approximately 125–150% of the recommended dietary allowance. Whenever possible, oral feeding is preferred, but may be insufficient to optimize the nutritional status of neonates and infants with prolonged cholestasis. Nocturnal enteral feeding improves nutritional indices of patients with chronic cholestatic disease.[122]

Gastrostomy tubes are generally less often used, because of iatrogenic bleeding risks with portal hypertensive gastropathy and the development of gastric varices. Medium chain triglyceride (MCT) oil-containing diets may reduce steatorrhea, improve energy balance and promote growth in children with chronic cholestasis.[123] MCT is relatively water-soluble, does not require bile acid micelles for solubilization and is directly absorbed into the portal circulation in the absence of bile secretion. Branched chain amino acid enriched formulas and TPN may improve nutritional status and body composition in infants with

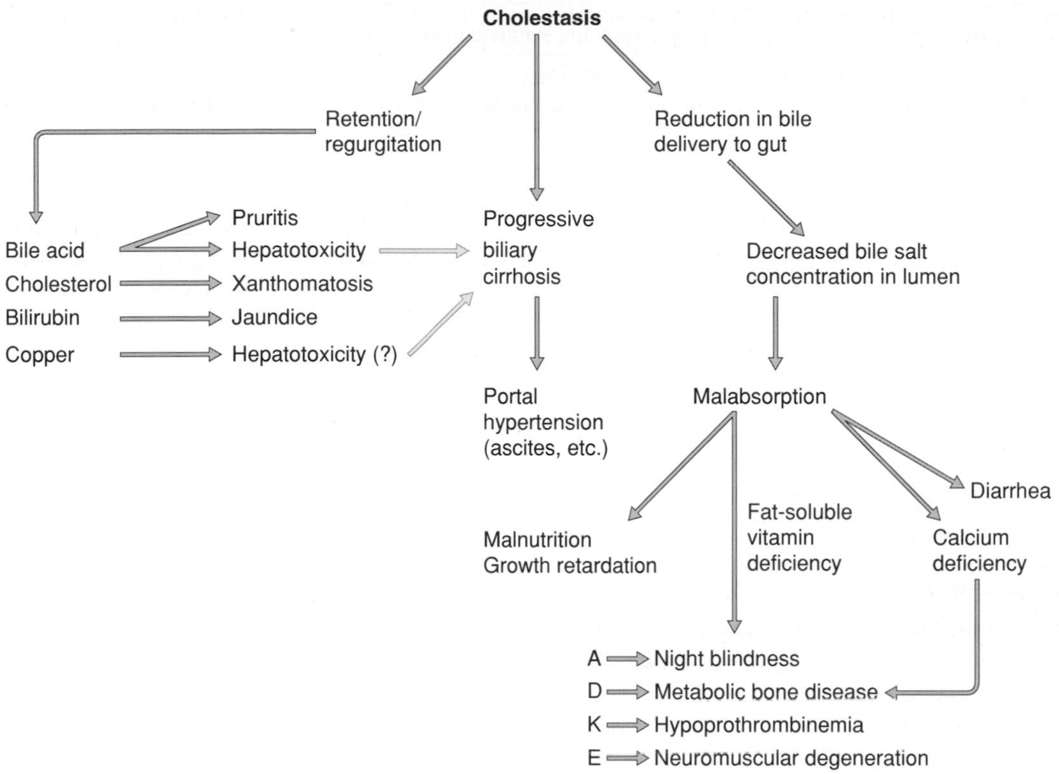

Cholestasis
Retention/ regurgitation
Reduction in bile delivery to gut
Bile acid → Pruritis
Bile acid → Hepatotoxicity
Cholesterol → Xanthomatosis
Bilirubin → Jaundice
Copper → Hepatotoxicity (?)
Progressive biliary cirrhosis
Portal hypertension (ascites, etc.)
Decreased bile salt concentration in lumen
Malabsorption
Malnutrition Growth retardation
Fat-soluble vitamin deficiency
Diarrhea
Calcium deficiency
A → Night blindness
D → Metabolic bone disease
K → Hypoprothrombinemia
E → Neuromuscular degeneration

Figure 58.4: Clinical sequelae of chronic cholestasis. The multiple consequences of cholestasis are the clinical manifestations and result of retention of substances normally excreted in bile, reduction of bile acid delivery to the intestine and progressive damage to the liver. (From: Balistreri WF. Liver disease in infancy and childhood. In: Schiff E, Sorrell MF, Maddrey WC, eds. Diseases of the Liver, Vol 2, 8th edn. Philadelphia, PA: Lippincott-Raven; 1999:1357–1512.)

cholestasis.[124] Adequate amounts of essential fatty acids should also be provided in order to prevent deficiency.[125] Supplementation with corn oil, safflower oil or lipid emulsions (such as Microlipid) can be added to formula to provide additional linoleic acid, if needed.[125] Essential fatty acid deficiency must be evaluated for in the cholestatic child with poor growth, dry scaly rash or thrombocytopenia. Monitoring effects of nutritional rehabilitation in infants and children with chronic cholestasis may be more accurately reflected by anthropometric measurements rather than the conventional serial weight-for-age or height-for-age parameters used in children with without chronic liver disease.[126] Dietary interventions should be made in consultation with an experienced pediatric dietitian.

Vitamin and micronutrient deficiencies

Table 58.4 summarizes the oral regimens for supplementation of fat-soluble vitamins in infants with chronic cholestasis, with the features of deficiency and toxicity of each vitamin. The impaired secretion of bile acids during cholestasis results in malabsorption of the fat-soluble vitamins, A, D, E and K. Appropriate supplementation should be initiated promptly when cholestasis begins in infancy, as depletion of meager body stores present at birth occurs rapidly, resulting in biochemical and clinical features of fat-soluble vitamin deficiency as early as 4–12 months of age. Deficiencies in fat-soluble vitamins and micronutrients may occur despite the use of 'routine' supplemental doses. Fat-soluble vitamin deficiency is associated with significant symptoms. Therefore, periodic assessment and appropriate monitoring of serum levels of these nutrients is needed, even during therapy to detect and prevent clinical manifestations of deficiencies. Serum levels of vitamin A and vitamin E may not accurately reflect hepatic stores. The most reliable index of vitamin E status is the ratio of serum vitamin E (mg/dl) to total serum lipids (g/dl), because elevated lipid levels in chronic cholestasis allow vitamin E to partition into the nonpolar phase (plasma lipoprotein fraction) and hence, artificially raise serum vitamin E concentration. In infants, a ratio of less than 0.6 mg/g indicates vitamin E deficiency.[127] The use of the molar ratio of serum retinol to retinal binding protein (retinol:RBP) accurately reflects hepatic stores of vitamin A non-invasively.[128]

Little is known about the nutritional status of water-soluble vitamins during chronic cholestasis in infants. However, deficiency of vitamins B_1, B_6, C and folic acid have been described in adults with cholestasis.[129] Recommending standard appropriate-for-age pediatric multivitamins supplements daily to supplement vitamins normally present in the diet are probably not unreasonable. As these supplements also contain additional

Vitamin	Features of deficiency	Supplement and standard dosage	Features of toxicity
A	Ocular findings and potential vision impairment (i.e. night blindness, xerophthalmia etc)	5000–25 000 IU/day Water miscible retinol preparation	Bony lesions Desquamative dermatitis Hepatotoxicity Pseudotumor cerebri
D	Cranial bossing Persistently open fontanelle Hypocalcemia Hypophosphatemia Tetany Osteomalacia Rickets	Oral vitamin D_3 at 3–10 × RDA dosage for age 25-OH-vitamin D_3 at 3–4 μg/kg per day	Hypercalcemia Depression of central nervous system Ectopic calcification Nephrocalcinosis and nephrolithiasis Cardiac arrhythmia
E	Areflexia/hyporeflexia Truncal and limb ataxia Depressed vibratory and position sensation, Impaired balance and coordination Peripheral neuropathy Proximal muscle weakness Ophthalmoplegia Retinal dysfunction Cognitive and behavioral abnormalities	d-alpha tocopheryl polyethylene glycol-1000 succinate (TPGS): 20–25 IU/kg per day given as a single morning oral dose (when bile flow is maximal)	None known
K	Coagulopathy Hemorrhagic manifestations	2.5–5 mg/day	Isolated cases of hemolytic anemia and thrombocytopenia

Table 58.4 Fat-soluble vitamins in infants with chronic cholestasis

amounts of the fat-soluble vitamins, this should be taken into account when calculating supplemental dose amounts of fat-soluble vitamins.

Attention to deficiency of minerals and trace element levels in chronic cholestasis to childhood is recommended. Hypocalcemia, hypophosphatemia and hypomagnesemia may develop with ensuing symptoms. Imbalance of trace minerals with major excretory pathways through the biliary route, such as copper, manganese and aluminum, may occur in children with chronic cholestasis.

Pruritus

The mechanisms underlying elevated serum levels of bile acids, cholesterol and triglyceride are complex. However, the end results of pruritus, fatigue, hyperlipidemia and cutaneous xanthomas are severe and debilitating complications. Pruritus often complicates cholestasis, yet there appears to be a lack of correlation between the severity of cholestasis and the apparent intensity with which pruritus is perceived. The best way to reverse pruritus associated with cholestasis is to effectively treat the cause of the cholestasis. However, complete reversal of the functional impairment causing cholestasis is often not possible. Pruritus complicating cholestasis remains a challenging management problem. Since the mechanisms which mediate pruritus of cholestasis remain to be definitively determined, the use of empirical therapies continues (Table 58.3).

One approach to therapy is to remove putative pruritogenic substances from the body, which is the rationale for the use of the anion-exchange resins, such as cholestyramine and colestipol. These drugs are postulated to bind pruritogens in the intestine and may be more effective if there is adequate biliary drainage to allow bile acids to reach the gut lumen. Administration of hepatic enzyme-inducing drugs, such as rifampicin and phenobarbital, may increase the metabolism of pruritogens and thereby enhance their removal.[130,131] Antihistamines are often administered in an attempt to reverse the effects of putative pruritogens, despite the fact that no skin changes consistent with histamine-mediated effects are found in the pruritus of cholestasis. Ursodeoxycholic acid appears to be effective in resolving or improving the liver function and the clinical status of a significant proportion of children with intrahepatic cholestasis.[132] Further, it may also reduce markedly elevated cholesterol levels and diminish the density of cutaneous xanthomata concurrently seen in some patients with intrahepatic cholestasis, particularly in those with Alagille syndrome.[132]

Recent evidence suggests that altered neurotransmission in the brain contributes to the pruritus of cholestasis, with studies supporting the hypothesis that there is an increase in central opioidergic tone.[133] However, the role of opiate antagonists such as naloxone has not been evaluated in children.[134] Some drugs with a sedative effect, such as phenobarbital, benzodiazepines, carbamazepine and antihistamines, may provide a nonspecific beneficial effect with the added benefit of improving sleep at night. The obvious down-side is the sedative effect on the infant's concentration and ability to learn during the day. The previous use of phototherapy with ultraviolet light lacks a clear rationale and is not efficacious. In case reports, plasma perfusion using charcoal-coated glass beads to remove bile acids and bilirubin has been reported to improve pruritus.

Selected patients with refractory pruritus failing maximal medical therapy have benefited from partial external diversion of bile. This represents a more extreme example of attempts to decrease the concentration of one or more unspecified and unknown pruritogens in patients with intractable pruritus of cholestasis.[135,136]

Progressive liver disease (portal hypertension)

In some patients with intrahepatic cholestasis, progressive hepatic fibrosis and cirrhosis ultimately leads to the development of portal hypertension with sequelae of ascites and variceal hemorrhage. The medical management of ascites needs to consider patient comfort and the relative risk of peritoneal bacterial infection. Judicious use of sodium restriction and diuretic therapy may help control the accumulation of ascites. Refractory ascites with respiratory compromise is best managed by therapeutic paracentesis with concomitant administration of intravenous colloid, such as albumin. Portal hypertension and its attendant complications are discussed in Chapter 64.

Family and psychological support

A multi-disciplinary team approach of care for these infants may prove beneficial. Physiotherapy can improve gross motor development while infant stimulation programs may enhance the neurodevelopmental status for infants who require frequent and recurrent hospitalizations. Family education and support are essential, particularly in aiding the family coping with the stress, social and emotional effects of chronic liver disease in attempts to optimize quality of life. Ongoing dialog with the family about the indications for liver transplantation is reasonable and discussed in detail in Chapter 65. Optimization and adherence to pretransplant medical management enhances the chances for a successful outcome from liver transplantation.

SUMMARY

The outcome of patients with neonatal hepatitis is variable and depends on the extent of the underlying parenchymal injury and accompanying hepatic fibrosis. Meticulous medical management to nutritional support, supplementation with fat-soluble vitamins and the use of choleretic agents may minimize adverse effects. In the future, additional diagnostic tools, using either protein or genetic markers, should increase the differential diagnosis entities and decrease the percentage of infants requiring the default diagnosis of idiopathic neonatal hepatitis.

ACKNOWLEDGEMENT

I thank Dr Ernest Cutz, Professor of Pathology and Dr Bo Ngan, Assistant Professor of Pathology, from the Department of Pathology and Laboratory Medicine at the Hospital for Sick Children and University of Toronto, for providing the photomicrographs.

References

1. Roberts EA. Neonatal hepatitis syndrome. Semin Neonatology 2003; 8(5):357–374.
2. Balistreri WF. Liver disease in infancy and childhood. In: Schiff E, Sorrell MF, Maddrey WC, eds. Diseases of the Liver, Vol 2, 8th edn. Philadelphia, PA: Lippincott-Raven; 1999:1357–1512.
3. Markowitz J, Daum F, Kahn EI, et al. Arteriohepatic dysplasia. I. Pitfalls in diagnosis and management. Hepatology 1983; 3(1):74–76.
4. Lai MW, Chang MH, Hsu SC, et al. Differential diagnosis of extrahepatic biliary atresia from neonatal hepatitis: a prospective study. J Pediatr Gastroenterol Nutr 1994; 18(2):121–127.
5. Maggiore G, Bernard O, Hadchouel M, et al. Diagnostic value of serum gamma-glutamyl transpeptidase activity in liver diseases in children. J Pediatr Gastroenterol Nutr 1991; 12(1):21–26.
6. Jansen PL, Sturm E. Genetic cholestasis, causes and consequences for hepatobiliary transport. Liver Int 2003; 23(5):315–322.
7. Bove KE. Liver disease caused by disorders of bile acid synthesis. Clin Liver Dis 2000; 4(4):831–848.
8. Franken EA. Jr., Smith WL, Siddiqui A. Noninvasive evaluation of liver disease in pediatrics. Radiol Clin North Am 1980; 18(2):239–252.
9. Park WH, Choi SO, Lee HJ. Technical innovation for noninvasive and early diagnosis of biliary atresia: the ultrasonographic 'triangular cord' sign. J Hepatobiliary Pancreat Surg 2001; 8(4):337–341.
10. Gilmour SM, Hershkop M, Reifen R, et al. Outcome of hepatobiliary scanning in neonatal hepatitis syndrome. J Nucl Med 1997; 38(8):1279–1282.
11. Rosenthal P, Miller JH, Sinatra FR. Hepatobiliary scintigraphy and the string test in the evaluation of neonatal cholestasis. J Pediatr Gastroenterol Nutr 1989; 8:292–296.
12. Zerbini MC, Gallucci SD, Maezono R, et al. Liver biopsy in neonatal cholestasis: a review on statistical grounds. Mod Pathol 1997; 10(8):793–799.
13. Montgomery CK, Ruebner BH. Neonatal hepatocellular giant cell transformation: a review. Perspect Pediatr Pathol 1976; 3:85–101.
14. Peng SS, Li YW, Chang MH, et al. Magnetic resonance cholangiography for evaluation of cholestatic jaundice in neonates and infants. J Formos Med Assoc 1998; 97(10):698–703.
15. Meyers RL, Book LS, O'Gorman MA, et al. Percutaneous cholecysto-cholangiography in the diagnosis of obstructive jaundice in infants. J Pediatr Surg 2004; 39(1):16–18.
16. Wilkinson ML, Mieli-Vergani G, Ball C, et al. Endoscopic retrograde cholangiopancreatography in infantile cholestasis. Arch Dis Child 1991; 66(1):121–123.
17. Watkins JB, Sunaryo FP, Berezin SH. Hepatic manifestations of congenital and perinatal disease. Clin Perinatol 1981; 8(3):467–480.
18. Schlossberg D. Syphilitic hepatitis: a case report and review of the literature. Am J Gastroenterol 1987; 82(6):552–553.
19. Chawla V, Pandit PB, Nkrumah FK. Congenital syphilis in the newborn. Arch Dis Child 1988; 63(11):1393–1394.

20. Herman TE. Extensive hepatic calcification secondary to fulminant neonatal syphilitic hepatitis. Pediatr Radiol 1995; 25(2):120–122.
21. Daaboul JJ, Kartchner W, Jones KL. Neonatal hypoglycemia caused by hypopituitarism in infants with congenital syphilis. J Pediatr 1993; 123(6):983–985.
22. Report of the Committee on Infectious Diseases. Red Book, 26th edn. Elk Grove Village, IL: American Academy of Pediatrics; 2003.
23. Sugiura H, Hayashi M, Koshida R, et al. Nonsyndromatic paucity of intrahepatic bile ducts in congenital syphilis. A case report. Acta Pathol Jpn 1988; 38(8):1061–1068.
24. Long WA, Ulshen MH, Lawson EE. Clinical manifestations of congenital syphilitic hepatitis: implications for pathogenesis. J Pediatr Gastroenterol Nutr 1984; 3(4):551–555.
25. Venter A, Pettifor JM, Duursma J, et al. Liver function in early congenital syphilis: does penicillin cause a deterioration? J Pediatr Gastroenterol Nutr 1991; 12(3):310–314.
26. Berk DR, Sylvester KG. Congenital tuberculosis presenting as progressive liver dysfunction. Pediatr Infect Dis J 2004; 23(1):78–80.
27. Foo AL, Tan KK, Chay OM. Congenital tuberculosis. Tuber Lung Dis 1993; 74(1):59–61.
28. Chou YH. Congenital tuberculosis proven by percutaneous liver biopsy: report of a case. J Perinat Med 2002; 30(5):423–425.
29. Balakrishnan S, Sharma S. Hepatic lesions in childhood tuberculosis. Indian J Child Health 1962; 11:365–371.
30. Becroft DM, Farmer K, Seddon RJ, et al. Epidemic listeriosis in the newborn. Br Med J 1971; 3(777):747–751.
31. Marino P, Maggioni M, Preatoni A, et al. Liver abscesses due to Listeria monocytogenes. Liver 1996; 16(1):67–69.
32. Hamilton JR, Sass-Kortsak A. Jaundice associated with severe bacterial infection in young infants. J Pediatr 1963; 63:121–132.
33. Bernstein J, Brown AK. Sepsis and jaundice in early infancy. Pediatrics 1962; 29:873–882.
34. Moseley RH. Sepsis and cholestasis. Clin Liver Dis 2004; 8(1):83–94.
35. Nolan JP. Intestinal endotoxins as mediators of hepatic injury–injuan idea whose time has come again. Hepatology 1989; 10(5):887–891.
36. Moseley RH, Wang W, Takeda H, et al. Effect of endotoxin on bile acid transport in rat liver: a potential model for sepsis-associated cholestasis. Am J Physiol 1996; 271(1):G137–G146.
37. Trauner M, Fickert P, Stauber RE. Inflammation-induced cholestasis. J Gastroenterol Hepatol 1999; 14(10):946–959.
38. Rooney JC, Hill DJ, Danks DM. Jaundice associated with bacterial infection in the newborn. Am J Dis Child 1971; 122(1):39–41.
39. Ng SH, Rawstron JR. Urinary tract infections presenting with jaundice. Arch Dis Child 1971; 46(246):173–176.
40. Sarici SU, Kul M, Alpay F. Neonatal jaundice coinciding with or resulting from urinary tract infections? Pediatrics 2003; 112(5):1212–1213.
41. Leung AK, Sauve RS, Davies HD. Congenital cytomegalovirus infection. J Natl Med Assoc 2003; 95(3):213–218.
42. Lai MW, Chang MH, Lee CY, et al. Cytomegalovirus-associated neonatal hepatitis. Zhonghua Min Guo Xiao Er Ke Yi Xue Hui Zhi 1992; 33(4):264–272.
43. Levy I, Shohat M, Levy Y, et al. Recurrent ascites in an infant with perinatally acquired cytomegalovirus infection. Eur J Pediatr 1989; 146(6):531–532.
44. Boppana SB, Pass RF, Britt WJ, et al. Symptomatic congenital cytomegalovirus infection: neonatal morbidity and mortality. Pediatr Infect Dis J 1992; 11(2):93–99.
45. Finegold MJ, Carpenter RJ. Obliterative cholangitis due to cytomegalovirus: a possible precursor of paucity of intrahepatic bile ducts. Hum Pathol 1982; 13(7):662–665.
46. Vanstapel MJ, Desmet VJ. Cytomegalovirus hepatitis: a histological and immunohistochemical study. Appl Pathol 1983; 1(1):41–49.
47. Shackelford GD, Kirks DR. Neonatal hepatic calcification secondary to transplacental infection. Radiology 1977; 122(3):753–757.
48. Nigro G, Scholz H, Bartmann U. Ganciclovir therapy for symptomatic congenital cytomegalovirus infection in infants: a two-regimen experience. J Pediatr 1994; 124(2):318–322.
49. Kimberlin DW, Lin CY, Sanchez PJ, et al. Effect of ganciclovir therapy on hearing in symptomatic congenital cytomegalovirus disease involving the central nervous system: a randomized, controlled trial. J Pediatr 2003; 143(1):16–25.
50. Benador N, Mannhardt W, Schranz D, et al. Three cases of neonatal herpes simplex virus infection presenting as fulminant hepatitis. Eur J Pediatr 1990; 149(8):555–559.
51. Ishak KG, Sharp HL. Developmental abnormalities and liver disease in childhood. In: MacSween R, Burt AD, Portmann BC, et al., eds. Pathology of the Liver, 4th edn. London: Harcourt; 2002:107–154.
52. Whitley R, Arvin A, Prober C, et al. A controlled trial comparing vidarabine with acyclovir in neonatal herpes simplex virus infection. Infect Dis Collab Antiviral Study Group N Engl J Med 1991; 324(7):444–449.
53. Egawa H, Inomata Y, Nakayama S, et al. Fulminant hepatic failure secondary to herpes simplex virus infection in a neonate: A case report of successful treatment with liver transplantation and perioperative acyclovir. Liver Transpl Surg 1998; 4(6):513–515.
54. Lee WS, Kelly DA, Tanner MS, et al. Neonatal liver transplantation for fulminant hepatitis caused by herpes simplex virus type 2. J Pediatr Gastroenterol Nutr 2002; 35(2):220–223.
55. Esterly JR, Slusser RJ, Ruebner BH. Hepatic lesions in the congenital rubella syndrome. J Pediatr 1967; 71:676–685.
56. Strauss L, Bernstein J. Neonatal hepatitis in congenital rubella. A histopathological study. Arch Pathol 1968; 86(3):317–327.
57. Sanchez PJ. Viral infections of the fetus and neonate. In: Feigin RD, Cherry JD, Demmler GJ, Kaplan SL, eds. Textbook of Pediatric Infectious Diseases, Vol 1, 5th edn. Philadelphia, PA: Saunders; 2004:866–909.
58. Yen HR, Lien R, Fu RH, et al. Hepatic failure in a newborn with maternal peripartum exposure to echovirus 6 and enterovirus 71. Eur J Pediatr 2003; 162(9):648–649.
59. Bryant PA, Tingay D, Dargaville PA, et al. Neonatal coxsackie B virus infection-a treatable disease? Eur J Pediatr 2004; 163(4/5):223–228.
60. Abzug MJ. Presentation, diagnosis and management of enterovirus infections in neonates. Paediatr Drugs 2004; 6(1):1–10.
61. Kawashima H, Ryou S, Nishimata S, et al. Enteroviral hepatitis in children. Pediatr Int 2004; 46(2):130–134.
62. Balistreri WF, Tabor E, Gerety RJ. Negative serology for hepatitis A and B viruses in 18 cases of neonatal cholestasis. Pediatrics 1980; 66(2):269–271.
63. Urganci N, Arapoglu M, Akyildiz B, et al. Neonatal cholestasis resulting from vertical transmission of hepatitis A infection. Pediatr Infect Dis J 2003; 22(4):381–382.

64. Friedt M, Gerner P, Lausch E, et al. Mutations in the basic core promotor and the precore region of hepatitis B virus and their selection in children with fulminant and chronic hepatitis B. Hepatology 1999; 29:1252–1258.
65. Roberts EA, Yeung L. Maternal-infant transmission of hepatitis C virus infection. Hepatology 2002; 36(5):S106–S113.
66. Zanetti AR, Ferroni P, Magliano EM, et al. Perinatal transmission of the hepatitis B virus and of the HBV-associated delta agent from mothers to offspring in northern Italy. J Med Virol 1982; 9(2):139–148.
67. Mast EE, Krawczynski K, Hepatitis E. an overview. Annu Rev Med 1996; 47:257–266.
68. Persaud D, Bangaru B, Greco MA, et al. Cholestatic hepatitis in children infected with the human immunodeficiency virus. Pediatr Infect Dis J 1993; 12(6):492–498.
69. Witzleben CL, Marshall GS, Wenner W, et al. HIV as a cause of giant cell hepatitis. Hum Pathol 1988; 19(5):603–605.
70. Tajiri H, Nose O, Baba K, et al. Human herpesvirus-6 infection with liver injury in neonatal hepatitis. Lancet 1990; 335(8693):863.
71. Asano Y, Yoshikawa T, Suga S, et al. Fatal fulminant hepatitis in an infant with human herpesvirus-6 infection. Lancet 1990; 335(8693):862–863.
72. Anand A, Gray ES, Brown T, et al. Human parvovirus infection in pregnancy and hydrops fetalis. N Engl J Med 1987; 316(4):183–186.
73. Metzman R, Anand A, DeGiulio PA, et al. Hepatic disease associated with intrauterine parvovirus B19 infection in a newborn premature infant. J Pediatr Gastroenterol Nutr 1989; 9(1):112–114.
74. Rieger-Fackeldey E, Aumeier S, Genzel-Boroviczeny O. Disseminated adenovirus infection in two premature infants. Infection 2000; 28(4):237–239.
75. Abzug MJ, Levin MJ. Neonatal adenovirus infection: four patients and review of the literature. Pediatrics 1991; 87(6):890 896.
76. Bagaglio S, Sitia G, Prati D, et al. Mother-to-child transmission of TT virus: sequence analysis of non-coding region of TT virus in infected mother-infant pairs. Arch Virol 2002; 147(4):803–812.
77. Tajiri H, Tanaka T, Sawada A, et al. Three cases with TT virus infection and idiopathic neonatal hepatitis. Intervirology 2001; 44(6):364–369.
78. Lin HH, Kao JH, Lee PI, et al. Early acquisition of TT virus in infants: possible minor role of maternal transmission. J Med Virol 2002; 66(2):285–290.
79. Steele MI, Marshall CM, Lloyd RE, et al. Reovirus 3 not detected by reverse transcriptase-mediated polymerase chain reaction analysis of preserved tissue from infants with cholestatic liver disease. Hepatology 1995; 21(3):697–702.
80. Tyler KL, Sokol RJ, Oberhaus SM, et al. Detection of reovirus RNA in hepatobiliary tissues from patients with extrahepatic biliary atresia and choledochal cysts. Hepatology 1998; 27(6):1475–1482.
81. Phillips MJ, Blendis LM, Poucell S, et al. Syncytial giant-cell hepatitis. Sporadic hepatitis with distinctive pathological features, a severe clinical course and paramyxoviral features. N Engl J Med 1991; 324(7):455–460.
82. Hicks J, Barrish J, Zhu SH. Neonatal syncytial giant cell hepatitis with paramyxoviral-like inclusions. Ultrastruct Pathol 2001; 25(1):65–71.
83. Roberts E, Ford-Jones EL, Phillips MJ. Ribavirin for syncytial giant cell hepatitis. Lancet 1993; 341(8845):640–641.
84. Guerina NG, Hsu HW, Meissner HC, et al. Neonatal serologic screening and early treatment for congenital Toxoplasma gondii infection. N Engl J Med 1994; 330(1858)
85. Nicol KK, Geisinger KR. Congenital toxoplasmosis: diagnosis by exfoliative cytology. Diagn Cytopathol 1998; 18(5):357–361.
86. Choo-Kang LR, Sun CC, Counts DR. Cholestasis and hypoglycemia: manifestations of congenital anterior hypopituitarism. J Clin Endocrinol Metab 1996; 81(8):2786–2789.
87. Sheehan AG, Martin SR, Stephure D, et al. Neonatal cholestasis, hypoglycemia and congenital hypopituitarism. J Pediatr Gastroenterol Nutr 1992; 14(4):426–430.
88. Kumura D, Miller JH, Sinatra FR. Septo-optic dysplasia: recognition of causes of false-positive hepatobiliary scintigraphy in neonatal jaundice. J Nucl Med 1987; 28(6):966–972.
89. Leblanc A, Odievre M, Hadchouel M, et al. Neonatal cholestasis and hypoglycemia: possible role of cortisol deficiency. J Pediatr 1981; 99(4):577–580.
90. Lacy DE, Nathavitharana KA, Tarlow MJ. Neonatal hepatitis and congenital insensitivity to adrenocorticotropin (ACTH). J Pediatr Gastroenterol Nutr 1993; 17(4):438–440.
91. Lee WS, Lum LC, Harun F. Addisonian-like crisis in congenital hypopituitarism and cholestatic jaundice. Med J Malaysia 2003; 58(2):279–281.
92. Puri P, Guiney EJ. Intrahepatic biliary atresia in Down's syndrome. J Pediatr Surg 1975; 10(3):423–424.
93. Lee LA, Sokol RJ, Buyon JP. Hepatobiliary disease in neonatal lupus: prevalence and clinical characteristics in cases enrolled in a national registry. Pediatrics 2002; 109(1):E11.
94. Kanagasegar S, Cimaz R, Kurien BT, et al. Neonatal lupus manifests as isolated neutropenia and mildly abnormal liver functions. J Rheumatol 2002; 29(1):187–191.
95. Lee LA, Reichlin M, Ruyle SZ, et al. Neonatal lupus liver disease. Lupus 1993; 2(5):333–338.
96. Lautt WW, Greenway CV. Conceptual review of the hepatic vascular bed. Hepatology 1987; 7(5):952–963.
97. Mace S, Borkat G, Liebman J. Hepatic dysfunction and cardiovascular abnormalities. Occurrence in infants, children and young adults. Am J Dis Child 1985; 139(1):60–65.
98. Cohen JA, Kaplan MM. Left-sided heart failure presenting as hepatitis. Gastroenterology 1978; 74(3):583–587.
99. Sivan Y, Nutman J, Zeevi B, et al. Acute hepatic failure after open-heart surgery in children. Pediatr Cardiol 1987; 8(2):127–130.
100. Peltenburg HG, Hermens WT, Willems GM, et al. Estimation of the fractional catabolic rate constants for the elimination of cytosolic liver enzymes from plasma. Hepatology 1989; 10(5):833–839.
101. Garland JS, Werlin SL, Rice TB. Ischemic hepatitis in children: diagnosis and clinical course. Crit Care Med 1988; 16(12):1209–1212.
102. Kelly DA. Liver complications of pediatric parenteral nutrition–epidemiology. Nutrition 1998; 14(1):153–157.
103. Heine RG, Bines JE. New approaches to parenteral nutrition in infants and children. J Paediatr Child Health 2002; 38(5):433–437.
104. Moss RK, Amii LA. New approaches to understanding the etiology and treatment of total parenteral nutrition-associated cholestasis. Semin Pediatr Surg 1999; 8:140–147.
105. Craig JM, Landing BH. Form of hepatitis in neonatal period simulating biliary atresia. AMA Arch Pathol 1952; 54(4):321–333.

106. Gray OP, Saunders RA. Familial intrahepatic cholestatic jaundice in infancy. Arch Dis Child 1966; 41(217):320–328.
107. Lawson EE, Boggs JD. Long-term follow-up of neonatal hepatitis: safety and value of surgical exploration. Pediatrics 1974; 53(5):650–655.
108. Danks DM, Campbell PE, Smith AL, et al. Prognosis of babies with neonatal hepatitis. Arch Dis Child 1977; 52(5):368–372.
109. Deutsch J, Smith AL, Danks DM, et al. Long term prognosis for babies with neonatal liver disease. Arch Dis Child 1985; 60(5):447–451.
110. Dick MC, Mowat AP. Hepatitis syndrome in infancy–infanan epidemiological survey with 10 year follow up. Arch Dis Child 1985; 60(6):512–516.
111. Odievre M, Hadchouel M, Landrieu P, et al. Long-term prognosis for infants with intrahepatic cholestasis and patent extrahepatic biliary tract. Arch Dis Child 1981; 56(5):373–376.
112. Chang MH, Hsu HC, Lee CY, et al. Neonatal hepatitis: a follow-up study. J Pediatr Gastroenterol Nutr 1987; 6(2):203–207.
113. Jacquemin E, Lykavieris P, Chaoui N, et al. Transient neonatal cholestasis: origin and outcome. J Pediatr 1998; 133(4):563–567.
114. Cohran VC, Heubi JE. Treatment of Pediatric Cholestatic Liver Disease. Curr Treat Options Gastroenterol 2003; 6(5):403–415.
115. Holt RI, Baker AJ, Miell JP. The pathogenesis of growth failure in paediatric liver disease. J Hepatol 1997; 27(2):413–423.
116. Weisdorf SA, Freese DK, Fath JJ, et al. Amino acid abnormalities in infants with extrahepatic biliary atresia and cirrhosis. J Pediatr Gastroenterol Nutr 1987; 6(6):860–864.
117. Munro HN, Fernstrom JD, Wurtman RJ. Insulin, plasma aminoacid imbalance and hepatic coma. Lancet 1975; 1(7909):722–724.
118. Pierro A, Koletzko B, Carnielli V, et al. Resting energy expenditure is increased in infants and children with extrahepatic biliary atresia. J Pediatr Surg 1989; 24(6):534–538.
119. O'Keefe SJ, El-Zayadi AR, Carraher TE, et al. Malnutrition and immuno-incompetence in patients with liver disease. Lancet 1980; 2(8195):615–617.
120. Bucuvalas JC, Cutfield W, Horn J, et al. Resistance to the growth-promoting and metabolic effects of growth hormone in children with chronic liver disease. J Pediatr 1990; 117(3):397–402.
121. Stewart SM, Uauy R, Kennard BD, et al. Mental development and growth in children with chronic liver disease of early and late onset. Pediatrics 1988; 82(2):167–172.
122. Moreno LA, Gottrand F, Hoden S, et al. Improvement of nutritional status in cholestatic children with supplemental nocturnal enteral nutrition. J Pediatr Gastroenterol Nutr 1991; 12(2):213–216.
123. Burke V, Danks DM. Medium-chain triglyceride diet: its use in treatment of liver disease. Br Med J 1966; 2(521):1050–1051.
124. Chin SE, Shepherd RW, Thomas BJ, et al. Nutritional support in children with end-stage liver disease: a randomized crossover trial of a branched-chain amino acid supplement. Am J Clin Nutr 1992; 56(1):158–163.
125. Socha P, Koletzko B, Swiatkowska E, et al. Essential fatty acid metabolism in infants with cholestasis. Acta Paediatr 1998; 87(3):278–283.
126. Sokol RJ, Stall C. Anthropometric evaluation of children with chronic liver disease. Am J Clin Nutr 1990; 52(2):203–208.
127. Sokol RJ, Heubi JE, Iannaccone ST, et al. Vitamin E deficiency with normal serum vitamin E concentrations in children with chronic cholestasis. N Engl J Med 1984; 310(19):1209–1212.
128. Mourey MS, Siegenthaler G, Amedee-Manesme O. Regulation of metabolism of retinol-binding protein by vitamin A status in children with biliary atresia. Am J Clin Nutr 1990; 51(4):638–643.
129. Rossouw JE, Labadarios D, Davis M, et al. Water-soluble vitamins in severe liver disease. S Afr Med J 1978; 54(5):183–186.
130. Cynamon HA, Andres JM, Iafrate RP. Rifampin relieves pruritus in children with cholestatic liver disease. Gastroenterology 1990; 98(4):1013–1016.
131. Bloomer JR, Boyer JL. Phenobarbital effects in cholestatic liver diseases. Ann Intern Med 1975; 82(3):310–317.
132. Narkewicz MR, Smith D, Gregory C, et al. Effect of ursodeoxycholic acid therapy on hepatic function in children with intrahepatic cholestatic liver disease. J Pediatr Gastroenterol Nutr 1998; 26(1):49–55.
133. Jones EA, Bergasa NV. Evolving concepts of the pathogenesis and treatment of the pruritus of cholestasis. Can J Gastroenterol 2000; 14(1):33–40.
134. Wolfhagen FH, Sternieri E, Hop WC, et al. Oral naltrexone treatment for cholestatic pruritus: a double-blind, placebo-controlled study. Gastroenterology 1997; 113(4):1264–1269.
135. Whitington PF, Whitington GL. Partial external diversion of bile for the treatment of intractable pruritus associated with intrahepatic cholestasis. Gastroenterology 1988; 95(1):130–136.
136. Ng VL, Ryckman FC, Porta G, et al. Long-term outcome after partial external biliary diversion for intractable pruritus in patients with intrahepatic cholestasis. J Pediatr Gastroenterol Nutr 2000; 30(2):152–156.

Chapter 59
Biliary atresia and neonatal disorders of the bile ducts

Giorgina Mieli-Vergani and Nedim Hadžić

Children with primary disorders of the bile ducts present early in life with classic signs of prolonged conjugated jaundice, pale stools and dark urine. They represent an important group within the so-called neonatal cholestasis syndrome. Disorders of the bile ducts can be due to developmental anomalies, an inflammatory process or genetic causes. If corrective surgical treatment is available, it should be instituted early in order to minimize the progression of chronic liver disease.[1]

SURGICALLY CORRECTABLE DISORDERS

Biliary atresia

Biliary atresia is the most common surgically correctable liver disorder in infancy, affecting around 1 in 16 000 liveborns.[2] It is characterized by complete obstruction to the bile flow due to progressive destruction and obliteration of part or all of the extrahepatic biliary tree. Studies of bile duct remnants, removed at surgery and from serial sectioning and reconstruction of surgical and necropsy liver specimens, indicate that biliary atresia arises from a sclerosing inflammatory process affecting previously formed bile ducts.[3] Comparative anatomic studies have suggested that, at least in some cases, biliary atresia may be caused by failure of the intrauterine remodeling process at the hepatic hilum, with persistence of fetal bile ducts poorly supported by mesenchyme. As bile flow increases perinatally, bile leakage from these abnormal ducts may trigger an intense inflammatory reaction, with consequent obliteration of the biliary tree.[4] The extrahepatic ducts are primarily affected, whereas the intrahepatic bile ducts remain patent in early infancy but then also become affected, obliterated and eventually disappear. Cirrhosis with complications such as portal hypertension may appear at any time from 2 months of age; few unoperated children survive beyond 18 months of age.

Etiology

The cause of biliary atresia is unknown. It is conceivable that the condition may represent a final phenotypic pathway of neonatal liver injury caused by diverse etiologies, including developmental, vascular or infectious factors, which may be operational antenatally or within the first 3 months of life. It is also tempting to speculate that aberrant host immune reactivity, related to physiologic immune incompetence at this age, may play a role in this condition, unique to early infancy. Histologic features similar to the inherited group of disorders termed 'ductal plate malformation' syndrome, which include congenital hepatic fibrosis and Caroli syndrome, have been reported in some cases of biliary atresia and have been interpreted as suggesting a developmental abnormality.[5] The presence of various inflammatory markers can be demonstrated in the biliary tissue excised at corrective surgery.[6] Recently, a predominance of the type 1 T helper cell (Th1) response was demonstrated by upregulation of genes regulating γ-interferon and osteopontin in 14 liver biopsies of infants with biliary atresia using DNA microarrays technique.[7]

Some 10–20% of patients with biliary atresia have other congenital anomalies, including splenic abnormalities (asplenia, polysplenia), total or partial situs inversus, mediopositioned liver, intestinal malrotation, atretic inferior vena cava, preduodenal portal vein and congenital heart defects. They may represent a separate etiologic subgroup – biliary atresia splenic malformation (BASM) syndrome.[8] It has been suggested that the precarious blood supply to the biliary tree may be further jeopardized with such abnormalities. An increased incidence of maternal diabetes mellitus has been associated with the BASM syndrome.[8] Children with this syndrome appear to have an increased frequency of infection, possibly leading to their poorer long-term prognosis compared with classic biliary atresia, including after liver transplantation, although no formal defect in their humoral immunity has been identified.[9]

It is possible that defective embryogenesis may play a part in the pathogenesis of the BASM syndrome, so this subgroup of biliary atresia has been termed 'congenital' or 'embryonic', in contrast to 'perinatal' or 'acquired'. The diagnosis of biliary atresia can occasionally be suspected prenatally in the presence of dilated bile ducts at ultrasonography performed at around 20 weeks of gestation.[10] Interestingly, however, of nine children with biliary atresia identified prenatally, only one had features of the BASM syndrome and none had histologic appearances of the 'ductal plate malformation'.[10] The 'perinatal' or 'acquired' form of biliary atresia is thought to occur following exposure to possible infectious triggers in susceptible infants, in whom an uncontrolled inflammatory response, as demonstrated by upregulation of various inflammatory markers, leads to the obstructive cholangiopathy.[6] Several viruses have been suspected of triggering this response in biliary

liver transplantation if this becomes necessary subsequently.

There are three macroscopic types of biliary atresia:

- Type I – affecting the distal part of the common duct
- Type II – affecting the common hepatic duct but sparing the gallbladder and common bile duct
- Type III – affecting right and left hepatic ducts and the gallbladder.

The most common form is type III (85–90% of cases), which is often referred to as 'uncorrectable'; surgical reconstruction (portoenterostomy) is most challenging is this form.

After surgery, the authors use phenobarbital at a dose of 10–15 mg/kg daily for long-term induction of the microsomal enzymes of the hepatocyte endoplasmic reticulum.[33] If the jaundice reappears, the dose could be doubled, following exclusion of a mechanical problem with the Roux-en-Y loop. Choleretic treatment with ursodeoxycholic acid (20–30 mg/kg daily) could also be considered. If the portoenterostomy is performed by an experienced surgeon, good bile flow with normal serum bilirubin values can be achieved in more than 80% of children operated on by 60 days of age, but in only 20–30% with later surgery.[1,33,34] If bilirubin returns to normal, a 90% 15-year survival rate has been reported,[34] with a good quality of life into the fourth decade.[35] Up to 11% of children could be completely free of clinical and biochemical signs of liver disease after 10-year follow-up.[36] If the bilirubin level is not reduced, the rate of progression of cirrhosis is not slowed and survival beyond the second birthday is unusual. If partial bile drainage is obtained, development of end-stage chronic liver disease may be delayed, but liver replacement usually becomes unavoidable by puberty. There are uncontrolled studies suggesting that the use of anti-inflammatory drugs such as steroids could have a beneficial role after Kasai portoenterostomy.[37–39] A prospective placebo-controlled double-blind study on the short-term use of prednisolone after Kasai portoenterostomy is ongoing at the authors' unit. After surgery, all children should be supplemented with fat-soluble vitamins.

An important postoperative complication is cholangitis. This is due to a wide range of micro-organisms and occurs in more than 50% of patients in the first 2 years after surgery.[40] It is characterized by fever, recurrence or aggravation of jaundice, and, frequently, features of septicemia. Blood culture, ascitic aspirate or liver biopsy to identify the organism responsible should precede intravenous antibiotic therapy, which is continued for 14 days if a pathogen is identified. Often, however, the diagnosis of cholangitis is not obvious and unexplained fever may be the only symptom. Intravenous antibiotics are then started empirically, after taking a blood culture and assessing liver function, C-reactive protein level and full blood count. If the fever responds to the antibiotics, these are continued for 5 days. Should the fever recur after stopping them, a liver biopsy is performed for histologic examination and culture. Amoxicillin and ceftazidime are currently the authors' initial choice pending *in vitro* sensitivities. Long-term prophylaxis with rotating antibiotics may be indicated for recurrent cholangitis.[33]

A degree of portal hypertension is present in almost all patients at the time of initial surgery. Approximately 50% of all survivors aged 5 years, even those with normal bilirubin levels, have esophageal varices, but only 10–15% have gastrointestinal bleeding. For these, variceal banding or injection sclerotherapy is the treatment of choice. In approximately 10% of patients in whom the serum bilirubin level returns to normal, intrahepatic cholangiopathy progresses and complications of biliary cirrhosis ultimately develop.[41] For these patients, and those for whom surgery has not been effective, liver transplantation should be considered.[42] With 1-year survival rates approaching 90%, and 5-year survival rates of over 80%,[43,44] liver transplantation is now a standard therapeutic option, although it remains a formidable surgicomedical procedure. The recipient is likely to have one or more life-threatening complications in the perioperative or postoperative period. Lifelong immunosuppressive therapy is required, with a high risk of opportunistic and community-acquired infections and malignancies, requiring close medical and surgical supervision. Most of the survivors have a good quality of life and attend school, although the long-term medical and psychologic effects of liver transplantation in childhood are as yet unknown. The supply of donors of suitable size and blood group, even with an increased use of split grafts where one donor liver is used for two recipients (usually one child and one adult), remains a major limiting factor in liver transplantation. Segmental graft transplant from living relatives has given survival rates of 90% in infants in whom Kasai portoenterostomy was unsuccessful.[45] The results are better in children transplanted when heavier than 10 kg (or after the age of 1 year) and when the procedure is done electively.[42] The precise indications and timing, and the optimal management of some of the intraoperative and postoperative problems, including the control of rejection, remain the subject of ongoing assessment and research. Liver transplantation in patients with biliary atresia should be complementary to portoenterostomy, except for infants in whom decompensated cirrhosis has developed because of delayed diagnosis. The combination of Kasai portoenterostomy followed by transplantation in case of failure has considerably improved the survival of children with biliary atresia. The reported 4-year actuarial survival rate with native liver is 51%, and an overall (with native liver and post liver transplant) 4-year actuarial survival rate is 89%.[44]

Choledochal cysts

Choledochal cysts are congenital dilations of the biliary ducts that may be associated with intermittent biliary obstruction (Fig. 59.4). If the condition is unrecognized and uncorrected, the impaired bile ouflow can lead to chronic hepatic injury, fibrosis and, ultimately, biliary cirrhosis with ensuing portal hypertension. Choledochal cysts can present at any age. Their inheritance is sporadic with an unexplained female prevalence. In the newborn period the presentation may be indistinguishable from the

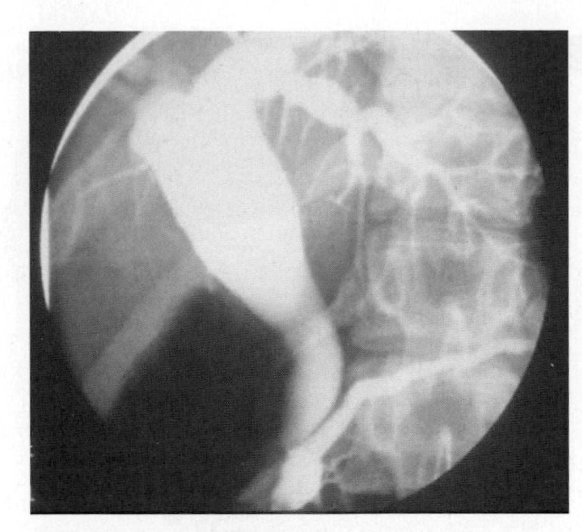

Figure 59.4: Percutaneous transhepatic cholangiography demonstrating a fusiform choledochal cyst affecting common, right and left bile ducts.

syndrome of neonatal cholestasis, including biliary atresia. A cystic echo-free mass demonstrated in the biliary tree by ultrasonography is strong evidence for this diagnosis. The intrahepatic bile ducts may be dilated due to the distal stasis. There are five types of choledochal cyst, affecting various segments of the biliary tree (Fig. 59.5). The most difficult for surgical management is type V, the most proximal type, in which the intrahepatic ducts are primarily affected. Classically, cystic and fusiform macroscopic types are described.

Choledochal cysts can be diagnosed prenatally on routine ultrasonography.[46,47] Children in whom a prenatal diagnosis of choledochal cyst is made should be referred promptly to a specialized pediatric hepatology center, as this can also be the mode of presentation of biliary atresia.[10,47] The cyst can be diagnosed by magnetic resonance cholangiopancreatography (MRCP), but often ERCP or percutaneous transhepatic cholangiography (PTC) is needed. Percutaneous liver biopsy is contraindicated owing to risks of biliary injury and peritonitis. Clinical examination of the abdomen should be restrained as there is a risk of perforation. Radionucleotide scanning adds little to direct and indirect cholangiography.

Up to two-thirds of children with choledochal cyst have a longer common pathway between the pancreatic and common bile ducts.[46] This anatomic variant may give rise to a reflux of proteolytic pancreatic enzymes into the bile structures, possibly playing a role in the pathogenesis of choledochal cyst by facilitating the initial injury of the biliary mucosa.

The definitive treatment is surgical removal with biliary drainage via a Roux-en-Y loop (hepaticojejunostomy).[48] With adequate surgery the long-term prognosis is good.[46] Cholangitis, rupture, pancreatitis and gallstones are important complications of choledochal cysts, and may occur even in early infancy, whereas chronic cholecystitis and carcinoma of the cyst wall may be a long-term complication.

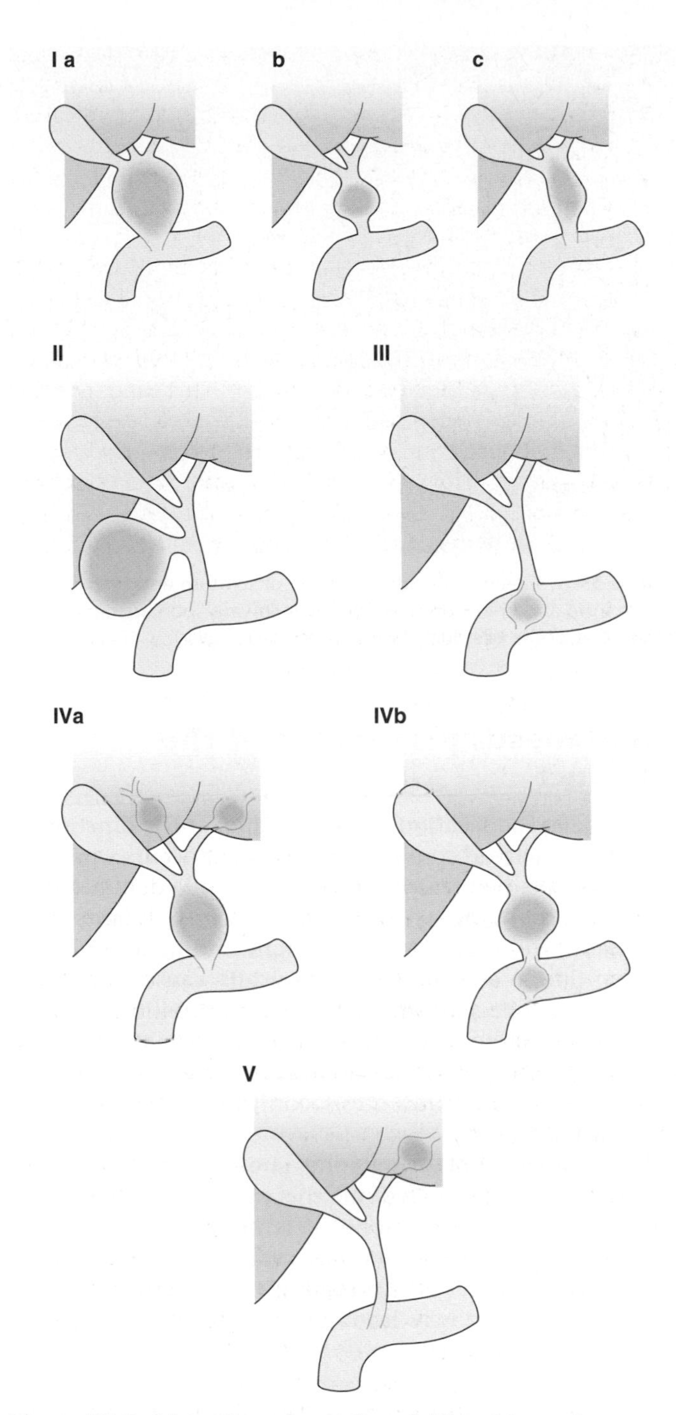

Figure 59.5: Schematic representation of different types of choledochal cyst.

Widespread use and improved quality of ultrasonography, both prenatally and postnatally, has led to increased detection of minor bile duct dilations early in infancy.[25] These dilations rarely, if ever, cause biochemical abnormalities and further increase of the bile duct caliber on follow-up ultrasonography is exceptional. Whether they represent incidental findings or 'forme fruste' of choledochal cysts remains to be established. Ursodeoxycholic acid is often used as a choleretic, without documented evidence for its benefits.

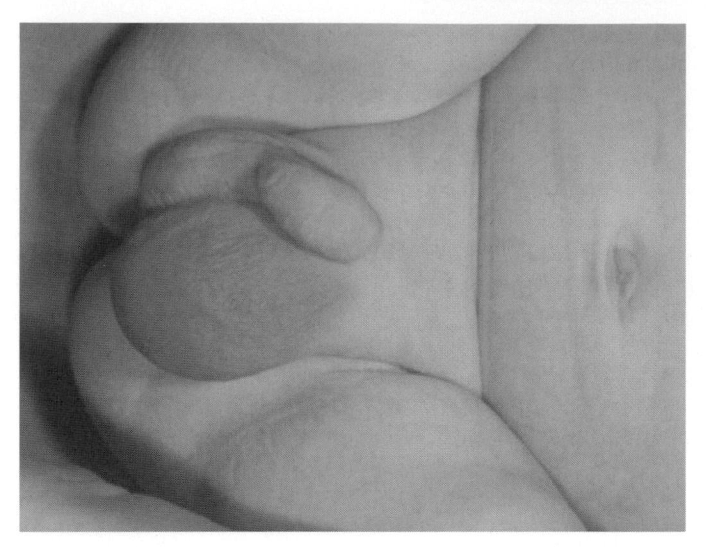

Figure 59.6: Green-yellow discoloration of scrotum and umbilicus due to intra-abdominal presence of bile following spontaneous perforation of the bile duct. (*See plate section for color*).

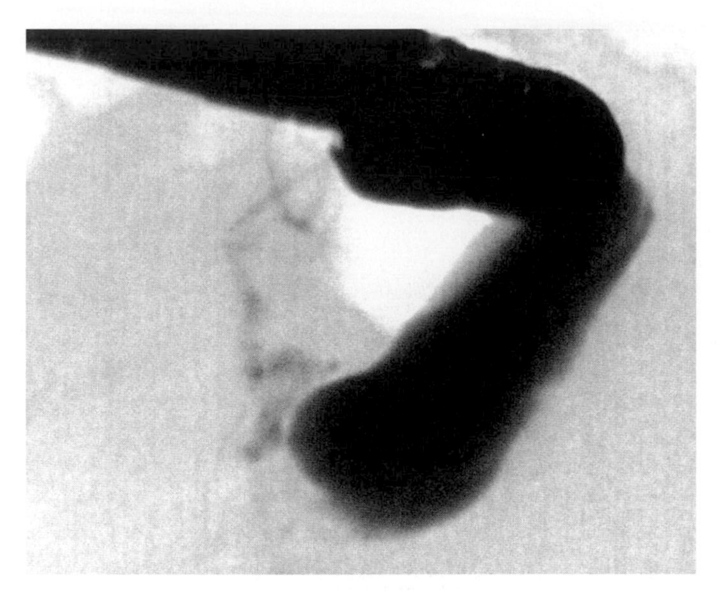

Figure 59.7: Endoscopic retrograde cholangiopancreatography demonstrating a patent biliary system in a 2-month-old infant with suspected biliary atresia.

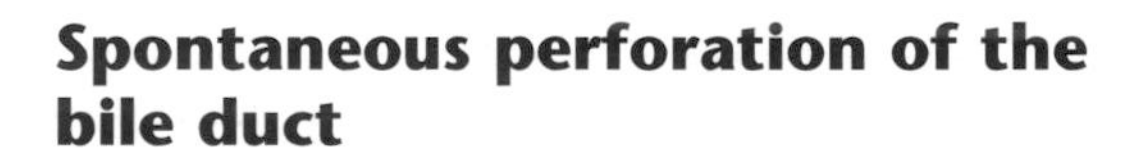

Spontaneous perforation of the bile duct

Spontaneous perforation of the bile duct at the junction of the cystic duct and common hepatic duct occurs when, for some unexplained reason, the common bile duct becomes blocked, usually at its distal end. Affected infants have mild jaundice, failure to gain weight and abdominal distension due to ascites, which classically causes the development of bile-stained inguinal or umbilical herniae (Fig. 59.6). The stools are white or cream in color, the urine is dark, and the biochemical markers of obstruction may be mildly abnormal. Paracentesis confirms the presence of bile-stained ascites.[49]

If operative cholangiography shows free drainage of contrast into the duodenum, the ruptured duct may be sutured, but more commonly it is necessary to establish cholecystojejunostomy drainage via a Roux-en-Y loop. With effective surgery the prognosis is excellent.[49] Delay in instituting surgery may lead to severe malnutrition, peritonitis and septicemia.

Neonatal sclerosing cholangitis

This condition is increasingly recognized as a result of the wider use of direct cholangiography (ERCP, PTC) in this age group.[29] The infants present with conjugated jaundice, hepatosplenomegaly and dark urine, but, in contrast to biliary atresia, the stools are pigmented.[50] Affected infants are usually not dysmorphic and have no associated extrahepatic anomalies. The histologic features are indistinguishable from those of large bile duct obstruction. Dynamic radionucleotide imaging – di-isopropyl-acetanilido-IDA (DISIDA), hepatic IDA (HIDA) and methyl-brom-IDA – can be helpful if it demonstrates the presence of contrast in the gut. ERCP is a 'golden' diagnostic standard, but requires a degree of technical expertise (Fig. 59.7).

Familial occurrence has been described[51] and there is a candidate locus for the genetic identification of this condition (R. Thompson, personal communication). Medical treatment is restricted to the enhancement of choleresis with ursodeoxycholic acid (25–35 mg/kg daily) and medical management of cholestasis with fat-soluble vitamin supplements and MCT-based milk formula. The response is variable and some children need liver replacement because of the development of biliary cirrhosis during early childhood.

Paucity of interlobular bile ducts (Alagille syndrome, intrahepatic biliary hypoplasia)

This is a histopathologic diagnosis where there is a decrease in the number of interlobular bile ducts, frequently seen in hypoplastic portal tracts. It is found in many conditions causing hepatitis in infancy (Table 59.1). When it occurs with cardiovascular, skeletal, renal, ocular, vascular and other anomalies (Table 59.2) it is called Alagille syndrome (syndromic paucity of the intrahepatic bile ducts; arteriohepatic dysplasia).[52] The inheritance is

- Alagille's syndrome
- Non-syndromic paucity of bile ducts
- α_1-Antitrypsin deficiency
- Prematurity
- Down syndrome
- Chronic rejection after liver transplantation
- Hepatic graft *vs* host disease
- Drugs
- Advanced phase of any chronic cholangiopathy
- Idiopathic

Table 59.1 Conditions associated with paucity of bile ducts

Cardiac
Peripheral pulmonary stenosis Tetralogy of Fallot Ventricular septal defect Atrial septal defect Aortic coarctation Pulmonary atresia
Skeletal
Short stature Butterfly vertebrae Fused vertebrae Rib anomalies Spina bifida occulta Thin cortical bones
Ocular
Posterior embryotoxon Axenfeld anomaly Optic disk drusen Shallow anterior chamber Microcornea
Vascular
Renal artery stenosis Intracranial bleeding CNS malformations
Other
Renal developmental abnormalities Renal tubulopathies Pancreatic exocrine and endocrine insufficiency High-pitched voice Microcolon

Table 59.2 Extrahepatic manifestations of Alagille's syndrome

autosomal dominant with variable expression. The estimated incidence is 1 in 100 000 live births. Alagille syndrome is caused by mutations in the human *Jagged 1* gene on chromosome 20p12.[53,54] Jagged 1 is a ligand in the Notch signalling pathway that has ubiquitous activity. However, mutations in this gene could also be present in asymptomatic individuals and in other liver conditions, including biliary atresia,[55] and some patients with Alagille syndrome do not have mutations.[56] The liver biopsy may not be diagnostic if performed early. The diagnostic difficulties at histologic examination may include physiologic hypoplasia of bile ducts in early infancy, but also expanded portal tracts and bile duct reduplication, reminiscent of biliary atresia.

The long-standing cholestasis causes jaundice, pruritus, failure to thrive, hypercholesterolemia and xanthomas. The severity of the cholestasis varies. Mild cases may have pruritus only. The majority have jaundice from the neonatal period, which in severe cases may persist but in others clears in late childhood or early adult life.[28] Diagnosis is supported by the finding of the typical facies: deep-set eyes, mild hypertelorism, overhanging forehead, a straight nose that in profile is in the same plane as the forehead, a small pointed chin, posterior embryotoxon (a centrally positioned prominent Schwalbe ring at the junction of corneal endothelium and uvea) on slit-lamp examination, and vertebral arch or rib defects on spinal radiography (Fig. 59.8). Increased serum cholesterol levels support the diagnosis. Renal abnormalities have been reported in 19% of patients.[28] Growth failure is universal, and pancreatic insufficiency, developmental delay and increased incidence of intracranial bleeding have been reported in some studies. Potentially life-threatening episodes of CNS bleeding in Alagille's syndrome are difficult to explain on the basis of classically unremarkable coagulation parameters and platelet count. One possibility is that the *Jagged 1* mutation in the Notch signalling pathway may play a role in the integrity of vascular endothelium, akin to association of the human Notch 3 receptor defect and adult-onset cerebral autosomal dominant arteriopathy with subcortical infarcts and leukoencephalopathy (CADASIL).

The treatment is that of chronic cholestasis, with particular emphasis on the control of pruritus and adequacy of vitamin D, E, K and A supplementation (Table 59.3).[26] In spite of maximal nutritional support, which often includes overnight nasogastric feeding, the majority of children will remain thin and short for age.

The long-term prognosis is unknown, but some 15% may go on to develop cirrhosis and 5–10% die from liver disease.[57] In one series 25% of patients died from cardiac involvement, classically a peripheral pulmonary stenosis, or infection.[52] Liver transplantation has improved the overall outcome, although postoperative recovery may be additionally complicated by cardiac problems and long-term survival affected by added chronic calcineurin inhibitor-related renal impairment.[58] Although hypercholesterolemia could represent a significant risk factor for cardiovascular disease in Alagille's syndrome, no macroscopic injury to the arterial intima has been reported at transplantation, in contrast to observations in familial hypercholesterolemia.

Neonatal gallstones

Cholelithiasis is an uncommon condition in children, but as a result of better ultrasonographic surveillance there is an increase in its detection.[59] In the neonatal age group, improved survival of premature and small-for-gestational age children has led to an increased recognition of children with biliary sludge or 'inspissated bile syndrome' following sepsis, exposure to total parenteral nutrition (TPN), dehydration or prolonged use of diuretics. Some of these children present with clinical signs of obstructive jaundice, but the majority are asymptomatic.[60] Some may have an underlying hemolytic condition, dyslipoproteinemia or a family history of gallstones. A female prevalence is not observed until adolescence.[60] It is important to exclude familial disorders of biliary transport, such as bile salt

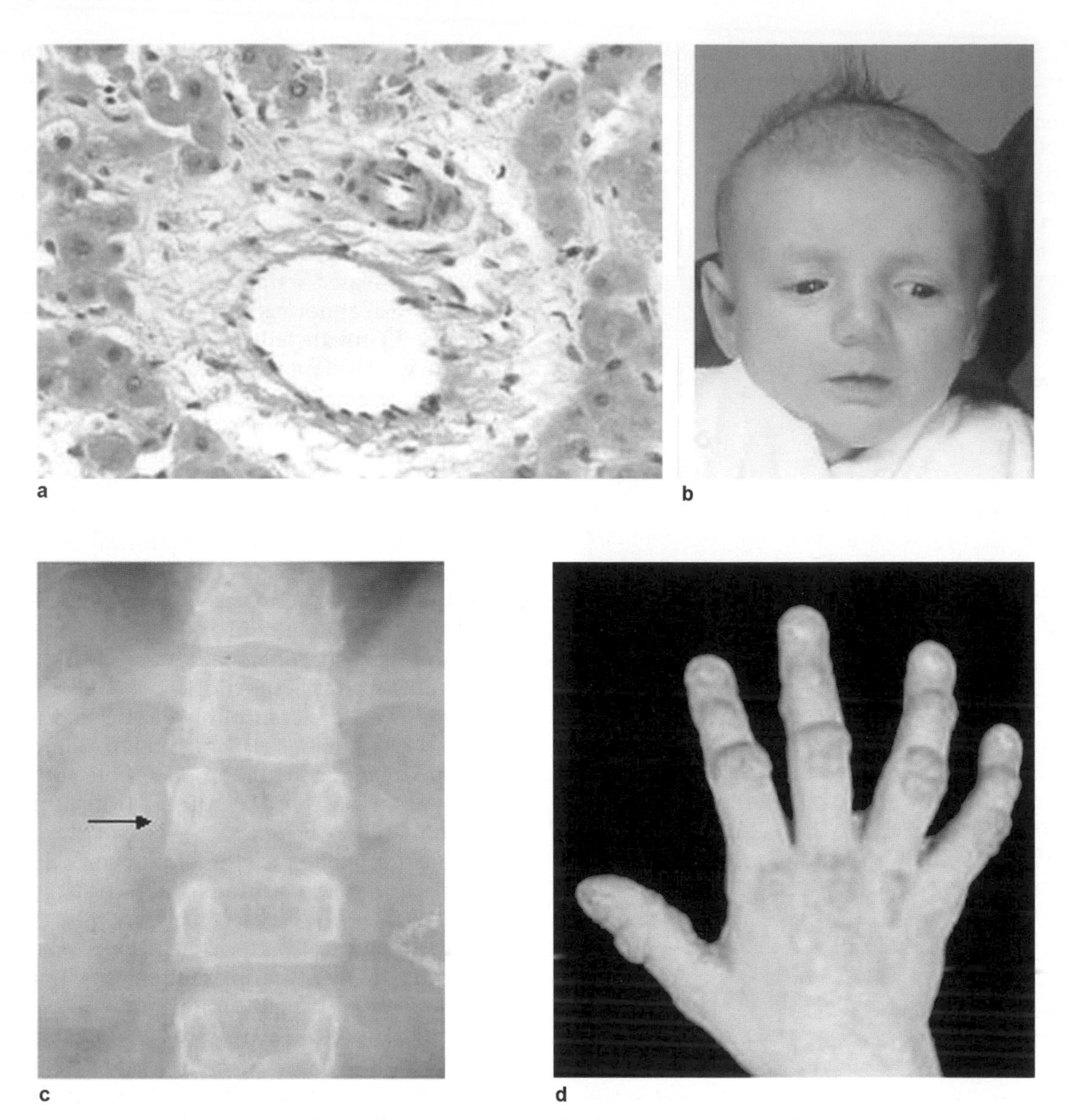

Figure 59.8: Alagille's syndrome. (**a**) Liver biopsy showing absence of bile duct in the portal tract (hematoxylin and eosin stain, ×320). (**b**) Classic facial appearance – triangular face, deep-set eyes, mild hypertelorism, prominent forehead, small pointed chin, low set ears. (**c**) Typical appearance of a 'butterfly' vertebra (arrow) on spinal radiography. (**d**) Disfiguring xanthomas on the hand. (Reproduced from Francavilla R, Mieli-Vergani G. Liver and biliary disease in infancy. Medicine 2002; 30:45–47 with permission from The Medicine Publishing Company.) (See plate section for color)

export pump (BSEP) deficiency and multidrug resistance (MDR) 3 deficiency, which may both present with infantile gallstones. It is noteworthy that about 50% of pediatric patients have black pigment stones.[61]

Percutaneous cholangiography with biliary drainage is an effective means of both diagnosis and treatment of infants with dilated intrahepatic ducts and common bile duct obstruction due to sludge or small stones.[59] Positive centrifugal pressure at cholangiography flushes the retained bile and improves the drainage. Formal biliary surgery can then be restricted to a limited number of patients, particularly those with congenital anomalies and/or associated strictures of the bile ducts. Ursodeoxycholic acid is a valuable addition to the radiologic management.

The natural history of asymptomatic gallstones and sludge in children is largely unknown.

Progressive familial cholestasis

Over the past decade, different types of progressive familial intrahepatic cholestasis (PFIC) syndromes, associated with a low or high γ-glutamyltranspeptidase (GGT) phenotype, have been characterized.[62] These autosomal recessive

Vitamin	Dosage
D	Ergocalciferol 800 IU per day, cholecalciferol 10 000 IU/kg per month or α-calcidol 100 ng/kg per day
K	Phytomenadione (Konakion) 1 mg daily
A	Retinol 2500 IU daily
E	α-Tocopherylacetate 100 mg/kg per day

Table 59.3 Recommended doses of fat-soluble vitamin supplements in chronic cholestasis

conditions can present with prolonged conjugated jaundice in infancy. GGT in the liver is normally bound to the canalicular membrane and to the biliary epithelium of cholangiocytes. Under cholestatic conditions, the detergent effect of the bile acids liberates GGT from the membrane. When this is combined with a poor bile flow, GGT leaks back into the circulation, where raised levels can be detected. In the absence of bile acids in the bile, even when there is a poor bile flow, GGT is not released and the serum levels remain normal. Therefore, in the presence of cholestasis, a normal serum level of GGT correlates well with low levels of biliary bile acids. These patients usually have low biliary, but high serum levels of bile acids in the absence of a primary defect in bile acid synthesis.

The original patients described with this phenotype were amongst the Old Order Amish in North America.[63] One of the original families was called Byler, and this condition has become widely known as Byler disease. Byler disease, or FIC-1, represents a third of the patients with low GGT PFIC and maps to chromosome 18.[64] The gene is termed *FIC1* and encodes FIC-1 or ABCB-8 protein. These patients may present with neonatal hepatitis of variable severity. The *FIC1* gene is widely expressed, with only relatively low-level expression in the liver. Patients with FIC-1 disease may have extrahepatic manifestations. Expression of *FIC1* is particularly high in the small intestine and pancreas. Thus, patients with FIC-1 may have pancreatic insufficiency and many have significant malabsorption, which is not improved by liver transplantation. A proportion will have abnormal sweat test and conductive deafness. The condition historically described as benign recurrent intrahepatic cholestasis (BRIC) and the clinically more severe Greenland Eskimo infantile cholestasis also map to the chromosome 18 locus and probably represent a different phenotype of FIC-1 disease.[64,65] Histologically, these patients usually have features of a bland cholestasis with no major inflammatory features. The disease frequently progresses to end-stage liver disease in childhood. The outcome of transplantation, however, is not satisfactory owing to a number of problems not corrected by liver replacement such as continuing malabsorption, rapid secondary fatty liver infiltration and failure to thrive. External or internal ('ileal bypass') diversion of biliary flow by preventing enterohepatic recirculation of the bile may represent one therapeutic option with unknown long-term outcome.[66,67] It is often used to treat intractable pruritus.

A third of patients with low GGT PFIC have an isolated defect in bile acid transport owing to deficiency of the BSEP. The condition maps to chromosome 2 and is due to mutations of the *ABCB11* gene.[68] These patients usually present in the first few months of life with a mild neonatal hepatitis. Initial histologic appearances are those of giant cell hepatitis. Immunohistochemical staining with anti-BSEP antibodies is negative, pointing to this diagnosis even in the absence of genuine clinical symptoms, such as pruritus, which are often not present in early infancy. The disease progresses and pruritus usually becomes a prominent problem towards the end of the first year. The rate of progression is variable, resulting in end-stage liver disease between 2 and 10 years of age, or possibly even later. No treatment apart from transplantation has shown to be of benefit, and it is particularly noteworthy that these patients appear to be incapable of excreting ursodeoxycholic acid.[69] Treatment with modest doses of ursodeoxycholic acid, however, may have a beneficial effect by further suppressing endogenous bile acid production. As expression of the gene appears to be limited entirely to the liver, liver transplantation has proved to be curative.

Appearances of bile at electromicroscopy could help differentiate between FIC-1 disease and BSEP deficiency. In BSEP deficiency the bile is amorphous, whereas in FIC-1 it has a coarse granular appearances (Byler bile) (Fig. 59.9), which could be due to ongoing microvillus damage.[70] The genetic basis of the remaining third of the patients within the spectrum of low GGT PFIC has not yet been clarified.

A form of high GGT PFIC is associated to MDR-3 deficiency resulting from mutations of the *ABCB4* gene.[71] It is believed that the *MDR3* gene product plays a critical role in the excretion of phosphatidylcholine, the major lipid component of human bile. A defect in phosphatidylcholine excretion is likely to result in the production of highly detergent bile, which can cause considerable tissue damage. Indeed, children with MDR-3 deficiency have marked portal inflammation and bile duct proliferation. Some patients, particularly those who have some residual protein function, show a good clinical response to

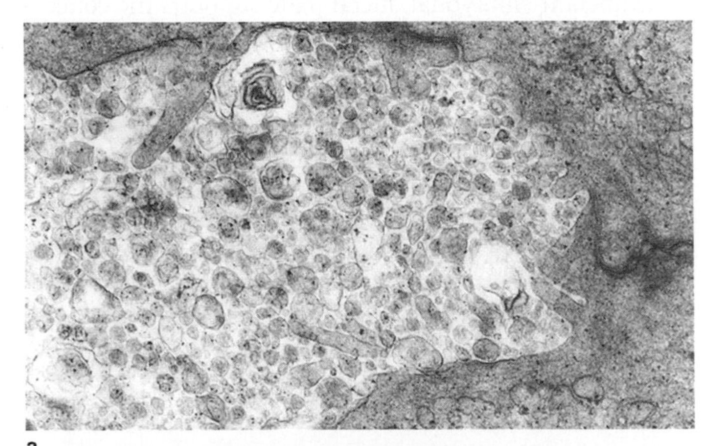

a

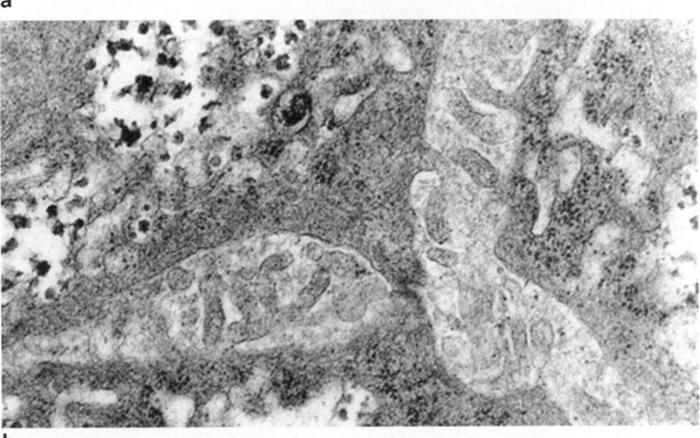

b

Figure 59.9: (**a**) Coarsely granular bile (Byler bile) seen in FIC-1 disease, with a normal canaliculus (**b**) normal, for comparison (electron microscopy, ×10 000).

ursodeoxycholic acid, based on its effect in reducing the hydrophobicity of the bile. The diagnosis is confirmed by low concentration of phospholipids in the bile, sampled at ERCP, or by mutation analysis. Preliminary data from a murine model showed that transplanted hepatocytes are capable of ameliorating the phenotype, suggesting that such transport defects in humans are good candidates for hepatocyte transplantation or gene therapy.[72]

Fibrocystic liver disease

This group of rare disorders includes three clinical entities: congenital hepatic fibrosis (CHF), Caroli disease and Caroli syndrome.[73] Caroli disease is characterized by a cystic dilation of the intrahepatic bile ducts that can affect the entire liver or be segmental or lobar. The grossly dilated ducts could be detected with ultrasonography, computed tomography, percutaneous cholangiography, ERCP or, more recently, MRCP.[74] More commonly, the disease is associated with CHF and then termed Caroli syndrome.

The term ductal plate malformation (DPM) refers to the histologic changes seen in the liver of a heterogeneous group of genetic disorders in which segmental dilations of the intrahepatic bile ducts are associated with fibrosis. They represent a merging spectrum of microscopic and/or macroscopic cystic lesions often associated with fibrocystic anomalies in the kidneys. Close histologic resemblance to an exuberant embryonal ductal plate supports the concept that an aberrant remodeling during organogenesis is the pathogenic mechanism common to these inherited disorders (Fig. 59.10).[5]

Patients may present with an incidental finding of bile duct dilation or with symptoms of recurrent cholangitis at any time in life, but frequently in childhood, including the neonatal period.[75] There is recurrent fever and abdominal pain with signs of systemic infection. When CHF is associated, portal hypertension is likely to be present. Complications include abscess formation, septicemia and

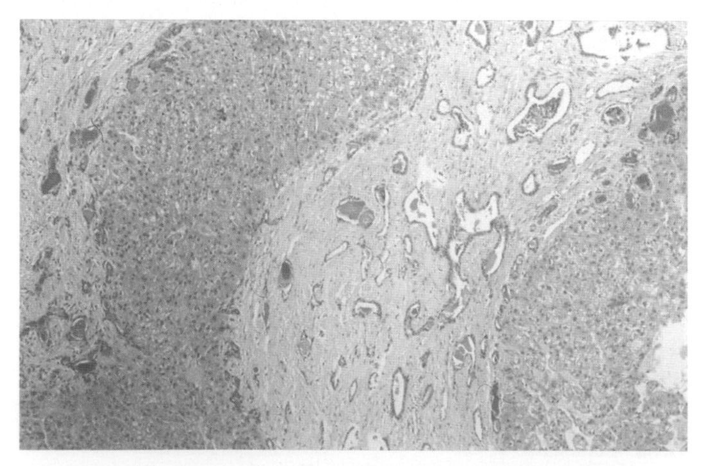

Figure 59.10: Liver biopsy in the ductal plate malformation; loose fibrous tissue containing small irregular bile ducts, some of them dilated and containing bile (hematoxylin and eosin stain, ×125). (See plate section for color)

- Firm hepatomegaly
- Abdominal distension
- Splenomegaly/hypersplenism
- Sudden gastrointestinal bleeding
- Renal polycystic disease
- Other vascular malformations

Table 59.4 Clinical manifestations of congenital hepatic fibrosis

- Autosomal recessive (infantile) and autosomal dominant (adult) polycystic kidney disease
- Nephronophthisis
- Ivemark syndrome
- Gruber syndrome
- Jeune syndrome
- Laurence–Moon–Biedl syndrome
- Tuberous sclerosis
- Ellis–van Creveld syndrome
- Meckel syndrome
- Senior–Loken syndrome

Table 59.5 Syndromes described in association with ductal plate malformation

intrahepatic lithiasis. Late development of adenocarcinoma has been reported in a few adult patients. Autosomal recessive polycystic kidney disease (ARPKD) or some form of renal tubular ectasia is often associated with Caroli syndrome. Recently, an interesting yet unexplained link was described between congenital hepatic fibrosis and carbohydrate glycoprotein deficiency type Ib.[76]

Recently, the gene for ARPKD has been identified and termed *PKDH1*. This gene is large, with 67 exons, and about 120 different mutations have been described. Some genotype–phenotype relationship appears to exist for severity of renal disease, with truncated mutations seen in more severe renal phenotypes with neonatal presentation. Fibrocystin is a protein present in the collecting ducts of the kidney and in the biliary epithelium. It is believed that fibrocystin expression is regulated by the *PKDH1* gene and that its absence could explain a link between renal and liver pathology.

Morphologically, the liver contains rounded or lanceolated bile duct cysts, some with characteristic fibrovascular bridges across their cavity. Inspissated bile, soft and friable bilirubin calculi, or muco-pus may be present in the lumen. Histologically, the cysts are lined by cubic or tall columnar epithelium, which may be ulcerated or focally hyperplastic. There is chronic and acute inflammation of the wall with fibrosis and, often, prominent mucus glands.[5] The lesion has to be distinguished from the pseudo-cystic lesions that develop secondary to a chronic obstructive cholangiopathy such as extrahepatic biliary atresia. In this situation inflammatory cholangiodestruction and the detergent power of extravasated bile operate to produce cystic cavities lined by inflamed granulation tissue and often filled with inspissated bile.

The severity of the renal lesions may overshadow the liver disease, as is observed in the early presentation of

ARPKD. Conversely, portal hypertension with a typically preserved liver function may dominate the delayed clinical presentation as seen in CHF[77] (Table 59.4). The management is for complications of portal hypertension, as described elsewhere (see Ch. 64). Cholangitis may develop, especially when the cysts communicate with the biliary system. Complications of portal hypertension and cholangitis are the main presenting features in children.[77] A liver biopsy may not be always indicated in the presence of convincing clinical and ultrasonographic information because of the risk of introducing infection in an abnormal biliary system. MRCP, a non-invasive investigation promising to reach sensitivity levels similar to those of direct cholangiography (PTC and ERCP),[74] is usually indicated.

Caroli's disease is managed with aggressive antibiotic therapy. Non-surgical approaches such as percutaneous biliary drainage, extracorporeal shockwave lithotripsy, and transhepatic or endoscopic decompression have been attempted with unconvincing results. Segmental or lobar forms have been treated by partial hepatectomy.

Isolated or combined kidney and liver transplants have become available for children with polycystic liver and kidney disease.[78] Immunosuppression after isolated renal transplantation may lead to an increased number of episodes of cholangitis and worsening liver condition. Therefore, a combined liver–kidney transplant may be required in children with established end-stage renal failure and advanced chronic liver disease.

References

1. Mieli-Vergani G, Howard ER, Portmann B, Mowat AP. Late referral for biliary atresia: missed opportunities for effective surgery. Lancet 1989; i:421–423.
2. McKiernan PJ, Baker AJ, Kelly DA. The frequency and outcome of biliary atresia in the UK and Ireland. Lancet 2000; 355:4–5.
3. Gautier M, Elliot N. Extrahepatic biliary atresia: morphological study of 94 biliary remnants. Arch Pathol Lab Med 1981; 105:397–402.
4. Tan CE, Driver M, Howard ER, Moscoso GJ. Extrahepatic biliary atresia: a first trimester event? Clues from light microscopy and immunohistochemistry. J Pediatr Surg 1994; 29:808–814.
5. Desmet VJ. Congenital diseases of intrahepatic bile ducts: variations on the theme 'ductal plate malformation'. Hepatology 1992; 16:1069–1083.
6. Davenport M, Gonde C, Redkar R, et al. Immunohistochemistry of the liver and biliary tree in extrahepatic biliary atresia. J Pediatr Surg 2001; 36:1017–1025.
7. Bezerra JA, Tiao G, Ryckman FC, et al. Genetic induction of proinflammatory immunity in children with biliary atresia. Lancet 2002; 360:1653–1659.
8. Davenport M, Savage M, Mowat AP, Howard ER. Biliary atresia splenic malformation syndrome: an etiological and prognostic subgroup. Surgery 1993; 113:662–667.
9. Taylor RM, Cheeseman P, Davenport M, et al. Humoral immunity in children with biliary atresia splenic malformation syndrome. Eur J Pediatr 2003; 162:539–540.
10. Hinds R, Davenport M, Mieli-Vergani G, Hadžić N. Antenatal diagnosis of biliary atresia. J Pediatr 2004; 144:43–46.
11. Tyler KL, Sokol RJ, Oberhaus SM, et al. Detection of reovirus RNA in hepatobiliary tissues from patients with extrahepatic biliary atresia and choledochal cysts. Hepatology 1998; 27:1475–1482.
12. Riepenhoff-Talty M, Gouvea V, Evans MJ, et al. Detection of group C rotavirus in infants with extrahepatic biliary atresia. J Infect Dis 1996; 174:8–15.
13. Fishler B, Ehrnst A, Forsgren M, Orvell C, Nemeth A. The viral association of neonatal cholestasis in Sweden: a possible link between cytomegalovirus infection and biliary atresia. J Pediatr Gastroenterol Nutr 1998; 27:57–64.
14. Drut R, Drut RM, Gomez MA, et al. Presence of human papilloma virus in extrahepatic biliary atresia. J Pediatr Gastroenterol Nutr 1998; 27:530–535.
15. Domiati-Saad R, Dawson DB, Margraf LR, et al. Cytomegalovirus and human herpesvirus 6, but not human papilloma virus, are present in neonatal giant cell hepatitis and extrahepatic biliary atresia. Pediatr Dev Pathol 2000; 3:367–373.
16. Morecki R, Glaser J. Reovirus 3 and neonatal biliary disease: discussion of divergent results. Hepatology 1989; 10:515–517.
17. Saito T, Shinozaki K, Matsunaga T, et al. Lack of evidence for reovirus infection in tissues from patients with biliary atresia and congenital dilatation of the bile duct. J Hepatol 2004; 40:203–211.
18. Silveira TR, Salzano FM, Howard ER, Mowat AP. Extrahepatic biliary atresia and twinning. Braz J Med Biol Res 1991; 24:67–71.
19. Silveira TR, Salzano FM, Donaldson PT, Mieli-Vergani G, Howard ER, Mowat AP. Association between HLA and extrahepatic biliary atresia. J Pediatr Gastroenterol Nutr 1993; 16:114–116.
20. Donaldson PT, Clare M, Constantini PK, et al. HLA and cytokine gene polymorphisms in biliary atresia. Liver 2002; 22:213–219.
21. Mowat AP. Hepatitis and cholestasis in infancy: intrahepatic disorders. In: Liver Disorders in Childhood, 3rd edn. London: Butterworths; 1994: 43–78.
22. Farrant P, Meire HB, Mieli-Vergani G. Improved diagnosis of extrahepatic biliary atresia by high frequency ultrasound of the gall bladder. Br J Radiol 2001; 74:952–954.
23. Choi SO, Park WH, Lee HJ, et al. 'Triangular cord': a sonographic finding applicable in the diagnosis of biliary atresia. J Pediatr Surg 1996; 31:363–366.
24. Kotb MA, Kotb A, Sheba MF, et al. Evaluation of the triangular cord sign in the diagnosis of biliary atresia. Pediatrics 2001; 108:416–420.
25. Farrant P, Meire HB, Mieli-Vergani G. The ultrasound features of the gallbladder in infants presenting with conjugated hyperbilirubinaemia. Br J Radiol 2000; 73:1154–1158.
26. Deprettere A, Portmann B, Mowat AP. Syndromic paucity of the intrahepatic bile ducts: diagnostic difficulty; severe morbidity throughout childhood. J Pediatr Gastroenterol Nutr 1987; 6:865–871.
27. Psacharopoulos HT, Mowat AP, Cook PJ, et al. Outcome of liver disease associated with alpha-1-antitrypsin deficiency (PiZ); implications for genetic counselling and antenatal diagnosis. Arch Dis Child 1983; 58:882–887.
28. Hoffenberg EJ, Narkewicz MR, Sondheimer JM, Smith DJ, Silverman A, Sokol RJ. Outcome of syndromic paucity of interlobular bile ducts (Alagille syndrome) with onset of cholestasis in infancy. J Pediatr 1995; 127:220–224.
29. Wilkinson ML, Mieli-Vergani G, Ball C, Portmann B, Mowat AP. Endoscopic retrograde cholangiopancreatography (ERCP) in infantile cholestasis. Arch Dis Child 1991; 66:121–123.

30. McClement JW, Howard ER, Mowat AP. Results of surgical treatment of extrahepatic biliary atresia in the United Kingdom. BMJ 1985; 290:345–349.
31. Markowitz J, Daum F, Kahn EI, et al. Arteriohepatic dysplasia. I. Pitfalls in diagnosis and management. Hepatology 1983; 3:74–76.
32. Kasai M, Kimura S, Asakura S, et al. Surgical treatment of biliary atresia. J Pediatr Surg 1968; 3:665–675.
33. Davenport M, Kerkar N, Mieli-Vergani G, Mowat AP, Howard ER. Biliary atresia: the King's College Hospital experience (1974–1995). J Pediatr Surg 1997; 32:479–485.
34. Ohi R, Nio M, Chiba T, et al. Long-term follow-up after surgery for patients with biliary atresia. J Pediatr Surg 1990; 25:442–445.
35. Chiba T, Ohi R, Nio M, Ibrahim M. Late complications in long term survivors of biliary atresia. Eur J Pediatr Surg 1992; 2:22–25.
36. Hadžić N, Davenport M, Tizzard S, et al. Long term survival following Kasai portoenterostomy: is chronic liver disease inevitable ? J Pediatr Gastroenterol Nutr 2003; 37:430–433.
37. Muraji T, Higashimoto Y. The improved outlook for biliary atresia with corticosteroid therapy. J Pediatr Surg 1997; 32:1103–1106.
38. Dillon PW, Owings E, Cilley R, et al. Immunosuppression as adjuvant therapy for biliary atresia. J Pediatr Surg 2001; 36:80–85.
39. Meyers RL, Book LS, O'Gorman MA, et al. High-dose steroids, ursodeoxycholic acid, and chronic intravenous antibiotics improve bile flow after Kasai procedure in infants with biliary atresia. J Pediatr Surg 2003; 38:406–411.
40. Ohkohchi N, Chiba T, Ohi R, Mori S. Long-term follow-up of patients with cholangitis after successful Kasai operation in biliary atresia: selection of recipients for liver transplantation. J Pediatr Gastroenterol Nutr 1989; 9:416–420.
41. Nietgen GW, Vacanti JP, Perez-Atayade A. Intrahepatic bile duct loss in biliary atresia despite portoenterostomy: a consequence of ongoing obstruction. Gastroenterology 1992; 102:2126–2133.
42. Nagral S, Muiesan P, Vilca-Melendez H, et al. Liver transplantation for extrahepatic biliary atresia. Tohoku J Exp Med 1997; 181:117–127.
43. Diem HV, Evrard V, Vinh HT, et al. Pediatric liver transplantation for biliary atresia: results of primary grafts in 328 recipients. Transplantation 2003; 75:1692–1697.
44. Davenport M, De Ville de Goyet J, Stringer MD, et al. Seamless management of biliary atresia in England and Wales (1999–2002). Lancet 2004; 363:1354–1357.
45. Ozawa K, Uemoto S, Tanaka K, et al. An appraisal of pediatric liver transplantation from living relatives. Initial clinical experience in 20 pediatric liver transplantations from living relatives as donors. Ann Surg 1992; 216:547–553.
46. Stringer MD, Dhawan A, Davenport M, et al. Choledochal cysts: lessons from a 20-year experience. Arch Dis Child 1995; 73:528–531.
47. Redkar R, Davenport M, Howard ER. Antenatal diagnosis of congenital anomalies of the biliary tract. J Pediatr Surg 1998; 33:700–704.
48. Tan KC, Howard ER. Choledochal cyst: a 14-year surgical experience with 36 patients. Br J Surg 1988; 75:892–895.
49. Howard ER, Johnstone DI, Mowat AP. Spontaneous perforation of the common bile duct in infants. Arch Dis Child 1976; 51:883–886.
50. Amedee-Manesme O, Bernard O, Brunelle F, et al. Sclerosing cholangitis with neonatal onset. J Pediatr 1987; 111: 225–229.
51. Baker A, Portmann B, Westaby D, et al. Neonatal sclerosing cholangitis in two siblings: a category of progressive intrahepatic cholestasis. J Pediatr Gastroenterol Nutr 1993; 17:317–322.
52. Alagille D, Estrada A, Hadchouel M, et al. Syndromic paucity of interlobular bile ducts (Alagille's syndrome or arteriohepatic dysplasia): review of eighty cases. J Pediatr 1987; 110:195–200.
53. Oda T, Elkahloun AG, Pike BL, et al. Mutations in the human *Jagged1* gene are responsible for Alagille syndrome. Nat Genet 1997; 16:235–242.
54. Li L, Krantz ID, Deng Y, et al. Alagille syndrome is caused by mutations in human *Jagged1*, which encodes a ligand for Notch1. Nat Genet 1997; 16:243–251.
55. Kohsaka T, Yuan ZR, Guo SX, et al. The significance of human *jagged 1* mutations detected in severe cases of extrahepatic biliary atresia. Hepatology 2002; 36:904–912.
56. Rand EB. The genetic basis of the Alagille syndrome. J Pediatr Gastroenterol Nutr 1998; 26:234–236.
57. Lykavieris P, Hadchouel M, Chardot C, Bernard O. Outcome of liver disease in children with Alagille syndrome: a study of 163 patients. Gut 2001; 49:431–435.
58. Aw MM, Samaroo B, Baker AJ, et al. Calcineurin-inhibitor related nephrotoxicity-reversibility in paediatric liver transplant recipients. Transplantation 2001; 724:746–749.
59. Debray D, Pariente D, Gauthier F, et al. Cholelithiasis in infancy: a study of 40 cases. J Pediatr 1993; 122:385–391.
60. Wesdorp I, Bosman D, de Graaf A, Aronson D, van der Blij F, Taminiau J. Clinical presentation and predisposing factors of cholelithiasis and sludge in children. J Pediatr Gastroenterol Nutr 2000; 31:411–417.
61. Stringer MD, Taylor DR, Soloway RD. Gallstone composition: are children different? J Pediatr 2003; 142:435–440.
62. Thompson RJ, Jansen PL. Genetic defects in hepatocanalicular transport. Semin Liver Dis 2000; 20:365–372.
63. Clayton RJ, Iber FL, Reubner BH, McKusick VA. Fatal familial intrahepatic cholestasis in an Amish kindred. Am J Dis Child 1969; 117:112–124.
64. Carlton VE, Knisely AS, Freimer NB. Mapping of a locus for progressive familial intrahepatic cholestasis (Byler disease) to 18q21-q22, the benign recurrent intrahepatic cholestasis region. Hum Mol Genet 1995; 4:1049–1053.
65. Bull LN, van Eijk MJ, Pawlikowska L, et al. A gene encoding a P-type ATPase mutated in two forms of hereditary cholestasis. Nat Genet 1998; 18:219–224.
66. Whitington PF, Freese DK, Alonso EM, Schwarzenberg SJ, Sharp HL. Clinical and biochemical findings in progressive familial intrahepatic cholestasis. J Pediatr Gastroenterol Nutr 1994; 18:134–141.
67. Kurbegov AC, Setchell KD, Haas JE, et al. Biliary diversion for progressive familial intrahepatic cholestasis: improved liver morphology and bile acid profile. Gastroenterology 2003; 125:1227–1234.
68. Strautnieks SS, Kagalwalla AF, Tanner MS, et al. Identification of a locus for progressive familial intrahepatic cholestasis PFIC2 on chromosome 2q24. Am J Hum Genet 1997; 61:630–633.
69. Jansen PL, Strautnieks SS, Jacquemin E, et al. Hepatocanalicular bile salt export pump deficiency in patients with progressive familial intrahepatic cholestasis. Gastroenterology 1999; 117:1370–1379.
70. Knisely AS. Progressive familial intrahepatic cholestasis: a personal perspective. Pediatr Dev Pathol 2000; 3:113–125.
71. de Vree JM, Jacquemin E, Sturm E, et al. Mutations in the *MDR3* gene cause progressive familial intrahepatic cholestasis. Proc Natl Acad Sci USA 1998; 95:282–287.

72. De Vree JM, Ottenhoff R, Bosma PJ, et al. Correction of liver disease by hepatocyte transplantation in a mouse model of progressive familial intrahepatic cholestasis. Gastroenterology 2000; 119:1720–1730.
73. D'Agata IDA, Jonas MM, Perez-Atayde AR, Guay-Woodford LM. Combined cystic disease of the liver and kidney. Semin Liver Dis 1994; 14:215–228.
74. Asselah T, Ernst O, Sergent G, L'hermine C, Paris JC. Caroli's disease: a magnetic resonance cholangiography diagnosis. Am J Gastroenterol 1998; 93:109–110.
75. Keane F, Hadžić N, Wilkinson ML, et al. Neonatal presentation of Caroli's disease. Arch Dis Child 1997; 77:F145–F146.
76. Nichues R, Hasilik M, Alton G, et al. Carbohydrate-deficient glycoprotein syndrome type 1b: phosphomannose isomerase deficiency and mannose therapy. J Clin Invest 1998; 191:1414–1420.
77. Samyn M, Hadžić N, Portmann B, et al. Fibropolycystic disease of the liver and kidneys in children. Hepatology 1999; 30:328A (Abstract).
78. Starzl TE, Reyes J, Tzakis A, et al. Liver transplantation for polycystic liver disease. Arch Surg 1990; 125:575–577.

Chapter 60
Fatty acid oxidation disorders

William R. Treem

INTRODUCTION

Disorders of fatty acid oxidation (FAO) comprise more than 20 distinct defects in the transport and metabolism of fatty acids in the mitochondria of the liver, muscle and other tissues (Table 60.1). During prolonged fasting or catabolic stress, the inability to fully metabolize fatty acids leads to continued reliance on glucose metabolism, a deficiency in intracellular energy that affects many other metabolic pathways, and the accumulation of toxic metabolites that further inhibit critical intracellular functions. These effects are evident not only in the tissues expressing the defective enzyme or transporter, but also in distant tissues, such as the brain, as a result of the cumulative actions of circulating toxic metabolites and energy deficiency.

The pediatric gastroenterologist will become involved with these patients because of several clinical features including hypoketotic hypoglycemia and liver dysfunction, fulminant hepatic failure with jaundice and markedly increased levels of aminotransferases, marked hepatomegaly with microvesicular and macrovesicular steatosis, acute fatty liver of pregnancy in the mother of an affected infant and, less commonly, pancreatitis, gastroesophageal reflux with poor feeding and failure to thrive and 'cyclic' vomiting. These presentations may dominate the picture or be overshadowed by cardiomyopathy, hypotonia and rhabdomyolysis, or even 'sudden infant death syndrome' (SIDS) or sudden cardiorespiratory arrest. A high index of suspicion is required to diagnose these disorders in young infants and children who present in the emergency room with a sudden decompensation during a presumed viral illness labeled 'possible sepsis'. Critical clues during the window of diagnostic opportunity can easily be missed if urine and blood samples are not collected initially at the time of presentation, before cellular metabolism is changed by the introduction of large quantities of intravenous dextrose. In these cases, what is often absent (ketones) is just as important as what is present (hypoglycemia, abnormal organic acids in the urine, and often unusual acylcarnitines in the plasma). Other pitfalls that prevent a timely diagnosis include ignoring a constellation of stereotypic and less dramatic findings, including mild acidosis and mild increases in the levels of creatine phosphokinase (CPK), aspartate aminotransferase (AST) and alanine aminotransferase (ALT), that may persist in these patients between metabolic crises.

The consequences of missing a diagnosis of a defect in FAO can be devastating, resulting in future episodes of hepatic failure, hypoglycemia, coma, cardiomyopathy and even sudden death. Although no specific treatment is available, preventive measures are usually effective. These include avoidance of fasting and prolonged catabolic states, the provision of co-factors to prevent the accumulation of toxic metabolites within the mitochondria, and the provision of fatty acid substrates that can bypass the metabolic block. This chapter reviews the physiology of FAO and describes the key enzymatic reactions that normally result in energy and ketone body production. The particular FAO disorders that may present with liver or gastrointestinal-dominant symptoms will be highlighted, with a review of their epidemiology, genetics, clinical presentations, diagnosis and treatment.

PHYSIOLOGY OF NORMAL FATTY ACID OXIDATION

The intramitochondrial β-oxidation of fatty acids provides a significant proportion of the energy needed in heart and muscle much of the time, but during prolonged fasting (when glycogen stores have been depleted) FAO becomes an essential metabolic pathway to sustain energy production.[1] In extrahepatic mitochondria, complete oxidation results in carbon dioxide production and is coupled to adenosine triphosphate (ATP) synthesis by supplying acetyl-coenzyme A (CoA) for the tricarboxylic acid (TCA) cycle and electrons for the mitochondrial respiratory chain. In the liver, long-chain fatty acids are oxidized to acetyl-CoA and then synthesized to ketone bodies and exported to extrahepatic tissues such as cardiac and skeletal muscle when the supply of glucose is limited. This pathway is activated by pancreatic secretion of glucagon in excess of insulin, that in turn provokes glycogenolysis, gluconeogenesis, adipose tissue lipolysis, the release of amino acids and lactate from skeletal muscle, and ketogenesis in the liver (Fig. 60.1). These adaptive mechanisms are designed to maintain blood glucose concentrations by allowing the consumption of alternative fuels by the bulk of body tissues, thereby preserving glucose for brain metabolism.[2] Under conditions of adequate availability of glucose (the fed state), fatty acids are repackaged into triglycerides and stored in the hepatocyte or exported as lipoproteins (very low density and low density lipoproteins).

In an adult man, fatty acids provide 80% of caloric requirements after a 24-h period of fasting.[3] During prolonged aerobic exercise, FAO accounts for 60% of muscle oxygen consumption. Cardiac muscle relies predominantly on fatty acid metabolism under almost all conditions.

Disorder (common name)	Abbreviation	First report (year)
Plasma membrane		
Long-chain fatty acid transporter defect		1998
Carnitine transporter defect	CT	1988
Carnitine cycle		
Carnitine palmitoyl transferase I deficiency (liver-type CPT deficiency)	CPT I	1988
Carnitine–acylcarnitine translocase deficiency	CACT	1992
Carnitine palmitoyl transferase II deficiency (neonatal onset)	CPT II	1988
Carnitine palmitoyl transferase II deficiency (late-onset muscle disease)	CPT II	1973
β-Oxidation cycle Inner mitochondrial membrane		
Very long-chain acyl-CoA dehydrogenase deficiency	VLCAD	1993
Trifunctional protein deficiency (α-subunit)	TFP-α	1992
Trifunctional protein deficiency (β-subunit)	TFP-β	1996
Long-chain 3-hydroxylacyl-CoA dehydrogenase deficiency	LCHAD	1990
Electron transport flavoprotein dehydrogenase deficiency (glutaric aciduria IIC)	ETFDH	1985
Mitochondrial matrix enzymes		
Medium-chain acyl-CoA dehydrogenase deficiency	MCAD	1982
Short-chain acyl-CoA dehydrogenase deficiency	SCAD	1987
Electron transport flavoprotein, α-subunit (glutaric aciduria IIA)	ETF-α	1985
Electron transport flavoprotein, β-subunit (glutaric aciduria IIB)	ETF-β	1990
Riboflavin-responsive glutaric aciduria II		1982
Short-chain 3-hydroxyacyl-CoA dehydrogenase deficiency (muscle)	SCHAD	1991
Short-chain 3-hydroxyacyl-CoA dehydrogenase deficiency (liver)	SCHAD	1996
Medium-chain 3-ketoacyl-CoA thiolase deficiency	MCKAT	1997
Unsaturated fatty acids		
2,4-Dienoyl-CoA reductase deficiency		1990
Ketone body synthesis		
3-Hydroxy-3-methylglutaryl-CoA synthase deficiency	HMG-CoA synthase	1997
3-Hydroxy-3-methylglutaryl-CoA lyase deficiency	HMG-CoA lyase	1976

From Treem, 2001.[73]

Table 60.1 Inherited disorders of intramitochondrial fatty acid oxidation

Reliance on FAO is even greater in infants, who generate ketones earlier than adults during a fasting period.[4] There are several reasons for this phenomenon:

- The infant's large ratio of surface area : body mass increases the basal energy needed to maintain body temperature.
- The developing brain is highly dependent on glucose and infants have a larger brain : body size ratio.
- The infant has decreased glycogen stores and muscle mass for glucose production.
- Enzymes involved in the gluconeogenic, glycogenolytic and carnitine synthesis pathways are less active in infants.

This increased reliance on effective ketogenesis for metabolic homeostasis during fasting renders infants particularly susceptible to disorders of FAO.

Figure 60.2 summarizes the uptake and transport of long-chain fatty acids into the hepatocyte, and subsequently across the mitochondrial membrane to enter the β-oxidation cycle, giving rise to acetyl-CoA which is converted to ketone bodies. The maintenance of adequate levels of intramitochondrial acetyl-CoA is critical to activating the gluconeogenic pathway via the enzyme pyruvate carboxylase.[5] Low intramitochondrial acetyl-CoA levels also contribute to hyperammonemia through an inhibition of the production of *N*-acetylglutamate, which is an allosteric activator of

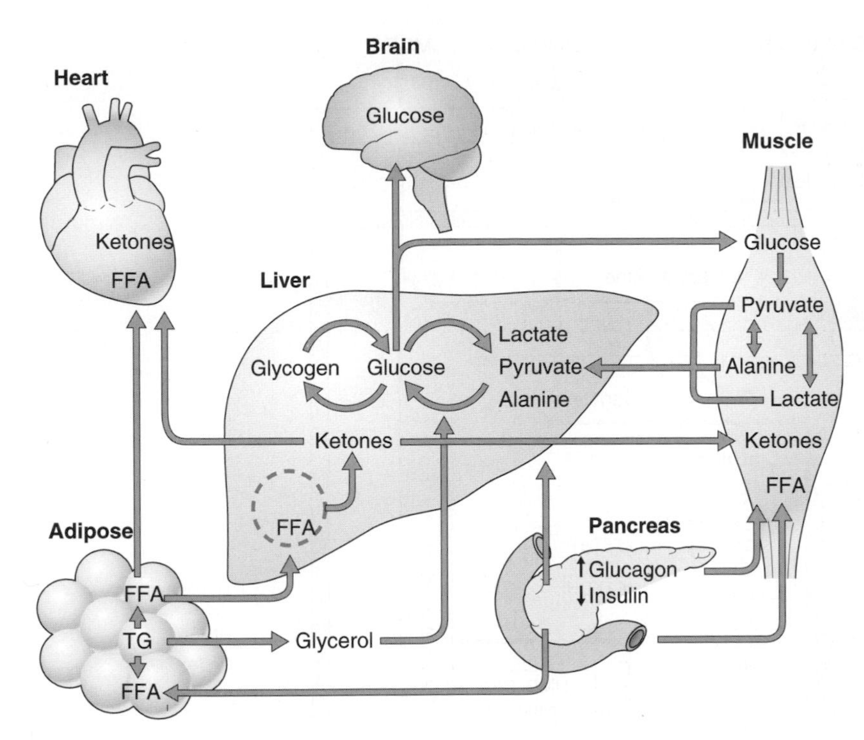

Figure 60.1: Organ and substrate interactions illustrating the normal adaptation to fasting. Under the influence of an increased circulating molar ratio of glucagon : insulin, enzymes are activated in the target organs to maintain glucose production, provide alternative fuels in tissues that can use them, and conserve glucose for brain metabolism. Glycogen is degraded to glucose in the liver. Glucose is newly synthesized from glycerol produced by lipolysis of triglycerides (TG) stored in adipose tissue. Free fatty acids (FFA) are mobilized from adipose tissue and exported directly to heart and skeletal muscle for complete oxidation to carbon dioxide. The liver becomes a ketogenic organ and oxidizes fatty acids to ketones. Ketones are exported to heart and skeletal muscle for catabolism in lieu of glucose. Glucose is conserved for the metabolic needs of the brain. (Adapted from Treem, 2003.)[72]

carbamyl phosphate synthetase, the first enzyme in the urea cycle. Decreased availability of acetyl-CoA would also be expected to depress ketone body production and flux through the TCA cycle and the generation of ATP.

The saturable uptake of long-chain fatty acids (LCFAs) by hepatocytes occurs by sodium-dependent active transport and is mediated by a family of tissue-specific fatty acid-binding transport proteins, some unique to the liver (FATP2) and others found in multiple tissues.[6] Inside the cell, fatty acids are esterified to CoA by the enzyme *acyl-CoA synthetase,* located on the outer aspect of the mitochondrial membrane. The resulting acyl-CoA esters can serve as substrates for triglyceride, phospholipids and cholesterol ester synthesis, but under fasting conditions they are directed largely toward mitochondrial β-oxidation. Like many other enzymes in the FAO pathway, the acyl-CoA synthetases differ in their specificities with respect to the chain lengths of fatty acid substrates. Their chain-length specificities are the basis for classifying them as short-, medium-, long- or very-long-chain *acyl-CoA synthetases.*

Carnitine cycle

After activation to their CoA esters, LCFAs are shuttled across the mitochondrial membrane by entering the carnitine cycle. In order to traverse the inner mitochondrial membrane, which is impermeable to CoA esters, long-chain acyl-CoA esters must first be transesterified to carnitine by the outer mitochondrial membrane enzyme *carnitine palmitoyltransferase I (CPT I)* to yield long-chain acylcarnitines. Three tissue-specific isoforms of *CPT 1* have been described, with the liver isoform designated *CPT I-A,* the muscle *CPT 1B,* and the brain *CPT1-C.*[7] *CPT I* is a key enzyme in the regulation of intramitochondrial FAO and is directly responsive to levels of malonyl-CoA, which rise during the fed state and suppress *CPT I* activity, and fall during fasting allowing increased enzyme activity and shunting of fatty acids into the β-oxidation pathway. The activity, immunoreactive protein, mRNA and transcription rate of *CPT I* are increased during high-fat feeding, starvation and diabetes, and by glucagon, cyclic adenosine monophosphate (cAMP), aspirin, hypolipidemic drugs and inflammatory cytokines.[8] A lipid-activated transcription factor, the peroxisome proliferators-activated receptor α (PPAR-α), plays a pivotal role in the cellular response to fasting, inducing the hepatic and cardiac expression of key intramitochondrial enzymes in the FAO pathway.[9] The mitochondrial transport system is highly specific for the transport of straight-chain fatty acids and restricts entry of branched-chain fatty acids (pristinic, phytanic acid), which are oxidized in the peroxisomes. In contrast to LCFAs (palmitate, oleate), medium- and short-chain fatty acids (octanoate, butyrate) can traverse the mitochondrial membrane as free acids without esterification to carnitine.

Carnitine (β-hydroxy-w-trimethylaminobutyric acid) is formed from lysine with *S*-adenosylmethionine specifically required as a methyl donor. The rate-limiting enzyme in the synthetic pathway is *γ-butyrobetaine hydroxylase,* found only in the cytosol of the liver and kidney. The activity of this enzyme in the livers of infants aged less than 3 months is only approximately one-tenth of that found in adults. This finding has led to the concept that carnitine is an essential nutrient during the neonatal period which must be supplied via breast milk or infant formula.[10] Later, rich sources of carnitine in the diet include dairy products and red meat.

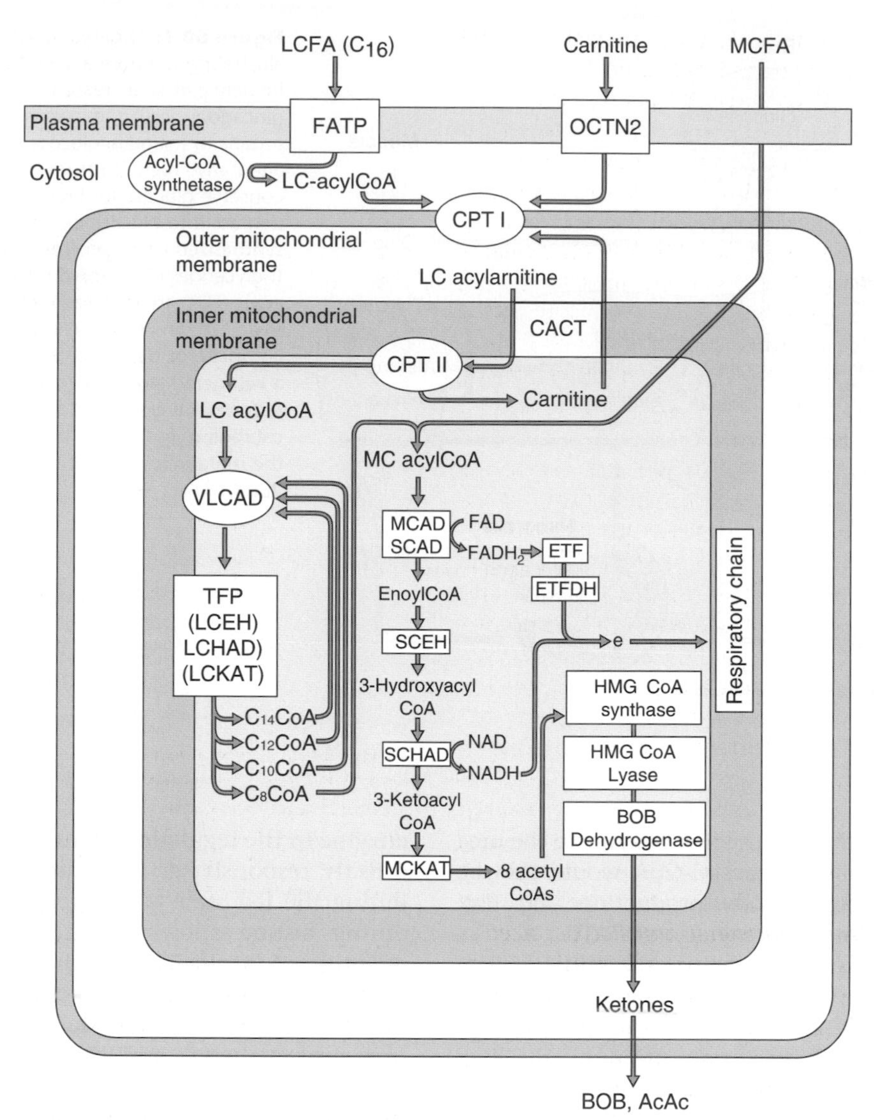

Figure 60.2: Pathway of hepatic mitochondrial fatty acid oxidation and ketogenesis showing steps for the oxidation of palmitate, a 16-carbon (C_{16}) long-chain fatty acid (LCFA). Note that eight-carbon medium-chain fatty acids (MCFA) enter the mitochondrion independent of the carnitine cycle. LCFAs are transported across the plasma membrane by a liver-specific LCFA-transporting polypeptide (FATP). Carnitine is supplied by a plasma membrane sodium-dependent carnitine transporter (OCTN2). On the outer mitochondrial membrane, carnitine palmitoyl transferase I (CPT I) is a major site of regulation that determines whether LCFAs are directed toward β-oxidation to ketones or to the resynthesis of triglycerides. LCFA-CoAs in the cytosol must first be transesterified to long-chain (LC) acylcarnitines by CPT I and then enter the carnitine cycle to be shuttled across the inner mitochondrial membrane. Once acrross the membrane, the acylcarnitine is re-esterified to a LC acyl-CoA and enters the β-oxidation cycle. All the relevant enzymes for LC acyl-CoAs are bound to the inner mitochondial membrane (VLCAD, TFP). At completion of the four reactions of the β-oxidation cycle, the LCFA has been shortened by two carbons, one molecule of acetyl-CoA has been generated for ketone body synthesis, and electrons have been transported to the respiratoary chain via flavin–adenine dinucleotide (FAD) and nicotinamide–adenine dinucleotide (NAD). As the LCFA is shortened, β-oxidation proceeds via enzymes located in the mitochondrial matrix (MCAD, SCAD, SCHAD, MCKAT). Enzymes and transporters are circled. CACT, carnitine acylcarnitine translocase; CPT II, carnitine palmitoyl transferase II; VLCAD, very-long-chain acyl-CoA dehydrogenase; TFP, trifunctional protein; LCAD, long-chain acyl-CoA dehydrogenase; MCAD, medium-chain acyl-CoA dehydrogenase; SCAD, short-chain acyl-CoA dehydrogenase; LCHAD, long-chain 3-hydroxyacyl-CoA dehydrogenase; LCEH, long-chain enoyl-CoA hydratase; LCKAT, long-chain ketothiolase; SCEH, short-chain enoyl-CoA dehydrogenase; MCKAT, medium-chain ketothiolase; HMG CoA, 3-hydroxy-3-methylglutaryl-CoA; AcAc, acetoacetate; BOB, β-hydroxybutyrate; ETF, electron transport flavoprotein; ETFDH, electron transport flavoprotein dehydrogenase; $FADH_2$, reduced flavin–adenine dinucleotide; NADH, reduced nicotinamide–adenine dinucleotide. (Adapted from Treem, 2001.)[73]

Because the muscle and heart must take up carnitine synthesized and exported from the liver and kidney, and because the concentration of carnitine is 20–40-fold higher in these tissues than in the blood, transport of carnitine must be mediated by an active transport mechanism that is driven by a sodium gradient. A recently cloned homolog of the organic cation transporter *OCTN1* (designated *OCTN2*) has sodium-dependent carnitine uptake properties, has been mapped to human chromosome 5q31.2-32, and is highly expressed in cultured human hepatoma cells.[11] Mutations in *OCTN2* have been identified in patients with systemic primary carnitine deficiency and in mice with juvenile visceral steatosis. Interestingly, through linkage analysis *OCTN2* pleomorphisms have recently been implicated as candidate genes in patients with Crohn's disease.[12] Evidence that there may be a connection between intracellular carnitine deficiency and inflammatory bowel disease comes from animal models, where induced abnormalities in FAO in intestinal epithelial cells result in enterocolitis. Carnitine transporters, like LCFA transporters, are tissue specific, which explains why those found in skeletal and cardiac muscle have a much higher K_m for the interaction of carnitine with *CPT I* compared with the liver isoform of this enzyme.[13] Thus, a defect in carnitine uptake and transport would be expected to have more severe consequences for cardiac and skeletal muscle than for other tissues.

Accumulating acylcarnitines in the plasma and urine reflect accumulating acyl-CoA esters within the mitochondria. During fasting, acetyl-CoA normally accumulates, and the ratio of acetyl-carnitine : free carnitine increases. However, in patients with FAO defects, the medium- and long-chain acylcarnitines that are excreted in the plasma and urine reflect the site of the metabolic block and are clues to the identification of the intramitochondrial defect. Detoxification of accumulating intramitochondrial acyl-CoAs by esterification to carnitine and transport out of mitochondria is crucial to the maintenance of the intramitochondrial free CoA pool upon which many of the other intramitochondrial metabolic pathways depend.[14] If not transported out of the mitochondria, accumulating long-chain acyl-CoA esters would inhibit specific enzymes and transporters such as *adenine nucleotide translocase*, needed for the transport of ATP from the mitochondria to the cytosol, and *pantothenic acid kinase*, a major regulator of free CoA synthesis in the heart, liver and kidney.[15]

After transesterification to carnitine, the resultant long-chain acylcarnitines are transported across the inner mitochondrial membrane by *carnitine–acylcarnitine translocase* (*CACT*). At the interface of the inner membrane with the mitochondrial matrix, acylcarnitines are re-esterified to regenerate acyl-CoA esters and free carnitine by *carnitine palmitoyltransferase II* (*CPT II*). The reconstituted acyl-CoA is delivered into the mitochondrial matrix and enters the β-oxidation cycle while the carnitine is reshuttled back across the inner mitochondrial membrane for transesterification with another long-chain acyl-CoA. Each turn of the β-oxidation cycle results in the progressive cleavage of two carbon fragments from the original LCFA in the form of acetyl-CoAs that are then directed into ketone body synthesis. An important byproduct of the β-oxidation cycle is the generation of electrons for the electron transport chain in the form of reduced flavin–adenine dinucleotide ($FADH_2$) and reduced nicotinamide–adenine dinucleotide (NADH). Transfer of these electrons to the intramitochondrial respiratory chain yields ATP via oxidative phosphorylation and maintains the normal intramitochondrial redox state.

β-Oxidation cycle

Figure 60.3 shows the four enzymes responsible for each turn of the β-oxidation cycle. In truth, each enzyme activ-

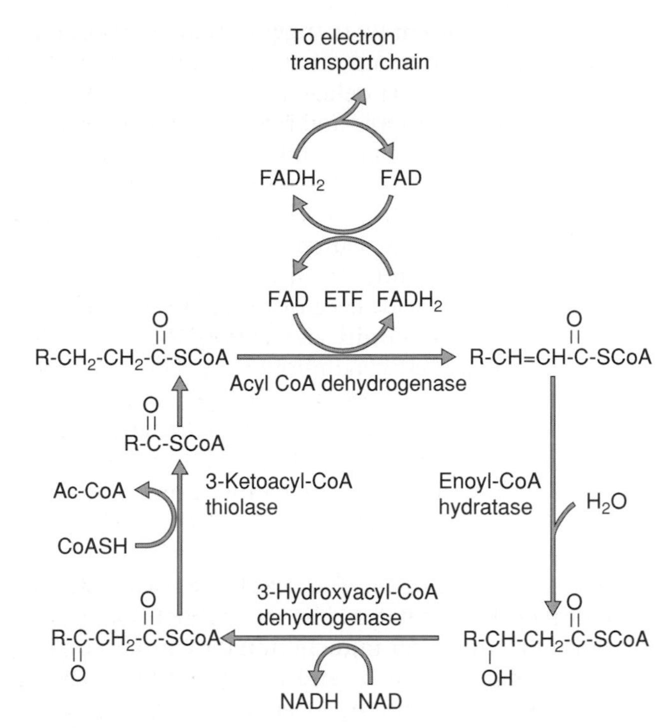

Figure 60.3: Spiral of fatty acyl-CoA β-oxidation in mitochondria. Acyl-CoA enters the spiral, whereupon acyl-CoA dehydrogenase inserts a double bond, forming an enoyl-CoA and transferring electrons to electron transfer flavoprotein (ETF). Enoyl-CoA hydratase adds water across the double bond to form 3-hydroxyacyl-CoA, which is oxidized by a nicotinamide–adenine dinucleotide (NAD)-linked 3-hydroxyacyl-CoA dehydrogenase to form a 3-ketoacyl-CoA. In the presence of free coenzyme A (CoASH), 3-ketoacyl-CoA thiolase cleaves the (α–β bond to yield acetyl-CoA and an acyl-CoA moiety, now two carbons shorter, which can then re-enter the spiral. $FADH_2$, reduced flavin–adenine dinucleotide. (Adapted from Treem, 2001.)[73]

ity is incorporated into a family of enzymes with different chain-length specificities for fatty acids with a 24-carbon-atom backbone down to four-carbon chain-length fatty acids. Enzymes responsible for the β-oxidation of longer chain-length species are associated with the inner mitochondrial membrane, whereas those responsible for the metabolism of medium- and short-chain species are located within the mitochondrial matrix. The metabolism of fatty acids with more than 24 carbon atoms starts in the peroxisomes and can be continued until the fatty acid is reduced to eight carbons (medium-chain acyl-CoAs). However, certain characteristics of peroxisomal oxidation limit its ability to compensate for intramitochondrial FAO.[16] Electrons generated by peroxisomal oxidation are passed to oxygen (forming hydrogen peroxide) instead of the respiratory chain; and peroxisomes lack a TCA cycle which, in mitochondria, is primed by acetyl-CoA from FAO.

The rate-limiting step in β-oxidation is the first reaction catalyzed by a family of *acyl-CoA dehydrogenases*. *Very-long-chain acyl-CoA dehydrogenase (VLCAD)* is bound to the inner mitochondrial membrane and accepts acyl-CoAs ranging from C24-CoA to C12-CoA with palmitoyl-CoA (C16) as the best substrate. The substrates for *long-chain acyl-CoA dehydrogenase (LCAD)* overlap with those of

VLCAD. However, recent work suggests that LCAD is much less important in humans than was once thought.[17] A mouse model of LCAD deficiency results in gestational loss, lipidosis, hypoglycemia and myocardial degeneration, a biochemical phenotype similar to human *VLCAD* deficiency. In humans, *LCAD* is present in heart tissue at low levels compared with *VLCAD*, whereas it is found in high levels in the kidney. Current thinking is that LCAD might play a major role in the metabolism of long branched-chain fatty acids because, as opposed to VLCAD, it apparently has high affinity and activity for 2-methyldecanoyl-CoA and 2-methylpalmitoyl-CoA. Located within the mitochondrial matrix are the other two *acyl-CoA dehydrogenases, medium-chain acyl-CoA dehydrogenase (MCAD)* with a broad chain-length specificity and optimal activity toward C6-CoA and C8-CoA (octanoyl-CoA), and *short-chain acyl-CoA dehydrogenase (SCAD),* which binds to four and six acyl-CoA esters.

For long-chain acyl-CoAs, the next three reactions of the β-oxidation cycle are catalyzed by the trifunctional protein (TFP) bound to the inner mitochondrial membrane. TFP is a hetero-octamer of four α- and four β-subunits. On the α-subunit of this protein is encoded the *enoyl-CoA hydratase* activity and the *long-chain 3-hydroxy-CoA dehydrogenase* (*LCHAD*) activity. The smaller β-subunit encodes the *long-chain 3-ketoacyl-CoA thiolase* (*LKAT*) activity.[18] Because of the complex association of the four α- and four β-subunits, mutations in either subunit may affect the intricate folding of the protein, rendering the entire complex unstable.

For medium- and short-chain acyl-CoAs, the relevant enzymes are located in the mitochondrial matrix rather than attached to the inner mitochondrial membrane, and they are synthesized as unrelated proteins and encoded by separate nucleur genes. These include two *acyl-CoA dehydrogenases* (*MCAD* and *SCAD*), a *short-chain enoyl-CoA hydratase* (*crotonase*), both *medium-* and *short-chain 3-hydroxy acyl-CoA dehydrogenases* (*MCHAD* and *SCHAD*), and *medium-chain 3-ketoacyl-CoA thiolase* (*MCKAT*). The intramitochondrial *short-chain ketothiolase* (*acetoacetyl CoA thiolase*) is active only with acetoacyl-CoA and 2-methylacetoacetyl-CoA, which makes it indispensable for isoleucine degradation and important in ketone body metabolism, but suggests no role in FAO. Riboflavin (vitamin B_2) is the major precursor for flavin coenzymes including flavin–adenine dinucleotide (FAD), which is linked to all three *acyl-CoA dehydrogenases* and acts as an electron transporter to the intramitochondrial respiratory chain. In experimental animals, riboflavin deficiency produces a rapid and selective decrease in FAO, and some patients with multiple *acyl-CoA dehydrogenase* deficiency (also called glutaric aciduria type II) are responsive to treatment with large doses of riboflavin.[19]

In the liver, acetyl-CoA liberated by FAO is targeted toward ketogenesis. *3-Hydroxy-3-methylglutaryl-CoA* (*HMG-CoA*) *synthetase* combines one molecule of acetyl-CoA and one of acetoacetyl-CoA to form HMG-CoA. This is then cleaved by *HMG-CoA lyase* to yield a molecule of acetoacetate, which is in redox equilibrium with D-3-hydroxybutyrate. Ketone bodies then enter the bloodstream and are taken up by tissues with a limited capacity to carry out β-oxidation, in particular the brain. There, acetoacetyl-CoA is cleaved into two molecules of acetyl-CoA and fed into the TCA cycle.

EPIDEMIOLOGY AND GENETICS OF DISORDERS IN FAO

The mitochondrial FAO defects so far described exhibit autosomal recessive inheritance of nuclear encoded genes. The exact incidence and prevalence data are lacking for most disorders of FAO owing to the lack of identification of a common mutation allowing for large-scale population screening. Other factors that hamper an accurate assessment include the lack of large numbers of described patients for most of the FAO disorders, and the finding of multiple mutations responsible for the same or at times a different phenotype. The best studied disorder is *MCAD* deficiency, in which a common point mutation accounts for approximately 80% of the cases, and no other mutation has been found in more than 1% of the mutant alleles. The best estimates of the prevalence of homozygosity for the common mutation in the general Caucasian population is approximately 1 in 12 000, but it appears to be higher in the USA (1 in 9000) and the UK (1 in 6000).[20] Because about 10% of affected individuals are compound heterozygotes, with one allele carrying the common mutation and the other a less frequent mutation, the prevalence of MCAD deficiency is actually slightly greater than these numbers suggest. In large neonatal screening programs, using tandem mass spectrometry, the incidence of detected cases of MCAD deficiency is 1 in 15 000 live births in the USA, 1 in 12 600 in the UK and 1 in 10 600 in Germany.[21]

The ability to determine the common mutation in MCAD deficiency, by using dried filter-paper blood spots to extract DNA, has led to large-scale screening studies of gene frequency in the general populations of various countries (the carrier state). Estimates range from as low as 1 in 68 in England, to 1 in 71 in Australia, about 1 in 100 in Denmark and The Netherlands, and approximately 1 in 107 in the USA. Two recent studies of patients with MCAD deficiency revealed that 159 of 161 were Caucasian.[22] For most, their country of origin was either the British Isles or Germany. In contrast, the frequency of the carrier state for the common mutation in Italy is only 1 in 333, and in Japan no carrier was identified in 500 Japanese neonates.[23] These data have led to the hypothesis that the common mutant allele for MCAD deficiency came from a small ancient population centered in Denmark or northern Germany, with subsequent spread to England, Ireland and later to the USA and Australia.

A common mutation has also been found for isolated LCHAD deficiency. This single base-pair change in the α-subunit of TFP has been found to account for as many as 87% of the mutant alleles in a study from Europe, but only approximately 65% of the mutations in the USA.[24] An analysis of the frequency of this G1528C mutation in Finland revealed a carrier frequency of 1 in 240.[25] In the USA, a carrier frequency of approximately 1 in 175 has been found, and in The Netherlands 1 in 680.[26] This mutation alters the NAD-binding site of LCHAD, leading to a loss of enzyme activity of LCHAD without affecting the other two enzyme acitivities in the TFP complex.

The situation with respect to SCAD deficiency is more complex. SCAD deficiency has a very heterogeneous clinical presentation, ranging from fatal metabolic decompensation in early life to subtle adult onset, with some patients even remaining asymptomatic. In many infants and children with mild presentations (poor feeding, vomiting, mild hypotonia, failure to thrive), isolated and repetitive bouts of ethylmalonic aciduria have been documented, provoked by fasting, fever or catabolic stress. Approximately 70% of these patients have been found to be homozygous or compound heterozygous for two polymorphisms in the *SCAD* gene (511C>T; 625G>A) in exons 5 and 6.[27] One of these variant alleles (625G>A) is present in homozygous form in 7% of the normal population in The Netherlands, and 14% of healthy European controls are either homozygous or compound heterozygous for these mutations. In the USA, these gene variants were detected in either homozygous or compound heterozygous form in 7% of a large cohort of neonatal blood spots collected at the Mayo Clinic.[28] However, in these patients the enzyme remains catalytically active but subject to thermal instability. This is the behavior of traditional temperature-sensitive folding mutations.[29]

Measurement of SCAD activity in cultured skin fibroblasts and muscle of patients with ethylmalonic aciduria who are homozygous for this polymorphism has yielded inconsistent results, with normal or variably decreased enzyme activity from 50% down to less than 10% of controls. Although plasma C4 acylcarnitine (butyrylcarnitine) levels are significantly higher in subjects homozygous for these polymorphisms when compared to those homozygous for wild-type SCAD, the concentration usually did not reach a level that would be consistent with a biochemical diagnosis of SCAD deficiency. These results have been interpreted to mean that these genetic variants confer disease susceptibility when combined with other genetic, cellular or environmental factors.

A number of the nuclear genes encoding for enzymes involved in the carnitine and β-oxidation cycles have been cloned, including genes for CPT I and CPT II deficiency, VLCAD, MCAD and SCAD deficiency, and LCHAD, TFP and SCHAD deficiency. This has led to the discovery of specific genetic mutations resulting in reduced enzyme activity, and the development of molecular probes to detect specific defects. Polymerase chain reaction-based assays are available commercially in a restricted number of laboratories to detect the common mutations in MCAD and LCHAD deficiencies. As all of these disorders are autosomal recessive, study of the implicated enzyme activity in cultured skin fibroblasts from the parents of index cases is revealing, and shows approximately 50% of control values.

CLINICAL PRESENTATIONS OF FAO DISORDERS

Heterogeneous clinical presentations are the rule rather than the exception in FAO disorders, and reflect a combination of the effects of energy depletion and endogenous toxicity from accumulating toxic metabolites (Table 60.2). The presentation in many patients predominantly affects organs outside the usual purview of the pediatric gastroenterologist. These patients usually present in infancy (as early as the first week of life) or early childhood to neonatologists or cardiologists with cardiomyopathy, arrhythmia, pericardial effusion and sudden cardiac death. They also may present later in childhood or even adolescence to neurologists with persistent hypotonia and developmental delay, or intermittent bouts of muscle pain, hypotonia and even rhabdomyolysis. The existence of different tissue isoforms of some of

Organ or system	Clinical manifestations
Liver	Hepatomegaly, steatosis (common); fibrosis, cirrhosis (rare)
	Aminotransferase 2–10 times normal (common); >1000 units/l (rare)
	Bilirubin level normal (common); moderately raised (rare)
	Coagulopathy (mild to moderate)
	Pruritus (rare); hepatic failure (rare)
Cardiac	Cardiomyopathy (hypertrophic and dilated)
	Congestive heart failure
	Cardiac arrhythmia
	Sudden infant death
	Increased CPK
Muscle	Hypotonic, weakness
	Muscle pain (exercise, stress)
	Rhabdomyolysis
	Increased CPK
Metabolic	Vomiting, lethargy, coma
	Encephalopathy
	Mild acidosis
	Increased lactate (LCHAD)
	Increased uric acid
Renal	Myoglobinuria
	Renal tubular acidosis (CPT, CPT II, MAD, LCHAD)
	Renal cysts, dysplasia (MAD, CPT II)
Non-specific	Failure to thrive
	Gastroesophageal reflux, vomiting
	Pancreatitis (CPT II)
	Retinitis pigmentosa (LCHAD, long term)
	Peripheral neuropathy (LCHAD)
	Hypoparathyroidism (LCHAD)
	Acute fatty liver of pregnancy (LCHAD, SCHAD, CPT I)
	Asymptomatic (MCAD)

CPK, creatine phosphokinase; CPT, carnitine palmitoyl transferase; LCHAD, long-chain 3-hydroxyacyl coenzyme A (CoA) dehydrogenase; MCAD, medium-chain acyl-CoA dehydrogenase; SCHAD, short-chain 3-hydroxy-acyl-CoA dehydrogenase.
Adapted from Treem, 2000.[74]

Table 60.2 Clinical manifestations of the fatty acid oxidation disorders

the enzymes in the FAO pathway (CPT I, carnitine transporter) encoded by different genes is responsible for some of this heterogeneity. In general, the more proximal the defect in the FAO pathway (i.e. at the level of the carnitine cycle or VLCAD), the earlier the presentation and the more likely it is to be dominated by cardiorespiratory arrest or cardiomyopathy and congestive heart failure. This chapter highlights the constellations of symptoms that are likely to provoke a gastroenterology consultation.

Hypoketotic hypoglycemia, hepatomegaly, liver dysfunction and encephalopathy

These dramatic findings in a 'previously healthy' infant or young child, usually in the first 2 years of life, will prompt a consult to the pediatric gastroenterologist for 'hepatic failure'. Diagnostic considerations will often include severe viral hepatitis, galactosemia (on a lactose-containing diet), glycogen storage disease (type I), hereditary fructose intolerance (on a sucrose-containing diet), hereditary tyrosinemia type I, neonatal iron storage liver disease, mitochondrial respiratory chain defects, inborn errors of bile acid synthesis and erythrophagocytic lymphohistiocytosis.

Most often, this constellation of symptoms is preceded by what appeared to be a routine viral infection with fever, upper respiratory symptoms and vomiting, or by a middle ear infection with a decreased appetite and fever. The common denominator is poor oral intake over several days, often with vomiting and a catabolic state (fever, fasting). Less frequently, young infants may present after weaning from the breast and sleeping for longer periods through the night without feeding. The most likely symptoms at the time of presentation are lethargy, emesis, apnea and even respiratory arrest, and seizures. Physical findings generally include marked hepatomegaly, no splenomegaly, hypotonia, and a gallop rhythm and poor perfusion if the heart is affected. Jaundice at the time of presentation is rare, thus contrasting FAO disorders from fulminant viral, drug-induced, sepsis-induced or ischemic hepatitis.[30] In certain disorders of FAO, a family history of SIDS, 'Reye' syndrome, sudden cardiac decompensation, or early infant death from presumed 'sepsis' or 'liver failure' can be elicited in approximately one-third of the patients.

Hypoketotic or non-ketotic hypoglycemia is a hallmark of most but not all FAO disorders. Hypoglycemia with fasting is likely the result of hepatic glycogen depletion and impaired gluconeogenesis. Patients with disorders that allow multiple turns of the β-oxidation cycle prior to the enzymatic block (SCAD and SCHAD deficiencies) still make some ketones, and these defects likely are responsible for some patients previously descriptively labeled as having ketotic hypoglycemia. Patients with MCAD deficiency or even more proximal defects in FAO make small amounts of β-hydroxybutyric acid, but the normal ratio of increased urinary ketones compared to dicarboxylic acids that is found in physiologic ketogenesis is reversed.[31]

The observation that alterations in mental status precede overt hypoglycemia in some of these patients has led to a search for accumulating neurotoxins (Fig. 60.4). Hyperammonemia is often present and arises from a secondary urea cycle dysfunction due to diminished availability of *N*-acetylglutamate, which in turn is secondary to raised propionyl-CoA and low acetyl-CoA concentrations. *In vivo* animal studies and *in vitro* cellular studies have implicated medium-chain fatty acids (octanoate), long-chain acyl-CoAs and long-chain dicarboxylic acids as direct brain mitochondrial toxins and inhibitors of brain energy metabolism.[32] Direct infusion of octanoate into normal rabbits, at concentrations reached in the blood of patients with MCAD deficiency during a metabolic crisis, results in coma, hyperammonemia, electroencephalographic changes, increased intracranial pressure, gross ultrastructural changes of brain

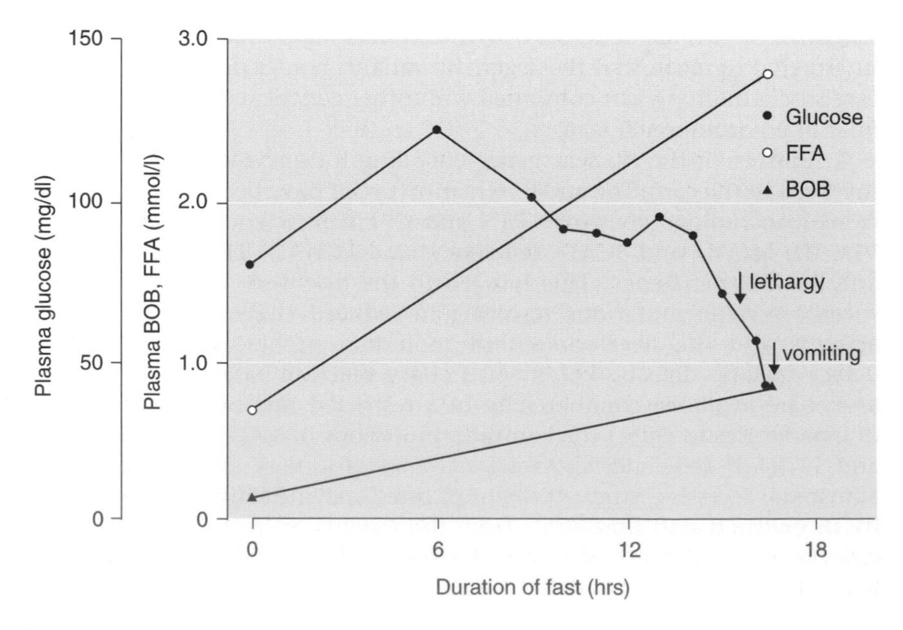

Figure 60.4: Consequences of prolonged fasting in a patient with MCAD deficiency. Normally, glucose concentration falls slightly and remains stable, while levels of ketones (β-hydroxybutyrate; BOB) rise steeply and free fatty acids (FFA) rise slightly and then stabilize. Here, because of the defect in FAO, glucose falls precipitously during a prolonged fast, with an inadequate ketogenic response and a marked rise in FFA levels. Note that lethargy and mental status changes precede actual hypoglycemia. In these disorders, the accumulations of toxic medium- and long-chain fatty acyl-CoAs and acylcarnitines mediate the central nervous system toxicity even before the hypoglycemia becomes critical. (Adapted from Treem, 2001.)[73]

mitochondria and depression of intramitochondrial ATP production.[33] In LCHAD deficiency, the accumulated metabolic intermediates include long-chain 3-hydroxy fatty acids, 3-hydroxyacylcarnitines, 3-hydroxyacyl-CoAs and 3-hydroxydicarboxylic acids. In high concentrations these can injure cell membranes, potentiate free radical-induced lipid peroxidation, inhibit Na^+–K^+ ATPase, uncouple mitochondrial oxidative phosphorylation and damage mitochondria.

Levels of aminotransferases are mildly increased in most patients with FAO defects, in the range of 2–10 times normal. Bilirubin concentration is usually normal or only mildly raised at the time of presentation. Although the clotting studies may be normal, at times the degree of coagulopathy appears incongruous with the minimal hepatocyte damage reflected in the mild increase in aminotransferase levels. Other accompanying abnormalities in basic laboratory parameters include mild to moderate increases in blood urea nitrogen (BUN), uric acid and CPK. Acidosis, if present, is usually mild. However, in some disorders, such as LCHAD, TFP and multiple acyl-CoA dehydrogenase (MAD) deficiencies, significant lactic acidemia may be present.[34]

Dramatic increases in liver size often develop over the first 48 h in a patient presenting with hypoketotic hypoglycemia and coma, even after intravenous dextrose has been provided and hypoglycemia ameliorated. The liver is brightly echogenic and homogeneous when examined with ultrasonography. Computed tomography (CT) shows a low-density liver characteristic of diffuse fatty infiltration. A liver biopsy performed at the time of the illness most often reveals diffuse marked macrovesicular steatosis. Some patients, particularly those with MCAD or SCAD deficiency, have only microvesicular fat accumulation, and these subtle changes can escape notice without the help of special stains (Oil Red-O) or electron microscopy. More severe changes with portal infiltrates, bile duct proliferation, hepatic fibrosis and even established cirrhosis have been noted in a minority of patients with LCHAD deficiency (Fig. 60.5a). Electron microscopy of liver tissue reveals an increase in the size and number of mitochondria, as well as mitochondrial damage manifested as swelling, irregular cristae and paracrystalline arrays (Fig. 60.5b).

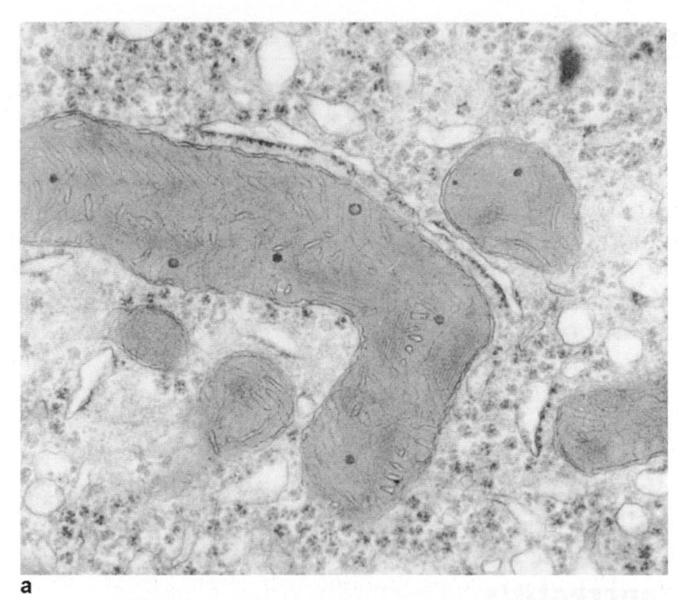

a

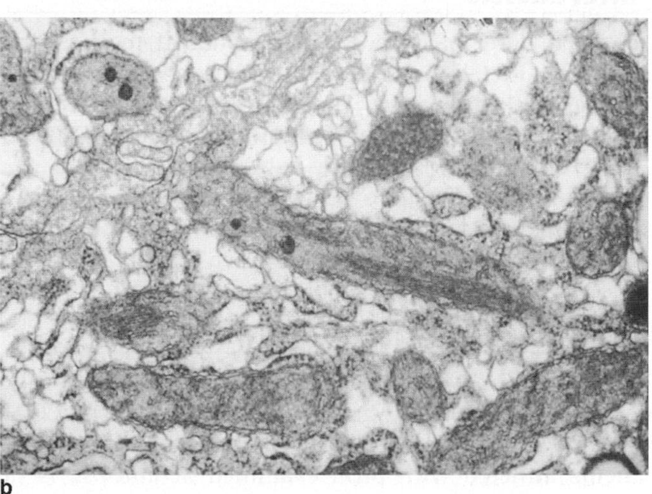

b

Figure 60.5: Electron micrographs of the liver from patients with (**a**) MCAD deficiency and (**b**) carnitine transport defect showing the elongated giant mitochondria with linear crystalline arrays in the matrix. (From Treem, 2001).[73]

Fulminant hepatic failure

A minority of patients with FAO defects present with true fulminant hepatic failure characterized by markedly increased levels of aminotransferases (more than 20 times normal), profound coagulopathy, hyperammonemia, hypoglycemia, coma and significant hyperbilirubinemia. Biopsies in these patients show significant confluent areas of hepatocyte necrosis and collapse. Although uncommon, patients with LCHAD, CACT and MCKAT deficiency have been described with this severe presentation.[35,36] Two patients with putative *in vitro* evidence of a defect of LCFA transport at the plasma membrane level have been reported with recurrent life-threatening episodes of acute liver failure that evolved into chronic severe liver disease necessitating transplantation.[37] However, other cases have not been confirmed and the exact mechanism of this defect remains to be elucidated.

Chronic vomiting, failure to thrive and gastroesophageal reflux

Some patients with SCAD deficiency may have a more indolent presentation of chronic vomiting and failure to thrive accompanied by other non-specific symptoms such as hypotonia, developmental delay and feeding aversion.[38] This constellation of findings often provokes a referral to the pediatric gastroenterologist. These patients can show an exacerbation of their chronic symptoms during times of metabolic stress, but may not have the hallmark features of hypoketotic hypoglycemia, coma and massive hepatomegaly. Although some ketones are present in the urine, other organic acids such as ethylmalonic acid often predominate and suggest the diagnosis.

Cyclic vomiting

Reported large series of children with cyclic vomiting syndrome (CVS) often include a few young patients subsequently discovered to have an underlying defect in FAO.[39] This presentation may reflect milder phenotypes of MCAD or SCAD deficiency. Lack of awareness of the relative hypoketonuria present, given the level of serum glucose at the time of a vomiting episode, may delay the diagnosis. A search for abnormal urine organic acids or plasma acylcarnitines may not be helpful even several hours after the initiation of intravenous fluids containing dextrose, thus re-emphasizing the need for prompt collection of blood and urine specimens at the time the patient presents in the emergency room. The alteration in mental status can be mistakenly interpreted as a possible indication of a migraine equivalent that is often associated with CVS.

Pancreatitis

Defects in FAO have recently been added to the list of underlying metabolic diseases in which repetitive episodes of pancreatitis dominate the clinical picture. Scattered case reports of patients with this presentation with LCHAD and CPT II deficiency have been published.[40] It is not clear whether this phenotype represents an example of the expression of a mutation of an isoform of the enzyme localized to one tissue but not another.

Sudden infant death syndrome

Recent studies have suggested that 1–5% of all cases of SIDS are due to abnormalities in FAO, including MCAD, VLCAD, MAD and LCHAD deficiencies.[41] Fatty change in the liver of patients afflicted with SIDS examined at autopsy is not uncommon. Various tissues and fluids are suitable for metabolite or enzyme analysis post mortem in infants with SIDS, including swabbed urine from the bladder, bile accumulated in the gallbladder, vitreous humor, and frozen liver, skeletal and cardiac muscle.[42] Post-mortem skin biopsies yield skin fibroblasts that can still be grown in tissue culture for later examination. Some of these cases have been discovered when a subsequent sibling is diagnosed with an FAO disorder years after the SIDS case. Recently, the use of polymerase chain reaction to amplify a small DNA fragment from genomic DNA in post-mortem paraffin-embedded or formalin-fixed tissued stored for as long as 18 years has allowed the diagnosis of MCAD deficiency in a SIDS victim.[43] A family history of SIDS or unexplained infantile death should always provoke a suspicion of the possibility of a defect in FAO in another child who later exhibits one of the clinical presentations described above.

Acute fatty liver of pregnancy in mothers carrying infants with FAO defects

Recently a number of published reports have established a link between acute fatty liver of pregnancy (AFLP) and FAO disorders, most notably LCHAD deficiency.[44–46] Women who carry a mutation in the α-subunit of TFP (thus reducing the synthesis of LCHAD by approximately 50%) and who are carrying a fetus affected by LCHAD deficiency (homozygous for the common mutation or a compound heterozygote) are at increased risk of developing AFLP in the last trimester of that pregnancy. Carrying an affected fetus appears to be a necessary condition for the development of AFLP, as these same women do not develop AFLP when carrying a heterozygous or completely unaffected fetus. This has led to the recommendation that the offspring who are the result of a pregnancy complicated by AFLP be tested for a defect in FAO. Retrospective studies of 35 families carrying heterogeneous mutations of the TFP have shown that 49% of women who carried affected fetuses had AFLP, and a further 11% had the syndrome of hemolysis, raised liver enzymes and low platelets (HELLP syndrome), or pre-eclampsia. All women with illnesses during pregnancy carried fetuses with isolated LCHAD deficiency. Approximately half of the affected pregnancies were also associated with premature delivery and intrauterine growth retardation.[47]

During the latter stages of pregnancy, the normal insulin resistance, increased activity of lipoprotein lipase and inhibition of the normal enzymes of FAO lead to increased LCFA substrate flux through a relatively inefficient pathway.[48] Pre-eclampsia, which is a common precursor of AFLP, further exaggerates these stressors and also results in a reduction of hepatic antioxidants to prevent lipid peroxidation and the generation of free radicals.

Recent studies have demonstrated that at least six different enzymes of the FAO pathway are active in the normal human placenta, and that their activity decreases with increasing gestational age during the second and third trimesters.[49] Trophoblast cells in culture oxidize the LCFAs palmitate and myristate in substantial amounts, indicating that the human placenta utilizes fatty acids as a significant metabolic fuel.[50] Placenta contains levels of FAO enzymes comparable to those present in mature, fatty acid-dependent tissues such as skeletal muscle, especially early in gestation. Contrary to the prevailing belief that glucose is the sole energy source in the placenta, these studies suggest that FAO is critical for normal growth and maturation of the placenta and for providing fuel for energy-consuming placental functions of ion, nutrient and waste transplacental transport. Thus, under certain circumstances, the 50% reduction in LCHAD activity in both the liver and the placenta that is normally inconsequential to female carriers of LCHAD deficiency may become critical, and contribute to metabolic decompensation in the third trimester of pregnancy and the development of AFLP. Although the fetus does not utilize fatty acids for energy production, the placental unit does, and so could be the source of the generation of liver-toxic metabolites of FAO in the LCHAD- deficient heterozygous mothers carrying fetuses affected by LCHAD deficiency. It is estimated that this situation may be responsible for as many as 20% of all cases of AFLP. Recent case reports have now linked other defects in FAO with AFLP, including TFP, SCAD, MCAD and CPT I deficiencies.[51,52]

DIAGNOSIS OF FAO DISORDERS

Fortunately, a number of signature metabolites in the urine and blood can point to the presence of a defect in FAO. Table 60.3 summarizes these diagnostic findings. These metabolites are most likely to be found at the time of presentation and before substantial amounts of intravenous dextrose have been given to correct hypoglycemia or for fluid resuscitation. The practice of obtaining extra urine and plasma and freezing it for later analysis in any patient presenting to the emergency room with a profile that fits one of the clinical scenarios described above may yield important clues for rapid diagnosis and appropriate treatment. This is critical because tissue enzyme analysis of liver, muscle or skin fibroblasts, or DNA analysis of known mutations, can often be delayed by the limitations associated with proper tissue handling and with laboratory availability.

Urine organic acids

Analysis of the urine organic acid profile is a powerful diagnostic tool. The presence of increased concentrations of dicarboxylic acids reflects the omega-oxidation of fatty acids in the liver through the action of a cytochrome P450-linked mixed-function oxygenase. The resulting dicarboxylic acids can then be transported back into the mitochondrial matrix or to peroxisomes for oxidation. Long-chain dicarboxylic acids are shortened by two carbon units via β-oxidation and transported into the blood as

Deficiency	Urinary organic acids	Plasma acylcarnitine	Diagnostic metabolites
MCAD	C_6–C_{10} DCA (saturated and unsaturated glycine conjugates)	Octanoylcarnitine Hexanoylcarnitine Decenoylcarnitine	Phenylpropionylglycine (urine) Hexanoylglycine (urine) Octanoic acid (plasma) *Cis*-4-decenoic acid
VLCAD	C_6–C_{10} DCA C_{12}–C_{14} DCA $C_{12:1}$ DCA	Acetylcarnitine (low) $C_{14:1}$, C_{16}, $C_{16:1}$, $C_{18:1}$, $C_{18:2}$ acylcarnitines	$C_{14:1}$ acylcarnitine (plasma)
SCAD	C_6–C_{10} DCA, ethylmalonic, butyric	Butyrylcarnitine	Butyrylglycine
HMG-CoA lyase	Butyric, 3-hydroxymethylglutaric, 3-methylglutaric, 3-methylglutaconic, 3-hydroxyisovaleric	3-Methylglutarylcarnitine 3-hydroxy-isovalerylcarnitine	3-Methylglutarylcarnitine
HMG-CoA synthase	Normal	Normal	Low β-hydroxybutyrate after fat load
ETF (mild)	C_6–C_{10} DCA, ethylmalonic		
ETF/ETF-DH (severe)	C_6–C_{10} DCA, glutaric, isovaleric	Glutarylcarnitine Octanoylcarnitine Butyrylcarnitine Isovalerylcarnitine	Glutarylcarnitine
LCHAD	C_6–C_{10} DCA, lactate C_6–C_{18} 3-hydroxy-DCA	Acrylylcarnitine ($C_{3:1}$) C_{10}–C_{18} acylcarnitines (saturated and unsaturated) C_{14}–C_{18} hydroxy-acylcarnitine	C_{12}–C_{14} 3-hydroxy-DCA > C_6 DCA C_{14}–C_{18} 3-hydroxy-acylcarnitine (plasma)
SCHAD	C_{12} 3-hydroxy-DCA, C_6–C_{10} DCA, ethylmalonic		
MCKAT	C_6–C_{12} DCA, lactic 3-hydroxy C_6–C_{14} DCA, 3-methylglutaconic		
Fatty acid transport	Minimal C_6–C_{12} DCA		High C_8–C_{18} FFA (plasma)
CPT II	Normal	Palmitoylcarnitine C_{18}, $C_{18:1}$, $C_{18:2}$ acylcarnitines	Very low free plasma carnitine; acylcarnitines 90% of total
CPT I	Normal	Normal	Free plasma carnitine level raised; absent long-chain acylcarnitines
CT	Normal	Normal	Total plasma carnitine <5% of normal (very low)
CACT	Normal	C_{16}, $C_{18:1}$ acylcarnitines	Very low free plasma carnitine; acylcarnitine 90% of total
2,4-Dienoyl-CoA reductase	Normal	$C_{10:2}$ acylcarnitine	

MCAD, medium-chain acyl-Co-A dehydrogenase; DCA, dicarboxylic acid; VLCAD, very-long-chain acyl-CoA dehydrogenase; SCAD, short-chain acyl-CoA dehydrogenase; HMG-CoA, hydroxymethylglutaryl coenzyme A; ETF, electron transport flavoprotein; LCHAD, long-chain 3-hydroxyacyl-CoA dehydrogenase; SCHAD, short-chain 3-hydroxyacyl-CoA dehydrogenase; MCKAT, medium-chain 3-ketoacyl-CoA thiolase; CPT, carnitine palmitoyl transferase; CT, carnitine transport; CACT, carnitine–acylcarnitine translocase; FFA, free fatty acids.
From Treem, 2001.[73]

Table 60.3 Characteristic urinary and plasma metabolites (during fasting or acute illness)

long-, medium- or short-chain dicarboxylic acids for eventual excretion in the kidney. Peroxisomal metabolism of dicarboxylic acids explains how patients with defects in mitochondrial β-oxidation may excrete dicarboxylic acids with a shorter chain length than would be predicted by the position of the defect.

Dicarboxylic acids are formed whenever there is increased flux through the β-oxidation spiral (i.e. diabetic ketoacidosis). They are also present in the urine of patients fed a diet high in medium-chain triglycerides (MCTs). Thus, infants fed some of the commercially available infant formulas that have approximately half of their fat in the form of MCTs invariably show the presence of dicarboxylic acids in their urine. However, in these infants the ratio of ketone bodies (β-hydroxybutyrate): dicarboxylic acids when fasting is greater than 1, whereas the ratio of urinary concentrations is reversed in infants presenting with symptoms of most FAO disorders.

Whereas the presence of increased levels of dicarboxylic acids is a useful sign in patients with enzymatic defects in the β-oxidation spiral, this is not the case in patients with disorders involving transport of LCFAs into mitochondria via the carnitine cycle (carnitine transport, CACT or CPT deficiencies). These defects are proximal to the entry of fatty acids into the β-oxidation cycle, and there is no accumulation of intermediates even though ketogenesis is impaired. Thus, the absence of dicarboxylic acids does not rule out a defect in FAO.

Other useful metabolites that appear in the urine of these patients are the glycine conjugates of acyl-CoA esters. Stable isotope dilution mass spectrometry is necessary to quantitate small amounts of these metabolites in the urine. The advantage of this technique is that small amounts of acylglycines appear to be consistently excreted in children with certain defects in FAO, even when they are well.[53] This technique has been particularly useful for the recognition of patients with mild or intermittent biochemical phenotypes, such as some patients with MCAD deficiency, MAD deficiency or with polymorphisms of the *SCAD* gene. Glycine conjugation is exclusively carried out in the mitochondria, with short- and medium-chain acyl-CoA esters acting as the preferred substrates. Therefore, the occurrence of glycine conjugates in a patient's urine reflects the intramitochondrial accumulation of acyl-CoA esters. This is the biochemical basis of the accumulation of suberylglycine, hexanoyl-glycine and phenylpropionyl-glycine in the urine of patients with MCAD deficiency.

Plasma acylcarnitine profiles

Excessive long-, medium- or short-chain acyl-CoAs that accumulate proximal to the metabolic block may be converted to acylcarnitines by chain length-specific carnitine acyltransferases. Acylcarnitines are then transported out of the mitochondria into the plasma, and are eventually filtered by the kidneys. They compete with free carnitine for renal tubular reabsorption and, because they have a higher affinity for the carnitine transporter, free carnitine will be excreted.[54] This accounts for the low levels of total plasma carnitine and the higher fraction of acylcarnitine compared with free carnitine in most patients with FAO defects, especially in the fasted but even in the fed state. Plasma acylcarnitine profiles are more informative than urinary levels because renal tubular absorption of long-chain acylcarnitines limits their appearance and detection in the urine. Also, under normoglycemic conditions, organic acids in the urine may revert to normal, but the plasma acylcarnitine profile remains abnormal and is informative regarding the defect. Pitfalls in the interpretation of abnormal acylcarnitine profiles include the presence of certain medications such as valproic acid and propofol, the consumption of high MCT-containing formulas, or the presence of a defect in the mitochondrial respiratory chain with an acylcarnitine profile that mimics that seen in certain FAO disorders.[55]

It is possible to analyze small amounts of plasma carnitine conjugates of abnormal intermediates using fast atom bombardment mass spectrometry (FAB-MS) or, more recently, FAB using two mass spectrometry instruments in tandem.[56] Another recent technologic breakthrough is the use of electrospray ionization.[57] These techniques have been adapted to neonatal blood spots and have become the dominant method for state neonatal screening programs designed to detect FAO defects at the time of birth.

Plasma free fatty acids and 3-hydroxy fatty acids

When available, the measurement of total plasma free fatty acids and β-hydroxybutyrate can signal a FAO disorder. Normal adaptation to prolonged fasting allows the increasing generation of ketones and the stabilization of plasma levels of free fatty acids (FFAs). However, when ketogenesis is disrupted, the ratio of β-hydroxybutyrate : FFAs is reversed. Plasma LCFAs, and even 3-hydroxy fatty acids, are found consistently in patients with LCHAD and TFP deficiency, even when they are asymptomatic and fed a low-fat diet. In other defects (VLCAD and MCAD deficiencies), the presence of long- or medium-chain FFAs in the plasma reflects the localization of the enzymatic defect. Target compounds in the plasma must first undergo derivitization of hydroxyl and carboxyl groups, and then analysis with gas chromatography/mass spectroscopy, which allows the simultaneous discovery of both FFAs and 3-hydroxy fatty acids.[58]

Tissue enzyme and molecular studies

Assays are available to measure the enzyme activity of virtually all the enzymes involved in FAO defects in various tissues, including the liver, muscle and skin fibroblasts. Skin fibroblasts are particularly useful as they can be cultured and kept alive indefinitely with assiduous tissue culture techniques, allowing future investigations as new information comes to light. These tissues can also be used to signal the presence of a disorder of FAO by incubating them with labeled LCFAs and measuring the rate of labeled carbon dioxide or water production, depending on whether the fatty acid was labeled with ^{14}C or ^{3}H. An alternative technique involves incubation of the target tissue with labeled acylcarnitines.[59]

Most of the genes encoding enzymes involved in the carnitine and β-oxidation cycles have been cloned. This has led to the discovery of specific genetic mutations responsible for the reduced enzyme activity in 15 of the 21 known FAO defects and the development of molecular probes to detect specific defects. Certain commercial laboratories offer examination of DNA from white blood cells to detect the common mutations responsible for most cases of MCAD and LCHAD deficiency.

TREATMENT OF DISORDERS OF FAO

Management of acute illness

Management of acute episodes of metabolic decompensation with hypoketotic hypoglycemia, coma, hepatic steatosis and liver dysfunction requires the rapid institution of intravenous dextrose, even when the blood glucose level is normal or only mildly reduced. The rate of glucose infusion should equal at least 10 mg per kg bodyweight per min in infants to raise insulin levels sufficiently to inhibit FAO and block further release of fatty acids from adipose tissue. Blood glucose levels should be maintained above 100 mg/dl (5.5 mmol/l). Drugs that inhibit FAO (e.g. valproate, salicylate and non-steroidal anti-inflammatory drugs), and those that increase FFA release (e.g. epinephrine), should be avoided. Intravenous fat emulsions, used in parenteral nutrition solutions, and intravenous propofol should not be given. Propofol is a soybean emulsion that provides a medium- and long-chain triglyceride load to the patient. Scattered case reports of 'propofol infusion syndrome' in children, characterized by metabolic acidosis, rhabdomyolysis, cardiac and renal failure, and the accumulation of intermediates of β-oxidation, mimic the phenotype of FAO and mitochondrial respiratory chain disorders.[60] Cold exposure leading to shivering thermogenesis with the liberation of FFAs should be avoided and fever should be controlled.

In certain patients presenting with coma and profound liver dysfunction, there may be a role for exchange transfusion or continuous venovenous hemofiltration to remove toxic metabolites.[61] This is particularly true in defects primarily affecting LCFA oxidation where there is little renal excretion of toxic long-chain acylcarnitines or long-chain dicarboxylic acids. Anecdotal reports documenting the disappearance of toxic metabolites from blood and urine, and the resolution of coma, have suggested a therapeutic role for these interventions.

L-Carnitine therapy (100 mg/kg daily) is recommended either intravenously or via a nasogastric tube if there is no vomiting or diarrhea. It is potentially life-saving in patients with the carnitine transport defect whose plasma carnitine levels are near zero and where flooding the system with carnitine will allow normalization of tissue carnitine levels in the liver and passive uptake of some carnitine into critically compromised tissues such as the myocardium. Its role in other defects is more controversial. Some investigators point to the increased concentrations of acylcarnitines in the urine and blood as evidence that exogenous carnitine supplementation is preventing the build-up of toxic long- and medium-chain acyl-CoAs in the mitochondria.[62] However, no controlled randomized trials have been conducted.

Preventive measures to reduce fasting-induced metabolic stress

Avoidance of fasting is the mainstay of therapy for disorders of FAO. In young infants, more than 6 h of fasting may be sufficient to provoke metabolic decompensation. In older infants, longer episodes are required or repetitive days of poor oral intake and catabolic stress. Thus, the prompt administration of intravenous dextrose in the early stages of any illness with fever, vomiting or diarrhea is mandatory even when there are no signs of dehydration. Waiting for the onset of hypoglycemia is a mistake, because at that time levels of FFAs and toxic metabolites are already high. Glucagon injections have no effect because glycogen stores are already depleted at the time of hypoglycemia. Prolonged aerobic exercise and cold exposure are other potential precipitating factors provoking early mobilization of FFAs. A high carbohydrate load prior to such activities is advisable.

Preventing overnight fasting in the well infant with some disorders of FAO may take the form of late night and early morning feedings. However, in infants with defects in LCFA oxidation (VLCAD, LCHAD, CPT, CACT or carnitine transport deficiencies), or in those with previous episodes of hypoketotic hypoglycemia and coma or cardiac decompensation, a more reliable preventive therapy is the placement of a gastrostomy tube and the institution of overnight feedings. We favor gastrostomy tube placement over nasogastric tube feedings because of enhanced stability, ease of infusion and a decreased likelihood that the gastrostomy tube will inhibit the development of normal oral motor skills and feeding behavior. In general, we recommend that patients with defects in the carnitine cycle and LCFA oxidation receive a high-carbohydrate, low-fat formula or diet with approximately 65% of the calories from carbohydrate, 15% from protein and 20% from fat. Formulas high in MCTs are recommended because medium-chain fatty acids do not require an intact carnitine cycle for entry into the mitochondria. MCAD- and SCAD-deficient patients do not appear to require a special formula, and there is no clear evidence that restricting long-chain fats is necessary. In spite of these generally agreed recommendations, there is no consensus among metabolic dieticians on the optimum dietary management of patients with defects in FAO, and little evidence supporting the protocols currently in use.[63]

In addition to dietary restrictions, the addition of MCT supplements and uncooked corn starch to the diet has been advocated by some clinicians. Theoretically, patients receiving large amounts of MCTs would incorporate this form of fat into adipose tissue stores that would later be available for mobilization, enhanced FAO and ketogenesis even in patients with defects in LCFA oxidation. No controlled trials of MCT oil supplementation in patients with FAO defects have been conducted. A recent survey of physicians caring for children with LCHAD deficiency suggested that a low-fat, MCT-supplemented diet reduced the incidence of hypoketotic hypoglycemia, and improved hypotonia, hepatomegaly, cardiomyopathy and lactic acidosis.[64] In 10 patients with LCHAD deficiency, a diet that provided approximatley 10% of energy as dietary LCFAs and 10–20% as MCTs, with 12% of energy coming from standard protein sources and 66% from carbohydrate, resulted in the maintenance of normal levels of hydroxypalmitoleic, hydroxyoleic and hydroxylinoleic carnitine esters and no episodes of metabolic decompensation. This diet should be supplemented with fat-soluble vitamins and vegetable oils as part of the 10% total LCFA intake to provide essential fatty acids.[65] MCT oil supplementation is contraindicated in patients with MCAD, SCAD, MCKAT and SCHAD deficiencies.

Treatment of patients with FAO disorders with oral L-carnitine restores normal levels of plasma carnitine but does not correct the basic enzymatic defect. The administration of large doses of L-carnitine (100 mg/kg daily) results in increased excretion of octanoyl carnitine in patients with MCAD deficiency; this is taken as evidence of detoxification of the inner mitochondrial milieu from accumulating medium-chain acyl-CoAs.[66] However, there have been no direct measurements of acyl-CoAs in tissue before and after treatment to support this hypothesis. There have been isolated published reports of small numbers of patients, primarily with LCFA oxidation defects, who appeared to tolerate fasting better and reduce the accumulation of plasma FFAs when supplemented with carnitine.[67] Most physicians caring for these patients supplement with L-carnitine to keep plasma levels within the normal range. However, recent studies in patients with LCHAD deficiency have found no correlation between carnitine supplementation and the levels of plasma hydroxyacylcarnitines, abnormal plasma organic acids or the frequency of metabolic decompensations.

Supplementation with riboflavin (300 mg/day) has been used in patients with MAD, MCAD and VLCAD deficiency, with reductions in the excretion of abnormal urinary metabolites and modest increases in enzyme activity of MCAD in cultured skin fibroblasts before and after therapy.[68] Riboflavin (vitamin B_2) is a major precursor for flavin coenzymes, including FAD which is a cofactor for the acyl-CoA dehydrogenases that catalyze the first reaction in the β-oxidation cycle.

New and experimental therapies

Several promising therapeutic approaches are currently under investigation. The first involves supplying anaplerotic odd-chain triglycerides (in the form of triheptanoin oil) to treat cardiomyopathy and rhabdomyolysis in LCFA disorders.[69] β-Oxidation of triheptanoin results in the formation of both acetyl-CoA and propionyl-CoA. Propionyl-CoA is an efficient substrate for citric acid cycle intermediates, the restoration of which would be expected to restore energy production and improve cardiac and skeletal muscle function. In three patients with VLCAD deficiency this treatment led to clinical improvement, including the permanent disappearance of chronic cardiomyopathy, rhabdymyolyis and muscle weakenss. No signs of propionic acid overload were observed. This therapy might also be effective in patients with deficiencies of CPT I, CACT, CPT II, VLCAD and LCHAD.

Agonists of PPAR-α, a promoter of FAO genes, such as bezafibrate have been shown to restore both CPT II activity and LCFA oxidation in fibroblasts from patients with the adult form of CPT II deficiency.[70] Another attractive target to upregulate genes regulating enzymes of fatty acid oxidation is *stearoyl-CoA desaturase 1* (*SCD1*), the rate-limiting enzyme in the biosynthesis of monounsaturated fatty acids. SCD1 knockout mice produce more ketones after a 4-h fast than wild-type mice, and genes for key enzymes in the FAO pathway are upregulated in these mice, including VLCAD and CPT I. Although these enzymes are known targets of PPAR-α and contain PPAR-α response regions in their promoters, the effect of knocking out SCD1 must be independent, because PPAR-α mRNA remains unchanged.[71]

References

1. Cahill G. Starvation in man. N Engl J Med 1970; 282:668–675.
2. McGarry J, Foster D. Regulation of hepatic fatty acid oxidation and ketone body production. Ann Rev Biochem 1980; 49:395–420.
3. Ahlborg G, Felig P, Hagenfeldt L, et al. Substrate turnover during prolonged exercise in man. Splanchnic and leg metabolism of glucose, free fatty acids, and amino acids. J Clin Invest 1974; 53:1080–1085.
4. Stanley C, Baker L. Hyperinsulinism in infancy; diagnosis by demonstration of abnormal response to fasting hypoglycemia. Pediatrics 1976; 57:702–711.
5. Denton E, McCormack J, Oviasu O. Short-term regulation of pyruvate dehydrogenase activity in the liver. In: Hue L, Van de Werve G, eds. Short-term Regulation of Liver Metabolism. Amsterdam: Elsevier; 1981:159–164.
6. Hirsch D, Stahl A, Lodish H. A family of fatty acid transporters conserved from mycobacterium to man. Proc Natl Acad Sci USA 1998; 95:8625–8629.
7. McGarry J, Woeltje K, Schroeder J, et al. Carnitine palmitoyltransferase structure/function/regulatory relationship. In: Tanaka K, Coates P, eds. Fatty Acid Oxidation: Clinical, Biochemical, and Molecular Aspects. New York: Alan R. Liss; 1990:193–208.
8. Wang L, Brady P, Brady L. Hormonal regulation of carnitine palmitoyltransferase synthesis in H4ITE cells. In: Tanaka K, Coates P, eds. Fatty Acid Oxidation: Clinical, Biochemical, and Molecular Aspects. New York: Alan R. Liss; 1990:209–216.
9. Leone T, Weinheimer C, Kelly D. A critical role for the peroxisome proliferators-activated receptor alpha (PPARalpha) in the cellular fasting reponse: the PPARalpha-null mouse as a model of fatty acid oxidation disorders. Proc Natl Acad Sci USA 1999; 96:7473–7478.
10. Rebouche C, Engel A. Tissue distribution of carnitine biosynthetic enzymes in man. Biochim Biophys Acta 1980; 630:472–475.

11. Nezu J, Tamai I, Oku A, et al. Primary systemic carnitine deficiency is caused by mutations in a gene encoding sodium ion-dependent carnitine transporter. Nat Genet 1999; 21:91–94.
12. Peltkova VD, Wintle RF, Rubin LA, et al. Functional variants of OCTN cation transporter genes are associated with Crohn's disease. Nat Genet 2004; 36:471–475.
13. Bonnefont JP, Djouadi F, Prip-Buus C, et al. Carnitine palmitoyltransferases 1 and 2: biochemical, molecular, and medical aspects. Mol Aspects Med 2004; 25:495–520.
14. Sobol S, Seitz H, Sies J, et al. Effect of long-chain fatty acylCoA on mitochondrial and cytolsolic ATP/ADP ratios in intact liver cell. Biochem J 1984; 220:371–376.
15. Fisher M, Robishaw J, Neely J. The properties and regulation of pantothenate kinase from rat heart. J Biol Chem 1985; 260:15745–15751.
16. Tolbert N. Metabolic pathways in peroxisomes and glycoxysomes. Annu Rev Biochem 1981; 50:133–157.
17. Kurtz D, Rinaldo P, Rhead W, et al. Targeted disruption of mouse long-chain acyl-CoA dehydrogenase gene reveals crucial roles for fatty acid oxidation. Proc Natl Acad Sci USA 1998; 95:15592–15597.
18. Kamijo T, Aoyama T, Komiyama A, et al. Stuctural analysis of cDNAs for subunits of human mitochondrial fatty acid beta-oxidation trifunctional protein. Biochem Biophys Res Commun 1994; 199:818–825.
19. Roettger V, Marshall T, Amendt B, et al. Multiple acyl coenzyme-A dehydrogenation disorder (MAD) responsive to riboglavin: biochemical studies in fibroblasts. In: Tanaka K, Coates P, eds. New Developments in Fatty Acid Oxidation. New York: Wiley-Liss; 1992:317–326.
20. Zladeh R, Hoffman E, Finegold D, et al. Medium-chain acyl CoA dehydrogenase deficiency in Pennsylvania: neonatal screening shows high incidence and unexpected mutation frequencies. Pediatr Res 1995; 37:675–678.
21. Klose D, Kolker S, Heinrich B, et al. Incidence and short-term outcome of children with symptomatic presentation of organic acid and fatty acid oxidation disorders in Germany. Pediatrics 2002; 110:1204–1211.
22. Gregerson N, Winter V, Curtis D, et al. Medium-chain acyl-CoA dehydrogenase (MCAD) deficiency: the prevalent mutation G985 (K304E) is subject to strong founder effect from northwestern Europe. Hum Hered 1993; 43:342–350.
23. Yokota I, Coates P, Hale D, et al. Molecular survey of prevalent mutation, A985 to G transition, and identification of five infrequent mutations in the medium-chain acyl-CoA dehydrogenase deficiency. In: Tanaka K, Coates P, eds. New Developments in Fatty Acid Oxidation. New York: Wiley-Liss; 1992:425–440.
24. Strauss A, Bennett M, Rinaldo P, et al. Inherited long-chain 3-hydroxyacyl-CoA dehydrogenase deficiency and a fetal–maternal interaction cause maternal liver disease and other pregnancy complications. Semin Perinatol 1999; 23:100–112.
25. Tyni T, Pihko H. Long-chain 3-hydroxyacyl-CoA dehydrogenase deficiency. Acta Paediatr 1999; 88:237–245.
26. Dinesh R, Bennett M, Rogers, B. Long-chain L-3-hydroxyacyl-coenzyme A dehydrogenase deficiency: a molecular and biochemical review. Lab Invest 2002; 82:815–824.
27. Gregerson N, Winter V, Corydon M, et al. Identificiation of four new mutations in the short-chain acyl-CoA dehydrogenase (*SCAD*) gene in two patients; one of the variant alleles, 511C-T, is present at an unexpectedly high frequency in the general population, as was the case for 625G-A, together conferring susceptibility toethylmalonic aciduria. Hum Mol Genet 1998; 7:619–627.
28. Narasimhan N, Kruckeberg K, Taucher A, et al. The frequency of short-chain acyl-CoA dehydrogenase gene variants in the US population and correlation with the C4 acylcarnitine concentration in newborn blood spots. Mol Genet Metab 2003; 78:239–246.
29. Mitraki A, Danner M, King J, et al. Temperature-sensitive mutations and second-site suppressor substitutions affect folding of the P22 tailspike protein *in vitro*. J Biol Chem 1993; 268:20071–20075.
30. Treem W, Witzleben C, Piccoli D, et al. Medium-chain and long-chain acyl-CoA dehydrogenase deficiency: clinical, pathologic, and ultrastructural differentiations from Reye's syndrome. Hepatology 1986; 6:1270–1278.
31. Bonnefont J, Specola N, Vassault A, et al. The fasting test in pediatrics; applications to the diagnosis of pathological hypo and hyperketotic states. Eur J Pediatr 1990; 150:80–85.
32. Parker W, Haas R, Stumpf D, et al. Effects of octanoate on rat brain and liver mitochondria. Neurology 1983; 33:1374–1377.
33. Trauner D, Adams H. Intracraniaal pressure elevations during octanoate infusion in rabbits: an experimental model of Reye syndrome. Pediatr Res 1981; 15:1097–1099.
34. Tyni T, Palotie A, Vlinikka L, et al. Long-chain 3-hydroxyacyl coenzyme A dehydrogenase deficiency with the G1528C mutation: clinical presentation of thirteen patients. J Pediatr 1997; 130:67–76.
35. Saudubray J, Martin D, DeLonlay P, et al. Recognition and management of fatty acid oxidation defects: a series of 107 patients. J Inherit Metab Dis 1999; 22:488–502.
36. VanMaldergren I, Tuerlinckx D, Wanders R. Long-chain 3-hydroxyacyl CoA dehydrogenase deficiency and early-onset cirrhosis in two siblings. Eur J Pediatr 2000; 159:108–112.
37. Odaib A, Schneider B, Bennett M, et al. A defect in the transport of long-chain fatty acids associated with acute liver failure. N Engl J Med 1998; 339:1752–1757.
38. Amendt B, Greene C, Sweetman L, et al. Short-chain acyl-coenzyme A dehydrogenase deficiency. Clinical and biochemical studies in two patients. J Clin Invest 1987; 79:1303–1309.
39. Rinaldo P. Mitochondrial fatty acid oxidation disorders and cyclic vomiting syndrome. Dig Dis Sci 1999; 44(Suppl):97–102.
40. Tein I, Christodoulou J, Donner E, et al. Carnitine palmitoyltransferase II deficiency: a new cause of recurrent pancreatitis. J Pediatr 1994: 124:938–940.
41. Boles R, Buck E, Blitzer M, et al. Retrospective biochemical screening of fatty acid oxidation disorders in postmortem livers of 418 cases of sudden death syndrome in the first year of life. J Pediatr 1998; 132:924–933.
42. Rinaldo P, Hye-Ran Y, Yu C, et al. Sudden and unexpected neonatal death; a protocol for the postmortem diagnosis of fatty acid oxidation disorders. Semin Perinatol 1999; 23:204–210.
43. Lundemose J, Kolvraa S, Gregerson N, et al. Fatty acid oxidation disorders as primary cause of sudden and unexpected death in infants and young children: an investigation performed on cultured fibroblasts from 79 children who dies aged between 0–4 years. Mol Pathol 1997; 59:212–217.
44. Treem W, Shoup M, Hale D, et al. Acute fatty liver of pregnancy, hemolysis, elevated liver enzymes, and low platelets syndrome, and long-chain 3-hydroxyacyl coenzyme A dehydrogenase deficiency. Am J Gastroenterol 1996; 91:2293–2300.
45. Tyni T, Ekkolm E, Pihko H. Pregnancy complications are frequent in long-chain 3-hydroxyacyl-coenzyme A dehydrogenase deficiency. Am J Obstet Gynecol 1998; 178:603–608.

46. Ibdah J, Bennett M, Rinaldo P, et al. A fetal fatty-acid oxidation disorder as a cause of liver disease in pregnant women. N Engl J Med 1999; 340:1723–1731.
47. Yang Z, Zhao Y, Bennett M, et al. Fetal genotypes and pregnancy outcomes in 35 families with mitochondrial trifunctional protein mutations. Am J Obstet Gynecol 2002; 187:715–720.
48. Treem W. Microvesicular fatty liver disorders: inborn defects in mitochondrial fatty acid oxidation? In: Reyes H, Leuschner U, Arias I, eds. Pregnancy, Sex Hormones, and the Liver. Falk Symposium. Dordrecht: Kluwer Academic; 1995:136–150.
49. Rakheja D, Bennett M, Foster B, et al. Evidence for fatty acid oxidation in human placenta, and the relationship of fatty acid oxidation enzyme acitivities with gestational age. Placenta 2002; 23:447–450.
50. Shekhawat P, Bennett M, Sadovsky Y, et al. Human placenta metabolizes fatty acids: implications for fetal fatty acid oxidation disorders and maternal liver diseases. Am J Physiol Endocrinol Metab 2003; 284:E1098–E1105.
51. Matern D, Hart P, Murtha AP, et al. Acute fatty liver of pregnancy associated with short-chain acyl-coenzyme A dehydrogenase deficiency. J Pediatr 2001; 138:585–588.
52. Innes A, Seargeant L, Balachandra K, et al. Hepatic carnitine palmitoyltransferase I deficiency presenting as maternal illness in pregnancy. Pediatr Res 2000; 47:43–45.
53. Rinaldo P, O'Shea J, Coates P, et al. Medium-chain acyl-CoA dehydrogenase deficiency: diagnosis by stable-isotope dilution measurement of urinary *n*-hexanoylglycine and 3-phenyl-propionylglycine. N Engl J Med 1988; 319:1308–1313.
54. Treem W, Stanley C, Finegold D, et al. Primary carnitine deficiency due to a failure of carnitine transport in kidney, muscle, and fibroblasts. N Engl J Med 1988; 319:1331–1336.
55. Sim K, Carpenter K, Hammond J, et al. Acylcarnitine profiles in fibroblasts from patients with respiratory chain defects can resemble those from patients with mitochondrial fatty acid oxidation disorders. Metabolism 2002; 51:366–371.
56. Millington D, Norwood D, Kodo N, et al. Application of fast atom bombardment with tandem mass spectrometry and liquid chromatography/mass spectrometry to the analysis of acylcarnitines in human urine, blood, and tissue. Anal Biochem 1989; 180:331–339.
57. Rashed M, Bucknall M, Little D, et al. Screening blood spots for inborn errors of metabolism by electrospray tandem mass spectrometry with a microplate batch process and a computer algorithm for automated flagging of abnormal results. Clin Chem 1997; 43:1129–1141.
58. Roe C, Millington D, Maltby D, et al. Recognition of medium chain acyl-CoA dehydrogenase deficiency in asymptomatic siblings of children dying of sudden infant death syndrome or Reye-like syndromes. J Pediatr 1986; 108:13–18.
59. Sim K, Hammond J, Wilcken B. Strategies for the diagnosis of mitochondrial fatty acid B-oxidation disorders. Clin Chim Acta 2002; 323:37–58.
60. Wolf A, Potter F. Propofol infusion in children: when does an anesthetic tool become an intensive care liability? Pediatr Anesth 2004; 14:435–439.
61. Thompson G, Butt W, Shann F, et al. Continuous venovenous hemofiltration in the management of acute decompensations of inborn errors of metabolism. J Pediatr 1991; 118:870–884.
62. Duran M, Loof N, Ketting D, et al. Secondary carnitine deficiency. J Clin Chem Clin Biochem 1990; 28:359–363.
63. Solis J, Singh R. Management of fatty acid oxidation disorders: a survey of current treatment strategies. J Am Diet Assoc 2002; 102:1800–1803.
64. Gillingham M, Van Calcar S, Ney D, et al. Dietary management of long-chain 3-hydroxyacyl-CoA dehydrogenase deficiency – a case report and survey. J Inherit Metab Dis 1999; 22:123–131.
65. Gillingham M, Connor W, Matern D. Optimal dietary therapy of long-chain 3-hydroxyacyl-CoA dehydrogenase deficiency. Molec Genet Metab 2003; 79:114–123.
66. Treem W, Stanley C, Goodman S. Medium-chain acyl-CoA dehydrogenase deficiency: metabolic effects and therapeutic efficacy of long-term L-carnitine supplementation. J Inherit Metab Dis 1989; 12:112–119.
67. Schwenk W, Hale D, Haymond M. Decreased fasting free fatty acids with L-carnitine in children with carnitine deficiency. Pediatr Res 1988; 23:491–494.
68. Duran M, Cleutjens B, Ketting L, et al. Diagnosis of medium-chain acyl-CoA dehydrogenase deficiency in lymphocytes aqnd liver by a gas chromatographic method: the effect of oral riboflavin supplementation. Pediatr Res 1992; 31:39–42.
69. Roe C, Sweetman L, Roe D, et al. Treatment of cardiomyopathy and rhabdomyolysis in long-chain fat oxidation disorders using an anaplerotic odd-chain triglyceride. J Clin Invest 2002; 110:259–269.
70. Djouadi F, Bonnefont J, Thullier L, et al. Correction of fatty acid oxidation in carnitine palmitoyl transferase II-deficient cultured skin fibroblasts by bezafibrate. Pediatr Res 2003; 54:446–451.
71. Ntambi J, Miyazaki M, Stoehr J, et al. Loss of stearoyl-CoA desaturase-1 function protects mice against adiposity. Proc Acad Am Sci 2002; 99:11482–11486.
72. Treem WR. Inborn errors in fasting adaptation. In: Walker A, Watkins JB, eds. Nutrition in Pediatrics: Basic Science and Clinical Application, 3rd edn. Paris: Decker; 2003:591–688.)
73. Treem WR. Inborn defects in michondrial fatty acid oxidation. In: Suchy F, Sokal E, Balistreri W, eds. Liver Disease in Children, 2nd edn. Philadelphia, PA: Lippincott, Williams & Wilkins; 2001:735–785.
74. Treem WR. New developments in the pathophysiology, clinical spectrum, and diagnosis of disorders of fatty acid oxidation. Curr Opin Pediatr 2000; 12:263-268.

Chapter 61
Abnormalities of hepatic protein metabolism

H. Hesham A-Kader and Fayez K. Ghishan

INTRODUCTION

Three disorders will be discussed in this chapter, including α_1-antitrypsin deficiency, tyrosinemia and urea-cycle enzyme defects.

α_1-ANTITRYPSIN DEFICIENCY

The description of α_1-antitrypsin deficiency and its association with lung disease was reported 40 years ago by Laurell and Eriksson.[1] The association between α_1-antitrypsin deficiency and hepatic cirrhosis in children was initially identified in 1969 by Sharp and co-workers.[2] Since these original observations, it is clear now that α_1-antitrypsin deficiency is a relatively common genetic disorder, affecting 1 in 1600 to 1 in 2000 live births and resulting in liver disease in infants, children and adults as well as lung disease primarily in adults.[3]

The characteristics of the α_1-antitrypsin protein

α_1-Antitrypsin is a 52 kD glycoprotein that is secreted by the hepatocytes and, to a minor extent, by lung epithelial cells and macrophages.[4] The half-life of α_1-antitrypsin is approximately 4–5 days.[5] The function of α_1-antitrypsin protein is to inhibit chymotrypsin, pancreatic elastase, skin collagenase, renin, urokinase, Hageman factor/co-factor and the neutral proteases of neutrophils.[6] α_1-Antitrypsin protein belongs to a large gene family of serine protease inhibitors referred to as serpins.[7,8]

α_1-Antitrypsin is composed of 394 amino acids arranged into three β-sheets (A, β and C), nine α-helices (A–I) and immobile inhibitory reactive center loop. The interaction between α_1-antitrypsin and proteases occurs by the formation of a 1-1 complex.[9] α_1-Antitrypsin protein is present in tears, duodenal fluid, saliva, nasal secretions, cerebral spinal fluid, pulmonary secretions and mother's milk. α_1-Antitrypsin acts as an acute phase reactant and increases in the setting of inflammation, neoplastic disease and pregnancy.

However, in patients with α_1-antitrypsin deficiency, these stimuli do not induce α_1-antitrypsin protein.[10]

Phenotyping of α_1-antitrypsin

The serum level of α_1-antitrypsin in the plasma ranges from 100 to 200 mg/dl. This plasma level is determined by both α_1-antitrypsin gene alleles, which are codominantly inherited. Several techniques including protein electrophoresis on starch gels and isoelectric focusing have contributed to our understanding of the variation in α_1-antitrypsin.[11,12] α_1-Globulins appear in this system as a series of characteristic bands of variable intensity. The α_1-antitrypsin variants included in an allelic system are called the Pi (protease inhibitor) system and are named based on their migration velocity in the starch-gel electrophoresis. Faster moving protein complexes are identified by earlier letters in the alphabet and the slowest moving protein is labeled Z. Thus, the variants of α_1-antitrypsin are labeled as M (medium), S (slow), F (fast), or Z (very slow).[13]

Three major categories of α_1-antitrypsin variants have been identified as useful clinical markers:[14]

1 Normal, in this category includes the four more common M variants (M_1–M_4)
2 Deficient, those are characterized by the α_1-antitrypsin variants Z and S and a number of less-frequent variants, such as M_{Malton}, $M_{Procida}$
3 Null, in which no detectable α_1-antitrypsin level is seen.

There are currently at least 100 different alleles of α_1-antitrypsin that have been described. The normal allele is PiM type with overall allelic frequency of 0.95. The next two most common alleles in the USA are PiS at 0.03 and PiZ at 0.01. Blacks have lower frequencies of these alleles. The highest prevalence of PiZ variant has been reported in Northern and Western European countries, peaking in Southern Scandinavia, Denmark, The Netherlands, the UK and Northern France.[15] Table 61.1 depicts the relationship between Pi phenotypes and serum concentration of α_1-antitrypsin.

Genetics of α_1-antitrypsin deficiency

The gene encoding α_1-antitrypsin has been cloned and is located on chromosome 14q31-32.2.[16–19] The α_1-antitrypsin gene is 12.2 kb in length and consists of seven exons, designated I_A, I_B, I_C, I (noncoding) and II, III, IV and V (coding). Exons II–IV are translated into 52 kD protein. The same gene is responsible for the α_1-antitrypsin production in the liver, lung and macrophages. The first two exons (I_A, I_B) and a short 5′ segment of I_C are included in the primary transcript in the macrophages, but not in hepatocytes.[20] The protein has three asparagine-linked branched oligosaccharide moieties. The basis for the

Phenotype	Serum concentration (%)
MM	100
MZ	60
SS	60
FZ	60
M-	50
PS	40
SZ	42.5
ZZ	15
Z-	10
–	0

Table 61.1 Relationship between Pi phenotypes and serum concentrations of α1-antitrypsin

genetic defect in the PiZ type of α_1-antitrypsin deficiency is the substitution of lysine for glutamic acid at position 342 from the carboxy terminus in the Z-type protein.[21,22]

The prevalence of the three major α_1-antitrypsin variants (PiM, PiZ and PiS) is reported as gene frequencies (the frequency of a variant in homozygotes). The highest prevalence of the PiZ variant has been recorded in European populations with a peak in Southern Scandinavia, Denmark, The Netherlands, UK and Northern France.[23–25] Most recent surveys indicate that α_1-antitrypsin deficiency is also prevalent in populations in the Middle East and North Africa, Central and Southern Africa and Central and Southeast Asia.[26] However, in Far East Asia, the gene frequency of α_1-antitrypsin deficiency is rather rare, especially in Japan and Far Eastern populations.[26]

Clinical manifestations of α_1-antitrypsin deficiency

Liver disease in children

Neonatal cholestasis is the first manifestation of α_1-antitrypsin deficiency and is commonly seen in the first few weeks of life.[27,28] The affected babies are generally small for gestational age and clinically, the liver is mildly enlarged. Acholic stools and dark urine may be seen. Biochemically, these patients appear to have elevated conjugated bilirubin and mildly elevated serum amino transferase levels. Alkaline phosphatase and gamma-glutamyl transpeptidase is also elevated. The jaundice usually disappears during the second to the fourth months of life. Neonates may rarely present with liver cirrhosis[29] or bleeding diathesis.[30]

The histological picture of the liver may be helpful in predicting the outcome of the liver disease. A picture similar to neonatal hepatitis, portal fibrosis with bile duct proliferation, or intrahepatic duct hypoplasia may be noted in the biopsies. Patients with portal fibrosis and bile duct proliferation appear to have worse outcomes.[31] However, the hallmark of the liver biopsy in these patients is the deposition of the PAS (Periodic Acid Schiff) stain positive diastase resistant α_1-antitrypsin depositions in the periportal hepatocytes.[32]

The number of infants presenting with neonatal cholestasis was addressed in a large prospective study of 200 000 Swedish newborns in which 120 PiZ patients were identified.[33–35] Fourteen of the 120 PiZ infants had prolonged obstructive jaundice and nine had severe clinical laboratory evidence of liver disease. Five patients had only laboratory evidence of liver disease. Eight other PiZ infants had minimal abnormalities in serum bilirubin and hepatic enzyme activity and variable hepatosplenomegaly. Approximately 50% of the remaining patients with PiZ had only abnormal aminotransferase levels. Follow-up studies of these patients at 18 years of age showed that more than 85% had persistently normal serum transaminase levels. A total of 48 patients with the phenotype PiSZ were identified in this study. None of these infants had clinical liver disease, but 10 of 42 patients at 3 months and 1 of 22 at 6 months of age had abnormal serum aminotransferases.

In the USA, screening of 107 038 newborns had shown that 21 infants were found to have the phenotype PiZ. Of the 18 infants followed, only one had neonatal cholestatic jaundice and five had hepatomegaly and biochemical abnormalities or both. At 3 to 6 years of age, none of the children had evidence of hepatic cirrhosis.[36] Other reports indicate that patients with PiZ who present with neonatal cholestasis are more likely to develop serious liver disease in the future compared to those infants without a history of neonatal cholestatic jaundice.[37] The overall risk of death from liver disease in PiZ children during childhood is estimated at 2–3%. Boys are at higher risk than girls. Why some patients with PiZ have worse liver disease than others is not known. However, genetic and/or environmental factors may play a role.[38]

Liver disease in adults

Single case reports and retrospective studies have suggested that adult patients with PiZ are likely to develop liver disease and hepatocellular carcinoma.[39–41] Therefore, it does appear that α_1-antitrypsin deficiency should be considered in the differential diagnosis of any adult patient with abnormal serum aminotransferases, cirrhosis, portal hypertension or hepatocellular carcinoma. It is estimated that the risk of developing cirrhosis in adults with α_1-antitrypsin deficiency is about 10%.[42]

A retrospective study on 17 autopsied cases of α_1-antitrypsin deficiency identified in Sweden indicated a strong relation between α_1-antitrypsin deficiency, cirrhosis and primary liver cancer.[39] However, the study suggests that male patients are the ones who are at higher risk of development of liver cirrhosis and hepatoma in α_1-antitrypsin deficiency.

The relationship between cirrhosis and partial deficiency or heterozygotic phenotype of α_1-antitrypsin has not been addressed on a larger scale in the literature. A number of case reports indicate the association of adult onset cirrhosis with PiSZ.[43–45] In one study, there was an increased prevalence of phenotype MZ in patients with cryptogenic cirrhosis and with non-B chronic hepatitis.[46] However, in another prospective study, the heterozygote state occurred with approximately equal frequencies in patients with and without hepatobiliary disease.[47]

In general, there is a suggestion that a partial deficiency of α_1-antitrypsin is more likely to predispose these patients to liver injury. What is clear is that patients with cirrhosis and α_1-antitrypsin deficiency are at risk of developing hepatocellular carcinoma. Indeed, Eriksson found six hepatomas in the nine cirrhotic adults who were phenotypically PiZ patients. Four of these tumors were hepatocellular carcinoma and two were cholangiocarcinoma.[42,48]

Liver disease has also been associated with several other allelic variants of α_1-antitrypsin deficiency, such as PiM_{Malton}, Pi_{FZ}, Pi_W, PiM_{Duarte} and PiS_{Iiyama}.[38]

Lung disease

The development of lung disease in the pediatric patient is exceedingly rare, despite several reports that suggest that these patients do have increased respiratory infections. However, it is clear that adults who are smokers will most likely develop emphysema.[49,50] Autopsy studies indicate that approximately 60% of patients with PiZ develop clinically significant lung injury.

Pathophysiology of liver disease in α_1-antitrypsin deficiency

The mutation in the PiZ α_1-antitrypsin leads to the deposition of globules of an amorphous material within the hepatocyte, particularly in the periportal areas. These globules, which have been shown to enlarge as the infant matures, are seen by positive PAS staining after treatment of the liver biopsy specimen with diastase. These globules are formed secondary to the accumulation of the mutated α_1-antitrypsin molecule and occur in the endoplasmic reticulum. Studies have suggested that the proper folding or assembly of the polypeptides is a prerequisite for their exit from the endoplasmic reticulum. Mis-folding of the α_1-antitrypsin variants allows the protein to be retained. The substitution of glutamine 342 for lysine in the α_1-antitrypsin Z variant results in reducing the stability of the molecule in its monomeric form to a polymeric form by way of a mechanism termed loop-sheet insertion.[32,51,52]

It appears that the mutation in the PiZ α_1-antitrypsin that is located at the head of the strand 5A and at the base of the mobile reactive loop would open the β-sheet A between strands 3 and 5 to favor the incorporation of the reactive loop from a second α_1-antitrypsin molecule to produce the dimer, which then extends to form chains of loop-sheet polymers. The demonstration of spontaneous polymerization of the PiZ α_1-antitrypsin at 37°, whereas the normal M variant remains in its native confirmation, supported the observations by Lomas' group.[38] Thus, within the hepatocyte, the PiZ α_1-antitrypsin is degraded by both proteasomes dependent and independent pathways and it appears that the clearing mechanism in those patients is inefficient.[52]

Indeed, this polymerization of the α_1-antitrypsin is not unique, as it does occur in other members of the serine proteinase inhibitor (serpin) family, such as antithrombin, C1 inhibitor and α_1-antichymotrypsin, to cause deficiency in the plasma level of these molecules, resulting in thrombosis, angioedema and emphysema, respectively. These serpin family disorders have been called conformational diseases.[53]

Pathology of liver disease in α_1-antitrypsin deficiency

The hallmark of α_1-antitrypsin deficiency is the distinctive accumulation of periodic acid-Schiff positive, diastase-resistant globules in the endoplasmic reticulum in the periportal hepatocytes. These globules enlarge with increasing age. With the hematoxylin-eosin (H&E) staining, they appear as eosinophilic deposits in the cytoplasm of the hepatocytes. These globules have also been observed in heterozygous individuals.

The absence of liver disease in the few Pi null individuals who have no deposits of these globules indicate that the deposition of the abnormal α_1-antitrypsin in the liver has a significant role in the pathogenesis of liver disease.[54] Electronmicroscopy studies show that these amorphous deposits are primarily within the dilated rough endoplasmic reticulum.[55] Liver biopsies in neonates with α_1-antitrypsin deficiency have shown three morphological patterns of hepatic alteration, including hepatocellular damage with a picture compatible with neonatal hepatitis portal fibrosis with biliary duct proliferation and biliary duct hypoplasia.[31]

Diagnosis of α_1-antitrypsin deficiency

Circulating levels of α_1-antitrypsin is between 100 and 200 mg/dl. However, a low serum level *per se* does not indicate the presence of α_1-antitrypsin deficiency, since this level could be low secondary to losses of α_1-antitrypsin in the gastrointestinal tract or in the lung. Therefore, determination of the α_1-antitrypsin phenotype by isoelectric focusing or by agarose electrophoresis at acid pH is indicated. α_1-Antitrypsin deficiency should be suspected in neonates with picture of neonatal hepatitis or in children and adults with unexplained chronic liver disease. Liver biopsies should be stained with periodic acid-Schiff followed by diastase treatment to determine the presence of α_1-antitrypsin globules in the periportal hepatocytes.

Treatment of α_1-antitrypsin deficiency

The two major clinical problems in α_1-antitrypsin deficiency are emphysema and liver disease resulting in cirrhosis. Therefore, avoidance of smoking is the most important preventative steps in the development of emphysema, because smoking accelerates the destructive lung disease. Once the patient develops cirrhosis, liver transplantation is the only viable option for these patients.[56] Replacement therapy of α_1-antitrypsin deficiency has been done in emphysema patients and found to be effective in raising the concentration of α_1-antitrypsin in the serum and in the lung.[57] The α_1-antitrypsin in the lung has been shown to be active in neutralizing the neutrophil elastases. A recombinant α_1-antitrypsin has been produced in *E. coli* and in yeast and was noted to be functional as an elastase inhibitor.[58,59] However, because the recombinant α_1-antitrypsin lacks the carbohydrate side chain, this product is unstable with a short half-life.

family. It is possible that patients with a larger mass of reverted hepatocytes may have the mild form of the disease. However, this remains to be further defined.

Treatment

Dietary restriction of phenylalanine and tyrosine has been the traditional treatment for patients with tyrosinemia. Dietary management has been shown to be effective for the renal tubular disease and the metabolic bone disease. However, there is no evidence that it prevents the development of cirrhosis or HCC.

NTBC (2-(2-nitro-4-trifluoromethylbenzoyl)-1.3-cyclohexamedione) belongs to a class of compounds developed in the 1980s as bleaching herbicidal. During animal studies it was noted that rats treated with NTBC developed corneal ulceration, a hallmark of elevated tyrosine level in rats and humans. It was then found out that NTBC is an inhibitor of 4-hydroxyphenylpyruvate dioxygenase (HPD). In 1992 Lindstedt et al.[93] proposed that the inhibition of HPD by NTBC can prevent the accumulation of maleylacetoacetate and fumarylacetoacetate and their derivatives (SAA and SA).

Recently the results of treating over 300 patients with NTBC were reviewed.[94,95] Marked hepatic improvement was seen in more than 95% of the patients. Renal functions also improved and Fanconi syndrome is avoided. A large number of patients have been on the drug more than 5 years (up to 9 years) without significant side effects. Typically NTBC is started at an oral dose of 1 mg/kg per day and the dose can be adjusted depending on clinical response and biochemical parameters. It is important that patients on NTBC remain on protein-restricted diet that is low in tyrosine and phenylalanine since NTBC will increase the blood tyrosine level. Biochemical monitoring of plasma amino acids, blood and urinary succinylacetone and liver functions is mandatory during therapy with NTBC. Recurrent ophthalmologic evaluation and hepatic imaging are also important. Measurement of α-fetoprotein is particularly important since few late-treated patients developed HCC despite NTBC therapy.[95] Although NTBC is still an investigational drug it can be obtained through research protocols in USA, Canada and Europe. Further follow-up is needed in order to assess the long-term effects and safety of NTBC therapy taking into consideration that some patients developed cancer despite therapy and the facts that patients with HPD deficiency develop neurologic problems[96,97] and mental retardation is seen in 50% of tyrosinemia type II patients.[98]

At the time being the definitive treatment for patients with tyrosinemia with end-stage liver disease is orthotopic liver transplantation (OLT) normalizing FAH activity and correcting the metabolic derangement and hepatic function.[76,99] OLT also has a marked beneficial effect on the renal function with improvement in the tubular dysfunction.[100] However, patients with severe renal disease prior to OLT may continue to have borderline renal function and poor growth even after transplant.

UREA CYCLE DEFECTS

Catabolism of amino acids produces ammonia, which is a potent neurotoxin unless inactivated by the liver. Animal studies have shown that hyperammonemia is toxic to the immature nervous system producing alterations in the level of consciousness. The neuropathologic changes involve the astrocytes and not the neurons, which suggests that the changes may be reversible.[101] However, repeated prolonged episodes of hyperammonemia can lead to permanent neurologic impairment.[102]

Detoxification of ammonia occurs through a series of reactions known as the Krebs-Henseleit or urea cycle (Fig. 61.2). Besides converting ammonia into urea, the cycle produces arginine, which becomes an essential amino acid in all urea cycle defects except arginase deficiency. Five enzymes are involved in the formation of urea: Carbamyl phosphate synthetase (CPS), ornithine transcarbamylase transferase (OTC), argininosuccinate synthetase (AS), argininosuccinate lyase (AL) and arginase. In addition a sixth enzyme, N-acetylglutamate synthetase is also needed for the formation of N-acetylglutamate. Four enzymes operate in a cyclic manner using ornithine as a substrate, which is regenerated. On the other hand, CPS, which is produced by a series of enzymatic reactions, enters the cycle by combining with ornithine. The other nitrogen atom of urea is derived from aspartate, which combines with citrulline.

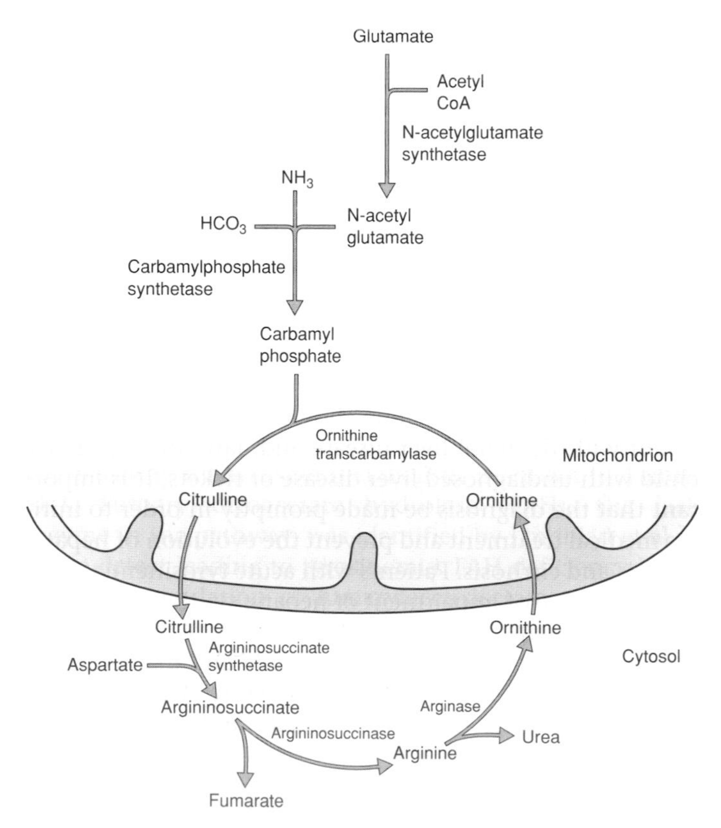

Figure 61.2: The urea cycle.

Clinical features

Symptoms may start early in life or be delayed until late childhood or adulthood. Newborns may have rapid clinical deterioration resembling sepsis usually after a few days of protein feedings. Symptoms include: refusal to eat, vomiting, tachypnea, seizure and lethargy progressing to coma. Increased intracranial pressure may be evident. Later in life hyperammonemia may present with vomiting and multiple neurological abnormalities including: irritability, mental confusion, ataxia, combativeness alternating with periods of drowsiness and coma. Delayed physical growth as well as development may be seen and the patients may elect to consume a low-protein diet in order to avoid the symptoms.

Diagnosis

Hyperammonemia is the characteristic feature of urea cycle defect. The degree of elevation in plasma ammonia varies according to the severity of the disorder and protein intake. Values up to 20–30 times normal may be seen during the neonatal period. Patients with late onset may have plasma ammonia levels around twice the normal values. A direct relation exits between the duration of the hyperammonemia and subsequent intellectual ability of the child.[102] However, there is no relation between the severity of hyperammonemia and later intelligence or neurologic development.[77]

Patients with CPS and OTC deficiencies do have specific abnormalities of plasma amino acids beside elevated alanine, glutamine and aspartic acid secondary to hyperammonemia. Plasma Citrulline level may serve as an initial screening tool in patients with urea cycle defects. Plasma citrulline, which is very low in OTC and CPS deficiencies, exceeds 1000 μmol/l in AS deficiency (citrullinemia) and is usually in the range of 100–300 μmol/l in AL deficiency. Urinary orotic acid level may help to differentiate CPS and NAGS deficiencies, which are characterized by low orotic acid levels from OTC deficiency which is associated with high urinary orotic acid levels.

Serum transaminases are elevated during the acute exacerbations and may remain high between the episodes. Prothrombin time may be markedly prolonged. Respiratory alkalosis is transiently present in acute attacks. Hepatic histology is usually nonspecific and unremarkable.[77] However, fibrosis has been noted in patients with several disorders of the urea cycle.[103,104] Heterozygote OTC deficiency females may exhibit several histological abnormalities including steatosis, focal necrosis and portal fibrosis.[103]

After the clinical condition stabilizes the diagnosis should be confirmed by measurement of enzyme activity in an appropriate tissue (Table 61.3). Besides the liver, OTC is expressed in the intestinal mucosa and therefore the diagnosis can be made by enzyme assays in duodenal and rectal biopsies.[105] However, the gold standard is measuring the enzyme activity in liver tissue in males with OTC deficiency as the enzyme activity may be virtually absent.[106,107] Males with partial variants may have enzyme activity that ranges from 5 to 25% of normal.[108,109] In symptomatic heterozygous females levels of activity range from 4 to 25% of normal.[107] Heterozygous mothers of affected children may have levels as high as 97% of normal activity. It has to be noted that the *in vitro* measurement of the enzyme activity may not accurately reflect the *in vivo* activity of the enzyme.

Disorder	Tissue diagnosis	Urine orotic acid
Carbamyl phosphate synthetase (CPS) deficiency	Liver	Normal
Ornithine transcarbamylase (OTC) deficiency	Liver	Very high
Argininosuccinate synthetase deficiency	Fibroblasts	High
Argininosuccinate lyase deficiency	Erythrocytes	High
Arginase deficiency	Erythrocytes	High
N-acetylglutamate synthetase (NAGS) deficiency	Liver	High

Table 61.3 Diagnostic tests in urea cycle defect

Differential diagnosis

The differential diagnosis of hyperammonemia is summarized in Table 61.4. In the neonatal period it is important to differentiate transient hyperammonemia (THA) of the newborn (THN) from inborn error of metabolism, namely urea cycle defects and organic acidemias. Differentiation may be made using an algorithm suggested by Hudak and

- Deficiencies of the urea cycle enzyme
  - Carbamyl phosphate synthetase deficiency
  - Ornithine transcarbamylase deficiency
  - Argininosuccinate synthetase deficiency
  - Argininosuccinate lyase deficiency
  - Arginase deficiency
  - N-acetylglutamate synthetase deficiency
- Lysinuric protein intolerance
- Organic acidemias
  - Propionic acidemia
  - Methylmalonic acidemia
  - Isovaleric acidemia
  - Glutaric acidemia type II
  - Multiple carboxylase deficiencies
  - 3-Hydroxy-3-methylglutaric acidurias
  - β-ketothiolase deficiency
  - Medium chain fatty acid acyl CoA dehydrogenase deficiency
- Systemic carnitine deficiency
- Hyperammonemia – hyperornithinemia – homocitrullinemia syndrome
- Transient hyperammonemia of the newborn
- Severe systemic illness
- Reye's syndrome
- Liver failure

Table 61.4 Differential diagnosis of hyperammonemia

12. Allen RC, Harley RA, Talamo RC. A new method for determination of $\alpha 1$ AT phenotypes using isoelectric focusing on polyacrylamide gel slabs. Am J Clin Pathol 1974; 62:732.
13. Fagerhol MK, Laurell CB. The Pi system-inherited variants of serum alpha-1-antitrypsin. Prog Med Genet 1970; 96:96–111.
14. American Thoracic Society/European Respiratory Society Statement. Standards for the diagnosis and management of individuals with alpha-1-antitrypsin deficiency. Am J Respir Crit Care Med 2003; 168:818–900.
15. Luisetti M, Seersholm N. Alpha-1-Antitrypsin deficiency -1: Epidemiology of alpha-1-antitrypsin deficiency. Thorax 2004; 59:164–169.
16. Kurachi K, Chandra T, Degen SJF, et al. Cloning and sequence of cDNA coding for alpha-antitrypsin. Proc Natl Acad Sci USA 1981; 78:6826–6830.
17. Long G, Chandra T, Woo S, et al. Complete sequence of cDNA for human alpha-1-antitrypsin and the gene for the S variant. Biochemistry 1984; 23:4878.
18. Schroeder WT, Miller MF, Woo SLC, Saunders GF. Chromosomal localization of the human α_1-antitrypsin gene (Pi) to 14q 31-32. Am J Hum Genet 1985; 37:868.
19. Rabin M, Watson M, Kidd V, et al. Regional localization of α_1-antichymotrypsin and α_1-antitrypsin genes on human chromosome 14. Somat Cell Mol Genet 1986; 12:209.
20. Perlino E, Cortese R, Ciliberto G. The human $\alpha 1$-antitrypsin gene is transcribed from two different promoters in macrophages and hepatocytes. EMBO J 1987; 6:2767.
21. Jeppson JO. Amino acid substitution Glu→Lys in α_1-antitrypsin PiZ. FEBS Lett 1976; 65:195.
22. Yoshida A, Lieberman J, Giadulis L, et al. Molecular abnormality of human alpha-1-antitrypsin variant (PiZZ) associated with plasma activity deficiency. Proc Natl Acad Sci USA 1976; 73:1324.
23. Hjalmarsson K. Distribution of alpha-1-antitrypsin phenotypes in Sweden. Hum Hered 1988; 38:37–30.
24. Arnaud P, Koistien JM, Wilson GB, et al. Alpha-1-antitrypsin (Pi) phenotypes in a Finnish population. Scand J Clin Lab Invest 1977; 37:339–343.
25. Thymann M. Distribution of alpha-1-antitrypsin (Pi) phenotypes in Denmark determined by separator isoelectric focusing in agarose gel. Hum Hered 1986; 36:19–23.
26. Serres FJ de. Worldwide racial and ethnic distribution of alpha-1-antitrypsin deficiency. Summary of an analysis of published genetic epidemiology surveys. Chest 2002; 122:1818–1829.
27. Porter CA, Mowat AP, Cook PJK, et al. α_1-Antitrypsin deficiency and neonatal hepatitis. Br Med J 1972; 3:435.
28. Mowat AP, Psacharopoulos HT, Williams R. Extrahepatic biliary atresia versus neonatal hepatitis. Arch Dis Child 1976; 51:763.
29. Ghishan FR, Gray GF, Greene HL. α_1-Antitrypsin deficiency presenting with ascites and cirrhosis in the neonatal period. Gastroenterology 1983; 85:435–438.
30. Hope PL, Hall MA, Millward-Sadler GH, et al. Alpha-1-antitrypsin deficiency presenting as a bleeding diathesis in the newborn. Arch Dis Child 1982; 57:68–70.
31. Hadchouel M, Goutier M. Histopathologic study of the liver in the early cholestatic phase of alpha-1-antitrypsin deficiency. J Pediatr 1976; 89:211.
32. Lomas DA, Evans DL, Finch JJ, et al. The mechanism of Z alpha-1-antitrypsin accumulation in the liver. Nature 1992; 357:605–607.
33. Sverger T. Liver disease in alpha-1-antitrypsin deficiency detected by screening of 200,000 infants. N Engl J Med 1976; 294:1316
34. Sveger T. α_1-Antitrypsin deficiency in early childhood. Pediatrics 1978; 62:22.
35. Sveger T. The natural history of liver disease in α_1-antitrypsin deficient children. Acta Paediatr Scand 1988; 77:847.
36. O'Brien ML, Buist NRM, Murphey H. Neonatal screening for alpha-1-antitrypsin deficiency. J Pediatr 1978; 92:1006.
37. Ghishan FK, Greene HL. Liver disease in children with PiZZ α_1-antitrypsin deficiency. Hepatology 1988; 8:307.
38. Crowther DC, Belorgey D, Miranda E, et al. Practical genetics: alpha-1-antitrypsin deficiency and the serpinopathies. Eur J Hum Genet 2004; 12(3):167–172.
39. Eriksson S, Carlson J, Velez R. Risk of cirrhosis and primary liver cancer in alpha-1-antitrypsin deficiency. N Engl J Med 1986; 314:736–739.
40. Ishak KG, Jenas EH, Marshall ML, et al. Cirrhosis of the liver associated with alpha-1-antitrypsin deficiency. Arch Pathol 1972; 94:445.
41. Berg NO, Eriksson S. Liver disease in adults with alpha-1-antitrypsin deficiency. N Engl J Med 1972; 287:1264.
42. Eriksson S, Hagerstrand I. Cirrhosis and malignant hepatoma in α_1-antitrypsin deficiency. Acta Med Scand 1974; 195:451.
43. Campra JL, Craig JP, Peters RL, et al. Cirrhosis associated with partial deficiency of alpha-1-antitrypsin in adults. Ann Intern Med 1973; 78:233.
44. Brand B, Bezahler GH, Gould R. Cirrhosis and heterozygous FZ alpha-1-antitrypsin deficiency in an adult. Case report and review of the literature. Gastroenterology 1974; 66:264.
45. Rawlings W, Moss J, Cooper HS, et al. Hepatocellular carcinoma and partial deficiency of alpha-1-antitrypsin (MZ). Ann Intern Med 1974; 81:771.
46. Hodges JR, Millwand-Sadler GH, Barbatis C, et al. Heterozygous MZ alpha-1-antitrypsin deficiency in adults with chronic active hepatitis and cryptogenic cirrhosis. N Engl J Med 1981; 304:557.
47. Fisher RL, Taylor L, Sherlock S. α_1-Antitrypsin deficiency in liver disease: the extent of the problem. Gastroenterology 1976; 71:646.
48. Eriksson S, Carlson J, Velez R. Risk of cirrhosis and primary liver cancer in alpha-1-antitrypsin deficiency. N Engl J Med 1986; 314:736.
49. Janus ED, Phillips NT, Carrell RW. Smoking, lung function and alpha-1-antitrypsin deficiency. Lancet 1985; I:152–154.
50. Piitulainen E, Eriksson S. Decline in FEV1 related to smoking status in individuals with severe alpha-1-antitrypsin deficiency. Eur Resp J 1999; 13:247–251.
51. Janciauskiene S, Dominaitiene R, Sternby NH, et al. Detection of circulating and endothelial cell polymers of Z and wildtype alpha-1-antitrypsin by a monoclonal antibody. J Biol Chem 2002; 277:26540–26546.
52. Wu Y, Swulius MT, Moremen KW, et al. Elucidation of the molecular logic by which misfolded alpha-1-antitrypsin is preferentially selected for degradation. Proc Natl Acad Sci USA 2003; 100:8229–8234.
53. Carrell RW, Lomas DA. Conformational disease. Lancet 1997; 350:134–138.
54. Brantly M, Nukiwa T, Crystal RG. Molecular basis of alpha-1-antitrypsin deficiency. Am J Med 1988; 84(suppl 6A):13–31.
55. Yunis EJ, Agostini RM, Glen RH. Fine structural observations of the liver in α-1-antitrypsin deficiency. Am J Pathol 1976; 82:265.
56. Hood JM, Koep LJ, Peters RL, et al. Liver transplantation for advanced liver disease with alpha-1-antitrypsin deficiency. N Engl J Med 1980; 302:272.

57. Courtney M, Jallat S, Tessier L-H, et al. Synthesis in E. coli of α_1-antitrypsin variants of therapeutic potential for emphysema and thrombosis. Nature 1985; 313:149.
58. Courtney M, Buchwalder A, Tessier L-H, et al. High-level production of biologically active human α_1-antitrypsin in Escherichia coli. Proc Natl Acad Sci USA 1984; 81:669.
59. Rosenberg S, Barr PJ, Najarian RC, Hallewell RA. Synthesis in yeast of a functional oxidation-resistant mutant of human α_1-antitrypsin. Nature 1984; 312:77.
60. Wewers MD, Gadek JE, Keogh BA, et al. Evaluation of danazol therapy for patients with PiZZ α_1-antitrypsin deficiency. Am Rev Respir Dis 1986; 134:476.
61. Flotte TR, Brantly ML, Spencer LT, et al. Phase 1 trial of intramuscular injection of recombinant adeno-associated virus alpha-1-antitrypsin gene vector for AAT-deficiency. Hum Gene Ther 2004; 15(1):93.
62. Mitchell GA, Grompe M, Lambert M, et al. Hypertyrosinemia. In: Scriver CR, Beaudet AL, Sly W, Valle D, eds. The Metabolic and Molecular Basis of Inherited Disease, 9th edn. New York: McGraw-Hill; 2001:1777–1805.
63. Levine SZ, Marples E, Gordon HH. A defect in the metabolism of aromatic amino acids in premature infants. The role of vitamin C. Science 1939; 90:620.
64. Sakai K, Kitagawa T. An atypical case of tyrosinosis. Part 1. Clinical and laboratory findings. Jikeikai Med J 1957; 4:1.
65. Sakai K, Kitagawa T. An atypical case of tyrosinosis. Part 2. A research on the metabolic block. Jikeikai Med J 1957; 4:11.
66. Sakai K, Kitagawa T, Yoshioka K. An atypical case of tyrosinosis. Part 3. The outcome of the patient. Jikeikai Med J 1959; 6:15.
67. Gentz J, Jagenburg R. Zetterstroem R. Tyrosinemia. J Pediatr 1965; 66:670–696.
68. Halvorsen S, Pande H, Loken AC, Gjessing LR. Tyrosinosis. A study of 6 cases. Arch Dis Child 1966; 41:238.
69. Gaul GE, Rassin DK, Solomon GE, et al. Biochemical observations on so-called hereditary tyrosinemia. Pediatr Res 1970; 4:337.
70. Strife DF, Zuroweste EL, Emmett EA, et al. Tyrosinemia with acute intermittent porphyria: aminolevulinic acid dehydratase deficiency related to elevated urinary aminolevulinic acid levels. J Pediatr 1977; 90:400.
71. Gentz J, Johansson S, Lindblad B, et al. Excretion of delta-aminolevulinic acid in hereditary tyrosinemia. Clin Chim Acta 1969; 23:257.
72. Lindblad B, Lindstedt S, Steen G. On the enzymic defects in hereditary tyrosinemia. Proc Natl Acad Sci USA 1977; 74:4641.
73. Spronsen FJ Van, Thomasse Y, Smith GPA, et al. Hereditary tyrosinemia: A new classification with difference in prognosis on dietary treatment. Hepatology 1994; 25:1187–1195.
74. Mitchell G, Larochelle J, Steen G, et al. Neurologic crisis in hereditary tyrosinemia. New Eng J Med 1990; 322:432–437.
75. Weinberg AG, Mize CE, Worthen HG. The occurrence of hepatoma in the chronic form of hereditary tyrosinemia. J Pediatr 1976; 88:434–439.
76. Paradis K, Weber A, Seidman EG, et al. Liver transplantation for hereditary tyrosinemia. The classic Quebec experience. Am J Hum Genet 1990; 47:338–343.
77. Balistreri WF. Liver diseases in infancy and childhood. In: Schiff E, Schiff L, eds. Diseases of the Liver, 7th edn. Philadelphia, PA: Lippincott; 1993:1099–1201.
78. Prive L. Pathological findings in patients with tyrosinemia. Can Med Assoc J 1967; 97:1054–1056.
79. Scriver CR, Larochelle J, Silverberg M. Hereditary tyrosinemia and tyrosyluria in French Canadian geographical isolate. Am J Dis Child 1967; 113:446.
80. Braekeleer M De, Larochelle J. Genetic epidemiology of hereditary tyrosinemia in Quebec and in Saguenay-Lac-St-Jean. Am J Hum Genet 1990; 47:302–307.
81. Phanuel D, Labelle Y, Berube D, et al. Cloning and expression of cDNA encoding human fumarylacetoacetate hydrolase. The enzyme deficient in hereditary tyrosinemia: assignment of the gene to chromosome 15. Am J Hum Genet 1991; 48:525–535.
82. St-Louis M, Leclere B, Laine J, et al. Identification of a stop mutation in five French patients suffering from hereditary tyrosinemia type I. Hum Mol Genet 1994; 2:941–946.
83. Grompe M, St-Louis M, Demera SI, et al. A single mutation of the fumarylacetoacetate hydrolase gene in French Canadians with hereditary tyrosinemia type I. N Engl J Med 1994; 331:353–357.
84. Poudrier J, Lettre F, Streiver CR, et al. Different clinical forms of hereditary tyrosinemia (type I) in patients with identical genotypes. Mol Genet Metab 1998; 64:119–225.
85. Jakobs C, Stellaard F, Kvittingen EA, et al. First-trimester prenatal diagnosis of tyrosinemia type I by amniotic fluid succinylacetone determination. Prenat Diagn 1990; 10:133–134.
86. Gremier A, Cederboum S, Laberge C, et al. A case of tyrosinemia type I with normal succinylacetone in the amniotic fluid. Prenat Diagn 1996; 16:239–242.
87. Kvittingen EA, Steinman B, Gitzelmann R, et al. prenatal diagnosis of hereditary tyrosinemia by determination of fumarylacetoacetase in cultured amniotic fluid cells. Pediatr Res 1985; 19:334–337.
88. Demers SI, Phaneuf D, Tanguay RM. Hereditary tyrosinemia type I: strong association with haplotype 6 in French Canadians permits simple carrier detection and prenatal diagnosis. Am J Hum Genet 1994; 55:327–333.
89. Rootwelt H, Kvittingen EA, Hole K, et al. The human fumarylacetoacetase gene: characterization of restriction fragment length polymorphisms and identification of haplotypes in tyrosinemia type 1 and pseudodeficiency. Hum Genet 1992; 89:229–233.
90. Demers SI, Phaneuf D, Tanguay RM. TaqI RFLP for the human fumarylacetoacetate hydrolase (FAH) gene. Nucl Acids Res 1991; 19:1352.
91. Kvittingen EA, Rootwelt H, Brandberg P, et al. Hereditary tyrosinemia type I. self-induced correction of the fumarylacetoacetase defect. J Clin Invest 1993; 91:1816–1821.
92. Kvittingen EA, Rootwelt H, Berger R, et al. self-induced correction of the defect in tyrosinemia type I. J Clin Invest 1994; 94:1657–1661.
93. Lindstedt S, Holme E, Locke E, et al. Treatment of hereditary tyrosinemia type I by inhibition of 4-hyroxyphenylpyruvate dioxygenase. Lancet 1992; 340:813–818.
94. Holme E, Lindstedt S. Tyrosinemia type I and NTBC (2-(2-nitro-4-trifluoromethylbenzoyl0-1.3-cyclohexamedione). J Inherit Met Dis 1999; 21:507–517.
95. Holme E, Lindstedt S. Pediatric liver: Helping adults by treating children. Nontransplant treatment of tyrosinemia. Clin Liver Dis 2000; 4:805–814.
96. Origuchi Y, Cantani A, Kennaway NG, et al. Sural nerve lesions in a case of Hypertyrosinemia. Brain Dev 1982; 4:463.
97. Giardini O, Cantani A, Kennaway NG, et al. Chronic tyrosinemia associated with 4-hydroxyphenylpyruvate dioxygenase deficiency with acute intermittent ataxia and

Chapter 62
Abnormalities of carbohydrate metabolism and the liver

Shikha S. Sundaram and Estella M. Alonso

INTRODUCTION

The liver is the central organ responsible for carbohydrate metabolism. The liver stores carbohydrates in the form of glycogen and synthesizes glucose through glycogen breakdown and gluconeogenesis. Glucose is an essential nutrient for the function of both the central nervous system and muscle. Disorders of carbohydrate metabolism may be acquired or inborn. This chapter highlights the molecular basis, clinical presentation, diagnosis and therapy of the most common errors in carbohydrate metabolism. Non-alcoholic fatty liver disease, galactosemia, hereditary fructose intolerance, fructose 1,6-bisphosphatase deficiency and glycogen storage disease will be discussed.

NON-ALCOHOLIC FATTY LIVER DISEASE

Non-alcoholic fatty liver disease (NAFLD) represents a spectrum of diseases, ranging from simple steatosis to steatohepatitis (NASH) or cirrhosis. It is speculated that NAFLD is the most common liver condition in the United States. In an autopsy study, Wanless and Lentz found steatosis in 70% of obese and 35% of lean individuals and non-alcoholic steatohepatitis (NASH) in 18.5% of obese and 2.7% of lean individuals.[1] These conditions are also increasingly common in pediatrics. Sixty percent of adolescents with increased transaminases are either overweight or obese.[2] Additionally, it is estimated that 1–2% of adolescents have NAFLD, including a sub-group with cirrhosis.[3,4] This astounding pediatric prevalence parallels the rise in obesity in children, with concurrent increases in hyperlipidemias and type 2 diabetes mellitus.

Type 2 diabetes mellitus is a presumed risk factor for the development of NAFLD. Up to 75% of those with type 2 diabetes mellitus have fatty liver disease.[5,6] Type 2 diabetes mellitus is a key component of the metabolic syndrome, which includes hypertension and NAFLD. The distribution of NAFLD among adult men and women is similar. It is our clinical impression, however, that NAFLD may be more common in male adolescents. Ethnic variation also exists, with a relative paucity of NAFLD in African Americans, compared with Caucasians and Hispanics.[5–7] Up to 20% of adults with NASH will develop cirrhosis.[8,9] The incidence of NASH induced cirrhosis in children remains unknown.

NAFLD and its progression to NASH, are clearly of multifactorial etiology (Fig. 62.1). Central to the development of fatty liver disease is abnormal lipid homeostasis. This can involve increased hepatic uptake of free fatty acids from peripheral adipocytes and dietary sources, impaired mitochondrial and peroxisomal beta-oxidation within the

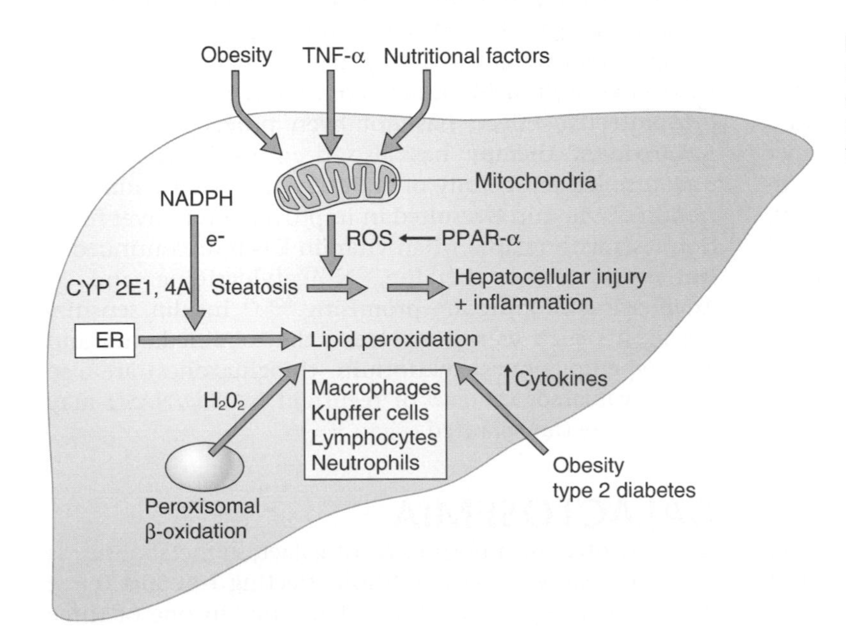

Figure 62.1: The etiopathogenesis of NASH. NADPH, reduced nicotinamide adenine dinucleotide phosphate; ER, endoplasmic reticulum; CYP, cytochrome; TNF-α, tumor necrosis factor alpha; ROS, reactive oxygen species. (Adapted from Chitturi 2001, with permission from Thieme.)[10]

hepatocyte or impaired triglyceride excretion through the formation of VLDL. Insulin resistance is strongly associated with NASH and contributes to the accumulation of hepatocellular fat by mobilizing free fatty acids from adipocytes and increasing their uptake by the liver.[10] In addition, excess free fatty acids and cytokines such as TNF-α and leptin may contribute to insulin resistance via downregulation of insulin receptor substrates and impaired insulin signaling.[4] Mesenteric fat is a large source of both TNF-α and leptin. TNF-α levels correlate well with body fat mass and may provide an important link between insulin resistance and adiposity.[4] Leptin is a regulator of body weight and energy expenditure. Leptin is crucial in preventing lipid accumulation in non-adipose tissue such as myocardial and skeletal muscle and liver.[11] Leptin likely has a role in the shunting of fat towards beta oxidation and away from triglyceride synthesis. The progression of liver disease may also be affected by increased oxidative stress. Numerous studies have demonstrated increased markers of oxidative stress in patients with NASH. This occurs through the generation of reactive oxygen species (ROS) formed by lipid peroxidation and peroxisomal beta-oxidation. The upregulation of various cytochrome P450 systems, particularly CYP2E1 and CYP4A, also support the role of oxidative stress in the pathogenesis of NASH. CYP2E1 and CYP4A are key enzymes responsible for microsomal lipoxygenation. Peroxisome proliferator activated receptor alpha (PPAR-α), a transcription factor that regulates microsomal and peroxisomal lipid peroxidation, may also contribute to the development of NASH through the formation of ROS.[4,11] Although much has been learned about the pathophysiology of NAFLD and its progression to NASH and cirrhosis, many questions remain unanswered and are under active investigation.

Clinical presentation

The clinical symptoms of NAFLD are quite variable. Most children are asymptomatic. Elevated transaminases or hepatic fat on an abdominal ultrasound are often discovered during testing performed for unrelated reasons. The typical patient is overweight or obese, though NAFLD may occur in lean individuals. Patients may complain of mild abdominal pain, sometimes localized to the right upper quadrant. Some have vague complaints of fatigue and constipation. Physical exam may be completely normal, demonstrate obesity, mild-moderate hepatomegaly and acanthosis nigricans (a sign of insulin resistance). Some patients may have normal BMIs with central adiposity.[11] Laboratory evaluation reveals mild elevations of transaminases, typically less than 1.5 times normal. Transaminase elevation cannot reliably confirm the diagnosis of NAFLD, nor predict the presence of fibrosis. In fact, it is possible to have significant liver disease from NAFLD with completely normal transaminases.[4] Laboratory evaluation may reveal hyperglycemia and hyperlipidemia, in particular increased triglyceride levels. Physicians should consider evaluation for insulin resistance with an oral glucose tolerance test given the high preponderance of type 2 diabetes in patients with NAFLD. An abdominal ultrasound or MRI can further identify steatosis, but cannot identify fibrosis. Patients suspected of having NAFLD should have other causes of fatty liver excluded, including Wilson's disease, glycogen storage disease, medications such as amiodarone, drugs, or alcohol.

Prognosis of this condition varies, with some patients remaining stable for years with only simple steatosis. Others develop progressive hepatitis and up to 20% of adults develop cirrhosis. NASH and the resultant cirrhosis are increasingly common reasons for liver transplantation.[9,12]

Diagnosis/treatment

The role of liver biopsy in the diagnosis of NAFLD/NASH remains controversial. It is the only modality available for assessing the presence and extent of necro-inflammation and fibrosis. Three components are necessary for a liver biopsy to be consistent with NASH: steatosis (macrovesicular greater than microvesicular), a mild, mixed lobular inflammation (polymorphonuclear cells and mononuclear cells) and hepatocyte ballooning.[4] Biopsies usually also have perisinusoidal fibrosis and glycogenated nuclei, though these are not necessary for diagnosis. In pediatrics, fibrosis is more characteristically portal, compared with perisinusoidal in adults.[3,4] Mallory's hyaline or scattered amounts of iron may also be observed. Currently, the need and utility of liver biopsy must be assessed individually for each patient.

Treatment of fatty liver disease necessitates lifestyle modifications. Weight loss is the only therapy proven to be beneficial.[13,14] Even a 10–15% weight loss can have positive effects on health. This goal can be achieved by increased exercise and decreased caloric intake. In addition to decreasing calories, some advocate the incorporation of a low glycemic index diet, high in fruits, vegetables, whole grain and fiber.[15] Aerobic exercise, initiated with the help of a physician, can decrease insulin resistance and contribute to improved liver disease. In adult populations, bariatric surgery has also improved fatty liver disease, though rapid weight loss may actually worsen NASH.[16,17] Ursodeoxycholic acid, though commonly prescribed for its cytoprotective effect, has not been proven beneficial.[18] Anti-oxidant therapy has also been used. In a small, uncontrolled pilot study of children with NASH, administration of Vitamin E resulted in improvement in liver function tests with relapse when vitamin E was discontinued.[19] Initial studies of betaine, N-Acetylcysteine and S-Adenosylmethionine are promising.[4,20,21] Insulin sensitizing agents such as sulfonylureas, thiazolidinediones and anti-hyperlipidemics (metformin, thioglitazones) are also being evaluated. *De novo* or recurrent NAFLD/NASH may occur in the transplanted organ.[12,22,23]

GALACTOSEMIA

Galactosemia, an inborn error of galactose metabolism, is an autosomal recessive condition affecting 1 of 50000 live births.[24] It is due to a cellular deficiency in one of three enzymes in the pathway of glucose to galactose conversion. The classic form of galactosemia, presenting with malnutrition, growth failure and progressive liver disease, results from deficiency in galactose-1-phosphate uridyl transferase (GALT). A much more rare deficiency in uridine diphosphate galacotse-4-epimerase results in a similar clinical presentation to GALT deficiency.[25,26] Lastly, galactokinase deficiency results primarily in cataract formation.[25] GALT is a 43 kD protein encoded by a 4 kb gene on chromosome 9p18. A majority of patients with galactosemia have missense mutations, of which greater than 150 have been identified.[27,28] The Q188R mutation, affecting 60–70% of Caucasians, where arginine is substituted for glutamine, results in no enzymatic activity.[28,29] The milder Duarte variant (N314D mutation), involves a change from asparagine to aspartate, with a resulting decrease in enzymatic activity.[30]

Galactose is a monosaccharide derived from the hydrolysis of milk sugar, lactose. Lactose is converted to glucose and galactose by the enterocyte brush border enzyme lactase. Galactose is then transported across the enterocyte by a Na-glucose/galactose transporter. Galactose is metabolized to glucose by a series of reactions that begins with the phosphorylation of galactose to galactose-1-phosphate (Fig. 62.2). This is further converted to glucose-1-phosphate by GALT. In the absence of GALT, alternative pathways overproduce galactitol and galactonate, potentially toxic metabolites.[31]

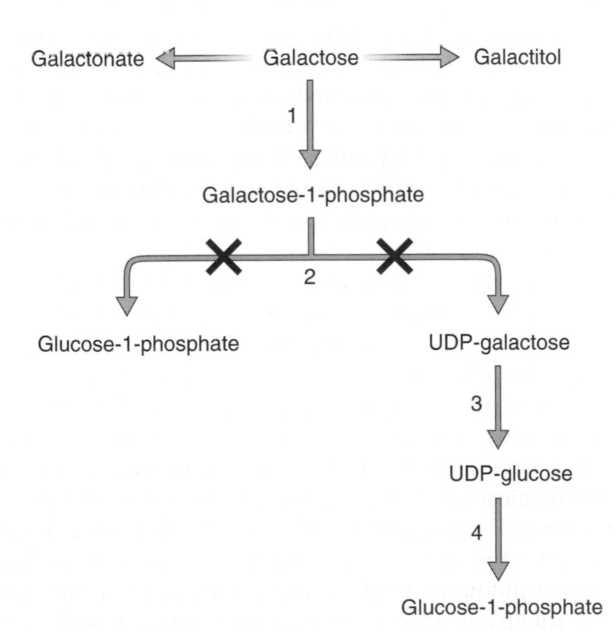

Figure 62.2: Galactose metabolism. Galactose is phosphorylated to galactose-1-phosphate, by galactokinase (1). This is then further converted to uridine diphosphate (UDP) galactose and glucose-1-phosphate by galactose-1-phosphate uridyl transferase (GALT) (2). UDP-galactose is converted to UDP-glucose by uridine diphosphate galactose-4-epimerase (3). UDP-glucose is converted to glucose-1-phosphate by uridine diphosphate glucose pyrophosphorylase (4). In the absence of GALT, galactitol and galactonate are overproduced.

Clinical presentation

The clinical presentation of galactosemia varies from an acute illness with hypoglycemia, vomiting, diarrhea and encephalopathy to a sub-acute illness. Patients most commonly present with failure to thrive, weight loss and emesis after initiation of lactose. Vomiting and diarrhea are almost universally present.[26] Patients may present with hypoglycemia and encephalopathy in the first few days of life. Some may present several days later with jaundice, ascites, hepatomegaly, splenomegaly and liver failure.[32,33] Hemolytic anemia can also be observed. Cataracts may be present at birth if the mother ingested large amounts of dairy late in pregnancy or develop postnatally. Cataracts are formed because of increased oncotic pressure exerted by the accumulation of galactitol in the lens.[34] Levy et al. discovered a strong correlation between galactosemia and neonatal *E. coli* sepsis.[35] Thus, the presence of *E. coli* sepsis in the neonate should prompt evaluation of galactosemia. Renal tubular dysfunction with albuminuria, aminoaciduria and galactosuria can also occur.[26] Furthermore, patients may manifest increased blood and urinary galactose levels and hyperchloremic acidosis.[36]

Long-term prognosis is good for patients with early diagnosis and intervention. Acute symptoms and biochemical changes regress rapidly upon withdrawal of lactose products. Long-term follow-up data of those treated show some variability. Growth and liver function revert to normal. Mental retardation is the most devastating result of toxicity. Intelligence, as measured by IQ, appears highly correlated with adequate dietary control. Some patients manifest residual defects in mental functioning, despite dietary restrictions and normal IQ. These include language delays, spatial and mathematic learning disabilities, short attention spans, abnormal visual perceptions and ataxia.[37,38] Additionally, there is a high incidence of postnatal hypergonadotropic hypogonadic ovarian failure.[39,40]

Diagnosis/treatment

A diagnosis of galactosemia should be suspected in patients with any of the above described constellation of symptoms. The presence of urinary reducing substances in the absence of glucosuria is suggestive of galactosemia, but neither is very sensitive nor specific.[26] False negatives may occur with poor lactose intake or intermittent excretion of galactose. False positives may occur with severe liver disease and some medications. Diagnosis of galactosemia should be confirmed by measuring GALT activity in red blood cells, which will be decreased.[26,36,41] Prenatal diagnosis is possible by measuring enzymatic activity of tissue or cells obtained by chorionic villus sampling or amniocentesis.[42] Most patients are detected by newborn screening programs conducted in a majority of states in the USA.

Treatment of galactosemia is based on elimination of dietary galactose. In infants, this is achieved by feeding soy or protein hydrosylate formulas.[26] In older children and adults, dietary avoidance of dairy products, with special attention to food additives is needed. Some concern exists regarding galactose toxicity from certain grains, fruits and vegetables.[43] Controversy also exists regarding safe or acceptable levels of galactose. In addition to dietary manipulation, close monitoring of neurodevelopment in children and yearly ophthomologic exams to evaluate for cataracts are also recommended.[26]

HEREDITARY FRUCTOSE INTOLERANCE

Hereditary fructose intolerance is an autosomal recessive metabolic disorder occurring in approximately 1:20 000 live births. This disorder is caused by a deficiency of fructose-1,6-bisphosphate aldolase (Aldolase B), one of a set of enzymes that converts fructose to intermediate constituents of the glycolytic-gluconeogenic pathway. These intermediary products are then further metabolized to glucose and glycogen (Fig. 62.3). Aldolase B is the product of a 14.5 kB gene on chromosome 9q22.3 that encodes a 364 amino acid polypeptide. More than 20 different mutations and 5 polymorphisms have been described.[44] Among people of northern European descent, the A149P allele is most common. The A174D allele is predominant in central and southern Europeans, whereas the N334K allele is predominant among those of central and eastern European descent.[45–47]

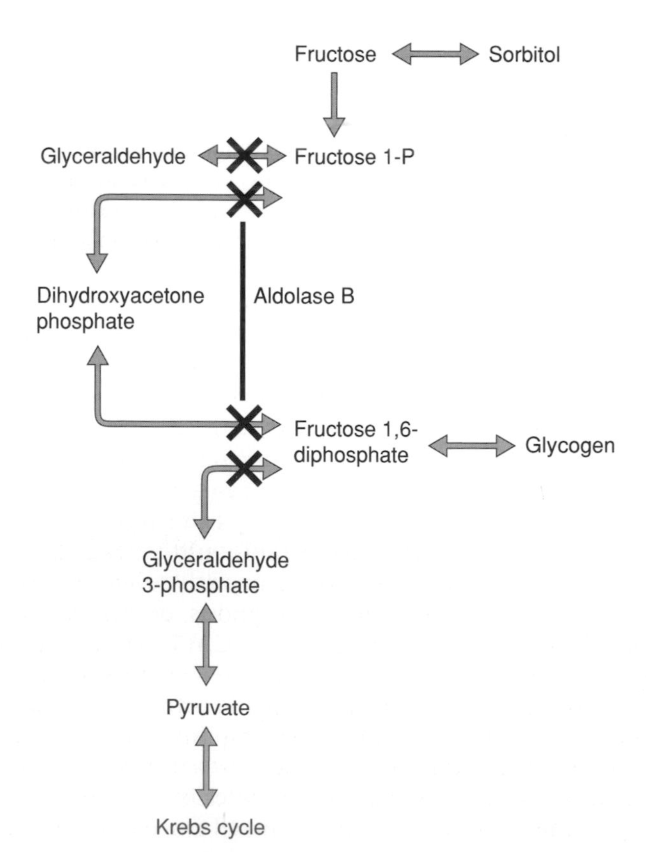

Figure 62.3: Fructose metabolism. Fructose is metabolized to glycogen or to components of the Krebs cycle. A deficiency in Aldolase B, as in hereditary fructose intolerance, results in the accumulation of fructose-1-phosphate.

Fructose is transported into hepatic and intestinal cells via GLUT 5, a sodium independent transporter. It is then phosphorylated into fructose-1-phosphate by fructokinase. Fructose-1-phosphate is cleaved by aldolase B into D-glyceraldehyde phosphate and dihydroxyacetone phosphate. These intermediates may then directly enter the glycolytic pathway, the gluconeogenesis pathway or become synthesized into glycogen (Fig. 62.2). Accumulation of fructose-1-phosphate results in hypoglycemia secondary to impaired glycogenolysis, as glycogen phosphorylase is inhibited, and impaired gluconeogenesis as glyceraldehyde-3-phosphate and dihydroxyacetone phosphate cannot be converted. Additionally, the formation and sequestration of large quantities of fructose-1-phosphate result in ATP and GTP depletion with impaired protein synthesis.[45,48]

Clinical presentation

Patients affected by this disorder remain completely asymptomatic unless they consume fructose containing foods. Newborns fed breast milk do not manifest symptoms, as breast milk contains lactose (made of glucose and galactose). Symptoms occur as infants are weaned and receive either sucrose containing formulas or begin baby foods. The most common symptoms are poor feeding and vomiting. Other gastrointestinal symptoms include diarrhea and abdominal pain. In addition, severe hypoglycemia with sweating, trembling, pallor and metabolic acidosis can occur.[49,50] Irritability, apathy and anuria/oliguria are also seen. A large fructose load may even cause seizures.[51] Chronic exposure to fructose leads to failure to thrive, signs of liver disease (hepatomegaly, splenomegaly, ascites, edema) and proximal renal tubular dysfunction (renal tubular acidosis, hypophosphatemia and rickets).[49,50] Occasionally, affected patients remain undiagnosed into adolescence or adulthood because of self-imposed dietary restrictions.[49] These individuals develop aversions to fructose containing foods, exhibiting unusual feeding behaviors such as eating the peel, but avoiding the fruit pulp.

Laboratory abnormalities are consistent with the affected organ systems. Patients may have elevations in liver transaminases, increased prothrombin times, hypoproteinemia, hypokalemia and hypophosphatemia. Urine studies reveal increased reducing substances, proteinuria, amino aciduria, organic aciduria and fructosuria. Patients may also have anemia and thrombocytopenia. Histology from liver biopsies shows steatosis with scattered hepatocyte necrosis and interlobular or periportal fibrosis. Electron microscopy reveals intracellular deposits of fructose-1-phosphate with polymorphous, electron dense, cytoplasmic inclusions in concentric membranous arrays.[50,51]

Diagnosis/treatment

Definitive diagnosis of hereditary fructose intolerance requires a tissue enzyme assay.[52,53] Diagnosis can also be made using an intravenous fructose tolerance test after several weeks of fructose withdrawal.[50,54] DNA mutation analysis has also been used for diagnosis, though it is available primarily as a research tool.[55] Treatment of acutely ill patients consists of supportive care to correct metabolic derangements, hypoglycemia and coagulopathy. The mainstay of long-term management is complete avoidance of fructose and sucrose. Special attention should be given to food additives and medications, as sucrose or sorbitol are often used as food additives, pill coatings and medication suspensions.[45] Long-term abstinence from fructose results in reversal of organ dysfunction, normal intelligence and catch up growth. Hepatomegaly may, however, persist for years.[51,56]

FRUCTOSE 1,6-BISPHOSPHATASE DEFICIENCY

Fructose 1,6-bisphosphatase deficiency is an autosomal recessive disease that results in disordered gluconeogenesis. It is a genetically heterogeneous disorder that affects females more than males (1.5:1).[57] Parental consanguinity has been reported in several families. Fructose 1,6-bisphosphatase deficiency results in inhibition of gluconeogenic substrates (Fig. 62.4).[58] Therefore, normoglycemia depends on adequate glucose intake or degradation of hepatic glycogen. If glycogen stores are limited, like in newborns, or exhausted during fasting, hypoglycemia results and gluconeogenic precursors (lactate, glycerol and alanine) accumulate. The enzyme deficiency is also present in liver, jejunum and kidney tissue. Muscle levels, however, are normal as muscle fructose 1,6-bisphophatase is encoded by a different gene.[49]

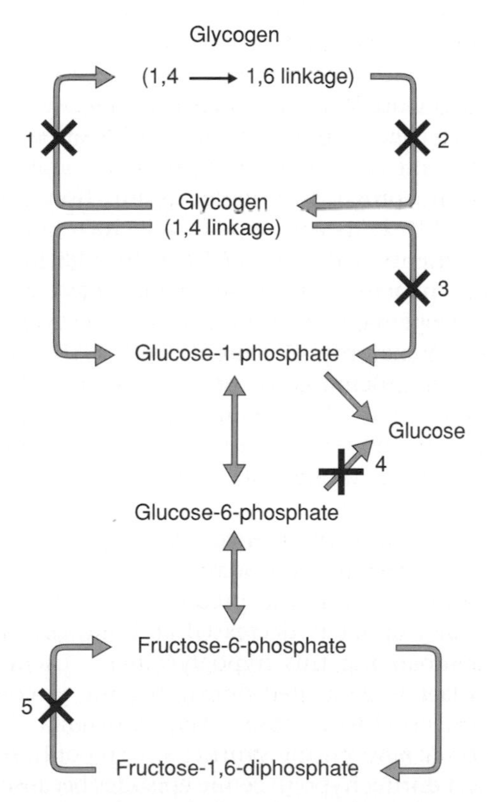

Figure 62.4: Glycogen metabolism. (1) Branching enzyme, deficient in glycogen storage disease (GSD) type IV; (2) debranching enzyme, deficient in GSD type III; (3) phosphorylase deficiency, defective in GSD type VI; (4) glucose-6-phophatase, deficient in GSD type 1; (5) fructose-1,6-biphosphatase. (Adapted from Ghishan FK, Ballew MP. Inborn errors of carbohydrate metabolism. In: Suchy FJ, Sokol RK and Balistreri WF, eds. Liver Disease in Children, with permission of Lippincott, Williams and Wilkins, 2001.)[58]

Clinical presentation

Fructose 1,6-bisphophatase deficiency should be suspected in newborns presenting with hypoglycemia, hyperventilation and metabolic acidosis. Approximately half of affected patients will develop symptoms in the first 4 days of life. The remainder develop symptoms in the first few months of life. In addition to the symptoms described above, patients may have dyspnea or apnea, tachycardia, irritability, seizures, coma, hypotonia or hepatomegaly. Later disturbances are often triggered by febrile illnesses with concurrent refusal to feed and emesis. Unlike hereditary fructose intolerance, patients do not develop an aversion to sweet foods. Additionally, disturbances in liver function are rare and kidney function is normal. These patients do, however, have a reduced tolerance to fructose and sorbitol. This intolerance is less severe than in patients with hereditary fructose intolerance. Laboratory studies show elevations in blood and urine lactate, ketones, alanine and uric acid.[50] Histologic examination of liver biopsies shows fatty infiltration without fibrosis.[50]

Diagnosis/treatment

Definitive diagnosis is established by observing a deficiency of fructose 1,6-bisphophatase in liver biopsy specimens. Whether this enzyme defect may be detected in leukocytes remains a matter of debate. Intravenous dextrose and sodium bicarbonate infusions are needed for the acute management of hypoglycemia and acidosis. Additionally, fasting should be avoided, with careful attention to periods when children are febrile. Fructose and sucrose should be limited, though complete elimination is unnecessary.[49]

GLYCOGEN STORAGE DISEASE

Glycogen storage diseases (GSD) are caused by deficiencies of enzymes in the glycogenolytic pathways (Fig. 62.4).[58] Ten different types of glycogen storage disease have been reported, each with unique clinical features. Type I, III, IV and VI primarily affect the liver. Glycogen production and breakdown are controlled by several factors through glycogen synthetase and phosphorylase. Both of these enzymes exist in active and inactive forms. After meals, sinusoidal glucose concentration is high, allowing glucose to bind to phosphorylase. This changes the active enzyme to its inactive form, halting glycogenolysis. Additionally, the active form of phosphorylase normally inhibits glycogen synthetase; the inactive phosphorylase allows glycogen synthesis to occur. During fasting, glucagon mediated increases in cyclic AMP allow phosphorylase conversion from inactive to active, with subsequent glycogenolysis. High glycogen levels also allow glycogenolysis to occur by glycogen synthetase breakdown.[59]

Glycogen storage disease, type I

Glycogen storage disease (GSD) type I, glucose-6-phosphatase deficiency, was previously considered to be a single entity. It is now recognized that three distinct clinical forms exist: types Ia, Ib and Ic. Glucose-6-phosphatase, located in the endoplasmic reticulum, catalyzes the terminal reaction of both glycogenolysis and gluconeogenesis (conversion of glucose-6-phosphate to glucose).[60] It is composed of a catalytic subunit and three distinct transport systems (Fig. 62.5).[58] The catalytic subunit has six endoplasmic reticulum transmembrane domains.[24] There is a polypeptide stabilizing protein that transports glucose-6-phosphate, known as T1, two polypeptides responsible for phosphate transport (T2) and a glucose transporter (T3), also called GLUT-7.[60] *Type Ia*, the classic form of GSD, results from mutations in the catalytic subunit. The gene for this entity is located on chromosome 17q21 and is 12.5 kb, encoding a 357 amino acid protein.[61] More than 30 distinct mutations have been identified in this gene, the most common being R83C and Q347X.[62] *Type Ib* GSD is caused by defects in the T1 translocase.[60] Normal phosphatase activity exists in fully disrupted microsomal preparations, but not in intact microsomal vesicles. The mutation for this disease is on chromosome 11q23.3.[63,64] The same genetic defect is seen in the liver, kidney and leukocytes of affected patients.[65] *Type Ic* GSD is caused by a defective T2 translocase (161), the gene for which is 11q23.3-24.2. Translocase 2 (T2) is a microsomal phosphate and pyrophosphate transport protein. These patients also have

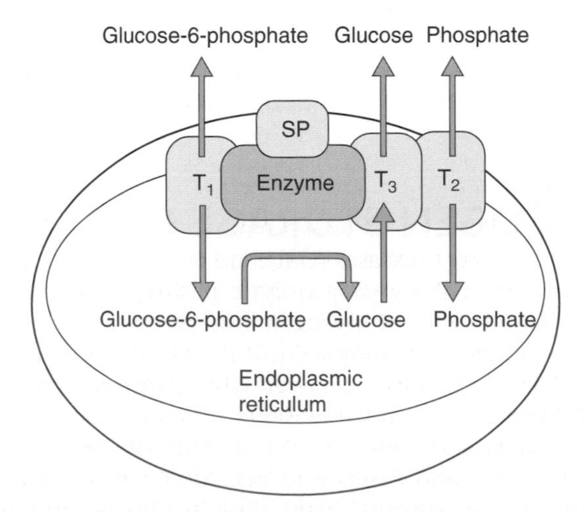

Figure 62.5: Hepatic microsomal glucose-6-phosphatase. (Adapted from Ghishan FK, Ballew MP. Inborn errors of carbohydrate metabolism. In: Suchy FJ, Sokol RJ and Balistreri WF, eds. Liver Disease in Children, with permission of Lippincott, Williams and Wilkins, 2001.)[58]

impaired insulin secretion as T2 is also located in the kidney and pancreas.[66,67]

Clinical presentation

The clinical presentation of this disease can be quite varied. Type Ia GSD is considered the classic form of glycogen storage disease. It affects approximately 1:200 000 births. Patients commonly present with severe hypoglycemia and metabolic acidosis 3–4 hours after a feeding. Symptoms often begin after the first several weeks of life, when the interval between feeds increases, infants begin sleeping through the night or when inter-current illness disrupts feeds. Hypoglycemia is accompanied by a metabolic acidosis with increases in lactic acid, triglycerides and uric acid. Some children present with failure to thrive because of peripheral starvation from lack of glucose, along with a protuberant abdomen and lordosis secondary to hepatomegaly. Untreated patients may develop failure to thrive, cushingoid facies and delayed motor development. Their social and cognitive development is not affected unless they suffer neurologic injury from recurrent episodes of hypoglycemia.[60] Untreated patients may develop high serum triglycerides, moderate increases in cholesterol, phospholipids, free fatty acids and apolipoprotein III. They may also develop xanthomas on the knees, elbows and buttocks in adolescence.[68] There may also be impaired platelet function secondary to metabolic derangements, with resultant epistaxis and oozing.[60] Liver transaminase elevation is typically mild and regresses to normal as glucose levels stabilize. Liver biopsy shows only increased glycogen. Adolescent and adult patients may also develop hepatic adenomas or carcinomas, nephrolithiasis, nephropathy, progressive renal dysfunction and gouty arthritis.[69–74] Patients with type Ib GSD have similar symptoms to patients with type Ia GSD. In addition to these symptoms, patients with type 1b may have constant or cyclic neutropenia, with recurrent mild to severe bacterial infections. A majority of patients with GSD type Ib will also develop inflammatory bowel disease (IBD). IBD is underdiagnosed in this population and requires a high index of suspicion.[75,76] Patients with type Ic present with classic symptoms along with signs of impaired insulin secretion.

The metabolic consequences of GSD type I are profound. Hypoglycemia, secondary to an inability to mobilize glycogen, remains the predominant feature. Insulin levels are appropriately decreased and glucagon levels are high accompanying this hypoglycemia.[77] Lactic acidosis occurs as lactate generated during hepatic glycolysis cannot be converted to glucose.[78] Hyperuricemia also occurs because of *de novo* purine synthesis.[79] Hypophosphatemia is common during hypoglycemic episodes because glucose-6-phospate cannot be converted to glucose. Phosphate is trapped intracellularly, causing a shift of extracellular phosphate into the cell. Hyperlipidemia also occurs, with high serum triglycerides and moderate increases in cholesterol, phospholipids and free fatty acids.[60] Abnormal platelet function, both aggregation and adhesiveness, cause recurrent oozing and epistaxis.[80]

Diagnosis/treatment

The diagnosis of GSD Type I should be considered in all children presenting with hypoglycemia and acidosis. Definitive diagnosis is made by assay of enzymatic activity of glucose-6-phophatase on liver biopsy specimens. Histologic exam of the liver shows hepatocytes filled with glycogen that is periodic acid-Schiff positive, diastase sensitive (Fig. 62.6).

Management of patients with GSD Type I requires a continuous dietary source of glucose to keep glucose levels greater than 70 mg/dl.[60] In infants, this can be accomplished by providing feedings every 2–3 hours while awake and at least every 3 hours while asleep.[60] It may be necessary to institute nocturnal nasogastric infusions of glucose.[81] When small frequent feedings or overnight nasogastric feedings are no longer feasible, raw cornstarch feedings may be used.[82,83] Cornstarch acts as a reservoir for glucose that can slowly be absorbed into the circulation and utilized as a glucose source for up to 6 hours. This therapy also restores hyperuricemia and hyperlipidemia to normal. Lipid lowering agents are rarely needed.[60] Treatment with recombinant G-CSF has been important in managing patients with neutropenia.[84]

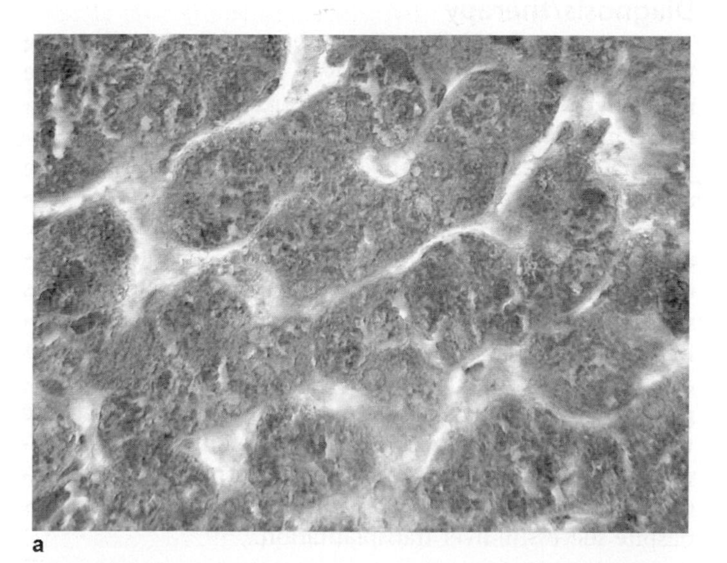
a

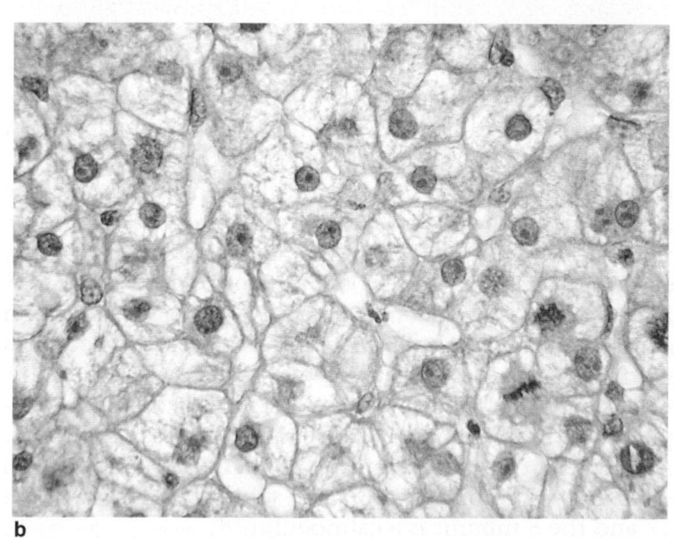
b

Figure 62.6: Type 1 Glycogen Storage Disease. (**a**) Glycogen filled hepatocytes seen on periodic acid-Schiff stain. (**b**) Plant like mosaic pattern of hepatic lobules on hematoxylin and eosin stain. (Courtesy of Dr H. Melin-Aldana.)

Glycogen storage disease Type III

Glycogen storage disease Type III (GSD Type III), also known as Forbe's disease, is an autosomal recessive condition due to deficiency of the glycogen debranching enzyme. In order for glucose to be released from glycogen stores, glycogen phosphorylase and glycogen debranching enzyme must work together. This enzyme is composed of 2 independent catalytic subunits on one polypeptide chain, oligo-1,4-1,4 glucan transferase and amylo-1,6-glucosidase. The phosphorylase initially works on the outermost branches of the glycogen molecule. The transferase then moves glucose residues from one short outer branch to another. Finally, glucosidase works on the inner chain 1,6 linkages. A lack of the debrancher enzyme results in accumulation of abnormal glycogen, called phosphorylase limit dextrin.[60] The 85 kB gene for the debrancher enzyme is located on chromosome 1p21 and encodes a 268 kD protein. The same gene encodes the debrancher enzyme in liver and muscle, but differential RNA transcription results in 2 separate isoforms.[85,86] GSD Type III is further subdivided into IIIa, in which both liver and muscle are involved and IIIb, involving only the liver.[87] In the USA, GSD Type IIIa predominates.[60]

Clinical presentation

Significant clinical heterogeneity exists among individual patients with GSD Type III. Initially, symptoms in infants and young children appear very similar to GSD Type I. They experience fasting hypoglycemia with a ketosis, hepatomegaly, hyperlipidemia and growth retardation.[60] Patients typically have moderate increases in liver transaminases, though decreasing levels with a concomitant decrease in hepatomegaly has been reported beginning in puberty.[88] By 4–6 years of age, however, some patients may develop hepatic fibrosis with resultant splenomegaly and later develop liver failure.[89] Because gluconeogenesis remains intact and glucose can be cleaved from the outermost branches, GSD Type III patients tolerate longer fasts than GSD Type I patients. They are less likely to experience difficulty as long as they remain on a frequent feeding schedule typical of infants. They do not have difficulty when experiencing infections or stress.[60]

Those with GSD Type IIIa have minimal muscle weakness in childhood. In the third to fourth decade, however, slow, progressive weakness of proximal and occasionally smaller distal muscles occurs.[60] Cardiac disease also develops because of limit dextrin accumulation in cardiac muscle. Some patients develop cardiomyopathy, while others manifest only sub-clinical disease with ventricular hypertrophy detected on echocardiogram or EKG.[90,91] The long-term prognosis for patients is variable, with some showing decreased hepatomegaly over time, while others develop fibrosis, cirrhosis and worsening myopathy. In addition, hepatocellular adenomas have been found in patients.[72]

Biochemically, patients with GSD Type III have normal lactate and uric acid levels and less severe hyperlipidemia. In addition, they develop a more rapid ketonemia than those with GSD Type I. Liver biopsy specimens have significantly increased glycogen content. Unlike GSD Type I, however, fibrous septa and a paucity of fat are seen on biopsy. Ultrastructural examination reveals small, lipid filled vacuoles.[60,92]

Diagnosis/therapy

Diagnosis of GSD Type III is made by assaying the debrancher enzyme in liver or muscle tissue. An elevated level of creatinine phosphokinase can suggest muscle involvement, though it may be normal.[60] Therapy is aimed at preventing hypoglycemia. Similar to GSD Type I, a continuous source of glucose by feedings of uncooked cornstarch is helpful in maintaining normoglycemia, achieving good growth and decreasing transaminases elevation.[93] In patients with severe growth retardation or myopathy, a diet high in oligosaccharides and protein has been beneficial.[94] Because of the risk of hepatocellular adenomas, annual α-feto protein and ultrasound may be useful. Patients with myopathy should also have annual echocardiograms and electrocardiograms.[60]

Glycogen storage disease Type IV

Glycogen storage disease Type IV (GSD Type IV) is an extremely rare condition, representing only 0.3% of all glycogenoses.[95] Also known as Andersen's disease or amylopectinosis, it is caused by a deficiency in the glycogen branching enzyme, α-1,4-glucan: α-1,4-glucan 6-glucosyltransferase. This enzyme usually creates branch points in the normal glycogen molecule. It is necessary for packing and degrading stored glycogen. Without this enzyme, a less soluble form of glycogen, similar to amylopectin, the plant starch, accumulates. This glycogen is less soluble and has longer outer and inner chains, with less branch points.[95,96] GSD Type IV is an autosomal recessive condition, due to a gene defect on chromosome 3p14.[97] The 3 kB cDNA encodes a 702 amino acid protein.[97]

Clinical presentation

Significant clinical variability exists among patients with GSD Type IV. Patients with the classic form of the disease are normal at birth and then develop failure to thrive, abdominal distension with hepatosplenomegaly, followed by progressive liver failure and death by age 3 to 5.[95] Patients with a non-progressive form of this liver disease have also been described.[87,98,99] Affected individuals may have concurrent abnormal neuromuscular development because of polysaccharide deposition. They may have neuronal involvement, severe hypotonia and muscle atrophy at birth or present later in childhood with a progressive myopathy.[100] Finally, cardiomyopathy and cardiac failure have been described secondary to myofibrillar damage resulting from cardiac amylopectin deposits.[101–103] These cardiac and neuromuscular symptoms may accompany or predominate the clinical picture.

Unlike other types of glycogen storage disease, hypoglycemia is rarely observed in GSD Type IV.[98] Patients have a normal glycemic response to glucose, fructose and galactose. Additionally, their response to glucagon and epinephrine is most often normal.[104,105] Affected individuals have moderate elevations in hepatic transaminases and alkaline phosphatase. They have normal levels of both lactate and pyruvate, though their cholesterol may be slightly increased. As liver disease progresses, however, hypoglycemia and hypercholesterolemia became more prominent symptoms. Histologically, liver biopsy specimens may show both micronodular and macronodular cirrhosis. Hepatocytes contain strongly periodic acid-Schiff positive and partially diastase sensitive deposits in the cytoplasm.[96] Ultra structure evaluation by electron microscopy may show glycogen particles, amylopectin-like fibrils and fine granular material.[95] Similar cytoplasmic deposits may be seen in cardiac, skeletal and neurologic muscle.

Diagnosis/therapy

The diagnosis of GSD Type IV can be made prenatally using PCR-based DNA mutation analysis. Diagnosis can also be made by evaluation of branching enzyme activity of cultured amniocytes or chorionic villi.[106,107] Glycogen branching enzyme deficiency can be demonstrated in liver biopsy specimens, erythrocytes, leukocytes and fibroblasts.[108–110]

Liver transplantation is the only effective therapeutic modality currently available for GSD Type IV patients.[96] This therapeutic modality is recommended only for individuals with progressive liver disease.[87] Some liver transplant recipients have improvement of abnormal glycogen in other affected organs such as heart or skeletal muscle after transplantation. This may be due to the development of systemic microchimerism that occurs after transplant, with lymphocytes and macrophages acting as migrating enzyme carriers.[95,111] Other patients, however, succumb to cardiac failure, despite successful liver transplantation.[112,113]

Glycogen storage disease Type VI and IX

Glycogen storage disease Type VI and glycogen storage disease Type IX are distinct, yet clinically similar disorders. GSD Type VI is an extremely rare deficiency of glycogen phosphorylase, necessary to breakdown glycogen. The defect leading to this disorder occurs on chromosome 14.[114] GSD Type IX is a more heterogeneous disorder, caused by a deficiency of phosphorylase kinase.[115] Phosphorylase kinase deficiency is the most common glycogen storage disease, representing 25% of all patients with a glycogen storage disease. Phosphorylase kinase is necessary to activate glycogen phosphorylase. It is composed of four subunits, encoded by different chromosomes. The α subunit is encoded by chromosome X, the β subunit by chromosome 16, the γ subunit by chromosome 17 and the δ subunit is a calmodulin.[116]

Clinical presentation

There are several variations of GSD Type IX, depending on the inheritance pattern and affected tissue. The most common subtype is x-linked and affects only the liver. The next most common group is an autosomal recessive variant that also only affects the liver. Several other exceedingly rare subtypes, all autosomal recessive, also exist. They affect liver and muscle together, isolated muscle or heart.[116] GSD Type VI and IX present with similar symptoms in infancy and early childhood. Most children have growth retardation, hepatomegaly and protuberant abdomen. Some children have slight motor developmental delay. They often have mild increases in triglycerides, cholesterol and transaminases.[117] Metabolic acidosis is rare and lactic and uric acid are normal. Hepatomegaly resolves around puberty and final height is usually normal. Most adults are completely asymptomatic, despite a persistent enzyme defect.[60]

Diagnosis/therapy

After an overnight fast, a glucagon stimulation test will show a normal glycemic response with increases in blood lactate. This will not, however, differentiate between phosphorylase and phosphorylase kinase deficiency.[118] Diminished phosphorylase kinase activity in erythrocytes can establish the diagnosis of liver and muscle disease. Normal activity, however, does not exclude these diagnoses. Therefore, study of enzymatic activity in tissue samples is ideal. Most patients require no specific therapy. Avoidance of prolonged fasting is recommended.[60,116]

References

1. Wanless IR, Lentz JS. Fatty liver hepatitis (steatohepatitis) and obesity: an autopsy study with analysis of risk factors. Hepatology 1990; 12:1106–1110.
2. Strauss RS, Pollack HA. Epidemic increase in childhood overweight, 1986-1998. JAMA 2001; 286:2845–2848.
3. Rashid M, Roberts EA. Nonalcoholic steatohepatitis in children. J Pediatr Gastroenterol Nutr 2000; 30:48–53.
4. Neuschwander-Tetri BA, Caldwell SH. Nonalcoholic steatohepatitis: summary of an AASLD Single Topic Conference. Hepatology 2003; 37:1202–1219.
5. Silverman JF, O'Brien KF, Long S, et al. Liver pathology in morbidly obese patients with and without diabetes. Am J Gastroenterol 1990; 85:1349–1355.
6. Marchesini G, Brizi M, Morselli-Labate AM, et al. Association of nonalcoholic fatty liver disease with insulin resistance. Am J Med 1999; 107:450–455.
7. Caldwell SH, Harris DM, Patrie JT, Hespenheide EE. Is NASH underdiagnosed among African Americans? Am J Gastroenterol 2002; 97:1496–1500.
8. Matteoni CA, Younossi ZM, Gramlich T, et al. Nonalcoholic fatty liver disease: a spectrum of clinical and pathological severity. Gastroenterology 1999; 116:1413–1419.
9. Roberts EA. Nonalcoholic steatohepatitis in children. Curr Gastroenterol Rep 2003; 5:253–259.
10. Chitturi S, Farrell GC. Etiopathogenesis of nonalcoholic steatohepatitis. Semin Liver Dis 2001; 21:27–41.
11. Chitturi S, Abeygunasekera S, Farrell GC, et al. NASH and insulin resistance: Insulin hypersecretion and specific association with the insulin resistance syndrome. Hepatology 2002; 35:373–379.
12. Contos MJ, Cales W, Sterling RK, et al. Development of nonalcoholic fatty liver disease after orthotopic liver transplantation for cryptogenic cirrhosis. Liver Transpl 2001; 7:363–373.
13. Vajro P, Franzese A, Valerio G, Iannucci MP, Aragione N. Lack of efficacy of ursodeoxycholic acid for the treatment of liver abnormalities in obese children. J Pediatr 2000; 136:739–743.
14. Baldridge AD, Perez-Atayde AR, Graeme-Cook F, Higgins L, Lavine JE. Idiopathic steatohepatitis in childhood: a multicenter retrospective study. J Pediatr 1995; 127:700–704.
15. Pawlak DB, Ebbeling CB, Ludwig DS. Should obese patients be counselled to follow a low-glycaemic index diet? Yes. Obes Rev 2002; 3:235–243.
16. Luyckx FH, Desaive C, Thiry A, et al. Liver abnormalities in severely obese subjects: effect of drastic weight loss after gastroplasty. Int J Obes Relat Metab Disord 1998; 22:222–226.
17. Silverman EM, Sapala JA, Appelman HD. Regression of hepatic steatosis in morbidly obese persons after gastric bypass. Am J Clin Pathol 1995; 104:23–31.
18. Lindor KD, Kowdley KV, Heathcote EJ, et al. Ursodeoxycholic acid for treatment of nonalcoholic steatohepatitis: results of a randomized trial. Hepatology 2004; 39:770–778.
19. Lavine JE. Vitamin E treatment of nonalcoholic steatohepatitis in children: a pilot study. J Pediatr 2000; 136:734–738.
20. Alvaro D, Gigliozzi A, Piat C, et al. Effect of S-adenosyl-L-methionine on ethanol cholestasis and hepatotoxicity in isolated perfused rat liver. Dig Dis Sci 1995; 40:1592–1600.
21. Abdelmalek MF, Angulo P, Jorgensen RA, Sylvestre PB, Lindor KD. Betaine, a promising new agent for patients with nonalcoholic steatohepatitis: results of a pilot study. Am J Gastroenterol 2001; 96:2711–2717.
22. Ong J, Younossi ZM, Reddy V, et al. Cryptogenic cirrhosis and posttransplantation nonalcoholic fatty liver disease. Liver Transpl 2001; 7:797–801.
23. Carson K, Washington MK, Treem WR, Clavien PA, Hunt CM. Recurrence of nonalcoholic steatohepatitis in a liver transplant recipient. Liver Transpl Surg 1997; 3:174–176.
24. Burchell A. The molecular basis of the type 1 glycogen storage diseases. Bioessays 1992; 14:395–400.
25. Bosch AM, Bakker HD, Gennip AH van, et al. Clinical features of galactokinase deficiency: a review of the literature. J Inherit Metab Dis 2002; 25:629–634.
26. Walter JH, Collins JE, Leonard JV. Recommendations for the management of galactosaemia. UK Galactosaemia Steering Group Arch Dis Child 1999; 80:93–96.
27. Reichardt JK, Packman S, Woo SL. Molecular characterization of two galactosemia mutations: correlation of mutations with highly conserved domains in galactose-1-phosphate uridyl transferase. Am J Hum Genet 1991; 49:860–867.
28. Tyfield L, Reichardt J, Fridovich-Keil J, et al. Classical galactosemia and mutations at the galactose-1-phosphate uridyl transferase (GALT) gene. Hum Mutat 1999; 13:417–430.
29. Reichardt JK, Woo SL. Molecular basis of galactosemia: mutations and polymorphisms in the gene encoding human galactose-1-phosphate uridylyltransferase. Proc Natl Acad Sci USA 1991; 88:2633–2637.
30. Wang BB, Xu YK, Ng WG, Wong LJ. Molecular and biochemical basis of galactosemia. Mol Genet Metab 1998; 63:263–269.
31. Novelli G, Reichardt JK. Molecular basis of disorders of human galactose metabolism: past, present and future. Mol Genet Metab 2000; 71:62–65.

glycogen phosphorylase) maps to chromosome 14. Am J Hum Genet 1987; 40:351–364.

115. Chen Y. Glycogen Storage Diseases. The Metabolic Basis of Inherited Disease. 2001:

116. Van De berg I. Phosphorylase b kinase Deficiency in Man: A Review. J Inher Metab Dis 1990; 13:442–451.

117. Willems PJ, Gerver WJ, Berger R, Fernandes J. The natural history of liver glycogenosis due to phosphorylase kinase deficiency: a longitudinal study of 41 patients. Eur J Pediatr 1990; 149:268–271.

118. Dunger DB, Leonard JV. Value of the glucagon test in screening for hepatic glycogen storage disease. Arch Dis Child 1982; 57:384–389.

Chapter 63
Acute and chronic hepatitis

Harpreet Pall and Maureen M. Jonas

INTRODUCTION

Hepatitis is defined as inflammatory liver injury regardless of cause. Recent discoveries in the field of molecular biology, microbiology, metabolism and immunology have greatly expanded the viral 'hepatitis alphabet' and our understanding of many of these diseases. New questions have also been raised, and the body of information has become more complex.

This chapter concentrates on acute and chronic hepatitis caused by viruses that affect the liver (the 'hepatotropic' viruses), as well as autoimmune hepatitis and non-alcoholic fatty liver disease, also known as non-alcoholic steatohepatitis (NASH). Other causes of hepatitis (e.g. chemical and non-viral infectious agents) are listed, to provide the reader with a comprehensive differential diagnosis.

EVALUATION OF THE CHILD WITH HEPATITIS

Hepatitis in pediatric patients can result from a diverse number of causes and present with a variety of signs and symptoms. The evaluation may be divided into assessment of the clinical presentation, serologic testing and imaging, and histopathologic examination. A list of the most common differential diagnoses of hepatitis in childhood is provided in Table 63.1.

Clinical presentation

Some children with hepatitis are asymptomatic and the disease is discovered fortuitously while they are being investigated for unrelated illness or during a routine well-child examination. This would be a typical presentation for chronic hepatitis B or C. Some present with the typical signs of symptoms of acute hepatic damage, such as jaundice, abdominal pain and malaise. Other children may present with signs of cirrhosis or hepatic failure. Among these extremes lies a spectrum of presentations.

A detailed history in a child with hepatitis should include an effort to determine the possible etiologic agent, such as exposure to hepatotoxic drugs, or mode of transmission, such as intravenous drug abuse or a family history of inherited or acquired liver disease. A complete physical examination should look for scleral, mucosal or cutaneous icterus, hepatosplenomegaly, ascites, edema, clubbing, petechiae, ecchymosis, spider angiomas and mental state changes. Non-hepatic causes of increased levels of aminotransferases, such as congestive heart failure or myopathy, should be considered.

Serologic testing and imaging

Blood tests have become the basis on which the diagnosis of hepatitis and the determination of its cause are made. Often the history and clinical examination provide important clues and guidelines in the choice of appropriate tests. Imaging studies such as ultrasonography or computed topography have become important tools in the evaluation of patients with liver dysfunction. They must be ordered judiciously and are not indicated in all patients.

Histopathologic examinations

Histologic examination of liver tissue is an important adjunct in the evaluation of children with hepatitis. It is not required in all patients, especially those with acute hepatitis in whom the etiologic diagnosis is known and who are expected to have a good prognosis. However, when the etiology and/or the outcome are uncertain, examination of liver tissue may be critical in the determination of diagnosis and prognosis. Guidelines for the histopathologic interpretation of liver biopsy specimens in children with viral and autoimmune hepatitis are provided in Table 63.2.

HEPATOTROPIC VIRUSES

Hepatitis A

Biology and pathogenesis

The virus responsible for hepatitis A (hepatitis A virus; HAV) is a 27-nm non-enveloped spherical endovirus with a single-stranded RNA genome.[1] Humans are the only natural host, although certain primates can be infected experimentally.[2] Hepatitis is the result of direct cytolytic and immune-mediated activities of HAV.[3]

Epidemiology

Hepatitis A is widespread and can be found throughout the world. The reported incidence of hepatitis A in the United States is approximately 25 000 cases per year;[4] however, this is an underestimate because most patients are asymptomatic and do not come to medical attention. HAV is spread primarily by the fecal–oral route. The disease may be acquired from direct fecal contact (e.g. daycare centers) or indirectly through ingestion of contaminated water or food. There is no carrier state or chronic infection.

High rates of HAV infection have been associated with low socioeconomic status, both in the USA and other countries.[5,6] In developing nations, under poor living conditions,

Infectious
Hepatotropic viruses
• HAV • HBV • HCV • HEV • HDV • Hepatitis non-A–E viruses • Systemic infection that may include hepatitis • Adenovirus • Arbovirus • Coxsackievirus • Cytomegalovirus • Enterovirus • Epstein–Barr virus • 'Exotic' viruses (e.g. yellow fever) • Herpes simplex virus • Human immunodeficiency virus • Paramyxovirus • Rubella • Varicella zoster • Other
Non-viral liver infections
• Abscess • Amebiasis • Bacterial sepsis • Brucellosis • Fitz–Hugh–Curtis syndrome • Histoplasmosis • Leptospirosis • Tuberculosis • Other
Autoimmune
• Chronic autoimmune hepatitis • Other (e.g. systemic lupus erythematosus, juvenile rheumatoid arthritis)
Metabolic
• α1-Antitrypsin deficiency • Glycogen storage disease • Tyrosinemia • Wilson's disease • Other
Toxic
• Iatrogenic or drug induced (e.g. acetaminophen) • Environmental (e.g. pesticides)
Anatomic
• Choledochal cyst • Biliary atresia • Other
Hemodynamic
• Shock • Congestive heart failure • Budd–Chiari syndrome • Other
Non-alcoholic fatty liver disease
• Idiopathic • Sclerosing cholangitis • Reye's syndrome • Other

Continued

Table 63.1 Causes and differential diagnosis of hepatitis in children

HAV, like other enteroviral infections, is a childhood disease. In these countries, 92–100% of 18 year olds show serologic evidence of past infection.[6] In developed countries the disease is acquired at a later age (20% by age 20, 50% by age 50 in the USA). As the disease is more severe in older patients, it poses a greater health problem in developed countries.[2,5,6]

Favorable conditions for endemic infections include crowding, poor sanitation and poor personal hygiene practices. Specific risk factors include contact with an infected person (26% of cases), homosexual activity (15%), foreign travel (14%), contact with children attending a daycare center (11%) and illicit drug use (10%). In 40% of patients no risk factor can be identified.[2] Well-documented high-risk areas include households with an infected individual, prisons, military camps, residential centers for the disabled and daycare centers.

Daycare centers are likely settings for transmission, especially if they have a large proportion of young children with orocentric behaviors or those not yet toilet trained. Under these conditions, the disease usually comes to medical attention from an infected adult staff member or an infected older household contact, rather than the asymptomatic daycare vector.[7,8]

There are geographic variations in the incidence of HAV in the USA.[9] Over the past several years it has become apparent that decreasing the public health burden of HAV involves widespread vaccination of children because they serve as the reservoir of HAV in the community.

Clinical course and outcomes

The clinical and serologic course of a typical HAV infection is shown in Figure 63.1. The average incubation period is 28 days (range 14–49 days).[10,11] Fecal shedding can occur for 2–3 weeks before and for 1 week after the onset of jaundice. It is during this period and while the patient is asymptomatic that the virus is most likely to be transmitted. Increased serum aminotransferase levels may persist for several months, and rarely for as long as a year.[2]

The clinical expression of HAV infection is age dependent, and there are no pathognomonic clinical signs that allow it to be differentiated from other forms of acute hepatitis. Examination may be remarkable for jaundice, evidence of

Type	Inflammation Portal	Periportal	Lobular	Portal lymphoid aggregates	Steatosis	Mallory bodies	Bile duct damage
HAV	1+	1+	±	–	–	–	–
HBV	2+	2+	2+	±	–	–	–
HCV	2+	1+	1+	2+	2+	1+	2+
HDV	2+	2+	2+	±	–	–	–
HEV	1+	1+	±	–	–	–	–
EBV	2+	1+	2+	1+	–	–	–
CMV	1+	±	–	±	–	–	–
NASH	1+	1+	2+	–	3+	1+	–
AIH	3+	3+	3+	1+	–	–	1+

HAV	Hepatitis A virus often causes periportal inflammation, possible pericentral cholestasis but without significant lobular inflammation.
HBV	Hepatitis B virus causes lymphocytic inflammation in and around the portal area; with increasing severity, inflammation and/or necrosis extends toward the centrolobular area.
HCV	The characteristic histologic appearance of HCV is portal inflammation with lymphoid aggregates, often disproportionate to the minimal lobular inflammation. Steatosis and mild bile duct injury are common.
HDV	HDV is essentially indistinguishable from HBV, although some studies have suggested higher levels of inflammation and more rapid progression to cirrhosis.
HEV	The minimal information available for HEV infection suggests it is similar to HAV.
EBV	Epstein–Barr virus infection in infectious mononucleosis typically causes a diffuse lymphocytic infiltrate in the sinusoids. Any part, or all, of the lobule may be affected.
CMV	In immunocompetent individuals, CMV produces a mononucleosis-like picture with characteristic intracytoplasmic and nuclear inclusions. In the neonatal period, giant cell transformation occurs. In immunocompromised individuals, inflammation may be minimal and necrosis is variable.
NASH	The primary defining features of NASH include macrovesicular steatosis, parenchymal lymphocyte-predominant inflammation, Mallory hyaline bodies and ballooning hepatocyte degeneration.
AIH	Autoimmune hepatitis often produces a severe necroinflammatory injury with dense mononuclear infiltration of portal tracts and periportal areas. Plasma cells may be conspicuous.

Prepared with assistance of Ken Barwick MD.

Table 63.2 Histopathologic features of hepatitis by type

dehydration, and a mildly enlarged, tender liver. Occasionally, splenomegaly is noted. Serum aminotransferase values usually peak around the time that jaundice occurs. These values are often 20–100 times the upper limit of normal, and decrease rapidly within the first 2–3 weeks, although minor increases may persist for months. Hyperbilirubinemia most often resolves within 4 weeks. Infants and toddlers are more likely to be asymptomatic ('anicteric hepatitis'), whereas the majority of adults develop clinically evident hepatitis ('icteric hepatitis').[7,8,12] Only 1 in 12 young children is likely to develop jaundice.[13] Children are more likely than adults (60% *vs* 20%) to have diarrhea, often leading to the mistaken diagnosis of infectious gastroenteritis. Asymptomatic HAV infection among children facilitates transmission to their adult contacts, who are more likely to experience symptomatic and severe infection. The outcome of hepatitis A infection in general is excellent. There are no reported cases of chronic infection. Most complications are rare, and the fatality rate from fulminant hepatitis in children younger than 14 years of age is 0.1%, compared with 1% in adults older than 40 years.[2,14] The complications and extraintestinal manifestations of HAV infection are outlined in Table 63.3.[15–25]

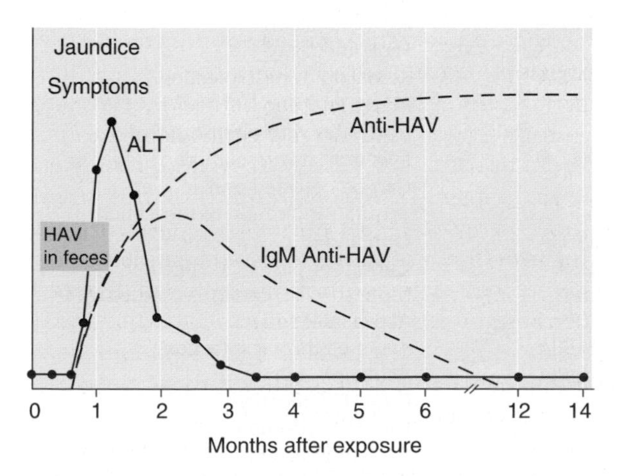

Figure 63.1: Typical clinical and serologic course of symptomatic hepatitis A. ALT, alanine aminotransferase; HAV, hepatitis A virus. (Reproduced from Hoofnagle JH, Di Bisceglie AM: Serologic diagnosis of acute and chronic viral hepatitis. Semin Liver Dis 1991; 11:73-83, with permission.)[26]

Diagnosis

The diagnosis of HAV infection may be suspected if the child becomes symptomatic, but is confirmed by specific serologic markers. A positive anti-HAV test indicates acute

Complication	Comments	References
Prolonged jaundice	May last 12 weeks; pruritus is frequent	16
Relapse	3–20% of cases; most often a single benign episode	17, 18
Meningoencephalitis		19, 20
Arthritis/rash		21, 22, 23
Cryoglobulinemia		22
Pancreatitis		24
Autoimmune hepatitis	Rare	23, 25
Fulminant hepatitis	0.1% in children	26

Table 63.3 Complications of HAV infection

infection, immunity from past infection, passive antibody acquisition (e.g. transfusion, serum immune globulin infusion) or vaccination. The diagnosis of acute or recent HAV infection in the presence of a positive anti-HAV finding requires determination of anti-HAV IgM. Anti-HAV IgM is present at the onset of disease but persists for only 3–12 months. Detection of HAV antigen in stool, and HAV-RNA in stool, liver and serum of infected individuals, is rarely required for the diagnosis.[26] Serologic markers of HAV infection are outlined in Table 63.4.

Passive immunoprophylaxis

Serum immune globulin can be given before exposure (e.g. travelers to endemic areas) or after exposure to an index case. The most frequent example in the latter situation occurs in the daycare setting or in household contacts. The recommended dose is 0.02 ml/kg bodyweight, given as soon as possible but no more than 2 weeks after exposure. Exact dosing and administration regimens are provided elsewhere.[27–29]

Active immunoprophylaxis

In 1995, the USA became the 41st country to license a vaccine against HAV. Two preparations are currently available, both made from formalin-inactivated virus grown in culture.[30] Dosages are prescribed in proprietary unit measurements, with both pediatric and adult formulations available. Recommended schedules include two injections 6–12 months apart, with 99% of children developing protective levels of antibody.[29–31] The vaccine is safe, with no serious complications having been reported. The most frequent side-effects reported in children are pain and tenderness at the injection site.[29,31] The lower age limit for administration is 2 years.

Routine immunization has been recommended for children living in communities with high rates of hepatitis A and periodic outbreaks.[29,31] Persons traveling to regions of endemic disease and those who belong to groups at high risk of acquiring HAV (see epidemiology of HAV) should also be immunized. Vaccines should replace serum immune globulin for use in pre-exposure cases and may be active in interrupting epidemics.[29] It may be reasonable in such situations to pair both active and passive immunization. The impact of the vaccination strategy has been dramatic. The incidence of hepatitis A has been falling since

Virus	Marker	Definition	Method	Significance
HAV	Anti-HAV	Total antibodies to HAV	RIA/EIA	Current or past infection
	Anti-HAV-IgM	IgM antibody to HAV	RIA/EIA	Current or recent infection
HBV	HBsAg	Hepatitis B surface antigen	RIA/EIA	Ongoing HBV infection or carrier state
	Anti-HBS	Antibody to HBsAg	RIA/EIA	Resolving or past infection Protective immunity Immunity from vaccination
	HBeAg	Nucleocapsid-derived Ag	RIA/EIA	Active infection High infectivity
	Anti-HBe	Antibody to HBeAg	RIA/EIA	Resolving or past infection
	HBV DNA	HBV viral DNA	PCR	Active infection Correlates with disease activity Loss indicates resolution
	HBcAg	Core Ag of HBV		Can be detected only in liver Sensitive indication of replication
	Anti-HBc	Antibody to HBcAg	RIA/EIA	Ongoing or past infection
HCV	Anti-HCV	Antibody to multiple HCV antigens	ELISA	Current or past HCV infection
			RIBA	More specific; confirms positive ELISA
	HCV-RNA	HCV viral RNA	PCR	Active infection
HDV	Anti-HDV	IgG/IgM to HDV antigen	EIA/RIA	Acute or chronic infection
	Anti-HDV IgM	IgM to HDV antigen	EIA/RIA	Acute infection
HEV	Anti-HEV IgM	IgM to HEV protein	EIA	Early HEV infection
	Anti-HEV IgG	IgG to HEV protein		Late HEV infection
HGV	HGV-RNA	RNA of HGV	PCR	Current infection

EIA, electroimmunoassay; ELISA, enzyme-linked immunosorbent assay; PCR, polymerase chain reaction; RIA, radio-immunoassay; RIBA, radio-immunobinding assay.

Table 63.4 Serologic markers of hepatitis infection

1998, commensurate with the increasing use of hepatitis A vaccination. In fact, the incidence in the USA reached its lowest level in 2002.[9]

Hepatitis B

Biology and pathogenesis

Despite a reduction in newly acquired hepatitis B virus (HBV) infections since the mid-1980s, HBV remains an important cause of liver disease in the USA. HBV is a 42-nm diameter spherical virus.[32] It is a member of the hepadnavirus family (hepatotropic DNA viruses) – the only member of this family capable of causing hepatitis in humans and non-human primates.

The intact virus (the Dane particle) has a double-shelled structure. The external shell, or envelope, expresses the 'Australia antigen', the hepatitis B surface antigen (HBsAg). An inner shell termed the core or nucleocapsid expresses a second antigen, hepatitis B core antigen (HBcAg). The presence of a viral shell has been associated with the development of chronicity and carcinoma.[33] Inside the core resides the viral genome, a reverse transcriptase (DNA polymerase) and a third antigen, hepatitis B e antigen (HBeAg). The significance of these three antigens is described in Table 63.4.

The HBV genome is a double-stranded DNA circle with a unique single-stranded area. It is 3200 nucleotide bases in length.[33] Viral replication, in a fashion similar to that of retroviruses, involves reverse transcription of an intermediate RNA template.[34] Although there is only one serotype, there are seven genotypes, A through G, that vary by 8% at the nucleotide level over the entire genome. Genotype predominance varies with geographic location.[35] There are important pathogenic and therapeutic differences among the genotypes. Genotype C is associated with more severe liver disease than genotype B,[36] and genotype D with more severe liver disease than genotype A.[37] Genotypes C and D are less responsive to interferon therapy than types A and B.[38,39] Mutations of the HBV genome have been described and may determine outcomes such as the development of a fulminant course, latency or response to treatment.[40–42] Two types of mutant have been described: pre-core mutants and pre-S/S mutants.

Pre-core mutant strains are responsible for 'e-minus' HBV infections in which HBeAg is absent, the result of a single point mutation causing a premature stop codon. HBV-DNA and anti-HBe remain detectable. E-minus infections can be responsible for a more severe course or outbreaks of fulminant hepatitis.[40,43] This contrasts to 'wild-type' (i.e. absence of mutation) infections in which lack of detectable HBeAg signifies cessation of viral replication.

The pre-S1, S2 and S genes are responsible for envelope protein synthesis, including HBsAg. Mutations in these genes have been found in chronically HBV-infected persons who are HBsAg negative. This has raised concerns regarding safety and screening of blood supplies. These individuals have detectable HBV-DNA, HBeAg and anti-HBs antibody.[42,44] The clinical significance of HBV mutations in pediatric liver disease is unclear; the study of these mutations is still ongoing and pediatric reports are rare.[45,46] It is likely that these mutations do not appear commonly in childhood because they represent a late stage of HBV, often seen after decades of infection.

Although HBV can infect other organs, such as the spleen, kidney or pancreas, its replication has been demonstrated only in the liver.[47,48] Replication produces not only complete viruses but also smaller 22-nm spherical and variable-length (50–1000 nm) filamentous particles. These latter particles are rich in HBsAg and are thought to be incomplete viral coats. All three forms can be detected in the blood.

Clinical expression of HBV is polymorphic and thought to be determined by the body's immune response to infection rather than a direct cytotoxic effect of the virus. The factors that determine a specific response, whether it is viral eradication, chronic persistent infection or fulminant hepatitis, are incompletely defined.

Study of the pathogenesis of chronically acquired HBV infection is ongoing. It is thought that neonates are predisposed to chronic HBV infection as a result of their immature immune systems. This is supported by the observation that these children most often demonstrate little, if any, hepatic inflammatory injury. It has been shown that the passive transplacental transfer of anti-HBc IgG may interfere with the recognition of HBcAg on the hepatocyte by cytotoxic T cells.[49] Additionally, two studies have shown that in both humans and transgenic mice HBeAg crosses the placental barrier and may induce immune tolerance.[50,51] This tolerance is achieved through neonatal T-cell unresponsiveness to HBeAg and HBcAg, both antigens sharing similar amino acid sequences.

Epidemiology

HBV is a major health problem throughout the world: 350 million people are infected chronically, with 250 000 deaths annually.[52] In the USA, however, the incidence has declined steadily since 1985.[4] The true incidence of childhood infection is unknown because 85–90% of infections in this age group are asymptomatic.[52]

The development of chronic infection is the most important consequence of infection acquired in childhood.[53] Ten percent of patients with initial infection across all age groups will become chronically infected. Even though children younger than 5 years of age represent only 1–3% of all new HBV infections in the USA, they account for 30% of all chronic infections.[4,52] The epidemiology of hepatitis B is strongly influenced by age, geographic location and mode of transmission.

The age at the time of initial infection influences both the development of symptoms and chronicity. A 1985 study by McMahon et al.[54] followed 1280 seronegative Eskimos in an endemic area of Alaska for 5 years. Their results, summarized in Table 63.5, show that the age of infection is inversely related to the development of an asymptomatic infection and the development of a chronic infectious state. These results have been confirmed by others and underline the significant influence of age on the epidemiology of HBV infections.[52,55,56] Age at the time of initial infection is believed to be the most important factor

Age (years)	No. tested	Clinical hepatitis (%)	Chronic infection (%)
0–4	21[b]	10	29
5–9	61[b]	10	16
10–19	58[b]	10	7
20–29	22[b]	14	14
>30	27[b]	33	8

[a] Based on 189 (15%) of 1280 Yupik Eskimos who seroconverted for HBV infection between 1971 and 1976.
[b] $n = 26$ for those tested for chronicity.
Adapted from McMahon et al., 1985, with permission of University of Chicago Press.[54]

Table 63.5 HBV infection: effect of age in the development of clinically evident hepatitis and chronicity[a]

affecting prevalence. In areas where prevalence rates are high, the disease is acquired perinatally or at a very young age when it is most likely to become persistent. Chronically infected individuals represent a persistent reservoir for infection and contribute significantly over their lifespans to the maintenance of high endemicity. In areas of low endemicity, the infection is acquired in adulthood and is less likely to become chronic and generate high prevalence rates.

Hepatitis B virus has a worldwide distribution, but prevalence rates vary significantly from areas of high endemicity, mainly in developing countries, to areas of low endemicity in developed countries (Fig. 63.2).[52] Small pockets of high prevalence exist and may be associated with minority ethnic groups (e.g. Alaskan Yupik Eskimos). In a mobile society it is important to recognize these geographic differences because it is not unusual to care for patients emigrating from areas of high endemicity. In a recent study of a mid-western US community, chronic HBV infection was predominantly seen in immigrants from endemic parts of the world. It is likely that targeted screening of high-risk populations will be effective in identifying subjects who are at risk for complications of long-term HBV infection such as hepatocellular carcinoma (HCC), as well as susceptible individuals who are at risk of acquisition and thus most likely to benefit from vaccination.[57] Furthermore, prevalence of HBV genotypes varies in different regions of the USA. There is a strong correlation between HBV genotypes and ethnicity. These genotypes may account for the heterogeneity in disease manifestations among patients with chronic HBV infection.[35]

There are no environmental reservoirs (e.g. food, water) for HBV such as those for HAV. Also, there are no natural animal reservoirs, and humans are the principal source of HBV infection. The traditional route of transmission is parenteral, through contaminated transfused blood products or intravenous drug abuse. Transmission may also occur percutaneously or transmucosally from exposure to blood or other contaminated body fluids. Although HBsAg has been found in virtually every body fluid (e.g. feces, bile, breast milk, sweat, tears, vaginal secretions, urine), only blood, semen and saliva have been shown to contain infectious HBV particles.[58] Transmission from infected human bites has been documented, whereas transmission from feces has not.[59,60] The lack of fecal–oral transmission and the types of close contact required for transmission probably explain the infrequent appearance of epidemics.

The route of acquisition within the pediatric population can be divided into three relevant age groups: perinatal, infancy–childhood and adolescent–young adult.

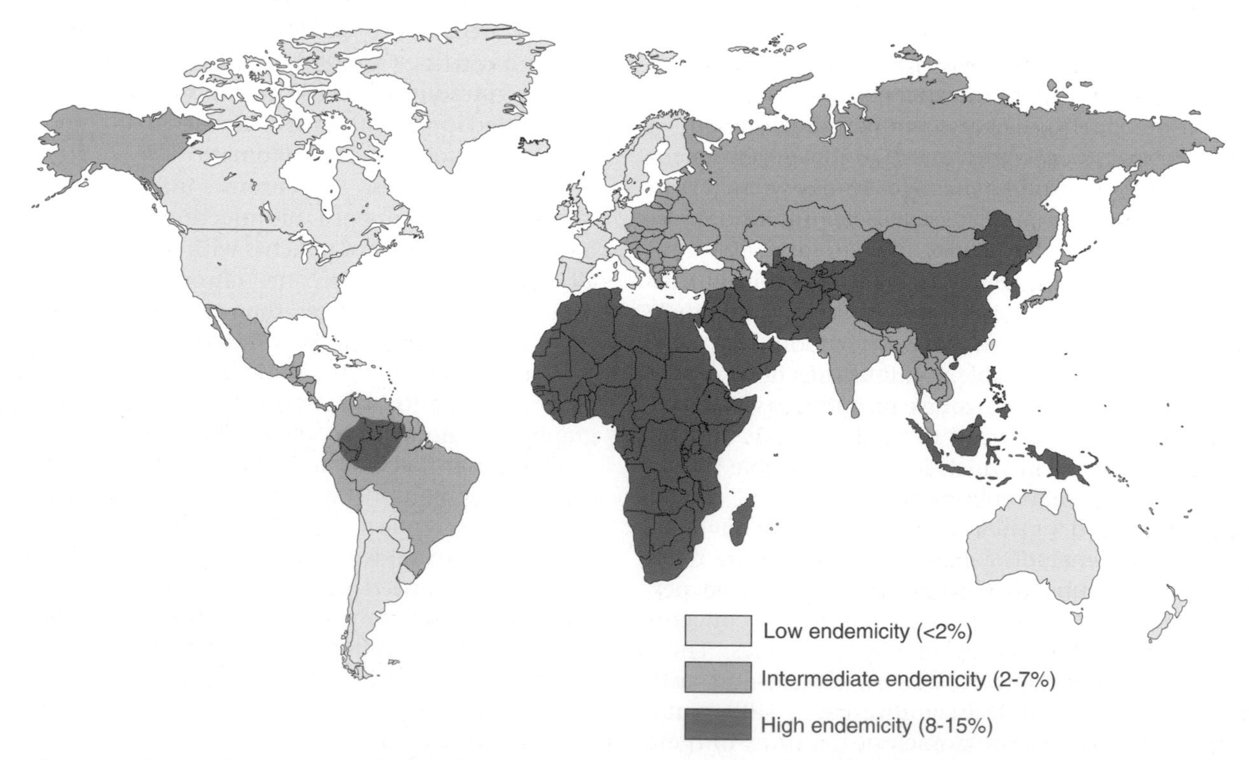

Figure 63.2: Geographic distribution of hepatitis B. (Adapted from Margolis HS et al., 1991, with permission.)[52]

Each year in the USA, 22 000 HBsAg-positive mothers give birth. Selective prenatal testing, based on the identification of known risk factors, is difficult and has shown an unacceptably low sensitivity (< 50%).[52] The failure of selective prenatal screening prompted recommendations for universal HBV screening of all pregnant women to identify at-risk newborns. The risk of perinatal or vertical transmission can be further defined by the mother's full serologic profile: mothers who are HBeAg positive have the highest rates of transmission (70–90%), whereas infants of mothers who are HBsAg positive but HBeAg negative have a lower risk (10–67%).[61–63] The presence of anti-HBe antibody in an HBsAg-positive mother does not always confer safety to her child; even though in most instances it signifies resolving disease, it may in rare cases predispose the newborn to fulminant hepatitis.[64–67] Acute maternal infection during the third trimester carries the highest risk of perinatal transmission.[55] *In utero* infections are rare, but have been described.[68] Perinatal acquisition is thought to occur during the birthing process because infection in newborns cannot be detected serologically for the first 1–3 months of age. It is postulated that during birth the infant comes into contact with infected maternal body fluids (most likely blood), although whether the virus crosses through the infant's mucosal membranes, intestinal tract or minor skin abrasions is still not known.

Infants and children who do not become infected perinatally from their HBsAg-positive mothers still remain at high risk of infection during the first 5 years of life.[69–71] This risk has been estimated in Asian children as 60% if the mother is HBeAg positive and as 40% if she is HBeAg negative.[69] Transmission in these instances was found to occur horizontally between children within the family.[71] HBsAg can be detected in breast milk, but whether infection can be transmitted through ingested breast milk or from swallowed maternal blood from injured nipples is unclear.[67]

Available data suggest that the risk of HBV transmission within the daycare setting, either between children or between caregivers and children, is low.[4,72,73] Current recommendations allow HBV-infected children to attend daycare unless they have other medical conditions or behaviors that would increase the risk of transmission.[73]

Nine percent of all cases of acute HBV reported to the Centers for Disease Control and Prevention occur in adolescents and young adults between 10 and 19 years of age.[4] In 60% of reported cases, no source of infection can be found. However, among the 40% with a reported source of infection, 50% of these are from sexual contact and 47% from intravenous drug abuse. The male : female ratio in adolescents is 0.7 : 1, but in adults it is 2 : 1.[4,52] The reasons for this ratio reversal are unclear, but perhaps reflect the earlier age of sexual activity in females.

The epidemiology of HBV infection allows the identification of certain high-risk groups, which are listed in Table 63.6.

Age (years)	Group
<11	Children of HBsAg-positive mothers (especially ages 0–5 years)
	Children of immigrants from highly endemic areas
	Adoptees from highly endemic areas
	Minority inner-city children
	Household contacts of HBV carriers
	Institutionalized children
≥11	Immigrants from highly endemic areas
	Sexually active adolescents, especially if multiple partners
	Intimate contacts of HBV carriers
	Intravenous drug abusers
	Homosexual males
	Prisoners
	Occupational exposure (e.g. healthcare)
	Travelers to highly endemic areas

Table 63.6 Groups at high risk for HBV infection

Acute HBV infection

Clinical course The clinical expression of acute HBV infection depends on the age at acquisition. The clinical course of a typically icteric and self-limiting acute HBV infection is portrayed in Figure 63.3. The incubation period ranges from 28 to 180 days (mean 80 days), after which the patient may develop a prodrome consisting of fever, anorexia, fatigue, malaise and nausea. In addition, during this period the child may present with immune-mediated extrahepatic manifestations, including migratory arthritis, angioedema, or a maculopapular or urticarial rash. Papular acrodermatitis of childhood or Gianotti–Crosti syndrome has been associated with HBV and may become evident during this period. The syndrome includes a characteristic 'lenticular, flat, erythematopapular' rash of the extremities, face and buttocks, and lymphadenitis associated with hepatitis.[74] It can be associated with other viral infections and is reported rarely in North America.[75] It is thought to be the result of circulating immune complexes.

After 1–2 weeks, most of the prodromal symptoms subside and clinically evident hepatitis develops, including, in many cases, jaundice, hepatosplenomegaly and pruritus.

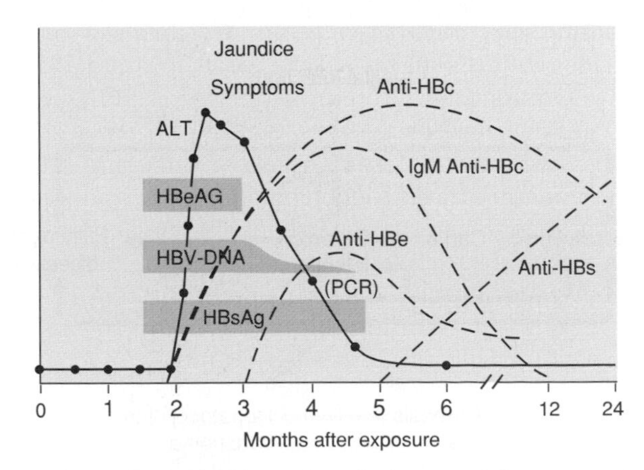

Figure 63.3: Typical clinical and serologic course of symptomatic acute hepatitis B. ALT, alanine aminotransferase; HBV, hepatitis B virus; HBsAg, hepatitis B surface antigen; HBeAg, hepatitis B e antigen; anti-HBc, anti-hepatitis B core antigen; PCR, polymerase chain reaction. (Reproduced from Hoofnagle JH, Di Bisceglie AM: Serologic diagnosis of acute and chronic viral hepatitis. Semin Liver Dis 1991; 11:73-83, with permission.)[26]

Intense fatigue is a common complaint during this period. Symptoms may persist for 1–2 months, and longer in a minority of patients.

Outcomes The potential outcomes of an acute HBV infection are outlined in Figure 63.4. The complications that may result from an acute infection with HBV include fulminant hepatitis or development of chronic infection. Chronic HBV infection is discussed below, along with the development of HCC. Any child with an acute fulminant HBV infection or a biphasic course should be investigated for concomitant HDV co-infection.

Chronic HBV infection

Chronic infection with HBV should be characterized as: HBeAg+ or HBeAg–, with or without detectable HBV-DNA, with or without raised levels of alanine aminotransferase (ALT), and activity and degree of fibrosis.

Terms such as 'asymptomatic' or 'healthy carrier state' are discouraged. 'Inactive carrier state' refers to a patient who is HBsAg+, HBeAg–, with a normal ALT concentration and HBV-DNA of less than 100 000 copies/ml. Resolved HBV should include normal ALT levels, absence of HBsAg and presence of anti-HBc (with or without anti-HBs) in serum.[76]

Clinical course Chronic HBV infections in children may present clinically in a variety of ways. Often, the infection is detected during the screening of asymptomatic children of HBV-positive mothers or other close household contacts. At other times the fortuitous discovery of raised aminotransferase levels in a child evaluated for an unrelated illness may lead to the diagnosis. Rarely, the infection may present initially in a child who already has well-established cirrhosis and end-stage liver disease, or the initial presentation may be that of HCC. Finally, chronic HBV infection should be included in the differential diagnosis of any child with hepatomegaly, jaundice or other signs of liver disease. Hepatitis D virus superinfection should be suspected in any patient with stable chronic HBV infection whose condition deteriorates suddenly.

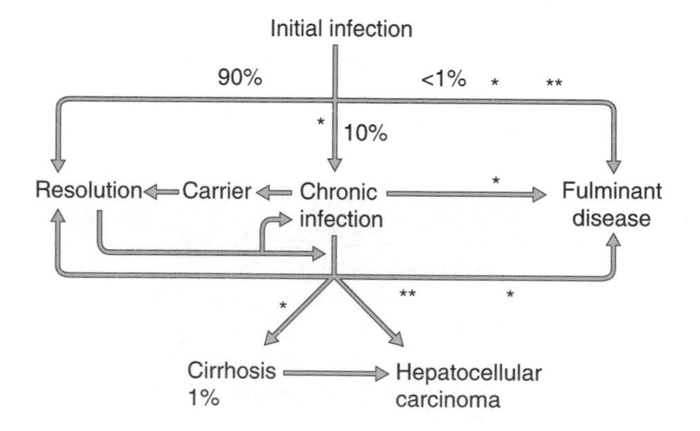

Figure 63.4: Potential outcomes of hepatitis B across all age groups.

Outcomes Cirrhosis, liver failure or HCC develops in approximately 15–40% of infected patients.[77] The natural history of chronic HBV infection in children has been partially defined. In a Chinese study of 51 asymptomatic HBsAg+ children followed for up to 4 years (mean 30 months), persistently high levels of viral replication were found but were associated with mild and stable liver disease.[78] Over the study period, 7% cleared HBeAg but all continued to be HBsAg+. In contrast, an Italian study observed 76 HBsAg+ children for up to 12 years (mean 5 years).[79] These researchers found that 70% of the study population lost serologic evidence of viral replication, with most of these (92%) normalizing liver function. Five patients became HBsAg–. These results are more favorable than those of the earlier Chinese study, but may reflect confounding variables such as differing epidemiologic backgrounds. Other pediatric reports have described a 10–14% annual seroconversion rate from HBeAg to anti-HBe, progression of liver disease over a longer follow-up period, and reactivation of viral replication after conversion to anti-HBe status in some chronically infected children.[80–83] It is difficult, owing to the number of variables, to compare these studies and draw broad conclusions.

Several studies in children with chronic HBV infection have shown cirrhosis in 3–5% of initial liver biopsy specimens.[79,84,85] In chronically infected adults with cirrhosis the estimated 5-year survival rate is 50%.[86] HBV-infected individuals with persistently normal aminotransferase levels carry little risk of developing cirrhosis.

Hepatocellular carcinoma

It is estimated that 320 000 new cases of HCC occur worldwide annually.[87] This is an important complication from the pediatric perspective, not only because it is a major cause of childhood malignancy in certain parts of the world such as Asia,[88] but also because the initial HBV infection in most patients with HCC occurred in childhood. Risk factors for the development of HCC include chronic infection with HBV, long duration of infection, male sex and the presence of cirrhosis.

The higher incidence of HBsAg positivity in the mothers than in the fathers of patients with HCC suggests that primary infection occurs perinatally or in early infancy.[89] This and other observations imply that the mean duration from primary infection to the development of HCC is 35 years.[90] However, reported cases in children, some as young as 8 months, raise the issue of different oncogenic mechanisms from those in adults.[91] A recent study following 426 children with chronic HBV infection revealed that, in 6250 person-years, two boys developed HCC. Both had e antigen seroconversion in early childhood and cirrhosis. Early e antigen seroconversion and/or cirrhosis may be risk factors for the development of HCC.[92]

Extrahepatic manifestations

Circulating immune complexes including HBsAg–anti-HBs complexes are reported to be responsible for the appearance of extrahepatic manifestations. Essential mixed cryoglobulinemia, polyarteritis nodosa and glomerulonephritis have been described in association with chronic HBV infection[93–96] and may even be the presenting signs of infection.

Diagnosis of acute and chronic hepatitis B

HBsAg is the first serologic marker to appear and, when sensitive assays are used, may be detected within 1–2 weeks after exposure. It precedes the development of symptoms by an average of 4 weeks.[97] The presence of HBsAg indicates ongoing infection. Qualitative but not quantitative methods are used by most clinical laboratories, because the amount of antigen does not correlate with disease activity or with the presence of an acute or chronic infection.[26] Some symptomatic patients may have self-limiting acute HBV infection without detectable HBsAg. These patients, up to 9% in some studies, have other detectable markers of infection.[97] HBeAg appears virtually simultaneously, peaks, and then declines in parallel with HBsAg. It usually disappears before HBsAg. Adult patients who remain persistently positive for HBcAg for more than 10 weeks are likely to become chronically infected. HBeAg indicates a high level of viral replication and infectivity. Most patients with undetectable HBeAg have either resolving, minimal or no active liver disease.[26] Pre-core mutants of HBV do not express HBeAg; they may be responsible for a more severe course and, in some cases, fulminant disease. Serum aminotransferase levels become raised, but are non-specific. They begin to increase just before the development of symptoms and then peak (sometimes 20 times or more higher than normal) with the development of jaundice.

The diagnosis of chronic HBV infection is based on the persistence of appropriate markers for at least 6 months or on detection of these markers in a child who on initial presentation has historic or physical evidence of longstanding infection. This information is summarized in Figures 63.3 and 63.5 and in Tables 63.4 and 63.7.

The third marker of disease to appear is HBV viral DNA (HBV-DNA), which appears with HBsAg, peaks with the onset of symptoms and then declines. Its quantitative value is also useful in determining disease activity, 'viral load' and potential response to therapy. Anti-HBc is the fourth serologic marker to appear. It can usually be detected 3–5 weeks after the appearance of HBsAg, but before the onset of symptoms; it persists for life. Detection of anti-HBc indicates ongoing or past infection. Anti-HBc does not appear after HBV vaccination and can be helpful in distinguishing between immunity from vaccination and that from natural infection.

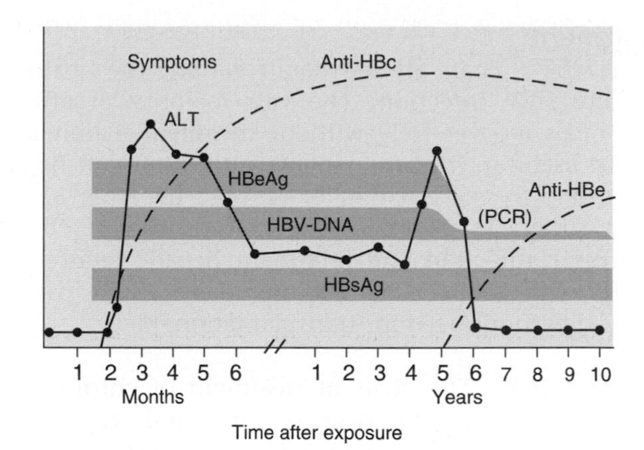

Figure 63.5: Typical clinical and serologic course of chronic hepatitis B. ALT, alanine aminotransferase; HBV, hepatitis B virus; HBsAg, hepatitis B surface antigen; HBeAg, hepatitis B e antigen; anti-HBc, anti-hepatitis B core antigen; PCR, polymerase chain reaction. (Reproduced from Hoofnagle JH, Di Bisceglie AM: Serologic diagnosis of acute and chronic viral hepatitis. Semin Liver Dis 1991; 11:73-83, with permission.)[26]

Anti-HBs confers protective immunity and indicates resolving or past infection. In the majority of patients with self-limiting infection it can be detected only after HBsAg becomes undetectable. In a minority of patients with serum sickness-like symptoms (arthralgia, rash), it may appear before the onset of clinical symptoms.[98,99] A 'window' of variable duration has been described in some patients, during which HBsAg has disappeared and anti-HBs cannot yet be detected.[97] The determination of anti-HBc may be helpful in these instances.

Antibody to HBeAg (anti-HBe) appears after HBeAg becomes undetectable and persists for 1–2 years after the resolution of hepatitis. The various markers of HBV are summarized in Table 63.4.

HBsAg	HBeAg	Anti-HBs	Anti-HBc	Anti-HBe	Interpretation
+	±	−	−	−	Early acute disease or carrier state
+	±	−	+	−	Acute disease, chronic disease or carrier state
+	−	−	+	−	Late acute disease or carrier state
+	−	−	+	+	Early resolution or 'e-minus' disease
−	−	−	+	−	Early resolution or 'window' period
−	−	+	+	+	Resolution
−	−	+	+	−	Immunity from past infection
−	−	+	−	−	Immunity from HBV vaccine

[a] Exceptions are described in the text.
HBV-DNA is of limited usefulness in this context, except in specific circumstances (see text).

Table 63.7 Guidelines for the serologic diagnosis and staging of HBV infections[a]

Treatment

Acute HBV There are few data regarding the treatment of acute HBV infection. The vast majority of affected individuals recover fully without treatment. Lamivudine may be useful in treating patients with fulminant hepatic failure due to exacerbation of chronic hepatitis B. In a recent study, 24 patients with exacerbation of chronic hepatitis B infection and fulminant hepatic failure were treated with lamivudine 100 mg daily. Eight patients survived without need for transplantation.[100]

Chronic HBV The goals of treatment of chronic HBV include cessation or decrease in viral replication, normalization of aminotransferase levels and liver histopathology, as well as prevention of cirrhosis and HCC. None of the medications currently licensed in the USA fulfills these goals for all children. For this reason, appropriate patient selection is critical so those children who are most likely to benefit from therapy are identified. Children to be treated must display evidence of chronic HBV infection, that is, detectable serum HBsAg for at least 6 months, and evidence of active viral replication, i.e. HBeAg and/or HBV-DNA. In addition, children most likely to respond to treatment are those with consistently abnormal ALT values. Before starting treatment, a liver biopsy is helpful to establish the extent and stage of liver disease, and to rule out any other potential disease processes. 'Background rates' of seroconversion must also be considered in making a decision regarding whom and when to treat. There are currently two licensed medications for treatment of chronic HBV infection in children in the USA: interferon-α (IFN-α) and lamivudine.

Since the first report in 1976 of treatment with pharmacologic doses of interferon, a number of studies in adults using mainly IFN-α have been published. They have used a variety of treatment regimens in terms of dosage, length of treatment and use of adjuvant therapies, such as 'steroid priming'.[101] Adult studies have shown that the greatest effectiveness was achieved at doses of 5–10 MU three times a week.[102] Most studies define a favorable response to therapy as the sustained loss of HBeAg and HBV-DNA and normalization of aminotransferase levels. In many patients who eventually clear HBeAg and HBV-DNA, a transient increase in serum aminotransferase levels may occur between the first and third months of treatment. It is thought that this increase corresponds to activation of the host immune response and early clearance of HBV-DNA. Approximately half of the 'responders' will eventually clear HBsAg and acquire anti-HBs. The duration of therapy is variable, with at least 6 months in most studies.

In adults, predictors of a beneficial response to treatment have been identified and include raised serum aspartate aminotransferase levels and low HBV-DNA levels.[103] Other positive predictive factors include a short duration of infection, histologically active disease and immunocompetency.[101] Our understanding of the benefits of IFN-α in the treatment of adults with chronic HBV infection is best summarized in a report by Wong et al.[104] In this meta-analysis of 15 previously published randomized controlled trials, the authors showed that 36% of 498 treated patients lost HBV-DNA and 32% lost HBeAg, compared with 16% of 339 controls who lost HBV-DNA and 12% who lost HBeAg.

The results of therapy in 330 children have now been reported in eight separate pediatric trials.[102,105] Comparison of the study parameters among these studies has shown a great degree of variability. These parameters have included choice of the study population (European or Chinese children), IFN dosage regimen (range 3–10 MU/m^2 subcutaneously, thrice weekly) and duration of therapy (range 12–48 weeks). In the studies of European children, 36% of treated children (n = 124; range 20–50%) lost HBeAg, compared with 14% of controls (n = 92; range 9–25%). These results are comparable to those found in adults. In Chinese children the response rate was much lower: 9% in 72 treated children *vs* 5% in 42 controls. Genetic factors, the presence of mutant strains, perinatally acquired disease and a long duration of infection in these Chinese children have all been postulated to justify these striking differences. The poorer response rate of Chinese children to IFN therapy is not well understood, but may be an artifact of the inclusion of a large number of children with normal ALT values. In Asian children with consistently abnormal ALT values, response rates may be similar to those of Western children.

Children rarely need to discontinue IFN-α therapy because of side-effects. Almost all children have an initial and transient influenza-like syndrome (fever, myalgia, headache, arthralgia and anorexia). Starting at a low dose and increasing over a week to the recommended dose of 6 MU/m^2 can ameliorate these side-effects. Other side-effects include bone marrow suppression, especially neutropenia. Changes in personality and irritability are reported more frequently in children than in adults. These changes are reversible on withdrawal of treatment. Other reported side-effects are febrile seizures and markedly increased levels of aminotransferases.

Lamivudine is an orally administered nucleoside analog. A clinical trial in children showed that the rate of virologic response after 52 weeks of treatment was higher among children who received lamivudine than among those who received placebo (23% *vs* 13%, P = 0.04). Lamivudine therapy was well tolerated, and also associated with higher rates of seroconversion from hepatitis B e antigen to hepatitis B e antibody, normalization of ALT levels and suppression of HBV-DNA.[106] As with IFN, children with higher ALT values have a higher likelihood of virologic response to lamivudine. Response rates to lamivudine are independent of previous IFN-α therapy. Adverse events to lamivudine are rare. However, the long-term use of lamivudine is limited by the development of viral resistance. The optimal duration of lamivudine therapy for children is unclear. It should be used for at least 1 year, and probably for at least 6 months after HBeAg to anti-HBe seroconversion.

Passive prophylaxis

A detailed discussion of HBV immunoprophylaxis is given in the American Academy of Pediatrics Red Book.[107] Hepatitis B serum immune globulin (HBIG) is prepared from pooled plasma from donors seropositive for anti-HBS. It has a high titer of anti-HBS (> 1 : 100 000). Its protective value is excellent when given as soon as possible after exposure and persists for 3–6 months. Its effect is doubtful, however, when given more than 7 days after exposure. HBIG is indicated for single instances of exposure, such as needlestick accidents, sexual contact and perinatal exposure. It should be paired with HBV vaccine in cases of repeated or prolonged exposure, such as in healthcare employees, intimate household contacts and neonates of infected mothers.

Active prophylaxis

The first vaccine against hepatitis B was prepared from human plasma of chronic HBV carriers and released in the USA in 1982. It has since been replaced by recombinant vaccines prepared by introducing an HBsAg gene-containing plasmid into baker's yeast (*Saccharomyces cerevisiae*). Recommended schedules involve three intra-deltoid injections over a 6-month period.[199] Combination vaccines for children that will include the HBV vaccine are under development. The vaccine is considered very safe; rare complications include anaphylaxis and Guillain–Barré syndrome.[29] The vaccine induces the production of anti-HBs, and the vaccine manufacturers report protective titers in 95–99% of healthy children who receive the full schedule of injections.

Initial immunization policies in the USA targeted individuals at high risk, such as newborns of seropositive mothers, illicit drug abusers and homosexual males. However, it became apparent that this strategy was ineffective in reducing the incidence of hepatitis B, and in 1991 the Centers for Disease Control and Prevention issued new recommendations.[108] This new three-part strategy recommends prevention of mother to infant transmission through prenatal testing of all pregnant women, universal vaccination of all infants and children by the age of 11 years, and immunization of adolescents and adults in high-risk groups such as teenagers with multiple sexual partners and homosexual males. The long-term effectiveness of HBV vaccine, even in those who have lost detectable anti-HBs, does not support the administration of late booster doses; however, when exposure is clearly documented and titers are low, it is reasonable to administer HBIG and a booster dose of HBV vaccine.[31]

A mass hepatitis B vaccination program, conducted by the government of Taiwan, was started in 1984. The success of this program has led to a decline in hepatitis B carrier rates among children in Taiwan, from 10% to less than 1%. Furthermore, the mortality rate of fulminant hepatitis in infants and the annual incidence of childhood hepatoma have also decreased significantly. This is a remarkable success story in public health.[109]

Hepatitis C

A third form of infectious hepatitis, not due to hepatitis A or B ('non-A, non-B hepatitis'; NANB), was first recognized epidemiologically in 1974 and was linked to transfused blood products in 1975.[99,110] In 1989, the cloned complementary DNA (cDNA) of RNA recovered from chimpanzees infected with post-transfusion NANB hepatitis was isolated.[111] This cDNA and its expressed antigen were linked etiologically to post-transfusion NANB hepatitis through the development of an antigen–antibody assay;[112] this long-suspected virus is now called the hepatitis C virus (HCV). This immunologic assay against HCV (anti-HCV) allowed the demonstration that HCV was the major cause of post-transfusion NANB and sporadic NANB hepatitis.[113]

Biology and pathogenesis

It has been suggested, based on its physical properties and similarity to other viruses, that HCV be considered a new genus within the flavivirus family. HCV is a 55-nm diameter lipid-enveloped virus with a 33-nm inner nucleocapsid. The genome is a linear, single-stranded, positive-sense RNA approximately 9400 nucleotides in length. *In vitro* translation of the genome results in three structural and four nonstructural proteins.

The genome is highly susceptible to mutations, and comparison of different HCV isolates has shown nucleotide sequence variation confined to specific areas. This has allowed the identification of six major genotypes and a number of subtypes based on major and minor genomic differences.[114,115] Genotype determination has already provided useful information with regard to prognosis and response to therapy. Type 1 has been shown to be particularly resistant to antiviral therapy.[114,116] Mapping of the geographic distribution of the known genotypes shows that types 1 (a and b) and 2 are the most prevalent genotypes in North America and western Europe.[114,116] This may have clinical significance for the development of effective vaccines.

Chronic HCV infection is not the consequence of the direct destruction of hepatic cells by the virus. Rather, it results from an intermediate immune response that is large enough to induce hepatic cell destruction and fibrosis, but not sufficient to eradicate the virus.[117] Patients with a poor response in the acute phase are often asymptomatic and are more likely to become chronic carriers than are those with a good response.

Epidemiology

The distribution of HCV, like that of HAV and HBV, is worldwide, but the prevalence rates appear to be evenly distributed, ranging from 0.3% to 1.5% when assessed among adult volunteer blood donors.[118] In the USA, HCV is associated with 40% of cases of chronic liver disease and with 8000 to 10 000 deaths each year.[119] Only a small proportion of HCV-infected individuals are children, and there are few, if any, manifestations of this infection during childhood. The incidence of HCV-associated disease has been declining since 1989, which corresponds to the development of the first serologic screening tools.[120]

The majority of cases of NANB hepatitis in adults (50–90%) have been attributed to HCV.[118,121,122] Bortolotti et al.[123] have compiled data to show that anti-HCV prevalence rates in children with NANB hepatitis are 60–65% in children with thalassemia, 59–95% in those with hemophilia and 52–72% in survivors of leukemia. As the transmission of HCV via transfusion of blood and blood products has been virtually eliminated, these rates have substantially decreased in developed countries.

Although infection with HCV is far less common on a worldwide basis than infection with HAV or HBV, its propensity to become chronic has resulted in HCV becoming a major cause of chronic hepatitis. In the USA, it is responsible for 65% of all cases of chronic viral hepatitis and 35% of all cases of chronic liver disease and cirrhosis.[120] Most HCV-infected children develop chronic hepatitis, and, although rare, cirrhosis and end-stage liver disease can occur during childhood.

There does not appear to be an epidemiologically relevant reservoir for HCV other than humans. The typical route of transmission is parenteral. Transmission may be divided into percutaneous (e.g. blood transfusions, intravenous drug abuse) and non-percutaneous (e.g. intrafamilial and sexual routes).

Historically, the transmission of HCV has been associated with the transfusion of blood and blood products. With the advent of routine blood screening for HCV antibodies (in 1991 in most countries), transfusion-related HCV has almost disappeared. Blood products such as factor concentrates have also been made safer through the development of improved inactivation procedures. However, this route of transmission is no longer a factor and perinatal transmission has become the major route of HCV acquisition in childhood.[124]

The proportion of cases attributable to intravenous drug abuse has been increasing and may be as high as 60% of new HCV infections.[125] This is due in part to the declining risk of transmission from blood products, but also to the increasing frequency of drug abuse. The prevalence of anti-HCV among intravenous drug abusers ranges from 60% to 90%.[118] Intravenous drug abuse in mothers also imposes a significant risk to their children; in one study this association was found in 6% of pediatric HCV cases.[126]

Occupational exposure in healthcare professionals occurs from percutaneous transmission of contaminated blood in instances of accidental needlestick injury. The risk of infection from a single needlestick from an HCV-RNA-positive patient is 10% and the disease is usually symptomatic.[127] Skin tattooing has become increasingly popular among adolescents and has been associated with the transmission of HCV.[128]

Non-percutaneous transmission This mode of transmission pertains to all cases that cannot be attributed to percutaneous transfer of HCV. This includes cases of perinatal and sexual transmission, intrafamilial and occupational spread, and sporadic cases in which no mode of transmission can be found. Although transmission of HCV through contaminated blood has been well established, the role of other body fluids as vehicles of transmission has not. Several studies have failed to detect the presence of HCV-RNA in the semen, saliva, urine, stool or vaginal secretions of patients with chronic HCV infection, leaving uncertainty surrounding the mechanism of transmission in cases of non-percutaneously transmitted infection.[129,130]

Acute HCV

Clinical course Acute hepatitis due to HCV appears to be an uncommon presentation in childhood, with most cases diagnosed once the chronic state has already been well established.[123] This implies that the majority of initial HCV infections in children are asymptomatic. When it presents acutely, HCV infection cannot be distinguished on clinical grounds from other forms of viral hepatitis. Acute self-limiting disease is the outcome in 15–50% of adults;[26,131] the percentage of resolving disease in children is unknown. Some individuals infected with HCV experience multiple episodes of acute hepatitis. Results of primate experimentation have shown that 'relapse' may be the result of re-infection with a different strain of HCV or lack of complete protective immunity resulting in re-infection (or reactivation) with a homologous strain.[132,133]

Outcomes and complications Evolution of acute HCV to fulminant hepatitis is rare, but co-infection with other hepatropic viruses (e.g. HBV) may accelerate progression.[127,134] The most common complication of a primary infection with HCV is the development of a chronic infection.

Chronic HCV

Clinical course The natural history of HCV disease in children remains incompletely defined. HCV infection is usually asymptomatic in children, and most HCV-infected children develop chronic hepatitis. The characteristics and evolution of HCV were studied retrospectively in 224 children with HCV at seven European centers.[135] Of 200 children followed for a mean of 6.2 years, only 12 (6%) achieved sustained viremia clearance and normalization of the ALT level. Older adolescents and young adults had a significantly higher rate of fibrosis than did younger children. Extrahepatic manifestations were rare. As in adults, HCV is a mild disease in children, independent of the source of infection. Severe activity and cirrhosis account for approximately 2% of cases. The relatively benign natural history of HCV infection in childhood may, however, cause significant morbidity and mortality later in life due to chronic inflammation and hepatic damage. Given the chronicity of this infection and the long-term risk of developing cirrhosis and HCC, children with HCV need to be identified and followed up regularly. However, no pediatric studies to date have evaluated the effect of treatment on outcomes of cirrhosis or HCC.

Diagnosis of acute and chronic HCV

Virus-specific serology is required for the accurate diagnosis of HCV infection. The serologic course of HCV disease is shown in Figure 63.6. Serum aminotransferase levels begin to rise with the development of symptoms and jaundice. They rise rapidly and then decline in a fashion that may be either monophasic and rapid or multiphasic, with wide fluctuations and a more protracted course. The multiphasic pattern may portend more severe disease or progression to a chronic state.[118,127] Assays for the detec-

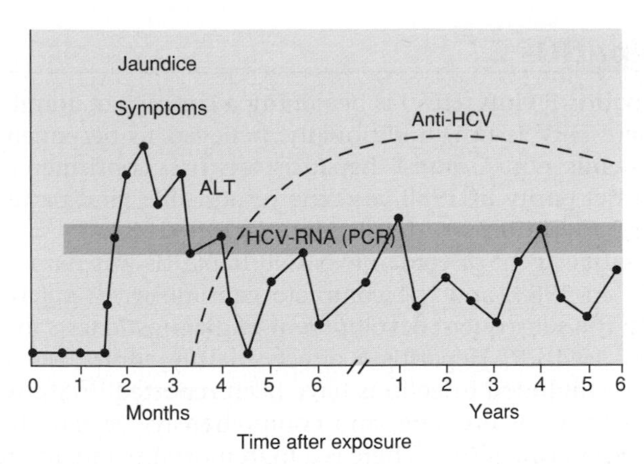

Figure 63.6: Typical clinical and serologic course of symptomatic acute hepatitis C. ALT, alanine aminotransferase; HCV, hepatitis C virus; PCR, polymerase chain reaction. (Reproduced from Hoofnagle JH, Di Bisceglie AM: Serologic diagnosis of acute and chronic viral hepatitis. Semin Liver Dis 1991; 11:73-83, with permission.)[26]

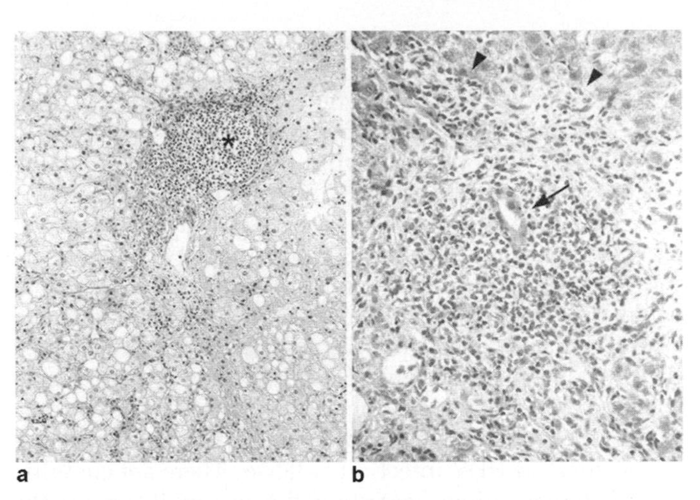

Figure 63.7: Histologic findings of HCV infection. Photomicrograph of the liver from a child with chronic hepatitis C. The characteristic histopathologic lesions include portal lymphoid aggregates or follicles (asterisk), sinusoidal lymphocytes and steatosis (**a**). Necrosis and inflammation are usually mild. At higher power (**b**) the typical bile duct injury is seen (arrow). Interface hepatitis (arrowheads) is present in this case.

tion of HCV antigens are not available, owing to the low concentrations of virus in the blood; diagnosis depends on the detection of antibodies to viral proteins (anti-HCV) and the viral genome (HCV-RNA) (see Table 63.4).

A third-generation enzyme-linked immunosorbent assay (ELISA) detects antibodies to multiple, immunodominant, structural and non-structural proteins of HCV. A positive anti-HCV finding indicates current or past infection. A negative anti-HCV finding does not exclude infection in its early stages, and neither does it exclude past infection because it may disappear in patients whose disease has resolved. False-positive results are seen in patients with autoimmune disorders. HCV-RNA is the earliest detectable marker in the blood of patients with hepatitis C. It can be detected during the incubation period, before the development of symptoms. It is detected by the polymerase chain reaction (PCR), which can detect as few as 1 to 10 molecules of nucleic acid.[26] PCR testing for HCV-RNA is the primary method available for direct assay of the presence of HCV, which is the most reliable measure of active infection;[136] in the absence of anti-HCV, this may be the only test to detect early acute hepatitis C or infection in individuals who cannot mount an antibody response (e.g. immunocompromised patients). Persistence of HCV-RNA beyond 6 months indicates chronic infection, and its loss correlates with resolved disease. Quantitation of HCV-RNA is helpful primarily in determining the response to therapy.

Histologic features of chronic hepatitis C infection are similar to those reported in adults. Necrosis and inflammation are usually mild; however, fibrosis is common and appears to progress with increasing age and duration of infection[137] (Fig. 63.7).

Treatment

Acute HCV Treatment of acute hepatitis C in adults with interferon-α-2b prevents chronicity in nearly all cases when therapy is initiated within 3 months of exposure.[138]

Chronic HCV All patients with chronic HCV are potential candidates for treatment.[139] Treatment is recommended in patients with detectable HCV-RNA and at least moderate inflammation with bridging or portal fibrosis on biopsy. However, children with less advanced liver disease may be considered for treatment to prevent progression, if they are at least 3 years of age, have documented chronic infection and no contraindications to therapy.

Combination therapy with pegylated interferon-α and ribavirin, a nucleoside analog, is now the standard of care in adults. The long-term sustained virologic response (SVR) rates are 40–50%.[140] Combination therapy with interferon-α-2b (Intron-A®) and ribavirin (Rebetol®) has recently been approved in the USA for use in children as young as 3 years of age. Suoglu et al.[141] reported a combination trial in children (IFN- -2b plus ribavirin for 12 months) that was associated with a SVR of 41.7%.

Predictors of SVR include short duration of infection, low HCV-RNA concentration, absence of cirrhosis and favorable genotype (i.e. types 2 and 3).[142] Contraindications to IFN include decompensated cirrhosis, illicit drug use, alcohol use, autoimmune disease, and other medical or neuropyschiatric conditions. Contraindications to ribavirin include renal failure, anemia, hemoglobinopathies and severe heart disease. IFN causes influenza-like symptoms early in the course of treatment. Depression and thyroid hyperfunction or hypofunction are also common. Neutropenia can be seen with IFN.[143,144] Ribavirin causes hemolytic anemia, which may be mild or severe.[145]

Hepatitis D

The hepatitis D virus (HDV), a small defective RNA virus, is dependent on HBV and can cause simultaneous infection in individuals with HBV or superinfection in chronic HBV carriers (Figs 63.8 & 63.9). Superinfection by HDV leads to acute hepatitis and causes progression to liver cirrhosis in a significant proportion of HBsAg carriers. Although HDV has been shown to have a direct cytopathic effect on liver cells, this alone is inconsistent with the existence of a well-described HDV carrier state.[146,147] Immune-mediated mechanisms of hepatocyte injury are also suspected. The outcomes for both the acute and chronic forms of HDV infection are more severe than for HBV alone. The mortality rate from acute HDV infections ranges from 2% to 20%, compared with less than 1% for acute HBV infections.[148] Cirrhosis may develop rapidly (within 2 years) in 15%, and in 70–80% over the long term, compared with 10% in patients with chronic hepatitis B infection.[148] The only agent that has had a beneficial effect in HDV infection is IFN-α. There are currently no recommendations regarding the use of IFN-α for the treatment of chronic HDV infection in children.

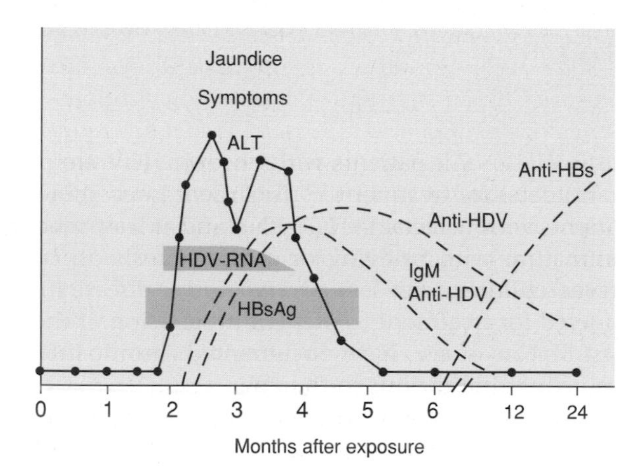

Figure 63.8: Typical clinical and serologic course of hepatitis D co-infection. ALT, alanine aminotransferase; HDV, hepatitis D virus; HBsAg, hepatitis B surface antigen. (Reproduced from Hoofnagle JH, Di Bisceglie AM: Serologic diagnosis of acute and chronic viral hepatitis. Semin Liver Dis 1991; 11:73-83, with permission.)[26]

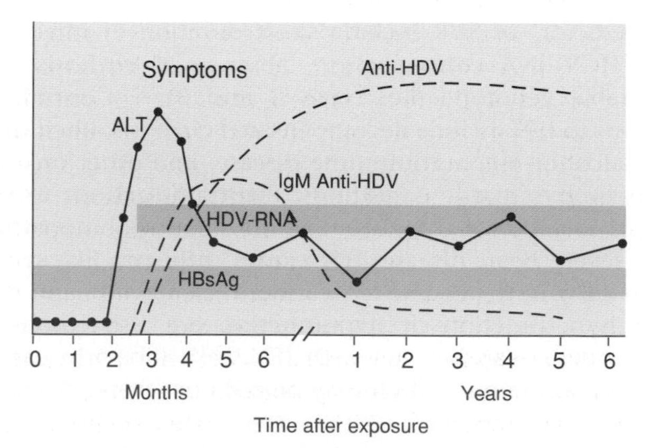

Figure 63.9: Typical clinical and serologic course of hepatitis D superinfection. ALT, alanine aminotransferase; HDV, hepatitis D virus; HBsAg, hepatitis B surface antigen. (Reproduced from Hoofnagle JH, Di Bisceglie AM: Serologic diagnosis of acute and chronic viral hepatitis. Semin Liver Dis 1991; 11:73-83, with permission.)[26]

Hepatitis E

Hepatitis E virus (HEV) is becoming a concern in countries where HEV is not, traditionally, believed to be endemic. Epidemic non-A, non-B hepatitis was first confirmed as a distinct entity in 1982, and the responsible viral particles were identified in fecal material in 1983.[149,150] The causative agent of epidemic NANB hepatitis was named as HEV in 1988, and the complete genome was sequenced with the subsequent development of diagnostic tests in the early 1990s.[151] Hepatitis E affects mainly adults, but isolated childhood infections have been reported.[152] Study of this disease is ongoing, and comprehensive reviews have been published.[153,154] There is a high mortality rate in pregnant women.

Hepatitis non-A–E

In one study of 79 patients with post-transfusion-associated hepatitis, ten (13%) failed to show evidence of any of the known hepatitis viruses.[155] It is clear that other, still to be identified, agents can be responsible for clinically evident hepatitis. Consequently, it can be expected, especially with further refinements in molecular biology techniques, that the 'hepatitis alphabet' will continue to expand, as will our knowledge of infectious hepatitis.

Epstein–Barr virus

Epstein–Barr virus (EBV) is a gamma-herpesvirus in the family of Herpesviridae. It is the principal cause of infectious mononucleosis, but it is also responsible for significant disease in immunocompromised patients such as children with the acquired immune deficiency syndrome (AIDS) or those who have undergone organ transplantation. EBV has also been linked to the development of tumors and lymphoproliferative disorders, especially in the immunosuppressed post-transplant patient.

Infectious mononucleosis in otherwise healthy children is generally a mild disease.[156] In addition to generalized symptoms of malaise, fatigue, pharyngitis and nausea, hepatitis is common, with hepatomegaly found in 10–15%. Serum aminotransferase levels are raised in 80% of children, but jaundice becomes apparent in less than 5%. Major symptoms typically persist for 2–4 weeks and then gradually recede. The prognosis is generally excellent; once the diagnosis is established, the hepatic component need be followed only clinically. Diagnosis is strongly suspected based on clinical findings of exudative pharyngitis, lymphadenopathy, hepatosplenomegaly and peripheral atypical lymphocytosis. The diagnosis is confirmed by the detection of heterophil and/or EBV-specific antibodies. EBV, like other herpesviruses, establishes a persistent latent infection after the primary illness.

Cytomegalovirus

Cytomegalovirus (CMV) is the largest of the herpesviruses, with a diameter of 200 nm. Infection with CMV can be acquired by intrauterine, perinatal, intrafamilial or sexual transmission, as well as by transfusion or organ transplantation.[157] CMV-DNA persists after primary infection, and multiple reactivations can occur that are normally con trolled by a host cell-mediated immune response. In immunocompetent individuals the primary infection and subsequent reactivations are generally asymptomatic but may be responsible for an infectious mononucleosis-type picture with mild hepatic involvement.

From a pediatric perspective, congenital CMV infections and infections in immunocompromised children are especially important. In these instances a severe and/or chronic condition can ensue. Newborns with congenital CMV infection frequently have hepatic involvement, with hepatosplenomegaly in 60%, jaundice in 67% and purpura in 13%.[158] The degree of jaundice is attributed to both the hepatitis and hemolytic anemia. The hepatitis may persist. but rarely progresses to cirrhosis.[157]

The prototypical CMV infection in immunocompromised children occurs in those who have received an organ transplant. The source of infection may be the grafted organ, transfused blood products or reactivation of a latent infection. CMV infection in this instance may cause hepatitis, which in the liver transplant patient, for example, may be difficult to distinguish from rejection or vascular compromise of the graft. In these children the infection may become persistent and lead to liver failure.[159]

Diagnosis is best established by isolation of CMV from urine, saliva or biopsy tissues, or from other body secretions. Total antibodies against CMV may also be assayed, but results may be confounded in the polytransfused child and in the neonate from circulating 'foreign' IgG antibodies. Antibodies directed against CMV may be helpful in diagnosing a primary infection by determining the presence of IgM and seroconversion from IgM to IgG. In limited instances, PCR to detect the CMV genome may be helpful. In the presence of hepatitis, and when clinically indicated, characteristic intranuclear inclusion bodies can be found on histologic examination of liver biopsy specimens.

AUTOIMMUNE HEPATITIS

Definition and classification

In children there are three liver diseases in which damage is likely to result from an autoimmune attack: autoimmune hepatitis (AIH), autoimmune sclerosing cholangitis overlap syndrome and *de novo* autoimmune hepatitis after liver transplantation. AIH, which has been described since the early 1950s, is a chronic necroinflammatory hepatitis of unknown etiology. It is characterized histologically by dense mononuclear and plasma cell infiltrates in the portal tracts, and serologically by autoantibodies targeted against liver- or organ-specific antigens.

Two main types of AIH have been described: type I or classic (AIH-I), and type II or anti-liver–kidney microsome-1 (anti-LKM-1) autoimmune hepatitis (AIH-II). The distinction is made according to differing profiles of circulating autoantibodies (Table 63.8). A third type of autoimmune hepatitis, characterized by antibodies against soluble liver antigens, has been proposed (AIH-III),[160] but has not been universally accepted, and many include this third type as a subset of AIH-I.[161] An overlapping syndrome between AIH and sclerosing cholangitis has been reported in both children and adults. In fact, one study showed that 40% of patients with sclerosing cholangitis had clinical, biochemical, immunologic and histologic features that are indistinguishable from those of AIH.[162]

Type	Characteristic autoantibodies	Occasionally present autoantibodies
I. Classic AIH	Antinuclear	Antimitochondrial
	Anti-smooth muscle	Anti-soluble liver antigen
	Antiactin	Anti-liver–pancreas protein
	Anti-asialoglyco-protein receptor	Anti-neutrophil cytoplasmic
II. Anti-LKM-1 AIH	Anti-LKM-1	Anti-liver cytosol[a]
	Anti-liver cytosol-1	Antinuclear[a]

[a] Rare.
LKM-1, liver–kidney microsome-1.
Adapted from Krawitt, 1996, with permission.[161]

Table 63.8 Classification of autoimmune hepatitis (AIH)

Pathogenesis

A conceptual framework for the pathogenesis of AIH has been proposed and involves a genetically predisposed individual exposed to an environmental agent. This agent triggers an autoimmune response targeted against liver antigens and results in a chronic hepatic necroinflammatory response, leading to fibrosis and cirrhosis.[161]

The search for predisposing genetic factors has focused on the major histocompatibility complex on chromosome 6, and in particular on the HLA-DR region. Susceptibility to AIH has been linked to two histocompatibility genes, *DR3* and *DR4*. It has been shown that the association with HLA-DR3 predisposes to more severe disease, which appears at an earlier age and results more frequently in liver transplantation.[163] A partial deficiency of the complement component C4, which is coded at the HLA-DR3 locus, has been described in some children with AIH. C4 plays a role in virus neutralization, and this type of deficiency may lead to the development of autoimmunity.[164]

The environmental triggers presumed to initiate AIH are unknown, but several viral candidates have been proposed based on reported evidence. These include rubella, Epstein–Barr virus and the hepatotropic viruses A, B and C.

The target antigen for AIH-I has not been identified, and none of the diagnostic autoantibodies for AIH-I appears to be pathogenic. Anti-LKM-1 antibodies recognize the cytochrome mono-oxygenase P450IID6 expressed on hepatocyte membrane surfaces, and this protein is the pathogenic autoantigen in AIH-II.[160]

Clinical course and outcomes

AIH affects both children and adults, with two peaks of incidence at 10–20 and 45–70 years of age.[164] AIH-I represents 80% of all cases in adults.[160] AIH-II usually affects children and young adults. AIH was originally described as a disease of young women, but more recent reports have identified a broad range among patients. AIH-II is almost exclusively a disease of younger women. Half of the patients with AIH present between 10 and 20 years of age. Its course can be particularly severe and rapidly progressive. More recently, cases of fulminant hepatitis in young children have been ascribed to AIH.[165]

Although AIH may present acutely, it always becomes chronic and it is not necessary to wait for 6 months to confirm chronicity.[164] The clinical features are heterogeneous and cover the spectrum from asymptomatic patients in whom hepatitis is an incidental biochemical finding to patients with fulminant hepatitis and liver failure.[161] The differential diagnosis between AIH, acute viral hepatitis, and other acute or chronic liver disorders may not be straightforward.[166] There may be no correlation between the clinical findings, or lack thereof, and the often severe histologic lesion seen on liver biopsy.[161]

The clinical course in adults has been well described and may be benign in some cases.[160,161] This does not appear to be the case for AIH presenting in childhood. A 20-year experience in 52 children with a median follow-up of 5 years has been reported.[167] The results indicated that AIH-II presents at an earlier age, with a more severe initial presentation, including fulminant hepatitis, and a poorer response to immunosuppressive therapy (Table 63.9). Long-term outcome between both groups, however, appears to be similar. A significant number of associated immune-related disorders have been found in patients and/or their first-degree relatives (21% and 40%, respectively), including inflammatory bowel disease, thyroiditis and nephrosis. Bilirubin level and prothrombin time at initial presentation appeared to be good predictors of outcome. Similar results in children with AIH were reported in two other studies,[168,169] but cirrhosis was present on biopsy in a larger proportion of patients (up to 89%), emphasizing the severity of this disease in the pediatric population. In children, recurrence after transplantation may occur.

	AIH-I	AIH-II
Demographics		
No. of patients	32 (62)	20 (38)
No. of females	24 (75)	15 (75)
Age (range) at diagnosis (years)	10 (2–15)	7 (0.3–19)
Initial presentation		
Acute hepatitis	16 (50)	13 (65)
Insidious onset	12 (38)	5 (25)
Hepatosplenomegaly	15 (47)	8 (40)
Cirrhosis on biopsy	18/26 (69)	5/13 (38)
Fulminant hepatitis	1 (3)	5 (25)
Response to immunosuppressive therapy		
Initial remission	31 (97)	13 (65)
Stopped after 3 years	6 (19)	0 (0)
Liver transplant	2 (6)	2 (10)
Death	1 (3)	2 (10)

Values in parentheses are percentages unless stated otherwise.

Table 63.9 Characteristics, clinical course and outcomes in 52 children with autoimmune hepatitis (AIH) followed for a median of 5 years (Reproduced from Gregorio GV, Portmann B, Reid F, et al. Autoimmune hepatitis in childhood: a 20-year experience. Hepatology 1997;25: 541-547, with permission of Wiley–Liss, Inc. a subsidiary of John Wiley & Sons, Inc).[167]

Diagnosis

The diagnosis of AIH in childhood must take into consideration clinical features, histologic findings and the detection of autoantibodies. A severe presentation with deep jaundice, dark urine and coagulopathy, along with accompanying immune-related disorders (e.g. thyroiditis, ulcerative colitis), may be important diagnostic clues, allowing the differentiation from other liver diseases with which it may be easily confused. A histologic picture of severe necroinflammatory hepatocellular injury and dense portal triad mononuclear cell infiltrates including plasma cells and parenchymal collapse is also helpful in differentiating AIH from viral or drug-induced hepatitis (Fig. 63.10). In addition, AIH in adolescents should be distinguished from the acute or chronic hepatitis presentation of Wilson's disease.

Delineation of a patient's autoantibody profile is important for diagnostic, typing and prognostic purposes (see Table 63.8). Patients with AIH-I typically present with cir-

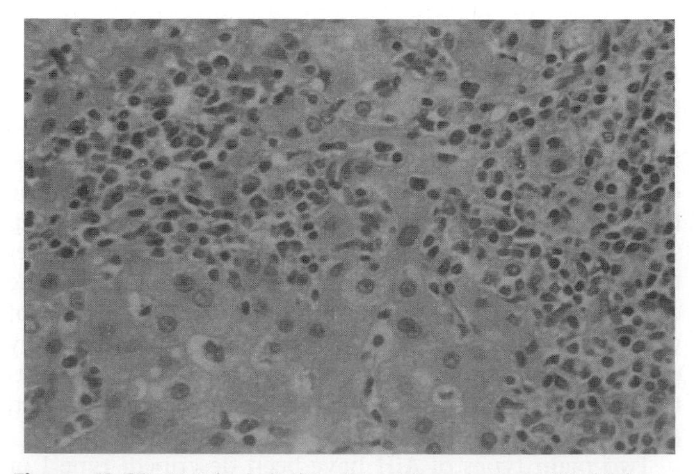

Figure 63.10: Histologic findings in autoimmune hepatitis. High-power micrograph of the liver from a child with autoimmune hepatitis demonstrating severe necroinflammatory hepatocellular injury and dense portal triad mononuclear cell infiltrates that include plasma cells. Parenchymal collapse is also common.

culating antinuclear, anti-smooth muscle and/or anti-actin antibodies. Although anti-actin antibodies are more specific than anti-smooth muscle antibodies, testing for them is not performed in most clinical laboratories. In AIH-II, antibodies against liver–kidney microsome-1 (anti-LKM-1) are characteristically present. A large proportion of adult patients with anti-LKM-1 show positivity for markers of HCV infection. This association is rare in children, and most likely represents a reactivity different from that found in AIH-II.[164,170] In some patients with AIH-II, anti-liver cytosol-1 antibodies can be present alone or with anti-LKM-1. Several pediatric patients with this profile and asymptomatic disease have been described.[171]

Autoantibodies can be found in low titers in adults with a variety of non-autoimmune disorders. In children who are healthy or who have non-autoimmune diseases, however, this is rare, and the presence of autoantibodies even in low titers is sufficient for the diagnosis of AIH.[164] Some patients with all the features of autoimmune hepatitis but without detectable autoantibodies have been reported, and are included in a group labeled as having 'cryptogenic cirrhosis'.[161]

Since its initial description, hyperproteinemia and hyperglobulinemia have been described in association with AIH. The hyperglobulinemia may lead to false-positive screening results for hepatitis C, but more specific HCV testing (see Hepatitis C) and detection of non-organ-specific and liver-specific autoantibodies should lead to the correct diagnosis.

Treatment

Chronic AIH generally responds to immunosuppressive therapy, of which corticosteroids have become the mainstay. Immunosuppressive therapy for AIH can be divided into two phases: (1) induction of remission and (2) maintenance of remission. There are no widely accepted guidelines for initial dosage and withdrawal of immunosuppressive agents. One pediatric regimen begins with prednisolone 2 mg/kg daily (maximum 60 mg) and is gradually decreased over a period of 4–6 weeks to the minimum dose capable of maintaining normal aminotransferase levels.[164] If excessive doses of corticosteroids are required to maintain normal aminotransferase levels, or if the child does not achieve remission, then azathioprine at a dose of 0.5 mg/kg daily is started. Based on the patient's response and presence or lack of drug-induced toxicity, the dose of azathioprine may be increased to 2 mg/kg daily. 6-Mercaptopurine, a related purine analog, can be substituted for azathioprine at a lower dose and, in some cases, has facilitated induction of remission when azathioprine has failed.[172] Results of this treatment protocol are shown in Table 63.9. The time necessary to achieve normalization of aminotransferase levels may be prolonged. In this protocol, normalization was reached after a median of 0.5 (range 0.2 to 7) years in AIH-I and 0.8 (range 0.2–3.2) years in AIH-II.[164]

Immunosuppressive therapy may be withdrawn in some patients, allowing a prolonged 'disease-free' period. Other children will require chronic, low maintenance doses of corticosteroids and a purine analog, alone or in combination, to maintain remission. Alternate-day or pulsed corticosteroid regimens have been disappointing.[161]

Forty percent of children will have at least one episode of relapse while on treatment, and many will progress to cirrhosis.[164] The risk of relapse is greater if prednisone is administered on alternate days. Poor indicators of response to therapy include cirrhosis at initial biopsy, diagnosis at a young age, long duration of disease, and presence of the HLA-B8 or DR3 phenotype.[161] Empiric non-steroidal treatments including ursodeoxycholic acid, ciclosporin and tacrolimus have been used in limited studies to treat recalcitrant disease or corticosteroid intolerance. Of all alternative agents, the greatest experience to date has been with ciclosporin. A pilot multinational multicenter clinical trial of ciclosporin involving 32 children with AIH was published recently.[173] Ciclosporin alone was administered for 6 months, followed by combined low doses of prednisone and azathioprine for 1 month, after which ciclosporin was discontinued. Of 30 patients, 25 had normal ALT levels by 6 months and all had normal levels by 1 year of treatment. In a recent series, five patients with refractory AIH responded to mycophenolate mophetil.[174]

Patients with AIH who have failed medical therapy or who presented initially with end-stage liver disease have been referred for liver transplantation with success. The disease may recur after transplantation despite aggressive immunosuppression, or several years after grafting when immunosuppression is reduced.[161]

NON-ALCOHOLIC FATTY LIVER DISEASE

Introduction and definitions

The epidemic of obesity in adults, children and adolescents has many significant consequences for the health of the population. The high prevalence of obesity has led to the recognition and characterization of types of chronic liver disease previously thought to be uncommon and limited to selected adult patients. This term is called non-alcoholic fatty liver disease (NAFLD) when alcohol is excluded as the etiology. NAFLD is increasingly recognized in children and adolescents, and may be the most common form of chronic liver disease in this population. Fatty liver, also referred to as hepatic steatosis, refers to accumulation of fat in the parenchymal cells of the liver. A more severe form of the disease is non-alcoholic steatohepatitis (NASH). NASH is now thought to be responsible for much of the non-infectious end-stage liver disease in the USA. NAFLD is a spectrum of types and severity of hepatic steatosis. As the name implies, it must be distinguished from alcoholic liver disease. In addition, NAFLD should be distinguished from microvesicular steatosis of the liver, which is seen in association with a variety of inherited or acquired disorders that have a final common pathway of defective oxidation of free fatty acids. Progression of NASH to chronic liver disease with significant fibrosis and cirrhosis is well documented. NAFLD is a histologic diagnosis: it may be associated with or caused by a variety of underlying diseases or drugs (Table 63.10).

Acquired metabolic conditions
Obesity Diabetes mellitus Rapid weight loss Total parenteral nutrition Acute starvation
Genetic metabolic conditions
Wilson's disease Hereditary tyrosinemia Abetalipoproteinemia
Surgical procedures
Jejunoileal bypass Gastroplasty Extensive small bowel resection
Drugs/toxins
Glucocorticoids Amiodarone Synthetic estrogens Isoniazid Others
Miscellaneous
Small bowel bacterial overgrowth
Adapted from Reid AE, 2001, © AGA, with permission.[179]

Table 63.10 Causes of NAFLD and NASH

Histologic features

Once the histologic lesion has gone beyond simple steatosis, the liver disease is classified as NASH. The primary defining features of NASH include macrovesicular steatosis, parenchymal lymphocyte-predominant inflammation and ballooning hepatocyte degeneration (Fig. 63.11). Other features observed with variable frequency include perisinusoidal fibrosis (predominantly in zone 3, the hepatocytes around the central veins), Mallory's hyaline, glycogenated nuclei, lipogranulomas, steatonecrosis and iron accumulation. The extent of fibrosis varies considerably, but fibrosis has been found in a higher prevalence of pediatric patients with NASH at presentation, compared with adults.[175] Well-established cirrhosis is found on initial biopsies in 7–16% of adult patients with NASH.

Prevalence and risk factors

The prevalence of NAFLD in the general population is not known because the majority of affected individuals are asymptomatic. Autopsy studies and studies of general populations have demonstrated rates of approximately 20% for NAFLD and 2–3% for NASH, but rates are substantially higher in obese and diabetic subjects. In a study of non-alcoholic adult patients referred for evaluation of abnormal aminotransferase levels, in whom no other etiology could be identified, NASH was found at biopsy in 26%.[176]

Prevalence rates for children and adolescents are not available because there are no large series of liver biopsies for abnormal aminotransferase values. However, some estimate of the magnitude of NAFLD in childhood has been made from data gathered in NHANES cycle III database

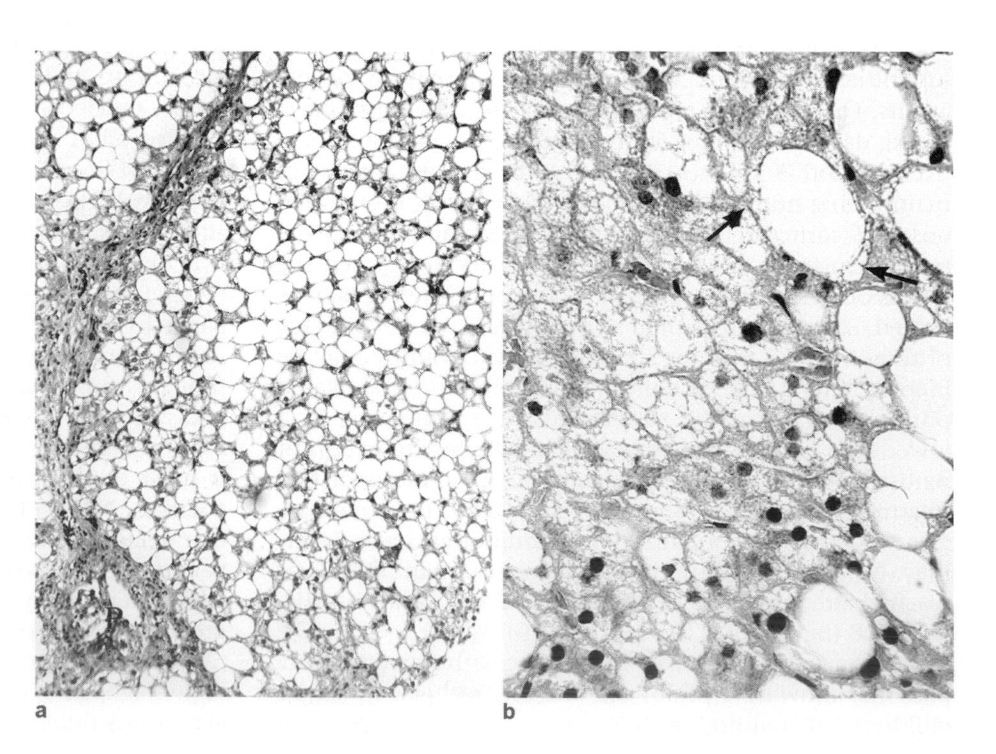

Figure 63.11: Histologic findings in NAFLD. Photomicrograph of the liver in NASH. **(a)** At low power, large lipid droplets can be seen in many of the enlarged hepatocytes. Bridging fibrosis and some inflammation in the portal areas are also noted. **(b)** At higher magnification, the large lipid vacuoles are seen to be compressing the cellular organelles and nuclei to the periphery of the hepatocytes (arrows).

(1988–1994). Abnormal ALT values were noted in 1.5% of adolescents of normal weight, in 5% of the overweight and in 9.5% of the obese. When children referred to obesity programs are studied, the prevalence of ALT abnormality increases to 12–25%, and the presence of fatty liver increases to 53%.[177]

Risk factors for NAFLD in adults include obesity, type II diabetes mellitus, hyperlipidemia and female sex, although men with this disorder are being recognized with increasing frequency. Although NAFLD is occasionally seen in lean individuals, a parallel rise in the frequency of obesity, NAFLD and type II diabetes mellitus has been noted. For these reasons, the primary risk factors for NAFLD in childhood are thought to be overweight/obesity and insulin resistance.

Pathogenesis

The pathogenesis of NAFLD has not been completely elucidated. Fat deposition in the liver occurs when the degree of lipogenesis is greater than the rate of lipolysis. This may result from delivery of fatty acids to the liver in greater amounts than is needed for the processes of mitochondrial oxidation for energy and synthesis of necessary lipids and phospholipids. This mechanism might explain the hepatic steatosis in obesity, acute starvation, excessive dietary fat intake and total parenteral nutrition. Alternatively, decreased use of fatty acids within the liver, either by disturbed mitochondrial oxidation or decreased synthesis, might also cause fat accumulation.

It is becoming clear that insulin resistance plays an important role in the generation of NAFLD. Insulin promotes the retention of triglycerides in hepatocytes. It has now been demonstrated repeatedly that most patients with NAFLD or NASH have raised insulin levels or insulin resistance, even in the absence of obesity or hypoglycemia. This association has been noted in children as well.

The first inciting factor in the development of NAFLD and NASH is the accumulation of triglycerides in hepatocytes. It is now generally accepted that a 'second hit' is necessary once hepatic steatosis is established, to promote progression to hepatocellular injury associated with inflammation and then fibrosis (Fig. 63.12). The resultant hepatocyte damage may then stimulate the influx of inflammatory cells, initiating an inflammatory cytokine cascade and leading to further tissue injury.

Clinical features

NAFLD and NASH are asymptomatic in the majority of patients. Symptoms such as fatigue, malaise and vague right upper-quadrant pain may be more common in adolescents. In most patients, NAFLD is discovered when hepatomegaly or abnormal ALT concentration is detected on routine testing or evaluation for another problem. Hepatomegaly, although sometimes difficult to appreciate owing to obesity, is present frequently, and not all patients have abnormal ALT values. Obese young adults with a high degree of abdominal wall fat are more likely to have

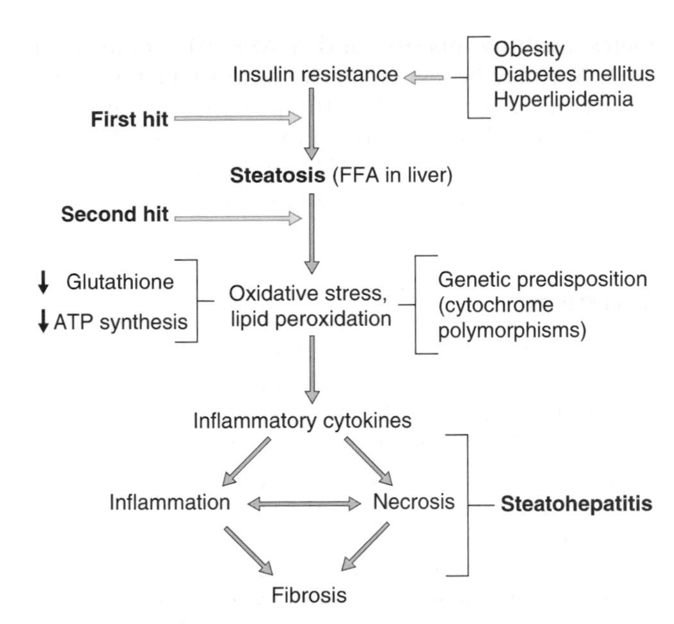

Figure 63.12: Two-hit hypothesis of NASH. Current understanding of the pathogenesis of hepatic steatosis and NASH. Insulin resistance associated with a variety of conditions causes accumulation of free fatty acids (FFA) in hepatocytes, the 'first hit' of hepatic steatosis. A 'second hit' injury caused by or associated with steatosis and mediated through lipid peroxidation causes release of inflammatory cytokines. The resultant inflammation and cell necrosis stimulate fibrogenesis, leading to the full-blown picture of steatohepatitis. ATP, adenosine triphosphate.

NAFLD. Acanthosis nigricans is commonly found on the neck and axillae of children and adolescents with insulin resistance. Ultrasonography may reveal a granular-appearing echogenic liver that is difficult to penetrate.

Laboratory findings in NAFLD and NASH are non-specific. Typically, aspartate aminotransferase (AST) and ALT levels are increased 2–5-fold, although greater increases are sometimes seen. Bilirubin, albumin and prothrombin time values are normal until the very latest stages of disease.

Natural history

The natural history of NAFLD is variable. Hepatic steatosis alone may have a benign or indolent course for many years. Once inflammation and tissue damage have developed, progressive liver disease ensues. In particular, the findings of inflammatory infiltrates and hepatocyte balloon degeneration suggest a high likelihood of progression to fibrosis and cirrhosis.[178]

Although no direct comparative studies have been done, fibrosis may be more common at the time of diagnosis of NAFLD in children and adolescents. One report described some degree of fibrosis in all 14 children with NASH discovered on a retrospective clinicopathologic review.[179] Instances of advanced liver disease and cirrhosis have been described during childhood and adolescence. NAFLD and NASH must be recognized as potential causes of serious liver disease in this population.

Risk factors for the progression of liver disease due to NAFLD have been identified in adults. These include age,

35. Chu C-J, Keeffe EB, Han S-H, et al. Prevalence of HBV precore/core promoter variants in the United States. Hepatology 2003; 38:619–628.
36. Kobayashi M, Arase Y, Ikeda K, et al. Clinical characteristics of patients infected with hepatitis B virus genotypes A, B, and C. J Gastroenterology 2002; 37:35–39.
37. Devarbhavi H, Cohen A, Patel R, et al. Preliminary results: outcome of liver transplantation for hepatitis B virus varies by hepatitis B virus genotype. Liver Transpl Surg 2002; 8:550–555.
38. Kao J-H, Chen P-J, Lai M-Y, Chen D-S. Hepatitis B genotypes correlate with clinical outcomes in patients with chronic hepatitis B. Gastroenterology 2000; 118:554–559.
39. Hou J, Shilling R, Janssen H, et al. Molecular characteristics of hepatitis B virus genotype A confer a higher response rate to interferon treatment. J Hepatol 2001; 34(Suppl 1):15.
40. Liang TJ, Hasegawa K, Rimon N, et al. A hepatitis B virus mutant associated wtih an epidemic of fulminant hepatitis. N Engl J Med 1991; 324:1705–1709.
41. Santantonio T, Jung MC, Monno L, et al. Long-term response to interferon therapy in chronic hepatitis B: importance of hepatitis B virus heterogeneity. Arch Virol 1993; 8(Suppl):171–178.
42. Carman WF, Zanetti AR, Karayiannis P, et al. Vaccine-induced escape mutant of hepatitis B virus. Lancet 1990; 336:325–329.
43. Naoumov NV, Schneider R, Grotzinger T, et al. Precore mutant hepatitis B virus infection and liver disease. Gastroenterology 1992; 102:538–543.
44. Yamamoto K, Horikita M, Tsuda F, et al. Naturally occurring escape mutants of hepatitis B virus with various mutations in the S gene in carriers seropositive for antibody to hepatitis B surface antigen. J Virol 1994; 68:2671–2676.
45. Raimondo G, Tanzi E, Brancatelli S, et al. Is the course of perinatal hepatitis B virus infection influenced by genetic heterogeneity of the virus? J Med Virol 1993; 40:87–90.
46. Terazawa S, Kojima M, Yamanaka T, et al. Hepatitis B virus mutants with pre-core region defects in two babies with fulminant hepatitis B virus and their mothers positive for antibody to hepatitis B e antigen. Pediatr Res 1991; 29:5–9.
47. Honigwachs J, Faktor O, Dikstein R, Shaul Y, Laub O. Liver-specific expression of hepatitis B virus is determined by the combined action of the core gene promoter and the enhancer. J Virol 1989; 63:919–924.
48. Mason A, Wick M, White H, Perrillo R. Hepatitis B virus replication in diverse cell types during chronic hepatitis B virus infection. Hepatology 1993; 18:781–789.
49. Pignatelli M, Waters J, Lever A, et al. Cytotoxic T-cell responses to the nucleocapsid proteins of HBV in chronic hepatitis. J Hepatol 1987; 4:15–21.
50. Milich DR, Jones JE, Hughes JL, et al. Is a function of the secreted hepatitis B e antigen to induce immunologic tolerance in utero? Proc Natl Acad Sci 1990; 87:6599–6603.
51. Hsu H, Chang M, Hsieh K, et al. Cellular immune response to HBcAg in mother-to-infant transmission of hepatitis B virus. Hepatology 1992; 15:770–776.
52. Margolis HS, Alter MJ, Hadler SC. Hepatitis B: evolving epidemiology and implications for control. Semin Liv Dis 1991; 11:84–92.
53. Maynard JE. Hepatitis B: Global importance and need for control. Vaccine 1990; 8(Suppl):S18–S20.
54. McMahon BJ, Alward WLM, Hall DB, et al. Acute hepatitis B virus infection: relation of age to the clinical expression of disease and subsequent development of the carrier state. J Infect Dis 1985; 151:599–603.
55. Tong M, Thursby M, Rakela J, et al. Studies of the maternal–infant transmission of the viruses which cause acute hepatitis. Gastroenterology 1981; 80:999–1003.
56. Stevens C, Beasley R, Tsui J, et al. Vertical transmission of hepatitis B antigen in Taiwan. N Engl J Med 1975; 292:771–774.
57. Kim W, Benson J, Therneau T, Torgerson H, et al. Changing epidemiology of hepatitis B in a US community. Hepatology 2004; 39:811–816.
58. Alter H, Purcell J, Gerin J. Transmission of hepatitis B to chimpanzees by hepatitis B surface antigen-positive saliva and semen. Infect Immun 1977; 16:928–933.
59. Centers for Disease Control. Hepatitis transmitted from a human bite. MMWR Morbid Mortal Weekly Rep 1974; 23:24.
60. Neefe J, Stokes J, Rheinhold J. Oral administration to volunteers of feces from patients with homologous serum hepatitis and infectious (epidemic) hepatitis. Am J Med Sci 1945; 210:29–32.
61. Dupruy J, Giraud P, Dupruy C, et al. Hepatitis B in children: II. Study of children born to chronic HBsAg carrier mothers. J Pediatr 1978; 92:200–204.
62. Xu ZY, Liu CB, Francis DP, et al. Prevention of perinatal acquisition of hepatitis B virus carriage using vaccine: preliminary report of a randomised, double blind placebo controlled and comparative trial. Pediatrics 1985; 76:713–718.
63. Stevens CE, Neurath RA, Beasley RP, et al. HBeAg and antiHBe detection by radioimmunoassay: correlation with vertical transmission of hepatitis B in Taiwan. J Med Virol 1979; 3:237–241.
64. Heijtink R, Boender P, Schalm S, et al. Hepatitis B virus DNA in serum of pregnant women with HBsAg and HBeAg or antibodies to HBe. J Infect Dis 1984; 150:462–470.
65. Sinatra F, Shah P, Weissman J, et al. Perinatal transmitted acute icteric hepatitis B in infants born to hepatitis surface antigen-positive and anti-hepatitis B e-positive mothers. Pediatrics 1982; 70:557–560.
66. Beath S, Boxall E, Watson R, et al. Fulminant hepatitis in infants born to anti-HBe hepatitis B carrier mothers. BMJ 1992; 304:1169–1170.
67. Shimuzu H, Mitsuda T, Fujita S, et al. Perinatal hepatitis B infection caused by anti-hepatitis B e-positive maternal mononuclear cells. Arch Dis Child 1991; 66:718–721.
68. Ohto H, Lin H, Kawana T, et al. Intrauterine transmission of hepatitis B virus is closely related to placental leakage. J Med Virol 1987; 21:1–6.
69. Beasley RP, Hwang LY. Postnatal infectivity of hepatitis B surface antigen carrier mothers. J Infect Dis 1983; 147:185–190.
70. Hurie MB, Mast EE, Davis JP. Horizontal transmission of hepatitis B virus infection to United States-born children of Hmong refugees. Pediatrics 1992; 89:269–273.
71. Franks AL, Berg CJ, Kane MA, et al. Hepatitis B infection among children born in the United States to southeast Asian refugees. N Engl J Med 1989; 321:1301–1305.
72. Shapiro CN, McCaig LF, Gensheimer KF, et al. Hepatitis B virus transmission between children in day care. Pediatr Infect Dis J 1989; 8:870–875.
73. Hurwitz E, Deseda C, Shapiro C, et al. Hepatitis infections in the day care setting. Pediatrics 1994; 94:1023–1024.
74. Gianotti F. Papular acrodermatitis of childhood: an Australian antigen disease. Arch Dis Child 1973; 48:794–799.
75. Draelos Z, Hansen R, James W. Gianotti–Crosti syndrome associated with infections other than hepatitis B. JAMA 1986; 256:2386–2388.

76. Lok A, Heathcote J, Hoofnagle J. Management of hepatitis B: 2000 – summary of a workshop. Gastroenterology 2001; 120:1828–1853.
77. Lok AS. Chronic hepatitis B. N Engl J Med 2002; 346:1682–1683.
78. Lok ASF, Lai CL. A longitudinal follow-up of asymptomatic hepatitis B surface antigen-positive Chinese children. Hepatology 1988; 8:1130–1133.
79. Bortolotti F, Cadrobbi P, Crivellaro C, et al. Long-term outcome of chronic type B hepatitis in patients who acquire hepatitis B virus infection in childhood. Gastroenterology 1990; 99:805–810.
80. Ruíz-Moreno M, Camps T, Aguado JG, et al. Serological and histological follow up of chronic hepatitis B infection. Arch Dis Child 1989; 64:1165–1169.
81. Moyes CD, Milne A, Waldon J. Liver function of hepatitis B carriers in childhood. Pediatr Infect Dis J 1993; 12:120–125.
82. Mengoli M, Balli ME, Tolomelli S, et al. Long-term outcome of chronic type B hepatitis in childhood. Arch Virol 1992; 4(Suppl):263–264.
83. Bortolotti F, Vajro P, Cadrobbi P, et al. Cryptogenic chronic liver disease and hepatitis C virus infection in children. J Hepatol 1992; 15:73–76.
84. Zancan L, Chiaramonte M, Ferrarese N, Zacchelllo F. Pediatric HBsAg chronic liver disease and adult asymptomatic carrier status: two stages of the same entity. J Pediatr Gastroenterol Nutr 1990; 11:380–384.
85. Bortolotti F, Calzia R, Cadrobbi P, et al. Liver cirrhosis associated with chronic hepatitis B virus infection in childhood. J Pediatr 1986; 108:224–227.
86. Weissberg J, Andres L, Smith C, et al. Survival in chronic hepatitis B: an analysis of 379 patients. Ann Intern Med 1984; 101:613–616.
87. Parkin D, Laara E, Muir C. Estimates of the worldwide frequency of sixteen major cancers in 1989. Int J Cancer 1988; 41:184–197.
88. Chang MH, Chen PJ, Chen JY, et al. Hepatitis B virus integration in hepatitis B virus-related hepatocellular carcinoma in childhood. Hepatology 1991; 13:316–320.
89. Larouze B, London W, Saimot G, et al. Host responses to hepatitis B infection in patients with primary hepatic carcinoma and their families: a case–control study in Senegal, West Africa. Lancet 1976; ii:534–538.
90. Steiner P. Cancer of the liver and cirrhosis in trans-Saharan Africa and the United States of America. Cancer 1960; 13:1085–1166.
91. Chung JL, Kao JH, Kong MS, Yang CP, Hung IJ, Lin TY. Hepatitis C and G virus infections in polytransfused children. Eur J Pediatr 1997; 156:546–549.
92. Wen W, Chang M, Hsu H, et al. The development of hepatocellular carcinoma among prospectively followed children with chronic hepatitis B virus infection. J Pediatr 2004; 144:397–399.
93. Willson R. Extrahepatic manifestations of chronic viral hepatitis. Am J Gastroenterol 1997; 92:4–17.
94. Hogg R. Hepatitis B surface antigenemia in North American children with membranous glomerulonephropathy. J Pediatr 1985; 106:571–578.
95. Gower RG, Sausker WF, Kohler PF, et al. Small vessel vasculitis caused by hepatitis B virus immune complexex. J Allergy Clin Immunol 1978; 62:222–228.
96. Levo Y, Govervic PD, Kassab HJ, et al. Association between hepatitis B virus and essential mixed cryoglobulinemia. N Engl J Med 1977; 296:1501–1504.
97. Hoofnagle J, Seef L, Bales Z, et al. Serologic responses in hepatitis B. In: Vyas GN, Cohen SN, Schmidt R, eds. Viral Hepatitis: A Contemporary Assessment of Etiology, Epidemiology, Pathogenesis and Prevention. Philadelphia, PA: Franklin Institute Press; 1978:278.
98. Gocke D. Extrahepatic manifestations of viral hepatitis. Am J Med Sci 1975; 270:49–52.
99. Prince A, Brotman B, Grady G, et al. Long-incubation post-transfusion hepatitis without serological evidence of exposure to hepatitis B serum. Lancet 1974; ii:241–246.
100. Tsang S, Chan H, Leung N, et al. Lamivudine treatment for fulminant hepatic failure due to acute exacerbation of chronic hepatitis B infection. Aliment Pharmacol Ther 2001; 15:1737–1744.
101. Perrillo RP. Interferon in the management of chronic hepatitis B. Dig Dis Sci 1993; 38:577–593.
102. Jonas M. Interferon-a for viral hepatitis. J Pediatr Gastroenterol Nutr 1996; 23:93–106.
103. Brook MG, Karayiannis P, Thomas HC. Which patients with chronic hepatitis B virus infection will respond to alpha interferon therapy? A statistical analysis of predictive factors. Hepatology 1989; 10:761–763.
104. Wong DKH, Cheung AM, O'Rourke K, et al. Effect of alpha-interferon treatment in patients with hepatitis B e antigen-positive chronic hepatitis B. Ann Intern Med 1993; 119:312–323.
105. Barbera C, Bortolotti F, Crivellaro C, et al. Recombinant interferon-alpha 2a hastens the rate of HBeAg clearance in children with chronic hepatitis B. Hepatology 1994; 20:287–290.
106. Jonas MM, Kelly DA, Mizerski J, et al. Clinical trial of lamivudine in children with chronic hepatitis B. N Engl J Med 2002; 346:1706–1713.
107. American Academy of Pediatrics. Hepatitis B. In: Peter G, ed. 1994 Red Book: Report of the Committee on Infectious Diseases, 24th edn. Elk Grove Village, IL: American Academy of Pediatrics; 1997:247–260.
108. Immunization Practices Advisory Committee, Centers for Disease Control. Hepatitis B virus: a comprehensive strategy for eliminating transmission in the United States through universal childhood vaccination. MMWR Mortal Morbid Wkly Rep 1991; 40:1–25.
109. Chan C, Lee S, Lo K. Legend of hepatitis B vaccination: the Taiwan experience. J Gastroenterol Hepatol 2004; 19:121–126.
110. Feinstone S, Kapikian A, Purcell R, et al. Transfusion-associated hepatitis not due to viral hepatitis type A or B. N Engl J Med 1975; 292:767–770.
111. Choo Q-L, Kuo G, Weiner AJ, et al. Isolation of a cDNA derived from a blood-borne non-A,non-B viral hepatitis genome. Science 1989; 244:359–362.
112. Kuo G, Choo Q-L, Alter HJ, et al. An assay for circulating antibodies to a major etiologic virus of human non-A, non-B hepatitis. Science 1989; 244:362–364.
113. Alter HJ, Purcell RH, Shih JW, et al. Detection of antibody to hepatitis C virus in prospectively followed transfusion recipients with acute and chronic non-A,non-B hepatitis. N Engl J Med 1989; 321:1494–1500.
114. Brechot C. Hepatitis C virus: molecular biology and genetic variability. Dig Dis Sci 1996; 41(Suppl):6–21.
115. Simmonds P. Variability of hepatitis C virus. Hepatology 1995; 21:570–583.
116. Cooreman M, Scoondermark-Van de Ven E. Hepatitis C: biological and clinical consequences of genetic heterogeneity. Scand J Gastroenterol 1996; 31(Suppl 218):106–115.

117. Heydtmann M, Shields P, McCaughan G, Adams D. Cytokines and chemokines in the immune response to hepatitis C infection. Curr Opin Infect Dis 2001; 14:279–287.
118. Alter HJ. Descartes before the horse: I clone, therefore I am: the hepatitis C virus in current perspective. Ann Intern Med 1991; 115:644–649.
119. Centers for Disease Control and Prevention. Recommendations for prevention and control of hepatitis C virus (HCV) infection and HCV-related chronic disease. MMWR Mortal Morbid Wkly Rep 1998; 47 (no. RR-19).
120. Di Bisceglie A, Hoofnagle J. Chronic viral hepatitis. In: Zakim D, Boyer TD, eds. Hepatology: A Textbook of Liver Disease, 3rd edn. Philadelphia, PA: WB Saunders; 1996:1299–1329.
121. Aach R, Stevens C, Hollinger F. Hepatitis C virus infection in post-transfusion hepatitis. N Engl J Med 1991; 325:1325–1329.
122. Alter MJ, Hadler SC, Judson FN, et al. Risk factors for acute non-A, non-B hepatitis in the United States and association with hepatitis C virus infection. JAMA 1990; 264:2231–2235.
123. Bortolotti F, Vajro P, Barbera C, et al. Hepatitis C in childhood: epidemiological and clinical aspects. Bone Marrow Transplant 1993; 12(Suppl):s21–s23.
124. Bortolotti F, Resti M, Giacchino R, et al. Changing epidemiologic pattern of chronic hepatitis C virus infection in Italian children. J Pediatr 1998; 133:378–381.
125. Sullivan L, Fiellin D. Hepatitis C and HIV infections: implications for clinical care in injection drug users. Am J Addict 2004; 13:1–20.
126. Bortolotti F, Jara P, Diaz C, et al. Posttransfusion and community-acquired hepatitis C in childhood. J Pediatr Gastroenterol Nutr 1994; 18:279–283.
127. Nowicki MJ, Balistreri WF. The hepatitis C virus: identification, epidemiology and clinical controversies. J Pediatr Gastroenterol Nutr 1995; 20:248–274.
128. Ko Y, Ho M, Chiang T, et al. Tattooing as a risk of hepatitis C infection. J Med Virol 1992; 38:288–291.
129. Hsu HH, Wright TL, Luba D, et al. Failure to detect hepatitis C virus genome in human secretions with the polymerase chain reaction. Hepatology 1991; 14:763–767.
130. Fried MW, Shindo M, Fong T-L, et al. Absence of hepatitis C viral RNA from saliva and semen of patients with chronic hepatitis C. Gastroenterology 1992; 102:1306–1308.
131. Seef L. Diagnosis, therapy and prognosis of viral hepatitis. In: Zakim D, Boyer TD, eds. Hepatology: A Textbook of Liver Disease, 3rd edn. Philadelphia, PA: WB Saunders; 1996:1067–1145.
132. Prince A, Brotman B, Huima T, et al. Immunity in hepatitis C infection. J Infect Dis 1992; 165:438–443.
133. Farci P, Alter HJ, Govindarajan S, et al. Lack of protective immunity against reinfection with hepatitis C virus. Science 1992; 258:135–140.
134. Feray C, Gigou M, Samuel D, et al. Hepatitis C virus RNA and hepatitis B virus DNA in serum and liver of patients with fulminant hepatitis. Gastroenterology 1993; 104:549–555.
135. Jara P, Resti M, Hierro L, et al. Chronic hepatitis C virus infection in childhood: clinical patterns and evolution in 224 white children. Clin Infect Dis 2003; 36:275–280.
136. Garson J, Tedder R, Briggs M, et al. Detection of hepatitis C viral sequences in blood donations by 'nested' polymerase chain reaction and prediction of infectivity. Lancet 1990; 335:1419–1422.
137. Jonas M. Children with Hepatitis C. Hepatology 2002; 36:S173–S178.
138. Jaeckel E, Cornburg M, Wedemeyer H, et al. Treatment of acute hepatitis C with interferon alfa-2b. N Engl J Med 2001; 345:1452–1457.
139. Emerick K. Treatment of hepatitis C in children. Pediatr Infect Dis J 2004; 23:257–258.
140. Fried MW, Shiffman ML, Reddy KJ, et al. Peginterferon alfa-2a plus ribavirin for chronic hepatitis C virus infection. N Engl J Med 2002; 347:975–892.
141. Suoglu O, Elkabes B, Sokucu S, et al. Does interferon and ribavirin combination therapy increase the rate of treatment response in children with hepatitis C? J Pediatr Gastroenterol Nutr 2002; 34:199–206.
142. Conjeevaram H, Everhart J, Hoofnagle J. Predictors of a sustained beneficial response to interferon alpha therapy in chronic hepatitis C. Hepatology 1995; 22:1326–1329.
143. Afdhal N, Geahigan T. Supporting the patient with chronic hepatitis during treatment. In: Koff R, Wu G, eds. Clinical Gastroenterology: Diagnosis and Therapeutics. Totawa, NJ: Humana Press; 211–232.
144. Maddrey W. Safety of combination interferon alfa-2b/ribavarin therapy in chronic hepatitis C-relapsed and treatment-naive patients. Semin Liv Dis 1999; 19(Suppl 1):57–65.
145. Bunn S, Kelly D, Murray KF, et al. Safety, efficacy and pharmacokinetics of interferon-alfa-2b and ribavirin in children with chronic hepatitis C (abstract). Hepatology 2000; 32:350A.
146. Cole S, Gowans E, MacNaughton T, et al. Direct evidence for cytotoxicity associated with expression of hepatitis delta antigen. Hepatology 1991; 13:845–851.
147. Gowans EJ, Bonino F. Hepatitis delta virus pathogenicity. Prog Clin Biol Res 1993; 382:125–130.
148. Hoofnagle J. Type D (delta) hepatitis. JAMA 1989; 261:1321–1325.
149. Tandon B, Joshi Y, Jain S, et al. An epidemic of non-A/non-B hepatitis in North India. Indian J Med Res 1982; 75:739–744.
150. Balayan M, Andjaparidze A, Savinskaya S, et al. Evidence for a virus in non-A/non-B hepatitis transmitted via the fecal–oral route. Intervirology 1983; 20:23–28.
151. Reyes G, Purdy MA, Kim JP, et al. Isolation of a cDNA from the virus responsible for enterically transmitted non-A, non-B hepatitis. Science 1990; 247:1335–1339.
152. Hyams KC, Purdy MA, Kaur M, et al. Acute sporadic hepatitis E in Sudanese children: analysis based on a new Western blot assay. J Infect Dis 1992; 165:1001–1005.
153. Krawczynski K. Hepatitis E. Hepatology 1993; 17:932–941.
154. Robinson W. Biology of human hepatitis viruses. In: Hepatology: A Textbook of Liver Disease. Philadelphia, PA: WB Saunders; 1996:1146–1206.
155. Alter HJ, Nakatsuji Y, Melpolder J, et al. The incidence of transfusion-associated hepatitis G virus infection and its relation to liver disease. N Engl J Med 1997; 336:747–754.
156. Sumaya C, Ench Y. Epstein–Barr virus infectious mononucleosis in children: I. Clinical and general laboratory findings. Pediatrics 1985; 75:1003–1010.
157. Griffiths PD, Ellis DS, Zuckerman AJ. Other common types of viral hepatitis and exotic infections. Br Med Bull 1990; 46:512–532.
158. Bopanna S, Pass R, Stagno S, et al. Symptomatic congenital cytomegalovirus infection: neonatal mortality and morbidity. Pediatr Infect Dis J 1992; 11:93–99.
159. Wiesner R, Marin E, Porayko M, et al. Advances in the diagnosis, treatment and prevention of cytomegalovirus

infections after liver transplantation. Gastroenterol Clin North Am 1993; 22:351–366.

160. Czaja A. Autoimmune hepatitis and viral infection. Gastroenterol Clin North Am 1994; 23:547–566.

161. Krawitt E. Autoimmune hepatitis. N Engl J Med 1996; 334:897–903.

162. el-Shabrawi M, Wilkinson M, Portmann B, et al. Primary sclerosing cholangitis in childhood. Gastroenterology 1987; 92(Pt 1):1226–1235.

163. Scully L, Toze C, Sengar D, et al. Early-onset autoimmune hepatitis is associated with a C4A gene deletion. Gastroenterology 1993; 104:1478–1484.

164. Mieli-Vergani G, Vergani D. Progress in pediatric autoimmune hepatitis. Semin Liver Dis 1994; 14:282–288.

165. Squires R. Autoimmune hepatitis in children. Curr Gastroenterol Rep 2004; 6:225–230.

166. Paradis K, Alvarez F, Seidman E, et al. Pitfalls in the diagnosis of autoimmune hepatitis associated with liver and kidney microsomal proteins. J Pediatr Gastroenterol Nutr 1994; 19:453–459.

167. Gregorio G, Portmann B, Reid F, et al. Autoimmune hepatitis in childhood: a 20-year experience. Hepatology 1997; 25:541–547.

168. Vajro P, Hadchouel P, Hadchouel M, et al. Incidence of cirrhosis in children with chronic hepatitis. J Pediatr 1990; 117:392–396.

169. Maggiore G, Veber F, Bernard O, et al. Autoimmune hepatitis associated with antiactin antibodies in children and adolescents. J Pediatr Gastroenterol Nutr 1993; 17:376–381.

170. Lunel F, Abuaf N, Frangeul L, et al. Liver/kidney microsome antibody type 1 and hepatitis C virus infection. Hepatology 1992; 16:630–636.

171. Klein C, Philipp T, Greiner P, et al. Asymptomatic autoimmune hepatitis associated with anti-LC-1 autoantibodies. J Pediatr Gastroenterol Nutr 1996; 23:461–465.

172. Pratt D, Flavin D, Kaplan M. The successful treatment of autoimmune hepatitis with 6-mercaptopurine after failure with azathioprine. Gastroenterology 1996; 110:271.

173. Alvarez F, Ciocca M, Canero-Velasco C, et al. Short-term cyclosporine induces a remission of autoimmune hepatitis in children. J Hepatol 1999; 30:222–227.

174. Devlin S, Swain M, Urbanski S, Burak K. Mycophenolate mofetil for the treatment of autoimmune hepatitis in patients refractory to standard therapy. Can J Gastroenterol 2004; 18:321–326.

175. Baldridge A, Perez-Atayde A, Graeme-Cook F, et al. Idiopathic steatohepatitis in childhood: a multicenter retrospective study. J Pediatr 1995; 127:700–704.

176. Daniel S, Ben-Menachem T, Vasudevan G, et al. Prospective evaluation of unexplained chronic liver transaminase abnormalities in asymptomatic and symptomatic patients. Am J Gastroenterol 1999; 94:3010–3014.

177. Franzese A, Vajro P, Argenziano A, et al. Liver involvement in obese children. Ultransonography and liver enzyme levels at diagnosis and during follow-up in an Italian population. Dig Dis Sci 1997; 42:1428–1432.

178. Matteoni C, Younossi Z, Gramlich T, et al. Nonalcoholic fatty liver disease: a spectrum of clinical and pathological severity. Gastroenterology 1999; 116:1413–1419.

179. Reid A. Nonalcoholic steatohepatitis. Gastroenterology 2001; 121:710–723.

180. Lin J, Smith M, Pagano J. Prolonged inhibitory effect of 9-(1,3-dihydroxy-2-popoxymethyl)guanine against replication of Epstein–Barr virus. J Virol 1984; 50:50–55.

171. Klein C, Philipp T, Greiner P, et al. Autoimmune [illegible] autoimmune hepatitis associated with anti-LKM [illegible] autoantibodies. J Pediatr Gastroenterol Nutr 1994; [illegible] 1-465.

172. [illegible] J, [illegible] D, Kapila [illegible] autoimmune [illegible] with [illegible]

173. Ahmed [illegible] cytomegalovirus [illegible] children. J Hepatol 1999; 30 [illegible]

174. [illegible]

[illegible] infection and liver transplantation. Gastroenterol Clin North Am 1993; 22:[illegible]

160. Czaja A. Autoimmune hepatitis and viral infection. Gastroenterol Clin North Am 1994; 23:[illegible]

161. Krawitt EL. Autoimmune hepatitis. N Engl J Med 1996; 334:897–903.

162. [illegible] M, [illegible] M, [illegible] R, et al. [illegible] in children [illegible] 1229–1235.

163. [illegible] C, Senger D, et al. Early-onset autoimmune hepatitis [illegible] C4A gene deletion. [illegible] 1993; [illegible]

164. [illegible]

Chapter 64
Portal hypertension

Vera F. Hupertz and Charles Winans

INTRODUCTION

The portal system drains the capillaries of the mesenteric and splenic veins and ends in the hepatic capillaries (Fig. 64.1). The portal vein supplies partially oxygenated blood flow to the liver, supplementing the highly oxygenated blood flow of the hepatic artery to the liver. Blood flow to the liver is finely tuned such that any disturbance to flow in one of these vessels can be offset to a certain degree by increased flow through the other vessel. This is known as the hepatic arterial buffer response. Blood from both the portal venous system and the hepatic arterial system combine within the sinusoids.

Portal hypertension occurs when there is increased portal resistance or an increased portal blood flow (Fig. 64.2). Generally, the portal venous system has a low baseline portal pressure of 7–10 mmHg and the hepatic venous pressure gradient (HVPG) ranges from 1 to 4 mmHg. Portal hypertension is defined as a portal pressure greater than 10 mmHg or a gradient greater than 4 mmHg. Pressure gradients above 10 mmHg have been associated with esophageal varices, and those above 12 mmHg are associated with ascites and variceal bleeding in adult patients.[1] To obtain a measurement of the portal pressure gradient, a catheter can be wedged into the hepatic vein via the femoral or transjugular approach and a wedged hepatic venous pressure (WHVP) measurement made. The catheter is then retracted into a free-flowing hepatic vein and free hepatic venous pressure (FHVP) is measured. The HVPG is the difference between the WHVP and the FHVP. Causes of portal hypertension can be suggested by the HVPG. In presinusoidal obstruction, the HVPG is normal but the WHVP is raised, whereas in cirrhosis both the WHVP and the HVPG are increased (Table 64.1).

Clinically, portal hypertension causes splenomegaly with resulting hypersplenism and the formation of collateral circulation. Collaterals form in the junctions between

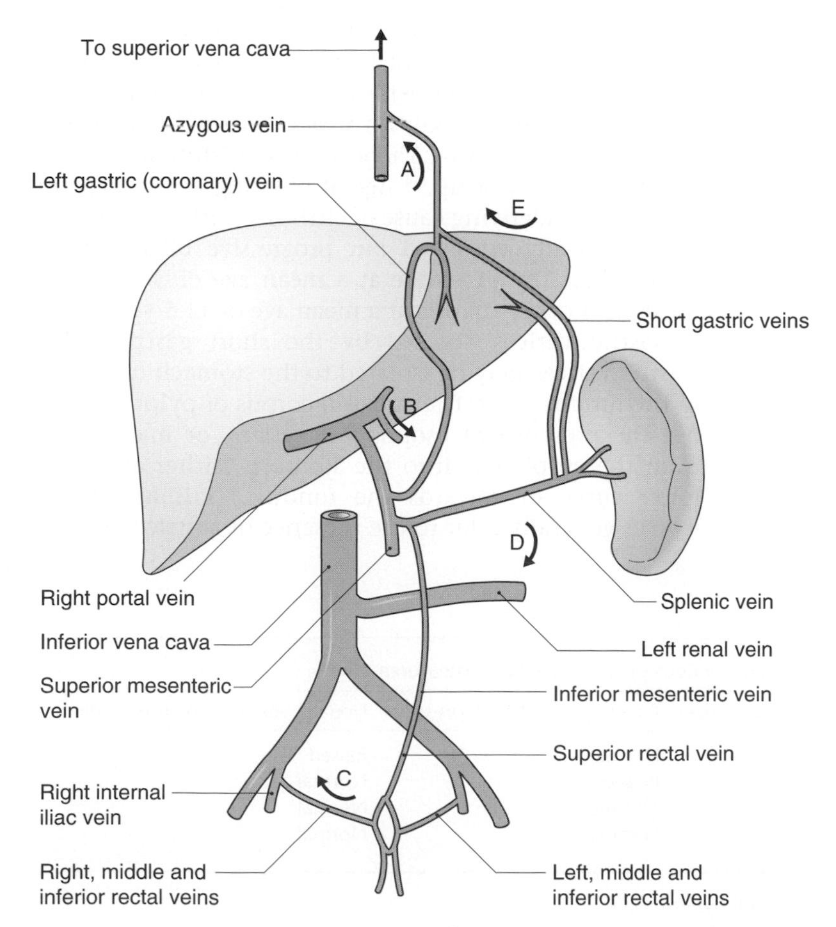

Figure 64.1: Diagram of portal circulation. The normal vascular anatomy and most common sites for the development of portal systemic collaterals are shown. A, Esophageal submucosal veins, which are supplied by the left gastric vein and drain into the superior vena cava via the azygous vein. B, Paraumbilical veins, which are supplied by the umbilical porton of the left portal vein and drain into the abdominal wall veins near the umbilicus. These veins may form a caput medusae. C, Rectal submucosal veins, which are supplied by the inferior mesenteric vein through the superior rectal vein and drain into the internal iliac veins through the middle rectal veins. D, Splenorenal shunts, which are created spontaneously or surgically. (From Feldman et al., 2002, with permission.)[108]

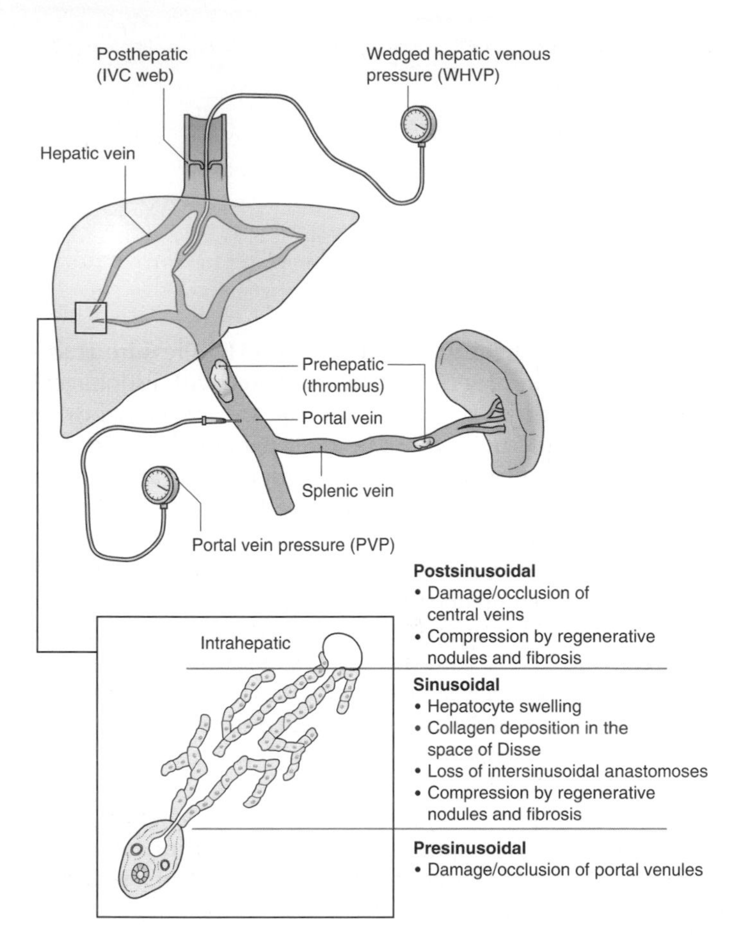

Figure 64.2: Sites of obstruction to portal venous flow and measurement of portal pressure, illustrating the major locations of extrahepatic (prehepatic and posthepatic) and intrahepatic (presinusoidal, sinusoidal and postsinusoidal) obstruction. A catheter tip is also shown wedged into a small hepatic vein (HV) for the measurement of the wedged hepatic venous pressure (WHVP). When the catheter tip is withdrawn into the hepatic vein the free hepatic vein pressure (FHVP) is obtained. Hepatic venous pressure gradient (HVPG) = WHPV – FHVP. Direct measurement of the portal venous pressure (PVP) is accomplished during surgery by catheterization of either the umbilical vein or the portal vein via the transjugular or transhepatic approach. IVC, inferior vena cava. (From Feldman et al., 2002, with permission.)[108]

protective epithelium and absorptive epithelium, such as in the cardia of the stomach, the anus, in the falciform ligament through remnants of the fetal umbilical circulation, abdominal organ contact with retroperitoneal tissues, and into the left renal vein. In extrahepatic obstruction, collaterals also form and attempt to bypass the blockage and enter directly into the liver at the porta hepatis. This is known as cavernous transformation.

Despite the formation of a significant collateral network, portal hypertension persists. This is a result of an increase in cardiac output and a decrease in splanchnic arteriolar tone. Retention of sodium and water via a hepatorenal reflex increases the circulating blood volume. There is also production of vasodilatory factors that cause arterial vasodilation of the splanchnic circulation. Several factors have been cited as possible mediators of splanchnic vasodilation, including glucagon, bile acids, nitric oxide,[2] prostaglandins and others. The above theories account for the increased portal flow. Increases in intrahepatic resistance could be due to hepatocyte swelling, fibrosis and inflammation within the portal tracts.

CLINICAL FEATURES

Gastrointestinal bleeding

Hematemesis and melena are the most frequent presentation of portal hypertension. Variceal bleeding is the most common cause. Esophageal varices occur in the distal esophagus, which is supplied by the anterior branch of the left gastric vein. Valves in the penetrating veins of the distal esophagus become incompetent and allow blood to flow in a retrograde fashion into the deep intrinsic veins of the esophagus. The risk of first-time bleeding from pediatric studies in children with cirrhosis is 22%, but rises to 38% in children with known varices over a 5-year period. Bleeding occurs in 15–25% of patients with biliary atresia in long-term follow-up.[3,4] Age at bleeding is also dependent on the underlying cause of cirrhosis, with patients who have surgically corrected but progressive biliary atresia bleeding for the first time at a mean age of 3 years and those with cystic fibrosis at a mean age of 11.5 years.[5]

Gastric varices are fed by the short gastric veins. Gastric varices may be isolated to the stomach (generally in the fundus, or in the antrum, corpus or pylorus) without the presence of esophageal varices, or may extend from the esophagus into the stomach (either along the lesser curve or towards the fundus).[6] Primary gastric varices generally refer to the presence of gastric varices at

	Hepatic venous pressure gradients measurements		
Cause of portal hypertension	Wedged hepatic venous pressure	Free hepatic venous pressure	Hepatic venous pressure gradient
Intrahepatic: sinusoidal (cirrhosis)	Raised	Normal	Raised
Posthepatic: hepatic venous obstruction	Raised	Raised	Normal
Intrahepatic: presinusoidal	Normal	Normal	Normal
Prehepatic: portal venous obstruction	Normal	Normal	Normal

Table 64.1 Hepatic venous pressure gradients in various forms of portal hypertension

initial examination in someone who has never had treatment for esophageal varices. Secondary gastric varices refers to the development of gastric varices after endoscopic therapy for esophageal varices. Gastric varices tend to lie deeper within the submucosa under the gastric mucosa, compared with the more superficial esophageal varices that form in the lamina propria and submucosa.

Rectal bleeding may occur as a result of inferior mesenteric–internal iliac venous collaterals. Hemorrhoids do not seem to be more common in patients with portal hypertension, but anorectal varices and portal colopathy are found more frequently.[7] Sites within the small intestine may also bleed,[8,9] and may respond only to surgical correction. Gallbladder varices have also been reported and seem to be more common in children with portal hypertension from extrahepatic portal vein obstruction (EHPVO). Gallbladder varices can be easily diagnosed by ultrasonography of the biliary tract.[10]

Portal hypertensive gastropathy can result in bleeding and is secondary to increased submucosal arteriovenous communications and increased gastric perfusion. Portal hypertensive gastropathy (PHG) can appear as discrete cherry-red spots assuming a mosaic pattern, or may be more confluent, and can occur over large areas of the stomach. Gastric antral vascular ectasia may be seen as linear streaks (watermelon stomach).[11] Bleeding may be worsened by the ingestion of gastric irritants such as nonsteoidal anti-inflammatory drugs (NSAIDs). PHG can occur prior to variceal eradication but is more common in patients who have undergone variceal obliteration. Venous congestion may also occur in the small intestine, making the mucosa edematous and friable. Duodenal erosions are often seen in portal hypertensive duodenopathy.[12] Bleeding also occurs more frequently at sites of mucocutaneous junctions such as stomas. Bleeding distal to the esophagus may be increased after successful esophageal variceal sclerotherapy and may respond only to reducing portal pressure.

Patients with portal hypertension can bleed from other gastric lesions such as ulcers and gastritis not secondary to portal hypertension. Coagulation problems may exacerbate bleeding. Patients with cirrhosis may have abnormalities of the prothrombin time due to decreased factor production. Coagulation abnormalities similar to a mild disseminated intravascular coagulation picture have been reported in teenagers with extrahepatic portal venous obstruction and in adults with noncirrhotic portal fibrosis. Abnormality of the international normalized ratio (INR), decreased fibrinogen and decreased platelet aggregation may be due to low circulating levels of endotoxin and increased cytokine activation.[13]

Variceal bleeding in children often follows an acute upper respiratory infection. The combination of factors including increased abdominal pressure from coughing or sneezing, increased cardiac output from fever, and possibly medications such as NSAIDs or aspirin contribute to the rupture of varices. Prolonged gastroesophageal reflux could also be associated with erosions over the varices that could lead to bleeding.

Esophageal varices can be graded;[14] the severity of the grading is considered to be a risk factor for bleeding:

- Grade I varices are flattened by insufflation.
- Grade II varices are not flattened by insufflation and are separated by areas of healthy mucosa.
- Grade III varices are confluent and not flattened by insufflation.

Patients with no varices or grade I varices are significantly less likely to bleed than patients with grade II or III varices. Other signs of increased bleeding risk include red wale markings.[15]

The risk of esophageal variceal bleeding in children with portal vein obstruction was thought to decrease in adolescence due to the development of spontaneous portosystemic collaterals. Lykavieris et al.[14] followed 44 children from age 12 years for a mean of 8 years. At the time of diagnosis of portal venous obstruction, no child had abnormal liver enzymes or function. The actuarial probability of bleeding was 49% at age 16 years and 76% at age 24 years. If the child had bled before the age of 12 years, the probability of bleeding was higher than in those who had not bled. As patients with grade II or III varices are at such a high risk of bleeding and unlikely to have regression of the varices, more effective treatment needs to be determined in the adolescent patient before significant bleeding occurs. In addition, there was no variceal regression but rather progression of varices in the majority of children, suggesting a lack of *significant* collateral formation (Fig. 64.3).[16]

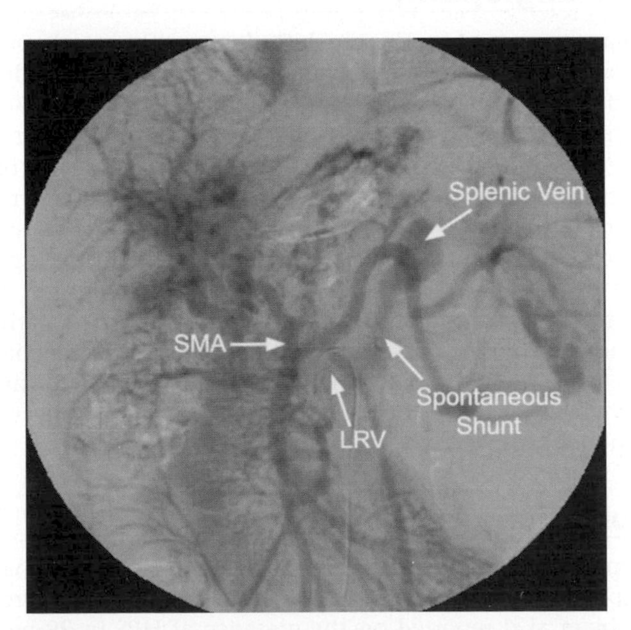

Figure 64.3: Angiogram from a 16-year-old patient with neonatal extrahepatic portal vein obstruction with persistent variceal bleeding despite the large patent spontaneous shunt shown above. LRV, left renal vein; SMA, superior mesenteric artery.

Splenomegaly

The enlarged spleen may be picked up incidentally on routine physical examination or by laboratory work showing changes consistent with hypersplenism. Hypersplenism can result in anemia as well as leukopenia and thrombocytopenia. Thrombocytopenia could result in frequent nose bleeds or petechiae. Hypersplenism rarely requires surgical intervention, except when the symptoms of anemia or physical discomfort are severe.[17]

Abdominal venous patterning

Portal hypertension-induced collateral formation can reperfuse the umbilical veins and lead to increased abdominal venous markings. If the level of obstruction is within the inferior vena cava, the flow in these vessels is cephalad. If the level of obstruction is not in the inferior vena cava, the flow is caudad in those vessels located below the umbilicus. Prominent periumbilical collaterals, caput medusae, may form on the abdominal wall with an audible venous hum, producing a Cruveilhier–Baumgarten murmur.

Ascites

Increased sodium retention and raised portal pressure may cause accumulation of fluid within the abdomen. Impaired lymphatic drainage may compound this. Treatment entails the use of diuretics. Albumin infusions can also be used to increase intravascular osmotic pressure. Paracentesis has been used safely in children as well, when the ascites is difficult to control.[18,19]

Cholangiopathy

Changes can occur in the bile ducts with extrahepatic venous obstruction. In several series including children and adults, biliary changes were reported in 80–100% of patients.[20–23] The common bile duct is most frequently affected, but changes may involve the intrahepatic bile ducts. The abnormalities include strictures, luminal irregularity, segmental dilation, ectasia, external compression by collateral veins, displacement of ducts and pruning of the intrahepatic ducts. Some of these changes are reversible after shunt surgery, suggesting that the pathogenesis is due to compression by collaterals.[20] Other changes were not reversible, indicating that the lesions may have been due to ischemic changes, possibly secondary to venous thrombosis.

Pulmonary complications

Hepatopulmonary syndrome (HPS) and portopulmonary hypertension are probably underdiagnosed in children. Barbe et al.[24] reported on the presence of HPS in 29 pediatric patients, 26 of whom had cirrhosis and 3 had extrahepatic causes of portal hypertension. HPS seems to progress more rapidly in patients with biliary atresia associated with polysplenia.[25] In an adult study of 31 noncirrhotic portal hypertensive patients compared with 46 patients with liver cirrhosis, HPS as diagnosed by contrast echocardiography and lung perfusion scans were equally common.[26] Patients with HPS have a higher incidence of dyspnea, cyanosis, platypnea (dyspnea that worsens in the upright position), clubbing and spider nevi.[24,27,28] There are two forms of HPS. In type I, the vessels enlarge such that the red blood cells traveling through the center of the vessel do not have significant contact time with the oxygen-rich alveoli. In type II HPS, the diffusion–perfusion mismatch is presumed to be due to arteriovenous communications completely bypassing alveoli.[29,30] HPS is thought to occur as a result of shunting of vasodilatory mediators from the mesentery away from the liver in portal hypertension. It is not related to the duration or severity of liver dysfunction. Liver transplantation may reverse HPS in more than 80% of patients, but if large shunts are present and the arterial partial pressure of oxygen is less than 50 mmHg on 100% oxygen, a poorer outcome may be expected.

Portopulmonary syndrome eventually leads to right-sided heart failure. Histologically there is pulmonary arteriopathy with concentric laminar intimal fibrosis consistent with a vasoconstrictive etiology. Pediatric cases have been reported.[31,32] The condition is defined by a pulmonary arterial pressure greater than 25 mmHg at rest and above 30 mmHg with exercise, raised pulmonary vascular resistance with pulmonary arterial occlusion pressure, or a left-ventricular end-diastolic pressure of less than 15 mmHg.[33] The most common symptom of pulmonary hypertension is exertional dyspnea. Other symptoms may include fatigue, palpitations, syncope or chest pains. Physical findings may include an accentuated second heart sound and systolic murmur of tricuspid regurgitation. Mild to moderate pulmonary hypertension may be reversible after liver transplantation, but severe pulmonary hypertension is not reversible and is associated with a very high mortality rate.

DISORDERS ASSOCIATED WITH PORTAL HYPERTENSION (TABLE 64.2)

Prehepatic disorders

Most cases of portal hypertension in children are due to extrahepatic obstruction of the portal vein, although splenic vein thrombosis can also lead to segmental portal hypertension. Portal vein thrombosis is idiopathic in the majority of cases (65%),[16] but could be secondary to neonatal omphalitis and/or catheterization of the umbilical vein (4.8%),[34] or pyelophlebitis secondary to appendicitis or other intra-abdominal infections in older children. Ando et al.[35] determined that many cases were caused by an embryologic malformation resulting in a tortuous, abnormal portal vein. There is also a rare association noted with cartilage–hair hypoplasia syndrome.[36] Malignancies, such as neuroblastoma and non-Hodgkin's

Prehepatic disorders
Portal vein thrombosis
Arteriovenous fistula
Splenic vein thrombosis
Splenomegaly
Posthepatic disorders
Budd–Chiari syndrome
Congestive heart failure
Inferior vena cava obstruction
Intrahepatic disorders (hepatocellular)
Autoimmune hepatitis
Hepatitis B
Hepatitis C
α_1-Antitrypsin deficiency
Wilson's disease
Steatohepatitis
Glycogen storage disease type IV
Toxins
• Methotrexate
• 6-Mercaptopurine
• Valproate
• Dilantin
• Vitamin A
• Arsenic
• Alcohol
Intrahepatic disorders (biliary)
Biliary atresia
Primary sclerosing cholangitis
Cystic fibrosis
Congenital hepatic fibrosis
Caroli's disease
Choledochal cyst
Familial cholestasis
• Progressive familial intrahepatic cholestasis type 1
• Alagille's syndrome
• Non-syndromic paucity syndrome
Primary biliary cirrhosis
Intrahepatic disorders (other)
Veno-occlusive disease
Schistosomiasis
Gaucher's disease
Idiopathic portal hypertension
Peliosis hepatis
• Anabolic steroids
• Azathioprine

Table 64.2 Causes of portal hypertension in children

lymphoma, have been reported as rare causes of portal vein thrombosis.[37,38]

Intrinsic clotting disorders have rarely been reported to play a role in EHPVO in children. A prospective randomized study of 20 patients with EHPVO showed that, despite lower levels of protein C, protein S and antithrombin III, there was no genetic basis and it was hypothesized to be due to increased clearance of activated clotting factors or to passive adsorption on the endothelium.[39]

Portal hypertension can result from increased portal flow, although rarely in children. Causes include arteriovenous fistula and splenomegaly. Arteriovenous fistulae have resulted from blunt or penetrating trauma to the liver (including diagnostic procedures such as liver biopsy and percutaneous cholangiography), hepatocellular carcinomas, hepatic artery aneurysms and congenital malformations.[40] Diagnosis is based on aortoportography. Splenoportography is not helpful as the flow in the portal vein is hepatofugal.

Posthepatic disorders

Budd–Chiari syndrome (hepatic venous outflow obstruction) results from obstruction of the posthepatic veins including the inferior vena cava and/or hepatic veins. This can be due to webs or thrombi in these vessels, although it has also been associated with pregnancy, contraceptive pills, myeloproliferative states, tumors and hypercoagulable states.[11] Congestive heart failure can cause chronic congestion in the liver that can progress to cirrhosis. Liver biopsy may show centrizonal congestion and necrosis. Presenting symptoms usually include abdominal pain, distention, jaundice and upper gastrointestinal bleeding. Hepatosplenomegaly, ascites and pedal edema may be present.

Intrahepatic disorders

In developed countries, intrahepatic causes are more frequent than extrahepatic causes of portal hypertension. Cirrhosis is the most common cause of intrahepatic portal hypertension, and may develop as a hepatocellular or biliary process. Hepatocellular causes of cirrhosis include α_1-antitrypsin deficiency, autoimmune hepatitis, infectious hepatitis, metabolic disease and toxins. Biliary causes include uncorrected or partially corrected biliary atresia, cystic fibrosis, primary sclerosing cholangitis, congenital hepatic fibrosis (CHF), Caroli's disease and progressive familial intrahepatic cholestasis.

Portal hypertension has been reported to occur in 35–75% of patients with biliary atresia due to progressive cirrhosis.[42] Caroli's disease is due to faulty remodeling of the early ductal plate with the formation of sac-like dilations of the larger intrahepatic bile ducts. These changes can generally be determined by ultrasonography.[43] CHF is due to a progressive necroinflammatory process of immature bile ducts causing presinusoidal intrahepatic portal hypertension. It is often associated with autosomal recessive polycystic kidney disease. Biliary inflammation leads to hepatic venule compression. Classically, children are asymptomatic until the age of 5–6 years and present at that time with symptoms of portal hypertension or cholangitis. Other associated disorders with CHF include medullary sponge kidney, Ivemark's familial dysplasia, vaginal atresia,

medical center. Long-term reduction of splanchnic pressures may help to reduce the risk of bleeding.

Most of the data regarding beta-blockade as primary prophylaxis against first-time bleeding come from adult studies. In meta-analyses,[59] beta-blockade resulted in a significant decrease in first-time bleeding and in some studies a possible reduction in the mortality rate.[84] Two non-placebo-controlled trials of propranolol in children with portal hypertension (primarily secondary to cirrhosis) as primary prophylaxis have been reported.[85,86] Use of propranolol, when treatment was adjusted to reduce the resting heart rate by 25%, was associated with a decreased risk of first-time bleeding of 15.6–19%. It was well tolerated with mild, transient side-effects. Some of these side-effects were eliminated by changing to long-acting preparations. Of the children who did bleed during therapy, compliance was an issue, as well as not being able to obtain a 25% reduction in heart rate. Twice-daily dosing was associated with bleeding more often than a three times a day dosing schedule, as were total daily doses of less than 1 mg/kg. Whether this was a truly significant decrease in first-time bleeding will need to be determined by future multicenter trials. Using transvenous portal pressure measurements before and during therapy with beta-blockers, a reduction of 20% in the HVPG has been shown to be associated with a decreased risk of bleeding to 10% in adult patients. Dropping the HVPG to less than 12 mmHg eliminated the risk of initial and recurrent variceal bleeding.[87]

There are few studies on the use of sclerotherapy in children to prevent first-time bleeding. Goncalves et al.[88] reported the long-term results of a prospective randomized controlled trial of sclerotherapy *vs* clinical monitoring. Prophylactic sclerotherapy significantly reduced the incidence of the first episode of esophageal variceal bleeding compared with that in controls without sclerotherapy (6% *vs* 42% respectively) and did not result in any significant complications. It did not increase the incidence of gastric varices, but, when varices were present, patients with prophylactic sclerotherapy had a higher risk of bleeding. Congestive hypertensive gastropathy occurred at a higher rate in patients with prophylactic sclerotherapy and was associated with a higher risk of bleeding. This increase in congestive hypertensive gastropathy may be associated with higher morbidity in the prophylactic sclerotherapy group overall, and would possibly require beta-blockade as therapy. Prophylactic sclerotherapy does not affect the survival rate. A meta-analyses of 19 adult studies[59] showed conflicting results. Studies that demonstrated high bleeding rates in control groups receiving only medical therapy but no beta-blockade demonstrated benefit of sclerotherapy for both bleeding and death. Studies that had low bleeding rates among the control populations did not show any benefit for sclerotherapy. EST actually resulted in a higher mortality rate in one study, and higher bleeding rates in another study. With this information, sclerotherapy as primary prophylaxis does not seem warranted, although further studies need to be performed to evaluate variceal banding as an option.

Secondary prophylaxis against rebleeding is important, especially in extrahepatic portal hypertension. Variceal obliteration has been shown to limit the chance of rebleeding. Beta-blocker therapy along with nitrates has been shown to decrease the risk of rebleeding in adult studies. Beta-blockers lower portal pressure through β_2 blockade of the splanchnic vascular supply. α-Adrenergic stimulation is then unopposed and there is a net decrease in splanchnic and portal perfusion. The goal of therapy is a 25% reduction in resting heart rate. Beta-blocker therapy may mask significant hypotension and is contraindicated in patients with asthma or heart block. Few studies have been performed in children, but those that have been done suggest that it is safe as well as effective.

Esophageal variceal sclerotherapy and band ligation have been used in children to avoid rebleeding after the initial bleeding episode. Repeated sessions every 2–4 weeks after the first episode has been shown to eradicate varices in 85–90% of patients, generally by five sessions (range 4.5–5.9).[34,60,89] In Poddar's large study of 207 children who underwent sclerotherapy for varices due to extrahepatic portal venous obstruction, complications included ulcers (17%), strictures (8%) and perforation (1.4%).[34] EVL may be associated with faster variceal eradication and fewer complications.[73,89] After sclerotherapy or band ligation, acid suppression or sucralfate should be instituted to promote ulcer healing. Follow-up endoscopy should be done yearly once variceal eradication has been achieved to re-evaluate for recurrence of varices, which may occur in up to 17% of patients.[34] The addition of a beta-blocker to sclerotherapy shortened the time to variceal eradication but did not affect rebleeding significantly.[90]

Surgical management is rarely needed in the acute situation but may be useful in long-term management for the prevention of rebleeding. In patients with normal liver function, such as those with extrahepatic portal vein thrombosis, appropriate surgical shunting is associated with a low risk of encephalopathy and markedly improves the long-term morbidity and mortality of recurrent bleeding. In patients with intrinsic liver disease whose varices cannot be obliterated and continue to bleed, surgical shunting may be the best approach if liver transplantation is not expected to be necessary in the near future. Indications for shunting include bleeding gastric or other non-esophageal varices, severe hypersplenism and continued acute bleeding despite the use of other non-surgical methods.

Shunt surgery

TIPS connect the portal vein with the hepatic vein via radiographic techniques. In adult studies it decreases the portal pressure by about 50% and encephalopathy is a complication in only 20% of patients who have underlying severe liver disease. The shunt can occlude or stenose in 20–50% of patients, necessitating frequent monitoring. Mortality from the procedure is low. Indications for the procedure in pediatric patients have included recurrent variceal bleeding not responsive to more conservative therapy, hypersplenism, ascites, Budd–Chiari syndrome,[91] hepatorenal syndrome and hepatopulmonary syndrome (Table 64.4).[92] Variceal bleeding is stopped after successful TIPS insertion in the majority of patients.[93,94] If rebleeding occurred, it was associated with shunt restenosis. Hypersplenism did not change significantly in the study by Huppert et al.[95] In veno-occlusive disease, early TIPS insertion led to a reduction in the portosystemic pressure gradient and improvement in arterial and portal flow to the liver, but the mortality rate remained extremely high from multiorgan system failure.[96,97] The procedure in pediatric patients may require general anesthesia, a longer procedure time and modification of the equipment. Limitations for the procedure in pediatrics may be due to vascular anomalies, which may be a relative contraindication.[98] Biliary atresia may also lead to increased difficulty with TIPS placement due to periportal fibrosis and small portal veins.[95] Scheduled re-evaluations of the shunts need to be carried out via physical examinations, laboratory testing and Doppler ultrasonography. If necessary, shunt revision can be performed using the transjugular approach for balloon angioplasty and shunt replacement. Reinterventions may be necessary in more than 50% of patients prior to more definitive surgery such as liver transplantation or surgical shunt placement.[95,98] Long-term shunt patency has been achieved, reaching durations of up to 6 years. Complications with TIPS placement include portal vein leakage, encephalopathy, perforation, hemolysis, infection and restenosis. Fever is common within the first 24–48 h after the procedure. Serum aspartate aminotransferase and alanine aminotransferase levels may also rise immediately after the procedure and then return to baseline.[99]

TIPS has been proven very effective in acute refractory variceal bleeding because it is a minimally invasive radiologic intervention that can possibly be performed under local anesthesia in adult patients. If the TIPS fails or is not possible, a surgical shunt can be performed. The type of shunt selected should be determined by the prognosis of the underlying liver disease, likelihood of liver transplantation, anatomy and surgical experience. Maintaining adequate hepatopedal flow following shunt surgery lowers the risk of encephalopathy and liver deterioration (Fig. 64.6).

Indication	Value
Prophylaxis of variceal bleeding	Effective
Refractory ascites in cirrhosis	Effective
Portal hypertensive gastropathy	Effective
Gastric antral vascular ectasia	Ineffective
Hepatic hydrothorax	Effective
Hypersplenism	Possibly effective
Acute hepatorenal syndrome	Possibly effective
Budd–Chiari syndrome	Effective
Chronic hepatorenal syndrome	Effective
Hepatopulmonary syndrome	Possibly effective
Veno-occlusive disease	Possibly effective

Table 64.4 TIPS: indications and effectiveness

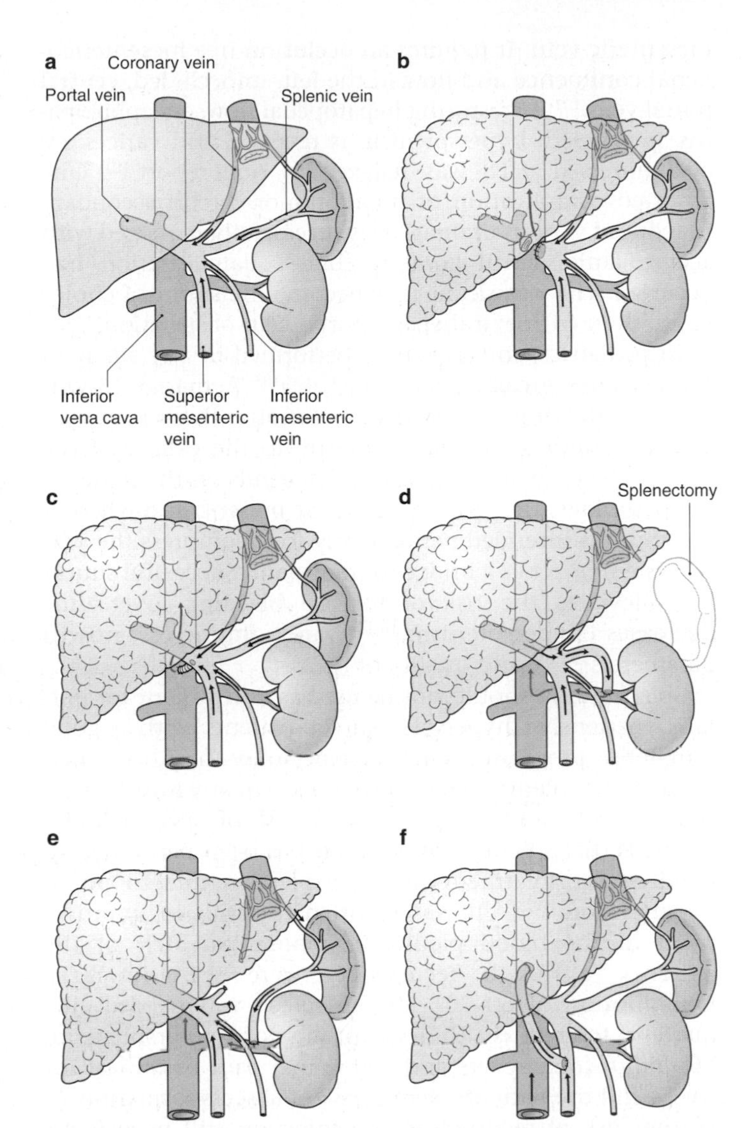

Figure 64.6: Types of portosystemic shunt. (**a**) Normal anatomy. (**b**) End-to-side portacaval shunt with ligation of portal vein at the liver. (**c**) Small-diameter portacaval H-graft. (**d**) Central splenorenal shunt requiring splenectomy. (**e**) Distal splenorenal shunt. (**f**) Superior mesenterico-left intrahepatic portal vein (Rex) shunt using the internal jugular as a graft.

Hepatopedal flow has been maintained most consistently with a selective splenorenal shunt (distal splenorenal shunt; DSRS), partial small-caliber portocaval or mesocaval interposition shunt.[100] In the long term, surgical shunts achieve variceal hemorrhage control in more than 90% of patients. Surgical shunts are preferred in patients with non-cirrhotic portal hypertension due to schistosomiasis, non-cirrhotic portal fibrosis, idiopathic portal hypertension, CHF, EHPVO, Budd–Chiari syndrome and veno-occlusive disease. In patients with non-cirrhotic portal hypertension, a DSRS is optimal as the risk of encephalopathy is low and a splenectomy is not needed.

The 'Rex shunt' (mesenterico-left portal bypass) restores hepatopetal flow by using a jugular venous autograft between the intrahepatic left portal vein and the superior mesenteric vein. It requires an occlusion-free mesenterico-lienal confluence and flow in the left, unoccluded, central portal vein.[101] By restoring hepatopedal flow, encephalopathy is avoided; hypersplenism is reversed and varices are decompressed. HPS was relieved in one report.[101] One reported complication of pseudotumor cerebri secondary to reduced venous drainage was successfully managed with acetazolamide until good cerebral collateralization had occurred. The Rex shunt may become the shunt of choice in children with extrahepatic portal vein obstruction.

In pediatrics, shunts can be performed in any age with success rates greater than 90%.[63,102,103] Actuarial 15-year survival rates of 95% have been noted after shunt surgery.[16] Shunt thrombosis is related mostly to the caliber of the shunt. The type of shunt selected depends on the underlying pathology, the vascular anatomy present, and whether the shunt is intended permanently to decompress the portal system or act as a bridge to transplant. Successful shunting alleviates the risk of variceal bleeding, over time decreases hypersplenism,[16,104] and improves growth parameters[102,105] and quality of life.

Splenectomy should not be used as a treatment for portal hypertensive hypersplenism in patients with a good long-term prognosis. Once splenectomy has been performed, the splenic vein cannot be used in any future shunt procedures,[100] and the patient is at risk of overwhelming sepsis. Partial splenic embolization has been performed in children for treatment of hypersplenism due to portal hypertension.[106,107] It was reported to result in improvement in the blood picture in more than 70% of the patients, although recurrences were seen in 30%. Embolization of 60–70% of the spleen was needed adequately to reduce the symptoms of hypersplenism. Morbidity from fevers and abdominal pain could last for weeks and the patients were at risk of abscess formation.[106] Further risk of recurrences and infection still need to be studied. This type of procedure should be performed only on patients with normal liver function and before the spleen size is too massive. This procedure does not correct the underlying portal hypertension.

References

1. Reddy SI, Grace ND. Liver imaging. A hepatologist's perspective. Clin Liver Dis 2002; 6:297–310, ix.
2. Shams V, Erkan T, Gumustas MK, et al. The role of nitric oxide in pediatric patients with portal hypertension. J Trop Pediatr 2003; 49:33–36.
3. van Heurn LW, Saing H, Tam PK. Portoenterostomy for biliary atresia: long-term survival and prognosis after esophageal variceal bleeding. J Pediatr Surg 2004; 39:6–9.
4. Karrer FM, Price MR, Bensard DD, et al. Long-term results with the Kasai operation for biliary atresia. Arch Surg 1996; 131:493–496.
5. Debray D, Lykavieris P, Gauthier F, et al. Outcome of cystic fibrosis-associated liver cirrhosis: management of portal hypertension. J Hepatol 1999; 31:77–83.
6. Ryan BM, Stockbrugger RW, Ryan JM. A pathophysiologic, gastroenterologic, and radiologic approach to the management of gastric varices. Gastroenterology 2004; 126:1175–1189.
7. Misra SP, Dwivedi M, Misra V. Prevalence and factors influencing hemorrhoids, anorectal varices, and colopathy in patients with portal hypertension. Endoscopy 1996; 28:340–345.
8. Astfalk W, Huppert PE, Schweizer P, Plinta-Zgrabczynski A. Recurrent intestinal bleeding from jejunojejunostomy caused by portal hypertension following hepatoportojejunostomy in extra hepatic biliary atresia (EHBA) – successful treatment by transjugular intrahepatic portosystemic shunt (TIPS). Eur J Pediatr Surg 1997; 7:147–148.
9. Hasegawa T, Tazuke Y, Ishikawa S, et al. Portal hypertensive enteropathy in biliary atresia. Pediatr Ssurg Int 1998; 13:602–604.
10. West MS, Garra BS, Horii SC, et al. Gallbladder varices: imaging findings in patients with portal hypertension. Radiology 1991; 179:179–182.
11. Sarin SK, Shahi HM, Jain M, Jain AK, Issar SK, Murthy NS. The natural history of portal hypertensive gastropathy: influence of variceal eradication. Am J Gastroenterol 2000; 95:2888–2893.
12. Shudo R, Yazaki Y, Sakurai S, Uenishi H, Yamada H, Sugawara K. Duodenal erosions, a common and distinctive feature of portal hypertensive duodenopathy. Am J Gastroenterol 2002; 97:867–873.
13. Bajaj JS, Bhattacharjee J, Sarin SK. Coagulation profile and platelet function in patients with extrahepatic portal vein obstruction and non-cirrhotic portal fibrosis. J Gastroenterol Hepatol 2001; 16:641–646.
14. Lykavieris P, Gauthier F, Hadchouel P, Duche M, Bernard O. Risk of gastrointestinal bleeding during adolescence and early adulthood in children with portal vein obstruction. J Pediatr 2000; 136:805–808.
15. Beppu K, Inokuchi K, Koyanagi N, et al. Prediction of variceal hemorrhage by esophageal endoscopy. Gastrointest Endosc 1981; 27:213–218.
16. Orloff MJ, Orloff MS, Girard B, Orloff SL. Bleeding esophagogastric varices from extrahepatic portal hypertension: 40 years' experience with portal-systemic shunt. J Am Coll Surg 2002; 194:717–728, discussion 728–730.
17. Triger DR. Extrahepatic portal venous obstruction. Gut 1987; 28:1193–1197.
18. Arikan C, Ozgenc F, Akman SA, Yagci RV, Tokat Y, Aydogdu S. Large-volume paracentesis and liver transplantation. J Pediatr Gastroenterol Nutr 2003; 37:207–208.
19. Kramer RE, Sokol RJ, Yerushalmi B, et al. Large-volume paracentesis in the management of ascites in children. J Pediatr Gastroenterol Nutr 2001; 33:245–249.
20. Dhiman RK, Puri P, Chawla Y, et al. Biliary changes in extrahepatic portal venous obstruction: compression by collaterals or ischemic? Gastrointest Endosc 1999; 50:646–652.
21. Dilawari JB, Chawla YK. Pseudosclerosing cholangitis in extrahepatic portal venous obstruction. Gut 1992; 33:272–276.
22. Khuroo MS, Yattoo GN, Zargar SA, et al. Biliary abnormalities associated with extrahepatic portal venous obstruction. Hepatology 1993; 17:807–813.
23. Nagi B, Kochhar R, Bhasin D, Singh K. Cholangiopathy in extrahepatic portal venous obstruction. Radiological appearances. Acta Radiol 2000; 41:612–615.
24. Barbe T, Losay J, Grimon G, et al. Pulmonary arteriovenous shunting in children with liver disease. J Pediatr 1995; 126:571–579.
25. Kimura T, Hasegawa T, Sasaki T, Okada A, Mushiake S. Rapid progression of intrapulmonary arteriovenous shunting in polysplenia syndrome associated with biliary atresia. Pediatr Pulmonol 2003; 35:494–498.

26. Kaymakoglu S, Kahraman T, Kudat H, et al. Hepatopulmonary syndrome in noncirrhotic portal hypertensive patients. Dig Dis Sci 2003; 48:556–560.
27. Anand AC, Mukherjee D, Rao KS, Seth AK. Hepatopulmonary syndrome: prevalence and clinical profile. Indian J Gastroenterol 2001; 20:24–27.
28. Yap FK, Aw MM, Quek SC, Quak SH, Quak SC. Hepatopulmonary syndrome: a rare complication of chronic liver disease in children. Ann Acad Med 1999; 28:290–293.
29. Yuan HC, Wu TC, Huang IF, Liu CS, Chern MS, Hwang BT. Hepatopulmonary syndrome in a child. J.Chin.Med Assoc 2003; 66:127–130.
30. Krowka MJ, Wiseman GA, Burnett OL, et al. Hepatopulmonary syndrome: a prospective study of relationships between severity of liver disease, PaO_2 response to 100% oxygen, and brain uptake after ^{99m}Tc MAA lung scanning. Chest 2000; 118:615–624.
31. Rossi SO, Gilbert-Barness E, Saari T, Corliss R. Pulmonary hypertension with coexisting portal hypertension. Pediatr Pathol 1992; 12:433–439.
32. Krowka MJ, Plevak DJ, Findlay JY, Rosen CB, Wiesner RH, Krom RA. Pulmonary hemodynamics and perioperative cardiopulmonary-related mortality in patients with portopulmonary hypertension undergoing liver transplantation. Liver Transpl 2000; 6:443–450.
33. Hoeper MM, Krowka MJ, Strassburg CP. Portopulmonary hypertension and hepatopulmonary syndrome. Lancet 2004; 363:1461–1468.
34. Poddar U, Thapa BR, Singh K. Endoscopic sclerotherapy in children: experience with 257 cases of extrahepatic portal venous obstruction. Gastrointest Endosc 2003; 57:683–686.
35. Ando H, Kaneko K, Ito F, Seo T, Watanabe Y, Ito T. Anatomy and etiology of extrahepatic portal vein obstruction in children leading to bleeding esophageal varices. J Am Coll Surg 1996; 183:543–547.
36. Fryns JP. Hypersplenism and portal hypertension with vena porta thrombosis in cartilage–hair hypoplasia (metaphyseal chondrodysplasia, McKusick type, MIM *250250). Genet Counsel 2000; 11:277–278.
37. Yule SM, Anderson J. Hepatic cirrhosis and portal hypertension in neuroblastoma. Pediatr Hematol Oncol 2000; 17:457–461.
38. Kauffman WM, Ribeiro RC. Cavernous transformation of the portal vein in a child with non-Hodgkin's lymphoma. Med Pediatr Oncol 1997; 29:143–145.
39. Dubuisson C, Boyer-Neumann C, Wolf M, Meyer D, Bernard O. Protein C, protein S and antithrombin III in children with portal vein obstruction. J Hepatol 1997; 27:132–135.
40. Heaton ND, Davenport M, Karani J, Mowat AP, Howard ER. Congenital hepatoportal arteriovenous fistula. Surgery 1995; 117:170–174.
41. Singh V, Sinha SK, Nain CK, et al. Budd–Chiari syndrome: our experience of 71 patients. J Gastroenterol Hepatol 2000; 15:550–554.
42. Narkewicz MR. Biliary atresia: an update on our understanding of the disorder. Curr Opin Pediatr 2001; 13:435–440.
43. Gorka W, Lewall DB. Value of Doppler sonography in the assessment of patients with Caroli's disease. J Clin Ultrasound 1998; 26:283–287.
44. Bansal D, Patwari AK, Logani KB, Jain R, Anand VK. Congenital hepatic fibrosis. Indian Pediatr 1998; 35:170–172.
45. Lebrec D, Benhamou JP. Noncirrhotic intrahepatic portal hypertension. Semin Liver Dis 1986; 6:332–340.
46. D'Antiga L, Baker A, Pritchard J, Pryor D, Mieli-Vergani G. Veno-occlusive disease with multi-organ involvement following actinomycin-D. Eur J Cancer 2001; 37:1141–1148.
47. Nakanuma Y, Hoso M, Sasaki M, et al. Histopathology of the liver in non-cirrhotic portal hypertension of unknown aetiology. Histopathology 1996; 28:195–204.
48. Dhiman RK, Chawla Y, Vasishta RK, et al. Non-cirrhotic portal fibrosis (idiopathic portal hypertension): experience with 151 patients and a review of the literature. J Gastroenterol Hepatol 2002; 17:6–16.
49. Poddar U, Thapa BR, Puri P, et al. Non-cirrhotic portal fibrosis in children. Indian J Gastroenterol 2000; 19:12–13.
50. Lachmann RH, Wight DG, Lomas DJ, et al. Massive hepatic fibrosis in Gaucher's disease: clinico-pathological and radiological features. Quart J Med 2000; 93:237–244.
51. Perel Y, Bioulac-Sage P, Chateil JF, et al. Gaucher's disease and fatal hepatic fibrosis despite prolonged enzyme replacement therapy. Pediatrics 2002; 109:1170–1173.
52. Bezerra Alves JG, Ulisses Montenegro FM. Portal hypertension due to schistosomiasis. Indian Pediatr 2001; 38:1416–1418.
53. Runyon BA, Montano AA, Akriviadis EA, Antillon MR, Irving MA, McHutchison JG. The serum–ascites albumin gradient is superior to the exudate–transudate concept in the differential diagnosis of ascites. Ann Intern Med 1992; 117:215–220.
54. Yu AS, Hu KQ. Management of ascites. Clin Liver Dis 2001; 5:541–568, viii.
55. Teo EL, Strouse PJ, Prince MR. Applications of magnetic resonance imaging and magnetic resonance angiography to evaluate the hepatic vasculature in the pediatric patient. Pediatr Radiol 1999; 29:238–243.
56. Glassman MS, Klein SA, Spivak W. Evaluation of cavernous transformation of the portal vein by magnetic resonance imaging. Clin Pediatr 1993; 32:77–80.
57. Santamaria F, Sarnelli P, Celentano L, et al. Noninvasive investigation of hepatopulmonary syndrome in children and adolescents with chronic cholestasis. Pediatr Pulmonol 2002; 33:374–379.
58. Teisseyre M, Szymczak M, Swiatek-Rawa E, et al. Scintiscanning in diagnostics of hepatopulmonary syndrome in children. Med Sci Monitor 2001; 7(Suppl 1):255–261.
59. D'Amico G, Pagliaro L, Bosch J. The treatment of portal hypertension: a meta-analytic review. Hepatology 1995; 22:332–354.
60. Howard ER, Stringer MD, Mowat AP. Assessment of injection sclerotherapy in the management of 152 children with oesophageal varices. Br J Surg 1988; 75:404–408.
61. Sarin SK, Misra SP, Singal AK, Thorat V, Broor SL. Endoscopic sclerotherapy for varices in children. J Pediatr Gastroenterol Nutr 1988; 7:662–666.
62. Yachha SK, Sharma BC, Kumar M, Khanduri A. Endoscopic sclerotherapy for esophageal varices in children with extrahepatic portal venous obstruction: a follow-up study. J Pediatr Gastroenterol Nutr 1997; 24:49–52.
63. Maksoud JG, Goncalves ME, Porta G, Miura I, Velhote MC. The endoscopic and surgical management of portal hypertension in children: analysis of 123 cases. J Pediatr Surg 1991; 26:178–181.
64. Brown JB, Emerick KM, Brown DL, Whitington PF, Alonso EM. Recombinant factor VIIa improves coagulopathy caused by liver failure. J Pediatr Gastroenterol Nutr 2003; 37:268–272.
65. Ryckman FC, Alonso MH. Causes and management of portal hypertension in the pediatric population. Clin Liver Dis 2001; 5:789–818.
66. Karrer FM, Narkewicz MR. Esophageal varices: current management in children. Semin Pediatr Surg 1999; 8:193–201.
67. Sokal EM, Van Hoorebeeck N, Van Obbergh L, Otte JB, Buts JP. Upper gastro-intestinal tract bleeding in cirrhotic children

candidates for liver transplantation. Eur J Pediatr 1992; 151:326–328.

68. Lobritto SJ. Endoscopic considerations in children. Gastrointest Endosc Clin North Am 2001; 11:93–109.
69. Eroglu Y, Emerick KM, Whitingon PF, Alonso EM. Octreotide therapy for control of acute gastrointestinal bleeding in children. J Pediatr Gastroenterol Nutr 2004; 38:41–47.
70. McKiernan PJ. Treatment of variceal bleeding. Gastrointest Endosc Clin North Am 2001; 11:789–812, viii.
71. Stringer MD, Howard ER. Longterm outcome after injection sclerotherapy for oesophageal varices in children with extrahepatic portal hypertension. Gut 1994; 35:257–259.
72. Karrer FM, Holland RM, Allshouse MJ, Lilly JR. Portal vein thrombosis: treatment of variceal hemorrhage by endoscopic variceal ligation. J Pediatr Surg 1994; 29:1149–1151.
73. Zargar SA, Javid G, Khan BA, et al. Endoscopic ligation compared with sclerotherapy for bleeding esophageal varices in children with extrahepatic portal venous obstruction. Hepatology 2002; 36:666–672.
74. Gimson AE, Ramage JK, Panos MZ, et al. Randomised trial of variceal banding ligation versus injection sclerotherapy for bleeding oesophageal varices. Lancet 1993; 342:391–394.
75. D'Amico G, Pietrosi G, Tarantino I, Pagliaro L. Emergency sclerotherapy versus vasoactive drugs for variceal bleeding in cirrhosis: a Cochrane meta-analysis. Gastroenterology 2003; 124:1277–1291.
76. Patch D, Sabin CA, Goulis J, et al. A randomized, controlled trial of medical therapy versus endoscopic ligation for the prevention of variceal rebleeding in patients with cirrhosis. Gastroenterology 2002; 123:1013–1019.
77. Villanueva C, Minana J, Ortiz J, et al. Endoscopic ligation compared with combined treatment with nadolol and isosorbide mononitrate to prevent recurrent variceal bleeding. N Engl J Med 2001; 345:647–655.
78. Banares R, Albillos A, Rincon D, et al. Endoscopic treatment versus endoscopic plus pharmacologic treatment for acute variceal bleeding: a meta-analysis. Hepatology 2002; 35:609–615.
79. Turler A, Wolff M, Dorlars D, Hirner A. Embolic and septic complications after sclerotherapy of fundic varices with cyanoacrylate. Gastrointest Endosc 2001; 53:228–230.
80. Greenwald BD, Caldwell SH, Hespenheide EE, et al. *N*-2-butyl-cyanoacrylate for bleeding gastric varices: a United States pilot study and cost analysis. Am J Gastroenterol 2003; 98:1982–1988.
81. Datta D, Vlavianos P, Alisa A, Westaby D. Use of fibrin glue (Beriplast) in the management of bleeding gastric varices. Endoscopy 2003; 35:675–678.
82. Fuster S, Costaguta A, Tobacco O. Treatment of bleeding gastric varices with tissue adhesive (Histoacryl) in children. Endoscopy 1998; 30:S39–S40.
83. Uno Y, Munakata A, Ishiguro A, Fukuda S, Sugai M, Munakata H. Endoscopic ligation for bleeding rectal varices in a child with primary extrahepatic portal hypertension. Endoscopy 1998; 30:S107–S108.
84. Hayes PC, Davis JM, Lewis JA, Bouchier IA. Meta-analysis of value of propranolol in prevention of variceal haemorrhage. Lancet 1990; 336:153–156.
85. Shashidhar H, Langhans N, Grand RJ. Propranolol in prevention of portal hypertensive hemorrhage in children: a pilot study. J Pediatr Gastroenterol Nutr 1999; 29:12–17.
86. Ozsoylu S, Kocak N, Demir H, Yuce A, Gurakan F, Ozen H. Propranolol for primary and secondary prophylaxis of variceal bleeding in children with cirrhosis. Turk J Pediatr 2000; 42:31–33.
87. Feu F, Garcia-Pagan JC, Bosch J, et al. Relation between portal pressure response to pharmacotherapy and risk of recurrent variceal haemorrhage in patients with cirrhosis. Lancet 1995; 346:1056–1059.
88. Goncalves ME, Cardoso SR, Maksoud JG. Prophylactic sclerotherapy in children with esophageal varices: long-term results of a controlled prospective randomized trial. J Pediatr Surg 2000; 35:401–405.
89. Ganguly S, Dasgupta J, Das AS, Biswas K, Mazumder DN. Study of portal hypertension in children with special reference to sclerotherapy. Trop Gastroenterol 1997; 18:119–121.
90. Sokucu S, Suoglu OD, Elkabes B, Saner G. Long-term outcome after sclerotherapy with or without a beta-blocker for variceal bleeding in children. Pediatr Int 2003; 45:388–394.
91. Murad SD, Valla DC, de Groen PC, et al. Determinants of survival and the effect of portosystemic shunting in patients with Budd–Chiari syndrome. Hepatology 2004; 39:500–508.
92. Paramesh AS, Husain SZ, Shneider B, et al. Improvement of hepatopulmonary syndrome after transjugular intrahepatic portasystemic shunting: case report and review of literature. Pediatr Transplant 2003; 7:157–162.
93. Wroblewski T, Rowinski O, Ziarkiewicz-Wroblewska B, et al. TIPS: a therapy to prevent variceal rebleeding in patients listed for liver transplantation. Transplant Proc 2002; 34:635–637.
94. Chui AK, Rao AR, Shi LW, et al. Liver transplantation in patients with transjugular intrahepatic portosystemic shunts. Transplant Proc 2000; 32:2204–2205.
95. Huppert PE, Goffette P, Astfalk W, et al. Transjugular intrahepatic portosystemic shunts in children with biliary atresia. Cardiovasc Intervent Radiol 2002; 25:484–493.
96. Azoulay D, Castaing D, Lemoine A, Hargreaves GM, Bismuth H. Transjugular intrahepatic portosystemic shunt (TIPS) for severe veno-occlusive disease of the liver following bone marrow transplantation. Bone Marrow Transpl 2000; 25:987–992.
97. Zenz T, Rossle M, Bertz H, Siegerstetter V, Ochs A, Finke J. Severe veno-occlusive disease after allogeneic bone marrow or peripheral stem cell transplantation – role of transjugular intrahepatic portosystemic shunt (TIPS). Liver 2001; 21:31–36.
98. Heyman MB, LaBerge JM, Somberg KA, et al. Transjugular intrahepatic portosystemic shunts (TIPS) in children. J Pediatr 1997; 131:914–919.
99. Boyer TD. Transjugular intrahepatic portosystemic shunt: current status. Gastroenterology 2003; 124:1700–1710.
100. Wolff M, Hirner A. Current state of portosystemic shunt surgery. Langenbecks Arch Surg 2003; 388:141–149.
101. Fuchs J, Warmann S, Kardorff R, et al. Mesenterico-left portal vein bypass in children with congenital extrahepatic portal vein thrombosis: a unique curative approach. J Pediatr Gastroenterol Nutr 2003; 36:213–216.
102. Alvarez F, Bernard O, Brunelle F, Hadchouel P, Odievre M, Alagille D. Portal obstruction in children. II. Results of surgical portosystemic shunts. J Pediatr 1983; 103:703–707.
103. Bismuth H, Franco D, Alagille D. Portal diversion for portal hypertension in children. The first ninety patients. Ann Surg 1980; 192:18–24.
104. Shilyansky J, Roberts EA, Superina RA. Distal splenorenal shunts for the treatment of severe thrombocytopenia from portal hypertension in children. J Gastrointest Surg 1999; 3:167–172.
105. Kato T, Romero R, Koutouby R, et al. Portosystemic shunting in children during the era of endoscopic therapy: improved

postoperative growth parameters. J Pediatr Gastroenterol Nutr 2000; 30:419–425.

106. Petersons A, Volrats O, Bernsteins A. The first experience with non-operative treatment of hypersplenism in children with portal hypertension. Eur J Pediatr Surg 2002; 12:299–303.

107. Nio M, Hayashi Y, Sano N, Ishii T, Sasaki H, Ohi R. Long-term efficacy of partial splenic embolization in children. J Pediatr Surg 2003; 38:1760–1762.

108. Feldman M, Friedman LS, Sleisenger MH, eds. Sleisenger and Fordtran's Gastrointestinal and Liver Disease, 7th edn. Philadelphia, PA: WB Saunders; 2002.

109. Feldman M, Scharschidt BF, Sleisenger MH. Sleisinger and Fordtran's Gastrointestinal and Liver Disease, Vol. 2, 6th edn. Philadelphia, PA. WB Saunders; 1998.

Chapter 65
Liver failure and transplantation

Deirdre Kelly

INTRODUCTION

Successful pediatric liver transplantation has been established since the 1990s and has changed the prognosis for many children dying from acute or chronic liver failure. The many advances in both medical and surgical management have led to international 1-year survival rates after pediatric liver transplantation of more than 90% and 5–10-year survival rates of 80%.[1]

The improved survival rates are related to improved preoperative and postoperative management in association with the development of innovative surgical techniques to expand the donor pool. These techniques have not only reduced deaths on the waiting list and improved survival overall but have extended the range of indications for liver transplantation to include transplantation for inborn errors of metabolism. As short-term survival rates have improved, interest in research has focused on evaluating quality of life in long-term survivors.

CHRONIC LIVER FAILURE

Chronic liver failure is the end-result of many different diseases discussed in previous chapters, many of which may result in cirrhosis (Table 65.1), including reduced bile secretion or bile duct obstruction (cholestasis), infections, toxins, metabolic, vascular and nutritional disorders. Hepatic dysfunction and cholestasis lead to malnutrition, impaired protein synthesis, coagulopathy, portal hypertension, hepatorenal and hepatopulmonary syndromes, encephalopathy and ascites. Cholestasis is also associated with pruritus and malabsorption. Many children with chronic liver disease are immunosuppressed with resulting bacterial infection. Hepatocellular carcinoma may complicate cirrhosis in childhood, particularly in chronic hepatitis B and tyrosinemia type I.

Chronic liver disease may be either *compensated,* when there are no clinical or laboratory features of liver failure, or *decompensated*, at which time transplantation is required.

Clinical presentation

Some diseases, such as autoimmune hepatitis type 1, cystic fibrosis and α_1-antitrypsin deficiency, may present with compensated cirrhosis, and the first sign of liver disease may be hepatosplenomegaly, splenomegaly alone, increased hepatic transaminases or increased alkaline phosphatase levels. The liver is small and impalpable, but it may be enlarged, hard or nodular with splenomegaly. Cutaneous features such as spider angiomata, prominent periumbilical veins and palmar erythema are all signs of chronic liver disease. The presence of prominent veins radiating from the umbilicus (caput medusa) is an indication of portal hypertension. Other cutaneous features include easy bruising, fine telangiectasia on the face and upper back, and clubbing of the fingers.

In contrast, children with cholestatic liver disease have persisting jaundice and pruritus, as in biliary cirrhosis. The liver is usually enlarged, and xanthelasma, malnutrition and deficiency of fat-soluble vitamins (particularly vitamins D and K) may be prominent features. Clubbing is more likely to occur in biliary cirrhosis, and malnutrition and decompensation occur earlier in this form of liver disease.

Decompensated liver disease is characterized by clinical and laboratory findings of liver synthetic failure, and the occurrence of complications such as malnutrition, ascites, peripheral edema, coagulopathy, gastrointestinal bleeding and hepatic encephalopathy. Malnutrition with reduced lean tissue and fat stores and poor linear growth is an important sign of chronic liver disease in children.[2] Spontaneous bruising caused by reduced synthesis of clotting factors and thrombocytopenia due to hypersplenism is a sign of advanced disease. There may also be changes in the systemic and pulmonary circulations, with arteriolar vasodilation, increased blood volume, a hyperdynamic circulatory state and cyanosis due to intrapulmonary shunting. Renal failure is a late but serious event. Laboratory

Chronic liver failure
Cholestatic liver disease
Biliary atresia
Idiopathic neonatal hepatitis
Alagille syndrome
Progressive familial intrahepatic cholestasis
Metabolic liver disease
α_1-Antitrypsin deficiency
Tyrosinemia type I
Wilson's disease
Cystic fibrosis
Glycogen storage type IV
Chronic hepatitis
Autoimmune
Idiopathic
Postviral (hepatitis B, C, other)
Cryptogenic cirrhosis
Fibropolycystic liver disease ± Caroli syndrome
Primary immunodeficiency

Table 65.1 Chronic liver failure

investigations may reveal increased levels of alkaline phosphatase, bilirubin, hepatic transaminases and ammonia, but in particular there is abnormal liver synthetic function, reflected by such findings as hypoalbuminemia and prolonged prothrombin time.

Diagnosis of the etiology of liver disease is based on clinical findings and the results of relevant investigations including the *liver biopsy* findings, which will confirm the extent of cirrhosis and possibly the cause of the liver disease.

Prevention and management of complications

The primary aims of management are:

- To prevent progressive liver damage by treating the cause
- To prevent or control the complications
- To consider liver transplantation prior to irreversible disease.

Malnutrition and nutritional support

The liver has a central role in regulating fuel and metabolism, nutrient homeostasis, and the absorption of a number of nutrients; malnutrition is thus a common complication of chronic liver failure, particularly in infants, because of their higher energy and growth requirements.[3] A wide range of nutrient deficits occurs in most chronic liver diseases in children and may be reversed with intensive nutritional supplementation and fat-soluble vitamins (Table 65.2).

Deficit	Management
Energy	Increase calorie intake
	Achieve 130–150% EAR
	Nocturnal enteral nutrition
	Continuous enteral nutrition
Protein	Provide adequate protein (3–4 g/kg daily)
	BCAA-enriched protein (32%)
	Albumin infusion (if serum albumin <25 g/l)
Fat	Improve fat absorption (MCT/LCT) 50 : 50
	Provide saturated fats high in EFA
	?Supplement DHA
Fat-soluble vitamins	Light exposure
	Vitamin $D_{1\alpha}$ (50 ng/kg)
	Vitamin K (2.5–5 mg/day)
	Vitamin E (50–400 IU/day) (as TPGS)
	Vitamin A (5000–10 000 IU/day)
Water-soluble minerals	Supplement vitamins
	Supplement as required

AAA, aromatic amino acids; BCAA, branched-chain amino acids; DHA, docosahexanoic acid; EAR, estimated average requirement; EFA, essential fatty acids; LCT, long-chain fatty acids; MCT, medium-chain fatty acids; PEM, protein-energy malnutrition; TPGS, tocopherol polyethyleneglycol-1000 succinate.

Table 65.2 Management of nutritional deficiency in pediatric liver failure

Portal hypertension

Portal pressure, or hepatic venous pressure gradient (HVPG), is the difference between wedged hepatic pressure and free hepatic venous pressure, which reflects inferior vena cava (IVC) pressure. HVPG should be less than 5 mmHg. A gradient of more than 12 mmHg indicates severe portal hypertension and is associated with an increased risk of variceal bleeding and the development of ascites in patients with chronic liver disease. Therapy with endoscopic sclerotherapy, band ligation and prophylactic beta-blockade therapy is discussed elsewhere.[4–6] Insertion of a transjugular intrahepatic portosystemic stent (TIPS) may be useful in intractable bleeding.[7]

Fluid balance and circulatory changes

Patients with chronic liver failure have fluid retention with ascites. This is managed with diuretics such as spironolactone or furosemide, with salt and water restriction. Peripheral vasodilation, dilation of the splanchnic vascular bed and arteriovenous shunting are common, as is intravascular depletion. Vigorous diuretic administration or therapeutic paracentesis may further decrease the circulating plasma volume, reducing renal perfusion and increasing sodium retention.[8]

Electrolyte changes and renal failure

Hypoglycemia (blood glucose level <40 mg/dl) is due to depletion of hepatic glycogen stores and impaired gluconeogenesis.[9] Contributing factors include raised serum insulin concentrations, as a result of decreased hepatic insulin catabolism, and abnormal levels of glucagon and growth hormone. Hyponatremia is frequently present because of decreased water excretion, increased renal sodium retention due to stimulation of the renin–angiotensin–aldosterone system, and decreased activity of the sodium–potassium pump.[10] Hypokalemia often accompanies hyponatremia and may be due to renal losses and hyperaldosteronism. With severe renal impairment, hyperkalemia may develop. Other electrolyte abnormalities include hypocalcemia and hypomagnesemia. Calcium levels should be corrected for corresponding albumin levels.

Renal excretion of sodium is significantly decreased in patients with well established cirrhosis and is an important pathophysiologic cause of ascites formation.[10] In addition to the development of hepatorenal syndrome characterized by redistribution of blood flow away from the renal cortex, renal changes in cirrhosis include glomerular sclerosis and membranoproliferative glomerulonephritis.[11] Acute tubular necrosis is also seen in patients with cirrhosis and is distinguished by a higher fractional excretion of sodium than seen with hepatorenal syndrome. Ascites should be managed with diuretics such as spironolactone or furosemide, and restriction of salt and water. Intervention with hemodialysis and hemofiltration should be considered if acute renal failure or hepatorenal failure develops.[12]

Hepatic encephalopathy

Chronic hepatic encephalopathy may be present in up to 50–70% of patients with cirrhosis.[13] Episodes of encephalopathy usually have a precipitating event such as gastrointestinal hemorrhage, infection and hypokalemia, which increase ammonia production; systemic alkalosis, which increases diffusion of ammonia across the blood–brain barrier; or hypoxemia, hypotension and dehydration. In addition, they may be due to portosystemic shunting, for example after the insertion of a TIPS for the management of esophageal varices.[13] Of children without encephalopathy but with chronic liver disease, those with early-onset liver disease (initial symptoms in the first year of life) have reduced intelligence quotient scores when compared with children with chronic liver disease of later onset.[14] This may be due to the vulnerability of an infant's brain to the metabolic abnormalities accompanying liver disease or to poor nutritional status, including vitamin E deficiency in young children with chronic liver disease.[11]

Although ammonia levels are typically raised in patients with chronic hepatic encephalopathy, especially those with portosystemic shunting, they correlate poorly with the degree of encephalopathy and are therefore not helpful in following the progression of encephalopathy.[13]

Treatment is directed at identifying and treating precipitating factors, avoiding fasting and sedatives, and reducing protein intake. Although protein restriction may be beneficial in the short term, this may result in growth failure and nutritional depletion in children. Thus, restriction of dietary and/or intravenous protein to 1–2 g/kg should be used in only acute or very symptomatic encephalopathy, and protein may be reintroduced as the encephalopathy subsides. A reduction in intestinal protein load and bacterial flora in the gastrointestinal tract can be achieved by enemas, particularly if an acute episode of encephalopathy is secondary to gastrointestinal hemorrhage, or by lactulose.

Nutritional supplements enriched with branched-chain amino acids (BCAAs) may be useful in hepatic encephalopathy by reducing muscle protein breakdown and normalizing plasma amino acid profiles.

Pulmonary disease

Pulmonary arteriovenous shunting with hypoxemia (hepatopulmonary syndrome) may be present in children with chronic liver disease and portal hypertension, and presents with dyspnea on exertion or with cyanosis. This condition is reversible after liver transplantation.[15]

Coagulopathy

The liver is responsible for the synthesis of factors II, V, VII, VIII, IX and X. Reduced levels of these factors, and of other proteins important in coagulation, reflect abnormalities of protein synthesis and impaired post-translational modification of vitamin K-dependent proteins (factors II, VII, IX, X; protein C, S) or malabsorption of vitamin K in cholestasis. Patients with coagulopathy secondary to liver disease may be asymptomatic or may have bleeding from the gastrointestinal tact, nasopharynx, retroperitoneum, tracheobronchial tree, genitourinary tract or subcutaneous tissues, or intracranial bleeding.[16] Petechiae from hypersplenism may cause epistaxis or exacerbate coagulopathy. Treatment consists of adequate vitamin K provision and use of fresh frozen plasma, cryoprecipitate and platelets as required.[16]

Indications for liver transplantation for chronic liver failure

Cholestatic liver disease

Chronic liver failure secondary to cholestatic liver disease is the main indication for liver transplantation in children with biliary atresia, and the commonest indication in children worldwide. Despite professional education about early referral for cholestatic disease, many children continue to be referred for treatment too late to benefit from a palliative Kasai portoenterostomy. Children who have an immediately unsuccessful Kasai portoenterostomy or who develop nutritional or hepatic complications[17] should be referred for urgent transplantation. Approximately 60% of children with biliary atresia will have a successful Kasai portoenterostomy, but even in these children cirrhosis and portal hypertension will develop and their need for liver transplantation will depend on the rate of development of hepatic complications.[18]

The outcome of cholestatic liver diseases such as Alagille syndrome and progressive familial intrahepatic cholestasis is variable. Many children have compensated liver disease for some time or are well maintained on supportive management. Liver transplantation is indicated when cirrhosis and portal hypertension develop, when malnutrition and growth failure are unresponsive to nutritional support, or when there is intractable pruritus that is resistant to maximal medical therapy, biliary diversion[19] or MARS (Molecular Absorbent Recirculating System), which anecdotally has improved pruritus for 6–12 months.

Some infants who present with giant cell hepatitis or neonatal hepatitis of unknown etiology develop persistent cholestasis and rapid progression to cirrhosis and portal hypertension, and become candidates for liver transplantation in the first 2–3 years of life.

Metabolic liver disease

α_1-Antitrypsin deficiency is the commonest form of inherited metabolic liver disease presenting in childhood in Europe and America. Although 50–70% of children in any population develop persistent liver disease progressing to cirrhosis, only a minority (approximately 20–30%) require liver transplantation in childhood.[20]

Tyrosinemia type I is an autosomal recessive disorder of tyrosine metabolism, secondary to deficiency of fumaryl acetoacetase, that prevents the metabolism of tyrosine leading to the development of toxic metabolites that damage liver, kidneys, heart and brain. The clinical presentation includes both acute and chronic liver disease and multiorgan failure with cardiac, renal and neurologic involvement. The management of this disorder has changed dramatically since the introduction of 2-(2-nitro-4-trifluoromethylbenzoyl)-1,3-cyclohexanedione (NTBC), which prevents the formation of toxic metabolites and produces rapid clinical and biochemical improvement. The widespread use of this drug in tyrosinemia type I has altered both the natural history of the disease and the indications for transplantation.[21,22] Prior to the introduction of NTBC, liver transplantation was indicated for acute or chronic liver failure or for hepatic dysplasia or hepatocellular carcinoma. Liver transplantation is now indicated only for those children who have a poor quality of life, who do not respond to NTBC, or in whom hepatic malignancy is thought to have developed.[22] Routine monitoring of children with tyrosinemia type I being treated with NTBC includes ultrasonography, computed tomography (CT) or magnetic resonance imaging (MRI) to detect the development of nodules and/or early hepatocellular carcinoma in association with regular determination of α-fetoprotein levels.[23,24]

Wilson's disease is a rare indication for liver transplantation in childhood. It is characterized by decreased serum copper and ceruloplasmin levels, raised 24-h urinary copper levels, hemolytic anemia, the presence of Kayser–Fleischer rings (a discoloration of Desçemet's membrane in the limbic area of the cornea seen by slit-lamp examination), and renal and neurologic abnormalities. Serum ceruloplasmin levels may be increased to normal levels in patients with Wilson's disease, and urinary copper excretion may be raised in patients with liver failure from other causes. Urinary copper excretion after penicillamine challenge with a low alkaline phosphatase level may be helpful in diagnosing Wilson's disease.[25,26] Early diagnosis and therapy with penicillamine, zinc or trientine should be curative, but many children present with established cirrhosis or fulminant liver failure. Liver transplantation is indicated for those children who present with advanced liver disease (Wilson's score >6) or fulminant liver failure (see below), or who have progressive hepatic disease despite penicillamine therapy.[27,28]

The short-term survival for children with cystic fibrosis has improved with increased attention on nutrition and appropriate management of pulmonary disease. Liver disease develops in approximately 20% of children, mainly in boys,[29] and is an important indication in the adolescent age group.[30] Referral for liver transplantation and the timing of transplantation are particularly difficult as many children present with compensated liver disease but with bleeding esophageal varices from portal hypertension.[31] In these children, management of portal hypertension by conservative means (sclerotherapy or band ligation of esophageal varices, or insertion of a TIPS) may be sufficient to control symptoms and improve quality of life.[31]

Liver transplantation is indicated if there is evidence of hepatic decompensation (falling serum albumin level or prolonged coagulation unresponsive to vitamin K), severe malnutrition unresponsive to nutritional therapy, or severe complications of portal hypertension that are unresponsive to medical management, such as ascites or uncontrolled variceal bleeding.[30,32] Careful assessment of pulmonary function is essential as severe lung disease (<50% predicted lung function) may indicate the necessity for heart, lung and liver transplantation.[30,32] In some children, the choice of timing of the liver transplantation is dependent on rapidly deteriorating pulmonary function. The management of pulmonary disease before transplantation should include vigorous physiotherapy, intravenous antibiotics and deoxyribonuclease (DNase).

Most children with glycogen storage disease type I do not develop liver failure if adequately managed by medical and nutritional treatment. Transplantation is indicated for children who develop multiple hepatic adenomas or in whom metabolic control has affected the quality of life. Children with glycogen storage disease types III and IV are more likely to progress to cirrhosis with portal hypertension and require transplantation because of hepatic dysfunction.[33]

The rare disorders of bile acid metabolism that present with persistent cholestasis may now respond to oral bile acids, reducing the need for transplantation.[34,35]

Chronic hepatitis

Autoimmune liver disease types I and II Autoimmune liver disease may present with either acute (see below) or chronic liver failure. The diagnosis is based on the dection of increased levels of immunoglobulins, particularly IgG, and reduced levels of complement (C3, C4) and non-specific autoantibodies (type I: anti-nuclear antibody (ANA) and anti-smooth muscle antibody (SMA); type II: anti-liver kidney microsomal (LKM) antibodies). Some children also present with autoimmune sclerosing cholangitis (overlap syndrome), which is more usually associated with type I disease and with positive anti-nuclear cytoplasmic antibodies (ANCA).[36] Liver transplantation is a rare indication for children with autoimmune liver disease type I or II, 80% of whom respond to immunosuppression with prednisolone or azathioprine, but is indicated in children who have not responded to immunosuppression despite alternative therapy such as cyclosporin A, mycophenolate mofetil or tacrolimus, and for those children who present with fulminant hepatic failure.[36] Fulminant hepatic failure is more likely in children with type II autoimmune hepatitis.

Chronic hepatitis B or C Chronic hepatitis B and C are important indications for transplantation in adults, but rare in children, who do not develop symptomatic liver disease in childhood. Recurrence of hepatitis B or C is likely in 90% of patients transplanted for chronic disease, unless appropriately prevented, but is less likely after transplantation for fulminant hepatitis.

Fibropolycystic liver disease

Fibropolycystic liver disease is an unusual indication for liver transplantation as liver function remains normal despite the development of severe portal hypertension. Liver transplantation is indicated if hepatic decompensation occurs or if it is associated with renal failure from infantile polycystic kidney disease, when both liver and kidney replacement may be required.[37]

Primary immunodeficiency

As bone marrow transplantation for primary immunodeficiency becomes increasingly successful, it has been recognized that some children have associated liver disease and may die from liver failure. The most common immunodeficiency is CD40 ligand deficiency – hyperimmunoglobulin M (hyper-IgM) syndrome – in which recurrent cryptosporidial infection of the gut and biliary tree leads to sclerosing cholangitis. In this group of children it is important to consider bone marrow transplantation before the development of significant liver disease, or to consider combined liver and bone marrow transplantation.[38]

Timing of transplantation for chronic liver failure

It may be difficult to plan the best time for liver transplantation for children with chronic liver failure as many children have compensated liver disease for years. Although it may be possible to predict biochemical decompensation by studying serial estimates of lidocaine metabolite formation and excretion,[39] this has not proved universally to be of value. The most useful guide to the timing of liver transplantation is provided by a variety of parameters that include:[40]

- A persistent rise in total bilirubin concentration to more than 150 μmmol/l (>9 mg/dl)
- Prolongation of the prothombin ratio (international normalized ratio (INR) >1.4)
- A persistent fall in serum albumin concentration to less than 35 g/l.

Serial evaluation of nutritional parameters is a useful guide to early hepatic decompensation. Progressive reduction of fat stores (measured by triceps skinfold or subscapular skinfold) or protein stores (measured by mid-arm circumference or mid-arm muscle area) despite intensive nutritional support is a good guide to hepatic decompensation.[41] Recently, development of the PELD (pediatric endstage liver disease) score has confirmed these observations.[42] McDiarmid et al.[42] evaluated data from the Studies of Pediatric Liver Transplantation (SPLIT), a consortium of 29 US and Canadian centers, to develop the PELD score. In the multivariate analyses, age, bilirubin, INR, growth failure and albumin were significant for outcome. A model using these five objective parameters has been developed and tested, and is now a useful tool for categorizing patients awaiting transplantation, although it may not improve selection.

An important consideration in the timing of liver transplantation is psychosocial development. Children with chronic liver disease have both social and motor developmental delay that increases with time unless reversed after early liver transplantation.[43,44]

Children with severe hepatic complications, such as chronic hepatic encephalopathy, refractory ascites, intractable pruritus or recurrent variceal bleeding despite appropriate medical management, should be referred immediately for transplantation. In some children, hepatopulmonary syndrome secondary to pulmonary shunting develops and is an important indication for liver transplantation.[45] It is essential that transplantation is performed before the development of severe pulmonary hypertension as this might preclude successful liver transplantation.[46]

For children with chronic liver disease to benefit from transplantation, it is essential that this procedure be considered before the complications of liver disease adversely impair the quality of their life, and before their growth and development are irreversibly retarded.

ACUTE LIVER FAILURE

Fulminant hepatic failure (FHF) or acute liver failure is a rare but fatal disease. It is a heterogeneous condition with many different etiologies in which the pathophysiology is unclear (Table 65.3).

The definition of FHF is the development of hepatic necrosis with hepatic encephalopathy and coagulopathy within 8 weeks of the onset of liver disease, and the absence of pre-existing liver disease in any form.[47] This definition is not useful in children because encephalopathy is difficult to detect or may not be a feature in infants. Secondly, acute liver failure may be the first presentation of an unrecognized autoimmune or metabolic liver disease (e.g. Wilson's disease or tyrosinemia type I). Thirdly, most hepatic failure in neonates is secondary to an inborn metabolic error or an intrauterine insult, which are pre-existing liver diseases.

The main pathologic feature is severe hepatic necrosis with failure of hepatic regeneration. The underlying mechanism for such profound hepatic damage is unknown but is multifactorial and depends on the age and susceptibility of the patient and the extent of hepatic injury.

The etiology of acute liver failure varies depending on the age of the child (Table 65.3). In neonates, an inborn error of metabolism or severe infection is likely, whereas viral hepatitis, autoimmune liver disease or drug-induced liver failure are common in older children.

Etiology	Disease
Neonates	
Infectious	Herpesviruses, echovirus, adenovirus, HBV
Metabolic	Galactosemia*, tyrosinemia*, neonatal hemochromatosis*, mitochondrial disease
Older children	
Infectious	HAV, HBV, NA-G, herpesviruses, sepsis*, other
Drugs	Valproate, isoniazid, acetaminophen, carbamazepine, halothane
Toxins	*Amanita phalloides*, carbon tetrachloride, phosphorus
Metabolic	Hereditary fructose intolerance*, Wilson's disease†
Autoimmune	Types 1 and 2

HAV, hepatitis A virus; HBV, hepatitis B virus; NA-G, non-A, non-G virus.
*Disease does not fulfil definition of FHF.
†Rare under 3 years of age.

Table 65.3 Causes of acute liver failure in children

Clinical presentation

The clinical presentation depends on the age of the patient and the etiology of acute liver failure, but the presentation may either be acute (within hours or days) or prolonged for up to 8–10 weeks, particularly if due to metabolic liver disease. The extent of jaundice and encephalopathy is variable in the early stages of acute liver failure, but all children have significant coagulopathy.

In neonates, encephalopathy is particularly difficult to diagnose. Vomiting and poor feeding may be an indication of encephalopathy due to metabolic liver disease, whereas irritability and reversal of day/night sleep patterns indicates more established hepatic encephalopathy. In older children, encephalopathy may present with aggressive behavior or convulsions.[48]

Neonatal acute liver failure

One of the common causes of acute liver failure in neonates is septicemia secondary to infection with *Escherichia coli*, *Staphylococcus aureus* or herpes simplex. Other causes of hepatitis include adenovirus, echovirus and Coxsackie virus. Acute liver failure secondary to hepatitis B usually presents at about 12 weeks of age, whereas hepatitis A is rare in neonates. Hepatitis C does not cause acute liver failure in neonates or infants.

Hepatitis B

Hepatitis B is vertically transmitted during pregnancy or delivery. The transmission rate is approximately 70% in mothers who are hepatitis B surface antigen (HBsAg) and hepatitis B e antigen (HBeAg) positive. Most infected infants become asymptomatic carriers. In contrast, infants born to mothers who are HBeAg negative have a high risk of developing fulminant hepatitis within the first 12 weeks of life unless successfully vaccinated.[49] The increased incidence of fulminant hepatitis B in these infants has now been demonstrated to be due to the transmission of a precore mutant hepatitis virus from mother to child.[50] Both the development of the carrier state and fulminant hepatitis B may be prevented by vaccination of all infants of hepatitis B carrier mothers, irrespective of their e antigen status.

Neonatal hemochromatosis

Neonatal hemochromatosis is a rare disorder that is associated with iron accumulation in liver, pancreas, heart and brain. It is not understood whether the disease is inherited with autosomal recessive inheritance or is an acquired defect of iron handling in pregnancy. Clinical presentation may be within hours or weeks of birth with jaundice, hypoglycemia and severe coagulopathy. Encephalopathy, although present, may not be obvious. The diagnosis is suggested by identifying raised ferritin levels (2000–3000 μg/l) and confirmed by demonstrating a high serum iron concentration with hypersaturation of iron-binding capacity (95–105%), and the demonstration of extrahepatic hemosiderosis. Because of the severe coagulopathy, liver biopsy is usually contraindicated, although extrahepatic siderosis may be demonstrated in salivary glands obtained by lip biopsy, or the accumulation of iron in the pancreas and brain on MRI. Intensive supportive management of the liver failure and the use of an antioxidant cocktail may be effective if begun within 24–48 h of birth, but liver transplantation is usually required within the first weeks of life.[51,52]

Tyrosinemia type I

Infants between 1 and 6 months of age may present with acute liver failure with mild jaundice, hypoglycemia, coagulopathy, encephalopathy, ascites and occasionally hyperinsulinism. The diagnosis is suggested by identifying increased plasma tyrosine, phenylalanine and methionine levels, and confirmed by identifying a toxic metabolite, succinyl acetone, in the urine. Management includes supportive management of acute liver failure and with NTBC, which prevents the formation of toxic metabolites and allows hepatic regeneration (see above). Liver transplantation is required for children who fail to respond to NTBC.[21,22]

Mitochondrial disorders

Mitochondrial disorders present with acute liver failure in the context of multiorgan disease. There are many different clinical phenotypes with varying modes of inheritance including transmission through maternal DNA. The disorders include deficiencies of the electron transport chain enzymes or depletion of mitochondrial DNA. Neonates and infants may present with jaundice, coagulopathy and neurologic features very similar to those of hepatic encephalopathy. The diagnosis is suggested by evidence of multiorgan failure (cardiac, renal, bone marrow involvement). Infants usually have metabolic acidosis with a increased blood lactate level, but this may be intermittent or non-specific. Other useful investigations are an increased plasma 3-hydroxybutyrate : acetoacetate ratio (>2) or detection of abnormal organic acids such as urinary 3-methylglutaconic acid. Evidence of multiorgan failure may be confirmed by muscle biopsy, which may demonstrate abnormal mitochondria, and an increased lactate concentration in the cerebrospinal fluid (CSF), or the presence of cerebral atrophy on CT or MRI may confirm neurologic involvement. Liver histology demonstrates microvesicular fatty infiltration, hepatocyte degeneration and micronodular cirrhosis. The diseases are fatal; liver transplantation is not indicated because of progressive neurologic disease and multiorgan failure.[53]

Familial hemophagocytic syndrome

Hemophagocytic syndrome is thought to be an autosomal recessive disorder due to a defect in immunomodulation. It may also be virally induced and the distinction may be difficult to make in neonates. Infants present with multiorgan failure with jaundice, hepatosplenomegaly, fever, skin rash and pancytopenia. The diagnosis is confirmed by the demonstration of erythrophagocytosis in bone marrow, liver and occasionally CSF. Confirmatory investigations are raised plasma triglycerides and increased serum ferritin levels. Treatment includes supportive management of acute liver failure, etoposide and corticosteroids. Cyclosporin and anti-T lymphocyte globulin have also been used with some effect in children who have achieved remission. Liver transplantation is not indicated, but bone marrow transplantation should be considered.[54]

Acute liver failure in older children

Viral hepatitis

Fulminant hepatitis secondary to hepatitis B is the commonest cause of fulminant hepatitis worldwide, but acute hepatitis A is more common in children and has a better prognosis. Hepatitis C and D rarely cause fulminant hepatic failure in childhood, whereas hepatitis E virus may be associated with fulminant hepatic failure, particularly in children returning from the Indian subcontinent. Viruses G and TTV (transfusion-transmitted virus), which are parentally transmitted viruses, have not been proven to cause liver disease. Hepatitis secondary to other viruses, such as Epstein–Barr virus (EBV) and parvovirus B19, occasionally lead to fulminant hepatitis. Approximately 50% of children with viral fulminant hepatic failure have no obvious etiology and are classified as having non non-A, non-G hepatitis.[48]

The survival associated with each type of infection varies; the highest spontaneous survival rates are found with acute hepatitis A infection, and lowest rates with non-A, non-G hepatitis.[55] The main causes of death are cerebral edema, renal failure, coagulopathy and infection.[56] Survival rates without liver transplantation are 67% when cerebral edema or renal failure is absent, 50% in patients with isolated cerebral edema, and 30% in those with coexisting cerebral edema and renal impairment.[57]

The clinical presentation includes a prodromal illness with anorexia, vomiting, lethargy, gradual onset of jaundice, coagulopathy and encephalopathy. The history may vary from 48 h to 6–8 weeks. The diagnosis is made by viral serology.

Autoimmune hepatitis

Both forms of autoimmune hepatitis (types I and II) may present with hepatic failure, although fulminant hepatitis is more common in type II. The clinical presentation is similar to that of viral hepatitis, or there may be a history of recurrent episodes of jaundice with lethargy, fatigue and weight loss.[36]

The diagnosis is confirmed, as indicated above, by identifying raised levels of immunoglobulins (particularly IgG), reduced levels of complement (C3, C4) and non-specific autoantibodies (type I: ANA and anti-SMA; type II: anti-LKM). Therapy includes supportive management and initiating immunosuppression with prednisolone (2 mg/kg). Encephalopathy may be exacerbated by high doses of steroids, and caution is required; 60 mg is the maximum dose. Liver transplantation is indicated for children who do not respond quickly to immunosuppression.

Drug-induced liver failure

In pediatric series, toxin- or drug-induced liver injury represents 15–20% of cases of FHF[55,58] (Table 65.3). Liver toxicity may be dose related, as seen with acetaminophen, aspirin, azathioprine and cyclosporin, or may represent an idiosyncratic reaction seen with valproic acid, phenytoin, isoniazid, chlorpromazine and halothane.[59,60] The most common cause of drug-related FHF in adolescents and young adults is intentional acetaminophen overdose,[61,62] with doses of more than 150 mg/kg. Maximal liver injury develops between 2 and 4 days after the overdose, and may be associated with metabolic acidosis and renal failure. The risk of significant acute liver failure is associated with ingestion of other drugs (e.g. anticonvulsant therapy), recreational drugs, such as ecstasy, or alcohol ingestion. Management includes estimation of serum acetaminophen levels, and prompt treatment with intravenous *N*-acetylcysteine to prevent massive hepatic necrosis. The median survival after acetaminophen ingestion for patients who ultimately die is 6–7 days, with a range of 3–56 days.[57] Poor prognostic factors include the presence of cerebral edema, oliguric renal failure and decompensated metabolic acidosis. The presence of cerebral edema alone decreases the survival rate to 71%; coexisting cerebral edema and renal failure decrease the survival rate to 53%. If decompensated metabolic acidosis is present, the survival rate decreases to 7%.[57]

The risk of acute liver failure with sodium valproate is particularly high in the first 3 years of life, but has been reported at any stage including adolescence and young adulthood. It may be the first presentation of an underlying metabolic disorder of fatty acid oxidation. The presentation may be atypical with jaundice, vomiting and increased frequency of convulsions, followed by edema and encephalopathy. Treatment is supportive. Liver transplantation is usually contraindicated, either because of an underlying metabolic disorder or the presence of multiorgan disease.[63]

Anticonvulsant medication with carbamazepine usually produces a cholestatic hepatitis, but may rarely cause fulminant hepatitis.

With some toxic reactions, damage may not resolve after medication withdrawal. Before the availability of liver transplantation, the survival rate for patients developing FHF with grade 3 or 4 encephalopathy due to idiosyncratic drug reactions or halothane hepatitis was 12.5%, compared with 53% for other causes.[57]

Metabolic liver disease

Wilson's disease is the commonest metabolic cause of fulminant hepatic failure in children over the age of 3 years. The presentation is variable and may be with similar features to those of viral hepatitis or hemolysis. The diagnosis is suggested by demonstrating hemolysis on a blood film, a relatively low alkaline phosphatase level (<600 IU/l), raised urinary copper concentration (before and after penicillamine challenge) and a low ceruloplasmin level. Kaiser–Fleisher rings may be absent, but there may be a response to D-penicillamine (20 mg/kg daily); liver transplantation is indicated for those who do not respond quickly or have advanced liver failure with severe coagulopathy and encephalopathy.[27]

Hepatoneurologic deterioration

Alpers' disease causes cerebral degeneration and disordered hepatic function, and may present with fulminant hepatic failure, which may be confused with primary hepatic failure if the characteristic neurologic symptoms are not obvious.[53] Disorders of fatty acid oxidation and of oxidative phosphorylation produce episodes of recurrent hepatic dysfunction and coma that may be confused with Reye's syndrome or severe hepatitis at any age.

Reye's syndrome

Reye's syndrome is characterized by acute encephalopathy and hepatic dysfunction. The cause is unknown but is thought to be due to a disorder of mitochondrial function. There is a prodromal illness, which may be precipitated by influenza or varicella if this is followed by vomiting, irritability, listlessness, evidence of cerebral edema and severe hepatic dysfunction. The administration of aspirin may play a role. Liver function abnormalities consist of markedly increased aminotransferase levels and prothrombin times, without a proportionate increase in serum bilirubin levels.[64,65] Ammonia levels may be increased and hypoglycemia may be present. Hepatomegaly may be found, and liver biopsy reveals a microvesicular steatosis, with swollen mitochondria on electron microscopy.[66] Management is directed to control of cerebral edema, while maintaining cerebral perfusion pressure.[67] There is a high case fatality rate due to cerebral herniation, and a high morbidity rate if the disorder is unrecognized and appropriate management is not initiated. Patients who survive show rapid improvement in liver function test results. Several inborn errors of metabolism such as medium and long-chain acyl coenzyme A dehydrogenase deficiency and organic acidemias mimic Reye's syndrome in presentation, and may preclude liver transplantation.[68]

Diagnosis

The diagnosis may be clear from the clinical presentation but it is important to establish a baseline by performing standard liver function tests and coagulation studies. Investigations will show a marked conjugated hyperbilirubinemia, raised aminotransferase levels (>10 000 IU/l), raised plasma ammonia concentration (>100 IU/l) and coagulopathy (prothrombin time >40 s). Liver biopsy is contraindicated because of abnormal coagulation, but can be performed by the transjugular route if essential for diagnosis.

Prevention and management of complications of acute liver failure

The clinical course is dominated by the complications of hepatic failure, and therapy should be focused on their prevention and management which includes early consideration for liver transplantation.

Hypoglycemia

Hypoglycemia (blood glucose <400 mg/l) develops in the majority of children. It may contribute to central nervous system impairment and other organ dysfunction. Factors contributing to hypoglycemia include:[69,70]

- Failure of hepatic glucose synthesis and release
- Hyperinsulinemia (due to failure of hepatic degradation)
- Increased glucose utilization.

Regular monitoring of blood glucose concentrations and the intravenous administration of glucose (10–50% dextrose) to maintain a blood glucose level above 4 mmol/l (60 mg/dl) are required. Profound refractory hypoglycemia is a poor prognostic sign and may be preterminal.

Coagulopathy and hemorrhage

The management of coagulopathy and hemorrhage is essential. Bleeding from needle puncture sites and line insertion is common, and pulmonary or intracranial hemorrhage may be terminal events. Major disturbances in hemostasis develop secondary to failure of hepatic synthesis of clotting factors and fibrinolytic factors, reduction in platelet numbers and function, or intravascular coagulation.[71] The coagulation factors synthesized by hepatocytes include Factors I (fibrinogen), II (prothrombin), V, VII, IX and X, and a reduction in synthesis leads to prolongation of prothrombin and partial thromboplastin times.

The prothrombin time is the most clinically useful measure of hepatic synthesis of clotting factors and determines the necessity for liver transplantation. Administration of parenteral vitamin K is important but may be ineffective.

Factor VII, which has a shorter half-life than other coagulation factors, is a sensitive indicator of hepatic function, as is Factor V, which is vitamin K independent.[72] Fibrinogen concentrations are usually normal unless there is disseminated intravascular coagulation (DIC). The level of Factor VIII may help differentiate between DIC and FHF, because Factor VIII is synthesized by vascular endothelium and its concentration is normal or increased in FHF. Decreased levels of Factor XIII may contribute to poor clot stabilization.

A reduction in platelet numbers (80×10^9/l) requires platelet transfusion and suggests hypersplenism, intravascular coagulation or aplastic anemia.

Once the need for liver transplantation has been established, coagulopathy should be corrected with fresh frozen plasma (FFP), cryoprecipitate and platelets as needed. Administration of recombinant factor VII (80 μg/kg) reliably corrects the coagulation defect in patients with FHF for a period of 6–12 h and may be useful in preparation for invasive procedures. Double-volume exchange transfusion may temporarily improve coagulation and DIC, and control hemorrhage. Hemofiltration may be necessary to control fluid balance to allow adequate coagulation support.[48]

Prevention of gastrointestinal hemorrhage

Gastrointestinal tract hemorrhage due to gastritis or stress ulceration may be life-threatening. High-dose H_2 antagonists (ranitidine 1–3 mg/kg every 8 h) or H-pump inhibitors (omeprazole 10–20 mg/kg daily) should be administered intravenously and sucralfate (1–2 g 4-hourly) may be given by nasogastric tube.[48]

Fluid balance and renal function

Acute liver failure is associated with a hyperdynamic circulation: a high cardiac output and a decrease in systemic vascular resistance and mean arterial pressure.[73] Vasodilation may trigger activation of neurohumoral factors that result in sodium retention, extracellular fluid volume expansion and the development of ascites.[73]

Renal failure is present in 40% of patients with acute liver failure and may be due to an imbalance between neurohumoral factors, renal vasoconstrictors and vasodilators.[58] Patients have marked renal vasoconstriction despite systemic vasodilation. Plasma renin activity is typically increased and renal prostaglandin activity is decreased in patients with acute liver failure. Acid–base disturbances may be present in up to 60% of children with FHF.[58] Acute tubular necrosis is present at autopsy in some children with FHF, although others appear to have 'functional renal failure' with normal histologic appearance.[59]

The aim of fluid balance is to maintain hydration and renal function while preventing cerebral edema. Maintenance fluids consist of 10% dextrose in 0.25 N saline, and intake should be 75% of normal maintenance requirements unless cerebral edema develops. A total sodium intake of 0.5–1 mmol/kg daily is usually adequate. Potassium requirements may be large, 3–6 mmol per kg per day, as guided by the serum concentration. As patients may become hypophosphatemic, intravenous phosphate may be given as potassium phosphate.[48]

Urinary output should be maintained using loop diuretics (furosemide at 1–3 mg/kg every 6 h), dopamine (2–5 μg per kg per min) and colloid/fresh frozen plasma (FFP) to maintain renal perfusion. Hemofiltration or dialysis may be required.

Cerebral edema and encephalopathy

Hepatic encephalopathy is graded from I to IV[74,75] (Table 65.4) and is variable in onset. Cerebral edema occurs in 45% or more of patients with FHF and is the major cause of morbidity and mortality. It may develop concurrently with other symptoms of hepatitis, or its development may be delayed.[76]

Cerebral blood flow adjusted for carbon dioxide levels (aCBF) correlates with cerebral swelling and mortality in patients with FHF. Patients with FHF may have hyperemia, normal flow or decreased cerebral blood flow. Increased cerebral blood flow may be associated with cerebral swelling on CT, but CT changes occur late and are absent in the majority of patients with increased intracranial pressure (ICP) on epidural monitoring.[77]

A baseline electroencephalogram (EEG) is helpful to stage coma and provide information on prognosis. CT may provide information on cerebral edema or irreversible brain damage later in the disease. Frequent evaluation of neurologic function and blood ammonia is essential to follow the progress of hepatic encephalopathy. The role of ICP monitoring remains controversial as there are significant complications, including bleeding, in patients with severe coagulopathy, but it may provide information on changes in ICP and improve selection for liver transplantation.[78]

Other therapy

The role of *N*-acetylcysteine (70 mg/kg 4-hourly) in the management of FHF other than paracetamol poisoning is

Stage	Clinical manifestations	Asterixis/reflexes	Neurologic signs	EEG changes
Subclinical	None	Absent/normal	Abnormalities on psychometric testing and proton magnetic spectroscopy in older patients	Usually absent
I	Confused, mood changes, altered sleep habits, loss of spatial orientation, forgetfulness	Absent/normal	Tremor, apraxis, impaired handwriting	May be absent or diffuse, slowing to theta rhythm, triphasic waves
II	Drowsy, inappropriate behavior, decreased inhibitions	Present/hyper-reflexive	Dysarthria, ataxia	Abnormal, generalized slowing, triphasic waves
III	Child is stuporous but obeys simple commands; infant is sleeping but arousable	Present/hyper-reflexive with positive Babinski sign	Muscle rigidity	Abnormal, generalized slowing, triphasic waves
IV	Child is comatose but arousable by painful stimuli (IVa) or does not respond to stimuli (IVb)	Absent	Decerebrate or decorticate	Abnormal, very slow delta activity

EEG, electroencephalography.
Data from Rogers, 1985,[74] and Devictor et al., 1995.[75]

Table 65.4 Stages of hepatic encephalopathy

unproven, but anecdotal results suggest that it may have a role. A multicenter study, supported by the US National Institutes of Health, of the role of *N*-acetylcysteine in the management of acute liver failure is in progress.

Antibiotic therapy

The results of surveillance cultures can be used to guide antibiotic therapy in the event of suspected infection, but broad-spectrum antibiotics (amoxicillin, cefuroxime, metronidazole and prophylactic fluconazole) are prescribed only if sepsis is suspected or liver transplantation is anticipated.[48]

Nutritional support

The role of parenteral nutrition in the management of patients with acute liver failure is controversial. The main aims of therapy are to maintain blood glucose and ensure sufficient carbohydrate for energy metabolism, reduce protein intake to 1–2 g/kg daily, and provide sufficient energy intake to reverse catabolism. Children who are mechanically ventilated should have parenteral nutrition, as it may be 7–10 days before full normal diet is resumed following transplantation.

Hepatic support

Many different measures have been used to support the liver while awaiting regeneration or transplantation, including a variety of experimental drugs such as prostaglandin E, insulin and glucagon, which have not been shown to be effective.

Methods to remove potential neuroactive toxins include double-volume exchange transfusion, plasmapheresis, charcoal hemoperfusion, liver assist devices containing chemical scrubbers[79] or cultured hepatocytes,[80] extracorporeal perfusion through human or animal livers[81] and cross-circulation with animals. Although these therapeutic maneuvers may provide support during liver regeneration or while awaiting a donor, none has been shown to have any benefit with regard to survival.

Double-volume exchange transfusion (in children weighing less than 15 kg) and plasmapheresis in older children may produce a transient improvement in coagulopathy and neurologic state, but may contribute to hemodynamic instability.[82]

Artificial liver support, using either porcine hepatocytes or a hepatoma cell line, has shown some benefit in improving coagulopathy and reducing encephalopathy in adults, acting as a 'bridge to transplantation', although long-term outcome and survival was not affected.[83] There is limited anecdotal experience in children.[84]

Molecular Absorbent Recirculating System (MARS)

MARS is an alternative form of hemodialysis that uses a specific filter to remove toxic products, but not albumin. It has a role in the management of both acute liver failure and acute-on-chronic liver failure in adults.[85] Use of MARS in the management of children is anecdotal, but it may have a role to play in creating a 'bridge to transplantation'.

Hepatocyte transplantation

Hepatocyte transplantation as therapy for acute liver failure using cell suspensions or synthetic constructs is at an early stage of research.[86]

Indications for liver transplantation for acute liver failure

The indications for liver transplantation for acute liver failure vary depending on whether the disease process is due to fulminant hepatitis or secondary to an inborn error of metabolism. In general, children with acute liver failure should be referred early to a specialist unit with facilities for transplantation in order to provide time for stabilization and to find an appropriate donor organ.

The factors known to imply a poor prognosis are:

- Non-A, non-G hepatitis
- Development of grade III or IV hepatic encephalopathy
  - the presence of cerebral edema carries a worse prognosis than renal failure, gastrointestinal bleeding or infection, and is present in 50% of non-survivors. Survival also correlates directly with the degree but not the duration of encephalopathy, with a 60% survival rate in those with grade I encephalopathy, decreasing to 5–25% in those with grade IV disease.[76] Jaundice of more than 7 days' duration before the development of hepatic encephalopathy is associated with a poor outcome.[56]
- Persistent severe coagulopathy (prothrombin time >50 s over control; INR >4).

In one pediatric series of FHF, only patients with a prothrombin time of less than 90 s survived, although 60% of non-survivors had a prothrombin time of less than 90 s.[76] In the case of acetaminophen overdose, the prothrombin time at admission is not helpful in differentiating survivors and non-survivors.[72]

Factor V levels are significantly decreased in non-survivors compared with survivors.[76] In children with FHF due to viral hepatitis or drug injury, Factor V levels were significantly higher in survivors without liver transplant (28 ± 11%) than in children who died (13 ± 7%) or who received a transplant (18±5%) ($P < 0.01$).[1] In patients with acetaminophen overdose, a Factor V level on admission of less than 10% predicted fatality.[72]

In infants with fulminant hepatitis, coagulopathy may be more severe than encephalopathy, and both are not required prior to listing for liver transplantation.[87,88]

It is essential that all children who have reached grade III hepatic coma or who have a persisting coagulopathy without evidence of irreversible brain damage from cerebral edema or hypoglycemia be listed for liver transplantation. It may be difficult to exclude underlying brain disease. Cerebral CT or MRI may demonstrate cerebral infarction, ischemia or hemorrhage, whereas EEG may indicate reduced voltage of brain waves. Although ICP monitoring has been demonstrated to improve selection for liver transplantation by excluding children with persistently raised ICP, it has not influenced survival.[89]

PRETRANSPLANTATION EVALUATION

The pretransplantation evaluation of the patient should include the following:

1 Assessment of the severity of the liver disease and the possibility for medical management
2 Consideration of any contraindications for transplantation
3 Psychologic preparation of the family and child.

The severity of liver disease should be assessed by evaluating the following.

Hepatic function

Listing for liver transplantation is based on evidence of deterioration in hepatic function as indicated by albumin concentration (>35 g/l), coagulation time (INR >1.4) and cholestasis as evidenced by a rise in bilirubin concentration (150 μmol/l, 8 mg/dl). In children with chronic liver failure, portal hypertension should be established by estimating the size of the spleen and portal vein by ultrasonography, and by diagnosing esophageal and gastric varices by gastrointestinal endoscopy.

Renal function

Children with acute or chronic liver failure have abnormalities of renal function, including renal tubular acidosis, glomerulonephritis, acute tubular necrosis and/or hepatorenal syndrome. Assessment of renal function is important to provide a baseline for the nephrotoxic effects of immunosuppressive drugs following transplantation and to consider the necessity for perioperative renal support or a renal-sparing immunosuppressive regimen. Children with fulminant hepatitis may develop hepatorenal syndrome with oliguria or anuria, and will need hemofiltration or dialysis.

Hematology

Baseline information on full blood count, platelets and coagulopathy are obtained. Determination of blood group is essential for organ donor matching.

Serology

Previous evidence of varicella, measles or infection with hepatitis A, B or C viruses, cytomegalovirus (CMV) or EBV is important information for postoperative management. Donor grafts are matched by CMV status if possible.

Radiology

The rapid development of Doppler ultrasonographic techniques has greatly improved the pretransplantation assessment of vascular anatomy and the patency of hepatic vessels. Evidence of retrograde flow and/or a reduction in size of the portal vein (<4 mm at the porta hepatis) suggests advancing portal hypertension and is an indication for early transplantation.[90] Children with biliary atresia have an increased incidence of abnormal vasculature, the hypovascular syndrome, which consists of an absent inferior vena cava, preduodenal or absent portal vein, azygous drainage from the liver, and polysplenia syndrome.[91] This may be associated with situs inversus, dextrocardia or left atrial isomerism. As these abnormalities may increase the technical risk associated with liver transplantation, it is important to diagnose these before transplantation.[92]

Cardiac and respiratory assessment

Liver transplantation is associated with significant hemodynamic changes during the operative and anhepatic phases, and information on both cardiac and respiratory function is needed. Electrocardiography, echocardiography and oxygen saturation provide most of the necessary information. Children with biliary atresia have an increased incidence of congenital cardiac disease, particularly atrial and ventricular septal defects, whereas peripheral pulmonary stenosis is a known feature of Alagille syndrome. Cardiomyopathy may develop secondary to tyrosinemia type I and the organic acidemias, and children with malignant tumors who have received chemotherapy need particular cardiac assessment. Cardiac catheterization is required in some cases to determine whether cardiac function is adequate to sustain the hemodynamic effect of liver transplantation, or whether cardiac surgery is required before transplantation. If the cardiac defect is inoperable, liver transplantation occasionally may be contraindicated.[93]

The development of intrapulmonary shunts (hepatopulmonary syndrome) is detected by measuring serial arterial blood gases while breathing room air and 100% oxygen, ^{99m}Tc-macroaggregated albumin pulmonary scanning, measurement of the alveoloarterial partial pressure of oxygen gradient, or contrast echocardiography.[15]

Neurodevelopmental assessment

As the aim of liver transplantation is to improve quality of life, it is important to identify any pre-existing neurologic or psychologic defects, not only to consider whether they would be reversible following transplantation but also to evaluate the need for corrective management. This is particularly important in children with acute liver failure as irreversible brain damage may be a contraindication for transplantation.

Dental assessment

Advanced liver disease has an adverse affect on all aspects of growth and development, including dentition. Pretransplantation dental problems include hypoplasia with staining of the teeth and gingival hyperplasia. As gingival hyperplasia is a significant side-effect of cyclosporin immunosuppression, it is important to establish good dental hygiene in the patient prior to transplantation.[94]

CONTRAINDICATIONS FOR LIVER TRANSPLANTATION

With increasing experience, there are fewer contraindications to transplantation. Although historically considered difficult, age below 1 year and weight of less than 10 kg are no longer contraindications for transplantation. Portal vein thrombosis increases the technical risk of the surgery, but can now be managed with venous or prosthetic grafts. Vascular abnormalities such as the hypovascular syndrome are no longer considered contraindications. Although infection with human immunodeficiency virus (HIV) was a contraindication, the improvement in long-term prognosis with antiviral drugs means that this infection can be controlled before transplant. The following contraindications remain:

- Severe systemic sepsis (particularly fungal sepsis) at the time of operation. It is important that the operation be deferred until the infection has been treated appropriately.
- Severe extrahepatic disease that is not reversible following liver transplantation. This includes severe cardiopulmonary disease for which there is no possibility of corrective surgery or severe structural brain damage with a poor prognosis.
- Multiorgan failure, especially that due to mitochondrial cytopathy,[53] as liver transplantation is not curative unless the mitochondrial defect is confined to the liver.
- Alpers' disease and sodium valproate toxicity are related disorders in which defects in the respiratory chain have been identified in some patients. Liver transplantation is contraindicated because of the progression of neurodegeneration despite transplantation.[95]
- Recurrent disease. Hepatitis B and C have a recurrence rate of 90–100% after transplantation, but can now be treated with antiviral agents before and after transplantation.[96,97] Autoimmune liver disease recurs in 24% of cases, as does primary sclerosing cholangitis. Although liver transplantation is not contraindicated for these conditions, the rate of recurrence must form part of the counseling of families. Autoimmune hemolytic anemia in association with giant cell hepatitis is a rare and fatal disease in which there is a 100% recurrence rate following transplantation, and transplantation is not recommended.[98]

PREPARATION FOR LIVER TRANSPLANTATION

Immunization

Although it may be possible to use live vaccines after liver transplantation, it is best to complete normal immunizations before transplantation.[99] This includes diphtheria, tetanus, polio, pneumovax for protection from streptococcal pneumonia, and *Hemophilus influenzae* type b (HIB) vaccine for protection against *Hemophilus influenza*. In children older than 6 months, measles, mumps, rubella and varicella vaccinations should be offered in addition to hepatitis A and B vaccination. Children with functional asplenia or multiple spleens should have pneumovax and penicillin prophylaxis.

Management of hepatic complications

It is important to ensure that specific hepatic complications related to either acute or chronic liver failure are appropriately managed while the patient waits for transplantation, as described above.

Sepsis that includes ascending cholangitis and spontaneous bacterial peritonitis should be treated with broad-spectrum antibiotics. In children awaiting transplantation for acute liver failure, prophylactic antifungal therapy is essential.

Nutritional support

The main purpose of nutritional therapy is to prevent or reverse catabolism and the malnutrition associated with either acute or chronic liver disease (see Table 65.2) High-calorie feeds (150–200% estimated average requirement) with adequate fat-soluble vitamin supplementation and appropriate protein content may be effective. It is possible to provide this high-energy intake with standard feeds using calorie supplements, but a modular feed that can be adapted may be better for infants. Feeds are best given by nocturnal nasogastric enteral feeding or continuous enteral feeding. Occasionally, enteral feeding is not tolerated due to severe hepatic complications such as ascites and intractable variceal bleeding; in these circumstances, parenteral nutrition is necessary.[100]

Psychologic preparation

Liver transplantation is a major undertaking for the child and family, and so psychologic counseling, information giving and preparation of the child and family is crucial, using a skilled multidisciplinary team with play therapists, psychologists and schoolteachers. Parents of children who develop acute liver failure may be too stressed to appreciate fully the implications and consequences of liver transplantation. In these families, counseling – in particular, counseling of the child – should continue after surgery.

LIVER TRANSPLANT SURGERY

The organization of liver transplantation is complex and involves a large multidisciplinary team.

Organ procurement

Organ donation and procurement are handled regionally or nationally, depending on geographic variation, but all countries have a national network: United Networks for Organ Sharing (UNOS) in the USA, United Kingdom Transplant Support Service Authority (UKTSSA) in the UK, and Eurotransplant in Europe. Once patients have been accepted by the transplantation team, they are listed and prioritized according to the severity of liver disease. All countries recognize the priority system, which allows patients with acute FHF the greatest priority, followed by patients in intensive care, in hospitals, or at home. Liver grafts are matched by size, blood group and (for CMV-negative children) CMV status. There are no absolute age limits but, in general, malignancy (except localized brain tumors), uncontrolled bacterial sepsis and HIV positivity remain absolute contraindications for acceptance as donors.[93]

The development of reduction hepatectomy has extended the size range applicable to young children, but the donor shortage has led to the replacement of reduction hepatectomies with split-liver grafts or living-related liver transplantation.[101–103]

The transplant operation

Management of the transplant operation has been improved by an understanding of coagulation disorders, by improved monitoring, and by sophisticated hemostatic techniques that have reduced transfusion requirements and allowed better hemodynamic stability. Constant monitoring of electrolytes and blood gases, along with thromboelastography (to assess coagulation), is essential and allows adequate supplementation of bicarbonate, electrolyte solutions, coagulation products and platelets.

Living-related liver transplantation

The shortage of suitable organ donors for young infants led to the development of living-related liver transplantation.[103] This technique not only improves the supply of liver grafts for small children but allows optimal timing and reduces the stress of waiting for a suitable organ. In addition, the graft is obtained from a healthy individual with a minimal preservation time.

Although excellent results have been obtained, particularly in Japan, the case for living-related transplantation remains controversial as there are potential risks to the donor.[104,105] Even in healthy individuals, partial hepatectomy has an appreciable morbidity with an estimated risk of mortality of 1 in 250. It is important that the donors are not only carefully evaluated for anesthetic risk, blood group compatibility, liver size and anatomy, but also that they are fully informed about the dangers of the procedure and, more importantly, the prospect of finding a cadaver graft for their child. Current organ donor shortages mean that most units will continue to offer living-related transplantation.

Auxiliary liver transplantation

In auxiliary liver transplantation, part of the donor liver (usually segments 2 and 3) is implanted beside or in continuity with the native liver. The main purpose of this form of liver transplantation is to ensure that the native liver is retained in the event of graft failure or for the future development of gene therapy. This operation is advisable for patients with metabolic liver disease secondary to hepatic enzyme deficiency in whom the liver is functioning normally but for whom liver transplantation is considered because of the development of severe extrahepatic disease.

The role of auxiliary liver transplantation in the management of FHF is more controversial. The rationale for using this technique in this condition is that, with time, the native liver may regenerate. Two recent studies in adults[106,107] demonstrated that the native liver regenerates in approximately half of the patients.

POSTOPERATIVE MANAGEMENT AND COMPLICATIONS

Postoperative management

Immediate postoperative management is based on ensuring hemodynamic stability, respiratory function and fluid balance. Most patients remain in the intensive care unit for 24 or 48 h, until liver function is satisfactory with good hepatic artery and portal vein flow on Doppler ultrasonography.

The aim of fluid management is to maintain circulating volume with crystalloid while replacing wound losses with colloid. It is important to ensure that the urine output is greater than 1 ml per kg per h and that central venous pressure is satisfactory (>5–6 mmHg). To prevent postoperative hepatic artery thrombosis, the hemoglobin level should be maintained between 8 and 10 g/l.[108] Immunosuppression is started immediately after operation; the protocol will vary with the center and experience. The protocol now includes: (1) cyclosporin microemulsion (Neoral), prednisolone and azathioprine; or (2) tacrolimus combined with low-dose steroids. Mycophenolate mofetil is a new immunosuppressive agent that may replace azathioprine in time.[109,110] Recent studies, in which immunosuppression is induced with the recently developed interleukin 2 (IL-2) antibodies that selectively block the IL-2 receptors on T cells, have shown reduced nephrotoxicity, which is of value in children with pretransplant renal impairment.[111] Sirolimus, a macrolide antibiotic that prevents T-cell proliferation, is also sparing to the kidneys as it does not inhibit calcineurin. Experience with its use in children is increasing.[112]

Broad-spectrum antibiotics should be prescribed for 48 h unless there is persistent infection. Fluconazole or liposomal amphotericin is advisable in children with acute liver failure or in those who have a second laparotomy. Low-dose cotrimoxazole or trimethoprim is used for prophylaxis against *Pneumocystis carinii*, and oral nystatin and amphotericin are used for 6–12 months to prevent oral and esophageal candidiasis.

Most units use prophylaxis for CMV infection for CMV-negative recipients of a CMV-positive donor organ. Ganciclovir (5 mg/kg intravenously per day) usually prevents CMV infection in the short term.[113] Although there is no proven prophylaxis for EBV, many units use ganciclovir for this purpose.

Other medications include ranitidine (3 mg/kg), sucralfate (2–3 g four times daily) or omeprazole (10–20 mg intravenously twice daily) as prophylaxis against stress ulceration.

As vascular thrombosis is higher in children than in adults, prophylaxis with antiplatelet drugs such as aspirin (3 mg/kg daily) and dipyridamole (3–6 mg/kg daily in three divided doses) may be useful. Antihypertensive medication is usually necessary secondary to immunosuppressive treatment with steroids, tacrolimus or cyclosporin A. Nifedipine (5–10 mg 4–6 hourly) or atenolol (25–50 mg per day) may be required.[93]

Some children require parenteral nutrition perioperatively, but the majority begin enteral feeds between days 3 and 5 after surgery. It is important to maintain adequate calories and to encourage normal feeding.

Postoperative complications

Early postoperative complications include primary graft non-function, surgical complications (e.g. intra-abdominal hemorrhage), vascular thrombosis and venous outflow obstruction.

The most common cause of primary graft failure is primary non-functioning of the graft or thrombosis of the hepatic artery or portal vein.[114] Primary non-functioning of the transplanted liver occurs within 48 h. The cause is unknown and may be related to donor factors. The presentation is with prolonged coagulation (INR >3), raised aminotransferase levels (>5000– 10 000 IU/l), a rising bilirubin concentration and, ultimately, a rise in the serum potassium level (>6 IU/l). Primary graft function may occasionally be secondary to hyperacute rejection, the diagnosis of which can be made only by liver biopsy. The only appropriate management is retransplantation.

Hepatic artery thrombosis occurs in approximately 10% of pediatric liver grafts; its frequency has decreased considerably following the introduction of reduction hepatectomy and living-related transplantation, because of the increased size of the donor vessel.[115] The development of microsurgical techniques for hepatic arterial reconstruction has also been beneficial.[116]

Portal vein thrombosis is a less common complication, but its incidence has not been altered with reduction or split-liver techniques, although there are some advances in the management of this complication with innovative surgery.[117]

The diagnosis of hepatic artery or portal vein thrombosis is made by Doppler ultrasonography and confirmed by angiography. Both complications may be treated by emergency thrombectomy and the use of anticoagulants or infusion of thrombolytic agents such as streptokinase. If hepatic perfusion is not adequately re-established, retransplantation is required. Hepatic artery ischemia ultimately results in biliary complications, such as leaks and strictures, or hepatic abscesses.[118]

Hemorrhage from the cut surface of the liver is an occasional complication. It should be managed conservatively unless there is persistent bleeding or hemodynamic instability. Abdominal tamponade from hemorrhage may decrease blood flow and lead to renal failure.

Many factors may predispose to postoperative renal failure within the first week. Patients with impaired renal function before surgery may be further compromised by intraoperative cardiovascular instability or inotropic support. In addition, the administration of nephrotoxic immunosuppression such as cyclosporin or tacrolimus may precipitate renal failure.[93]

Oliguria (<1 ml/kg) is common and can be managed conservatively with fluid replacement or a furosemide challenge (1–2 mg/kg intravenously). The development of anuria with an increase in urea, creatinine and potassium levels necessitates renal dialysis or hemofiltration.

Rejection

Acute cellular rejection may occur between 7 and 10 days after the operation. The incidence of acute rejection varies. It is less common in infants (20%) but increases to 50–60% in older children and adults.[119,120] Clinical features include fever, irritability, abdominal discomfort and (occasionally) ascites. The diagnosis is confirmed by detecting a rise in the levels of bilirubin, alkaline phosphate, γ-glutamyl transpeptidase, and aspartate and alanine transaminases. Histologic confirmation is essential. Acute rejection is indicated by demonstration of a mixed inflammatory infiltrate, including eosinophils in portal tracts. There is usually a subendothelial lymphoid infiltration of blood vessels (endotheliitis) and inflammation and infiltration of the bile ducts.[93] Most units treat acute rejection initially by using intravenous methylprednisolone in doses varying from 20 mg/kg daily for 3 days to 45 mg/kg in total, in association with an increase in baseline immunosuppression. If there is insufficient histologic or biochemical response, treatment with methylprednisolone may be repeated. However, if the rejection is unresponsive to steroids, it is usual to convert to a more potent immunosuppressive drug such as tacrolimus or to add other agents such as mycophenolate mofetil or sirolimus.[121]

Cyclosporin A (Sandimmune) has been replaced by the partially water-soluble cyclosporin microemulsion (Neoral). Several studies in both adult and pediatric patients post-transplantation have indicated that Neoral is well absorbed, with a peak absorption at 2 h and a half-life of approximately 8–12 h[122–124] in patients immediately after transplantation and in stable patients in the long term. The incidence of side-effects with Neoral is similar to the range of side-effects with Sandimmune, namely gingival hyperplasia and hirsutism, whereas the incidence of hypertension and nephrotoxicity is lower. It is possible that monitoring C2 levels (concentration 2 h after dosing) may be more effective than through level monitoring for preventing rejection and reducing side-effects.[125]

Experience with tacrolimus (FK506) has increased,[110,121] and indicates that it is an extremely effective immunosuppressive drug in the prevention of acute rejection. Tacrolimus does not cause hirsutism or gingival hyperplasia, and with lower doses the initial increase in serious neurologic side-effects, lymphoproliferative disease and hypertrophic cardiomyopathy described in children taking high doses of tacrolimus has not been substantiated.[110]

Many units consider the withdrawal of prednisolone at postoperative intervals ranging from 3 to 12 months; this has proved easier to accomplish using tacrolimus therapy.[126]

Chronic rejection occurs in less than 10% of children after transplantation.[120] Clinical features include gradual onset of jaundice, pruritus and pale stools, indicating biliary obstruction. The diagnosis may be confirmed by detecting biochemical changes that include a relative increase in bilirubin, alkaline phosphatase and γ-glutamyl transpeptidase levels compared with aminotransferases. Liver histology demonstrates extensive damage and loss to bile ducts (vanishing bile duct syndrome with arterial obliteration and fibrosis). There may be a response to an increase in immunosuppression, such as a change to tacrolimus[127] or the addition of mycophenolate mofetil. Non-response to medical management requires retransplantation.[128]

Biliary complications

The range of biliary complications after transplantation includes biliary leaks and strictures, which have increased with the use of reduction hepatectomies.[118] Biliary strictures may develop secondary to an anastomotic stricture related to edema of the bile ducts or hepatic artery ischemia. Biliary leaks may be secondary to leakage from the cut surface of the reduction hepatectomy or from hepatic artery ischemia. The majority of biliary leaks settle with conservative management, but large leaks that cause biliary peritonitis, biliary abscess or sepsis should have surgical drainage and reconstruction. The management of biliary strictures should initially be conservative, with the use of ursodeoxycholic acid (20 mg/kg) to allow the edema to settle. Persistent strictures leading to biliary dilation should initially be managed radiologically, using percutaneous transhepatic cholangiography. The dilated biliary tree is cannulated and external biliary drainage is established. Once sepsis and edema of the biliary tree have reduced, biliary dilation may be performed using balloons and biliary stents. Surgical reconstruction is required for anastomotic or recurrent biliary strictures if interventional radiology is unsuccessful.

Other complications and sepsis

Persistent drain losses may be due to preoperative ascites or secondary to rejection, sepsis, hepatic obstruction or bacterial peritonitis. There will be acidosis and coagulopathy due to loss of bicarbonate and coagulation factors in the ascitic fluid. It is best to treat the primary cause if possible and to manage the condition conservatively with fluid restriction and diuretics.

Infection is still the main complication following liver transplantation.[129,130] Bacterial infections occur immediately after transplantation and are related to the high doses of immunosuppressive drugs and central line infections. The main bacteria identified are *Streptococcus fecalis* and *S. viridans*, *Pseudomonas aeruginosa* and *S. aureus*. Postoperative fungal infections are more likely in patients undergoing transplantation for acute liver failure or in children having laparotomies for technical complications post-transplantation.[131] The most common fungal infection is with *Candida albicans*, but aspergillosis may occur in 20% of patients.

More recently, vancomycin-resistant *Enterococcus* (VRE) has become a significant pathogen following both liver and small bowel–liver transplantation.[132] Risk factors for developing VRE are recurrent central line infections treated with vancomycin therapy, but it is important to differentiate between patients who are colonized and those who have systemic infection. Treatment with new drugs such as linezolid are effective.[93]

Late complications post-transplantation

Late complications may occur at any time after transplantation. They include CMV or EBV infection, the side-effects of immunosuppression, post-transplantation lymphoproliferative disease (PTLD), late biliary strictures, and hepatic artery or portal vein thrombosis. Chronic rejection may occur at any time.

Infection with CMV occurs between 5 and 6 weeks after liver transplantation. The risk of CMV disease is highest in CMV-negative recipients who receive an organ from a CMV-positive donor.[113,133] Although prophylaxis with intravenous ganciclovir (5 mg/kg daily) and intravenous immunoglobulins (IVIGs) is more effective than prophylaxis with ganciclovir alone, approximately 20% of patients will develop primary infection. Treatment with intravenous ganciclovir and IVIG is usually effective.[134]

The development of primary infection with the EBV is a significant problem in pediatric transplantation. As two-thirds of children undergoing liver transplantation are likely to be EBV-negative before transplantation, and 75% of this group will develop primary infection after transplantation, it is essential to diagnose primary EBV infection in order to reduce immunosuppression and thus prevent the development of lymphoproliferative disease.[134]

There is a well known association between primary EBV infection and the subsequent development of PTLD.[134] The clinical features are varied and include symptoms of infections, mononucleosis (tonsilitis and lymphadenopathy), isolated lymph node involvement, and EBV infiltration of the liver, gut and iris, ranging from isolated organ involvement to malignant lymphoma.[135,136]

Considerable efforts have been devoted to the early diagnosis of EBV infection and PTLD. It is now possible to measure EBV polymerase chain reaction (PCR) prospectively and to reduce immunosuppression when high levels are achieved.[137,138] Serologic confirmation of EBV infection (EBV IgM antibodies) is usually a late feature, and it may be more appropriate to measure EBV PCR sequentially. Patients who develop gut PTLD may present with diarrhea, weight loss and gastrointestinal bleeding. The diagnosis should be confirmed histologically by biopsy of the appropriate tissue (liver, gut).[137] First-line treatment for PTLD is reduction of immunosuppression. Aciclovir (1500 mg/m^2 daily) or ganciclovir (5 mg/kg daily) may also be prescribed, but there is no clear evidence that either drug is effective. Use of rituximab, a monoclonal antibody, or HLA-matched T-cell therapy directed against EBV are under investigation and may prove effective.[139,140] As reduction of immunosuppression leads inevitably to graft rejection, balancing treatment for PTLD and rejection may be difficult. If lymphoproliferative disease becomes overtly malignant, chemotherapy is required.[141]

Late biliary strictures may be due to hepatic artery ischemia or thrombosis, and may lead to recurrent cholangitis, hepatic abscess and the development of secondary biliary cirrhosis. Although they may be treated radiologically as described above, retransplantation may be required for the development of biliary cirrhosis.[142]

Portal vein stenosis due to anastomotic stricture may lead to portal hypertension with varices and splenomegaly. Initial treatment is radiologic by venoplasty, but surgical reconstruction with an intrahepatic mesoportal shunt may be required.[117,128,143]

Gastrointestinal perforation is an infrequent complication after liver transplantation. It is related to previous abdominal surgery and malnutrition.[144]

SURVIVAL

Current results from international centers indicate that the 1-year survival rate following liver transplantation may be in excess of 90%.[1,145] Long-term survival rates (5–10 years) range from 60% to 80%.[146] Preliminary results suggest that patients who undergo elective living-related transplantation have a higher 1-year survival rate (94%) than those of equivalent hepatic status receiving cadaveric grafts (78%).[147]

Many different factors influence survival. Reduction hepatectomy and living-related transplantation have reduced the waiting-list mortality rate[102] and extended liver transplantation to infants, but have also demonstrated that equivalent survival may be achieved in infants transplanted under the age of 1 year and in older children.[148]

Protein malnutrition at the time of liver transplantation has a significant influence on both morbidity and mortality.[2] The degree of malnutrition, in addition to the severity of liver disease, has a significant effect on short-term survival,[149] and a number of studies have demonstrated improved survival for children with metabolic liver disease compared with those with chronic liver disease or fulminant hepatitis.

In general, outcome is not related to diagnosis, although children with FHF are less likely to survive the initial transplant.[142] An important aspect contributing to improved survival has been the increase in surgical and medical experience,[150] particularly with the development of innovative surgery and better immunosuppressive drugs.

There has also been an improvement in the rate of retransplantation for technical problems or graft failure secondary to chronic rejection,[142,151] but survival following retransplantation is considerably less. Children receiving more than one graft have a 50% 1-year survival rate, compared with 90% in children receiving only one graft. This may be related to the factors contributing to the necessity for retransplantation, such as primary graft non-function, technical problems and the development of multiorgan failure.

In some instances, survival may be affected by recurrence of the original disease. Recurrence of hepatitis B virus infection is 100% in patients who were positive for hepatitis B virus (HBV), DNA or hepatitis B e (HBe) antigen at the time of the initial operation.[152] The recurrence rate of chronic hepatitis B post-transplantation has been much reduced by therapy with the nucleoside analogs lamivudine and adefovir, and the use of hepatitis immune globulin.[153]

Chronic hepatitis C is a rare indication for transplantation in children, but recurrence is inevitable in those who were infected preoperatively before screening for hepatitis C virus became available[154] and in those who were infected perioperatively.[155] The outcome for these children is varied, with the majority developing non-specific hepatitis. However, a minority develop rapidly progressive liver failure. Treatment for hepatitis C infection has improved with the combination of interferon and ribavirin, which achieves a 45% sustained remission rate overall.[156]

The rate of recurrence of autoimmune hepatitis both immunologically and histologically post-transplantation is about 25%. The recurrence may be more severe than the original disease,[157] and it is important to ensure that immunosuppression with steroids is continued in this group of patients.

DE NOVO AUTOIMMUNE HEPATITIS

Several studies have documented the development of autoantibodies (ANA, SMA and rarely LKM) following transplantation in both child and adult recipients who had no autoimmune disease before transplantation,[158,159] associated with a graft hepatitis and progressive fibrosis. The hepatitis resolves with steroid therapy or azathioprine.[160]

LONG-TERM RENAL FUNCTION

The calcineurin inhibitors cyclosporin and tacrolimus both produce a 30% reduction in renal function, which initially remains constant, but only 4–5% of patients develop severe chronic renal failure in the long term, requiring renal transplantation.[161,162] The use of anti-IL-2 inhibitors with low-dose calcineurin inhibitors as induction therapy, or renal-sparing drugs such as mycophenolate mofetil or sirolimus for maintenance immunosuppression, prevents significant renal dysfunction.[111] Acute postoperative hypertension is seen in 65% of children, but persists long term in only 28%.[163]

HYPERLIPIDEMIA

As children survive longer, it is important to remember that both cyclosporin and sirolimus increase serum lipid levels, particularly that of cholesterol, and that high levels may require a change to tacrolimus or mycophenolate mofetil.[121]

TRANSPLANT TOLERANCE

It is now thought that 20% of adults will develop tolerance to the graft and can be withdrawn from immunosuppression.[164] Complete withdrawal of immunosuppression in children has not been documented.

QUALITY OF LIFE AFTER TRANSPLANTATION

Children who survive liver transplantation can expect to achieve a normal lifestyle despite the necessity for continuous monitoring of immunosuppressive treatment. An important aspect in achieving normal quality of life is nutritional rehabilitation after transplantation. Recent studies have demonstrated that, with appropriate nutritional support, 80% of survivors achieve normal growth patterns and body habitus.[17,165] Linear growth may be delayed for between 6 and 24 months, and is directly related to steroid dosage and preoperative stunting.[166]

Future growth may depend on the etiology of the pretransplantation disease. For instance, 50% of children who were transplanted for the hepatic complications of Alagille syndrome and who were growth retarded before transplantation did not achieve normal height.[167]

Additional factors in the etiology of post-transplant growth failure may be behavioral feeding problems and the difficulties in establishing normal feeding. Before transplantation, many children will have been fed unpalatable feeds, often by nasogastric tube, and may have missed their normal developmental milestones for chewing, swallowing and feeding. A significant proportion of these patients will have difficulty establishing normal feeding regimens after transplantation and will require nocturnal enteral feeding for 1–2 years.[166]

An important aspect of long-term survival is the development of puberty. A long-term study from France has demonstrated that there are no differences between the sexes in attaining puberty and developing secondary sexual characteristics.[168] Girls develop menarche, and successful pregnancies have been reported for females receiving both cyclosporin and tacrolimus immunosuppression.[169]

SIDE-EFFECTS OF IMMUNOSUPPRESSION

The side-effects of immunosuppression are well known (Table 65.5). Hypertension is common with steroids, cyclosporin and tacrolimus, but tends to be short term and related to the intensity of immunosuppression. Growth failure and stunting related to steroids may have a significant effect on the ability to regain normal height.

Immunosuppressive therapy	Complications
Steroids	Stunting Hypertension Cushingoid facies Salt and water retention Weight gain
Cyclosporin A	Hirsuitism Gingival hyperplasia
Cyclosporin A–tacrolimus	Nephrotoxicity Hypertension Neurotoxicity ?Lymphoproliferative disease ?Skin cancer
Tacrolimus	Hyperglycemia ?Cardiomyopathy
Sirolimus	Delayed wound healing Hepatic artery thrombosis Hyperlipidemia Bone marrow depression

Table 65.5 Immunosuppressive complications after transplantation

Hirsutism and gingival hyperplasia are recognized side-effects of cyclosporin that are dose related and, although cosmetic, have an important effect on quality of life, particularly in adolescence.

There remains a long-term risk of PTLD, skin cancer and other tumors.

PSYCHOSOCIAL DEVELOPMENT

Previous studies have demonstrated that there is an initial deterioration in psychosocial development in the first year after transplantation, as noted by a deterioration in social skills, language development and eye–hand coordination,[170] presumably related to the stress of the operation, the high doses of immunosuppression and prolonged hospitalization. Nevertheless, most children achieve normal psychosocial development within 1–2 years, although the rate of improvement is related to age at onset of liver disease and age at time of transplantation.[14] Risk factors for persistent developmental delay include malnutrition at the time of transplantation, length of hospital stay and age at transplantation, with younger children at particular risk of developmental delay.[14,171]

The stress of liver transplantation on family structure and dynamics is well known, although most parents indicate improved psychologic symptoms following successful liver transplantation. A longer-term study indicated that 20% of marriages failed and that 30% of families were considered to be functioning outside the normal range.[172]

NON-ADHERENCE WITH THERAPY

Non-compliance or non-adherence with immunosuppressive therapy is likely in most teenage patients and may be a significant cause of late graft loss.[146,173] Management is difficult and requires a non-judgmental approach.

SUMMARY

Liver transplantation for acute or chronic liver failure, or for metabolic liver disease, is an effective therapy that restores good quality of life in more than 80% of recipients. Considerable advances in medical and surgical expertise and immunosuppression have improved not only survival but also the quality of life for the majority of liver transplant recipients. It is essential to encourage both child and family to return to a normal life as far as possible, although continued counseling and support by a multidisciplinary team is essential. The long-term outlook for children receiving liver transplantation in the twenty-first century is likely to be limited by organ donor shortages, the side-effects of immunosuppressive drugs, and the potential development of PTLD or other tumors. It is hoped that the advances in molecular genetics will lead to effective gene therapy or hepatocyte transplantation and reduce the need for solid-organ transplantation.

References

1. Kelly DA. Current results and evolving indications for liver transplantation in children. J Pediatr Gastroenterol Nutr 1998; 27:214–221.
2. Chin SE, Sepherd RW, Cleghorn GJ. Survival, growth and quality of life in children after orthotopic liver transplantation: a 5 year experience. J Pediatr 1994; 124:368–373.
3. Sokol RJ, Stall C. Anthropometric evaluation of children with chronic liver disease. Am J Clin Nutr 1990; 52:203–208.
4. Howard ER, Stringer MD, Mowat AP. Assessment of injection sclerotherapy in the management of 152 children with oesophageal varices. Br J Surg 1988; 75:404–408.
5. Fox VL, Carr-Locke DL, Connors PJ, Leichtner AM. Endoscopic ligation of esophageal varices in children. J Pediatr Gastroenterol Nutr 1995; 20:202–208.
6. Stringer MD. Pathogenesis and management of esophageal and gastric varices. In: Surgery of the Liver, Bile Ducts and Pancreas in Children. Stringer MD, Howard ER, Colombani PM, eds. London: Arnold; 2002:297–314.
7. Johnson SP, Leyendecker JR. Transjugular portosystemic shunts in paediatric patients awaiting liver transplantation. Transplantation 1996; 62:1178–1181.
8. Sherlock S, Dooley J. Ascites. In: Diseases of the Liver and Biliary System, 10th edn. Sherlock S, Dooley J, eds. Oxford: Blackwell Science; 1997:119–134.
9. Russell GJ, Fitzgerald JF, Clark JH. Fulminant hepatic failure. J Pediatr 1987; 111:313–319.
10. Wyllie R, Arasu TS, Fitzgerald JF. Ascites: pathophysiology and management. J Pediatr 1980; 97:167–176.
11. Crawford DH, Endre ZH, Axelsen RA, et al. Universal occurrence of glomerular abnormalities in patients receiving liver transplants. Am J Kidney Dis 1992; 19:339–344.
12. Ellis D, Avner E, Starzl TE. Renal failure in children with hepatic failure undergoing liver transplantation. J Pediatr 1989; 108:393–398.
13. Riordan SM, Williams R. Treatment of hepatic encephalopathy. N Engl J Med 1997; 337:473–479.
14. Stewart SM, Uauy R, Kennard BD, et al. Mental development and growth in children with chronic liver disease of early and late onset. Pediatrics 1988; 82:167–172.
15. Barbe T, Losay J, Grimon G, et al. Pulmonary arteriovenous shunting in children with liver disease. J Pediatr 1995; 126:571–579.
16. Kelly DA. Fulminant hepatitis and acute liver failure. In: Buts JP, Sokal EM, eds. Management of Digestive and Liver Disorders in Infants and Children. Amsterdam: Elsevier Science; 1993:577–593.
17. Beath SV, Brook GD, Kelly DA, et al. Successful liver transplantation in babies under 1 year. BMJ 1993; 307:825–828.
18. Gauthier F, Chardot C, Branchereua S, et al. Urgent liver transplantation for biliary atresia. Tohoku J Exp Med 1997; 181:129–138.
19. Whitington PF, Freese SK, Alonso EM. Clinical and biochemical findings in progressive familial intrahepatic fibrosis. J Pediatr Gastroenterol Nutr 1994; 18:134–141.
20. Filipponi F, Soubrane O, Labrousse F. Liver transplantation for end stage liver disease associated with alpha-1-antitrypsin deficiency in children. Pre-transplant natural history, timing and results of transplantation. J Hepatol 1994; 20:72–78.
21. Lindstetd S, Holme E, Lock EA, et al. Treatment of hereditary tyrosinaemia type I by inhibition of 4-hydroxyphenyl-pyruvate dioxygenase. Lancet 1992; 340:813–817.
22. Mohan N, McKiernan P, Preece MA, et al. Indications and outcome of liver transplantation in tyrosinemia type1. Eur J Pediatr 1999; 158:S49–S54.
23. Macvicar D, Dicks-Mireaux C, Leonard JV, et al. Hepatic imaging with computed tomography of chronic tyrosinaemia type I. Br J Radiol 1990; 63:605–608.
24. Manowski Z, Silver MM, Roberts EA, et al. Liver cell dysplasia and early liver transplantation in hereditary tyrosinaemia. Mod Pathol 1990; 36:694–701.
25. Martins da Costa C, Baldwin D, Portmann B, et al. Value of urinary copper excretion after penicillamine challenge in the diagnosis of Wilson's disease. Hepatology 1992; 15:609–615.
26. Berman DH, Leventhal RI, Gavaler JS, et al. Clinical differentiation of fulminant Wilsonian hepatitis from other causes of hepatic failure. Gastroenterology 1991; 100:1129–1134.
27. Nazer H, Ede RJ, Mowat AP, et al. Wilson's disease: clinical presentation an dose of prognostic index. Gut 1986; 27:1377–1381.
28. Rela M, Heaton ND, Vougas V, et al. Orthotopic liver transplantation for hepatic complications of Wilson's disease. Br J Surg 1993; 80:909–911.
29. Scott-Jubb R, Lama M, Tanner MS. Prevalence of liver disease in cystic fibrosis. Arch Dis Child 1991; 66:698–701.
30. Milkiewicz P, Skiba G, Kelly D, et al. Transplantation for cystic fibrosis. Outcome following early liver transplantation. J Ped Gastroenterol Nutr 2002; 17:208–213.
31. Debray D, Lykavieris P, Gauthier F, et al. Outcome of cystic fibrosis associated liver cirrhosis: management of portal hypertension. J Hepatol 1999; 31:77–83.
32. Couetil JP, Soubrane O, Hussin DP, et al. Combined heart–lung–liver, double lung–liver, and isolated liver transplantation for cystic fibrosis in children. Transpl Int 1997; 10:33–39.
33. Sokal EM, Van Hoof F, Alberti D, et al. Progressive cardiac failure following orthotopic liver transplantation for type IV glycogenosis. Eur J Pediatr 1992; 151:200–203.
34. Balistreri WF. Inborn errors of bile acid metabolism; clinical and therapeutic aspects. In: Hofmann AF, Paumgartner G, Stiehl A, eds. Bile Acids in Gastroenterology: Basic and Clinical Advances. London: Kluwer Academic; 1993: 333–353.

35. Setchell KDR, O'Connell NA. Inborn errors of bile acid biosynthesis: update on biochemical aspects. In: Hofmann AF, Paumgartner G, Stiehl A, eds. Bile Acids in Gastroenterology: Basic and Clinical Advances. London: Kluwer Academic; 1998:129–136.
36. Gregorio GV, Portmann B, Reid F, et al. Autoimmune hepatitis in childhood: a 20-year experience. Hepatology 1997; 25:541–547.
37. Li D-Y, Schwarz KB. Congenital and structural abnormalities of the liver. In: Kelly DA, ed. Diseases of the Liver and Biliary System in Children. London: Blackwell Science; 2003:162–182.
38. Khawaja K, Genner AR, Flood TJ, et al. Bone marrow transplantation for CD40 ligand deficiency: a single center experience. Arch Dis Child 2001; 84:508–511.
39. Oellerich M, Burdelski M, Lautz HU, et al. Lidocaine metabolite formation as a measure of liver function in patients with cirrhosis. Ther Drug Monit 1990; 12:219–226.
40. Malatack JJ, Schald DJ, Urbach AH, et al. Choosing a paediatric recipient of orthotopic liver transplantation. J Pediatr 1987; 112:479–489.
41. Beath SV, Booth I, Kelly DA. Nutritional support in liver disease. Arch Dis Child 1993; 69:545–547.
42. McDiarmid SV, Anand R, Lindbald AS. The Principal Investigators and Institutions of the Studies of Pediatric Liver Transplantation (SPLIT) Research Group. Development of a pediatric end-stage liver disease score to predict poor outcome in children awaiting liver transplantation. Transplantation 2002; 74:173–181.
43. Beath SV, Brook GA, Cash AJ, et al. Quality of life after paediatric liver transplantation. Liver Transpl Surg 1995; 6:429.
44. Wayman KI, Cox KL, Esquivel CO. Neurodevelopmental outcome of young children with extrahepatic biliary atresia 1 year after liver transplantation. J Pediatr 1997; 131:894–898.
45. Uemoto S, Vinomarta Y, Tanarka A, et al. Living related liver transplantation in children with hypoxaemia related to intrapulmonary shunting. Transpl Int 1996; 9:S157–S159.
46. Losay J, Piot D, Bougaran J, et al. Early liver transplantation is crucial in children with liver disease and pulmonary artery hypertension. J Hepatol 1998; 28:337–342.
47. Trey C, Lipworth L, Davidson CS. Parameters influencing survival in the first 318 patients reported to the fulminant hepatic failure surveillance study. Gastroenterology 1970; 58:306 (abstract).
48. Whitington PF, Alonso EM. Fulminant hepatitis and acute liver failure. In: Kelly DA, ed. Diseases of the Liver and Biliary System in Children. London: Blackwell Science; 2003:107–126.
49. Beath SV, Boxall EH, Watson RM, et al. Fulminant hepatitis B in infants born to anti-HBe hepatitis B carrier mothers. BMJ 1992; 304:1169–1170.
50. Friedt M, Gerner P, Lausch E, et al. Mutations in the basic core promotor and the precore region of hepatitis B virus and their selection in children with fulminant and chronic hepatitis B. Hepatology 1999; 29:1252–1258.
51. Sigurdsson L, Reyes J, Kocoshis SA, et al. Neonatal hemochromatosis: outcome of pharmacologic and surgical techniques. J Pediatr Gastroenterol Nutr 1998; 26:85–89.
52. Flynn DM, Mohan N, McKiernan PJ, et al. Progress in therapy and outcome for neonatal haemochromatosis. Arch Dis Child 2003; 88:124–127.
53. Thomson M, McKiernan P, Buckels J, et al. Generalised mitochondrial cytopathy is an absolute contraindication to orthotopic liver transplantation in childhood. J Pediatr Gastroenterol Nutr 1998; 26:478–481.
54. Jabado N, de Graeff-Meeder ER, Cavazzana-Calvo M, et al. Treatment of familial hemophagocytic lymphohistiocytosis with bone marrow transplantation from HLA genetically nonidentical donors. Blood 1997; 90:4743–4748.
55. Rivera-Penera T, Moreno J, Skaff C, et al. Delayed encephalopathy in fulminant hepatic failure in the pediatric population and the role of liver transplantation. J Pediatr Gastroenterol Nutr 1997; 24:128–134.
56. Tandon BN, Joshi YK, Tandon M. Acute liver failure. Experience with 145 patients. J Clin Gastroenterol 1986; 8:664–668.
57. O'Grady JG, Gimson AE, O'Brien CJ, et al. Controlled trials of charcoal hemoperfusion and prognostic factors in fulminant hepatic failure. Gastroenterology 1988; 94:1186–1192.
58. Devictor D, Tahiri C, Rousset A, et al. Management of fulminant hepatic failure in children – an analysis of 56 cases. Crit Care Med 1993; 21:S348–S349.
59. Lee WM. Drug-induced hepatotoxicity. N Engl J Med 1995; 333:1118–1127.
60. Konig SA, Siemes H, Blaker F, et al. Severe hepatotoxicity during valproate therapy: an update and report of eight new fatalities. Epilepsia 1994; 35:1005–1015.
61. Rivera-Penera T, Gugig R, Davis J, et al. Outcome of acetaminophen overdose in pediatric patients and factors contributing to hepatotoxicity. J Pediatr 1997; 130:300–304.
62. Makin AJ, Wendon J, Williams R. A 7-year experience of severe acetaminophen-induced hepatotoxicity (1987–1993). Gastroenterology 1995; 109:1907–1916.
63. Kelly DA. Liver transplantation: to do or not to do? Pediatr Transpl 2000; 4:170–172.
64. Osterloh J, Cunningham W, Dixon A, et al. Biochemical relationships between Reye's and Reye's-like metabolic and toxicological syndromes. Med Toxicol Adverse Drug Exp 1989; 4:272–294.
65. Glasgow JF, Moore R. Reye's syndrome 30 years on. BMJ 1993; 307:950–951.
66. Hou JW, Chou SP, Wang TR. Metabolic function and liver histopathology in Reye-like illnesses. Acta Paediatr 1996; 85:1053–1057.
67. Jenkins JG, Glasgow JF, Black GW, et al. Reye's syndrome: assessment of intracranial monitoring. BMJ (Clin Res Ed) 1987; 294:337–338.
68. Smith ET Jr, Davis GJ. Medium-chain acylcoenzyme-A dehydrogenase deficiency. Not just another Reye syndrome. Am J Forensic Med Pathol 1993; 14:313–318.
69. Clark SJ, Shojaee-Moradie F, Croos P, et al. Temporal changes in insulin sensitivity following the development of acute liver failure secondary to acetaminophen. Hepatology 2001; 34:109–115.
70. Harry R, Auzinger G, Wendon J. The clinical importance of adrenal insufficiency in acute hepatic dysfunction. Hepatology 2002; 36:395–402.
71. O'Grady JG, Langley PG, Isola LM, et al. Coagulopathy of fulminant hepatic failure. Semin Liver Dis 1986; 6:159–163.
72. Pereira LM, Langley PG, Hayllar KM, et al. Coagulation factor V and VIII/V ratio as predictors of outcome in paracetamol induced fulminant hepatic failure: relation to other prognostic indicators. Gut 1992; 33:98–102.
73. Navasa M, Garcia-Pagan JC, Bosch J, et al. Portal hypertension in acute liver failure. Gut 1992; 33:965–968.
74. Rogers EL. Hepatic encephalopathy. Crit Care Clin 1985; 1:313–325.
75. Devictor D, Tahiri C, Lanchier C, et al. Flumazenil in the treatment of hepatic encephalopathy in children with fulminant liver failure. Intens Care Med 1995; 21:253–256.

76. Psacharopoulos HT, Mowat AP, Davies M, et al. Fulminant hepatic failure in childhood: an analysis of 31 cases. Arch Dis Child 1980; 55:252–258.

77. Munoz SJ, Robinson M, Northrup B, et al. Elevated intracranial pressure and computed tomography of the brain in fulminant hepatocellular failure. Hepatology 1991; 13:209–212.

78. Keays RT, Alexander GJ, Williams R. The safety and value of extradural intracranial pressure monitors in fulminant hepatic failure. J Hepatol 1993; 18:205–209.

79. Mitzner SR, Stange J, Klammt S, et al. Extracorporeal detoxification using the molecular absorbent recirculating system for critically ill patients with liver failure. J Am Soc Nephrol 2001; 12:S75–S82.

80. Sussman NL, Chong MG, Koussayer T, et al. Reversal of fulminant hepatic failure using an extracorporeal liver assist device. Hepatology 1992; 16:60–65.

81. Horslen SP, Hammel JM, Fristoe LW, et al. Extracorporeal liver perfusion using human and pig livers for acute liver failure. Transplantation 2000; 70:1472–1478.

82. Singer AL, Olthoff KM, Kim H, et al. Role of plasmapheresis in the management of acute hepatic failure in children. Ann Surg 2001; 234:418–424.

83. Hughes RD, Williams R. Use of bioartificial and artificial liver support devices. Semin Liver Dis 1996; 16:435–444.

84. Okamoto K, Kurose M, Ikuta Y, et al. Prolonged artificial liver support in a child with fulminant hepatic failure. ASAIO J 1996; 42:233–235.

85. Schmidt LE, Sorensen V, Swendsen L, et al. Hemodynamic changes during a single treatment with the molecular absorbents recirculating system in patients with acute on chronic liver failure. Liver Transpl 2001; 12:1034–1039.

86. Kobayashi N, Fujiwara T, Westerman KA, et al. Prevention of acute liver failure in rates with reversibly immortalized human hepatocytes. Science 2000; 287:1258–1262.

87. Goss JA, Shackleton CR, Maggard M, et al. Liver transplantation for fulminant hepatic failure in the pediatric patient. Arch Surg 1998; 133:839–844.

88. Bonatti H, Muiesan P, Connolly S, et al. Liver transplantation for acute liver failure in children under 1 year of age. Transplant Proc 1997; 29:434–435.

89. Lidofsky SD, Bass NM, Prager MC, et al. Intracranial pressure monitoring and liver transplantation for fulminant hepatic failure. Hepatology 1992; 6:1–7.

90. Badger IL, Czerniak A, Beath S, et al. Hepatic transplantation in children using reduced size allografts. Br J Surg 1989; 24:77–82.

91. Lilly JR, Starzl TE. Liver transplantation in children with biliary atresia and vascular anomalies. J Pediatr Surg 1974; 9:707–714.

92. Varela-Fascinetto G, Castaldo P, Fox IJ, et al. Biliary atresia–polysplenia syndrome: surgical and clinical relevance in liver transplantation. Ann Surg 1998; 227:583–589.

93. Kelly DA, Mayer ADM. Liver transplantation. In: Kelly DA, ed. Diseases of the Liver and Biliary System in Children. London: Blackwell Science; 2003:378–401.

94. Hosey MT, Gordon G, Kelly DA, et al. Oral findings in children with liver transplants. Int J Paediatr Dent 1995; 5:29–34.

95. Thomson MA, Lynch S, Strong R, Shepherd RW, Marsh W. Orthotopic liver transplantation with poor neurologic outcome in valproate-associated liver failure: a need for critical risk–benefit appraisal in the use of valproate. Transplant Proc 2000; 32:200–203.

96. Lucey MR, Graham DM, Martin P, et al. Recurrence of hepatitis B and delta hepatitis after orthotopic liver transplantation. Gut 1992; 33:1390–1396.

97. Ferrell LD, Wright TL, Roberts J, et al. Hepatitis C viral infection in liver transplant recipients. Hepatology 1995; 21:30–34.

98. Horsmans Y, Galant C, Nicholas ML, et al. Failure of ribavirin or immunosuppressive therapy to alter the course of post-infantile giant-cell hepatitis. J Hepatol 1995; 22:382.

99. Rand EB, McCarthy CA, Whitington PF. Measles vaccination after orthotopic liver transplantation. J Pediatr 1993; 123:87–89.

100. Protheroe S, Kelly DA. Cholestasis and end-stage liver disease. Ballieres Clin Gastroenterol 1998; 12:823–841.

101. Broelsch CE, Emond JC, Thistlethwaite JR, et al. Liver transplantation, including the concept of reduced-size liver transplants in children. Ann Surg 1988; 208:410–420.

102. de Ville de Goyet J, Hausleithner V, Reding R, et al. Impact of innovative techniques on the waiting list and results in pediatric liver transplantation. Transplantation 1993; 56:1130–1136.

103. Broelsch CE, Whitington PF, Edmond JC, et al. Liver transplantation in children from living related donors. Ann Surg 1991; 214:428–437.

104. Fujita S, Kim ID, Uryuhara K, et al. Hepatic grafts from live donors: donor morbidity for 470 cases of live donation. Transpl Int 2000; 13:333–339.

105. Hayashi M, Cao S, Concepcion W, et al. Current status of living-related liver transplantation. Pediatr Transpl 1998; 2:16–25.

106. Pereira SP, McCarthy M, Ellis AJ, et al. Auxiliary partial orthotopic liver transplantation for acute liver failure. J Hepatol 1997; 26:1010–1017.

107. Sudan DL, Shaw BW Jr, Fox IJ, et al. Long-term follow up of auxiliary orthotopic liver transplantation for the treatment of fulminant hepatic failure. Surgery 1997; 122:777–778.

108. Buckels JAC, Tisone G, Gunsen BK, et al. Low haematocrit reduces hepatic artery thrombosis after liver transplantation. Transplant Proc 1989; 21:2460–2461.

109. Renz JF, Lightdale J, Mudge C, et al. Mycophenolate mofetil, microemulsion cyclosporine, and prednisone as primary immunosuppression for pediatric liver transplant recipient. Liver Transpl Surg 1999; 5:136–143.

110. Kelly D, Jara P, Burkhard R, et al. Tacrolimus and steroids versus ciclosporin microemulsion, steroids, and azathioprine in children undergoing liver transplantation: randomised European multicentre trial. Lancet 2004; 364:1054–1061.

111. Ganschow R, Broering DC, Stuerenburg I, et al. First experience with basiliximab in paediatric liver graft recipients. Pediatr Transpl 2001; 5:353–358.

112. Pappas PA, Weppler D, Pinna AD, et al. Sirolimus in paediatric gastrointestinal transplantation: the use of sirolimus for paediatric transplant patients with tacrolimus-related cardiomyopathy. Pediatr Transpl 2000; 4:45–49.

113. Davison SM, Murphy MS, Adeodu OO, et al. Impact of cytomegalovirus and Epstein–Barr virus infection in children following liver transplantation.Gut 1993; 24:S32.

114. Brant de Carvalho F, Reding R, Falchetti D, et al. Analysis of liver graft loss in infants and children below 4 years. Transplant Proc 1991; 23:1451–1455.

115. Rela M, Muiesan P, Bajtnagar V, et al. Hepatic artery thrombosis after liver transplantation in children under 5 years of age. Transplantation 1996; 61:1355–1357.

116. Shackleton CR, Goss JA, Swenson K, et al. The impact of microsurgical hepatic arterial reconstruction on the outcome

of liver transplantation for congenital biliary atresia. Am J Surg 1997; 173:431–435.

117. Chardot C, Herrera JM, Debray D, et al. Portal vein complications after liver transplantation for biliary atresia. Liver Transpl Surg 1997; 3:351–358.

118. Chardot C, Candinas D, Mirza D, et al. Biliary complications after paediatric liver transplantation: Birmingham's experience. Transplant Int 1995; 8:133–140.

119. Edmond JC, Whitington P, Broelsch C, et al. Rejection in liver allograft recipients, clinical characterisation and management. Clin Transplant 1987; 1:143–150.

120. Murphy MS, Harrison R, Davies P, et al. Risk factors for liver rejection: evidence to suggest enhanced allograft tolerance in infancy. Arch Dis Child 1996; 75:502–506.

121. Egawa H, Coso SK, Cox K. FK506 conversion therapy in paediatric liver transplantation. Transplantation 1994; 57:1169–1173.

122. Loss GE Jr, Brady L, Grewal HP, et al. Cyclosporine versus cyclosporine microemulsion in pediatric liver transplant recipients. Transplant Proc 1998; 30:1435–1436.

123. Van Mourik IDM, Melendez HV, Thomson M, et al. Efficacy of neoral in the immediate postoperative period in children post liver transplantation. Liver Transpl Surg 1998; 4:491–498.

124. Van Mourik IDM, Thomson M, Kelly DA. Comparison of pharmacokinetics of Neoral and Sandimmune in stable pediatric liver transplant recipients. Liver Transpl Surg 1999; 5:107–111.

125. Keown P. Optimization of cyclosporine therapy with new therapeutic drug monitoring strategies: report from the International Neoral TDM Advisory Consensus Meeting. Transplant Proc 1998; 30:1645–1649.

126. Abe M, Fuchinoue S, Koike T, et al. Successful prednisone withdrawal after living-related liver transplantation. Transplant Proc 1998; 30:1441–1442.

127. Sher LS, Cosenza CA, Michel J, et al. Efficacy of tacrolimus as rescue therapy for chronic rejection in orthotopic liver transplantation: a report of the US. Transplantation 1997; 64:258–263.

128. Nicolette LA, Reichard KW, Falkenstein K, et al. Results of transplantation for acute and chronic hepatic allograft rejection. J Pediatr Surg 1998; 33:909–912.

129. Garcia S, Roque J, Ruza F, et al. Infection and associated risk factors in the immediate postoperative period of pediatric liver transplantation: a study of 176 transplants. Clin Transplant 1998; 12:190–197.

130. Gladdy RA, Richardson SE, Davies HD, et al. *Candida* infection in pediatric liver transplant recipients. Liver Transpl Surg 1999; 5:16–24.

131. Gray J, Darbyshire PJ, Beath SV, et al. Experience with quinupristin/dalfopristin in treatment infections with vancomycin-resistant *Enterococcus faecum* in children. Pediatr Infect Dis J 2000; 19:234–238.

132. Mellon A, Shephead RW, Faoagali JL, et al. Cytomegalovirus infection after liver transplantation in children. J Gastroenterol Hepatol 1993; 8:540–544.

133. Green M, Kaufmann M, Wilson J, et al. Comparison of intravenous ganciclovir followed by oral acyclovir with intravenous ganciclovir alone for prevention of cytomegalovirus and Epstein–Barr virus disease and liver transplantation in children. Clin Infect Dis 1997; 25:1344–1349.

134. Newell KA, Alonso EM, Whittington PF, et al. Posttransplant lymphoproliferative disease in paediatric liver transplantation. Interplay between primary Epstein–Barr virus infection and immunosuppression. Transplantation 1996; 62:370–375.

135. Robinson R, Murray PI, Willshaw HE, Raafat F, Kelly D. Primary ocular post-transplant lymphoproliferative disease. J Paediatr Ophthalmol 1995; 32:393–394.

136. Younes BS, Ament ME, McDiarmid SV, Martin MG, Vargas JH. The involvement of the gastrointestinal tract in posttransplant lymphoproliferative disease in pediatric liver transplantation. J Pediatr Gastroenterol Nutr 1999; 28:380–385.

137. Cacciarelli TV, Reyes J, Mazariegos GV, et al. Natural history of Epstein–Barr viral load in peripheral blood of pediatric liver transplant recipients during treatment for post transplant lymphoproliferative disorder. Transplant Proc 1999; 31:488–489.

138. Pinkerton CR, Hann I, Weston CL, et al. Immunodeficiency-related lymphoproliferative disorders: prospective data from the United Kingdom Children's Cancer Study Group Registry. Br J Haematol 2002; 118:456–461.

139. Haque T, Taylor C, Wilkie GM, et al. Complete regression of posttransplant lymphoproliferative disease using partially HLA-matched Epstein–Barr virus-specific cytotoxic T cells. Transplantation 2001; 72:1399–1402.

140. Gross TG, Hinrichs SH, Winner J, et al. Treatment of post transplant lymphoproliferative disease (PTLD) following solid organ transplantation with low-dose chemotherapy. Ann Oncol 1998; 9:339–340.

141. Achilleos OA, Mirza D, Talbot D, et al. Outcome of liver retransplantation in children. J Liver Transplant 1999; 5:401–406.

142. de Ville de Goyet J, Alberti D, Clapuyt P, et al. Direct bypassing of extrahepatic portal venous obstruction in children: a new technique for combined hepatic portal evascularization and treatment of extrahepatic portal hypertension. J Pediatr Surg 1998; 33:597–601.

143. Beierle EA, Nicoletter LA, Billmire DF, et al. Gastrointestinal perforation after pediatric orthotopic liver transplantation. J Pediatr Surg 1998; 33:240–242.

144. McDiarmid SV. The SPLIT Research Group. Studies of Pediatric Liver Transplantation. Update from studies in pediatric liver transplantation. Transplant Proc 2001; 33:3604–3605.

145. Sudan DL, Shaw BW Jr, Langnas AN. Causes of late mortality in pediatric liver transplant recipients. Ann Surg 1998; 227:289–295.

146. Kuang AA, Rosenthal P, Roberts JP, et al. Decreased mortality from technical failure improves results in paediatric liver transplantation. Arch Surg 1996; 131:887–892.

147. Zitelli BJ, Gartner B, Malatack JJ, et al. Pediatric liver transplantation: patient evaluation and selection, infectious complications, and life-style after transplantation. Transplant Proc 1987; 19:3309–3316.

148. Van der Werf WJ, D'Alessandro AM, Knectle SJ, et al. Infant pediatric liver ttransplantation results equal those for older pediatric patients. J Pediatr Surg 1998; 33:20–23.

149. Rodeck B, Melter M, Kardoff R, et al. Liver transplantation in children with chronic end stage liver disease; factors influencing survival after transplantation. Transplantation 1996; 62:1071–1076.

150. Talbot D, Achielleos OA, Gunson BK, et al. Progress in pediatric liver transplantation – the Birmingham experience. J Pediatr Surg 1997; 32:710–713.

151. Newell KA, Millis JM, Bruce DS, et al. An analysis of hepatic retransplantation in children. Transplantation 1998; 65:1172–1178.

152. O'Grady JG, Smith HM, Davies SE, et al. Hepatitis B virus reinfection after orthotopic liver transplantation. J Hepatol 1992; 14:104–111.

153. Mutimer D. Long term outcome of liver transplantation for viral hepatitis: is there a need to re-evaluate patient selection? Gut 1999; 45:475–476.
154. Nowicki MJ, Ahmad N, Heubi JE, et al. The prevalence of hepatitis C virus (HC) in infants and children after liver transplantation. Dig Dis Sci 1994; 39:2250–2254.
155. Pastore M, Willems M, Cornu C, et al. Role of hepatitis C virus in chronic liver disease occurring after orthotopic liver transplantation. Clinical transplantation. Arch Dis Child 1995; 72:403–407.
156. Kelly DA, Bunn S. Safety, efficacy and pharmacokinetics of interfeon alfa 2B plus ribavirin in children with chronic hepatitis C. Hepatology 2001; 34:342A.
157. Birnbaum AH, Benkov KJ, Pittman NS, et al. Recurrence of autoimmune hepatitis in children after liver transplantation. J Pediatr Gastroenterol Nutr 1997; 25:20–25.
158. Kerkar N, Hadzi N, Davies ET, et al. *De-novo* autoimmune hepatitis after liver transplantation. Lancet 1998; 351:409–413.
159. Andries S, Casamayou L, Sempoux M, et al. Posttransplant immune hepatitis in pediatric liver transplant recipients: incidence and maintenance therapy with azathioprine. Transplantation 2001; 72:267–272.
160. Salcedo M, Vaquero J, Banares R, et al. Response to steroids in *de novo* autoimmune hepatitis after liver transplantation. Hepatology 2002; 35:349–356.
161. Arora-Gupta N, Davies P, McKiernan P, et al. The effect of long-term calcineurin inhibitor therapy on renal function in children after liver transplantation. Pediatr Transpl 2004; 8:145–150.
162. Berg UB, Ericzon BG, Nemeth A. Renal function before and long after liver transplantation in children. Transplantation 2001; 27:561–562.
163. Bartosh SM, Alonso EM, Whittington PF. Renal outcomes in pediatric liver transplantation. Clin Transplant 1997; 11:354–360.
164. Riordan SM, Williams R.Tolerance after liver transplantation: does it exist and can immunosuppression be withdrawn. J Hepatol 1999; 31:1106–1119.
165. Holt RI, Broide E, Buchanan CR, et al. Orthotopic liver transplantation reverses the adverse nutritional changes of end-stage liver disease in children. Am J Clin Nutr 1997; 65:534–542.
166. Kelly DA. Post-transplant growth failure in children. Liver Transplant Surg 1997; 3:S32–S39.
167. Cardona A, Houssin D, Gauthier F, et al. Liver transplantation in children with Alagille syndrome – a study of 12 cases. Transplantation 1995; 60:339–342.
168. Codoner-Franch P, Bernard O, Alvarez F. Long-term follow up of growth in height after successful liver transplantation. J Pediatr 1994; 124:368–373.
169. Jain A,Venkataramanan R, Fung JJ, et al. Pregnancy after liver transplantation under tacrolimus. Transplantation 1997; 64:559–565.
170. van Mourik ID, Beath SV, Brook GA, et al. Long-term nutritional and neurodevelopmental outcome of liver transplantation in infants aged less than 12 months. J Pediatr Gastroenterol Nut 2000; 30:269–275.
171. Bucuvalas JC, Britto M, Krug S, et al. Health-related quality of life in pediatric liver transplant recipients: a single-center study. Liver Transplant 2003; 9:62–71.
172. Tarbell SE, Kosmach B. Parental psychosocial outcomes in pediatric liver and/or intestinal transplantation: pretransplantation and the early postoperative period. Liver Transplant Surg 1998; 4:378–387.
173. Molmenti E, Mazariegos G, Bueno T, et al. Noncompliance after paediatric liver transplantation. Transplant Proc 1999; 31:408.

Chapter 66
Diseases of the gallbladder

Mark A. Gilger

INTRODUCTION

Gallbladder disease in children has become more common over the past 20 years. Improved diagnostic modalities, such as abdominal ultrasound, has led to 'incidental' or 'silent' gallstones being detected more often in children, even *in utero*. Hemolytic disease remains the single most common cause of gallstones, but there is an increasing likelihood of finding gallstones in patients with other conditions such as prematurity, necrotizing enterocolitis, cystic fibrosis, conditions necessitating total parenteral nutrition (TPN) and obesity.

EPIDEMIOLOGY OF GALLSTONE DISEASE

Over 20 million adults in the USA have gallstones and approximately 300 000 cholecystectomies are performed yearly.[1] Predominantly a disease of adulthood, gallstone disease ranges in prevalence from 4% to 11% in Western societies, with wide variations along racial and ethnic lines.[2–8] The incidence in adults is approximately 1–3%.[9] The incidence and prevalence of gallstone disease is influenced by age, sex, culture, ethnicity and a variety of medical factors,[6,10–14] and it varies geographically. For instance, members of the Masai tribe of East Africa, whose bile is only half saturated with cholesterol, do not develop gallstones, whereas the Pima Indians of Arizona have an 80% prevalence.[5,15] Investigations into gallstone formation using a mouse model suggest that genetic factors, such as presence of genes known as Lith1 and Lith2 may determine susceptibility to gallstone formation.[16] MDR3 is the physiologic translocator of phospholipids across the canalicular membrane of the hepatocyte. Mutations of the gene MDR3 have been described in adults with cholesterol gallstones.[17]

The earliest reported case of cholelithiasis in a child was by Gibson in 1737.[18] Attempts to estimate the frequency of childhood gallstones included an extensive review of 5037 cases in 1959, in which a prevalence of 0.15% in children younger than 16 years of age was noted.[19] The prevalence of gallbladder disease in children since the 1960s appears to be increasing.[20–28] For example, in a review in 1984, of 708 infants referred for cholestasis between 1970 and 1981, an incidence of 1.4% was found,[25] whereas a review in 2000 of 4200 children who underwent abdominal ultrasound between 1988 and 1998, estimated a prevalence of gallstones at 1.9%.[26] Other reports have noted that 4% of all cholecystectomies are performed in patients younger than 20 years of age.[29,30] In a review of 693 cases of childhood gallstones reported since 1968, early infancy and adolescence were the most common ages for diagnosis.[31] Infants younger than 6 months of age represented 10% of all cases in which the age was known. Children from 6 months to 10 years of age accounted for 21% and adolescents (mostly female) 11–21 years of age represented 69% of all cases.[31] Most gallstones in children have an underlying predisposing condition, such as hemolytic disease, pregnancy and TPN. Gallstones of infancy are typically found in 'ill' infants receiving TPN. Stones found in children from the ages of 1–5 years are usually secondary to hemolysis and stones found in adolescents are most likely associated with menarche, pregnancy, obesity and the use of oral contraceptives.[17,31]

PATHOPHYSIOLOGY OF GALLSTONE DISEASE

Bile is composed of five major components: water, bilirubin, cholesterol, bile pigments and phospholipids. Lecithin is the primary phospholipid. Calcium salts and some proteins are minor components of bile. Stone formation occurs owing to the precipitation of the insoluble constituents of bile, which are cholesterol, bile pigments and calcium salts. Gallstones are classically divided into either cholesterol stones or pigment stones (Table 66.1). Chemically pure gallstones are rare and in any single stone the composition varies from the core to the crust. Most stones are 'mixed' in composition and the formation patterns of both cholesterol and pigment stones share many characteristics.

Cholesterol, the major sterol in bile, is nearly insoluble in water. It is made soluble in aqueous bile by aggregation with bile salts or lecithin. When cholesterol is no longer soluble, cholesterol monohydrate crystals precipitate from solution, a process known as *nucleation*.[32,33]

The interplay among the major bile components cholesterol, lecithin and bile salts is depicted in Figure 66.1.[34] When the composition of bile lies in the micellar zone, the bile can solubilize additional cholesterol. As the cholesterol concentration continues to increase, the likelihood of cholesterol crystallization and hence gallstone formation, increases. A decrease in bile salt concentration or lecithin also predisposes to gallstones.

There appear to be three primary conditions that must be met to permit the formation of cholesterol gallstones.[35] First, the bile must be supersaturated with cholesterol, which then acts as the driving force behind crystal precipitation. Second,

		Pigment stones	
Characteristics	Cholesterol stones	Black	Brown
Color	Yellow-white (often with dark core)	Black to brown	Brown to orange
Consistency	Hard	Hard, shiny	Soft, greasy 50% amorphous; rest crystalline, inorganic salts
	Crystalline	Crystalline	
	Layered		
Number and morphology	Multiple: 2–25 mm faceted, smooth	Multiple: <5 mm	Multiple: 10–30 mm
	Solitary: 2–4 cm (~10%) round, smooth	Irregular or smooth	Round, smooth
Composition	Cholesterol monohydrate >50%	Bile pigment polymer ~40%	Calcium bilirubinate ~60%
	Glycoprotein	Calcium carbonate or phosphate salts ~15%	Calcium palmitate and stearate soaps ~15%
	Calcium salts	Cholesterol ~5%	Cholesterol ~15%
		Mucin glycoprotein ~20%	Mucin glycoprotein ~10%
Radiopaque	No	Yes ~50%	No
Location	Gallbladder ± common bile duct	Gallbladder	Common bile duct, intrahepatic ducts
Clinical associations	Hyperlipidemia	Hemolytic anemia	Bacterial infection (*Escherichia coli*)
	Obesity	Cirrhosis	Parasitic infection
	Clofibrate	Total parenteral nutrition	Bile duct anomaly
	Pregnancy	Ileal disease (after puberty)	
	Birth control pills	Ceftriaxone	
	Cystic fibrosis		
	Octreotide		
Recurrent	Yes	No	Yes
Sex	Female >male	No difference	No difference
Age	Pubertal; increases with age	Any; increases with age	Any; increases with age
Bacteria	No	No	Yes (consistently found at core)
Soluble	Yes	No	No (minimally)

Table 66.1 Characteristics of gallstones in children[25,59,60]

bile kinetics must be such as to allow nucleation, the transition to solid cholesterol crystals. Finally, gallbladder stasis must exist to allow agglomeration of cholesterol crystals into stones.[36] Two secondary conditions also appear to be critical in lithogenesis: gallbladder hypersecretion of mucus and excess arachidonyl lecithin (Fig. 66.2).[37–40]

Cholesterol supersaturation can result from the following conditions:

1 An increased delivery of cholesterol to the liver via increased lipoprotein (low-density lipoprotein and chylomicrons). This occurs in women secondary to estrogen or oral contraceptive use or to increased dietary cholesterol intake.[37,41]
2 An increased endogenous cholesterol synthesis secondary to 3-hydroxy-3-methylglutaryl coenzyme A (HMG-CoA) reductase activity. Obesity and hypertriglyceridemia are causes of increased HMG-CoA reductase activity.[42,43]
3 A decrease in 7-α-hydroxylase activity, thus decreasing the conversion of cholesterol to bile acids.[44] This defect occurs most commonly with increasing age.
4 A decrease in the conversion of cholesterol to cholesterol esters from inhibited acyl-CoA cholesterol acyltransferase activity (ACAT).[37] Progesterone, either pregnancy induced or exogenous and clofibrate are examples of ACAT inhibitors.

The potential defects leading to cholesterol supersaturation are thus numerous and overlapping.

Nucleation is not as well understood as cholesterol supersaturation. Nucleation times are strikingly different between gallstone patients and control subjects. Gallbladder hypomotility seems to be involved in the crystallization process, because agitation prevents aggregation. Animal studies support hypomotility as an important causative factor.[45,46] Technetium-99m-dimethyl iminodiacetic acid gallbladder emptying studies in adult gallstone patients have documented diminished gallbladder emptying after meals.[47]

Biliary sludge, or tumefacient sludge, a collection of mucus, calcium bilirubinate and cholesterol crystals, appears to precede the formation of gallstones in animal models.[32,33,48] However, some clinical studies in children do not support sludge as being a precursor of gallstones.[26] Mucin hypersecretion appears to be a primary event in sludge formation and evidence suggests that prostanoids, such as arachidonyl lecithin, mediate the hypersecretion.[37–39] Mucin may serve as the nidus for nucleation and subsequent sludge formation owing to its hydrophobic domain, which binds phospholipid and cholesterol.[49]

Figure 66.2 summarizes the current understanding of the formation of cholesterol gallstones and, perhaps, of

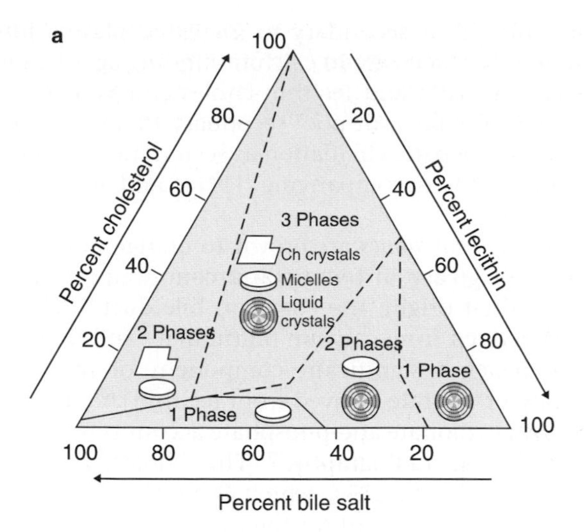

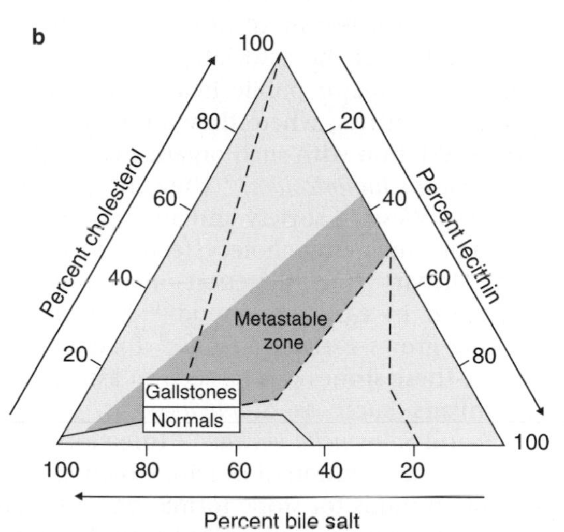

Figure 66.1: (**a**) Triangular phase diagram showing phases present at equilibrium in biles of differing compositions. In the micellar zone (the area in the lower left of the triangle), all the cholesterol is held in solution as micelles. Biles with a composition outside the micellar zone, if allowed to come to equilibrium, would form liquid and/or solid cholesterol crystals (as depicted schematically in each of the zones). The micellar zone is larger for gallbladder bile (a 10% lipid solution shown here) than for hepatic bile (a 3% lipid solution not shown). (**b**) Triangular phase diagram with schematic representations of ranges of lipid compositions found in gallbladder biles of normals and gallstone patients. Bile with a composition that falls in the metastable zone takes a prolonged time to come to equilibrium and thus appears to be stable. Excess cholesterol is 'carried' in the metastable zone by cholesterol-rich unilamellar vesicles. The boundaries of the physiologically relevant metastable zone are approximate.[33] (From Carey MC, Cohen DE. Biliary transport of cholesterol in micelles and liquid crystals. In: Paumgartner G, Stiehl A, Gerak W, eds. Bile Acids and the Liver. Lancaster: MTP Press; 1987:287–300, with permission.)[34]

any gallstone. The process must have a supersaturated solution (either cholesterol or bilirubin pigment); a 'still' environment, or gallbladder stasis; and crystal agglomeration or nucleation. The initial nucleating event creates the core of the stone, from which a self-perpetuating process ensues.

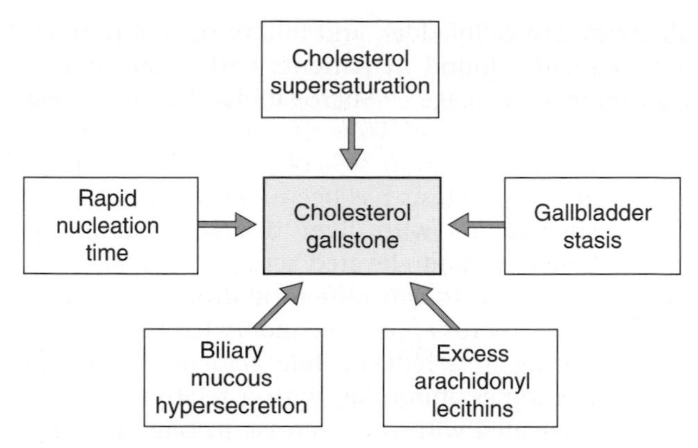

Figure 66.2: Current understanding of cholesterol gallstone formation. Cholesterol supersaturation is an essential prerequisite, which combined with a more rapid nucleation time and gallbladder stasis allows crystal formation. Excess biliary mucus provides a structural nidus for crystal growth, driven by increased dietary arachidonyl lecithins. (Adapted from Hay DW, Carey MC. Pathophysiology and pathogenesis of cholesterol gallstone formation. Semin Liver Dis 1990; 10:159–170, with permission.)[40]

CHOLESTEROL STONES

Cholesterol gallstones are yellowish-white in appearance, hard, crystalline and layered. They frequently have a brownish core, with a variety of substances found there, including calcium salts. 'Rings' of protein (glycoproteins) and calcium salts (calcium bilirubinate, calcium hydroxyapatite and calcium carbonate) form around the core, resulting in the layered appearance. The cholesterol content is higher than 50%, with minimal calcium salt content. This composition is not radiopaque; thus, the stones are rarely seen on plain film radiographs. Cholesterol stones form within the gallbladder and are frequently multiple, ranging in size from approximately 2 to 25 mm in diameter. The presence of cholesterol stones in the biliary tree is the result of migration. Cholesterol gallstones account for approximately 70% of all stones found in Western populations. The prevalence of cholesterol gallstones in children is unknown, but increases slowly with age in both sexes.[50] Pubertal changes, in particular early menarche, cause a dramatic increase in the incidence of cholesterol gallstones.[50,51] This phenomenon has been attributed to the effect of estrogen and progesterone surges that occur during puberty; it has also been seen in pregnancy and with the use of oral contraceptives, although investigation suggests no relationship between oral contraceptives and gallstones.[52] Sex hormones appear to induce biliary stasis and cause cholesterol hypersecretion by the liver.[53] It remains unclear whether estrogen, the progestins, or a combination of both, are responsible. There clearly are genetic influences, with high prevalence rates seen in both children and adult Native Americans. Studies of the Pimas of Arizona have demonstrated the development of lithogenic bile containing excess cholesterol during adolescence.[51] Obesity has been shown to increase the likelihood of cholesterol gallstone formation, apparently from excessive hepatic cholesterol secretion secondary to increased cholesterol synthesis.[54]

Gallstones and gallbladder, and biliary tract abnormalities are frequently found in patients with cystic fibrosis and they increase with age.[55] 'Microgallbladders' have been identified in as many as 16% of adult cystic fibrosis patients radiologically and in 30% of patients at autopsy.[56] Common bile duct stenosis has been identified in 96% of cystic fibrosis patients with liver disease, resulting in enlarged gallbladders and elevated serum bile acid levels, which may predispose to gallstone formation.[55] Gallstones in cystic fibrosis patients appear secondary to excessive bile acid loss resulting in a reduced bile acid pool. The bile composition becomes abnormal, with a relative excess of cholesterol associated with the decrease in bile salts, thus making the bile lithogenic. The bile acid malabsorption and reduced bile salt pool respond to pancreatic enzyme therapy. Gallstones have not been found without pancreatic insufficiency.[57,58]

PIGMENT STONES

Pigment stones account for a much higher percentage of stones in prepubertal children, whereas cholesterol stones are predominant in adolescence and adulthood. Two types of pigment gallstones are found in children and are referred to as *black* and *brown*. In both black and brown stones, the pigment present is calcium bilirubinate, which interacts with mucin glycoproteins to form stones (Table 66.1).[59]

Black pigment stones are black to dark brown in color and small (usually <5 mm), occur multiply and are typically hard, shiny and crystalline.[60] They are composed primarily of highly cross-linked polymers of bilirubin with mucin glycoproteins and calcium salts of phosphate and carbonate.[61,62] The high concentration of calcium salts (as compared with brown and cholesterol stones) accounts for the 50–75% radiopacity seen on plain radiographs. Black stones typically form within the gallbladder and do not recur after resection. They are usually associated with hemolytic diseases, of which sickle cell disease and hereditary spherocytosis are the most common. The duration of the hemolytic disease appears to be a significant risk factor for stone formation. Children younger than 10 years of age with sickle cell disease have a 14% prevalence of stones, whereas children 11 to 20 years of age have a 36% prevalence. Older adults with sickle cell disease have more than a 50% prevalence.[63,64] Other disease states, such as thalassemia, Wilson's disease and mechanical shearing of erythrocytes associated with artificial heart valves, have all been associated with black pigment stones. Black pigment stones form within the gallbladder and their presence in the common bile duct is the result of migration. Black stones are found in sterile bile and are not associated with infection.[65]

The formation of black stones results from altered gallbladder bile homeostasis and supersaturation of the bile. This process could occur by at least three mechanisms: an increase in bilirubin anions, an increase in unbound Ca^{2+} and a decrease in factors that solubilize bilirubin and calcium.[60] An increase in bilirubin anions has been shown to occur secondary to hemolysis.[60,66] Increased unbound calcium could occur secondary to increased plasma ionized calcium or to a decrease in calcium-binding agents, such as micellar bile salts and lecithin-cholesterol vesicles.[66] The decrease in the bile salt pool secondary to an interruption of the enterohepatic circulation as seen in ileal resection or the NPO status accompanying TPN could result in this phenomenon.

Brown pigment stones are brown to orange in color, soft, soap-like or greasy in texture and commonly assume the shape of their origin, the common bile duct.[60] The stone color is derived from calcium bilirubinate and their greasy texture belies a significant component of fat (calcium palmitate or stearate derived from lecithin).[67] The scarcity of calcium carbonate and phosphate accounts for their lack of opacity on radiography.[59] The cholesterol content ranges from 2% to 28%, which is higher than in black stones and allows in part for their increased solubility. The most distinct clinical feature of brown gallstones in both adults and children is the association with infection.[25,68] These stones are a major public health problem in rural areas of Asian countries, where they are found secondary to parasitic infestation with such organisms as *Opisthorchis sinensis* and *Ascaris lumbricoides*.[69] They are an uncommon type of stone in Western society and are typically found in the common bile duct after cholecystectomy when the bile is infected. Urinary tract infections may predispose to stone formation in early childhood.[70] In some 85% of cases, the bile grows *Escherichia coli*.[71] In children, especially infants, these stones can be seen in association with other organisms such as *Staphylococcus, Enterobacter, Citrobacter*,[68] and *Salmonella virchow*.[72] Infection with stasis results in excessive secretion of mucin, which may serve as the glycoprotein nidus for stone formation.[66] Bacteria also release beta-glucuronidase, phospholipase A_1 and conjugated bile salt hydrolase, which hydrolyze bilirubin glucuronides, lecithin and conjugated bile salts, producing unconjugated bilirubin, free saturated fatty acids, lysolecithin and free bile acids.[73] With the exception of lysolecithin, these products precipitate with calcium to form stones.[66] Biliary tree abnormalities, such as stenosis, also may predispose to brown stone formation.

GALLSTONES IN INFANTS

Infants younger than 12 months of age may be predisposed to gallstone formation, as compared with older children[68] (Table 66.2). For example, the bile of infants is more dilute than that of older children, with a lower bile salt concentration, a shorter nucleation time and a higher cholesterol saturation index.[74] These factors may help explain the increased tendency of infants to produce sludge and gallstones.[31] Table 66.2 demonstrates the likelihood (nearly one half of reported cases) for spontaneous resolution of gallstones during infancy.[75–85] Such information deserves special consideration concerning therapeutic intervention in infants and suggests that, unless symptomatic, gallstones during infancy do not require surgical intervention and often resolve without treatment.[26]

Author	Number of infants	Spontaneous resolution	Surgical treatment[a]	Persistent asymptomatic	Follow-up data NA	Recurrence
Keller (1985)[78]	5	5				
Jacir (1986)[79]	4	3	1			
Jonas et al. (1990)[80]	7	2	5			
Ljung et al. (1992)[81]	5	1	1	3		
Debray et al. (1993)[77]	40	15	21	4		2
Roman et al. (1994)[82]	1	1				
Johart (1995)[83]	2	1		1		
Monnerie (1995)[84]	1	1				
Morad (1995)[76]	14	8			6	
Ishitani et al. (1996)[85]	1		1			
Stringer et al. (1996)[75]	3	2		1		
Totals	83	39 (46%)	29 (35%)	9 (11%)	6 (6%)	2 (2%)

[a] Includes therapeutic ERCP.

Table 66.2 Gallstones in infancy (<12 months old)

TOTAL PARENTERAL NUTRITION-ASSOCIATED STONES

The association between TPN and cholelithiasis is clearly established.[86] Gallstone formation in premature infants and neonates receiving TPN appears to have four stages: decreased hepatobiliary flow due to immaturity, stasis within the biliary tree, sludge formation and finally, stone formation. Cholestasis, which increases with decreasing gestational age, is found in at least 50% of infants with a birthweight less than 1000 g.[87] After 2 months on TPN, 80% of infants have cholestasis.[87] This predisposition to cholestasis in infancy is multifactorial. Bile acid transport, bile secretion and basal and stimulated bile salt flow rates all are immature.[88,89] Bile salt-dependent and -independent flow are decreased, approximating only 50% of that in adults.[86,88] The absence of oral feeding reduces the enterohepatic circulation of bile acids.[86] Fasting also inhibits the release of gut and biliary tree hormones, such as cholecystokinin, gastrin, secretin, motilin and glucagon. The formation of echogenic, thick, 'molasses-like' biliary sludge within the gallbladder has been documented in both adults and children receiving TPN.[86,90,91] Serial ultrasound examinations of adults receiving continuous TPN infusion show sludge formation increasing from 6% of patients in the first week to 50% in the fourth week and 100% after 6 weeks.[92] Gallbladder enlargement may be the first physical sign of sludge formation in the infant. Stagnant bile in a dilated gallbladder provides an ideal milieu for the development of both acalculous cholecystitis and cholelithiasis. TPN-induced gallstones are pigment stones, typically black and usually found in the gallbladder. They often have a high calcium phosphate or carbonate content; however, stone analysis indicates that they are of a mixed bilirubin-cholesterol composition and perhaps belong to a special group of TPN-induced pigment stones.

ILEAL DISEASE AND ILEAL RESECTION-ASSOCIATED STONES

The enterohepatic circulation constantly replenishes the bile acid pool, which in turn governs the rate of bile salt secretion. The terminal ileum serves as the site of nearly 98% of bile acid resorption. Terminal ileal disease, typically Crohn's disease, or surgical resection of the ileum can result in an interruption of this bile acid recycling. The bile salt pool is subsequently reduced, thus altering the balance of bile components and favoring cholesterol supersaturation and increased bile lithogenicity. The formation of gallstones secondary to ileal disease has been reported in both adults and children. However, it appears that ileal resection only increases the tendency to gallstone formation after puberty.[93] After puberty, cholesterol secretion increases, whereas bile salt secretion declines, predisposing to cholesterol supersaturation and, hence, stone formation.[93]

DRUG-ASSOCIATED STONES

The use of several drugs, furosemide, octreotide, ceftriaxone, ciclosporin and tacrolimus, has been associated with an increased tendency to form gallstones. In reported cases associated with furosemide administration, numerous other contributing factors, such as prematurity, sepsis and small bowel disease, were also noted. Whether furosemide alone contributes to gallstone formation remains unclear.[94–97]

Octreotide has a wide range of biologic activities, including several clinically useful applications such as treatment of upper gastrointestinal bleeding, secretory diarrhea, acromegaly and gastroenteropancreatic endocrine tumors.

Gallstone formation has been found in about half of patients who receive chronic octreotide therapy.[98–100] It is believed that this may be related to octreotide-induced gallbladder stasis or a direct effect of octreotide on gallbladder absorption.[101]

Ceftriaxone can induce gallbladder concretions. Ceftriaxone is excreted in bile and has the ability to displace bilirubin from albumin-binding sites. Reports in both adults and children have noted biliary echo densities or sludge often causing symptoms of cholecystitis with right upper quadrant pain, nausea and vomiting. Analysis of the sludge reveals high concentrations of a calcium salt of ceftriaxone, with traces of bilirubinate and cholesterol, thus resembling pigment stone composition.[102] Fasting and age older than 24 months are risk factors associated with this so-called 'pseudolithiasis'.[95,103] The process of bile concretion and the related symptoms are reversible when the drug is discontinued.[95,104]

Ciclosporin usage in children undergoing bone marrow and solid organ transplant has been implicated in gallstone formation, possibly related to elevated drug levels and hepatic toxicity.[105,106] However, underlying sepsis, total parenteral nutrition and nil per os status are also likely contributors. Heart transplant in infants under 3 months of age appears to confer the greatest risk of cholelithiasis,[107] substantially higher than that seen in kidney or liver graft recipients.[96] Children undergoing bone marrow transplant also have been reported to have a higher likelihood of cholelithiasis.[97]

DIAGNOSIS OF GALLSTONE DISEASE

The classic symptom complex of right upper quadrant pain and vomiting is usually associated with stones only in older children and adolescents. Younger children tend to present with nonspecific symptoms. Jaundice is frequently encountered in 'symptomatic' infants.[31] The most likely age for silent stones is infancy through the pre-school years. Intolerance to fatty food is rarely reported in children. Fever is an unusual finding at any age and, if present, indicates associated cholecystitis. Complications of gallstone disease include cholecystitis, choledocholithiasis, cholangitis and gallbladder perforation, but these occur rarely in children. Pancreatitis has been identified in 8% of children with gallstone disease and may represent the most common complication in children.[108]

Laboratory evaluation is usually unrewarding. Occasional patients will have a leukocytosis as well as mildly elevated hepatic transaminase levels. Plain film radiography is more useful in children than in adults, because about 50% of stones in children are radiopaque. Ultrasonography is the diagnostic procedure of choice, because it is noninvasive, sensitive and specific. Ultrasonography also allows examination of the surrounding abdominal viscera, such as the pancreas and the biliary tree. Annual biliary ultrasonography has been suggested in children with known predisposition to gallstones, such as those with hereditary spherocytosis and sickle cell anemia.[109,110] Oral cholecystography has been largely replaced by ultrasound, but it can occasionally be useful in the evaluation of gallbladder function. Endoscopic retrograde cholangiopancreatography (ERCP) is particularly useful in the evaluation of ductal stones. Percutaneous cholangiograms offer another approach, but are seldom used in children.

TREATMENT OF GALLSTONE DISEASE

Observation may be the most prudent treatment in infants with asymptomatic gallstone disease (Table 66.2). As the infant ages, the hepatobiliary enzyme systems mature and the potential for spontaneous stone dissolution exists. Spontaneous stone resolution also has been observed in TPN-induced gallstones. In children for whom the duration of TPN is expected to be limited and the stones are asymptomatic, observation is indicated. However, in children who are chronically dependent on TPN, such as in Crohn's disease, pseudo-obstruction syndrome and the short bowel syndrome, stones should be removed.[111]

Gallstones in older children should be removed, because spontaneous resolution seldom occurs. Cholecystostomy is indicated for acute drainage of the gallbladder and perhaps in seriously ill patients for whom only simple stone extraction is needed. Laparoscopic cholecystectomy is rapidly becoming the surgical procedure of choice, in both adults and children.[112–114]

Options for nonsurgical treatment of gallstone disease continue to proliferate. Despite the growing popularity of medical therapy for adults, there is no such approved medical treatment for gallstones in children (Table 66.3). Two bile acids currently exist for oral gallstone dissolution: chenodeoxycholic acid (chenodiol) and ursodeoxycholic acid (ursodiol). Both agents occur naturally and are present in bile. Chenodiol works by inhibiting HMG-CoA reductase, which suppresses hepatic cholesterol synthesis.[115,116] Side-effects such as diarrhea and hepatotoxicity have limited its widespread use. The mechanism of action of ursodiol is similar to chenodiol, inhibiting HMG-CoA reductase and additionally, blocking intestinal absorption of cholesterol.[115] It has no hepatotoxicity and is currently under experimental use in chronic cholestatic diseases for treatment of pruritus and fatigue in both adults and children.[116] Diarrhea is rarely encountered. Combination use of both chenodiol and ursodiol appears more effective and allows a 50% reduction in dosage with fewer side-effects.[117] Drawbacks to the use of such therapy include the long duration of therapy, recurrence after stopping, low success rate and high cost. Only cholesterol stones are amenable to this therapy, thereby limiting its use in children.

Extracorporeal shock-wave lithotripsy (ESWL) was first used successfully in humans to fragment renal calculi. ESWL generates high-amplitude pressure waves that are focused on the stone by computerized ultrasonography. Only symptomatic stones that are radiolucent can be

Type	Comments	Approved in children
Cholecystectomy	Method of choice in most cases	Yes
Cholecystostomy	Effective for acute gallbladder drainage (i.e. acalculous cholecystitis)	Yes
Laparoscopic cholecystectomy	Effective with severely ill patients, shortens hospitalization (e.g. cystic fibrosis)	Yes
ERCP		
Basket removal	Bile duct stone removal	Yes
Mechanical basket lithotripsy	Stone crushing within bile ducts	No
Laser lithotripsy	Stone destruction within bile ducts (experimental)	No
ESWL	Limited experience (unpublished), only for cholesterol stones currently	No
Dissolution		
Oral	Ursodeoxycholic acid and chenodeoxycholic acid	
	Blocks HMG-CoA reductase, decreases cholesterol synthesis	No
Contact	Methyl *tert*-butyl-ether (for cholesterol stones only)	No
	Bile acid EDTA (for pigment stones; experimental)	No
Preventive		
Enteral feeds	Even small amounts during TPN decrease stone risk	Yes
Weight loss	For obesity–gradual weight loss	Yes
Lovastatin and simvastatin	Block HMG-CoA reductase, decrease cholesterol synthesis (experimental)	No
Cholecystokinin	Stimulates gallbladder contraction while NPO (experimental)	No

EDTA, ethylene diaminetetraacetic acid; ERCP, endoscopic retrograde cholangiopancreatography; ESWL, extracorporeal shock-wave lithotripsy.

Table 66.3 Treatment alternatives for gallstones in children

treated with this method, again limiting its use in children. Best results are obtained with solitary stones, with success rates of 95–100% reported.[118] Oral dissolution therapy appears to be a rational addition to lithotripsy to achieve complete stone dissolution.[119] The two major complications of lithotripsy are cholecystitis and pancreatitis, reported in 1–2% of patients.[118,119] Successful treatment of gallstones in children has been accomplished.[120,121]

Cholesterol gallstones can be dissolved using methyl *tert*-butyl ether (MTBE). The procedure first requires placement of a percutaneous transhepatic catheter into a contrast-enhanced gallbladder. A greater than 95% success rate in stone dissolution has been reported.[122] Complications include leakage of the MTBE, causing nausea, vomiting and duodenitis and intravascular hemolysis if the MTBE enters the vascular system, which has limited its application in both adults and children.[122] Chemical dissolution of calcified cholesterol stones and brown pigment stones has been tried experimentally with bile acid ethylenediaminetetraacetic acid, but has shown only limited success.

The prevention of gallstones in children entails recognition of risk factors and an understanding of the pathophysiology of stone disease. The use of limited enteral feedings during TPN therapy, for example, stimulates gallbladder contraction, thus decreasing gallbladder stasis. Early use of pancreatic enzyme supplements in patients with cystic fibrosis decreases the propensity to stone formation. Informed use of contraceptives other than birth control pills, particularly in women with known gallstone risk factors, would seem advisable. Weight control in obese patients is advisable to decrease the risk of gallstone disease, but rapid weight loss programs in obese patients may actually promote gallstone formation secondary to increased bile cholesterol saturation and gallbladder stasis.[123,124] Medical therapy with cholesterol-lowering agents, such as lovastatin and simvastatin, may be considered in high-risk patients, although no data exist for the use of this therapy in children (Table 66.3).

CHOLECYSTITIS

Cholecystitis is a disease that results from inflammation of the gallbladder, typically secondary to gallstone obstruction of the cystic duct. Cholecystitis may be acute or chronic. Most cholecystitis in children is chronic and is associated with gallstones. The presentation of 'acute' cholecystitis in children most likely represents a significant episode of an ongoing process of gallbladder distention and mucosal damage that culminated in cholecystitis.

The pathophysiology of cholecystitis parallels that of gallstone formation, with gallbladder stasis as the initiating event. The stasis is usually secondary to obstruction of the cystic duct by a gallstone or to local edema secondary to a stone. Other causes include external compression of the cystic duct by swollen lymph nodes, torsion of the gallbladder, congenital ductal abnormalities and trauma. The basis for the inflammation is unclear, although mechanical distention, ischemia, bacteria and lysolecithins have been implicated.

The typical presenting symptom is right upper quadrant abdominal pain, occasionally radiating to the back and associated with vomiting. When distended and inflamed, the gallbladder lies on the anterior abdominal wall between the 9th and 10th costal cartilages, causing localized tenderness on palpation and giving rise to the diagnostic Murphy's sign. Jaundice and fever are seen in 25–30% of children and are more common in young infants. The onset of symptoms is usually over a period of

1 week, but lesser symptoms of biliary colic may occur over several years. The differential diagnosis should include hepatitis, hepatic abscess, tumor, gonococcal perihepatitis (Fitz-Hugh-Curtis syndrome), pancreatitis, appendicitis, peptic ulcer disease, pneumonia, pyelonephritis and kidney stones.

Laboratory evaluation should include a complete blood count and differential; serum bilirubin, alkaline phosphatase or gamma-glutamyltransferase, serum aminotransferases, amylase levels; and urinalysis. Leukocytosis is frequently found. Elevated aminotransferase levels and mild hyperbilirubinemia are seen in 20% of patients. Elevated amylase levels are common even without pancreatitis. Marked elevation of the bilirubin, alkaline phosphatase, or γ-glutamyltransferase levels may indicate stones in the biliary tree. The characteristic ultrasound finding is a discrete echo density indicating a stone, usually occupying a dependent position in the gallbladder, which changes or moves when the patient is moved and is associated with acoustic shadowing (Fig. 66.3). Gallbladder dilation, a thickened gallbladder wall, the presence of sludge and biliary tree anomalies also may be seen (Fig. 66.4). Cholescintigraphy can be helpful to evaluate gallbladder function, revealing normal hepatic uptake, but non-visualization of the gallbladder at 1 h.[125] False-positive results may occur with prolonged fasting, TPN and hepatocellular disease. Oral cholecystography is used less frequently, owing to several inherent drawbacks, such as failure to concentrate the dye (particularly if hyperbilirubinemia exists), a 6–8% false-negative rate, hypersensitivity to the dye and radiation exposure.

Hospitalization with institution of intravenous fluids, cessation of oral feeding, gastric decompression and analgesics is appropriate. Antibiotics are not needed in simple cases, but if fever persists or the condition worsens, their use is indicated. Ampicillin, gentamicin and clindamycin are a common combination used to cover enteric organisms and provide good biliary excretion. Cefoperazone also is a logical choice owing to its excellent biliary excretion and broad spectrum of bacterial sensitivity.

Cholecystectomy is the procedure of choice in calculous cholecystitis. In children with sickle cell disease, hypertransfusion should be performed prior to surgery. Children with certain medical disorders, such as congenital heart disease, appear to have an increased risk of death after urgent cholecystectomy and elective cholecystectomy may be advisable.[126] Cholecystostomy with stone removal can be done in those patients for whom a functioning gallbladder is important, such as in patients with Crohn's disease. Table 66.3 lists the possible treatment options in children.

Most cases of cholecystitis usually resolve over several days. Complications occur in 30% of cases and include gallbladder perforation, abscess, or empyema formation. When fever persists or exceeds 102°F and pain or tenderness worsens, perforation is likely. Such perforations typically occur in the fundus of the gallbladder. A local perforation may wall off as an abscess, extend into the peritoneum as peritonitis, or lead to a cholecystoenteric fistula. Surgical intervention with vigorous antibiotic support is essential.

Chronic obstruction of the cystic duct may lead to the interesting finding of the 'milk of calcium' gallbladder or 'limy bile' syndrome. In this situation, complete obstruction of the cystic duct leads to a hydropic gallbladder. Bile pigments are deconjugated to colorless compounds and excess calcium is secreted, opacifying the bile to a white appearance both visually and radiographically. Calcium accumulating in the wall of the gallbladder secondary to chronic cystic duct obstruction may produce the 'porcelain gallbladder'. This condition appears secondary to chronic cholecystitis and in adults leads to carcinoma in as many as 50% of cases.[127] Courvoisier's gallbladder is a markedly enlarged gallbladder secondary to chronic, often malignant obstruction of the common bile duct.[128] This condition is unusual in adults and has not been reported in children.

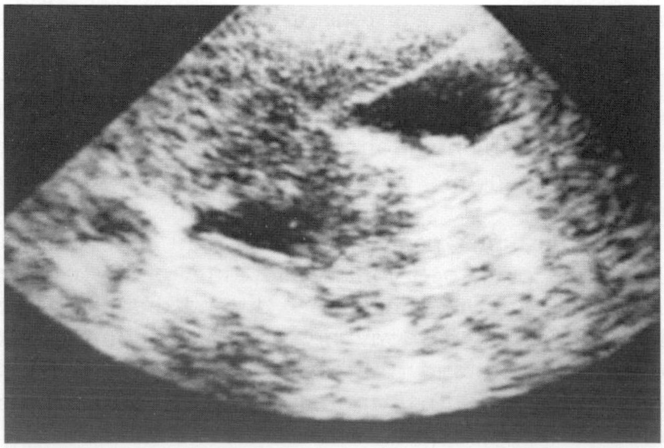

Figure 66.3: Ultrasound of gallstone within the gallbladder showing acoustic shadowing. (Courtesy of Dr Robert V. Dutton.)

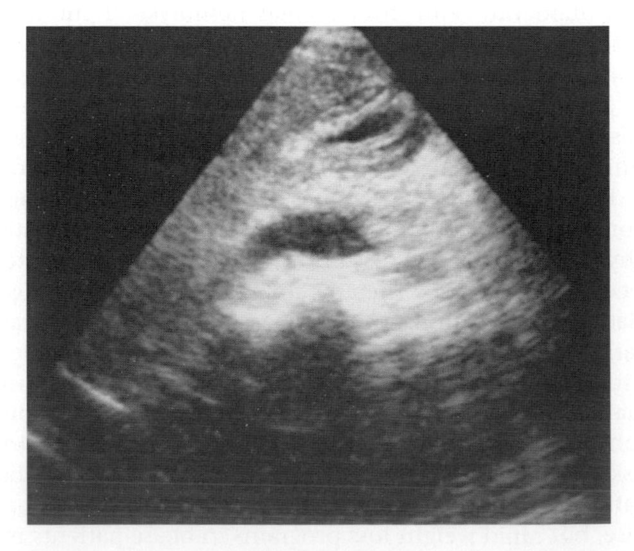

Figure 66.4: Ultrasound of dilated gallbladder with a thickened wall. (Courtesy of Dr Robert V. Dutton.)

CHOLEDOCHOLITHIASIS (COMMON BILE DUCT STONES)

Common bile duct stones are an unusual occurrence in children. Most ductal stones in children are black pigment stones, although cholesterol stones have been found. Both of these types of stones originate from the gallbladder. Less common are brown pigment stones, which form within the common bile duct secondary to infection.[68] Most ductal stones in children are believed to lodge within the common bile duct because of congenital narrowing or stenosis.[129] The usual clinical presentation of common bile duct stones in children is jaundice, progressing to symptoms similar to those of cholecystitis. Right upper quadrant pain with fever is common.

Laboratory evaluation may reveal leukocytosis, elevated aminotransferase levels and specific elevations of biliary tract enzymes such as alkaline phosphatase and γ-glutamyltransferase. If fever is present, blood cultures may be positive. Abdominal ultrasound is indicated to detect the presence of stones or ductal dilation. Magnetic resonance cholangiography is a new diagnostic tool that is useful in viewing the biliary tree, especially if suspected stones are not detected by ultrasound.[130,131]

The presence of fever requires broad-spectrum antibiotic coverage, as with cholecystitis. A dilated biliary tree with accompanying fever necessitates prompt surgical intervention, with drainage and stone removal. ERCP is an excellent tool for both diagnosis and therapy, including stone removal, dilation of a stenosis, or placement of a stent. The use of ERCP has become much more common in children, even infants.[132–134]

ACALCULOUS CHOLECYSTITIS

Cholecystitis can occur without the presence of gallstones. This condition is rare in adults, but occurs with surprising frequency in pediatrics, usually in extremely ill children in intensive care units. The cause is not known but is associated with the immediate postoperative state, trauma, or burns. Sepsis from a variety of organisms, including *Leptospira*, group B streptococci, *Shigella*, Salmonella and *E. coli*, has been associated with this condition, although no organism has emerged as the definitive cause.[135] A variety of other conditions are also associated with acalculous cholecystitis, including congestive heart failure, diabetes, malignant disease and abdominal vasculitis.[136] Because no obstructing stone is present, gallbladder stasis likely plays an important role. The stasis may be due to fever, dehydration, prolonged fasting, ileus, or TPN, which are common in the severely-ill child.[135]

The clinical findings are usually fever, abdominal pain and jaundice. Physical examination reveals a palpable abdominal mass, quite tender to touch. Laboratory studies are usually not helpful, but may reveal leukocytosis and elevated bilirubin levels. Diagnosis is aided by ultrasound identification of a large, distended gallbladder with a thickened wall and tenderness during the procedure (the ultrasonographic Murphy's sign). Biliary scintigraphy also is accurate, revealing normal liver uptake but no visualization of the gallbladder. Unfortunately, false-negative results of both ultrasound and scintigraphy occur in as many as 20% of cases when no stone is seen.[137]

In most instances, the treatment of choice is emergency laparotomy, with either cholecystostomy or cholecystectomy. Because the incidence of gallbladder gangrene is rare in children as compared with adults, simple drainage may be the method of choice. If gangrene is suspected on inspection of the gallbladder at laparotomy, resection is necessary.

ACUTE HYDROPS OF THE GALLBLADDER

Hydrops of the gallbladder is characterized by distention without inflammation. The distinction between acalculous cholecystitis and hydrops is therefore one of histology. Clinically, the differentiation of these two entities may be difficult. Most cases of acalculous cholecystitis are in severely ill patients, whereas hydrops tends to occur in a more benign setting, frequently involving a systemic vasculitis. The mucocutaneous lymph node syndrome (Kawasaki syndrome) is the commonest cause of gallbladder hydrops.[138] Hydrops also has been associated with other vascular disorders, such as Sjögren's disease, systemic sclerosis and Henoch-Schönlein purpura, as well as nephrotic syndrome, familial Mediterranean fever, mesenteric adenitis, leptospirosis, Epstein–Barr virus and bacterial infection with *Staphylococcus* and *Streptococcus*.[135,139,140] The cause is unknown, although local lymph node enlargement around the cystic duct and local vasculitis causing gallbladder ischemia are possibilities.

The clinical presentation is acute right upper quadrant abdominal pain, nausea and vomiting. Examination reveals upper abdominal tenderness, often with a palpable mass. Diagnosis is aided by ultrasound findings of a distended gallbladder with normal wall thickness and no echo densities. Biochemical studies are usually of little help. Surgical consultation should be obtained in all cases of suspected hydrops, although surgical intervention is rarely indicated. Medical management is supportive, with vigilant surgical observation. The development of fever or an increasingly tender abdomen suggests perforation and requires surgery. Most cases show steady resolution over about 2 weeks, with no known long-term sequelae.

UNUSUAL DISEASES OF THE GALLBLADDER

Carcinoma of the gallbladder has been reported in children, but is rare.[141] In adults, gallbladder carcinoma is usually associated with gallstones. Although commoner than gallbladder carcinoma in children, benign gallbladder tumors also are rare. Adenomatous polyps have been described associated with Peutz–Jeghers syndrome.[142]

Adenomyomatosis, or hyperplastic gallbladder, denotes hyperplasia of the mucous membrane, thickening of the muscularis and deep diverticular formations known as *Rokitansky–Aschoff sinuses*.[54] Odd deformities of the gallbladder, such as the phrygian cap, fish-hook anomaly and Hartmann's pouch, are associated with adenomyomatosis of the gallbladder.[1] The cause of the hyperplasia is unknown, although increased intraluminal gallbladder pressure has been implicated. No specific symptoms have ever been attributed to this condition; therefore, no specific therapy is advised.

Cholesterolosis is characterized by accumulation of cholesterol esters in the mucosa and submucosa of the gallbladder. After resection, these areas are visible as yellow spots on a red mucosal background, giving the appearance of a strawberry, thus the term *strawberry gallbladder*. Occasionally, these areas enlarge and become polypoid, leading to cystic duct obstruction. Typically though, no symptoms are directly attributed to this condition and thus no therapy is indicated. If symptoms do occur, cholecystectomy is indicated.

Metachromatic leukodystrophy, or sulfatide lipidosis, is an autosomal recessive disorder of sphingolipid metabolism. The biochemical defect in this disorder is the inability to degrade sphingolipid sulfatide or galactose-3 sulfate ceramide. The absence or deficiency of the lysosomal enzyme arylsulfatase A results in the accumulation of sulfatide in both neural and non-neural tissues, in particular the gallbladder. Gallstones have been reported in association with this disorder. The cause may involve gallbladder hypomotility secondary to sulfatide accumulation in the wall of the gallbladder or sulfatide granules serving as 'seeds' for gallstone formation.[143]

Polypoid gastric heterotopia in the gallbladder is extremely rare in children, consisting of polyps within the gallbladder with ectopic gastric mucosa.[144] Gallbladder polyps are usually asymptomatic and occur in association with other diseases such as Crohn's disease, Peutz-Jeghers syndrome, or leukodystrophy.[145,146] The presence of ectopic gastric mucosa may allow acid secretion, causing mucosal inflammation leading to cholecystitis.

Gallstones have been noted in pseudohypoaldosteronism,[147] presumed secondary to dehydration and electrolyte abnormalities. Wildervanck's syndrome (cervico- oculoacoustic syndrome) also has been found to include gallstones,[148] although the cause is unknown.

References

1. Way LW, Sleisenger MH. Cholelithiasis: chronic and acute cholecystitis. In: Sleisenger MH, Fordtran JS, eds. Gastrointestinal Disease: Pathophysiology, Diagnosis, Management. Philadelphia: WB Saunders; 1989:1691.
2. Holland C, Heaton KH. Increasing frequency of gallbladder operations in the Bristol area. Br Med J 1972; 3:672.
3. Friedman GD, Kamel WB, Dawber TR. The epidemiology of gallbladder disease: observations in the Framingham Study. J Chron Dis 1966; 19:273.
4. The Coronary Drug Project Research Group. the Coronary Drug Project: design, methods and baseline results. Circulation 1973; 47(suppl 1):1.
5. Sampliner RE, Bennet PH, Comess LJ, et al. Gallbladder disease in the Pima Indians: demonstration of high prevalence and early onset by cholecystography. N Engl J Med 1970; 283:1358.
6. Bainton D, Davies GT, Evans KT, et al. Gallbladder disease: prevalence in a South Wales industrial town. N Engl J Med 1976; 294:1147.
7. Maurer KR, Everhart JE, Exxati TM, et al. Prevalence of gallstone disease in Hispanic populations in the United States. Gastroenterology 1989; 96:487.
8. Bates GC, Brown CH. Incidence of gallbladder disease in chronic hemolytic anemia (spherocytosis). Gastroenterology 1952; 21:104.
9. Barbara L, Festi D, Frabboni R, et al. Incidence and risk factors for gallstone disease: the Sirmione study (abstract). Hepatology 1988; 8:1256.
10. Barker DJP, Gardner MJ, Power C, et al. Prevalence of gallstones at necropsy in nine British towns: a collaborative study. Br Med J 1979; 2:1389.
11. Bateson MC, Bouchier IAD. Prevalence of gallstones in Dundee: necropsy study. Br Med J 1975; 4:4271.
12. Layde PM, Vessey MP, Yeatles D. Risk factors for gallbladder disease: a cohort study of young women attending family planning clinics. J Epidemiol Commun Health 1982; 36:274.
13. Lindstrom CG. Frequency of gallstone disease in a well-defined Swedish population: a prospective necropsy study in Malmo. Scand J Gastroenterol 1977; 12:341.
14. Rome Group for the Epidemiology and Prevention of Cholelithiasis. (GREPCO): prevalence of gallstone disease in an Italian adult female population. Am J Epidemiol 1984; 119:796.
15. Biss K, Ho KJ, Mikkelson B, et al. Some unique biologic characteristics of the Masai of East Africa. N Engl J Med 1971; 284:694.
16. Khanuja B, Cheah YC, Hunt M, et al. Lithil, a major gene affecting cholesterol gallstone formation among inbred strains of mice. Proc Natl Acad Sci USA 1995; 92:7729–7733.
17. Rosmorduc O, Hermelin B, Poupon R. MDR3 gene defect in adults with symptomatic intrahepatic and gallbladder cholesterol cholelithiasis. Gastroenterol 2001; 120:1459–1467.
18. Gibson J. An extraordinary large gallbladder and hydropic cystis: medical essays and observations. Philos Soc Edin 1737(2):352.
19. Glenn F. 25-years experience in the surgical treatment of 5037 patients with non-malignant biliary tract disease. Surg Gynecol Obstet 1959; 109:591–606.
20. Andrassy RJ, Treadwell TA, Ratner IA, et al. Gallbladder disease in children and adolescents. Am J Surg 1976; 132:10.
21. Shafer AD, Ashley JV, Goodwin CD, et al. A new look at the multifactorial etiology of gallbladder disease in children. Am Surg 1983; 49:314.
22. Lau GE, Andrassy RJ, Mahour GH. A 30-year review of the management of gallbladder disease at a children's hospital. Am Surg 1983; 49:411.
23. Henschue CI, Littlewood-Teele R. Cholelithiasis in children: recent observations. J Ultrasound Med 1983; 2:481.
24. Holcomb GW. Gallbladder disease. In: Welch KJ, Randolph JA Jr, Rowe MI, ed. Pediatric Surgery, Vol 2. Chicago: Year Book Publications; 1986:1060.
25. Descos B, Bernard O, Brunelle F, et al. Pigment gallstones of the common bile duct in infancy. Hepatology 1984; 4:678.
26. Wesdorp I, Bosman D, Graaff A de, et al. Clinical presentation and predisposing factors of cholelithiasis and sludge in children. J Pediatr Gastroenterol Nutr 2000; 31:411–417.

27. Kumar R, Nguyen K, Shun A. Gallstones and common bile duct calculi in infancy and childhood. Asut N Z J Surg 2000; 70:188–191.
28. Lobe TE. Cholelithiasis and cholecystitis im children. Semin Pediatr Surg 2000; 9:170–176.
29. Calabrese C, Pearlman DM. Gallbladder disease below the age of 21 years. Surgery 1971; 70:413.
30. Honore LH. Cholesterol cholelithiasis in adolescent females. Arch Surg 1980; 114:62.
31. Friesen CA, Roberts CC. Cholelithiasis: clinical characteristics in children, case analysis and literature review. Clin Pediatr 1989; 28:294.
32. Holan KR, Holzbach RT, Hermann RE, et al. Nucleation time: a key factor in the pathogenesis of cholesterol gallstone disease. Gastroenterology 1979; 77:611–617.
33. Donovan JM, Carey MC. Separation and quantitation of cholesterol 'carriers' in bile. Hepatology 1990; 12:945–1045.
34. Carey MC, Cohen DE. Biliary transport of cholesterol in micelles and liquid crystals. In: Paumgartner G, Stiehl A, Gerak W, eds. Bile Acids and the Liver. Lancaster: MTP Press; 1987:287–300.
35. Carey MC. Formation of cholesterol gallstones: the new paradigms. In: Paumgartner G, Stiehl A, Gerok W, eds. Trends in Bile Acid Research. Dordrecht, Netherlands: Kluwer; 1989:259–281.
36. Forgacs IC. Pathogenesis of cholesterol gallstone disease: the motility defect. In: Northfield T, Jazrawi R, Zentler-Munro P, eds. Bile Acids in Health and Disease. Dordrecht, Netherlands: Kluwer; 1988:135–153.
37. Carey MC, Cahalane MC. Whither biliary sludge? Gastroenterology 1988; 95:508–523.
38. Booker ML, Scott TE, LaMorte WW. Effect of dietary cholesterol on phosphatidylcholines and phosphatidylethanolamines in bile and gallbladder mucosa in the prairie dog. Gastroenterology 1989; 97:1261–1267.
39. Kajiyama G, Kubota S, Sasaki H, et al. Lipid metabolism in the development of cholesterol gallstones in hamsters: I. Study on the relationship between serum and biliary lipids. Hiroshima J Med Sci 1980; 29:133–141.
40. Hay DW, Carey MC. Pathophysiology and pathogenesis of cholesterol gallstone formation. Semin Liver Dis 1990; 10:159–170.
41. Lee DWT, Gilmore CJ, Bonorris G, et al. Effect of dietary cholesterol on biliary lipids in patients with gallstones and normal subjects. Am J Clin Nutr 1985; 42:414–420.
42. Angelin B, Backman L, Einarsson K, et al. Hepatic cholesterol metabolism in obesity: activity of microsomal 3-hydroxy-3-methylglutaryl coenzyme A reductase. J Lipid Res 1981; 23:770–773.
43. Ahlberg J, Angelin B, Bjorkhem I, et al. Hepatic cholesterol metabolism of normal and hyperlipidemic patients with cholesterol gallstones. J Lipid Res 1979; 20:107–115.
44. Einarsson K, Nilsel K, Leijd B, et al. Influence of age on secretion of cholesterol and synthesis of bile acids by the liver. N Engl J Med 1985; 313:277–282.
45. Pellegrini CA, Ryan T, Broderick W, et al. Gallbladder filling and emptying during cholesterol gallstone formation in the prairie dog. Gastroenterology 1986; 90:143–149.
46. Li YF, Weisbrodt NW, Moody FG, et al. Calcium-induced contraction and contractile protein content of gallbladder smooth muscle after high-cholesterol feeding of prairie dogs. Gastroenterology 1987; 92:746–750.
47. Behar J, Lee KY, Thompson WE, et al. Gallbladder contraction in patients with pigment and cholesterol stones. Gastroenterology 1989; 97:1479–1484.
48. Lee SP, Maher K, Nicholls JF. Origin and fate of biliary sludge. Gastroenterology 1988; 94:170.
49. Smith BF. Human gallbladder mucin binds biliary lipids and promotes cholesterol crystal nucleation in model bile. J Lipid Res 1987; 28:1088.
50. Nilsson S. Gallbladder disease and sex hormones. Acta Chir Scand 1966; 132:275.
51. Bennion LJ, Knowler WC, Mott DM, et al. Development of lithogenic bile during puberty in Pima Indians. N Engl J Med 1979; 300:873.
52. Vessey M, Painter R. Oral contraceptive use and benign gallbladder disease revisited. Contraception 1994; 50:167–173.
53. Kern F, Everson GT. Contraceptive steroids in cholesterol in bile: mechanisms of actions. J Lipid Res 1987; 28:828.
54. Warren KW, Williams CI, Tan EGC. Diseases of the gallbladder and bile ducts. In: Schiff L, Schiff ER, eds. Diseases of the Liver. Philadelphia: JB Lippincott; 1987:1289–1335.
55. Gaskin KJ, Waters DLM, Howman-Giles R, et al. Liver disease and common-bile-duct stenosis in cystic fibrosis. N Engl J Med 1988; 318:340.
56. Isenberg J, L'Heureux PR, Warwick W, et al. Clinical observations on the biliary system in cystic fibrosis. Am J Gastroenterol 1976; 65:134.
57. Weber AM, Roy CC, Morin CL, et al. Malabsorption of bile acids in children with cystic fibrosis. N Engl J Med 1973; 289:1001.
58. Watkins JB, Tercyak AM, Szczepanik P, et al. Bile salt kinetics in cystic fibrosis. Gastroenterology 1974; 67:385.
59. Crowther RS, Soloway RD. Pigment gallstone pathogenesis: from man to molecules. Semin Liver Dis 1990; 10:171.
60. Ostrow JD. The etiology of pigment gallstones. Hepatology 1984; 4:215S.
61. Black BE, Carr SH, Ostrow JD, et al. Equilibrium swelling of pigment gallstones: evidence for network polymer structure. Biopolymers 1882(21):601.
62. Burnett W, Dwyer KR, Kennard CHL. Black pigment in polybilirubinate gallstones. Ann Surg 1981; 193:331.
63. Sarnaik S, Slovis TI, Corbett DP, et al. Incidence of cholelithiasis in sickle cell anemia using the ultrasonic gray-scale technique. J Pediatr 1980; 96:1005.
64. Lackman BS, Lazerson J, Stashak RJ, et al. The prevalence of cholelithiasis in sickle cell disease as diagnosed by ultrasound and cholecystography. Pediatrics 1979; 64:501.
65. Tabata M, Nakayama F. Bacteria and gallstones: etiological significance. Dig Dis Sci 1981; 26:218.
66. Cahalane MJ, Neubrand MW, Carey MC. Physical-chemical pathogenesis of pigment gallstones. Semin Liver Dis 1988; 8:317.
67. Wosiewitz U, Schenk J, Sabinski F, et al. Investigations on common bile duct stones. Digestion 1983; 26:43.
68. Treem WR, Malet PF, Gourley GR, et al. Bile and stone analysis in two infants with brown pigment gallstones and infected bile. Gastroenterology 1989; 96:519.
69. Hikasa Y, Nagase M, Tanimura H, et al. Epidemiology and etiology of gallstones. Arch Jpn Chir 1980; 49:555.
70. Hes FJ, Jong TP de, Bax NM, Houwen RH. Urinary tract infections and cholelithiasis in early childhood. J Pediatr Gastroenterol Nutr 1995; 21:319–321.
71. Tabata M, Nakayama F. Bacteria and gallstones: etiological significance. Dig Dis Sci 1981; 26:218.
72. Beiler HA, Kuntz C, Eckstein TM, Daum R. Cholecystolithiasis and infection of the biliary tract with Salmonella Virchow – a very rare case in early childhood. Eur J Pediatr Surg 1995; 5:369–371.

73. Akiyoshi T, Nakayama F. bile acid composition in brown pigment stones. Dig Dis Sci 1990; 35:27–32.
74. Halpern Z, Vinograd Z, Laufer H, et al. Characteristics of gallbladder bile of infants and children. J Pediatr Gastroenterol Nutr 1996; 23:147–150.
75. Stringer MD, Lim P, Cave M, et al. Fetal gallstones. J Pediatr Surg 1996; 31:1589–1591.
76. Morad Y, Zin N, Merlob P. Incidental diagnosis of asymptomatic neonatal cholelithiasis: a case report and a literature review. J Perinatol 1995; 15:314–317.
77. Debray D, Pariente P, Gauthier F, et al. Cholelithiasis in infancy: a study of 40 cases. J Pediatr 1993; 122:385–391.
78. Keller MS, Markle BM, Laffey PA, et al. Spontaneous resolution of cholelithiasis in infants. Radiology 1985; 157:345.
79. Jacir NN, Anderson KD, Eichelberger M, et al. Cholelithiasis in infancy: resolution of gallstones in three of four infants. J Pediatr Surg 1986; 21:567.
80. Jonas A, Yahav J, Fradkin A, et al. Choledocholithiasis in infants: diagnostic and therapeutic problems. J Pediatr Gastroenterol Nutr 1990; 11:513–517.
81. Ljung R, Ivarsson S, Nilsson P, Solvig J. Cholelithiasis during the first years of life: a case report and literature review. Acta Paediatr 1992; 81:69–72.
82. Roman B, Chiappa JL, Formantici F, et al. Neonatal choledocholithiasis: a case report. Pediatr Med Chir 1994; 16:595–597.
83. Johart G. Congenital cholelithiasis. Orv Hetil 1995; 136:67–70.
84. Monnerie JL, Soulard D. Cholelithiasis in infants with spontaneously favorable course. Arch Pediatr 1995; 2:654–656.
85. Ishitani MB, Shaul DB, Padua EA, McAlpin CA. Choledocholithiasis in a premature infant. J Pediatr 1996; 128:853–855.
86. Suchy FJ, Mullick FG. Total parenteral nutrition-associated cholestasis. In: Balistreri WF, Stocker JT, eds. Pediatric Hepatology. New York: Hemisphere; 1990:29–40.
87. Beale EF, Nelson RM, Buccarelli RL, et al. Intrahepatic cholestasis associated with parenteral nutrition in premature infants. Pediatrics 1979; 64:347.
88. Suchy FJ, Bucavalas JC, Novak DA. Determinants of bile formation during development: ontogeny of hepatic bile acid metabolism and transport. Semin Liver Dis 1987; 7:77.
89. Suita S, Ikeda K, Naito K, et al. Cholelithiasis in infants: association with parenteral nutrition. J Parenter Enteral Nutr 1984; 8:569.
90. Enzenauer RW, Montrey JS, Barcia PJ, et al. Total parenteral nutrition cholestasis: a cause of mechanical biliary obstruction. Pediatrics 1985; 76:905.
91. Lilly JR, Sokol RJ. On the bile sludge syndrome or is total parenteral nutrition cholestasis a surgical disease? Pediatrics 1985; 76:992.
92. Benjamin DR. Hepatobiliary dysfunction in infants and children associated with long-term total parenteral nutrition: a clinicopathologic study. Am J Clin Pathol 1980; 81:276.
93. Heubi JE, O'Connell NC, Setchell KD. Ileal resection/dysfunction in childhood predisposes to lithogenic bile only after puberty. Gastroenterology 1992; 103:636–640.
94. Callahan J, Haller JO, Cacciarelli AA, et al. Cholelithiasis in infants: association with total parenteral nutrition and furosemide. Pediatr Radiol 1982; 143:437.
95. Prince JS, Senae MO Jr. Ceftriaxone-associated nephrolithiasis and biliary pseudolithiasis in a child. Pediatr Radiol 2003; 33:64–561.
96. Granschow R. Cholelithiasis in pediatric organ transplantation: detection and management. Pediatr Transplant 2002; 6:91–96.
97. Safford SD, Safford KM, Martin R, et al. Management of cholelithiasis in pediatric patients who undergo bone marrow transplant. J Pediatr Surg 2002; 36:86–90.
98. Trendle MC, Moertel CG, Kvois LK. Incidence and morbidity of cholelithiasis in patients receiving chronic octreotide for metastatic carcinoid and malignant islet cell tumors. Cancer 1996; 79:830–834.
99. Redfern JS, Fortuner WJII. Octreotide-associated biliary tract dysfunction and gallstone formation: pathophysiology and management. Am J Gastroenterol 1995; 90:1042–1052.
100. McKnight JA, McCance DR, Sheridan B, Atkinson AB. Four years' treatment of resistant acromegaly with octreotide. Eur J Endocrinol 1995; 132:429–432.
101. Moser AJ, Abedin MZ, Giurgiu DI, Roslyn JJ. Octreotide promotes gallbladder absorption in prairie dogs: a potential cause of gallstones. Gastroenterology 1995; 108:1547–1555.
102. Park HZ, Lee SP, Schy AL. Ceftriaxone-associated gallbladder sludge. Gastroenterology 1991; 100:1665.
103. Kong MS, Chen CY. Risk factors leading to ceftriaxone-associated biliary pseudolithiasis in children. Chang Keng i Hsueh-Chang Gung Medical J 1996; 19:50–54.
104. Robertson FM, Crombleholme TM, Barlow SE, et al. Ceftriaxone choledocholithiasis. Pediatrics 1996; 98:133–135.
105. Weinstein S, Lipsitz EC, Addonizio L, Stolar CJ. Cholelithiasis in pediatric cardiac transplant patients on cyclosporine. J Pediatr Surg 1995; 30:61–64.
106. Pitcher GJ, Azmy AF. Cholelithiasis in paediatric renal transplant patients: implications for screening and management. Br J Urol 1996; 78:316–317.
107. Sakopoulos AG, Gundry S, Razzouk AJ, et al. Cholelithiasis in infant and pediatric heart transplant patients. Pediatr Transplant 2002; 6:231–234.
108. Reif S, Sloven DG, Lebenthal E. Gallstones in children: characteristics by age, etiology and outcome. Am J Dis Child 1991; 146:105.
109. Tamary H, Aviner S, Freud E, et al. High incidence of early cholelithiasis detected by ultrasonography in children and young adults with hereditary spherocytosis. J Pediatr Hematol Oncol 2003; 25:952–954.
110. Al-Salem AH, Qaisruddin S. The significance of biliary sludge in children with sickle cell disease. Pediatr Surg Int 1998; 13:14–16.
111. Thompson JS. The role of prophylactic cholecystectomy in the short bowel syndrome. Arch Surg 1996; 131:556–559.
112. Kim PC, Wesson D, Superina R, Filler R. Laparoscopic cholecystectomy versus open cholecystectomy in children: which is better? J Pediatr Surg 1995; 30:971–973.
113. Holbling N, Pilz E, Feil W, Schiessel R. Laparoscopic cholecystectomy-a meta analysis of 23,700 cases and status of a personal patient sample. Wien Klin Wochenschr 1995; 107:158–162.
114. Holcomb GW. III, Naffis D: Laparoscopic cholecystectomy in infants. J Pediatr Surg 1994; 29:86–87.
115. Salen G, Tint GS, Shefer S. Oral dissolution treatment of gallstones with bile acids. Semin Liver Dis 1990; 10:181.

116. Leuschner U, Leuschner M, Sieratzki J, et al. Gallstone dissolution with ursodeoxycholic acid in patients with chronic active hepatitis and two years follow-up: a pilot study. Dig Dis Sci 1985; 30:642.
117. Podda M, Zuin M, Battezzati M, et al. Efficacy and safety of a combination of chenodeoxycholic and ursodeoxycholic acid for gallstone dissolution: a comparison with ursodeoxycholic acid alone. Gastroenterology 1989; 96:222.
118. Sackman M, Delius M, Sauerbruch T, et al. Shock-wave lithotripsy of gallbladder stones-the first 175 patients. N Engl J Med 1988; 318:393.
119. Albert MB, Fromm H. Extracorporeal shock-wave lithotripsy of gallstones with the adjuvant use of cholelitholytic bile acids. Semin Liver Dis 1990; 10:197.
120. Ziegenhagen DJ, Wedel S, Kruis W, Zehnter E. Successful extracorporeal lithotripsy of gallbladder stones in a 12 year old girl. Padiatr Padol 1993; 28:55–56.
121. Sokal EM, Bilderling G De, Clapuyt P, et al. Extracorporeal shock-wave lithotripsy for calcified lower choledocholithiasis in an 18 month old boy. J Pediatr Gastroenterol Nutr 1994; 18:391–394.
122. Thistle JL, Peterson BT, Bender CE, et al. Percutaneous dissolution of gallstones using methyl tert-butyl ether. Can J Gastroenterol 1990; 4:625.
123. Weinsier RL, Wilson LJ, Lee J. Medically safe rate of weight loss for the treatment of obesity: a guideline based on risk of gallstone formation. Am J Med 1995; 98:115–117.
124. Gebhard RL, Prigge WF, Ansel HJ, et al. The role of gallbladder emptying in gallstone formation during diet-induced rapid weight loss. Hepatology 1996; 24:544–548.
125. Pare P, Shaffer EA, Rosenthall L. Nonvisualization of the gallbladder by 99mTc-HIDA cholescintigraphy as evidence of cholecystitis. Can Med Assoc J 1978; 118:384.
126. Miltenberg DM, Schaffer R, Breslin, et al. Changing indications for pediatric cholecystectomy. Pediatr 2000; 105:1250–1253.
127. Freund MC. Images in clinical medicine: porcelain gallbladder. N Engl J Med 1994; 330:402.
128. Bromley PJ, Keller FS. Courvoisier's gallbladder. N Engl J Med 2001; 345:1542.
129. Lilly JR. Common bile duct calculi in infants and children. J Pediatr Surg 1980; 15:577.
130. Ishizaki Y, Wakayama T, Okada Y, Kobayashi T. Magnetic resonance cholangiography for evaluation of obstructive jaundice. Am J Gastroenterol 1993; 88:2072–2077.
131. Meakem TJ, Schnall MD. Magnetic resonance cholangiography. Gastroenterol Clin North Am 1995; 24:221–238.
132. Gilger MA. The role of ERCP in children. Pr Gastroenterol 1996; 20:11–20.
133. Werlin SL. Endoscopic retrograde cholangiopancreatography in children. Gastrointest Endosc Clin North Am 1994; 4:161–178.
134. Guelrud M, Mendoza S, Zager A. ERCP and endoscopic sphincterotomy in infants and children with jaundice due to common duct stones. Gastrointest Endosc 1992; 39:450–453.
135. Ternberg JL, Keating JP. Acute acalculous cholecystitis: complication of other illnesses in childhood. Arch Surg 1975; 110:543.
136. Barie PS, Eachempati SR. Acute acalculous cholecystitis. Curr Gastroenterol Rep 2003; 5:302–309.
137. Shuman WP, Rogers JV, Rudd TG, et al. Low sensitivity of sonography and cholescintigraphy in acalculous cholecystitis. Am J Roentgenol 1984; 142:531.
138. Grisoni E, Fisher R, Izant R. Kawasaki syndrome: report of four cases with acute gallbladder hydrops. J Pediatr Surg 1984; 19:9–11.
139. Amemoto K, Nagita A, Aoki S, et al. Ultrasonographic gallbladder wall thickening in children with Henoch-Schonlein purpura. J Pediatr Gastroenterol Nutr 1994; 19:126–128.
140. Dinulos J, Mitchell DK, Egerton J, Pickering LK. Hydrops of the gallbladder associated with Epstein-Barr virus infection: a report of two cases and review of the literature. Pediatr Infect Dis J 1994; 13:924–929.
141. Iwai N, Goto Y, Taniguchi H, et al. Cancer of the gallbladder in a 9-year-old girl. Kinderchir 1985; 40:106.
142. Foster DR, Foster DBE. Gallbladder polyps in Peutz-Jeghers syndrome. Postgrad Med J 1980; 56:373.
143. McKhann GM. Metachromatic leukodystrophy: clinical and enzymatic parameters. Neuropediatrics 1984; 15(suppl):4.
144. Schimpl G, Schaffer G, Sorantin E, et al. Polypoid gastric heterotopia in the gallbladder: clinicopathological findings and review of the literature. J Pediatr Gastroenterol Nutr 1994; 19:129–131.
145. Sears HF, Golden GT, Horseley J. Cholecystitis in childhood and adolescence. Arch Surg 1973; 106:651–653.
146. Warfel KA, Hull MT. Villous papilloma of the gallbladder in association with leukodystrophy. Hum Pathol 1984; 15:1192–1194.
147. Hanaki K, Ohzeki T, Itisuka T, et al. An infant with pseudohypoaldo steronism accompanied by cholelithiasis. Biol Neonate 1994; 65:85–88.
148. Kose G, Ozkan H, Ozdamar F, et al. Cholelithiasis in cervico-oculo-acoustic (Wildervanck's) syndrome. Acta Paediatr 1993; 82:890–891.

SECTION SEVEN
THE PANCREAS

Chapter 67
Developmental anatomy and physiology of the pancreas

Aaron Turkish and Elyanne Ratcliffe

DEVELOPMENT OF THE PANCREAS

Overview of pancreatic development

The pancreas develops from dorsal and ventral pancreatic buds that arise in the caudal foregut (the primordial proximal duodenum; Fig. 67.1). The dorsal pancreatic bud, the larger of the two buds, appears by the fifth week of human gestation. Dorsal pancreatic cells grow out of the primordial duodenum and invade the dorsal mesentery. The ventral pancreatic bud develops from the duodenal wall close to the bile duct. As the duodenum and stomach rotate, the ventral pancreatic bud is carried dorsally with the common bile duct. As a result of this motion, the ventral pancreatic bud moves to the dorsal mesentery, posterior and inferior to the dorsal pancreatic bud within the mesentery. The two buds fuse to form the pancreas by the seventh week of gestation. Although uncommon, occasionally the ventral pancreas consists of two lobes; if the lobes migrate around the duodenum in opposite directions to fuse with the dorsal pancreatic bud, an annular pancreas is formed.

The ventral pancreatic bud is responsible for the formation of the uncinate process and the inferior part of the head of the pancreas, which either completely or partially surrounds the common bile duct. The dorsal pancreatic bud is responsible for the formation of the bulk of the pancreas. Despite its smaller size, the ventral pancreatic bud forms the main pancreatic duct (of Wirsung), which opens to the major duodenal papilla (ampulla of Vater). The duct of the dorsal pancreas usually connects to the main pancreatic duct, but may remain separate in a common anomaly known as a persistent dorsal or accessory duct (of Santorini) that opens into a minor accessory papilla, located about 2 cm above the main duct. The two ducts often communicate with each other, but in about 9% of people the pancreatic duct systems fail to fuse and the original ducts persist in a condition known as pancreas divisum.[1]

The formation of the exocrine and endocrine components of the pancreas will be later discussed in detail. In overview, the acinar cells begin as clusters along the primordial pancreatic ducts during the third month of gestation. Endocrine cells, which also originate from ductal epithelium, start to differentiate earlier than the acinar cells, during the eighth week. During the tenth to fourteenth weeks of gestation, the islets start to form clumps and eventually detach from the ducts.[2]

Molecular biology of pancreatic development

Specification of the pancreas

The morphogenesis and development of the pancreas has been well studied and a large number of markers that can be used to define pancreatic cells at different developmental stages have been identified. Most of the information about molecules that control pancreatic organogenesis has been derived from genetic analysis of transcription factors (Table 67.1; see also Jensen, 2004, for a comprehensive recent review).[3] These transcription factors play critical roles in the various processes required for normal development, including the specification, growth and differentiation of the pancreas.

Prior to and during the formation of the dorsal and ventral pancreatic buds, the organ primordium expresses pancreatic and duodenal homeobox 1/insulin promoter factor 1/somatostatin transactivating factor 1 (Pdx1/Ipf1/Stf1, referred to as Pdx1 in this chapter). All pancreatic cell types derive from *Pdx1*$^{+}$ progenitors (Fig. 67.2).[4,5] When *Pdx1* is mutated, pancreatic development is arrested after budding,[6,7] suggesting that factors other than *Pdx1* promote pancreatic specification.

Advances in identifying factors involved in pancreatic specification have been accomplished by studying various developmental models including zebrafish, chick and mice. For example, studies in zebrafish have identified several factors that are involved in pancreatic specification; these factors include retinoic acid (RA), bone morphogenetic protein (BMP) and Hedgehog (Hh).[8–11] In zebrafish, when either RA, BMP or Hh is inhibited, the pancreas fails to develop. Conversely, if the pathways of either of these factors is excessively active, the pancreas develops abnormally in size and/or location. RA and BMP have also both been demonstrated to regulate anterior-posterior patterning in the zebrafish endoderm.[10,11] Hh is a good example of the complexity of these signaling factors. In mice, the Hh pathway is active in the developing stomach and duodenum but is suppressed in pancreatic tissue; ectopic activation of Hh signaling at the onset of pancreatic development inhibits the organ formation.[12,13] More recent studies involving the secreted Hh ligands Sonic (Shh) and Indian (Ihh) hedgehog have shown that even at later stages of pancreatic development, ectopic Hh signaling can cause pancreatic defects.[14] Thus factors that are critical in early pancreatic

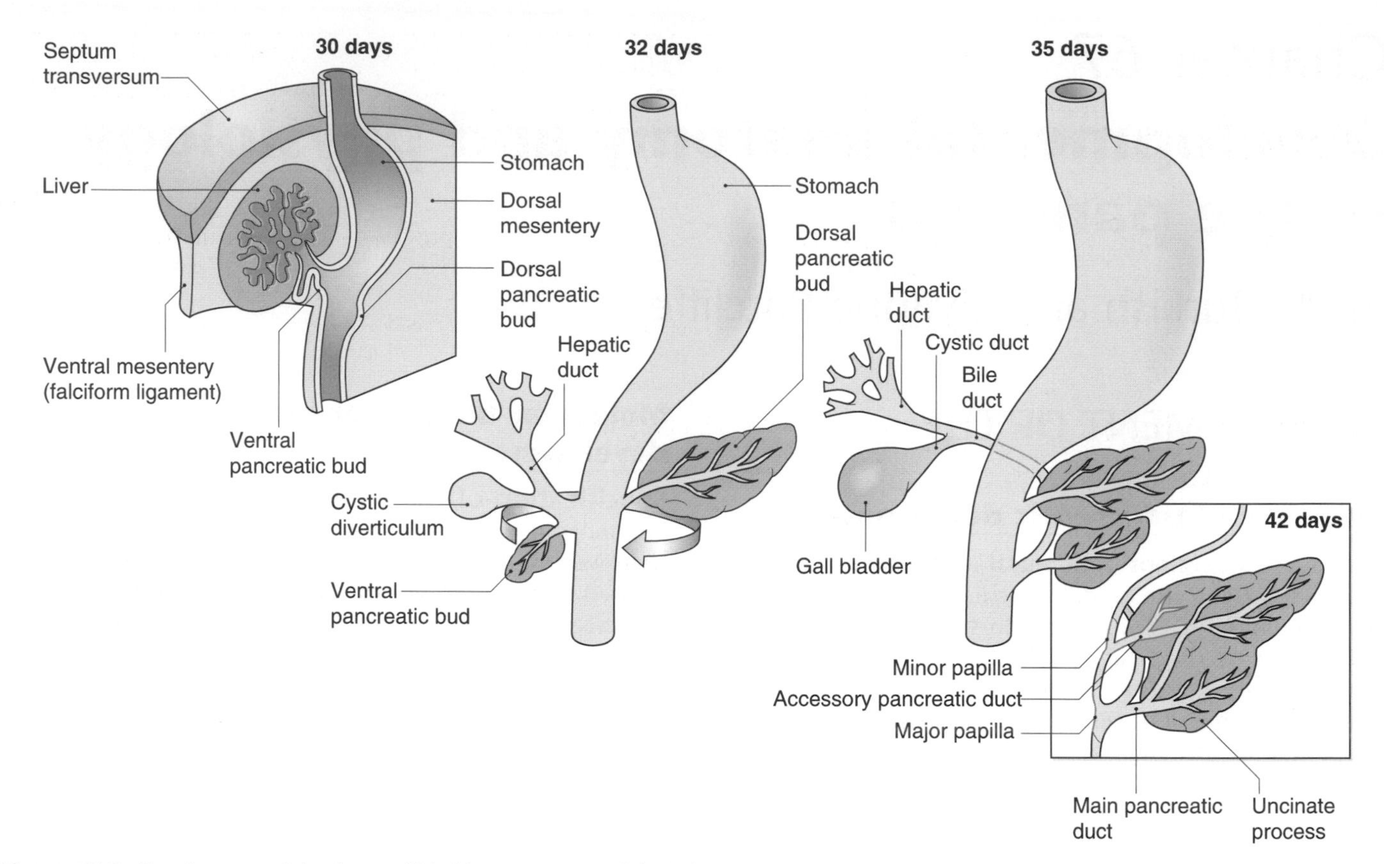

Figure 67.1: Development of the liver, gallbladder, pancreas and their duct systems from endodermal diverticula of the duodenum. The liver bud sprouts during the fourth week and expands in the ventral mesentery. The cystic diverticulum and ventral pancreatic bud also grow into the ventral mesentery, whereas the dorsal pancreatic bud grows into the dorsal mesentery. During the fifth week, the ventral pancreatic bud migrates around the posterior (former right side) of the duodenum to fuse with the dorsal pancreatic bud. The main duct of the ventral bud ultimately becomes the major pancreatic duct, which drains the entire pancreas. (Adapted from Larson, 2001, with permission.)[152]

morphogenesis can have continued involvement throughout development.

Studies in mice have revealed that *Sox17*, a member of the Sry-related HMG box gene family, may also be required for pancreas specification. *Sox17* is expressed throughout the endoderm after gastrulation and is one of the earliest specific markers of the definitive endoderm.[15] In order to better study the function of the *Sox17* gene, the phenotype of *Sox17* null mutant mice was examined. In these mice, the definitive endoderm lining the developing gut was deficient. Furthermore, *Pdx1* expression, which is essential for pancreatic outgrowth and differentiation, was not detected at the sites of the primordial pancreatic buds, suggesting that *Sox17* activity may also be important in the formation of the pancreas.[15]

As the pancreatic buds form, one becomes dorsal and the other ventral. Both early pancreatic buds express the homeobox gene *Hlxb9*, which encodes the homeoprotein Hb9.[16,17] However, in the dorsal bud, *Hlx9* expression precedes *Pdx1* expression; thus in knockout mice where *Hlbx9* is absent, the dorsal pancreas is also absent and *Pdx1* is not expressed.[17] The remaining ventral pancreas does form, but has small islets of Langerhans with reduced numbers of β cells.[16] It is unclear as to why Hb9 has different effects in the dorsal *vs* the ventral pancreas, but it is possible that Hb9 has an indirect effect via its expression in the notochord, which is known to promote dorsal pancreatic development.[18] In contrast to *Hlxb9* knockout mice, mice lacking *Ptf1a/p48*, a basic helix–loop–helix (bHLH) transcription factor, exhibit normal dorsal bud formation, whereas the ventral pancreas not only fails to bud but also becomes integrated into the surrounding duodenum.[19] Mutations in *PTF1A* have recently been described to cause pancreatic and cerebellar agenesis in a consanguineous family.[20]

In summary, the position and extent of the pancreatic buds is determined not only by specific inductive interactions with neighboring tissues, but also by the ability of the pancreatic endoderm to respond to these inductive signals. Appropriate pancreatic development depends on the position of the pancreas; this positional information is interpreted by transcription factors, which ultimately specify pancreatic fate.

Growth of the pancreatic primordium

Once the pancreatic buds have formed, the developing pancreas enters a stage of rapid growth and branching; this process is referred to as branching morphogenesis. Pioneering work on the development of the pancreas was accomplished during the 1960s, when Golosow and Grobstein[21] and Wessells and Cohen[22] carried out classic embryologic experiments to study aspects of pancreatic specification, growth and morphogenesis. Golosow and Grobstein were the first to show that, as in other developing organs, development of the pancreas is dependent on endodermal–mesenchymal interactions.

Factor	Family	Expression	Downstream pancreatic genes	Mouse mutations[a]	Human mutations
Neurogenin 3	bHLH	Fetal pancreas (endocrine progenitor cells) and CNS	neuroD1/BETA2, pax4, nkx2.2	Diabetes, no islet cells	
NeuroD1/BETA2	bHLH	Islet, gut endocrine cells, CNS	Insulin	Diabetes, decreased islet cells	Het: late-onset diabetes
P48/PTF	bHLH	Exocrine pancreas, CNS	Exocrine enzyme genes	Exocrine pancreatic agenesis, islets in spleen	
Mist1	bHLH	Exocrine pancreas, serous exocrine cells		Exocrine pancreas disorganization	
PDX1/IPF1	Parahox homeodomain	β and δ cells, duodenum, stomach, CNS	Insulin, IAPP, glucokinase, glut2	Pancreatic agenesis	Het: MODY4 Hom: pancreatic agenesis
HB9	Parahox homeodomain	β cells, gut, lymphoid, CNS	glut2 genesis	Dorsal pancreatic agenesis	Het: sacral agenesis
Pax2	Paired domain	Islet, urogenital tract and CNS	Glucagon	Defects in optic nerve, CNS and urogenital tract	Het: renal-coloboma syndrome
Pax4	Paired-homeodomain	Fetal pancreas and CNS	pax4 (autorepression)	Decreased β and δ cells	Het: late-onset diabetes Hom: early diabetes
Pax6	Paired-homeodomain	Islet, gut endocrine cells, CNS	Glucagon, insulin, somatostatin glucagon	Decrease in all islet cells, decreased	Het: Aniridia
Nkx2.2	NK-homeodomain	β, α and PP cells, and CNS	nkx6.1 insulin, glut2, GK	Diabetes, no insulin	
Nkx6.1	NK-homeodomain	β cells and CNS		Decreased β cells, postnatal lethal	
Cdx2/3	Caudal-homeodomain	Islet and gut	Glucagon	Het: gut tumors Hom: embryonic lethal	
Isl1	LIM-homeodomain	Islet and CNS	Somatostatin, glucagon	No islet cells, embryonic lethal	Het: late-onset diabetes
Lmx1.1	LIM-homeodomain	β cells and CNS	Insulin	Dreher: roof plate, cerebellum defects	
Brn4	Pou-homeodomain	α cells and CNS	Glucagon		Hom: congenital neurogenic deafness
HNF1α	Pou-homeodomain	Islet, liver, kidney	pax4, neurogenin3, glut2, rat insulin I	Diabetes, impaired β-cell glucose sensing	Het: MODY3
HNF1β	Pou-homeodomain	Islet, pancreatic duct, liver, kidney	pax4, PDX1	Embryonic lethal	Het: MODY5
HNF6	Cut-homeodomain	Pancreatic duct, liver	Neurogenin 3	IGT, small islets	
Foxa1/HNF3α	Forkhead/Winged Helix	Islet, gut, liver	Glucagon	Hypoglycemia	
Foxa2/HNF3β	Forkhead/Winged Helix	Islet, pancreatic duct, gut, liver, CNS	PDX1, neurogenin 3, Kir6.2, SUR1	Embryonic lethal	
Foxa3/HNF3γ	Forkhead/Winged Helix	Islet, gut, liver	Glucagon	No pancreatic phenotype	
HNF4α	Nuclear receptor	Liver, islet, kidney	HNF1α, glycolytic enzymes, pax4	Embryonic lethal	Het: MODY1
MafA	bZip	β cells, eye and thymus	Insulin		
c-Maf	bZip	α cells, eye	Glucagon		

het, heterozygous; hom, homozygous; CNS, central nervous system; GK, glucokinase; IAPP, islet amyloid polypeptide.
[a] All mouse phenotypes are for homozygous mutant animals unless stated otherwise.
Adapted from Wilson et al., 2003.[156]

Table 67.1 Pancreas transcription factors

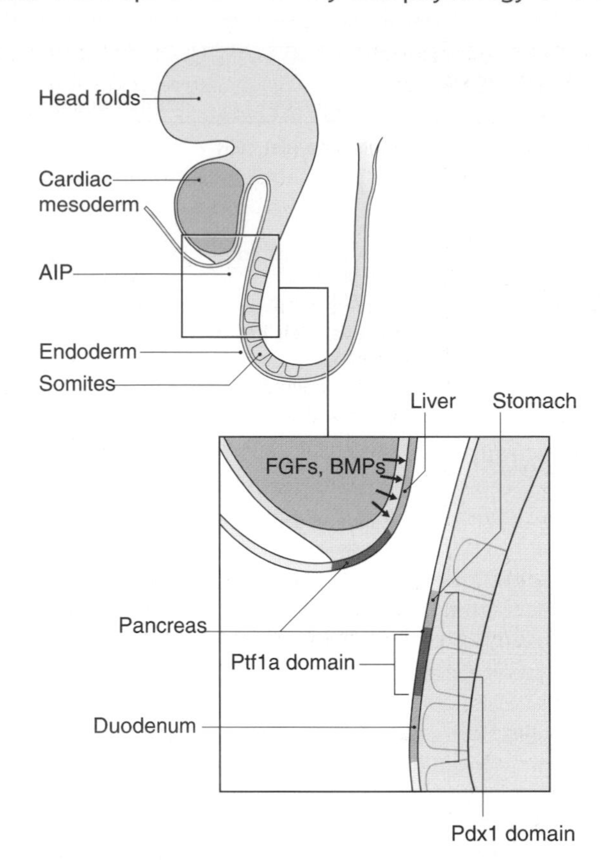

Figure 67.2: Competing induction of neighboring organs. A schematic representation of an E8.5 mouse embryo during foregut formation; embryo viewed from the side, anterior towards top, ventral to the left. The expression of *Ptf1a* within the *Pdx1* domain may define those cells that will adopt a pancreatic fate.[19] AIP, anterior intestinal portal; BMP, bone morphogenetic protein; FGF, fibroblast growth factor. (Adapted from Kumar and Melton, 2003, with permission.)[153]

During embryogenesis the pancreatic endoderm in exposed to a sequence of distinct mesodermal cell populations that participate, for example, in the formation of the two distinct pancreatic buds. The dorsal endoderm has sequential contact with the notochord, aorta and pancreatic mesenchyme, while the early ventral pancreatic endoderm forms adjacent to the septum transversum and cardiogenic mesoderm and then to the ventral (vitelline) veins and mesenchyme.[23] It is in response to signals from the varying surrounding mesodermal tissues that the dorsal bud forms first. Signals for induction come from two major sources: the mesenchyme and the notochord.

The role of the mesenchyme The importance of the mesenchyme in pancreatic organogenesis is demonstrated by the impaired dorsal pancreatic development observed in *Isl1*$^{-/-}$ mice (the *islet1* gene encodes a LIM homeodomain protein).[24] Normally, during bud formation, *Isl1* is expressed in the dorsal pancreatic mesenchyme; in *Isl1*$^{-/-}$ mice, this dorsal mesenchyme does not form. Moreover, when studied *in vitro*, the dorsal bud from *Isl1*$^{-/-}$ animals fails to undergo exocrine differentiation. This failure can be rescued by recombining the *Isl1*$^{-/-}$ dorsal pancreas with embryonic wild-type mesenchyme, demonstrating the importance of mesenchymal *Isl1*.

Similar phenotypes are seen in mice lacking N-cadherin[25] and pre B-cell leukemia transcription factor 1 (*Pbx1*).[26] N-cadherin, like *Isl1*, is expressed and functionally required in the dorsal pancreatic mesenchyme.[25] A less severe phenotype is seen in mice lacking *Pbx1*, a member of the three-amino loop extension (TALE) class of homeodomain transcription factors, which is expressed in pancreatic mesenchyme and epithelium. In *Pbx1* mutant mice, the pancreas overall is hypoplastic with the dorsal pancreas being particularly malformed. These mice also exhibit marked defects in exocrine and endocrine differentiation; the exocrine differentiation can be rescued following recombination with wild-type mesenchyme.[26]

The mesenchyme is also involved in promoting epithelial growth. For example, in mutant mice lacking one of the fibroblast growth factors (FGF), *Fgf10*, the dorsal and ventral pancreatic buds are hypoplastic, possibly secondary to decreased epithelial proliferation.[27] Other mesenchymal signals that promote epithelial proliferation include Pdx1 protein[28] and possibly members of the epidermal growth factor (EGF) family.[29,30]

Signals from the notochord The dorsal endoderm is in direct contact with the notochord during the period in which pancreatic fate is determined. Thus, the notochord is in an ideal position to be a signaling source that promotes induction of the dorsal pancreas. *In vitro* experiments carried out on cultures of early chick endoderm in the absence or presence of the notochord have demonstrated the role of the notochord in promoting pancreatic development by producing signals that repress *Shh* expression in the dorsal endoderm.[18] Notochord factors that repress endodermal *Shh* include FGF2 and activin-βB.[12]

Specification and differentiation of endocrine and exocrine cell types

The pancreas is made up of acinar (exocrine) cells, ducts and, embedded within the acinar structures, islets of endocrine cells. Each islet is composed of distinct α, β, δ and PP cells, which secrete glucagon, insulin, somatostatin and pancreatic polypeptide respectively. Endocrine islets, exocrine acini and pancreatic ducts are all derived from the endodermal epithelium. Although progress had been made in identifying the factors involved in endocrine and exocrine differentiation, little is known about ductal differentiation.

As discussed previously, all adult pancreatic cells derive from *Pdx1*-expressing progenitors. While the expression of *Pdx1* has been shown to persist throughout development,[31,32] its direct involvement has been unclear. In order to study the roles of Pdx1 in later stages of fetal pancreatic development, mice were created in which *Pdx1* expression could be suppressed at any time. These studies revealed that the inhibition of *Pdx1* before cell differentiation blocked the formation of acini and islets, demonstrating the importance of *Pdx1* in pancreatic cellular differentiation.[28]

The bHLH protein Neurogenin 3 (Ngn3) is a significant regulator of endocrine development with exclusive expression in endocrine precursor cells and subsequent downregulation during differentiation.[5,33] Cells which express *Ngn3* have been demonstrated to be islet progenitors[5] and ectopic expression of *Ngn3* is sufficient to turn endodermal cells into endocrine cells that, for example, form islets expressing glucagon.[34]

The *Ngn3* misexpression data, together with studies of mice lacking the ligand *Delta1*,[35] the Notch DNA-binding partner *RBPJκ*,[35] the Notch target gene Hairy-and-Enhancer-of-split 1 (*Hes1*)[36] or *Ngn3*,[37] collectively show that Notch signaling is critical for the decision between endocrine and progenitor/exocrine cell fates in the developing pancreas. Studies have shown that by blocking Notch receptor activation in early pancreatic progenitors, *Ngn3* expression increases and subsequently promotes the precocious differentiation of endocrine cells, thereby limiting the overall potential of pancreatic cell differentiation.[35,36] Therefore, the activation of Notch can be seen as preventing the premature differentiation of pancreatic progenitor cells, thus allowing their subsequent proliferation and morphogenesis.[38]

Ngn3 is also regulated by hepatocyte nuclear factor 6 (Hnf-6), which is part of class of cut homeodomain transcription factors. In mice lacking *Hnf-6*, the exocrine pancreas appears to be normal, while endocrine differentiation is impaired.[39] These investigations have further revealed that without *Hnf-6*, *Ngn3* expression is almost abolished and have demonstrated that Hnf-6 binds to and stimulates the Ngn3 gene promoter. However, the block of endocrine differentiation in *Hnf-6*$^{-/-}$ mice seems to be temporary; in postnatal stages, the number of endocrine cells increases and islets begin to appear.[39]

Factors that influence the differentiation of β cells include members of the mammalian NK2 homeobox transcription factor family, Nkx2.2 and Nkx6.1.[40,41] *Nkx.2.2* is expressed in α, β and PP cells, but not in δ cells in the developing pancreas.[40] In transgenic *Nkx2.2*$^{-/-}$ mice, the β cells fail to undergo their final differentiation and are instead arrested in a pre-β cell state; the α and PP cells are also markedly decreased.[40] In contrast to *Nkx2.2*, *Nkx6.1* expression is limited to β cells, and in *Nkx6.1* mutant mice, there is a profound defect in β-cell formation, which is particularly evident after the onset of the secondary transition.[41] Since islet development in *Nkx6.1*/*Nkx2.2* double mutant mice is identical to that in *Nkx2.2* homozygous mutants, *Nkx6.1* can be considered as acting downstream of *Nkx2.2* in the pathway of β cell formation.[41] Studies in transcription factor deficient mice have revealed that *Ngn3* expression is not dependent on either *Nkx2.2* or *Nkx6.1*, suggesting that both these factors act downstream of *Ngn3*.[33]

Since both endocrine and exocrine cells ultimately arise from early *Pdx1+* progenitors, it is unclear as to the timing during development at which an either endocrine or exocrine fate is determined. An *in vitro* study using retroviral labeling has revealed that a common pancreatic progenitor cells does exist, which gives rise to both endocrine and exocrine cells.[42] It is possible that early *Pdx1+* cells are indeed bipotential and that their expansion and later endocrine or exocrine differentiation can be influenced by a combination of intrinsic and extrinsic signals. The exact pathways that promote either an endocrine or exocrine fate are an area of further study.

While progress has been made in understanding the transcriptional control of differentiation within the endocrine and exocrine lineages, similar progress has yet to be made in understanding the earlier events in which the epithelial cells interact with the surrounding mesenchyme and form elaborate branches.[43] Recent research has demonstrated a novel role for netrin-1, an axon guidance molecule, in cell adhesion and cell migration at the developmental stages when the pancreatic epithelium branches into the surrounding mesenchyme (Fig. 67.3).[44] In this study, netrin 1 was shown to be expressed together with two integrins, $\alpha_6\beta_4$ and $\alpha_3\beta_1$, in fetal pancreatic epithelium. Pancreatic cells were demonstrated to adhere, spread and migrate on netrin-coated substrata by interacting with $\alpha_6\beta_4$; $\alpha_3\beta_1$ was shown to mediate hepatocyte growth factor (HGF)-simulated cell migration on netrin-coated substrata.

Recent work has also demonstrated the importance of netrin 1 in the formation of pancreatic ganglia.[45] Netrin 1 immunoreactivity was shown to be concentrated in the basolateral cytoplasm of acinar cells, and a subset of enteric crest-derived cells expressed the netrin receptor, deleted in colorectal cancer (*DCC*). In *in vitro* studies, crest-derived cells were found to migrate away from explants of bowel in the direction of co-cultured pancreatic buds; this migration was inhibited by the addition of antibodies to *DCC* to the culture media. Transgenic mice that lack *DCC* were investigated to test the hypothesis that chemoattractants secreted by the pancreas induce *DCC*-expressing crest-derived cells in the small intestine to deviate from their proximodistal path to enter the pancreas. Pancreatic neurons were not present in *DCC*$^{-/-}$ mice, consistent with the idea that netrins, secreted by the pancreas, participate in the formation of pancreatic ganglia.

Pancreatic stem cells

Studies in pancreatic organogenesis are not only important in furthering the field of congenital anomalies and genetic disorders, but also in developing new therapies for human disease. In order to generate functional β cells that are suitable for transplantation into diabetic patients, it is critical to identify factors that control the generation of functional β cells as well as to isolate markers of pancreatic stem cells. Progress has already been made in identifying, for example, *Pdx1*, which is not only highly expressed in adult β cells, but is also crucial for β-cell function in both mice and humans.[46–48] Heterozygosity for a nonsense mutation in the human *IPF1* gene has been linked to maturity-onset diabetes of the young (MODY),[48] a monogenetic form of diabetes in humans that results from β-cell dysfunction. Similarly, inactivation of *Pdx1* in the β cells of adult mice leads to the development of diabetes.[46,47] Knowledge of organogenesis and of key intrinsic and extrinsic factors in pancreatic cell development will eventually contribute to the efficient and reproducible generation of stable, fully functional β cells.

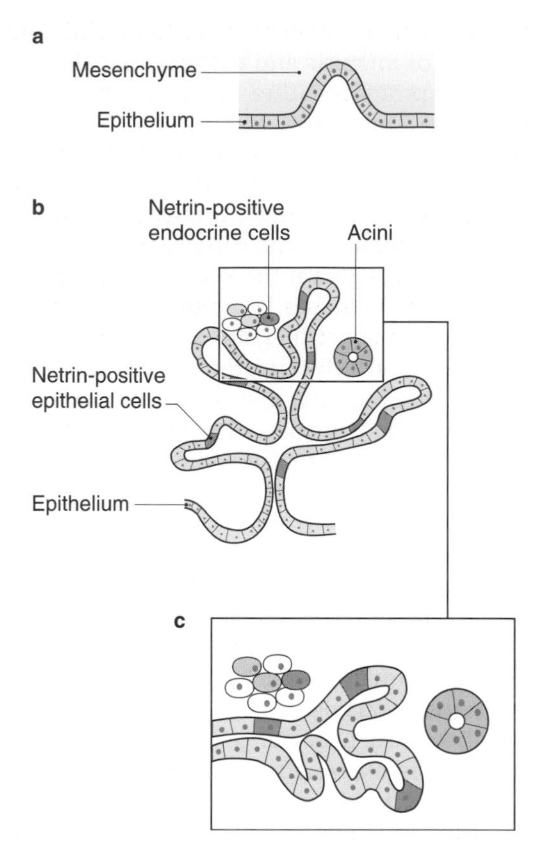

Figure 67.3: Pancreas morphology and distribution of netrin 1. (**a**) At early stages of pancreas organogenesis, the endodermal epithelium buds into the surrounding mesenchyme. (**b**) During later stages, the epithelium undergoes elaborate branching morphogenesis and the mature cell types of the exocrine and endocrine lineage start to emerge. The exocrine component comprises acinar cells that produce and secrete digestive enzymes into an elaborate system of interconnected channels formed by the other main exocrine cell type, the duct cell. In addition to providing digestive enzymes, the pancreas also contains an endocrine portion located in islets of Langerhans, clusters of hormone-producing cells interspersed within the exocrine matrix. (**b,c**) Netrin-1 protein is distributed in a subset of epithelial as well as differentiated endocrine and acinar cells. In addition, expression is localized to the basement membrane that separates the epithelial and mesenchymal layers. (Adapted from Hebrok M, Reichardt LF. Brain meets pancreas: netrin, an axon guidance molecule, control epithelial cell migration. Trends Cell Biol 2004; 14:153–155, with permission).[154]

PANCREATIC SECRETION AND EXOCRINE FUNCTION

Overview of pancreatic physiology

The pancreas is a vital endocrine and exocrine organ responsible for the release of hormones and the secretion of fluid, electrolytes and various enzymes that are intricately involved in the digestion of food. Although pancreatic secretion has traditionally thought to be under distinct hormonal and neuronal regulation, there is increasing evidence that its regulation is mediated by a complex neuroendocrinologic interplay.[49] Within this milieu, a variety of stimulatory and inhibitory factors regulate pancreatic secretion.

Functional anatomy of the exocrine pancreas

More than 80% of the exocrine pancreas is composed of clusters of acini lobules within a network of connective tissue[49–51] (Fig. 67.4). The acinus, a spherical or tubular group of pyramidal cells arranged with their apices towards its center, synthesizes, stores and releases pancreatic digestive enzymes.[49] The basal region of the acinar cell contains the nucleus and endoplasmic reticulum, where proteins are synthesized.[50,52] The rate of synthesis is 10 million enzyme molecules per acinar cell per minute.[53] These enzymes are then packaged into secretory (zymogen) granules in the Golgi complex, and stored in the apical region of the cell until their release.[50] The entire process from enzymatic synthesis to the point at which enzymes are ready for secretion is about 50 min.[53]

The basolateral membrane of the acinar cell harbors multiple receptors for secretagogs such as cholecystokinin (CCK) and for neurotransmitters such as acetylcholine and vasoactive intestinal peptide (VIP).[49] Centroacinar (proximal ductular) cells that extend into the acinar lumen and pancreatic duct cells modify pancreatic juice by secretion of water and bicarbonate (HCO_3^-).[49,53] Intercalated ducts that empty into intralobular ducts drain these cells. Intralobulular ducts drain into extralobular ducts that eventually drain into the main pancreatic duct, which, in combination with the common bile duct, enters the duodenum.

The endocrine cells of the pancreas are distributed within the islets of Langerhans. They are composed of A cells, which produce glucagon, B cells, which produce insulin, D cells, which secrete the largely inhibitory hormone, somatostatin, and F cells, which secrete pancreatic polypeptide[49] in response to vagal stimulation. Acinar cells are exposed to endocrine secretions (in a reciprocal relationship) via cell-to-cell contact between exocrine and endocrine tissue, as well as direct capillary connections between the islets and acini within the insulinoacinar portal system.[54,55] Islet cell hormones enter the systemic circulation via pancreatic blood flow. The pancreas also falls under the influence of a complex neuronal network

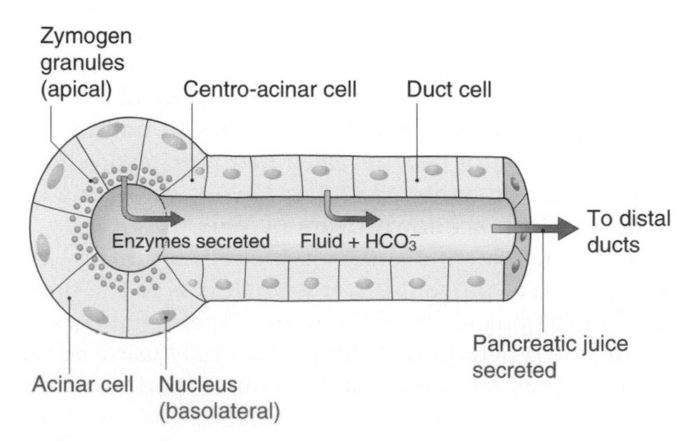

Figure 67.4: The acinus and cross-sectional appearance of the pancreatic ductule.

composed of parasympathetic (vagal), sympathetic, peptidergic and sensory innervates of glandular cells and vessels. The pancreas also has its own intrinsic nerve plexus, comparable to the enteric nervous system.[56]

Formation of pancreatic juice

About 1 liter of pancreatic juice is secreted into the small intestine per day;[51,57] it is a clear, isotonic and colorless alkaline fluid composed of water, electrolytes and enzymes important in the digestion of protein, fat and starch.[58] The centroacinar and ductal cells are responsible for secretion of the HCO_3^--rich fluid that transports the digestive enzymes synthesized and secreted by the acinar cells into the small intestine (Fig. 67.5).

Fluid and electrolytes

Utilizing an osmotic gradient created by the active secretion of electrolytes such as sodium (Na^+), potassium (K^+), bicarbonate (HCO_3^-) and chloride (Cl^-), water enters pancreatic juice via passive diffusion[51] into the pancreatic duct lumen. There are two means by which HCO_3^- enters the cell: (1) the Na^+–HCO_3^- co-transporter on the basolateral membrane;[59,60] (2) carbon dioxide (CO_2) is produced in the cell as a metabolic product or enters the cell via diffusion from the extracellular fluid by the action of H^+ on plasma HCO_3^-. Carbonic anhydrase hydrates CO_2 and produces carbonic acid (H_2CO_3), which then dissociates into HCO_3^- and H^+.[51]

There are several channels, transporters and exchangers on the basolateral membrane that are responsible for creating the pH and ionic gradients that drive HCO_3^- into the cell. Some animal studies have shown that the Na^+ gradient created by the Na^+/ K^+-ATPase pump greatly contributes to HCO_3^- influx via the Na^+–HCO_3^- co-transporter.[61] Other evidence has revealed that an H^+-ATPase actively moves H^+ out of the cell, driving HCO_3^- back into the cell.[62] This vacuolar ATPase merges with the basolateral membrane via exocytosis in response to secretin. A Na^+/H^+ exchanger appears to play a minor role in H^+ efflux induced HCO_3^- entry into the cell.[62] The gastrointestinal hormone secretin binds to its receptor on the basolateral membrane and activates adenylate cyclase to produce cyclic adenosine monophosphate (cAMP). A rise in cAMP concentration activates the cystic fibrosis transmembrane conductance regulator (CFTR) Cl^- channel on the luminal membrane, resulting in increased Cl^- secretion into the duct lumen.[63,64] This, in turn, induces an increase in HCO_3^- efflux into the lumen via the Cl^-/HCO_3^- exchanger. The resulting net luminal electronegative potential pulls Na^+ and K^+ into the lumen intercellularly, with a burst of water following this osmotic gradient.[51] HCO_3^- in pancreatic juice can then provide the necessary pH for digestion and absorption of protein, lipids and carbohydrates within the small intestine.

At rest, pancreatic juice is secreted at a rate of 0.2 ml/min and the bicarbonate concentration equals that of plasma. During secretin-induced stimulation, the rate of secretion increases to about 4.0 ml/min, and bicarbonate concentration increases asymptotically to a maximum of 140 mEq/l, creating a pH of about 8.2 in pancreatic juice.[57,58] The sum of Cl^- and HCO_3^- concentrations remains constant, because the Cl^- concentration falls with

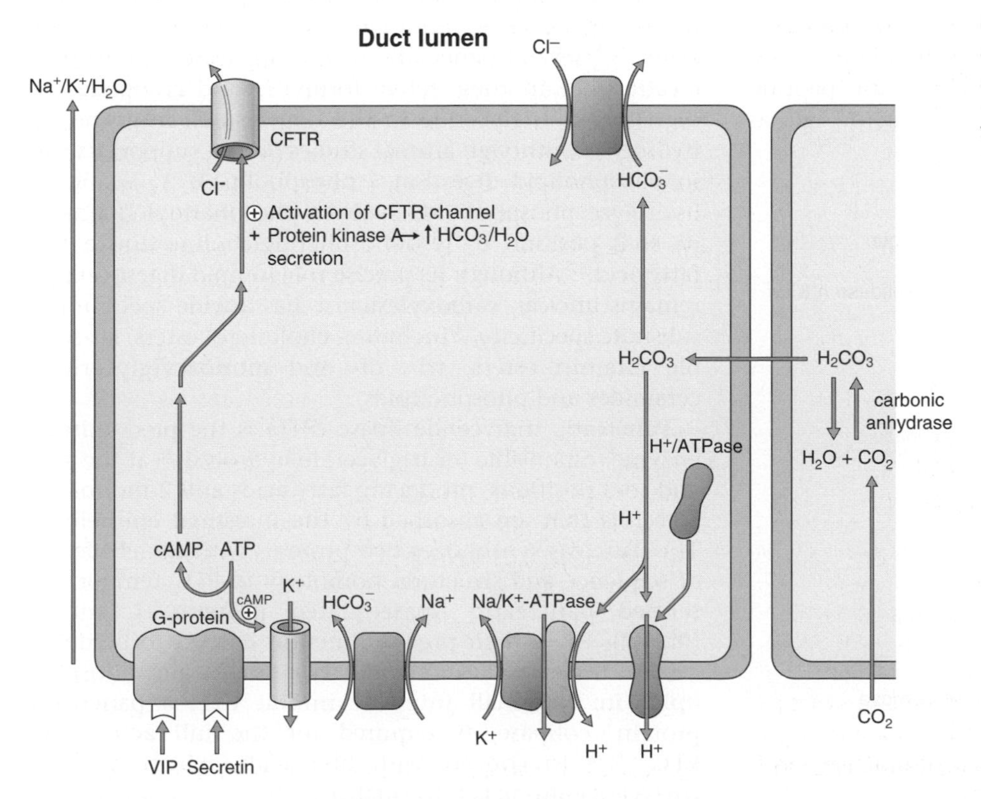

Figure 67.5: Model of fluid and bicarbonate secretion in a pancreatic duct cell. ATP, adenosine triphosphate; cAMP, cyclic adenosine monophosphate; CFTR, cystic fibrosis transmembrane conductance regulator; VIP, vasoactive intestinal peptide.

increasing secretion rates. Pancreatic juice also contains calcium (Ca^{2+}) and small amounts of magnesium (Mg^{2+}), zinc (Zn^{2+}), phosphate (HPO_4^{2-}) and sulfate (SO_4^{2-}).[51]

Pancreatic enzymes

Some 0.7–10% of pancreatic juice is composed of various proteins synthesized and secreted by the pancreas, including the digestive enzymes and pro-enzymes, plasma proteins, trypsin inhibitors and mucoproteins.[51]

The digestive enzymes secreted by the pancreas are responsible for about half of the overall digestion of nutrients in the gastrointestinal tract[49,51] and are comprised of proteolytic, lipolytic and amylolytic enzymes (Fig. 67.6). Many are synthesized and stored in zymogen granules as inactive pro-enzymes prior to secretion in pancreatic juice, and must be activated in the duodenum in order to possess activity. This also provides a degree of autoprotection by preventing pancreatic autodigestion by these proteins. Enzymes within the zymogen granules are in a solid form and solubilize once they enter the alkaline environment in the pancreatic ducts. In turn, these acid-sensitive enzymes are protected by the bicarbonate-rich pancreatic fluid in which they are transported.[52,57,65,66]

The proteolytic enzymes account for most enzymes in pancreatic juice and are secreted as inactive precursor enzymes.[51] Trypsinogen is a pro-enzyme that undergoes hydrolysis of its amino-terminal fragment via enterokinase at the intestinal brush border, and is activated by its conversion to trypsin. Trypsin then catalyzes the activation of other proteolytic enzymes, such as chymotrypsinogen, proelastase, pro-carboxypeptidase A and B, and trypsinogen itself. Carboxypeptidase cleaves peptide bonds at the carboxy-terminal ends of proteins. Trypsin cleaves interior peptide bonds involving basic amino acids. Chymotrypsin acts on interior peptide bonds involving aromatic amino acids, leucine, glutamine and methionine. Elastase cleaves peptide bonds at neutral aliphatic amino acids. The combined action of gastric pepsin and pancreatic proteases digests proteins into oligopeptides and amino acids, which are further digested by intestinal brush border enzymes prior to absorption.[57,65,67] The pancreas also secretes pancreatic secretory trypsin inhibitor, SPINK1, which acts as a first-line of defense against pancreatic autodigestion by small amounts of active trypsin by binding to and inactivating 20% of trypsin.[68,69]

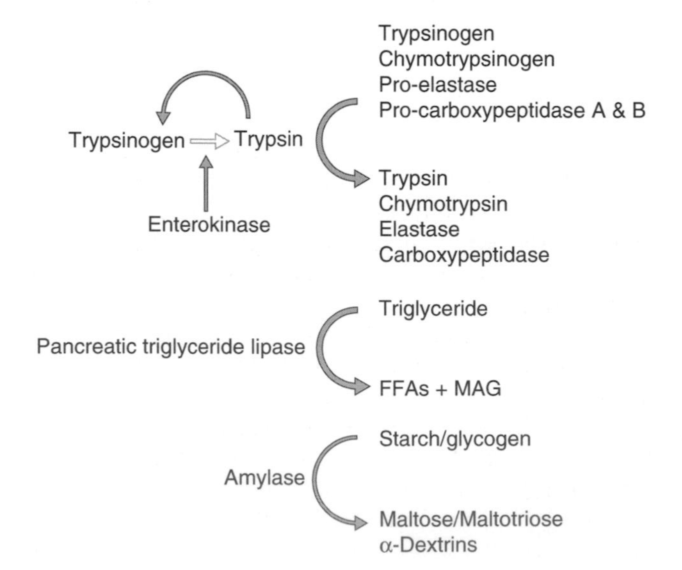

Figure 67.6: Digestive enzymes secreted by the pancreas. FFA, free fatty acids; MAG, monoacylglycerol.

The intestinal epithelium is able to absorb carbohydrates only as monosaccharides, and depends on α-amylase to hydrolyze dietary starch into glucose. α-Amylase is secreted by the salivary glands and the pancreatic acinus in its active form, and digests dietary starch from plants and glycogen from animal sources. The major dietary starches are amylose, a straight-chain α-1,4-linked glucose polymer, and amylopectin, which has α-1,4-glucose linkages and α-1,6-linked branches. α-Amylase hydrolyzes α-1,4-glucose linkages but not α-1,6 linkages, nor terminal glucose residues of starch and glycogen. The products of amylase digestion are short-chain α-1,6-linked polysaccharides, termed α-limit dextrins, composed of maltose (an α-1,4-linked glucose dimer), maltotriose (a trimer of α-1,4-linked glucose molecules) and branched oligosaccharides with α-1,4 and α-1,6 linkages. Sucrase, glycoamylase and isomaltase complete the digestion of dextrins at the intestinal brush border, allowing for glucose absorption by intestinal epithelial cells.[57,65,67]

Triglycerides account for the overwhelming majority of dietary lipid[70] and must be digested into fatty acids and monoacylglycerols prior to absorption by the intestine. Following emulsification of dietary lipids, gastric lipase begins the process and cleaves 15–20% of the fatty acids.[71,72] Several pancreatic lipases are secreted into pancreatic juice in their active forms[51,57] and complete the digestion of triglyceride in the upper small intestine via hydrolysis. Although animal studies do not support its role in phospholipid digestion,[73] phospholipase A_2 is able to hydrolyze phospholipids such as phosphatidylcholine at its sn-2 position to lysophosphatidylcholine and a free fatty acid.[57] Although its precise role in lipid digestion also remains unclear, carboxylesterase has a wide spectrum of substrate specificity,[74] including cholesterol esters, fat-soluble vitamin esters, tri-, di- and monoacylglycerides, ceramides and phospholipids.

Pancreatic triglyceride lipase (PTL) is the predominant enzyme responsible for triglyceride hydrolysis[75] at the sn-1 and sn-3 positions, producing fatty acids and 2-monoacylglycerols that are absorbed by the intestinal epithelium. The pancreas synthesizes two proteins with a high degree of sequence and structural homology to PTL, temporarily termed pancreatic lipase-related proteins 1 and 2 (PLPR2),[75,76] as their precise function has yet to be determined. Because bile salts, dietary proteins and phospholipids in the small intestine inhibit PTL, a pancreatic protein, colipase, is required for the full activity of PTL.[75,77,78] In concert with bile acids, which emulsify triglyceride droplets into smaller particles, colipase forms a complex with PTL to increase greatly the surface area upon which PTL can act.[57,75]

Regulation of pancreatic secretion

Regulation of pancreatic secretion is mediated by a complex interplay of several stimulatory and inhibitory gastrointestinal hormones and neuronal pathways (Table 67.2). There is an increasing body of evidence that other novel regulatory peptide hormones and neurotransmitters are also involved in pancreatic secretion. Pancreatic juice is secreted during basal, fasting states (the interdigestive period) and the postprandial (digestive) period.

Interdigestive pancreatic secretion

The interdigestive phase is cyclic and closely follows the pattern of the migrating myoelectric complex (MMC) in the intestine.[49,57] Phase I of the MMC is characterized by a lack of motility, with phases II and III possessing increasingly more activity. During phase I, pancreatic secretion of enzymes and bicarbonate is at its nadir (about 10% and 2% of maximum rates respectively).[51] Every 60–120 min there is a surge in intestinal motility associated with phase II and III of the MMC in the duodenum and a progressive increase in gastric acid, bile and pancreatic secretion.[66,79,80] It is thought that this cyclic secretion of pancreatic juice is important in digestion of residual food, cellular debris and pathogens in the duodenum during the interdigestive period. Although the mechanism of this process remains to be determined, it appears that the gastrointestinal hormones motilin and pancreatic polypeptide, as well as the autonomic nervous system, are involved with the regulation of MMC cycling.[49,79,81–83] Administration of motilin prematurely activates the MMC and shortens the frequency between peaks.[83] It appears that pancreatic polypeptide is an inhibitory hormone in this process. MMC blockade following the administration of atropine implicates a vagal cholinergic stimulatory role during the interdigestive period.[51]

Stimulatory
Cholecystokinin (CCK)
Secretin
Vasoactive intestinal pepitde (VIP)
Gastrin-Releasing Peptide (GRP)
Insulin
Gastrin
Nitric oxide
Serotonin
Substance P
Pancreatic phospholipase A_2
Inhibitory
Somatostatin
Pancreatic polypeptide (PP)
Peptide YY
Neuropeptide Y
Calcitonin gene-related peptide (CGRP)
Glucagon
Serotonin
Enkephalins
Leptin

Table 67.2 Pancreatic stimulatory and inhibitory factors

Postprandial pancreatic secretion

Exocrine pancreatic secretion begins almost immediately after ingestion of a meal and is associated with an increase in the concentration of several pancreatic stimulatory and inhibitory hormones in plasma as well as neural stimulation via the vagus nerve. Postprandial pancreatic secretion is divided into three phases: the cephalic, gastric and intestinal phases, which contributes 20%, 10% and 70% respectively to the overall postprandial response.[84]

The cephalic phase is mediated by the vagus nerve in response to sight, smell, taste and thought of food, and accounts for a significant amount of pancreatic enzyme secretion and a smaller portion of HCO_3^- secretion.[49,51] This is accompanied by a rise in plasma gastrin, CCK, a minor rise in plasma secretin, and increased levels of the inhibitory hormones pancreatic polypeptide and leptin.[49,85] Sham feeding studies, in which subjects smell, taste and chew but do not swallow food, suggest that direct vagal stimulation of acinar cells is the major stimulant during the cephalic phase.[86] Because subjects with achlorhydria continue to secrete pancreatic juice during sham feeding, it is now thought that gastric acid secretion does not contribute substantially to the cephalic phase.[51] Sham feeding experiments that revealed an incomplete block of pancreatic secretion during atropine administration suggest that peptidergic neurons from the vagus nerve may directly activate acinar cells via release of stimulatory peptides such as vasoactive intestinal peptide (VIP) and gastrin-releasing peptide (GRP).[57] VIP is known to stimulate acinar cells and duct epithelial cells.[57,87]

The gastric phase begins when food enters the stomach, increasing the rate of pancreatic secretion of enzymes as the stomach distends.[88–90] Stimulation of mechanoreceptors in the body of the stomach activates the vagovagal cholinergic reflex that leads to a low-volume, enzyme-rich secretion from the pancreas.[57] The precise contribution of the gastric phase in postprandial pancreatic secretion has not been determined.

When gastric juice and food in the form of chyme enters the duodenum, the most important and final phase of postprandial pancreatic secretion, the intestinal phase, begins. The intestinal phase is neurohormonally regulated and produces the largest contribution to pancreatic secretion, with increases in both acinar and ductal secretions.[49,51] The major hormonal mediators of the intestinal phase are secretin and cholecystokinin (CCK). A vasovagal cholinergic neural input also contributes to secretion during this phase.[56]

neurotransmitters are involved in these processes. Adrenergic innervation of the pancreas occurs through postganglionic neurons whose cell bodies are in the celiac and superior mesenteric ganglia, and is distributed primarily amongst the pancreatic vasculature.[56] Inhibition of fluid and bicarbonate secretion is achieved by sympathetic stimulation and subsequent pancreatic vasoconstriction.[51] Neurons in ganglia from the myenteric plexuses of the upper gastrointestinal tract also innervate the pancreas, and have cholinergic and serotoninergic characteristics.[143,144] Neurons containing VIP are the most common of the pancreatic peptidergic nervous system. VIP released from vagal neurons can stimulate both acinar cells to secrete enzymes, and ductal cells to secrete fluid and HCO_3^-.[51] Other peptidergic neurotransmitters with possible roles in pancreatic secretion include GRP,[134–136] substance P,[145] neuropeptide Y,[49] enkephalins[57] and calcitonin gene-related peptide.[146,147] Similar to the enteric nervous system, the pancreas has its own intrinsic innervation whose precise physiological function has yet to be clarified.[56]

Cellular regulation of pancreatic secretion

There are generally two pathways in the intracellular regulation of pancreatic secretion (Fig. 67.8). VIP and secretin bind to their respective receptors on the pancreatic acinus, which then couple to a G protein. This coupling leads to the activation of adenylate cyclase, production of cAMP and subsequent activation of protein kinase A. Protein kinase A alters the phosphorylation of several proteins, leading to pancreatic bicarbonate and fluid secretion. The second intracellular pathway begins with the binding of gastrin-releasing protein, CCK and acetylcholine to their respective receptors, leading to coupling with G proteins and activation of phospholipase C. Phospholipase C then hydrolyzes phosphatidylinositol 4,5-bisphosphate (PI-P2) to inositol 1,4,5-trisphosphate (IP_3) and diacylglycerol (DAG). IP_3 releases Ca^{2+} from endoplasmic reticulum stores and ushers in a Ca^{2+} influx into the cell through activated plasma membrane Ca^{2+} channels. Ca^{2+} binds to calmodulin (CAM), which activates several protein kinases and one protein phosphatase. DAG, in combination with Ca^{2+}, activates protein kinase C. These protein kinases and phosphatases also alter the phosphorylation of several proteins and induce secretion of pancreatic enzymes via the exocytosis and fusion of zymogen granules with the apical membrane of the acinus.[51,57,148]

Pancreatic secretion inhibitors

Much less is known about the mechanisms of pancreatic secretory inhibition, although there are several known hormones and neural regulators involved in this process. It appears that the hormones and neurotransmitters do not act directly on pancreatic acinar cells, but modulate cholinergic influences on pancreatic secretion.[51,56]

Pancreatic polypeptide (PP) is a peptide hormone found in the islets of Langerhans and between the acinar cells that inhibits pancreatic secretion of fluid, bicarbonate and enzymes.[51,57] Plasma levels of PP increase after sham feed-

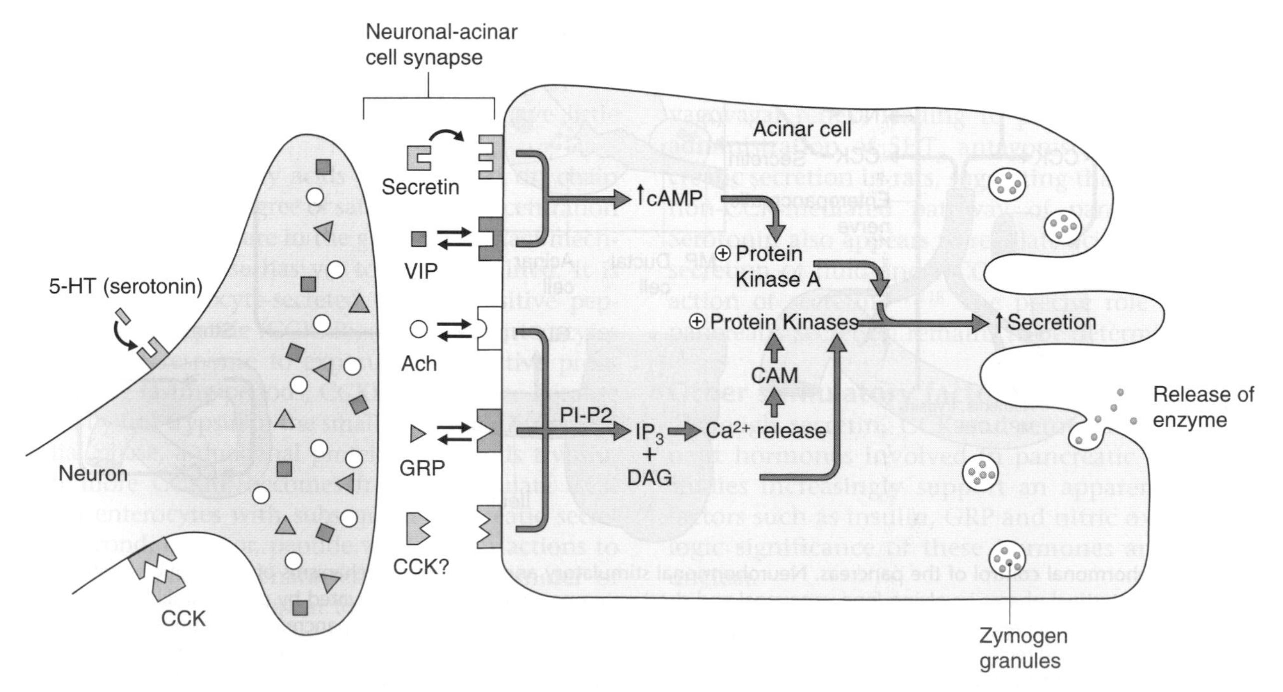

Figure 67.8: Mechanism of intracellular regulation of secretion in acinar cells. Ach, acetylcholine; CAM, calmodulin; cAMP cyclic adenosine monophosphate; CCK, cholecystokinin; DAG, diacylglycerol; GRP, gastrin-releasing peptide; IP_3, inositol 1,4,5-trisphosphate; PI-P2, phosphatidylinositol 4,5-bisphosphate; VIP, vasoactive intestinal peptide.

ing, eating and duodenal acidification.[57] Although vagal cholinergic activation is the most powerful stimulant to PP secretion,[149] exposure to CCK, secretin, VIP, gastrin and GRP also results in its release.[57] PP probably modulates cholinergic transmission to the pancreas by interfering with acetylcholine release by presynaptic neurons in the pancreas.[150] The discovery of PP receptors within the central nervous system suggests a central target of PP in the negative feedback of pancreatic secretion.[51]

Peptide YY is a small peptide predominantly released in response to fat in the distal ileum and colon; it significantly attenuates HCO_3^- and enzyme secretion by decreasing pancreatic responses to CCK and secretin.[79] Peptide YY likely inhibits release of acetylcholine and mucosal CCK as its primary mechanism of action.[57]

Somatostatin is a pancreatic hormone produced in the gastric and duodenal mucosa as well as the D cells in the islets of Langerhans.[57,79] Its release is stimulated by cholinergic activation in response to exposure to fat and amino acids in the intestinal tract.[57,79] Somatostatin may act directly on pancreatic acinar cells, but the prevailing thought is that it inhibits pancreatic secretion through a cholinergic mechanism in the central nervous system.[151]

Although its mechanism of action is still unknown, pancreatic glucagon inhibits pancreatic secretion stimulated by CCK, secretin, or both, to decrease fluid, bicarbonate and enzyme release.[51] It appears that other hormones and peptides, such as pancreastatin, calcitonin gene-related peptide and enkephalins, inhibit pancreatic secretion by modulation of cholinergic stimulation at central vagal sites.[51,57]

References

1. Moore KL. Clinically Oriented Anatomy, 4th edn. Baltimore, MD: Lippincott Williams & Wilkins; 1999.
2. Kozu T, Suda K, Toki F. Pancreatic development and anatomical variation. Gastrointest Endosc Clin N Am 1995; 5:1–30.
3. Jensen J. Gene regulatory factors in pancreatic development. Dev Dyn 2004; 229:176–200.
4. Ohlsson H, Karlsson K, Edlund T. IPF1, a homeodomain-containing transactivator of the insulin gene. EMBO J 1993; 12:4251–4259.
5. Gu G, Dubauskaite J, Melton DA. Direct evidence for the pancreatic lineage: NGN3+ cells are islet progenitors and are distinct from duct progenitors. Development 2002; 129:2447–2457.
6. Ahlgren U, Jonsson J, Edlund H. The morphogenesis of the pancreatic mesenchyme is uncoupled from that of the pancreatic epithelium in IPF1/PDX1-deficient mice. Development 1996; 122:1409–1416.
7. Offield MF, Jetton TL, Labosky PA, et al. PDX-1 is required for pancreatic outgrowth and differentiation of the rostral duodenum. Development 1996; 122:983–995.
8. Roy S, Qiao T, Wolff C, Ingham PW. Hedgehog signaling pathway is essential for pancreas specification in the zebrafish embryo. Curr Biol 2001; 11:1358–1363.
9. diIorio PJ, Moss JB, Sbrogna JL, Karlstrom RO, Moss LG. Sonic hedgehog is required early in pancreatic islet development. Dev Biol 2002; 244:75–84.
10. Stafford D, Prince VE. Retinoic acid signaling is required for a critical early step in zebrafish pancreatic development. Curr Biol 2002; 12:1215–1220.
11. Tiso N, Filippi A, Pauls S, Bortolussi M, Argenton F. BMP signalling regulates anteroposterior endoderm patterning in zebrafish. Mech Dev 2002; 118:29–37.
12. Hebrok M, Kim SK, Melton DA. Notochord repression of endodermal Sonic hedgehog permits pancreas development. Genes Dev 1998; 12:1705–1713.
13. Hebrok M, Kim SK, St Jacques B, McMahon AP, Melton DA. Regulation of pancreas development by hedgehog signaling. Development 2000; 127:4905–4913.
14. Kawahira H, Scheel DW, Smith SB, et al. Hedgehog signaling regulates expansion of pancreatic epithelial cells. Dev Biol 2005; 280:111–121.
15. Kanai-Azuma M, Kanai Y, Gad JM, et al. Depletion of definitive gut endoderm in *Sox17*-null mutant mice. Development 2002; 129:2367–2379.
16. Harrison KA, Thaler J, Pfaff SL, Gu H, Kehrl JH. Pancreas dorsal lobe agenesis and abnormal islets of Langerhans in *Hlxb9*-deficient mice. Nat Genet 1999; 23:71–75.
17. Li H, Arber S, Jessell TM, Edlund H. Selective agenesis of the dorsal pancreas in mice lacking homeobox gene *Hlxb9*. Nat Genet 1999; 23:67–70.
18. Kim SK, Hebrok M, Melton DA. Notochord to endoderm signaling is required for pancreas development. Development 1997; 124:4243–4252.
19. Kawaguchi Y, Cooper B, Gannon M, Ray M, MacDonald RJ, Wright CV. The role of the transcriptional regulator *Ptf1a* in converting intestinal to pancreatic progenitors. Nat Genet 2002; 32:128–134.
20. Sellick GS, Barker KT, Stolte-Dijkstra I, et al. Mutations in *PTF1A* cause pancreatic and cerebellar agenesis. Nat Genet 2004; 36:1301–1305.
21. Golosow N, Grobstein C. Epitheliomesenchymal interaction in pancreatic morphogenesis. Dev Biol 1962; 4:242–255.
22. Wessells NK, Cohen JH. Early pancreas organogenesis: morphogenesis, tissue interactions and mass effects. Dev Biol 1967; 15:237–270.
23. Kim SK, MacDonald RJ. Signaling and transcriptional control of pancreatic organogenesis. Curr Opin Genet Dev 2002; 12:540–547.
24. Ahlgren U, Pfaff SL, Jessell TM, Edlund T, Edlund H. Independent requirement for ISL1 in formation of pancreatic mesenchyme and islet cells. Nature 1997; 385:257–260.
25. Esni F, Johansson BR, Radice GL, Semb H. Dorsal pancreas agenesis in *N*-cadherin-deficient mice. Dev Biol 2001; 238:202–212.
26. Kim SK, Selleri L, Lee JS, et al. Pbx1 inactivation disrupts pancreas development and in *Ipf1*-deficient mice promotes diabetes mellitus. Nat Genet 2002; 30:430–435.
27. Bhushan A, Itoh N, Kato S, et al. Fgf10 is essential for maintaining the proliferative capacity of epithelial progenitor cells during early pancreatic organogenesis. Development 2001; 128:5109–5117.
28. Holland AM, Hale MA, Kagami H, Hammer RE, MacDonald RJ. Experimental control of pancreatic development and maintenance. Proc Natl Acad Sci USA 2002; 99:12236–12241.
29. Miettinen PJ, Huotari M, Koivisto T, et al. Impaired migration and delayed differentiation of pancreatic islet cells in mice lacking EGF-receptors. Development 2000; 127:2617–2627.
30. Cras-Meneur C, Elghazi L, Czernichow P, Scharfmann R. Epidermal growth factor increases undifferentiated pancreatic embryonic cells *in vitro*: a balance between proliferation and differentiation. Diabetes 2001; 50:1571–1579.

31. Guz Y, Montminy MR, Stein R, et al. Expression of murine STF-1, a putative insulin gene transcription factor, in beta cells of pancreas, duodenal epithelium and pancreatic exocrine and endocrine progenitors during ontogeny. Development 1995; 121:11–18.
32. Jensen J, Heller RS, Funder-Nielsen T, et al. Independent development of pancreatic alpha- and beta-cells from neurogenin3-expressing precursors: a role for the notch pathway in repression of premature differentiation. Diabetes 2000; 49:163–176.
33. Schwitzgebel VM, Scheel DW, Conners JR, et al. Expression of neurogenin3 reveals an islet cell precursor population in the pancreas. Development 2000; 127:3533–3542.
34. Grapin-Botton A, Majithia AR, Melton DA. Key events of pancreas formation are triggered in gut endoderm by ectopic expression of pancreatic regulatory genes. Genes Dev 2001; 15:444–454.
35. Apelqvist A, Li H, Sommer L, et al. Notch signalling controls pancreatic cell differentiation. Nature 1999; 400:877–881.
36. Jensen J, Pedersen EE, Galante P, et al. Control of endodermal endocrine development by *Hes-1*. Nat Genet 2000; 24:36–44.
37. Gradwohl G, Dierich A, LeMeur M, Guillemot F. Neurogenin3 is required for the development of the four endocrine cell lineages of the pancreas. Proc Natl Acad Sci USA 2000; 97:1607–1611.
38. Edlund H. Pancreatic organogenesis – developmental mechanisms and implications for therapy. Nat Rev Genet 2002; 3:524–532.
39. Jacquemin P, Durviaux SM, Jensen J, et al. Transcription factor hepatocyte nuclear factor 6 regulates pancreatic endocrine cell differentiation and controls expression of the proendocrine gene *ngn3*. Mol Cell Biol 2000; 20:4445–4454.
40. Sussel L, Kalamaras J, Hartigan-O'Connor DJ, et al. Mice lacking the homeodomain transcription factor Nkx2.2 have diabetes due to arrested differentiation of pancreatic beta cells. Development 1998; 125:2213–2221.
41. Sander M, Sussel L, Conners J, et al. Homeobox gene *Nkx6.1* lies downstream of *Nkx2.2* in the major pathway of beta-cell formation in the pancreas. Development 2000; 127:5533–5540.
42. Fishman MP, Melton DA. Pancreatic lineage analysis using a retroviral vector in embryonic mice demonstrates a common progenitor for endocrine and exocrine cells. Int J Dev Biol 2002; 46:201–207.
43. Hebrok M, Reichardt LF. Brain meets pancreas: netrin, an axon guidance molecule, controls epithelial cell migration. Trends Cell Biol 2004; 14:153–155.
44. Yebra M, Montgomery AM, Diaferia GR, et al. Recognition of the neural chemoattractant netrin-1 by integrins $alpha_6beta_4$ and $alpha_3beta_1$ regulates epithelial cell adhesion and migration. Dev Cell 2003; 5:695–707.
45. Jiang Y, Liu MT, Gershon MD. Netrins and DCC in the guidance of migrating neural crest-derived cells in the developing bowel and pancreas. Dev Biol 2003; 258:364–384.
46. Ahlgren U, Jonsson J, Jonsson L, Simu K, Edlund H. beta-cell-specific inactivation of the mouse *Ipf1/Pdx1* gene results in loss of the beta-cell phenotype and maturity onset diabetes. Genes Dev 1998; 12:1763–1768.
47. Hart AW, Baeza N, Apelqvist A, Edlund H. Attenuation of FGF signalling in mouse beta-cells leads to diabetes. Nature 2000; 408:864–868.
48. Stoffers DA, Ferrer J, Clarke WL, Habener JF. Early-onset type-II diabetes mellitus (MODY4) linked to IPF1. Nat Genet 1997; 17:138–139.
49. Konturek SJ, Pepera J, Zabielski K, et al. Brain–gut axis in pancreatic secretion and appetite control. J Physiol Pharmacol 2003; 54:293–317.
50. Gorelick FS, Jamieson JD. The pancreatic acinar cell. In: Johnson LR, Alpers DH, Christensen J, Jacobson ED, Walsh JH, eds. Physiology of the Gastrointestinal Tract, Vol 2, 3rd edn. New York: Raven Press; 1994:1353–1376.
51. Owyang C, Williams JA. Pancreatic secretion. In: Yamada T, Alpers DH, eds. Textbook of Gastroenterology, Vol 1, 4th edn. Philadelphia, PA: Lippincott Williams & Wilkins; 2003:340–366.
52. Scheele GA, Kern HF. Cellular compartmentation, protein processing, and secretion in the exocrine pancreas. In: Go VLW, DiMagno EP, Gardner JD, Lebenthal E, Reber HA, Scheele GA, eds. The Pancreas: Biology, Pathobiology, and Disease, 2nd edn. New York: Raven Press; 1993:121–150.
53. Case RM. Pancreatic secretion; cellular aspects. In: Duthe HL, Wormsley KG, eds. Scientific Basis of Gastroenterology. Edinburgh: Churchill Livingstone; 1979:163–173.
54. Henderson JR, Daniel PM. Portal circulations and their relation to counter-current systems. Q J Exp Physiol Cogn Med Sci 1978; 63:355–369.
55. Henderson JR, Daniel PM. A comparative study of the portal vessels connecting the endocrine and exocrine pancreas, with a discussion of some functional implications. Q J Exp Physiol Cogn Med Sci 1979; 64:267–275.
56. Niebergall-Roth E, Singer MV. Central and peripheral neural control of pancreatic exocrine secretion. J Physiol Pharmacol 2001; 52:523–538.
57. Henderson JM. Pancreatitis. In: Henderson JM, ed. Gastrointestinal Pathophysiology. Philadelphia, PA Lippincott Williams & Wilkins; 1996:124–132, 188–201.
58. Argent BE, Case RM. Pancreatic ducts: cellular mechanism and control of bicarbonate secretion. In: Johnson LR, Alpers DH, Christensen J, Jacobson ED, Walsh JH, eds. Physiology of the Gastrointestinal Tract, Vol 2, 3rd edn. New York: Raven Press; 1994:1473–1498.
59. Marino CR, Jeanes V, Boron WF, Schmitt BM. Expression and distribution of the $Na^+–HCO_3^-$ cotransporter in human pancreas. Am J Physiol 1999; 277:G487–G494.
60. Abuladze N, Lee I, Newman D, et al. Molecular cloning, chromosomal localization, tissue distribution, and functional expression of the human pancreatic sodium bicarbonate cotransporter. J Biol Chem 1998; 273:17689–17695.
61. Smith ZD, Caplan MJ, Forbush B 3rd, Jamieson JD. Monoclonal antibody localization of Na^+-K^+-ATPase in the exocrine pancreas and parotid of the dog. Am J Physiol 1987; 253:G99–G109.
62. Veel T, Villanger O, Holthe MR, Cragoe EJ Jr, Raeder MG. Na^+-H^+ exchange is not important for pancreatic HCO_3^- secretion in the pig. Acta Physiol Scand 1992; 144:239–246.
63. Shumaker H, Amlal H, Frizzell R, Ulrich CD 2nd, Soleimani M. CFTR drives Na^+-nHCO_3^- cotransport in pancreatic duct cells: a basis for defective HCO_3^- secretion in CF. Am J Physiol 1999; 276:C16–C25.
64. Gray MA, Greenwell JR, Argent BE. Secretin-regulated chloride channel on the apical plasma membrane of pancreatic duct cells. J Membr Biol 1988; 105:131–142.
65. Lowe ME. The structure and function of pancreatic enzymes. In: Johnson LR, Alpers DH, Christensen J, Jacobson ED, Walsh JH, eds. Physiology of the Gastrointestinal Tract, Vol 2. New York: Raven Press; 1994:1531–1542.
66. DiMagno EP, Scheele GA. Human exocrine pancreatic enzyme secretion. In: Go VLW, DiMagno EP, Gardner JD, Lebenthal E, Reber HA, Scheele GA, eds. The Pancreas: Biology,

Pathobiology, and Disease, 2nd edn. New York: Raven Press; 1993:275–300.

67. Alpers DH. Digestion and absorption of carbohydrates and proteins. In: Johnson LR, Alpers DH, Christensen J, Jacobson ED, Walsh JH, eds. Physiology of the Gastrointestinal Tract, Vol 2, 3rd edn. New York: Raven Press; 1994:1531–1543.
68. Marchbank T, Freeman TC, Playford RJ. Human pancreatic secretory trypsin inhibitor. Distribution, actions and possible role in mucosal integrity and repair. Digestion 1998; 59:167–174.
69. Marchbank T, Chinery R, Hanby AM, Poulsom R, Elia G, Playford RJ. Distribution and expression of pancreatic secretory trypsin inhibitor and its possible role in epithelial restitution. Am J Pathol 1996; 148:715–722.
70. Carey M, Hernell O. Digestion and absorption of fat. Semin Gastrointest Dis 1992; 3:189–208.
71. Carriere F, Barrowman JA, Verger R, Laugier R. Secretion and contribution to lipolysis of gastric and pancreatic lipases during a test meal in humans. Gastroenterology 1993; 105:876–888.
72. Carriere F, Renou C, Lopez V, et al. The specific activities of human digestive lipases measured from the *in vivo* and *in vitro* lipolysis of test meals. Gastroenterology 2000; 119:949–960.
73. Richmond BL, Boileau AC, Zheng S, et al. Compensatory phospholipid digestion is required for cholesterol absorption in pancreatic phospholipase A_2-deficient mice. Gastroenterology 2001; 120:1193–1202.
74. Hui DY, Howles PN. Carboxyl ester lipase: structure–function relationship and physiological role in lipoprotein metabolism and atherosclerosis. J Lipid Res 2002; 43:2017–2030.
75. Lowe M. The triglyceride lipases of the pancreas. J Lipid Res 2002; 43:2007–2016.
76. D'Agostino D, Lowe ME. Pancreatic lipase-related protein 2 is the major colipase-dependent pancreatic lipase in suckling mice. J Nutr 2004; 134:132–134.
77. Verger R. Pancreatic lipase. In: Borgstrom B, Brockman HL, eds. Lipases. Amsterdam: Elsevier; 1984:84–150.
78. D'Agostino D, Cordle RA, Kullman J, Erlanson-Albertsson C, Muglia LJ, Lowe ME. Decreased postnatal survival and altered body weight regulation in procolipase-deficient mice. J Biol Chem 2002; 277:7170–7177.
79. Owyang C, Achem-Karam SR, Vinik AI. Pancreatic polypeptide and intestinal migrating motor complex in humans. Effect of pancreaticobiliary secretion. Gastroenterology 1983; 84:10–17.
80. Solomon TE. Control of pancreatic secretion. In: Johnson LR, Alpers DH, Christensen J, Jacobson ED, Walsh JH, eds. Physiology of the Gastrointestinal Tract, Vol 2, 3rd edn. New York: Raven Press; 1994:1499–1530.
81. Konturek SJ, Thor PJ, Bilski J, Bielanski W, Laskiewicz J. Relationships between duodenal motility and pancreatic secretion in fasted and fed dogs. Am J Physiol 1986; 250:G570–G574.
82. Keane FB, DiMagno EP, Dozois RR, Go VL. Relationships among canine interdigestive exocrine pancreatic and biliary flow, duodenal motor activity, plasma pancreatic polypeptide, and motilin. Gastroenterology 1980; 78:310–316.
83. Magee DF, Naruse S. The role of motilin in periodic interdigestive pancreatic secretion in dogs. J Physiol 1984; 355:441–447.
84. Chey WY. Neurohumoral control of the exocrine pancreas. Curr Opin Gastroenterol 1997; 13:375–380.
85. Konturek SJ, Bielanski W, Solomon TE. Effects of an antral mucosectomy, L-364,718 and atropine on cephalic phase of gastric and pancreatic secretion in dogs. Gastroenterology 1990; 98:47–55.
86. Anagnostides A, Chadwick VS, Selden AC, Maton PN. Sham feeding and pancreatic secretion. Evidence for direct vagal stimulation of enzyme output. Gastroenterology 1984; 87:109–114.
87. Fahrenkrug J, Schaffalitzky de Muckadell OB, Holst JJ, Jensen SL. Vasoactive intestinal polypeptide in vagally mediated pancreatic secretion of fluid and HCO_3. Am J Physiol 1979; 237:E535–E540.
88. Blair EL, Brown JC, Harper AA, Scratcherd T. A gastric phase of pancreatic secretion. J Physiol 1966; 184:812–824.
89. White TT, McAlexander RA, Magee DF. The effect of gastric distension on duodenal aspirates in man. Gastroenterology 1963; 44:48–51.
90. Vagne M, Grossman MI. Gastric and pancreatic secretion in response to gastric distention in dogs. Gastroenterology 1969; 57:300–310.
91. Fahrenkrug J, Schaffalitzky de Muckadell OB, Rune SJ. pH threshold for release of secretin in normal subjects and in patients with duodenal ulcer and patients with chronic pancreatitis. Scand J Gastroenterol 1978; 13:177–186.
92. Rune SJ. pH in the human duodenum. Its physiological and pathophysiological significance. Digestion 1973; 8:261–268.
93. Chang TM, Chang CH, Wagner DR, Chey WY. Porcine pancreatic phospholipase A_2 stimulates secretin release from secretin-producing cells. J Biol Chem 1999; 274:10758–10764.
94. Li P, Lee KY, Chang TM, Chey WY. Mechanism of acid-induced release of secretin in rats. Presence of a secretin-releasing peptide. J Clin Invest 1990; 86:1474–1479.
95. Osnes M, Hanssen LE, Flaten O, Myren J. Exocrine pancreatic secretion and immunoreactive secretin (IRS) release after intraduodenal instillation of bile in man. Gut 1978; 19:180–184.
96. Watanabe S, Chey WY, Lee KY, Chang TM. Secretin is released by digestive products of fat in dogs. Gastroenterology 1986; 90:1008–1017.
97. Owyang C. Physiological mechanisms of cholecystokinin action on pancreatic secretion. Am J Physiol 1996; 271:G1–G7.
98. You CH, Rominger JM, Chey WY. Effects of atropine on the action and release of secretin in humans. Am J Physiol 1982; 242:G608–611.
99. Park HS, Lee YL, Kwon HY, Chey WY, Park HJ. Significant cholinergic role in secretin-stimulated exocrine secretion in isolated rat pancreas. Am J Physiol 1998; 274:G413–G418.
100. Meyer JH, Kelly GA. Canine pancreatic responses to intestinally perfused proteins and protein digests. Am J Physiol 1976; 231:682–691.
101. Liddle RA, Goldfine ID, Rosen MS, Taplitz RA, Williams JA. Cholecystokinin bioactivity in human plasma. Molecular forms, responses to feeding, and relationship to gallbladder contraction. J Clin Invest 1985; 75:1144–1152.
102. Meyer JH, Kelly GA, Jones RS. Canine pancreatic response to intestinally perfused oligopeptides. Am J Physiol 1976; 231:678–681.
103. Meyer JH, Jones RS. Canine pancreatic responses to intestinally perfused fat and products of fat digestion. Am J Physiol 1974; 226:1178–1187.
104. Malagelada JR, DiMagno EP, Summerskill WH, Go VL. Regulation of pancreatic and gallbladder functions by

intraluminal fatty acids and bile acids in man. J Clin Invest 1976; 58:493–499.

105. Li Y, Owyang C. Peptone stimulates CCK-releasing peptide secretion by activating intestinal submucosal cholinergic neurons. J Clin Invest 1996; 97:1463–1470.

106. Li Y, Hao Y, Owyang C. High-affinity CCK-A receptors on the vagus nerve mediate CCK-stimulated pancreatic secretion in rats. Am J Physiol 1997; 273:G679–G685.

107. Owyang C, Logsdon CD. New insights into neurohormonal regulation of pancreatic secretion. Gastroenterology 2004; 127:957–969.

108. Li Y, Owyang C. Vagal afferent pathway mediates physiological action of cholecystokinin on pancreatic enzyme secretion. J Clin Invest 1993; 92:418–424.

109. Konturek S. Physiology of pancreatic secretion. J Physiol Pharmacol 1993; 46:5–24.

110. Bozkurt T, Adler G, Koop I, Arnold R. Effect of atropine on intestinal phase of pancreatic secretion in man. Digestion 1988; 41:108–115.

111. Adler G, Beglinger C, Braun U, et al. Interaction of the cholinergic system and cholecystokinin in the regulation of endogenous and exogenous stimulation of pancreatic secretion in humans. Gastroenterology 1991; 100:537–543.

112. Soudah HC, Lu Y, Hasler WL, Owyang C. Cholecystokinin at physiological levels evokes pancreatic enzyme secretion via a cholinergic pathway. Am J Physiol 1992; 263:G102–G107.

113. Gabryelewicz A, Kulesza E, Konturek SJ. Comparison of loxiglumide, a cholecystokinin receptor antagonist, and atropine on hormonal and meal-stimulated pancreatic secretion in man. Scand J Gastroenterol 1990; 25:731–738.

114. de Weerth A, Pisegna JR, Huppi K, Wank SA. Molecular cloning, functional expression and chromosomal localization of the human cholecystokinin type A receptor. Biochem Biophys Res Commun 1993; 194:811–818.

115. Li Y, Hao Y, Zhu J, Owyang C. Serotonin released from intestinal enterochromaffin cells mediates luminal non-cholecystokinin-stimulated pancreatic secretion in rats. Gastroenterology 2000; 118:1197–1207.

116. Kato M, Ohkuma S, Kataoka K, Kashima K, Kuriyama K. Characterization of muscarinic receptor subtypes on rat pancreatic acini: pharmacological identification by secretory responses and binding studies. Digestion 1992; 52:194–203.

117. Suzuki A, Naruse S, Kitagawa M, et al. 5-Hydroxytryptamine strongly inhibits fluid secretion in guinea pig pancreatic duct cells. J Clin Invest 2001; 108:749–756.

118. Li JP, Chang TM, Chey WY. Roles of 5-HT receptors in the release and action of secretin on pancreatic secretion in rats. Am J Physiol Gastrointest Liver Physiol 2001; 280:G595–G602.

119. Kanno T, Saito A. The potentiating influences of insulin on pancreozymin-induced hyperpolarization and amylase release in the pancreatic acinar cell. J Physiol 1976; 261:505–521.

120. Park HJ, Lee YL, Kwon HY. Effects of pancreatic polypeptide on insulin action in exocrine secretion of isolated rat pancreas. J Physiol 1993; 463:421–429.

121. Saito A, Williams JA, Kanno T. Potentiation of cholecystokinin-induced exocrine secretion by both exogenous and endogenous insulin in isolated and perfused rat pancreata. J Clin Invest 1980; 65:777–782.

122. Singh J. Mechanism of action of insulin on acetylcholine-evoked amylase secretion in the mouse pancreas. J Physiol 1985; 358:469–482.

123. Singh J, Adeghate E. Effects of islet hormones on nerve-mediated and acetylcholine-evoked secretory responses in the isolated pancreas of normal and diabetic rats. Int J Mol Med 1998; 1:627–634.

124. Singh J, Adeghate E, Salido GM, Pariente JA, Yago MD, Juma LO. Interaction of islet hormones with cholecystokinin octapeptide-evoked secretory responses in the isolated pancreas of normal and diabetic rats. Exp Physiol 1999; 84:299–318.

125. Singh J, Yago MD, Adeghate E. Involvement of cellular calcium in exocrine pancreatic insufficiency during streptozotocin-induced diabetes mellitus. Arch Physiol Biochem 2001; 109:252–259.

126. Juma LM, Singh J, Pallot DJ, Salido GM, Adeghate E. Interactions of islet hormones with acetylcholine in the isolated rat pancreas. Peptides 1997; 18:1415–1422.

127. Lee KY, Zhou L, Ren XS, Chang TM, Chey WY. An important role of endogenous insulin on exocrine pancreatic secretion in rats. Am J Physiol 1990; 258:G268–G274.

128. Lee YL, Kwon HY, Park HS, Lee TH, Park HJ. The role of insulin in the interaction of secretin and cholecystokinin in exocrine secretion of the isolated perfused rat pancreas. Pancreas 1996; 12:58–63.

129. Iwabe C, Shiratori K, Shimizu K, Hayashi N. Role of endogenous insulin in pancreatic secretion in rats. Pancreatology 2001; 1:300–305.

130. Ferrer R, Medrano J, Diego M, et al. Effect of exogenous insulin and glucagon on exocrine pancreatic secretion in rats *in vivo*. Int J Pancreatol 2000; 28:67–75.

131. Patel R, Singh J, Yago MD, Vilchez JR, Martinez-Victoria E, Manas M. Effect of insulin on exocrine pancreatic secretion in healthy and diabetic anaesthetised rats. Mol Cell Biochem 2004; 261:105–110.

132. Berry SM, Fink AS. Insulin inhibits secretin-stimulated pancreatic bicarbonate output by a dose-dependent neurally mediated mechanism. Am J Physiol 1996; 270:G163–G170.

133. Howard-McNatt M, Simon T, Wang Y, Fink AS. Insulin inhibits secretin-induced pancreatic bicarbonate output via cholinergic mechanisms. Pancreas 2002; 24:380–385.

134. Konturek SJ, Krol R, Tasler J. Effect of bombesin and related peptides on the release and action of intestinal hormones on pancreatic secretion. J Physiol 1976; 257:663–672.

135. Knuhtsen S, Holst JJ, Jensen SL, Knigge U, Nielsen OV. Gastrin-releasing peptide: effect on exocrine secretion and release from isolated perfused porcine pancreas. Am J Physiol 1985; 248:G281–G286.

136. McDonald T. The gastrin-releasing polypeptide (GRP). Adv Metab Dis 1988; 11:199–250.

137. Erspamer V, Improta G, Melchiorri P, Sopranzi N. Evidence of cholecystokinin release by bombesin in the dog. Br J Pharmacol 1974; 52:227–232.

138. Bilski J, Konturek SJ. Role of nitric oxide in the control of pancreatic secretion. In: Pierzynowsky SG, Zabielski R, eds. Biology of the Pancreas in Growing Animals. Amsterdam: Elsevier; 1999:193–212.

139. Zoucas E, Nilsson C, Ihse I. Differential roles of endogenous nitric oxide on neural regulation of basal exocrine pancreatic secretion in intact and denervated pancreas. Pancreatology 2001; 1:96–101.

140. Konturek JW, Hengst K, Kulesza E, Gabryelewicz A, Konturek SJ, Domschke W. Role of endogenous nitric oxide in the control of exocrine and endocrine pancreatic secretion in humans. Gut 1997; 40:86–91.

141. Bilski J, Konturek JW, Konturek SJ, Domschke W. The involvement of endogenous nitric oxide in vagal-cholinergic stimulation of exocrine and endocrine pancreas in dogs. Int J Pancreatol 1995; 18:41–49.

142. Konturek SK, Konturek PC. Role of nitric oxide in the digestive system. Digestion 1995; 56:1–13.

143. Kirchgessner AL, Gershon MD. Presynaptic inhibition by serotonin of nerve-mediated secretion of pancreatic amylase. Am J Physiol 1995; 268:G339–G345.

144. Kirchgessner AL, Gershon MD. Innervation of the pancreas by neurons in the gut. J Neurosci 1990; 10:1626–1642.

145. Larsson LI. Innervation of the pancreas by substance P, enkephalin, vasoactive intestinal polypeptide and gastrin/CCK immunoractive nerves. J Histochem Cytochem 1979; 27:1283–1284.

146. Jaworek J, Konturek SJ, Szlachcic A. The role of CGRP and afferent nerves in the modulation of pancreatic enzyme secretion in the rat. Int J Pancreatol 1997; 22:137–146.

147. Li Y, Kolligs F, Owyang C. Mechanism of action of calcitonin gene-related peptide in inhibiting pancreatic enzyme secretion in rats. Gastroenterology 1993; 105:194–201.

148. Williams JA. Intracellular signaling mechanisms activated by cholecystokinin-regulating synthesis and secretion of digestive enzymes in pancreatic acinar cells. Annu Rev Physiol 2001; 63:77–97.

149. Schwartz TW. Pancreatic polypeptide: a hormone under vagal control. Gastroenterology 1983; 85:1411–1425.

150. Jung G, Louie DS, Owyang C. Pancreatic polypeptide inhibits pancreatic enzyme secretion via a cholinergic pathway. Am J Physiol 1987; 253:G706–G710.

151. Li Y, Owyang C. Somatostatin inhibits pancreatic enzyme secretion at a central vagal site. Am J Physiol 1993; 265:G251–G257.

152. Larson WJ. Human Embryology, 3rd edn.. Philadelphia, PA: Churchill Livingstone; 2001.

153. Kumar M, Melton D. Pancreas specification: a budding question. Curr Opin Genet Dev 2003; 13:401–407.

154. Hebrok M, Reichardt LF. Brain meets pancreas: netrin, an axon guidance molecule, control eptithelial cell migration. Trends Cell Biol 2004; 14:153–155.

155. Konturek SJ, Zabielski R, Konturek JW, Czarnecki J. Neuroendocrinology of the pancreas; role of the brain–gut axis in pancreatic secretion. Eur J Pharmacol 2003; 481:1–14.

156. Wilson ME, Scheel D, German MS. Gene expression cascades in pancreatic development. Mech Dev 2003; 120:65–80.

Chapter 68
Cystic fibrosis and congenital anomalies of the exocrine pancreas

Arthur B. Atlas and Joel R. Rosh

CYSTIC FIBROSIS

Cystic fibrosis (CF) is the most common inherited life-shortening disease in Caucasians. It is a disease that affects pancreatic exocrine gland function, involves numerous organs and presents with varied clinical symptoms. Even though pulmonary disease is the major cause of morbidity and mortality, most patients have insufficient pancreatic function and suffer from gastrointestinal symptoms. The majority of patients are diagnosed by 6months of age and may present with failure to thrive, chronic diarrhea or recurrent respiratory symptoms. Diagnosis is confirmed by a raised sweat chloride test result or the identification of two abnormal mutations of the CF gene. The average life expectancy is approximately 33years, but significantly higher in patients with sufficient pancreatic function.

Cystic fibrosis transmembrane regulator

CF is caused by an autosomal recessive gene found on the long arm of chromosome7 (7q31 region), spanning 250kb and coding for a single-chain polypeptide of 1480 amino acids called the cystic fibrosis transmembrane regulator (CFTR).[1] CFTR is a cyclic adenosine monophosphate (cAMP)-regulated chloride channel, which probably also regulates other ion channels. It is similar to a family of proteins called ATP-binding cassette (ABC) proteins, which are involved with ATP hydrolysis-mediated solute transport function.[2] CFTR contains two membrane-spanning domains (MSD1 and MSD2), two nucleotide-binding domains (NBD1 and NBD2) and a central intracellular regulatory domain, or R region, with multiple phosphorylation sites (Fig. 68.1).[1,3] The MSDs form the channel pore. Phosphorylation of the R domain determines channel activity, and ATP hydrolysis by NBDs controls gaiting.[3]

Abnormal CFTR function can be divided into five or six major classes reflecting known or predicted molecular dysfunction (Fig. 68.2).[4] There is little or no protein synthesis in class I mutations due to premature termination signals. Class II mutations are characterized by defective processing or trafficking of CFTR protein. DF508, a class II mutation – and the most common CF mutation – has a three-nucleotide deletion of phenylalanine; this prevents normal glycosylation. The partially glycosylated protein is retained in the endoplasmic reticulum, where it is degraded instead of being transported and inserted into the apical cellular membrane.[5] In class III mutations, proteins are processed properly, but owing to a mutation in the NBD region the chloride channel lacks sensitivity to stimulations of intracellular cAMP. Class IV mutations are characterized by alterations of conductance, and have reduced cAMP-regulated currents in the chloride channel. Class V mutations affect splicing of mRNA, producing extra or skipped exons. The stability of the protein and mRNA are affected by these mutations. Class VI mutations may also affect the regulatory function of CFTR on other ion channels. Individual mutations can have characteristics of more than one class.[6]

ΔF508 is the most common mutation of CFTR, found in 70% of chromosomes in American Caucasians with CF, although there are ethnic and regional variations. ΔF508 is found in approximately 45% of the chromosomes of African Americans,[7] approximately 30% of Ashkenazi Jews,[8] and in less than 5% of Native Americans.[9] Currently, more than 1200 mutations of CFTR have been described, accounting for 92–94% of abnormalities in CF.

The CFTR protein has variable expression, and probably functions differently in the epithelium of different organs. There is clinical variability among patients with the same CFTR genotype, suggesting that environmental and heredity factors can modify the disease phenotype. Evidence is accumulating that phenotypic heterogeneity is influenced by genes at one or more unlinked loci in the human genome, which act as modifier genes of CFTR.[10–12]

CFTR function in the pancreas

In the pancreas, CFTR is found predominantly in the cell membrane of centroacinar and intralobular duct epithelium,[13] which is responsible for secreting fluid with a high concentration of sodium bicarbonate. Normally, chloride excreted into the lumen is exchanged for bicarbonate, with sodium and water following. In CF, the abnormal CFTR limits this exchange, and also limits apical trafficking of zymogen, resulting in a more viscous, sodium bicarbonate-depleted fluid.[14] Owing to ductal inspissation, the fluid is unable to carry pancreatic enzymes adequately and efficiently from the pancreas to the duodenum, where normal digestion occurs.[15]

There are progressive histologic findings in the CF pancreas, correlating to the severity and age of the patient. Initially, focal intraluminal eosinophilic concentrations with dilation of pancreatic ducts are present. There is progression of acinar atrophy, and fibrosis with ductal ectasia. Late in the disease there is total loss of acinar tissue and

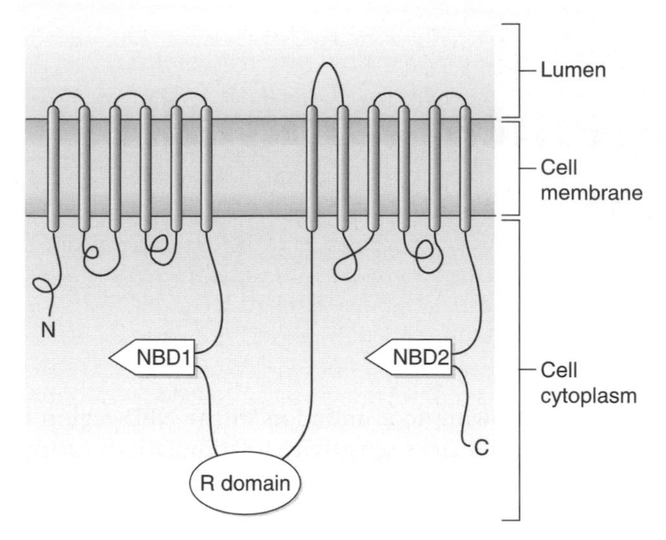

Figure 68.1: Schematic of the cystic fibrosis transmembrane regulator protein. NBD, nucleotide-binding domain; R domain, regulatory domain. (Redrawn from http://www.tripod.com/cellbiology).

ductal obliteration. Islets of Langerhans are diminished, but not totally destroyed.[16] The preserved islets have decreased glucagon-secreting α cells, insulin-secreting β cells and pancreatic polypeptide-secreting cells.[17] Autopsy studies show that pancreatic nesidioblastosis is common in children with CF, but not in adolescents and adults.[18] Diabetes increases in prevalence with age, but is rare in young children with CF, possibly because of children's ability to form new islets.

Pancreatic sufficiency

Approximately 15% of patients with CF retain enough residual pancreatic secretion for normal digestion, and are termed pancreatic sufficient. Of all CF phenotypes, pancreatic function has the strongest correlation to CFTR genotype. Mutations that are associated with pancreatic sufficiency are considered 'mild' mutations. Patients who have one or two mild mutations are typically pancreatic sufficient, and have class IV or V defects of CFTR. Patients who remain pancreatic sufficient have less enzyme secretion, and lower concentrations of bicarbonate in pancreatic fluid compared with the normal finding.[15] Their growth is usually normal or close to normal, and so as a group they are diagnosed with CF later than patients with pancreatic insufficiency, except when CF newborn screening is utilized. Generally, pancreatic sufficient patients have less severe disease, lower sweat chloride levels, and their life expectancy is substantially longer than those of pancreatic insufficient patients.

Pancreatic insufficiency

'Severe mutations' identify genotypes specifically associated with pancreatic insufficiency, and do not necessarily correlate with severity of lung function or disease. Mutations associated with pancreatic insufficiency are usually class I–III defects, which affect CFTR function more severely. Clinical signs of pancreatic insufficiency develop when less than 10% of normal pancreatic enzyme activity is present in the duodenum.[19]

CF is the major cause of pancreatic exocrine failure in children. Approximately 85% of patients with CF are pancreatic insufficient. At birth approximately 65% of infants with CF are pancreatic insufficienct. Of the remaining pancreatic sufficient infants, approximately 15–20% will have progressive loss of pancreatic function by 3 years of age.[20] CF is usually diagnosed before 6 months of age in pancreatic insufficient infants due to failure to thrive and malnutrition. The calorie and protein losses in the stool prevent normal weight gain, growth and development, and may be associated with hypoalbuminemia, edema and normochromic, normocytic anemia.[21]

Pancreatic function testing

Even though most infants and children with CF have pancreatic insufficiency, pancreatic function testing (Table 68.1) should be obtained before beginning replacement

Figure 68.2: Classes I–VI of *CFTR* mutation. The subdivision reflects the known or predicted biosynthetic and functional consequences. ATP, adenosine triphosphate; NBD, nucleotide-binding domain; RD, regulatory domain. (Redrawn from Witt, 2003.)[184]

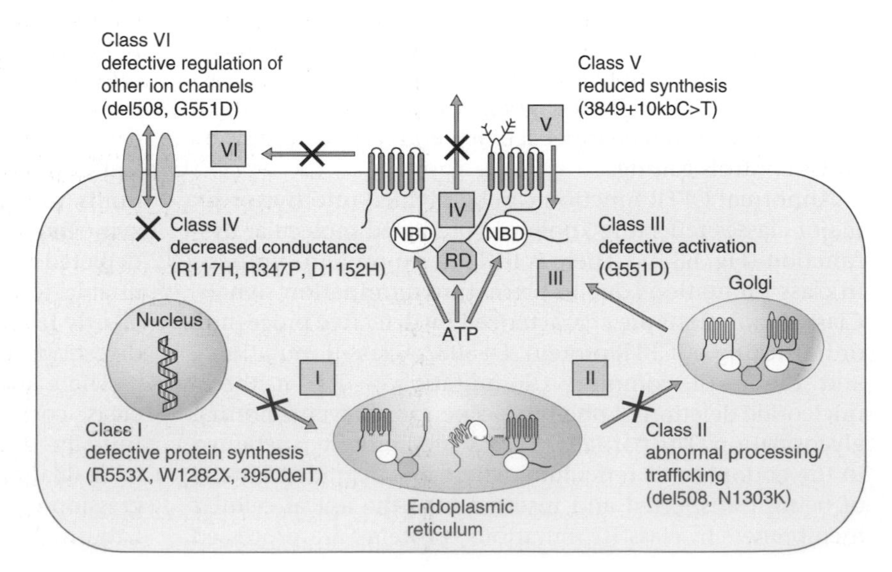

Direct stimulation of pancreatic secretions
Pancreozymin–secretin test
Lundh test
Fecal studies
Titrimetric method
Fat absorption coefficient
Steatocrit method
Microscopic examination using Sudan III staining
Near-infrared reflectance spectroscopy
Fecal enzyme studies
Fecal chymotrypsin
Fecal elastase
Fecal immunoreactive lipase
Stool nitrogen excretion
Blood levels
Immunoreactive trypsin (IRT)
Pancreatitis-associated protein
These and other tests of pancreatic function are outlined in detail in Leus et al.[22]

Table 68.1 Testing of pancreatic function

pancreatic enzymes. The best method for measuring pancreatic exocrine function is direct stimulation of pancreatic secretions. This is done using exogenous hormones, secretin/cholecystokinin or endogenous nutrients to stimulate pancreatic secretions, which are collected through a tube placed at the ligament of Treitz and analyzed for pH, bicarbonate, chymotrypsin, trypsin, lipase, colipase, amylase and carboxypeptidase output.[22] Although this is the best test for evaluating pancreatic function, because of the invasive nature and expense it is seldom used in clinical practice. Indirect analysis of pancreatic function is less accurate, but more practical in clinical practice. A 72-h quantitative fecal fat evaluation compares the amount of fat ingested to that excreted, and the percentage of fat absorbed correlates with the degree of pancreatic function; fat absorption of less than 90% is abnormal. This is a non-invasive test, but is laborious and unpleasant for patients, parents and staff.

Detection of fecal enzymes is also helpful in determining pancreatic function and does not require prolonged stool collections. The fecal enzyme levels can be influenced by pancreatic enzyme supplements, with the exception of fecal elastase, which is not found in enzyme supplements. Fecal immunoreactive lipase and fecal elastase measurements have a high level of sensitivity and specificity for pancreatic insufficiency.[23,24] Immunoreactive trypsin (IRT) detected in serum is not as sensitive or specific as the fecal enzyme studies. However, most state newborn CF screening programs combine IRT levels with DNA screening because of the ease of testing blood on a Guthrie filter card. Decreased fat-soluble vitamin levels, and low β-carotene levels indirectly suggest pancreatic insufficiency.

Pancreatic enzyme replacement

Pancreatic insufficiency in CF is treated with oral exogenous pancreatic enzyme replacement derived from processed porcine pancreas. Initially, powdered supplemental enzymes were routinely used; these improved fat absorption, but many patients continued to have steatorrhea or needed numerous capsules per meal. Skin and mucous membrane irritation secondary to the powdered enzymes was common, and because of the high purine content of the powdered enzymes hyperuricosemia and hyperuricosuria were seen.[25,26] IgE-mediated hypersensitivity has been reported rarely in individuals exposed to powdered and enteric-coated pancreatic preparations.[27,28] Gelatin capsules with enteric-coated enzyme beads, or microspheres, encased in an acid-resistant coating is the current standard, and has all but replaced the use of powdered enzymes. These capsule preparations result in improved fat and protein absorption, and easier administration of the enzymes. The capsules can be swallowed whole, or opened and the beads sprinkled on non-alkaline foods. Once the beads have been swallowed, the coating dissolves at a pH above 5.5, allowing enzyme activation to occur in the proximal small bowel. With appropriate enzyme replacement, most patients are able to achieve normal or close to normal fat absorption and resolution of abdominal complaints.

Supplemental enzyme therapy is initiated once pancreatic insufficiency has been diagnosed. In infants, preparations with the smallest microspheres, either mixed in a small amount of fruit or applied to the tongue just before offering the bottle or breast, work well. Powdered enzymes are still occasionally used in infants, but increase the risk of oral and perianal excoriation. In infants, dosing of enzymes can be based on food intake, but for the older child weight-based dosing is better. The National Cystic Fibrosis Foundation guidelines on pancreatic enzyme dosing (Table 68.2) should be used when starting or adjusting therapy. The goals of therapy are to promote weight gain, growth and development, and limit abdominal symptoms. There is a wide individual variation in response to supplemental enzyme dosing. The lower range of the recommended dosage should be started and adjusted upward based on stool pattern and weight gain. To decrease the risk of fibrosing colonopathy, enzyme doses should be less than 2500 lipase units/kg per meal, or less than 4000 lipase units/g fat per day.[29]

Once on adequate pancreatic enzyme replacement, a rapid improvement in the degree of steatorrhea should be seen, with decreased stool frequency, abdominal pain and bloating, and reduced appetite. However, some patients continue to be symptomatic with abnormal fat absorption, despite taking appropriate enteric-coated enzymes. Many of these patients benefit from reducing gastric acid secretion with H_2-receptor antagonists or proton pump inhibitors, which serve to optimize the intraluminal action

Age	Recommended dose
Infant	2000–4000 lipase units per 4 oz formula or per breast-feed
4 years and younger	1000 lipase units per kg per meal 500 lipase units per kg per snack
4 years and older	500 lipase units per kg per meal 250 lipase units per kg per snack
Adolescents and adults	Lower enzyme doses can be tried as intake of fat/kg declines with age

There is individual patient variability with enzyme dosing. These recommended doses for enzyme replacement should be used as a 'starting point' and adjustments made as necessary to control signs and symptoms of malabsorption. Doses greater than 2500 lipase units per kg per meal should be used with caution, and only if there is documented improved fat absorption by 72-h fecal fat measurement. Doses greater than 6000 lipase units per kg per meal have been associated with colonic stricture in children aged less than 12 years.[31]

Table 68.2 Current recommended pancreatic enzyme dosing in cystic fibrosis[31]

of the supplemental enzymes.[30] Other common causes of diminished response to enzyme replacement include non-adherance, taking enzymes after eating, and decreased enzyme potency as a result of either exposure to heat or use past the expiry date (Table 68.3). There is a tendency for clinicians to continue to increase the enzyme dosage when a patient complains of increased abdominal symptoms. However, patients on high-dose enzymes and antacid therapy who continue to have persistent abdominal symptoms require a fecal fat absorption study and evaluation for other causes of malabsorption, including celiac disease, Crohn's disease, lactose intolerance, parasitic disease and bacterial overgrowth (Table 68.4).

Fibrosing colonopathy

Fibrosing colonopathy is a potentially significant complication of supplemental enzyme therapy and is associated with prolonged doses of lipase greater than 6000 units lipase per kg per meal.[29,31] Symptoms include abdominal pain, vomiting, bloody or persistent diarrhea, and poor weight gain or weight loss. Thickening of the bowel wall can be seen by ultrasonography, and predates stricture formation.[32] Barium enema can show focal or generalized narrowing, with the ascending colon most frequently affected, although total colonic involvement has been reported.[33] Many patients show clinical improvement with decreasing supplemental enzymes and parenteral nutrition, but some require surgical resection of the narrowed section of colon. The pathophysiology of the colonic damage in fibrosing colonopathy is not clear, but is associated with high-dose supplemental pancreatic enzymes. The Cystic Fibrosis Foundation recommends that enzyme doses should be less than 2500 lipase units per kg per meal, or less than 4000 lipase units per g of fat per day.[29,31] The association of high-dose enzyme use with fibrosing colonopathy led to a commercial recall of high-potency enzymes. Since the recall there has been a decreased incidence of fibrosing colonopathy.

Non-adherence to prescribed dosing
Expired enzymes
Inactivated enzymes due to prolonged exposure to heat
High acidic small intestinal environment
Prolonged exposure of microspheres to alkaline foods
Taking enzymes after eating
'Grazing'
Generic enzymes with lower potency
Chewed or crushed microspheres
Inadequate dose of enzymes reaching the small intestine
Glycine-conjugated bile acids limit micelle formation

Table 68.3 Factors that can reduce the effects of supplemental pancreatic enzymes

Causing steatorrhea
Hepatobiliary disease with portal hypertension
Cholestatic liver disease
Celiac disease
Giardiasis
Short gut syndrome
Bacterial overgrowth of small intestine
Without steatorrhea
Recurrent abdominal pain
Inflammatory bowel disease
Irritable bowel syndrome
Lactose intolerance
Infectious enteritis
Esophagitis
Gastroesophageal reflux
Fibrosing colonopathy
Eating disorders
Digestive tract cancers

Table 68.4 Potential confounding gastrointestinal conditions in cystic fibrosis

Meconium ileus

Meconium ileus (MI) is the earliest clinical manifestation of CF. Infants with CF are at risk for delayed passage of meconium, intestinal plugging with meconium, and meconium ileus. In CF, meconium has an increased concentration of albumin and decreased water and mineral concentrations, resulting in a thicker, more viscous, texture.[34,35] Increased mucus production from goblet cell secretions, combined with gelatinous meconium, contributes to inspissation of meconium, resulting in partial or total intestinal obstruction. MI occurs almost exclusively in patients with pancreatic insufficiency, and is influenced by the presence of a modifier gene found on chromosome 19.[12] The incidence of MI in CF ranges between 10% and 18%. When a child with CF develops MI, the occurrence rate significantly increases in subsequent siblings with CF.[36–38] Most infants with MI are diagnosed with CF, but there are reports of rare exceptions.[37,39] Neonatal intestinal obstruction can be diagnosed with prenatal ultrasonography. A hyperechoic pattern with dilated bowel, with or without ascites, has a high specificity for CF.[40]

Clinical symptoms of MI are present at birth or soon after birth, with signs of intestinal obstruction. There is absence of passage of meconium in the first 48 h. Abdominal radiography shows distended bowel loops, usually without air–fluid levels, with a bubbly ground-glass density at the terminal ileum (Fig. 68.3a). Contrast enema is diagnostic, showing an unused microcolon and filling defects from inspissated meconium in the distal small bowel (Figs 68.3b,c). Hyperosmolar contrast enema successfully relieves the obstruction in 50–90% of uncomplicated cases.[40,41] Approximately 50% of cases of MI are complicated by intestinal perforation, peritonitis, necrosis, volvulus, meconium cysts or intestinal atresia, and require laparotomy.[40] Intraoperative bowel infusion with acetylcysteine, or hyperosmolar contrast, has been shown to decrease the need for surgical resection.[41,42] If intraoperative infusions are unsuccessful, or there are complications, resection of the affected bowel with primary anastomosis or side-by-side enterostomy is performed.[40]

Current surgical and nutritional modalities have significantly decreased the formerly high mortality rate in infants with MI.[42] However, MI in CF is associated with a higher mortality rate when diagnosed late and skilled care is delayed.[43] Prognostically, it has been shown that children with CF who are born with MI have similar nutritional outcomes but go on to have more clinically significant pulmonary disease[44] and a shorter life expectancy[45] than those who did not have neonatal MI.

Other abnormalities due to meconium can occur in CF. Meconium plug syndrome (MPS) is seen in infants with CF as well as those with Hirschsprung's disease, hypotonia and prematurity. The presenting signs and symptoms of MPS are similar to those of MI, but there is distal obstruction at the level of the colon rather than the ileum. A contrast enema shows a normal-caliber colon with filling defects from inspissated meconium, and is usually diagnostic and therapeutic. Surgical intervention is usually not indicated.[39]

Distal intestinal obstruction syndrome

Distal intestinal obstruction syndrome (DIOS), once called meconium ileus equivalent, occurs at all ages but is more common in adolescents and adults. It is seen almost exclusively in patients with pancreatic insufficiency, but has been reported in pancreatic sufficient patients.[46] Patients with prior MI may be at increased risk for DIOS,[47] and DIOS may be a risk factor for developing liver disease.[48] The exact incidence varies considerably, and has been reported as between 4% and 40%.[47,49] Since the introduction of enteric-coated microsphere preparations of pancreatic enzymes, the frequency of DIOS has decreased.[49] DIOS is believed to result from a combination of retained mucofeculent material, abnormal intestinal secretions and abnormal intestinal motility, leading to impaction of stool in the terminal ileum, cecum and proximal colon.[50,51] Precipitating causes of DIOS are frequently not identified, but non-compliance with supplemental pancreatic enzyme, dehydration, change in diet, opiates and anticholinergics have all been implicated. Symptoms include crampy lower abdominal pain, abdominal distention, vomiting and anorexia. A palpable mass in the lower right quadrant can be felt on physical examination. During episodes of DIOS, normal stooling patterns may continue, but progression to complete obstruction, intussusception or volvulus can occur.[16] A diagnosis of DIOS is made by the

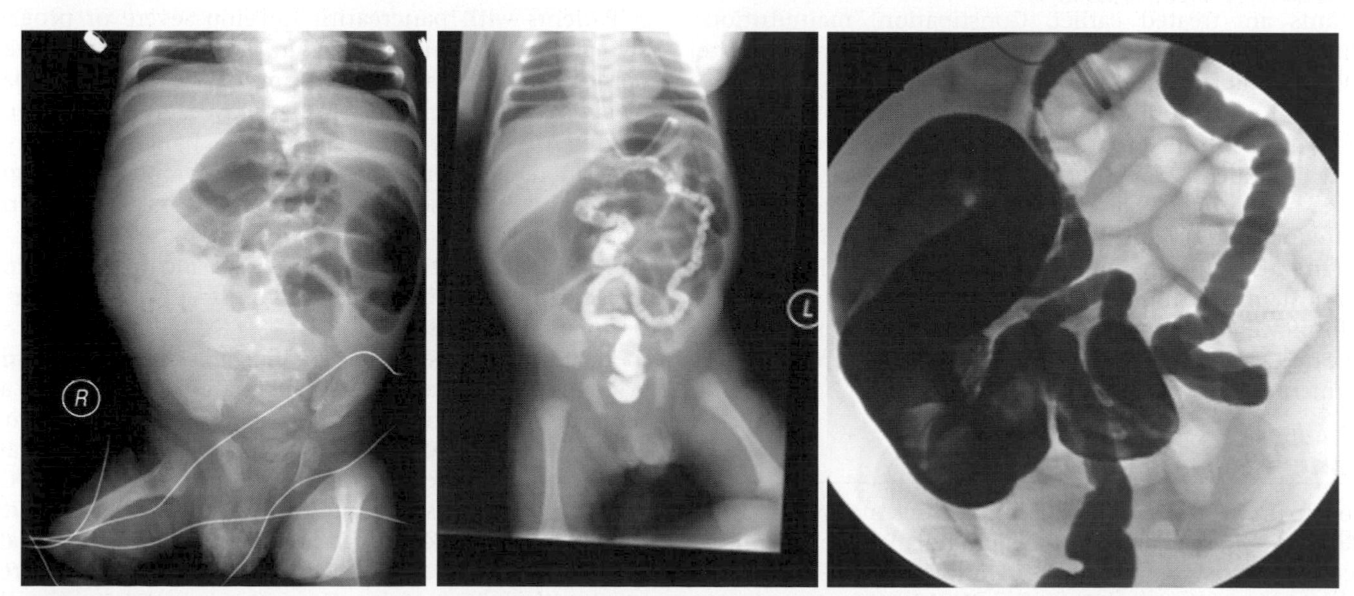

Figure 68.3: (**a**) Abdominal radiograph of meconium ileus with a 'bubbly' fullness in the right lower quadrant and dilated proximal small bowel loops. (**b**) Contrast enema in meconium ileus with dilated small bowel and unused microcolon. (**c**) Contrast enema in meconium ileus showing a huge dilated distal ileum with filling defects due to inspissated meconium. Dilated loops of small bowel and unused microcolon can also be seen. (Courtesy of Robin C. Murphy MD.)

history and physical examination. Abdominal radiography shows retained stool in the ileum and cecum, which can appear as 'bubbly' granular opacities. Air–fluid levels can be seen. The differential diagnosis includes intussusception, volvulus, pancreatitis, gallbladder disease, appendicitis, peptic ulcer disease and esophagitis.

In the absence of complete bowel obstruction, the preferred treatment is gastrointestinal lavage with a balanced isotonic solution containing polyethylene glycol (Golytely™), administered orally or through a nasogastric tube.[50] The endpoint of therapy is to relieve the partial obstruction, which is determined by passage of stool, resolution of pain, and resolution of the palpable lower right quadrant mass. Follow-up radiography may be helpful in documenting resolution. Therapeutic enemas using water-soluble contast under radiologic control, as with as enemas containing *N*-acetylcysteine, are used less frequently owing to the success of antegrade intestinal lavage. Once the acute episode has been managed, dose optimization or improved compliance with pancreatic enzymes, increasing fluid intake and additional dietary fiber help to prevent recurrence. Osmotic laxatives including lactulose and chronic polyethylene glycol (Miralax™) may decrease the risk of recurrence.

Rectal prolapse

The most common cause of rectal prolapse in children is severe constipation. However, rectal prolapse can be a presenting sign of CF, and a sweat test should therefore be considered in this setting. Rectal prolapse occurs in up to 20% of patients with CF, usually between 6 months and 2 years of age.[51] It is uncommon in patients with CF diagnosed and treated with pancreatic enzymes prior to 3 months of age. Rectal prolapse may become even less common as newborn screening becomes more widespread and infants are treated earlier. Constipation, malnutrition, chronic cough and pelvic muscle weakness increase the risk of rectal prolapse.

Rectal prolapse initially starts as intussusception of the rectum, and then progresses.[52] The prolapse can involve only the mucosa (mucosal prolapse) or all layers of the rectum – a complete prolapse or procidentia. Rectal prolapse is frequently recurrent in CF, and initially noticed by the parents. Usually the parents can easily reduce it. Rarely is surgical intervention required. Recurrence of prolapse is minimized by improved nutrition and decreased malabsorption, and appropriate use of pancreatic enzyme supplementation.

Pancreatitis

Approximately 15% of pancreatic sufficient patients with CF develop pancreatitis in their lifetime. Pancreatitis in CF occurs almost exclusively in older pancreatic sufficient patients, but has been described in infants and may be the presenting symptom of CF.[53] Pancreatitis can occur in patients with severe CF mutations, prior to the complete loss of pancreatic function. The exact pathophysiology of pancreatitis in patients with CF is not clear, but preservation of acinar tissue function is required.

The CFTR protein is found at the apical cell membrane of the ductal epithelial cells and maintains normal pancreatic secretions by controlling the movement of chloride into the duct, with water following; this alkalizes and dilutes the fluid as it flows through the pancreatic duct. In CF, abnormal CFTR causes low acinar luminal pH, which inhibits endocytosis of secretory granule proteins and reduces the solubility of the concentrated fluid.[54] Accordingly, patients with CF have pancreatic secretions that are highly concentrated and proteinaceous. Physical obstruction of the pancreatic ducts from these proteinaceous plugs, or alteration of acinar function, develops from the concentrated pancreatic secretions. Pancreatic proteolytic enzymes are subsequently activated, leading to pancreatic autodigestion.[16,54] Early destruction of functional acinar tissue leading to acinar atrophy presumably protects pancreatic insufficient patients from autodigestion and pancreatitis.

The natural history of pancreatitis in CF is characterized by the onset of acute pancreatitis that recurs and can develop into chronic pancreatitis over time.[55] Compound heterozygote genotypes, containing one severe mutation and one mild-variable mutation of CFTR, are at greatest risk for CF-related pancreatitis. 5T mutations, which are associated with inefficient splicing of exon 10 leading to non-functional copies of the CFTR, are frequently found in patients with CF and pancreatitis.[56] The pancreatic secretory trypsin inhibitor (*PSTI*) gene produces proteins in the acinar granules. The risk of pancreatitis is greatly increased in patients with CF who are CFTR compound heterozygotes and also carry mutations of PSTI. Patients may also be at increased risk of progression from acute to chronic pancreatitis, with abnormalities of both genes.[57]

Patients with pancreatitis develop severe or progressive abdominal pain, with vomiting, and epigastric tenderness. Serum and urinary amylase and serum lipase levels are raised. Imaging studies may be normal, but narrowing of the pancreatic duct on pancreatography,[58] peripancreatic edema on abdominal computed tomography[53] and increased pancreatic echogenicity on ultrasonography have been described. Acute episodes of pancreatitis can be precipitated by alcohol ingestion, tetracycline or fatty meals, but most episodes appear to occur spontaneously.

Recurrent acute episodes are typical, but pseudocyst and systemic complications of CF-related pancreatitis are unusual. As patients with recurrent acute episodes may eventually develop pancreatic insufficiency, pancreatic function should be monitored closely. Treatment for CF-related pancreatitis consists of intravenous fluids, nutritional support and analgesics. Supplemental pancreatic enzymes may provide a negative feedback to the pancreas by limiting endogenous enzyme secretions, thereby decreasing autodigestion and pain. In patients with frequent attacks, supplemental enzymes may prevent or increase the interval between episodes.

Cystic fibrosis-related diabetes mellitus

Diabetes mellitus is a well recognized complication of CF. In CF, the total pancreatic mass decreases due to progressive fibrosis of the pancreas, producing a decrease in glucagon-secreting α cells and insulin-secreting β cells. As the proportion of β cells decreases, glucose intolerance increases and diabetes mellitus may develop. Pancreatic insufficiency is a prerequisite for CF-related diabetes (CFRD). Glucose intolerance is present in a substantial number of young children with CF,[59] and approximately 75% of adults with CF have some degree of glucose intolerance.[60] CFRD rarely develops before the age of 10 years, and average onset is at approximately 20 years, with prevalence increasing with age. Females may be more susceptible, and develop diabetes at a younger age.[61] A significant deterioration in lung function and growth may occur years before CFRD is diagnosed.[62,63] Development of CFRD is estimated to increase the mortality rate by as much as six-fold.[62,64]

In CFRD, stimulated insulin secretion is impaired and there is debate regarding insulin sensitivity. It is likely that insulin sensitivity increases initially, but insulin resistance ensues as glucose tolerance deteriorates.[65] Insulin resistance is increased with glucocorticosteroid use, pregnancy and acute infections. CFRD is not autoimmune mediated and is rarely associated with ketoacidosis. Microvascular complications may be seen in CFRD, usually after 10 years' duration. Macrovascular complications have not been reported.[65]

Patients with CFRD complain of lethargy and have difficulty maintaining weight. There is calorie loss from glycosuria, with subsequent loss of weight loss and muscle mass. Lung function typically deteriorates, and there is an increased risk of pulmonary infection due to impairment of immune system function. The progression from glucose intolerance to diabetes is a slow, indolent process, and there is no way to predict which patients with glucose intolerance will develop CFRD. Monitoring hemoglobin A_{1c} is not useful for screening for CFRD owing to shortened erythrocyte survival, but can be used to monitor diabetes control.[65] Adolescent patients with CF should be screened with annual oral glucose tolerance testing. Patients younger than 10 years who demonstrate unexplained lung function deterioration or weight loss should also be considered for oral glucose tolerance testing. The goal of treatment for CFRD is maintenance of glucose homeostasis, normal growth and good nutrition. Carbohydrates are not restricted, but foods and drinks with concentrated simple sugars are discouraged. Fats are encouraged as an important source of calories, and calories typically are not restricted. Exogenous insulin administration is used to maintain glucose homeostasis in CFRD. Insulin may be needed intermittently with acute infections in patients with glucose intolerance.

Nutrition

Malnutrition and growth retardation are common problems in children with CF. Malnutrition results from a combination of increased energy expenditure, decreased caloric intake, chronic infection and inflammation, and caloric and nutrient losses due to malabsorption in pancreatic insufficient patients. Optimal dietary intake is an essential component of CF care. The nutritional recommended daily allowance (RDA) is 120–140% of that of healthy children. Most patients with CF obtain only 80–100% of the RDA. Patients with CF often require 35–40% of calories from fat and 15% of calories from protein, which are higher than the levels recommended for the healthy population.[66] There is a negative correlation between the degree of malnutrition and the degree of illness, pulmonary function and survival. Equally concerning are data demonstrating that prolonged malnutrition in young children with CF is associated with decreased cognitive function.[67]

Pancreatic function has a direct influence on nutritional status and is a strong predictor of outcome. However, obtaining full genetic height potential is a strong indicator of nutritional status. Growth, pulmonary function and survival is better in cohorts of patients with higher height and weight percentiles, compared with those with lower percentiles.[68] When nutrition improves, height and weight percentiles increase, and the differences between the two groups disappear.[69] Early nutritional intervention in patients diagnosed with CF by neonatal screening results in a sustained improvement in growth parameters.[70]

Nutritional deficiencies in CF affect body stores of fat-soluble vitamins, essential fatty acids, prealbumin, albumin, trigycerides, cholesterol and some trace metals. All water-soluble vitamins are well absorbed, except vitamin B_{12}, which is absorbed normally with adequate pancreatic enzyme supplementation.[71] However, even with appropriate pancreatic enzyme replacement and supplemental fat-soluble vitamins (Table 68.5), serum vitamin levels may remain decreased.

	0–12 months	1–3 years	>8 years	
Vitamin A (IU)	1500	5000	5000–10000	10 000
Vitamin E (IU)	40–50	80–150	100–200	200–400
Vitamin D (IU)	400	400–800	400–800	400–800
Vitamin K (mg)	At least 0.3 mg	At least 0.3 mg	At least 0.3 mg	At least 0.3 mg
Calcium (mg/day)	0–6 months: 210			
	7–12 months: 270	500	800	1300

Table 68.5 Recommendations for vitamin supplementation and calcium intake in cystic fibrosis

Vitamin A

Vitamin A is required for normal vision, immunity, epithelial cell integrity and proliferation. Pancreatic lipase is needed to digest retinyl esters to allow absorption, placing pancreatic insufficient patients at risk of vitamin A deficiency. Decreased vitamin A levels are associated with decreased retinol-binding protein, due to decreased vitamin A absorption from the gut.[72] In spite of vitamin A and pancreatic enzyme replacement, low serum vitamin A levels are common, although clinical signs of deficiency are rare. However, dark-field adaptation deficits have been described in as many as 18% of adolescent and adult patients with CF. This risk is greatest in patients with liver disease and those non-compliant with enzyme supplementation.[73] A normal serum vitamin A to retinol-binding protein ratio is the goal, to ensure adequate levels. As vitamin A is an acute-phase reactant, and can be negatively influenced by infections, levels can be misleading during hospitalization for acute illness.[74]

Vitamin D

Calcium absorption is dependent on vitamin D. Decreased vitamin D levels lead to decreased calcium absorption and are associated with osteoporosis, increased bone fracture and delayed tooth eruption. Sun exposure is an important source of vitamin D, but skin cancer concerns have led to a limiting of sun exposure and increased use of sunscreen. As a result, inadequate 25-hydroxyvitamin D levels are frequently found in patients with CF. Vitamin D deficiency has been demonstrated in 10–40% of patients with CF, and is seen more commonly in the very ill and patients living in northern latitudes.[75]

Vitamin E

Vitamin E (α-tocopherol) is an antioxidant that has been shown to act as a free radical scavenger and to have positive effects on immune function. Vitamin E deficiency develops early in life in pancreatic insufficient patients and is present in almost all pancreatic insufficient patients with CF who are not receiving tocopherol supplementation.[76] It has also been shown that 5–10% of patients continue to have low serum levels of vitamin E, even with supplementation.[77]

Supplementation with multivitamins and pancreatic enzymes in infants diagnosed with CF has been shown to have a more profound effect in correcting corrected levels of vitamin A and D than vitamin E. Most infants with vitamin E deficiency continue to be deficient for a prolonged period of time.[75]

Despite supplementation, sporadic or recurrent deficiencies of all fat-soluble vitamins occur throughout childhood, but are seen more frequently with vitamin E. Plasma levels of α-tocopherol below 300 mg/dl are associated with cell membrane instability, erythrocyte destruction and risk of hemolytic anemia.[67] Neurologic findings associated with vitamin E deficiency include decreased vibratory sensation and proprioception, decreased deep tendon reflexes, muscle weakness and ataxia. Neurodevelopment and cognitive function are significantly reduced in patients with CF and vitamin E deficiency, compared with those with normal vitamin E levels.[67]

Vitamin K

Vitamin K is required for the biosynthesis of clotting factors. Some authorities suggest that in patients with CF who are supplemented with pancreatic enzymes, vitamin K deficiency is uncommon;[78] however, there have been reports of vitamin K deficiency.[79] Patients with liver disease are at greatest risk; this can be corrected with higher doses of vitamin K.[80] It is widely believed that chronic antibiotic use reduces vitamin K levels because of disruption of the enteric flora. However, Beker et al.[81] were unable to find significant changes of serum levels with antibiotic use. PIVKA-II (protein induced by vitamin K absence or antagonism) concentration is a sensitive assay for the measurement of vitamin K deficiency, but is not practical owing to the lack of clinical availability.[77] Therefore, prothrombin time is used as an indirect measure, even though when prolonged it is a late indicator of vitamin K deficiency.

Calcium

There is a high prevalence of osteopenia and osteoporosis, and an increased risk of fractures in patients with CF. Bone mineral density decreases with advancing age in CF due to chronic inflammation, inactivity, steroid use, and chronic malabsorption of vitamin D and calcium. Calcium absorption is augmented by pancreatic enzyme supplementation, but calcium supplementation (Table 68.5) is frequently needed to improve bone density. Dual-energy X-ray absorptiometry (DEXA) is helpful in evaluating bone density, but is still limited by lack of standardized normal ranges in children.

Iron

The prevalence of iron deficiency anemia in CF increases with age. Serum ferritin is frequently used to monitor iron status. When interpreting this result, it should be kept in mind that ferritin is an acute-phase reactant and, as a result, the measurement can be affected by acute inflammation. Serum transferrin receptors are not affected by inflammation and may be a more reliable indicator of iron deficiency, but are of limited use in clinical practice; this is not a commercially available test.[82] Annual hemoglobin and hematocrit levels are often used to monitor iron status, even though they are less sensitive.

Trace metals

Normal zinc metabolism is critical for normal growth and immune function. Approximately 30% of young infants diagnosed with CF by newborn screening have been shown to have low plasma zinc levels; this was significantly improved with pancreatic enzyme supplementation.[83] Zinc homeostasis is dependent on the absorption of exogenous zinc, and the secretion and excretion of endogenous zinc through the gastrointestinal tract. Endogenous zinc is, at least in part, found in pancreatic secretions. Zinc absorption from the gastrointestinal tract is influenced by physiologic demand, zinc load and the presence of dietary enhancers including human milk and animal proteins.[84] Zinc deficiency can affect vitamin A status, and supplementation with zinc should be considered in patients with suboptimal vitamin A levels.[84] Severe zinc deficiency is more common in malnutrition, and can be associated with an acrodermatitis enteropathica-like rash. Plasma zinc concentration is used to monitor zinc status, but is not a sensitive marker. The best assessment of zinc status is the response to a trial of approximately 1 mg elemental zinc per kg per day. A plasma zinc concentration of less than 80 mg/dl has been used as a predictor of a significant growth response to zinc supplementation.[84]

Malabsorption of magnesium can occur in CF, but symptomatic hypomagnesemia is usually due to exogenous factors. Paresthesias, muscle weakness, carpopedal spasms and other symptoms of hypomagnesemia should be treated with magnesium replacement.

Copper deficiency occurs in CF, possibly due to abnormal copper metabolism. The exact mechanism is not clear, but may be related to low activity levels of superoxide dismutase and plasma diamine oxidase, enzymes involved in copper metabolism. Zinc deficiency can have a negative impact on copper status. Copper supplementation does not readily correct the deficiency, even when supplemented with zinc.[85] Ceruloplasmin is an acute-phase reactant and it concentration may be raised in CF.[86] Selenium serum levels in CF can be decreased, and at one time selenium was considered by some to be significant. However, clinically significant selenium deficiency has not been reported in CF.

Essential fatty acids

Essential fatty acid deficiency in CF is well described, and until recently was thought to be due to malabsorption.[87] More recent studies support the hypothesis that essential fatty acid abnormalities in CF may be due to CFTR dysfunction. CFTR has been shown to have a potential role in cellular fatty acid metabolism.[88,89] Chronic inflammation affects fatty acid metabolism, but CFTR-regulated tissue levels may not reflect plasma fatty acid levels.[89] Linoleic acid and docosahexaenoic acid levels are decreased in CF, and eicosatrienoic acid concentration is increased.[87,88] Linoleic and arachidonic acid (a metabolite of eicosatrienoic acid) are n-6 fatty acids, and docosahexaenoic acid is an n-3 fatty acid. The biologic effects of fatty acids depend not only on the absolute levels, but also on the ratio of n-6 to n-3 fatty acids. In CF there is an increased ratio of arachidonic to docosahexaenoic acid. Metabolites of arachidonic acid are proinflammatory agents, and metabolites of docosahexaenoic acid are potent anti-inflammatory agents. The altered ratio may play a role in increased inflammation in CF. High doses of docosahexaenoic acid fed to CF-knockout mice not only corrects the fatty acid deficiency, but also reverses the histologic inflammatory changes in the pancreas and ileum.[89,90] Studies on the efficacy of high-dose docosahexaenoic acid administration in humans are ongoing.

Nutritional management

In spite of all the improvements in CF care, undernutrition and malnutrition continue to be problematic in patients with CF, and influence morbidity and mortality. Numerous studies have shown the value of improved nutrition on longevity and lung health,[68,91,92] but maintaining optimal nutrients and calories is not easily done. There are numerous factors that contribute to the nutritional status in CF. Chronic coughing, post-tussive emesis and tachypnea add to calorie losses and anorexia. As well as calorie and nutrient loss from malabsorption, and losses due to CFRD, patients with CF have increased basal metabolic rates and total daily energy expenditures.[93,94] Even when aggressive dietary intervention is employed, maintenance of the required high-energy levels may not be met.[92,95]

Growth may also be affected by factors unrelated to energy absorption and requirements. Chronic inflammation results in increased levels of interleukin 6 (IL-6), which can decrease levels of insulin-like growth factor 1 (IGF-1) and growth.[96] Synthetic growth hormone increases IGF-1, decreases protein degradation, and improves growth and nutritional status in CF.[96,97] Reduced stores of essential fatty acids result in increased eicosanoid synthesis in CF, which increases inflammation. Administration of essential fatty acids, and n-3 fatty acids in particular, decreases inflammation and can also improve nutrition and growth.[98,99] Chronic respiratory infections have been the assumed culprit for the chronic inflammation seen in CF. Improved airway clearance and antibiotics are the cornerstone of care for pulmonary infections, which has a positive effect on nutritional status. However, the pathophysiology of growth disturbance in chronic inflammatory states such as CF is poorly understood and requires further research.

Stunting of growth occurs when malnutrition exists for at least 4 months.[96] Early detection of suboptimal growth allows for early evaluation and intervention. To detect early signs of nutritional failure, growth and nutritional status should be monitored routinely at 3-month intervals. Accurate sequential measurements for height, length, weight and head circumference are obtained and plotted on the 2000 NCHS/CDC growth chart. Assessment of 'weight for height proportions,' using percentage ideal bodyweight (IBW) by the Moore method,[77] is also plotted as a percentile, using NCHS/CDC growth charts. Patients may be showing early signs of nutritional failure even if their percentage IBW is 90% or higher, but demonstrate a plateau of weight or loss of weight. If a child's height is below the predicted genetic potential, or the weight for length is below the 25th percentile, evaluation should be considered, because the patient is at risk for nutritional failure. Children whose height is below the fifth percentile for age or whose weight for height is below the 10th percentile, or who are below the 10th percentile for ideal body weight (IBW), are considered as having nutritional failure.[77]

Body mass index (BMI) is an estimate of body fat; it should remain fairly constant throughout adulthood, but varies in childhood. Therefore, BMI percentiles, also available on a CDC growth chart, may be an early indicator of nutritional problems when there is variation from a consistent percentile. For children under the age of 2 years, weight for length percentiles are used, because percentiles for BMI are not available. Children with CF are at risk of nutritional failure when their BMI is below the 25th percentile; they are exhibiting nutritional failure if they fall below the 10th percentile.[77]

Children with CF are frequently unable consistently to consume the volume of food needed to obtain their energy requirements. Their desire and ability to eat further decreases with acute exacerbations of infections, when energy requirements increase. In infants with CF, breastfeeding is preferred, although commercial formulas can be used. When additional calories are needed to maintain optimal growth, fortification of breast milk, concentrating formula, or adding oil or carbohydrates to the fluid increases the number of calories without significantly changing the volume. Solid foods should be introduced according to the recommendations of the American Academy of Pediatrics. Carbohydrate polymers, vegetable oil or medium-chain triglyceride oil can provide additional calories without significantly affecting taste or volume. In older children calorie-dense foods and liquid supplements are added to a balanced diet to boost energy intake. High-calorie snackbars are useful in school and for active children 'on the run' who don't find the time for between-meal snacks. The ability or desire to maintain a consistently high-calorie diet with oral supplementation is limited. Nasogastric or gastrostomy tube feedings are the most effective method of providing consistent nutritional supplementation. Percutaneous placement of a gastrostomy tube reduces morbidity and has less effect on body image. Continuous nighttime feedings allow for a normal daytime lifestyle and eating pattern. Gastrostomy tube feedings also remove the battles that frequently develop over constant prodding to eat more.

If there is limited response to nutritional supplementation, further evaluation for the etiology of growth failure need to be considered. Behavior feeding issues are more common in early childhood, but may be present at any age. School-aged children and adolescents may try to hide their disease from peers, and not take enzymes in school. Adolescents are at greatest risk for eating disorders, and also are the most resistant to gastrostomy tubes, owing to change of body image. The older patient with CF is also at a greater risk than the general population for intestinal cancer;[100] this may also contribute to weight loss or nutritional failure.

Hepatobiliary complications of cystic fibrosis

Hepatobiliary complications of CF are a well recognized component of the disease (Table 68.6).[101] Recognition of liver disease in CF has led to increased surveillance with a possible increase in its diagnosis.[102] Improved longevity in patients with CF has served to increase the prevalence of this usually slow-moving process. In fact, liver complications are now the leading non-pulmonary cause of mortality in patients with CF.[103]

Neonatal cholestasis
Hepatomegaly
Raised levels of liver enzymes
Hepatic steatosis
Focal biliary cirrhosis
Multilobular cirrhosis with portal hypertension

Table 68.6 Manifestations of cystic fibrosis-associated liver disease

Pathophysiology

CF-associated liver disease begins in the biliary tree. CFTR is not found in hepatocytes, but is located in the apical portion of the biliary epithelial cell in the bile ducts and gallbladder.[104] It is thought that in CF the impaired secretory function of the biliary epithelium affects water and solute composition of the bile.[105] The adverse effects on bile flow and alkalinization allow for cholestasis, bile plugging in small biliary radicals, and damage to the biliary tree by cytotoxins and bacteria.[106] Periportal fibrosis can be a secondary complication. Over many years, this process can progress toward bridging fibrosis, and ultimately focal biliary and multilobular cirrhosis with portal hypertension.

Unlike CF-associated pancreatic disease, a solid genotype–phenotype relationship has not yet been established in CF-associated liver disease. As a spectrum of liver disease is seen in patients who share the same CFTR defect, there are likely to be disease-modifying environmental factors, such as nutritional status.[107] Recently, there has also been interest in potential disease-modifying genetic factors, including the histocompatibility complex (HLA).[108] This has raised the possibility that the immune response may be playing a role in the development of liver disease in CF. Patients who are heterozygotes for α_1-antitrypsin deficiency may also have an increased risk of developing hepatic complications.[109]

Spectrum of disease

Several clinical realities make it difficult to assess the true prevalence of hepatobiliary disease in CF.[110] This probably accounts for a published incidence that ranges from one-third to more than 90% of patients with CF. Physical findings may be absent, or include only hepatomegaly, which may be dismissed in the light of pulmonary hyperinflation. It has been recognized for some time that liver chemistry may not be indicative of liver involvement, even in documented cases of cirrhosis.[111] Percutaneous liver biopsy has also been shown to be subject to sampling error and false-negative results.[112] There has been recent evidence that ultrasonography may be a useful modality for the screening and staging of liver involvement in CF.[113] These diagnostic issues have been addressed by consensus in the statement from the Cystic Fibrosis Foundation, which recommends yearly physical examination and determination of liver chemistries as initial screening, and further evaluation for persistent or marked (three times normal) increased in liver chemistries[102].

Neonatal cholestasis is certainly one of the more obvious modes of presentation of CF-associated liver disease.[114] It is estimated that as many as 5% of patients with CF suffer from this complication. Many authors have questioned whether neonatal cholestasis can lead to a higher incidence of cirrhosis, although one study has not supported this concern.[112]

The most common pathologic change seen in the liver of patients with CF is hepatic steatosis. Fatty change probably occurs in more than one-third of patients with CF, and can be seen independent of nutritional status and body habitus. The etiology of hepatic steatosis in CF is not fully known. It is as common early in life as in older patients. The relationship between steatosis and the development of fibrosis and cirrhosis in CF is unknown.

As described above, there is a potential progression from focal biliary cirrhosis to multilobular cirrhosis with portal hypertension. Varices and portal hypertension are treated in the usual manner, with endoscopic band ligation or sclerotherapy. Beta-blockade may be problematic due to its effect on pulmonary bronchoconstriction. Cirrhosis can lead to end-stage liver failure and the need for liver transplantation. Good results with liver replacement are possible in patients without severe pulmonary compromise who are nutritionally replete and in whom careful attention has been paid to colonization with potential infectious pathogens.[115] Lung function may be improved after liver transplantation in CF, but the etiology for the improvement is unclear.

Extrahepatic biliary complications are also seen in patients with CF (Table 68.7). Asymptomatic gallbladder abnormalities can be seen on imaging of the biliary system.[116] Micro-gallbladder and absence of the gallbladder can also be seen in biliary atresia that has been diagnosed in patients with CF.[101] Cholelithiasis is seen in as many as 10% of patients with CF, but is often asymptomatic. The gallstones are composed primarily of calcium bilirubinate, and are not responsive to medical treatment with ursodeoxycholic acid.[117] Extrahepatic strictures, including a beading of the extrahepatic ducts reminiscent of primary sclerosing cholangitis (PSC), has been reported. This is of interest because patients with PSC have an increased incidence of CFTR mutations.[118]

Ursodeoxycholic acid (urso) therapy is choluretic and cytoprotective, and has been shown to have an immunomodulatory effect.[119] In CF, improvement in liver chemistries has been shown with urso therapy, especially at increased doses of 20 mg/kg daily.[120] Although it is not clear whether this treatment has an effect on the long-term outcome and progression of liver involvement, a 10-year study has suggested improvement in ultrasonographic findings.[121] The recommendation of the Cystic Fibrosis Foundation consensus statement is to use such therapy in the presence of liver disease.[102]

Biliary complications
Asymptomatic cholelithiasis
Cholecystitis – acute and chronic
Micro or absent gallbladder
Biliary strictures (primary sclerosing cholangitis-like)
Biliary atresia

Table 68.7 Biliary complications of cystic fibrosis

STRUCTURAL ABNORMALITIES OF THE PANCREAS

Structural abnormalities of the pancreas originate from the complex embryologic development of the gland. Failure of normal pancreatic development *in utero* can result in anomalies of the pancreatic duct system as well as the parenchyma of the gland. The resultant congenital anomalies can then be classified in terms of ductal abnormalities, abnormalities in location (migration) of pancreatic tissue, and abnormalities in the amount of pancreatic tissue (Table 68.8).

Embryology

By the end of the first month of gestation, two outpouchings – one dorsal and the other ventral – arise from the caudal aspect of the embryonic foregut.[122] The dorsal primordium arises from the posterior wall of the duodenum and becomes the tail, body and part of the head of the pancreas. The ventral bud develops from the hepatic diverticulum and commonly has a bilobed origin. The right and left lobes of the ventral portion later fuse to form the unci-

Ductal abnormalities
Pancreas divisum
Anomalous pancreaticobiliary union
Defects in pancreatic migration
Ectopic pancreas
Annular pancreas
Fatty replacement of pancreatic tissue
Shwachman–Diamond syndrome
Johanson–Blizzard syndrome
Pancreatic fibrosis
Pearson's marrow–pancreas syndrome
Juene's syndrome
Abnormalities in pancreatic volume
Pancreatic hypoplasia
Pancreatic agenesis

Table 68.8 Congenital pancreatic abnormalities

nate process and remaining portion of the head of the pancreas (Fig. 68.4).[123,124]

A critical aspect of normal pancreatic development occurs by the end of the second month of gestation when the ventral bud rotates in a clockwise manner and comes to lie in an inferior and posterior location, where it then joins the dorsal bud. There are separate ducts associated with the dorsal and ventral portions of the embryonic pancreas. These independent ducts undergo subsequent division and merge to become the drainage system of the mature pancreas.

The dorsal duct arises from the duodenum along with the dorsal tissue. The proximal portion of this duct becomes the accessory duct, or duct of Santorini. The accessory duct drains a portion of the head of the pancreas and enters the duodenum via the minor papilla in 70% of individuals.[125] The distal portion of the embryonic dorsal duct merges with the duct from the ventral bud of the pancreas. This merged structure becomes the duct of Wirsung, or main pancreatic duct. The main duct drains the tail, body and remaining head of the pancreas, and enters the duodenum via the ampulla of Vater in the main papilla. It should be noted that the common bile duct shares this entrance. Therefore, the common entrance into the duodenum of the common bile duct and the duct of Wirsung results from the hepatic origins of the ventral pancreatic bud and its associated duct.[123,126]

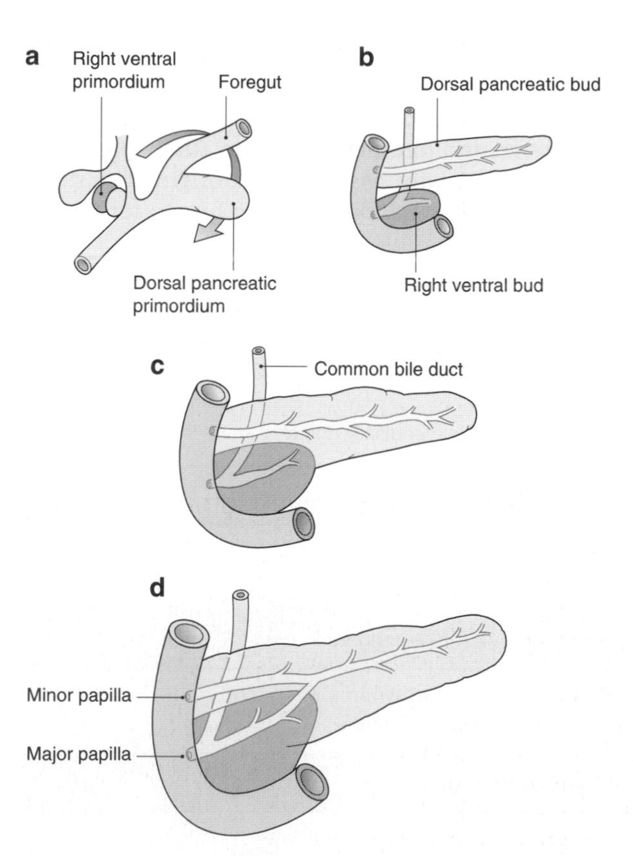

Figure 68.4: Embyrologic development of the pancreas. (**a**) 4 weeks' gestation–formation of the dorsal and ventral pancreatic buds. (**b**) 6 weeks' gestation–rotation of the ventral bud bringing it alongside the dorsal bud. (**c**) 7–8 weeks' gestation–fusion of the dorsal and ventral pancreatic buds. (**d**) final arrangement of the pancreatic ducts with the accessory duct draining part of the head of the pancreas via the minor papila (above). The common bile duct meets the main pancreatic duct which drains the majority of the pancreas via the main papilla (below).

Ductal abnormalities

Various abnormalities in the anatomy of the pancreatic ducts can occur; these find their roots in the complex embryology described above. Pancreas divisum, for example, results when the embryonic dorsal and ventral ducts do not merge.[127]

Pancreas divisum

More than 90% of individuals undergo normal development of the main pancreatic duct via fusion of the ducts associated with the dorsal and ventral pancreatic buds. When the ducts fail to fuse *in utero*, the result is two separate drainage systems known as pancreas divisum.[125,128–133] In individuals with pancreas divisum, the head of the pancreas drains independently through the major papilla. The minor papilla then drains the body and tail, which is the majority of the pancreatic tissue. It is postulated that the flow of a relatively high volume of pancreatic secretions through this smaller opening can allow pancreatic enzymes to inflame the papilla, leading to stasis, stenosis and recurrent pancreatitis.[133]

Diagnosis of pancreas divisum is most commonly made by means of endoscopic retrograde cholangiopancreatography (ERCP).[131–133] There are now reports demonstrating that this anomaly can be diagnosed using endoscopic ultrasonography, as well as magnetic resonance cholangiopancreatography (MRCP) (Fig. 68.5).[134] Administration of secretin

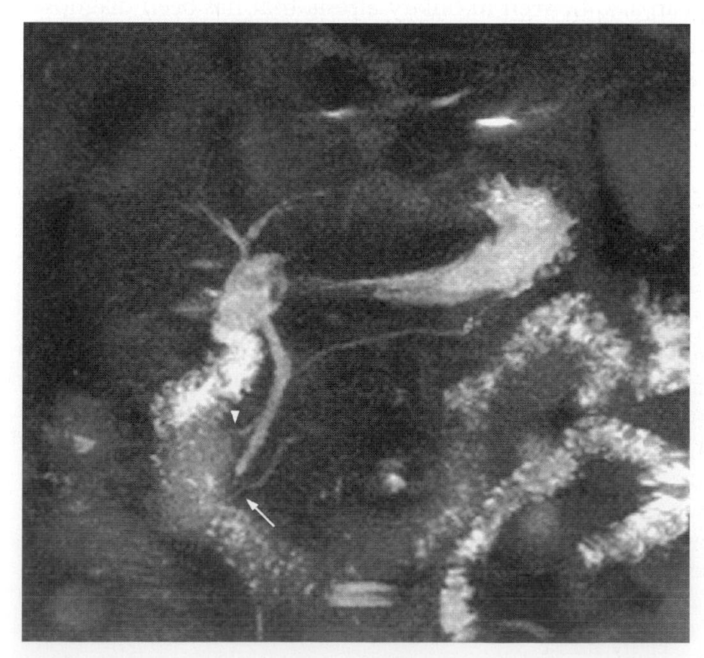

Figure 68.5: Magnetic resonance cholangiopancreatogram showing the separate ventral duct (arrow) and dorsal duct (arrowhead) of pancreas divisum. (Courtesy of Brian Herts MD.)

has been shown to increase the potential yield of such an MRCP examination by increasing the secretions in the ducts, thereby allowing clearer delineation of the anatomy.[135–137]

It remains controversial whether pancreas divisum is simply a normal anatomic variant[138,139] or whether it increases the risk of recurrent pancreatitis.[133,140–142] Successful therapeutic trials are usually used as evidence for the argument that pancreas divisum is a cause of recurrent pancreatitis. There are studies looking at surgical[143–145] and endoscopic[146–149] interventions, including sphincterotomy and stent placement across the minor papilla. Many experts point out potential selection bias in these studies and urge caution in interpreting the results.[150]

Anomalous pancreaticobiliary union

Anomalous pancreaticobiliary union (APBU) describes an abnormality in the junction between the common bile duct and the main pancreatic duct. In APBU, this confluence occurs outside the duodenal wall, forming a channel more than 15 mm in length.[151] It is believed that APBU arises from an uneven proliferation of bile duct epithelium during fetal development,[152] perhaps explaining the development of some choledochal cysts. APBU interferes with normal flow of pancreatic and biliary secretions, possibly causing recurrent pancreatitis,[153,154] and may increase the risk of cholangiocarcinoma. When associated with a choledochal cyst, treatment includes removal of the cyst with Roux-en-Y reconstruction of the remaining biliary tree. When there is no cyst, prophylactic cholecystectomy is recommended in light of the increased risk of cholangiocarcinoma.[155]

Abnormalities of migration

As already described, embryologic development of the pancreas requires migration of parenchymal tissue to the site of the gland's normal anatomic location. There are several recognized congenital abnormalities in the location, volume and structure of the pancreatic parenchyma that can result from a disordered progression of this aspect of pancreatic development.

Ectopic pancreas

Ectopic pancreatic tissue is most commonly referred to as a pancreatic rest. Other terms in the literature include heterotopic, aberrant and accessory pancreatic tissue. Consistent with its embryologic origins, the majority of ectopic pancreatic tissue is found in the foregut, with 75% being found in the stomach, including the prepyloric gastric antrum.[156,157] Duodenal and proximal jejunal sites have also been reported. Ectopic pancreatic tissue has also been seen in the ileum, Meckel's diverticulum, gallbladder, common bile duct, splenic hilum, umbilicus, lung, and in perigastric and periduodenal tissue.[158] In autopsy series, the average frequency of ectopic pancreas is between 1% and 2% (range 0.55–13%).[159]

By definition, such tissue has no physical or vascular continuity with the pancreatic gland. Pancreatic rests are frequently functional but are usually asymptomatic and discovered as an incidental finding on upper gastrointestinal contrast study.[160] Upper endoscopy can also demonstrate these lesions, which appear as a round, smooth, submucosal mass with a central umbilication, most commonly found in the antrum and gastric outlet.

There have been reports of clinical symptoms associated with large (>1.5 cm) pancreatic rests.[161] The most common symptoms were abdominal pain, dyspepsia and gastrointestinal bleeding. Biliary and pyloric obstruction may occur.[162] Pancreatitis in the ectopic tissue has also been described, and there are reported cases of cancer occurring in the ectopic pancreas.[163] As ectopic pancreatic tissue is usually asymptomatic, management is usually observational with operative treatment reserved for complicated cases.[164] The submucosal location of pancreatic rests makes endoscopic removal unattractive, owing to the perforation risk.

Annular pancreas

During its migration in the second month of gestation, the ventral portion of the pancreas can become misaligned, encircle the second portion of the duodenal sweep, and then fuse with the dorsal aspect of the developing pancreas.[165] This anatomy is known as annular pancreas (Fig. 68.6). The most common clinical presentation of annular pancreas is a neonatal bowel obstruction proximal to the ampulla of Vater. This anatomic abnormality can occur in isolation or together with other congenital malformations. The most commonly associated malformations are usually gastrointestinal, including intestinal malrotation, duodenal abnormalities such as web, stenosis and atresia, tracheoesophageal fistula, imperforate anus and Hirschsprung's disease. Annular pancreas can occur with congenital heart disease, and has an increased incidence in patients with trisomy 21.[166]

Annular pancreas has a variety of clinical presentations. In infancy, it can present as upper gastrointestinal obstruction with a classic 'double bubble' sign on abdominal radiography. It may be asymptomatic or present in adulthood with duodenal obstruction, chronic pancreatitis or ulceration. As

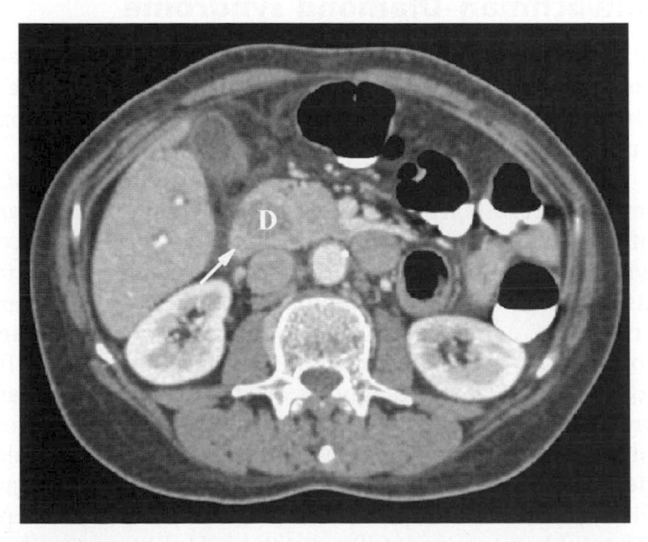

Figure 68.6: Annular pancreas. Contrast-enhanced axial computed tomogram showing pancreatic tissue (arrow) lateral to and surrounding the duodenum (D). (Courtesy of Brian Herts MD.)

duodenal malformation frequently accompanies annular pancreas, the treatment of choice is surgical bypass of the lesion, usually with a duodenoduodenostomy.

Abnormalities in volume

Both pancreatic agenesis and hypoplasia have been reported in isolation and with other congenital abnormalities.[167] Endocrine and exocrine insufficiency may occur, and appropriate hormone and enzyme replacement therapy can lead to improved survival if diagnosed in a timely manner. Intrauterine growth retardation can be a consequence of lack of fetal insulin *in utero*. Hypoplasia may result from agenesis of the dorsal bud of the pancreas which normally supplies 90% of the pancreatic tissue.[168] Such a short gland has been reported to occur with other congenital abnormalities, including polysplenia.[169] Fatty replacement of the gland has also been reported and can be considered a form of pancreatic hypoplasia.[170]

Epithelium-lined congenital pancreatic cysts have also been described. The mode of presentation of these rare cysts includes gastrointestinal obstruction, biliary obstruction and the finding of an asymptomatic mass. Treatment is by surgical excision.

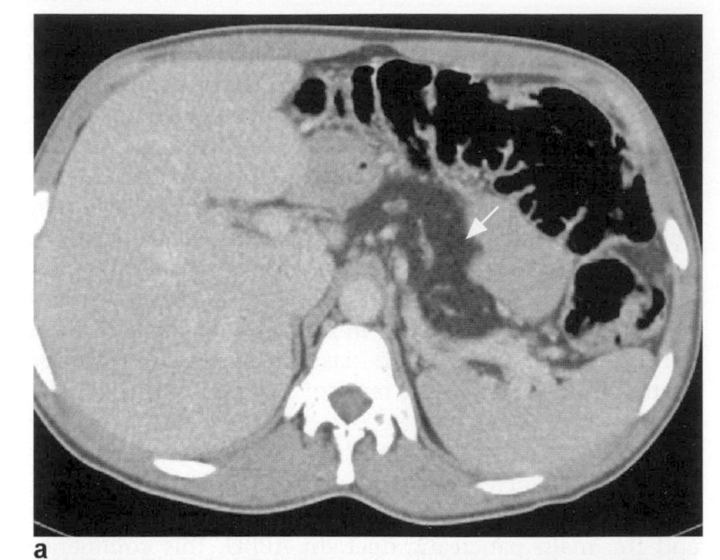

a

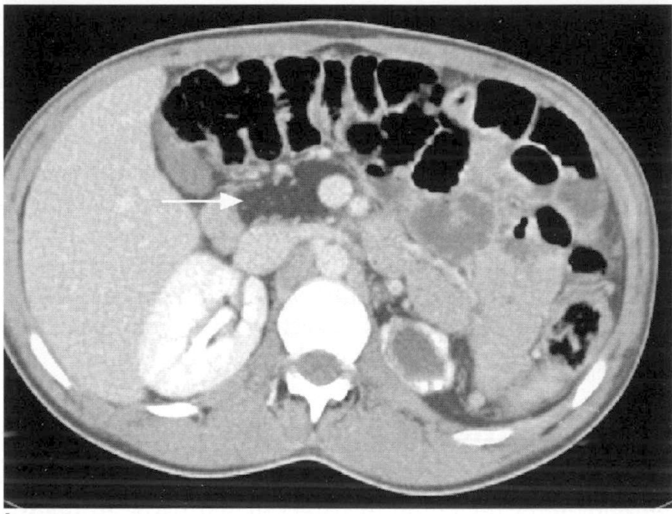

b

Figure 68.7: Shwachman–Diamond syndrome. Contrast-enhanced axial computed tomograms through (**a**) the body and (**b**) the head of the pancreas showing complete fatty replacement of the gland (arrows). (Courtesy of Brian Herts MD.)

FUNCTIONAL ABNORMALITIES OF THE PANCREAS

Several syndromes have been described that include congenital exocrine pancreatic insufficiency and other anomalies, including the bone marrow and skeletal systems. In these syndromes pancreatic insufficiency results from an inadequate volume of acinar cells due to fibrosis or fatty replacement of parenchymal tissue. The most common of these is the Shwachman–Diamond syndrome (SDS).

Shwachman–Diamond syndrome

SDS is the second most common inherited cause of pancreatic insufficiency. This autosomal recessive syndrome is characterized by exocrine pancreatic insufficiency, bone marrow dysfunction and skeletal abnormalities.[171]

The pathogenesis of pancreatic insufficiency in SDS probably results from the failure of normal development of acinar tissue *in utero*. The normal tissue is replaced with fatty deposition (Fig. 68.7).[172] Pancreatic lipomatosis accounts for the distinctive appearance of the pancreas on abdominal ultrasonography. Computed tomography can be even more sensitive and is a useful test to establish the diagnosis of SDS.[173] Clinically, pancreatic insufficiency that results in steatorrhea is most prominent early in life. Subsequent malabsorption, calorie loss and failure to thrive are treated with appropriate dietary intervention, including pancreatic enzyme and fat-soluble vitamin supplementation. Unlike cystic fibrosis, which leads to obstruction and damage to the pancreatic ducts, SDS affects the acinar tissue, and the ductal elements remain intact. Over time, pancreatic hypoplasia is reversed, and there is an increase in normal pancreatic tissue volume. Improved pancreatic function has been reported in several series of patients with SDS. Approximately half of patients can establish pancreatic sufficiency by 4 years of age.[174,175] In managing patients with SDS, potential improvement in pancreatic function over time should be kept in mind. Accordingly, pancreatic function and clinical tests of fat absorption are followed serially, and pancreatic enzyme replacement therapy adjusted accordingly.

Bone marrow dysfunction is another hallmark component of SDS. Persistent or non-cyclic but recurrent neutropenia is the most common abnormality seen. Infectious complications, especially in young patients with neutropenia, become a clinical concern leading to significant morbidity and mortality in some patients.[174] Prophylactic antibiotics have been a mainstay of therapy, but successful use of bone marrow transplantation has been reported.[176] The advent of human granulocye colony-stimulating factor has improved the treatment of neutropenia in patients with SDS.[177] In addition to neutropenia, both the red cell and platelet lines can be affected separately or in combination. Patients with SDS also have an increased risk of developing myelodysplasia and a variety of leukemias that may be treatment resistant.[174] Bone marrow surveillance is prudent in these patients.

Skeletal abnormalities are also seen in patients with SDS. Progressive long-bone dysostosis or metaphyseal chondrodysplasia is the most common finding seen over time in approximately half of patients with SDS. Abnormalities of the thoracic cage are seen in as many as one-third of patients.[174]

Research into the genetics of SDS has focused on a region on chromosome 7. In 2003, Boocock et al.[178] reported their genetic findings after studying 156 unrelated patients with SDS. Some 89% of these patients had mutations in a previously uncharacterized gene mapped to chromosome 7q11, which the authors labeled the *SDS* (Shwachman–Diamond) or *SBDS* (Shwachman–Bodian–Diamond syndrome) gene. This genetic breakthrough should help further the understanding of the pathogenesis of SDS. Genetic testing will also aid in the diagnosis of SDS. Currently, SDS is a clinical diagnosis that can prove difficult in this syndrome, which has variable clinical manifestations.

Johanson–Blizzard syndrome

This is a syndrome of exocrine pancreatic insufficiency with multiple congenital anomalies including deafness, imperforate anus, urogenital malformations and dental anomalies.[179] As with SDS, pancreatic insufficiency results from fatty replacement of the gland. Multiple endocrine abnormalities have been associated with Johanson–Blizzard syndrome, including hypothyroidism, growth hormone deficiency, diabetes and panhypopituitarism.[180]

The syndrome is characterized by typical facies including nasal hypoplasia leading to a 'beak-shaped' appearance, small or misshapen teeth, and sparse, dry hair.

Pearson's marrow–pancreas syndrome

Similar to SDS, Pearson's syndrome involves the bone marrow and pancreas, and results from deletions in mitochondrial DNA.[181,182] Patients with Pearson's syndrome present with a profound and frequently refractory sideroblastic anemia. The bone marrow examination is distinctive, showing vacuolization of bone marrow precursors and ringed sideroblasts. Ultimately other blood cell lines may be involved. There is pancreatic exocrine insufficiency, and autopsy data have demonstrated significant pancreatic fibrosis. As a mitochondrial disease there is a resultant defect in oxidative phosphorylation, explaining the often persistent and even fatal lactic acidosis that has been reported in patients with Pearson's syndrome. Ultimately, there can be renal, endocrine and other multiorgan involvement and failure. Death frequently ensues in infancy or early childhood due to sepsis or metabolic disarray.

Jeune's syndrome

This rare syndrome is characterized by pancreatic insufficiency and fibrosis with anomalies of the skeletal structure of the upper thorax that lead to respiratory compromise.[183]

References

1. Riordan JR, Rommens JM, Kerem B, et al. Identification of cystic fibrosis gene: cloning and characterization of complementary DNA. Science 1989; 245:1066–1073.
2. Riordan JR. The cystic fibrosis transmembrane conductance regulator. Annu Rev Physiol 1993; 55:609–630.
3. Sheppard DN, Welsh MJ. Structure and function of the CFTR chloride channel. Physiol Rev 1999; 79:523–545.
4. Mickle JE, Cutting GR. Genotype–phenotype relationship in cystic fibrosis. Med Clin North Am 2000; 84:597–607.
5. Cheng SH, Gregory RJ, Marshall J, et al. Defective intracellular transport and processing of CFTR is the molecular basis of most cystic fibrosis. Cell 1990; 63:827–834.
6. Fulmer SB, Schwiebert EM, Morales MM, Guggino WB, Cutting GR. Two cystic fibrosis transmembrane conductance regulator mutations have different effects on both pulmonary phenotype and regulation of outwardly rectified chloride currents. Proc Natl Acad Sci USA 1995; 92:683–686.
7. McColley SA, Rosenstein BJ, Cutting GR. Differences in expression of cystic fibrosis in blacks and whites. Am J Dis Child 1991; 145:94–97.
8. Gasparini P, Nunes V, Savoia A, et al. The search for South European cystic fibrosis mutations: identification of two new mutations, four variants and intronic sequences. Genomics 1991; 10:193–200.
9. Mercier B, Raguenes O, Estivill X, et al. Complete detection of mutations in cystic fibrosis patients of Native American origin. Hum Genet 1994; 94:629–632.
10. Dean M, Santis G. Heterogeneity in the severity of cystic fibrosis and the role of CFTR gene mutations. Hum Genet 1994; 3:364–368.
11. Zielenski J, Tsui LC. Cystic fibrosis: genotypic and phenotypic variations. Annu Rev Genet 1995; 29:777–807.
12. Zielenski J, Corey M, Rozmahel R, et al. Detection of a cystic fibrosis modifier locus for meconium ileus on human chromosome 19q13. Nat Genet 1999;22:128–129.
13. Marino C, Matovcik L, Gorelick F, Cohn J. Localization of the cystic fibrosis transmembrane conductance regulator in pancreas. J Clin Invest 1991; 88:712–716.
14. Scheele G, Fukuoka S, Kern H, Freedman S. Pancreatic dysfunction in cystic fibrosis occurs as a result of impairments in luminal pH apical trafficking of zymogen granule membranes and solubilization of secretory enzymes. Pancreas 1996; 12:1–9.
15. Kopelman H, Durie P, Gaskin K, Weizman Z, Forstner G. Pancreatic fluid secretion and protein hyperconcentration in cystic fibrosis. N Engl J Med 1985; 312:329–334.
16. Shepherd RW, Cleghorn GJ. Cystic Fibrosis: Nutritional and Intestinal Disorders. Boca Raton, FL: CRC Press; 1989.
17. Iannucci A, Mukai K, Johnson D, Burke B. Endocrine pancreas in cystic fibrosis: an immunohistochemical study: Hum Pathol 1984; 15:278–284.

18. Brown RE, Madge GE. Cystic fibrosis and nesidioblastosis. Arch Pathol 1971; 92:53–57.
19. DiMagno EP, Go VL, Summerskill WH. Relationship between pancreatic enzyme outputs and malabsorption in severe pancreatic insufficiency. N Engl J Med 1973; 288:813–817.
20. Bronstein M, Sokol R, Abrams S, et al. Pancreatic insufficiency growth and nutrition in infants identified by newborn screening as having cystic fibrosis. J Pediatr 1992; 120:533–540.
21. Fleisher D, DiGeorge A, Barness L, Cornfeld D. Hypoproteinemia and edema in infants with cystic fibrosis of the pancreas. J Pediatr 1964; 64:341–348.
22. Leus J, Van Biervliet S, Robberecht E. Detection and follow-up of exocrine pancreatic insufficiency in cystic fibrosis; a review. Eur J Pediatr 2000; 159:563–568.
23. Durie PR, Forstner GG, Gaskin KJ, et al. Age related alterations of immunoreactive pancreatic cationic trypsinogen in sera from cystic fibrosis patients with and without pancreatic insufficiency. Pediatr Res 1986; 20:209–213.
24. Wallis C, Leung T, Cubitt D, Reynolds A. Stool elastase as a diagnostic test for pancreatic function in children with cystic fibrosis. Lancet 1997; 350:1001.
25. Davidson GP, Hassel FM, Crozier D, Corey D, Corey M, Forstner GG. Iatrogenic hyperuricemia in children with cystic fibrosis. J Pediatr 1978; 93:976–978.
26. Stapleton FB, Kennedy J, Noursia, Arvanitakis S, Linshaw MA. Hyperuricosuria due to high dose pancreatic extract therapy in cystic fibrosis. N Engl J Med 1976; 295:246–248.
27. Twarog FJ, Weinstein SF, Khaw KT, Strieder DJ, Colten HR. Hypersensitivity to pancreatic extracts in parents of patients with cystic fibrosis. J Allergy Clin Immunol 1977; 59:35–40.
28. Chamarthy LM, Reinstein I, Schnapf B, Good RA, Bahna SL. Desensitization to pancreatic enzyme intolerance in a child with cystic fibrosis. Pediatrics 1998; 102:e13.
29. FitzSimmons SC, Burkhart GA, Borowitz D, et al. High dose pancreatic enzyme supplements and fibrosing colonopathy in children with cystic fibrosis. N Engl J Med 1997; 336:1283–1289.
30. Rothbaum R. Improving digestion in children with cystic fibrosis. Contemp Pediatr 1996; 13:39–54.
31. Borowitz DS, Grand RJ, Durie PR. Use of pancreatic enzyme supplements for patients with cystic fibrosis in the context of fibrosing colonopathy. Consensus Committee. J Pediatr 1995; 127:681–684.
32. MacSweeney E, Oades PJ, Buchdahl RM, Phelan M, Bush A. Relationship between ultrasonic colonic thickening and pancreatic enzymes. Pediatr Pulmonol 1994; 10(Suppl):274.
33. Pettei MJ, Leonidas JC, Levine JJ, Gorvoy JD. Pancolonic disease in cystic fibrosis and high dose pancreatic enzyme therapy. J Pediatr 1978; 93:976–978.
34. Kopito L, Shwachman H. Mineral composition of meconium. J Pediatr 1966; 68:313–314.
35. Green MN, Shwachman H. Presumptive tests for cystic fibrosis based on serum protein in meconium. Pediatrics 1968; 41:989–992.
36. Kerem E, Corey M, Kerem B, Durie P, Tsui LC, Levison H. Clinical and genetic comparisons of patients with cystic fibrosis with or without meconium ileus. J Pediatr 1989; 114:767–773.
37. FitzSimmons SC. The changing epidemiology of cystic fibrosis. J. Pediatr 1993; 122:1–9.
38. Allan JL, Robbie M, Phelan PD, Danks DM. Familial occurrence of meconium ileus. Eur J Pediatr 1981; 135:291–292.
39. Olsen M, Luch S, Lloyd-Still J, Raffensperger J. The spectrum of meconium disease in infancy. J Pediatr Surg 1982; 17:479–481.
40. Casaccia G, Trucchi A, Nahom A, et al. The impact of cystic fibrosis on neonatal intestinal obstruction: the need for prenatal/neonatal screening. Pediatr Surg Int 2003; 19:75–78.
41. Rescola FJ, Grosfeld JL, West KJ, Vane DW. Changing patterns of treatment and survival in neonates with meconium ileus. Arch Surg 1989; 42:837–840.
42. Del Pin CA, Czyrko C, Ziegler MM, Scanlin TF, Bishop HC. Management and survival of meconium ileus: a thirty year review. Ann Surg 1992; 215:179–185.
43. Oliveira MCLA, Reis FJC, Monteiro APAF, Penna FJ. Effect of meconium ileus on the clinical prognosis of patients with cystic fibrosis. Braz J Med Biol Res 2002; 35:31–38.
44. Evan AKC, Fitzgerald DA, McKay KO. The impact of meconium ileus on the clinical course of children with cystic fibrosis. Eur Respir J 2001; 18:784–789.
45. Lai HJ, Cheng Y, Cho H, Kosorok MR, Farrell PM. Association between initial disease presentation, lung disease outcomes and survival in patients with cystic fibrosis. Am J Epidemiol 2004; 159:537–546.
46. Davidson AC, Harrison K, Steinfort CL, Geddes DM. Distal intestinal obstruction syndrome in cystic fibrosis treated with oral intestinal lavage and a case of recurrent obstruction despite normal pancreatic function. Thorax 1987; 42:538–541.
47. Rubenstein S, Moss R, Lewiston N. Constipation and meconium ileus equivalent in patients with cystic fibrosis. Pediatrics 1986; 78:473–479.
48. Colombo C, Apostolo MG, Ferrari M, et al. Analysis of risk factors for the development of liver disease associated with cystic fibrosis. J Pediatr 1994; 124:393–393.
49. Anderson HO, Hjelt K, Waever E, Overgaard K. The age-related incidence of meconium ileus equivalent in a cystic fibrosis population: the impact of high-energy intake. J Pediatr Gastroenterol Nutr 1990; 11:356–360.
50. Koletzko S, Stringer DA, Cleghorn GJ, Durie PR. Lavage treatment of distal intestinal obstruction syndrome in children with cystic fibrosis. Pediatrics 1989; 83:727–733.
51. Stern RC, Izant RJ, Boat TF, Wood RE, Matthews LW, Doershuk CF. Treatment and prognosis of rectal prolapse in cystic fibrosis. Gastroenterology 1982; 82:707–710.
52. Siafakas C, Vottle TP, Anderson JM. Rectal prolapse in pediatrics. Clin Pediatr 1999; 38:63–72.
53. Atlas AB, Orenstein SR, Orenstein DM. Pancreatitis in young children with cystic fibrosis. J Pediatr 1992; 120:756–759.
54. Durno C, Corey M, Zielenski, J, Tullis E, Tsui LC, Durie P. Genotype and phenotype correlation in patients with cystic fibrosis and pancreatitis. Gastroenterology 2002; 123:1857–1864.
55. Frulloni L, Castellani C, Bovo P, et al. Natural history of pancreatitis associated with cystic fibrosis gene mutations. Digest Liver Dis 2003; 35:179–185.
56. Noone, PG, Zhaoqing A, Silverman LM, Jowell PS, Knowles MR, Cohn JA. Cystic fibrosis gene mutations and pancreatic risk: relation to epithelial ion transport and trypsin inhibitor gene mutations. Gastroenterology 2001; 121:1310–1319.
57. Cohn JA, Noone PG, Jowell PS. Idiopathic pancreatitis related CFTR: complex inheritance and identification of a modifier gene. J Invest Med 2002; 50:247S–255S.
58. Shwachman H, Lebenthal E, Khaw K. Recurrent acute pancreatitis in patients with cystic fibrosis with normal pancreatic enzymes. Pediatrics 1975; 55:86–95.
59. Moran A. Diagnosis screening and management of cystic fibrosis related diabetes. Curr Diabetes Rep 2002; 2:111–115.
60. Hardin D, Moran A. Diabetes mellitus in cystic fibrosis. Pediatr Endocrinol 1999; 28:787–801.

61. Rosenecker J, Eichler I, Kuhn L, Harms HK, von der Hardt H. Genetic determination of diabetes mellitus in patients with cystic fibrosis. J Pediatr 1995; 127:441–443.
62. Finkelstein SM, Wielinski CL, Elliot GR, et al. Diabetes mellitus associated with cystic fibrosis. J Pediatr 1998; 112:373–377.
63. Lanng S, Thorsteinsson B, Nerup J, Koch C. Influence of the development of diabetes mellitus on clinical status in patients with cystic fibrosis. Eur J Pediatr 1992; 151:684–687.
64. Cystic Fibrosis Foundation Registry. Annual Data Report. Bethesda, MD: Cystic Fibrosis Foundation; 1998.
65. Makie ADR, Thornton SJ, Edenborough FP. Cystic fibrosis related diabetes: Diabetes UK. Diabetic Med 2003; 20:425–436.
66. Ramsey BW, Farrell PM, Pencharz P. Nutritional assessment and management in cystic fibrosis: a consensus report. Am J Clin Nutr 1992; 55:108–116.
67. Koscik RL, Farrell PM, Kosorok MR, et al. Cognitive function of children with cystic fibrosis: deleterious effect of early malnutrition. Pediatrics 2004; 113:1549–1558.
68. Corey M, McLaughlin FJ, Williams M, Levison H. A comparison of survival growth and pulmonary function in patients with cystic fibrosis in Boston and Toronto. J Clin Epidemiol 1998; 41:583–591.
69. Lai HC, Corey M, Fitzsimmons S, Kosorok MR, Farrell PM. Comparison of growth status of patients with cystic fibrosis between the United States and Canada. Am J Clin Nutr 1999; 69:531–538.
70. Farrell PM, Kosorok MR, Laxova A, et al. Nutritional benefits of neonatal screening for cystic fibrosis. Wisconsin Cystic Fibrosis Neonatal Screening Study Group. N Engl J Med 1997; 337:963–969.
71. Lindermans J, Neijens HJ, Kerrebijn KF, Abaels J. Vitamin B_{12} absorption in cystic fibrosis. Acta Paediatr Scand 1984; 3:537–540.
72. Ahmed F, Murphy J, Wootton S, Jackson AA. Excessive faecal losses of vitamins A (retinol) in cystic fibrosis: Arch Dis Child 1990; 65:589–593.
73. Rayner RJ, Tyrell JC, Hiller EJ, et al. Night blindness and conjunctival xerosis caused by vitamin A deficiency in patients with cystic fibrosis. Arch Dis Child 1989; 64:1151–1156.
74. Duggan C, Collin AA, Agil A, Higgin L, Rifai N. Vitamin A status in acute exacerbations of cystic fibrosis: Am J Clin Nutr 1996; 64:635–639.
75. Feranchak AP, Sontag MK, Wagener JS, Hammond KB, Accurso FJ, Sokol RJ. Prospective long-term study of fat-soluble vitamin status in children with cystic fibrosis identified by newborn screen. J Pediatr 1999; 135: 601–610.
76. Farrell PM, Bieri JG, Frantantoni JF, Wood RE, di Saint'Agnese PA. The occurrence and effects on human vitamin E deficiencies. J Clin Invest 1977; 60:233–241.
77. Borowitz D, Baker RD, Stallings V. Concensus report on nutrition for pediatric patients with cystic fibrosis. J Pediatr Gastroenterol Nutr 2002; 35:246–259.
78. Cornelissen EAM, van Lieburg AF, Motobara K, van Oostrom CG. Vitamin K status in cystic fibrosis. Acta Paediatr 1992; 81:658–661.
79. Rashid M, Durie P, Andrew M, et al. Prevalence of vitamin K in cystic fibrosis. Am J Clin Nutr 1999; 70:378–382.
80. Blanchard RA, Furie BC, Jorgensen M, Kruger SF, Furie B. Vitamin dependent carboxylation dependent deficiency in liver disease. N Engl J Med 1981; 305:242–248.
81. Beker LT, Ahrens RA, Fink RJ, et al. Effect of vitamin K1 supplementation on vitamin K status in cystic fibrosis patients. J Pediatr Gastroenterol Nutr 1997; 24:512–517.
82. Keevil B, Rowlands D, Burton I, Webb AK. Assessment of iron status in cystic fibrosis patients. Ann Clin Biochem 2000; 37:662–665.
83. Krebs NF, Sontag M, Accurso F, Hambidge KM. Plasma zinc concentrations in young infants with cystic fibrosis. J Pediatr 1998; 133:761–764.
84. Krebs NF, Westcott JE, Arnold TD, et al. Abnormalities in zinc homeostasis in young infants with cystic fibrosis: Pediatr Res 2002; 48:256–261.
85. Best K, McCoy K, Gemma S, Disilvestro RA. Copper enzyme activities in cystic fibrosis before and after copper supplementation plus or minus zinc. Metabolism 2004; 53:37–41.
86. Solomons NW, Wagonfield JB, Rieger C. Some biochemical indices of nutrition in treated patients with cystic fibrosis. Am J Clin Nutr 1981; 34:462–474.
87. Farrell PM, Mischler EH, Engle MJ, Brown J, Lau SM. Fatty acid abnormalities in cystic fibrosis. Pediatr Res 1985; 19:104–109.
88. Roulet M, Frascarolo P, Rappas I, Pilet M. Essential fatty acid deficiency in well nourished young cystic patients. Eur J Pediatr 1997; 156:952–956.
89. Freedman SD, Blanco PG, Zaman MM, et al. Association of cystic fibrosis with abnormalities in fatty acid metabolism. N Engl J Med 2004; 350:560–569.
90. Freedman SD, Katz MH, Parker EM, Laposata M, Urman MY, Alvarez JG. A membrane lipid imbalance plays a role in the phenotypic expression of cystic fibrosis in $CFTR^{(-/-)}$ mice. Proc Natl Acad Sci USA 1999; 96:3995–4000.
91. Kawchak DA, Ahao H, Scanlin TF, Tomezsko JL, Cnaan A, Stallings JA. Longitudinal prospective analysis of dietary intake in children with cystic fibrosis. J Pediatr 1996; 129:119–129.
92. Walkowiak J, Przyslawski J. Five-year prospective analysis of dietary intake and clinical status in malnourished cystic fibrosis patients. J Hum Nutr Diet 2003; 16:225–231.
93. Vaisman N, Pencharz P, Corey M, Canny GJ, Hahn E. Energy expenditure of patients with cystic fibrosis. J Pediatr 1987; 111:496–500.
94. Tomezsko JL, Stallings VA, Kawchak DA, Goin JE, Diamond G, Scanlin TF. Energy expenditure and genotype of children with cystic fibrosis. Pediatr Res 1994; 35:451–460.
95. Powers SW, Patton SR. A comparison of nutrient intake between infants and toddlers with and without cystic fibrosis. J Am Diet Assoc 2003; 103:1620–1625.
96. Hankard R, Munck A, Navaro J. Nutriton and growth in cystic fibrosis. Horm Res 2002; 58(Suppl 1):16–20.
97. Hardin DS, Sy JP. Effects of grwoth hormone treatment in children with cystic fibrosis: the National Cooperative Growth Study Experience. J Pediatr 1997; 131: 565–569.
98. Steinkamp G, Demmelmair H, Ruhl-Bagheri I, von der Hardt H, Koletzko B. Energy supplements rich in linoleic acid improve body weight and essential fatty acid status of cystic fibrosis patients. J Pediatr Gastroenterol Nutr 2000; 318:418–423.
99. Van Egmond AW, Kosorok MR, Koscik R, Laxova A, Farrell PM. Effect of linoleic acid intake on growth of infants with cystic fibrosis. Am J Clin Nutr 1996; 63:746–752.
100. Neglia J, FitzSimmons S, Maisonneuve P, et al. and the Cystic Fibrosis and Cancer Study Group. The risk of cancer among patients with cystic fibrosis. N Engl J Med 1995; 332:494–499.

101. Feranchak AP. Hepatobiliary complications of cystic fibrosis. Curr Gastroenterol Rep 2004; 6:231–239.

102. Sokol RJ, Durie PR. Recommendations for management of liver and biliary tract disease in cystic fibrosis. Cystic Fibrosis Foundation Hepatobiliary Disease Consensus Group. J Pediatr Gastroenterol Nutr 1999; 28(Suppl 1):S1–S13.

103. Cystic Fibrosis Foundation. Patient Registry 1997, Annual Data Report. Bethesda, MD: Cystic Fibrosis Foundation; 1999.

104. Cohn JA, Strong TV, Picciotto MR, Nairn AC, Collins FS, Fitz JG. Localization of the cystic fibrosis transmembrane conductance regulator in human bile duct epithelial cells. Gastroenterology 1993; 105:1857–1864.

105. Grubman SA, Fang SL, Mulberg AE, et al. Correction of the cystic fibrosis defect by gene complementation in human intrahepatic biliary epithelial cell lines. Gastroenterology 1995; 108:584–592.

106. Colombo C, Battezzati PM, Strazzabosco M, Podda M. Liver and biliary problems in cystic fibrosis. Semin Liver Dis 1998;18:227–235.

107. Lepage G, Levy E, Ronco N, Smith L, Galeano N, Roy CC. Direct transesterification of plasma fatty acids for the diagnosis of essential fatty acid deficiency in cystic fibrosis. J Lipid Res 1989; 30:1483–1490.

108. Duthie A, Doherty DG, Daonaldson PT, et al. The major histocompatilbility complex influences the development of chronic liver disease in male children and young adults with cystic fibrosis. J Hepatol 1995; 23:532–537.

109. Friedman KJ, Ling SC, Macek M, et al. Complex multigenic inheritance influences the development of severe CF liver disease. Pediatr Pulmonol 2001; 22:340.

110. Narkewicz MR. Markers of cystic fibrosis-associated liver disease. J Pediatr Gastrenterol Nutr 2001; 32:421–422.

111. Roy CC, Weber AM, Morin CL, et al. Hepatobiliary disease in cystic fibrosis: a survey of current issues and concepts. J Pediatr Gastroenterol Nutr 1982; 1:469–478.

112. Gaskin KJ, Waters DL, Howman-Giles R, et al. Liver disease and common-bile-duct stenosis in cystic fibrosis. N Engl J Med 1988; 318:340–346.

113. Lenaerts CM, Lapierre C, Patriquin H, et al. Surveillance for cystic fibrosis-associated hepatobiliary disease: early ultrasound changes and predisposing factors. J Pediatr 2003; 143:343–350.

114. Lykavieris P, Bernard O, Hadchouel M. Neonatal cholestasis as the presenting feature in cystic fibrosis. Arch Dis Child 1996; 75:67–70.

115. Fridell JA, Bond GJ, Mazariegos GV, et al. Liver transplantation in children with cystic fibrosis: a long-term longitudinal review of a single center's experience. J Pediatr Surg 2003; 38:1152–1156.

116. Quillin S, Siegel M Rothbaum R. Hepatobilary sonography in cystic fibrosis. Pediatr Radiol 1993; 23:1–3.

117. Colombo C, Bertolini E, Assaisso ML, et al. Failure of usodeoxycholic acid to dissolve radiolucent gallstones in patients with cystic fibrosis. Acta Paediatr 1993; 82:562–565.

118. Sheth S, Shea JC, Bishop MD, et al. Increased prevalence of *CFTR* mutations and variants and decreased chloride secretion in primary sclerosing cholangitis. Hum Genet 2003; 113:286–292.

119. Caetecher JS, Jazrawi RP, Petroni ML, et al. Ursodeoxycholic acid in chronic liver disease. Gut 1991; 32:1061–1065.

120. van de Meeberg PC, Houwen RH, Sinaasappel M, et al. Low dose versus high-dose ursodeoxycholic acid in cystic fibrosis-related cholestatic liver disease: results of a randomized study with 1-year follow-up. Scand J Gastroenterol 1997; 32:369–373.

121. Nousia-Arvanitakis S, Fotoulaki M, Economou H, Xefteri M, Galli-Tsinopoulou A. Long-term prospective study of the effect of usodoxycholic acid on cystic fibrosis-related liver disease. J Clin Gastroenterol 2001; 32:324–328.

122. Parker HW. Congenital anomalies of the pancreas. In: Sivak MV, ed. Gastroenterologic Endoscopy. Philadelphia, PA: WB Saunders; 1987:770–779.

123. Freeny PC, Lawson TL. Embryology of the pancreas and biliary tract. In: Freeny PC, Lawson TL, eds. Radiology of the Pancreas. New York: Springer; 1982:98–144.

124. Moore KL. The Developing Human, 3rd edn. Philadelphia, PA: WB Saunders; 1980.

125. Kleisch WP. Anatomy of the pancreas: a study with special reference to the duct system. Arch Surg 1955; 71:795.

126. Kozu T, Sude K, Toki F. Panacreatic development and anatomical variation. Gastrointest Endosc Clin North Am 1995; 5:1–30.

127. Dawson W, Langman J. An anatomical–radiological study on the pancreatic duct pattern in man. Anat Rec 1961; 139:59–68.

128. Lehman GA, Sherman S. Pancreas divisum: diagnosis, clinical significance and management alternatives. Gastrointest Endosc Clin North Am 1995; 5:145–170.

129. Dawson W, Langman V. An anatomical–radiological sudy of the pancreatic duct pattern in man. Anat Rec 1961; 139:59.

130. Smanio T. Proposed nomenclature and classification of the human pancreatic ducts and duodenal papillae. Study based on 200 post mortems. Int Surg 1969; 52:125–141.

131. Sahel J, Cros RC, Bourry J, Sarles H. Clinico-pathological conditions associated with pancreas divisum. Digestion 1982; 23:1–8.

132. Delhaye M, Engelholm L, Cremer M. Pancreas divisum: congenital anatomic variant or anomaly. Gastroenterology 1985; 89:951–958.

133. Cotton PB. Congenital anomaly of pancreas divisum as cause of obstructive pain and pancreatitis. Gut 1980; 21:105–114.

134. Bret PM, Reinhold C, Taourel P, Guibaud L, Atri M, Barkun AN. Pancreas divisum: evaluation with MR cholangiopancreatography. Radiology 1996; 199:99–103.

135. Matos C, Metens T, Deviere J, Delhaye M, LeMoine O, Cremer M. Pancreas divisum: evaluation with secretin-enhanced magnetic resonance cholangiopancreatography. Gastrointest Endosc 2001; 53:728–733.

136. Matos C, Metens T, Deviere J, et al. Pancreatic duct: morphologic and functional evaluation with dynamic MR pancreatography after secretin stimulation. Radiology 1997; 203:435–441.

137. Manfredi R, Costamagna G, Brizi MG, et al. Severe chronic pancreatitis versus suspected pancreatic disease: dynamic MR cholangiopancreatography after secretin stimulation. Radiology 2000; 214:849–855.

138. Sugawa C, Walt AJ, Nunez DC, Masuyama H. Pancreas divisum: is it a normal anatomic variant? Am J Surg 1987; 153:62–67.

139. Burtin P, Person B, Charneau J, Boyer J. Pancreas divisum and pancreatitis: a coincidental association? Endoscopy 1991; 23:55–58.

140. Cotton PB. Congenital anomaly of pancreas divisum as cause of obstructive pain and pancreatitis. Gut 1980; 21:105–114.

141. Richter JM, Schapiro RH, Mulley AG, Warshaw AL. Association of pancreas divisum and pancreatitis and its treatment by sphincteroplasty of the accessory ampulla. Gastroenterology 1981; 81:1104–1110.

142. Bernard JP, Sahel J, Giovannini M, Sarles H. Pancreas divisum is a probable cause of acute pancreatitis: a report of 137 cases. Pancreas 1990; 5:248–254.

143. Bradley EL 3rd, Stephan RN. Accessory duct sphincteroplasty is preferred for long-term prevention of recurrent acute pancreatitis in patients with pancreas divisum. J Am Coll Surg 1996; 183:65–70.

144. Warshaw AL, Simeone JF, Schapiro RH. Evaluation and treatment of dominant dorsal duct syndrome. Am J Surg 1990; 159:59–64.

145. Richter JM, Schapiro RH, Mulley AG, Warshaw AL. Association of pancreas divisum and pancreatitis and its treatment by sphincteroplasty of the a accessory ampulla. Gastroenterology 1981; 81:1104–1110.

146. Ertan A. Long-term results after endoscopic pancreatic stent placement without pancreatic papillotomy in acute recurrent pancreatitis due to pancreas divisum. Gastrointest Endosc 2000; 52:9–14.

147. Coleman SD, Eisen GM, Troughton AB. Endoscopic treatment in pancreas divisum. Am J Gastroenterol 1994; 89:1152–1155.

148. Lans JI, Geenen JE, Johanson JF. Endoscopic therapy in patients with pancreas divisum and acute pancreatitis: a prospective, randomized, controlled clinical trial. Gastrointest Endosc 1992; 38:430–434.

149. Lehman GA, Sherman S, Nizi R. Pancreas divisum: results of minor papilla sphincterotomy. Gastrointest Endosc 1993; 39:1–8.

150. Delhaye M, Matos C, Deviere J. Acute relapsing pancreatitis: congenital variants, diagnosis, treatment, outcome. J Pancreas 2001; 2:373–381.

151. Guelrud M, Morera C, Rodriguez M, Prados JG, Jaen D. Normal and anomalous pancreaticobiliary union in children and adolescents. Gastrointest Endosc 1999; 50:189–193.

152. Misra SP, Dwivedi M. Pancreaticobiliary ductal union. Gut 1990; 31:1144–1149.

153. Sugiyama M, Atomi Y, Kuroda A. Pancreatic disorders associated with anomalous pancreaticobiliary junction. Surgery 1999; 126:492–497.

154. Guelrud M, Morera C, Rodriguez M, Jaen D, Pierre R. Sphincter of Oddi dysfunction in children with recurrent pancreatitis and anomalous pancreaticobiliary union: an etiologic concept. Gastrointest Endosc 1999; 50:194–199.

155. Sugiyama M, Atomi Y. Anomalous pancreaticobiliary junction without congenital choledochal cyst. Br J Surg 1998; 85:911–916.

156. Grendell JH, Ermak TH. Anatomy, histology, embriology, and developmental anomalies of the pancreas. In: Sleisenger & Fordtran's Gastrointestinal and Liver Disease. Philadelphia, PA: WB Saunders; 1998:761–771.

157. Milosavljevic T, Perisic V, Opric D, et al. Ectopic pancreas in the gastric wall. Arch Gastroenterohepatol 2000; 19:24–27.

158. Kopelman HR. The pancreas: congenital anomalies. In: Walker WA, Durie PR, Hamilton RJ, Walker-Smith JW, Watkins JB, eds. Pediatric Gastrointestinal Disease. St Louis, MI: Mosby; 1996:1427–1436.

159. Dolan RV, ReMine WH, Dockerty MB. The fate of heterotopic pancreatic tissue. Arch Surg 1974; 109:762–765.

160. Kilman W, Berk R. The spectrum of radiographic features of aberrant pancreatic rests involving the stomach. Radiology 1977; 123:291–296.

161. Matsushita M, Hajiro K, Okazaki K, Takakuwa H. Gastric aberrant pancreas: EUS analysis in comparison with the histology. Gastrointest Endosc 1999; 49:433–439.

162. Masi C, Benvenuti P, Freschi G, et al. Frequency and clinical significance of ectopic pancreas. Minerva Chir 1990; 45:5–10.

163. Maklouf HR, Almeida JL, Sobin LH. Carcinoma in jejunal pancreatic heterotopia. Arch Pathol Lab Med 1999; 123:707–711.

164. Pang LC. Pancreatic heterotopia: a reappraisal and clinicopathologic analysis of 32 cases. South Med J 1988; 81:1264–1275.

165. Glazer GM, Margulis AR. Annular pancreas: etiology and diagnosis using endoscopic retrograde cholangiopancreatography. Radiology 1979; 133:303–308.

166. Torfs CP, Christianson RE. Anomalies in Down syndrome individuals in a large population-based registry. Am J Med Genet 1998; 77:431–438.

167. Lemons JA, Ridenour R, Orshi EN. Congenital absence of the pancreas and intrauterine growth retardation. Pediatrics 1979; 64:255–257.

168. Stoffers DA, Zinkin NT, Stanojevic V, et al. Pancreatic agenesis attributable to a single nucleotide deletion in the human *IPF1* gene coding sequence. Nat Genet 1997; 15:106–110.

169. Herman TE, Siegal MJ. Polysplenia syndrome with congenital short pancreas. AJR Am J Roentgenol 1991; 156:799–800.

170. Park CM, Han JK, Kim TK, et al. Fat replacement with absence of acinar and ductal structure in the pancreatic body and tail. J Comput Assist Tomogr 2000; 24:893–895.

171. Shwachman H, Diamond LK, Oski FA, Khaw KT. The syndrome of pancreatic insufficiency and bone marrow dysfunction. J Pediatr 1964; 65:645–663.

172. Bodian M, Sheldon W, Lightwood R. Congenital hypoplasia of the exocrine pancereas. Acta Paediatr 1964; 53:282–293.

173. Berrocal T, Simon MJ, al-Assir I, et al. Shwachman–Diamond syndrome: clinical, radiological and sonographic aspects. Pediatr Radiol 1995; 25:289–292.

174. Mack DR, Forstner GG, Wilschanski M, Freedman MH, Durie PR. Shwachman syndrome: exocrine pancreatic dysfunction and variable phenotypic expression. Gastroenterology 1996; 111:1593–1602.

175. Ginzberg H, Shin J, Ellis L, et al. Shwachman syndrome: phenotypic manifestations of sibling sets and isolated cases in a large patient cohort are similar. J Pediatr 1999; 135:81–88.

176. Hsu JW, Vogelsang G, Jones RJ, Brodsky RA. Bone marrow transplantation in Shwachman–Diamond syndrome. Bone Marrow Transplant 2002; 30:255–258.

177. Welte K, Boxer LA. Severe chronic neutropenia: pathophysiology and therapy. Semin Hematol 1997; 34:267–278.

178. Boocock GR, Morrison JA, Popovic M, et al. Mutations in SBDS are associated with Shwachman–Diamond syndrome. Nat Genet 2003; 33:97–101.

179. Johanson AJ, Blizzard RM. A syndrome of congenital aplasia of the alae nasi, deafness, hypothyroidism, dwarfism, absent permanent teeth, and malabsorption. J Pediatr 1971; 79:982–987.

180. Sandu BK, Brueton MJ. Concurrent pancreatic and growth hormone insufficiency in Hohanson–Blizzard syndrome. J Pediatr Gastroenterol Nutr 1989; 9:535–538.

181. Pearson HA, Lobel, JS, Kocoshis SA, et al. A new syndrome of refractory sideroblastic anemia with vacuolization of marrow precursors and exocrine pancreatic dysfunction. J Pediatr 1979; 95:976–984.

182. Rotig A, Cormier V, Koll F, et al. Site-specific deletions of the mitochondrial genome in the Pearson marrow–pancreas syndrome. Genomics 1991; 10:502–504.

183. Turkel SB, Diehl EJ, Richmond JA. Necropsy findings in neonatal asphyxiating thoracic dystrophy. J Med Genet 1985; 22:112–118.

184. Witt H. Chronic pancreatitis and cystic fibrosis. Gut 2003; 52(Suppl 2):ii31–ii41.

Chapter 69
Pancreatitis

Kadakkal Radhakrishnan and James L. Sutphen

ACUTE AND CHRONIC PANCREATITIS

Pancreatitis affects both children and adults. It is difficult to estimate the true incidence and prevalence of pancreatitis in children because the pediatric literature is limited to a few series, and most of these series contain few patients.[1–4] Most large pediatric centers see an average of five to ten patients with acute pancreatitis each year. More cases of pancreatitis are now being diagnosed in children due to increased awareness among pediatricians about this clinical problem. Biliary tract disease and alcoholism are the two most common etiologic factors associated with pancreatitis in adults, whereas infection, trauma, multisystem disorders and congenital anomalies of the pancreatic duct are the most common causes of pancreatitis in children. In some children, there are no clear etiologic factors. Most children with pancreatitis have a single self-limiting episode; chronic pancreatitis is rare in this population. Recent advances in the genetics of hereditary pancreatitis and recurrent pancreatitis, and a better understanding of the pathogenesis and pathophysiology, will help us develop more effective treatments for pancreatitis in both children and adults.

Definition and classification

Acute pancreatitis is defined as an acute inflammatory process of the pancreas with variable involvement of other regional tissues or remote organ systems.[5,6] Unless findings from endoscopic retrograde cholangiopancreatography (ERCP) or computed tomography (CT) suggest chronicity, all episodes should be considered acute. The severity of the disease varies from mild to severe. In mild disease, there is minimal organ dysfunction and the pancreas recovers completely. Severe disease is characterized by multisystem organ failure or local complications such as necrosis, abscess and/or pseudocyst.

There is no clear consensus on the definition of chronic pancreatitis; the most accepted definitions are based on histologic changes. Chronic pancreatitis involves a chronic inflammatory process that irreversibly destroys the exocrine pancreatic tissue and subsequently leads to fibrosis and, in some patients, loss of endocrine pancreatic function.[5,7] Definitions have also been proposed based on ERCP and changes seen on ultrasonography and CT, but these findings and changes can take years to develop.

Chronic pancreatitis can be classified into three categories based on histologic changes:[5,8]

- *Chronic calcific pancreatitis* is associated with calcification and patchy inflammation.
- *Chronic obstructive pancreatitis* is seen in association with obstruction of the main pancreatic duct.
- *Chronic inflammatory pancreatitis* is characterized by fibrosis, mononuclear cell infiltrates and atrophy.

ACUTE PANCREATITIS

Pathogenesis

Exposure to a causal factor initiates a cascade of pathologic events that ultimately lead to acute pancreatitis.[9] Initially, trypsinogen is converted to trypsin in quantities that override the body's innate protective mechanisms.[10] Trypsin, in turn, activates certain pro-enzymes (e.g. trypsinogen) and inactive precursors of elastase, carboxypeptidase and phospholipase A_2. These active enzymes auto-digest the gland and further activate enzyme precursors. Under normal conditions, a small amount of trypsinogen is activated spontaneously and quickly inactivated by protective mechanisms. Some 20% of the trypsin that is secreted is inactivated by pancreatic secretory trypsin inhibitor.[11] Other protective mechanisms involve mesotrypsin, enzyme Y and trypsin itself, which splits and inactivates trypsin.[9] Antiproteases such as α_1-antitrypsin and α_2-macroglobulin may also play a protective role. The pancreatic enzymes are normally sequestered within the intracellular compartments during synthesis and transport; this prevents lysosomal hydrolases such as cathepsin B from activating trypsinogen, providing yet another protective mechanism. In addition, a small amount of activated zymogen is retained in the cellular acini, also preventing cell injury.

An intact cytoskeleton is required for secretion from the pancreatic acinar cell.[11] In animal experiments, hyperstimulation with cholecystokinin (CCK) or carbachol disrupts the apical cytoskeleton of the cells, leading to zymogen activation within the pancreatic acinar cells and thereby causing injury.[12] However, bombesin, a secretogog, leads to zymogen activation but does not disrupt the cytoskeleton, resulting in release of enzymes from the cells.[13] Whenever the pancreatic cells and interstitium are disrupted, pancreatic enzymes are discharged, thereby inducing interstitial edema and increasing the amount of pancreatic enzymes in the serum.

Several stimulatory pathways are believed to activate zymogens in the acinar cells. However, the auto-activation of trypsinogen and cathepsin B has received most attention.[14] It is unclear which of these mechanisms plays the

and includes the conditioning agents, immune suppressants, infections and graft *vs* host disease. Acute pancreatitis in varying severity is seen after solid organ transplant, including liver transplant.[39,69]

Metabolic

Acute pancreatitis is associated with a variety of metabolic disorders. These disorders are generally rare causes of pancreatitis in children and are listed in Table 69.1.

Hyperlipidemia Acute pancreatitis and hyperlipidemia have a well documented association. Types I, IV and V hyperlipoproteinemia are more commonly associated with acute pancreatitis.[70] Adults with hyperlipidemia have a 25% chance of developing pancreatitis, but this statistic is confounded by the fact that alcoholism, the leading cause of chronic pancreatitis in adults, is also associated with hyperlipidemia. Type V hyperlipidemia, the most prevalent type in adults, is associated with diabetes, obesity and hyperuricemia. Hyperlipidemia has been documented as a cause of pancreatitis in children,[58] and there has been a case report of familial lipoprotein lipase deficiency (type I) causing pancreatitis in a neonate.[71] It is important to test for hyperlipidemia during quiescent pancreatitis because increased lipid levels may be due to active pancreatitis and not represent a precursor condition.

Hypercalcemia Hypercalcemia is a well documented cause of pancreatitis in adults. Research suggests that calcium activates trypsinogen in the pancreatic parenchyma and is deposited in the pancreatic ducts.[72] Hyperparathyroidism accounts for 0.5% of all cases acute pancreatitis, and 0.23–1.5% of cases of hyperparathyroidism are associated with acute pancreatitis.[73] Rarely, pancreatitis occurs with other causes of hypercalcemia such as hypervitaminosis D, sarcoidosis, parenteral nutrition and metastatic bone disease.

Metabolic disorders Although generally rare, organic acidemias have been associated with acute pancreatitis.[74] Other metabolic disorders associated with pancreatitis include glycogen storage disease type I, carnitine palmitoyltransferase II deficiency, mitochondrial cytopathy and lactic acidosis. Metabolic crisis can trigger pancreatitis and vice versa. It is possible that some cases of idiopathic pancreatitis have an underlying metabolic disorder.

Malnutrition and refeeding In severe malnutrition the pancreatic glands atrophy; this compromises enzyme synthesis and secretion. Raised levels of cationic trypsin correlate with the severity of malnutrition and appear to reflect pancreatic damage.[75] Pancreatitis can be induced during vigorous refeeding in malnourished patients.[76] The same phenomenon has also been reported during refeeding of anorexic patients. Serum amylase levels may also rise when there is salivary gland inflammation associated with malnutrition.

Diabetes mellitus

Severe diabetic ketoacidosis has been associated with acute pancreatitis. In general, children with ketoacidosis complain of abdominal pain. The increased amylase concentration typically seen in these patients stems from the salivary glands.

Hereditary pancreatitis

Mutations in cationic trypsinogen and in the serine protease inhibitor Kazal type 1 (SPINK-1) are associated with hereditary pancreatitis. The first episode in these patients cannot be differentiated from any other cause of acute pancreatitis. Acute pancreatitis also occurs in patients with cystic fibrosis who are pancreas sufficient. These two topics are discussed in detail in the section on Chronic pancreatitis below.

Idiopathic

In 20–25% of children with acute pancreatitis, no etiologic factor can be identified. Unlike adults, children with idiopathic pancreatitis have a higher chance of recurrence. Some of these patients have been diagnosed with *CFTR* or cationic trypsinogen mutations. Further advancements in gene testing will help elucidate mechanisms of disease for these conditions.

Clinical presentation

Acute pancreatitis in children has a wide spectrum of presentations, which are often non-specific. The clinical course is usually mild (Table 69.3). A high index of suspicion is needed to make the diagnosis in some instances. Clinical features and biochemical abnormalities supported by imagining techniques are often needed to diagnose acute pancreatitis.

Children with acute pancreatitis often complain of epigastric and left upper quadrant pain and discomfort. On rare occasions, pain is absent. These patients also complain of anorexia, nausea and vomiting. Occasionally, the pain

	Common	Uncommon
Symptoms	Abdominal pain	Back pain
	Nausea	Dypsnea
	Vomiting	Altered sensorium or coma
	Anorexia	
Signs	Abdominal tenderness	Renal failure
	Low-grade fever	Hypotension
	Diminished or absent abdominal bowel sounds	Grey Turner's sign
	Abdominal distension	Cullen's sign
		Ascites
		Pleural effusion, predominantly left sided
		Fluid retention

Table 69.3 Signs and symptom of acute pancreatitis

radiates to the back and lower abdomen. Often, the pain and vomiting worsen after eating. The patient may appear acutely ill and may lie on the side curled in a knee–chest position. In children who are unable to express themselves verbally, irritability and listlessness with vomiting are usually the presenting symptoms. The diagnosis of pancreatitis should be considered in any child with the above clinical presentations. Pain and vomiting increase in severity during the initial 24–48 h of the attack and warrant hospitalization for fluid and electrolyte replacement. Otherwise, shock may occur and exacerbate the process greatly.

On physical examination, patients may appear completely asymptomatic or may have some degree of direct mid-abdominal, generalized or epigastric tenderness. They may have mild icterus, fever and tachycardia. The abdomen may be distended. Guarding and rebound tenderness may be present, suggesting peritonitis. Some patients may have tenderness posteriorly on the left, adjacent to the T12, L1 vertebrae. The bowel sounds are decreased or absent.

Severe acute pancreatitis is rare in children. In these children, jaundice, ascites and pleural effusion may occur. These children are severely ill with intractable nausea, vomiting and abdominal pain. The pancreas could be hemorrhagic or necrotic, and could transform into an abscess. Cullen's sign (bluish periumbilical discoloration) and Grey Turner's sign (bluish discoloration of the flanks) may be seen. Both are non-specific signs that can be seen with any intra-abdominal hemorrhage. The mortality rate associated with severe pancreatitis in adults ranges from 20% to 50%. The high mortality rates are secondary to shock, renal failure, infection, massive gastrointestinal bleeding and other causes. The classification system that is used to predict the outcome in adult patients with severe pancreatitis is generally not applicable to children.

Diagnosis

Initial evaluation

The initial evaluation should begin with a careful history with an eye towards possible etiologic factors such as a family history of any inherited conditions, medications and recent illnesses, trauma or procedures. The patient should be queried about any unexplained episodes of abdominal pain or vomiting. The clinical presentation varies from mild disease mimicking gastritis to severe disease mimicking acute abdomen or small bowel obstruction. Thus, acute pancreatitis should be considered in any child presenting with upper or diffuse abdominal pain or acute abdomen. Acute pancreatitis should also be considered in a child with unexplained vomiting. The first episode of recurrent pancreatitis in a child is often attributed to gastroenteritis. Gastroenteritis can cause dehydration, which may lead to a spurious mild increase in serum amylase levels that promptly disappears with rehydration.

The child who has renal disease with an increased creatinine level offers a special diagnostic challenge, because the concentration of pancreatic enzymes is often raised and peritonitis often occurs in children receiving ambulatory peritoneal dialysis. Serum amylase levels are seldom increased above 500 IU/l unless actual pancreatitis exists. Radiographic assessment of these patients with CT or ultrasonography may be necessary.

Laboratory investigations

There is no single 'gold standard' test to diagnose pancreatitis. A large number of tests are recommended; therefore, careful interpretation of the test results is required, along with a strong index of suspicion. The two most commonly used tests are determination of serum amylase and serum lipase levels.[77–79]

Amylase α-Amylase, which hydrolyzes the 1–4 glucosidic linkage in starch, is one of the most commonly used biochemical tests in the diagnosis of pancreatitis. This enzyme is synthesized in several organs, but the bulk of the production occurs in the pancreas and salivary glands. Small measurable amounts of amylase normally enter the circulation: 33–45% is from the pancreas and the rest comes mainly from the salivary glands.

Serum amylase levels rise within hours of inflammation of the pancreas and remain increased for 3–5 days. The specificity of the serum amylase assay is highest when the increase is at least 3-fold. A persistent increase suggests a local complication of the pancreas, such as a pseudocyst, pancreatic tumor or macroamylasemia. There is no correlation between the degree of increase in the serum level of amylase or other pancreatic enzymes and the severity of the pancreatic inflammation.

Although serum amylase is used to diagnose pancreatitis, both false-positive and false-negative results occur. About 20% of adults with acute pancreatitis have normal serum amylase levels.[80] Normal amylase levels usually indicate that the inflammation in the pancreas has resolved, but normal levels may be seen in half of the adults with alcoholic pancreatitis or biliary lithiasis (18%). Hemorrhagic or necrotizing pancreatitis may also be associated with normal amylase levels.

A long list of extrapancreatic conditions has been associated with hyperamylasemia, for instance diabetic ketoacidosis, salpingitis, acute abdominal emergencies, renal failure and in patients with burns (Table 69.4). The production of salivary amylase is increased in acute parotitis, trauma and salivary duct obstruction.

Fractionation of serum amylase isoenzymes into salivary and pancreatic enzymes may help to delineate the source of the amylase. Sternby et al.[77] reported a sensitivity of 90% and a specificity of 92% for pancreatic isoamylase in the diagnosis of acute pancreatitis. There is no evidence to suggest that the pancreatic isoamylase assay has a higher sensitivity and specificity than the conventional measurement of serum amylase and lipase.

Macroamylasemia is a benign condition in which the enzyme forms enzymatically active complexes that are too large for normal glomerular filtration.[81] Patients with this

Pancreatic amylase
Biliary obstruction
Bowel obstruction
Perforated duodenal ulcer
Acute appendicitis
Mesenteric ischemia or infarction
Peritonitis
Salivary amylase
Salivary: parotitis (mumps), trauma, surgery, salivary duct obstruction
Diabetic ketoacidosis
Anorexia nervosa, bulimia
Ovarian: malignancy, ruptured ecotpic pregnancy, cysts
Malignancy
Mixed or unknown
Renal failure
Head trauma
Burns
Postoperative
Macroamylasemia

Adapted from Werlin, 1999.[138]

Table 69.4 Non-pancreatic causes of hyperamylasemia in children

condition do not have pancreatitis. Macroamylasemia occurs in 1% of healthy people and in 2.5% of adults with hyperamylasemia. The diagnosis should be suspected when serum amylase levels are raised but all test results for pancreatitis are normal, including lipase levels and the urinary amylase : creatinine ratio. The urinary amylase : creatinine ratio has not proved to be of major diagnostic value except in the diagnosis macroamylasemia.

Lipase Improvements to the serum lipase assay have increased its specificity in acute pancreatitis, so that it is now probably more specific than the measurement of serum amylase concentration. The specificity of the test is increased when the serum lipase level is increased 3-fold. Lipase cleared by the kidney is reabsorbed by the tubules, and this keeps the lipase serum levels raised for up to 14 days.[82] The sensitivity of serum lipase assay is higher than that of serum amylase 24 h after the illness, and the overall sensitivity of serum lipase determination is between 85% and 95%.[78,82]

Other tests Although numerous tests have been evaluated for the diagnosis of acute pancreatitis, none has proven to be superior to the serum amylase and lipase assays. The tests that have been evaluated include serum pancreatic elastase, fecal elastase, phospholipase A_2, urinary trypsinogen, trypsinogen activation peptide (TAP) and pancreatitis-associated protein (PAP).[83,84] TAP is probably the earliest pancreatic enzyme to be detected in pancreatitis.

In adults, several tests have been shown to be useful in predicting the severity of pancreatitis, including C-reactive protein (CRP), phospholipase A_2, TAP, interleukin (IL) 6 and IL-8, trypsinogen 2, SPINK-1 and TNF-α receptor. At 48 h, CRP is the best available laboratory marker of severity, but IL-6 and -8, SPINK-1 and TNF-α receptor may be better predictors than CRP.[83,84] Trypsinogen 2 may be useful in diagnosing pancreatitis induced by ERCP.

Hypocalcemia is detected in about 30–50% of patients with pancreatitis, but usually causes no symptoms. Transient hypoglycemia is commonly seen in the initial phase of acute pancreatitis. Minor increases in serum bilirubin concentration may be seen secondary to compression of the intrapancreatic portion of common bile duct. A rise in unconjugated bilirubin should make one suspect obstruction to the bile duct, possibly choledocholithiasis. Serum aspartate amino transferase concentration is increased to the mild to moderate range in up to 50% of patients. Moderate hypoalbuminemia may be found, especially after replenishing the intravascular space with fluids.

Imaging in acute pancreatitis

Conventional radiography Conventional radiography has a limited role in the diagnosis of acute pancreatitis and has been surpassed by other imaging modalities. Nevertheless, some of the soft signs seen on plain abdominal radiography are worth mentioning. A sentinel loop is a distended small bowel loop adjacent to the pancreas. The colon cutoff sign shows air in the splenic or hepatic flexure with a paucity of air in the distal colon. These findings are not specific for pancreatitis. Calcifications in the pancreas indicate chronic pancreatitis. A barium upper gastrointestinal series may show the effects of pancreatic enlargement, but newer radiographic techniques have superseded this relatively insensitive and non-specific finding.

Sonography Sonography is the most frequently used investigative modality for pancreatitis in children because it does not require radiation and can be performed without sedation. Its usefulness is limited by poor image quality when air is present in the bowel overlying the pancreas. The findings of pancreatitis on ultrasonography include diffuse or local enlargement of the pancreas, poorly defined borders, decreased echogenicity, dilated pancreatic ducts and pseudocyst[84] (Fig. 69.3a). Ultrasonography is also helpful when evaluating the gallbladder for cholelithiasis or choledocholithiasis; both of these factors cause obstruction and pancreatitis. Percutaneous aspiration of a pancreatic pseudocyst can be done using ultrasonographic guidance.

Computed tomography Abdominal CT is generally used when sonography is technically difficult or more anatomic details are needed. It is a useful imaging modality in abdominal trauma, but sedation is required for young or frightened children. The findings seen on CT include diffuse enlargement of the pancreas, hemorrhage, necrosis, traumatic damage and complications such as pseudocyst (Figs 69.3b). A rapid bolus CT can identify areas of

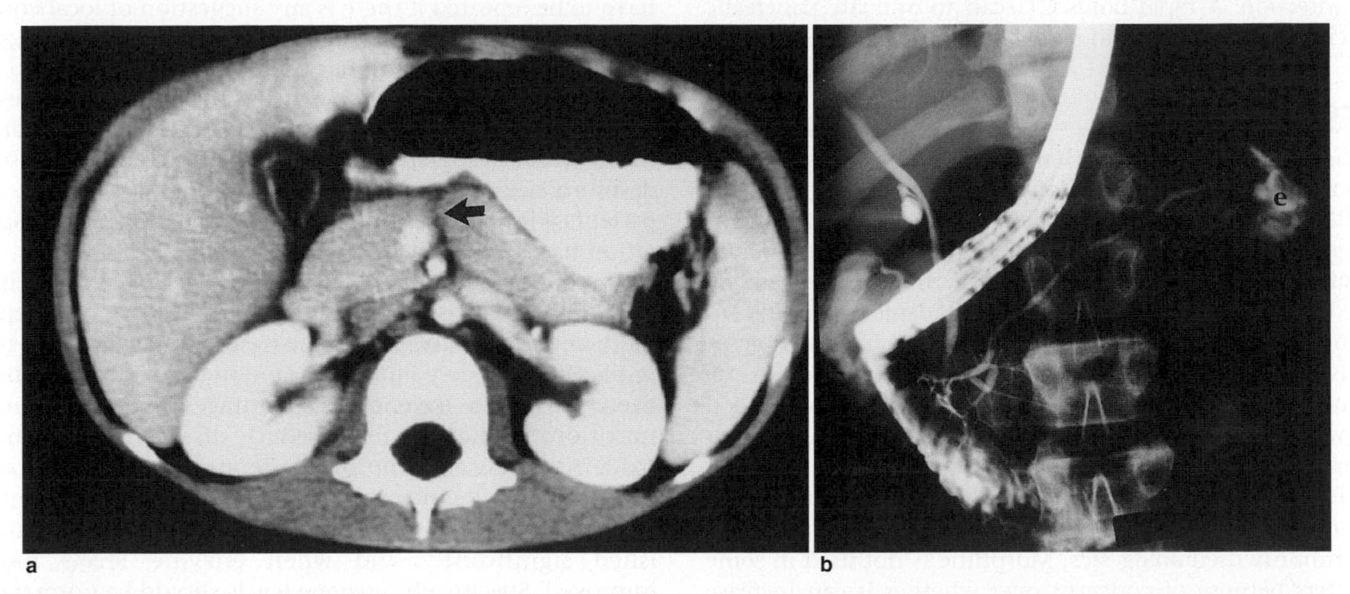

Figure 69.3: Ruptured duct. (**a**) Computed tomogram showing enlarged linear low attenuation area at the neck of the pancreas (arrow), compatible with a panceatic laceration. (**b**) ERCP examination showing extravasation at the pancreatic dut tail compatible with pancreatic duct laceration (**e**).

pancreatic necrosis. A normal CT finding does not exclude pancreatitis; up to 20% of patients with acute pancreatitis have normal CT findings.[85]

Magnetic resonance cholangiopancreatography Magnetic resonance cholangiopancreatography (MRCP) is a new non-invasive method of obtaining images of the pancreaticobiliary tract. Recent advances in MR technology and image quality have made it easy to diagnose structural abnormalities of the pancreaticobiliary tract in children.[86,87] In addition to being non-invasive, MRCP requires no radiation and has a lower complication rate than ERCP. The main disadvantage of MRCP is its poor ability to define the peripheral biliary tree.[87] The current indication for MRCP in acute pancreatitis is unsuccessful ERCP. It can also be used to create a road map for therapeutic intervention. A normal MRCP finding may obviate the need for more invasive studies. The authors almost always perform MRCP first when indicated, and ERCP only when the MRCP is inconclusive or when a papilotomy or stent might be necessary.

Endoscopic retrograde cholangiopancreatography This procedure has a more prevalent role in chronic than in acute pancreatitis, and it is a well accepted technique in children.[44–46] The indications for ERCP in children include recurrent pancreatitis (more than two discrete episodes of pancreatitis), prolonged episode of pancreatitis (more than 1 month), MRCP suggesting structural abnormalities, first episode of pancreatitis in a child with a family history of pancreatitis, pancreatitis following liver transplantation and pancreatitis associated with cystic fibrosis.[44–46, 88–90] It is also indicated in pancreatic trauma (see Fig. 69.2) and preoperative evaluation of non-resolving or enlarging pseudocyst or other pancreatic masses. It may also be used to extract gallstones and for endoscopic sphincterotomy.[89–91]

ERCP is currently the most sensitive and specific mode of investigation available to diagnose congenital abnormalities of the ducts such as choledochal cyst and pancreas divisum. It is also the only test that can diagnose sphincter of Oddi dysfunction (by sphincter manometry) and anomalous pancreatobiliary union.[64,65]

The complications of ERCP in children are similar to those in adults and include pancreatitis, cholangitis, post-procedure pain requiring analgesics, intramural dye injection, perforation, ileus and fever. Fewer than 5% of children develop complications. The procedure has been performed in children with acute pancreatitis and has been found to be safe.

Indicators of severity

There is no prognostic scoring system for evaluating the severity of pancreatitis in children. Ranson's score, which is used widely in adult patients, is not applicable to children. The severity can be assessed using results from clinical, laboratory and imaging tests. Certain clinical features are suggestive of severe disease: an alteration of sensorium, hypotension, renal failure, pulmonary edema, shock and hemorrhage.[91] A rupture or hemorrhage from the pancreatic pseudocyst and the presence of a pancreatic abscess increase the risk of mortality. Laboratory indicators of severe disease include hypocalcemia, hyperglycemia, hypoxemia, hypoproteinemia, elevated blood urea nitrogen (BUN) and creatinine levels, leukocytosis and a decreased hematocrit. Multiple other markers have been studied (discussed above), but the CRP level at 48 h is the one used most widely.[82,83] There appears to be a direct correlation between the amount of necrosis and the severity of the disease and susceptibility to infection. A rapid bolus CT scan to evaluate pancreatic necrosis may be useful in patients with severe disease.

Treatment

Mild disease Patients with mild pancreatitis are stable and do not exhibit any sign of local or systemic complications. Mild pancreatitis has an excellent prognosis. The treatment is mainly supportive and includes intravenous fluid resuscitation and pain management. In addition, enteral feedings are usually withheld. Fluid depletion occurs in pancreatitis from vomiting, third space loss and diaphoresis. It is generally believed that hypovolemia can worsen the pancreatic microcirculation by compromising the blood flow to the already inflamed pancreas. Most patients recover completely without any complications.

Pain management is an important aspect in the treatment of pancreatitis. Meperidine (Demerol) is one of the commonly used analgesics. Morphine is not used in some centers because of concerns over whether it can increase pressure inside the sphincter of Oddi. The current trend at some centers is to avoid using meperidine owing to concerns about seizures, especially in patients with renal disease. All opiates, including meperidine, have been shown to increase sphincter pressures intermittently, and small increases in basal sphincter pressures are seen with high doses of morphine.[91,92] There is no clear advantage of using meperidine over morphine, and no comparative study between the two agents has been published. A patient-controlled anesthesia pump is a reasonable option for chronic narcotic medication because it controls pain more effectively, lowers the total narcotic requirement and facilitates weaning. Dosing of the pain medications should be monitored carefully and the daily dosage adjusted according to the patient's ongoing needs.

Nasogastric tubes are not usually required in mild disease. The indications include intestinal or gastric ileus, or severe nausea or vomiting. There is no role for prophylactic antibiotics in mild disease. Refer to the section below for a discussion on enteral feeding and antibiotic use.

Severe disease In severe pancreatitis, patients show signs of hemodynamic instability and are at risk for systemic and local complications. These patients tend to have necrotizing rather than interstitial pancreatitis. The aim of treatment is to address local, systemic and septic complications while providing supportive care.

Supportive care is the mainstay of treatment in pancreatitis of any severity. This includes careful monitoring of vital signs, ensuring bedrest, providing adequate analgesia, and correcting intravascular fluid depletion and acidosis. Patients must be observed carefully for pulmonary complications, acute renal failure and metabolic complications such as hyperglycemia, acidosis and hypocalcemia. Chest and abdominal radiography, ultrasonography, CT and MRCP can be used to image the pancreas and are generally helpful. CT and MRCP should be ordered early because of the usual difficulties in scheduling and coordinating anesthesia for younger children. Imaging of the pancreas will have to be repeated if there is any suggestion of local complications. Pain control is an important part of management in pancreatitis, and has been discussed above.

Nasogastric decompression helps the pancreas to rest. The gastric contents are aspirated, so reducing pancreatic stimulation. Nasogastric decompression is commonly used despite a lack of clinical trials showing that it is helpful. In patients with vomiting or paralytic ileus, nasogastric aspiration has a proven role.

Nutritional support is important in patients with severe pancreatitis. Patients can be fed either nasojejunally or parenterally.[93] With the nasojejunal route, the tip is placed at or beyond the ligament of Trietz; this has been shown to have clear advantages over parenteral nutrition.[94,95] Enteral feeds reduce disease severity and oxidative stress and improve patient outcome. There are no specific guidelines about refeeding in these patients. In general, oral feeds can begin when the pain has diminished significantly and when enzyme levels have improved. Specifically, enzyme levels should be normal or near normal when the feedings begin. The lipase level is often disproportionately high, and does not necessarily need to be within normal limits for feedings to begin. Patients may be fed jejunally while still symptomatic as long as there is adequate motility and no clear exacerbation of the symptoms associated with the feedings. Intravenous feedings can be implemented at any time but are more expensive, increase the risk of infection and are difficult to utilize in a home setting. The use of intravenous lipids in acute pancreatitis is safe. The authors' center recommends a low-fat diet when the enteral route is used, to reduce pancreatic stimulation.

Infection is probably the leading cause of death in patients with severe pancreatitis. Bacterial translocation has been shown to occur in severe pancreatitis.[27] Early use of antibiotics may prevent infection and multiorgan failure.[96] Some studies have found early use of antibiotics to be helpful in patients with severe disease, especially in those with necrotizing pancreatitis, although one recent study has questioned the use of antibiotics in pancreatitis.[96, 97]

Several antiproteases have been used in animal and human studies to prevent the progression of pancreatitis. Aprotinin and gabexate mesilate reduced injury in experimental pancreatitis, although there was no clear benefit in human trials.[98] Lexipafant, an inhibitor of platelet-activating factor, showed promise in preventing multiorgan failure in small trials, but the results of major trials have not been conclusive.[99,100]

Some researchers have attempted to suppress pancreatic secretions with glucagons, somatastain and octreotide. Octreotide has been used most commonly, but several trials – including one large German multicenter trial – have not shown any major clinical benefits.[101]

Surgery

Indications for surgery in acute pancreatitis are controversial. Suggested indications include infected pancreatic necrosis and traumatic pancreatitis with ductal rupture. Relative surgical indications include persistent pancreatitis despite optimal medical therapy, clinical deterioration with multiorgan failure, and sterile pancreatic necrosis involving more than 50% of the gland. Improved imaging techniques have reduced the need for diagnostic laparotomy in acute pancreatitis.

In adults with severe necrotic pancreatitis, therapeutic surgery has been advocated to remove necrotic tissue in and around the pancreas and to remove infected tissue.[102] The belief is that removal of the necrotic or infected tissue improves survival in these patients. The criteria for selection of patients are not clear, however. In one study, patients who underwent surgery 2 weeks or more after the onset of acute pancreatitis had a lower mortality rate than those who had the operation in the 2 weeks immediately after the attack.[103] The surgical experience in children with severe pancreatitis is limited, and the advantages of therapeutic surgery are unclear. Endoscopic stone removal is preferred over surgery in the treatment of most cases of biliary pancreatitis, followed by elective cholecystectomy after the acute episode resolves.

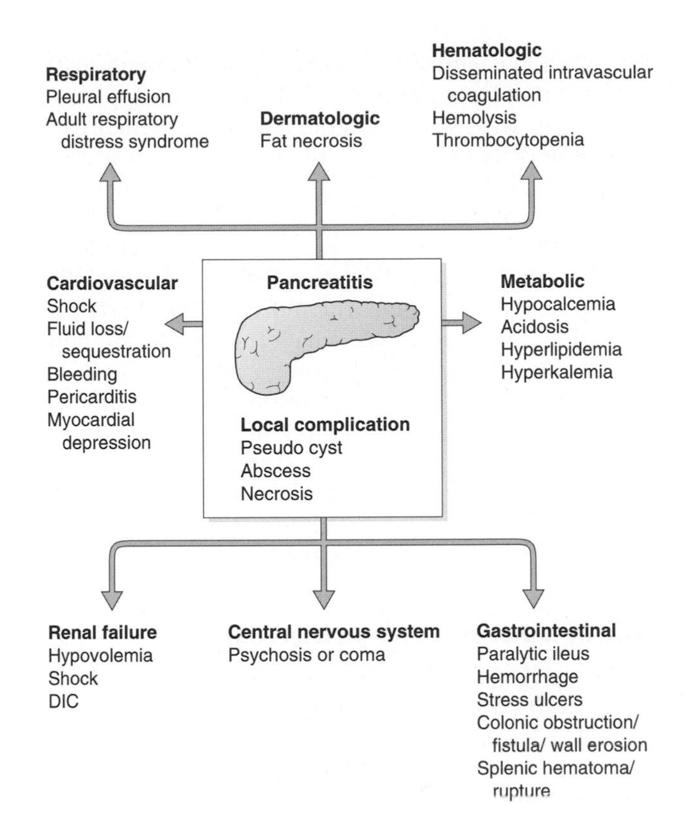

Figure 69.4: Complications of acute pancreatitis.

Complications

Systemic complications

Systemic complications (Fig. 69.4) are uncommon in children. The metabolic changes associated with pancreatitis include hypocalcemia, hyperglycemia, hyperlipidemia, acidosis and hyperkalemia. These metabolic changes are due to organ system failure. Circulatory failure occurs secondary to fluid loss from emesis and third space loss, bleeding from disseminated intravascular coagulation, sepsis and pericarditis. Renal failure may be seen secondary to hypovolemia, shock and disseminated intravascular coagulopathy. Respiratory failure secondary to adult respiratory distress syndrome is seen in adults, and pleural effusion (left sided or bilateral) can occur in pancreatitis. Gastrointestinal complications include paralytic ileus, hemorrhage, gastritis, duodenitis and stress ulcers. Other complications have been reported as well, including obstruction at the splenic flexure due to edema, fistula and hemorrhage as a result of colonic wall erosion.[104] Rarely, significant intra-abdominal hemorrhage has been seen secondary to erosion of the splenic or gastroduodenal artery. Splenic hematoma, splenic rupture and splenic vein thrombosis have also been reported with acute pancreatitis.[105] Subcutaneous fat necrosis is rare in acute pancreatitis.[106]

Local complications

Pseudocyst is usually a local sequela of necrotic pancreatitis and is generally uncommon. These cysts consist of fluid collections in the lesser sac of the peritoneum; they can enlarge and expand in any direction. A pseudocyst is suspected when an acute episode fails to resolve, when an abdominal mass develops after an episode of pancreatitis or when pancreatitis recurs after clinical improvement. Clinically, the patient presents with pain, nausea, vomiting and jaundice. Ultrasonography is the most useful investigation, and can be used for serial follow-up. CT (Fig. 69.5) and ERCP also have a diagnostic role. Sequential imaging studies have shown that pseudocysts are more common than previously thought; most remain asymptomatic and resolve without intervention.

Infection, hemorrhage and rupture are complications associated with pseudocyst. Complications are not common in children.[107] Infection of a pseudocyst is generally rare and should be suspected when the patient presents

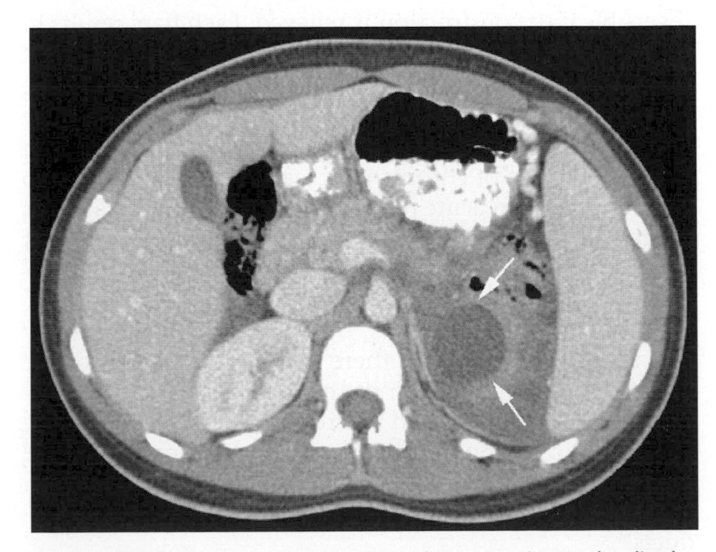

Figure 69.5: Pseudocyst (indicated by white arrows) near the distal body and tail of the pancreas in a 14-year-old girl with pancreatitis.

with high fever, chills and leukocytosis. Patients with a pseudocyst that has ruptured into the peritoneal space generally present with signs of acute abdomen, which can be fatal. Pseudocysts rarely erode blood vessels causing hemorrhage. When the hemorrhage does occur, it may manifest as rapid enlargement of a previously diagnosed cyst, gastrointestinal hemorrhage or, very rarely, direct bleeding into the peritoneum resulting in massive hemorrhage.

Most pseudocysts resolve in children without any active intervention.[108] Pseudocysts smaller than 4 cm almost always resolve spontaneously. Some cysts erode and drain into the stomach or colon, and resolve without any complications. Symptomatic cysts may be drained endoscopically, radiologically or surgically.[108,109] Pseudocysts should be allowed to mature for 4–6 weeks if surgery is required. In children, this duration can be extended further if the child is asymptomatic and the cyst is stable or decreasing in size.

Clinical course and prognosis

The clinical course of acute pancreatitis varies from very mild disease that is indistinguishable from gastritis to fulminant disease with severe systemic manifestation. Severe disease in adults is associated with a mortality rate of 15–50%, but the overall reported mortality rate is 5–10%. There are no accurate data for mortality in children. A 22% fatality rate was noted in one study (13 of 61), but the authors were from a tertiary care center and therefore the study could have suffered from referral bias.[1] In general, the overall mortality rate in children is probably lower than that for adults. The disease tends to run a milder course in children, and systemic complications are rare.

CHRONIC PANCREATITIS

In chronic pancreatitis there is continuous destruction of the pancreatic gland resulting in irreversible scarring of the acinar and ductal cells. The exception is chronic obstructive pancreatitis, where some or all changes may be reversible if the obstruction is relieved. Each flare results in further damage and eventually leads to exocrine and endocrine dysfunction. The pancreas generally has a large reserve capacity. About 90% of the gland must be destroyed before clinical signs of pancreatic dysfunction occur. A flare-up of chronic pancreatitis may be difficult to differentiate from acute pancreatitis because the symptoms of chronic pancreatitis sometimes do not cause the patient to seek medical attention until signs of pancreatic dysfunction or diabetes occur for the first time.

With chronic pancreatitis, the disease is initially patchy and focal, and eventually there is complete fibrosis of the gland. There is infiltration of the glandular tissue by lymphocytes, plasma cells and macrophages, in contrast to the neutrophilic response that occurs in acute pancreatitis.[24] Pancreatic ducts show fibrosis, stricture and dilation. Calcification may be seen in the gland and within the ducts.

Pathophysiology

The pathophysiology of chronic pancreatitis is not known completely. The two main forms of chronic pancreatitis are calcific and obstructive, and both are rare in children. Some 95% of adults with chronic calcific pancreatitis are chronic alcohol abusers. Chronic alcohol abuse leads to the secretion of low-volume pancreatic juice, which is high in protein and low in bicarbonate. This may lead to precipitation of protein in the duct with secondary calcification.

Hereditary pancreatitis, tropical pancreatitis, idiopathic pancreatitis and, in adults, alcoholic pancreatitis are associated with pancreatic ductal stones. Lithostatine is a protein that is secreted into the pancreatic duct and inhibits calcium carbonate precipitation. Lithostatine levels are diminished in patients with alcoholic and calcific chronic pancreatitis, but the role of this protein in inhibiting pancreatic calculi is controversial.[110] GP-2 (glycosyl phosphatidyl inositol) is another compound that is secreted into the duct in response to inflammation. It readily precipitates, thereby facilitating the formation of calculi.[111] The role this compound plays in pancreatitis is not clear, however. Toxins such as alcohol can induce chronic pancreatitis in adults. Repeated episodes of acute pancreatitis that causes cellular damage in these patients will eventually lead to chronic pancreatitis.

Obstruction of the pancreatic duct from a congenital anomaly or acquired condition such as a tumor, fibrosis or stricture can cause pancreatitis. The pancreas in these patients is inflamed and may be replaced with fibrous tissue, but the ductal system remains intact or is amenable to dilation. Calcifications and protein plug formation in these patients are rare. Deficiency of antioxidants and/or increased free radicals may contribute to the injury and progression of the disease in chronic pancreatitis.[112]

CFTR mutations have been associated with chronic pancreatitis, and some patients with idiopathic chronic pancreatitis have been diagnosed later with mutations in the *CFTR* gene.[113,114] The lack of CFTR in the ductal apical cell membrane prevents alkalization and inspissation, and increases the viscosity of the pancreatic secretion. This can cause stasis and pancreatic enzyme activation. Functional mutations in the cationic trypsinogen gene lead to enzyme activation and destruction of the pancreatic acini and eventual fibrosis.[21–23] α_1-Antitrypsin is of interest in chronic pancreatitis because it may prevent auto-digestion of the pancreas by inhibiting protease activity. Current evidence does not favor the theory that α_1-antitrypsin mutations cause chronic pancreatitis.[112]

Etiology (Table 69.5)

Chronic calcific pancreatitis

Hereditary pancreatitis Hereditary pancreatitis is a genetic condition first described in 1952. The cationic trypsinogen gene mutation – also referred to as serine protease 1 (*PRSS1*) – is a well recognized cause of this

Obstructive
• Congenital ductal anomalies Pancreas divisum Choledochal cyst Stricture • Trauma • Sclerosing cholangitis • Idiopathic fibrosing cholangitis • Autoimmune pancreatitis • Secondary to other autoimmune disorders
Calcific
• Hereditary or genetic causes of pancreatitis Cationic trypsin mutation *SPINK1* *CFTR* mutations ?Mesotrypsin mutation ?Anionic trypsin mutation • Tropical pancreatitis • Hyperlipidemia • Hypercalcemia • Organic acidemias
Miscellaneous
• Idiopathic • Mitochondrial cytopathy • Inflammatory bowel disease
Modified from Werlin, 1999.[138]

Table 69.5 Etiology of chronic pancreatitis in children

condition. This condition has an 80% penetrance rate and variable expressivity, and is the second most common cause of hereditary chronic pancreatitis. Several groups[115] have mapped the cationic trypsinogen gene to chromosome 7q35. R112H appears to be the most prevalent mutation worldwide. The other mutations include N29I and A16V. These mutations are associated with a gain in function of the trypsinogen molecule, causing activation to trypsin and eventually, pancreatitis.

Symptoms usually begin at 10–12 years of age, and up to 75% of patients are symptomatic by 20 years of age. There is usually a positive family history. The initial presentation is similar to that of acute pancreatitis. Severe hemorrhagic pancreatitis, although rare, can occur with the initial episodes. Patients with hereditary pancreatitis typically experience recurrent episodes of pancreatitis, each lasting 4–8 days. Patients are generally well for intervals of months to years between episodes, but may experience recurrent abdominal pain. Each episode is associated with further damage to the pancreas. Amylase and lipase levels may remain normal even during each episode as chronicity develops. The pancreas eventually becomes fibrotic, calcified and shrunken. There is a long-term risk of diabetes and pancreatic adenocarcinoma.

SPINK-1, also known as pancreatic secretory trypsin inhibitor, is a specific inactivator of intrapancreatic trypsin activity.[115] SPINK-1 inhibits up to 20% of the trypsin activity in the pancreas. This protein is also synthesized in the liver, lung, kidney, ovary and breast. It occurs as an acute-phase reactant and may protect the gastric mucosa from excessive digestion and promote mucosal repair after injury. This gene has been localized to chromosome 5, and N34S is the most common mutation that has been identified. In one series, 22 of 96 patients had *SPINK1* mutations; other series have confirmed this high frequency.[115–117] Approximately 1% of the general population is heterozygous for the N34S mutation, and 25–45% of patients with idiopathic chronic pancreatitis carry this mutation on at least one allele. This mutation causes chronic pancreatitis in an autosomal recessive pattern, a multigenetic (combination of *SPINK1* and yet unidentified genes) pattern and an autosomal dominant pattern. A positive family history is generally absent.

Other candidate genes are being investigated. A locus at short arm of chromosome 12 may be associated with pancreatitis. Other possible genes include the gene for anionic trypsinogen and mesotrypsinogen. Mesotrypsin is an inhibitor of trypsin and is itself activated by trypsin. Pancreatic stone protein or lithostathine may play a role in the etiology of chronic pancreatitis.

Cystic fibrosis Between 20% and 40% of patients with idiopathic chronic pancreatitis may eventually be found to be compound heterozygotes for *CFTR* mutations.[113] The *CFTR* gene is expressed in the ductal tissue of the pancreas.[118] *CFTR* genotypes associated with milder impairment of CFTR function (less than 10% of function) cause pancreatitis and a congenital absence of the vas deferens. Evidence indicates that idiopathic chronic pancreatitis is closely associated with the compound heterozygote *CFTR* (one mild and one severe mutation) genotype. These patients exhibit abnormal CFTR function in their nasal mucosa. This makes it likely that the CFTR function would be abnormal in other tissues where the gene is expressed, such as the pancreatic ductal tissue.[114] Chronic pancreatitis may also be caused by two mild mutations or a combination of *CFTR* mutation and other gene mutations.[113,114,119]

More than 1000 mutations have been described in the *CFTR* gene. The most common mutation that causes severe reduction in *CFTR* expression is the deltaF508. By contrast, the allele most commonly responsible for a mild loss of CFTR function is an abnormally short polythymidine tract (5T), causing abnormal splicing between the eighth and ninth exons.[118] Three variants seen at the splice junction are 5T, 7T and 9T. Two major studies demonstrated that the frequency of *CFTR* mutations was four to six times higher and the frequency of 5T allele mutations were twice as high in patients with idiopathic chronic pancreatitis.[114,120] More comprehensive gene testing may identify compound heterozygotes in patients with idiopathic chronic pancreatitis who are now considered carriers.

Tropical chronic pancreatitis This is a juvenile form of chronic calcific pancreatitis that is seen almost exclusively in developing tropical countries. Some of the features of this disorder are young age of onset, an accelerated disease course causing steatorrhea or diabetes, the presence of large intraductal calculi and a high susceptibility to pancreatic cancer.[118] Diabetes in these patients is severe but ketosis is rare, and most patients need insulin. Most of these patients are malnourished, and micronutrient deficiency may have a role in the pathogenesis of this condition. Associations between *SPINKl* mutations[121] – and to a lesser extent *CFTR* mutations[122] – have been reported in this disorder. Consumption of cassava, a tuber, was thought to have an etiologic factor, but this hypothesis lacks evidence.

Metabolic Patients with triglyceride levels of 1000 mg/dl may develop chronic pancreatitis. About 30% of cases of type I hyperlipidemia, 30–40% of type V and 15% of type IV may be associated with pancreatitis.[70] Because patients with acute pancreatitis tend to have raised triglyceride levels, the levels have to be remeasured after the acute episode. Chronic pancreatitis may also be associated with organic acidemias and hypercalcemia.

Chronic obstructive pancreatitis

Pancreas divisum The embryologic basis and incidence of this pancreatic anomaly have been discussed above. The clinical relevance of this anomaly remains controversial. The duct of Santorini, which becomes the main draining duct in patients with this condition, may become obstructed, leading to pancreatitis. The consensus is that this disorder may be associated with chronic pancreatitis. *CFTR* mutations may also be associated with pancreatitis in pancreas divisum.[118] The diagnosis can be made by MRCP or ERCP (Fig. 69.6). The management of pancreas divisum associated with chronic pancreatitis is controversial. Endoscopic sphincterotomy or surgical sphincteroplasty may be beneficial in selected groups of patients. Endoscopic placement of stents into the minor papilla may help some patients.

Idiopathic fibrosing pancreatitis This is a rare cause of chronic pancreatitis; just over 40 cases have been reported in the literature. Patients usually present with abdominal pain or obstructive jaundice, the latter of which is caused by the head of the pancreas blocking the common bile duct.[123] The gland is diffusely infiltrated by fibrous tissue, and inflammation may or may not be present. Mutations in the *PRSS1*, *SPINK1* and *CTFR*-5T genotype may be associated with this condition.

Abdominal trauma Unsuspected ductal damage after abdominal trauma can lead to stricture formation, chronic pancreatitis and pseudocyst formation.[124] Abdominal trauma is usually associated with a self-limiting acute pancreatitis.

Congenital anomalies A few congenital anomalies other than pancreas divisum have been associated with chronic pancreatitis. These include choledochal cyst, pancreatic ductal duplication and anomalous pancreaticobiliary union.

Immunologic Autoimmune pancreatitis has been recognized as a cause of chronic pancreatitis, and is characterized by ductal and periductal infiltration by lymphocytes, plasma cells and granulocytes.[125] The disorder can be primary, where it is limited to the pancreas, or secondary and associated with other autoimmune disorders such as Sjögren's disease or lupus. Irregular narrowing of the pancreatic duct and a diffuse enlargement of the pancreas are common. Autoimmune pancreatitis is associated with hypergammaglobulinemia, which responds favorably to steroids.[126] Sclerosing cholangitis has been associated with chronic pancreatitis.[127] The underlying mechanism causing pancreatitis is not clear, but it is believed to be due to obstruction of the common ductal channels.

Idiopathic The data on this group in children are not clear, but it is assumed that idiopathic pancreatitis accounts for one-third of all cases of chronic pancreatitis.

Clinical presentation and course

Patients commonly present with repeated bouts of pancreatitis. Chronic abdominal pain may be the only manifestation in some patients; acute episodes are absent in this group. In some, the onset is insidious and pain is absent or negligible. These patients present with diabetes, malabsorption or obstructive jaundice of undetermined etiology.

Pain is the major cause of morbidity in chronic pancreatitis. The intensity and frequency of pain improves in most patients with the duration of the disease. The improvement in pain is believed to be secondary to the glands 'burning out' from the chronic inflammation. This generally coincides with exocrine and endocrine pancreatic insufficiency and, in some patients, intrapancreatic calcifications. It may take 10–20 years for the glands to 'burn out', but the time course is generally variable.

The pancreas generally has a great reserve capacity, and exocrine pancreatic failure does not manifest until approximately 98% of the reserve capacity is lost. Patients generally present with hyperphagia to compensate for the gastrointestinal malabsorptive losses and secondary growth failure. These patients have bulky, malodorous and greasy stools, and frequently complain of abdominal discomfort after eating. Because the pancreas can no longer digest carbohydrates, the production of salivary amylase and intestinal brush border enzymes increases. Patients with chronic pancreatitis develop severe malabsorption of protein and fat. Some fat digestion occurs with the help of lingual lipase. Often, protein maldigestion is the most prominent deficiency because there are no compensatory non-pancreatic protein digestion pathways with the exception of pepsin. Thus, there is a pronounced kwashiorkor flavor to pancreatic insufficiency. Biochemical and clinical deficiencies of fat-soluble vitamins and essential fatty acids

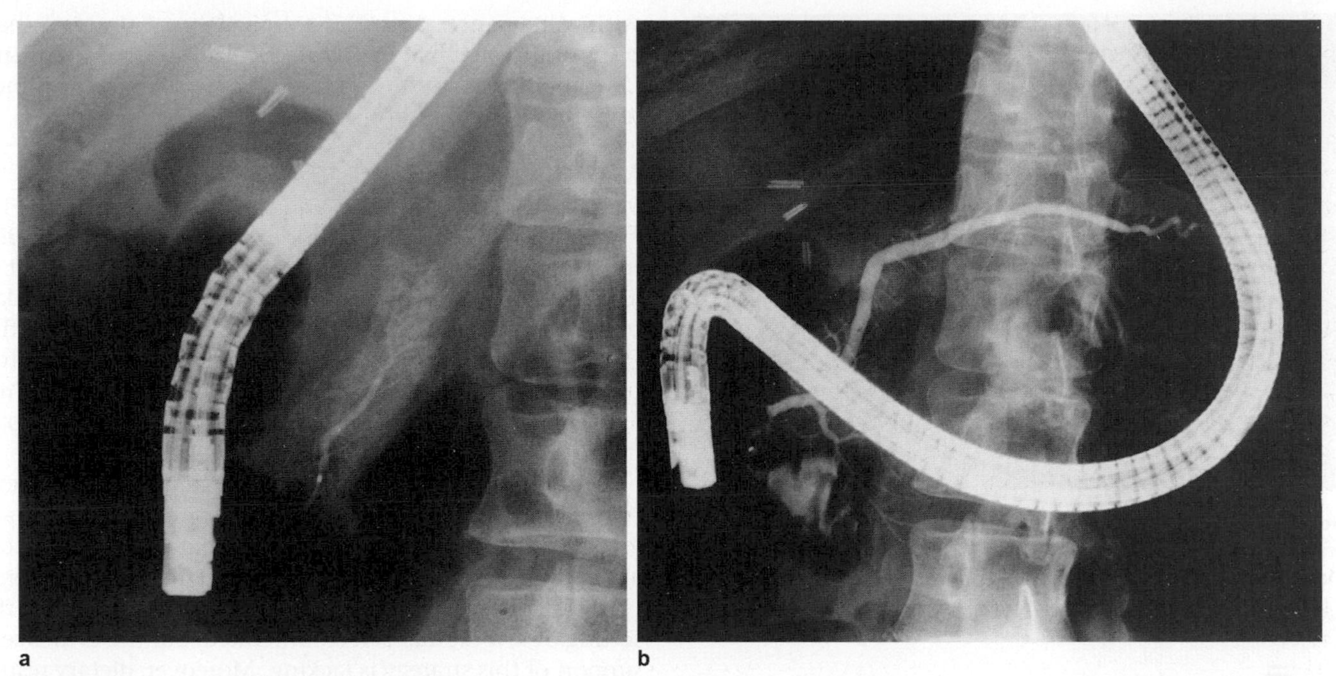

Figure 69.6: ERCP in pancreas divisum. (**a**) Injection into the major papilla (Wirsung) fills only the ventral pancreas. (**b**) In the same patient, injection into the minor papilla (Santorini) fills the dorsal pancreatic duct.

may develop in these patients. Biochemical evidence of vitamin B_{12} deficiency secondary to reduced degradation of cobalamin R binding protein complex by the pancreatic proteases may be seen. A reduced bile acid pool due to increased fecal loss secondary to steatorrhea is also seen in patients with chronic pancreatitis, which increases the lithogenicity of the bile. A loss of endocrine pancreatic function leads to diabetes. This complication is generally delayed until adulthood or adolescence. Diabetic ketoacidosis is generally rare.

Diagnosis

A diagnosis of chronic pancreatitis can be made when (1) a patient presents with acute or recurrent episodes of pancreatitis and (2) the imaging study demonstrates signs of chronicity. The diagnosis is more difficult in patients who have painless disease or mild symptoms. Poor growth and malnutrition may be seen in patients with exocrine dysfunction and malabsorption. There are no specific physical findings. Clinical signs of fat-soluble vitamins deficiency are rare.

Laboratory studies

Routine laboratory results are generally normal in patients with chronic pancreatitis, with the exception of serum amylase and lipase levels. Glucose intolerance, hypoalbuminemia, deficiency of fat-soluble vitamins and/or raised liver function test results may be seen late in the disease. Serum amylase and lipase levels may eventually normalize in chronic pancreatitis when sufficient pancreatic mass is lost. However, early in the disease, patients present with bouts of acute pancreatitis with increased enzyme levels, and those with a pseudocyst have persistently raised amylase and lipase levels. Once a diagnosis of chronic pancreatitis is established, patients should be followed up based on their symptoms and not on their enzyme levels.

Pancreatic function tests Pancreatic function tests, both direct and indirect, are discussed in Chapter 67. Invasive tests are normally not required, especially when there is clinical evidence and stool studies that suggest malabsorption along with radiologic signs of pancreatic calcification. In patients with suspected chronic pancreatitis, the need for invasive testing of pancreatic function is controversial.

Radiology

Calcifications in the pancreas on CT or plain radiography of the abdomen confirm the diagnosis of chronic pancreatitis. Abdominal CT may also show a dilated pancreatic duct (Fig. 69.7). MRCP is useful in defining the anatomy of the pancreatic duct and may obviate the need for ERCP in some patients (Fig. 69.8). Secretin MRCP may increase the sensitivity of the study.[128]

Endoscopic retrograde cholangiopancreatography This procedure plays an important role in the diagnosis and management of chronic pancreatitis. It is indicated in patients who are newly diagnosed with chronic pancreatitis and in the diagnosis of congenital or structural abnormalities of the pancreatic or biliary tree. In early disease, the ERCP findings may be normal. In advanced disease, however, the ducts appear beaded with narrowing and

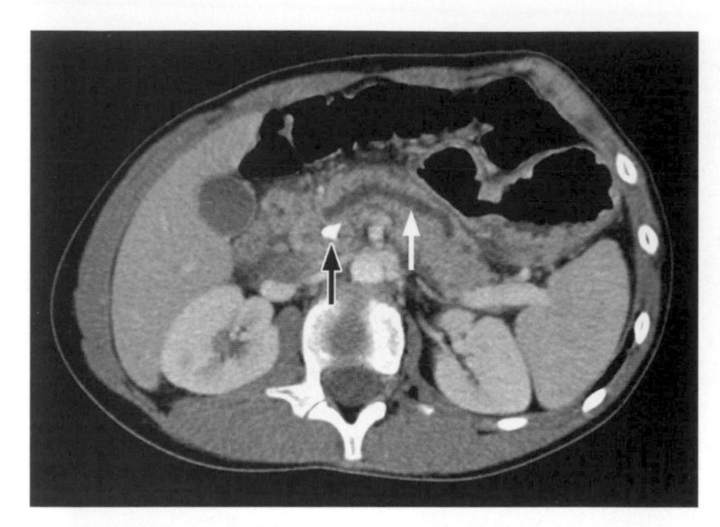

Figure 69.7: Chronic pancreatitis. Computed tomogram showing calcification in the head of the pancreas (black arrow) and dilated pancreatic duct (white arrow) in a 12-year-old patient. (Courtesy of Dr. Janet Reid.)

dilation. This procedure may also be used for therapeutic intervention such as stricture dilation, stone extraction, sphincterotomy and stent insertion. Preoperative ERCP also helps the surgeon to define the anatomy of the ductal system and evaluate surgically correctable lesions.

Treatment

Exacerbations of chronic pancreatitis are severe in the initial phase of the disease but become milder as the disease progresses. Flare-ups should be treated like those associated with acute pancreatitis; these management strategies have been outlined above in the section on Acute pancreatitis. Uncomplicated chronic pancreatitis is usually treated medically.

Management of pain

Pain can be debilitating in chronic pancreatitis. The etiopathogenesis is multifactorial and complex. According to the pancreatic compartment theory, pain is caused by an increase in interstitial and ductal pressures, secondary to a chronic fibrosing reaction. The neural inflammation theory explains pain based on a chronic fibro-inflammatory process that affects the visceral pancreatic nerves, which are abundant in the pancreatic parenchyma and peripancreatic tissue.

Because eating can exacerbate pain, many patients reduce their food intake, which leads to weight loss and growth failure. Judicious use of non-narcotic and narcotic analgesic may be needed in these patients.[129] Input from a chronic pain management team would be valuable in this setting. A low-fat diet is recommended, but the evidence in support of this strategy is lacking. Moreover, dietary restriction may worsen growth failure. Patients in their teens should be advised to avoid alcohol.

Taking pancreatic enzyme supplements with meals may help reduce the frequency and severity of pain. Cholecystokinin stimulates pancreatic secretion and bile, and intestinal proteases inhibit pancreatic secretion by inhibiting CCK secretion. Feedback inhibition of CCK is mediated through a trypsin-sensitive, CCK-releasing peptide.[130] The oral enzymes are believed to degrade this protein and thus reduce the CCK-mediated enzyme release from the pancreas. Some clinicians question the

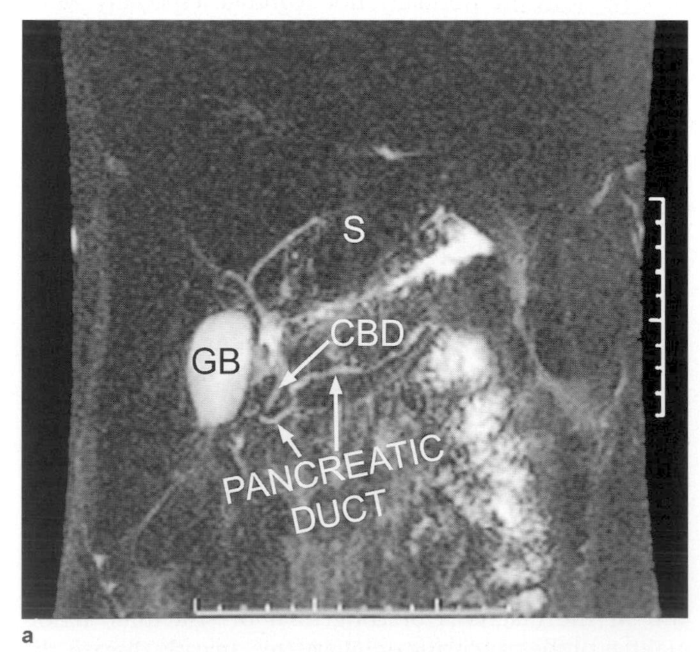

a

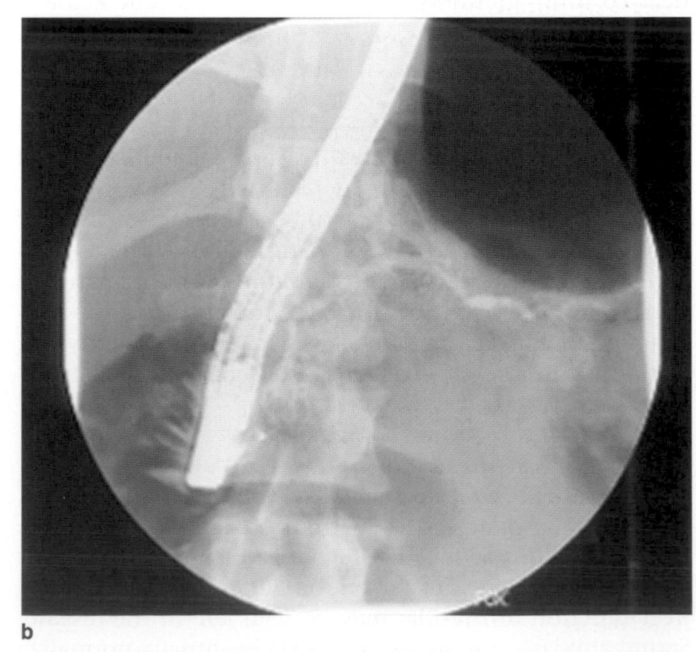

b

Figure 69.8: Chronic pancreatitis. (**a**) MRCP (T2-weighted image reconstruction) showing dilated, irregular pancreatic duct. Also labeled are the common bile duct (CBD), gallbladder (GB) and stomach (S). (**b**) ERCP of the same patient showing dilated, irregular pancreatic duct. (Courtesy of Dr. Janet Reid.)

efficacy of pancreatic enzyme supplementation in chronic pancreatitis, but it is used routinely in the authors' institution.

Octreotide has been shown to reduce pancreatic secretion. The routine use of octreotide in chronic pancreatitis is controversial, however, and some studies have not shown an improvement in pain.[131]

Surgical attempts to control pain should be considered only after all medical therapies have been exhausted. The decision to operate is generally delayed because the gland eventually burns out, which lessens the pain. ERCP may be helpful and may obviate the need for surgery. It can also be used in combination with sphincterotomy and/or stent placement to reduce pain and relieve obstructions. The pancreatic ducts can be drained using a variety of surgical procedures, which may help relieve pain in the long term.[132] A pancreatic ductal dilation of 7 mm is preferred when performing some form of lateral drainage. In the Puestow procedure, the pancreas and the main pancreatic duct are sectioned longitudinally and oversewn with a segment of similarly filleted jejunum so that the pancreatic juice drains directly into the intestine. Anatomic resection of the gland, either proximal or distal pancreatectomy, is another surgical option.

Preferred surgical techniques in children are not clear owing to a lack of adequate patient data. Some retrospective surgical series indicate that distal pancreatectomy with pancreaticojejunostomy may be effective.[133] Longitudinal drainage is preferred in some centers over anatomic resection, especially in children with chronic relapsing pancreatitis.[134] In adult patients, resection of the pancreatic head relieves pain in 80% of patients, whereas the Puestow procedure relieves pain in about 60%.[135]

Islet cell autotransplantation

This is an evolving treatment modality that can help manage pain and prevent diabetes in patients with chronic pancreatitis. With this technique, a total resection of the pancreas is performed, and the islet cells are isolated and reinfused into the patient.[135] The liver is the most frequent site of islet cell implantation. Although significant advances have been made in this area, most patients may require insulin at some point after transplantation. Studies indicate that initially patients have better glycemic control on insulin after the transplant compared with total pancreatic resection. At least 50% of these patients may become insulin independent at 1 year after transplant.[136] Currently, islet cell yield and processing are major limiting factors.[137] Segmental autotransplantation of the pancreas to the iliac fossa after denervation is another therapeutic option. This procedure was designed to provide pain relief while trying to maintain islet cell function.

Nutrition

Nutritional support is important in patients with chronic pancreatitis to prevent malnutrition and maintain adequate growth. A transpyloric feeding tube placed in the jejunum will bypass the pancreas. This way, adequate caloric intake can be ensured while minimizing pancreatic stimulation as the pancreas burns out. Patients with chronic pancreatitis need a high-calorie diet with adequate protein and fat supplementation to compensate for the fecal loss secondary to malabsorption.

Malabsorption

Malabsorption becomes problematic when most of the pancreatic reserves are destroyed. The goal of treatment is to improve growth and absorption without increasing pain. Prior to therapy, a fecal fat estimation should be considered to quantify the extent of fecal fat loss. A well balanced diet with vitamin supplementation, especially fat-soluble vitamins, should be prescribed. Pancreatic enzyme supplementation was discussed above.

Diabetes

Diabetes mellitus may be seen in up to 25% of patients with long-standing chronic pancreatitis. Diabetes associated with chronic pancreatitis generally is mild, and ketoacidosis is rare. Hypoglycemia is common in patients with chronic pancreatitis because of decreased pancreatic secretion of glucagon.

References

1. Weizman Z, Diurie PR. Acute pancreatitis in childhood. J Pediatr 1988; 113:24–29.
2. Haddock G, Coupar G, Youngson GG, et al. Acute pancreatitis in children: a 15 year review. J Pediatr Surg 1994; 29:719–722.
3. Yeung CY, Lee HC, Huang FY, et al. Pancreatitis in children – experience with 43 cases. Eur J Pediatr 1996; 155:458–463.
4. Mathew P, Wyllie R, Caulfield M, Steffen R, Kay M. Chronic pancreatitis in late childhood and adolescence. Clin Pediatr 1994; 33:88–94.
5. Sarles H. Definition and classification of pancreatitis. Pancreas 1991; 6:470–474.
6. Bradley EL. A clinic based classification of system for acute pancreatitis. Arch Surg 1993; 128:586–590.
7. Chari ST, Singer MV. The problem of classifying and staging chronic pancreatitis. Proposal based on current knowledge of its natural history. Scand J Gastroenterol 1994; 29:949–960.
8. Sarles H. Etiopathogenesis and definition of chronic pancreatitis. Dig Dis Sci 1986; 31:91S–107S.
9. Karne S, Gorelick FS. Etiopathogenesis of acute pancreatitis. Surg Clin North Am 1999; 79:699–710.
10. Norman J. The role of cytokines in the pathogenesis of acute pancreatitis. Am J Surg 1998; 175:76–83.
11. Marks WH, Ohlsson K. Isolation and partial characterization of the pancreatic secretory trypsin inhibitor in the rat. Biochim Biophys Acta 1982; 717:91–97.
12. O'Konski MS, Pandol SJ. Cholecystokinin JMV-180 and caerulein effects on the pancreatic acinar cell cytoskeleton. Pancreas 1993; 8:638–646.
13. Muallem S, Kwiatlowska K, Xu X, et al. Actin filament disassembly is sufficient final trigger for exocytosis in non excitable cells. J Cell Biol 1995; 128:589–598.
14. Figarella C, Miszczuk-Jamska B, Barret A. Possible lysosomal activation of pancreatic zymogens: activation of both human trypsinogen by cathepsin B and spontaneous acid

activation of human trypsinogen 1. Biol Chem 1988; 369:293–298.

15. Lerch MM, Adler G. Experimental animal models of acute pancreatitis. Int J Pancreatol 1994; 15:159–170.
16. Grady T, Saluja A, Kaiser A, Steer M. Edema and intrapancreatic trypsinogen activation precede glutathione depletion during caerulein pnacreatitis. Am J Physiol 1996; 271:G20–G26.
17. Saluja AK, Donovan EA, Yamanaka K, et al. Cerulein-induced *in vitro* activation of trypsinogen in rat pancreatic acini is mediated by cathepsin B. Gastroenterology 1997; 113:304–310.
18. Steer ML. The early intraacinar cell events that occur during acute pancreatitis. Pancreas 1998; 17:31–37.
19. Roxvall LI, Bengstrom LA, Heidman JMI. Anaphylatoxin and terminal complement complexes in pancreatitis. Arch Surg 1990; 125:918–921.
20. Lasson A, Ohlsson K. Protease inhibitor in acute pancreatitis: correlation between biochemical changes and clinical course. Scand J Gastroenterol 1984; 17:776–786.
21. Gorry MC, Gabbaaizeseh D, Furey W, et al. Mutation in the cationic trypsinogen are associated with recurrent acute and chronic pancreatitis. Gastroenterology 1997; 113:1063–1068.
22. Whitcomb DC, Gorry MC, Preston RA, et al. Hereditary pancreatitis is caused by a mutation in the cationic trypsinogen gene. Nat Genet 1996; 14:141–146.
23. Cohn JA, Friedman KJ, Noone PG, et al. Relationship between mutation of the cystic fibrosis gene and idiopathic pancreatitis. N Engl J Med 1998; 339:653–658.
24. Koppel G, Maillet B. Pathology of acute and chronic pancreatitis. Pancreas 1993; 8:659–670.
25. Prinz RA. Mechanism of acute pancreatitis: vascular etiology. Int J Pancreatol 1991; 9:31–38.
26. Toyama MT, Lewis MP, Kusske AM, et al. Ischaemia–reperfusion mechanisms in acute pancreatitis. Scand J Gastroenterol Suppl 1996; 219:20–23.
27. Schmid SW, Uhl W, Freiss H, et al. The role of infection in acute pancreatitis. Gut 1999; 46:311–316.
28. Agarwal N, Pitchumoni CS. Acute pancreatitis: a multisystem disorder. Gastroenterology 1993; 1:115–128.
29. Huang JL, Huang CC, Chen CY, et al. Acute pancreatitis: an early manifestation of systemic lupus erythematosus. Pediatr Emerg Care 1994; 10:291–293.
30. Lanting WA, Muinos WI, Kamani NR. Pancreatitis heralding Kawasaki's disease. J Pediatr 1992; 121:743–744.
31. Grodinsky S, Telmesani A, Robson WLM, et al. Gastrointestinal manifestation of hemolytic uremic syndrome: recognition of pancreatitis. J Pediatr Gastroenterol Nutr 1990; 17:286–291.
32. Robitaille P, Gonthier M, Grignon A, et al. Pancreatic injury in hemolytic uremic syndrome. Pediatr Nephrol 1997; 11:631–632.
33. Weber P, Seibold F, Jenss H. Acute pancreatitis in Crohn's disease. J Clin Gastroenterol 1993; 17:286–291.
34. Huang C, Lichenstein DR. Pancreatic and biliary tract disorders in inflammatory bowel disease. Gastrointest Endosc Clin North Am 2002; 12:535–539.
35. Keljo DJ, Sugerman KS. Pancreatitis in patients with inflammatory bowel disease. J Pediatr Gastroenterol Nutr 1997; 25:108–112.
36. Eghtesad B, Reyes EB, Ashrafi M, et al. Pancreatitis after liver transplantation in children: a single-center experience. Transplantation 2003; 75:190–193.
37. Benefla M, Weizman Z. Acute pancreatitis in childhood: analysis of literature data. J Clin Gastroenterol 2003; 37:100–102.
38. Werlin SL, Kugathasan S, Frautschy BC. Pancreatitis in children. J Pediatr Gastroenterol Nutr 2003; 37:591–595.
39. Smego DR, Richardson JD, Flint LM. Determinants of outcome in pancreatic trauma. J Trauma 1985; 25:771–776.
40. Ryan S, Sandler A, Trenhaile S, et al. Pancreatic enzyme elevation after blunt trauma. Surgery 1994; 116:622–627.
41. Wilson RH, Moorehead RJ. Current management of trauma to the pancreas. Br J Surg 1991; 78:1196–1202.
42. Ziegler DW, Long JA, Philippart AI. Pancreatitis in childhood. Ann Surg 1988; 207:257–261.
43. Karjoo M, Luisiri A, Silberstein M, et al. Duodenal hematoma and acute pancreatitis after upper gastrointestinal endoscopy. Gastrointest Endosc 1994; 40:493–495.
44. Brown CW, Werlin SL, Geenen JE, et al. The diagnostic and therapeutic role of endoscopic retrograde cholangiopancreatography. J Pediatr Gastroenterol Nutr 1993; 27:19–23.
45. Guelrud M. Endoscopic therapy of pancreatic disease in children. Gastrointest Endosc Clin North Am 1998; 8:195–219.
46. Werlin SL. Endoscopic retrograde cholangiopancreatography in children. Gastrointest Endosc Clin North Am 1994; 4:161–178.
47. Parenti DM, Steinberg W, Kang P. Infectious causes of acute pancreatitis. Pancreas 1996; 13:356–371.
48. Mishra A, Saigal S, Gupta R, et al. Acute pancreatitis associated with viral hepatitis: a report of six cases with review of literature. Am J Gastroenterol 1999; 94:2292–2295.
49. De La Rubia L, Herrera MI, Cebrero M, De Jong JC. Acute pancreatitis associated with rotavirus infection. Pancreas 1996; 12:98–99.
50. Niemann T, Trigg ME, Winick N, et al. Disseminated adenoviral infection presenting as acute pancreatitis. Hum Pathol 1993; 24:1145–1149.
51. Glassman M, Tahan S, Hillemeier C. Pancreatitis in patients with Reye's syndrome. J Clin Gastroenterol 1981; 3:165–169.
52. Murthy UK, DeGregorio F, Oates RP, et al. Hyperamylasemia in patients with the acquired immunodeficiency syndrome. Am J Gastroenterol 1992; 87:332–336.
53. Miller TL, Winter HS, Luginbuhl LM, et al. Pancreatitis in pediatric human immunodeficiency virus infection. J Pediatr 1992; 120:223–227.
54. Yabut B, Werlin SL, Havens P, et al. Endoscopic retrograde cholangiopancreatography in children with HIV infection. J Pediatr Gastroenterol Nutr 1993; 17:19–23.
55. Wilmink T, Frick TW. Drug induced pancreatitis. Drug Saf 1996; 14:406–423.
56. Bartholomew C. Acute scorpion bite pancreatitis in Trinidad. BMJ 1970; 1:666–667.
57. Weizman Z, Sofer S. Acute pancreatitis in children with acute anticholinesterase insecticide intoxication. Pediatrics 1992; 90:203–206.
58. Hillemeier C, Gryboski JD. Acute pancreatitis in infants and children. Yale J Biol Med 1984; 57:149–159.
59. Cotton PB. Congenital anomaly of pancreatic divisum as a cause of obstructive pain and pancreatitis. Gut 1980; 21:105–114.
60. Delhaye M, Engelholm L, Cremer M, et al. Pancreas divisum: congenital anatomic variant or anomaly? Contribution of endoscopic retrograde dorsal pancreatography. Gastroenterology 1985; 89:951–958.

61. Guelrud M. The incidence of pancreas divisum in children. Gastrointest Endosc 1996; 43:83–84 (Letter).
62. Lehman GA, Sherman S. Sphincter of Oddi dysfunction. Int J Pancreatol 1996; 20:11–25.
63. Linder JD, Geels W, Wilcox CM. Prevalence of sphincter of Oddi dysfunction: can results from specialized centers be generalized. Dig Dis Sci 2002; 47:2411–2415.
64. Guelrud M, Morera C, Rodriguez M, et al. Sphincter of Oddi dysfunction in children with recurrent pancreatitis and anomalous pancreaticobiliary union: an etiologic concept. Gastrointest Endosc 1999; 50:194–199.
65. Guelrud M, Morera C, Rodriguez M, et al. Normal and anomalous pancreaticobiliary union in children and adolescents. Gastrointest Endosc 1999; 50:189–193.
66. Choi BH, Lim YJ, Yoon CH, et al. Acute pancreatitis associated with biliary disease in children. J Gastroenterol Hepatol 2003; 18:915–921.
67. Lee SP, Nicholls JF, Park HZ. Biliary sludge as a cause of acute pancreatitis. N Engl J Med 1992; 326:589–593.
68. Werlin S, Casper J, Antonson D, et al. Pancreatitis associated with bone marrow transplantation in children. Bone Marrow Transplant 1992; 10:199–201.
69. Hagopian E, Chabot J, Oluwale S, et al. Allograft rejection and corticosteroids in acute pancreatitis following renal and cardiac transplantation. Transplant Proc 1997; 29:583–583.
70. Toskes PP. Hyperlipidemic pancreatitis. Gastroenterol Clin North Am 1990; 19:783–791.
71. Saifakas GG, Brown MR, Miller TL. Neonatal pancreatitis associated with familial lipoprotein lipase deficiency. J Pediatr Gastroenterol Nutr 1999; 29:95–98.
72. Ward JB, Petersen OH, Jenkins SA, et al. Is an elevated concentration of acinar cytosolic free ionized calcium the trigger for acute pancreatitis? Lancet 1995; 346:1016–1019.
73. Shearer MG, Imrie CW. Parathyroid hormone levels, hyperparathyroidism, and pancreatitis. Br J Surg 1986; 73:282–284.
74. Kahler SG, Sherwood WG, Woolf D, et al. Pancreatitis in patients with organic acidemias. J Pediatr 1994; 124:239–243.
75. Durie PR, Forstner GG, Gaskin KJ, et al. Elevated immunoreactine pancreatic cationic trypsinogen in acute malnutrition: evidence of pancreatic damage. J Pediatr 1985; 106:233–238.
76. Gryboski J, Hillemeier C, Kocoshis S, et al. Refeeding pancreatitis in malnourished children. J Pediatr 1980; 97:441–443.
77. Sternby B, O'Brien JF, Zinsmeister AR, et al. What is the best test to diagnose acute pancreatitis? A prospective clinical study. Mayo Clin Proc 1996; 71:1138–1144.
78. Tietz NW, Shuey DF. Lipase in serum – the elusive enzyme: an overview. Clin Chem 1993; 39:746–756.
79. Orebaugh SL. Normal amylase levels in the presentation of acute pancreatitis. Am J Emerg Med 1994; 12:8–20.
80. Kleiman DS, O'Brien JF. Laboratory medicine – macroamylase. Mayo Clin Proc 1986; 45:669–670.
81. Agarwal N, Pitchumoni CS, Sivaprasad AV. Evaluating tests for acute pancreatitis. Am J Gastroenterol 1990; 85:356–366.
82. Yadav D, Agarwal N, Pitchumoni CS. A critical evaluation of laboratory tests in acute pancreatitis. Am J Gastroenterol 2002; 97:1309–1318.
83. Frossard J-L, Hadengue A, Pastor CM. New serum markers for the detection of severe acute pancreatitis in humans. Am J Respir Crit Care Med 2001; 164:152–170.
84. Fleischer AC, Parker P, Kirchner SG, James AE Jr. Sonographic findings of pancreatitis in children. Radiology 1983; 146:151–155.
85. Lawson TL. Acute pancreatitis and its complications. Computed tomography and sonography. Radiol Clin North Am 1983; 21:495–513.
86. Arcement CM, Meza MP, Arumanla S, Towbin RB. MRCP in the evaluation of pancreaticobiliary disease in children. Pediatr Radiol 2001; 31:92–97.
87. Shimizu T, Suzuki R, Yamashiro Y, et al. Magnetic resonance cholangiopancreatography in assessing the cause of acute pancreatitis in children. Pancreas 2001; 22:196–199.
88. Hsu RK, Draganov P, Leung WJ, et al. The therapeutic ERCP in the management of pancreatitis in children. Gastrointest Endosc 2000; 51:396–400.
89. Pfau PR, Chelimsky GG, Kinnard MF, et al. Endoscopic retrograde cholangiopancreatography in children and adolescents. J Pediatr Gastroenterol Nutr 2002; 35:619–623.
90. Guelrud M. Endoscopic retrograde cholangiopancreatography. Gastrointest Endosc Clin North Am 2001; 11:585–601.
91. Robertson MA. Acute and chronic pancreatitis. In: Walker A, Durie PR, Hamilton JR, Walker-Smith JA, Watkins JB, eds. Pediatric Gastrointestinal Disease. Hamilton, Ontario: BC Decker, 2000:1321–1344.
92. Thompson DR. Narcotic analgesic effects on the sphincter of Oddi: a review of the data and therapeutic implications in treating pancreatitis. Am J Gastroenterol 2001; 96:1266–1272.
93. McClave SA, Spain DA, Snider HL. Nutritional management in acute and chronic pancreatitis. Gastroenterol Clin North Am 1998; 27:421–434.
94. Kalferentzos F, Kehagais J, Mead N, et al. Enteral nutrition is superior to parenteral nutrition in severe acute pancreatitis. Br J Surg 1997; 84:1665–1669.
95. McClave SA, Dryden GW. Issues of nutritional support for the patient with acute pancreatitis. Semin Gastrointest Dis 2002; 13:154–160.
96. Runzi M, Layer P. Nonsurgical management of acute pancreatitis. Use of antibiotics. Surg Clin North Am 1999; 79:759–765, ix.
97. Golub R, Siddiqi F, Pohl D. Role of antibiotics in acute pancreatitis: a meta-analysis. J Gastrointest Surg 1998; 2:496–503.
98. Messori A, Rampazzo R, Scroccaro G, et al. Effectiveness of gabexate mesilate in acute pancreatitis. A meta-analysis. Dig Dis Sci 1995; 40:734–738.
99. Imrie CW, McKay CJ. The scientific basis of medical therapy of acute pancreatitis. Could it work, and is there a role for lexipafant? Gastroenterol Clin North Am 1999; 28:591–599, ix.
100. Johnson CD, Kingsnorth AN, Imrie CW, et al. Double blind, randomized, placebo controlled study of a platelet activating factor antagonist, lexipafant, in the treatment and prevention of organ failure in predicted severe acute pancreatitis. Gut 2001; 48:62–69.
101. Uhl W, Büchler MW, Malfertheiner P, et al. A randomized, double-blind, multicentre trial of octreotide in moderate to severe acute pancreatitis. Gut 1999; 45:97–104.
102. D'Egidio A, Schein M. Surgical strategies in the treatment of pancreatic necrosis and infection. Br J Surg 1991; 78:133–137.
103. Mier J, Leon EL, Castillo A. Early versus late necrosectomy in severe necrotizing pancreatitis. Am J Surg 1997; 173:71–75.
104. Aldridge MC, Francis ND, Glazer G, et al. Colonic complications of severe acute pancreatitis. Br J Surg 1989; 76:362–367.

105. Lankisch PG. The spleen in inflammatory pancreatic disease. Gastroenterology 1990; 98:509–516.
106. Bem J, Bradley EL. Subcutaneous manifestations of severe acute pancreatitis. Pancreas 1998; 16:551–555.
107. Ford EG, Hardin WD Jr, Mahour GH, et al. Pseudocysts of the pancreas in children. Am Surg 1990; 56:384–387.
108. Haluszka O, Campbell A, Horvath K. Endoscopic management of pancreatic pseudocyst in children. Gastrointest Endosc 2002; 55:128–131.
109. Pitchumoni CS, Agarwal N. Pancreatic pseudocyst. When and how should drainage be performed? Gastroenterol Clin North Am 1999; 28:615–639.
110. Patard L, Lallemand JY, Stoven V. An insight into the role of human pancreatic lithostathine. J Pediatr 2003; 4:92–103.
111. Freedman SD, Sakamoto K, Venu RP. GP2, the homologue to the renal cast protein uromodulin, is a major component of intraductal plugs in chronic pancreatitis. J Clin Invest 1993; 92:83–90.
112. Witt H, Becker M. Genetics of chronic pancreatitis. J Pediatr Gastroenterol Nutr 2002; 34:125–136.
113. Sharer N, Schwartz M, Malone G, et al. Mutation of the cystic fibrosis gene in patients with chronic pancreatitis. N Engl J Med 1998; 339:645–652.
114. Marino CR, Matovick LM, Gorelick FS, et al. Localization of the cystic fibrosis transmembrane conductance regulator in pancreas. J Clin Invest 1991; 88:712–716.
115. Witt H, Luck W, Hennies HC, et al. Mutation in the gene encoding the serine protease inhibitor, Kazal type I are associated with chronic pancreatitis. Nat Genet 2000; 25:213–216 (Letter).
116. Pfutzer RH, Barmada MM, Brunskill AP, et al. SPINK1/PSTI polymorphisms act as disease modifiers in familial and idiopathic chronic pancreatitis. Gastroenterology 2000; 119:615–623.
117. Cohn J, Friedman KJ, Noone PG, et al. Relation between mutation of the cystic fibrosis gene and idiopathic pancreatitis. N Engl J Med 1998; 339:653–658.
118. Barman KK, Premalatha G, Mohan V. Tropical calcific pancreatitis. Postgrad Med J 2003; 79:606–615.
119. Cohn J, Bornstein J, Jowell J. Cystic fibrosis mutations and genetic predisposition to idiopathic chronic pancreatitis. Med Clin North Am 2000; 34:621–631.
120. Truninger K, Malik N, Ammann RW, et al. Mutations of the cystic fibrosis gene in patients with chronic pancreatitis. Am J Gastroenterol 2001; 96:2657–2661.
121. Bhatia E, Choudhuri G, Sikora SS, et al. Tropical calcific pancreatitis: strong association with *SPINK1* trypsin inhibitor mutations. Gastroenterology 2002; 123:1020–1025.
122. Bhatia E, Durie P, Zielenski J, et al. Mutations in the cystic fibrosis transmembrane regulator gene in patients with tropical calcific pancreatitis. Am J Gastroenterol 2000; 95:3658–3659 (Letter).
123. Sclabas G, Kirschstein T, Uhl W, et al. Juvenile idiopathic fibrosing pancreatitis. Dig Dis Sci 2002; 47:1230–1235.
124. Bradley EL. Chronic obstructive pancreatitis as a delayed complication of pancreatic trauma. HPB Surg 1991; 5:49–60.
125. Kloppel G, Luttges J, Lohr M, et al. Autoimmune pancreatitis: pathological, clinical, and immunological features. Pancreas 2003; 27:14–19.
126. Borkje B, Vetvik K, Odegaard S, et al. Chronic pancreatitis in patients with sclerosing cholangitis and ulcerative colitis. Scand J Gastroenterol 1985; 20:539–542.
127. Okazaki K, Chiba T. Autoimmune related pancreatitis. Gut 2002; 51:1–4.
128. Manfredi R, Lucidi V, Gui B, et al. Idiopathic chronic pancreatitis in children: MR cholangiopancreatography after secretin administration. Radiology 2002; 224:675–682.
129. Singh VV, Toskes PP. Medical therapy for chronic pancreatitis pain. Curr Gastroenterol Rep 2003; 5:110–116.
130. Liddle RA. Regulation of cholecystokinin secretion by intraluminal releasing factors. Am J Physiol 1995; 269:G319–G327.
131. Malfertheiner P, Mayer D, Buchlr M, et al. Treatment of pain in chronic pancreatitis by inhibition of pancreatic secretion with octreotide. Gut 1995; 36:450–454.
132. Sakorafas GH. Farnell MB. Nagorney DM, et al. Surgical management of chronic pancreatitis at the Mayo Clinic. Surg Clin North Am 2001; 81:457–465.
133. Weber TR, Keller MS. Operative management of chronic pancreatitis in children. Arch Surg 2001; 136: 550–554.
134. Petersen C, Goetz A, Burger D, et al. Surgical therapy and follow-up of pancreatitis in children. J Pediatr Gastroenterol Nutr 1997; 25:204–209.
135. Watkins GL, Krebs A, Rossi RL. Pancreatic autotransplantation in chronic pancreatitis. World J Surg 2003; 27:1235–1240.
136. White S, Davies J, Pollard C, et al. Pancreas resection and islet autotransplantation for end stage chronic pancreatitis. Ann Surg 2001; 233: 423–431.
137. Morrison C, Wemyss-Holden S, Dennison A, et al. Islet cell yield remains a problem in islet autotransplantation. Arch Surg 2002; 137:80–83.
138. Werlin SL. Pancreatitis. In: Wyllie R, Hyams J, eds. Pediatric Gastrointestinal and Liver Disease. Philadelphia, PA: WB Saunders; 1999:681–694.

Chapter 70
Secretory neoplasms of the pancreas

Hillel Naon and Daniel W. Thomas

INTRODUCTION

Pancreatic neoplasms are exceedingly rare in children. The majority of childhood pancreatic tumors are benign endocrine neoplasms that secrete hormonally active peptides.[1,2] A case of insulinoma was first described in 1927 by Wilder et al.[3] in an adult with a metastatic islet cell carcinoma and profound hypoglycemia. Islet cell adenoma in a neonate was described by Sherman[4] in 1947 and was the first reported case of a secretory type of pancreatic neoplasm in pediatrics. The focus in this chapter is on functioning neoplasms of the pancreas occurring in childhood.

Functioning pancreatic neoplasms are composed primarily of islet cells that elaborate various endocrine secretory products. More than 50% of pancreatic endocrine neoplasms are multihormonal. However, clinical manifestations are nearly always derived primarily from hypersecretion of only one of the hormones that is produced.[5–7] The diagnosis of pancreatic islet cell neoplasms with excessive hormone production depends on the recognition of clinical syndromes associated with autonomous endocrine product secretion. The pancreatic islet A cells secrete glucagon; the B cells secrete insulin; the D cells secrete somatostatin; the F cells secrete vasoactive intestinal polypeptide (VIP), substance P and possibly secretin; and the G cells secrete gastrin.[7,8]

Great progress has been made regarding our understanding of congenital hyperinsulinism, formerly known as nesidioblastosis. The development of highly specific and sensitive radioimmunoassays for detection of circulating peptides in the blood has facilitated the recognition and diagnosis of hormone-secreting neuroendocrine tumors and their associated syndromes. In children, the most common secretory pancreatic neoplasm comparatively is insulinoma associated with islet B-cell adenoma, which is a benign tumor, or hyperplasia. Zollinger–Ellison syndrome (ZES) associated with gastrinoma, VIPoma (Verner–Morrison syndrome) and multiple endocrine neoplasia (MEN) have been described in children and are often malignant.[9] Glucagonoma and somatostatinoma have not been reported in children.[10] Table 70.1 lists these tumors and their characteristics.

MULTIPLE ENDOCRINE NEOPLASIA

Three distinct types of multiple endocrine neoplasms have been identified (MEN-I, MEN-IIA and MEN-IIB).[11] MEN-I, or Wermer's syndrome, is associated with islet cell tumors of the pancreas, hyperparathyroidism and non-functional adenomas of the pituitary. The MEN-II syndromes are not associated with pancreatic tumors but include thyroid (medullary carcinoma) and adrenal (pheochromocytoma) tumors. MEN-IIA, or Sipple's syndrome, is distinguished by its association with parathyroid hyperplasia, and MEN-IIB is associated with multiple mucosal and alimentary tract neuromas. Each of these syndromes has autosomal dominant inheritance. MEN-I and -IIA usually occur in adults, whereas MEN-IIB may present in childhood. MEN-I rarely presents in childhood. Both sexes are affected with equal frequency.[9,12] The disorder is inherited in a dominant mode with a high degree of penetrance.[13,14] The *MENI* gene has been mapped to chromosome 11[15] and genetic markers have been identified.[16] The *MENII* gene has been mapped to chromosome 10.[17] Evidence suggests that tumor formation is associated with loss of a specific gene, which possibly unmasks a recessive mutation at this locus.

The clinical manifestations of MEN-I are heterogeneous and depend on the endocrine organ involved and the functional nature of the secretory neoplasm. An extensive review of 88 patients, only seven of whom were pediatric patients, by Ballard et al.[9] provided much of the early knowledge concerning the various features of MEN-I. These include parathyroid gland hyperfunction (84%), pituitary neoplasms (65%), adenomas and hyperplasia of the adrenal cortex (38%), thyroid disease (19%) (thyrotoxicosis, thyroid carcinoma and non-functioning adenomas) and peptic ulcers (58%). Ulcers were multifocal in more than half of the patients. Some patients had watery diarrhea or bronchial carcinoids. Pancreatic neoplasms were found in more than 75% of all the patients with MEN-I. These neoplasms were almost always multiple and consisted of both B cells, giving rise to insulinoma, and non-B cells, resulting in ZES. Other associated neoplasms included glucagonoma, VIPoma and somatostatinoma. Genetic counseling, confirmatory genetic testing[18] and screening of family members with careful follow-up are important aspects in the management of patients with MEN-I. Treatment of pancreatic neoplasms associated with MEN-I is discussed below in the section dealing with insulinoma.

Children with MEN-IIB may have a distinctive phenotype with a marfanoid habitus, muscle wasting, growth failure, everted eyelids, thick lips and multiple mucosal neuromas. Thickened lips and everted eyelids are secondary to the development of neuromas and tend to be more prominent over time.[19] The importance of recognizing MEN-IIB early is in the detection of medullary carcinoma

Neoplasm	Hormone secreted	Islet cell type	Major clinical features	Malignant (%)	Treatment
Insulinoma (adenoma, hyperplasia, congenital hyperinsulinism)	Insulin	B	Hypoglycemia	10	Diazoxide combined with frequent feedings, octreotide acetate, surgery
Gastrinoma	Gastrin	G	Peptic ulcers, diarrhea, excessive acid secretion	65	Gastric acid antagonists/blockers, surgery
VIPoma	VIP	F	Secretory diarrhea, hypokalemia, hypochlorhydria	50	Fluid and electrolyte replacement, octreotide acetate, corticosteroids, surgery
Glucagonoma	Glucagon	A	Rash, stomatitis, diabetes	75	Octreotide acetate, surgery

VIP, vasoactive intestinal peptide.

Table 70.1 Secretory neoplasms of the pancreas

of the thyroid, which tends to occur early in patients with MEN-IIB with rapid metastasis.

The gastrointestinal manifestations of MEN-IIB range from mild constipation to symptoms mimicking Hirschsprung's disease or episodes of pseudo-obstruction. Histologic examination of intestinal biopsies demonstrates diffuse proliferation of nerves and ganglion cells throughout the small and large intestine. In children who have growth failure or physical stigmata of MEN-IIB, rectal suction biopsy often demonstrates hyperplasia of nerve fibers. Serum calcitonin levels confirm the diagnosis.

INSULINOMA

Insulinomas, although rare, are by far the most common form of hormone-secreting tumors of the pancreas in children and adults.[20] They are discrete pancreatic endocrine neoplasms composed mainly or exclusively of islet B cells. Insulinomas have been recognized as a cause of inappropriate insulin secretion for more than half a century. Whipple[21] described the typical triad of symptoms associated with this syndrome: insulin shock with fasting, a fasting blood sugar level less than half the normal value, and relief of symptoms with the administration of glucose. More than 100 cases of insulinoma, including islet B-cell adenoma and hyperplasia, were compiled by Tudor in the Childhood Disease Registry.[22] The number of reports has increased considerably since a radioimmunoassay for insulin became available for clinical use. Published cases of insulinoma indicate that an islet cell adenoma or hyperplasia may become manifest at any age during childhood, but there are two periods of peak incidence: (1) the neonatal period through the first year of life, and (2) after age 4 years, with a peak from age 8 to 13 years.[12] Insulinomas are more frequent in females.[22,23] Eighty percent are solitary neoplasms, and more than 90% are benign.[22,24] Malignant insulinomas are exceedingly rare in children.[2] Patients with insulinomas and the MEN-I syndrome often have multiple insulinomas and are usually diagnosed at 15–25 years of age.[12] They account for about 10% of adult patients with insulinoma. In neonates, diffuse islet adenomatosis is frequently the cause of hyperinsulinemia.[25]

Insulinomas vary in size from lesions that are difficult to find even under dissection to huge tumors that are over 1500 g.[23] Ninety percent of insulinomas are less than 20 mm in diameter. Solitary tumors that are smaller than 5 mm in diameter are seldom associated with hypoglycemia.[23] They are usually encapsulated, firm, yellow-brown nodules that are composed histologically of cords and nests of well-differentiated B islet cells. Regardless of their size, insulinomas can be located anywhere in the pancreas and are rarely found outside the pancreas. Distinction between a benign or malignant insulinoma is difficult on the basis of histologic appearance alone. Because MEN-I is the most common condition associated with multiple benign insulinomas, the presence of genetic markers for MEN-I may alert the physician to the possibility of multiple insulinomas.[15] The α chain of human chorionic gonadotropin (hCG-a) has been reported as a marker for malignancy in functioning endocrine neoplasms, including insulinomas.[26]

Symptoms of hypoglycemia such as headaches, visual disturbances, confusion, weakness, sweating and palpitations are characteristic; convulsions and coma are features of significant sustained hypoglycemia. Most symptoms occur after fasting and are often confused with neurologic or psychiatric disease. The finding of hypoglycemia that can be provoked with fasting remains the keystone in the recognition of the possibility of an insulinoma. Significant hypoglycemia can be demonstrated after a 12-h overnight fast in more than 90% of patients with proven insulinoma.[23] Plasma insulin levels are inappropriately raised during hypoglycemia. Patients with insulinoma have insulin-connecting peptide (C-peptide) concentrations that parallel the increased plasma insulin levels. Normally, when insulin is cleared from its precursor pro-insulin, the C-peptide is released into the portal vein in a 1 : 1 ratio with insulin. Because insulinoma cells often process pro-insulin incompletely, the serum often has a high ratio of pro-insulin to insulin.[23] In normal subjects, serum insulin concentrations decrease to less than 5 μU/ml when the blood sugar level falls to 40 mg/dl or lower, and the ratio of plasma insulin concentration (μU/ml) to serum glucose concentration (mg/dl) remains less than 0.3. In patients with insulinomas, this ratio is usually greater than 0.4 and increases with fasting.[24] Hypoglycemia in the absence of urinary ketones and the presence of low plasma β-hydroxybutyrate is consistent with the diagnosis of insulinoma.

It is often difficult to localize insulinomas once the diagnosis has been made on clinical and laboratory grounds. Non-invasive studies, such as computed tomography, ultrasonography and magnetic resonance imaging, are usually helpful when the insulinoma is greater than 2 cm. Insulinomas that are less than 2 cm in diameter can sometimes be visualized before surgery by endoscopic ultrasonography.[27,28] The sensitivity of somatostatin receptor scintigraphy is less than 60% for insulinomas that express the somatostatin receptor subtype that can be recognized by the current radionuclide-labeled somatostatin analog.[29,30] Selective arteriography is usually performed if the non-invasive studies are negative. A hypervascular insulinoma can be detected by selective arteriography in 50–80% of cases.[31] In patients with negative non-invasive studies and non-diagnostic arteriography, portal venous sampling of blood for insulin is performed before surgery. Tumors that cannot be identified before surgery can be either palpated during surgery or detected by intraoperative ultrasonography.[32,33]

The treatment of choice for insulinoma is surgical ablation, which carries an excellent prognosis in most infants and children. At surgery, the islet cell tumor is often pink and firmer than the surrounding gland. The tumor is usually discrete and well encapsulated. The majority of these neoplasms can be simply enucleated. If the neoplasm cannot be localized, distal pancreatectomy with careful examination of sequential frozen sections of the gland is advisable. Resection of more than 80% of the gland is rarely required.[10]

In patients with MEN-I syndrome who have extensive pancreatic microadenomatosis, a 95% subtotal pancreatectomy is needed to achieve a cure.[1] The residual pancreatic tissue mass is usually sufficient to maintain normal exocrine and endocrine function. Transient hyperglycemia is frequent in the immediate postoperative period.[34,35] Diabetes mellitus with refractory hyperglycemia and ketonemia may develop immediately after massive subtotal pancreatectomy,[35,36] but may occur years after subtotal pancreatectomy.[37] Improved medical treatment has facilitated postponement of blind pancreatectomy until the tumor can be identified. Regularly scheduled feedings combined with diazoxide therapy can be used to manage some patients for a prolonged period of time. Octreotide acetate (Sandostatin®; Novartis Pharmaceuticals) is an eight-amino-acid synthetic peptide that possesses pharmacologic effects similar to those of the native hormone somatostatin but has much longer duration of action. Octreotide has an apparent elimination half-life of 1.7 h in plasma, compared with 1–3 min for the natural hormone somatostatin. The duration of action of subcutaneously administered Sandostatin® is variable, but extends up to 12 h, necessitating multiple daily doses. Sandostatin LAR® Depot is long acting and designed to be injected intramuscularly once every 4 weeks. Lanreotide (Sandostatin® SR) is a new depot formulation of somatostatin receptor-specific peptide that can be administered once weekly. Octreotide effectively suppresses insulin release in approximately half the patients with insulinoma.[38] The agent most frequently used in the chemotherapy of malignant insulinoma is streptozotocin.[23,39]

CONGENITAL HYPERINSULINISM

Congenital hyperinsulinism, formerly termed nesidioblastosis, or diffuse proliferation of nesidioblasts, was first described and named by Laidlaw in 1938.[40] Infants with congenital hyperinsulinism present in the neonatal period with symptomatic hypoglycemia, which may cause seizures or permanent brain damage. In the past, these infants were believed to have a disturbance in pancreatic development associated with persistence of the fetal pattern of islet cell formation, termed nesidioblastosis.[41] This concept of congenital hyperinsulinism has been discarded, owing to the recognition in many infants of specific genetic defects in the regulation of insulin secretion. The recessive mutations of sulfonylurea receptor 1 (*SUR1*) and potassium inward rectifier, the two adjacent genes on chromosome 11p that comprise the β-cell plasma membrane ATP-sensitive potassium channels, are responsible for the most common form of this congenital hyperinsulinism.[41,42] Dominant hyperinsulinism mutations have been identified in the gene for glucokinase on 7p and the gene for glutamate dehydrogenase on 10q. In addition, some infants with congenital hyperinsulinism were found to have isolated focal lesions of islet adenomatosis.[41,42] Affected infants have the same broad spectrum of clinical manifestations as described for insulinoma, and are equally refractory to medical therapy. They have a relatively high plasma insulin : glucose ratio.

The treatment of choice is 95% pancreatectomy, which is successful in 80–90% of infants with this disorder.[41] Medical therapy with diazoxide or octreotide is used for preoperative management, as well as in infants who fail surgery.[38,41] Providing permanent brain damage from hypoglycemia has not occurred, the prognosis of congenital hyperinsulinism is good.

GASTRINOMA: ZOLLINGER–ELLISON SYNDROME (ZES)

In 1955, Zollinger and Ellison[43] described one adult patient and a 16-year-old girl who presented with the triad of gastric hypersecretion, fulminant and intractable peptic ulcer disease, and a non-B-cell neoplasm of the pancreas. The hormone produced by the pancreatic tumor in this syndrome was recognized as gastrin more than 10 years later.[44,45] Tumors producing gastrin may be associated with symptoms other than those of ZES, such as diarrhea, steatorrhea and malabsorption.[46] Gastrinomas can originate in organs other than the pancreas, but they occur in the pancreas more often than any other site. The duodenum is the second most common site of origin.[47,48]

There are at least four major peptide forms of gastrin that differ in the length of their polypeptide chains but have identical C-terminal peptide amides. The C-terminal tetrapeptide amide has been shown to constitute the physiologically active site of the gastrin molecule.[49] Each of the peptide forms of the gastrin molecule exists in sulfated and non-sulfated forms; this appears to confer no differences in physiologic activity or potency of the molecule. The principal form of gastrin in gastrinoma is a heptadecapeptide (G-17), which contains 17-amino-acid residues.[50,51]

ZES can develop at any age. It occurs most frequently, however, between the ages of 35 and 65 years and is more common in men than in women. Forty-six cases of childhood gastrinomas have been reported in the Childhood Disease Registry,[22] 43 of which occurred in boys. The youngest patient reported was a 5-year-old girl who also had Marden–Walker syndrome.[52] The age range of ZES reported in children is 5 to 16 years. Thirty-seven children had documented neoplasms, and hyperplasia was observed in six. Sixty-five percent of the tumors were malignant. This is similar to the findings in adults, in whom 60% are malignant, and most patients have liver metastases at the time of diagnosis.[53] Twelve cases of gastrinoma in childhood were associated with islet cell carcinoma.[22] Although many adult patients with ZES have accompanying diseases, especially MEN-I syndrome,[54] similar cases have not been reported in the pediatric age group.[10]

Symptoms in ZES are due to the high circulating serum gastrin levels, which cause proliferation of the gastric parietal cell mass and stimulation of excessive gastric acid secretion. Children with ZES invariably have volumes of gastric secretions ranging from 600 to 2000 ml/day or more, with total acid production of 23–164 mEq/l.[55] Abdominal pain due to peptic ulcer disease is the most common clinical finding. Ulcers usually occur in the first portion of the duodenum or in the stomach. The ulcers are usually single but can be multiple. When multiple ulcers occur, they are frequently located not only in the first portion of the duodenum but also in the remainder of the duodenum, or even the jejunum. Diarrhea is a frequent problem; it may precede ulceration in some patients or occur without ulcers in others. The diarrhea is due to the excessive amount of hydrochloric acid released into the duodenum. In addition to an osmotic diarrhea, the increased amounts of acid and pepsin entering the small bowel produce inflammatory changes of the intestinal mucosa. Steatorrhea is less common than diarrhea. Acidity of the duodenum and small intestine causes inactivation of pancreatic lipase, reduction of conjugated bile acids, and the previously mentioned mucosal damage.

The diagnosis of ZES is based on the presence of gastric acid hypersecretion and hypergastrinemia.[56] Raised fasting serum gastrin levels can also occur with massive small intestinal resection, pernicious anemia with gastric achlorhydria, renal failure, chronic gastritis, peptic ulcer disease and antral G-cell hyperplasia. Basal acid output greater than 15 mEq/h in the unoperated patient should prompt suspicion of gastrinoma. There is a smaller increase between basal acid output and pentagastrin-stimulated gastric acid secretion in patients with gastrinoma. This test by itself cannot establish or exclude the diagnosis of ZES because of the overlap in values with normal and peptic ulcer patients. Acid output is difficult to measure after ulcer surgery because it is difficult to recover all the acid, and because bile and pancreatic juice often reflux into the stomach. Therefore, decreased acid secretion after partial gastric resection does not exclude the diagnosis of ZES.

By using radioimmunoassay for gastrin, the upper limit of normal is 100–150 pg/ml. Gastrin levels greater than 500 pg/ml in a patient with acid hypersecretion are diagnostic of gastrinoma.[56] Several provocative tests have been used to evaluate patients with possible gastrinoma, especially those who do not exhibit serum gastrin levels higher than 500 pg/ml. These tests use measurements of serum gastrin levels in response to intravenous secretin, calcium infusion or ingestion of a standard meal. The secretin stimulation test is by far the most valuable provocative test in identifying patients with ZES.[56] Secretin, at a dose of 1–2 units per kg bodyweight, is given intravenously over 30–60 s. Gastrin is measured in serum samples obtained before the injection of secretin and at 5-min intervals thereafter for 30 min. In normal individuals and patients with peptic ulcer disease, achlorhydria or antral G-cell hyperplasia, the infused secretin has little effect. In patients with ZES, intravenous secretin induces a substantial and prompt increase of serum gastrin by at least 200 pg/ml, usually at 5 min, gradually returning to basal levels by 30 min. In patients with gastrinoma, intravenous calcium infusion produces an increase in serum gastrin concentration of more than 400 pg/ml above the basal serum concentration. However, because this test does not add to the sensitivity or specificity of the secretin stimulation test and calcium infusion is potentially more hazardous, this test is not recommended. The third provocation test involves the feeding of a meal. In patients with gastrinoma, serum gastrin levels increase little or not at all after a meal, but an increase in serum gastrin level of more than 200% is observed in individuals with antral G-cell hyperplasia.

Gastrinomas are difficult to localize. In almost half of the patients with clinical and laboratory evidence, the tumor cannot be identified at surgery.[48] Upper gastrointestinal series, computed tomography, magnetic resonance imaging, duodenography, selective angiography and transhepatic portal venous sampling have been employed to locate gastrinomas before surgery. It has been recommended that somatostatin receptor scintigraphy should be the initial imaging study of choice in patients with gastrinomas because of the test's high sensitivity and specificity, and the results may affect clinical management[57] (Fig. 70.1). Endoscopic ultrasonography is highly effective in localizing gastrinomas.[58]

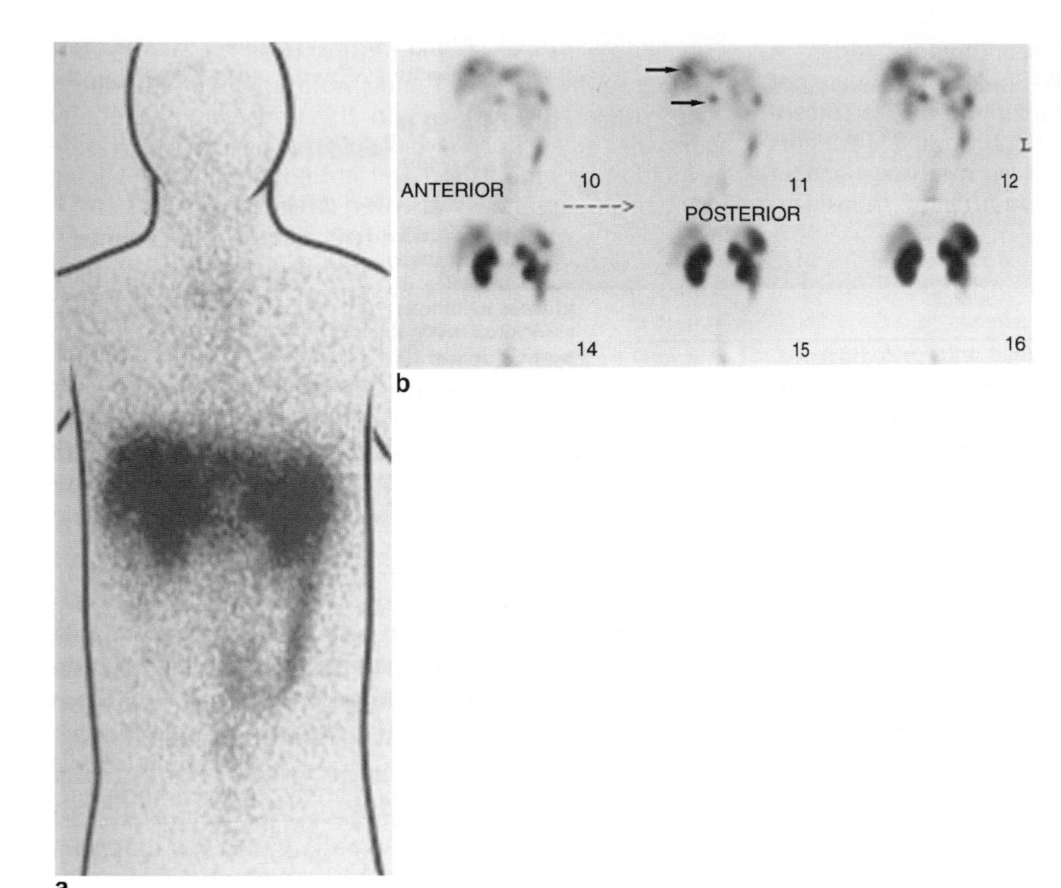

Figure 70.1: Gastrinoma. (**a**) Anterior view obtained at 24 h on an ^{111}indium-labeled octreotide (somatostatin) scan does not demonstrate any obvious abnormalities. Hepatobiliary excretion into the bowel and renal activity limit interpretation. (**b**) Multiple coronal single-photon emission computed tomography (SPECT) images from anterior to posterior clearly demonstrate an intrahepatic lesion as well as an anterior lesion in the region of the epigastrium (arrows). (From Mettler and Guiberteau, 1998, with permission.)[106]

Treatment of ZES centers upon control of the effects of hypergastrinemia, in particular peptic ulcer disease, as well as surgical treatment of the tumor, which is often malignant. Treatment should be individualized. In selecting the best therapy, the biologic behavior of these neoplasms and the clinical manifestations in each patient must be taken into consideration. A high dose of proton pump inhibitors given twice daily is the most effective way to reduce gastric acid secretion and induce ulcer healing in patients with ZES.[59,60] Massive doses of oral histamine (H_2)-receptor antagonists must be used every 4–6 h to control acid hypersecretion in patients with ZES[9,56,61] and should be restricted to the intravenous form in fasting patients. However, in ZES an intravenous proton pump inhibitor (pantoprazole or lansoprazole) may be more effective.[62,63] The dose of H_2-receptor antagonist or proton pump inhibitor that is required to maintain a satisfactory reduction in gastric acid secretion can be assessed by measuring the basal gastric acid output during the hour immediately before the next scheduled dose. The goal is to reduce gastric acid output to less than 10 mEq/h during this interval.[56] This approach is based on endoscopic evidence that duodenitis and ulceration are absent when acid secretion is kept below 10 mEq/h.[59] Data demonstrate that medically induced achlorhydria may lead to malabsorption of vitamin B_{12} and iron, both of which require acid for optimal absorption.[64] In one study, researchers reported that 3% of patients with ZES receiving long-term treatment with a proton pump inhibitor developed low serum vitamin B_{12} levels.[65]

Complete surgical resection of the tumor should be performed when possible. Full surgical removal of gastrinoma with cure has been achieved in approximately 30% of all patients with ZES.[66–69] Forty percent of patients with sporadic gastrinoma who have no evidence of metastatic disease have occult neoplasms, which are found most often in the duodenal wall and are frequently no greater than 2 mm in diameter.[49] These microgastrinomas can be detected only after duodenotomy and intraluminal exploration.[48] Pancreatic gastrinomas are not completely resectable in most cases. When a metastatic or irresectable gastrinoma is present, control of the ulcer disease may be accomplished in most cases by treatment with acid production inhibitors, in conjunction with parietal cell vagotomy,[70] and in some patients by total gastrectomy.[53,71,72] Total gastrectomy is not a preferred option in the management of gastric hypersecretion in patients with ZES, except in the minority of patients who are non-compliant or unable to take medication.[73] There is no convincing evidence that tumor progression is influenced by gastrectomy.[74] The routine use of selective parietal cell vagotomy at the time of surgical exploration has been recommended, whereas aggressive resections such as the Whipple resection are not advised.[75] Success with chemotherapy using streptozotocin, 5-fluorouracil and doxorubicin is limited.[69] Patients with metastatic liver disease given interferon-α and octreotide in combination with chemotherapy showed an improved outcome.[76,77]

VIPOMA

Pancreatic cholera,[78] also called watery diarrhea, hypokalemia and achlorhydria (WDHA) syndrome or Verner–Morrison syndrome,[79] is a secretory diarrheal disorder associated with pancreatic neoplasms. Secretory diarrhea in conjunction with a pancreatic islet non-B-cell tumor in adults was first described by Verner and Morrison in 1958.[80] One of the patients they reported was a 19-year-old woman. It is now widely accepted that VIP is the principal mediator involved in the pathogenesis of the diarrhea.[81] In adults, about 50% of VIP-producing tumors are malignant and the remainder are due to pancreatic adenomas, hyperplasia or non-pancreatic ganglioneuromas.[82] Most VIP-producing neoplasms in children are of neurogenic origin and include ganglioneuroblastomas, ganglioneuromas and neuroblastomas.[22,83,84] Rare occurrences have been reported in association with neurofibromatosis and pheochromocytoma.[22] Sixty-four cases of childhood VIPoma have been reported.[22] Primary pancreatic islet cell lesions were evident in only two of these children. In 1979, Ghishan et al.[85] were the first to report on the association between sustained watery diarrhea and increased levels of plasma VIP and pancreatic islet non-B-cell hyperplasia. Their patient was a 3-month-old infant presenting with secretory diarrhea beginning at 2 weeks of age. After a 95% pancreatectomy, plasma VIP levels returned to normal. Brenner et al.[86] described a 15-year-old girl with massive watery and protein-losing diarrhea who was found to have an islet cell tumor secreting high levels of VIP. A subtotal pancreatectomy was required to remove the tumor. There was no recurrence for up to 6 years later.

VIP is composed of 28 amino acids. Because the amino acid sequence of VIP is similar to that of secretin and glucagon,[87] VIP has endocrine functions similar to secretin, such as increased pancreatic bicarbonate excretion and inhibition of gastric acid secretion stimulated by pentagastrin and histamine. VIP also has a glucagon-like action of abnormal glucose tolerance. It stimulates cyclic adenosine monophosphate in intestinal epithelial cells, resulting in increased secretion of water and electrolytes into the small bowel that exceeds the normal reabsorptive capacity of the colon.[88] General physiologic effects of VIP include vasodilation in the systemic and splanchnic vascular beds, bronchodilation, immunosuppression, hormonal secretion and increased gastric motility. VIP has pivotal roles in the regulation of sleep, circadian rhythm and neuroendocrine control of the hypothalamic–pituitary–adrenal axis.[89] Localization of VIP is widespread throughout the body, being found normally in the ganglion cells of the autonomic nervous system, adrenal medulla, brain, bladder and predominantly in the gastrointestinal tract.[90] Since the first cloning of the VIP gene[91] and chromosomal localization,[92] many important advances in the understanding of the molecular biology of VIP have been made, including gene regulation by innervation and hormonal control, splicing mechanisms and newly discovered regulatory sites.

Clinically, the most prominent features of VIPoma are profuse diarrhea, hypochlorhydria, hypokalemia and metabolic acidosis. Other described features include spontaneous cutaneous flushing, hypokalemic renal failure, reduced or absent gastric acid secretion, diabetes mellitus, hypomagnesemia, hypercalcemia and excessive tearing.[90]

Diagnosis of VIPoma is made based on the clinical picture associated with increased plasma concentrations of VIP by radioimmunoassay. Confirmatory laboratory findings include hypokalemic acidosis, prerenal azotemia and decreased gastric secretion. Table 70.2 summarizes the symptoms and laboratory findings in VIPoma. Catecholamine levels should be obtained. Once the diagnosis of VIPoma has been confirmed, it is necessary to determine whether the tumor is situated in the pancreas or in another location such as a paraspinal ganglioneuroma. Computed tomography and somatostatin receptor scintigraphy are indicated in the evaluation (Fig. 70.2). If the pancreas is the suspected organ of origin, selective arteriography may localize the tumor. Transhepatic portal venous sampling for VIP may help localize the tumor before surgery.[93] Surgical exploration is often necessary for diagnostic purposes. Confirmation of the diagnosis is made by the immunocytochemical detection of neuron-specific enolase, VIP in the neoplasm, and electron microscopy for secretory granules.[1,82]

It is important that dehydration and electrolyte imbalance be corrected before surgery. Many palliative agents for symptomatic relief have been used with some success

Symptom or laboratory finding	Frequency (%)
Watery diarrhea	100 (31/31)
Dehydration	100 (31/31)
Weight loss	100 (31/31)
Flushing	33 (9/27)
Flaccid paralysis	20 (5/25)
Acidosis	35 (9/26)
Skin rash (chest, back, upper limb)	3 (1/31)
Multiple adenomatous polyps of colon	32 (1/31)
Hypokalemia	68 (21/31)
Achlorhydria	64 (16/25)
Hyperglycemia	28 (7/25)
Vasoactive intestinal peptide	100 (15/15)
Pancreatic peptide	50 (1/2)
Calcitonin	50 (1/2)
Somatostatin	100 (2/2)
5-Hydroxytryptamine	0 (0/3)
Human chorionic gonadotropin	67 (2/3)

From Peng et al., 2004, with permission.[108]

Table 70.2 Symptoms and laboratory findings in VIPomas

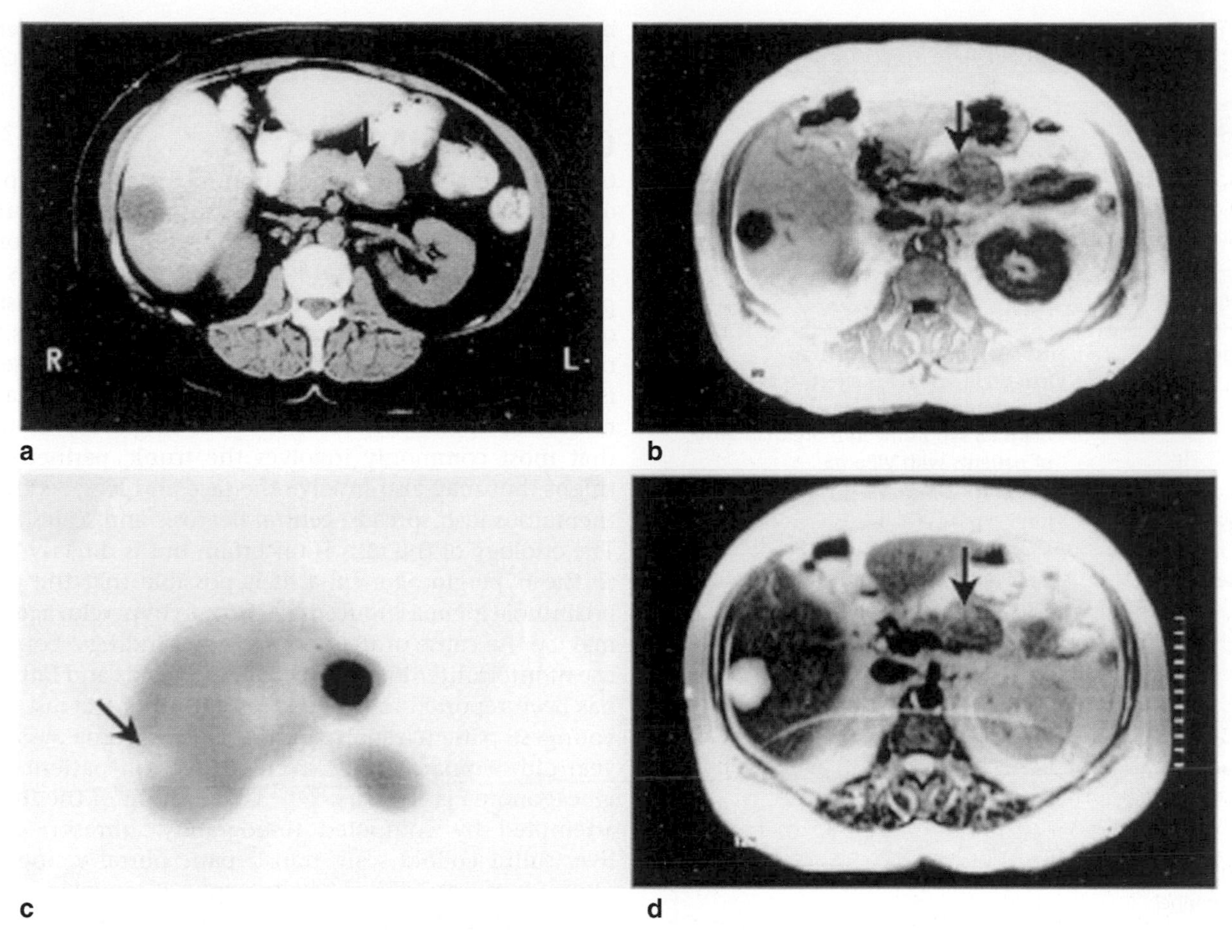

Figure 70.2: VIPoma. (**a**) On a non-contrasted computed tomogram, a 4.5-cm mass with a solitary calcification is seen in the midline (arrow). This mass is in the inferior portion of the pancreas and corresponds to the lesion seen on the magnetic resonance imaging (MRI) and somatostatin receptor scintigraphy (SRS) scans. A poorly characterized lesion in the right lobe of the liver is also visible. On MRI, T1 gradient echo (**b**) and T2 (**c**) images show an approximately 5-cm pancreatic mass that is partially exophytic and corresponds to the results of the nuclear medicine study (arrow). A cyst-like density is seen again in the right lobe of the liver and is low signal on T1 and high signal on T2. (**d**) With SRS, an axial SPECT image shows an area of intense accumulation of octreotide in the anterior aspect of the pancreas. No accumulation of the radiopharmaceutical was seen in the region of the liver or adrenal glands. Note the small photopenic area in the right lobe of the liver, now clearly representing a cyst rather than metastatic disease (arrow). (From Thomason et al., 2000, with permission.)[107]

(Table 70.3) and may allow time for further diagnostic studies to localize the tumor. The most potent pharmacologic antagonist of VIPomas is the long-acting somatostatin analog octreotide acetate. This drug has been given successfully to patients with VIPoma to suppress peptide secretion and watery diarrhea.[38,81] The mechanism of action of this somatostatin analog is to inhibit the release of VIP from the tumor and to inhibit intestinal secretion at the level of the enterocyte. The plasma concentrations of VIP in patients treated with octreotide acetate usually decline, but normalize in only 30% of treated patients.[94] Although all patients treated with octreotide acetate responded initially with an improvement in diarrhea and lower VIP plasma levels, some patients have had a short-term effect. In other cases, a rebound situation was observed for the diarrhea as well as VIP levels.[94] In such cases, increased dosage of octreotide acetate in combination with corticosteroids has proved to be helpful. Indometacin may be useful in cases of VIPoma associated with raised prostaglandin E_2 levels.[95] Other pharmacologic agents, including clonidine, phenothiazine, lithium carbonate, propranolol and interferon, may be helpful in selected patients in whom other therapies have failed.

The most definitive treatment of VIPoma is surgery. Because most VIPomas in children are of neurogenic origin, they are usually found in the adrenals or retroperitoneal area. Removal of the tumor with or without adjunctive chemotherapy is indicated. The infant with VIPoma reported by Ghishan et al.[85] died from sepsis after a 95% pancreatectomy. Histopathologic examination revealed non-B islet cell hyperplasia. The 15-year-old girl with VIPoma described by Brenner et al.[86] was found to have a large tumor of the body and tail of the pancreas. Microscopic examination revealed a tumor of islet cells. Because the tumor was found in 1 of 25 perisplenic lymph nodes and also in a small pancreatic vein, the diagnosis was islet cell carcinoma. An 85% distal pancreatectomy achieved complete cure in this patient. Because the experience with primary pancreatic VIPoma is extremely limited in children, information concerning this type of pancreatic

Modality	Comment
Acute supportive	
Intravenous fluids	May require >6 l/day
Correct hypokalemia, metabolic acidosis	350 mEq K^+/day often required
Peptide/peptidomimetic	
Octreotide	First-line symptomatic therapy Octreotide acetate is effective in the symptomatic improvement of watery diarrhea syndrome in more than 90% of patients with VIPoma
Pharmacotherapy	
Corticosteroids	All enhance absorption; corticosteroids most effective. All inhibit secretion; lithium carbonate and phenothiazines may be slightly more effective. All are effective only transiently
α_2Agonists	
Angiotensin II	
Indometacin	
Lithium carbonate	
Phenothiazines	
Opiates	
Propranolol	
Calcium channel blockers	
Adenylate cyclase inhibitors	
Surgery	Considered as both definitive therapy and, when possible, debulking therapy
Chemotherapy	
Streptozotocin	Combination therapy is useful but does not produce permanent remission
5-Fluorouracil	Renal impairment can be very serious and is usually drug limiting
Chlorozotocin	
Dacarbazine (DTIC)	
Interferon-α with chemotherapy	

Modified from O'Dorisio et al., 1989, with permission.[81]

Table 70.3 Treatment regimens for VIPoma syndromes

neoplasm is derived from the adult literature. This type of secretory neoplasm is usually found in the distal two-thirds of the pancreas. Isolated, single tumors have been reported in 80% of the patients. About half of all VIPomas are benign. Twenty-five percent of the tumors consist of islet cell hyperplasia.[90] A complete cure can be expected with subtotal (85%) pancreatectomy for biopsy-proven islet cell hyperplasia.[1,90] Excision of the primary malignancy, even in the presence of liver metastasis, is indicated to reduce the bulk of the tumor for subsequent chemotherapy. The combination of 5-fluorouracil, streptozotocin and interferon-α is reported to have a response rate of more than 65%.[76,77,96]

OTHER TUMORS

Glucagonoma and somatostatinoma have been reported only in adults. Glucagonoma is associated with increased levels of glucagon due to islet A cell tumors of the pancreas. Mallinson et al.[97] reported nine patients with pancreatic tumors who had a clinical complex consisting of diabetes mellitus, stomatitis, anemia, weight loss, diarrhea and rash. Although the rash is not always present, it is the most characteristic feature of a glucagonoma. The rash is described as necrolytic with migratory erythema that most commonly involves the trunk, perineum and thighs, but may also involve the face and legs. As the erythematous rash spreads, central necrosis and scales appear. The etiology of the rash is uncertain but is directly related to the hyperglucagonemia. It is possible that the panhypoaminoacidemia induced by chronic hyperglucagonemia may be the cause of the dermatologic findings. Long-term use of intermittent infusions of amino acids and fatty acids has been reported to produce resolution of the rash.[98] The youngest patient reported with glucagonoma was a 19-year-old woman;[99] the average age of patients with glucagonoma is 56 years.[100,101] Localization of the tumor is attempted by computed tomography, ultrasonography, liver sulfur colloid scan, transhepatic portal venous sampling for glucagon, and arteriography if knowledge of the tumor vascular supply is desired before surgery. Somatostatin receptor scintigraphy is the best technique to visualize the tumor preoperatively. The majority of the tumors are found in the body and tail of the pancreas, are at least 3 cm in diameter and have distinctive characteristics.[101] Surgery is the treatment of choice. Chemotherapy for metastatic glucagonomas includes streptozotocin, with or without 5-fluorouracil. Occasionally, dacarbazine (DTIC) is used.[102]

Somatostatinoma has been designated the 'inhibitory syndrome' because of its physiologic and pharmacologic effects of suppression of insulin, glucagon, gastrin and cholecystokinin release.[1] Clinical findings include diabetes, cholelithiasis, steatorrhea, indigestion, hypochlorhydria and, occasionally, anemia.[103] The majority of tumors are found coincidentally at the time of cholecystectomy for cholelithiasis. However, the appearance of gallstones and steatorrhea in a diabetic patient should alert the physician to the remote possibility of a somatostatinoma, necessitating exploration of the foregut organs for a tumor during cholecystectomy. When found, the tumor is usually single, although it may metastasize to the liver. The diagnosis can be confirmed by radioimmunoassay for an increased plasma concentration of somatostatin. Treatment is surgical removal of the tumor. Chemotherapy consists of streptozotocin and 5-fluorouracil.[1]

SUMMARY

Endocrine pancreatic tumors in children are rare. The dominant peptide they secrete and the resulting clinical syndromes have determined classification of these tumors. Most, because they are insulinomas, are benign, tend to grow slowly and are difficult to localize. Resection of a localized tumor is usually curative, and a variety of potent drugs facilitates medical management in advanced cases. More advanced diagnostic techniques will make the diagnosis of such tumors much easier once the condition is suspected. The application of a somatostatin receptor scanning technique using a labeled analog of octreotide as a radionuclide for the imaging of most of somatostatin receptor-positive tumors and their metastases has proved to be highly successful.[29,30,57,104,105] This technique is based on evidence that the majority of endocrine neoplasms responding to octreotide therapy do so because they have abundant somatostatin receptors. The development of other radionuclide-labeled somatostatin analogs that recognize other subtypes of the somatostatin receptor will further improve the usefulness of this technique. The ability to target receptors on tumor cells raises the possibility of selectively directed chemotherapy or radiation therapy for inoperable or advanced tumors.

References

1. Friesen SR. Update on the diagnosis and treatment of rare neuroendocrine tumors. Surg Clin North Am 1987; 67:379–393.
2. Grosfeld JL, Clatworthy HW, Hamoudi AB. Pancreatic malignancy in children. Arch Surg 1970; 101:370–375.
3. Wilder RM, Allan FN, Powell MH, et al. Carcinoma of islands of pancreas with hyperinsulinism and hypoglycemia. JAMA 1927; 89:348–355.
4. Sherman H. Islet cell tumor of pancreas in a newborn infant. Am J Dis Child 1947; 74:58–79.
5. Baylin SB, Mendelson G. Ectopic (inappropriate) hormone production by tumors: mechanisms involved and the biological and clinical implications. Endocr Rev 1980; 1:45–77.
6. Polak JM, Bloom SR, Adrian TE, et al. Pancreatic polypeptide in insulinomas, gastrinomas, VIPomas and glucagonomas. Lancet 1976; i:328–330.
7. Larsson LI, Schwartz T, Lundgrist G. Occurrence of human pancreatic polypeptide in pancreatic endocrine tumors. Am J Pathol 1976; 85:675–684.
8. Unger RH, Orci L. Glucagon and the cell: physiology and pathophysiology. N Engl J Med 1981; 304:1518–1524.
9. Ballard HS, Frame B, Hartsock RJ. Familial multiple endocrine adenoma–peptic ulcer complex. Medicine 1964; 43:481–516.
10. Grosfeld JL, Vane DW, Rescorla FJ, et al. Pancreatic tumors in childhood. J Pediatr Surg 1990; 25:1057–1062.
11. Wick MJ. Clinical and molecular aspects of multiple endocrine neoplasia. Clin Lab Med 1997; 17:39–57.
12. Rasbach DA, Van Harden JA, Telander RL, et al. Surgical management of hyperinsulinism in the multiple endocrine neoplasia type 1 syndrome. Arch Surg 1985; 120:584–589.
13. Wermer P. Genetic aspects of adenomatosis of the endocrine glands. Am J Med 1954; 16:363–371.
14. Schimke RN. Genetic aspects of multiple endocrine neoplasia. Annu Rev Med 1984; 35:25–31.
15. Larson C, Skogseid B, Oberg K, et al. Multiple endocrine neoplasia type I gene maps to chromosome 11 and is lost in insulinoma. Nature 1988; 332:85–87.
16. Manickam P, Guru SC, Debelenko LV et al. Eighteen new polymorphic markers in the multiple endocrine neoplasm type 1 (MEN1) region. Hum Genet 1997; 101:102–108.
17. Gardner DG. Recent advances in multiple endocrine neoplasia syndromes. Adv Intern Med 1997; 42:597–627.
18. Burgess JR, Nord B, David R, et al. Phenotype and phenocopy: the relationship between genotype and clinical phenotype in a single large family with multiple endocrine neoplasia type 1. Clin Endocrinol 2000; 53:205–211.
19. Griffiths AM, Mack DR, Byard RW, et al. Multiple endocrine neoplasia IIb: an unusual cause of chronic constipation. J Pediatr 1990; 116:285–288.
20. Buchanan KD. Johnston CF, O'Hare MT, et al. Neuroendocrine tumors: a European review. Am J Med 1986; 81(Suppl 6B):14.
21. Whipple AO. Adenoma of islet cells with hyperinsulinism. Ann Surg 1935; 101:1299–1355.
22. Tudor RB. Childhood Disease Registry. Bismarck, ND: Q & R Clinic; 1997.
23. Marks V. Hypoglycemia due to pancreatic causes. In: Samols E. ed. The Endocrine Pancreas. New York: Raven Press; 1991:207–227.
24. Liu TH, Tseng HC, Zhu Y, et al. Insulinoma: an immunocytochemical and morphologic analysis of 95 cases. Cancer 1985; 56:1420–1429.
25. Aynsley-Green A, Polak JM, Bloom SR, et al. Nesidioblastosis of the pancreas: definition of the syndrome and management of the severe neonatal hyperinsulinemic hypoglycemia. Arch Dis Child 1981; 56:496–508.
26. Kloppet G, Heitz PU. Pancreatic endocrine tumors. Pathol Res Pract 1988; 183:155–168.
27. Palazzo L, Roseau G, Salmeron M. Endoscopic ultrasonography in the preoperative localization of pancreatic endocrine tumors. Endoscopy 1992; 24:350–353.
28. Ueno N, Tomiyama T, Tano S, et al. Utility of endoscopic ultrasonography with color Doppler function for the diagnosis of islet cell tumor. Am J Gastroenterol 1996; 91:772–776.
29. Van Eijck C, Lambert S, Lemaire L, et al. The use of somatostatin receptor scintigraphy in the differential diagnosis of pancreatic duct cancers and islet cell tumors. Ann Surg 1996; 224:119–124.
30. Virgolini I, Traub T, Novotny C, et al. Experience with indium-111 and yttrium-90-labled somatostatin analogs. Curr Pharm Des 2002; 8:1781–1807.
31. Boden G. Glucagonomas and insulinomas. Gastroenterol Clin North Am 1989; 18:831–845.
32. Grant CS, Van Heerden J, Charboneau JW, et al. Insulinoma: the value of intraoperative ultrasonography. Arch Surg 1988; 123:843–848.
33. Norton JA, Cromack DT, Shawker TH, et al. Intraoperative ultrasonographic localization of islet cell tumors: a prospective comparison to palpation. Ann Surg 1988; 207:160–168.
34. Thomas CG, Underwood LE, Carney CN, et al. Neonatal and infantile hypoglycemia due to insulin excess: new aspects of diagnosis and surgical management. Ann Surg 1977; 185:505–517.
35. Dunger DB, Burns C, Ghale GK, et al. Pancreatic exocrine and endocrine function after subtotal pancreatectomy for nesidioblastosis. J Pediatr Surg 1988; 23:112–115.
36. Greene SA. Aynsley-Green A, Soltesz G, et al. Management of secondary diabetes mellitus after total pancreatectomy in infancy. Arch Dis Child 1984; 59:356–359.
37. Labrune P, Lechevallier S, Rault M, et al. Diabetes mellitus 14 years after a subtotal pancreatectomy for neonatal hyperinsulinism. J Pediatr Surg 1990; 25:1246–1247.

38. Maton PN. The use of the long-acting somatostatin analogue, octreotide acetate, in patients with islet cell tumors. Gastroenterol Clin North Am 1989; 18:897–922.
39. Burns AR, Dackiw AP. Insulinoma. Curr Treat Options Oncol 2003; 4:309–317.
40. Laidlaw GF. Nesidioblastoma, the islet cell tumor of the pancreas. Am J Pathol 1938; 14:175–134.
41. Stanley CA. Advances in diagnosis and treatment of hyperinsulinism in infants and children. J Clin Endocrinol Metab 2002; 87:4857–4859.
42. Thornton PS, MacMullen C, Ganguly A, et al. Clinical and molecular characterization of a dominant form of congenital hyperinsulinism caused by mutation in the high-affinity sulfonylurea receptor. Diabetes 2003; 52:2403–2410.
43. Zollinger RM, Ellison EH. Primary peptic ulcerations of the jejunum associated with islet cell tumors of the pancreas. Ann Surg 1955; 142:709–728.
44. Gregory RA. Grossman MI, Tracy HJ, et al. Nature of the gastric secretagogue in Zollinger–Ellison syndrome tumors. Lancet 1967; ii:543–544.
45. Gregory RA, Tracy HJ, Agarwal KL, et al. Amino acid constitution of two gastrins isolated from Zollinger–Ellison tumor tissue. Gut 1969; 10:603–608.
46. Ellison EH, Wilson SD. The Zollinger–Ellison syndrome: reappraisal and evaluation of 260 registered cases. Ann Surg 1964; 160:512–530.
47. Creutzfeldt W, Arnold R, Creutzfeldt C, et al. Pathomorphologic, biochemical and diagnostic aspects of gastrinomas (Zollinger–Ellison syndrome). Hum Pathol 1975; 6:47–76.
48. Thompson NW, Vinik AI, Eckhauser FE. Microgastrinomas of the duodenum: a cause for failed operations for the Zollinger–Ellison syndrome. Ann Surg 1989; 209:396–404.
49. Tracy HJ, Gregory RA. Physiological properties of a series of synthetic peptides structurally related to gastrin 1. Nature 1964; 204:935–977.
50. Dockray GJ, Taylor IL. Heptadecapeptide gastrin: measurement in blood by specific radioimmunoassay. Gastroenterology 1976; 71:971–977.
51. Power DM, Bunnett N, Turner AJ, et al. Degradation of endogenous heptadecapeptide gastrin by endopeptidase 24.11 in the pig. Am J Physiol 1987; 253:G33–G39.
52. Abe K, Niikawa N, Sasaki H. Zollinger–Ellison syndrome with Marden–Walker syndrome. Am J Dis Child 1979; 133:735–738.
53. Thompson JC, Lewis BG, Wiener I, et al. The role of surgery in Zollinger–Ellison syndrome. Ann Surg 1983; 197:594–605.
54. Gibril F, Schumann M, Pace A, et al. Multiple endocrine neoplasia type 1 and Zollinger–Ellison syndrome: a prospective study of 107 cases and comparison with 1009 cases from the literature. Medicine 2004; 83:43–83.
55. Schwartz DL, White JJ, Saulsbury F, et al. Gastrin response to calcium infusion: an aid to the improved diagnosis of Zollinger–Ellison syndrome in children. Pediatrics 1974; 54:599–602.
56. Deveney CW, Deveney KE. Zollinger–Ellison syndrome (gastrinoma): current diagnosis and treatment. Surg Clin North Am 1987; 67:411–423.
57. Termanini B, Gibril F, Reynolds J, et al. Value of somatostatin receptor scintigraphy: a prospective study in gastrinoma of its effect on clinical management. Gastroenterology 1997; 112:335–347.
58. Anderson MA, Carpenter S, Thompson NW, et al. Endoscopic ultrasound is highly accurate and directs management in patients with neuroendocrine tumors of the pancreas. Am J Gastroenterol 2000; 95:2271–2277.
59. McArthur KE, Collen MJ, Maton PN, et al. Omeprazole: effective, convenient therapy for Zollinger–Ellison syndrome. Gastroenterology 1985; 88:939–944.
60. Maton P, McArthur K, Wank S, et al. Long-term efficacy and safety of omeprazole in patients with Zollinger–Ellison syndrome. Gastroenterology 1986; 90:1537.
61. Raufman JP, Collins SM, Pandol SJ, et al. Reliability of symptoms in assessing control of gastric acid secretion in patients with Zollinger–Ellison syndrome. Gastroenterology 1983; 84:108–113.
62. Lew EA, Pisegna JR, Starr JA, et al. Intravenous pantoprazole rapidly controls gastric hypersecretion in patients with Zollinger–Ellison syndrome. Gastroenterology 2000; 118:696–704.
63. Metz DC, Forsmark C, Lew EA, et al. Replacement of oral proton pump inhibitors with intravenous pantoprazole to effectively control gastric acid hypersecretion in patients with Zollinger–Ellison syndrome. Am J Gastroenterol 2001; 96:3274–3280.
64. Marcuard SP, Albernaz L, Khazanie PG. Omeprazole therapy causes malabsorption of cyanocobalamin (vitamin B_{12}). Ann Intern Med 1994; 120:211–215.
65. Stewart CA, Termanini B, Gibril F, et al. Prospective study of the effect of long-term gastric acid antisecretory treatment on serum vitamin B_{12} levels in patients with Zollinger–Ellison syndrome. Gastroenterology 1995; 108:A226.
66. Wolfe MM, Jensen RT. Zollinger–Ellison syndrome: current concepts in diagnosis and management. N Engl J Med 1987; 317:1200–1209.
67. Vogel SB, Wolfe MM, McGuigan JE, et al. Localization and resection of gastrinomas in Zollinger–Ellison syndrome. Ann Surg 1987; 200:550–555.
68. Norton JA, Fraker DL, Alexander HR, et al. Surgery to cure the Zollinger–Ellison syndrome. N Engl J Med 1999; 341: 635–644.
69. Li ML, Norton JA. Gastrinoma. Curr Treat Options Oncol 2001; 2:337–346.
70. Richardson CT, Peters MN, Feldman M, et al. Treatment of Zollinger–Ellison syndrome with exploratory laparotomy, proximal gastric vagotomy and H_2-receptor antagonists. Gastroenterology 1985; 89:357–367.
71. Rothenberg RE, Radulescu OV, LaRaja RD, et al. The surgical treatment of the Zollinger–Ellison syndrome: an update. Am Surg 1987; 53:573–574.
72. Vinik AI, Thompson N. Controversies in the management of Zollinger–Ellison syndrome. Ann Intern Med 1986; 105:956–959.
73. Maton PN, Gardner JD, Jensen RT. Recent advances in the management of gastric acid hypersecretion in patients with Zollinger–Ellison syndrome. Gastroenterol Clin North Am 1989; 18:847–863.
74. Morowitz DA, Levine AE. Malignant Zollinger–Ellison syndrome: remission of primary metastatic pancreatic tumor after gastrectomy: report of a case and review of the literature. Am J Gastroenterol 1986; 81:471–473.
75. Jensen RT. Should the 1996 citation for Zollinger–Ellison syndrome read: 'Acid-reducing surgery in, aggressive resection out'? Am J Gastroenterol 1996; 91:1067–1070.
76. Frank M, Klose KJ, Wied M, et al. Combination therapy with octreotide and alpha-interferon: effect on tumor growth in metastatic endocrine gastroenteropancreatic tumors. Am J Gastroenterol 1999; 95:1381–1387.
77. Fjallskog ML, Sundin A, Westlin JE, et al. Treatment of malignant endocrine pancreatic tumors with a combination of alpha-interferon and somatostatin analogs. Med Oncol 2002; 19:[illegible]

78. Matsumoto KK, Peter JB, Schultze RG, et al. Watery diarrhea and hypokalemia associated with pancreatic islet cell adenoma. Gastroenterology 1966; 50:231–242.

79. Marks IH, Banks S, Louw JH. Islet cell tumor of the pancreas with reversible watery diarrhea and achlorhydria. Gastroenterology 1967; 52:695–708.

80. Verner JV, Morrison AB. Islet cell tumor and a syndrome of refractory watery diarrhea and hypokalemia. Am J Med 1958; 25:374–380.

81. O'Dorisio TM, Mekhjian HS, Gaginella TS. Medical therapy of VIPomas. Endocrinol Metab Clin North Am 1989; 18:545–556.

82. Capella C, Polak JM, Buffa R, et al. Morphologic patterns and diagnostic criteria of VIP-producing endocrine tumors. Cancer 1983; 52:1860–1874.

83. Jansen-Goemans A, Engelhardt J. Intractable diarrhea in a boy with vasoactive intestinal peptide-producing ganglioneuroblastoma. Pediatrics 1977; 59:710–716.

84. Mitchell CH, Sinatra FR, Crast FW, et al. Intractable watery diarrhea, ganglioneuroblastoma and vasoactive intestinal peptide. J Pediatr 1976; 89:593–595.

85. Ghishan FK, Soper RT, Nassif EG, et al. Chronic diarrhea of infancy: non-beta islet cell hyperplasia. Pediatrics 1979; 64:46–49.

86. Brenner RW, Sank LI, Kemer MB, et al. Resection of a VIPoma of the pancreas in a 15-year-old girl. J Pediatr Surg 1986; 21:983–985.

87. Mutt V. Isolation and structure of vasoactive intestinal polypeptide from various species. In: Said SI, ed. Vasoactive Intestinal Peptide. New York: Raven Press; 1982:1–10.

88. Racusen LC, Binder HJ. Alteration of large intestinal electrolyte transport by vasoactive intestinal polypeptide in the rat. Gastroenterology 1977; 73:790–796.

89. Brenneman DE, Hill JM, Gozes I. Vasoactive intestinal peptide in the central nervous system. In: Psychophamacology: The Fourth Generation of Progress. Nashville, TN: American College of Neuropsychopharmacology; 2000. Online. Available: http://www.acnp.org/g4/GN01000057/Default.htm 7 Feb 2005

90. Krejs GJ. VIPoma syndrome. Am J Med 1987; 82(Suppl 5B):37–48.

91. Bodner M, Fridkin M, Gozes I. Coding sequences for vasoactive intestinal peptide and PHM-27 peptide are located on two adjacent exons in the human genome. Proc Natl Acad Sci 1985; 82:3548–3551.

92. Gozes I, Avidor R, Yahav Y, et al. The gene encoding vasoactive intestinal peptide is located on human chromosome 6p21-6qter. Hum Genet 1987; 75:41–44.

93. Parkman HP, Malet PF, Ogorek CP, et al. Preoperative localization of a vasoactive intestinal peptide-secreting tumor by transhepatic portal venous sampling. Am J Gastroenterol 1988; 83:559–563.

94. Koelz A, Kraenzlin M, Gyr K, et al. Escape of the response to a long-acting somatostatin analogue (SMS 201-995) in patients with VIPoma. Gastroenterology 1987; 92:527–531.

95. Jaffe BM, Kopen DF, DeSchryver-Kecskemeti K, et al. Indomethacin-responsive pancreatic cholera. N Engl J Med 1977; 297:817–821.

96. Moertel CG, Hanley JA, Johnson LA. Streptozotocin alone compared with streptozotocin plus fluorouracil in the treatment of advanced islet cell carcinoma. N Engl J Med 1980; 303:1189–1194.

97. Mallinson CN, Bloom SR, Warin AP, et al. A glucagonoma syndrome. Lancet 1974; ii:1–5.

98. Alexander EK, Robinson M, Staniec M, Dluhy RG. Peripheral amino acid and fatty acid infusion for the treatment of necrolytic migratory erythema in the glucagonoma syndrome. Clin Endocrinol 2002; 57:827–831.

99. Riddle MC, Golper TA, Fletcher WS, et al. Glucagonoma syndrome in a 19-year-old woman. West J Med 1978; 129:68–72.

100. Stacpoole PW. The glucagonoma syndrome: clinical features, diagnosis and treatment. Endocrinol Rev 1981; 2:347.

101. Higgins GA, Recant L, Fischman AB. The glucagonoma syndrome: surgically curable diabetes. Am J Surg 1979; 137:142–148.

102. Prinz RA, Badrinath K, Banerji M, et al. Operative and chemotherapeutic management of malignant glucagon-producing tumors. Surgery 1981; 90:713–719.

103. Konomi K, Chijiiwa K, Katsuta T, et al. Pancreatic somatostatinoma: a case report and review of the literature. J Surg Oncol 1990; 43:259–265.

104. Lamberts SWJ, Bakker WH, Reubi JC, Krennig EP. Somatostatin-receptor imaging in the localization of endocrine tumors. N Engl J Med 1990; 323:1246–1249.

105. Laznicck M, Laznickova A, Trejtnar F, et al. Lanreotide labeled with ^{99m}Tc: preparation, preclinical testing and comparison with $^{(111)}$In-DTPA–octreotide. Anticancer Res 2002; 22:2125–2130.

106. Mettler FA Jr, Guiberteau MJ. Essentials of Nuclear Medicine Imaging, 4th edn. Place: WB Saunders; 1998.

107. Thomason JW, Martin RS, Fincher ME. Somatostatin receptor scintigraphy. The definitive technique for characterizing vasoactive intestinal peptide-secreting tumors. Clin Nucl Med 2000; 25:661–664.

108. Peng SY, Li JT, Liu YB, et al. Diagnosis and treatment of VIPoma in China (case report and 31 cases review). Pancreas 2004; 28:93–97.

Nutrient—cont'd	Age	RDA	AI	UL
Vitamin B_6 (mg/day) (pyridoxine)	0–6 months		0.1	ND
	7–12 months	0.5	0.3	ND
	1–3 years	0.6		30
	4–8 years			40
Vitamin B_{12} (μg/day) (cobalamin)	0–6 months		0.4	
	7–12 months	0.9	0.5	
	1–3 years	1.2		
	4–8 years			
Vitamin C (mg/day) (ascorbic acid)	0–6 months		5	25
	7–12 months		5	25
	1–3 years		5	50
	4–8 years		5	50
Vitamin D (μg/day) (calciferol) 1{ts}μg calciferol = 40 IU vitamin D	0–6 months		5	25
	7–12 months		5	25
	1–3 years		5	50
	4–8 years		5	50
Arsenic	0–6 months	ND	ND	
	7–12 months	ND	ND	
	1–3 years	ND	ND	
	4–8 years	ND	ND	
Boron (mg/day)	0–6 months	ND	ND	ND
	7–12 months	ND	ND	ND
	1–3 years	ND	ND	3
	4–8 years	ND	ND	6
Calcium (mg/day)	0–6 months		210	ND
	7–12 months		270	ND
	1–3 years		500	2500
	4–8 years		800	2500
Chromium (μg/day)	0–6 months		0.2	
	7–12 months		5.5	
	1–3 years		11	
	4–8 years		15	
Copper (μg/day)	0–6 months		200	ND
	7–12 months	340	220	ND
	1–3 years	440		1000
	4–8 years	1300		3000
Fluoride (mg/day)	0–6 months		0.01	0.7
	7–12 months		0.5	0.9
	1–3 years		0.7	1.3
	4–8 years		1	2.2
Iodine (μg/day)	0–6 months		110	ND
	7–12 months	90	130	ND
	1–3 years	90		200
	4–8 years			300
Iron (mg/day)	0–6 months		0.27	40
	7–12 months	11		40
	1–3 years	7		40
	4–8 years	10		
Magnesium (mg/day)	0–6 months		30	ND
	7–12 months	80	75	ND
	1–3 years	130		65
	4–8 years			110
Manganese (mg/day)	0–6 months		0.003	ND
	7–12 months		0.6	ND
	1–3 years		1.2	2
	4–8 years		1.5	3
Molybdenum (μg/day)	0–6 months		2	ND
	7–12 months	17		ND
	1–3 years	22		300
	4–8 years			600
Nickel (mg/day)	0–6 months	ND	ND	ND
	7–12 months	ND	ND	ND
	1–3 years	ND	ND	0.2
	4–8 years	ND		0.3

Table 71.3 Dietary Reference Intakes

(Continued)

Nutrient—cont'd	Age	RDA	AI	UL
Phosphorus (mg/day)	0–6 months		100	ND
	7–12 months	460	275	ND
	1–3 years	500		3000
	4–8 years			3000
Selenium (μg/day)	0–6 months		15	45
	7–12 months	20	20	60
	1–3 years	30		90
	4–8 years			150
Silicon	0–6 months	ND	ND	
	7–12 months	ND	ND	
	1–3 years	ND	ND	
	4–8 years	ND	ND	
Vanadium (mg/day)	0–6 months	ND	ND	
	7–12 months	ND	ND	
	1–3 years	ND	ND	
	4–8 years	ND	ND	
Zinc (mg/day)	0–6 months		2	4
	7–12 months	3		5
	1–3 years	3		7
	4–8 years	5		12

ND, PUFA, polyunsaturated fatty acid.

Table 71.3 Dietary Reference Intakes

nutritional, health and social reasons for this recommendation. Initial studies on the health benefits of breast-feeding were criticized for failings in study design and data analysis. More recent research has been rigorous, and studies performed in developed countries show that breast-feeding provides benefits for infants. Infants who are exclusively breast-fed have fewer episodes of infections, such as otitis media,[15–20] lower rates of respiratory tract illness,[21] less gastrointestinal illnesses during the first year of life[22] and fewer urinary tract infections,[23,24] and human milk may confer protection against specific infectious agents, such as *Haemophilus influenza* type b[25,26] and botulism.[27]

Human milk is dynamic. Nutrient concentrations vary over time (months, and within a single day), within a single feed, and among women. The tremendous variability of human milk contents makes it difficult to assume average nutrient content, as the IOM has in establishing AI for nutrients.[28] Human milk is generally considered as colostrum, transitional milk and mature milk.

Colostrum is the fluid secreted by the mammary gland for the first 7 days after birth. The volume varies from 2 to 20 ml per feeding, and colostrum consists of a mixture of mammary duct contents, newly secreted milk and immunologically active cells.[29] Colostrum is recognized by its intense yellow color, due to a high concentration of carotenoids, α-carotene, β-carotene, β-crytoxanthin, lutein and xeaxanthin,[30] its high levels of vitamin E, protein and immunoglobulin, especially IgA,[31] and its low fat levels.[28]

Transition milk is that produced between colostrum and mature milk, from about 7 to 10 days postpartum. Its nutrient content gradually changes from that of colostrum to mature milk. The protein, immunoglobulin and fat-soluble vitamin content decreases, while the lactose, water-soluble vitamin, fat and total caloric content increases. Interestingly, the total fat content may have predictive value as 90% of women whose milk contained 20 g or more fat per feeding on the seventh day of lactation successfully breast-fed for at least 3 months, whereas those whose milk contained 5–10 g of fat had an 80% dropout rate by 3 months.[32]

In general, mature human milk is a reliable source of all nutrients for healthy, term infants, except for vitamin D[33]

	Age (months) At birth	1	2	3	4	5	6	7	8	9	10	11	12
Weight (kg)	3.6	4.4	5.2	6.0	6.8	7.4	8.0	8.4	8.8	9.2	9.6	10.0	10.4
Weight increase (kg)	0.8	0.8	0.8	0.8	0.8	0.6	0.6	0.4	0.4	0.4	0.4	0.4	0.4
% increase	22	18	15	13	12	8	8	5	4.7	4.5	4.3	4.2	4

Table 71.4 Growth in weight for an infant born at the 50th percentile and growing at the 50th percentile

(and some argue iron[34]) for the first 4–6 months. Exclusively breast-fed infants must be supplemented with vitamin D to prevent rickets,[33] and infants of vegan mothers must be supplemented with vitamin B_{12}.

At 4–6 months the concentrations of calories, iron and zinc may become limiting. The WHO and UNICEF recommend exclusive breast-feeding for the first 6 months of life. The AAP supports exclusive breast-feeding for approximately 6 months, but recognizes that infants are developmentally ready to accept complementary foods between 4 and 6 months.[35] A systematic review of the literature examining the length of time for which exclusive breast-feeding can provide the nutritional needs of infants was recently published[36] and reviewed.[37]

There are few contraindications to breast-feeding. The AAP lists the following contraindiations: galactosemia, women with human immunodeficiency virus (HIV) and T-cell lymphotrophic virus (TCLV) infection in developed countries, herpetic lesions on the breast (not the vagina), untreated miliary tuberculosis, women receiving antimetabolite drugs and those using drugs of abuse.[38]

Human milk is not without risks, however. The AAP's *Nutirition Handbook*,[39] Tables B-1 through B-7, lists medications and environmental agents that may have an effect on human milk, are excreted in human milk or may have an effect on infants. The impact of environmental factors on human milk is discussed in depth by the AAP[40] and the National Research Council.[41]

The Centers for Disease Control maintains a website (http://www.cdc.gov/breastfeeding/) that contains information on breast-feeding promotion, support for breast-feeding activities and national policies on breast-feeding.

FORMULA FEEDING

Infant formulas are liquids or reconstituted powders fed to infants and young children to serve as substitutes for human milk. They are safe and efficacious complete foods. No vitamin or mineral supplementation is necessary for healthy infants who are solely formula-fed. Infant formulas are regulated under the Federal Food, Drug and Cosmetic Act of 1938, the Federal Meat Inspection Act of 1907 and the Poultry Products Inspection Act of 1957. The Federal Drug Administration (FDA), an agency in the Department of Health and Human Services, regulates infant formulas and evaluates the safety of food and color additives. This information is outlined and updated at http://www.cfsan.fda.gov/~dms/inf-regu.html on a regular basis.

Formula feeding is indicated if the infant or mother has a medical problem (e.g. galactosemia, HIV infection), the family chooses not to breast-feed or the infant fails to thrive on exclusive breast-feeding. For breast-fed infants who develop failure to thrive, infant formula should be provided as a supplement and not a replacement for human milk. It is important to note, however, that if formula replaces breast-feeding, the mother's milk supply will decrease, making it likely that complete cessation of breast-feeding will occur. If an infant is formula-fed, the formula should be provided to the infant for the full first year to avoid malnutrition.[42]

Infant formulas have undergone considerable changes in the recent past and they continue to be re-evaluated and reformulated in the light of new knowledge. While the makers of infant formulas have sought to replicate the content of human milk in their formulas, more recently infant formula-makers have sought to replicate the performance of human milk. In making this concept shift, they have recognized that it is not possible to replicate all the contents of human milk; moreover, it is not possible to reconstruct the complex matrix in which nutrients and other factors interact to alter absorption, bioavailability and function.

Formulas can be grouped according to protein, carbohydrate or fat content.[43] With respect to protein, there are four types of formula: cow's milk based, soy, hydrolyzed cow's milk, and chemically defined. Only cow's milk formula is available with low iron content, and no indication exists for its use.[44] Formulas are produced with and without lactose, with sucrose, hydrolyzed cornstarch, glucose polymers, with and without fiber, tapioca, and maltodextrins. Formulas can contain more or less medium-chain triglycerides, soybean oil, safflower oil, sunflower oil, canola oil, structured lipids, lecithin, corn oil and coconut oil.

Standard, iron fortified, cow's milk formula is the formula of choice when breast-feeding is not used or is stopped before 1 year of age. The AAP *Nutrition Handbook* notes that cow's milk formulas from different producers have similarities, but differ substantially from one another in the quality and quantity of nutrients. Although manufacturers offer rationales for the composition of their formula, the AAP notes that physiologically significant differences have not been clearly demonstrated among the various products. Appendices E, F and G of the AAP handbook list the formulas and their composition as of 2003.[43] It is important to note that the content of infant formulas is in constant flux, and for up to date information it is best to contact the formula-maker.

Soy formulas were developed during the 1960s for infants who could not tolerate milk proteins or lactose. Currently soy formulas constitute about 25% of the sales of all infant formulas in the USA. Soy formulas support growth and development equivalent to that of breast-fed and cow's milk-based formula-fed infants.[45–47] Soy formulas have added methionine to compensate for the low concentration of this essential amino acid in soy protein, and a trypsin inhibitor is added. Soy formulas have sucrose, cornstarch hydrolysates or mixtures as the carbohydrate source, and palm olein, soy, coconut and high-oleic safflower oils as the fat source. Minerals and vitamins are added, as are taurine and carnitine. Soy formulas contain phytoestrogens that have physiologic activity in rodents, but to date no significant effects have been found on growth or pubertal development in humans.[48] The AAP recommends the use of soy formulas for term infants whose nutritional needs are not met from breast milk, term infants with galactosemia or hereditary lactase deficiency, term infants with documented transient lactase deficiency, infants with documented IgE-associated allergy to cow's milk, and parents who wish to feed a vegetarian diet to their term infant.[49] Soy formulas are contraindicated for pre-term infants with birth weights of less than 1800 g, for infants with cow's milk protein-induced entercolitis or enteropathy, or for the prevention of colic or allergy.[49]

Protein hydrolysate formulas were developed for infants who could not digest or were intolerant to intact cow's milk protein, and are recommended for infants intolerant to cow's milk and soy proteins and for those with significant malabsorption due to gastrointestinal or hepatobiliary disease such as cystic fibrosis, short gut, biliary atresia, cholestasis or protracted diarrhea. The hydrolysates have the disadvantage of poor taste due to the presence of sulfated amino acids, high cost and high osmolality. There are several protein hydrolysates available.[43] To produce the hydrolysate, either casein or whey is heat-treated and enzymatically hydrolyzed. The resulting hydrolysate consists of free amino acids and peptides of various lengths. In some instance the peptides are so small that they are incapable of eliciting an immunologic response in infants. The formula is then fortified with amino acids to compensate for the amino acids lost in the manufacturing process. The various products contain differing amounts of peptides of various chain lengths. These formulas are free of lactose and contain sucrose, tapioca starch, corn syrup solids and cornstarch as the carbohydrate source. The formulas contain varying amounts of medium-chain triglycerides and polyunsaturated vegetable oil to supply essential fatty acids.

Chemically defined formulas are those produced from single amino acids and formulated specifically for infants with extreme protein hypersensitivity whose symptoms persist on hydrolyzed protein formulas.

There are no definitive *in vitro* tests that quantify the allergenicity of a formula. Studies of antigenicity in animals are not indicative of antigenicity in human infants. The only way to test the allergenicity accurately is in studies in infants.

Long-chain polyunsaturated fatty acids, those with a chain length of more than 18 carbons and two or more double bonds, particularly arachidonic acid (AA) and docosahexaenoic acid (DHA), are found in breast milk. Some studies on cognitive development in term babies have suggested that there might be a difference in development between infants fed formulas supplemented with AA and DHA, and those who were not supplemented; other studies have shown no differences.[50–53] For these reasons, the AAP has no official position on the supplementation of term infant formulas with AA and DHA. DHA and AA supplements offer an advantage to premature infants.[54]

Cow's milk, full-fat, skim, 1%, 2% fat, goat milk, evaporated milk and other 'milks' not specifically formulated to meet infant nutritional requirements are not recommended for use during the first 12 months of life.[55] Infants fed these milks are at risk of iron deficiency anemia because of low iron concentration, low bioavailability of iron and possible intestinal blood loss.[56,57] These milks also contain higher protein, sodium, potassium and chloride concentrations, and increase renal solute load.[58] The essential fatty acids, vitamin E and zinc are so low that deficiency may result. Low-fat milks may cause the infant to consume excessive amounts of protein to satisfy caloric needs.[59]

COMPLEMENTARY FEEDING

The optimal age at which complementary feedings should be introduced is controversial. Some health organizations recommend exclusive breast-feeding for 6 months, whereas others recommend exclusive breast-feeding for 4–6 months. The dilemma is to provide the best and safest nutrition for infants. Longer exclusive breast-feeding protects against the exposure to potentially contaminated and/or low-nutrient dense foods that put infants at risk for diarrhea and malnutrition. If a safe supply of water and complementary foods exist, then the focus for the timing of introduction of complementary foods is on nutrients themselves. Exclusively breast-fed infants are at risk of developing iron, zinc and calorie deficiency after 4–6 months of age and may benefit from the introduction of complementary feedings at that time. There is no evidence that prolonged exclusive breast-feeding protects against allergy. There are no studies that compare neurocognitive development or behavior in exclusively breast-fed infants and those on mixed feedings. No information exists on the optimal time at which to introduce complementary foods for formula-fed infants. Developmentally, infants are ready to receive complementary foods when they have some hand–eye coordination and the extrusion reflex abates (Table 71.5).

As breast-fed infants are at risk of developing iron and zinc deficiency, complementary foods high in these minerals, such as meats, should be introduced as the first food. Iron-fortified infant cereal is often recommended as the initial solid food; however, the absorption and bioavailability of iron from fortified cereals is low[32,60] and they do not provide zinc.

Juice is sometimes recommended in the first year of life and parents often provide it without consulting their doctors. Historically, pediatricians recommended fruit juice as a source of vitamin C when scurvy was a serious concern for infants. Fruit juice is marketed as a healthy, natural source of vitamins and, in some instances, calcium. Because juice tastes good, children readily accept it. There is no nutritional indication to feed juice to infants younger than 6 months of age. Offering juice before solid foods are introduced into the diet could risk having juice replace breast milk or infant formula in the diet. This can result in reduced intake of protein, fat, vitamins and minerals such as iron, calcium and zinc.[61] Malnutrition has been associated with excessive consumption of juice.[62]

Because foods high in iron are recommended as weaning foods, beverages that contain vitamin C do not offer a nutritional advantage for iron-sufficient individuals. The AAP recommends that juice not be offered to infants younger than 6 months and for those older than 1 year it be provided in limited amounts.[63]

	Newborn	Head up	Supported sitter	Independent sitter	Crawler	Beginning to walk	Independent toddler
Physical skills	Needs head support	More skillful head control with support emerging	Sits with help or support On tummy, pushes up on arms with straight elbows	Sits independently Can pick up and hold small object in hand Leans toward food or spoon	Learns to crawl May pull self to stand	Pulls self to stand Stands alone Takes early steps	Walks well alone Runs
Eating skills	Baby establishes a suck–swallow–breathe pattern during breast- or bottle-feeding	Breast- or bottle-feeds Tongue moves forward and back to suck	May push food out of mouth with tongue; this gradually decreases with age Moves puréed food forward and backward in mouth with tongue to swallow Recognizes spoon and holds mouth open as spoon approaches	Learns to keep thick purées in mouth Pulls head downward and presses upper lip to draw food from spoon Tries to rake foods toward self into fist Can transfer food from one hand to the other Can drink from a cup held by feeder	Learns to move tongue from side to side to transfer food around mouth and push food to the side of the mouth so food can be mashed Begins to use jaw and tongue to mash food Plays with spoon at mealtime, may bring it to mouth, but does not use it for self-feeding yet Can feed self finger foods Holds cup independently Holds small foods between thumb and first finger	Feeds self easily with fingers Can drink from a straw Can hold cup with two hands and take swallows More skillful at chewing Dips spoon in food rather than scooping Demands to spoon-feed self Bites through a variety of textures	Chews and swallows firmer foods skillfully Learns to use a fork for spearing Uses spoon with less spilling Can hold cup in one hand and set it down skillfully
Baby's hunger and fullness cues	Cries or fusses to show hunger Gazes at caregiver; opens mouth during feeding indicating desire to continue Spits out nipple or falls asleep when full Stops sucking when full	Cries or fusses to show hunger Smiles, gazes at caregiver, or coos during feeding to indicate desire to continue Spits out nipple or falls asleep when full Stops sucking when full	Moves head forward to reach spoon when hungry May swipe the food toward the mouth when hungry Turns head away from spoon when full May be distracted or notice surroundings more when full	Reaches for spoon or food when hungry Points to food when hungry Slows down in eating when full Clenches mouth shut or pushes food away when full	Reaches for food when hungry Points to food when hungry Shows excitement when food is presented when hungry Pushes food away when full Slows down in eating when full	Expresses desire for specific foods with words or sounds Shakes head to say 'no more' when full	Combines phrases with gestures, such as 'want that' and pointing Can lead parent to refrigerator and point to a desired food or drink Uses words like 'all done' and 'get down' Plays with food or throws food when full

Appropriate foods and textures	Breast milk or infant formula	Breast milk or infant formula	Breast milk or infant formula Infant cereals Thin puréed foods	Breast milk or infant formula Infant cereals Thin puréed baby foods Thicker puréed baby foods Soft mashed foods without lumps 100% juice	Breast milk or infant formula 100% juice Infant cereals Puréed foods Ground or soft mashed foods with tiny soft noticeable lumps Foods with soft texture Crunchy foods that dissolve (such as baby biscuits or crackers) Increase variety of flavors offered	Breast milk, infant formula, or whole milk 100% juice Coarsely chopped foods, including foods with noticeable pieces Foods with soft to moderate texture Toddler foods Bite-sized pieces of foods Bites through a variety of textures	Whole milk 100% juice Coarsely chopped foods Toddler foods Bite-sized pieces of foods Becomes efficient at eating foods of varying textures and taking controlled bites of soft solids, hard solids, or crunchy foods by 2 years

Table 71.5 Development and eating skills in infants and toddlers. Butte N, Cobb K, Dwyer J. The healthy feeding guidelines for infants and toddlers. Journal of the American Dietetic Association 1994; 104:452 with permission from the American Dietetic Association.

SUPPLEMENTS

As noted above, exclusively breast-fed infants require supplementation with vitamin D to prevent rickets. Exclusively breast-fed infants of vegan mothers require supplementation with vitamin B_{12}. Healthy, term, formula-fed infants do not require vitamin or mineral supplements as all of the formulas, except the low-iron formulas, are complete foods. Infants aged 6 months or more may benefit from fluoride supplementation if their water is not fluoridated.[64] No information is available on the fluoride content of bottled water.

TODDLERS

There is no widely accepted definition of 'toddler'. The term is taken from the wide-based gait seen in children who are just learning to walk. It is generally agreed that 'toddlerhood' begins at the age of 12 months; the upper boundary of this age bracket is poorly defined. In this discussion it is assumed that toodlerhood ends at 36 months. Thus, a child aged less than 12 months is an infant and after 36 months a toddler becomes a 'pre-schooler'. Because many of the data in the literature are given for children aged 2–5 years, 'pre-schoolers' are often included in the discussion.

Growth and therefore nutritional requirements peak during the first year of life. Growth rate during the second 12 months of life continues to be high. The second year of life is one of transition from an infant diet to a modified adult diet, yet there is a paucity of studies and guidelines on toddlers' nutrition. There are a number of studies that describe what toddlers eat.[65–70] There have been studies documenting change in eating patterns of toddlers[71,72] and reports on the psychologic and behavioral aspects of toddler nutrition.[73–75] However, few studies have been performed to determine the nutritional requirements of toddlers.[76,77] There are also few published guidelines,[78,79] and those that are available often use data extrapolated from other age groups.

Barker hypothesis

This hypothesis proposes that 'a baby's nourishment before birth and during infancy' programs the development of raised blood pressure, fibrinogen concentration, factor VIII concentration and glucose tolerance, and so is an important determinant of future coronary artery disease.[80,81] The Barker hypothesis, as originally stated, was limited to fetal and infant nutrition and the subsequent development of coronary artery disease. The hypothesis has been broadened to include any adult ailment that may have its beginning during childhood, such as osteoporosis and renal disease. The Barker hypothesis continues to be debated, but to the extent that it proves true, early nutrition gains tremendous importance. It is during toddler years that dietary patterns are established for life.[82]

DESCRIPTIVE INFORMATION

A number of cross-sectional national studies as well as some longitudinal studies are presently available for analysis. The major national cross-sectional studies are the National Health and Nutrition Examination Survey (NHANES I, II and III) and the present continuous NHANES study. There are four Continuous Survey of Food Intake by Individuals studies (CSFII, 1998; 1994–1996; 1989–1991; 1985–1986). Data on toddlers are also available from the National Food Consumption Survey (1977–1978). Additionally, there is one recent industry-sponsored survey addressing toddler nutrition, the Feeding Infants and Toddlers Study (FITS) conducted and supported by Gerber Products.[83] The FITS data include 3022 infants and toddlers aged from 4 to 24 months. FITS does not provide information on the older toddler. All of these studies point to consistency in energy intake and in the relative proportions of macronutritients across the country, across racial and ethnic groups, and over the years. This consistency lends support to the long-held notion that toddlers, when presented with adequate nutrition, self-regulate their intake to a remarkable extent.[84–86] In counterdistinction to this consistency, a number of trends in toddler nutrition have been documented over the past 30 years. As with other segments of the population, in children less than 5 years of age there has been an increased prevalence of overweight from 7.2% in the NHANES II to 10.4% in the most recent NHANES continuous survey[87] (Fig. 71.1). Snacking has always been an important source of nutrition for toddlers. Recent surveys have shown an increase in the importance of snacking as

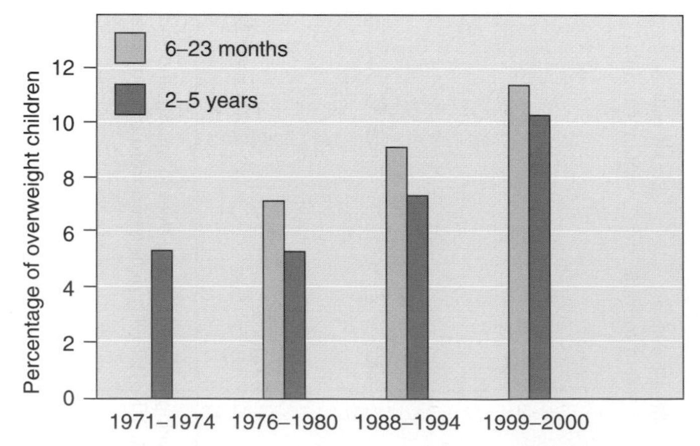

Figure 71.1: Percentage of overweight children aged 6–60 months, as reported by the National Health and Nutrition Examination Surveys (NHANES).

a component of toddlers' diets. Snacks now represent 24% of total caloric intake by 2–5-year-olds (Fig. 71.2).[71] The change is attributed to an increase in the number of snacks (rather than larger portion size) and a shift to higher-calorie, higher-fat snacks.

EXPERIMENTAL INFORMATION

Energy

Energy needs are variable in toddlers, as they are for other age groups, and depend on basal metabolic rate, rate of growth, physical activity and body size. Energy requirements also depend on whether the child is overweight or underfed. The reader is directed to the most recent Dietary Reference Intakes (DRIs) for a thorough discussion of the various factors that influence energy requirements.[6,88–92]

Energy needs can be determined experimentally in a number of ways: indirect calorimetry, doubly labeled water and the factorial method. Of these, doubly labeled water, the most accurate method, has the advantage of measuring energy consumption in a free-living individual over a prolonged period of time. Its disadvantages are expense and lack of availability. Indirect calorimetry determines oxygen consumed and carbon dioxide produced by careful measurement of inspired and expired gases. Accurate measurements are difficult in the toddler age range. The factorial method sums the contributions of basal metabolic rate, physical activity, thermic effect of food, growth and any known losses. The factorial method is the least accurate, but was the method most frequently used in the past.

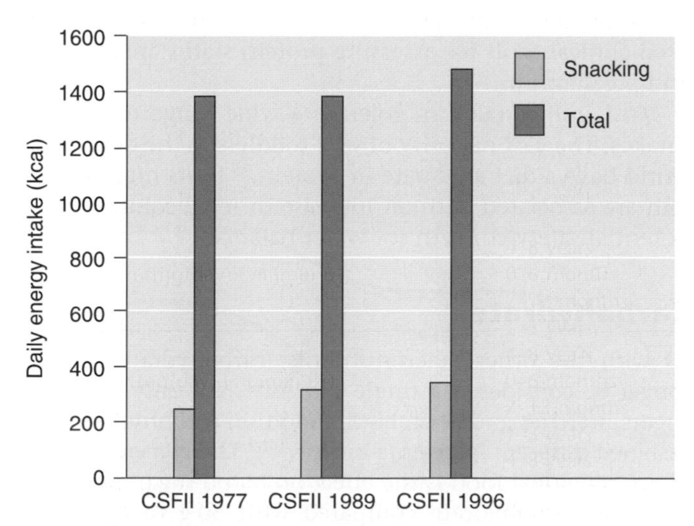

Figure 71.2: Contribution of snacking to total energy intake by 2–5-year-old children, as reported by Continuous Survey of Food Intakes by Individuals (CSFII).

It is now generally believed that previous estimates of toddlers' energy needs were erroneously high. The 10th edition of the Recommended Dietary Allowances (RDAs) set the energy requirements of 1–3-year-olds at 103 kcal per kg bodyweight per day.[92]

Prentice et al.,[93] using doubly labeled water, determined the energy expenditure of children aged 12, 24 and 36 months at 83, 84 and 85 kcal per kg per day respectively. The most recent DRIs, depending on doubly labeled water measurements, set the estimated energy requirement for 12-month-old boys at 844 kcal/day and that for 12-month-old girls at 768 kcal/day. The estimated energy requirements of boys aged 24 months are 1050 kcal/day and those for girls 997 kcal/day. For 35-month-old boys the estimated energy requirement is 1184 kcal/day and for girls 1139 kcal/day. Assuming a weight at the 50th percentile for age, these numbers translate into 81.2 kcal/kg daily for 12-month-old boys and 80.6 kcal/kg daily for girls, and 82.7 and 83.1 kcal/kg daily for 24-month-old boys and girls respectively. For 35-month-old boys the estimated energy requirement is 84.0 kcal/kg daily and that for girls is 83.8 kcal/kg daily. The new DRIs are in line with the measurements of Prentice et al.[93] and significantly lower than the previous RDAs.

Fats

The principle of any diet for children must be that it adequately supports growth and development. Particularly with fats, this principle has led to controversy. Limiting fat intake should not jeopardize a toddler's growth and neurologic development, but excess fat might lead to obesity and future athrosclerotic disease. There has been a strong recommendation from the AAP not to limit fat in the diet of toddlers until 24 months of age. It is feared that a fat-restricted diet might be deficient in energy or other nutrients. Between 24 months and 18 years of age, the recommendation calls for a child to be taking not more than 30% but not less than 20% of calories from fat; of this, not more than 10% should be from saturated fats. The recommendations say that average daily cholesterol intake should be less than 300 mg.[94] With emphasis on decreasing the amount of fat in the diet of adults, there has been a steady decline in the amount of fat that toddlers consume: the latest FITS reports that fat intake for many toddlers is less than that recommended.[95]

Essential fatty acids (EFAs)

For humans, α-linoleic acid, an omega-6 polyunsaturated fatty acid, and linolenic acid of the omega-3 series of polyunsaturated fatty acids are essential. Approximately 1–2% of dietary calories must come from these two EFAs to avoid deficiencies. α-Linoleic acid is a precursor of arachidonic acid (AA), whereas linolenic acid is metabolized to docosohexanoic acid (DHA). AA and DHA are prominent fatty acids of neural tissue, and DHA is found in high concentration in the retina. Humans can synthesize both AA and DHA, but recent studies have suggested that premature infants and possibly full-term infants may synthesize inadequate quantities of these fatty acids (conditionally essential). AA and DHA are present in human milk and have been added to some infant formulas. Whether the addition of these fatty acids to infant formulas will improve vision and cognition, as claimed, is the subject of a number of studies with diverse results.[50,53,54,96,97] Nevertheless, this debate over AA and DHA for infants has led to speculation as to whether AA and DHA are required by toddlers. Toddlers continue to lay down significant amounts of neural tissue and, hence, DHA. Whether toddlers synthesize adequate amounts of AA and DHA from precursors is not known. Improvement with administration of DHA has been reported in children known to have illnesses associated with disordered fat metabolism, such as cystic fibrosis[98] and peroxomal disease.[99] Low levels of red blood cell DHA have been demonstrated in malnourished Pakistani children.[100,101]

Trans-fats

In an unsaturated fatty acid, the carbon atoms on either side of the double bond can be in either a *cis* or a *trans* configuration. The higher the concentration of *trans* fatty acids, the more solid the fat. So oils are generally high in *cis* fatty acids, and margarine and lard are high in *trans* fatty acids. Fatty acids can be changed from the *cis* to the *trans* form by processes such as heating, baking and frying. *Trans* fatty acids are implicated in cardiovascular disease in adults.[102] The importance of *cis vs trans* fatty acids for toddlers is entirely unknown, but, by extrapolation from adult data and invoking the extended Barker hypothesis, it is important to study this question carefully.

Proteins

Proteins are essential for all metabolic functions in the body and serve as the main structural element of the body, as biochemical catalysts and as regulators of gene expression. Proteins are complex and their function is influenced by energy and nutrients, such as minerals, vitamins and trace elements. Proteins consist of amino acids that have been categorized as essential (or indispensable) and nonessential (or dispensable). The nine essential amino acids cannot be synthesized from precursors and hence must be provided. However, as more information on protein and intermediary metabolism is understood, the definition of essential becomes blurred. Laidlaw and Kopple[103] propose adding a third category of amino acid: conditionally indispensable. Conditionally indispensable amino acids are those that are synthesized from other amino acids or that have limited synthesis under special physiologic conditions.[103–105] Protein quality is determined by digestibility and the indispensable amino acid composition of the protein. If the content of a single indispensable amino acid is less than the requirement, that amino acid limits the utilization of other amino acids, preventing normal rates of protein synthesis even when the total nitrogen is adequate.

Unlike energy and other nutrients, the body has little in the way of protein that can be mobilized during times of insufficient intake. In a 70-kg adult the 'reservoir' of labile protein is estimated at about 1% of total body protein. More than half of the body protein is present as skeletal muscle, skin and blood. The liver and kidney are metabolically active tissues that contain about 10% of total body protein. Brain, heart, lung and bone account for about 15% of whole body protein. The distribution of protein among these organs varies with age. The toddler has proportionately more brain and visceral tissue and less muscle. When exogenous protein is inadequate, functional body proteins are used. The body can adapt to a wide range of protein intakes; however, pathologic conditions such as infection or trauma can cause substantial protein loss, either as demand for amino acids increases or as amino acid carbon skeletons are used to meet energy demands. If these extra needs are not met, a serious depletion of body protein mass occurs. Skeletal muscle is the largest single contributor to protein loss.

Protein requirements are based on the assumptions that adequate energy is provided, so that the carbon skeletons of amino acids are not needed as an energy source and the protein quality is high. Estimates of protein requirements for toddlers range from 0.88 g/kg daily[88] to 1.2 g/kg daily.[106] Proposed amino acid requirements of the nine indispensable amino for children and adults have been reviewed.[107]

The most reliable method to assess the adequacy of dietary protein is nitrogen balance: the difference between nitrogen intake and the amount excreted in urine, feces, skin and sweat. This measurement is not practical clinically, especially for children. There is no reliable clinical measure of protein nutritional status. Failure to gain weight or length can be used to assess the overall nutritional adequacy of a diet, and failure to gain length occurs with borderline inadequate protein intake.[108] Other anthropometrics are less sensitive. The most commonly used clinical tools for assessing protein status are albumin and prealbumin.

Most individuals can tolerate a wide range of protein intakes. The vast majority of well toddlers in the developed world have a diet adequate in protein.[95] Diets high in protein are associated with an increase in renal solute load, a potential safety concern for water balance.

Carbohydrates

As with the other macronutrients, carbohydrate can no longer be considered a single category. Not only are there sugars, starches and fiber, but in addition carbohydrates are assigned different 'glycemic indices'.[109] The glycemic index of an individual food is the effect on blood sugar of 50 g of available carbohydrate compared with 50 g of a control food. From the glycemic indices, the glycemic load of a diet can be calculated. Glycemic load has been shown to be an independent risk factor for type 2 diabetes,[110,111] for cancer[112] and for cardiovascular disease in women.[113] Relatively few studies have been done to determine glycemic load in children.[114] There are no recommendations for carbohydrate intake in toddlers; however, carbohydrate accounts for 52% of the energy intake of children aged 1–5 years.[92,115] Fiber and non-absorbable starch are important carbohydrate components of the diet. They change the viscosity of the small bowel content, thus altering transit time and the absorption of nutrients. After entering the large intestine, these substances are not 'inert' but regulate colonic bacterial bulk as well as changing the composition of the flora. Bacteria produce short-chain fatty acids through fermentation. These short-chain fatty acids are used for fuel by colonocytes, but are also absorbed into the circulation. These actions of fiber and non-absorbable starch promote defecation, a desirable effect, as constipation is a major problem among toddlers.[116] Toddlers in the USA ingest a mean of 8.5 g fiber per day.[95] The Institute of Medicine recommends that toddlers have 19 g fiber daily.[88]

SPECIFIC NUTRIENT DEFICITS

Iron

Despite a demonstrable decline in prevalence, iron deficiency anemia remains the most common cause of anemia in young children.[117] However, perhaps more important than anemia itself, is the suggestion that iron deficiency alters long-term development and behavior, and that some of these effects may not be reversible. There have been an overwhelming number of studies linking iron deficiency with neurodevelopmental and motor delays, and indicating the benefits of iron supplementation. These studies are the subject of a Cochrane Database Review.[118] The conclusion of the review was that there was no firm evidence for a short-term (2 weeks) beneficial effect of iron supplementation on neurologic and motor development, but there did appear to be a long-term (3 months) effect. Even more concerning than the evidence that iron deficiency is adversely affecting development is that these adverse effects can be documented 10 years after the deficiency has been corrected, and so are likely permanent.[3]

Iron is present in the body in association with hemoglobin, myoglobin and as a co-factor for enzymes (functional iron), or as a part of ferritin and hemosiderin (stored iron).

Depleted iron stores

If there is a negative iron balance, iron stores are depleted and serum ferritin levels decrease. Because ferritin levels are affected by mechanisms other than iron depletion, such as inflammation, ferritin alone cannot be used to determine iron status. Measured levels of serum transferring receptors (TfRs) increase early with depletion of iron stores. TfR levels are not affected by inflammation, but experience with this measurement in children is limited.[119]

Iron deficiency without anemia

As iron stores become more limiting, there is disordered erythropoiesis leading to increased erythrocyte protoporphyrin and decreased transferrin saturation.

Iron deficiency anemia

When hemoglobin levels and the hematocrit begin to decrease, iron deficiency anemia is present. There are a number of conditions that mimic iron deficiency anemia, such as anemia of chronic disease, lead poisoning, thalasemia minor or other mild hereditary anemias. These other conditions need to be considered and excluded. The WHO recently recommended using hemoglobin, ferritin and transferrin receptor levels to identify iron deficiency anemia, and hemoglobin, ferritin and C-reactive protein to monitor anemia (personal communication).

Comparison of the NHANES III and the present NHANES data suggests that the prevalences of iron deficiency and iron deficiency anemia have decreased. National data place the prevalence of iron deficiency at 9% and iron deficiency anemia at 3% of toddlers.[120] Looking at disadvantaged areas, the prevalence is reported to be as high as 24% for iron deficiency and 11% for iron deficiency anemia.[121] Presently, two types of screening programs are recommended: universal and selective screening. Universal screening at 9–12 and 15–18 months of age is used in communities with a high incidence of iron deficiency. In communities where iron deficiency is not common, selective screening uses the same schedule, but screens only children thought to be at risk. At-risk children include pre-term babies, those with a low birthweight, those not receiving iron-fortified formula and breast-fed children over the age of 6 months not consuming a diet with adequate iron. Confirmation of a positive screen with a second test will eliminate most false positives.[122]

There are a number of possible approaches to dealing with the problem of iron deficiency in the toddler years: selective treatment, universal supplementation and food fortification. At present, selective treatment based on the screening programs outlined above is recommended. Oral supplementation (3–6 mg/kg daily of elemental iron) is given for 4 weeks, and hemoglobin and hematocrit are then remeasured. An appropriate rise in the hemoglobin concentration (1 g/dl) confirms iron deficiency anemia. An insufficient rise should trigger further investigations, including adherence, blood loss, hemoglobinopathy and lead poisoning. This selective treatment approach is certain to miss a proportion of children with iron deficiency and iron deficiency anemia. In view of the long-term sequelae associated with iron deficiency, including behavioral and developmental changes, we may want to consider another approach.

Zinc

Zinc is essential for growth. It is involved in chromosome replication, regulation of the translation of genetic information, provides structure for 'zinc-finger' proteins, stabilizes ribosomes and membranes, and is a component of a number of enzymes.[123] Zinc deficiency in humans impairs cell-mediated immunity. Signs of zinc deficiency include dermatitis, alopecia, diarrhea and immune deficiency. Severe, parenteral nutrition-associated zinc deficiency mimics acrodermatitis enteropathica.[124,125] With zinc deficiency, relatively more fat accrues than lean tissue.[126] Zinc status is difficult to monitor. Stress, infections and trauma all alter circulating zinc levels. Despite these shortcomings, serum zinc is commonly used to monitor zinc nutriture. Zinc is lost from the body through urine, sweat and stool. Zinc status should be assessed and corrected, if necessary, in the face of extra losses – as in the case of diarrhea or high ostomy output. Studies using the RDAs from 1989 found the zinc intake of toddlers to be too low;[127] however, using the new DRI recommendations, the FITS found that the majority of toddlers achieved the recommended intakes.[95] Whether the new standards are too low needs to be monitored carefully.

Vitamin E

Vitamin E deficiency has been associated with spinocerebellar disorders.[128] As an antioxidant, vitamin E has an unsubstantiated but potential role in the long-term prevention of oxidative damage, including cardiovascular disease, osteoarthritis and others. The vitamin E status of toddlers is of concern. A number of studies have documented intakes of vitamin E less than the recommendations.[78,95,129] However, none of these studies has identified any signs or symptoms of vitamin E deficiency.

TODDLERS' NUTRITON AND STOOLING

Toddlers are going through a time of transition. As the diet changes from a predominantly milk-based one to a modified adult diet, the colonic flora also changes from an infant-type to more adult flora. Eating behavior is also in transition, going from being fed to self-feeding. All of these factors lead to extreme variation in stooling patterns. Many toddlers suffer from constipation, sometimes made worse by withholding behavior.[116] Some toddlers have diarrhea and some alternate between the two. Toddlers tend not to chew their food well and it is not uncommon for food particles to appear in the feces apparently unchanged.

Diarrhea

Toddler's diarrhea is defined as diarrhea in a toddler who is otherwise healthy and for whom no other cause of diarrhea can be identified. Experience shows that this type of diarrhea eventually resolves.[130] Merely normalizing the toddler's diet and following the recommendations of the AAP to limit the quantity of juice result in resolution or improvement.[63]

Constipation

There is general agreement that functional constipation is extremely common among toddlers. The exact prevalence, however, is not known. Toddlers with constipation account for 3% of visits to the general pediatrician and for 25% of visits to pediatric gastroenterologists.[131] At least a part of the reason for the high prevalence of constipation among toddlers may be the low-fiber content of their diet. Toddlers consume an average of 8.5 g fiber a day, whereas the IOM recommends 19 g per day. There is little experimental evidence that increasing the fiber intake improves symptoms of constipation, except in those with developmental disabilities.[132,133]

PSYCHOLOGY OF TODDLERS' NUTRITION

The parent–child interaction around eating behavior is extremely complex and varies with the special needs of the child and the parents. The family make-up, economic, social, ethnic and other factors influence this relationship. No rigid rules can be given, but some general principles apply. Structure and consistency are all important. Parents should identify what is acceptable to them and contrive ways to stay within the acceptable limits. Power struggles are to be avoided. Although a parent may win the battle ('You will not leave the table until every bit of broccoli is gone from your plate'), the war will probably be lost as the child may develop a lifelong loathing of broccoli. Bribery, especially with food, is not a good idea.

Eating the right amount

The toddler years are marked by transition to an adult-like diet. Although growth remains high, this is a time of decelerating growth and growth velocity. Toddlers are also becoming increasingly independent in their feeding skills and vocal in their likes and dislikes. There is often a perception that toddlers do not eat enough and are 'picky eaters'.[134] The FITS reports that by 24 months of age 50% of children are identified as 'picky eaters' by their caregivers. However, the study found that picky eaters were no more likely than non-picky eaters to have inadequate diets. Further, the study found that picky eaters were less likely to be overweight.[135]

Toddlers frequently exhibit 'food neophobia', that is, a reluctance to try new foods. Sullivan and Birch[136] found that repeated exposures (five to ten) to a new food increased the likelihood of a toddler accepting it. However, parents and caregivers questioned in the FITS identified a food as not liked by their toddler if refused an average of three times.

Meals and snacks

For the toddler, both meals and snacks are important opportunities for nutrition. They are also a time to learn skills, values and interact with others. For all toddlers, but especially for the younger toddler aged 12–24 months, all meals and snacks should be supervised. The danger of choking on small, hard foods is significant throughout toddlerhood. By 12 months of age the pattern of breakfast, lunch and dinner plus snacks is well established. In the FITS, toddlers ate an average of seven times per day. Snacks provided 25% of the toddlers' energy intake. Snacks tended to be of lower nutritional quality compared with meals.[137] Snacking, as a component of the toddler's diet, has increased over time. In 1977, the average number of snacks per day consumed by children aged 2–5 years was 1.7. By 1996, the average had increased to 2.3. During the same time-frame, the energy provided by snacking increased by 100 kcal/day.[71] Snacks, like meals, should be a planned part of the toddler's nutrition.

References

1. Lucas A, Morley R, Isaacs E. Nutrition and mental development. Nutr Rev 2001; 59:S24–S33.
2. Algarin C, Peirano P, Garrido M, Pizarro F, Lozoff B. Iron deficiency anemia in infancy: long-lasting effects on auditory and visual system functioning. Pediatr Res 2003; 53:217–223.
3. Lozoff B, Jimenez E, Hagen J, Mollen E, Wolf AW. Poorer behavioral and developmental outcome more than 10 years after treatment for iron deficiency in infancy. Pediatrics 2000; 105:E51.
4. Fomon SJ. Nutrition of Normal Infants. St Louis, MI: Mosby; 1993.
5. Institute of Medicine. Dietary Reference Intakes Applications in Dietary Assessment. Washington, DC: National Academy Press; 2000.
6. Institute of Medicine. Dietary Reference Intakes for Calcium, Phosphorus, Magnesium, Vitamin D and Fluoride. Washington, DC: National Academy Press; 1997.
7. Allen JC, Keller RP, Archer P, Nevelle MC. Studies in human lactation: milk composition and daily secretion rates of macronutrients in the first year of lactation. Am J Clin Nutr 1991; 54:69–80.
8. Butte NF, Garza C, Smith EO, Nichols BL. Human milk intake and growth in exclusively breast-fed infants. J Pediatr 1984; 104:187–195.
9. Heinig MJ, Nommsen LA. Peerson JM, Lonnderal B, Dewey KG. Energy and protein intakes of breast-fed and formula-fed infants during the first year of life and their association with growth velocity: the DARLING study. Am J Clin Nutr 1993; 58:152–161.
10. Dewey KG, Peerson JM, Brown KH, et al. World Health Organization Working Group on Infant Growth. Growth of breast-fed infants deviates from current reference data: a pooled analysis of US, Canadian and European data sets. Pediatrics 1995; 96:495–503.
11. Kramer MS, Guo T, Platt RW, et al. Breastfeeding and infant growth: biology or bias? Pediatrics 2002; 110:343–347.
12. Motil KJ, Sheng H-P, Montandon C, Wong WW. Human milk protein does not limit growth of breast-fed infants. J Pediatr Gastroenterol Nutr 1997; 24:10–17.
13. Ogden CL, Kuczmarski RJ, Flegel KM, et al. Centers for Disease Control and Prevention 2000 growth charts for the United States: improvements to the 1977 National Center for Health Statistics version. Pediatrics 2002; 109:45–60.
14. Kleinman RE, ed. Nutrition Handbook. Elk Grove Village, IL: American Academy of Pediatrics; 2004:55.
15. Duncan B, Ey J, Holberg CJ, Wright AL, Martinez RFD, Taussig LM. Exclusive breast-feeding for at least 4 months protects against otitis media. Pediatrics 1993; 91:867–872.
16. Aniansson G, Alm B, Andersson B, et al. A prospective cohort study on breast-feeding and otitis media in Swedish infants. Pediatr Infect Dis J 1994; 13:183–188.
17. Owen MJ, Baldwin CD, Swank PR, Pannu AK, Johnson DL, Howie VM. Relation of infant feeding practices, cigarette smoke exposure, and group child care to the onset and duration of otitis media with effusion in the first two years of life. J Pediatr 1993; 123:702–711.
18. Teele DW, Klein JO, Rosner B. Epidemiology of otitis media during the first seven years of life in children in greater Boston: a prospective, cohort study. J Infect Dis 1989; 160:83–94.
19. Paradise JL, Elster BA, Tan L. Evidence in infants with cleft palate that breast milk protects against otitis media. Pediatrics 1994; 94:853–860.
20. Dewey KG, Heinig MJ, Nommsen-Rivers LA. Differences in morbidity between breast-fed and formula-fed infants. J Pediatr 1995; 126:696–702.
21. Wright AL, Holberg CJ, Martinez FD, Morgan WJ, Taussig LM. Breast feeding and lower respiratory tract illness in the first year of life. Group Health Medical Associates. BMJ 1989; 299:946–949.
22. Howie PW, Forsyth JS, Ogston SA, Clark A, Florey CD. Protective effect of breast feeding against infection. BMJ 1990; 300:11–16.
23. Marild S, Jodal U, Hanson LA. Breastfeeding and urinary-tract infection. Lancet 1990; 336:942.
24. Pisacane A, Graziano L, Mazzarella G, Scarpellino B, Zona G. Breast-feeding and urinary tract infection. J Pediatr 1992; 120:87–89.
25. Arnold C, Makintube S, Istre GR. Day care attendance and other risk factors for invasive *Haemophilus influenzae* type b disease. Am J Epidemiol 1993; 138:333–340.
26. Petersen GM, Silimperi DR, Chiu CY, Ward JI. Effects of age, breast feeding, and household structure on *Haemophilus influenzae* type b disease risk and antibody acquisition in Alaskan Eskimos. Am J Epidemiol 1991; 134:1212–1221.
27. Arnon SS, Damus K, Thompson B, Midura TF, Chin J. Protective role of human milk against sudden death from infant botulism. J Pediatr 1982; 100:568–573.
28. Hibberd CM, Brooke OG, Carter ND, Haug M, Harzer G. Variation in the composition of breast milk during the first 5 weeks of lactation: implications for the feeding of preterm infants. Arch Dis Child 1982; 57:658–662.
29. Parmely MJ, Williams SB. Selective expression of immunocompetence in human colostrums: preliminary evidence for the control of cytotoxic T lymphocytes including those specific for paternal alloantigens. In: Ogra PI, Dayton D, eds. Immunology of Breast Milk. New York: Raven Press; 1979:173–183.
30. Subcommittee on Nutrition During Lactation, Institute of Medicine. Nutrition during lactation. Washington, DC: National Academy Press; 1991.
31. Ogra SS, Ogra PL. Immunologic aspects of human colostrums and milk. I. Distribution characteristics and concentrations of immunoglobulins at different times after the onset of lactation. J Pediatr 1978; 92:546–549.
32. Hytten FE. Clinical and chemical studies in human lactation. VII. The effect of differences in yield and composition of milk on the infant's weight gain and duration of breastfeeding. BMJ 1954; 1:1410.
33. Lawrence M, Gartner, FR. Section on Breastfeeding and Committee on Nutrition (1 Apr 2003) Prevention of rickets and vitamin D deficiency: new guidelines for vitamin D intake. Pediatrics 2003; 111:908–910.

34. Fomon SJ. Nutrition of Normal Infants. St Louis, MI: Mosby; 1993:250–256.
35. Kleinman RE, ed. Nutrition Handbook. Elk Grove Village, IL: American Academy of Pediatrics; 2004:104–105.
36. Kramer MS, Kakuma R. Optimal duration of exclusive breastfeeding. Cochrane Database Syst Rev 2002; (1)CD003517.
37. Kleinman RE, ed. Nutrition Handbook. Elk Grove Village, IL: American Academy of Pediatrics; 2004:105–108.
38. Kleinman RE, ed. Nutrition Handbook. Elk Grove Village, IL: American Academy of Pediatrics; 2004:65.
39. Kleinman RE, ed. Nutrition Handbook. Elk Grove Village, IL: American Academy of Pediatrics; 2004:886–896.
40. Committee on Environmental Health, American Academy of Pediatrics. Handbook of Pediatric Environmental Health. Elk Grove, IL: American Academy of Pediatrics; 1999.
41. Committee on Pesticides in the diets of infants and children, National Research Council. Pesticides in the Diets of Infants and Children. Washington, DC: National Academy Press; 1993.
42. Kleinman RE, ed. Nutrition Handbook. Elk Grove Village, IL: American Academy of Pediatrics; 2004:87.
43. Kleinman RE, ed. Nutrition Handbook. Elk Grove Village, IL: American Academy of Pediatrics; 2004:938–960.
44. American Academy of Pediatrics, Committee on Nutrition. Iron-fortified infant formulas. Pediatrics 1999; 104:119–123.
45. Graham GG, Placko RP, Morales E, Acevedo G, Cordano A Dietary protein quality in infants and children. VI. Isolated soy protein milk. Am J Dis Child. 1970; 120:419–423.
46. Fomon SJ, Ziegler EE. Soy protein isolates in infant feeding. In: Wilcke HL, Hopkins DT, Waggle DH, eds. Soy Protein and Human Nutrition. New York: Academic Press; 1979:79–86.
47. Kohler L, Meeuwisse G, Mortensson W. Food intake and growth of infants between six and twenty-six weeks of age on breast milk, cow's milk formula, or soy formula. Acta Paediatr Scand 1984; 73:40–48.
48. Strom BL, Schinnar R, Ziegler EE, et al. Follow-up study of a cohort fed soy-based formula during infancy. Endocrinol Metab 2000; 7:Abstract LB 39.
49. American Academy of Pediatrics, Committee on Nutrition. Soy protein-based formulas: recommendations for use in infant feeding. Pediatrics 1998; 101:148–153.
50. Auestad N, Halter R, Hall RT, et al. Growth and development in term infants fed long-chain polyunsaturated fatty acids: a double-masked, randomized, parallel, prospective, multivariate study. Pediatrics 2001; 108:372–381.
51. Lucas A, Stafford M, Morley R, et al. Efficacy and safety of long-chain polyunsaturated fatty acid supplementation of infant-formula milk: a randomized trial. Lancet 1999; 354:1948–1954.
52. Makrides M, Neumann MA, Simmer K, Gibson RA. A critical appraisal of the role of dietary long-chain polyunsaturated fatty acids on neural indices of term infants: a randomized, controlled trial. Pediatrics 2000; 105:32–38.
53. Birch EE, Garfield S, Hoffman DR, Uauy R, Birch DG. A randomized controlled trial of early dietary supply of long-chain polyunsaturated fatty acids and mental development in term infants. Dev Med Child Neurol 2000; 42:174–181.
54. O'Connor DL, Jacobs J, Hall R, et al. Growth and development of premature infants fed predominantly human milk, predominantly premature infant formula, or a combination of human milk and premature formula. J Pediatr Gastroenterol Nutr 2003; 37:437–446.
55. American Academy of Pediatrics, Committee on Nutrition. The use of whole cow milk in infancy. Pediatrics 1992; 89:1105–1109.
56. Penrod JC, Anderson K, Acosta PB. Impact on iron status of introducing cow's milk in the second six months of life. J Pediatr Gastroenterol Nutr 1990; 10:462–467.
57. Tunnesson WW Jr, Oski FA. Consequences of starting whole cow milk at 6 months of age. J Pediatr 1987; 111:813–816.
58. Zeigler EE, Fomon SJ. Potential renal solute load of infant formulas. J Nutr 1989; 119:1785–1788.
59. Ryan AS, Martinez GA, Drieger FW. Feeding low-fat milk during infancy. Am J Phys Anthropol 1987; 73:539–548.
60. Hurrell RF, Furniss DE, Burri J, Whittaker P, Lynch SR, Cook JD. Iron fortification of infant cereals: a proposal for the use of ferrous fumarate or ferrous succinate. Am J Clin Nutr 1989; 49:1274–1282.
61. Smith MM, Lifshitz F. Excess fruit juice consumption as a contributing factor in nonorganic failure to thrive. Pediatrics 1994; 93:438–443.
62. Gibson SA. Non-milk extrinsic sugars in the diets of pre-school children: association with intakes of micronutrients, energy, fat and NSP. Br J Nutr 1997; 78:367–378.
63. American Academy of Pediatrics, Committee on Nutrition. The use and misuse of fruit juice in pediatrics. Pediatrics 2001; 107:1210–1213.
64. Online. Available: http://www.cdc.gov/mmwr/PDF/RR/RR5014.pdf
65. Tippett KS, Mickle SJ, Goldman JD, et al. Food and Nutrient Intake by Individuals in the United States, 1 Day, 1989–91. Continuing Survey of Foods Intakes by Individuals, 1989–91. US Department of Agriculture, Agricultural Research Service, NSF Report; 1995:91–92.
66. Tippett KS, Cypel YS. Design and Operation: Continuing Survey of Foods Intakes by Individuals and the Diet and Health Knowledge Survey, 1994–1996. US Department of Agriculture, Agricultural Research Service; NSF Report; 1998:96–91.
67. Nationwide Food Consumption Survey, 1977–1978. US Department of Agriculture, Agricultural Research Service, Food Surveys Research Group, NTIS, Report No. 1–2, Accession No. PB91-105858; 1984.
68. National Health and Nutrition Examination Survey (NHANES I), US Department of Health, Education and Welfare, Public Health Service, National Center for Health Statistics, DHEW Publication No. (PHS), 79–1310; 1973.
69. National Health and Nutrition Examination Survey, 1976–1980 (NHANES II), US Department of Health, Education and Welfare, Public Health Service, National Center for Health Statistics, DHEW Publication No. (PHS) 81 I317; 1981.
70. National Health and Nutrition Examination Survey, 1988–1994 (NHANES III), National Center for Health Statistics, Centers for Disease Control and Prevention; 1996.
71. Jahns L, Siega-Riz AM, Popkin BM. The increasing prevalence of snacking among US children from 1977 to 1996. J Pediatr 2001; 138:493–498.
72. McConahy KL, Smiciklas-Wright H, Birch LL, Mitchell DC, Picciano MF. Food portions are positively related to energy intake and body weight in early childhood. J Pediatr 2002; 140:340–347.
73. Rolls BJ, Engell D, Birch LL. Serving portion size influences 5-year-old but not 3-year-old children's food intakes. J Am Diet Assoc 2000; 100:232–234.
74. Sullivan S, Birch LL. Pass the sugar; pass the salt: experience dictates preference. Dev Psychol 1990; 26:546–551.
75. Abramowitz BA, Birch LL. Five-year-old girls' ideas about dieting are predicted by mothers' dieting. J Am Diet Assoc 2000; 100:1157–1163.
76. Kaskoun MC, Johnson RK, Goran MI. Comparison of energy intake by semiquantitative food frequency questionnaire with

total energy expenditure by doubly labeled water method in young children. Am J Clin Nutr 1994; 60:43–47.

77. Goran MI, Poehlman ET, Johnson RK. Energy requirements across the life span: new findings based on measurement of total energy expenditure with doubly labeled water. Nutr Res 1995; 15:115–120.

78. Picciano MF, Smiciklas-Wright H, Birch LL, Mitchell DC, Murray-Kolb L, McConahy KL. Nutritional guidance is needed during dietary transition in early childhood. Pediatrics 2000; 106:109–114.

79. Butte N, Cobb K, Dwyer J, Graney L, Heird W, Rickard K. The start healthy feeding guidelines for infants and toddlers. J Am Diet Assoc 2004; 104:442–454.

80. Fall CHD, Osmond C, Barker DJP, et al. Fetal and infant growth and cardiovascular risk factors in women. BMJ 1995; 310:428–432.

81. Paneth N, Susser M. Early origin of coronary heart disease (the 'Barker Hypothesis'). BMJ 1995; 310:411–412.

82. Singer MR, Moore LL, Garrahie EJ, Ellison RC. The tracking of nutrient intake in young children: the Framingham Children's Study. Am J Public Health 1995; 85:1673–1677.

83. Feeding Infants and Toddlers Study (FITS). J Am Diet Assoc 2004; 104(Suppl 1):S1–S79.

84. Davis CM. Self selection of diet by newly weaned infants: an experimental study. Am J Dis Child 1928; 36:651–679.

85. Davis CM. Results of self selection diets by young children. Can Med Assoc J 1939; 41:257–261.

86. Birch LL, Johnson SL, Anderson G, Peters JC, Schulte MC. The variability of young children's energy intake. N Engl J Med 1991; 324:232–235.

87. Ogden CL, Flegal K, Carroll MD, Johnson CL. Prevalence and trends of overweight among US children and adolescents, 1999–2000. JAMA 2002; 288:1728–1732.

88. Institute of Medicine, Food and Nutrition Board. Dietary reference intakes: energy, carbohydrate, fiber, fat, fatty acids, cholesterol, protein and amino acids. Washington, DC: National Academy Press; 2002.

89. Institute of Medicine, Food and Nutrition Board. Dietary Reference Intakes for Vitamin A, Vitamin K, Arsenic, Boron, Chromium, Copper, Iodine, Iron, Manganese, Molybdenum, Nickel, Silicon, Vanadium and Zinc. Washington, DC: National Academy Press; 2002.

90. Institute of Medicine, Food and Nutrition Board. Dietary Reference Intakes for Vitamin C, Vitamin E, Selenium and Carotenoids. Washington, DC: National Academy Press; 2002.

91. Institute of Medicine, Food and Nutrition Board. Dietary Reference Intakes for Thiamine, Riboflavin, Niacin, Vitamin B_6, Folate, Vitamin B_{12}, Pantothenic Acid, Biotin and Choline. Washington, DC: National Academy Press; 2002.

92. Food and Nutrition Board. Recommended Dietary Allowances, 10th edn. Washington, DC: National Academy Press; 1989.

93. Prentice AM, Lucas A, Vasquez-Velasquez L, Davies PS, Whitehead RG. Are current dietary guidelines for young children a prescription for overfeeding? Lancet 1988; ii:1066–1069.

94. American Academy of Pediatrics, Committee on Nutrition. Cholesterol in childhood. Pediatrics 1998; 101:141–144.

95. Devaney B, Ziegler P, Pac S, Karwe V, Barr SI. Nutrient intakes of infants and toddlers, (FITS). J Am Diet Assoc 2004; 104:S14–S21.

96. SanGiovanni JP, Berkey CS, Dwyer JT, Colditz GA. Dietary essential fatty acids, long-chain polyunsaturated fatty acids, and visual resolution acuity in healthy fullterm infants: a systematic review. Early Hum Dev 2000; 57:165–188.

97. SanGiovanni JP, Parra-Cabrera S, Colditz GA, Berkey CS, Dwyer JT. Meta-analysis of dietary essential fatty acids and long-chain polyunsaturated fatty acids as they relate to visual resolution acuity in healthy preterm infants. Pediatrics 2000; 105:1292–1298.

98. De Vizia B, Raia V, Spano C, Pavlidis C, Coruzzo A, Alessio M. Effect of an 8-month treatment with omega-3 fatty acids (eicosapentaenoic and docosahexaenoic) in patients with cystic fibrosis. JPEN J Parenter Enteral Nutr 2003; 27:52–57.

99. Martinez M, Vazquez E. MRI evidence that docosahexaenoic acid ethyl ester improves myelination in generalized peroxisomal disorders. Neurology 1998; 51:26–32.

100. Smit EN, Muskiet FA, Boersma ER. Docosahexaenoic acid (DHA) status of breastfed malnourished infants and their mothers in North Pakistan. Adv Exp Med Biol 2000; 478:395–396.

101. Smit EN, Woltil HA, Boersma ER, Muskiet FA. Low erythrocyte docosahexaenoic acid in malnourished, often breast-fed, Pakistani infants: a matter of concern? Eur J Pediatr 1999; 158:525–526.

102. de Roos NM, Schouten EG, Katan MB. *Trans* fatty acids, HDL-cholesterol, and cardiovascular disease. Effects of dietary changes on vascular reactivity. Eur J Med Res 2003; 8:355–357.

103. Laidlaw SA, Kopple JD. Newer concepts of the indispensable amino acids. Am J Clin Nutr 1987; 46:593–605.

104. Chipponi JX, Bleier JC, Santi MT, Rudman D. Deficiencies of essential and conditionally essential nutrients. Am J Clin Nutr 1982; 5:1112–1116.

105. Harper AE. Dispensable and indispensable amino acid relationships. In: Blackburn GL, Grant JP, Young VR, eds. Amino Acids. Metabolism and Medical Applications. Boston, MA: John Wright-PSG; 1983:105–121.

106. ASPEN Board of Directors and the Clinical Guidelines TaskForce. Guidelines for the use of parenteral and enteral nutrition in adult and pediatric patients. JPEN J Parenter Enteral Nutr 2002; 26(Suppl 1):1SA–138SA.

107. Standing Committee on the Scientific Evaluation of Dietary Reference Intakes, Food and Nutrition Board, Institute of Medicine. Dietary Reference Intakes for Energy, Carbohydrate, Fiber, Fat, Fatty Acids, Cholesterol, Protein and Amino Acids (Macronutrients). Washington, DC: National Academy Press; 2002.

108. Jelliffe DB. The Assessment of the Nutritional Status of the Community. WHO Monograph Series No. 53. Geneva: World Health Organization; 1966.

109. Foster-Powell K, Holt SH, Brand-Miller JC. International table of glycemic index and glycemic load values: 2002. Am J Clin Nutr 2002; 76:5–56.

110. Salmeron J, Ascherio A, Rimm EB, et al. Dietary fiber, glycemic load, and risk of NIDDM in men. Diabetes Care 1997; 20:545–550.

111. Salmeron J, Manson JE, Stampfer MJ, Colditz GA, Wing AL, Willett WC. Dietary fiber, glycemic load, and risk of non-insulin-dependent diabetes mellitus in women. JAMA 1997; 277:472–477.

112. Franceschi S, Dal Maso L, Augustin L, et al. Dietary glycemic load and colorectal cancer risk. Ann Oncol 2001; 12: 173–178.

113. Liu S, Willett WC, Stampfer MJ, et al. A prospective study of dietary glycemic load, carbohydrate intake, and risk of coronary heart disease in US women. Am J Clin Nutr 2000; 71:1455–1461.

114. Scaglioni S, Stival G, Giovannini M. Dietary glycemic load, overall glycemic index, and serum insulin concentrations in healthy schoolchildren. Am J Clin Nutr 2004; 79:339–340.

115. *Continuing survey of food intake by individuals.* US Department of Agriculture Research Service. Human Nutrition Research Center. National Technical Information Service 2004.
116. Baker SS, Liptak GS, Colletti RB, et al. Constipation in infants and children: evaluation and treatment. J Pediatr Gastroenterol Nutr 1999; 29:612–626.
117. Dallman PR, Yip R. Changing characteristics of childhood anemia, J Pediatr 1989; 114:161–164.
118. Martins S, Logan S, Gilbert R. Iron therapy for improving psychomotor development and cognitive function in children under the age of three with iron deficiency anaemia. Cochrane Database Syst Rev 2001; (2)CD001444.
119. Malope BI, MacPhail AP, Alberts M, Hiss DC. The ratio of serum transferrin receptor and serum ferritin in the diagnosis of iron status. Br J Haematol 2001; 115:84–89.
120. Anonymous. Iron deficiency – United States, 1999–2000. MMWR Morbid Mortal Wkly Rep 2002; 51:897–899.
121. Sargent JD, Stukel TA, Dalton MA, Freeman JL, Brown MJ. Iron deficiency in Massachusetts communities: socioeconomic and demographic risk factors among children. Am J Public Health 1996; 86:544–550.
122. American Academy of Pedaitrics, Committee on Nutrition. Iron deficiency. In: Kleinman R, ed. Pediatric Nutrition Handbook, 5th edn. Elk Grove Village, IL: American Academy of Pedaitrics. 2004:299–313.
123. Beck FW, Prasad AS, Kaplan J, Fitzgerald JT, Brewer GJ. Changes in cytokine production and T cell subpopulations in experimentally induced zinc-deficient humans. Am J Physiol 1997; 272:E1002–E1007.
124. Anonymous. Acrodermatitis enteropathies–hereditary zinc deficiency. Nutrition Reviews 1975; 33:327–329.
125. Main AN, Hall MJ, Russell RI, Fell GS, Mills PR, Shenkin A. Clinical experience of zinc supplementation during intravenous nutrition in Crohn's disease: value of serum and urine zinc measurements. Gut 1982; 23:984–991.
126. Golden BE, Golden MH. Plasma zinc, rate of weight gain, and the energy cost of tissue deposition in children recovering from severe malnutrition on a cow's milk or soya protein based diet. Am J Clin Nutr 1981; 34:892–899.
127. Nolan K, Schell LM, Stark AD, Gomez MI. Longitudinal study of energy and nutrient intakes for infants from low-income, urban families. Public Health Nutr 2002; 5:405–412.
128. Westermarck T, Aberg L, Santavuori P, Antila E, Edlund P, Atroshi F. Evaluation of the possible role of coenzyme Q10 and vitamin E in juvenile neuronal ceroid-lipofuscinosis (JNCL). Mol Aspects Med 1997; 18(Suppl):S259–S262.
129. Nitzan Kaluski D, Basch CE, Zybert P, Deckelbaum RJ, Shea S. Calcium intake in preschool children – a study of dietary patterns in a low socioeconomic community. Public Health Rev 2001; 29:71–83.
130. Hoekstra JH. Toddler diarrhoea: more a nutritional disorder than a disease. Arch Dis Child 1998; 79:2–5.
131. Molnar D, Taitz LS, Urwin OM, Wales JK. Anorectal manometry results in defecation disorders. Arch Dis Child 1983; 58:257–261.
132. Tse PW, Leung SS, Chan T, Sien A, Chan AK. Dietary fibre intake and constipation in children with severe developmental disabilities. J Paediatr Child Health 2000; 36:236–239.
133. Staiano A, Simeone D, Del Giudice E, Miele E, Tozzi A, Toraldo C. Effect of the dietary fiber glucomannan on chronic constipation in neurologically impaired children. J Pediatr 2000; 136:41–45.
134. Saarilehto S, Lapinleimu H, Keskinen S, Helenius H, Talvia S, Simell O. Growth, energy intake, and meal pattern in five-year-old children considered as poor eaters. J Pediatr 2004; 144:363–367.
135. Carruth BR, Ziegler PJ, Gordon A, Barr SI. Prevalence of picky eaters among infants and toddlers and their caregivers' decisions about offering a new food (FITS). J Am Diet Assoc 2004; 104:S57–S64.
136. Sullivan SA, Birch LL. Pass the sugar, pass the salt: experience dictates preference. Dev Psychol 1990; 26:546–551.
137. Skinner JD, Ziegler P, Pac S, Devaney B. Meal and snack patterns of infants and todders (FITS). J Am Diet Assoc 2004; 104:S65–S70.

Chapter 72
Nutritional assessment

Kathleen J. Motil, Sarah M. Phillips and Claudia A. Conkin

INTRODUCTION

Nutritional assessment is an essential component of the history and physical examination of children with gastrointestinal disorders. Protein-energy malnutrition, linear growth failure, overweight and iron deficiency anemia frequently complicate the clinical course of common gastrointestinal problems in childhood. The clinician should have an understanding of the normal and abnormal patterns of growth and the changes in body composition during childhood, as well as a working knowledge of the clinical and research techniques available to assess the nutritional status of the child. Technical skills to accurately perform a nutritional assessment and the ability to interpret the information obtained from the nutritional evaluation are crucial.

EPIDEMIOLOGY OF NUTRITIONAL DISORDERS IN PEDIATRIC PATIENTS

Our clinical experience indicates that three nutritional disorders, protein-energy malnutrition (PEM), linear growth failure and overweight, occur frequently in the practice of pediatric gastroenterology. Malnutrition and growth failure occur as a consequence of poor dietary intake in conjunction with loss of appetite and the presence of abdominal symptoms, increased intestinal losses secondary to diarrhea or malabsorption and increased nutrient requirements associated with the inflammatory or infectious complications of gastrointestinal diseases. On the other hand, overweight is more likely to be identified in children who use medications such as corticosteroids, which may be prescribed for specific gastrointestinal disorders.

To determine the prevalence of common nutritional disorders in children, particularly those with gastrointestinal disorders, and to identify the clinical factors that placed these children at nutritional risk, nutritional assessments on newly hospitalized children and on children evaluated in our outpatient clinics were performed. Our survey documented that 44% ($n = 288$) of all patients ($n = 655$) had evidence of PEM, growth failure, or overweight. Of those children, 20% were acutely malnourished, 13% were overweight and 31% were chronically malnourished. Infants and toddlers, the age group most frequently admitted to the hospital, were at greatest risk for acute and chronic PEM. However, as a proportion of each age group, acute malnutrition, as well as overweight, was found most frequently among adolescents, whereas chronic malnutrition was distributed evenly across all age groups, with an average prevalence of 30% (Fig. 72.1). Gender or racial and ethnic differences did not influence the prevalence of PEM, growth failure, or overweight in these children. Although nutritional problems were identified across a broad spectrum of clinical disorders, children hospitalized with general pediatric problems that included failure to thrive were at greatest risk for acute malnutrition, while children diagnosed with gastrointestinal disease, followed by renal or cardiac disease, were at greatest risk for chronic malnutrition (Fig. 72.2).

In the outpatient setting, 35% ($n = 221$) of all children ($n = 632$) were diagnosed with PEM, growth failure, or overweight. Of those children with gastrointestinal disorders, 23% were acutely malnourished, 14% were overweight and 26% were chronically malnourished. The pattern of nutritional disorders among the children with gastrointestinal diseases paralleled the distribution of nutritional abnormalities of hospitalized children with respect to age, gender and racial or ethnic features. These observations suggest that there is no single group of children in whom nutritional disorders prevail. Nevertheless, children with gastrointestinal diseases rank high with respect to the frequency of poor nutritional status among children with chronic illness.

CLINICAL SIGNIFICANCE OF NUTRITIONAL ASSESSMENT

Nutritional assessment is an important tool used in the clinical care of children with gastrointestinal disorders because it allows the clinician to characterize the patterns

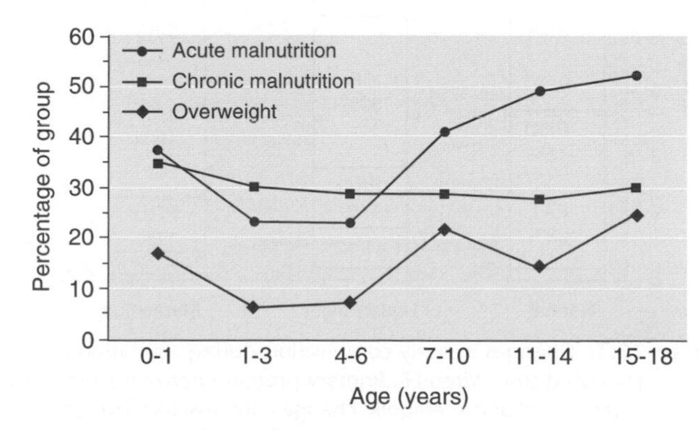

Figure 72.1: Prevalence of acute and chronic malnutrition and overweight by age in hospitalized children.

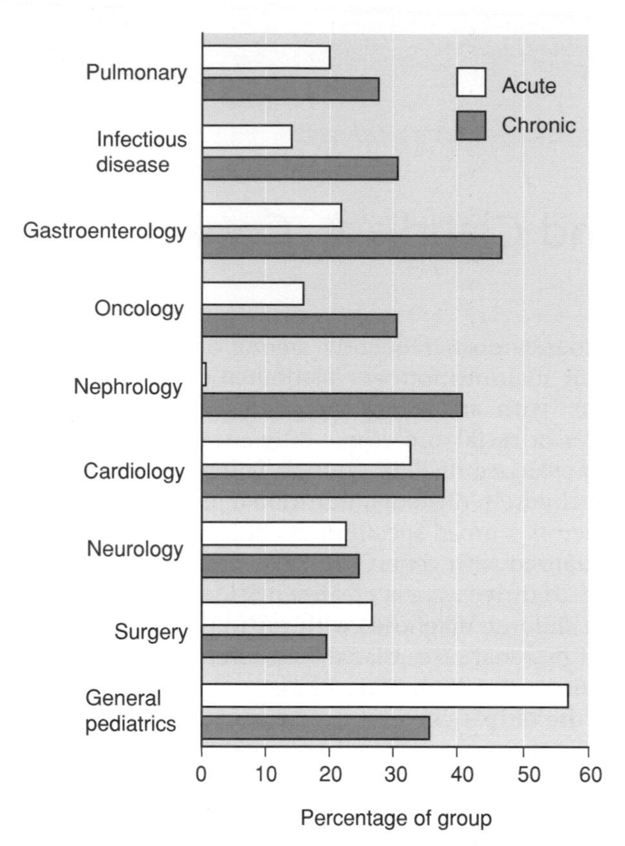

Figure 72.2: Prevalence of acute and chronic malnutrition by admitting diagnosis in hospitalized children.

of growth and the changes in the body composition of the child in response to altered dietary intakes or poor appetite. For example, Figure 72.3 illustrates the changes in weight and body composition that occur during starvation in infancy.[1] In the healthy infant, 22% of bodyweight is composed of fat, 15% of protein and 60% of body water. As the infant become progressively more malnourished, bodyweight loss occurs. The absolute amount of body fat, as well as the proportion of body fat that composes bodyweight, decreases markedly. The absolute amount of body protein also decreases, although the proportion of body protein stores relative to overall bodyweight is unchanged. The pattern of weight loss in the older child with chronic gastrointestinal disease may differ from that of the child with simple starvation. For example, children with Crohn's disease may have substantial weight deficits relative to their age-matched peers.[2] However, the absolute amount of lean body mass generally is reduced to a much greater extent than body fat. The significance of these changes in body composition is that a loss of 40% or more of bodyweight is associated with an increased risk of morbidity and mortality.

Nutritional assessment also is used to determine the changes in growth or body composition that occur in response to infectious or inflammatory processes concurrent with underlying disease. For example, a febrile illness promptly initiates a catabolic response that results in negative body nitrogen balance because of the increased urinary loss of body nutrients (Fig. 72.4).[3] Negative nitrogen balance persists until the febrile illness resolves. The cumulative urinary nitrogen losses are of significant magnitude and persist well beyond the period of the acute febrile illness. The recovery process may require as long as three weeks to replenish depleted body stores. Failure to pay

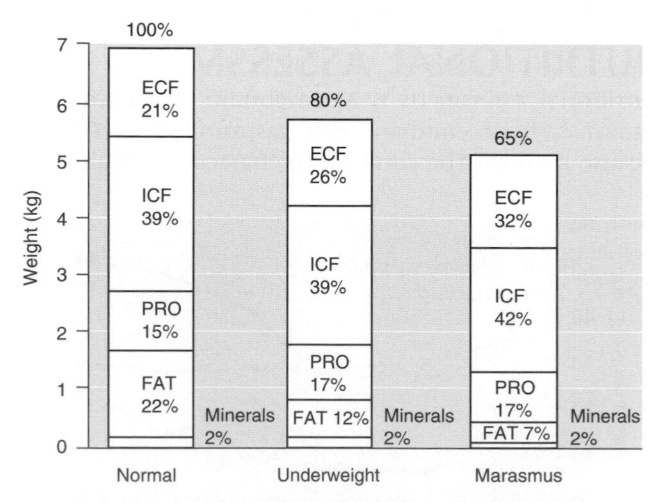

Figure 72.3: Changes in body composition during starvation in infancy. (Adapted from Viteri FE. Primary protein-energy malnutrition: clinical, biochemical and metabolic changes. In: Suskind RM, ed. Textbook of Pediatric Nutrition. New York: Raven Press; 1981:189–215, with permission.)[1]

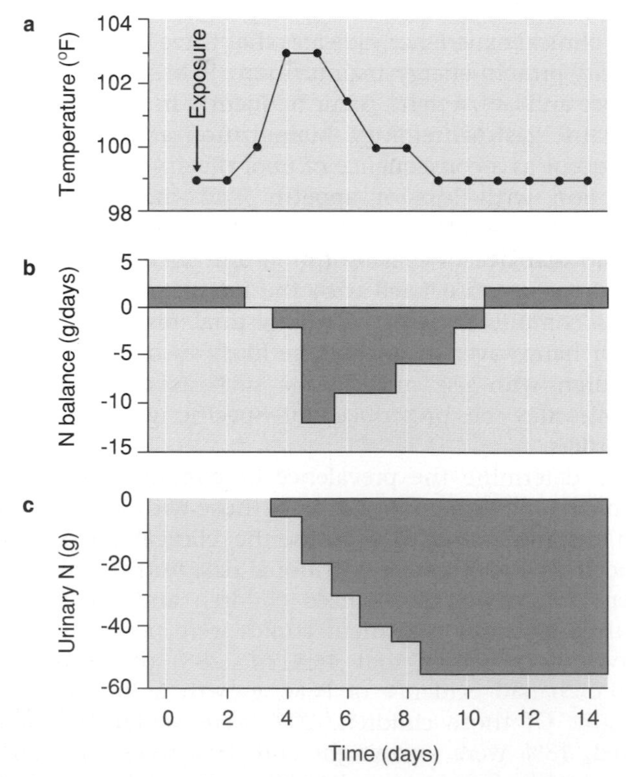

Figure 72.4: Consequences of a febrile illness on nitrogen (N) balance. (Adapted from Beisel WR. Interrelated changes in host metabolism during generalized infectious illness. Am J Clin Nutr 1972; 25:1254–1260, with permission.)[3]

attention to brief episodes of nutritional depletion leads to a vicious cycle in which the nutritional status of the child worsens with each repeated illness and becomes a factor contributing to morbidity.

CLINICAL FEATURES OF NORMAL GROWTH AND BODY COMPOSITION IN CHILDREN

Normal patterns of growth in children

Growth is most rapid in healthy children during early infancy and adolescence (Table 72.1).[4] The average gain in length during the first year of life is 25 cm. This rate declines abruptly to 11 cm/year during the second and third years and then slows again to 6 cm/year in the pre-school- and school-age child. The average gain in weight during the first year of life is 7 kg. This rate declines abruptly to 2.2 kg/year in toddlers, then 2.5 kg/year in the preschool- and school-age child. During the adolescent growth spurt, peak weight velocities average 3 kg per 6 months, but may be as high as 6–7 kg per 6 months in females and males, respectively. Estimates of height and weight velocities are essential to quantify because these measurements predict the energy needs for normal growth. For example, if we estimate that the energy cost of tissue deposition averages 5.5 kcal/g and that tissue deposition is 75% lean and 25% fat, then an additional 15 200 kcal/year is required to support the growth process in the pre-school and school-age child.[5]

Age group	Height velocity	Weight velocity
Infancy (1st year)	25 cm/year	7 kg/year
Toddler (2nd/3rd year)	11 cm/year	2.2 kg/year
Pre-school/school age	6 cm/year	2.8 kg/year
Adolescent	3–4 cm/6 months	6–7 kg/6 months

Table 72.1 Normal growth rates in children

Normal patterns of body composition in children

The clinical features of body composition have been much more difficult to characterize because of the biologic complexity of the human body. From a theoretical perspective, the body has been represented as a two-compartment model or multicompartment models.[6] In the two-compartment model, the body is divided into the fat and fat-free mass (FFM) (Fig. 72.5).[7] The fat mass is composed entirely of fat, as opposed to adipose tissue, which contains body fat and its supporting cellular and extracellular tissues. The FFM is composed of the lean body mass (LBM) plus the nonfat components of adipose tissue. In clinical practice, the two-compartment model is useful because of the ease with which body fat and FFM can be measured and the simplicity with which their changes during health and disease can be assessed. Nevertheless, the two-compartment model is subject to error because the methods used to measure body fat and FFM are based on the assumption that the chemical composition of these tissue stores remains constant across a broad range of ages and disease states.

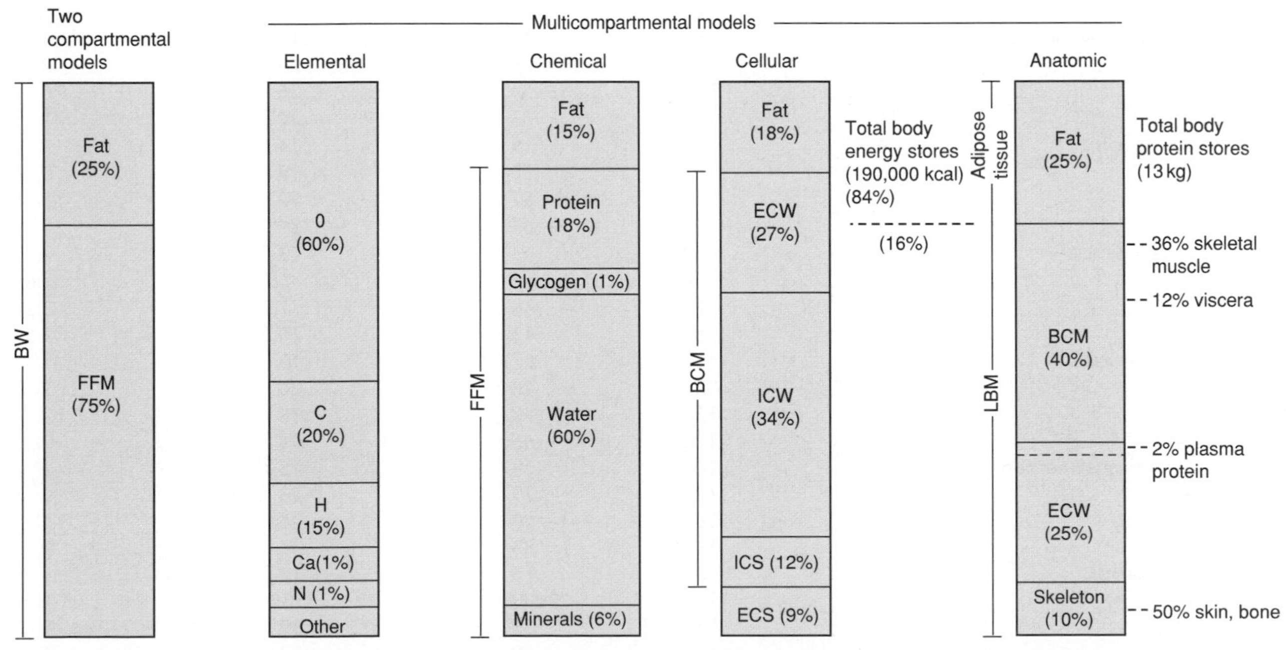

Figure 72.5: Multicompartment models of body composition. BW, bodyweight; FFM, fat-free mass; BCM, body cell mass; ECW, extracellular water; ICW, intracellular water; ICS, intracellular solids; ECS, extracellular solids. (Adapted from Wang Z-M, Pierson RN, Heymsfield SB. The five-level model: a new approach to organizing body-composition research. Am J Clin Nutr 1992; 56:19–28,[6] with permission; and Heymsfield SB, Waki M. Body composition in humans: advances in the development of multicompartment clinical models. Nutr Rev 1991; 49:97–108, with permission from the International Life Sciences Institute.)[7]

Other techniques that characterize multicompartment models of body composition have been developed to reduce the errors inherent in the two-compartment model.[8] The multicompartment models derived from these techniques include elemental, chemical, cellular and tissue models (Fig. 72.5).[7] The elemental model describes body composition in terms of the most common elements of the body (oxygen, carbon, hydrogen, nitrogen, calcium, phosphorus, sodium, potassium and chloride), whereas the chemical model characterizes body composition on the basis of its water, mineral (osseous and non-osseous) and organic (protein, glycogen and fat) components and the cellular model describes the body on the basis of its cell mass and body water compartments. The tissue model provides the most useful information about body composition because it integrates the elemental, chemical and cellular aspects of body composition into functional units that can be measured routinely in the clinical setting. For example, in this model the functional integrity of body fat and skeletal muscle can be measured by anthropometry and 24-h urinary creatinine excretion and that of the viscera, by serum albumin. Abnormalities in these clinical measurements suggest the presence of alterations in the functional adequacy of these compartments of the body and hence, altered nutritional status.

The body composition of children from birth to 16 years of age, which has been derived from a multicompartment model, is summarized in Table 72.2.[8–10] The estimates of lean body mass and body fat increase with increasing age throughout childhood, but vary at any given age depending on gender and race or ethnicity. These estimates serve as reference values for healthy children and may be useful comparative indices to assess the degree of nutritional deficits of children with gastrointestinal disorders.

Methods to measure body composition

Body composition can be determined from a number of direct (e.g. ^{18}O dilution) and indirect (e.g. total body electrical conductance, TOBEC) methods, most of which, however, are carried out only in research facilities. Direct methods quantify a specific component of the body, whereas indirect methods estimate body compartments on the basis of assumed relationships among body constituents. All of these methods have limitations, both theoretical and practical. In general, the estimates of body

Gender	Race/ethnicity	Age (years)	Height (cm)	Weight (kg)	Lean body mass (kg)	Fat mass (kg)
Female	Multiracial	Birth	50	3.3	2.8	0.5
		0.5	66	7	5.1	1.9
		1	74	9	6.8	2.2
		2	85	12	9.6	2.4
	Caucasian	4	107	18	14	4
		8	127	28	20	7
		12	151	44	30	12
		16	164	56	38	15
	African-American	4	106	18	14	4
		8	133	33	23	9
		12	157	54	36	16
		16	162	63	40	21
	Hispanic	4	106	19	14	4
		8	124	30	19	8
		12	153	57	32	17
		16	161	67	39	25
Male	Multiracial	Birth	52	3.5	3.0	0.5
		0.5	68	8	6.0	2.0
		1	76	10	7.8	2.2
		2	87	13	10.5	2.5
	Caucasian	4	103	17	13	3
		8	126	26	20	5
		12	157	52	38	12
		16	174	67	54	10
	African-American	4	105	18	15	2
		8	127	29	23	4
		12	161	60	46	13
		16	176	83	66	8
	Hispanic	4	99	16	12	1
		8	127	30	21	4
		12	158	56	39	9
		16	172	69	54	6

Data from references[7–9].

Table 72.2 Body composition of healthy children

composition in children are highly dependent on their age, gender and race or ethnicity.

Anthropometry is the method used routinely for estimating body composition in the clinical setting. A metal tape measure and calibrated skinfold calipers are the only instruments needed. In clinical practice, the upper-arm muscle circumference (or area) is determined most commonly because this value can be compared with reference standards to determine the degree of muscle wasting in children of various ages and gender.[11] The triceps skinfold thickness is the site most frequently selected as a measure of body fat because it can be compared with reference standards to determine the degree of overweight in children of various ages and gender.[11] However, no single skinfold site is entirely representative of the combined subcutaneous and deep fat stores of the body. Hence, a method that uses multiple skinfold thickness measurements, such as biceps, triceps, subscapular and suprailiac sites, may provide a better estimate of body fat and its regional distribution.[12,13] Nevertheless, this method fails to incorporate measurements of the thigh and lower leg, sites that may contribute substantially to changes in body composition during periods of weight loss or gain. Accurate estimates of body fat mass using anthropometry are difficult to obtain in morbidly overweight children or in children with generalized edema because of altered relationships between body tissue water and fat in these conditions.

Duel-energy X-ray absorptiometry (DXA) has been developed recently to estimate FFM, body fat and bone mineral density, a relative measure of bone mass.[14,15] This technique is rapidly becoming available as a useful clinical test for children.[16] In this method, the child is scanned with an X-ray source of two different energy levels, the difference in the absorption being proportional to the type of tissue scanned. Although the child is exposed to radiation, this technique is considered to be safe because the average radiation dose to the skin is only 1–3 mrem per scan. The precision and reproducibility of the DXA instruments are at least 99.5% and 98%, respectively. Because of their overall performance, DXA scans are quickly becoming accepted as a standard procedure in clinical practice.[17]

Bone mineral measurements can be made of the whole body as well as regions such as the lumbar spine, hip and distal radius. The choice of site may be important because of differences in the proportions of trabecular and cortical bone that may be affected. For example, corticosteroid-induced bone mineral loss primarily affects trabecular, rather than cortical, bone. Two types of DXA machines are available, the pencil beam and the fan beam.[18] The fan beam machine scans more rapidly, but the radiation doses are greater, making this technique impractical in healthy children. Different machines give different results, depending on the hardware and software used. For example, machines calibrated against ashed bone provide values for bone mineral content that are higher than those calibrated against hydroxyapatite. Detection of the edge of the bone being measured and magnification errors may occur with fan beam machines if the distance between the bone and X-ray source is calibrated for adults rather than for children or the type of tissue surrounding the bone varies. Two potential errors in interpreting the DXA scans are the use of T-scores and bone mineral density (BMD) to report loss of bone mineral content.[15,19] T-score values represent standard deviation (SD) scores for young adults which cannot be applied to children because there is no adjustment for their smaller size. Furthermore, DXA machines measure the mass of mineral within a bone, i.e. bone mineral content (BMC) and bone area (BA), then calculate the ratio of these terms as bone mineral density (BMD). BMD is a misnomer because it is a two-dimensional, rather than a three-dimensional, unit that does not distinguish which of the two components of bone mass is being assessed, bone size (volume) or density. BMD is affected by the person's size and tends to underestimate bone density in small individuals and overestimate it in larger individuals. Because consensus on the most appropriate way to report DXA results corrected for bone size has not been achieved, the mass of mineral within the bones of children commonly is reported as BMC and should be interpreted in the context of the child's body (bone) size, pubertal stage, pubertal tempo, age, gender and racial or ethnic group.[15]

Other methods used to measure bone mineral mass and density include quantitative computed tomography, which has the disadvantage of a high radiation dose, making this technique unsuitable for use in healthy children and peripheral quantitative computed tomography, which provides a three dimensional assessment of the structure of the appendicular skeleton with lower radiation exposure. Ultrasound techniques that measure the speed and attenuation of sound through appendicular bone have been developed, but have not been tested systematically in children.[20]

All other methods used to measure body composition are, for practical purposes, limited currently to the research setting. In general, body fat and lean body mass can be measured by densitometry or derived from measures of total body water. Underwater weighing, the oldest method to determine body composition, is used to estimate body density by dividing the individual's actual weight by the weight lost while under water. This method assumes that the density of the fat-free mass remains constant across a broad range of ages, an assumption known to be invalid and therefore requiring correction factors to determine actual body composition. Underwater weighing is not feasible in many children because the child being weighed must be submerged totally under water and must be able to hold his or her breath for a period of time to determine body density. More recently, air displacement plethysmography, a density technique that directly measures body composition from body mass and volume within an air-filled chamber, has been developed for use in infants, children and adolescents.[21,22] This test procedure is non-invasive, can be performed quickly, does not require the infant to be sedated and is environmentally comfortable for the child. Air displacement plethysmography is a reliable and accurate method to measure body fat and has the potential to provide an alternative approach to determine the body composition of children in the future.

Total body water is measured directly by isotope dilution using the stable isotopes of deuterium (^2H_2O) or oxygen ($H_2{}^{18}O$)[23] and indirectly by TOBEC[24] or bioelectrical impedance analysis (BIA).[25] With TOBEC and BIA methods, total body water is estimated based on the principle that body fluids in lean tissue conduct a high-frequency electrical current more readily than body fat. Both of these methods require that the child rest quietly without movement for a short period of time, no small feat for a toddler or young child. BIA and TOBEC also are sensitive to changes in body shape. Because body shape varies among children of the same height, especially during growth, the measurement of body composition using these methods is imprecise.[26] Furthermore, because TOBEC and BIA are indirect methods, the instruments must be calibrated against an independent estimate of total body water such as isotope dilution. Once total body water has been determined, the fat-free mass of the body must be calculated, based on the assumption that the hydration of lean tissue is constant across a broad range of ages and gender. Because this assumption is invalid, correction factors must be used to convert total body water to fat-free body mass.

Total body potassium counting is a method that measures the natural abundance of radioactive potassium (^{40}K) in the body.[27] ^{40}K emits a characteristic gamma ray which in turn serves as a marker for lean body mass, based on the assumption that the potassium content of the FFM remains constant with respect to tissue nitrogen content. This method is noninvasive and safe, but limited in availability. Neuron activation analysis is a method in which exposure to a given dose of neutrons generates a known amount of radioactivity within a given mass.[28] The particular element being examined, such as nitrogen, calcium, or phosphorus, can be identified by the characteristic energy of the electromagnetic radiation it emits and its decay rate. Nevertheless, radiation exposure makes this technique generally prohibitive in children. Imaging techniques such as ultrasonography, computerized axial tomography and nuclear magnetic resonance imaging display a visual image of body fat and fat-free mass throughout the body.[29] Although it is possible to estimate total body fat from these images, the inaccuracy of some of the methods, the high level of radiation exposure and the cost and maintenance of the equipment preclude their use in children.

INDICATIONS FOR NUTRITIONAL ASSESSMENT

A nutritional assessment is warranted if a child with newly diagnosed gastrointestinal disease meets the screening criteria for the risk of developing PEM, growth failure, or overweight. This recommendation assumes that the child has not been evaluated previously by the physician and that the availability of antecedent growth information is unlikely to be obtained. As a general guideline: (1) any child whose height-for-age is less than the 10th percentile is at risk for chronic malnutrition; (2) any child younger than 2 years of age whose weight-for-height is less than the 10th percentile or any child age 2 years or older whose body mass index (BMI) is less than the 10th percentile is at risk for acute malnutrition and (3) any child age 2 years or older whose BMI is greater than the 85th percentile is at risk for overweight (Table 72.3). These screening criteria do not imply categorically that the child has nutritional deficits, but that the child whose growth measurements plot at the extremes of the growth curves merit closer scrutiny to determine if nutritional deficits or excesses truly are present.

Serial height and weight measurements provide additional information on which nutritional risk can be identified. In this setting, a nutritional assessment is warranted if a child who is older than 2 years fails to demonstrate appropriate linear or ponderal gains during a 6-month to 1-year interval. Thus, a height velocity less than 5 cm/year after 2 years of age may be consistent with linear stunting or chronic malnutrition (Table 72.3). A prepubertal weight velocity less than 1 kg/year or a pubertal peak weight velocity less than 1 kg every 6 months may be consistent with acute malnutrition. In clinical practice, growth velocity measurements may be the most sensitive factors for elucidating which children are at risk for nutritional disorders.

COMPONENTS OF NUTRITIONAL ASSESSMENT

Nutritional assessment is defined as the comprehensive approach to characterizing quantitatively the nutritional status of the child.[30–32] A comprehensive nutritional assessment has four components: (1) dietary, medical and medication history; (2) physical examination; (3) growth and anthropometric measurements and (4) laboratory tests.

Dietary history

A dietary history that determines the actual quality and quantity of the child's pattern of food consumption and the eating behaviors and beliefs of the family is an important component of the nutritional assessment. The physician should ask about the type of food that is provided to

Risk criteria (NCHS, CDC)	Risk
Ht-for-age <10th percentile Ht velocity <5 cm/year after age 2 years	Chronic malnutrition
Wt-for-ht <10th percentile before age 2 years BMI <10th percentile after age 2 years Wt velocity <1 kg/year (prepubertal) Wt velocity (peak) <1 kg/6 months (prepubertal)	Acute malnutrition
BMI >85 percentile after age 2 years	Obesity

NCHS, National Center for Health Statistics; CDC, Centers for Disease Control and Prevention; Ht, height; Wt, weight; BMI, body mass index.

Table 72.3 Indications for nutritional assessment

the child, the number of meals and snacks per day, the use of a special diet, the consistency with which vitamin and mineral supplements are given, food allergies, food intolerances or avoidances and unusual feeding behaviors. Although the physician may review the child's dietary history by 24-h recall, this method of analysis frequently is misleading because it may not be representative of habitual food consumption patterns, particularly when illness intervenes. In general, a 3-day food record, performed while the infant or child is at home, is a more valid tool to quantify actual dietary intake.[33] However, even in this setting, dietary intakes may be doubtful because anxious parents tend to overestimate or underestimate the child's food consumption depending on the nature of the nutritional problem. Despite these difficulties, every effort should be made to document the possibility that altered dietary intakes contribute to the child's nutritional problem. Once food records have been obtained, the help of a dietitian is invaluable in converting food servings into nutrient content using either the Atwater conversion factors (1 g of protein, carbohydrate and fat equals 4, 4 and 9 kcal/g, respectively), to estimate the energy content of the diet or a computerized nutrient database to provide a more complete list of nutrient intakes. The estimate of the nutrient content of the diet should be compared with age- and gender-specific Dietary Reference Intakes, with the caveat that these standards meet the nutrient needs of healthy children but do not take into account the nutrient needs of children diagnosed with acute or chronic illness.[34]

The assessment of the dietary intake of infants with gastrointestinal illness should be rigorous because of the rapidity with which failure to thrive may develop in this age group. However, the assessment of the dietary intake of the breast-fed infant may be difficult to obtain because the feeding pattern of the nursing infant is highly variable. General guidelines to determine the adequacy of intake include the frequency and duration of breast-feeding, the frequency of urination and the infant's weight gain. The breast-fed infant generally nurses every 2–3 h, or 8–12 times/day. The average duration of each nursing is 5–15 min per breast. As a rule, the breast-fed infant gains 30 g/day during the first 6 months of life.[4] The assessment of the dietary intake of the formula-fed infant is much easier to obtain than that of the breast-fed infant. General guidelines to determine the adequacy of the dietary intake include the frequency of feeding, the volume of milk consumed which on average ranges from 150 to 180 ml/kg per day, the energy density of the formula, a comparison of the actual dietary energy intake with age- and gender-specific Dietary Reference Intakes,[34] and a weight gain of 30 g/day during the first 6 months of life.[4] In the presence of nutritional deficits, the physician should anticipate increased energy intakes in the range of 150–180 kcal/kg per day and higher weight gains of 50–60 g/day to reverse the adverse nutritional consequences associated with gastrointestinal disorders.

The assessment of the dietary intake of children 2 years of age or older should follow the guidelines of the prudent diet.[35] Total daily fat intake should comprise less than 30%

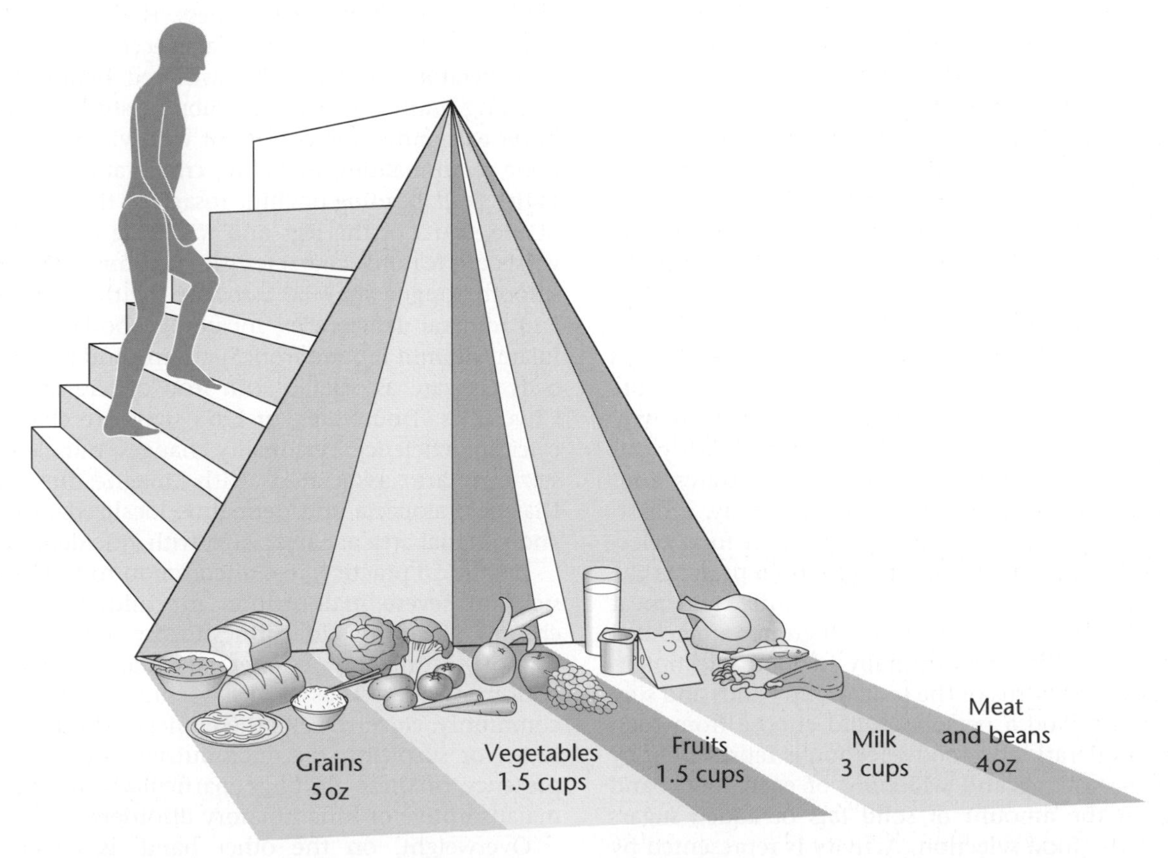

Figure 72.6: Food Guide Pyramid, from http://www.usda.gov/cnpp. (Accessed date: 1 August, 2004.)[38]

Food	Age (years)		
	1–3	4–6	7–10
Milk, yogurt (c)	1/2	3/4	1
Cheese (oz)	1/2	1	1–1/2
Meat, poultry, fish (oz)	1	1–1/2	3
Eggs	1	1–1/2	2
Peanut butter (tbsp)	1	2	3
Vegetables – cooked or raw (c)	3T	1/3	1/2
Fruits			
Canned (c)	3T	1/3	1/2
Fresh (small)	1/2	1	1 medium
Juice (c)	1/3	1/2	3/4
Bread (slice)	1/2	1	1
Dry cereal (c)	1/2	3/4	1
Pasta, rice (c)	1/3	1/2	3/4

(c) = cup.

Table 72.4 Daily serving sizes of food

of total daily energy intake. Saturated and polyunsaturated fats should comprise less than 10% each of total daily energy intakes. Cholesterol intake should be limited to 300 mg/day. Total daily carbohydrate intake should comprise 60% or more of total daily energy intake. Complex carbohydrates, such as starch, should comprise more than 50% and simple sugars should comprise less than 10% of the total daily energy intake. A high-fiber diet should be encouraged; a useful guideline is the child's age in years plus 5 equals the grams of fiber per day, where one serving of fruit, vegetable, or cereal each contains 2–3 g of fiber.[36] Table salt should not be readily available. The diet should be nutritionally complete, include a variety of foods and be adequate for normal growth and physical activity. In those conditions where dietary modifications may be necessary to ameliorate bothersome gastrointestinal symptoms, careful attention to appropriate nutrient substitutes or supplements should be given to prevent specific nutrient deficiencies, imbalances, or toxicities.

The new revision of the Food Guide Pyramid is the practical tool to assess the prudent diet across all age groups (Fig 72.6)[37,38] The United States Department of Agriculture has published the new MyPyramid (http://www.mypyramid.gov) to symbolize a personal approach to healthy eating and physical activity. MyPyramid illustrates four concepts related to healthy eating habits: variety, proportionality, moderation, and activity. Variety in food selection is symbolized by the 6 color bands and represents the 5 food groups; grains, vegetables, fruits, milk, and meat and beans, as well as oils. Foods from all groups are needed daily for good health. Proportionally in food selection is symbolized by the widths of the food group bands and suggests how much food a person should choose from each food group. Moderation in food selection is represented by the vertical narrowing and widening of each food band depending on the amount of solid fats or added sugars contained in the food selection. Activity is represented by the steps and the person climbing them as a reminder of the importance of daily physical activity. The kinds and amounts of food to eat each day based on age, gender, and physical activity, can be determined for any individual by connecting to the website.

Physical examination

Protein-energy malnutrition includes two clinical entities: marasmus and kwashiorkor. Marasmus is characterized by the wasting of muscle mass and the depletion of body fat stores, whereas kwashiorkor is characterized by generalized edema (anasarca) and flaky, peeling skin rashes. Children with PEM may manifest a broad spectrum of clinical features. Children with malnutrition may be irritable or apathetic. The flag sign (i.e. loss of hair color) is associated with a period of malnutrition followed by recovery. Follicular hyperkeratosis and night blindness are characteristic of vitamin A deficiency. Weakness of the leg muscles, pedal edema, tachycardia, congestive heart failure and seizures are associated with thiamine deficiency (beriberi). Angular stomatitis, cheilosis and seborrheic dermatitis of the lips and nose are associated with riboflavin deficiency, whereas dry, cracked skin in areas exposed to sunlight, such as the neck, hands and feet, is associated with niacin deficiency (pellagra). Weakness, nervousness, insomnia, a hypochromic, microcytic anemia and seizures are associated with pyridoxine deficiency, whereas a macrocytic anemia is associated with folate and vitamin B_{12} deficiency. A peripheral neuropathy, consisting of loss of vibratory sensation and proprioception, paresthesias and motor weakness, is characteristic of vitamin B_{12} deficiency. Petechiae and ecchymoses of the skin, hyperkeratotic hair follicles with red hemorrhagic halos, bleeding gums and painful, subperiosteal bleeding of the lower extremities are consistent with vitamin C deficiency. Bone abnormalities, including craniotabes, frontal bossing of the skull, beading (rachitic rosary) of the rib cage, bowing of the shafts of the legs and widening of the radii at the wrists are features characteristic of vitamin D deficiency. A smooth tongue may be associated with multiple vitamin and mineral deficiencies, including riboflavin, pyridoxine, folate, vitamin B_{12} and iron. Spooning and pallor of the nail beds also are associated with iron deficiency. Tetany and Chvostek's, Trousseau's, or Erb's signs are characteristic of calcium deficiency. Personality changes, muscle spasms and seizures are associated with magnesium deficiency. Diarrhea, alopecia and dermatitis localized to the perioral and perianal area are associated with zinc deficiency.

In clinical practice, it is uncommon to find many of the signs of severe malnutrition in children with acute or chronic gastrointestinal illnesses. In general, a combination of wasting and peripheral edema, signifying a combination of marasmus and kwashiorkor, is found most commonly. Nevertheless, the clinician should have a high index of suspicion for micronutrient deficiencies in the presence of these findings, particularly in children with malabsorptive or inflammatory disorders.

Overweight, on the other hand, is characterized by increased deposition of truncal and peripheral body fat.

Increased fatness is associated with several other effects on growth including increased lean body mass, increased height, advanced bone age and the early onset of menarche. Overweight children may be hypertensive and often display dysfunctional behaviors because of poor self-esteem. Morbid overweight is associated with metabolic complications, such as diabetes mellitus and hyperlipidemia; gallbladder disease, such as cholecystitis and cholelithiasis; orthopedic disorders, including slipped capital femoral epiphysis and bowing of the tibia and femur; and cardiopulmonary problems, including congestive heart failure and obstructive sleep apnea. Whereas simple, exogenous overweight is a national epidemic, the type of overweight that occurs secondary to medications (e.g. prednisone) is more difficult to manage because these drugs ameliorate inflammatory conditions but lead to voracious appetites.

Growth and anthropometric measurements

Growth measurements are the most important components of the nutritional assessment because normal growth patterns are the gold standard by which physicians assess the health and well-being of the child. Growth measurements inherently are not useful unless the physician is able to convert the absolute values to relative standards and to interpret correctly the information provided by these measurements.[4] A normal growth pattern is not a guarantee of overall health, but the child with an atypical growth pattern is more likely to manifest the nutritional complications of gastrointestinal disease. Altered growth patterns are a relatively late consequence of nutritional insult. Thus, surveillance is an important component of the nutritional assessment of the child with gastrointestinal disease.

Height and weight measurements are the mainstay of the nutritional assessment of the child. The use of appropriate measurement techniques is essential to assess the adequacy of growth in children. The only appropriate way to measure length or height is to use a flat, horizontal or vertical surface with perpendicular surfaces at each end (Fig. 72.7).[43] Weight measurements should be obtained on a scale that has been calibrated properly. The head circumference should be measured at the maximum diameter through the glabella and occiput (Fig. 72.8).[43] Growth measurements, including length or height, weight and head circumference should be plotted on the growth charts from the National Center for Health Statistics which can be accessed readily from the website for the Centers for Disease Control and Prevention (http://www.cdc.gov/growthcharts). Any length, height, or weight measurement that falls below the 5th percentile, is greater than the 95th percentile, or crosses two major growth channels is considered to represent an abnormal growth pattern. Serial measurements must be obtained to determine if the growth pattern is truly abnormal or if these findings merely represent constitutional short stature or the re-channeling of normal growth curves. Radiographic studies of bone age may help to clarify the presence of abnormal growth patterns because chronic undernutrition is one of the causes of delayed bone maturation and hence, delayed linear growth.[44]

Incremental growth measurements that characterize height and weight velocities over a 6-month interval may be valuable in assessing the growth response of children with chronic illness.[45] Any prepubertal child whose weight velocity is less than 1 kg/year, or any pubertal child whose peak weight velocity is less than 1 kg every 6 months, may be at risk for developing the nutritional complications of chronic illnesses.

Height velocity measurements may be the most sensitive measure to detect growth abnormalities early in the course of chronic gastrointestinal illnesses.[46] Any child older than 2 years of age whose height velocity is less than

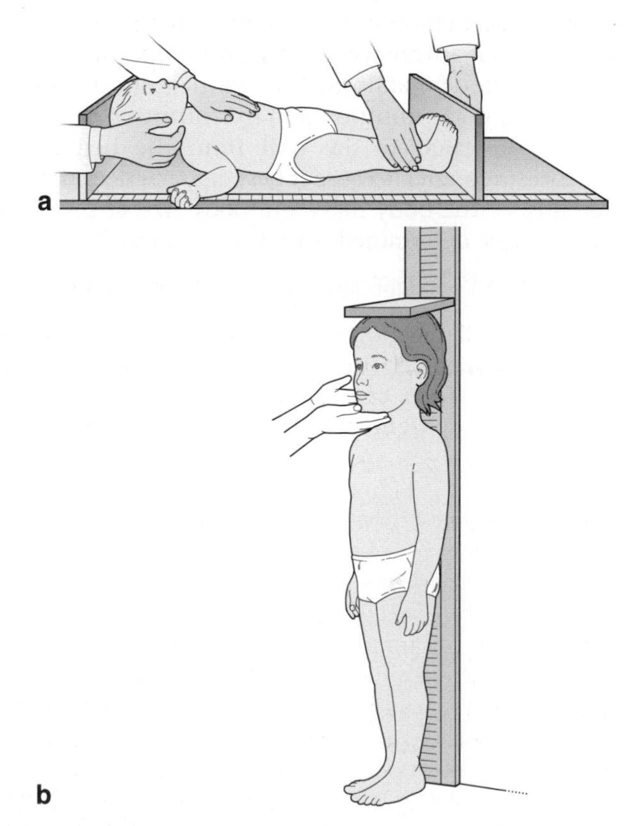

Figure 72.7: Technique for measuring (**a**) recumbent length of (**b**) height. (Adapted from Jelliffe DB. The assessment of the nutritional stature of the community. Geneva: World Health Organization; 1966: Monograph Series No. 53, with permission.)[43]

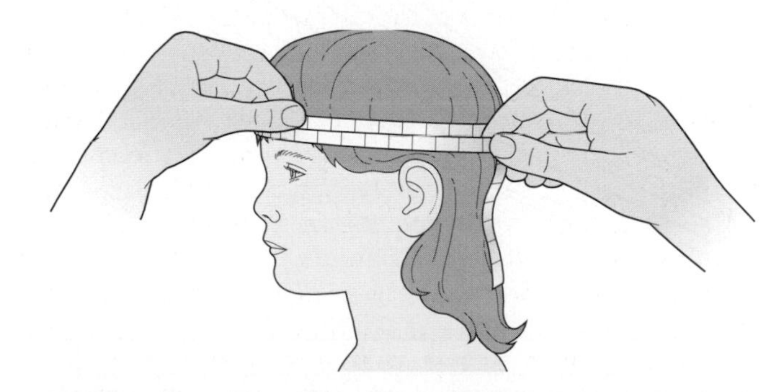

Figure 72.8: Technique for measuring head circumference. (Adapted from Jelliffe DB. The assessment of the nutritional stature of the community. Geneva: World Health Organization; 1966: Monograph Series No. 53, with permission.)[43]

5 cm/year should be monitored carefully for progressive nutritional deficits.

Height and weight measurements may be converted to Z-scores, or values that represent standard deviations from the median height and weight values for age. Any child whose height or weight Z-score is less than –1.64 (i.e. below the 5th percentile) is considered to have an abnormal growth pattern; height and weight Z-scores more than 2 SD below the median are considered to represent significant nutritional abnormalities. Most clinicians do not use Z-scores routinely because growth abnormalities can be identified readily by plotting height and weight measurements on the growth charts. The use of Z-scores is helpful primarily when assessing growth information in the research setting.

The BMI is an anthropometric measure that can be used to screen children for abnormalities in their nutritional status, including undernutrition and overnutrition.[47] The clinician should calculate the BMI from the height and weight measurements because it best characterizes the proportionality of the body mass and body size of the child. The BMI can be determined from the equation:[48]

$$\text{BMI (kg/m}^2\text{)} = \text{weight (kg)}/[\text{height (cm)}/100\ \text{(cm/m)}]^2$$

The BMI should be plotted on the gender-appropriate BMI charts from the National Center for Health Statistics (Fig. 72.9a, b) which can be accessed readily from the website for the Centers for Disease Control and Prevention (http://www.cdc.gov/growthcharts). Although the BMI is an indirect measure of body fatness, it correlates well with other more direct measures of body composition such as those obtained by underwater weighing and DXA.[49] The BMI is gender-specific and age-specific for children.[50] In contrast to adults, the BMI in children increases in a nonlinear fashion with increasing age. Consequently, the BMI-for-age is the measure that relates BMI values in childhood to those obtained in adults. For children older than 6 years, BMI-for-age predicts underweight and overweight better than weight-for-height measurements.[51] For children younger than 6 years, BMI-for-age and weight-for-height estimates equally predict discrepancies in body fatness. The BMI is useful because it can be used to track body size throughout the life cycle. In addition, the BMI-for-age is important to measure in childhood because it correlates well with the clinical risk factors for cardiovascular disease in adulthood, including hyperlipidemia, hyperinsulinemia and hypertension.[52] Thus, BMI-for-age in adolescence is associated directly with the risk of developing these chronic diseases in adulthood.[53] Currently, the Centers for Disease Control and Prevention recommend that: (1) the BMI-for-age be used routinely to screen children for overweight and underweight, (2) children be classified as underweight if their BMI is less than the 5th percentile and (3) children be classified at risk for overweight if

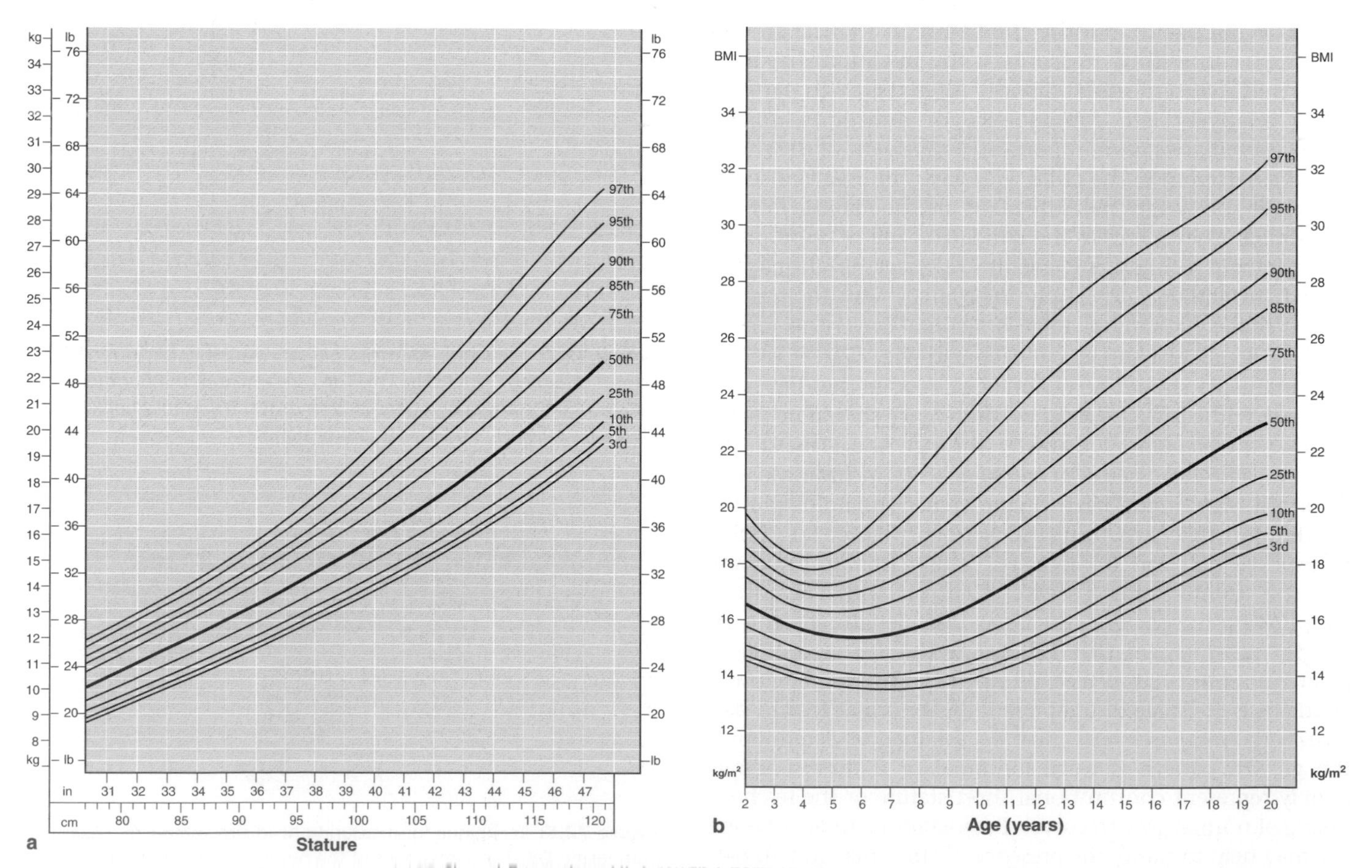

Figure 72.9: Centers for Disease Control (CDC) and Prevention US Growth Charts (**a**) for girls: 2–20 years, (**b**) for boys: 2–20 years (from http://www.cdc.gov/growthcharts.)[4]

their BMI-for-age is between the 85th and 95th percentiles and as overweight if their BMI-for-age is greater than the 95th percentile.

Once children have been screened, using the BMI and found to be undernourished, the degree of acute and chronic malnutrition, characterized as ponderal wasting and linear stunting, respectively, can be assessed clinically using Waterlow criteria.[54,55] This method assumes that during periods of nutritional deprivation, weight deficits initially occur followed by length or height deficits. An arrest of head growth is spared unless compromised by severe starvation. The Waterlow criteria also assume that the expected height and weight measurements of the child fall along the 50th percentile of the growth curves. This assumption is necessary because prior height and weight measurements usually are not available when evaluating the child for the first time. Under these circumstances, the genetic growth potential of the child may not be known. The birthweight or the current head circumference percentile may provide a clue to the true growth potential of the child. Nevertheless, in some instances, the genetic growth potential may be determined only in retrospect after aggressive nutritional intervention has been implemented.

Acute malnutrition, measured in terms of weight deficit, can be determined from the equation

$$\text{Weight deficit (\%)} = [\text{actual weight (kg)}/\text{expected weight for actual height (kg)}] \times 100$$

In this case, the expected weight measurement is determined by drawing a horizontal line from right to left between the child's measured height and the point at which the actual height measurement falls on the 50th percentile line, then connecting this point by means of a vertical line with the point at which the weight measurement falls on the 50th percentile line for a child of the same chronologic age (Fig. 72.10a).

Chronic malnutrition, measured in terms of a height or length deficit, can be determined from the equation

$$\text{Height deficit (\%)} = [\text{actual height (cm)}/\text{expected height at 50th percentile for chronologic age (cm)}] \times 100$$

In this case, the expected height is derived by plotting the height measurement at the 50th percentile for the child's actual chronologic age (Fig. 72.10b). However, if the child's

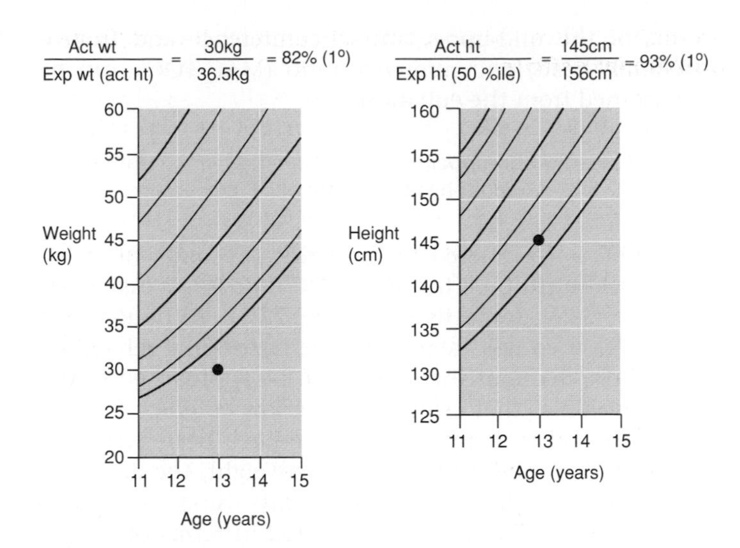

Figure 72.10: Clinical application of Waterlow criteria. Act. wt. = actual weight; Exp. wt. = expected weight; Act. ht. = actual height; Exp. ht. = expected height.

true height potential has been documented previously from serial height measurements, then the adjusted value should be used to estimate the true height deficit.

The nutritional assessment of a malnourished child using Waterlow criteria is illustrated in Table 72.5. A child is considered to have first-, second-, or third-degree acute malnutrition if the weight-for-height estimate is less than 90%, 80%, or 70% of expected, respectively. Likewise, a child is considered to have first-, second-, or third-degree chronic malnutrition if the height-for-age estimate is less than 95%, 90%, 85%, of expected, respectively. The significance of these estimates is that they provide a useful guideline for the nutritional rehabilitation of the child with gastrointestinal disease. Thus, aggressive nutritional rehabilitation should be implemented by the oral route for first-degree acute and chronic malnutrition. Aggressive enteral refeeding using a nasogastric tube or button gastrostomy should be considered in the presence of second-degree malnutrition, while total parenteral nutrition may be required for third-degree malnutrition.

An alternative method to estimate the degree of acute malnutrition in children younger than 4 years of age is the McLaren criteria.[56] This method is useful when accurate length measurements are difficult to obtain. This method assumes that a malformation of the head, such as microcephaly, is not present. Acute malnutrition, measured in

	Degree of malnutrition				Degree of overweight			
Criteria	0 (Normal)	1 (Mild)	2 (Moderate)	3 (Severe)	Normal	Mild	Moderate	Morbid
Wt-for-ht (%)	≥90	<90	<80	<70	≤110	>110	>120	>140
Ht-for-age (%)	≥95	<95	<90	<85				
MAC/FOC	≥0.31	<0.31	<0.28	<0.25				

Wt, weight; Ht, height; MAC, mid-upper arm circumference; FOC, frontal-occipital head circumference. Data from references[52–54].

Table 72.5 Criteria for malnutrition and overweight

terms of the mid-upper arm circumference and fronto-occipital (head) circumference ratio (MAC/FOC), can be determined from the equation

MAC/FOC = Mid-upper arm circumference (cm) / frontal-occipital head circumference (cm)

The child is considered to have first-, second-, or third-degree malnutrition if the MAC/FOC ratio is less than 0.31, 0.28, or 0.25, respectively (Table 72.5). Although this method is used less frequently, the nutritional rehabilitation of the malnourished child can be approached in the same fashion as that using the Waterlow criteria.

On the other hand, if children have been screened, using the BMI and found to be overweight, the degree of overweight can be accessed clinically using weight-for-height criteria. Overweight, measured in terms of weight excess, can be determined from the equation

Weight excess (%) = [actual weight (kg)/ideal weight for actual height (kg)] × 100

where ideal weight is the actual weight-for-age found at the percentile that matches the actual height-for-age percentile. Moderately overweight is defined as an ideal weight-for-height measurement greater than 120% of expected and morbidly overweight is defined as a weight-for-height measurement greater than 140% of expected (Table 72.5). The significance of these estimates is that they serve as a useful guideline for the approach to diet modification in the overweight child. Thus, an energy-deficit diet can be implemented in the child with moderate overweight, whereas a more restrictive diet, such as the protein-sparing modified fast, may be necessary for morbid overweight.[57]

Alternative anthropometric measurements that can be used to assess body fatness are the mid-upper arm circumference and triceps skinfold thickness. The technique for measuring the mid-upper arm circumference includes the following steps (Fig. 72.11): (1) the child's right arm should be flexed to a 90° angle; (2) the midpoint between the tip of the olecranon and acromion should be marked; (3) the child's arm should hang freely; (4) the circumference of the arm should be measured to the nearest 0.1 cm at the midpoint with a flexible metal tape.[43] The technique for measuring the triceps skinfold thickness includes the following steps (Fig. 72.12): (1) the child's right arm should hang freely; (2) using the thumb and forefinger of the left hand, the upper arm skinfold (skin and fat minus the underlying muscle) should be pulled out 1 cm above midpoint; (3) using the right hand, the calipers should be applied 1 cm in depth at the measured midpoint; (4) the calipers should be released and the reading should be obtained to the nearest 1 mm as soon as the needle is steady; (5) the average value of duplicate measurements should be recorded.[43] The mid-arm circumference (MAC, cm), in conjunction with the triceps skinfold thickness (TSF, cm), can be used to estimate the mid-arm muscle circumference (MAMC, cm) as follows[11]:

$$MAMC = MAC - [p^{*} TSF]$$

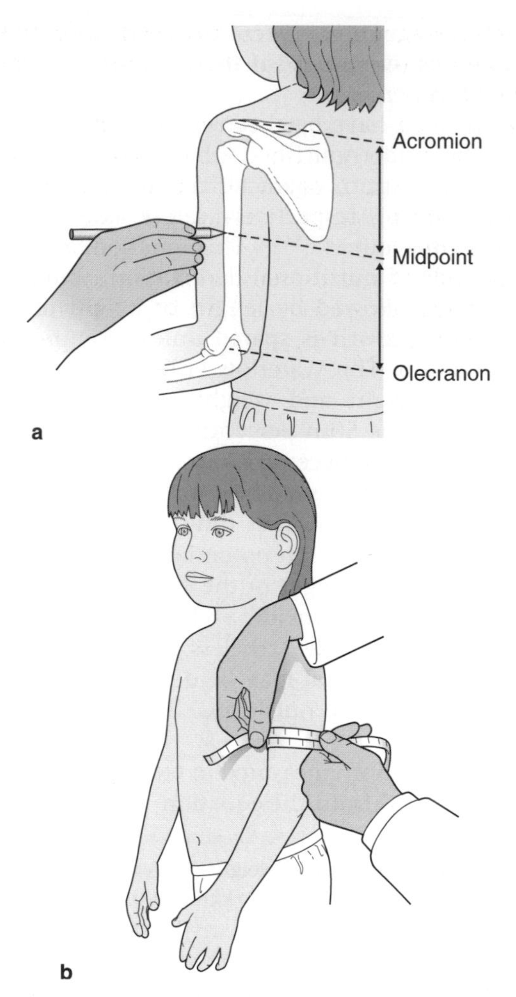

Figure 72.11: Technique for measuring (**a**) mid-upper arm length and (**b**) circumference. (Adapted from Jelliffe DB. The Assessment of the Nutritional Stature of the Community. Geneva: World Health Organization; 1966: Monograph Series No. 53, with permission.)[43]

where *p* equals 3.1416. The values obtained for arm muscle area and triceps skinfold thickness should be compared with reference values to assess the nutritional status of the child.[11] In general, values less than the 5th percentile for

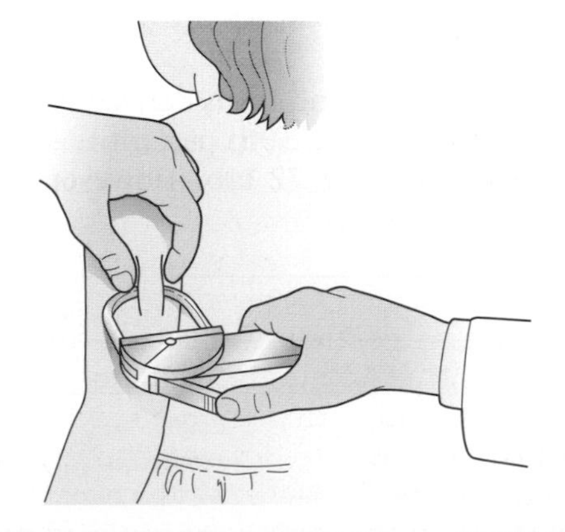

Figure 72.12: Technique for measuring triceps skinfold thickness (Adapted from Jelliffe DB. The Assessment of the Nutritional Stature of the Community. Geneva: World Health Organization; 1966: Monograph Series No. 53, with permission.)[43]

age are consistent with the diagnosis of acute malnutrition and values greater than the 95th percentile are consistent with the diagnosis of overweight.

Thigh and lower leg circumferences and skinfold thicknesses are secondary measurements that may be useful to assess the regional distribution of muscle wasting and loss or gain of peripheral body fat depots using the same calculations as described for the upper arm. In addition, four skinfold sites – biceps, triceps, subscapular and suprailiac – have been measured collectively to provide a better estimate of body fat using the following age- and gender-specific equations:[12]

Gender	Age (years)	Body density (*y*)
Male	2–18	$y = [1.1315 + 0.0018\,(a - 2)] - \{0.0719 - [0.0006\,(a - 2) \times \log x]\}$
Female	2–10	$y = [1.1315 + 0.0004\,(a - 2)] - \{0.0719 - [0.0003\,(a - 2) \times \log x]\}$
	11–18	$y = [1.1350 - 0.0031\,(a - 10)] - \{0.0719 - [0.0003\,(a - 2) \times \log x]\}$

where y equals body density, a equals age (year), x equals the sum of the triceps, biceps, subscapular and suprailiac skinfold thicknesses (mm) and:

$$BF = [(4.95/y) - 4.5] \times 100$$

where BF equals the proportion (%) of bodyweight that is composed of body fat. The absolute body fat mass can be calculated as the multiple of BF and bodyweight and the absolute lean body mass can be calculated as the difference between bodyweight and the absolute body fat mass. Although these measurements can be made readily in the clinical setting, anthropometric measurements may not provide substantially greater additional information about the nutritional status of the child than height and weight measurements.

Laboratory tests

Selected laboratory tests may be useful to assess the nutritional status of the child with gastrointestinal disease, although in the current era of managed care and cost containment, judicious use of these tools is warranted (Table 72.6). Laboratory tests may identify deficiencies before clinical findings are evident, may confirm the presence of selected nutrient deficiencies that are commonly associated with specific gastrointestinal entities, or may be helpful to monitor the clinical recovery from malnutrition when it occurs as a complicating feature of specific gastrointestinal diseases. Nevertheless, laboratory tests have limited usefulness over and above the clinical findings determined from growth and anthropometric measurements.

Malnutrition is associated with global nutrient deficits, but these deficiencies generally are not severe enough to be reflected in blood plasma or serum values. A complete blood count and serum ferritin level may be useful to confirm the diagnosis of iron deficiency anemia. Tests for urine specific gravity, serum electrolytes and carbon dioxide, or blood urea nitrogen (BUN) may be useful to determine the hydration, electrolyte and acid-base status of the child. Low BUN or serum transthyretin levels suggest poor dietary intake of recent onset, whereas low albumin levels suggest poor dietary intake of long-standing duration. Low serum values of vitamin A, E, or 25-hydroxyvitamin D may be present in fat malabsorption disorders. Magnesium or zinc deficiencies may be found in chronic diarrheal illnesses. Elevated serum cholesterol and triglyceride levels, impaired glucose tolerance and increased insulin levels may occur in conjunction with drug-associated overweight.

Although all laboratory tests may be of clinical importance, the most valuable tests of nutritional status in children with gastrointestinal disease are hemoglobin concentrations and red cell indices (mean corpuscular volume, mean corpuscular hemoglobin), as well as serum potassium, phosphorus, transthyretin and albumin levels. Iron deficiency anemia is the most common nutritional anemia associated with chronic gastrointestinal diseases and should be assessed routinely. Hypochromic, microcytic, red cell morphology suggests iron deficiency anemia. Serum ferritin is the most sensitive measure of the adequacy of body iron status. Depressed serum folate levels may be the consequences of drug-nutrient interactions (e.g. sulfasalazine) or diffuse inflammation of the gastrointestinal tract. On the other hand, low vitamin B_{12} levels occur in response to localized disease of the terminal ileum. Potassium and phosphorus are labile serum minerals that should be monitored carefully early in the course of aggressive nutritional rehabilitation of children with malnutrition. Serum potassium and phosphorus levels may decline rapidly during the early refeeding period because of intracellular ion shifts and can lead to unwanted complications such as cardiac arrhythmias. Transthyretin, a rapidly turning-over protein with a half-life of 2 days, is a good predictor of the adequacy of the diet and serves to corroborate the details of the diet history obtained from the parent. If dietary intakes have been poor, serum transthyretin levels fall rapidly.[58] If adequate refeeding has been re-instituted, serum transthyretin levels will rise to low normal levels within 10 days after initiating nutritional therapy, whereas serum albumin, a slowly turning-over protein, may not be restored to normal levels for at least 3 weeks after nutritional therapy has commenced (Fig. 72.13).[59] On the other hand, the serum albumin level serves as a good predictor of gastrointestinal tolerance to enteral feedings,[60] with the likelihood that higher protein and energy intakes can be provided when serum albumin levels are greater than 30 g/l. The serum albumin level also is a good predictor of morbidity and mortality; when serum albumin levels fall below 10–15 g/l, the mortality rate of malnourished children approximates 40%.[61]

Tests	Age and sex group			
	Neonate (Birth–1 month)	Infant (1–12 months)	Child (1–9 years)	Child (9–18 years)
Protein				
Blood				
Serum albumin (g/dl)	≥2.5	≥3	≥3.5	≥3.5
Retinol-binding protein (mg/dl)	2–3	2–3	2–3	3–6
Blood urea nitrogen (mg/dl)	7–22	7–22	7–22	7–22
Thyroxine-binding protein (mg/dl)	20–50	20–50	20–50	20–50
Transferrin (mg/dl)	170–250	170–250	170–250	170–250
Fibronectin (mg/dl)	30–40	30–40	30–40	30–40
Urine				
Creatinine/height index	>0.9	>0.9	>0.9	>0.9
3-Methyl histidine (μmol/kg)	4.2 ± 1.3	–	–	3.2 ± 0.6
3-Methyl histidine (μmol/kg creatinine)	253 ± 78	–	–	126 ± 32
Hydroxyproline index	>2	>2	>2	>2
Vitamin A				
Plasma retinol (μg/dl)	≥30	≥30	≥30	≥30
Plasma retinol-binding protein (mg/dl)	2–3	2–3	2–3	2–3
Vitamin D				
25-OH-D_3 (ng/ml)	≥20	≥20	≥20	≥20
Riboflavin				
Red cell glutathione reductase stimulation effect (%)	<20	>20	>20	<20
Vitamin B_6				
Red cell transaminases	Not readily available, not practical in children younger than 9 years of age			
Plasma pyridoxal phosphate				
Xanthurenic acid excretion				
Folacin				
Serum folate (ng/ml)	>6	>6	>6	>6
Red blood cell folate (ng/ml)	>160	>160	>160	>160
Vitamin K				
Prothrombin time (sec)	11–15	11–15	11–15	11–15
Vitamin E				
Plasma α-tocopherol (mg/dl)	≥0.7	≥0.7	≥0.7	≥0.7
Red blood cell hemolysis test (%)	≤10	≤10	≤10	≤10
Vitamin C				
Plasma (mg/dl)	>0.2	>0.2	>0.2	>0.2
Leukocyte (μg/10^8 cells)	Difficult to perform on infants and children owing to sample requirements			
Thiamine				
Red blood cell transketolase stimulation effect (%)	>15	>15	>15	>15
Vitamin B_{12}				
Serum vitamin B_{12} (pg/ml)	≥200	≥200	≥200	≥200
Absorption test	Excretion of more than 7.5% of the orally ingested labeled vitamin B_{12}			
Iron				
Hematocrit (%)	31	33	36	36
Hemoglobin (g/dl)	12	12	13	13
Serum ferritin (ng/ml)	>10	>10	>10	>10
Serum iron (μg/dl)	>30	>40	>50	>60
Serum total iron-binding capacity (μg/dl)	350–400	350–400	350–400	350–400
Serum transferrin saturation (%)	>12	>12	>15	>16
Serum transferrin (mg/dl)	170–250	170–250	170–250	170–250
Erythrocyte protoporphyrin (μg/dl red blood cells)	<80	<75	<70	<70
Zinc				
Serum zinc (μg/dl)	80–120	80–120	80–120	80–120
Erythrocyte zinc	Erythrocytes contain approximately 10 times more zinc than plasma			

Table 72.6 Normal values: biochemical measurements of specific nutritional status

The assessment of specific nutrient deficiencies may be necessary in gastrointestinal diseases in which malabsorption or inflammation is a prominent feature of the clinical course. Fat-soluble vitamin (A, D, E, K) levels should be monitored at 6-month to yearly intervals in children with fat malabsorption disorders of the gastrointestinal tract such as cystic fibrosis or biliary atresia. In these conditions, low serum vitamin A, E and 25-

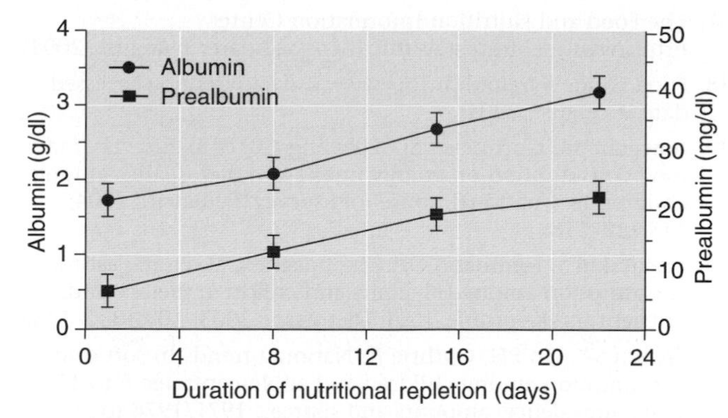

Figure 72.13: Response of serum albumin and prealbumin to refeeding in malnourished children. (Data from Helms RA, Dickerson RN, Ebbert ML, et al. Retinol-binding protein and prealbumin: useful measures of protein repletion in critically ill, malnourished infants. J Pediatr Gastroenterol Nutr 1986; 5:586–592,[59] and Ingenbleek Y, De Visscher M, De Nayer P. Measurement of prealbumin as index of protein-calorie malnutrition. Reproduced with permission from The Lancet 1972; 2:106–109.)[58]

hydroxyvitamin D levels or a prolonged prothrombin time indicate the need for supplemental therapy. Serum folate and vitamin B_{12} levels should be monitored at similar time intervals in gastrointestinal disorders associated with inflammatory processes of the terminal ileum (e.g. necrotizing enterocolitis, short gut syndrome, Crohn's disease). Although water-soluble vitamin deficiencies have been described, the subclinical abnormalities that may occur in children with chronic gastrointestinal diseases remain difficult to diagnose and are of questionable significance.

SUMMARY

Nutritional assessment is an essential component of the evaluation of children with gastrointestinal diseases because the clinical course of these individuals frequently is complicated by nutritional disorders such as malnutrition, growth failure, drug-induced overweight and iron deficiency anemia. Although a complete nutritional assessment includes a review of the diet history, physical examination, anthropometric measurements and selected laboratory testing, accurate height and weight measurements and their transformation to relative indices of overnutrition or undernutrition, serve as the mainstay of the nutritional assessment of the child with gastrointestinal disorders. The maintenance of a favorable nutritional status is essential to minimize disease-associated morbidity and maximize the child's quality of life.

ACKNOWLEDGEMENTS

The authors thank I. Tapper for secretarial support, L.A. Loddeke for editorial assistance and A. Gillum for illustrations. This chapter is a publication of the USDA/ARS Children's Nutrition Research Center, Department of pediatrics, Baylor College of Medicine, Houston, Texas and has been funded in part with federal funds from the US Department of Agriculture, Agricultural Research Service, under Cooperative Agreement Number 58-6250-1-003. The contents of herein do not necessarily reflect the views or policies of the US Department of Agriculture, nor does mention of trade names, commercial products, or organizations imply endorsement by the US government.

References

1. Viteri FE. Primary protein-energy malnutrition: clinical, biochemical and metabolic changes. In: Suskind RM, ed. Textbook of Pediatric Nutrition. New York: Raven Press; 1981:189–215.
2. Motil KJ, Grand RJ, Matthews DE, et al. Whole body leucine metabolism in adolescents with Crohn's disease and growth failure during nutritional supplementation. Gastroenterology 1982; 82:1359–1368.
3. Beisel WR. Interrelated changes in host metabolism during generalized infectious illness. Am J Clin Nutr 1972; 25:1254–1260.
4. Centers for Disease Control and Prevention. United States Growth Charts Body Mass Index, http://www.cdc.gov/growthcharts (Accessed date: 1 August, 2004).
5. Spady DW, Payne PR, Picou D, et al. Energy balance during recovery from malnutrition. Am J Clin Nutr 1976; 29:1073–1088.
6. Wang Z-M, Pierson RN, Heymsfield SB. The five-level model: a new approach to organizing body-composition research. Am J Clin Nutr 1992; 56:19–28.
7. Heymsfield SB, Waki M. Body composition in humans: advances in the development of multicompartment clinical models. Nutr Rev 1991; 49:97–108.
8. Fomon SJ, Haschke F, Ziegler EE, et al. Body composition of reference children from birth to 10 years. Am J Clin Nutr 1982; 35:1169–1175.
9. Ellis KJ, Abrams SA, Wong WW. Body composition of a young, multiethnic female population. Am J Clin Nutr 1997; 65:724–731.
10. Ellis KJ. Body composition of a young multiethnic male population. Am J Clin Nutr 1997; 66:1323–1331.
11. Frisancho AR. New norms of upper limb fat and muscle areas for assessment of nutritional status. Am J Clin Nutr 1981; 34:2540–2545.
12. Westrate JA, Deurenberg P. Body composition in children: proposal for a method for calculating body fat percentage from total body density or skinfold thickness measurements. Am J Clin Nutr 1989; 50:1104–1115.
13. Slaughter MH, Lohman TG, Boileau RA, et al. Skinfold equations for estimation of body fatness in children and youth. Hum Biol 1988; 60:709–723.
14. Lukaski HC. Soft tissue composition and bone mineral status: evaluation by dual-energy X-ray absorptiometry. J Nutr 1993; 123:438–443.
15. Fewtrell MS, British Paediatric and Adolescent Bone Group. Bone densitometry in children assessed by dual X-ray absorptiometry: uses and pitfalls. Arch Dis Child 2003; 88:795–798.
16. Rauch F, Plotkin H, Zeitlin L, et al. Bone mass, size and density in children and adults with osteogenesis imperfecta: effect of intravenous pamidronate therapy. J Bone Miner Res 2003; 18:610–614
17. Svendsen OL, Haarbro J, Hassager C. Accuracy of measurements of total-body-soft-tissue composition by dual energy X-ray absorptiometry in vivo. In: Ellis KJ,

Eastman JD, eds. Human Body Composition: In vivo Methods, Models and Assessment. Basic Life Science V edn., No. 60. New York: Plenum Press, 1993:381–383.

18. Koo WW, Hammami M, Hockman EM. Interchangeability of pencil-beam and fan-beam dual-energy X-ray absorptiometry measurements in piglets and infants. Am J Clin Nutr 2003; 78:236–240.
19. Gafni I, Baron J. Overdiagnosis of osteoporosis in children due to misinterpretation of dual-energy X-ray absorptiometry (DEXA). J Pediatr 2004; 144:253–257.
20. Brukx LJ, Waelkens JJ. Evaluation of the usefulness of a quantitative ultrasound device in screening of bone mineral density in children. Ann Hum Biol 2003; 30:304–315.
21. Ma G, Yao M, Liu Y, et al. Validation of a new pediatric air-displacement plethysmograph for assessing body composition in infants. Am J Clin Nutr 2004; 79:653–650.
22. Radley D, Gately PJ, Cooke CB, Carroll S, Oldroyd B, Truscott JG. Estimates of percentage body fat in young adolescents: a comparison of dual-energy X-ray absorptiometry and air displacement plethysmography. Eur J Clin Nutr 2003; 57:1402–1410.
23. Schoeller DA, van Santen E, Peterson DW, et al. Total body water measurement in humans with ^{18}O and ^{2}H labeled water. Am J Clin Nutr 1980; 33:2686–2693.
24. Fiorotto M. Application of the TOBEC measurement for determining fat and fat-free mass of the human infant. In: Klish WJ, Kretchmer N, eds. Body Composition Measurements in Infants and Children. Report of the 98th Ross Conference on Pediatric Research, Columbus, OH: Ross Laboratories; 1989:57.
25. Segal KR, Burastero S, Chun A, et al. Estimation of extracellular and total body water by multiple frequency bioelectrical-impedance measurement. Am J Clin Nutr 1991; 54:26–29.
26. Forbes GB, Simon W, Amatruda JM. Is bioimpedance a good predictor of body composition change? Am J Clin Nutr 1992; 56:4–6.
27. Ellis KJ, Nichols BL. Body composition. Adv Pediatr 1993; 40:159.
28. Heymsfield SB, Wang Z, Baumgartner RN, et al. Body composition and aging: a study by in vivo neutron activation analysis. J Nutr 1993; 123:432–437.
29. Baumgartner RN, Rhyne RL, Garry PJ, et al. Imaging techniques and anatomical body composition in aging. J Nutr 1993; 123:444–448.
30. Hubbard VS. Clinical assessment of nutritional status. In: Walker WA, Watkins JB, eds. Nutrition in Pediatrics: Basic Science and Clinical Application, 2nd edn. Toronto, BC: Decker; 1997:7.
31. Lo C. Laboratory assessment of nutritional status. In: Walker WA, Watkins JB, eds. Nutrition in Pediatrics: Basic Science and Clinical Application, 2nd edn. Toronto, BC: Decker; 1997:29.
32. Puig M. Body composition and growth. In: Walker WA, Watkins JB, eds. Nutrition in Pediatrics: Basic Science and Clinical Application, 2nd edn. Toronto, BC: Decker; 1997:44.
33. Rockett HR, Colditz GA. Assessing the diets of children and adolescents. Am J Clin Nutr 1997; 65(suppl):1116S–1122S.
34. National Academies. http://www.nap.edu (Accessed date: 1 August, 2004).
35. US Department of Health and Human Services. Dietary Guidelines for Americans, 4th edn. Washington, DC: US Government Printing Office; 1995.
36. Hampl JS, Betts NM, Benes BA. The 'age +5' rule: comparisons of dietary fiber intake among 4- to 10-year-old children. J Am Diet Assoc 1998; 98:1418–1423.
37. The Food and Nutrition Information Center. http://www.nal.usda.gov/fnic (Accessed date: 1 August, 2004).
38. Food Guide Pyramid. http://www.usda.gov/cnpp (Accessed date: 1 August, 2004).
39. Bowman SA, Gortmaker SL, Ebbeling CB, et al. Effects of fast-food consumption on energy intake and diet quality among children in a national household survey. Pediatrics 2004; 113:112–118.
40. Paeratakul S, Ferdinand DP, Champagne CM, et al. Fast-food consumption among US adults and children: dietary and nutrient intake profile. J Am Diet Assoc 2003; 103:1332–1338.
41. French SA, Lin BH, Guthrie JF. National trends in soft drink consumption among children and adolescents age 6 to 17 years: prevalence, amounts and sources, 1977/1978 to 1994/1998. J Am Diet Assoc 2003; 1003:1326–1331.
42. Herbert V. Toxicity of 25,000 IU vitamin A supplements in 'health' food users. Am J Clin Nutr 1982; 36:185–186.
43. Jelliffe DB. The assessment of the nutritional status of the community. Geneva: World Health Organization; 1966:Monograph Series No 53.
44. Greulich WW, Pyle SI. Radiographic Atlas of Skeletal Development of the Hand and Wrist, 2nd edn. Stanford, CA: Stanford University Press; 1959.
45. Roche AF, Himes JH. Incremental growth charts. Am J Clin Nutr 1980; 33:2041–2052.
46. Kanof ME, Lake AM, Bayles TM. Decreased height velocity in children and adolescents before the diagnosis of Crohn's disease. Gastroenterology 1988; 95:1523–1527.
47. Barlow SE, Dietz WH. Obesity evaluation and treatment: expert committee recommendations. The Maternal and Child Health Bureau, Health Resources and Services Administration and the Department of Health and Human Services. J Pediatr 1998; 102:E29.
48. Keys A, Fidanza F, Karvonen MJ, et al. Indices of relative weight and obesity. J Chronic Dis 1972; 25:329–343.
49. Peitrobelli A, Faith MS, Allison DB, et al. Body mass index as a measure of adiposity among children and adolescents: a validation study. J Pediatr 1998; 132:204–210.
50. Hammer LD, Kraemer HC, Wilson DM, et al. Standardized percentile curves of body-mass index for children and adolescents. Am J Dis Child 1991; 45:259–263.
51. Mei Z, Grummer-Strawn LM, Pietrobelli A, et al. Validity of body mass index compared with other body-composition screening indexes for the assessment of body fatness in children and adolescents. Am J Clin Nutr 2002; 75:978–985.
52. Freedman DS, Dietz WH, Srinivasan SR, et al. The relation of overweight to cardiovascular risk factors among children and adolescents: the Bogalusa Heart Study. Pediatrics 1999; 103:1175–1182.
53. Must A, Jacques PF, Dallal GE, et al. Long-term morbidity and mortality of overweight adolescents. N Engl J Med 1992; 327:1350–1355.
54. Waterlow JC. Classification and definition of protein-calorie malnutrition. BMJ 1972; 3:566–569.
55. Waterlow JC. Note on the assessment and classification of protein-energy malnutrition in children. Lancet 1973; 2:87–89.
56. Kanawati AA, McLaren DS. Assessment of marginal malnutrition. Nature 1970; 228:573–575.
57. Figueroa-Colon R, Franklin FA, Lee JY, et al. Feasibility of a clinic-based hypocaloric dietary intervention implemented in a school setting for obese children. Obes Res 1996; 4:419–429.

58. Ingenbleek Y, De Visscher M, De Nayer P. Measurement of prealbumin as index of protein-calorie malnutrition. Lancet 1972; 2:106–109.

59. Helms RA, Dickerson RN, Ebbert ML, et al. Retinol-binding protein and prealbumin: useful measures of protein repletion in critically ill, malnourished infants. J Pediatr Gastroenterol Nutr 1986; 5:586–592.

60. Ford EG, Jennings M, Andrassy RJ. Serum albumin (oncotic pressure) correlates with enteral feeding tolerance in the pediatric patient. J Pediatr Surg 1987; 22:597–599.

61. Waterlow JC. Protein-energy malnutrition: challenges and controversies. Proc Nutr Soc India 1991; 37:59–87.

Chapter 73
Tubes for enteric access

Donald E. George and Maryanne L. Dokler

There are a multitude of tubes available to allow access to the gastrointestinal tract, but only two reasons for using them: to remove or add contents. Decompression with suction is required when there is obstruction, ileus or pernicious vomiting. Nasogastric tubes also are used to remove stomach contents after ingestion of a toxic substance or to examine the contents, for example gastric aspirate for blood. These tubes are generally larger in diameter and stiffer, and do not collapse when suction is applied. Tubes also may be used to introduce content, usually nutrients or medications, into the gastrointestinal tract. There are numerous tubes made with a myriad of differences all based on the desired use. Of greatest interest are the tubes for feeding.

Ideally all patients receive nutrition by mouth. However, when a child is unable to eat normally or when oral intake fails to meet nutritional needs for any reason, alternative modes of nutrient delivery are considered. When gut failure is present, intravenous routes are used. Conversely it is axiomatic that 'if the gut works, use it'. Enteral feedings by tube have multiple advantages in maintaining gut function, promoting mucosal integrity and reducing infection.[1] There are clear advantages in terms of cost and ease of use. However, it should not be assumed that enteral nutrition is safer than parenteral nutrition in all patients.[2–4]

Tube feedings have been used for centuries. The Ancient Egyptians used nutrient enemas. Silver, leather and rubber tubes placed in the stomach were used in the seventeenth and eighteenth centuries.[5] Use of tubes for gavage feeding of pediatric patients was first described in the late 1800s. Over the past two decades a multitude of formulas, supplements, tubes and other enteral access devices have been developed to allow delivery of enteral nutrition to neonates, infants and children.[6] Many different techniques have been described, all with particular indications, advantages and disadvantages. It is important to consider the specific needs of each patient and therapy to ensure the desired outcomes.

EVALUATION

The decision to use an enteric tube requires a thoughtful analysis of the clinical situation, nutritional needs and prognosis (Fig. 73.1). Careful evaluation of the patient is of paramount importance. The indications, risks, potential benefits and possible alternatives should be reviewed for each patient. Several parameters should be assessed including nutritional status, etiology and prognosis of the underlying disease and respiratory status. All patients should have an evaluation to document ability to protect the airway. Other factors to be considered include size of the patient, medical condition, surgical history, presence of gastroesophageal reflux disease and potential risk of aspiration. The probable duration of treatment and proposed type of feed should also be considered. Attention must be paid to the child's developmental abilities, social situation and growth potential (Table 73.1). The evaluation is enhanced when a team of professionals is available to assess the child. The team may include oromotor specialists, dietitians, nurses and social workers as well as gastroenterologists, surgeons and the child's primary doctor. If the tube feedings are to be relatively short term and take place while the child is in the hospital, the issues are often straightforward. If tube feedings are to be longer in duration and used at home or an alternative site, the issues may be more complex. It is crucial to include the parents (and the patient if appropriate) in the decision process.[7]

In pediatrics, the provision of enteral feedings is often required because of an inability to swallow or progressive dysphagia. Some common indications and contraindications are noted in Tables 73.2 and 73.3 respectively. Patients with neurologic and neuromuscular disorders, head and neck malignancy, major trauma or congenital anomalies often have normal gastrointestinal tracts, but are unable to take adequate feeds orally.[8] Supplemental enteral feeding may also be needed when the patient is unable to consume adequate nutrition orally because of illness or choice. Gastrostomy tube feeds provide a means of delivering continuous feedings or unpalatable diets, which may be needed in a wide variety of disorders including cystic fibrosis,[9] short bowel syndrome, severe gastrointestinal allergy, metabolic disorders, anorexia associated with malignancy,[10] chronic diarrhea, intestinal hypomotility, chronic renal failure, intestinal lymphangiomatosis, Crohn's disease,[11,12] chronic cholestasis[13] or congenital heart disease.[14] Feedings by tube pose risks to the child (Table 73.4), and the potential benefits of nutrition must be evaluated in each patient. Careful patient selection and evaluation will minimize complications.

Selection of enteral tubes is guided by patient comfort and tube performance. Multiple tubes are available and the choice is often influenced by product availability and cost. Tubes vary by composition, inner and outer diameter, presence or absence of weighted tip, tip size and shape, and location and number of access ports and egress ports. Some tubes have a stylet to aid insertion (Figs 73.2 and 73.3). Feeding tubes may be placed into the stomach or advanced

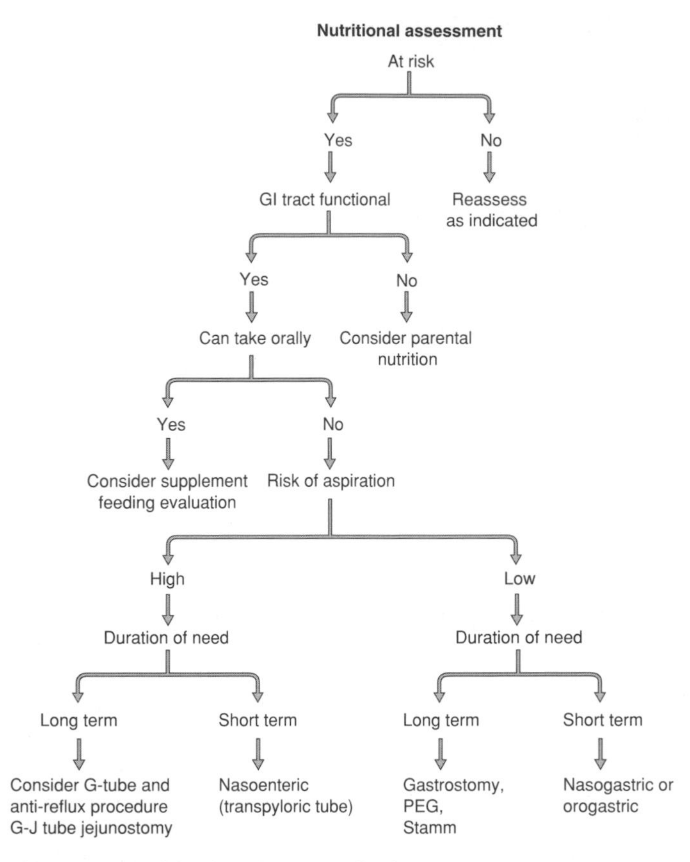

Figure 73.1: Algorithim for enteric feeding.

- Underlying condition and reason for feeding
- Co-morbidities (e.g. craniofacial defects, vomiting, aspiration, cardiac defects)
- Age and size of patient
- Nutritional needs and volume of feeding
- Ease of administration and location of care (home, hospital)
- Projected duration of support (for how long will it be needed?)
- Patient activity, cooperation and comfort
- Tube composition (polyvinyl chloride, polyurethane, Silastic)
- Tube length, diameter, style, weighted tip, end or side port

Table 73.1 Considerations in enteral feeding

beyond the pylorus. Transpyloric feeds are suggested when there is vomiting, gastroparesis or a risk of aspiration.

The anticipated duration of need for the tube is another consideration in selecting the route and type of enteral tube (Table 73.5). Tubes can be divided arbitrarily into those best suited for short-term and those for long-term use. For short-term feedings, tubes are most often passed through the nose into the gastrointestinal tract. In special situations orally placed tubes are also used. They are readily available and do not require surgery to place them. They are relatively easy to place, less invasive and less costly than surgically placed tubes. However, they are easily displaced and must be positioned and monitored carefully.[15,16] If long-term use is anticipated – percutaneous endoscopic gastrostomy (PEG), gastrostomy, jejunostomy, etc. – a more permanent enterostomal tube is preferred. These are generi-

Condition	Indication
Dysphagia	
Anatomic	ENT abnormalities
	Pierre–Robin sequence
	Cleft lip and/or cleft palate
Neurologic	Head trauma, cerebral palsy
	Hypoxic encephalopathy
Esophageal disease	Atresia, stricture
	Caustic ingestion
Failure to grow	Cholestasis, chronic liver disease
	AIDS, chronic renal failure
	Food refusal, chronic diarrhea, malignancy
	Congenital heart disease
	Cystic fibrosis, bronchopulmonary dysphasia
Bowel disease	Short bowel syndrome, intestinal dysmotility
	Inflammatory bowel disease, eosinophilic gastroenteritis
	Malabsorption
Inability to eat for other reasons	Trauma, burns, prematurity, chemotherapy
	Bone marrow transplant
Special nutrient needs	Inborn errors of metabolism

Table 73.2 Indications for enteral feeds

- Ileus
- Bowel obstruction
- Peritonitis or intra-abdominal sepsis
- Necrotizing pancreatitis
- High-output gastrointestinal fistulae

Table 73.3 Relative contraindications to enteral feeds

Mechanical
Tracheobronchial intubation
Erosive tissue damage
Tube occlusion
Metabolic
Increased blood glucose level
Electrolyte abnormality
Refeeding syndrome
Pulmonary
Aspiration
Cough
Gastrointestinal
Nausea and vomiting
Diarrhea
Abdominal pain
Bowel necrosis

Table 73.4 Complications of tube feedings

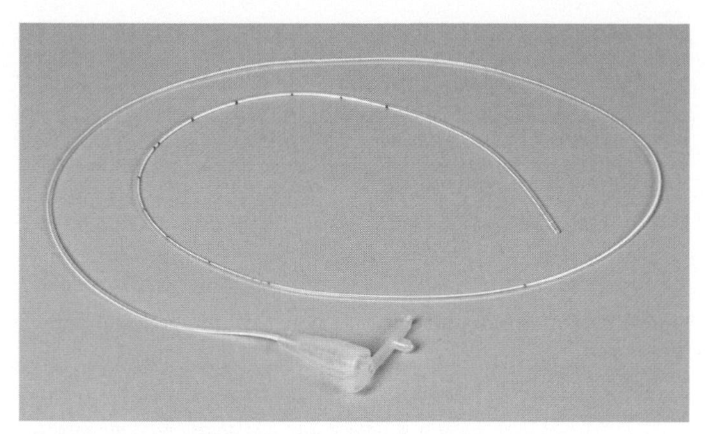

Figure 73.2: Typical 'fine-bore' nasoenteric tube without stylus. The single-lumen marking helps to assess placement.

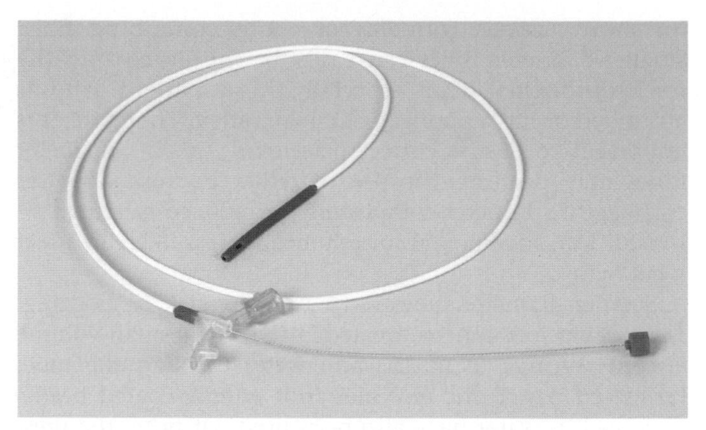

Figure 73.3: Nasoenteric tube with stylet and weighted tip.

ally placed through the skin into the desired area of the gastrointestinal tract; a surgical procedure is required for placement. There is no consensus as to what is long term *vs* short term, although most agree that less than 4 weeks is short term and more than 8–12 weeks long term.[1,17,18]

CONSIDERATIONS FOR SHORT-TERM ACCESS

The gastric route is generally the preferred route for feeding. This allows normal mixing of nutrients with bile and pancreatic secretions, and maintains the physiologic digestive process. Feeding into the stomach allows bolus feedings and the use of hypertonic formulas. In patients with a high risk of aspiration or gastroparesis, or after some gastric surgical procedures, post-pyloric feeding is indicated.

The size of the tube influences both performance and tolerability. Tube length is determined by the size of the patient and whether it is positioned in the stomach, duodenum or jejenum. Tube diameter is measured in 'French (1 Fr = 0.33 mm), and both inner and outer diameters are important. Large-bore tubes are used for decompression or suction. For patient comfort, the smallest diameter tube that allows flow of formula is used for feeding. Smaller-diameter tubes, 5–8 Fr can be used with most commercially available formulas. Larger-diameter tubes may be needed

	Indications	Benefits	Considerations
Orogastric	Used mainly in premature infants or patients with no nasal access	Relatively inexpensive, easy to place, generally available	Risk of pulmonary aspiration due to misplacement or GER. Impaired swallowing
Nasogastric	Short-term feedings in patients without vomiting or failure to protect airway	As for orogastric	Visible on face; irritation to nares, sinusitis. May interfere with oro-motor development. Impairs patient mobility
Nasoenteric (beyond pylorus)	Useful when aspiration, GER and/or gastroparesis are present. Short-term feedings	Reduces vomiting and aspiration risk. NJ feed may allow earlier feeds in pancreatitis or early after surgery	Visable on face. Requires continuous rather than bolus feeds. Requires a pump. Placement more cumbersome and time consuming. Frequently dislodged. Risk of perforation or necrosis of intestine
Gastrostomy (Stamm or PEG)	Useful for long-term feedings	Relatively more expensive and requires a procedure for placement. Less likely to dislodge. Greater patient comfort and mobility. No tube visible during day	Stoma care needed. Risk of pulmonary aspiration or GER; stomal infection; scar
G-J	Placed when there is a high risk of aspiration	Allow drainage of stomach and enteral feeds. Useful when stomach function is impaired	May dislodge or migrate to stomach. Small-bore tubes clog. Requires monitoring and continuous infusion. Requires fluoroscopic or endoscopic placement. Risk of perforation
Jejunostomy	Useful for long-term feeds	Allows drainage of stomach and enteral feeds. Useful when stomach function is impaired. Usually stable and less likely to dislodge	May dislodge or migrate to stomach. Small-bore tubes clog. Requires monitoring and continuous infusion. Requires fluoroscopic or endoscopic placement. Increased risk of perforation. Requires surgery

GER, gastroesophageal reflux; G-J, gastrojejunostomy; NJ, nasojejunal; PEG, percutaneous endoscopic gastrostomy.

Table 73.5 Enteral feeding routes

for more viscous formulas or those containing fiber. Smaller-diameter tubes can easily be misplaced into the tracheobronchial tree, especially in a patient who is obtunded or has a poor gag or cough reflex. Therefore, it is important to ensure correct placement. Smaller-diameter tubes may decrease the risk of reflux because of lower esophageal sphincter compromise or reduced gagging.[19–21] In addition, smaller and softer tubes are less likely to affect swallowing.

Smaller-diameter tubes have a greater risk of clogging. Tube occlusion can be treated by using a small-volume (10 ml) syringe to flush warm water through the tube. Powdered pancreatic enzymes (not enteric-coated beads) dissolved in water have also been used. Of note, the pressure that can be generated is sufficient to rupture the tube. There are commercial products available that either dissolve or mechanically remove the obstruction.[22]

The most commonly available tubes are made of polyvinylchloride (PVC), polyurethane or silicone polymers (Table 73.6). PVC is rather firm, and becomes less flexible and more brittle with exposure to gastric acid. The walls are not easily compressed or collapsed, and gastric content can be easily aspirated. PVC tubes are not recommended for tube feedings and are most often used for gastric decompression and drainage. Straight drainage tubes have a single lumen and multiple distal ports. They can be left open for venting or attached to intermittent suction. 'Sump type' (Fig. 73.4) tubes are used specifically for decompression and have a second lumen that allows air in during suction and thus prevents the gastric mucosa from being pulled into the tube ports. They are best used with continuous suction.

Polyurethane does not stiffen or discolor, and permits a thinner wall construction. Polyurethane tubes can be used for aspiration without collapsing. Silicone or silicone–elastomer tubes are very soft and generally collapse when suction is used. They frequently require a stylet to facilitate placement.

Many nasoenteric tubes have weights on the distal tip (see Fig. 73.3). They come in several sizes, styles and materials. Weighted tips are thought to be advantageous when advancing a tube past the pylorus, but similar rates of passage are achieved using unweighted tubes.[23] Further, it is not clear whether weighted tubes stay in place longer than unweighted tubes.[24] Unless a nasogastric or nasoenteric feeding tube has been placed under direct vision endoscopically or with fluoroscopic guidance, there is a risk of misplacement into the bronchial tree. This is especially important when using fine-bore tubes for feeding. Tip position cannot be ensured by auscultation of air injected through the tube. Radiographic confirmation of distal tip placement must be obtained before initiating feedings because of the severe consequences of aspiration or feeding into the lungs. Checking the pH of aspirate has been recommended to confirm tube position between feedings,[15] but radiography remains the most accurate method.[14]

Material	Comments
Polyvinylchloride	Stiff, and gets stiffer with long-term placement. Useful for aspiration of stomach
Polyurethane	Thinner walled. Large internal diameter. Can aspirate without collapsing the tube.
Silicone	Very flexible and soft. Collapses with suction. Often requires a stylet for positioning

Table 73.6 Tube composition

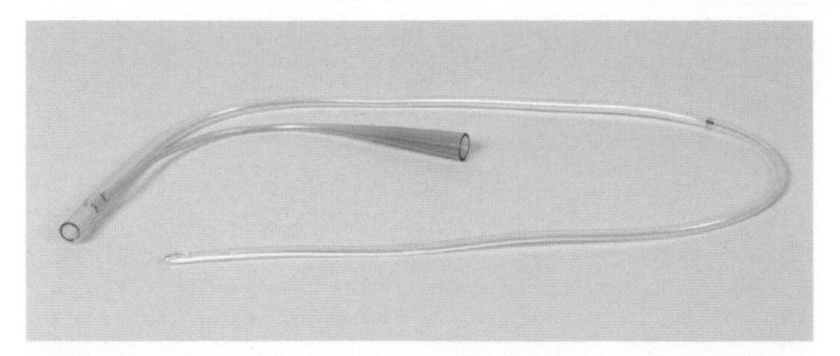

Figure 73.4: Tube for nasogastric suction. Note the thick wall and 'sump' port.

CONSIDERATIONS FOR LONG-TERM ACCESS

Tubes suitable for short-term use are usually not used for long-term access because of patient comfort, complications (e.g. sinusitis), malposition or mechanical failure. Further, they require careful monitoring because of the risk of inadvertent displacement, and need to be replaced frequently. Many techniques for placement of more stable and longer-lasting tubes are available: laparotomy, laparoscopy, endoscopy, radiographically or any combination. All require particular skills and experience to accomplish safely, and expertise and facilities for each may not be available in all institutions. Gastrostomy and jejunostomy are most often done by surgeons, usually at the time of laparotomy for another reason. Endoscopic and radiologic techniques are considered less invasive, although morbidity and complication rates are similar[25,26] (Table 73.7).

Gastrostomy, the operative creation of a fistulous tract between the stomach and the abdominal surface, is a common way of providing enteral access for patients. The Stamm gastrostomy is the most common surgical gastrostomy. A tube is inserted through the abdominal wall into the stomach and secured to the wall of the stomach with a purse-string suture. Many types of catheter can be used, including dePezzar, Melecot and Foley catheters. All have a balloon or mushroom tip to hold the stomach to the anterior abdominal wall (Fig. 73.5). It is important that the tube be anchored to the abdominal wall (external bolster) to prevent it from migrating into the small bowel and causing obstruction. Latex catheters erode with prolonged exposure to gastric juices; silicone or PVC catheters last longer. Gastrostomy tubes can be used for feeding or decompression.[27]

The percutaneous endoscopic gastrostomy (PEG) was developed by Gauderer and Ponsky utilizing the idea of

	Early	Late
Major complications	Pneumoperitoneum	Enteroenteric fistulae
	Bleeding	Enterocutaneous fistula
	Enteroenteric fistula	Tube migration
	External migration	Volvulus, gastric ulceration
	Perforation	Intestinal obstruction
	Aspiration	Cutaneous necrosis
		Buried or extruded tube
		Gastric ulceration
Minor complications	Stomal infection	Stomal infection
	Neuralgia	Granulation tissue
	Diarrhea	Displacement, leakage
	Bleeding	Tube obstruction

Table 73.7 Complications of gastrostomy placement

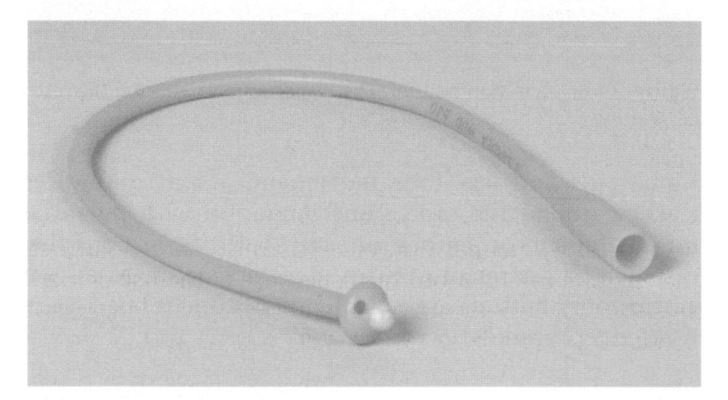

Figure 73.5: Gastrostomy tube with mushroom tip. These tubes are placed at operation.

sutureless approximation of the stomach to the abdominal wall with a catheter.[28] Over time, adhesions develop between the stomach and the peritoneum around the tract of the catheter. PEG has been used extensively in both adults and children to provide long-term enteral nutrition in a wide variety of clinical conditions. Currently more than 200 000 PEGs are performed in the USA annually,[29] and approximately 5000 of these procedures are done in children. PEGs are now widely available and have become a commonly used method of enteral access. Indeed, PEGs now represent the most utilized technique for long-term enteral access.

A PEG may be used for feeding, decompression, combined feeding and decompression, gastric access for esophageal dilation or medication administration, management of gastric volvulus, and multiple portals for intragastric surgical interventions.[27]

Contraindications to the placement of a PEG include the inability to perform upper endoscopy safely and to bring the anterior gastric wall in apposition to the abdominal wall. The inability to juxtapose the anterior gastric and abdominal walls should be considered in patients with ascites, hepatomegaly or obesity. Failure to identify transabdominal illumination or to visualize the indentation of the finger on the stomach wall should suggest this problem. A PEG should not be used for nutrition when obstruction of the gastrointestinal tract is present, although it may be used for decompression in some circumstances. The presence of gastric varices, although not an absolute contraindication, may make placement of any gastrostomy device more concerning. Depending on severity, relative contraindications to PEG placement include coagulopathy, inflammatory or infiltrative disease of the gastric or abdominal walls, and intra-abdominal infection. Young age and low weight are not contraindications to PEG.[28,30]

At times the trasverse colon may lie across the desired placement site. Concomitant fluoroscopy at the time of the PEG may identify the transverse colon, facilitating placement.

Except for gastric resection, prior abdominal surgical procedures are not an absolute contraindication to PEG placement.[31] Placement could be more difficult because of disruption of the normal anatomy by adhesions, and careful attention to preoperative contrast studies and intraoperative technique is important. Morbidity and types of complication following PEG are similar in previously operated and non-operated patients.[32] Elective placement of a PEG in patients with existing ventriculoperitoneal shunts has been accepted by neurosurgeons, although simultaneous placement of a shunt and PEG should be avoided.[33] PEG is not associated with a higher risk of infection than open gastrostomy, and may be associated with less morbidity. Careful attention should be paid to infection, and an intraoperative antibiotic is recommended (see below). Common alternatives to PEG are nasogastric or orogastric feeds, open gastrostomy, gastrostomy with anti-reflux procedure, and percutaneous endoscopic or open jejunostomy.

Several techniques have been described for the placement of a PEG. They share several basic elements (Table 73.8) and the published outcomes are similar.[34,35]

Non-endoscopic, radiologically controlled insertion of a gastrostomy tube has been described in adults but has not been widely adopted in children, because of the risk of pushing the stomach away from the abdominal wall and the small size of the catheters utilized. Gastrostomies can also be placed percutaneously utilizing a 'push' technique under laparoscopic guidance in conjunction with other

- Adequate gastric insufflation to bring gastric wall in apposition to abdominal wall
- Placement of cannula into stomach
- Passage of guidewire
- Placement of tube/button
- Verification of position

Table 73.8 Basic elements of PEG placement common to all techniques

abdominal procedures. A variety of percutaneous gastrostomy tubes are available. The original procedure utilized a dePezzer catheter threaded onto a tapered Medicut sheath. Similar tubes are now available made of Silastic and in a variety of sizes.

Because the tubes pass through the mouth, PEG procedures carry a substantial risk of infection, generally stomal infections with either oropharygeal or cutaneous bacteria; however, bacteremia may occur. Therefore, a single preoperative or postoperative dose of antibiotic is recommended to minimize the incidence of infection in uncomplicated procedures.[36,37] Cefazolin or cefotaxime is often used. Prophylaxis for subacute bacterial endocarditis, recommended by the American Heart Association, is utilized for patients at risk owing to congenital heart disease or implanted vascular devices. The duration of antibiotic therapy has not yet been defined; patients may receive one to several doses. Antibiotics are continued for a minimum of 24 h for patients with ventriculoperitoneal shunts.

In 1982, the gastrostomy button was introduced. This is a skin-level device with a one-way valve at the gastric opening of the shaft to prevent reflux of gastric contents externally (Fig.73.6). Some 2–3 months after placing a long gastrostomy tube percutaneously, the tube can be removed and replaced with a gastrostomy button. The low-profile devices are preferred by many patients and their parents because they are less obtrusive. They are not as effective for decompression. Some centers use the one-step button (Figs 73.7 and 73.8).[38] Complications of catheter removal and replacement are reduced. The one-step button can be placed as the initial gastric tube, allowing families to use a low-profile device immediately for feedings.[27,39] This obviates the need to change the long tube for a button at a later date, and training caregivers and obtaining supplies is somewhat easier. Use of a long gastrostomy tube is reserved for very small infants (less than 4 kg) or when a transpyloric tube is needed. The low-profile gastrostomy device has additional advantages. Because it is skin level, inadvertent displacement is less likely. The shorter shaft of the tube results in less clogging from feeds and less tube movement, which minimizes leakage around the tube. Tube migration with potential for obstruction or perforation, seen with the use of Foley catheters as gastrostomy tubes, does not occur. As all the gastrostomy buttons are made with silicone rubber, there is often less granulation tissue.

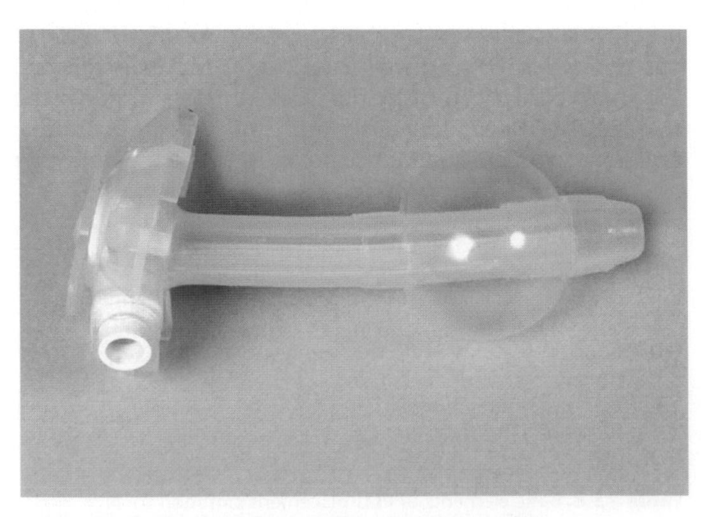

Figure 73.6: Skin-level (low profile) gastrostomy tube.

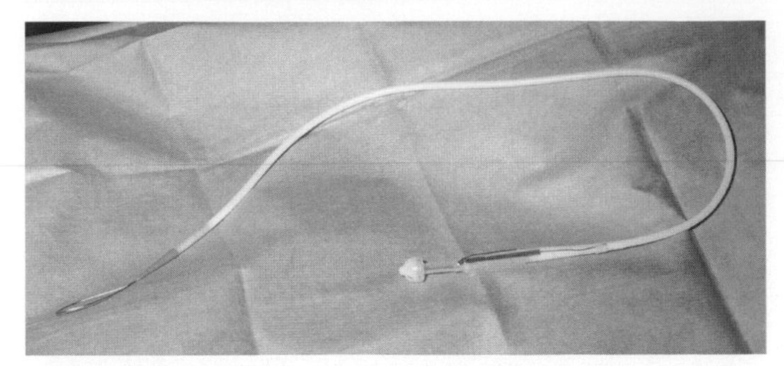

Figure 73.7: The 'one-step button' technique is similar to other PEG techniques.

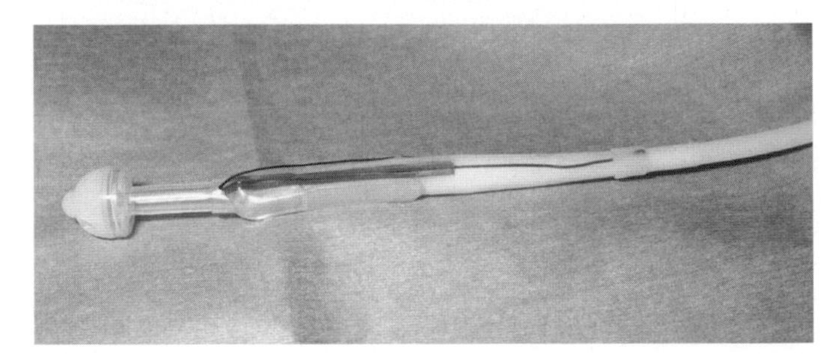

Figure 73.8: 'One-step button'. The button is released from the rest of the tube.

GASTROESOPHAGEAL REFLUX AND TUBES

Conditions for which feeding tubes are considered in children are frequently associated with a high rate of gastroesophageal reflux (GER). This can be manifested as recurrent vomiting, malnutrition, esophagitis or recurrent aspiration penumonia. Nasoenteric tubes are known to exacerbate GER.[19–21] Further, it is well accepted that Stamm-type open gastrostomy is associated with development of GER.[40,41] This finding has led many to propose anti-reflux surgery for all neurologically disabled children who need a feeding gastrostomy.[42] The recognition that anti-reflux surgery has both early and late complications (such as dumping syndrome, retching, aerophagia and gas-bloat), and a significant rate of recurrence of GER, has caused a rethinking of this approach.[43,44] No single preoperative study can reliably identify all the children who need an anti-reflux procedure.

The unmasking of GER may be less pronounced after PEG compared with operative gastrostomy. However, contradictory data exist about the effect of PEG on GER and the need for anti-reflux procedures.[45–47] The development or worsening of GER, or the need for subsequent conversion to an anti-reflux procedure, percutaneous gastrojejunostomy (PEJ) or jejunostomy is considered a complication of a PEG. Much attention has been paid to the role of PEG placement in the child with GER, and the possibility that the PEG procedure might promote reflux. Several factors may contribute to worsening of reflux, including volume of feeding, method of feeding (continuous or bolus) and type of formula. Malnutrition has a deleterious effect on GER, and nutritional rehabilitation may lessen vomiting attributed to GER.[48]

It is recommended that all children be evaluated clinically to determine the presence of GER and whether the GER can be controlled medically. If GER is absent or can be controlled by medical treatment, including proton pump inhibitors and/or prokinetic agents, PEG should be performed. In the presence of severe GER, especially with impaired pulmonary function, or the inability to tolerate nasogastric feeds, an anti-reflux procedure with gastrostomy, jejunostomy or gastrojejunostomy (G-J tube) may be appropriate. As a previous PEG does not make subsequent fundoplication more risky, it seems reasonable to suggest a trial of feedings via PEG in patients with mild symptoms or symptoms controlled by medication before embarking on a more extensive procedure.[49,50]

Jejunostomy is performed to reduce the risk of aspiration, or in patients with severe GER or those with a nonfunctioning stomach. Even though the risk of aspiration is reduced with jejunal feedings when compared to gastric feedings, it is important to note that aspiration is not completely avoidable. Multiple techniques using surgery, laporoscopy, endoscopy and radiology are available[1,26] and generally require surgery. They are all operator dependent, and the choice is based on experience and expertise available within an institution.

Complications of jejunal feedings are related to the small bowel location. Jejunal tubes are difficult to anchor and prone to dislodgment. Gastrointestinal complaints are common including abdominal distension, pain and diarrhea. Bolus feeds cannot be used and continuous feeds are often cumbersome. Small bowel ischemia and necrosis have been described.[26,51]

PEJ may be an alternative to surgery in selected cases (Fig. 73.9). This involves the placement of a jejunal feeding tube through a previously created gastrostomy tube, most often using fluoroscopy or endoscopy. Several systems are available commercially. Experience with PEJ in children is limited.[52] The initial enthusiasm to convert PEG to PEJ has waned as high rates of dysfunction without elimination of aspiration have been observed. There seems to be a tendency for the jejunal arm to migrate back into the stomach, and careful monitoring is essential. Further, these tubes are of small diameter and tend to clog.[53] Direct placement of a PEJ tube into the jejunum is described in adults, but has not been studied in children. The technique is similar to PEG, and the need for careful transillumination and visualization of the fingertip indentation on the wall of the intestine is emphasized.

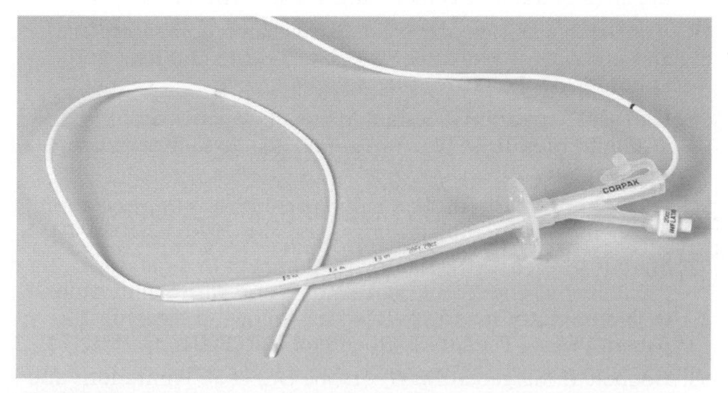

Figure 73.9: Gastrostomy tube with jejunal extender (PEJ). The smaller internal tube is placed into the jejunum either endoscopically or fluoroscopically through the gastrostomy.

SUMMARY

A wide variety of tubes are available to allow intubation of the gastrointestinal tract. Systematic evaluation of the child is the most important step in deciding which tube to use. Newer techniques of endoscopic tube placement have reduced the need for surgery in many patients. However, the contribution of GER to morbidity and mortality remains considerable. Careful patient selection and scrupulous attention to technique can minimize complications and improve outcomes.

References

1. Atten MJ, Skipper A, Kumar S, et al. Enteral nutrition support. Dis Mon 2002; 48:751–790.
2. Jeejeebhoy KN. Total parenteral nutrition: potion or poison. Am J Clin Nutr 2001; 74:160–163.
3. Lippman TO. Grains or veins: is enteral nutrition really better than parenteral nutrition? JPEN J Parenter Enteral Nutr 1978; 22:167–182.
4. Woodcock N, Zeigler D, Palmer M, et al. Enteral versus parenteral nutrition: a pragmatic study. Nutrition 2001; 17:1–12.
5. McCamish MA, Bounous G, Geraghty ME. History of enteral feeding: past and present perspectives. In: Rombeau JL, Rolandelli RH, eds. Clinical Nutrition: Enteral and Tube Feeding, 3rd edn. Philadelphia, PA: WB Saunders; 1997:1–11.
6. Harkness L. The history of enteral nutrition therapy: from raw eggs and nasal tubes to purified amino acids and early postoperative jejunal delivery. J Am Diet Assoc 2002; 102:399–404.
7. Scolapio JE, Picco MF, Tarrosa VB. Enteral *vs* parenteral nutrition: The patient's preference. JPEN JParenter Enteral Nutr 2002; 26:248–250.
8. Britton JE, Lipscomb G, Mohr PD, et al. The use of percutaneous endoscopic gastrostomy (PEG) feeding tubes in patients with neurological disease. J Neurol 1997; 244:431–434.
9. Williams SG, Ashworth F, McAlweenie A, et al. Percutaneous endoscopic gastrostomy feeding in patients with cystic fibrosis. Gut 1999; 44:87–90.
10. Bisgaard Pedersen A-M, Kok K, Petersen G, et al. Percutaneous endoscopic gastrostomy in children with cancer. Acta Paediatr 1999; 88:849–852.
11. Cosgrove M, Jenkins HR. Experience of percutaneous endoscopic gastrostomy in children with Crohn's disease. Arch Dis Child 1997; 76:141–143.

12. Mahajan L, Olive L, Wyllie R, et al. The safety of gastrostomy in patients with Crohn's disease. Am J Gastroenterol 1997; 92:985–988.
13. Duche M, Habes D, Lababidi A, et al. Percutaneous endoscopic gastrostomy for continuous feeding in children with cholestasis. J Pediatr Gastroenterol Nutr 1999; 29:42–45.
14. Hofner G, Behrens R, Koch A, et al. Enteral nutritional support by percutaneous endoscopic gastrostomy in children with congenital heart disease. Pediatr Cardiol 2000; 21:341–346.
15. Newman MJ, Meyer CT, Dutten JL, et al. Hold that x-ray: aspirate pH and auscultation prove enteral tube placement. J Clin Gastroenterol 1995; 20:293–295.
16. Huffman S, Piper, P, Jarczyk K, et al. Methods to confirm feeding tube placements: application of research in practice. Pediatr Nurs 2004; 30:10–13.
17. Vaneck VW. The ins and outs of enteral access, Part I: Short term access. Nutr Clin Pract 2002; 17:275–283.
18. Minard G. Enteral access. Nutr Clin Pract 1994; 9:172–182.
19. Noviski N, Yehuda YB, Serour F, et al. Does size of nasogastric tubes affect gastroesophageal reflux in children? J Pediatr Gastroenterol 1999; 29:448–451.
20. Peter CS, Beichers C, Bohwhorst B, et al. Influence of nasogastric tubes on gastroesophageal reflux in preterm infants: a multiple intraluminal impedence study. J Pediatr 2002; 141:277–279.
21. Kuo B, Castell DO. The effect of nasogastric intubation on gastroesophageal reflux: a comparison of different tubes sizes. Am J Gastroenterol 1995; 90:1804–1807.
22. Lord LM. Restoring and maintaining patency of enteral feeding tubes. Nutr Clin Pract 2003; 18:422–426.
23. Lord LM, Weiser-Maimowe A, Pulhamus M, et al. Comparison of weighted *vs* unweighted enteral feeding tubes for efficacy of transpyloric intubation. JPEN J Parenter Enteral Nutr 1993; 17:271–273.
24. Silk DB, Rees RG, Keohane PP, et al. Clinical efficacy and design changes of 'fine-bore' nasogastric feeding tubes. JPEN J Parenter Enteral Nutr 1987; 11:378–383.
25. Vaneck VW. The ins and outs of enteral access, Part II: Long term access: gastrostomy. Nutr Clin Pract 2003; 18:50–74.
26. Vaneck VW. The ins and outs of enteral access, Part III: Long term access jejunostomy. Nutr Clinc Pract 2003; 18:201–220.
27. George D, Dokler M. Percutaneous endoscopic gastrostomy in children. Techniques in Gastrointestinal Endoscopy 2002; 4:201–206.
28. Gauderer MW, Stellato TA. Gastrostomies: evolution, techniques, indications and complications. Curr Probl Surg 1986; 23:661–719.
29. Gauderer MW. Percutaneous endoscopic gastrostomy – 20 years later: a historical perspective. J Pediatr Surg 2001; 36:217–219.
30. Wilson L, Oliva-Hemker M. Percutaneous endoscopic gastrostomy in small medically complex infants. Endoscopy 2001; 33:433–436.
31. Eleftheriadis E, Kotzampassi K. Percutaneous endoscopic gastrostomy after abdominal surgery. Surg Endosc 2001;.15:213–216.
32. Foultch PE, Talbert GA, Waring JP. Percutaneous endoscopic gastrostomy in patients with prior abdominal surgery: virtues of a safe tract. Am J Gastroenterol 1988; 83:147–150.
33. Taylor AL, Carroll TA, Jakubowski J, et al. Percutaneous endoscopic gastrostomy in patients with ventriculoperitoneal shunts. Br J Surg 2001; 88:724–727.
34. Cosentini EP, Sautner T, Gnant M, et al. Outcomes of surgical percutaneous endoscopic and percutaneous radiologic gastrostomies. Arch Surg 1998; 33:1076–1083.
35. Ruckauer K, Salm R, Sontheimer J, et al. Nonendoscopic percutaneous gastrostomy. Surg Gynecol Obstet 1990; 171:339–341.
36. American Society for Gastrointestinal Endoscopy. Antibiotic prophylaxis for gastrointestinal endoscopy. Gastrointest Endosc 1995; 42:630–634.
37. Rey JR, Axon A, Budzynska A, et al. Guidelines of the European Society of Gastrointestinal Endoscopy (ESGE) antibiotic prophylaxis for gastrointestinal endoscopy. Endoscopy 1998; 30:318–324.
38. Evans JE. Should single stage PEG buttons become the procedure of choice for PEG placement in children? Second World Congress of Gastroenterology, Hepatology and Nutrition, Paris, 2004 (Abstract presentation).
39. Ferguson DR, Harig JM, Kozarek RA, et al. Placement of a feeding button ('one-step button') as the initial procedure. Am J Gastroenterol 1993; 88:501–504.
40. Mollitt DL, Golladay ES, Seibert JJ. Symptomatic gastroesophageal reflux in neurologically impaired patients. Pediatrics 1985; 75:1124–1126.
41. Berezin S, Schwarz SM, Halata MS, et al. Gastroesophageal reflux secondary to gastrostomy tube placement. Am J Dis Child 1986; 140:669–701.
42. Jolley SG, Smith EI, Tunell WP. Protective anti-reflux operation with feeding gastrostomy. Experience with chidlren. Ann Surg 1985; 201:736–740.
43. Sullivan PB. Gastrostomy feeding in the disabled child: when is an anti-reflux procedure required? Arch Dis Child 1999; 81:463–464.
44. Khoshoo V. Use of endoscopic gastrostomy for neurologically impaired children with and without GE reflux. J Pediatr Gastroenterol Nutr 1995; 20:467–469.
45. Launay V, Gottrand F, Turck D, et al. Percutaneous endoscopic gastrostomy in children: influence on gastroesophageal reflux. Pediatrics 1996; 97:726–728.
46. Razeghi S, Lang T, Behrens R. Influence of percutaneous endoscopic gastrostomy on gastroesophageal reflux: a prospective study in 68 children. J Pediatr Gastroenterol Nutr 2002; 35:27–30.
47. Sulaeman E, Udall JN, Brown RF, et al. Gastroesophageal reflux and Nissen fundoplication following percutaenous endoscopic gastrostomy in children. J Pediatr Gastroenterol Nutr 1998; 26:269–273.
48. LewisD, Khoshoo V, Pencharz PB, et al. Impact of nutritional rehabilitation on gastroesophageal reflux in neurologically impaired children. J Pediatr Surg 1994; 29:167–169.
49. Van Der Zee DC, Bax NM, Ure BM. Laparoscopic secondary antireflux procedure after PEG placement in children. Surg Endosc 2000; 14:1105–1106.
50. Liu DC, Flattmann GJ, Karam MT, et al. Laparoscopic fundoplication in children with previous abdominal surgery. J Pediatr Surg 2000; 35:334–337.
51. Raj J, Flint LM, Ferrara JJ. Small bowel necrosis in association with jejunostomy tube feedings. Am Surg 1996; 62:1050–1054.
52. Mathus-Vliegen EMH, Koning H, Taminiau JA, et al. Percutaneous endoscopic gastrostomy and gastrojejunostomy in psychomotor retarded subjects: a follow-up covering 106 patient years. J Pediatr Gastroenterol Nutr 2001; 33:488–494.
53. Godbole P, Margabanthu G, Crabbe DC, et al. Limitations and uses of gastrojejunal feeding tubes. Arch Dis Child 2002; 86:134–137.

Chapter 74
Parenteral nutrition

Maria R. Mascarenhas and Samantha Kim

INTRODUCTION

Parenteral nutrition (PN) is the intravenous administration of nutrients necessary for the maintenance of life. These nutrients include dextrose, amino acids, fat, electrolytes, multivitamins and trace elements. Clinicians caring for infants and children need to be concerned with the changing nutrient requirements with age; specialized needs of children; vascular access; the sometimes limited ability of infants, children and the critically ill to handle large amounts of fluid, protein, fat and carbohydrates.[1] In the 1960s, Dudrick and Wilmore showed that beagle puppies and subsequently an infant could be successfully nourished with the use of PN solutions and central venous access.[1,2] Since that time there have been exciting developments in the fields of intravenous access, PN solution components as well as an improved understanding of the needs of patients with various illnesses especially in neonates and adult patients. Normal growth and development has been shown in patients exclusively fed on PN.

INDICATIONS

PN may be used as primary therapy, adjunctive or supportive. The enteral route is the route of choice when the clinician is deciding how to provide nourishment for any patient. It is only in those instances when a patient cannot receive some or all of his or her nutrition enterally for a significant period of time, that the parenteral route should be used. When the patient's tolerance for enteral feeds improves, every attempt should be made to start and advance the delivery of enteral nutrition. PN is therefore used in patients who cannot be fed enterally for 5 or more days and should be used to support the patient until recovery from the underlying condition has occurred. In the very low birth weight (VLBW) or malnourished infant with limited nutritional reserves, PN should be given if the infant cannot be fed enterally for 2–3 days. In some neonatal intensive care units, a protein and glucose containing solution is started on the first day of life. Appropriate indications for initiating PN include severe burns, liver failure, severe diarrhea and malabsorption, chemotherapy-induced emesis and feeding intolerance. (Table 74.1). PN is especially important in the patient with pre-existing malnutrition or with a chronic disease. It may be used to supplement enteral intake in patients who have increased needs (e.g. patients with chronic diarrhea, malabsorption, short bowel syndrome, or cystic fibrosis) or those who are unable to tolerate adequate enteral feeds to support themselves nutritionally. Most patients with 25 cm of small bowel and an ileocecal valve will be able to ultimately tolerate enteral feeds and be able to discontinue PN.[2] The use of supplemental PN should also be considered when slow advancement of enteral feeds is anticipated. In addition to a supportive role, PN may be used to treat an underlying condition (e.g. chylothorax).

Primary	Gut failure, necrotizing enterocolitis, severe motility disorders, Crohn's disease
Supportive	Postoperative patients, burns, liver failure, renal failure, severe viral gastroenteritis, oncology and bone marrow transplant recipients, inflammatory bowel disease, trauma
Supplemental	Nutritional failure, feeding intolerance

Table 74.1 Indications for parenteral nutrition

ROUTE OF ADMINISTRATION

Parenteral nutrition can be administered via a central or peripheral venous route depending on the available access and the composition of the PN solution. Peripheral PN is generally used for patients whose nutritional status is normal, anticipated period of inadequate enteral feedings is less than two weeks and have normal fluid requirements.[3] It is often difficult to maintain peripheral access for longer than two weeks or to deliver adequate calories with solutions containing 10% or 12.5% dextrose solutions. When hyperosmolar solutions with dextrose concentrations higher than 12.5% are administered through a peripheral intravenous line there is a risk of phlebitis and thrombosis. In our institution, we use a maximum of 900 mmol to determine if a solution can be given via peripheral catheter in neonates. Solutions with high dextrose (>12.5% dextrose) and calcium concentrations may have increased risk for phlebitis. The concomitant administration of intravenous fat may help decrease phlebitis in a peripheral vein. Depending on the size of the vein, it may not be possible to infuse large volumes or run PN at a high rate.

The central venous route is used for the administration of large volumes at high infusion rates, hypertonic solutions and for chronic administration of PN solutions (more than 4–6 weeks).[4] PN may be administered via a peripheral inserted intravenous central catheter (CVC), a tunneled catheter (e.g. Broviac), or an implantable port (e.g. Portocath). It is recommended the tip of the catheter be placed at the junction of the superior vena cava and right atrium. The best place for a line associated with the least amount of complications is the right internal jugular vein with the tip of the catheter high in the superior vena cava. This position, corresponding to the level of thoracic vertebra level -T6, is at the level of the right main stem bronchus and the junction of the right atrium and superior vena cava. When femoral lines or umbilical venous catheters are used, the tip of the catheter should be placed above the level of the diaphragm. In our institution, we try to discontinue umbilical venous catheters as soon as possible. Malpositioned catheters, such as those at the level of the renal vessels and those in the liver, should not be used for PN administration due to the risk of thrombosis. It is not recommended PN be administered via umbilical arterial catheters because of the risk of sepsis. The incidence of peripheral venous access and thrombosis has been well described.[5] Measures to prevent thrombosis of vessels include making sure the vessel is not traumatized during insertion of the catheter, using correct tip placement, avoiding the subclavian and femoral veins, always using the smallest catheter possible, using the smallest vein possible and using an appropriate sized catheter for the vein.[6] Other measures utilized to prevent thrombosis include not administering PN into a small vessel, removing the CVC as soon as possible, treating CVC blockages early, preventing and treating all infections and venous occlusions, re-using previous access sites for CVC placement and not placing the CVC into a fibrin sheath. In a patient with poor access, the following sites for placing a CVC may need to be considered: translumbar inferior vena cava, re-cannulation of the central vein, transhepatic intravenous catheter, use of collateral veins, azygous and hemi-azygous veins, intercostal veins and putting the line directly into the right atrium. Long lines or peripheral inserted intravenous central catheter lines (PICC) are threaded into the heart through a large peripheral vein like the antecubital fossa. The success of placement is dependent on the patency of the vein chosen, the presence of valves and experience of the person placing the line. PICC lines have been used since the 1980s and are now quite popular because there are few limitations regarding their use related to age, gender, or diagnosis. They can remain in place for up to 1 year without complications. There is a low incidence of complications with PICC lines, less than 1% for infection, central vein thrombosis and catheter malposition. Additionally significant cost savings are associated with the use of this type of catheter. Contraindications to the placement of PICC lines include dermatitis, cellulitis, burns at or near the insertion site and previous ipsilateral venous thrombosis.

Patients receiving chronic PN benefit from the placement of a permanent CVC or tunneled Silastic catheter (e.g. Broviac, Hickman and Groshong) and subcutaneous portocaths.[7–9] A surgeon or an interventional radiologist using general anesthesia or conscious sedation generally places these catheters. Tunneled catheters can be placed either via a cut down or percutaneously and have a Dacron cuff located on the mid-portion of the catheter. This cuff stimulates the formation of dense fibrous adhesions, which anchor the catheter subcutaneously, to prevent dislodgment of the catheter. The cuff also acts as a barrier to bacteria migrating subcutaneously along the catheter surface. Sutures are needed to anchor the catheter at the exit site for several weeks after insertion to allow time for the formation of fibrous adhesions to the Dacron cuff.

Implantable ports are made of plastic or titanium with a compressed silicon disk designed for 1000 to 2000 insertions with a non-coring needle. They are inserted percutaneously into the jugular, subclavian, or cephalic vein and placed in a subcutaneous pocket over the upper chest wall. There are smaller ports available that are primarily used for arm placement and for children. These ports are generally used in situations in which the catheter is only periodically accessed. Patients at high risk for thrombosis of their catheter are those with cancer, those with infections and those receiving chemotherapeutic agents or PN.

PN can also be delivered via peritoneal or hemodialysis catheters. Intradialytic PN is the administration of PN during dialysis and has been shown to be useful in those patients with end-stage renal disease who do not respond to oral nutritional intervention.[10] PN can also be administered to patients who are on extracorporeal membrane oxygenation (ECMO). The dextrose/amino acid solution is administered through the ECMO circuit and intravenous fat is given through a peripheral line to avoid occlusion of the ECMO circuit.

PARENTERAL NUTRITION COMPONENTS AND REQUIREMENTS

Energy

A patient's enteral requirements are 20% higher than their parenteral requirements to account for the thermic effect of food and for the loss of some nutrients in the stool during the process of digestion and absorption. There are several ways to estimate energy requirements: World Health Organization (WHO) equation, Dietary Reference Intakes (DRI), prediction equations like the Schofield height/weight equation and those developed by Duro et al. and Pierro et al.[11–13] Demonstration of adequate weight gain in the absence of edema and normalization of certain nutritional markers (e.g. prealbumin) is the best way to determine if a patient's energy requirements have been accurately assessed. This response is sometimes hard to assess in the critically ill patient, patients with edema, renal failure or those on corticosteroids. It is also unclear whether one should expect normal rates of growth in the critically ill patient or just provide enough energy to prevent catabolism. The reader is referred to an excellent discussion of about energy requirements in patients on PN.[14] It has been our experience that predictive equations do not provide an accurate estimate of energy requirements.[15] In some instances, indirect calorimetry may be used to measure resting energy expenditure. Indirect calorimetry measures oxygen consumption and carbon dioxide production during respiratory gas exchange. Indirect calorimetry is increasingly available and is often helpful to determine the caloric requirements of patients who are nutritionally at risk such as infants and children with failure to thrive, those who are PN or enteral tube feed dependent, obese and those with an unusual response to their present nutrition therapy. This technology provides an accurate measure of resting energy expenditure (REE) in non-intubated patients. The technique is not accurate in intubated pediatric patients for various technical reasons. Unfortunately, it is this group of critically ill patients who would benefit the most from measurements of energy expenditure. REE can be measured in non-ventilated patients over 5 kg who are not receiving supplemental oxygen. Patients in the intensive care unit who have a pulmonary artery catheter can also have their REE calculated using cardiac output.[16]

Infants and children have higher per kg caloric requirements compared with adults, due to growth and development requirements.[17] For infants up to 1 year of age, a per kg caloric requirement that decreases with age is used.[17] This is based on their energy requirements and the need for catch-up growth. We use the World Health Organization (WHO) equation for determining the needs of children older than 1 year of age.[18] This equation, which provides an estimate of REE, is based on data from several thousand children and has been found to be accurate in children older than 1 year of age. Total energy needs may then be determined by multiplying the REE by a factor determined by the severity of underlying disease, activity level of the patient and need for catch-up growth. (Tables 74.2, 74.3).

The energy needs of obese patients are best determined by the Schofield height–weight equation.[15] Caloric needs and energy intake may be increased in a patient with head injury or sepsis. The paralyzed patient on a ventilator will have no physical activity and has lower energy needs. Often the 'stressed' patient will be given additional calories, but it is not clear whether this practice should be endorsed. Various studies have shown that the increased demands of illness are often counter balanced by decreased physical activity which keeps total energy expenditure the same whether the patient is well or sick.[19] While our concern has always been to not underfeed the patient and to prevent catabolism, it is equally important to not overfeed the patient and thereby increase the risk of complications from PN. It is important to provide not only calories but also protein in adequate amounts so the patient is in positive nitrogen balance, otherwise the patient will utilize protein for energy.

Age (years)	Male	Female
1–3	60.9 wt–54	61.0 wt–51
3–10	22.7 wt+495	22.5 wt+499
10–18	17.5 wt+651	12.2 wt+746
18–30	15.3 wt+679	14.7 wt+496

Wt, weight in kg. [a] Estimated daily energy requirements = REE × disease activity/stress factor. [b] Adapted from World Health Organization: Energy and protein requirements. Technical Report Series No. 734. Geneva: World Health Organization; 1985.[18]

Table 74.2 Estimated daily resting energy expenditure (kcal)[a,b]

1.1–1.3	Well-nourished child at rest with mild to moderate stress or after minor surgery
1.3–1.5	Normal active child with mild-to-moderate stress, inactive child with severe stress (trauma, cancer, extensive surgery), or malnourished child requiring catch-up growth or with severe stress
1.5–1.7	Active child requiring catch-up growth or with severe stress

[a] Estimated daily energy requirements = REE × disease activity/stress factor.

Table 74.3 Disease activity/stress factors[a]

Protein

The protein source in PN is provided by crystalline amino acids, which provides approximately 4 cal/g of protein.[20] Protein usually provides 10–15% of total PN calorie needs. Since the advent of these purer forms of amino acids the incidence of hyperammonemia and metabolic acidosis has been rare. It has also been shown that nitrogen retention is better with amino acid formulations when compared with protein hydrolysates. There are a variety of protein solutions available for use in children and adults and patients with hepatic disease, renal disease and metabolic disease. An example of a protein solution used in a metabolic disorder is the parenteral protein solution that has been designed for use in methylmalonic acidemia. In this instance, the amounts of certain amino acids can be dosed based on daily blood amino acid levels. The composition of protein solutions for infants, including pre-term, are different than those used in children and adults. Infant amino acid formulations, such as TrophAmine (B. Braun), provide essential amino acids like cysteine, histidine and tyrosine which are not found in adult formulations.[21] TrophAmine also contains taurine which is important for brain and retinal growth and this amino acid may be responsible for the decreased cholestasis seen in patients receiving PN regimens containing taurine.[22] The plasma amino acid pattern seen in infants receiving TrophAmine resembles normal 2-h post-prandial levels seen in one-month-old healthy full term breast-fed infants.[23] The low pH of TrophAmine allows for large amounts of calcium and phosphorus to be added to the PN solution without precipitation.[24] TrophAmine also contains a higher concentration of branched chain amino acids. Branched chain amino acids have been shown to improve nitrogen balance, protein synthesis and immunocompetence in septic or trauma patients.[20] TrophAmine is a better choice of protein for the neonate than Freamine III or Aminosyn PF. Improved weight gain, nitrogen retention and better amino acid profiles have been seen in patients receiving Trophamine as their protein source.[24] TrophAmine is used in patients under 6 months of age and an adult amino acid preparation is used in patients over 6 months of age. TrophAmine can be used for patients with end stage liver disease and cholestasis because of its branched chain amino acid profile. Aminosyn-PF is another amino acid formulation designed for neonates and it has similar beneficial properties for neonates when compared to the adult amino acid preparations. Novamine (Clintec Nutrition Co., Chicago) is a standard protein formulation given to patients older than 6 months of age. It is available in 1% to 15% solutions. The 15% solution is particularly useful in fluid-restricted patients. Specialized amino acid formulations are available for certain disease states (renal and hepatic failure). These solutions are expensive and studies have not demonstrated a clear beneficial survival effect when these solutions have been used in patients with renal and hepatic failure. The amino acid formulation designed for use in patients with severe liver failure and hepatic encephalopathy contains increased amounts of branched chain amino acids and reduced amounts of methionine and aromatic amino acids. However, study results using this formulation are mixed and have not demonstrated a clear beneficial survival effect in these patients.[25,26] Specialized formulations for renal failure have also been developed, but their use is not widespread in renal failure due to a lack of clear benefit (Table 74.4).[27,28]

There is a tendency to add albumin to PN solution in patients with hypoproteinemia. This is generally not recommended for a variety of reasons. Albumin has a short half-life and no nutritional value. Endogenous albumin has a half-life of 21 days, but exogenous albumin does not stay in circulation very long. Its sole value is to increase oncotic pressure. There is a significant amount of aluminum and sodium present in albumin solutions, which can be detrimental to the patient. The addition of albumin to PN solutions can result in the flocculation of albumin. There is also a concern that albumin may increase sepsis.[29]

In addition to providing calories to patients it is also important to include protein in adequate amounts. The most commonly used method for determining the protein needs of full-term infants less than 1 year of age and older children, is the Recommended Daily Allowances (RDA) or DRI (Dietary Reference Intakes) for age and gender.[30] The protein recommendations are derived from the minimum amount of protein intake required to maintain nitrogen balance. The protein needs for premature infants or children with chronic disease may be higher than the RDA.

Protein needs decline progressively with age. As a result, the protein needs of infants and children are higher than those of adults due to differing growth rates.[17] In certain conditions, protein intake needs to be higher than normal, due to increased protein losses. Increased protein needs may be found in conditions such as protein-losing enteropathy, protein-calorie malnutrition, sepsis or inflammatory bowel disease. Protein can be safely administered on the first or second day of life in pre-term infants. Protein is typically started at 2.0 g/kg of amino acids per day the first day PN is used and then increased to 3.0 g/kg on day 2, in most pre-term infants.[31] Some pre-term infants may need as much as 4 g/kg per day.[32] Exceptions to this rule may be in VLBW infants, critically ill patients with hepatic or renal insufficiency (not on dialysis)

	Troph-Amine®	Aminosyn®	Novamine®	Hepat-Amine®	Aminosyn® RF
Essential amino acids					
L-isoleucine	82	72	50	113	88
L-leucine	140	94	69	138	139
L-lysine	82	72	79	76	102
L-methionine	34	40	50	13	139
L-phenylalanine	48	44	69	13	139
L-threonine	42	52	50	56	63
L-tryptophan	20	16	17	8	31
L-valine	78	80	64	105	101
Non-essential amino acids					
L-alanine	54	128	145	96	–
L-arginine	120	98	98	75	115
L-aspartic acid	32	–	29	–	–
L-glutamic acid	50	–	50	–	–
L-glycine	36	128	69	113	–
L-histidine	48	30	60	30	82
L-proline	68	86	60	100	–
L-serine	38	42	39	63	–
L-taurine	2.5	–	–	–	–
L-tyrosine	24	44	3	–	–
% Branched chain amino acids	30	–	–	35	33
% Essential amino acids	53	47	45	52	80
% Non-essential amino acids	47	53	55	48	20

Adapted from The Children's Hospital of Philadelphia Pharmacy Handbook and Formulary 2003–2004. Department of Pharmacy Services. Hudson, OH: Lexi-Comp Inc; 2003.[28]

Table 74.4 Composition of crystalline amino acid solutions (mg amino acid/g protein)

and patients with disorders of protein metabolism (Table 74.5).[33] Older children and adolescents require protein intakes of 1–2 g/kg per day. At our institution, we use a maximum of 150 g protein/day. Unless the patient has hepatic or renal failure or a disorder of protein metabolism is suspected there is no evidence to suggest starting protein at the low end of the range and then advancing it to goal at a slow rate. The above practice only results in a delay of adequate nutrition. Protein needs in infants, children and adolescents vary from 0.75 g/kg per day to 2.5 g/kg per day.[34–36] Blood urea nitrogen (BUN) is a useful measure of adequate or excessive protein intake if nutritional status and hydration are within normal limits. A current concept that is gaining more support is the recommendation to provide protein enterally rather than parenterally in the patient with cholestasis in order to reduce liver disease.[37]

Cysteine is a conditionally essential amino acid in neonates and infants. Improved nitrogen retention has been seen with the administration of cysteine to PN solutions.[38] However, it is not present in significant amounts in amino acid solutions due to instability. Cysteine can be added to TrophAmine to reduce the pH of the PN, which allows for increased phosphorous and calcium solubility. Cysteine should not be added to the PN solution if the infant is acidotic, because cysteine may exacerbate metabolic acidosis. The recommended dose for cysteine is 40 mg/g of PN protein. Taurine can also be found in infant amino acid formulations and plays an integral role in brain and retinal membrane development as well as bile acid conjugation.[39] Glutamine was originally classified as a nonessential amino acid but is now currently classified as a conditionally essential amino acid.[40] Studies have shown supplementation with glutamine has improved nitrogen balance, immunocompetence, decreased sepsis and maintained protein synthesis in postoperative patients. Other studies have shown a beneficial effect of PN supplemented with glutamine in patients with short bowel syndrome, trauma, patients who have undergone bone marrow transplantation and critically ill burn patients.[41–44] Wischmeyer et al. gave intravenous glutamine to 26 burn patients and showed patients had less gram negative bacteremia accompanied by improvements in prealbumin and decreases in C-reactive-protein. However, other studies have not shown similar improvement.[45,46] Glutamine has also been found to be safe for use with preterm infants and preliminary studies show a benefit in glutamine supplemented PN.[47,48] Current amino acid formulations do not contain glutamine, as it is unstable in solution, although this can be avoided by the use of glutamine dipeptides.

Infants 0–5 kg	3–3.5
Children 5–20 kg	2–3
Children 20–40 kg	1–2
Children/adults >40 kg	0.8–2[a]

[a]A maximum of 150 g protein/day is recommended

Table 74.5 Guidelines for dosing intravenous protein (g/kg per day)

Carnitine is synthesized in the body from two essential amino acids, lysine and methionine and is required for the transport of long-chain fatty acids into the mitochondria.[49] Neonates and infants are unable to produce carnitine endogenously. They need an exogenous supply. Carnitine supplementation of PN solutions in premature infants has been suggested to correct low free and acylcarnitine levels. Although hereditary carnitine deficiency responds to carnitine supplementation, it is not clear whether the low levels seen in premature infants and patients with short bowel syndrome represent a true deficiency and need to be supplemented.[50] Indeed, while there have been studies showing improved levels, fat tolerance and some increase in growth and nitrogen retention, other studies have failed to show any significant effect or even a negative effect with high doses.[51–53] An intravenous form of L-carnitine is available and may be added to PN formulations. The recommended dose for L-carnitine is 50 mg/kg per day with a maximum dose of 300 mg/kg per day. It has been suggested that intravenous carnitine be added to the PN of VLBW infants to assist with triglyceride beta-oxidation, if triglyceride levels increase over 200 g/dl.[54] However, this practice is not widespread and has not been found to be beneficial in the short term.[55–57] Currently, there have been no studies looking at carnitine supplementation and levels in patients on chronic PN.

Choline is a precursor of acetylcholine and phosphatidylcholine. The major dietary source of choline is lecithin. Choline is widely distributed and so deficiency states are uncommon. The premature infant and the patient on long-term PN without sufficient enteral feeds is at risk for choline deficiency. Choline deficiency has been suggested as a cause of hepatic steatosis seen in patients on PN solutions that do not contain choline.[58,59] Buchman et al. showed a reduction in hepatic steatosis and increased plasma free choline levels after administration of 6 weeks of choline supplemented PN solution.[60] Buchman et al. also showed lower than normal plasma free choline levels in patients on home TPN. This observation was made in about 80% of home PN patients. The provision of oral lecithin caused increased plasma free choline levels as well as decreased hepatic steatosis.[61] Buchman was also able to show that low choline status was associated with fatty liver and elevated transaminases. Additionally in a pilot study Buchman et al. showed that choline supplemented PN reversed hepatic abnormalities in four patients.[60] In another trial, 15 patients were randomized to get standard PN or PN supplemented with 2 g of choline. An improvement in liver function tests was noted in the choline-supplemented group. After the choline supplementation was stopped there was a recurrence of steatosis.[62]

Carbohydrates

The majority of calories in PN are provided by the intravenous monohydrate form of dextrose, which provides 3.4 kcal/g and not the 4 kcal/g provided by the enteral form of carbohydrates. Carbohydrates usually provide 45–60% of total calorie intake. PN given through a peripheral vein should have a maximum concentration of 10% dextrose because more concentrated dextrose solutions can result in osmolalities greater than 900 mmol/l and an increased risk of phlebitis.[5] In special circumstances, a 12.5% dextrose solution may be used peripherally with caution but should not be used in neonates and infants due to the increased risk of extravasation and phlebitis. PN given through a centrally placed line allows for the infusion of higher dextrose concentrations, osmolalities greater than 900 mmol/l and is typically appropriate for patients requiring PN for greater than 7–10 days.

It is important to calculate glucose delivery or glucose infusion rate (GIR) in patients who receive PN. The GIR allows the practitioner to determine if glucose delivery will exceed glucose utilization rates. The GIR is usually expressed in mg/kg of bodyweight per min. If the GIR is higher than recommended, glucose utilization is decreased. The recommended GIR for infants is between 5 and 12 mg/kg per min. Glucose utilization is known to decrease when the GIR exceeds 14 mg/kg per min.[63] The initial rate of dextrose infusion should be approximately 5 mg/kg per min in infants. The GIR can then be increased by 2–5 mg/kg per min daily or 5–10% per day. In older children the recommend GIR is between 2 and 5 mg/kg per min. Urine should be monitored for glucose when PN is started and after changes in GIR. Serum glucose levels should be checked if a patient has positive glucosuria and the GIR should be reduced as appropriate. LBW infants, malnourished infants and children with small glycogen stores place them at increased risk of hypoglycemia when parenteral glucose is abruptly stopped.[64] It is recommended to taper down the rate of the PN solution when cycling PN with a dextrose concentration greater than 10% to decrease the risk of rebound hypoglycemia.

Unbalanced macronutrient regimens may have a role in PN-related liver disease. Excessive carbohydrate intake results in hyperglycemia, hepatic steatosis, infection, increased carbon dioxide production and can result in decreased respiratory function in ventilator dependent patients.[65–67] Increases in energy expenditure and respiratory quotient have been seen with regimens with high glucose infusion rates.[68,69] Indeed overfeeding itself may lead to increased carbon dioxide production with negative consequences.[70–72] Serum glucose levels should be maintained in the normal range for age. Hyperglycemia in critically ill patients on PN has been associated with increased mortality and morbidity. Patients receiving PN who have significant hyperglycemia may require an insulin infusion to help achieve and maintain euglycemia. Hyperglycemia is common in the stressed LBW and VLBW infant soon after birth. Insulin can be used to maintain serum glucose levels in the normal range and may be considered as an alternative to the use of a hypocaloric regimen.[73] It is preferable to run the insulin as a separate infusion as opposed to adding it to the PN solution, because the insulin may adhere to the tubing, resulting in lower amounts being delivered to the patient. It is also difficult to adjust the rate of the insulin infusion without affecting calorie intake and glucose homeostasis when insulin is mixed with the PN solution.

Lipids

Fat provides a concentrated form of both calories and essential fatty acids, which are required for prostaglandin and membrane lipid synthesis, brain and somatic growth, immune function, skin integrity and wound healing. Intravenous fat emulsions available in the USA are composed entirely of long-chain triglycerides, usually from soybean and safflower oils. There are two product types available; a soy-based emulsion (Intralipid) or a soy and safflower oil-based emulsion (Liposyn II). Intralipid is a commonly used intravenous fat and is available in 10%, 20% and 30% emulsions (Table 74.6).[74] The 20% emulsion is preferred due to its lower phospholipid content and improved triglyceride clearance.[75–77] The 10% solution may result in hyperlipidemia because of its high phospholipid: triglyceride ratio, so it used far less frequently. Phospholipids are thought to inhibit lipoprotein lipase, the main enzyme responsible for intravenous fat clearance. The 30% emulsion can only be used in a total nutrient admixture and cannot be infused alone into a peripheral vein.

The total daily dose of intravenous fat is usually delivered over 24 h, except when the PN is cycled. However, continuous 24-h infusions are better tolerated than intermittent infusions. There is a concern about the growth of bacteria in intravenous fat solutions when these solutions have been hung for more than 12 h. It has been suggested the hang time be 12 h or less and that unit doses be used so the bottle is only entered once in order to decrease the incidence of sepsis.[78] Intravenous fat is usually started at a relatively low initial dosage and increased over 1–3 days, if triglyceride clearance is within normal limits (Table 74.7). There are no clearly accepted values for serum triglycerides during PN administration for hypertriglyceridemia. While some authors have suggested in neonates intravenous

	Intralipid 10%	Intralipid 20%	Intralipid 30%
Purified soybean oil (g)	100	200	300
Purified egg phospholipids (g)	12	12	12
Glycerol (g)	22	22	16.7
Osmolality (mmol/l)	300	350	310
Kcal/ml	1.1	2	3

Table 74.6 Composition of intralipid emulsions (per liter)

	0–5 kg Infants	5–20 kg Children	20–40 kg Children	>40 kg Children/ adults
Initial dose	1–1.5	1–1.5	1–1.5	0.5–1
Dose increase	0.5–1	1	1	0.5–1
Maximum dose[a]	1–3	1–3	1–2.5	0.5–1.5

[a]Percentage of calories from fat should not exceed 60% of total caloric intake.

Table 74.7 Guidelines for dosing intravenous fat (g/kg per day)

lipids should be decreased if triglyceride levels are >200 mg/dl, we accept triglyceride levels up to 300 mg/dl in infants and young children. A rising triglyceride value in the face of sepsis would be a reason to decrease intravenous fat administration. In adults triglyceride levels greater than 400 mg/dl level have been suggested as a cut off value above which the intravenous fat dose should be decreased.[79] Triglyceride levels depend on the rate of clearance of the infused fat. This in turn is affected by nutritional status, degree of malnutrition, concurrent administration of medications and the clinical situation (stress, organ dysfunction and infection).[80] The impact of intravenous fat administration on lung function has been well discussed in two review articles.[81,82]

In general, when formulating a PN regimen the fat percentage should provide 30%–40% of total calories. There are some exceptions to this rule where fat percentage may be higher but should never exceed more than 60% of total calories. The maximum dose of intravenous fat in infants is 3–4 g/kg per day. The dosage of intravenous fat decreases with age. Patients requiring 100% of their caloric needs from PN need to receive intravenous fat in order to prevent essential fatty acid deficiency (EFAD), which develops in patients who are not receiving any long-chain fats. As a rule EFAD can be prevented with only 0.5–1.0 g/kg per day of intravenous fat, which equates to 2–4% of total calories from intravenous fat.[83,84] In the extremely LBW infant, EFAD can develop within 48–72 h if no intravenous fat is provided.[85] Pre-term infants on PN without intravenous fat and enteral feeds can develop EFAD biochemically within 7 days.[83] Clinical signs of EFAD include growth failure, flaky dry skin, alopecia, thrombocytopenia, increased infections and impaired wound healing. EFAD can be diagnosed by a triene-to-tetraene ratio >0.4.

The intravenous fat emulsions available in the USA contain only long-chain triglycerides (LCT). Structured lipids (LCT and medium-chain triglycerides (MCT) attached to a glycerol backbone), MCT emulsions, mixtures of MCT and LCT emulsions, olive oil containing emulsions, mixtures of soybean oil, MCT, olive oil and fish oil and mixtures of MCT, LCT and fish oil have been developed to prevent complications seen with conventional fat emulsions.[86–91] The latter emulsion is currently in use in Europe. Mixtures of MCT and LCT have been used for more than 20 years in Europe.[92] These emulsions have been studied in hospitalized patients as well as in home PN patients. The advantages of MCT containing lipid emulsions are that they are more soluble, are rapidly hydrolyzed by lipases, quickly eliminated from the circulation and are taken up by the peripheral tissue. They are not stored by the body, are ketogenic and are oxidized more rapidly than LCT. There is less elevation of liver enzymes with these emulsions. Emulsions containing MCT and LCT are more efficient, have less of a negative effect on the liver, immune system and reticuloendothelial system when compared with LCT containing intravenous fat emulsions. They produce a similar amount of prostaglandins and have been shown to be useful in patients with systemic inflammatory response syndrome. Structured lipids have been studied in the pediatric age group.[93,94] Studies in infants have been performed showing improved lipid levels in those receiving a mixture of MCT and LCT.[95] However, these new formulations are not currently available in the USA.

Electrolytes and minerals

Electrolyte requirements vary with age and are added to the PN solution in maintenance concentrations.[96,97] These requirements are derived from the Recommended Daily Allowance (RDAs) with allowances made for the efficiency of absorption. (Table 74.8) These include sodium, potassium, calcium, magnesium and phosphorus. Chloride and acetate are used to balance the PN solutions. It is recommended to obtain baseline serum electrolytes before ordering the PN solution and then add electrolytes accordingly. Periodic monitoring of serum electrolytes is required, especially in the critically ill and malnourished patient. In neonates and children with high calcium and phosphorus needs, the amounts added to a PN solution may be limited due to solubility issues. Increasing the amount of protein and adding cysteine (30–40 mg cysteine/g amino acid), thereby lowering the pH of the solution, can allow the addition of higher amounts of calcium and phosphorus to the PN solution without causing precipitation. In instances where the patient's calcium and phosphorus requirements cannot be met via the PN solution, a separate infusion of

		Children		
	Infants 0–5 kg	5–20 kg	20–40 kg	Adolescents/Adults >40 kg
Sodium	2–5 mEq/kg	2–6 mEq/kg	2–3 mEq/kg	80–150 mEq/day
Potassium	1–4 mEq/kg	2–3 mEq/kg	1.5–2.5 mEq/kg	40–60 mEq/day
Phosphorus	2–4 mEq/kg	1–2 mEq/kg	1–1.5 mEq/kg	30–60 mEq/day
Chloride	2–5 mEq/kg	2–5 mEq/kg	2–3 mEq/kg	80–150 mEq/day
Acetate	Balance	Balance	Balance	Balance
Calcium	1–4 mEq/kg	0.5–1 mEq/kg	10–25 mEq/day	10–20 mEq/day
Magnesium	0.3–0.5 mEq/kg	0.3–0.5 mEq/kg	0.3–0.5 mEq/kg	10–30 mEq/day

Initiate dose at lower end of range and increase based on individual needs. Dose ranges are suggested guidelines only. Specific clinical situations may require doses outside of these ranges. Use laboratory tests to adjust electrolyte dosing. (Adapted from The Children's Hospital of Philadelphia Pharmacy Handbook and Formulary 2003–2004. Department of Pharmacy Services. Hudson, OH: Lexi-Comp Inc; 2003.)[28]

Table 74.8 Intravenous requirements (daily) for electrolytes

calcium or phosphorus may need to be given. Patients with high calcium needs and those who cannot get all the calcium in their PN, may benefit from enteral calcium administration if tolerated. It should be noted that in patients with hypocalcemia and hypomagnesemia, magnesium status needs to be normalized before calcium levels will respond to calcium supplementation.

Vitamins

Guidelines for adult multivitamins formulations and dosing were revisited in 2000, but the pediatric guidelines have not been revised since 1988.[97,98] There are currently two types of multivitamin (MVI) preparations used in the USA: pediatric and adult formulations. The pediatric MVI was designed to meet the needs of preterm and term infants and children up to 10 years of age.[97,99] It is dosed on a per kilogram basis and pre-term infants receive 40% of a vial/kg of bodyweight. The adult and pediatric MVI preparations differ in the concentration of the different vitamins/ml. In general, the adult MVI has a greater concentration of vitamins, except it contains less vitamin D and has no vitamin K compared with the pediatric formulation. In children older than 10 years of age, the adult MVI is used with the addition of vitamin K. The new recommendation is for adult multivitamin preparations to contain vitamin K. (Table 74.9) The dosing recommendations for vitamins take into account the losses associated with administration. Some vitamins may adhere to the intravenous tubing, while others may be affected by light exposure while the PN solution is being administered.[100] It is recommended that the adult multivitamin preparation not be used for children because it contains propylene glycol and polysorbate additives which may be toxic to the premature infant.[101,102]

Vitamin A is an important mediator of cell differentiation and repair in the lung and other organs. Greene et al. demonstrated a higher incidence of BPD and low plasma retinol levels in VLBW infants with a birth weight less than 1000 g who were on PN for 1 month. These levels progressively decreased over time.[103] This was subsequently confirmed in seven infants (450–1360 g), who were receiving standard multivitamin supplements and despite parenteral vitamin A supplementation, all infants did not have complete normalization of retinol levels.[104] Shenai et al. showed that treatment with 400–450 µg/kg per day i.m. of vitamin A resulted in improved levels as well as decreased BPD.[105] Subsequently, it was shown that vitamin A supplementation resulted in a modest reduction in chronic lung disease and the recommendation was made to routinely supplement vitamin A in all infants below 1000 g who require respiratory support on the first day of life.[106] Vitamin A can adhere to tubing and can be destroyed by the effect of light and may result in decreased administration to the patient.

Trace elements

In addition to the previously discussed components, iron, zinc, copper, chromium, manganese, selenium and molybdenum need to be added to make the PN solution complete. However, molybdenum is not routinely added to PN solutions. These trace elements are dosed according to published guidelines.[97] There are no parenteral requirements for fluoride and iodine. The latter trace element is present as a contaminant in many trace element preparations and in other products used in association with PN solutions. Copper and manganese are excreted in the bile and selenium, molybdenum and chromium are excreted in urine. Increased copper losses occur in burns and increased zinc losses occur in diarrhea. Trace elements may need to be adjusted in patients with organ dysfunction because of altered elimination of certain trace elements (e.g. copper and manganese). Serum levels of trace elements eliminated from the PN solution need to be monitored. Trace elements such as zinc, copper, manganese and selenium can also be present as contaminants of the components of PN.

	Pre-term infants/kg	Term infants and Children >1 year	MVI® pediatric (5 ml)	MVI®-12[a] (5 ml)
Biotin (µg)	8	20	20	60
Folate (µg)	56	140	140	400
Niacin (mg)	4–6.8	17	17	40
Pantothenic acid (mg)	1–2	5	5	15
Riboflavin (mg)	0.15–0.2	1.4	1.4	3.6
Thiamine (mg)	0.2–0.35	1.2	1.2	3
Vitamin A (retinol) (IU)	700–1500	2300	2300	3300
Vitamin B_6 (mg)	0.15–0.2	1	1	4
Vitamin B_{12} (µg)	0.3	1	1	5
Vitamin C (mg)	15–25	80	80	100
Vitamin D (IU)	40–160	400	400	200
Vitamin E (tocopherol) (IU)	3.5	7	7	10
Vitamin K (mg)	0.3	0.2	0.2	[a]

[a] Patients receiving MVI®-12 will get 0.2 mg/day of vitamin K. New formulation of MVI-12R will contain Vitamin K and new levels of vitamins. (Adapted from The Children's Hospital of Philadelphia Pharmacy Handbook and Formulary 2003–2004. Department of Pharmacy Services. Hudson, OH: Lexi-Comp Inc; 2003.)[28]

Table 74.9 Intravenous vitamin requirement recommendations (daily) and products

There is some controversy whether iron should be routinely added to PN solutions as well as some controversy regarding the methods of administration of iron in PN solutions. Some practitioners may give iron to all patients on PN. Others advocate it should be administered on a weekly basis in a separate bag of intravenous fluids only in patients who receive PN for more than 3 months.[107–109] There are currently three forms of intravenous iron available: iron dextran, sodium ferric gluconate and iron sucrose. However, the experience of iron in PN solutions is with iron dextran. There is concern about compatibility issues of iron and PN solutions especially with total nutrient admixture solutions (TNA).[110] At our institution we give all patients maintenance doses of iron (0.1 mg/kg per day) after 2 months of age, with the exception of chronically transfused patients (e.g. those with inherited anemias, malignancies and bone marrow transplant recipients). Iron-deficient patients may receive additional amounts based on results of iron studies.

Additional zinc may be required in patients with zinc deficiency. As zinc is lost primarily through the gastrointestinal (GI) tract, patients with increased GI losses may need additional zinc supplementation. In addition, patients with poor wound healing and/or decubitus ulcers should have zinc status evaluated. Low serum alkaline phosphatase levels may be suggestive of zinc deficiency.

Copper and manganese are excreted in bile and so may need to be removed from the PN solutions of patients with cholestatic liver disease and/or liver failure to prevent toxicity.[111] If copper is removed from the PN solution secondary to cholestasis copper deficiency can develop in adult patients who receive PN.[112] Symptoms of copper deficiency include anemia, leukopenia, hypercholesterolemia, osteopenia and pigmentary changes in hair. The presence of high blood manganese levels in patients on PN supplementation has been associated with psychosis and extrapyramidal symptoms. Manganese deposition in the basal ganglia has been seen in head magnetic resonance imaging studies (MRI) and confirmed on autopsy in patients on long-term PN. In a study by Bertinet et al., 67% of patients showed evidence of manganese deposition on head MRI.[113] This improved when manganese was removed from the PN solution. There was also a decrease in blood levels within 1 year of stopping manganese in the PN solution. Erythrocyte manganese levels are a good way to evaluate manganese status. Takagi et al. showed that a dose of 1 μmol/day was an optimal dose for adults.[114] Inuma et al. showed in a group of six patients that whole blood manganese levels did not always correlate with the accumulation of manganese in the brain and recommended periodic head MRIs to check for toxicity.[115]

Glomerular filtration rate needs to be monitored annually when chromium is added to PN solutions. It has been suggested chromium and selenium be used with caution in patients with significant renal dysfunction since they are excreted in the urine. Molybdenum deficiency is extremely rare and need not be supplemented except in adolescent patients who receive 80% or more of their caloric requirements from PN for 3–6 months. Molybdenum is also excreted in the urine. Iodine is not added to PN solutions because patients usually receive adequate amounts of iodine from unavoidable contamination of PN solutions and from topical administration of iodine containing antiseptic solutions.

Additives

Commonly used medications like ranitidine and cimetidine may be added to the PN solution if they are compatible with the PN solution. When medications can be added to PN solutions, this can result in ease of care as well as a reduction of intravenous fluids which is beneficial to the fluid-restricted patient. Certain drugs are not compatible with PN and therefore cannot be run concurrently. See Table 74.10 for some commonly used medications and their compatibility with PN and intravenous lipids (Table 74.10)

Patients born with inborn errors of metabolism may need additional amounts of specific amino acids added to their PN. Hydrochloric acid may be added to PN solutions given to patients on extracorporeal membrane oxygenation (ECMO) to correct alkalosis. This has to be done through central access. When the patient comes off ECMO and PN is provided via peripheral access the hydrochloric acid must be discontinued. Insulin may also be added to PN solutions to assist with blood glucose control. Heparin is added to all PN solutions which results in less thrombosis formation, less fibrin sheath formation, sepsis

Drug	Parenteral nutrition	Intravenous lipid
Albumin	Compatible	No information – not recommended
Amikacin	Compatible	Incompatible
Amphotericin B	Incompatible	Incompatible
Ampicillin	Incompatible	Compatible up to 4 h
Ciclosporin	Incompatible	Compatible
Furosemide	Compatible up to 4 h	Compatible up to 4 h
Gentamicin	Compatible	Compatible up to 4 h
Imipenem	Compatible up to 4 h	Compatible
Iron Dextran	Compatible	Incompatible
Oxacillin	Compatible	Compatible up to 4 h
Penicillin	Compatible	Compatible up to 4 h
Phenobarbitol	Compatible	Incompatible
Phenytoin	Incompatible	Incompatible
Propofol	Compatible up to 4 h	No information – not recommended
Ranitindine	Compatible	Compatible
Ticarcillin	Compatible	No information – not recommended
Tobramycin	Compatible	Compatible up to 4 h
Vancomycin	Compatible	Compatible

Adapted from The Children's Hospital of Philadelphia Pharmacy Handbook and Formulary 2003–2004. Department of Pharmacy Services. Hudson, OH: Lexi-Comp Inc; 2003.[28]

Table 74.10 Compatibility of parenteral nutrition, intravenous lipid and commonly used intravenous medications

and enhanced triglyceride clearance by stimulating lipoprotein lipase release.[116,117]

MONITORING

Monitoring patients on PN is very important. This consists of monitoring the appropriateness of the regimen using serum chemistries and growth parameters (Table 74.11). Typically, a baseline nutritional assessment and check of serum chemistries should be completed before starting PN. Daily laboratory values should be obtained and the PN regimen adjusted accordingly until goal regimen is achieved. Laboratory values should be obtained after any changes in the PN regimen. Most patients in the hospital can have weekly laboratory blood tests to assess response to the PN regimen once a stable regimen is achieved. Growth monitoring is based on the age of the patient. Malnourished patients at risk for re-feeding syndrome must be closely monitored. Patients on long-term PN solutions, those with increased losses or increased needs, may need to have trace element and vitamin levels checked periodically.

COMPLICATIONS

Complications related to the use of PN can be divided into three main categories: mechanical, infectious and metabolic. With careful use of PN, these complications can be avoided or minimized.[118,119]

Laboratory tests[a]	
Baseline	Complete blood cell count, serum electrolytes, triglycerides, calcium, magnesium, phosphorus, alkaline phosphatase, total protein, albumin, blood urea nitrogen, creatinine, liver functions tests, iron studies, total bilirubin and prealbumin
Weekly	Serum electrolytes, triglycerides, calcium, magnesium, phosphorus, alkaline phosphatase, total protein, albumin, blood urea nitrogen, creatinine, liver functions tests, total bilirubin and prealbumin
Monthly	Complete blood cell count, reticulocyte count, iron studies
Bi-annually	Serum selenium, chromium, zinc, vitamin A, E, D (25-hydroxy), copper, ceruloplasmin, manganese, carnitine, prothrombin time or PIVKA II level
Growth measurement	
Baseline	Weight, height/length, head circumference (patients <3 years), arm anthropometrics
Daily	Weight (patients <2 years)
Weekly	Weight (patients >2 years and adolescents, height/length (<2 years)
Monthly	Height/length (>2 years), head circumference (patients <3 years), arm anthropometrics

[a] Serum electrolytes, calcium, magnesium, phosphorus, blood urea nitrogen should be monitored daily until goal regimen is reached.

Table 74.11 Monitoring of patients receiving parenteral nutrition

Mechanical complications

Mechanical complications seen with the use of PN include those associated with the initial insertion of a CVC and subsequent use of the catheter. These include arrhythmias, hemomediastinum, air embolism, pneumothorax, hemothorax, hydrothorax, intravascular and extravascular malpositioning, brachial plexus injury, arterial injury, catheter embolism, perforation of the heart, pericardium and thrombosis formation.[120,121] Introduction of an air embolus can occur at the time of CVC insertion, with defective catheters and with catheters with faulty connections. Symptoms of air embolism include shortness of breath, hypoxia, tachycardia, hypotension and neurologic changes. Pneumothorax, hydrothorax and hemothorax can occur at the time of CVC placement or as a result of delayed catheter perforation due to erosion of the blood vessel. Intravascular malpositioning refers to coiled catheters and those in the right atrium or ventricle. If the catheter tip is positioned in the right atrium, arrhythmias can occur due to irritation of the myocardium. Extravascular malpositioning results when the catheter gets lodged in the pleural space, in the mediastinum, or outside the vascular space.

Catheter breakage and occlusion can occur with chronic use of CVC. Small tears, pinholes, or breakage may occur in the silastic material of the catheter. Damage to the septum of the implantable port may occur if an inappropriate needle is used, resulting in leakage of fluid into the surrounding tissue. Extravasation of fluid can also occur with tunneled catheters with fluid leaking into the surrounding tissue. The complication rate for any line placement should be less than 8%.[122] Catheter occlusion can occur as a result of an intramural thrombus, extraluminal fibrin sleeve, mural thrombosis, development of a biofilm, or a build-up of precipitate from drugs or components of the PN solution. The occlusion can range from a withdrawal problem such as an inability to aspirate blood but fluids infuse without difficulty to a complete occlusion when nothing can be infused through the catheter. The development of thrombi may occur as a result of a vascular injury during the catheter placement or from contact with the tip of the catheter. These thrombi can develop either within the catheter (intramural thrombi) or at the site of the vascular injury (mural thrombi). Over time, mural thrombi can become large veno-occlusive thrombi. Fibrin sleeves also develop from the catheter's contact with blood. As with the development of a thrombus, platelets and fibrin adhere to the catheter, causing a 'sleeve' to form that encapsulates the catheter.

Solutions used to flush the catheter are intended to maintain catheter patency and include heparin and normal saline. The results of prophylactic heparin therapy preventing occlusion in PN solutions remain questionable. The risk of potential adverse effects and optimal dosage regimen are unclear. Currently, a dose of 0.5 U/ml PN solution is recommended for neonates under 1500 g and 1 U/ml of PN solution for neonates over 1500 g, infants, children and adolescents. With intraluminal blockages, urokinase, ethanol, hydrochloric acid and sodium bicarbonate may be instilled in the catheter. Occasionally, a combination of fibrinolytic agents and guidewire manipulation is needed to restore patency. Embolization of occluding compounds may occur in such settings. Warfarin or other anticoagulants may need to be used.[123]

Infectious complications

The use of CVC is frequently complicated by either local or systemic infections. These include sepsis (bacterial and fungal), line contamination and infective thrombophlebitis. Common infectious agents are Staphylococcus epidermidis, Staphylococcus aureus, enterococci, gram negative rods and Candida albicans.[124] The majority of infections start with a local infection of the catheter site where the patient's own cutaneous flora invades the intracutaneous tract at the time the catheter is placed or sometime thereafter. Children with abnormal gastrointestinal tracts such as in short bowel syndrome also have a significant incidence of gram negative infection, presumably by blood invasion of bowel bacteria. In pediatric oncology patients, PN appears to increase the risk of CVC infections. The infection rate increased from 0.06/100 days to 0.5/100 days when PN was administered using Hickman–Broviac catheters.[125] Other risk factors include age, underlying disease, site of the CVC, environmental factors, length of use and frequency of line entry for blood drawing.[126] The majority (70–85%) of infections can be treated safely without line removal. Treatment consists of initial antibiotic therapy to cover common organisms pending cultures.[127] Once the organism has been identified, then the appropriate antibiotic is chosen and given for 7 to 14 days, depending on the clinical situation. Persistent fevers, positive blood cultures and tunnel infections may require removal of the line. The Centers for Disease Control and Prevention have made recommendations for intravenous catheter care.[128]

Metabolic complications

Metabolic complications related to PN solution include electrolyte and mineral imbalances, hyperammonemia, hyperglycemia, hypoglycemia, bone disease and cholestasis.[129] Hyperammonemia was initially reported in infants who received casein hydrolysate containing PN solutions and is no longer noted with the currently available amino acid solutions. Hyperglycemia can occur with high infusion rates, especially in the presence of sepsis, trauma, surgery and the use of corticosteroids. Hypoglycemia occurs when total parenteral nutrition (TPN) is abruptly stopped. Excessive glucose administration can lead to excessive carbon dioxide production and ventilator dependence. Hyponatremia can result from inadequate sodium intake, excessive free water, excess sodium loss and renal disease. Hypernatremia can occur with excessive sodium intake and fluid restriction. Hyperkalemia may be noted with excessive intake and renal disease. Hypokalemia may result from increased losses, inadequate replacement or from increased requirements, as is seen with refeeding syndrome. Hypocalcemia occurs with osteopenia of prematurity, diuretics, excessive phosphate intake, severe vitamin D deficiency, inadequate calcium intake and magnesium deficiency. Hypophosphatemia can result with re-feeding syndrome, inadequate intake, use of amphotericin B, hypomagnesemia and increased renal excretion of phosphorus. Hypomagnesemia occurs with decreased intake, increased losses as seen with diarrhea and renal disease and use of certain drugs like amphotericin B and ciclosporin A. Rapid infusions of intravenous fat can result in hypertriglyceridemia and elevated free fatty acid levels due to saturation of lipoprotein lipase and subsequent accumulation of atypical lipoproteins. Hypertriglyceridemia occurs when there is decreased triglyceride clearance and is seen with excessive intravenous fat intake, sepsis and overfeeding. Fat overload syndrome occurs with extremely high fat infusions over a short period. This is characterized by a decrease in oxygenation, thrombocytopenia and tachypnea. If PN solutions without intravenous fat are administered, essential fatty acid deficiency can occur with deleterious effects on energy metabolism, membrane structure, prostaglandin synthesis and fat tissue storage. There has been evidence suggesting an association between intravenous fat administration and the incidence of chronic lung disease and death in neonates, but a meta-analysis did not find any significant effect on death or chronic lung disease.[130–133] The oxidation of intravenous fat by phototherapy and ambient lights results in the formation of lipid hydroperoxides. Decreased hydroperoxide levels have been shown when intravenous fat emulsions were protected from light.[134,135] These hydroperoxides lead to the formation of free radicles and injury in various organs. Allergy to intravenous fat is rare.[136,137] It is recommended that patients with potential allergies be given a test dose of intravenous fat after appropriate skin testing has been performed. An allergy consultation may be valuable in these cases. PN-related bone disease can occur in up to 3% of adult patients on long-term PN. It is also seen in children receiving home PN.[138–140] It is characterized by bone pain, pathologic fractures and hypercalciuria. Symptoms usually improve after discontinuation of PN. The exact etiology is unknown, but possible factors include abnormal vitamin D metabolism, aluminum toxicity, hypercalciuria, inadequate phosphate administration and abnormal calcium-to-phosphorus ratio.[141,142] Premature infants are at high risk for developing osteopenia. Care must be taken to administer adequate calcium and phosphorus intake as well as to maintain an optimal calcium to phosphorus ratio.[143]

Aluminum contamination of PN solutions is a well-known complication of PN solutions. On 3 June, 2004, the Food and Drug Administration (FDA) is issued a new safety mandate regarding aluminum content in large volume parenterals (LVPs), small volume parenterals (SVPs) and pharmacy bulk packaging (PBPs).[144,145] Some LVPs include amino acids, concentrated dextrose and parenteral lipids and some SVPs include calcium, potassium and sodium. The FDA is recommending aluminum exposure in intravenous solutions not exceed 5 μg/kg per day. Pediatric populations are particularly at risk for developing aluminum toxicity, including metabolic bone disease, encephalopathy and impaired neurologic development. The pediatric patients most at risk are premature infants, patients with renal disorders and those on long term PN.[146] Bishop et al. showed neonates in a neonatal intensive care unit in the UK who were given an aluminum depleted PN solution had a higher Bayley mental development index.[147] For those infants who did not have neuromotor impairment, increasing aluminum exposure reduced Bayley mental development index by 1 point for each day of PN.[147,148] Impaired neurologic development and decreased bone density are among the toxic effects of increased aluminum levels. The FDA mandate will require manufacturers to state the aluminum content on the labels of all LVPs , SVPs and PBPs and has determined the safe upper limit for aluminum in all LVPs, SVPs and PBPs is 25 μg/l or less.

Re-feeding syndrome occurs when malnourished patients receive aggressive nutritional rehabilitation via the enteral or parenteral route.[149] Patients with protein-calorie malnutrition commonly maintain normal serum electrolyte levels in the presence of intracellular depletion of these same electrolytes. Administration of carbohydrate calories results in the stimulation of insulin secretion, which drives phosphorus and potassium into the cell, with resultant hypokalemia, hypophosphatemia and hypomagnesemia. Vitamin deficiency and abnormalities in glucose metabolism can also occur. Increased metabolic rate and anabolism further decrease potassium and phosphorus levels and also induce hypomagnesemia. Re-feeding syndrome can be fatal if not recognized and treated appropriately. It is prudent to start calories at 75% of a patient's resting energy expenditure (REE) or at a previously tolerated level of calories. Calories should then be increased by 10–20% per day provided serum electrolyte levels are normal and congestive heart failure or significant edema is not evident.[150]

Hepatobiliary complications are associated with PN and can occur as early as 2 weeks after the initiation of PN.[151–154] The earliest signs are elevated serum y-glutamyltransferase and cholylglycine levels. The exact incidence is not known, but may vary from 7.4% to 84%. The highest incidence occurs in the LBW premature infant with necrotizing enterocolitis, short bowel syndrome, multiple bouts of sepsis or multiple periods of not being fed. The etiology is unknown, but the following factors have been implicated: excessive protein and carbohydrate intake, amino acid composition, relative carbohydrate-to-nitrogen imbalance, intravenous fat, carnitine, taurine or serine deficiency, excessive phytosterol intake, EFAD, bacterial overgrowth, lack of enteral stimulation, alteration in canalicular membrane transport proteins, effects of ambient light and photo-oxidation on PN constituents and continuous delivery of PN.[155,156] Adults on chronic PN appear to get steatosis, whereas neonates and children develop cholestasis, cirrhosis and portal hypertension. Acalculous cholecystitis, biliary sludge and gallstones can also be seen in patients on chronic PN. Ursodeoxycholic acid has been used to treat this hepatobiliary damage, but there have been no controlled trials demonstrating efficacy. Prevention of PN associated liver disease consists of the following measures: avoiding overfeeding, excessive protein and carbohydrate intake, cycling of PN, using an appropriate amino acid solution and institution of some enteral feeds even if only trophic feeds. Copper and manganese should be decreased or discontinued from the PN solution and copper, ceruloplasmin and manganese levels should subsequently be monitored. All episodes of sepsis should be treated promptly and in the future choline administration may be useful.[60,157,158]

TOTAL NUTRIENT ADMIXTURES

PN admixtures may be administered in one of two forms: (1) a 2-in-1 solution in which the dextrose and amino acid solution is delivered in one bag and the intravenous fat is administered separately as a piggyback infusion, or (2) a 3-in-1 solution or total nutrient admixture (TNA) where the intravenous fat is added directly to the dextrose and amino acid solution. This obviates the need for separate infusion lines and pumps. TNAs simplify PN administration and are particularly useful in the pediatric home PN patient. In 1995, the Food and Drug Administration issued a safety alert after the death of two patients related to microvascular pulmonary thrombi containing calcium phosphate precipitates.[159] Several recommendations were made regarding the amount of calcium and phosphorus added to the PN solution, the order the components of the PN are added when mixed and the use of a filter.[160–162] With a TNA it is difficult to meet the high calcium and phosphorus needs of neonates without resulting precipitation of the solution. The emulsion may also separate out with high electrolyte concentrations. TNAs are associated with a possible increased risk of thrombosis, pulmonary emboli, shorter catheter life and infection since a standard 0.2 μm filter cannot be used. Additionally, precipitates may not be noticed in a TNA because it is an opaque or cloudy solution. Some of the advantages of a TNA solution is that it costs less, is easier to use since only one pump is required both at home or in the hospital and requires less tubing. Other advantages of TNAs are less risk of contamination and growth of bacteria because there is only one system and it requires less nursing time and pharmacy preparation time. Disadvantages are that it is difficult to see particulate material because the solution is opaque, there could be more growth of bacteria and the stability of the intravenous fat may be affected when high concentrations of electrolytes are used. Typically water-soluble additives are added first, the fat-soluble vitamins are then added to the intravenous fat and finally the two are mixed together. All TNA solutions need to be refrigerated similar to the 2-in-1 solutions. An inline filter of 1.2 μm has to be used with a TNA and this is different from the 0.22 μm filter that is used for the 2-in-1 solution.[160] It is recommended that TNA solutions not be used in neonates and infants.[163] In our institution we do not use TNA for hospitalized patients. Patients on home PN are given TNAs for ease of care. If home PN patients are on solutions that contain high electrolyte concentrations and a TNA will result in precipitation, then the patient is prescribed a 2-in-1 solution.

FORMULATING A REGIMEN

Once the decision has been made to start the patient on PN, it is important to determine whether the patient will require central or peripheral PN. The patient who will require PN for a short time, who has low to average energy, protein and electrolyte needs and has adequate nutritional status should be given PN administered through a peripheral intravenous catheter or peripheral PN. The patient with increased fluid, caloric, protein and energy needs, who is malnourished and who will need PN for more than one week should be given PN which is administered through a central line. Fluid requirements can be calculated using bodyweight or surface area. Fluid needs are not only influenced by age and weight, but also by insensible losses, as well as the underlying medical condition or disease state. Allowances will need to be made for ongoing losses. Some patients such as those with renal failure, or fluid overload and neonates with bronchopulmonary dysplasia and patent ductus arteriosus may need fluid restriction. These patients benefit from concentrated PN administered via a central line. In general, patients receive maintenance fluids from their PN. PN should not be used as a replacement solution for the patient with excessive fluid losses since this will result in the excessive delivery of some nutrients. In these circumstances, we recommend using specifically designated replacement solutions. A common method for determining fluid requirements is as follows: 100 ml/kg for each of the first 10 kg of bodyweight, then an additional 50 ml/kg for the each of the next 10 kg of bodyweight, up to 20 kg. Patients whose weight is >20 kg have an additional 20 ml/kg for every kg over 20 kg. Alternatively, 1600 cc/m^2 can be used if body surface area can be determined. Whatever the method chosen, the patient should always be examined for excessive or inadequate fluid intake by evaluating fluid intake and output data, weight, urine specific gravity and physical examination. The next step in formulation a PN regimen is to determine the goal for the patient's caloric and protein needs. Depending on the patient's nutritional status, a patient can usually receive calories equaling the REE or 75–85% of goal calories and then have caloric delivery increased to goal calories over the next 2–3 days. Patients at risk for re-feeding syndrome should have their PN regimen advanced more slowly. A dextrose solution of 10% is used initially; and if it is tolerated and central access is present, then a more concentrated dextrose solution of up to 30–35% can be used if needed. Most patients receive dextrose concentrations of less than 20%. Once the fat and protein calories have been calculated, the balance of calories is provided as intravenous carbohydrate. It is important to make sure the final PN solution is balanced to prevent complications of overfeeding as well as excessive administration of carbohydrate, protein and fat. We try to provide carbohydrate calories in the range of 50–55%, fat calories in the range of 30–35%, with protein calories making up the balance of calories. It is also important to calculate the GIR and make sure it does not exceed the recommended ranges. After a baseline chemistry panel is reviewed, appropriate amounts of electrolytes and minerals are added. Serum electrolyte levels should initially be monitored daily, until a stable regimen has been reached. A triglyceride level should be checked whenever intravenous fat intake is increased. Additionally, patients with sepsis may have problems with triglyceride clearance and need to have values checked periodically. Prealbumin is a useful test of protein status and the caloric adequacy of the PN regimen and weekly values are helpful in assessing adequacy of the PN regimen.

CYCLIC PARENTERAL NUTRITION

The administration of cyclic PN allows for the provision of PN over a specified period of time each day.[164] Cycling allows for a more normal daytime routine and increased mobility of the patient. Cycling is not usually initiated until a patient is on a stable PN regimen and/or can tolerate a large volume of fluid and nutrients over a short period of time. PN can be cycled from 24 h/day to as low as 8 h/day, but most cycled TPN runs for 10–12 h in children over 4–6 months of age. Reductions in the number of hours a patient is receiving PN can be done in 4–6-h increments. Infants under 4–6 months of age who receive all their nutrition parenterally may only be able to tolerate being off of PN for up to 4 h.[15] There are many benefits to cycling PN. Cycling PN may help to decrease the risk of PN-associated steatosis by allowing time for the mobilization of hepatic fat stores.[16,17] When cycling PN, the rate is cut in half during the last hour of the infusion to prevent hypoglycemia. However, some patients may require tapering over 2 h.[18,64] It is important to monitor for the presence of glucosuria during the PN cycle, since this may be indicative of a lack of tolerance to the regimen. There is the occasional patient who does not tolerate cycling and develops nausea and vomiting. Lengthening the cycle usually allows for improvement of these symptoms. An easy way to calculate the cycling rate is to divide the total volume of PN to be infused by the number of hours the PN will run, minus one half hour, and then half the rate for the last half hour (e.g. a total PN volume of 1500 cc is to be infused over 12 h. 1500/11.5 = 130.4 cc/h for 11 h and 65.2 cc/h for the last hour). Another more precise way to calculate the rates has been described by Longhurst et al.[20] Some institutions also start the PN infusion at half the goal rate for the first half hour.

HOME PARENTERAL NUTRITION

Home PN refers to the administration of PN solutions to patients at home. These are usually patients who cannot maintain normal nutritional status through enteral feeds, patients who require chronic PN administration, or patients who only need to be hospitalized to receive PN.[21] Patients usually receive a combination of enteral and parenteral feeds and every attempt is made to increase enteral feeds and wean PN as soon as possible. This potentially helps with decreasing bacterial translocation and improving enteral tolerance due to intestinal stimulation. Home PN patients have central access and are usually on cycled PN for ease of care, the achievement of a more normal lifestyle and to decrease long-term complications of PN. Patients who fail to tolerate sufficient enteral regimens and wean off PN in the hospital are often sent home on PN. Common patient diagnoses include the patient with short bowel syndrome following surgical resection, oncology patients with vomiting and poor oral intake who cannot tolerate tube feeds, patients with significant small bowel damage from villous atrophy, Crohn's disease, intestinal pseudo-obstruction and other motility disorders and patients with severe pancreatitis with pseudocyst formation. It is important to make sure the patient, parent or guardian gets adequate training and is selected carefully. Contraindications to home PN include a poor home situation where the parent/guardian cannot or is not willing to learn care and administration of PN and the central line. In some instances nursing services at home may be provided to assist the family.

A team is usually required for the management of these patients. This includes a physician, nurse practitioner, dietitian, social worker, pharmacist and psychologist. Members of the home PN team assist with the determination of eligibility for home PN, training, developing the home regimen prior to discharge and education of the family. They also meet with the inpatient team and primary care physician and discuss objectives and goals for the patient at home. Parents and guardians need to document competency with line care, PN set up, an understanding of pumps and infusion rates and addition of vitamins and other additives to the PN solution. A nurse form the home care company usually visits the family the first night the PN is infused at home to assist the family with the set up and technique. It is essential the patient have good central access with either a Broviac or PICC line that is centrally placed. The patients PN may be cycled for 8–16 h, depending on their needs, tolerance and size.

Complications are similar to those described in the above section on metabolic complications. Common complications include line sepsis, line malfunction including occlusion, tunnel infections, PN associated liver disease, bone disease and abnormal micronutrient status: either deficiency or excessive levels depending on the patient and underlying disease state.[60,114,139,140,153,165,166]

Sepsis can be a difficult complication to manage in certain home PN patients. All patients with possible line sepsis need to be evaluated and blood cultures obtained from the line as well as from a peripheral vein. Additionally patients need to have their line site examined and other possible sources of infection excluded. Other laboratory tests that need to be performed include a complete blood count with differential, clotting function, comprehensive metabolic panel, triglyceride level and an evaluation for disseminated intravascular coagulation. Most line infections can be treated through the line, but in the case of persistent bacterial or fungal sepsis the line may need to be removed. Once the sepsis has been cleared the line will need to be replaced. Catheter related thrombosis and occlusion of vessels in patients on home PN has been described.[167]

MONITORING THE HOME PN PATIENT

All home PN patients need to be monitored closely for growth and nutritional status, advancement of enteral feeds and laboratory status. Guidelines have been developed and labs are usually obtained weekly after discharge until a stable regimen has been achieved.[33,168] Thereafter the frequency of laboratory testing is gradually decreased to once per month. Vitamin, trace element and carnitine levels are checked every 3–6 months. Bone densitometry evaluations should be obtained at the initiation of PN and then every 1–2 years depending on the presence and severity of bone disease.

Normal long-term growth can be achieved in patients on home PN who receive enteral and parenteral nutrition. Those on primarily PN may not grow as well.[169] Improved growth has been seen with correction of essential fatty acid and trace element deficiency, correction of a co-existing endocrine disorder and supplementation of alpha-ketoglutarate deficiency.[170] Some studies have shown normal developmental function in patients on home PN and defects in perceptual motor function, but overall normal functioning can be achieved.[171]

SUMMARY

There have been several developments in the field of parenteral nutrition for neonatal and pediatric patients. However, much work needs to be done. Continuing efforts need to be made to improve the safety and efficacy of parenteral nutrition. Future studies also need to assist in better defining the nutritional requirements of parenteral nutrition as well as effectiveness of parenteral nutrients and additives.

References

1. Klein S, Kinney J, Jeejeebhoy K, et al. Nutrition support in clinical practice: Review of published data and recommendations for future research directions. J Parenter Enteral Nutr 1997; 21:133–156.
2. Dudrick SJ, Wilmore DW, Vars HM. Long-term total parenteral nutrition with growth in puppies and positive nitrogen balance in patients. Surg Forum 1967; 18:356–357.
3. Wilmore, DW, Dudrick SJ. Growth and development of an infant receiving all nutrients exclusively by vein. JAMA 1968; 203:140–144.
4. Dorney SF et al. Improved survival in very short bowel of infancy with use of long-term parenteral nutrition. J Pediatr 1985; 107:521.
5. Everitt NJ, McMahon MJ. Peripheral intravenous nutrition. Nutrition 1994; 10:49–57.

6. Moukarzel AA, Haddad ME, Ament ME, et al. Two hundred and thirty patient years of experience with long-term parenteral nutrition in childhood: natural history and life of central venous catheters. J Pediatr Surg 1994; 29:1324.
7. Allen A et al. Venous thrombosis associated with the placement of peripherally inserted central catheters. J Vasc Interv Radiol. 2000; 11(10):1309–1314.
8. Jacobs BR. Central venous catheter occlusion and thrombosis. Crit Care Clin 2003; 19:489–514.
9. Hickman RO, Buchner CD, Clift RA, et al. A modified right atrial catheter for access to the venous system in marrow transplant recipients. Surg Gynecol Obstet 1979; 166:295–301.
10. Denny DF. Placement and management of long-term central venous access catheters and ports. Am J Radiol 1993; 161:385–393.
11. Gullo SM. Implanted ports: technological advances and nursing care issues. Nursing Clin North Am 1993; 28:859–871.
12. Brewer ED. Pediatric experience with intradialytic parenteral nutrition and supplemental tube feeding. Am J Kidney Dis 1999; 33:205–207.
13. Schofield W. Predicting basal metabolic rate, new standards and review of previous work. Hum Nutr Clin Nutr 1985; 39(suppl 1):5–41.
14. Duro D, Rising R, Cole C, Valois S, Cedillo M, Lifshitz F. New equations for calculating the components of energy expenditure in infants. J Pediatr 2002; 140:534–539.
15. Kaplan As, Zemel BS, Neiswinder KM, Stallings VA. Resting energy expenditure in clinical pediatrics: measured versus prediction equations. J Pediatr 1995; 127:200–205.
16. Liggett SB, St. John RE, Lefrak SS. Determination of resting energy expenditure utilizing the thermodilution pulmonary artery catheter. Chest 1987; 91(4):562–566.
17. Heird WC. Amino acid and energy needs of pediatric patients receiving parenteral nutrition. Pediatr Clin North Am. 1995; 42(4): 765–789.
18. World Health Organization: Energy and protein requirements. Technical Report Series No. 734. Geneva: World Health Organization; 1985.
19. Stokes MA, Hill GL. Total energy expenditure in patients with Crohn's disease: measurement by the combined body scan technique. J Parenter Enteral Nutr 1993; 17(1):3–7.
20. Gardiner K, Barbul A. Amino acid as specific therapy in human disease. In: Torosian M, ed. Nutrition for the Hospitalized Patient: Basic Science and Principles of Practice. New York: Marcel Decker; 1995:183–205.
21. Heird RA, Christersen ML, Mauer EC, et al. Comparison of a pediatric verses standard amino acid formulation in preterm neonates requiring parenteral nutrition. J. Pediatr 1987; 110:466–470.
22. Cooper A, Betts JM, Periera GR. Taurine deficiency in the severe hepatic dysfunction complicating total parenteral nutrition. J Pediatr Surg 1984; 19:462.
23. Wu PYK, Edwards NB, Strom MC. Characterization of the plasma amino acid pattern of normal term breast-fed infants. J Pediatr 1986; 109:347.
24. Fitzgerald KA, MacKay MW. Calcium and phosphate solubility in neonatal parenteral nutrient solutions containing TrophAmine. Am J Hosp Pharm 1986; 43:88.
25. Chin SE, Shepherd RW, Thomas BJ et al. Nutritional support in children with end-stage liver disease: a randomized crossover trail of a branched-chain amino acid supplement. Am J Clin Nutr 1992; 56:158–163.
26. Marchesani G, Bianchi G, Rossi B et al. Nutritional treatment with branched-chain amino acids in advanced liver cirrhosis. J Gastroenterol 2000; 35 suppl12:7–12.
27. Heyman MB, General and specialized parenteral amino acid formulations for nutrition support. J Am Diet Assoc 1990; 90; 401–408.
28. Department of Pharmacy Services. The Children's Hospital of Philadelphia Pharmacy Handbook and Formulary 2003–2004. Hudson, OH: Department of Pharmacy Services, Lexi-Comp Inc; 2003.
29. Acra SA, Rollins C. Principles and guidelines for parenteral nutrition in children. Pediatr Ann 1999; 28(2):113–120.
30. Panel on Macronutrients, Subcommittees on Upper Reference Levels of Nutrients and Interpretation and Uses of Dietary Reference Intakes and the Standing Committee on the Scientific Evaluation of Dietary Reference Intakes. Dietary Reference Intakes for Energy, Carbohydrate, Fiber, Fat, Fatty Acids, Cholesterol, Protein and Amino Acids (Macronutrients) A Report; 2002.
31. Van Goudoever JB, Colen T, Wattimena JLD, et al. Immediate commencement of amino acid supplementation in preterm infants: effect on serum amino acid concentrations and protein kinetics on the first day of life. J Pediatr 1995; 127:456–465.
32. Porcelli PJ, Sisk PM. Increased parenteral amino acid administration to extremely low-birth-weight infants during early post-natal life. J Pediatr Gastroenterol Nutr 2002; 34:174–179.
33. ASPEN Board of Directors and The Clinical Guidelines Task Force. Guidelines for the use of parenteral and enteral nutrition in adult and pediatric patients. J Parenteral and Enteral Nutr 2002; 1(Suppl):27SA.
34. Heird WC, Amino acids in pediatric and neonatal nutrition. Curr Opin Clin Nutr Metab Care 1998; 1:73–78.
35. Bruton JA, Ball RO, Pencharz PB. Current total parenteral nutrition solutions for the neonate are inadequate. Curr Opin Nutr Metab Care 2000; 3:299–304.
36. National Advisory Group on Standards and Practice Guidelines for Parenteral Nutrition. Safe practices for parenteral nutrition formulations. J Parenteral Enteral Nutr 1998; 22:49–46; Tables 59.52 and 59.53.
37. Brown MR, Thumberg BJ, Golub L et al. Decreased cholestasis with enteral instead of intravenous protein in the very low-birth-weight infant. J Pediatr Gastroenterol Nutr 1989; 9:21–27.
38. Kashyap S, Abildskov K, Heird WC. Cysteine supplementation of very-low-birth-weight infants receiving parenteral nutrition. II. Pediatr Res 1992; 31:290A.
39. Groff, J, Gropper, S, Hunt, S. Advanced Nutrition and Human Metabolism. St Paul, MN: West Publishing Co 1995; 175.
40. Andrews FJ, Griffiths RD. Glutamine: essential for immune nutrition in the critically ill. Br J Nutr 2002; 87(suppl 1):S3–S8.
41. Byrne TA, Persinger RC, Young LS et al. A new treatment for patients with short-bowel syndrome. Ann Surg 1995; 222:243–255.
42. Ziegler TR, Young LS, Benfell K et al. Clinical and metabolic efficacy of glutamine-supplemented parenteral nutrition after bone marrow transplantation. Ann Intern Med 1992; 116:821–828.
43. Wischmeyer PE, Lynch J, Leidel J et al. Glutamine administration reduced gram-negative bacteremia in severely burned patients; a prospective, randomized, double-blind trial versus isonitrogenous control. Crit Care Med 2001; 29:2075–2080.

44. Gore DC. Deficiency in peripheral glutamine production in pediatric patients with burns. J Burn Care Rehabil 2000; 21:171–177.

45. Scolapio JS, Camilleri M, Fleming CR et al. Effects of growth hormone, glutamine and diet on adaptation in short bowel syndrome: a randomized, controlled trial. Gastroenterol 1997; 113:1074–1081.

46. Poindexter BB. Ehrenkranz RA, Stoll BJ et al. Parenteral glutamine supplementation in ELBW infants: a multicenter randomized clinical trial. Pediatr Res 2002; 51(Pt 2):317A.

47. Thompson SW, McClure BG, Tubman TR. A randomized, controlled trial of parenteral glutamine in ill, very low birth-weight neonates. J Pediatr Gastroenterol Nutr. 2003; 37(5): 550–553.

48. Lacey JM, Crouch JB, Benfell K, et al. The effects of glutamine supplemented parenteral nutrition in premature infants. J Parenter Enteral Nutr 1996; 20:74–79.

49. Hoppel C. The role of carnitine in normal and altered fatty acid metabolism. Am J Kidney Dis 2003; 41(Suppl 4): S4–12.

50. Bonner CM, DeBrie KL, Hug G, Landrigan E, Taylor BJ. Effects of parenteral L-carnitine supplementation on fat metabolism and nutrition in premature neonates. J Pediatr 1995; 126(2): 287–292.

51. Helms RA, Borum PR, Hay WW et al. Intravenous (IV) carnitine during parenteral nutrition (PN) in infants. J parenteral Enteral Nutr 1987; 11(Suppl):9.

52. Stahl GE, Spear ML, Hamosh M. Intravenous administration of lipid emulsions to premature infants. Clin Perinatol 1986; 13:133.

53. Sulkers EJ et al. Effects of high carnitine supplementation on substrate utilization in low-birth-weight infants receiving total parenteral nutrition. Am J Clin Nutr 1990; 52:889.

54. Schmidt-Sommerfield E, Penn D, Wolf H. Carnitine deficiency in premature infants receiving total parenteral nutrition: Effect of L-carnitine supplementation. J Pediatr 1983; 102:931.

55. Whitfield J, Smith T, Sollohub H et al Clinical effects of L-carnitine supplementation on apnea and growth in very low birth weight infants. Pediatr 2003; 111:477–482.

56. Meyburg J, Schulze A, Kohlmueller D et al. Acylcarnitine profiles of preterm infants over the first four weeks of life. Pediatr Res 2003; 52:720–723.

57. Cairns PA, Stalker DJ. Carnitine supplementation of parenterally fed neonates. Cochrane Database Syst Rev 2000; (4):CD000950.

58. Buchman Al, Moukarzel AA, Jenden DJ et al. Hepatic transaminase abnormalities are associated with low plasma free choline in patients receiving long-term parenteral nutrition. Clin Nutr 1993; 12:38–42.

59. Buchman AL, Dubin M, Jenden D, et al. Lecithin increases plasma free choline and decreases hepatic steatosis in long term total parenteral nutrition patients. Gastroenterol 1992; 102:1363–1370.

60. Buchman Al, Dubin MD, Moukarzel AA et al. Choline deficiency: a cause of hepatic steatosis during parenteral nutrition that can be reversed with intravenous choline supplementation. Hepatol 1995; 22:1399–1403.

61. Buchman AL, Dubin M, Jenden D, et al. Lecithin increases plasma free choline and decreases hepatic steatosis in long term total parenteral nutrition patients. Gastroenterol 1992; 102:1363–1370.

62. Buchman AL, Ament ME, Sohel M, et al. Choline deficiency causes reversible hepatic abnormalities in patients receiving parenteral nutrition: proof of a human choline requirement: a placebo-controlled trial. J Parenter Enteral Nutr 2001; 25(5):260–268.

63. Jones MO, Pierro A, Hammond P, et al. Glucose utilization in the surgical newborn receiving TPN. J Pediatr Surg 1993; 8:1121–1125.

64. Krzywda EA, Andris DA, Whipple JK, Street CC, Ausman RK, Schulte WJ, Quebbeman EJ. Glucose response to abrupt initiation and discontinuation of total parenteral nutrition. J Parenter Enteral Nutr 1993; 17(1): 64–67.

65. Tulikoura I, Huikuri K. Morphological fatty changes and functions of the liver, serum fatty acids and triglycerides during parenteral nutrition. Scan J Gastroenterol 1982; 17:177–185.

66. Gore DC, Chinkes D, Heggers J. Association of hyperglycemia with increased mortality after severe burn injury. J Trauma 2001; 51:540–544.

67. Khaodhiar L, McCowen K, Bistrian B. Perioperative hyperglycemia, infection or risk? Curr Opin Clin Nutr Metab Care 1999; 2:79–82.

68. Elwyn Dh, Askanazi J, Kiney JM et al. Kinetics of energy substrates. Acta Chir Scand Suppl 1981; 507:209–219.

69. Nose O, Tipton JR, Ament ME. Effect of the energy source on changes in energy expenditure, respiratory quotient and nitrogen balance during total parenteral nutrition in children. Pediatr Res 1987; 21:538–541.

70. Shikora SA, Benotti PN. Nutritional support of the mechanically ventilated patient. Respir Care Clin N Am 1997; 3:69–90.

71. Klien CJ, Stanek GS, Wiles CE. Overfeeding macronutrients to critically ill adults: metabolic complications. J Am Diet Assoc 1998; 98:795–806.

72. Rodriguez JL, Askaazi J, Weissman C, et al. Ventilatory and metabolic effects of glucose infusions. Chest 1985; 88:512–518.

73. Colins JW et al. A controlled trial of insulin infusion and parenteral nutrition in extremely-low-birth-weight infants with glucose intolerance. J Pediatr 1991; 118:921–926.

74. Nordenstrom J, Thorne A. Comparative studies on a new concentrated fat emulsion: Intralipid 30% vs. 20%. Clin Nutr 1993; 12:160–167.

75. Garcia-de-Lorenzo A, Lopez-Martinez J, Planas M, et al. Safety and metabolic tolerance of a concentrated long-chain triglyceride lipid emulsion in critically ill septic and trauma patients. J Parenter Enteral Nutr 2003; 27(3):208–215.

76. Haumont D, Deckelbaum RJ, Richelle M, et al. Plasma lipid and plasma lipoprotein concentrations in low birth weight infants given parenteral nutrition with twenty or ten percent lipid emulsion. J Pediatr 1989; 115:787–793.

77. Haumont D, Richelle M, Deckelbaum RJ, et al. Effect of liposomal content of lipid emulsions on plasma lipid concentrations in low birth weight infants receiving parenteral nutrition. J Pediatr 1992; 121:759–763.

78. Sacks G, Driscoll D. Does lipid hang time make a difference? Time is of the essence. NCP 2002; 17:284–290.

79. Koretz Rl, Lipman TO, Klein S. AGA Technical Review on parenteral nutrition. Gastroenterol 2001; 121:970–1001.

80. Shulman RJ, Phillips S. Parenteral Nutrition in infants and children. J Pediatr Gastroenterol Nutr 2003; 36:421–441.

81. Skeie B, Askanazi J, Rothkopf MM. Intravenous fat emulsions and lung function: a review. Crit Care Med 1988; 16:183–194.

82. Hageman JR, Hunt CE. Fat emulsions and lung function. Clin Chest Med 1986; 7:69–77.

83. Gutcher GR, Farrell PM. Intravenous infusions of lipid for the prevention of essential fatty acid deficiency in premature infants. Am J Clin Nutr 1991; 54:1024–1028.

84. Friedman Z. Essential fatty acids revisited. Am J Dis Child 1980; 134:397–408.

85. Friedman Z, Danon A, Stahlamn MT etal. Rapid onset of essential fatty acid deficiency in the newborn. Pediatr 1976; 58:640.

86. Dahn MS, Structured lipids: An alternative energy source. Nutr Clin Pract 1995; 10:89–90.

87. Carpentier YA, Dupont IE. Advances in intravenous lipid emulsions. World J Surg 2000; 24(12): 1493–1497.

88. Ok E, Yilmaz Z, Karakucuk I, Akgun H, Sahin H. Use of olive oil based emulsions as an alternative to soybean oil based emulsions in total parenteral nutrition and their effects on liver regeneration following hepatic resection in rats. Ann Nutr Metab 2003; 47(5): 221–227.

89. Pscheidl E, Schywalsky M, Tschaikowsky K, Boke-Prols T. Fish oil-supplemented parenteral diets normalize splanchnic blood flow and improve killing of translocated bacteria in a low-dose endotoxin rat model. Crit Care Med 2000; 28(5):1489–1496.

90. Koch T, Duncker HP, Klein A, Schlotzer E, Peskar BM, van Ackern K, Neuhof H. Modulation of pulmonary vascular resistance and edema formation by short-term infusion of a 10% fish oil emulsion. Infusionsther Transfusionsmed 1993; 20(6):291–300.

91. Gadek JE, DeMichele SJ, Karlstad MD, et al. Effect of enteral feeding with eicosapentaenoic acid, gamma-linolenic acid and antioxidants in patients with acute respiratory distress syndrome. Enteral Nutrition in ARDS Study Group. Crit Care Med. 1999; 27(8):1409–1420.

92. Adolph M. Lipid emulsions in total parenteral nutrition – state of the art and future perspectives. Clin Nutr 2001; 20 (suppl 4):11–14.

93. Bresson JL, Narcy P, Sachs C, et al. Energy substrate competition: comparative study of LCT and MCT utilization during continuous TPN in infants. Clin Nutr 1986; 5(suppl):54(A).

94. Goulet O, De Potter S, Postaire M, et al. Long term TPN in children: utilization of medium chain triglycerides. Nutrition 1992; 8:333–337.

95. Lima LAM, Murphy JF, Stansbie D et al. Neonatal parenteral nutrition with a fat emulsion containing medium chain triglycerides. Acta Paediatr Scan 1988; 77; 332–339.

96. ASPEN Board of Directors and The Clinical Guidelines Task Force. Guidelines for the use of parenteral and enteral nutrition in adult and pediatric patients. J Parenter and Enteral Nutr 2002; 1(Suppl):26SA.

97. Greene HL, Hambidge M, Schanler R, Tsang RC. Guidelines for the use of vitamins, trace elements, calcium, magnesium and phosphorus in infants and children receiving total parenteral nutrition: report of the subcommittee on pediatric parenteral nutrient requirements from the Committee on Clinical Practice Issues of the American Society for Clinical Nutrition. Am J Clin Nutr 1988; 48:1324–1342.

98. Department of Health and Human Service Food and Drug Administration. Parenteral multivitamin products: Drugs for Human Use; Drug efficacy study implementation; Amendment. Federal Register. April 2000; 56:21200–21201.

99. Multivitamin preparation for parenteral use: a statement by the nutrition advisory group. J Parenteral Enteral Nutr 1975; 3:258–262.

100. Gillis J, Jones G, Pencharz P. Delivery of vitamins A, D and E in parenteral nutrition solutions. J Parenter Enteral Nutr 1983; 7:11.

101. Alade SL, Brown RE, Paquet A. Polysorbate 80 and E-Ferol toxicity. Pediatr 1986; 77:593–597.

102. Mac Donald MG, Getson PR, Glasgow AM et al. Propylene glycol: increased incidence of seizures in low birth weight infants. Pediatr 1987; 79:622–625.

103. Greene HL, Phillips BL, Franck L, et al. Persistently low blood retinol levels during and after parenteral feeding of very low birth weight infants: examination of losses into intravenous administration sets and a method of prevention by addition to a lipid emulsion. Pediatr 1987; (6):894–900.

104. Baeckert PA, Greene HL, Fritz I, Oelberg DG, Adcock EW. Vitamin concentrations in very low birth weight infants given vitamins intravenously in a lipid emulsion: measurement of vitamins A, D and E and riboflavin. J Pediatr 1988; 113(6):1057–1065.

105. Shenai JP, Kennedy KA, Chytil F, Stahlman MT. Clinical trial of vitamin A supplementation in infants susceptible to bronchopulmonary dysplasia. J Pediatr 1987; 111(2): 269–277.

106. Tyson JE, Wright LL, Oh W, et al. Vitamin A supplementation for extremely-low-birth-weight infants. National Institute of Child Health and Human Development Neonatal Research Network. N Engl J Med. 1999; 340(25):1962–1968.

107. Norton JA, Peters ML, Wesley R et al. Iron supplementation of TPN : a prospective study. J Parenter Enteral Nutr 1983:7:457–461.

108. Fleming CR. Trace element metabolism in adult patients requiring TPN. Am J Clin Nutr 1989; 49:573–579.

109. Khaodhiar L, Keane-Ellison M, Tawa N, et al. Iron deficiency anemia in patients receiving home TPN. J Parenter Enteral Nutr 2002; 26:114–119.

110. Kumpf VJ. Update on parenteral iron therapy. Nutr Clin Pract 2003; 18:318–326.

111. Fok TF, Chui KK, Cheung R, Ng PC, Cheung KL, Hjelm M. Manganese intake and cholestatic jaundice in neonates receiving parenteral nutrition; a randomized controlled study. Acta Paediatr 2001; 90:1009–1015.

112. Spiegel JE, Willenbucher RF. Rapid development of severe copper deficiency in a patient with Crohn's disease receiving parenteral nutrition. J Parenter Enteral Nutr 1999; 23(3):169–172.

113. Bertinet DB, Tinivella M, Balzola FA, et al. Brain manganese deposition and blood levels in patients undergoing home parenteral nutrition. J Parenter Enteral Nutr 2000; 24(4):223–227.

114. Takagi Y, Okada A, Sando K, Wasa M, Yoshida H, Hirabuki N. Evaluation of indexes of in vivo manganese status and the optimal intravenous dose for adult patients undergoing home parenteral nutrition. Am J Clin Nutr 2002; 75(1):112–118.

115. Iinuma Y, Kubota M, Uchiyama M, et al. Whole-blood manganese levels and brain manganese accumulation in children receiving long-term home parenteral nutrition. Pediatr Surg Int 2003; 19(4):268–272.

116. Bailey MJ. Reduction of catheter-associated sepsis in parenteral nutrition using low-dose intravenous heparin. BMJ 1979; 1:1671.

117. Berkow SE, Spear ML, Stahl GE, et al. Total parenteral nutrition with intralipid in premature infants receiving TPN with heparin: effect on plasma lipolytic enzymes, lipids and glucose. J Pediatr Gastroenterol Nutr 1987; 6:581–588.

118. Collins E, Lawson L, Lau M, et al. Care of central venous catheters for total parenteral nutrition. Nutr Clin Pract 1996; 11(3):109–114.

119. Bilodeau J, Poon C, Mascarenhas MR. Parenteral nutrition/care of central lines. In: Altschuler SM, Liacouras CA, eds. Pediatric Gastroenterology. London: Churchill Livingstone; 1998.

120. Dollery CM, Sullivan ID, Bauraind O, et al. Thrombosis and embolism in long-term central venous access for parenteral nutrition. Lancet 1994; 344:1043–1045.

121. Mehta S, Connors AF Jr, Danish EH et al. Central venous catheters and risk of thrombosis in newborns. J Pediatr Surg 1992; 27:18–22.
122. Lewis Ca et al. Quality improvement guidelines for central venous access. J Vascular Interventional Radiol 2003; 14:S231–2350.
123. Newall F, Barnes C, Savoia H, Campbell J, Monagle P. Warfarin therapy in children who require long-term total parenteral nutrition. Pediatrics 2003; 112(5):e386.
124. Hospital Infection Control Practices Advisory Committee. Guideline for prevention of intravascular device-related infections: I. Intravascular device-related infections: an overview. Am J Infect Control 1996; 24:262–293.
125. Christenson ML, Hancock ML, Gattuso J, et al. Parenteral nutrition associated with increased infection rate in children with cancer. Cancer 1993; 72:2732–2738.
126. Mulloy RH, Jadavji T, Russell ML. Tunneled central venous catheter sepsis: risk factors in a pediatric hospital. J Parenter Enteral Nutr 1991; 15:460–463.
127. Nahata MC, King DR, Powell DA, et al. Management of catheter-related infections in pediatric patients. J Parenter Enteral Nutr 1988; 12:58–59.
128. O'Grady N, et al. Guidelines for the prevention of intravascular catheter-related infections. Morbidity and Mortality Weekly Report 2002; 51 (RR–10):1–29.
129. Ament ME, Misra S, Vargas J, Reyen L. Complications of total parenteral nutrition and long-term outcome. Ann Nestle 1996; 54(2):61–69.
130. Cooke RWI. Factors associated with chronic lung disease in preterm infants. Arch Dis Child 1991; 66:776.
131. Alwaidh MH, Bowden L, Shaw B, Ryan SW. Randomized trial of effect of delayed intravenous lipid administration on chronic lung disease in preterm neonates. J Pediatr Gastroenterol Nutr 1996; 22:203.
132. Sosenko IRS, Rodriguez-Pierce M, Bancalari E. Effect of early initiation of intravenous lipid administration on the incidence and severity of chronic lung disease in premature infants. J Pediatr 1993; 123:975.
133. Fox GF, Wilson DC, Ohlsson A. Effect of early vs. late introduction of intravenous fat to preterm infants on death and chronic lung disease (CLD)-results of a meta-analysis. Pediatr Res 1998; 43:214A.
134. Neuzil J, Darlow BA, Inder TE, Sluis KB, Winterbourn CC, Stocker R. Oxidation of parenteral lipid emulsion by ambient and phototherapy lights: potential toxicity of routine parenteral feeding. J Pediatr 1995; 126:785–790.
135. Helbok HJ, Motchnik PA, Ames BN. Toxic hydroperoxides in intravenous lipid emulsions used in preterm infants. Pediatr 1993; 91–83.
136. Market AD, Lew DB, Schropp KP, Hak EB. Parenteral nutrition-associated anaphylaxis in a 4–year old child. J Pediatr Gastroenterol Nutr 1998; 26:229–231.
137. Buchman Al, Ament ME. Comparative hypersensitivity in intravenous lipid emulsion. J Parenter Enteral Nutr 1991; 15:345–346.
138. Verhage AH, Cheong WK, Allard JP, Jeejeebhoy KN. Increase in lumbar spine bone mineral content in patients on long-term parenteral nutrition without vitamin D supplementation. J Parenter Enteral Nutr 1995; 19:431–436.
139. Koo WWK. Parenteral nutrition-related bone disease. J Parenter Enteral Nutr 1992; 16:386–394.
140. Hurley DL, McMahon MM. Long-term parenteral nutrition and metabolic bone disease. Endocrinol Metabol Clin North Am 1990; 19:113–131.
141. Lipkin EW. Metabolic bone disease in the long-term parenteral nutrition patient. Clin Nutr 1995; 14(Suppl 1):65–69.
142. Seidner Dl and Licata A. Parenteral Nutrition-associated metabolic bone disease: Pathophysiology, evaluation and treatment. Nutr Clin Pract 2000; 15:163–170.
143. Trissel, LA. Trissel's Calcium and Phosphate Compatibility in Parenteral Nutrition. Houston, TX: TriPharma Communications; 2001.
144. Federal Register – Proposed Rules 2000; 65:4103–4111.
145. Department of Health and Human Services. Aluminum in large and small volume parenteral used in total parenteral nutrition; amendment: delay of effective date. Federal Register 2002; 67:70691–70692.
146. Advenier E, Landry C, Colomb V, et al. Aluminum loading in children on long-term parenteral nutrition. J Pediatr Gastroenterol Nutr 2003; 36(4)448–453.
147. Bishop NJ, Morley R, Day JP, Lucas A. Aluminum neurotoxicity in preterm infants receiving intravenous-feeding solutions. N Engl J Med 1997; 336:1557–1561.
148. Baluarte HJ, Gruskin AB, Hiner LB, Foley CM, Grover WD. Encephalopathy in children with chronic renal failure. Proc Clin Dial Transplant Forum 1977; 7; 95–98.
149. Solomon SM, Kirby DF. The refeeding syndrome: a review. J Parenter Enteral Nutr 1990; 14:90–97.
150. Dunn R, Stettler N, Mascarenhas M. Refeeding syndrome in hospitalized pediatric patients. NCP 2003; 18: 327–332.
151. Merritt RJ. Cholestasis associated with total parenteral nutrition. J Pediatr Gastroenterol Nutr 1986; 5:9–22.
152. Quigley EMM, Marsh MN, Shaffer JL, Markin RS. Hepatobiliary complications of total parenteral nutrition. Gastroenterology 1993; 104:286–301.
153. Buchman A. Total parenteral nutrition associated liver disease. J Parent Enteral Nutr 2002; 26(5)Suppl: S43–S48.
154. Teitelbaum DH. Parenteral nutrition-associated cholestasis. Curr Opin Pediatr 199; 9:270–275.
155. Colomb V, Jobert-Giraud A, Lacaille F, Goulet O, Fournet JC, Ricour C. Role of lipid emulsions in cholestasis associated with long-term parenteral nutrition in children. J Parenter Enteral Nutr 2000; 24(6):345–350.
156. Bindl L, Lutjohann D, Buderus S, Lentze MJ, v Bergmann K High levels of phytosterols in patients on parenteral nutrition: a marker of liver dysfunction. J Pediatr Gastroenterol Nutr 2000; 31:313–316.
157. Kaufman SS. Prevention of parenteral nutrition-associated liver disease in children. Pediatr Transplantation 2002; 6(1): 37–42.
158. Wright K, Ernst KD, Gaylord MS et al. Increased incidence of parenteral nutrition-associated cholestasis with Aminosyn PF compared to TrophAmine. J Perinatology 2003; 23:444–450.
159. Hill SE, Heldman LS, Goo ED, Whippo PE, Perkinson JC. Fatal microvascular pulmonary emboli from precipitation of a total nutrient admixture solution. J Parenter Enteral Nutr 1996; 20(1):81–87.
160. Bethune K, Allwood M, Grainger C, Wormleighton C. Use of filters during the preparation and administration of parenteral nutrition: position paper and guidelines prepared by a British pharmaceutical nutrition group working party. Nutrition 2001; 17:403–408.
161. Driscoll DF, Bacon MN, Bistrian BR. Effects of in-line filtration on lipid particle size distribution in total nutrient admixtures. J Parenter Enteral Nutr 1996; 20:296–301.

162. McKinnon BT. FDA Safety Alert: Hazards of precipitation associated with parenteral nutrition. Nutr Clin Pract 1996; 11:59–65. (Erratum in: Nutr Clin Pract 1996; 11(3):120).

163. Pierro A, Jones MO, Hammond P, Donnell SC, Lloyd DA. A new equation to predict the resting energy expenditure of surgical infants. J Pediatr Surg 1994; 29:1103–1108.

164. Shulman RJ, Phillips S. Parenteral nutrition in infants and children. J Pediatr Gastroenterol Nutr 2003; 36:587–607.

165. Moukarzel AA, Song MK, Buchman Al et al. Excessive chromium intake in children receiving total parenteral nutrition. Lancet 1992; 339:385.

166. Moukarzel AA et al. Carnitine status of children receiving long term total parenteral nutrition: a longitudinal prospective study. J Pediatr 1992; 120:759.

167. Andrew M et al. A cross-sectional study of catheter related thrombosis in children on home parenteral nutrition. J Pediatr 1995; 126:358.

168. Board of Directors, American Society for Parenteral and Enteral Nutrition. Guidelines for use of home total parenteral nutrition. J Parent Enteral Nutr 1987; 11:342.

169. Dahlstrom KA Strandvik B, Kopple J, Ament ME. Nutritional status in children receiving home parenteral nutrition. J Pediatr 1985; 107:219.

170. Moukarzel AA, Goulet O, Salas JS, et al. Growth retardation in children receiving long-term total parenteral nutrition: effects of ornithine alpha-ketoglutarate. Am J Clin Nutr 1994; 60(3):408–413.

171. Howard L, Heaphey L, Fleming CR, Lininger L, Steiger E. Four years of North American registry home parenteral nutrition outcome data and their implications for patient management. J Parent Enteral Nutr 1991; 15:384.

Chapter 75
Enteral nutrition

Lesley Smith, Linda Casey and Marilyn Kennedy-Jones

INTRODUCTION

The normal route of entry for nutrients into the body is via the gastrointestinal tract. When it is not possible to maintain adequate growth and nutritional status by oral feeding alone, supplemental or sole feeding by the enteral route is preferred over the use of parenteral feeding when the gut is intact (and even sometimes when it is compromised).[1] Use of the gastrointestinal tract maintains gut integrity, utilizes and induces the specialized transport systems available for nutrients and increases intestinal cell mass.[2,3] Enteral feeding stimulates pancreatic enzymes and intestinal disaccharidases and promotes physiological neurohumoral mechanisms important in enhancing gut and hepatobiliary function including motility.[4–6] Enteral feeding also avoids the complications associated with parenteral nutrition (TPN) including cholestasis, sepsis and thrombosis and is considerably less expensive and time-consuming to administer.[7,8] Enteral feeding provides trophic nutrients such as glutamine, trace elements, short-chain fatty acids and fiber and stimulates epithelial growth factor and glucagon-like peptide II production, which are usually not present in TPN.[9] The addition of prebiotics such as oligosaccharides (to positively influence colonic flora) and fish oils (to reduce inflammation by prostaglandin modulation) to defined formulas is also currently of interest.[10–14] The goal of enteral feeding should be to support and maintain growth and development in the face of the metabolic challenges faced by children with acute or chronic disease who are unable or unwilling to maintain an adequate oral intake.

This chapter will summarize the indications for enteral nutrition support in childhood disease, the appropriate nutritional care of the hospitalized malnourished child, the types of enteral feeding available and their specific uses; the composition of enteral feeds for the pre-term and term neonate, infant, child and adolescent; practical issues of enteral feeding; complications pertaining to its use and the method of delivery and enteral nutrition support in the community.

MALNUTRITION IN THE HOSPITAL SETTING

Malnutrition in hospitalized children is recognized as common even in the developed world.[15] Malnutrition may occur quite rapidly in the face of acute disease necessitating hospital admission and is particularly of concern in critically ill patients nursed in the pediatric intensive care unit, post-surgical patients facing unforeseen complications, in traumatized patients with increased metabolic needs, on oncology units during and following chemotherapy or bone marrow transplantation and in the burn unit. Malnutrition may also occur on a chronic basis in patients who are hospitalized for weeks or months, often following a bout of critical illness. The significant occurrence of malnutrition in children in hospital has led to the concept of risk assessment at admission and on an ongoing basis during the hospital stay (see Ch. 72 for more on nutritional assessment).[16]

The global severity of this problem is addressed by the WHO in its manual for physicians and other senior health workers which provides a protocolized management tool for severely malnourished children, but deals mainly with the issue of primary malnutrition.[17] Malnutrition in hospitalized children in the developed world is usually of a secondary nature and contributes significantly to mortality in a variety of severe acute and chronic diseases of childhood, interferes with recovery from surgery and is economically costly.[18,19] It has been recommended that patients hospitalized with malnutrition not be discharged until the attainment of 90% of the median WHO/NCHS reference values for weight-for-height, a goal which is often difficult to achieve in the developed world with hospital bed pressures and which is often not practical or economically feasible in developing countries. Despite this, acknowledgement of the issue and the development of nutrition support teams within hospitals has influenced the incidence and prognosis of the condition.[20] The prevalence of malnutrition in hospitalized patients globally seems to have been consistently as high as 30% over the last 20 years.[21,22] Hendricks et al. showed that the incidence of acute malnutrition in hospitalized children fell from 33% to 25% from 1979 to 1995 and chronic malnutrition from 55% to 27%.[23] Despite the improvement, the issue of malnutrition in hospital remains significant. The early institution of enteral feeding in the face of inadequate oral intake in hospital has consistently been shown to improve outcomes following acute and chronic illnesses. Increasingly, community care teams (often called home enteral feeding teams) are being utilized to successfully care for children with a need for nutritional support in their own homes on a chronic basis.

INDICATIONS FOR ENTERAL FEEDING (Table 75.1)

Inadequate intake

Inadequate intake may be caused by any disease which disrupts the normal oral phase of ingestion for anatomical or functional reasons, chronic diseases which elaborate anorexia-inducing cytokines and psychogenic states causing food aversion. Severe head, neck and oral trauma may make it impossible to achieve significant oral intake and head and neck tumors particularly those which affect the nasopharynx or mouth may interfere with ingestion. Lesions affecting the brainstem may significantly impair mastication and swallowing mechanisms and chemotherapy or radiotherapy may induce severe mucositis. Caustic injuries to the mouth and esophagus may also acutely impair intake although sufficiently severe injury causing stricture may require long term feeding by nasogastric tube, or gastrostomy feeding. Congenital disorders of the palate, pharynx, larynx and esophagus may also impair ingestion and swallowing mechanisms. Children with cleft lip and palate and those with tracheo-esophageal fistula are particularly at risk. The latter frequently have esophageal strictures, esophageal motility disorders and are prone to gastroesophageal reflux. Generally such patients require relatively short-term support. Infants with swallowing dysfunction where no anatomical lesion or chronic neurological condition have been identified may also require temporary nutritional support whilst normal physiological mechanisms mature. Depending on the severity of the problem and the likely length of support required, this may be provided by means of nasogastric or gastrostomy feeding, or if there is a significant risk of aspiration, by jejunal feeding.

Many children with chronic systemic disease, particularly if these involve significant inflammation, may develop impaired intake which is largely due to the presence of circulating cytokines which are anorexigenic such as tumor necrosis factor alpha. Lastly, but importantly, anorexia nervosa in adolescents and food aversion states of a psychogenic nature which may occur in infancy or early childhood may also require supplemental enteral feeding, in some cases to preserve life. The care of such patients is often difficult and the intervention poorly tolerated by anorexic patients who may be non-compliant and controlling. Multidisciplinary care teams, inpatient care and intensive community support are essential in the usually long-term management of children and adolescents with these disorders.

- Inadequate intake
  - Severe head and neck trauma
  - Tumors of the oropharynx, head and neck
  - Severe mucositis
  - Brainstem injury or neoplasm
  - Caustic injury to mouth and esophagus
  - Cleft lip and palate
  - Tracheo-esophageal fistula
  - Other congenital and acquired disorders of oropharyngeal function
  - Anorexia of chronic disease
  - Psychogenic food aversion
  - Anorexia nervosa
- Gastrointestinal dysfunction, hepatobiliary disease and malabsorption
  - Short bowel syndrome
  - Chronic intestinal pseudo-obstruction
  - Inflammatory bowel disease
  - Autoimmune enteropathy
  - Allergic enteropathy
  - Intractable diarrhea
  - Celiac disease
  - Severe gastro-esophageal reflux
  - Acute pancreatitis
  - Chronic cholestasis and liver transplantation
- Critical illness
- Growth failure associated with chronic disease
  - Cardiac disease
    - Cyanotic congenital heart disease with pulmonary hypertension
  - Respiratory disease
    - BPD
    - Cystic fibrosis
    - Pulmonary disorders requiring lung transplantation
  - Renal failure
    - Chronic peritoneal dialysis
  - Neurological disease
    - Acute neurological dysfunction
    - Cerebral palsy
    - Neuromuscular disease
    - Degenerative disease
  - Oncologic disease and bone marrow transplantation
  - Hypermetabolic states
    - HIV/AIDS
    - Head injury, trauma and surgery
    - Burns
  - Metabolic disease
    - Glycogen storage disease type 1

Table 75.1 Indications for enteral feeding

Gastrointestinal disease, malabsorption and hepatobiliary disease

Short bowel syndrome occurring as a result of surgical treatment for congenital disorders of the GI tract in infancy (e.g. gastroschisis, intestinal atresias, Hirschsprung disease), acquired disease (e.g. volvulus, necrotizing enterocolitis) or intestinal failure caused by congenital disorders of absorption or chronic intestinal pseudo-obstruction (e.g. microvillus inclusion disease, megacystis-microcolon hypoperistalsis syndrome) usually require nutritional support. Initially this support may need to be provided by the parenteral route but gradually enteral feeding is introduced to the maximum tolerated, as this has been shown to promote intestinal adaptation and reduce TPN-associated cholestasis and sepsis. Careful attention must be paid to fluid and electrolyte balance as these patients may have significant vomiting, stomal losses or diarrhea and the choice of feeding in terms of its macronutrient composition and osmolality is important in management of these challenges. In general, long-chain triglycerides promote intestinal adaptation and thus defined formulas which include hydrolyzed protein, low-osmolality glucose polymers and long chain fat may optimize gut function.[24] However, limited absorptive capacity may make a formula containing a significant proportion of fat in the form of medium-chain triglyceride a more rational choice especially if there is significant hepatobiliary dysfunction as a result of TPN-associated cholestasis. Cycling of TPN in association with continuous and then intermittent enteral feeding is associated with a lower risk of TPN-associated liver failure. The period required for adaptation and thus nutritional support is highly variable depending on the length and function of the remaining bowel, but may be months or years.

Inflammatory bowel diseases such as Crohn's disease and ulcerative colitis often result in a requirement for supplemental nutrition.[25] Since Crohn's disease may involve the small bowel where significant nutrient absorption takes place, it more frequently requires nutrition support on a long-term basis.[26] Sole enteral feeding by nasogastric tube in Crohn's disease may be used to induce remission in mild to moderately active disease thus avoiding the systemic side-effects of steroids and both polymeric whole-protein and defined formula diets ('elemental' formulas) have been shown to have beneficial effects on acute inflammatory parameters and to promote weight gain and growth. Continuation of supplementation of calories by nocturnal enteral feeding after induction of remission may be associated with prolongation of remission. Children with small bowel disease seem to do better than those with colonic disease. Supplemental enteral feeding may be used during acute exacerbations to reverse catabolism and may be used chronically by nocturnal feeding via nasogastric tube or gastrostomy to reverse growth failure.[27] Supplemental enteral feeding can be useful in promoting anabolism in children with ulcerative colitis undergoing exacerbation or awaiting colectomy.

Children with autoimmune or allergic enteropathy may also require enteral nutrition to achieve appropriate weight gain and those with allergic disorders may need formulas which contain hydrolyzed protein.[28] In some cases, severe allergic enteropathy may require a peptide or amino-acid based formula. Depending on the severity of the mucosal injury, the fat may be provided in the form of long-chain triglycerides (LCT) to promote repair or a mix of MCT and LCT to promote absorption in the face of severe loss of villous surface area. When the prognosis is good for eventual reversal of the condition as in cow's milk protein hypersensitivity or where food elimination diets are effective, this support is only likely to be required in the short term. However patients with severe enteropathy which is poorly-controlled may require extensive and prolonged support which can usually be provided in the home. Patients with severe, intractable diarrhea who do not respond to a food elimination diet may recover more quickly if fed enterally compared with parenteral feeding, although severe monosaccharide intolerance may preclude this route of feeding. In such cases, an elemental feed is usually required and the protein may need to be fully hydrolyzed to amino acids. Enteral feeding supports a more rapid return of intestinal disaccharidase function.

In celiac disease, it is rare to require enteral feeding once a gluten-free diet has been instituted. However, from time to time and usually in infancy, nasogastric feeding with a lactose-free polymeric formula may be necessary for nutritional rehabilitation. Infants with severe gastroesophageal reflux and growth failure may also require enteral nutrition supplementation until their disease comes under control with medication or surgery.

Acute pancreatitis has been shown to increase the rate of protein catabolism by 80% and energy expenditure by 20%.[29] The standard of care for patients with acute pancreatitis requiring nutritional support is enteral rather than parenteral feeding and early support is advocated, safe and effective.[30] There is very little pediatric, but a wealth of adult, data to support this assertion. Evidence shows that enteral feeding, if provided distal to the ligament of Treitz, is superior to parenteral feeding in acute pancreatitis by meta-analyses and randomized, controlled clinical trials in adults. Jejunal feeding has been associated with a significantly lower incidence of infections, reduced surgical interventions to control pancreatitis, lower metabolic complication rate, improved gut barrier function, reduced oxidative stress, decreased length of hospital stay and is significantly less costly when compared to parenteral feeding.[31] Enteral feeding is safe even in instances of severe necrosis and is best provided early in the case of moderate to severe pancreatitis, although no specific benefits in terms of survival have been demonstrated.

Malnutrition associated with chronic cholestasis is common in children and is especially important in infancy when it can be associated with poor neurodevelopmental outcomes and with decreased survival following liver transplantation.[32,33] Specific micronutrient deficiencies especially of fat-soluble vitamins and essential fatty acids may occur.[34] Both nasogastric and gastrostomy feeding have been shown to be safe and effective in promoting catch-up growth, improving body composition, anthropometric parameters and weight gain without an effect specifically on growth factors such as IGF-1 and IGF binding proteins.[35–37] Enteral feeding does not result in an increase in ammonia concentration or the development of encephalopathy in such patients.[38] Severe portal hypertension has been felt to be a relative contra-indication to the placement of percutaneous endoscopic or radiological gastrostomy tubes particularly if there is hypersplenism and severe thrombocytopenia because of the risk of bleeding and organ trauma. Transplant surgeons should be consulted before a gastrostomy is placed since this may provide a challenge during the transplant operation with further upper abdominal adhesions.

Critical illness

Patients with critical illness in the PICU face significant metabolic stress as a result of shock, sepsis, trauma, burns, severe inflammation, organ failure, or other extensive tissue injury and elaborate cytokines which increase the resting energy expenditure by as much as 30% in mild to moderate stress and 50% in severe stress.[39] Pharmacologic neuromuscular paralysis and sedation may reduce this requirement. Despite this significant hypermetabolism, caloric intake is often limited in the early stages of illness due to fluid management and medications and paralysis may make enteral feeding difficult. Enteral nutrition during critical illness helps to maintain gastrointestinal form and function, enhances immunocompetence and attenuates the metabolic consequences of the stress response. Clinical studies have shown that early institution of enteral feeding within 24–48 h of hospital admission is beneficial in improving patient outcome and survival. Transpyloric feeding may be of benefit in the ventilated patient, especially if pharmacologic paralysis can be weaned and jejunal tubes can usually be placed by a simple bedside insufflation technique and failing that, endoscopically.[40,41] Once the patient is extubated and if the aspiration risk is deemed to be minimal, then nasogastric feeding and progression to bolus feeding can usually be achieved provided gastrointestinal function has not been compromised by the illness or its treatment.[42]

GROWTH FAILURE ASSOCIATED WITH CHRONIC DISEASE

Cardiac disease

Children and especially infants with chronic cardiac disease, either congenital or acquired, often require supplemental nutrition during acute exacerbations of their disease, such as heart failure or infection which increase their energy needs.[43] Growth impairment may occur also because of the nature of the hemodynamic lesion especially if there is chronic heart failure, tissue hypoxia, acidosis and increased metabolic needs due to stress, impaired intake due to dyspnea or associated gastroesophageal reflux and malabsorption due to lymphangiectasia or bowel edema. Cyanotic patients with pulmonary hypertension appear to be the most at risk for adverse nutritional outcomes.[44] The impaired intake may be improved by supplemental nasogastric feeding but because of limitations on fluid intake, the formula may need to be concentrated initially to 24 cal/oz and sometimes as much as 30 cal/oz. Judicious use of enteral feeding can promote anabolism in the infant with congenital heart disease awaiting surgery (where resting energy expenditures are often high) and improve surgical outcomes.[45] Continuous enteral feeding appears to be the most efficacious means of provision.[46] Care in the concentration of formulas may be required so as not to provide too high a renal solute load in the face of fluid restriction and use of diuretics. These children may also have impaired gastric motility and delayed gastric emptying which may decrease intake and increase gastroesophageal reflux. Gastrostomy feeding may be helpful if nutritional support is required on a chronic basis and continuous nocturnal feeding is the preferred means of provision, with children taking intermittent bolus feeding by mouth or by tube during the day.[47] Lymphangiectasia (which may be relatively common following the Fontan procedure) and chylous ascites/pleural effusion following surgery may require the use of formulas containing a large proportion of medium-chain triglyceride (such as Pregestimil® or Portagen®) for prolonged periods of support.

Respiratory illness

Pre-term infants with bronchopulmonary dysplasia may have growth failure for a variety of reasons including poor sucking and swallowing mechanisms, poor intake due to circulating inflammatory cytokines, increased work of breathing, hypoxia and oxygen dependence, hypercapnia and recurrent vomiting associated poor gastric emptying and reflux.[48] They may require hypercaloric supplementation up to 30 cal/oz best achieved by a mix of fat and carbohydrate modulars in equal amounts.[49] However, overzealous carbohydrate supplementation may aggravate existing hypercapnia and attention must be paid to electrolytes, particularly if diuretics are required for associated heart failure.

Children with cystic fibrosis (CF) have elevated caloric needs due to increased work of breathing and resting energy expenditures. They also frequently have decreased intake as a result of circulating cytokines from the chronic inflammatory processes in their lungs and increased caloric losses due to maldigestion and absorption from chronic pancreatic insufficiency and hepatobiliary dysfunction.[50] For this reason, early institution of a high calorie diet is an important component of the care of such children and supplementary enteral nutrition by nasogastric feeding may be required during acute exacerbations of pulmonary disease. However, the chronic nutritional care of children with CF is important in maintaining a positive energy balance, preventing respiratory muscle fatigue and preventing micronutrient deficiencies such as fat-soluble vitamin and essential fatty acid deficiency. Oral supplementation with a high calorie polymeric product is advocated first and if patients are still unable to ingest sufficient calories to maintain desirable growth parameters then supplemental nutrition with polymeric or defined enteral formulas by nasogastric tube (often provided nocturnally) may be instituted and on a short term basis has proved very beneficial. The long-term use of NG feeding often leads to non-compliance however and if supplemental nutrition is still required on a chronic basis, then consideration of placement of an enterostomy tube should be undertaken. Nocturnal gastrostomy or jejunostomy feeding of a long-term nature is being undertaken with benefit more frequently in malnourished patients with cystic fibrosis.[51] Gastrostomy tube feeding post double lung transplant for cystic fibrosis is associated with better weight gain than oral intake alone in the first year post transplant.[52]

Children with other severe chronic pulmonary diseases and especially those awaiting lung transplantation also require close nutritional observation and early institution of supplemental feeding by the enteral route if required.[53] Avoidance of parenteral nutrition is preferred because of the additional risks of sepsis and the contribution of highly concentrated intravenous glucose sources to hypercapnia. Maintenance of a positive energy balance pre-transplant is important in the clinical outcome of children following lung transplantation.[54]

Renal disease

Children with renal failure, particularly those in which the disease was congenital or acquired in infancy, frequently exhibit impaired nutritional status and developmental delay. This may occur because of metabolic acidosis, chronic electrolyte disturbances, protein-calorie malnutrition, endocrine abnormalities, osteodystrophy, gastroesophageal reflux and delayed gastric emptying. Nutritional supplementation during peritoneal dialysis (PD) and nasogastric or gastrostomy feeding have been safe and associated with improved outcomes including neurological development.[55–57] Gastrostomy tubes have often been placed at the same time as Tenckhoff catheter insertion for PD and need to be placed before cycling PD is started. Gastrostomy buttons may be placed safely as early as 4 weeks post PEG insertion,[58] though many clinicians prefer to wait longer (8–12 weeks). Nocturnal nasogastric feeding for up to 12 h a day has resulted in catch-up growth and normalization of weight parameters, especially if started before the age of 2 years.[59] The importance of early preventive intervention must be emphasized as it can be difficult to repair chronic deficits later.

Neurological disease

The nutritional impact of neurological disease is variable and depends on the severity and distribution of the disability involved. Determinants include the ability to orally feed and swallow, hyper or hypotonia, mobility, severity of impairment, cognitive ability and gastrointestinal complications of neurologic dysfunction including gastroesophageal reflux, delayed gastric emptying and constipation.[60] Children with cerebral palsy involving spastic quadriparesis and cognitive delay frequently are unable to achieve sufficient caloric intake to maintain growth and development and will thus require chronic enteral feeding via a permanent enterostomy.[61,62] Recent publications have emphasized the need for new methods of assessing resting energy expenditure in non-ambulatory tube-fed patients with severe neurodevelopmental disabilities and have led to a downward assessment of energy needs.[63] However increased energy needs may be seen in the face of choreoathetosis or with severe contractures. Chronic, progressive neurological diseases especially of a degenerative nature usually also require nutritional intervention and support for the duration of life. Feeding in these severe cases usually occurs via continuous nocturnal gastrostomy feeding with bolus supplements if tolerated in the daytime. The risk of aspiration from above due to swallowing dysfunction and from below due to GERD will determine the choice of feeding route. Considerations with regard to the composition of feeding include fluid intake (since often not enough free water is provided), caloric density, osmolality and fiber intake in such children. If it is anticipated that a transition to oral feeding may occur, then adequate oral stimulation, even of a non-nutritive nature, should be provided.

Oncologic disease and bone marrow transplantation

The systemic effects of malignant disease, the side effects of necessary treatment involving chemotherapy and radiotherapy and complications such as sepsis contribute to malnutrition in the pediatric oncology patient.[64] Cachexia with significant weight loss and growth failure may occur as a result of increased metabolic rate and circulating cytokines (TNF-α, interleukin-1 and interleukin-6) inducing anorexia, increased whole body protein breakdown, increased lipolysis and increased gluconeogenesis. Food intake may be reduced as a consequence of nausea, vomiting, dysgeusia, mucositis and xerostomia. Acute illnesses such as neutropenic fever and infections place further nutritional stress on the child with oncologic disease by increasing metabolic rate and catabolism. Some children may suffer palatal and pharyngeal dysfunction with subsequent swallowing difficulties as a result of radiotherapy to the head and neck. Children with intestinal lymphomas and other intestinal tumors may suffer malabsorption and subacute obstruction, which can often still be supported with enteral nutrition. Emphasis is now being placed on 'room service' for patients at significant risk, with good nutritional choices of whole foods available in a 'just-in-time' fashion on the oncology unit itself and where possible the fresh food itself cooked locally rather than centrally. Nutritional difficulties often stress the child and parents from a psychological perspective and a multidisciplinary approach to the support of the family is required, with careful preparation for supplemental enteral feeding by the nasal or enterostomal approach. Percutaneous endoscopic gastrostomy for chronic nutritional support is effective and safe if performed in oncology patients when they are not neutropenic, thrombocytopenic or septic.[65]

Nutritional insult after bone marrow transplantation is common since the conditioning and treatment regimes cause considerable gastrointestinal disturbance, nausea and vomiting and mucositis may be severe. Enteral feeding is both cheaper and easier to provide than parenteral nutrition and avoids venous catheter-related complications.[66,67] Intense multidisciplinary counseling is necessary to ensure success as tubes may need to be replaced and mucositis may cause significant pain requiring morphine infusion. Children undergoing bone marrow transplantation benefit from early enteral feeding with improved weight gain and anthropometric parameters.[68] Interestingly diarrhea does not seem to be more of a problem with enteral feeding compared with TPN and common micronutrient deficiencies such as hypomagnesemia, hypophosphatemia, zinc and selenium deficiency are not different between enteral and parenterally fed children.

HYPERMETABOLIC STATES

HIV/AIDS

Pediatric patients with human immunodeficiency virus infection/acquired immunodeficiency syndrome (HIV/AIDS) are often at risk nutritionally since inflammatory processes and sepsis associated with the condition elevate metabolic rate and the side effects of the drugs required for management of the disease often give rise to nausea, vomiting and diarrhea limiting intake. Protein-calorie malnutrition and malabsorption are relatively common in children with established AIDS and often require nutritional support via nasogastric or gastrostomy feeding.[69] In addition, such tubes may be required to administer the drugs since children frequently find them unpalatable. Malnutrition itself may further impair immune function. Micronutrient deficiencies including zinc, iron, selenium, B_2, B_6, B_{12}, carnitine, vitamin A, vitamin D and essential fatty acids may occur and vitamin B_{12} and vitamin A deficiency may influence the rate of mother-to-infant transmission of the disease in developing countries.[70] Micronutrient repletion may slow progression of the disease, increasing growth and T lymphocyte function in the case of zinc. Energy repletion may increase the CD4 count.[71] Antiviral treatment with protease inhibitors is important, as decreased viral load correlates with a positive outcome in nutritional support.[72]

Head injury, trauma and surgery

Children with uncomplicated severe, closed head injuries have been demonstrated to have resting energy expenditures similar to patients with burns and require appropriate enteral support usually given via nasojejunal tube in the ICU while ventilated, nasogastric tube on the ward once stable from a cardiorespiratory point of view, or by gastrostomy feeding if the duration is likely to exceed 2 months. In the surgical patient, postoperative enteral feeding has been associated with reduced sepsis, improved wound healing, enhanced gut mucosal barrier function and increased mass of gut-associated lymphoid tissue (GALT) as well as prevention of bacterial translocation. Post trauma surgical patients may benefit with improved nitrogen balance and nutritional status if fed early in the postoperative phase via the enteral route, although the choice of route and type of feeding is determined by the operative intervention. Early provision of enteral nutrition even in the face of gut resection by trans-pyloric and trans-anastomotic routes has been advocated for the neonate (premature or otherwise) undergoing gut resection for necrotizing enterocolitis, volvulus or congenital malformation.[73] The child undergoing orthopedic spinal manipulation is at risk for superior mesenteric artery syndrome, which may be obviated by feeding distal to the relative obstruction. Any child expected to have limited oral intake of greater than 5 days duration or sooner if at nutritional risk prior to surgery should have supplemental enteral nutrition provided as soon as feasible postoperatively.

Burns

Early enteral nutritional support is believed to improve gastrointestinal, immunological, nutritional and metabolic responses to critical injury in burned patients.[74] Enteral feeding has been shown to reduce caloric deficits and promote insulin secretion and protein retention.[75] Gut-derived endotoxemia and increased intestinal permeability are also improved by early feeding after thermal injury and reduce the rate of enterogenic sepsis.[76] Indeed, intolerance to enteral feeding has been seen as an early marker preceding overt sepsis.[77] In adult studies early successful enteral feeding after burn injury has been associated with significantly decreased mortality. In very young children with mild to moderate burns (8–25% BSA) who nevertheless had hypermetabolism with REEs averaging 130% of normal, early enteral feeding normalized protein status and significantly increased energy intake.[78] Immediate enteral feeding following burn injury even in ventilated patients has been shown to be safe and effective without an increase in aspiration through the judicious use of nasojejunal and nasogastric feeding.[79] Most severely burned children require frequent surgery for wound debridement and skin grafts and the promotion of enteral feeding through the extensive perioperative period has been associated with a reduction in caloric deficits, wound infections and requirement for exogenous albumin supplementation.[80] Early in the post-burn period a hydrolyzed defined formula may be helpful if a polymeric formula is not well tolerated, with emphasis on a high-protein, high-calorie intake.

Metabolic disease

Glycogen storage disease type 1 usually requires the institution of nocturnal supplementation, usually with cornstarch, to prevent hypoglycemia and to reduce hypertriglyceridemia. Other metabolic syndromes require specialized formulas to treat the disease and avoid the effects of accumulated toxic substrates. A team approach to the management of these children is advocated with strong input from the nutrition support service.

CHOICE OF ENTERAL FEEDING ROUTE

Oral feeding

The choice of feeding route depends upon the functional status of the child.[81] Even when adequate intake cannot be achieved in total by mouth, preservation of this route of feeding for even partial nutrition is recommended as it preserves normal physiology and function and is psychologically satisfying for the child and family. Coma, ventilation, head and neck trauma or tumors, severe mucositis following chemotherapy, impaired swallowing mechanisms and risk for aspiration may preclude this route of feeding.

Enteral feeding

Once the requirement has been established, enteral feeding may be provided for the patient with short-term needs, for example, after trauma or during a bout of severe pancreatitis. It may be necessary to continue nutrition support for prolonged periods of time such as with chronic renal or liver disease or indefinitely in the case of patients with chronic neurological dysfunction. The type of feeding required and the route by which it is provided, depend upon the individual circumstances of the child but in general the use of nasoenteric tubes is preferred where the time required for nutritional support is likely to be short (less than 8 weeks) and enterostomy tubes are preferred for long-term use. The gastric route is preferred over delivery into the jejunum to maintain gastric barrier function and the normal pulsatile delivery of nutrients to the small bowel. However, patients in coma, requiring ventilatory support and pharmacologically paralyzed, at risk of aspiration, with severe gastroesophageal reflux or delayed gastric emptying, or with pancreatitis may require jejunal feeding which must be given continuously to avoid over-distension and the metabolic equivalent of dumping syndrome. Long-term jejunal feeding is difficult from a practical perspective, especially at home, where tubes may be frequently dislodged accidentally.

Polyvinyl nasogastric tubes may only be used for a few days before they become stiff and traumatizing to the nares and thus should only be used for very short-term feeding, or changed frequently. Tubes made of silicone or polyurethane can be used for prolonged periods and are soft, comfortable and flexible.[82] Polyurethane tubes have a greater internal diameter than silicone tubes for the same external diameter and therefore may block less easily. Such tubes often have weighted tips theoretically to allow for easier onward passage into the duodenum or jejunum and to prevent easy dislodgement. However, studies have shown that such weighting is probably unnecessary and some weights may be too large to allow easy passage into the small bowel.[83] Tube sizes between 5–8 Fr are appropriate for most pediatric indications and patients and caregivers trained in their placement. With appropriate psychological support even very young children can be trained to place their own tubes.

Children with a chronic requirement for enteral nutrition support beyond two months should be considered for placement of a gastrostomy tube.[84] In most cases this may be achieved by placement of a percutaneous gastrostomy tube endoscopically (PEG) or radiologically and both types are generally associated with less complications than surgically-placed tubes.[85] Care should be exercised in patients with ventriculoperitoneal shunts and PEG should probably only be performed if the shunt is placed in the right side of the abdomen. Percutaneous gastrostomy placement may be contraindicated in patients who have had previous upper abdominal surgery, have significant ascites, portal hypertension, or hepatosplenomegaly, in the presence of an abdominal tumor or in obesity. The main complication of cellulitis occurring after PEG placement can be prevented by a single dose of intravenous broad-spectrum antibiotic given at the time of placement and avoidance of tension on the outer bolster. However, confirmation of the tube in the stomach, preferably endoscopically, should occur before it is used. Mechanical irritation of the stomach may occur with any tube and intermittent blockage of the pylorus may occur in those that can migrate such as Malechot or Foley catheters placed surgically.

Gastrostomy buttons may be placed usually 6–8 weeks after primary tube placement, sometimes without anesthesia if the tube is traction-removable. The time interval should probably be longer, up to 12 weeks, in patients who are significantly immunocompromised and may have poor wound healing. Button gastrostomies are preferred by most families since they lie flush to the skin and therefore cannot be easily pulled out and tubing is just attached by a locking method at the time of feeding. Those with inflatable internal bolsters are less traumatic to place and remove but are more prone to breakage than those with deformable internal bolsters which may tear, disrupt the tract or cause perforation (2%). Some children at significant risk of aspiration due to GERD, particularly those with neurological impairment, may require a surgical anti-reflux procedure with or without a pyloroplasty for delayed gastric emptying and a surgically-placed gastrostomy.[86] Such patients might also be successfully managed by placement of a gastro-jejunal tube but this is usually difficult to sustain on a long-term basis. However, unless the symptoms of GERD are severe and/or aspiration has already occurred, it is preferred to assess the patients first by way of a trial of nasogastric feeding. If this is tolerated, it is likely that fundoplication is not required at that time, although it may be in the future.

Jejunal tubes may be placed nasally, via a gastrostomy or directly into the jejunum by a percutaneous or surgical approach. The nasojejunal route is preferred for short-term feeding, but tubes are easily dislodged and difficult to replace. Placement of jejunal tubes through existing gastrostomy tubes is feasible either endoscopically or radiologically, but there are few products suitable for use in children and the jejunal tubes to fit within existing gastrostomy tubes are often too long without any easy method for shortening.[87] However, with sufficient ingenuity a solution can usually be fashioned. For long-term use, a surgically placed jejunostomy tube may be a good alternative.

CHOICE OF FEEDING METHOD (CONTINUOUS, NOCTURNAL OR BOLUS FEEDING)

In general, intermittent bolus feeding is preferred to continuous feeding, as it is more practical, more physiologic in providing a pulsatile delivery of nutrients to the GI tract and requires much less in the way of supplies. The feed is usually delivered over 15–20 min as if the food was being delivered orally and may be given at increasing time intervals as the volume of each feed is increased. It is also not unusual in transitional states to have the child continually fed nocturnally and to have bolus feeding or even oral feeding in the daytime, again mainly for practical reasons. Many studies have shown that patients often can tolerate bolus feeding more readily than appreciated and several studies in premature infants, in critically ill children and those who have undergone surgery have suggested that it is as well tolerated as continuous feeding without a significant difference in outcomes. Thus, bolus feeding should be attempted early and only abandoned if it is met with intolerance (vomiting, retching, increased gastric residuals, aspiration).

Continuous feeding is required for those patients who are intolerant of bolus feeding, or who may be transitioning from parenteral or jejunal feeding. Nocturnal continuous nasogastric feeding is frequently used for the patient with a requirement for chronic nutritional support as it may free them for oral or bolus feeding in the daytime. It is particularly useful for patients with significant intestinal dysfunction and malabsorption and those with protracted diarrhea. Patients on jejunal feeds also require continuous feeding as mentioned above. Continuous feeding requires more supplies in terms of feeding tubes and pumps for the delivery of the feed are more technologically demanding on the family and the nutrition support team. Care must be taken to ensure adequate support for families using pumps, as failures almost inevitably happen on nights or weekends. Continuous feeding is therefore both more resource-intensive and expensive than bolus feeding. The specifics of formula choice under different circumstances are covered in the next section (Fig. 75.1).

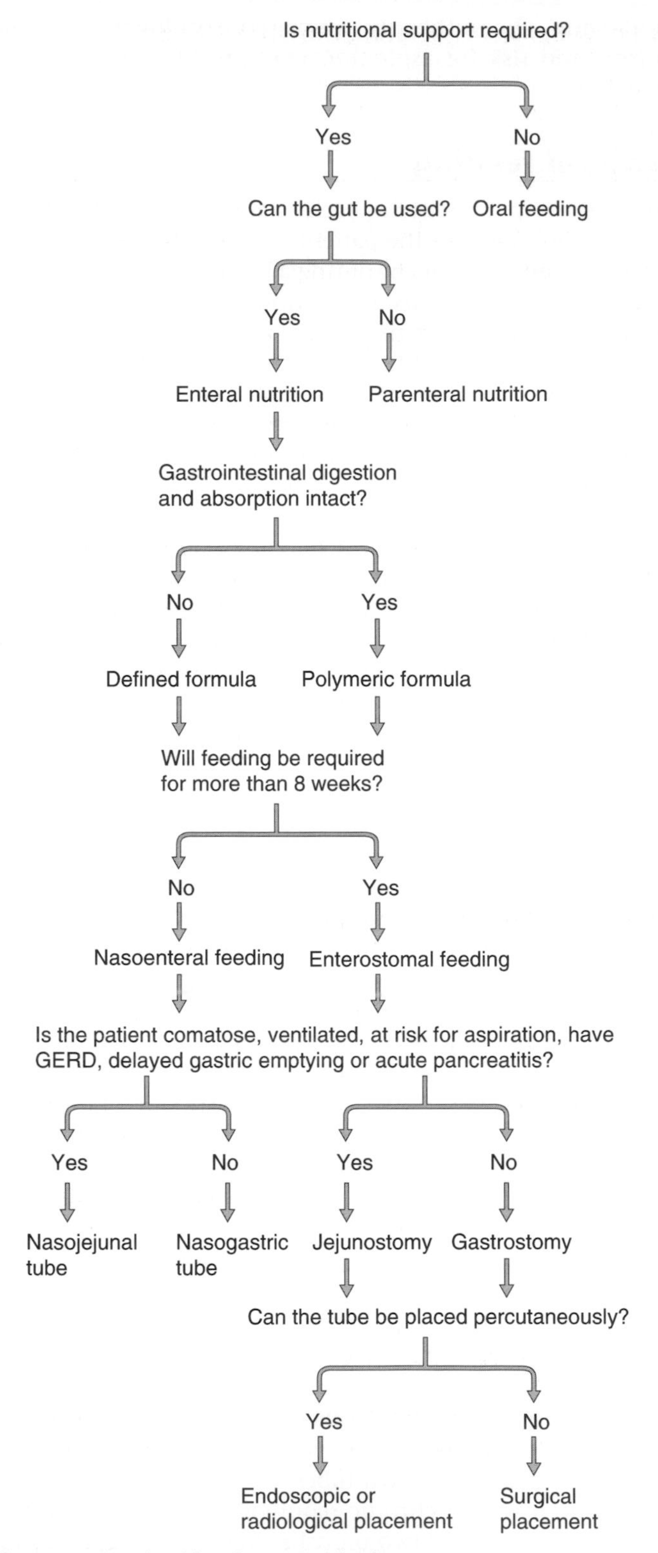

Figure 75.1: Algorithm for enteral feeding.

ENTERAL NUTRITION IN THE NEONATE

With the development of neonatal care over the past 30 years, increasing attention is being paid to the role of adequate nutrition on both short- and long-term outcomes. Enteral nutrition support is an important tool in the neonatal intensive care unit, delivering nutrients to the gastrointestinal tract when oral feeding is limited by prematurity or illness.[88–91]

Minimal enteral nutrition

The approach to enteral nutrition will vary depending on the gestational age and clinical status of the individual infant. Infants deemed too ill to begin regular, progressively increased feeds may receive 'priming' or 'minimal enteral feeds'. In this approach, infants receive very small volumes of milk – usually 10–20 ml/kg per day – either continuously or intermittently. Although these volumes contribute minimally to energy and macronutrient intake, they appear to be beneficial in improving later feeding tolerance and gut function.[92–94] This may be based on the maintenance of more normal mucosal architecture, motility or mucosal function. If an infant is unstable and unable to increase feeds, these low volume feeds may be maintained until clinical status improves.

Progression of enteral nutrition

Once the infant attains cardiorespiratory stability, enteral feeds are incrementally advanced by 10–50 ml/kg per day, depending on the birthweight of the infant, tolerance and clinical status.[95] In general, approximately 150 ml/kg per day will provide adequate energy and nutrients to support appropriate growth, but this is variable depending on the clinical status of the individual infant.[96]

Continuous *vs* bolus feeds

While both methods of administration may effectively deliver formula to the growing premature infant, theory and evidence exist to support each as the superior approach. Continuous feeds offer the advantage of using the smallest possible volume, resulting in less gastric and abdominal distention and potentially, less pulmonary compromise. Despite this potential benefit, some studies have demonstrated no adverse effects on pulmonary parameters during bolus feeds.[97] It has been postulated that episodes of apnea and bradycardia may be reduced during continuous compared with bolus feeds, but evidence is inconsistent.[98] It has also been argued that bolus feeds trigger a more physiologic series of events by stimulating hormonal responses that increase motility, gallbladder contraction and pancreatic enzyme release.[99,100] It is possible that this sequence of events results in more effective digestion and absorption of nutrients and may minimize the effects of complications such as neonatal cholestasis.[101] Although these issues have been examined by systematic review, the evidence was insufficient to support the benefits of one approach over the other.[98] Practice varies between neonatal units and may be based on experience within the unit and the clinical evaluation of individual infants. If continuous feeds are used for a prolonged period of time, the transition to bolus feeds may be achieved by gradually shortening the infusion time and lengthening the time between feeds. This may be useful in supporting a gradual increase in gastric volume and lessening the risk of intolerance, but this has not been scientifically evaluated.[102]

Choice of feeding

All neonatal units strongly support the use of expressed mother's milk as the food of choice for all neonates.[103] Mothers are encouraged and supported to begin milk expression as soon as possible after delivery. Milk may be used fresh, or may be refrigerated or frozen for later use. Mother's milk presents some unique challenges when it is delivered by tube. Fat separates readily and may adhere to syringes and tubing, decreasing the amount which reaches the baby.[104] Positioning the syringe with the tip directed upward and limiting the frequency of syringe and tubing changes (while maintaining standards consistent with bacteriologic safety) may be useful in decreasing fat loss, but optimal practice to maximize fat delivery has not yet been clarified.

Human milk fortifiers

Despite the many benefits of mother's milk, particularly to the vulnerable premature infant, it is clear that mother's milk alone is insufficient to meet the extremely high needs of the growing premature infant. In particular, protein, calcium and phosphorus and sodium needs exceed the availability in mother's milk at usual intakes. Human milk fortifiers have been developed to address this issue and, when added to expressed milk, support improved growth compared with that attained with unsupplemented mother's milk.[105,106] All preparations currently available are cow's milk based and may be liquid or powdered formulations. Although either preparation is acceptable, recently reported deaths due to infection related to use of powdered products have raised concerns regarding handling and administration procedures when using these products.[107] Initially, mother's milk alone is used to begin enteral feeding. Once the infant has become established at or near full-volume feeds, fortifier is added in a gradual fashion.

Formulas

If mother's milk is unavailable, infants will receive infant formula (Table 75.2). In addition to the standard infant formulas described, specially designed premature formulas which provide increased protein, calcium, phosphorus, sodium and variable micronutrients support superior growth outcomes in premature infants compared with standard term formula (Table 75.3). Furthermore, this improvement in growth may be accompanied by improved neurodevelopmental outcomes.[108–110] There is some evidence that feeding a formula with hydrolyzed protein may accelerate the gastrointestinal response to feeding in very

Formula type	Protein (g/l)	Carbohydrate (g/l)	Fat (g/l)
Term infant formula	17.8 (14–21)	71.6 (67–78)	35 (30–37)
Premature 20 kcal/oz formula	19 (18–20)	72.5 (72–73)	35.5 (34–37)
Premature 24 kcal/oz formula	23 (22–24)	86.5 (86–87)	42 (40–44)

Table 75.2 Comparison of macronutrient concentration of term formulas, premature 20 kcal/oz formulas and premature 24 kcal/oz formulas expressed as mean value (range)

Formula type	Na (mEq/l)	K (mEq/l)	Ca (mg/l)	PO4 (mg/l)	Mg (mg/l)	Vitamin D (IU/l)	Vitamin A (IU/l)	Fe (mg/l)
Term infant formula	11 (7–14)	20 (7–27)	664 (435–827)	457 (245–621)	65 (48–83)	395 (300–580)	2057 (1200–2727)	11.8 (10.2–12)
Premature 20 kcal/oz formula	15 (13–17)	19.5 (17–22)	1158 (1100–1216)	615 (553–676)	70 (60–80)	1307 (1014–1600)	8389 (8333–8445)	12.1 (12–12.2)
Premature 24 kcal/oz formula	17.5 (15–20)	23.5 (20–27)	1391 (1320–1463)	738 (664–813)	97 (96–98)	1569 (1219–1920)	10082 (10000–10163)	14.5 (14–15)

Table 75.3 Comparison of micronutrient concentration of term formulas, premature 20 kcal/oz formulas and premature 24 kcal/oz formulas expressed as mean value (range)

low-birthweight infants, but currently not enough evidence to change standard practice.[111,112] Standard infant formula and premature formula are compared below.

Transition to oral feeds

For the ill term infant in the intensive care unit, the transition to oral feeds will be directed by the clinical status of the infant. In order to initiate oral feeds, cardiorespiratory stability is mandatory. The infant must tolerate the handling associated with feeds without compromising this stability. Although infants may feed safely while receiving supplemental oxygen, it may be hazardous to do so if continuous positive airway pressure or high-flow oxygen are necessary to maintain oxygen saturations. These methods of respiratory support may compromise the ability of the infant to coordinate sucking, swallowing and breathing and increase the risk of pulmonary aspiration. Bolus feeds must be established prior to beginning oral feeds and the baby must demonstrate appropriate sucking behavior, be neurologically alert and ideally demonstrate appropriate hunger cues. Initial feedings in particular must be carefully observed by an experienced caregiver to determine the safety and efficacy of oral feeding.

Premature infants will most often be unable to begin oral feeds prior to approximately 32–34 weeks gestational age, due to immature coordination of sucking, swallowing and breathing. After that, the determination of feeding readiness will be based on clinical criteria as described above. The introduction of 'kangaroo care' (skin to skin handling between mother and infant) and nuzzling at a pumped breast may be useful in supporting successful breast-feeding and can begin whenever the infant can tolerate these activities.[113] Initially breast-feeding or bottle feeding must be introduced gradually (initially once or twice per day) to prevent exhaustion of the infant and facilitate progressive success. Once a significant volume of mother's milk or formula is consumed orally, enteral feeding may be reduced by a corresponding amount. Similarly, if the infant is unable to consume the expected volume orally, the remainder of the volume may be provided enterally to ensure sufficient energy intake to maintain growth.

ENTERAL FEEDING IN THE INFANT AND CHILD

One of the more challenging tasks in providing enteral nutrition support is to select from an ever-increasing variety of products those best suited to the needs of individual patients. The choice of enteral formulas should be the result of a systematic, detailed assessment of patient requirements based as much as possible on objective information. A thorough knowledge of available formulas is essential to facilitate a formula choice that most closely matches requirements. Additional modifications may be made when required to meet specialized requirements. This process can be approached in a stepwise fashion, as outlined below.

Patient evaluation

In order to provide appropriate enteral nutrition support, it is critical to begin with an analysis of the needs of the individual patient and goals of therapy. Although nutritional evaluation has previously been described in detail (Ch 72), it is worthwhile emphasizing two specific aspects relevant to enteral nutrition support. First, quantitative needs for energy, macro- and micro-nutrients and fluid must be estimated as accurately as possible to minimize the risks of under- or over-nutrition. Second, the patient's ability to digest and absorb nutrients must be determined in order to determine qualitative nutrient requirements and minimize the risk of adverse events related to enteral feeding.

Selecting the formula category to meet quantitative requirements

Formulas suitable for enteral feeding are categorized as infant, pediatric or adult. The first step in selecting a formula is to identify the formula category that most closely approximates the patient's needs. Infant formulas are intended to meet normal requirements of infants to 1 year of age, pediatric formulas are generally suitable for children from 1–10 years and adult formulas may be utilized thereafter. However, while these age ranges provide a useful guide for formula selection, they should not be rigidly adhered to. The most appropriate formula will be that which most closely meets the estimated needs of the individual patient, regardless of age.[114]

Within the infant and pediatric categories, the composition of formulas is quantitatively very similar across products. Much greater variation occurs among adult formulas, in order to meet the specialized needs of various patient groups. In general, progression from infant to adult formulas results in increasing protein and carbohydrate content and decreasing fat content, consistent with recommended dietary intakes across the lifespan. While this generalization holds true for 'standard' adult formulas, many exceptions occur within this category such as 'high protein' or low carbohydrate (and thus higher fat) 'diabetic' formulas. Caloric density is generally greater in formulas intended for pediatric or adult patients than in infant formulas and this results in a corresponding increase in osmolality. As caloric density increases, nutritional requirements may be met with smaller volumes of formula. While this may be a distinct advantage where fluid intake is restricted, it may also result in the need for additional fluids to be provided to meet daily fluid requirements. Table 75.4 shows the types of enteral formula available for infants and children and the conditions under which they may be used. This is meant to be illustrative rather than exhaustive. Composition of formulas may change rapidly and without notice and the reader is advised to consult the product monograph or manufacturer's website for precise details. Table 75.5 compares average energy density, macronutrient content and osmolalities of infant, pediatric and standard adult formulas as well as some specialty adult formulas.

Selecting the formula category to meet qualitative requirements

Enteral nutrition support in its simplest form is merely a delivery system to overcome limitations of oral intake. This implies that all other gastrointestinal functions, i.e. digestion, absorption, motility and elimination, are intact and will function normally when nutrients are delivered into the stomach. In fact, derangements of any or all of the above functions are extremely common in children requiring enteral nutrition support and these abnormalities may have implications for formula selection. In addition,

Infant formulas	Pediatric formulas	Adolescent formulas
Milk-based, whole protein (WP)	Milk-based, WP, lactose-free	Milk-based, WP, lactose-free
Enfamil (with and without Fe)	*PediaSure*	*Ensure*
Similac (with and without iron)	*PediaSure* with fiber	*Ensure* with fiber
Gerber infant formula (with and without Fe)	*Nutren Junior*	Isocal
Soy protein-based, lactose-free	Peptide-based with MCT	Nutren 1.0, 1.5 and 2.0
Enfamil ProSoBee	Peptamen Junior	Nutren with fiber
Similac Isomil	Amino-acid based with MCT	Jevity
Carnation Alsoy	Vivonex Pediatric	Osmolite
Gerber Soy	Elecare	Sustacal
Partially hydrolyzed whey protein (not for CMP allergy)	Amino-acid-based with LCT	Peptide-based
Carnation Good Start	Neocate One+	Peptamen
Casein hydrolysate+ LCT (CMP Allergy, SBS)		Criticare HN
Nutramigen		Reabilan
Casein hydrolysate + MCT (Malabsorption, SBS)		AlitraQ
Pregestimil		Impact (with fish oil)
Alimentum		Peptide-based with MCT
High MCT (lymphangiectasia, chylous ascites)		Peptamen
Portagen		Lipisorb
Amino-acid based (allergy, SBS)		Reabilan
Neocate (+LCT)		AlitraQ
Elecare (+MCT)		Amino-acid based
		Vivonex TEN
		Tolerex
		Amin-Aid
		Specialized adult formulas
		Pulmocare (lung disease)
		Glucerna (diabetes)
		Hepatic-Aid II (liver disease)
		Travasorb Renal (kidney disease)

NB: Some Mead Johnson infant formulas now include DHA and ARA in the form of LIPIL®, and Ross formulas with similar supplementation are marketed under the brand name Similac ADVANCE®. Nestle formula names include DHA and ARA. CMP Allergy, Cow's milk protein allergy; SBS, short bowel syndrome.

Table 75.4 Selected enteral feeding products available in North America, their composition and uses

Category	Protein (g/l)	Fat (g/l)	Carbohydrate (g/l)	Energy (kcal/100ml)	Osmolality (mmol/kg H_2O)
Infant	17.7 (14–28)	35 (30–37)	71.5 (67–78)	67	294 (200–375)
Pediatric	29.8 (24–38)	41.1 (24–50)	127.5 (104–146)	100 (80–106)	448 (290–820)
Standard adult	45 (34–56)	35.8 (17–46)	152.9 (135–170)	109 (100–120)	383 (270–600)
Adult low fat	44 (38–63)	17 (2.8–39)	173 (105–220)	101 (100–106)	493 (270–650)
Adult high calorie	70.7 (60–90)	64.9 (22.8–106)	188.7 (150–220)	159.8 (128–200)	567.2 (385–790)
Adult pulmonary	62.7 (62.4–63)	93.3 (92.8–93.7)	106 (105.5–106.4)	150	490
Adult diabetes	53 (42–64)	51 (47–55)	96 (95–97)	103 (100–106)	412.5 (375–450)
Adult renal	72 (70–74)	98 (96–100)	210 (200–220)	200	652 (665–700)

Table 75.5 Summary of macronutrient content, energy content and osmolality within categories of formulas suitable for enteral feeding expressed as mean value (range)

allergy or other adverse reaction may require that formula be selected to eliminate the suspected trigger. The most significant differences between formulas suitable for enteral administration is among the form in which macronutrients are provided.

Protein

Formulas may provide nitrogen in any of three forms: intact protein, peptides of varying chain length or free amino acids.

Intact protein

Often referred to as 'polymeric,' these formulas contain large intact protein molecules, which require digestion prior to absorption by the small intestine. Infant and adult formulas may be based on either cow's milk protein or soy protein. All currently available pediatric products are cow's milk-based. Because plant protein is partly contained within cell walls resistant to digestion by human digestive enzymes, soy protein bioavailability is reduced compared with that of cow's milk protein. For this reason, the protein content of soy-based formulas is slightly higher than that of cow's milk formulas to provide equivalent utilizable protein. This is most evident when comparing infant formulas, where there is otherwise little variability in protein content between products. Cow's milk is modified for use in all products and is often provided as calcium or sodium caseinates. Whey protein concentrate may also be included or may be the primary protein source. The inclusion of whey in infant formulas more closely resembles the protein profile found in human milk. In addition, whey-based formulas may enhance gastric emptying to a moderate degree.[115,116] Although whey protein is partially hydrolyzed, whey-protein-based formulas contain significant concentrations of intact cow's milk protein and have provoked serious reactions in many allergic infants.[117] Partially hydrolyzed whey-based formulas should therefore not be used in infants with documented cow's milk protein allergy.

Protein hydrolysates

Protein may also be provided in a 'partially digested' form consisting entirely or mainly of peptides. These formulas are referred to as 'extensively hydrolyzed' and contain small peptides of <1500 Da, equivalent to approximately 8–12 amino acid residues. These formulas meet established clinical criteria for hypoallergenicity and are appropriate for most children with cow's milk allergy. However, even these short peptides require digestion by pancreatic carboxypeptidases and/or mucosal aminopeptidases to produce free amino acids, di- and tri-peptides, which can then be transported into the enterocyte.

Free amino acid

These formulas contain only free amino acids and require no digestion prior to intestinal absorption. In addition, the absence of intact protein and peptides eliminates the possibility of allergic reaction in those children with cow's milk protein allergy.

Carbohydrate

Carbohydrate may be provided in formula as complex carbohydrate (starch), disaccharides or simple sugars (glucose or glucose polymers).

Complex carbohydrate (starch)

Complex carbohydrate may be included in formulas in a digestible form as a source of energy, or in a largely non-digestible form as a source of fiber. Digestible carbohydrates will most often be identified as starch (often cornstarch) or as maltodextrin, which is a modified starch with enhanced solubility and digestibility. These products will require the action of pancreatic amylase for initial digestion and mucosal oligosaccharidases for final digestion prior to absorption.

Non-digestible carbohydrates

Non-digestible carbohydrates in a variety of forms may be added to formulas primarily for their effect on intestinal motility. Fiber which is soluble and viscous in nature will form a gel within the stomach and will effectively delay gastric emptying and nutrient absorption, effects which may be used to advantage in various clinical settings. The fiber then passes undigested into the colon, but there is fermented by colonic bacteria to various short-chain fatty acids. These can be used as an energy source either locally by colonic cells, or transported for use elsewhere in the body. Thus soluble fiber, while classified as non-digestible carbohydrate, does make a small contribution to the energy provided by carbohydrate. Fiber which behaves in this way will be most commonly identified as a gum or pectin or soy fiber. Recently, formulas containing fructo-oligosaccharides (FOS) and/or gum arabic (a soluble, but non-viscous fiber) have become available. These compounds have no significant effect on gastric motility, but their presence in the colon influences the composition of colonic flora.[10] As *Bifidobacteria* and *Lactobacilli* possess the enzymes to utilize these compounds, their growth is promoted,[118] while the growth of *Escherichia coli* and *Clostridium perfringens* (which do not possess these enzymes) are suppressed. It is postulated that these additives may protect against gastrointestinal infection, or enhance recovery from antibiotic associated diarrhea, as has been shown in an animal model.[119] Insoluble fiber has no significant effect on upper intestinal motility but exerts its most significant effect in the colon. As it is resistant to digestion by colonic bacteria, it remains intact during its passage through the colon. This contributes bulk to the stools, but also increases their water content. These effects result in decreased colonic transit time and improvement in constipation.[120] Because insoluble fiber remains undigested, it makes no contribution to the energy content of formula. Fiber which acts in this way is most often identified as cellulose, lignin or hemicellulose. Many enteral products include a combination of soluble and insoluble fiber.

Fat

All fat included in formula is provided in the form of triglyceride and will be identifiable on product labels as oils. The oils most commonly found in formulas include high oleic sunflower, soybean, canola, corn, safflower and palm olein. All of these oils provide triglyceride composed of long-chain fatty acids and are a source of essential fatty acids. Although the specific fatty acid composition differs between the oils, these differences are not clinically significant. In addition, formulas may contain coconut oil or MCT (medium-chain triglyceride) oil, as a variable proportion of the total fat content. These oils are preferentially digested by pancreatic lipase and the resulting fatty acids are readily absorbed without the need for micellar solubilization. In addition, MCT may also be absorbed intact into the enterocyte, subsequently undergoing hydrolysis intracellularly. Thus MCT is utilized more effectively than long chain fat in the setting of pancreatic insufficiency and/or cholestasis. It must be recognized that essential fatty acid requirements cannot be met by MCT oil alone, as essential fatty acids are all of long chain length. A source of long chain fat must be included in order to prevent essential fatty acid deficiency. A recent development in infant formula production in North America has been the inclusion of *C. cohnii* oil and *M. alpina* oil. These oils are sources of docosahexanoic acid (DHA) and arachidonic acid (ARA), respectively. Although these fatty acids may be produced endogenously in older children and adults by elongation and desaturation of alpha linolenic and linoleic acids, their presence in human milk prompted questions as to the efficiency of this process in infants. Several studies have now demonstrated small but significant gains in developmental scores and visual acuity in infants receiving formula supplemented with docosahexanoic acid and arachidonic acid.[121–123]

Modular products

Despite the wide range of products currently available, it is sometimes useful to modify existing formulas to tailor them more specifically to individual patient requirements. Modular products – preparations of fat, carbohydrate or protein alone – are designed for this purpose. It should be emphasized that modular products are not nutritionally complete formulas, but merely provide an additional source of an individual macronutrient to be added to a complete formula. Protein modulars may contain intact protein as found in complete formulas, or free amino acids only. Amino acid preparations may contain either a full complement of amino acids, or essential amino acids alone. The amino acids arginine and glutamine are also available, either individually or in combination, although the clinical indications for their use remain to be clarified. Carbohydrate modulars may be used to increase the caloric density of formulas and consist mainly of glucose polymers. In addition either soluble or insoluble fiber may be added for specific clinical effects as described earlier. Additional fat may be provided by the addition of MCT oil or oils containing long-chain fatty acids. While a specialized preparation of safflower oil is available for tube feeding, formulas may also be supplemented with readily available cooking oils such as canola oil. While the addition of these products to formulas may allow very precise adaptation of enteral nutrition to patient needs, they should be used judiciously to ensure that the additional cost and labor required for preparation and administration are justified by patient outcome. Table 75.6 summarizes some of the currently available modular products and their constituents.

PRACTICAL ISSUES OF ENTERAL NUTRITION

Calculating formula needs

A thorough nutritional assessment of children who require enteral feeding should be performed by a pediatric registered dietitian along with a medical evaluation by the healthcare team.[124] Energy, protein and nutrient needs must first be determined. Energy and protein is required for both maintenance of body metabolism as well as for growth in children. Caloric requirements in children may be calculated in various ways, including a modification of the Harris-Benedict equation,[125,126] using the Dietary Reference Intakes (DRIs)[127,128] or FAO/WHO Tables.[129,130]

Category	Product Name	Manufacturer	Description	Concentration
Protein	Essential AA Module®	SHS International	Mixture of essential amino acids only	79 g protein equivalent (316 kcal)/100 g product
Protein	Complete AA Module®	SHS International	Mixture of essential and non-essential amino acids	82 g protein equivalent (328 kcal)/100 g product
Protein/ glutamine	GlutaSolve ®	Novartis	Glutamine and maltodextrin	15 g glutamine (90 kcal) in 22.5 g product
Protein	Casec®	Mead Johnson	Intact protein with small amount of fat and lactose	90 g protein (380 kcal)/100 g product
Protein	Resource Beneprotein Instant Protein Powder®	Novartis	Whey protein isolates	6 g protein (25 kcal)/7 g product
Protein	ProMod®	Ross	Whey protein	5 g protein (28 kcal)/6.6 g product
Lipid	Microlipid®	Mead Johnson	50% safflower oil emulsion	4.5 kcal/ml
Lipid	MCT Oil®	Mead Johnson	100% MCT oil	8.3 kcal/ml
Carbohydrate	Moducal®	Mead Johnson	Glucose polymers	3.8 kcal/g
Carbohydrate	Polycose®	Ross	Glucose polymers	4 kcal/g powder, 2 kcal/ml liquid
Carbohydrate	Caloreen®	Nestle	Maltodextrin	3.9 kcal/g powder

Adapted from Irving SY, Simone S, Derengowski S, Hicks F, Verger JT. Nutrition for the critically-ill child. AACN Clin Issues 2000; 11:541–548.[39]

Table 75.6 Modular macronutrient products available for supplementation of enteral feeds and their composition

Estimated energy and protein needs of infants and older children are shown in Tables 75.1 and 75.2. Other conditions that may alter the child's nutritional status must be taken into account, e.g. cardiac, renal and pulmonary diseases and activity level. Often the initial goal of nutrition therapy is 'catch-up growth', but this will need to be monitored so that children, starting out as underweight, do not become overweight.[124] A pediatric formula will often meet nutrient needs based on the DRI for age in children.[127,128]

Children with decreased energy needs may need a lower volume of formula with supplemental protein, vitamins and minerals, using the DRI as a guide. Children with developmental disabilities are at risk for malnutrition as a result of oropharyngeal dysphagia, interactions between nutrients and medications, altered energy and nutrient requirements and their reliance on others to feed them. A variety of proprietary formulas have been developed to provide these patients with nutritional support. The nutritional requirements of patients with developmental delay in general and cerebral palsy in particular are poorly understood. Studies using indirect calorimetry confirm that energy requirements are often much lower than standard predictive equations suggest. This has been hypothesized to be a result of decreased energy due to inactivity, decreased muscle tone, or lowered growth potential. As a result, the amount of energy provided in tube feedings is often reduced to match energy needs and this can be as low as 50% of the usual age-based recommended DRIs for energy.

Most formulas designed for children aged 1 to 10 years meet the DRIs for micronutrients when volumes between 980 ml/d and 1100 ml/d are given. Amino acid-based formulas generally have a lower concentration of micronutrients and therefore more volume must be given to meet the DRI. For children aged 4 to 10 years, this amount can be as high as 1400 ml/d to 2000 ml/d. When patients receive less than the DRI for energy, their micronutrient intake may be inadequate. Vitamin A, C and zinc deficiencies have been reported in such instances.[131] Tables 75.7 and 75.8 show the estimated energy and protein needs of infants and older children.

Calculating fluid requirements

Free water requirements may be altered by cardiac and renal dysfunction, drainage tubes and insensible water losses. Fluid requirements may be higher than the formula volume. Fluid requirements in children are based on bodyweight according to the Holliday-Segar method[132] as seen

Age (years)	kcal/kg bodyweight
0–1	90–120
1–7	75–90
7–12	60–75
12–18	30–60
>18	25–30

Data from ASPEN Board of Directors and the Clinical Guidelines Task Force. Guidelines for the use of parenteral and enteral nutrition in adult and pediatric patients. J Parenter Enteral Nutr 2002; Jan–Feb;26(Suppl 1): 1SA–138SA.[130]

Table 75.7 Estimated energy needs of infants and older children

Age	g protein/kg body weight
Low birthweight	3–4
Full term	2–3
1–10 years	1–1.2
Adolescent boy	0.9
Adolescent girl	0.8
Critically ill child/adolescent	1.5

Data from ASPEN Board of Directors and the Clinical Guidelines Task Force. Guidelines for the use of parenteral and enteral nutrition in adult and pediatric patients. J Parenter Enteral Nutr 2002; Jan–Feb;26(Suppl 1):1SA–138SA.[130]

Table 75.8 Estimated protein needs of infants and older children

Weight	Baseline daily fluid requirement
1–10 kg	100 ml/kg
11–20 kg	1000 ml + 50 ml/kg for each kg >10 kg
Over 20 kg	1500 ml + 20 ml/kg for each kg >20 kg

Adapted from Holliday MA, Segar WE. The maintenance need for water in parenteral fluid therapy. Pediatrics 1957; 19:823.[132]

Table 75.9 Calculating fluid requirements in children

in Table 75.9. All formulas provide water, but the level of free water varies based on the osmolality of each individual product. To calculate the additional free water required, the sodium-free water content of the tube feeding must be known. This varies from product to product and ranges from 600 to 923 ml free water/1000-ml tube feeding. Values can be found in the product literature. Otherwise, these guidelines are frequently used to calculate free water: ~90% of infant formula volume, ~85% of most other formula volume and ~72% for pediatric formulas providing 1.5 kcal/ml.[124] If the patient has no other source of hydration (i.e. intravenous fluids or medications), then the additional free water can be supplied as 'flushes' through the feeding tube that also serve to facilitate tube patency.[133] It can also be given in between feeds if larger bolus feeds are not well tolerated, or it can be mixed in to the formula.

Feeding schedules and mode of administration

Children starting on tube feedings may be started at full strength formula given at low volumes. Children should be fed with head elevated 30–45 degrees during feeding and for 1 h afterwards to limit risk of aspiration. The following is a sample schedule to initiate enteral feedings:

Infants <10 kg	10 ml/h
Children 10–20 kg	20 ml/h
Children 20–40 kg	30 ml/h
Children >40 kg	50 ml/h

The rate should be advanced as tolerated to meet the nutrition goal. The volume should then be increased every 4–12 h, monitoring for tolerance. Tolerance is defined as absence of diarrhea, abdominal distension, vomiting or gagging. If the formula is not tolerated, the formula volume or strength can be decreased and the child given longer time to adjust. After the child tolerates the formula and becomes accustomed to the volume, gradual adjustments to feeding schedule may be made to fit with the family lifestyle.[124] The method of delivery will depend on a variety of factors such as tolerance, volume requirements, safety and the family schedule. A schedule that works well in a hospital (with 24-h a day nursing care) may be impractical and exhausting for a parent to do at home.[134]

When possible, increments of formula should be delivered in user-friendly volumes. For example, if a can of formula can be used at one time, this is easier for the caregiver and leftovers are less of a problem. If syringe feeding, increments easy to measure in the syringe should be used, e.g. 60 ml *vs* 63 ml. Portable pumps can make life easier for caregivers, particularly when a child requires continuous feeds.[134] Viscosity, temperature and feeding tube size affect flow rate. The former two can be improved by diluting with free water and warming the formula.

Enteral pumps are accurate to plus or minus 10%. The more additives, i.e. protein, carbohydrate or fat powders/liquids, the less accurate the infusion. Caregivers should be instructed to give total prescribed volume versus rate calculated volume.[134] Children who suffer significant regurgitation, pulmonary gastroesophageal reflux disease (GERD) or bolus feeding induced retching may benefit from continuous feeds given over 12–24 h.[134,135]

Medications

Medications should never be added directly into the formula as drug/nutrient interactions and incompatibility with enteral feeds may occur.[134] For instance, iron added to a formula results in almost complete degradation of vitamin C if hung at room temperature for 12 h. This has led to scurvy in clinical situations.[136] Other recognized drug-nutrient interactions include vitamin C and Phenobarbital.[131]

SAFETY OF ENTERAL FEEDS

Closed *vs* open systems

Bacterial contamination may occur at any stage of preparation and infusion. For open systems, 27% are contaminated at the start and 67% by the end of an infusion. Coliforms, Enterococcus sp. and mesophilic aerobic organisms have been cultured.[137] Adding new formula to a bag already in use or adding modular components amplifies this risk. Closed systems which require only spiking onto the infusion system greatly reduce bacterial contamination risk.[138–140] Antimicrobial agents have been added to formula by some manufacturers but the long-term effects of these requires careful study in children.

Bacterial contamination of feeds

There is a growing body of information pertaining to *Enterobacter sakazakii* infections in premature infants and those with underlying medical conditions fed milk-based powdered infant formulas from various manufacturers and different countries.[141] The majority of cases of *E. sakazakii* infection occur in neonates. Sepsis, meningitis and necrotizing enterocolitis have been reported with a case-fatality rate as high as 33%. The pathogen is also a rare cause of bacteremia and osteomyelitis in adults. Powdered infant formulas are not guaranteed to be sterile. Powdered milk-based infant formulas are heat-treated during processing but, unlike liquid formula products, are not subjected to high temperature for sufficient time to guarantee sterility. A substantial percentage of premature neonates in neonatal intensive care units are fed powdered infant formula. In light of the epidemiological findings, the FDA has recommended that powdered infant formulas should not be used in neonatal intensive care settings, unless there is no alternative available.[142,143] If the only option available to address the nutritional needs of a particular infant is a powdered formula, the risk of infection in a tube-fed infant can be reduced by preparing only a small amount of reconstituted formula for each feeding to reduce the quantity and time that formula is held at room temperature for consumption, minimizing the holding time, whether at room temperature or while under refrigeration, before the formula is fed and minimizing the 'hang-time' (i.e. the amount of time a formula is at room temperature in the feeding bag and accompanying lines during enteral tube feeding), with no 'hang-time' exceeding 4 h.[144] Longer times should be avoided because of the potential for significant microbial growth in reconstituted infant formula.[142] An outbreak of Salmonella Saintpaul in a children's hospital was traced to contaminated enteral feeding formula.[145] Implementation of Hazard Analysis Critical Control Points systems have shown an improvement in the quality of feeds. Blenders used in reconstituting feeds may be a source of bacterial contamination.[137] Enteral feeding tubes and feeding sets represent another potential hazard in terms of bacterial contamination.[146–149]

Tubing

Safety with tubing is a concern for children that are active in their crib/bed. Some hospitals now have a device that encases the tubing, making it rigid and less able to become a strangling device. Also, guiding the tubing through the bottom of a child's pyjamas directs the tubing away from the neck.[131]

COMPLICATIONS

Complications of enteral tube feeding can largely be anticipated and prevented. If they occur, most are capable of being solved without stopping enteral nutrition. Complications can be dependent on the underlying disease state, the access to the intestinal tract (e.g. nasoenteric versus percutaneous-gastric *vs* small bowel), the feeding technique (e.g. type of formula, gravity *vs* pump feeding) and the metabolic state (e.g. anabolism, catabolism, postoperative stress). The reported frequency of these complications varies greatly. Gastrointestinal side-effects (including diarrhea) are most frequent. Individual assignment of feeding regimens to each patient and close monitoring are the best means of prevention, with monitoring by a specialist team. Awareness of the existence, frequency and etiological factors of complications represents the most important means of preventing them (Table 75.10).[150]

Diarrhea

Diarrhea (unformed stool, usually increased in number and changed from the usual stool habit of that person) may occur in a child receiving enteral nutrition. Since enteral feeding formulas are frequently low in residue, stool consistency is normally looser than with a normal full oral diet. A sudden onset of diarrheal stool requires investigation of all possibilities, including enteric infection

Complications
Gastrointestinal
Diarrhea
Nausea and vomiting
Constipation
Aspiration
Bloating/gas
Metabolic
Dehydration or overhydration
Hyperkalemia
Hypokalemia
Hypernatremia
Hypophosphatemia
Hypoglycemia
Refeeding syndrome
Microbial
Bacterial contamination of feed
Bacterial contamination of administration sets
Developmental
Food aversion due to inadequate oral stimulation
Mechanical
Perforation
Disruption of tract
Burial of bolster in stomach wall
Fistula formation
Pyloric obstruction
Leakage
Nasal/esophageal erosion
Tube blockage
Strangling with tubing
Equipment malfunction

Table 75.10 Complications of enteral feeding

(e.g. *C. difficile*, nosocomial viral infection), bacterial contamination of the feed, lactose content, enteral medications, systemic illness, maldigestion or malabsorption of the feed and anatomic peculiarities of the bowel. Enteral nutrition itself should not be cited as the cause of diarrhea without evidence and should be continued until the cause is identified.[151,152]

Nausea and vomiting

Nausea and vomiting often impede successful enteral nutrition. However, effective antiemetics and prokinetic agents (e.g. metoclopramide or low dose erythromycin) may be employed before turning to TPN.[153–155] The rate of feeding can be decreased until nausea subsides then gradually returned to full volume. Whey-based formulas induce faster gastric emptying than casein-based formulas. These are helpful for children who have poor weight gain secondary to volume intolerance as manifested by gagging, discomfort or emesis following bolus feeds.[156] Persistent true vomiting (*vs* gastroesophageal reflux) may indicate a gastric motility disorder and may require intestinal rather gastric feeding.

Constipation

Constipation may be related to inadequate fluid or fiber intake, side-effects of medications, inactivity, gastrointestinal dysmotility and bowel obstruction. A prophylactic bowel regimen should be discussed with a physician and dietitian ensuring adequate fluid and fiber intake and/or use of a stool softener or laxative. Where possible, regular exercise is encouraged and the physician should review the medications for possible constipating side-effects. This is a particular problem for children with cerebral palsy or neuromuscular disorders.

Metabolic complications

Care must be taken with the composition and reconstitution of enteral feeds. Underhydration is relatively common if insufficient free water is provided, or if the formula is over-concentrated. Overhydration may occur if large volumes are provided, or large volumes of water are used to flush the tube. Both hypo- and hyperkalemia may occur, particular if the patients have diarrhea or renal compromise. Hypoglycemia may occur if bolus feeding with too long a period between feeds after continuous feeding or TPN have preceded boluses, or attempted bolus feeding into the jejunum, occurs. Re-feeding syndrome has rarely been reported with enteral feeding and usually takes the form of profound hypophosphatemia.[157]

Mechanical complications

Perforation may occur at the time of placement or due to erosion of the tube through the bowel wall. Disruption of the tract most commonly occurs when button gastrostomy tubes with deformable internal bolsters are changed. It is also possible for an internal bolster to become buried in the stomach wall, often when the tube is cinched too tightly, usually requiring surgical removal. Pyloric obstruction occurs with migrating Foley and Malechot catheters and especially if tubes are mistakenly placed in the antrum. Leakage may occur because of infection in the tract or surrounding skin, granuloma formation at the tract, or because of cinching too tightly causing necrosis and skin breakdown. Nasal, esophageal and stomach irritation may occur as a result of movement or pulling on the tube. Equipment malfunction can occur at any time, but seems to have a predilection for nights, weekends and holidays.

Tube clogging

Tube clogging is a common complication especially in long, small-bore feeding tubes used frequently in acute care settings. Nasally placed gastric and jejunal tubes tend to clog more readily than gastrostomy tubes because of length and the smaller internal diameter. Minimizing the incidence of tube clogging decreases time off feeds, time and expense of reinsertion, radiography and child/parent frustration and trauma.[158] Feeding tubes can clog for a variety of reasons that include formation of a formula precipitate from contact with an acidic fluid, stagnant formula, feeding tube properties, contaminated formula and improper medication administration. Crushed insoluble medication (e.g. Metronidazole) are particularly likely to clog a tube.

Formula contact with gastric acid

Acid precipitates protein at its pK. For milk proteins, this is about pH 4.5. A feeding tube with intact casein containing formula will clog within seconds with the addition of acid at pH <4.6. The normal fasting gastric pH is 1.5–2.0. Any maneuver which increases the exposure of the formula within the tube to gastric acid will increase risk of tube clogging. This includes checking for gastric residuals, disconnecting the tube and allowing siphoning and stopping feeds without flushing the tube. Formulas with only amino acids and dipeptides greatly reduce the risk of clogging. Jejunal feeding tubes have the advantage of no exposure to acid, but the disadvantage of a longer tube.

Stagnant formula

Nutritional formulas can easily precipitate when they are infusing at slow rates, or paused without a water flush. This occurs because nutrition formulas are suspensions and the larger particles (sodium, calcium caseinate, soy protein) will settle in the tube if the flow rate is too slow or stops. Calorically dense or fiber-containing formulas are more viscous and further increase the risk for clogging. Feeding tubes should be flushed routinely with about 5–30 ml of water at least every 4 h during continuous feedings and at least 5–30 ml water flush after each intermittent or bolus feeding. The amount depends on size of the child and the internal diameter and length of the tube. Enteral infusion pumps should be used when slow infusion rates are ordered. The formula container should not be allowed to run dry and pump alarms should be responded to promptly.

Contaminated formula

A formula clog may be caused by significant bacterial contamination (bacterial count of >10^7 cfu/ml) Proper hand-washing and clean technique should be used when preparing and administering the formula to minimize contamination. Manufacturer's recommendations should be followed regarding formula hang times and proper use of the enteral delivery sets.[146]

Solutions for feeding tube flushes

Various solutions have been used to flush feeding tubes. These include water, carbonated beverages and cranberry juice. Cranberry juice (pH 2.6) has consistently been shown to be inferior to water in preventing tube clogging.[158] Coca Cola® showed no advantage over water. Water is the preferred solution for feeding tube flushes because it is easily obtainable at low cost, low neutral pH and no solution has been shown to be superior in maintaining tube patency.

Medication clogs

Tube clogging can be caused by inadequately crushed pills, congealed medications, formation of precipitate from medication with formula, or medication-medication interactions. Medications should not be mixed together or mixed with the nutritional formula, unless approved by a pharmacist. Feeding tubes should be flushed with at least 5 ml water before and after medication administration and medications should be administered separately with at least a 5 ml water flush between each one. Whenever possible, liquid medications should be used. Elixirs or suspensions are less likely to cause clogging compared with syrups that tend to be acidic. Pharmacies may be able to formulate a liquid solution or suspension from powders or tablets. If not, tablets should be crushed into a fine powder and dispersed well in warm water. A crushed tablet can be placed into a 60 ml syringe, 30 ml of warm water drawn up and the diluted medication can be administered through the feeding tube. It is wise to trial the administration through a similar tube first to check for obstruction risk. Enteric coated or timed-release tablets or capsules should be not be crushed. The administration of bulk-forming agents such as soluble fiber (e.g. psyllium) through feeding tubes should be avoided, as they quickly congeal when combined with water. Some fiber sources, e.g. Unifiber® by Novartis have instructions for tube feeding administration. Some formulas already contain insoluble fiber or a blend of soluble and insoluble fibers. These formulas should be shaken vigorously before administration to ensure that the fiber remains in solution.

Tube unclogging

Proper tube feeding administration and handling, medication administration and water flushes should minimize the incidence of tube clogging. In instances where it would be difficult to replace a clogged tube (e.g. newly placed jejunostomy tube, or gastro-jejunal tube), a solution of Viokase® in bicarbonate solution may be used (Viokase®: 1 tablet crushed or 1/4 tsp powder; sodium bicarbonate 324 mg tablet or 1/8 tsp baking soda in 5 ml tap water). The solution is injected into the tube and clamped for 30 min, then flushed well with water. This is done at home once or twice weekly for nasoenteric and gastrojejunal tubes. This practice successfully resolves sluggish infusions and prevents tube occlusions, possibly by clearing any residue buildup in the tube lumen. It frequently allows parents to unclog tubes at home without coming to the hospital. Tubes should be unclogged as soon as the obstruction is identified.

Aspiration

Children on tube feedings may aspirate oral secretions, formula and/or gastric contents. Pulmonary damage may be due to nutritional (e.g. lipid) or microbiological factors. Pulmonary aspiration may occur if the child has poor airway protection, usually associated with incoordinate swallowing, significant gastroesophageal reflux, delayed gastric emptying, or oral-positioning of the feeding tube itself. Gastric acid suppression increases the risk of bacterial overgrowth and bacterial aspiration pneumonia. Fundoplication and jejunal tube feeding (beyond the ligament of Treitz) may reduce the risk of aspiration of formula if gastroesophageal reflux is severe and the latter reduces gastric and duodenal secretions.[159] The progression from an aspiration event to aspiration pneumonia is very difficult to predict and several studies support oropharyngeal bacteria as a more significant factor in aspiration, or even the key factor, rather than colonization of gastric contents.[138] Body position can make a significant difference in the risk of aspiration. The head of the bed should be elevated at 20–30 degrees.

Monitoring

Initial monitoring parameters for a child on enteral feedings should include daily intake of calories, protein and electrolytes, fluid intake and output and the weight of the patient. Appropriate laboratory investigations, including but not limited to electrolytes, albumin or prealbumin, blood urea nitrogen (BUN) and glucose are done daily to weekly until stable. Vitamin, mineral and trace element intake should be evaluated at regular intervals. Once the formula feeding is tolerated and any complications managed, then growth can be monitored by weekly weight measurement. Once expected growth is realized, then review for tolerance, tube problems and growth (weight, length and head circumference) can be decreased to approximately monthly. In addition, laboratory monitoring will decrease concomitantly. Trace elements and vitamin assays should be performed twice annually and supplements provided if required.[131] When children are discharged home on tube feeding, the child and family should be seen again within 10 days to troubleshoot and to provide support. The frequency of subsequent visits will depend upon the abilities of the family and their needs and complexity of the case.

As the child grows, enteral feedings need to be adjusted. At each outpatient visit, the indications for and goals of enteral feeding should be re-evaluated, techniques of problem solving reinforced and signs and symptoms of complications identified.[160] Formula volume should be modified based on a child's rate of growth. For this reason, it is important to monitor a child's growth regularly. Changes in weight and height should be monitored at least every 3–6 months for a child who is tube-fed. This is especially important during periods of transitional feeding, i.e. when transitioning from fully tube feeding to oral feeding or from fully oral feeding to supplemental feeds.

Routine monitoring should include:

1 Weight measurement, length and head circumference
2 Intake (including enteral and oral)
3 Review of current medications for drug-nutrient interactions
4 Laboratory parameters
5 Psychological status: changes in lifestyle, home environment
6 Assessment of relevant organ function to evaluate feasibility of transitional feeding.

The frequency of monitoring children on home enteral nutrition depends upon the needs of the family and the complexity of the case.[161] Many decisions require health professionals' input, documentation or support. A team including a physician, nurse, occupational or speech therapist and dietitian works best for the child and family.[124]

Oral stimulation

Patients who have no contraindications to oral feeding should be encouraged to feed by mouth.[160] Feeding time is important to children and parents. It should be an enjoyable and relaxing time. This does not have to change while children are being tube-fed. Caretakers can hold, talk to and play with children during feeding. All children on tube feeding require oral stimulation for development of feeding skills. If the child is unable to take foods orally, some type of oral stimulation is needed such as offering a pacifier. This will help children develop the skills necessary to begin eating by mouth. For infants, the denial of oral stimulatory experiences because of gastrointestinal dysfunction may have significant deleterious side-effects such as appetite suppression, inability to distinguish hunger and satiety, food aversion, inadequate and uncoordinated sucking and swallowing, poor mother-child bonding and developmental delays in language and gross motor skills. The goal is to have children associate sucking or chewing with satiety in order to ease transition from tube to oral feeds. A speech language pathologist or occupation therapist with experience in feeding/swallowing disorders can outline an oral motor program to follow during feedings.[124]

TRANSITION FROM PARENTERAL TO ENTERAL/ORAL NUTRITION

As soon as the gut can be accessed and fluid safely infused, then enteral feeding should be started. Enteral feeding promotes bowel growth. Initial enteral feeding may be minute: 1–2 ml/h, but should be gradually advanced as tolerated. When 20% of required nutrients can be absorbed from the bowel, parenteral nutrition can start to be weaned. If oral feeds are progressing, parenteral nutrition may be given solely at night until no longer required.

Tube removal

Parents are often anxious to know when the tube can be removed. For nasoenteric tubes, the tube is removed as soon as oral feeding is fully adequate.[139] The tube can be replaced as required. For gastrostomy or gastrojejunal feeding tubes, a general rule of thumb (established only by expert opinion) is that if the tube has not been used for 90 days and the child continues to thrive, the tube can be removed. Some physicians prefer to also see if the child can manage to get through an illness without having to rely on the tube for feeds, oral rehydration therapy, or medications.[131]

Home enteral nutrition

Home enteral feeding should be considered for any patient whose sole reason for hospitalization is to receive enteral support.[162] The decision to provide enteral feeding in the patient's home must take into account medical needs as well as social, psychological and financial factors.[163] Enteral feeding offers a safe and cost-effective alternative to parenteral nutrition and can usually be carried out at home, preferably under the supervision of a nutritional care team.[164] The provision of nutritional support at home allows for a return to a comfortable environment, avoidance of the negative emotional effects of hospitalization, reduction of the risk of infection and reduction in costs.[160]

Home enteral nutrition is appropriate for children with diagnoses falling into several broad categories but which all relate to the child being unable to safely and voluntarily ingest adequate nutrition by mouth.[165] Enteral feeding has usually been started in hospital and is continued at home. However, when used as a supplement or primary therapy for conditions such as Crohn's disease, enteral feeding may be started in the outpatient clinic. Enteral feeding is started with the agreement of the parents with whom the objectives of treatment must be fully discussed. It is important that parents do not see tube feeding as a failure, but rather as a positive step which will free them from the worries of maintaining an adequate nutritional intake and allow them to devote more time to their child with activities that are less stressful and more rewarding than feeding.

An important element of home enteral nutrition is continuous parental support and regular follow-up of the patients by both the nutritional care team of the base hospital and the community medical and nursing staff.[166] Home-based care has been increasingly practiced in the care of children. It requires a multidisciplinary team that includes physicians, dietitian and nurses as well as occupational therapists, speech-language pathologists, physiotherapists and social workers and allows many children with multiple handicaps to be cared for at home.

SUMMARY

Enteral feeding provides the best solution to the nutritional support of the child with acute or chronic disease who is unable to maintain adequate growth and development with oral feeding alone, where the gut is intact and functional (and sometimes even when it is not). The malnourished, hospitalized child is a particular challenge, but children with a chronic need for nutritional support can often have it provided in the safety and comfort of their own homes. A variety of disease states may give rise to a requirement for nutritional supplementation by the enteral route including disorders which impair intake, gastrointestinal dysfunction and malabsorption, hepatobiliary disease, critical illness, chronic system-based disorders which impair growth and hypermetabolic states. Enteral feeding may be provided by nasoenteral or enterostomal approaches depending on individual circumstances and the choice of formula to be used, whether polymeric or defined, will depend on the digestive and absorptive capabilities of the child and the metabolic stressors involved at the time of provision of nutritional support. The complications of enteral feeding can largely be anticipated and avoided with appropriate care and monitoring of the patient. The nutritional care of the hospitalized patient may be transitioned appropriately into the community, to continue rehabilitation or long-term nutritional support. The importance of a multidisciplinary team-based approach to the care of children requiring enteral feeding, with appropriate psychosocial support, cannot be over-emphasized.

References

1. Marchand V, Baker SS, Baker RD. Enteral nutrition in the pediatric population. Gastrointest Endosc Clin N Am 1998; 8:669–703.
2. Hyman PE, Feldman EJ, Ament ME, Byrne WJ, Euler AR. Effect of enteral feeding on the maintenance of gastric acid secretory function. Gastroenterology 1983; 84:341–345.
3. Morin CL, Ling V, Van Caillie M. Role of oral intake on intestinal adaptation after small bowel resection in growing rats. Pediatr Res 1978; 12:268–271.
4. Aynsley-Green A, Lucas A, Lawson GR, Bloom SR. Gut hormones and regulatory peptides in relation to enteral feeding, gastroenteritis and necrotizing enterocolitis in infancy. J Pediatr 1990; 11: S24–S32.
5. Lucas A, Bloom SR, Green AA. Gastrointestinal peptides and the adaptation to extrauterine nutrition. Can J Physiol Pharmacol 1985; 63:527–537.
6. Levine GM, Deren JJ, Steiger E, Zinno R. Role of oral intake in maintenance of gut mass and disaccharidase activity. Gastroenterology 1974; 67:975–982.
7. Okada Y, Klein N, Saane HK, Pierro A. Small volumes of enteral feedings normalize immune function in infants receiving parenteral nutrition. J Pediatr Surg 1998; 33: 16–19.
8. Andrassy RJ. Preserving the gut mucosal barrier and enhancing immune response. Contemp Surg 1988; 32:1–40.
9. Johnson LR. The trophic action of gastrointestinal hormones. Gastroenterology 1976; 70:278–281.
10. Boehm G, Fanaro S, Jelinek J, Stahl B, Marini A. Prebiotic concept for infant nutrition. Acta Paediatr Suppl 2003; 91:64–67.
11. Boehm G, Lidestri M, Casetta P, Jelinek J, Negretti F, Stahl B, Marini A. Supplementation of a bovine milk formula with an oligosaccharide mixture increases counts of Bifidobacteria in preterm infants. Arch Dis Child Fetal Neonatal Ed 2002; 86:F178–F181.
12. Butel MJ, Waligora-Dupriet AJ, Szylit O. Oligofructose in an experimental model of neonatal necrotizing enterocolitis. Brit J Nutr 2002; 87(Suppl 2):S213–S219.
13. Minard G, Kudsk KA, Melton S, Patton JH, Tolley EA. Early versus delayed feeding with an immune-enhancing diet in patients with severe head injuries. J Parenter Enter Nutr 2000; 24:145–148.
14. Bower RH, Cerra FB, Bershadsky B, et al. Early enteral administration of a formula (Impact®) supplemented with arginine, nucleotides and fish oil in intensive care unit patients: Results of a multicenter, prospective, randomized, clinical trial. Crit Care Med 1995; 23:436–449.
15. Merritt RJ, Suskind RM. Nutritional survey of hospitalized pediatric patients. Am J Clin Nutr 1979; 32:1320–1325.
16. Fuchs GJ. Secondary malnutrition in children. In: Suskind R, Suskind L, eds. The Malnourished Child. New York: Raven Press, 1990:23–36.
17. WHO. Management of Severe Malnutrition: A Manual for Physicians and Other Senior Health Care Workers. Geneva, Switzerland: World Health Organization; 1999.
18. Moy RJD, Smallman S, Booth IW. Malnutrition in a UK Children's Hospital. Human Nutr Dietet 1990; 3:93–100.
19. Tucker HN, Miguel SG. Cost containment through nutrition intervention. Nutrition 1996; 54:111–121.
20. Brown RO, Carlson SD, Cowna GS Jr, Powers DA, Luther RW. Enteral nutrition support management in a university hospital: team vs nonteam. J Parenter Enter Nutr 1987; 11:52–56.
21. Parsons HG, Francoeur TE, Howland P, et al. The nutritional status of hospitalized children. Am J Clin Nutr 1980; 33:1140–1146.
22. LeLeiko NS, Luder E, Friedman M, Fersel J, Benkov K. Nutritional assessment of pediatric patients admitted to an acute-care pediatric service utilizing anthropometric measurements. J Parenter Enter Nutr1986; 10:166–168.
23. Hendricks KM, Duggan C, Gallagher L, et al. Malnutrition in hospitalized pediatric patients: current prevalence. Arch Pediatr Adolesc Med 1995; 149:1118–1122.
24. Bines J, Francis D, Hill D. Reducing parenteral requirement in children with short bowel syndrome: Impact of an amino-acid based complete formula. J Pediatr Gastroenterol Nutr 1998; 26:123–128.
25. Escher JC, Taminiau JA. Treatment of inflammatory bowel disease in childhood. Scand J Gastroenterol 2001(Suppl); 234:48–50.
26. Ruuska T, Savilahti E, Maki M, Ormala T, Visakorpi JK. Exclusive whole protein enteral diet versus prednisolone in the treatment of acute Crohn's disease in children. J Pediatr Gastroenterol Nutr 1994; 19:175–180.

27. Israel DM, Hassall E. Prolonged use of gastrostomy for enteral hyperalimentation in children with Crohn's disease. Am J Gastroenterol 1995; 90:1084–1088.
28. Walker-Smith JA. Nutritional management of enteropathy. Nutr 1998; 14:775–779.
29. Pisters P, Ranson JH. Nutritional support for acute pancreatitis. Surg Gynecol Obstet 1992; 175:275–284.
30. Marik PE, Zaloga GP. Meta-analysis of parenteral versus enteral nutrition in patients with acute pancreatitis. BMJ 2004:328:1407.
31. Gupta R, Patel K, Calder PC, Yaqoob P, Primrose JN, Johnson CD. A randomized clinical trial to assess the effect of total enteral and total parenteral nutritional support on metabolic, inflammatory and oxidative markers in patients with predicted severe pancreatitis. Pancreatology 2003; 3:406–413.
32. Wicks C, Somasundaram S. Comparison of enteral feeding and total parenteral nutrition after liver transplantation. Lancet 1994; 344:837–840.
33. Stewart SM, Uauy R, Waller DA, Benser M, Andrews WS. Mental development and growth in children with chronic liver disease of early and late onset. Pediatrics 1988; 82:167–172.
34. Heubi JE, Heyman MB, Shulman RJ. The impact of liver disease on growth and nutrition. J Pediatr Gastroenterol Nutr 2002; 35(Suppl 1): S55–S59.
35. Holt RI, Miell JP, Jones JS, Miele-Vergani G, Baker AJ. Nasogastric feeding enhances nutritional status in paediatric liver disease but does not alter circulating levels of IGF–1 and IGF binding proteins. Clin Endocrinol 2000; 52:217–224.
36. Duche M, Habes D, Lababidi A, Chardot C, Wenz J, Bernard O. Percutaneous endoscopic gastrostomy for continuous feeding in children with chronic cholestasis. J Pediatr Gastroenterol Nutr 1999; 29:42–45.
37. Moreno LA, Gotrand F, Hoden S, Turck D, Loeuille GA, Faariauz JP. Improvement of nutritional status in cholestatic children with supplemental nocturnal enteral nutrition. J Pediatr Gastroenterol Nutr 1991; 12:213–216.
38. Charlton CP, Buchanan E, Holden CE, Prece MA, Green A, Booth IW, Tarlow MJ. Intensive enteral feeding in advanced cirrhosis: reversal of malnutrition without precipitation of hepatic encephalopathy. Arch Dis Child 1992; 67:603–607.
39. Irving SY, Simone SD, Hicks FW, Verger JT. Nutrition for the critically ill child: enteral and parenteral support. AACN Clin Issues 2000; 11:541–558.
40. DaSilva PS, Paulo CS, de Oliveira Iglesias SB, de Carvalho WB, Santana e Meneses F. Bedside transpyloric tube placement in the pediatric intensive care unit: a modified insufflation air technique. Int Care Med 2002; 28:943–946.
41. Panadero E, Lopez-Herce J, Caro L, et al. Transpyloric feeding in critically ill children. J Pediatr Gastroenterol Nutr 1998; 26:43–48.
42. Horn D, Chaboyer W. Gastric feeding in critically ill children: a randomised controlled trial. Am J Crit Care 2003; 12:461–8
43. Forchielli, ML, McColl R, Walker WA, Lo C. Children with congenital heart disease: a nutrition challenge. Nutr Rev 1994; 52:348–353.
44. Varan B, Tokel K, Yilmaz G. Malnutrition and growth failure in cyanotic and acyanotic congenital heart disease with and without pulmonary hypertension. Arch Dis Child 1999; 81:49–52.
45. Hofner G, Behrens R, Koch A, et al. Enteral nutritional support by percutaneous endoscopic gastrostomy in children with congenital heart disease. Pediatr Cardiol 2000; 21:341–346.
46. Vanderhoof JA, Hofschire PJ, Baluff MA, et al. Continuous enteral feedings. An important adjunct to the management of complex congenital heart disease. Am J Dis Child 1982; 136:825–827.
47. Schwarz SM, Gewitz MH, See CC, et al. Enteral nutrition in infants with congenital heart disease and growth failure. Pediatrics 1990; 86:368–373.
48. Kurzner SI, Garg M, Bautista DB, Sargent CW, Bowman CM, Keens TG. Growth in bronchopulmonary dysplasia: elevated metabolic rates and pulmonary mechanics. J Pediatr 1988; 142:73–80.
49. Reimers KJ, Carlson SJ, Lombard KA. Nutritional management of infants with bronchopulmonary dysplasia. Nutr Clin Pract 1992; 7:127–132.
50. Walker SA, Gozal D. Pulmonary function correlates in the prediction of long-term weight gain in cystic fibrosis patients with gastrostomy feedings. J Pediatr Gastroenterol Nutr 1998; 27:53–56.
51. Boland MP, Patrick J, Stoski DS, Soucy P. Permanent enteral feeding in cystic fibrosis: advantages of a replaceable jejunostomy tube. J Pediatr Surg 1987; 22:843–847.
52. Fulton JA, Orenstein DM, Koehler AN, Kurland G. Nutrition in the pediatric double lung transplant patient with cystic fibrosis. Nutr Clin Pract 1995; 10:67–72.
53. Holcombe RJ, Resler R. Nutrition support for lung transplant patients. Nutr Clin Pract 1994; 9:235–239.
54. Dosanjh A. A review of nutritional problems and the cystic fibrosis lung transplant patient. Pediatr Transplant 2002; 6:388–391.
55. Ledermann SE, Spitz L, Moloney J, Rees L, Trompeter RS. Gastrostomy feeding in infants and children on peritoneal dialysis. Pediatr Nephrol 2002; 17:246–250.
56. Ledermann SE, Shaw V, Trompeter RS. Long-term enteral nutrition in infants and young children with chronic renal failure. Pediatr Nephrol 1999; 13:870–875.
57. Watson AR, Coleman JE, Taylor EA. Gastrostomy buttons for feeding children on continuous cycling peritoneal dialysis. Adv Perit Dial 1992; 8:391–395.
58. Kuizon BD, Nelson PA, Salusky IB. Tube feeding in children with end-stage renal disease. Miner Electrolyte Metab 1997; 23:306–310.
59. Claris-Appiani A, Ardissino GL, Dacco V, Funari C, Terzi F. Catch-up growth in children with chronic renal failure treated with long-term enteral nutrition. J Parenter Enteral Nutr 1995; 19:175–178.
60. Sullivan PB. Gastrointestinal problems in the neurologically impaired child. Bailliere's Clin Gastroenterol 1997; 11:529–546.
61. Saunders KD, Cox K, Cannon R, et al. Growth response to enteral feeding by children with cerebral palsy. J Parenter Enteral Nutr 1990; 14:23–26.
62. Samson-Fang L, Butler C, O'Donnell M. AACPDM. Effects of gastrostomy feeding in children with cerebral palsy: an AACPDM evidence report. Dev Med Child Neurol 2003; 45:415–426.
63. Dickerson RN, Brown RO, Hanna DL, William JE. Validation of a new method of estimating resting energy expenditure of non-ambulatory tube-fed patients with severe neurodevelopmental disabilities. Nutrition 2002; 18:681–683.
64. Andrassy RJ, Chwals WJ. Nutritional support of the pediatric oncology patient. Nutrition 1998; 14:124–129.
65. Skolin L, Hernell O, Larsson MV, et al. Percutaneous endoscopic gastrostomy in children with malignant disease. J Pediatr Oncol Nursing 2002; 19:154–163.
66. Langdana A, Tully N, Molloy E, Bourke B, O'Meara A. Intensive enteral nutrition support in paediatric bone marrow transplantation. Bone Marrow Transplant 2001; 27:741–746.

67. Szeluga DJ, Stuart RK, Brookmeyer R, Utermohlen V, Santos GW. Nutritional support of bone marrow transplant recipients: a prospective, randomized clinical trial comparing total parenteral nutrition to an enteral feeding program. Cancer Res 1987; 47:3309–3316.
68. Papadopoulou A, MacDonald A, Williams MD, Darbyshire PJ, Booth IW. Enteral nutrition after bone marrow transplantation. Arch Dis Child 1997; 77:131–136.
69. Buys H, Hendricks M, Eley B, Hussey G. The role of nutrition and micronutrients in paediatric HIV infection. SADJ; 57:454–456.
70. Singhal N, Austin J. A clinical review of micronutrients in HIV infection. J Int Assoc Physicians AIDS Care 2002; 1:63–75.
71. Guarino A, Spagnuolo MI, Giacomet V, et al. Effects of nutritional rehabilitation on intestinal function and CD4 cell number in children with HIV. J Pediatr Gastroenterol Nutr 2002; 34:366–371.
72. Miller TL, Mawn BE, Orav EJ, et al. The effect of protease inhibitor therapy on growth and body composition in human immunodeficiency virus type–typ1 infected children. Pediatrics 2001; 107: E77.
73. Bohnhorst B, Muller S, Dordelmann M, Peter CS, Petersen C, Poets CF. Early feeding after necrotizing enterocolitis in preterm infants. J Pediatr 2003; 143:484–487.
74. Gottschlich MM, Jenkins ME, Mayes T, Khoury J, Kagan RJ, Warden GD. The 2002 Clinical Research Award. An evaluation of the safety of early vs delayed enteral support and effects on clinical, nutritional and endocrine outcomes after severe burns. J Burn Care Rehabil 2002; 23:401–415.
75. McArdle AH, Palamson C, Brown HC, Williams HB. Early enteral feeding of patients with major burns: prevention of catabolism. Ann Plastic Surg 1984; 13:396–401.
76. Peng YZ, Yuan ZQ, Xiao GX. Effects of early enteral feeding on the prevention of enterogenic infection in severely burned patients. Burns 2001; 27:145–149.
77. Wolf SE, Jeschke MG, Rose JK, Desai MH, Herndon DN. Enteral feeding intolerance: An indicator of sepsis-associated mortality in burned children. Arch Surg 1997; 132:1313–1314.
78. Trocki O, Michelini JA, Robbins ST, Eichelberger MR. Evaluation of early enteral feeding in children less than 3 years old with smaller burns (8–25% TBSA). Burns 1995; 21:17–23.
79. McDonald WS, Sharp CW Jr, Deitch EA. Immediate enteral feeding in burn patients is safe and effective. Ann Surg 1991; 213:177–183.
80. Jenkins ME, Gottschlich MM, Warden GD. Enteral feeding during operative procedures in thermal injuries. J Burn Care Rehabil 1994; 15:199–205.
81. Wilson SE, Dietz WH Jr, Grand RJ. An algorithm for pediatric enteral alimentation. Pediatr Ann 1987; 16:233–234.
82. Sartori S, Trevisani L, Nielsen I, Tassinari D, Cecotti P, Abbasciano V. Longevity of silicone and polyurethane catheters in long-term enteral feeding via percutaneous endoscopic gastrostomy. Aliment Pharmacol Ther 2003; 17:853–856.
83. Lord LM, Weiser-Maimone A, Pulhamus M, Sax HC. Comparison of weighted versus unweighted enteral feeding tubes for efficacy of transpyloric intubation. J Parenter Enteral Nutr 1993; 17:271–273.
84. Sigmon RL Jr. Endoscopic placement of enteral feeding tubes: pediatric versus adult patients. Nutr Clin Pract 1997; 12 (Suppl 1):S4–S6.
85. Ho CS, Yee AC, McPherson R. Complications of surgical and percutaneous nonendoscopic gastrostomy: review of 233 patients. Gastroenterology 1988; 95:962.
86. Albanese CT, Towbin RB, Ulman I, Lewis J, Smith SD. Percutaneous gastrojejunostomy versus Nissen fundoplication for enteral feeding of the neurologically impaired child with gastroesophageal reflux. J Pediatr 1993; 123:371–375.
87. Godbole P. Margabanthu G, Crabbe DC, et al. Limitations and uses of gastrojejunal feeding tubes. Arch Dis Child 2002; 86:134–137.
88. Chan DK. Enteral nutrition of the very low birthweight infant. Ann Acad Med, Singapore 2001; 30:174–182.
89. Williams AF. Early enteral feeding of the preterm infant. Arch Dis Child Fetal Neonatal Ed 2000:83:F219–F220.
90. Newell SJ. Enteral feeding of the micropremie. Clin Perinatol 2000; 27:221–234.
91. Yu VY. Enteral feeding in the preterm infant. Early Hum Dev 1999; 56:89–115.
92. Troche B, Harvey-Wilkes K, Engle WD, et al. Early minimal feedings promote growth in critically ill premature infants. Biol Neonate 1995; 67:172–181.
93. Tyson JE, Kennedy KA. Minimal enteral nutrition for promoting feeding tolerance and preventing morbidity in parenterally fed infants. Cochrane Database Syst Rev 2000; 2:CD000504.
94. Schanler RJ, Shulman RJ, Lau C, Smith EO, Heitkemper MM. Feeding strategies for premature infants: randomized trial of gastrointestinal priming and tube-feeding method. Pediatrics 1999; 103:492–493.
95. Kuschel CA, Evans N, Askie L, Bredemeyer S, Nash J, Polverino J. A Randomized trial of enteral feeding volumes in infants born before 30 weeks gestation. J Paediatr Child Health 2000; 36:581–586.
96. Schanler RJ, Rifka M. Calcium, phosphorus and magnesium needs for the low birth weight infant. Acta Paediatrica Suppl 1994; 405:111–116.
97. Brar G, Geiss D, Brion LP, et al. Respiratory mechanics in very low birth weight infants during continuous versus intermittent gavage feeds. Pediatr Pulmonol 2001; 32:442–446.
98. Premji S, Chessell L. Continuous nasogastric milk feeding versus intermittent bolus milk feeding for premature infants less than 1500 grams (Cochrane Review). In: The Cochrane Library Issue 3; 2001.
99. Akintorin SM, Kamat M, Pildes RS, Kling P, Andes S, Hill J, Pyati S. A prospective randomized trial of feeding methods in very low birth weight infants. Pediatrics 1997; 100: E4.
100. Jawaheer G, Pierro A, Lloyd DA, Shaw NJ. Gallbladder contractility in neonates: effects of parenteral and enteral feeding. Arch Dis Child Fetal Neonatal Ed 1995:F200–F202.
101. Jawaheer G, Shaw NJ, Pierro A. Continuous enteral feeding impairs gallbladder emptying in infants. J Pediatr 2001; 138:822–825.
102. Berseth CL, Bisquera JA, Paje VU. Prolonging small feeding volumes early in life decreases the incidence of necrotizing enterocolitis in very low birthweight infants. Pediatrics 2003; 111:671–672.
103. O'Connor DL, Jacobs J, Hall R, et al. Growth and development of preterm infants fed predominantly human milk, predominantly preterm formula, or a combination of human milk and premature formula. J Pediatr Gastroenterol Nutr 2003; 37:437–446.
104. Brennan-Behm M, Carlson GE, Meier P, et al. Caloric loss from expressed mother's milk during continuous gavage infusion. Neonatal Network 1994; 13:27–32.
105. Kuschel CA, Harding M. Multicomponent fortification of human milk for premature infants. Cochrane Database; 1998.

106. Schanler RJ, Shulman RJ, Lau C. Feeding strategies for premature infants: beneficial outcomes of feeding fortified human milk versus preterm formula. Pediatrics 1999; 103:1150–1157.
107. Bar-Oz B, Preminger A, Peleg, et al. Enterobacter sakazakii infection in the newborn. Acta Paediatrica 2001; 90:356–358.
108. Lucas A, Morley R & Cole TJ. Randomised trial of early diet in preterm babies and later intelligence quotient. Brit Med J 1998; 317:1481–1487.
109. Bougle D, Denise P, Vimard F, Nouvelot A, Penneilo MJ, Guillois B. Early neurological and neuropsychological development of the preterm infant and polyunsaturated fatty acid supply. Clin Neurophysiol 1999; 111:1363–1370.
110. Billeaud C, Bougle D, Sarda P, et al. Effect of preterm infant formula supplementation with alpha-linolenic acid with a linoleate/alpha-linolenate ratio of 6: a multi-centric study. Eur J Clin Nutr 1997; 51:520–526.
111. Mihatsch WA, Franz AR, Hogel J, Pohlandt F. Hydrolyzed protein accelerates feeding enhancement in very low birth weight infants. Pediatrics 2002; 110:1199–1203.
112. Riezzo G, Indrio F, Montagna O, Tripaldi C, Laforgia N, Chiloio M, Mautone A. Gastric electrical activity and gastric emptying in preterm newborns fed standard and hydrolysate formulas. J Pediat Gastroenterol Nutr 2001; 33:290–295.
113. Kirsten GF, Bergman NJ, Hann FM. Kangaroo mother care in the nursery. Pediatr Clin N Am 2001; 48:443–452.
114. Johnson TE, Janes SJ, MacDonald A, Elia M, Booth IW. An observational study to evaluate micronutrient status during enteral feeding. Arch Dis Child 2002; 86:411–415.
115. Billeaud C, Guillet J, Sandler B. Gastric emptying in infants with or without gastro-oesophageal reflux according to type of milk. Eur J Clin Nutr 1990; 44:577–583.
116. Fried MD, Khoshoo V, Secker DJ, et al. Decrease in gastric emptying time and episodes of regurgitation in children with spastic quadriplegia fed a whey-based formula. J Pediatr 1992; 120:569–572.
117. Businco L, Cantani A, Longhi MA, et al. Anaphylactic reactions to a cow's milk whey protein hydrolysate (Alfa-Re, Nestle) in infants with cow milk allergy. Ann All 1989; 62:333–335.
118. Moro G, Minoli I, Mosca M, et al. Dosage-related Bifidogenic effects of galacto- and fructooligosaccharides in formula-fed term infants. J Pediatr Gastroenterol Nutr 2002; 34:291–295.
119. Correa-Matos NJ, Donovan SM, Isaacson RE, et al Fermentable fiber reduces recovery time and improves intestinal function in piglets following Salmonella typhimurium infection. J Nutr 133:1845–1852.
120. Liebl BH, Fischer MH, Van Calcar SC, Marlett JA. Dietary fiber and long-term large bowel response in enterally nourished nonambulatory profoundly retarded youth. J Parenter Enteral Nutr 1990; 14:371–375.
121. Uauy R, Hoffman DR, Mena P, et al. Term infant studies of CHA and ARA supplementation on neurodevelopment; results of randomized controlled trials. J Pediatr 2003; 143(Suppl 4): S17–S25.
122. O'Connor DL, Hall R, Adamkin D, et al. Growth and development in preterm infants fed long-chain polyunsaturated fatty acids: a prospective, randomized controlled trial. Pediatrics 2001; 108:359–371.
123. Koletzko B, Edenhofer S, Lipowsky G, Reinhardt D. Effects of a low birth weight infant Formula containing human milk levels of docosahexanoic acid and arachidonic acids. J Pediatr Gastroenterol Nutr 1995; 21:200–208.
124. Pederson A. Tube feeding update. Nutr Focus 2002; 17(6)1–8.
125. Baker J, Detsky A, Wesson D. Nutritional assessment: A comparison of clinical judgment and objective measurements. N Engl J Med 1982; 306:969.
126. Caldwell MD, Kennedy-Caldwell C. Normal Nutritional Requirements. Surg Clin N Am 1981; 61:491.
127. National Academy of Sciences. Dietary Reference Intakes: Applications in Dietary Planning. Washington, DC: The National Academies Press; 2003.
128. National Academy of Sciences. Dietary Reference Intakes: Guiding Principles for Nutrition Labeling and Fortification. Washington, DC: The National Academies Press; 2004.
129. World Health Organization. Energy and protein requirements. Report of a Joint FAO/WHO/UNU Expert Consultation. WHO Technical Report Series No. 724. Geneva: World Health Organization; 1985.
130. ASPEN Board of Directors and the Clinical Guidelines Task Force. Guidelines for the use of parenteral and enteral nutrition in adult and pediatric patients. J Parenter Enteral Nutr 2002; 26(Suppl 1):1SA–138SA.
131. Jones J, Campbell KA, Duggan C, et al. Multiple Micronutrient Deficiencies in a Child fed an Elemental Formula. J Pediatr Gastroenterol Nutr 2001; 33:602–605.
132. Holliday MA, Segar WE. The maintenance need for water in parenteral fluid therapy. Pediatrics 1957; 19:823.
133. American Gastroenterological Association. Medical Position Statement: Guidelines for the Use of Enteral Nutrition. 17 Sept 1994; 1–32. Online. Available at: http://www.us.elsevierhealth.com/gastro/policy/v108n4p1280.html
134. Frederick A. Practical tips for tube feeding. Nutr Focus 2003; 18(1):1–7.
135. Shang E, Geiger N, Sturm JW, et al. Pump-assisted versus gravity-controlled enteral nutrition in long-term percutaneous endoscopic gastrostomy patients: a prospective controlled trial. J Parenter Enteral Nutr 2003; 27(3):216–219.
136. Gorman SR, Armstrong G, Ellis J, et al. Scarcity in the midst of plenty: enteral tube feeding complicated by scurvy. J Pediatric Gastroenterol Nutr 2002; 35:93–95.
137. Oliviera MH, Bonelli R, Aidoo KE, et al. Microbiological quality of reconstituted enteral formulations used in hospitals. Nutrition 2000; 16(9):729–733.
138. Aspiration in patients on enteral tube feeding-how do we prevent it? Nutrition News from ASPEN. 2003; 19–22 Jan:1–9.
139. Papadopoulou A and Booth I. Home enteral nutrition in infants and children. In: Preedy H, Grimble G, Watson R, eds. Nutrition in the Infant – Problems and Practical Procedures. London: Greenwich Medical Media; 2001:69–78.
140. Bott L, Husson MO, Guimber D, et al. Contamination of gastrostomy feeding systems in children in a home-based enteral nutrition program. J Pediatr Gastroenterol Nutr 2001; 33(3):266–270.
141. CDC. Enterobacter sakazakii infections associated with the use of powdered infant formula – Tennessee, 2001. Morbidity and Mortality Weekly Report, 2002; 12 April, 51:297–300.
142. US Food and Drug Administration, Center for Food Safety and Applied Nutrition, Office of Nutritional Products, Labeling and Dietary Supplements. Health Professionals Letter on Enterobacter sakazakii Infections Associated With Use of Powdered (Dry) Infant Formulas in Neonatal Intensive Care Units. 2002; 11 April, Revised October 10.
143. Schwenk WF. Presidential Address. Specialized nutrition support: the pediatric perspective. J Parenter Enteral Nutr 2003; 27(3):160–167.
144. Freedland CP, Roller RD, Wolfe BM, Flynn NM. Microbial contamination of continuous drip feedings. J Parenter Enteral Nutr 1989; 13:18–22.

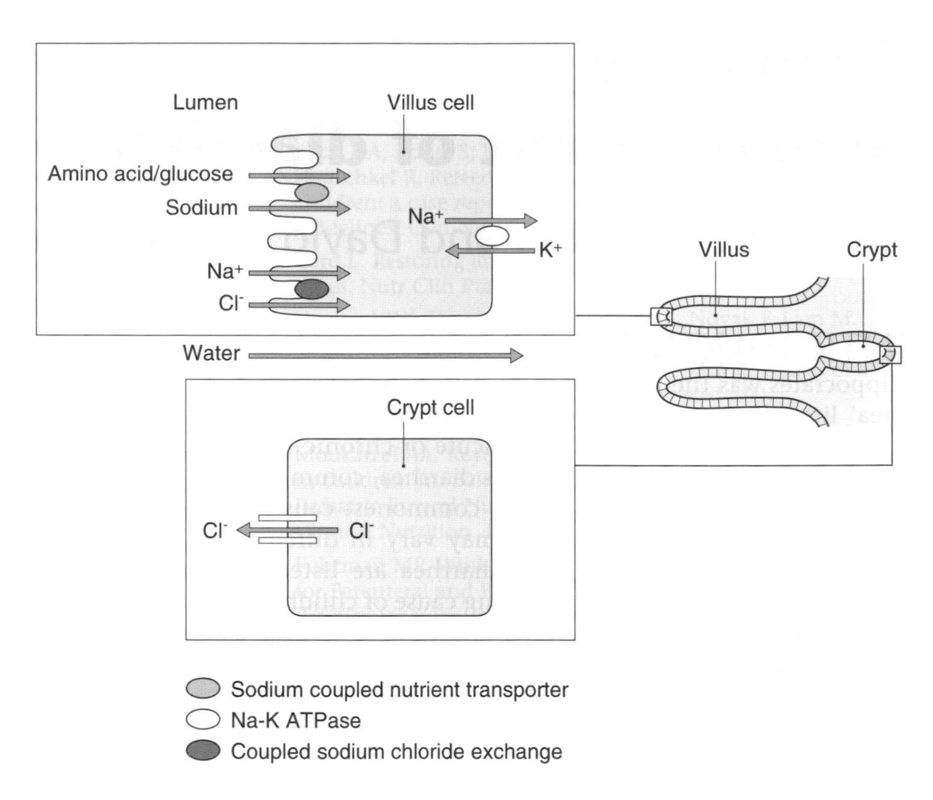

Figure 76.1: Absorptive and secretory processes in gut epithelium.

rationale for its use. The sodium concentration of the standard WHO-ORS, 90 mmol/l, was in part based on the fecal sodium concentration in adults with cholera.[10] This product with an osmolarity of 311 mmol/l has been used worldwide and has contributed substantially to the global reduction in mortality from diarrheal disease. Concerns that this solution which is slightly hyperosmolar when compared to plasma, may cause hypernatremia[11] in well-nourished children with non-cholera diarrhea in the developed world, resulted in the proliferation of ORS formulations with a range of sodium concentrations (30–60 mmol/l). Stools in children with Rotavirus infection, the commonest infective pathogen particularly in the developed world, have a lower concentration of sodium.[12] In the 1980s, the American Association of Pediatrics (AAP) recommended a solution containing 45 mmol/l sodium for American children for the correction of dehydration. In 1992, a working group on Acute Diarrhoea of the European Society of Paediatric Gastroenterology and Nutrition (ESPGHAN) considered the scientific evidence and published 'Recommendations for the composition of ORS for the children of Europe'.[13] ESPGHAN recommended a solution containing 60 mmol/l sodium and 70–110 mmol/l glucose with an osmolarity of 225–260 mmol/l. Various manufacturers of ORS took on board the recommendations and this solution has gradually replaced other solutions in Europe.

Super ORS

During the past 20 years there have been attempts to develop a super ORS by using rice powder, amino acids, glucose polymers, etc. instead of glucose. Laboratory studies were encouraging, but in a clinical setting, results were disappointing for amino acids[14] and harmful using a glucose polymer.[15] The initial results using rice powder and other cereals were more encouraging.[16] However, a meta analysis of 13 clinical trials of rice based ORS concluded that the benefit of rice-based ORS is 'sufficient to warrant use in patients with cholera but is considerably smaller in noncholera diarrhea'.[17] Furthermore, a study by Santhosham et al. showed that treatment with standard ORS and simultaneous feeding with boiled rice produced similar results to using rice based ORS.[18]

Hypo-osmolar ORS

In vitro experiments have shown that water absorption is increased from hypotonic ORS when compared to isotonic ORS.[19,20] Clinical trials have shown that in both the developing world and the developed world, hypotonic ORS with a sodium concentration of 50–70 mmol/l are safe and effective for rehydration and maintenance therapy of mild to severe dehydration from non-cholera diarrhea.[21,22] *In vitro* and *in vivo* data suggest that low osmolarity may be the key for enhancing the clinical effectiveness of ORS.[23] A recent meta analysis of randomized trials of reduced osmolarity ORS *vs* standard WHO ORS in children with non cholera diarrhea,[24] concluded that the use of a reduced osmolarity ORS was associated with: (a) a reduction in the need for unscheduled IV fluids, (defined as the clinical requirement for intravenous fluids once oral rehydration has commenced); (b) a trend toward reduced stool output (about 20%) and (c) reduction in the incidence of vomiting (about 30%). The incidence of hyponatremia (serum sodium 130 mEq/l at 24 h) was higher but this difference was not statistically significant. The accumulating evidence on hypo-osmolar ORS has resulted in a recent expert consultation on ORS formulation by the WHO/ UNICEF. This concluded that the efficacy of glucose based ORS for treatment of children with acute non cholera diarrhea is improved by reducing the sodium content to 60–75 mEq/l, glucose to 75–90 mmol/l and total osmolarity to 215–260 mmol/l.[25] The composition of the proposed New WHO ORS is listed on Table 76.2.

Oral therapy remains the mainstay of the WHO efforts to reduce the morbidity and mortality caused by acute diarrheal disease. In the developing world the uptake is still suboptimal. Simultaneous uptake of ORS in industrialized countries has been slow, despite many clinical trials having documented the safety and efficacy of this form of therapy. A major barrier to the wider uptake of ORS is that it is not perceived to be a medication. A WHO report estimates that less than 50% of acute diarrheal episodes are treated with ORS.[26] An American study that looked at practices compared with AAP recommendations found that less than 30% of responding physicians used a recommended solution to treat dehydration.[27] Another study showed that in the USA, several barriers among pediatricians exist to the use of oral rehydration, including its lack of convenience, the need for additional training for support staff and the question of reimbursement for intravenous *vs* oral rehydration.[28] Similar problems exist in Europe. A recent ESPGHAN survey reported that one in six doctors in Europe would not prescribe ORS.[29]

Early feeding

The primary goals in treating acute diarrhea are preventing and reversing ongoing dehydration and minimizing the nutritional consequences of mucosal injury. Diarrhea, malnutrition and intestinal integrity have a close complex relationship. Malnutrition leads to an increased susceptibility to GI infections and this vicious cycle leads to thousands of children dying everyday worldwide. It has been observed in animal models that starvation alters mucosal barrier function. In addition to the development of ORS, one other milestone has been the advent of early feeding and the avoidance of the so-called intestinal rest.

Historical review of published literature reveals that introduction of a period of starvation dates back to 1926 when Powers wrote his treatise on treatment of diarrhea.[30] There was no scientific basis to the recommendation of this practice. Following this, children were routinely starved during diarrhea and then gradually graded from quarter strength formula to full strength formula over 2–4 days. A study in 1948 showing that there was no scientific rationale for grading was ignored.[31] In 1979, Rees and Brook[32] and later Dugdale et al.[33] and Placzek and Walker Smith[34] showed that gradual grading of feed to full strength was not needed. In 1985, a study by Khin-Maung[35] showed that continued breast-feeding at the time of acute diarrhea was of benefit. Isolauri et al. in 1986, showed that in children older than 6 months after initial oral rehydration therapy, full feeding appropriate for age (including milk) is well tolerated with no adverse effects.[36] Brown et al. then published studies, which clearly showed advantages of continued feeding on clinical and nutritional outcomes.[37,38]

A community based study in the UK[39] and an Eastern European study[40] involving infants of 0–1 year of age further suggested that early feeding was safe, with no increase of lactose intolerance or vomiting and resulted in better weight gain.

The ESPGHAN Working Group on acute diarrhea conducted a large multicenter study, that compared the effect of ORS and early or late feeding on the duration and severity of diarrhea, weight gain and complications (carbohydrate intolerance and vomiting) in weaned European infants[41] and has made recommendations based on this.[42]

The conclusions of this study were as follows:

1 Complete resumption of a child's normal feeding including lactose containing formula after 4 h of rehydration with glucose ORS (ESPGHAN recommended composition) led to significantly higher weight gain after rehydration and during hospitalization (Fig. 76.2).
2 There was no worsening of diarrhea, no prolongation of diarrhea and no increased vomiting or lactose intolerance in the early-feeding group compared with the late feeding group (Figs 76.3, 76.4).

In malnourished children, the nutritional benefits of early feeding have been clearly established.[37] This study, involving a range of hospitals from around Europe, lends further credence to this practice and suggests that there are benefits for children who are not necessarily nutritionally compromised. Theoretical benefits of continuing feeding are minimizing protein loss and energy deficits and reduced functional hypotrophy associated with starving.[43] There is indirect evidence to support the strategy of early feeding, based on studies revealing the positive effects of luminal nutrition on regeneration and mucosal growth as seen in short bowel syndrome. Early re-feeding reduces

Component	Old WHO ORS	AAP ORS	ESPGHAN ORS	New WHO ORS
Sodium (mmol/l)	90	45	60	75
Glucose (mmol/l)	111	138	74–111	75
Osmolarity (mmol/l)	311	250	225–260	245
Chloride (mmol/l)	80	60	60	65
Potassium (mmol/l)	20	20	20	20
Citrate (mmol/l)	10	10	10	10

Table 76.2 The evolution of the Oral Rehydration Solution, ORS (Composition of WHO, AAP, ESPGHAN and new proposed WHO-ORS)

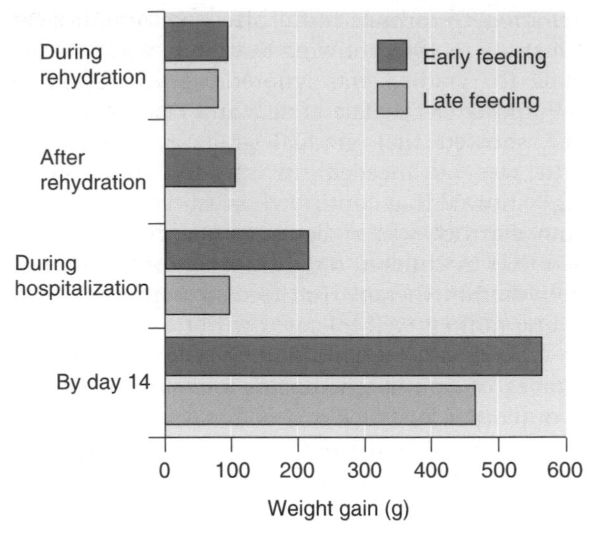

Figure 76.2: Espghan study on early feeding. Comparison of weight gain between early feeding group and late feeding group.

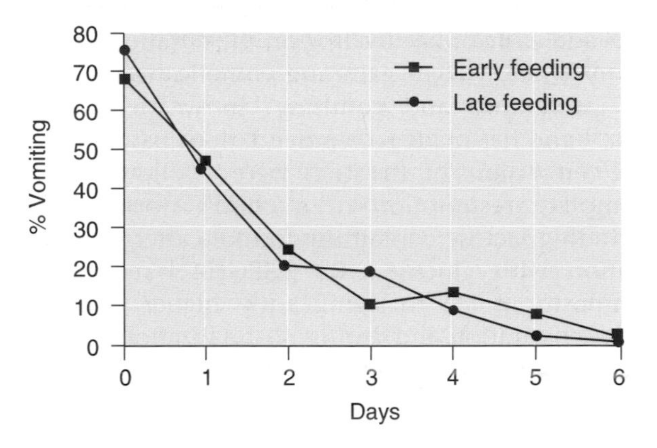

Figure 76.3: Frequency of vomiting between early feeding group and late feeding group (Espghan Study).

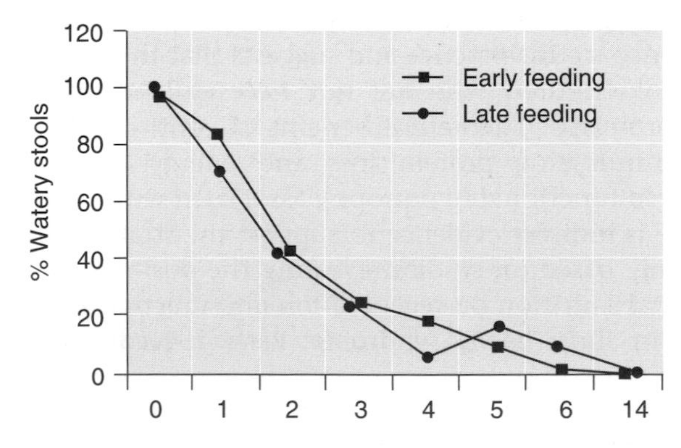

Figure 76.4: Frequency of watery stools between early feeding group and late feeding group (Espghan Study).

the abnormal increase in intestinal permeability that occurs in acute gastroenteritis and may promote recovery of the brush border membrane disaccharidase.[44,45] Early resumption of feeding is now recommended by the ESPGHAN,[42] the American Academy of Pediatrics (AAP)[46] and WHO.

Treatment strategies and practical guidelines

There is now general consensus among pediatric gastroenterologists that the optimum management of acute diarrhea of mild to moderately dehydrated children should consist of the following 'Six Pillars of Good Practice'.[29,46–49]

1 The use of Oral Rehydration Solution (ORS) to correct dehydration in the initial 4 h of management
2 The use of the hypo-osmolar solution (60 mmol/l sodium, 74–111 mmol/l glucose)
3 Breast-feeding should continue throughout
4 Early re-feeding, i.e. resumption of a normal diet once rehydration is complete
5 Prevention of further dehydration by supplementing maintenance fluids with ORS (10 ml/kg ORS for every watery stool)
6 Avoidance of routine use of medication.

Infants with acute diarrhea are more prone to dehydration than are older children because they have a higher body surface area to weight ratio. History and examination should guide the clinician to the severity of dehydration. The severity of dehydration is most accurately assessed in terms of weight loss as a percentage of total body weight. This is the gold standard against which other tests are measured.[48] In the absence of weight, clinical markers may be used to approximate the degree of dehydration (Table 76.3). A good correlation has been reported between capillary refill and fluid deficit.[50] Prolonged skin retraction time and deep breathing may also be reliable indicators of dehydration.[51] The other signs and symptoms are less reliable. If dehydration is less than 5%, the child can be managed at home. Indications for hospital admission include: (a) the child is more than 5% dehydrated; (b) parents unable to manage oral rehydration at home; (c) the child does not tolerate oral rehydration (severe vomiting, insufficient intake); (d) failure of treatment, worsening diarrhea and/or dehydration despite oral rehydration treatment; (e) other concerns, e.g. uncertain diagnosis, potential for surgery, child 'at risk', irritable or drowsy, or a child younger than 2 months.

Work-up and laboratory studies

Most cases of children with mild to moderate dehydration require no laboratory tests. Electrolyte, urea, creatinine and glucose levels should be obtained for severely dehydrated children or where intravenous therapy is deemed to be necessary. The American Academy of Pediatrics suggest in their practice parameter[46] that electrolyte levels should be measured in moderately dehydrated children whose histories or physical findings are inconsistent with straightforward diarrheal episodes and where a 'doughy' feel to the skin may indicate hypernatremia.

Stool microscopy and culture and electron microscopy or ELISA for rotavirus may be useful for etiological information but have little bearing on immediate management. Microscopy for leucocytes in the stool and gram staining of the stools may help in differentiating bacterial from non-bacterial diarrhea. Stool cultures are indicated for those that have bloody diarrhea.

Home management

Ideally, management of acute diarrhea should begin at home as early intervention can reduce complications. The child should be rehydrated using ORS. Effective teaching of the parent or the guardian of procedures for administering the solution and instructions about when to bring the child back for reassessment is absolutely crucial. The use of 'clear fluids' (water alone, cola or fruit juice) is inappropriate and maybe dangerous because they lack adequate sodium. Fruit juices and cola can potentially worsen diarrhea as they have a high osmolar load.

The calculated fluid deficit is replaced over 4 h. Thus, in a 10 kg child, with 5% dehydration, the deficit is 5% of 10 000 g, which equals 500 ml. This is given as ORS over 4 h. It is vital to emphasize the importance of adequate hydration with clear instructions to make up the ORS. If the child is breast-fed, this should continue. Ideally, a child should be reassessed 4 h after rehydration and if fully hydrated, normal feeding should be commenced. Ongoing fluid losses in the form of vomiting or diarrhea should be made up in addition to maintenance fluid requirements, by administering ORS 10 ml/kg for every loose stool or vomitus.

Hospital management

The child should be fully assessed in order to exclude other causes of acute diarrhea. An accurate estimate of the degree of dehydration should be made ideally by using current and previous weights and the child hydrated over 4 h. If moderately or severely dehydrated, investigations should include plasma urea and electrolytes, complete blood count and a stool analysis for viruses and bacteria. If the patient does not tolerate oral rehydration (refuses, vomits profusely or takes inadequate amounts), a nasogastric tube can be used to give ORS. The patient should be reviewed after 4 h and if sufficiently hydrated, a normal diet should be commenced and maintenance fluids continued (150 ml/kg per day for the first 6 kg, plus 50 ml/kg per day for the next 7–20 kg, plus 20 ml/kg per day for the remainder of weight over 20 kg). Supplement ORS, 10 ml/kg for every watery stool, should be continued to make up for on going losses. If dehydration persists, the degree of dehydration should be reassessed and the fluid deficit corrected with ORS over the following 4 h.

Intravenous therapy is only indicated if the child is 10% or more dehydrated, is in shock or if there is failure of oral replacement therapy. If the child is shocked, he should be first resuscitated with 20 ml/kg of normal saline. Deficits should be replaced with 0.9% saline or 0.45% saline in 5% dextrose and calculations based on uncorrected weight. Half the deficit should be replaced in 4 h and the remainder in the next 4 h. Once dehydration is corrected, *maintenance fluids should be continued,* oral feeding commenced and ongoing stool losses replaced with ORS (10 ml/kg per watery stool).

Hypernatremic dehydration

A child with hypernatremia (i.e. sodium of greater than 150 mmol/l) needs careful monitoring with frequent reassessment. Oral rehydration or nasogastric rehydration is by far the safest method. If this fails, resuscitation with i.v. fluid should be carried out slowly as the aim is a gradual reduction in the sodium as a sudden fall can be dangerous and lead to cerebral edema and convulsions. The calculated deficit should be replaced with 0.45% saline/5% dextrose over 8 h, with careful monitoring of the plasma sodium until the child becomes normonatremic. The management should then be as for non-hypernatremic dehydration.

Complications

If diarrhea continues for more than 10 days, parents should be advised to return with the child for a re-assessment and the stool checked for persistent infection. The recurrence of diarrhea each time with re-introduction of milk should alert the physician to the possibility that the child may have developed lactose intolerance. The stool

Signs and symptoms	General condition	Eyes	Tears	Mouth/ tongue	Thirst	Skin	Percentage bodyweight loss	Estimates fluid deficit (ml/kg)
No signs of dehydration	Well, alert	Normal	Present	Moist	Drinks normally, not thirsty	Pinch retracts immediately	<5	<50
Some dehydration	Restless, irritable	Sunken	Absent	Dry	Thirsty, drinks eagerly	Pinch retracts slowly	5–10	50–100
Severe dehydration	Lethargic, unconscious, floppy and dry	Very sunken	Absent	Very dry	Unable to drink	Pinch retracts very slowly	>10	>100

From: Sandhu BK. Practical Guidelines for the Management of Acute Gastroenteritis in Children. J Pediatr Gastroenterol Nutr 2001; 33:S36–S39.[49]

Table 76.3 Assessment of dehydration

pH should be checked and the stool reducing substances measured. This can be done at the bedside using CLINITAB or carried out by the laboratory. If the reducing substances are present at 1% or more, it is considered diagnostic of lactose malabsorption and the child should be placed on a lactose free diet for a 2-week period and then reassessed. Most lactose intolerance is temporary and caused by patchy villous damage and once the gut villi regenerate, lactase and other disaccharidases levels normalize. If the stool is negative to reducing substances and the diarrhea is related to milk protein intake, the child may have developed cow's milk protein intolerance and may require a protein hydrolysate formula.

Antimicrobial therapy

Since viral agents are the predominant cause of acute diarrhea, antibiotics play a limited role in its management. Treatment with appropriate antibiotics is indicated if there is evidence of systemic bacterial infection. Predisposing factors include a history of recent travel, immunodeficiency and history of recent antibiotic use (in which case *Clostridium difficile* should be suspected). Appropriate antibiotics have been shown to be effective in the treatment of Shigellosis, *Clostridium difficile* and Campylobacter. Randomized control trials have shown that in Shigellosis, appropriate antibiotic therapy shortens the duration of diarrhea by 2.4 days, decreases the duration of fever and reduces the excretion of infectious organisms.[52,53] Ciprofloxacin has been shown to be safe and effective in children with shigellosis.[54] Non-typhoidal salmonella gastroenteritis is usually self-limiting and studies have failed to show any benefit from antibiotic treatment.[55] Protozoal pathogens associated with diarrhea that persists for more than 7–10 days are *Giardia lamblia* and Cryptosporidium. Metronidazole or Tinidazole is used for treating proven *Giardia* infection, while Nitazoxanide, which was recently approved by the Food and Drug Administration for use in children,[56] is effective against cryptosporidium. Regardless of the causative agent, initial therapy should include rehydration.

Probiotics

Probiotics have been part of human nutrition for centuries, but in recent years there has been a growing interest in probiotics as a potential method of changing intestinal bacterial flora. Probiotics may potentiate host gastrointestinal defenses and stimulate non-specific host resistance to microbial pathogens. They may protect by increasing non-immunological defenses. The exact mechanisms by which probiotics carry this out is not known yet although the possible mechanisms include the synthesis of anti microbial substance and competition at substrate level.

Lactobacillus rhamnosus strain GG (ATCC 53103) has been the most common bacterial species used to counteract intestinal infections. It has been shown in trial settings to have a number of potentially beneficial effects in preventing and treating acute diarrhea.[57–60] A recent multicenter trial to evaluate the efficacy of Lactobacillus GG administered in the oral rehydration solution in children aged 1 month to 3 years with acute-onset diarrhea of all causes, was conducted by the ESPGHAN Working Group on acute diarrhea.[61] This showed that in rotavirus positive children, diarrhea lasted longer in children in the placebo arm of the trial and the risk of having diarrhea for more than 1 week was reduced nearly four-fold in the lactobacillus treated group. The study showed no benefit in children who were more likely to have had a bacterial cause of diarrhea. This is in concordance with previous reports.[62,63]

A systematic review of published randomized, double blind, placebo controlled trials reviewed 13 studies carried out between 1974 and 2000.[64] The outcome measures that were considered included duration of diarrhea, number of watery stools per day, risk of diarrhea lasting more than 7 days, duration of hospitalization and weight gain. The meta analysis concluded that the use of probiotics was associated with a significant reduced risk of diarrhea lasting more than 3 days. This observation was limited to Lactobacillus GG and there were no adverse outcome measures seen. However, based on WHO recommendations of using stool output rather than duration of diarrhea as a primary outcome measure when evaluating diarrhea treatment, no firm conclusions could be drawn on the effect of probiotics on stool output in acute diarrhea.[64] A Cochrane Library review is due to be published shortly on the use of probiotics in acute diarrhea and these results may impact future clinical practice. (S Allen et al., personal communication).

Antidiarrheal agents

Antidiarrheal agents are not indicated in the management of acute diarrhea. Opioids have an antimotility effect which may mask the severity of diarrhea. They can also have serious side-effects. Very few over the counter antidiarrheal products have been demonstrated to be effective in randomized, controlled trials. Because antimotility agents have been implicated in hemolytic-uremic syndrome in children infected with Shiga toxin producing *E. coli*,[65] these agents should be avoided in children with bloody diarrhea. There is insufficient data to support the routine use of adsorbents such as kaolin-pectin, activated charcoal and attapulgite. Despite the fact that pediatric guidelines discourage the use of antidiarrheal drugs in children,[46,49,66] various studies have highlighted the widespread use of drugs by caregivers in treating children with diarrhea. Easy availability of antidiarrheal drugs is an important factor in perpetuating their misuse.[67] The key strategy in regulating therapy would be to make antidiarrheal agents unacceptable to caregivers and physicians through appropriate education and training. Caregivers and physicians must realize that such drugs are not only unnecessary, but also potentially harmful. Simultaneously, confidence in the ORS needs to be boosted. Table 76.4 shows a summary of the evaluation of safety and efficacy of various antidiarrheal drugs.

Drug	Available evidence	Status
Loperamide (Imodium)	Well-designed trials have shown some benefit in reducing stool volume and duration of diarrhea	Not recommended
	Effects are statistically significant but not clinically significant	
	Unacceptably high rate of side-effects, e.g. lethargy, ileus, respiratory depression, coma	
Other opiates	Hardly any data supporting use	Not recommended
	High potential for toxicity including respiratory depression, paralytic ileus	
Anticholinergics	High toxicity especially in infants and children	Not recommended
Bismuth subsalicylate	No conclusive evidence to demonstrate decreased duration or frequency of diarrhea	Not recommended

From: American Academy of Pediatrics. Provisional committee on quality improvement, subcommittee on acute gastroenteritis. Practice parameter: the management of acute gastroenteritis in young children. Pediatrics 1996; 97:424–435.[46]

Table 76.4 Status of antidiarrheal drugs in children

In theory an antisecretory agent without antimotility effect or significant side-effects may have a role. Racecadotril (Acetorphan) has been proposed as such an agent. Unlike Loperamide and other opioids, it is said to have only antisecretory properties. A placebo-controlled trial showed that with Racecadotril there was a 46% reduction in stool output and reduction in the duration of diarrhea, with only minor adverse effects.[68] However, its peripheral antisecretory selectivity has been questioned,[69] and much further research is needed before reliable conclusions can be drawn on the role of Racecadotril in the treatment of acute diarrhea.

Prevention

Acute diarrhea is a preventable disease and properly applied measures aimed at decreasing its incidence lead to a considerable lowering of infant mortality and morbidity. This is particularly challenging in the developing nations. The obvious measures are improvement in sanitation, provision of clean drinking water, sewerage systems and garbage disposal, adequate housing, promotion of breast-feeding and safe weaning practices and education about basic principles of hygiene.

Prevention through effective vaccination is another possibility. Over the past few years, efforts have been put into the development, trial and production of vaccines against different causes of infectious diarrhea such as cholera, typhoid, shigella and rotavirus. Major factors that interfere with the massive utilization of vaccines are variability in antigenic determinants and the high cost of manufacturing. Rhesus-based rotavirus tetravalent vaccine was withdrawn voluntarily from the market in 1999 because of concerns about an increase in intussusception. A Cochrane database systematic review of 64 trials on efficacy and safety of three main types of rotavirus vaccines recently concluded that the rhesus rotavirus vaccine (particularly RRV-TV) and the human rotavirus vaccine 89-12 are effective in preventing diarrhea caused by rotavirus and all-cause diarrhea.[70] However, evidence about safety, mortality and prevention of severe outcomes was scarce and further research is needed.

Conclusion

In the last three decades, the development and use of scientifically based ORS has dramatically improved the management of children with acute diarrhea, although uptake is still suboptimal. More recently, the benefits of early feeding following rehydration have been recognized and are gaining wider acceptance. This combination of oral rehydration therapy and early feeding should be the mainstay of management of acute diarrhea. Future development of safe vaccines, improvement in public health, further optimization of ORS and perhaps development of safe antisecretory agents and probiotics may help further combat one of the most common public health problems in children worldwide.

MANAGEMENT OF CHRONIC DIARRHEA

Chronic diarrhea is defined as passing four or more watery stools per day for a period of 2 weeks or more. The etiology varies and a systematic approach to the assessment, investigation and management is needed. It is important to think of the child's age when establishing a differential diagnosis as particular conditions manifest for the first time at certain ages. A history of onset in the neonatal period, after excluding infection, suggests cows milk protein enterocolitis, Hirschsprung's disease, cystic fibrosis, adrenogenital syndrome, lymphangiectasia, congenital microvillous atrophy and inherited transport defects such as congenital chloridorrhea. Bloody diarrhea suggests necrotizing enterocolitis in the neonatal period and inflammatory bowel disease in the older child. In the age group, 6 months–2 years, the conditions to be considered are toddler diarrhea, post-enteritis syndrome and celiac disease. Associated recurrent respiratory tract infection may suggest cystic fibrosis or immunological deficiency. In countries where there is a high prevalence of HIV, this needs to be considered early. Clinical examination is important and may give clues to the diagnosis, for example an abdominal mass in phaeochromocytoma and erythema nodosum in Crohn's disease.

References

1. Guarino A, Albano F, Guandalini S, Working Group on Acute Gastroenteritis. Oral rehydration: toward a real solution. Review. J Pediatr Gastroenterol Nutr 200; 33(Suppl 2):S2–S12.
2. Davidson G, Barnes G, Barsey D, et al. Report of the working group on infectious diarrhea. In: Sokol RJ, ed. Report of the Working Groups of the World Congress of Pediatric Gastroenterology, Hepatology and Nutrition 2000. A Global Plan for the future. New York: McGraw Hill; 2000.
3. Tucker AW, Haddix AC, Bresee JS, et al. Cost effectiveness analysis of a rotavirus immunization program in the United States. JAMA 1998; 279:1371–1376.
4. Ho MS, Glass RI, Pinsky PF, et al. Diarrheal deaths in American children – are they preventable? JAMA 1988; 260:3281–3285.
5. Glass RI, Lew JF, Gangarosa RE, LeBaron CW, Ho MS. Estimates of morbidity and mortality rates for diarrheal diseases in American children. J Pediatr 1991; 118: S27–S33.
6. Schultz SG, Zalusky R. Ion transport in isolated rabbit ileum. II. The interaction between active sodium and active sugar transport. J Gen Physiol 1964; 47:1043–1059.
7. Hirschhorn N. The treatment of acute diarrhea in children. An historical and physiological perspective. Am J Clin Nutr 1980; 33:637–663.
8. Walker-Smith JA. Management of infantile gastroenteritis. Arch Dis Child 1990; 65(editorial):917–918.
9. Sunderland R, Emery JL. Apparent disappearance of hypernatraemic dehydration from infant deaths in Sheffield. Br Med J 1979; ii:575–576.
10. Phillips RA. Water and electrolyte losses in cholera. Fed Proc 1964; 23:705–712.
11. Paneth N. Hypernatremic dehydration of infancy: an epidemiologic review. Am J Dis Child 1980; 134:785–791.
12. Molla MA, Rahman M, Sarket A, et al. Stool electrolyte content and purging rates in diarrhea caused by rotavirus, enterotoxigenic E. coli and V. cholerae in children. J Pediatr 1981; 98:835–838 8.
13. Booth I, Cunha Ferreira R, et al. Recommendations for composition of oral rehydration solutions for the children of Europe. Report of ESPGAN Working Group. J Pediatr Gastroenterol Nutr 1992; 14:113–115.
14. Vesikari T, Isolauri G. Glycine supplemented oral rehydration solution for diarrhoea. Arch Dis Child 1986; 61:372–376.
15. Sandhu BK, Jones BJ, Brook CG, Silk DB, Oral rehydration in acute infantile diarrhoea with a glucose-polymer electrolyte solution. Arch Dis Child 1982; 57(2):152–154.
16. Molla AM, Sarker SA, Hussain M, et al. Rice powder electrolyte solution as oral therapy in diarrhea due to Vibrio cholerae and Escherichia coli. Lancet 1982; 1:1317–1319.
17. Gore SM, Fontaine O, Pierce NF. Impact of rice based oral rehydration solutions on stool output and duration of diarrhoea: Meta analysis of 13 clinical trials. Br Med J 1992; 304:287–291.
18. Santhosham M, Fayad M, Hashem M, Goepp JG, Refat M, Sack RB. A comparison of rice based oral rehydration solution and 'early feeding' for the treatment of acute diarrhea in infants. J Pediatr 1990; 116:868–875.
19. Wapnir RA, Lifshitz F. Osmolality and solute concentration – their relationship with oral rehydration solution effectiveness: an experimental assessment. Pediatr Res 1985; 19:894–898.
20. Sandhu BK, Christobal FI, Brueton MJ. Optimising oral rehydration solution composition in model systems: studies in normal mammalian small intestine. Acta Paediatr Scand 1989; 364: S17–S22.
21. Elliot EJ, Cunha-Ferreira R, Walker Smith JA, et al. Sodium concentration of oral rehydration solutions: a reappraisal. Gut 1989; 30:1610–1621.
22. International Study Group on Reduced Osmolality ORS. Multicenter evaluation of reduced osmolality oral rehydration salt solution. Lancet 1995; 345:282–285.
23. Thillainaygam AV, Hunt JB, Farthing MJG. Enhancing clinical efficacy of oral rehydration therapy: is low osmolality the key? Gastroenterology 1998; 114:197–210.
24. Hanh SK, Kim YJ, Garner P. Reduced osmolarity oral rehydration solution for treating dehydration due to diarrhoea in children: systematic review. Br Med J 2001; 323:81–85.
25. WHO/UNICEF. Expert Consultation on Oral Rehydration Salts (ORS) Formulation. New York: WHO/UNICEF; July 2001.
26. World Health Organisation. The State of the World's Children. Geneva: WHO; 1988–1997.
27. Snyder JD. Use and misuse of oral rehydration therapy for diarrhea: comparison of US practices with American Academy of Pediatrics recommendations. Pediatrics 1991; 87:28–33.
28. Reis EC, Goepp JG, Katz SK, et al. Barriers to use of oral rehydration therapy. Pediatrics 1994; 93:708–711.
29. Szajewska H, Hans Hoekstra J, Sandhu B, et al. Management of acute gastroenteritis in Europe and the impact of the new recommendations: a Multicentre study. J Pediatr Gastroenterol Nutr 2000; 30:522–527.
30. Powers GF. A comprehensive plan of treatment for the so-called intestinal intoxification of infants. J Dis Child 1926; 32:232–257.
31. Chung AW, Viscorova B. The effect of oral feeding versus early oral starvation on the course of infantile diarrhea. J Pediatr 1948; 33:14–22.
32. Rees L, Brook CGD. Gradual reintroduction of full strength milk after acute gastroenteritis in children. Lancet 1979; 2:770–771.
33. Dugdale A, Lovell S, Gibbs V, Ball D. Refeeding after acute gastroenteritis: a controlled study. Arch Dis Child 1982; 57:76–79.
34. Placzek M, Walker-Smith JA. Comparison of two feeding regimens following acute gastroenteritis in infancy. J Pediatr Gastroenterol Nutr 1984; 3:245–248.
35. Khin-Maung U, Nyunt-Nyunt-Wai, Myo Khin, Mu-Mu Khin, Tin-U, Thane-Tao. Effect on clinical outcome of breast feeding during acute diarrhoea. Br Med J 1985; 290:587–589.
36. Isolauri E, Vesikari T, Saha P, et al. Milk versus no milk in rapid refeeding after acute gastroenteritis. J Pediatr Gastroenterol Nutr 1986; 5:254–261.
37. Brown KH. Dietary management of acute childhood diarrhea: optimal timing of feeding and appropriate use of milks and mixed diets. J Pediatr 1991; 118: S92–S98.
38. Brown KH, Peerson JM, Fontaine O. Use of nonhuman milks in the dietary management of young children with acute diarrhea: a meta analysis of clinical trials. Pediatrics 1994; 93:17–27.
39. Hoghton MAR, Mittal NK, Mahdi G, Sandhu BK. Continuous modified feeding in acute gastroenteritis. J Gen Practice 1996; 46:173–175.
40. Nanulescu M, Condor M, Popa M, et al. Early re-feeding in the management of acute diarrhoea in infants of 0–1 year of age. Acta Paediatr 1995; 84:1002–1006.
41. EL-Matary W, Spray C, Sandhu BK. Irritable Bowel Syndrome: the commonest cause of recurrent abdominal pain in children. Eur J Paediatric 2004; 163: 584–588.
42. Walker-Smith J, Sandhu BK, Isolauri E, et al. Recommendations for feeding in childhood gastroenteritis. Medical position

paper on behalf of ESPGAN. J Ped Gastroenterol Nutr 1997; 24:619–620.

43. Levine GM, Deren JJ, Steiger E, et al. Role of oral intake in maintenance of gut mass and disaccharide activity. Gastroenterology 1974; 67:972–982.

44. Knudson KB, Bradley EM, Lecocq FR, et al. Effect of fasting and refeeding on the histology and disaccharidase activity of the human intestine. Gastroenterology 1968; 55:46–51.

45. Isolauri E, Juntunen M, Wiren S, et al. Intestinal permeability changes in acute gastroenteritis: effects of clinical factors and nutritional management. J Pediatr Gastroenterol Nutr 1989; 8:466–473.

46. American Academy of Pediatrics. Provisional committee on quality improvement, subcommittee on acute gastroenteritis. Practice parameter: the management of acute gastroenteritis in young children. Pediatrics 1996; 97:424–435.

47. Lifshitz FI, Maggiori A. The nutritional management of acute diarrhea in young infants. J Ped Gastroenterol Nutr 1994; 19:148–150.

48. Murphy MS. Guidelines for managing acute gastroenteritis based on a systematic review of published research. Arch Dis Child 1998; 79:279–284.

49. Sandhu BK. Practical Guidelines for the Management of Gastroenteritis in Children. J Pediatr Gastroenterol Nutr 2001; 33: S36–S39.

50. Saavendra JM, Harris GD, Li S, Finberg L. Capillary refilling (skin turgor) in the assessment of dehydration. Am J Dis Child 1991; 145:296–298.

51. Mackenzie A, Barnes G, Shann F. Clinical signs of dehydration in children. Lancet 1989; 2:605–607.

52. Tong MJ, Martin DG, Cunningham JJ, Gunning JJ. Clinical and bacteriological evaluation of antibiotic in Shigellosis. JAMA 1970; 214:1841–1844.

53. Bennish ML, Salam MA, Haider R, Barza M, Therapy for Shigellosis. II. Randomised, double blind comparison of ciprofloxacin and ampicillin. J Infect Dis 1990; 162:711–716.

54. Zimbabwe, Bangladesh, South Africa (Zimbasa) Dysentery Study Group. Multicenter, randomised, double blind clinical trial of short courses versus standard course oral ciprofloxacin for Shigella dysenteriae in children. Pediatr Infect Dis J 2002; 21:1136–1141.

55. Nelson JD, Kusmiesz H, Jackson LH, Woodman E. Treatment of salmonella gastroenteritis with ampicillin, amoxycillin or placebo. Pediatrics 1980; 65:1125–1130.

56. Rossignol JF, Ayoub A, Ayers MS. Treatment of diarrhea caused by Cryptosporidium parvum: a prospective randomised double-blind, placebo-controlled study of nitazoxanide. J Infect Dis 2001; 184:103–106.

57. DuPont HL. Lactobacillus GG in prevention of traveler's diarrhea: An encouraging first step. J Travel Med 1997; 4:1–2.

58. Hilton E, Kolakowoski P, Singer C, Smith M. Efficacy of Lactobacillus GG as a diarrheal preventive in travellers. J Travel Med 1997; 4:41–43.

59. Guandalini S. Probiotics in the treatment of diarrheal diseases in children. Gastroenterology Int 1998; 11:87–90.

60. Vanderhoof JA, Young RJ. Use of probiotics in childhood gastrointestinal disorders. J Pediatr Gastroenterol Nutr 1998; 27:323–332.

61. Guandalini S, Pensabene L, Zikri MA, et al. Lactobacillus GG administered in oral rehydration solution to children with acute diarrhea: a multicenter European trial. J Pediatr Gastroenterol Nutr 2000; 30(1):54–60.

62. Raza S, Graham SM, Allen SJ, Sultana S, Cuevas L, Hart CA. Lactobacillus GG promotes recovery from acute non bloody diarrhea in Pakistan. Pediatr Infect Dis J 1995; 14:107–111.

63. Pant AR, Graham SM, Allen SJ, et al. Lactobacillus GG and acute diarrhea in young children in the tropics. J Trop Pediat 1996; 42:162–165.

64. Szajewska H, Mrukowicz JZ. Probiotics in the Treatment of Acute infectious Diarrhea in Infants and Children: A systematic Review of Published Randomised, Double Blind, Placebo-Controlled Trials. J Pediatr Gastroenterol Nutr 2000; 33:S17–S25.

65. Cimolai N, Basalyga S, Mah DG, Morrison BJ, Carter JE. Continuing assessment of risk factors for the development of Escherichia coli O157:H7-associated haemolytic uremic syndrome. Clin Nephrol 1994; 42:85–89.

66. Armon K, Stephenson T, MacFaul R, Eccleston P, Werneke U. An evidence and consensus based guideline for acute diarrhoea management. Arch Dis Child 2001; 85:132–142.

67. SK Mittal, Mathew J. Regulating the use of drugs in diarrhea. J Pediatr Gastroenterol Nutr 2001; 33: S26–S30.

68. Salazar-Lindo E, Santisteban-Ponce J, Chea-Woo E, Gutierrez M. Racecadotril in the treatment of acute watery diarrhea in children. N Engl J Med 2000; 343(7):463–467.

69. Guandalini S; The treatment of acute diarrhea in the third millennium: a pediatrician's perspective. Acta Gastroenterol Belg 2002; 65(1):33–36.

70. Soares-Weiser K, Goldberg E, Tamimi G, Pitan O, Leibovici L, Rotavirus vaccine for preventing diarrhoea. Cochrane Database Syst Rev 2004; 1:CD002848.

71. Gracey M. Persistent childhood diarrheas: patterns, pathogenesis and prevention. J Gastroenterol Hepatol 1993; 8(3):259–266.

72. Karim AS, Akhter S, Rahamn MA, Nazir MF. Risk factors of persistent diarrhea in children below five years of age. Indian J Gastroenterol 2001; 20:59–61.

73. Roy SK, Tomkins AM, Mahalanabis D, et al. Impact of zinc supplementation on persistent diarrhea in malnourished Bangladeshi children. Acta Paediatr 1998; 87:1235–1239.

74. Penny ME, Peerson JM, Marin RM, et al. Randomised, community-based trial of the effect of zinc supplementation, with and without other micronutrients, on the duration of persistent childhood diarrhea in Lima, Peru. J Pediat 1999; 135:208–217.

75. Gupta SK, Chong SK, Fitzgerald JF, Disaccharidase activities in children: normal values and comparison based on symptoms and histologic changes. J Pediatr Gastroenterol Nutr 1999; 28:246–251.

76. Walker Smith JA, Cow's Milk Intolerance as a cause of postenteritis diarrhea. J Pediatr Gastroenterol Nutr1982; 1(2):163–173.

77. Fenton T R, Harries JT, Milla PJ. Disordered small intestinal motility: a rational basis for toddler's diarrhea. Gut 1983; 24:897–903.

78. Dodge JA, Hamdi IA, Burns GM, Yamashiro Y. Toddler diarrhoea and prostaglandins. Arch Dis Child 1981; 56:705–707.

79. Cohen SA, Hendrics KM, Mathis RK, et al. Chronic non-specific diarrhea: dietary relationships. Pediatrics 1979; 64:402–407.

80. Llyod-Still JD: Chronic diarrhea of childhood and the misuse of elimination diets. J Pediatr 1979; 95:10–13.

81. Hyams JS, Burke G, Davis PM, Treem WR, Shoup M. Characterization of symptoms in children with recurrent abdominal pain: resemblance to irritable bowel syndrome. J Pediatr Gastroenterol Nutr 1995; 20:209–214.

82. Larcher VF, Shepherd R, Francis DEM, Harries JT. Protracted diarrhea in infancy: analysis of 82 cases with particular reference to diagnosis and management. Arch Dis Child 1977; 52:597–605.
83. Sawczenko A, Sandhu BK, Newer diarrheal syndromes. Indian J Pediatr 1999; 66: S46–S51.
84. Phillips AD, Jenkins P, Raafat F, et al. Congenital microvillus atrophy specific diagnostic features. Arch Dis Child 1985; 60:730.
85. Unsworth J, Hutchins P, Mitchell J, et al. Flat small intestinal mucosal and autoantibodies against the gut epithelium. J Paediatr Gastroenterol Nutr 1982; 1:503–513.
86. Mirakian R, Richardson A, Milla P, et al. Protracted diarrhoea of infancy: evidence in support of an autoimmune variant. BMJ 1986; 293:1132–1136.
87. Guarino A, Spagnuolo MI, Russo S, Albano F, Guandilini S, Capano G. Etiology and risk factors of severe and protracted diarrhea. J Ped Gastroenterol Nutr 1995; 20(2):173–178.
88. Francis DEM: Diets for sick children. Blackwell Scientific Publications London, 1974.
89. Gunn T, Brown RS, Pencharz P, Colle T. Total parenteral nutrition in malnourished infants with intractable diarrhea. Can Med Assoc 1977; 117:357–360.
90. Goulet O, Jan D, Lacaille F, et al. Intestinal transplantation in children: preliminary experience in Paris. J Parenter Enteral Nutr 1999; 23(5 Suppl):S121–S125.
91. Lubani MM, Doudin KI, Sharda DC, et al. Congenital chloride diarrhoea in Kuwaiti children. Eur J Paediatr 1989; 148:333–336.
92. Aichbichler BW, Zerr CH, Santa Ana CA, Porter JL, Fordtran JS. Proton pump inhibition of gastric chloride secretion in congenital chloridorrhea. New Engl J Med 1997; 336:106–109.

Chapter 77

Effects of digestive diseases on bone metabolism

Francisco A. Sylvester

INTRODUCTION

Bone provides a supporting scaffold for organs and soft tissues in the body. Bone mass, the most important determinant of bone strength, is regulated by the activities of bone-forming cells (osteoblasts) and bone-resorbing cells (osteoclasts).[1] Bone tissue is formed when osteoblast function outpaces bone resorption. Bone loss occurs when osteoclast activity predominates over bone formation. Both osteoblasts and osteoclasts can respond to systemic and local signals, and their function can be altered in disease states. Therefore, it is not surprising that many gastrointestinal and liver diseases have an impact on bone mass. As growing children have actively remodeling bones, they may be particularly vulnerable to the effects of disease on the skeleton. However, restoration of health in children offers the hope of skeletal reconstitution, a characteristic that may be unique to pediatric patients. Current knowledge indicates that the response of children's bone metabolism to both disease and therapy is different to that in adults. Therefore, similar to other fields in pediatrics, observations on the impact of gastrointestinal and liver disease on the adult skeleton should not be directly extrapolated to children. This chapter points out differences in how digestive diseases affect bone in children and in adults. To achieve this goal, we will review basic bone biology, the assessment of bone mass and bone metabolic activity, current knowledge on the effects of digestive diseases on bone metabolism and bone mass in children, and available therapies to enhance bone mass. The reader is referred to excellent recent reviews on this subject that focus on the impact of these diseases on skeletal health of adult patients.[2,3]

BONE BIOLOGY IN CHILDREN

The bones of growing children increase in size and change shape ('bone modeling') until they reach pubertal maturity, when their growth plate closes and linear growth ceases. This normal physiologic process is regulated by an array of endocrine and paracrine factors.[4,5] These systems act on osteoblasts, cells derived from mesenchymal precursors, and osteoclasts, which develop from hematologic precursors (Fig. 77.1). Osteoblasts go through a defined sequence of events controlled by hormones and transcriptional factors that ensure the proper development of their mature phenotype and functional properties. The main function of osteoblasts is to form a protein matrix that is rich in type I collagen. Under normal circumstances this matrix becomes mineralized with calcium phosphate crystals to form mature bone tissue. Some osteoblasts become embedded in the mineralized matrix and become osteocytes. Osteocytes develop radiating processes that form a network that senses mechanical stress, which induces bone adaptation.[6] Other osteoblasts die by apoptosis, and others form lining cells over newly repaired bone.[7] These lining cells can become active osteoblasts when needed. The protein matrix is embedded with many other proteins besides type I collagen, some of which have regulatory functions, such as transforming growth factor β, osteonectin and osteopontin.[8] Osteoblasts have receptors for cytokines and parathyroid hormone,[9–11] and can secrete interleukin (IL) 6 and other regulatory factors[12–14] into the bone microenvironment. Normal osteoblast activity is essential for osteoclast formation and activation.

Osteoclasts require receptor activator of nuclear factor κ-ligand (RANKL) to differentiate and become active. RANKL is produced by osteoblasts and other cells, such as activated T cells, and serves as the final common mediator by which other factors affect osteoclast development.[15,16] RANKL can be bound to the osteoblast surface, or released into the extracellular fluid in a soluble form. RANKL binds to its receptor RANK on the osteoclast precursor surface, stimulating its proliferation, differentiation and activity. Mice lacking RANKL or RANK have abnormally dense bones owing to lack of osteoclasts. These mice also fail to develop lymph nodes, establishing a link between the immune system and bone cell biology.[16] Interestingly, cytokines associated with inflammation such as IL-6, IL-1β and tumor necrosis factor (TNF) α can increase osteoclast formation by stimulating RANKL synthesis.[17–20] However, interferon (INF) γ, IL-4 and IL-12 are potent inhibitors of osteoclast formation by inhibiting RANKL function.[21–23]

In bone modeling, periosteal bone is laid down by osteoblasts, while osteoclasts resorb endosteal bone. These activities result in relatively large increases in bone mass that are not coupled. In contrast, in bone remodeling, bone mass is maintained due to the coordinated osteoclast bone resorption and osteoblast formation (Fig. 77.2). Consequently, diseases that decrease osteoblast activity eventually result in decreased bone resorption, a state referred to as *low bone turnover*. In this state, bone mass is lost primarily due a decrease in osteoblast function. Conversely, when bone resorption is increased, osteoblast activity is induced. However, because bone formation

Figure 77.1: Osteoblasts are derived from pluripotent mesenchymal precursors preent in bone marrow. Bone morphogenetic protein (BMP) and other factors stimulate specific signal transduction pathways in stromal cells that lead to the transactivation of critical transcription factors. These regulate the expression of appropriate genes to direct the differentiation of immature cells into osteoblasts. Receptor activator of nuclear factor κ-ligand (RANKL) produced by osteoblasts can then stimulate osteoclastogenesis and osteoclast activation. RANKL activity can be blocked by a soluble decoy receptor osteoprotegerin (OPG). NF-κB, nuclear factor κB; M-CSF, macrophage colony-stimulating factor.

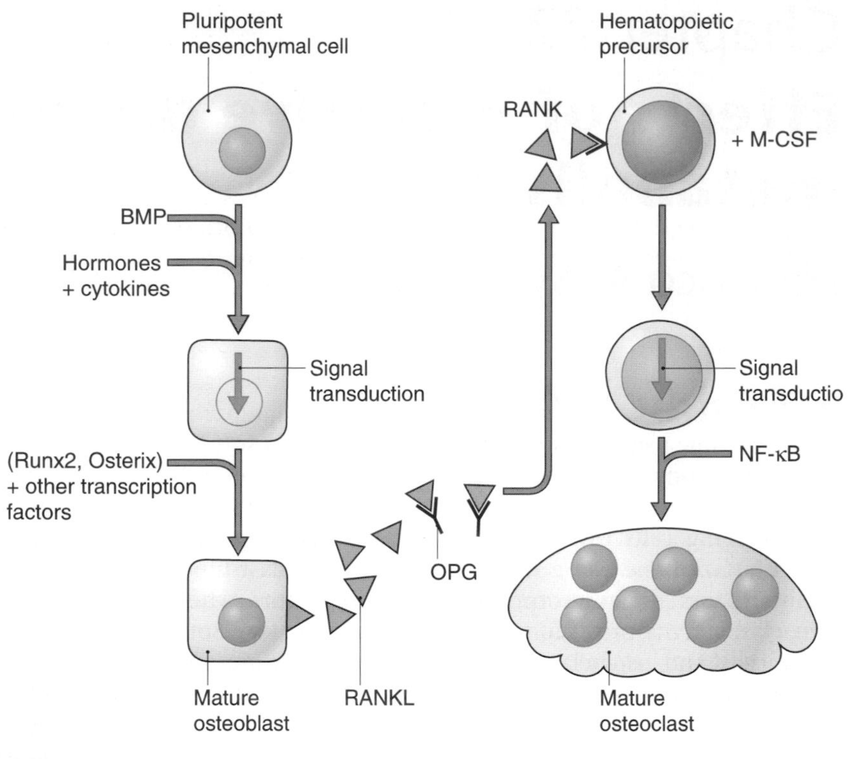

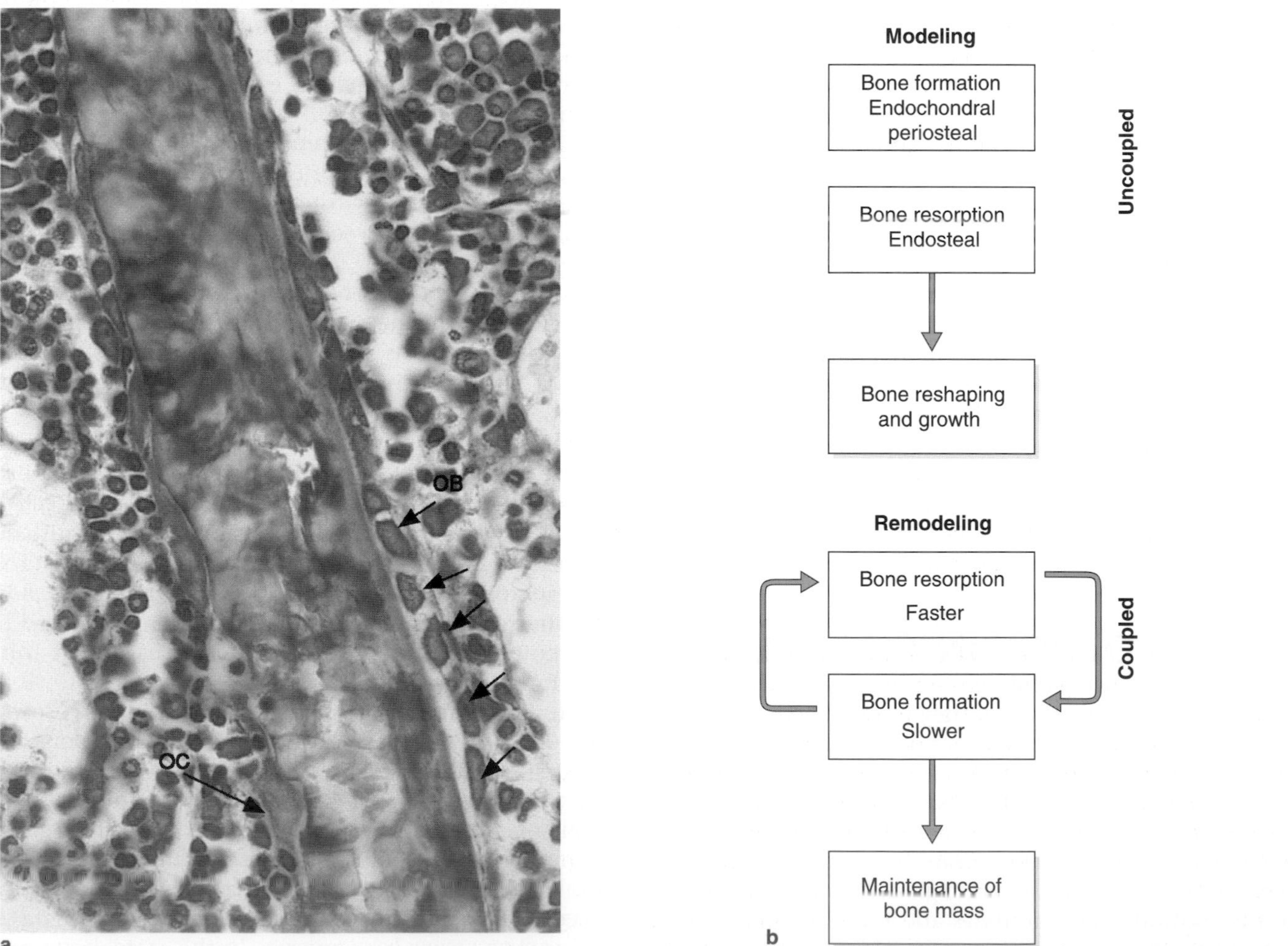

Figure 77.2: Bone mass is regulated by the balance between osteoblast and osteoclast activities. (**a**) Photomicrograph from a bone trabecula of mouse femur (×400) lined by osteoblasts (OB, short arrows) and osteoclasts (OC, long arrow). (**b**) Bone formation by osteoblasts lags behind bone resportion by osteoclasts. (Photomicrograph courtesy of Dr Ernesto Canalis). (See plate section for color).

normally lags behind bone resorption, this will result in loss of bone mass. This remodeling state is known as *high bone turnover*. In some diseases, the function of osteoblasts and osteoclasts can be uncoupled; for example, in adults with Crohn's disease decreased bone formation can be associated with increased bone resorption.[24] Digestive diseases in children in general tend to induce a state of low bone turnover,[25–27] rather than increased bone resorption, which is common in adult patients. This has important implications for the treatment of osteopenia associated with digestive diseases in children (see below).

Bones have a cortex of compact bone and an inner lattice of trabecular bone. Beyond their gross appearance, there are important structural and functional differences between these two types of bone. Cortical or compact bone constitutes approximately 80% of the bone mass. It is formed by an array of tightly packed mineralized cylinders, each with an axis formed by a nourishing blood vessel that runs parallel to the long axis of the bone. Each cylinder is made of concentric layers of mineralized matrix in which there are embedded osteocytes. However, trabecular bone is made from interconnecting mineralized elements, resembling the structure of a sponge. Each trabecula consists of mineralized matrix containing osteocytes, and lined by osteoblasts and osteoclasts. Trabecular bone is intimately associated with the bone marrow. It is the most metabolically active form, accounting for 80% of bone metabolic activity. Therefore, digestive diseases in children tend preferentially to affect bones that are rich in trabecular bone, such as vertebral bodies and ribs.

PEAK BONE MASS

Bone mass is the major determinant of bone strength over the life of the individual. Rapid gain of bone mass occurs throughout childhood, especially during puberty when bones grow rapidly in longitude, volume and strength. Eventually, newly formed matrix becomes fully mineralized, signaling the end of bone mass accretion, usually early in the third decade of life. At this time, an individual has finished bone modeling and has gained the maximum of bone tissue, called *peak bone mass*.[28,29] Peak bone mass is achieved earlier in women than in men because women complete their sexual maturation earlier. After late adolescence (about 20 years of age), bone mass is maintained by remodeling, but after a period that lasts approximately 1-2 decades it is lost at a steady rate for the rest of the person's life, predominantly at the expense of trabecular bone. Eventually, in some individuals, the remaining bone may not be able to sustain the stresses of daily living or trauma, fail structurally, and fracture. Therefore, the amount of bone that a child has built is the most important determinant of lifelong skeletal health.[30] Peak bone mass is determined primarily by heredity. A family history of osteoporosis and fractures is a major risk factor for decreased bone mass. Other factors that influence bone mass include bodyweight, physical activity, diet and ethnicity.[29,31] There is a narrow, fixed window of opportunity during puberty and early adulthood when peak bone mass can be acquired. If this time passes, the individual will not attain peak bone mass.[32] This has important practical implications for children with gastrointestinal and liver diseases in whom delayed puberty is common. Every effort should be made to minimize the impact of the underlying disease on pubertal maturation.

MEASUREMENT OF BONE METABOLISM AND BONE MASS IN CHILDREN

Bone biopsy can be used to assess bone remodeling and to diagnose bone metabolic disease in both children and adults. Although it is considered the 'gold standard', a major disadvantage of bone biopsy for routine pediatric use is its invasive nature. Bone biopsy is usually done in the iliac crest after timed administration of oral tetracycline to label the mineralizing front in the bone. The bone is then embedded in plastic, sectioned, stained and analyzed using quantitative histomorphometry. Normative data are limited in children for interpretation of these results.[33] Bone biopsy studies have not yet been performed in children with digestive diseases.

Several indirect markers of bone metabolism are used to assess bone formation and resorption. However, interpretation of their results is difficult because they depend on age, pubertal stage, growth velocity, mineral accrual, hormonal regulation, nutritional status, circadian variation, day-to-day variation specificity for bone tissue, sensitivity and specificity of assays.[34] Bone formation can be studied by measuring serum osteocalcin (a marker of mature osteoblasts), serum bone-derived alkaline phosphatase (an indicator of osteoblast activity) and pro-collagen extension peptides (a sign of bone matrix synthesis). For bone resorption, the products of type I collagen degradation can be measured as markers. These include N- and C-terminal telopeptides (NTx and CTx), and collagen crosslinks (urinary deoxypyridinoline). At this point, these markers should be used to compare bone metabolic trends between defined patient groups rather than in individual patients.

There are several methods to determine bone mineral mass, but in children two methods are most commonly used – dual energy X-ray absorptiometry (DXA) and quantitative computed tomography (qCT). In children, DXA is usually performed in the total body and lumbar spine, and is currently the best validated method. In DXA, an X-ray source generates beams of two different energies, which are differentially attenuated by bone and soft tissues. After traversing the body, the residual X-ray energy is measured by an array of detectors placed on a wand coupled with the X-ray source. A computer analyzes the data and reports them as bone mineral content (BMC, in g) and bone area (cm^2). Bone mineral density (BMD, in g/cm^2) is a calculated value (BMC divided by bone area). In addition, information on body composition (percentage fat and lean tissue) can be collected. Newer instruments can reconstruct an image of the lateral spine, and analyze vertebral bodies for compression fractures. DXA involves minimal radiation and time, and is reproducible; however, although its use has been validated in children, there is still a lack of standardized pediatric reference data, especially in children under 8 years of age.[35] DXA measured by different instruments is not interchangeable, and the different software packages that define the mineralized areas to be scanned can add an additional level of variability. The assessment of BMD by DXA is dependent on a two-dimensional projected area rather than a volumetric value, so these measurements are critically dependent on bone size. DXA does not measure the dimension of depth of bone; bone density by DXA will appear to increase in growing bones, even if the true volumetric density remains constant.[36] Therefore, special caution needs to be taken to interpret DXA measurements properly in children with growth retardation and/or delayed puberty,[37–39] a common complication of gastrointestinal and liver diseases in children. DXA tends to underestimate BMD in children who are small for their age, whereas it tends to overestimate BMD in children with larger skeletons. To overcome this limitation, the volumetric bone density can be calculated using geometric assumptions to generate a value called the bone *apparent* mineral density (BMAD).[40] For children with short stature or pubertal delay, it may be more appropriate to use height–age or Tanner stage rather than chronologic age to interpret DXA results. In children who have not yet reached peak bone mass, BMD should be expressed as a Z score, which measures the deviation of the observed BMD from normative values (Z score = Observed BMD – BMD for age, sex and race/standard deviation).[35] In adults, BMD is expressed as a T score, which measures the variance from mean BMD values of young healthy adults.[41] T scores should not be used in children. In addition to mineral content, other properties of bone are important in determining bone strength, including bone geometry, bone quality and material properties that are not examined by DXA.[42] For example, an equal amount of bone mineral distributed across a larger diameter will confer increased bone strength. The impact of childhood illness on these properties is not known.

Quantitative CT can measure true volumetric bone density, but involves more ionizing radiation and time. Peripheral qCT devices are being developed that measure volumetric bone density in the distal extremities with much less radiation. This technology is promising for use in children, and may be adapted more widely with standardization of measurements at different skeletal sites, improved precision and generation of normative data.[43]

Measurement of BMD should be considered in children on chronic corticosteroid therapy, with chronic disease, radiographic evidence of bone demineralization, or recurrent low impact fractures.

DEFINITION OF OSTEOPOROSIS IN CHILDREN

Based on epidemiologic data in postmenopausal women, the World Health Organization (WHO) established definitions for normal bone mass and for mild-to-moderate (osteopenia) and severe (osteoporosis) demineralization.[44] These definitions correlate BMD measured by DXA with fracture risk, and define a T score ≥ -1 as normal; <-1 but >-2.5 as osteopenia, and ≤ -2.5 as osteoporosis. There is no 'cutoff' value for fracture risk; instead, there is a continuous increase in fracture risk with each decrease in T score. Although these definitions were originally intended to be used in population studies, they are now widely applied to individual postmenopausal women and elderly men to estimate fracture risk and need for therapy. However, it is important to note that such *a relationship between BMD and fracture risk is not established in children*, with the exception of forearm fractures in healthy children.[45] Therefore, the WHO definitions cannot be extrapolated directly to children and should not constitute the sole basis by which a decision is based to start pharmacologic therapy. The International Society for Clinical Densitometry has recently stated that the WHO definitions of osteopenia and osteoporosis cannot be applied to children and that in this population it is more appropriate to talk in terms of mild-to-severe bone demineralization, depending on the child's Z score. A Z score <-2 should be reported, for example, as 'low bone density for chronologic age'.[35,43] As the clinical endpoint of osteopenia is bone fracture, the significance of low BMD in this age group remains uncertain and longitudinal studies are needed to determine the risk of fracture based on BMD and other factors in specific digestive diseases in children.[46]

COMMON MECHANISMS BY WHICH DIGESTIVE DISEASES AFFECT BONE MASS

Puberty is characterized by rapid longitudinal bone growth, volumetric expansion and bone mineralization.[47] These events require many endocrine and paracrine systems working in harmony. Chronic gastrointestinal and liver diseases can affect normal bone development by affecting these systems. For example, malnutrition due to lack of intake and/or malabsorption is common in children with these diseases. Protein malnutrition is associated with suboptimal bone development.[29,48,49] Malabsorption of luminal fatty acids in cholestatic states or enteropathies can bind calcium and prevent its absorption. In addition, it is possible that the inflamed intestine may leak calcium into the lumen and be lost in the stool. This can affect the pool of calcium available to mineralize bone. In addition, malabsorption of fat-soluble vitamins such as vitamin D and vitamin K can adversely affect bone metabolism. Vitamin D insufficiency can result in rickets. Children who are ill may spend more time indoors and limit their exposure to sunlight, thereby decreasing the cutaneous synthesis of vitamin D.[50] They may also limit their intake of vitamin D-fortified dairy products due to primary or secondary lactose intolerance, which will also decrease their calcium intake. The role of vitamin K in normal calcium homeostasis is being increasingly appreciated.[51–53] Vitamin K is a co-factor in the post-translational modification of osteocalcin and other proteins such as clotting factors. Osteocalcin is a marker of mature osteoblast activity, and plays a role in the regulation of bone mass.[54] Vitamin K serves as a co-factor in the γ-carboxylation of glutamic acid to form γ-carboxyglutamic acid residues that can bind calcium. Deficient osteocalcin carboxylation due to vitamin K deficiency leads to a markedly decreased affinity of osteocalcin for calcium. The presence of raised serum levels of uncarboxylated osteocalcin is a sensitive indicator of vitamin K deficiency, before changes in prothrombin time occur. Subclinical vitamin K deficiency has been reported in Crohn's disease[52] and cystic fibrosis.[55]

Delayed puberty is often a feature of chronic digestive diseases and can permanently affect the attainment of peak bone mass.[32] Estrogen is critical in maintaining bone mass in both males and females.[56,57] A relative estrogen deficiency, as seen in children with delayed sexual maturation, may therefore affect bone mass development in growing children. Normal bone development is stimulated by weight-bearing exercise. Children with chronic disease may have limitations in their endurance and prefer more sedentary activities. This can potentially decrease bone strength over time.

During puberty there is a marked increase in the magnitude and frequency of growth hormone release. This induces the expression of insulin-like growth factor (IGF)-I in the liver and other tissues, including the skeleton. IGF-I is a potent growth factor for bone. It stimulates longitudinal growth by chondrocytes and expansion of the outer cortical layer by periosteal osteoblasts. In the trabecular bone compartment, IGF-I may promote the recruitment of undifferentiated stromal cells into cells of the osteoblast lineage.[5,47] IGF-I is also essential for the activation of 1,25-dihydroxyvitamin D.[58] Active chronic diseases in childhood are frequently associated with decreased serum IGF-I levels, probably due to a combination of cytokine effects and nutritional deficiencies (e.g. protein and zinc). Serum IGF-I concentration tends to increase in parallel with clinical improvement, which may help to re-establish normal skeletal homeostasis.[59–61]

Cytokines and other factors released by inflamed tissues can influence the function of bone cells, and bone cells can secrete cytokines conventionally associated with inflammation (see above). For example, IL-6 is an acute-phase reactant and its concentration is commonly raised systemically in inflammatory diseases.[62] IL-6 can activate bone resorption by osteoclasts and may also inhibit some aspects of osteoblast function[63–68] and activate others.[10,11] INF-γ, a product of activated T helper type 1 (Th1) CD4+ cells found in inflamed tissues,[69,70] can inhibit both osteoclastogenesis and osteoblast function.[21,71–74] RANKL, a potent stimulus for osteoclast differentiation and activity, is synthesized by activated T cells.[75] The specific role of these and other factors in the regulation of bone mass is the subject of intense study.

Medications used to treat digestive disorders can also affect bone cell function. Corticosteroids decrease BMD and increase the risk of fractures in adults, an effect that occurs early in the course of therapy and can be observed even with small doses.[76] A recent large case–control study involving children who received four or more courses of oral corticosteroids (mean duration 6.4 days) found an increased risk of fracture among children who received the medication compared with controls.[77] Corticosteroids affect both osteoblasts and osteoclasts, although their initial effect is primarily on bone formation. They can directly inhibit osteoblast function and decrease osteoblast number. In addition, they can affect osteoblasts indirectly by decreasing the synthesis of anabolic sex steroids. Corticosteroids can also inhibit the activity of vitamin D and stimulate parathyroid hormone (PTH) activity, thus stimulating bone resorption. Increased PTH activity also impairs intestinal calcium absorption and promotes renal elimination of calcium and phosphate.[78] Calcineurin inhibitors such as ciclosporin and tacrolimus can inhibit osteoblast function.[79–82] However, under certain conditions tacrolimus may induce osteoblast differentiation from mesenchymal precursors.[83] Limited information on interferon (INF)-α suggests that it decreases the proliferation of human osteoblast precursors,[84] and treatment of chronic hepatitis C with INF-α and ribavarin may result in bone loss.[85] Cholestyramine, used to treat pruritus from cholestasis or diarrhea due to unconjugated bile acids, can adsorb vitamin D and prevent its absorption from the intestinal lumen. Loop diuretics for treatment of ascites can increase urinary calcium loss as a side-effect.

SELECTED GASTROINTESTINAL DISEASES ASSOCIATED WITH DECREASED BMD

Inflammatory bowel diseases

Both Crohn's disease and ulcerative colitis are associated with decreased bone mass. In adults, the prevalence of osteopenia ranges from 0% to 65%, depending on the population studied and the method used to determine bone mass; most large studies report a prevalence of low BMD of about 15%.[2] Some studies suggest that patients with Crohn's disease may be affected more severely than those with ulcerative colitis.[86–88] Children with inflammatory bowel disease (IBD) can also have decreased BMD,[89–91] even at the time of diagnosis before corticosteroid use.[92] Non-traumatic fractures have been reported in both adults and children with IBD, especially at sites rich in trabecular bone.[25,88,93–97] Several large studies have been conducted to estimate the risk of fracture in adults with IBD. In a retrospective population-based cohort study, Bernstein et al.[98] reported that Canadian patients with IBD had a 41% greater risk of fractures compared with the general population, with similar increases for Crohn's disease and ulcerative colitis. A case–control study in patients recruited from the Danish Colitis/Crohn's Association found a 2.5-fold increase of fracture only in females with Crohn's disease.[88] A subsequent study by the same group using a hospital discharge registry reported a modest increase in fracture risk in Crohn's patients, but not in those with ulcerative colitis.[99] Using a primary care-based nested case–control approach, a study from the UK showed that the risk of fracture was higher in patients with IBD than in controls, especially fracture of the hip in subjects with Crohn's disease.[96] However, Loftus et al.[100,101] did not detect an overall increased risk of fracture in adults with Crohn's disease or ulcerative colitis. Nevertheless, the true prevalence of fractures in patients with IBD may be underestimated, because a minority of vertebral fractures come to clinical attention.[95,102] Similar epidemiologic studies have not yet been conducted in children with IBD to establish fracture risk.

The pathogenesis of bone loss in IBD, as in other digestive disorders, is likely multifactorial, with roles for protein-calorie malnutrition,[90] vitamin deficiencies (e.g. vitamin D[50] and possibly vitamin K[52]), malabsorption, inactivity, hypogonadism,[103] corticosteroid use[104–106] and systemic inflammation.[107] Interestingly, endogenous overproduction of active vitamin D has been reported in Crohn's disease, resulting in hypercalcemia.[108] Biochemical markers of bone metabolism suggest that bone formation is reduced in both adults and children with longstanding Crohn's disease,[24,25,109–111] whereas bone resorption is increased in adults but not in children.[24,109,110] In animal models of colitis that mimic the physiologic situation in a growing child, decreased bone formation results in decreased bone mass.[112] Using an *in vitro* model of intact bone, Hyams et al.[113] showed that serum from children with newly diagnosed Crohn's disease decreases bone weight and calcium incorporation, with no increase in bone resorption. The serum of children with ulcerative colitis had no effect.[113] Antibody neutralization of serum IL-6 in part reverses the effects of Crohn's serum in this model.[68] Similar studies using primary osteoblast cultures showed that osteoblast function is impaired by serum from untreated children with newly diagnosed Crohn's disease.[114] These data suggest important differences in the pathogenesis of osteopenia between Crohn's disease and ulcerative colitis, and between children and adults with IBD, which have implications in how these children should be treated.

Inflammation is thought to play an important role in inducing bone loss in these patients. Specific cytokines have been implicated in the osteopenia associated with IBD. For example, Pollak et al.[115] observed that high serum IL-6 levels were associated with osteoporosis (spine or hip BMD T score <–2.5) in a cohort of adults with Crohn's disease and ulcerative colitis. In the skeleton, IL-1β stimulates bone resorption by increasing osteoclast activity. Nemetz et al.[116] found that an IL-1β polymorphism conferring a phenotype of increased IL-1β secretion was associated with decreased BMD in adults with IBD compared with healthy controls. Schulte et al.[117] observed that non-carriage of the 240-base-pair allele of the IL-1 receptor antagonist (IL-1ra) gene and carriage of the 130-base-pair allele of the IL-6 gene were independently associated with increased bone loss. These studies emphasize the need to control inflammation to promote skeletal reconstitution in patients with IBD.

A rare skeletal complication associated with IBD is chronic recurrent multifocal osteomyelitis. This condition is associated with sterile inflammation of the clavicles and long bones, and usually appears years before the onset of gastrointestinal symptoms. It is not specific to IBD, as it can occur in other chronic inflammatory diseases. It responds to treatment of the underlying disease.[118,119]

Celiac disease

Loss of bone mass can occur in patients with celiac disease, even in those who do not present with classic symptoms.[120–122] In adults, the prevalence of osteopenia at the spine is 28% and at the hip 15%.[123–125] The risk of fracture has been studied in adults with celiac disease. In a large population-based cohort study of middle-aged patients, West et al.[126] observed a modest increase in the overall risk ratio for any fracture of 1.30 (95% confidence interval 1.16–1.46). The most commonly affected sites were the hip, ulna and radius. In a cross-sectional case–control study, patients with 'classic' symptoms of celiac disease had a higher prevalence of fractures than patients with subclinical or 'silent' disease,[127] with fractures more common in the peripheral skeleton.[128] However, other studies have failed to detect an increase in the risk of fractures in these patients.[99,129] These apparent discrepancies may be due to patient selection and degree of compliance with a gluten-free diet.[124] Children who follow this diet strictly have an excellent chance of full skeletal repair 1 year after diagnosis.[122,130,131] There are reports of osteopenia in adolescents following a long-term gluten-free diet;[120,132] this may also be due to issues of compliance with the diet in this age group and decreased skeletal plasticity in older children.

The pathogenesis of bone loss in celiac disease is not well understood. Studies in children suggest that bone formation is reduced at the time of diagnosis, as judged by decreased serum levels of osteocalcin and C-terminal peptide of type I collagen (PICP).[26] Bone remodeling becomes significantly more active after the initiation of a gluten-free diet, as determined by biochemical indices of bone turnover.[26,121] Bone turnover may be inhibited by inflammation in untreated children. For example, raised serum levels of IL-6, a marker of active inflammation, and reduced levels of IL-1ra, an anti-inflammatory factor, correlate with decreased BMD in celiac disease at diagnosis.[133] Malnutrition could also adversely affect bone metabolism in celiac disease. Calcium deficiency can occur because calcium binds to unabsorbed fatty acids and forms indigestible soaps. Malabsorption of vitamin D can lead to hyperparathyroidism, with further impairment of calcium absorption in the intestine.[134–136] Clinical vitamin K deficiency with prolongation of prothrombin time has been observed in patients with celiac disease.[137] Vitamin K deficiency may also affect the post-translational γ-carboxylation of osteocalcin, a matrix protein that is an indicator of mature osteoblast function. Magnesium deficiency has been detected by sensitive methods in patients with celiac disease; it can decrease bone turnover and contribute to osteopenia.[132,138]

Currently it is not clear whether screening is indicated to detect osteopenia in children with celiac disease. This would be justified if children who strictly avoided gluten were at increased risk of fracture. This is currently not known. However, as children rapidly accelerate the accrual of bone mass after the institution of a gluten-free diet, it is unlikely that these patients are at higher fracture risk in the long term. The question of screening for celiac disease in adult patients with idiopathic osteoporosis has not yet been resolved.[129,139–142]

LIVER DISEASES

Cholestatic liver disease

Cholestatic liver disease is associated with decreased BMD in both children and adults. In adult patients, primary biliary cirrhosis (PBC) is the major cholestatic disease, but rarely (if ever) occurs in children.[143] Therefore, studies that considered patients with PBC will not be discussed here, as the mechanisms by which PBC affects bone metabolism may be different to those in childhood cholestatic disorders. The reader is referred to recent excellent reviews on bone loss associated with PBC for more information.[3,144,145] Studies in children with cholestatic diseases such as extrahepatic biliary atresia and Alagille syndrome have shown that osteopenia is prevalent, as judged by DXA.[146–152]

The nature of bone disease in children with cholestasis is not known precisely. In adults with cholestasis, bone histomorphometry suggests a decrease of both bone formation and osteoblast activity, consistent with a low bone turnover state,[153] although in women there may be uncoupling of bone remodeling with increased bone resorption.[154] In these patients, osteoporosis is more common than osteomalacia.[155] Such studies have not been conducted in children. Indirect biochemical markers of bone metabolism suggest decreased bone formation.[156–158] Although fragility fractures occur in cholestatic children,[149,159–161] their precise fracture risk is not known.

The pathogenesis of bone loss in cholestatic liver disease probably involves multiple factors. Vitamin D malabsorption is common and the serum concentration of 25-hydroxyvitamin D, which reflects vitamin D stores, needs to be followed carefully.[151,162–165] Radiologic changes of rickets are typically not present.[148,165] Adequacy of vitamin D stores can be difficult to ensure in children with cholestasis. Co-administration of vitamin D with an amphipathic form of vitamin E (D-α-tocopheryl polyethylene glycol-1000 succinate, or TPGS) can increase its absorption.[166] Calcium absorption is normal in cholestatic patients who have normal serum levels of vitamin D.[167] 7-Dehydrocholesterol, the precursor for the formation of vitamin D in the presence of ultraviolet light, is present in normal concentration in the skin of cholestatic patients, so skin photoconversion of vitamin D is probably normal.[168] IGF-I is a potent anabolic agent for bone growth. Interestingly, growth hormone concentration is increased in children with cholestasis, whereas serum levels of IGF-I and its binding protein 3 are both low. This suggests that in chronic cholestasis there is peripheral resistance to growth hormone and decreased production of IGF-I in the liver and other tissues.[61,169] Unconjugated bilirubin has direct negative effects on osteoblast proliferation and function *in vitro*, whereas the role of bile acids is not clear.[170] In addition, specific genetic defects associated with Alagille syndrome[171,172] may affect osteoblast differentiation and skeletal maturation.[173–177] Lastly, children with cholestatic liver disease who are receiving parenteral nutrition can develop hypercalcemia of unknown cause. Intravenous pamidronate, a bisphosphonate, has been used successfully to control this metabolic abnormality.[178]

Liver transplantation

The most common indication for liver transplantation in children is biliary atresia, and most of these children are transplanted in infancy. This is a very different population from adults who require transplantation, so there are significant differences in the post-transplantation bone biology between children and adults. In adults there is a rapid decline in bone mass and increased fracture risk after surgery, especially in the early postoperative period.[179,180] Histomorphometric examination of dual tetracycline-labeled bone biopsies obtained at the time of transplantation and 4 months later shows loss of bone volume and increased bone resorption at baseline and an increase in bone formation but continued high resorption after transplantation, with a net decrease in bone mass.[181] Bone histology has not been examined in children after liver transplantation. However, in contrast to adults, liver transplantation appears to have an anabolic effect on bone in children, with a significant increase in bone mass by 3 months after transplantation.[152,182] BMD becomes normal approximately 1 year after transplantation,[157,183] which may be due in part to increases in bone size associated with catch-up growth.[157] These data suggest that restoration of normal liver function, with consequent improvement in nutrient intake, absorption and physical activity, may outweigh the negative effects of immunosuppressive therapy on bone metabolism in these children. Although fragility fractures have been reported after liver transplantation in children,[184] more studies are needed to examine their precise risk, especially in the context of more refined post-transplantation medical therapy that reduces steroid exposure.[185,186] In addition, some patients receive liver grafts from living-related donors, which allows for earlier surgery and may prevent long-term complications from end-stage liver disease such as bone loss.

CYSTIC FIBROSIS

Osteopenia

Bone loss and fractures have been reported in both adults and children with cystic fibrosis (CF). Fractured ribs can make it more difficult to cough effectively and to perform chest physiotherapy, and chest deformities from kyphosis can further restrict lung capacity.[187] Approximately one-third of patients with CF have a significant decrease in bone mineral mass.[187–202] However, the precise prevalence of osteopenia in children is debated, because of methodologic limitations of studies (small sample sizes, mixed age groups, inclusion of severely ill adults) and because patients with CF can be short for their age, so their bone density may be underestimated by DXA.[201,203,204] It is also possible that there are regional differences in BMD in patients with CF. Fractures tend to occur in skeletal sites that are rich in trabecular bone.[187] In studies measuring bone density of the lumbar spine by qCT (which measures volumetric BMD), Gibbens et al.[205] showed a statistically significant decrease in mineral density in 57 patients with

CF aged less than 21 years compared with healthy controls, but using the same method Haworth et al.[200] reported only mild osteopenia in 151 adult patients. However, Buntain et al.[206] reported normal BMD measured by DXA in well nourished prepubertal children with CF, but decreased bone density after the onset of adolescence. This suggests that increased longevity in patients with CF may convey a higher risk of bone loss.

The pathogenesis of bone loss in CF is not known precisely. Histomorphometric data that have examined bone remodeling are very limited. A 25-year-old man with CF, who sustained a fragility fracture of the femoral neck and was treated with an oral bisphoshonate, had severe cortical and trabecular osteopenia with no osteomalacia.[199] Serum osteocalcin concentration is low in young patients with CF, suggesting decreased osteoblast activity and bone formation.[207–209] A longitudinal study of children and adults with CF showed failure to gain bone mineral at the expected rate.[27] As judged by balance studies using stable isotopes of calcium, rates of calcium deposition into bone are decreased, even in clinically stable patients.[209] Therefore, bone formation may be compromised in young individuals with CF. However, the specific contribution of the disease *vs* the impact of age, malnutrition, severity of lung disease, underlying inflammation, gonadal function, physical activity and corticosteroid use is not clear.[204] Interestingly, levels of undercarboxylated osteocalcin and plasma prothrombin in vitamin K absence (PIVKA-II) are increased in CF, indicating subclinical vitamin K deficiency,[55,210] which may negatively affect calcium balance. Vitamin D concentration can be normal[211] or low,[212,213] so serum 25-hydroxyvitamin D levels should be monitored periodically and supplemented.[200] Recent calcium balance data suggest that endogenous fecal losses of calcium occur in girls with CF, in spite of normal calcium absorption, suggesting that calcium is leaked abnormally into the intestinal lumen.[214,215]

Hypertrophic pulmonary osteoarthropathy

Patients with CF with advanced lung disease may develop joint swelling, pain and morning stiffness.[216] The etiology of this complication is not understood. It is usually controlled with non-steroidal anti-inflammatory drugs, physiotherapy and sometimes corticosteroids. Intravenous pamidronate, a bisphosphonate that inhibits bone resorption, has also been used.[217]

TREATMENT

In the vast majority of children with digestive diseases, measures that improve general well-being go a long way to promote bone health. For example, optimal nutrition (including adequate caloric and protein intake, vitamins D and K, calcium and magnesium), encouraging weight-bearing physical activities, control of the underlying inflammatory activity of the disease, and judicious use of medications that can affect bone metabolism such as corticosteroids should be considered in all children, regardless of their diagnosis. Clinical experience has demonstrated the potential for complete skeletal reconstitution in children treated for digestive diseases,[92] a feature that may be unique to patients who have not yet achieved skeletal maturity. As physicians, we have a responsibility to take advantage of this opportunity to optimize lifelong bone health.

In the absence of pediatric data, it is common to extrapolate indications and results obtained with therapeutic agents in adults. We need to be aware of the potential consequences of this assumption, given important physiologic differences. Consideration of this principle is important when deciding who to treat for decreased bone mineral mass. We cannot assume that drugs used to treat osteoporosis in adults are appropriate for use in children. Although there is strong evidence suggesting that decreased bone mass (as defined by reduced BMD) is common in pediatric gastrointestinal disorders, it is critical to remember that the important clinical endpoint for decreased bone mass is fracture. Therefore, reduced BMD alone should never be used as the sole criterion to start therapy in a child. In children in whom a fracture or fractures have occurred, risk factors for osteoporosis should be identified and, if possible, corrected. These children should probably be considered for pharmacologic therapy to try to prevent future fractures and alleviate bone pain.

Therapeutic options for children with decreased bone mass and fractures are limited. Bisphosphonates are derivatives of pyrophosphate that have been shown to increase BMD and decrease the risk of new fractures in postmenopausal women and patients receiving long-term corticosteroids. These drugs are potent anti-resorptive agents. Although oral forms are poorly absorbed, they accumulate in bone tissue where they can remain for several years. There is very limited published experience with these agents in patients who have digestive diseases and decreased bone mass,[92,218–220] and most experience in children is with intravenous pamidronate.[221] Before treatment with bisphosphonates can be recommended, it is important to remember that no trials have been conducted in this group of patients using reduced fracture risk as an endpoint, but rather increases in BMD. Increases in BMD do not necessarily result in decreased fracture risk. In addition, these agents have not been licensed for use or adequately studied in children. Although observational studies suggest that pamidronate reduces fractures and increases BMD in children, no randomized controlled trials have been performed to establish the safety, efficacy and optimal dosage of bisphosphonates for use in children.[222] In addition, one needs to consider that digestive diseases in children appear in general to retard bone formation rather than increasing bone resorption, suggesting that bisphosphonates may have a limited role. The administration of bisphophonates should be done in conjunction with a pediatric endocrinologist with experience in bone diseases.

Anabolic agents are being developed to promote osteoblast function. Teriparatide, a new recombinant human PTH(1–34), is the first US Food and Drug Administation-approved anabolic growth agent for bone,[223] but its use is contraindicated in individuals whose growth plate is not fused, because of the theoretical concern of promoting the development of osteosarcoma.[224] Other agents, such as intranasal calcitonin, have seen limited use in children.

References

1. Katagiri T, Takahashi N. Regulatory mechanisms of osteoblast and osteoclast differentiation. Oral Dis 2002; 8:147–159.
2. Bernstein CN, Leslie WD, Leboff MS. AGA technical review on osteoporosis in gastrointestinal diseases. Gastroenterology 2003; 124:795–841.
3. Leslie WD, Bernstein CN, Leboff MS. AGA technical review on osteoporosis in hepatic disorders. Gastroenterology 2003; 125:941–966.
4. Lian JB, Stein GS. Concepts of osteoblast growth and differentiation: basis for modulation of bone cell development and tissue formation. Crit Rev Oral Biol Med 1992; 3:269–305.
5. Yakar S, Rosen CJ, Beamer WG, et al. Circulating levels of IGF-1 directly regulate bone growth and density. J Clin Invest 2002; 110:771–781.
6. Buckwalter JA, Glimcher MJ, Cooper RR, Recker R. Bone biology. II: Formation, form, modeling, remodeling, and regulation of cell function. Instr Course Lect 1996; 45:387–399.
7. Jilka RL, Weinstein RS, Bellido T, Parfitt AM, Manolagas SC. Osteoblast programmed cell death (apoptosis): modulation by growth factors and cytokines. J Bone Miner Res 1998; 13:793–802.
8. Mundy GR, Boyce B, Hughes D, et al. The effects of cytokines and growth factors on osteoblastic cells. Bone 1995; 17(Suppl):71S–75S.
9. Bellido T, Stahl N, Farruggella TJ, Borba V, Yancopoulos GD, Manolagas SC. Detection of receptors for interleukin-6, interleukin-11, leukemia inhibitory factor, oncostatin M, and ciliary neurotrophic factor in bone marrow stromal/osteoblastic cells. J Clin Invest 1996; 97:431–437.
10. Franchimont N, Gangji V, Durant D, Canalis E. Interleukin-6 with its soluble receptor enhances the expression of insulin-like growth factor-I in osteoblasts. Endocrinology 1997; 138:5248–5255.
11. Franchimont N, Rydziel S, Delany AM, Canalis E. Interleukin-6 and its soluble receptor cause a marked induction of collagenase 3 expression in rat osteoblast cultures. J Biol Chem 1997; 272:12144–12150.
12. Ishimi Y, Miyaura C, Jin CH, et al. IL-6 is produced by osteoblasts and induces bone resorption. J Immunol 1990; 145:3297–3303.
13. Chaudhary LR, Spelsberg TC, Riggs BL. Production of various cytokines by normal human osteoblast-like cells in response to interleukin-1 beta and tumor necrosis factor-alpha: lack of regulation by 17 beta-estradiol. Endocrinology 1992; 130:2528–2534.
14. Lisignoli G, Toneguzzi S, Pozzi C, et al. Proinflammatory cytokines and chemokine production and expression by human osteoblasts isolated from patients with rheumatoid arthritis and osteoarthritis. J Rheumatol 1999; 26:791–799.
15. Yasuda H, Shima N, Nakagawa N, et al. Osteoclast differentiation factor is a ligand for osteoprotegerin/osteoclastogenesis-inhibitory factor and is identical to TRANCE/RANKL. Proc Natl Acad Sci USA 1998; 95:3597–3602.
16. Kong YY, Yoshida H, Sarosi I, et al. OPGL is a key regulator of osteoclastogenesis, lymphocyte development and lymph-node organogenesis. Nature 1999; 397:315–323.
17. Koseki T, Gao Y, Okahashi N, et al. Role of TGF-beta family in osteoclastogenesis induced by RANKL. Cell Signal 2002; 14:31–36.
18. Palmqvist P, Persson E, Conaway HH, Lerner UH. IL-6, leukemia inhibitory factor, and oncostatin M stimulate bone resorption and regulate the expression of receptor activator of NF-kappa B ligand, osteoprotegerin, and receptor activator of NF-kappa B in mouse calvariae. J Immunol 2002; 169:3353–3362.
19. Ritchlin CT, Haas-Smith SA, Li P, Hicks DG, Schwarz EM. Mechanisms of TNF-α- and RANKL-mediated osteoclastogenesis and bone resorption in psoriatic arthritis. J Clin Invest 2003; 111:821–831.
20. Romas E, Gillespie MT, Martin TJ. Involvement of receptor activator of NFkappaB ligand and tumor necrosis factor-alpha in bone destruction in rheumatoid arthritis. Bone 2002; 30:340–346.
21. Fox SW, Chambers TJ. Interferon-gamma directly inhibits TRANCE-induced osteoclastogenesis. Biochem Biophys Res Commun 2000; 276:868–872.
22. Horwood NJ, Elliott J, Martin TJ, Gillespie MT. IL-12 alone and in synergy with IL-18 inhibits osteoclast formation *in vitro*. J Immunol 2001; 166:4915–4921.
23. Moreno JL, Kaczmarek M, Keegan AD, Tondravi M. IL-4 suppresses osteoclast development and mature osteoclast function by a STAT6-dependent mechanism: irreversible inhibition of the differentiation program activated by RANKL. Blood 2003; 102:1078–1086.
24. Schoon EJ, Geerling BG, Van Dooren IM, et al. Abnormal bone turnover in long-standing Crohn's disease in remission. Aliment Pharmacol Ther 2001; 15:783–792.
25. Abitbol V, Roux C, Chaussade S, et al. Metabolic bone assessment in patients with inflammatory bowel disease. Gastroenterology 1995; 108:417–422.
26. Pratico G, Caltabiano L, Bottaro G, Palano GM, Rotolo N, Spina M. Serum levels of osteocalcin and type I procollagen in children with celiac disease. J Pediatr Gastroenterol Nutr 1997; 24:170–173.
27. Bhudhikanok GS, Wang MC, Marcus R, Harkins A, Moss RB, Bachrach LK. Bone acquisition and loss in children and adults with cystic fibrosis: a longitudinal study. J Pediatr 1998; 133:18–27.
28. Bonjour JP, Theintz G, Buchs B, Slosman D, Rizzoli R. Critical years and stages of puberty for spinal and femoral bone mass accumulation during adolescence. J Clin Endocrinol Metab 1991; 73:555–563.
29. Molgaard C, Thomsen BL, Michaelsen KF. Influence of weight, age and puberty on bone size and bone mineral content in healthy children and adolescents. Acta Paediatr 1998; 87:494–499.
30. Soyka LA, Fairfield WP, Klibanski A. Hormonal determinants and disorders of peak bone mass in children. J Clin Endocrinol Metab 2000; 85:3951–3963.
31. Bryant RJ, Wastney ME, Martin BR, et al. Racial differences in bone turnover and calcium metabolism in adolescent females. J Clin Endocrinol Metab 2003; 88:1043–1047.
32. Finkelstein JS, Neer RM, Biller BM, Crawford JD, Klibanski A. Osteopenia in men with a history of delayed puberty. N Engl J Med 1992; 326:600–604.
33. Glorieux FH, Travers R, Taylor A, et al. Normative data for iliac bone histomorphometry in growing children. Bone 2000; 26:103–109.

34. Szulc P, Seeman E, Delmas PD. Biochemical measurements of bone turnover in children and adolescents. Osteoporos Int 2000; 11:281–294.
35. Writing Group for the ISCD Position Development Conference. Diagnosis of osteoporosis in men, premenopausal women, and children. J Clin Densitom 2004; 7:17–26.
36. Compston JE. Bone density: BMC, BMD, or corrected BMD? Bone 1995; 16:5–7.
37. Herzog D, Bishop N, Glorieux F, Seidman EG. Interpretation of bone mineral density values in pediatric Crohn's disease. Inflamm Bowel Dis 1998; 4:261–267.
38. Ahmed SF, Horrocks IA, Patterson T, et al. Bone mineral assessment by dual energy X-ray absorptiometry in children with inflammatory bowel disease: evaluation by age or bone area. J Pediatr Gastroenterol Nutr 2004; 38:276–280.
39. Gafni RI, Baron J. Overdiagnosis of osteoporosis in children due to misinterpretation of dual-energy x-ray absorptiometry (DEXA). J Pediatr 2004; 144:253–257.
40. Carter DR, Bouxsein ML, Marcus R. New approaches for interpreting projected bone densitometry data. J Bone Miner Res 1992; 7:137–145.
41. Blake GM, Fogelman I. Application of bone densitometry for osteoporosis. Endocrinol Metab Clin North Am 1998; 27:267–288.
42. Heaney RP. Is the paradigm shifting? Bone 2003; 33:457–465.
43. Khan AA, Bachrach L, Brown JP, et al. Standards and guidelines for performing central dual-energy x-ray absorptiometry in premenopausal women, men, and children. J Clin Densitom 2004; 7:51–64.
44. Assessment of fracture risk and its application to screening for postmenopausal osteoporosis. Report of a WHO Study Group. World Health Organ Tech Rep Ser 1994; 843:1–129.
45. Bailey DA, Wedge JH, McCulloch RG, Martin AD, Bernhardson SC. Epidemiology of fractures of the distal end of the radius in children as associated with growth. J Bone Joint Surg Am 1989; 71:1225–1231.
46. Compston J. The skeletal effects of liver transplantation in children. Liver Transpl 2003; 9:371–372.
47. Rosen CJ. Insulin-like growth factor I and calcium balance: evolving concepts of an evolutionary process. Endocrinology 2003; 144:4679–4681.
48. Abrams SA, Silber TJ, Esteban NV et al. Mineral balance and bone turnover in adolescents with anorexia nervosa. J Pediatr 1993; 123:326–331.
49. Bonjour JP, Ammann P, Chevalley T, Rizzoli R. Protein intake and bone growth. Can J Appl Physiol 2001; 26(Suppl):S153–S166.
50. Sentongo TA, Semaeo EJ, Stettler N, Piccoli DA, Stallings VA, Zemel BS. Vitamin D status in children, adolescents, and young adults with Crohn disease. Am J Clin Nutr 2002; 76:1077–1081.
51. Knapen MH, Hamulyak K, Vermeer C. The effect of vitamin K supplementation on circulating osteocalcin (bone Gla protein) and urinary calcium excretion. Ann Intern Med 1989; 111:1001–1005.
52. Szulc P, Meunier PJ. Is vitamin K deficiency a risk factor for osteoporosis in Crohn's disease? Lancet 2001; 357:1995–1996.
53. van Hoorn JH, Hendriks JJ, Vermeer C, Forget PP. Vitamin K supplementation in cystic fibrosis. Arch Dis Child 2003; 88:974–975.
54. Lian JB, Stein GS, Stein JL, van Wijnen AJ. Osteocalcin gene promoter: unlocking the secrets for regulation of osteoblast growth and differentiation. J Cell Biochem Suppl 1998; 30–31:62–72.
55. Rashid M, Durie P, Andrew M, et al. Prevalence of vitamin K deficiency in cystic fibrosis. Am J Clin Nutr 1999; 70:378–382.
56. Riggs BL. The mechanisms of estrogen regulation of bone resorption. J Clin Invest 2000; 106:1203–1204.
57. Riggs BL, Khosla S, Melton LJ 3rd. Primary osteoporosis in men: role of sex steroid deficiency. Mayo Clin Proc 2000; 75(Suppl):S46–S50.
58. Kasukawa Y, Baylink DJ, Wergedal JE, et al. Lack of insulin-like growth factor I exaggerates the effect of calcium deficiency on bone accretion in mice. Endocrinology 2003; 144:4682–4689.
59. Kirschner BS, Sutton MM. Somatomedin-C levels in growth-impaired children and adolescents with chronic inflammatory bowel disease. Gastroenterology 1986; 91:830–836.
60. Donaghy A, Ross R, Gimson A, Hughes SC, Holly J, Williams R. Growth hormone, insulinlike growth factor-1, and insulinlike growth factor binding proteins 1 and 3 in chronic liver disease. Hepatology 1995; 21:680–688.
61. Bucuvalas JC, Horn JA, Slusher J, Alfaro MP, Chernausek SD. Growth hormone insensitivity in children with biliary atresia. J Pediatr Gastroenterol Nutr 1996; 23:135–140.
62. Bross DA, Leichtner AM, Zurakowski D, Law T, Bousvaros A. Elevation of serum interleukin-6 but not serum-soluble interleukin-2 receptor in children with Crohn's disease. J Pediatr Gastroenterol Nutr 1996; 23:164–171.
63. Devlin RD, Reddy SV, Savino R, Ciliberto G, Roodman GD. IL-6 mediates the effects of IL-1 or TNF, but not PTHrP or 1,25(OH)2D3, on osteoclast-like cell formation in normal human bone marrow cultures. J Bone Miner Res 1998; 13:393–399.
64. Dai J, Lin D, Zhang J, et al. Chronic alcohol ingestion induces osteoclastogenesis and bone loss through IL-6 in mice. J Clin Invest 2000; 106:887–895.
65. Deyama Y, Takeyama S, Suzuki K, Yoshimura Y, Nishikata M, Matsumoto A. Inactivation of NF-kappaB involved in osteoblast development through interleukin-6. Biochem Biophys Res Commun 2001; 282:1080–1084.
66. Fang MA, Hahn TJ. Effects of interleukin-6 on cellular function in UMR-106-01 osteoblastlike cells. J Bone Miner Res 1991; 6:133–139.
67. Grey A, Mitnick MA, Masiukiewicz U, et al. A role for interleukin-6 in parathyroid hormone-induced bone resorption *in vivo*. Endocrinology 1999; 140:4683–4690.
68. Sylvester FA, Wyzga N, Hyams JS, Gronowicz GA. Effect of Crohn's disease on bone metabolism *in vitro*: a role for interleukin-6. J Bone Miner Res 2002; 17:695–702.
69. Davidson NJ, Hudak SA, Lesley RE, Menon S, Leach MW, Rennick DM. IL-12, but not IFN-gamma, plays a major role in sustaining the chronic phase of colitis in IL-10-deficient mice. J Immunol 1998; 161:3143–3149.
70. Fais S, Capobianchi M, Pallone F, et al. Spontaneous release of interferon gamma by intestinal lamina propria lymphocytes in Crohn's disease. Kinetics of *in vitro* response to interferon gamma inducers. Gut 1991; 32:403–407.
71. Gowen M, MacDonald BR, Russell RG. Actions of recombinant human gamma-interferon and tumor necrosis factor alpha on the proliferation and osteoblastic characteristics of human trabecular bone cells *in vitro*. Arthritis Rheum 1988; 31:1500–1507.
72. Nanes MS, McKoy WM, Marx SJ. Inhibitory effects of tumor necrosis factor-alpha and interferon-gamma on deoxyribonucleic acid and collagen synthesis by rat osteosarcoma cells (ROS 17/2.8). Endocrinology 1989; 124:339–345.

73. Kurihara N, Roodman GD. Interferons-alpha and -gamma inhibit interleukin-1 beta-stimulated osteoclast-like cell formation in long-term human marrow cultures. J Interferon Res 1990; 10:541–547.
74. Takayanagi H, Kim S, Taniguchi T. Signaling crosstalk between RANKL and interferons in osteoclast differentiation. Arthritis Res 2002; 4(Suppl 3):S227–S232.
75. Kong YY, Feige U, Sarosi I, et al. Activated T cells regulate bone loss and joint destruction in adjuvant arthritis through osteoprotegerin ligand. Nature 1999; 402:304–309.
76. van Staa TP, Leufkens HG, Abenhaim L, Zhang B, Cooper C. Oral corticosteroids and fracture risk: relationship to daily and cumulative doses. Rheumatology (Oxf) 2000; 39:1383–1389.
77. van Staa TP, Cooper C, Leufkens HG, Bishop N. Children and the risk of fractures caused by oral corticosteroids. J Bone Miner Res 2003; 18:913–918.
78. Canalis E. Mechanisms of glucocorticoid action in bone: implications to glucocorticoid-induced osteoporosis. J Clin Endocrinol Metab 1996; 81:3441–3447.
79. Cvetkovic M, Mann GN, Romero DF, et al. The deleterious effects of long-term cyclosporine A, cyclosporine G, and FK506 on bone mineral metabolism *in vivo*. Transplantation 1994; 57:1231–1237.
80. McCauley LK, Rosol TJ, Capen CC. Effects of cyclosporin A on rat osteoblasts (ROS 17/2.8 cells) *in vitro*. Calcif Tissue Int 1992; 51:291–297.
81. Nacher M, Aubia J, Serrano S, et al. Effect of cyclosporine A on normal human osteoblasts *in vitro*. Bone Miner 1994; 26:231–243.
82. Fornoni A, Cornacchia F, Howard GA, Roos BA, Striker GE, Striker LJ. Cyclosporin A affects extracellular matrix synthesis and degradation by mouse MC3T3-E1 osteoblasts *in vitro*. Nephrol Dial Transplant 2001; 16:500–505.
83. Tang L, Ebara S, Kawasaki S, Wakabayashi S, Nikaido T, Takaoka K. FK506 enhanced osteoblastic differentiation in mesenchymal cells. Cell Biol Int 2002; 26:75–84.
84. Oreffo RO, Romberg S, Virdi AS, Joyner CJ, Berven S, Triffitt JT. Effects of interferon alpha on human osteoprogenitor cell growth and differentiation *in vitro*. J Cell Biochem 1999; 74:372–385.
85. Solis-Herruzo JA, Castellano G, Fernandez I, Munoz R, Hawkins F. Decreased bone mineral density after therapy with alpha interferon in combination with ribavirin for chronic hepatitis C. J Hepatol 2000; 33:812–817.
86. Ghosh S, Cowen S, Hannan WJ, Ferguson A. Low bone mineral density in Crohn's disease, but not in ulcerative colitis, at diagnosis. Gastroenterology 1994; 107: 1031–1039.
87. Martin JP, Tonge KA, Bhonsle U, Jacyna MR, Levi J. Bone mineral density in patients with inflammatory bowel disease. Eur J Gastroenterol Hepatol 1999; 11:537–541.
88. Vestergaard P, Krogh K, Rejnmark L, Laurberg S, Mosekilde L. Fracture risk is increased in Crohn's disease, but not in ulcerative colitis. Gut 2000; 46:176–181.
89. Cowan FJ, Warner JT, Dunstan FD, Evans WD, Gregory JW, Jenkins HR. Inflammatory bowel disease and predisposition to osteopenia. Arch Dis Child 1997; 76:325–329.
90. Boot AM, Bouquet J, Krenning EP, de Muinck Keizer-Schrama SM. Bone mineral density and nutritional status in children with chronic inflammatory bowel disease. Gut 1998; 42:188–194.
91. Gokhale R, Favus MJ, Karrison T, Sutton MM, Rich B, Kirschner BS. Bone mineral density assessment in children with inflammatory bowel disease. Gastroenterology 1998; 114:902–911.
92. Thearle M, Horlick M, Bilezikian JP, et al. Osteoporosis: an unusual presentation of childhood Crohn's disease. J Clin Endocrinol Metab 2000; 85:2122–2126.
93. Compston JE, Judd D, Crawley EO, et al. Osteoporosis in patients with inflammatory bowel disease. Gut 1987; 28:410–415.
94. Semeao EJ, Stallings VA, Peck SN, Piccoli DA. Vertebral compression fractures in pediatric patients with Crohn's disease. Gastroenterology 1997; 112:1710–1713.
95. Stockbrugger RW, Schoon EJ, Bollani S, et al. Discordance between the degree of osteopenia and the prevalence of spontaneous vertebral fractures in Crohn's disease. Aliment Pharmacol Ther 2002; 16:1519–1527.
96. van Staa TP, Cooper C, Brusse LS, Leufkens H, Javaid MK, Arden NK. Inflammatory bowel disease and the risk of fracture. Gastroenterology 2003; 125:1591–1597.
97. Card T, West J, Hubbard R, Logan RF. Hip fractures in patients with inflammatory bowel disease and their relationship to corticosteroid use: a population based cohort study. Gut 2004; 53:251–255.
98. Bernstein CN, Blanchard JF, Leslie W, Wajda A, Yu BN. The incidence of fracture among patients with inflammatory bowel disease. A population-based cohort study. Ann Intern Med 2000; 133:795–799.
99. Vestergaard P, Mosekilde L. Fracture risk in patients with celiac disease, Crohn's disease, and ulcerative colitis: a nationwide follow-up study of 16 416 patients in Denmark. Am J Epidemiol 2002; 156:1–10.
100. Loftus EV Jr, Crowson CS, Sandborn WJ, Tremaine WJ, O'Fallon WM, Melton LJ 3rd. Long-term fracture risk in patients with Crohn's disease: a population-based study in Olmsted County, Minnesota. Gastroenterology 2002; 123:468–475.
101. Loftus EV Jr, Achenbach SJ, Sandborn WJ, Tremaine WJ, Oberg AL, Melton LJ 3rd. Risk of fracture in ulcerative colitis: a population-based study from Olmsted County, Minnesota. Clin Gastroenterol Hepatol 2003; 1:465–473.
102. Klaus J, Armbrecht G, Steinkamp M, et al. High prevalence of osteoporotic vertebral fractures in patients with Crohn's disease. Gut 2002; 51:654–658.
103. Clements D, Compston JE, Evans WD, Rhodes J. Hormone replacement therapy prevents bone loss in patients with inflammatory bowel disease. Gut 1993; 34:1543–1546.
104. Bernstein CN, Seeger LL, Sayre JW, Anton PA, Artinian L, Shanahan F. Decreased bone density in inflammatory bowel disease is related to corticosteroid use and not disease diagnosis. J Bone Miner Res 1995; 10(2):250–256.
105. D'Haens G, Verstraete A, Cheyns K, Aerden I, Bouillon R, Rutgeerts P. Bone turnover during short-term therapy with methylprednisolone or budesonide in Crohn's disease. Aliment Pharmacol Ther 1998; 12:419–424.
106. Dear KL, Compston JE, Hunter JO. Treatments for Crohn's disease that minimise steroid doses are associated with a reduced risk of osteoporosis. Clin Nutr 2001; 20:541–546.
107. Bernstein CN, Leslie WD. Osteoporosis and inflammatory bowel disease. Aliment Pharmacol Ther 2004; 19:941–952.
108. Bosch X. Hypercalcemia due to endogenous overproduction of 1,25-dihydroxyvitamin D in Crohn's disease. Gastroenterology 1998; 114:1061–1065.
109. Robinson RJ, Iqbal SJ, Abrams K, Al-Azzawi F, Mayberry JF. Increased bone resorption in patients with Crohn's disease. Aliment Pharmacol Ther 1998; 12:699–705.
110. Schulte C, Dignass AU, Mann K, Goebell H. Reduced bone mineral density and unbalanced bone metabolism in patients with inflammatory bowel disease. Inflamm Bowel Dis 1998; 4:268–275.

111. Dresner-Pollak R, Karmeli F, Eliakim R, Ackerman Z, Rachmilewitz D. Increased urinary *N*-telopeptide cross-linked type 1 collagen predicts bone loss in patients with inflammatory bowel disease. Am J Gastroenterol 2000; 95:699–704.
112. Lin CL, Moniz C, Chambers TJ, Chow JW. Colitis causes bone loss in rats through suppression of bone formation. Gastroenterology 1996; 111:1263–1271.
113. Hyams JS, Wyzga N, Kreutzer DL, Justinich CJ, Gronowicz GA. Alterations in bone metabolism in children with inflammatory bowel disease: an *in vitro* study. J Pediatr Gastroenterol Nutr 1997; 24:289–295.
114. Varghese S, Wyzga N, Griffiths AM, Sylvester FA. Effects of serum from children with newly diagnosed Crohn disease on primary cultures of rat osteoblasts. J Pediatr Gastroenterol Nutr 2002; 35:641–648.
115. Pollak RD, Karmeli F, Eliakim R, Ackerman Z, Tabb K, Rachmilewitz D. Femoral neck osteopenia in patients with inflammatory bowel disease. Am J Gastroenterol 1998; 93:1483–1490.
116. Nemetz A, Toth M, Garcia-Gonzalez MA, et al. Allelic variation at the interleukin 1beta gene is associated with decreased bone mass in patients with inflammatory bowel diseases. Gut 2001; 49:644–649.
117. Schulte CM, Dignass AU, Goebell H, Roher HD, Schulte KM. Genetic factors determine extent of bone loss in inflammatory bowel disease. Gastroenterology 2000; 119:909–920.
118. Bousvaros A, Marcon M, Treem W, et al. Chronic recurrent multifocal osteomyelitis associated with chronic inflammatory bowel disease in children. Dig Dis Sci 1999; 44:2500–2507.
119. Carpenter E, Jackson MA, Friesen CA, Scarbrough M, Roberts CC. Crohn's-associated chronic recurrent multifocal osteomyelitis responsive to infliximab. J Pediatr 2004; 144:541–544.
120. Kalayci AG, Kansu A, Girgin N, Kucuk O, Aras G. Bone mineral density and importance of a gluten-free diet in patients with celiac disease in childhood. Pediatrics 2001; 108:E89.
121. Mora S, Barera G, Beccio S, et al. A prospective, longitudinal study of the long-term effect of treatment on bone density in children with celiac disease. J Pediatr 2001; 139:516–521.
122. Kavak US, Yuce A, Kocak N, et al. Bone mineral density in children with untreated and treated celiac disease. J Pediatr Gastroenterol Nutr 2003; 37:434–436.
123. Corazza G, Di Sario A, Cecchetti L, et al. Bone mass and metabolism in patients with celiac disease. Gastroenterology 1995; 109:122–128.
124. Bai JC, Gonzalez D, Mautalen C, et al. Long-term effect of gluten restriction on bone mineral density of patients with coeliac disease. Aliment Pharmacol Ther 1997; 11:157–164.
125. Cellier C, Flobert C, Cormier C, Roux C, Schmitz J. Severe osteopenia in symptom-free adults with a childhood diagnosis of coeliac disease. Lancet 2000; 355:806.
126. West J, Logan RF, Card TR, Smith C, Hubbard R. Fracture risk in people with celiac disease: a population-based cohort study. Gastroenterology 2003; 125:429–436.
127. Moreno ML, Vazquez H, Mazure R, et al. Stratification of bone fracture risk in patients with celiac disease. Clin Gastroenterol Hepatol 2004; 2:127–134.
128. Vasquez H, Mazure R, Gonzalez D, et al. Risk of fractures in celiac disease patients: a cross-sectional, case–control study. Am J Gastroenterol 2000; 95:183–189.
129. Thomason K, West J, Logan RF, Coupland C, Holmes GK. Fracture experience of patients with coeliac disease: a population based survey. Gut 2003; 52:518–522.
130. Mora S, Barera G, Beccio S, et al. A prospective, longitudinal study of the long-term effect of treatment on bone density in children with celiac disease. J Pediatr 2001; 139:516–521.
131. Szathmari M, Tulassay T, Arato A, Bodanszky H, Szabo A, Tulassay Z. Bone mineral content and density in asymptomatic children with coeliac disease on a gluten-free diet. Eur J Gastroenterol Hepatol 2001; 13:419–424.
132. Sdepanian VL, de Miranda Carvalho CN, de Morais MB, Colugnati FA, Fagundes-Neto U. Bone mineral density of the lumbar spine in children and adolescents with celiac disease on a gluten-free diet in Sao Paulo, Brazil. J Pediatr Gastroenterol Nutr 2003; 37:571–576.
133. Fornari MC, Pedreira S, Niveloni S, et al. Pre- and post-treatment serum levels of cytokines IL-1beta, IL-6, and IL-1 receptor antagonist in celiac disease. Are they related to the associated osteopenia? Am J Gastroenterol 1998; 93:413–418.
134. Keaveny AP, Freaney R, McKenna MJ, Masterson J, O'Donoghue DP. Bone remodeling indices and secondary hyperparathyroidism in celiac disease. Am J Gastroenterol 1996; 91:1226–1231.
135. Selby PL, Davies M, Adams JE, Mawer EB. Bone loss in celiac disease is related to secondary hyperparathyroidism. J Bone Miner Res 1999; 14:652–657.
136. Valdimarsson T, Toss G, Lofman O, Strom M. Three years' follow-up of bone density in adult coeliac disease: significance of secondary hyperparathyroidism. Scand J Gastroenterol 2000; 35:274–280.
137. Cavallaro R, Iovino P, Castiglione F, et al. Prevalence and clinical associations of prolonged prothrombin time in adult untreated coeliac disease. Eur J Gastroenterol Hepatol 2004; 16:219–223.
138. Rude RK, Olerich M. Magnesium deficiency: possible role in osteoporosis associated with gluten-sensitive enteropathy. Osteoporos Int 1996; 6:453–461.
139. Lindh E, Ljunghall S, Larsson K, Lavo B. Screening for antibodies against gliadin in patients with osteoporosis. J Intern Med 1992; 231:403–406.
140. Mather KJ, Meddings JB, Beck PL, Scott RB, Hanley DA. Prevalence of IgA-antiendomysial antibody in asymptomatic low bone mineral density. Am J Gastroenterol 2001; 96:120–125.
141. Nuti R, Martini G, Valenti R, Giovani S, Salvadori S, Avanzati A. Prevalence of undiagnosed coeliac syndrome in osteoporotic women. J Intern Med 2001; 250:361–366.
142. Gonzalez D, Sugai E, Gomez JC, et al. Is it necessary to screen for celiac disease in postmenopausal osteoporotic women? Calcif Tissue Int 2002; 71:141–144.
143. Dahlan Y, Smith L, Simmonds D, et al. Pediatric-onset primary biliary cirrhosis. Gastroenterology 2003; 125:1476–1479.
144. Heathcote EJ. Management of primary biliary cirrhosis. The American Association for the Study of Liver Diseases practice guidelines. Hepatology 2000; 31:1005–1013.
145. Levy C, Lindor KD. Management of osteoporosis, fat-soluble vitamin deficiencies, and hyperlipidemia in primary biliary cirrhosis. Clin Liver Dis 2003; 7:901–910.
146. Kobayashi A, Kawai S, Utsunomiya T, Obe Y. Bone disease in infants and children with hepatobiliary disease. Arch Dis Child 1974; 49:641–646.
147. Glasgow JF, Thomas PS. The osteodystrophy of prolonged obstructive liver disease in childhood. Acta Paediatr Scand 1976; 65:57–64.
148. Argao EA, Specker BL, Heubi JE. Bone mineral content in infants and children with chronic cholestatic liver disease. Pediatrics 1993; 91:1151–1154.

149. Hoffenberg EJ, Narkewicz MR, Sondheimer JM, Smith DJ, Silverman A, Sokol RJ. Outcome of syndromic paucity of interlobular bile ducts (Alagille syndrome) with onset of cholestasis in infancy. J Pediatr 1995; 127:220–224.

150. Ulivieri FM, Lisciandrano D, Gridelli B, et al. Bone mass and body composition in children with chronic cholestasis before and after liver transplantation. Transplant Proc 1999; 31:2131–2134.

151. Chongsrisawat V, Ruttanamongkol P, Chaiwatanarat T, Chandrakamol B, Poovorawan Y. Bone density and 25-hydroxyvitamin D level in extrahepatic biliary atresia. Pediatr Surg Int 2001; 17:604–608.

152. Pawlowska J, Matusik H, Socha P, et al. Beneficial effect of liver transplantation on bone mineral density in small infants with cholestasis. Transplant Proc 2004; 36:1479–1480.

153. Diamond T, Stiel D, Mason R, et al. Serum vitamin D metabolites are not responsible for low turnover osteoporosis in chronic liver disease. J Clin Endocrinol Metab 1989; 69:1234–1239.

154. Guichelaar MM, Malinchoc M, Sibonga J, Clarke BL, Hay JE. Bone metabolism in advanced cholestatic liver disease: analysis by bone histomorphometry. Hepatology 2002; 36(Pt 1):895–903.

155. Stellon AJ, Webb A, Compston J, Williams R. Lack of osteomalacia in chronic cholestatic liver disease. Bone 1986; 7:181–185.

156. Heubi JE, Higgins JV, Argao EA, Sierra RI, Specker BL. The role of magnesium in the pathogenesis of bone disease in childhood cholestatic liver disease: a preliminary report. J Pediatr Gastroenterol Nutr 1997; 25:301–306.

157. D'Antiga L, Moniz C, Buxton-Thomas M, et al. Bone mineral density and height gain in children with chronic cholestatic liver disease undergoing transplantation. Transplantation 2002; 73:1788–1793.

158. Klein GL, Soriano H, Shulman RJ, Levy M, Jones G, Langman CB. Hepatic osteodystrophy in chronic cholestasis: evidence for a multifactorial etiology. Pediatr Transplant 2002; 6:136–140.

159. Katayama H, Suruga K, Kurashige T, Kimoto T. Bone changes in congenital biliary atresia. Radiologic observation of 8 cases. Am J Roentgenol Radium Ther Nucl Med 1975; 124:107–112.

160. Katayama H, Shirakata A, Miyano T. Hepatic osteodystrophy in congenital biliary atresia. Nippon Igaku Hoshasen Gakkai Zasshi 1985; 45:455–461.

161. DeRusso PA, Spevak MR, Schwarz KB. Fractures in biliary atresia misinterpreted as child abuse. Pediatrics 2003; 112(Pt 1):185–188.

162. Dibble JB, Sheridan P, Hampshire R, Hardy GJ, Losowsky MS. Osteomalacia, vitamin D deficiency and cholestasis in chronic liver disease. Q J Med 1982; 51:89–103.

163. Sokol RJ, Farrell MK, Heubi JE, Tsang RC, Balistreri WF. Comparison of vitamin E and 25-hydroxyvitamin D absorption during childhood cholestasis. J Pediatr 1983; 103:712–717.

164. Bengoa JM, Sitrin MD, Meredith S, et al. Intestinal calcium absorption and vitamin D status in chronic cholestatic liver disease. Hepatology 1984; 4:261–265.

165. Heubi JE, Hollis BW, Specker B, Tsang RC. Bone disease in chronic childhood cholestasis. I. Vitamin D absorption and metabolism. Hepatology 1989; 9:258–264.

166. Argao EA, Heubi JE, Hollis BW, Tsang RC. D-Alpha-tocopheryl polyethylene glycol-1000 succinate enhances the absorption of vitamin D in chronic cholestatic liver disease of infancy and childhood. Pediatr Res 1992; 31:146–150.

167. Bucuvalas JC, Heubi JE, Specker BL, Gregg DJ, Yergey AL, Vieira NE. Calcium absorption in bone disease associated with chronic cholestasis during childhood. Hepatology 1990; 12:1200–1205.

168. Paterson CR, Moody JP, Pennington CR. Skin content of 7-dehydrocholesterol in patients with malabsorption. Nutrition 1997; 13:771–773.

169. Bucuvalas JC, Horn JA, Carlsson L, Balistreri WF, Chernausek SD. Growth hormone insensitivity associated with elevated circulating growth hormone-binding protein in children with Alagille syndrome and short stature. J Clin Endocrinol Metab 1993; 76:1477–1482.

170. Janes CH, Dickson ER, Okazaki R, Bonde S, McDonagh AF, Riggs BL. Role of hyperbilirubinemia in the impairment of osteoblast proliferation associated with cholestatic jaundice. J Clin Invest 1995; 95:2581–2486.

171. Li L, Krantz ID, Deng Y, et al. Alagille syndrome is caused by mutations in human *Jagged1*, which encodes a ligand for Notch1. Nat Genet 1997; 16:243–251.

172. Oda T, Elkahloun AG, Pike BL, et al. Mutations in the human *Jagged1* gene are responsible for Alagille syndrome. Nat Genet 1997; 16:235–242.

173. Pereira RM, Delany AM, Durant D, Canalis E. Cortisol regulates the expression of Notch in osteoblasts. J Cell Biochem 2002; 85:252–258.

174. Schnabel M, Fichtel I, Gotzen L, Schlegel J. Differential expression of *Notch* genes in human osteoblastic cells. Int J Mol Med 2002; 9:229–232.

175. Tezuka K, Yasuda M, Watanabe N, et al. Stimulation of osteoblastic cell differentiation by Notch. J Bone Miner Res 2002; 17:231–239.

176. Sciaudone M, Gazzerro E, Priest L, Delany AM, Canalis E. Notch 1 impairs osteoblastic cell differentiation. Endocrinology 2003; 144:5631–5639.

177. de Jong DS, Steegenga WT, Hendriks JM, van Zoelen EJ, Olijve W, Dechering KJ. Regulation of Notch signaling genes during BMP2-induced differentiation of osteoblast precursor cells. Biochem Biophys Res Commun 2004; 320:100–107.

178. Attard TM, Dhawan A, Kaufman SS, Collier DS, Langnas AN. Use of disodium pamidronate in children with hypercalcemia awaiting liver transplantation. Pediatr Transplant 1998; 2:157–159.

179. Haagsma EB, Thijn CJ, Post JG, Slooff MJ, Gips CH. Bone disease after orthotopic liver transplantation. J Hepatol 1988; 6:94–100.

180. Bjoro K, Brandsaeter B, Wiencke K, et al. Secondary osteoporosis in liver transplant recipients: a longitudinal study in patients with and without cholestatic liver disease. Scand J Gastroenterol 2003; 38:320–327.

181. Guichelaar MM, Malinchoc M, Sibonga JD, Clarke BL, Hay JE. Bone histomorphometric changes after liver transplantation for chronic cholestatic liver disease. J Bone Miner Res 2003; 18:2190–2199.

182. Okajima H, Shigeno C, Inomata Y, et al. Long-term effects of liver transplantation on bone mineral density in children with end-stage liver disease: a 2-year prospective study. Liver Transpl 2003; 9:360–364.

183. Argao EA, Balistreri WF, Hollis BW, Ryckman FC, Heubi JE. Effect of orthotopic liver transplantation on bone mineral content and serum vitamin D metabolites in infants and children with chronic cholestasis. Hepatology 1994; 20:598–603.

184. Hill SA, Kelly DA, John PR. Bone fractures in children undergoing orthotopic liver transplantation. Pediatr Radiol 1995; 25(Suppl 1):S112–S117.

185. Scolapio JS, DeArment J, Hurley DL, Romano M, Harnois D, Weigand SD. Influence of tacrolimus and short-duration prednisone on bone mineral density following liver

transplantation. JPEN J Parenter Enteral Nutr 2003; 27:427–432.

186. Segal E, Baruch Y, Kramsky R, Raz B, Tamir A, Ish-Shalom S. Predominant factors associated with bone loss in liver transplant patients – after prolonged post-transplantation period. Clin Transplant 2003; 17:13–19.
187. Aris RM, Renner JB, Winders AD, et al. Increased rate of fractures and severe kyphosis: sequelae of living into adulthood with cystic fibrosis. Ann Intern Med 1998; 128:186–193.
188. Mischler EH, Chesney PJ, Chesney RW, Mazess RB. Demineralization in cystic fibrosis detected by direct photon absorptiometry. Am J Dis Child 1979; 133:632–635.
189. Ross J, Gamble J, Schultz A, Lewiston N. Back pain and spinal deformity in cystic fibrosis. Am J Dis Child 1987; 141:1313–1316.
190. Lipnick RN, Glass RB. Bone changes associated with cystic fibrosis. Skeletal Radiol 1992; 21:115–116.
191. Henderson RC, Specter BB. Kyphosis and fractures in children and young adults with cystic fibrosis. J Pediatr 1994; 125:208–212.
192. Bachrach LK, Loutit CW, Moss RB. Osteopenia in adults with cystic fibrosis. Am J Med 1994; 96:27–34.
193. Shaw N, Bedford C, Heaf D, Carty H, Dutton J. Osteopenia in adults with cystic fibrosis. Am J Med 1995; 99:690–692.
194. Bhudhikanok GS, Lim J, Marcus R, Harkins A, Moss RB, Bachrach LK. Correlates of osteopenia in patients with cystic fibrosis. Pediatrics 1996; 97:103–111.
195. Henderson RC, Madsen CD. Bone density in children and adolescents with cystic fibrosis. J Pediatr 1996; 128:28–34.
196. Salamoni F, Roulet M, Gudinchet F, Pilet M, Thiebaud D, Burckhardt P. Bone mineral content in cystic fibrosis patients: correlation with fat-free mass. Arch Dis Child 1996; 74:314–318.
197. Haworth CS, Selby PL, Webb AK, Adams JE. Osteoporosis in adults with cystic fibrosis. J R Soc Med 1998; 91(Suppl 34):14–18.
198. Aris RM, Lester GE, Dingman S, Ontjes DA. Altered calcium homeostasis in adults with cystic fibrosis. Osteoporos Int 1999; 10:102–108.
199. Haworth CS, Freemont AJ, Webb AK, et al. Hip fracture and bone histomorphometry in a young adult with cystic fibrosis. Eur Respir J 1999; 14:478–479.
200. Haworth CS, Selby PL, Webb AK, et al. Low bone mineral density in adults with cystic fibrosis. Thorax 1999; 54:961–967.
201. Laursen EM, Molgaard C, Michaelsen KF, Koch C, Muller J. Bone mineral status in 134 patients with cystic fibrosis. Arch Dis Child 1999; 81:235–240.
202. Ujhelyi R, Treszl A, Vasarhelyi B, et al. Bone mineral density and bone acquisition in children and young adults with cystic fibrosis: a follow-up study. J Pediatr Gastroenterol Nutr 2004; 38:401–406.
203. Humphries IR, Allen JR, Waters DL, Howman-Giles R, Gaskin KJ. Volumetric bone mineral density in children with cystic fibrosis. Appl Radiat Isot 1998; 49:593–595.
204. Hardin DS, Arumugam R, Seilheimer DK, LeBlanc A, Ellis KJ. Normal bone mineral density in cystic fibrosis. Arch Dis Child 2001; 84:363–368.
205. Gibbens DT, Gilsanz V, Boechat MI, Dufer D, Carlson ME, Wang CI. Osteoporosis in cystic fibrosis. J Pediatr 1988; 113:295–300.
206. Buntain HM, Greer RM, Schluter PJ, et al. Bone mineral density in Australian children, adolescents and adults with cystic fibrosis: a controlled cross sectional study. Thorax 2004; 59:149–155.
207. Baroncelli GI, De Luca F, Magazzu G, et al. Bone demineralization in cystic fibrosis: evidence of imbalance between bone formation and degradation. Pediatr Res 1997; 41:397–403.
208. Greer RM, Buntain HM, Potter JM, et al. Abnormalities of the PTH–vitamin D axis and bone turnover markers in children, adolescents and adults with cystic fibrosis: comparison with healthy controls. Osteoporos Int 2003; 14:404–411.
209. Schulze KJ, O'Brien KO, Germain-Lee EL, Booth SL, Leonard A, Rosenstein BJ. Calcium kinetics are altered in clinically stable girls with cystic fibrosis. J Clin Endocrinol Metab 2004; 89:3385–3391.
210. Wilson DC, Rashid M, Durie PR, et al. Treatment of vitamin K deficiency in cystic fibrosis: effectiveness of a daily fat-soluble vitamin combination. J Pediatr 2001; 138:851–855.
211. Chavasse RJ, Francis J, Balfour-Lynn I, Rosenthal M, Bush A. Serum vitamin D levels in children with cystic fibrosis. Pediatr Pulmonol 2004; 38:119–122.
212. Hahn TJ, Squires AE, Halstead LR, Strominger DB. Reduced serum 25-hydroxyvitamin D concentration and disordered mineral metabolism in patients with cystic fibrosis. J Pediatr 1979; 94:38–42.
213. Donovan DS Jr, Papadopoulos A, Staron RB, et al. Bone mass and vitamin D deficiency in adults with advanced cystic fibrosis lung disease. Am J Respir Crit Care Med 1998; 157(Pt 1):1892–1899.
214. Schulze KJ, O'Brien KO, Germain-Lee EL, Baer DJ, Leonard A, Rosenstein BJ. Efficiency of calcium absorption is not compromised in clinically stable prepubertal and pubertal girls with cystic fibrosis. Am J Clin Nutr 2003; 78:110–116.
215. Schulze KJ, O'Brien K O, Germain-Lee EL, Baer DJ, Leonard AL, Rosenstein BJ. Endogenous fecal losses of calcium compromise calcium balance in pancreatic-insufficient girls with cystic fibrosis. J Pediatr 2003; 143:765–771.
216. Athreya BH, Borns P, Rosenlund ML. Cystic fibrosis and hypertrophic osteoarthropathy in children. Report of three cases. Am J Dis Child 1975; 129:634–637.
217. Garske LA, Bell SC. Pamidronate results in symptom control of hypertrophic pulmonary osteoarthropathy in cystic fibrosis. Chest 2002; 121:1363–1364.
218. Haworth CS, Selby PL, Webb AK, Mawer EB, Adams JE, Freemont TJ. Severe bone pain after intravenous pamidronate in adult patients with cystic fibrosis. Lancet 1998; 352:1753–1754.
219. Haworth CS, Selby PL, Webb AK, Adams JE, Freemont TJ. Oral corticosteroids and bone pain after pamidronate in adults with cystic fibrosis. Lancet 1999; 353:1886.
220. Brenckmann C, Papaioannou A. Bisphosphonates for osteoporosis in people with cystic fibrosis. Cochrane Database Syst Rev 2001(4):CD002010.
221. Batch JA, Couper JJ, Rodda C, Cowell CT, Zacharin M. Use of bisphosphonate therapy for osteoporosis in childhood and adolescence. J Paediatr Child Health 2003; 39:88–92.
222. Bachrach LK. Bare-bones fact– children are not small adults. N Engl J Med 2004; 351:924–926.
223. Neer RM, Arnaud CD, Zanchetta JR, et al. Effect of parathyroid hormone (1–34) on fractures and bone mineral density in postmenopausal women with osteoporosis. N Engl J Med 2001; 344:1434–1441.
224. Vahle JL, Long GG, Sandusky G, Westmore M, Ma YL, Sato M. Bone neoplasms in F344 rats given teriparatide [rhPTH(1–34)] are dependent on duration of treatment and dose. Toxicol Pathol 2004; 32:426–438.

Chapter 78
Nutrition and feeding for children with developmental disabilities

Stanley A. Cohen, Aruna Navathe and Cathleen C. Piazza

INTRODUCTION

Individuals with developmental disabilities are more likely to have problems with feeding and nutrition. As many as 60–90% of children with developmental disabilities have feeding problems, based on parental report,[1] report and observation,[2] and videofluoroscopy.[3] Often, feeding difficulties may precede and in fact herald the diagnosis of cerebral palsy in 60% of children whose mothers note poor sucking, vomiting and choking.[2,4] Many individuals with developmental disabilities may have significant oral motor dysfunction with medical sequelae such as (retching, choking and aspiration) and subsequent behavioral factors[5–7] that further impact upon their nutritional status.[2]

The nutritional goals for the individual with developmental disabilities may appear obvious and implicit: adequate nutritional substrates to maintain the individual's metabolic and fluid requirements, sufficient energy intake to perform those metabolic tasks, additional energy stores to withstand stress (e.g. infections) and optimize growth, rehabilitation of malnutrition, and the correction and prevention of nutrient deficiencies. The challenges that arise at the practical level are:

- How to best deliver that nutrition, account for the individual's needs and the caregiver's abilities
- How to modify the feedings to lessen potential risks and problems (e.g. aspiration and constipation)
- How do we assess and estimate the individual's status and real needs (e.g. what is optimal growth for a patient with developmental disabilities)?

Historically, severe malnutrition was accepted as a concomitant of these disabilities,[8] and aspiration pneumonia was often the expected mode of death.[9] Poor nutritional state was often marked by linear growth failure, decreased lean body mass and diminished fat stores.[10] Over the past two to three decades, enteral feedings and surgical intervention to protect the airway and provide these feedings have significantly improved the outcome for individuals with severe disabilities.[11] In addition, recognition of the complex interplay of gastroesophageal, oropharyngeal and neurobehavioral factors has driven the development of multidisciplinary feeding programs that provide comprehensive evaluation and treatment of feeding disorders in children with developmental disabilities, thereby improving nutritional status and reducing the hospitalization rate.[12]

The periods of greatest nutritional risk are in early infancy during the phase of rapid physical growth and brain development, and in the second decade of life when nutritional needs increase as a result of increasing size – with feeding time needing to increase concomitantly to meet caloric and nutritional needs. Oral feeding difficulties can result in decreased feeding efficiency and may become more problematic as the child grows, requiring increased oral intake[13] and skill as foods of greater complexity (variously textured solids and cupped liquids) are presented. Moreover, children with developmental disabilities seem to have a slow convalescence from illnesses because of their inability to increase their energy consumption during or following illness.

Studies on small groups of children with developmental disabilities have demonstrated that increased nutrient intake can improve weight for height, muscle mass, subcutaneous energy stores, peripheral circulation, the healing of decubitus ulcers and general well-being, while decreasing irritability and spasticity.[14–16] The weight gain is both lean body mass (15%) and body fat (85%). Importantly, earlier initiation of nutritional intervention leads to a significantly improved outcome.[16] However, this improved nutritional status may not translate into an increase in height or improved function. Children with mild cerebral palsy, who are not malnourished and able to walk, are still below average for height.[17] Even those receiving improved nutrition do not attain commensurate linear growth.[18] As a result, these children are smaller in height and weight than their, peers.[19]

Data on adults are limited, despite the fact that increased survival of low birthweight infants and increased longevity results in 65–90% of children with developmental disabilities surviving into adulthood, depending on the age at which survival is calculated.[20] In a study of 86 adult men and women recruited through a cerebral palsy center or participating in regional games sponsored by the US Cerebral Palsy Association, 40% had heights below the 5th percentile, although their body mass indices and mean body fat were within normal range compared with healthy individuals.[21] In a comparative study of 14 adults and 8 adolescents receiving enteral feedings, both groups had decreased bodyweight and height, although the adolescents were significantly more so (bodyweight 26.9 ± 4.9 *vs* 37.8 ±10.5 kg, and height 120 ±12 *vs* 149 ±11 cm). However, the calculated percentage of body fat and measured resting energy expenditures were similar for both groups.[22] These data suggest that these individuals do not necessarily 'grow out of' their feeding problems. That is, caloric intake may not improve with time, and intervention may be necessary to achieve adequate nutritional status if feeding problems are manifested early.

ETIOLOGY

There may be multiple factors complicating the ability of individuals with developmental disabilities to feed normally and obtain nutritional sufficiency by mouth.[23] Historically the classification of feeding was assigned to an organic or non-organic cause, with non-organic causes reflecting social and environmental antecedents[24–26] and comprising the majority of children hospitalized for failure to thrive.[27] More recent classification recognizes the complex overlap of these parameters with physical features and concurrent, often consequential, behavioral elements.[6] Gastrointestinal abnormalities,[28,29] neurologic conditions, structural/oromotor disorders and behavioral issues often contribute to aberrant eating dysfunction.[6,30]

A model to evaluate undernutrition (Fig. 78.1) can assist in understanding the issues involved in order to direct the assessment and approach the treatment of individuals with developmental disablities who have feeding problems and/or potential nutritional deficiency or impairment.

The *historical perspectives* include the genetic endowment provided by the biologic parents as well as any mutations that may modify the inherent potential growth of the individual. The model then accounts for the child's or adult's underlying illness. For example, a cardiorespiratory problem with tachypnea may not only increase caloric expenditure and need, but the rate of breathing may also complicate the issue of oral coordination and ability. Metabolic dysfunctions, such as phenylketonuria or fructose intolerance, may cause growth disturbances and vomiting if not recognized and appropriately treated. A multicenter study[29] of 14 children with lifelong feeding aversion, retching or vomiting, 11 of whom had cerebral palsy, demonstrated motility and sensory abnormalities of the gastrointestinal abnormalities that responded to treatment in 80% of the children involved.

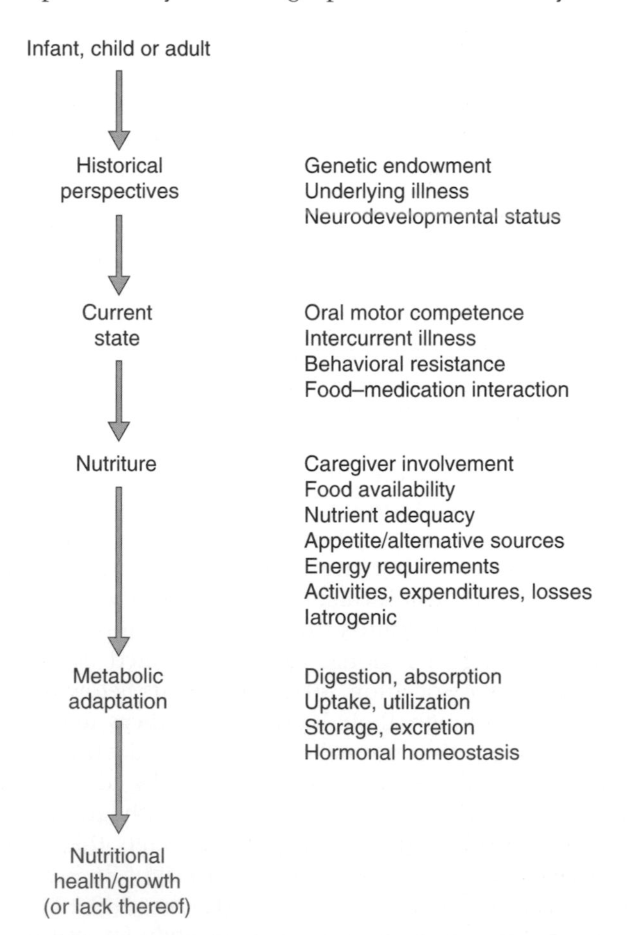

Figure 78.1: Conceptual model of the etiology of feeding disorders and undernutrition in children and adults with developmental disabilities. (Adapted from Cohen.)[99]

Neurodevelopmental status logically has the largest impact on children and adults with neurologic impairments. Knowledge of the natural history of the specific disease involvement is imperative in order to understand whether the individual's condition is degenerative, static or temporary, as this knowledge will guide therapy and nutritional counseling with the family. The degree of disability correlates with risk of malnutrition,[31] with lower nutrient levels associated more with the degree of mental retardation and learning of self-help skills than the motor handicaps imposed by cerebral palsy.[32]

As indicated above, *oral motor dysfunction* is a frequent concomitant and often one of the first signs of neuromuscular impairment.[1–3] Additionally, anatomic abnormalities such as cleft palate, laryngeal clefts and tracheo-esophageal fistula may accompany neurologic deficits as part of a congenital or genetic syndrome. These problems often manifest with difficult or unsuccessful feeding, nasopharyngeal regurgitation, aspiration, choking, persistent drooling, recurrent respiratory tract infections and/or poor weight gain.[1–3]

Normal feeding and swallowing are complex, sequential processes often taken for granted. Motor and/or sensory problems[33] may initiate a disturbance in any of these functional phases (Table 78.1), resulting in dysphagia.[30,34] Children with hypotonia or hypertonia may have difficulty using their tongue to move a food bolus through the mouth; others with motor problems may have choking or aspiration with incoordination of the larynx, as the vocal cords close to protect the airway and pharyngeal muscles propel food to the esophagus.[30]

These motor-based dysphagias often demonstrate greater difficulty with thin liquids, such as juice or water; difficulty with chewing; choking or gagging during or immediately after meals, with the meals often prolonged; gurgly vocal quality after meals; or respiratory compromise.[34]

Individuals with sensory-based problems often have more problems with foods that require chewing, and may separate foods of thicker texture and pocket them in their mouths. They often have a sensory integration defect with the texture and perhaps the taste of foods. This may be localized and associated with gastroesophageal reflux (GER), which may have lessened sensitivity in the

Phase	Description
Pre-oral	Appropriate food provided and presented
	Food introduced into oral cavity
Oral	Suck or mastication prepares bolus
	Passage of bolus into pharynx
Pharyngeal	Respiration ceases
	Elevation of larynx; glottic closure
	Opening of upper esophageal sphincter
	Pharyngeal peristalsis with clearance of pharynx
Esophageal	Esophageal peristalsis
	Opening of lower esophageal sphincter
Gastrointestinal	Receptive relaxation allows storage of food in stomach
	Controlled emptying of nutrients into small intestine
	Mixing with digestive enzymes and secretions
	Intestinal digestion and absorption of nutrients

Adapted from Rudolph and Link, 2002.[30]

Table 78.1 Phases of normal feeding

hypopharynx from inflammation, or it may be more global with sensory problems involving light, touch and noise.[35]

Intercurrent illnesses, with events as mundane as an upper respiratory infection, may temporarily impact feeding function, with more prolonged infections, such as respiratory syncytial virus bronchiolitis, interfering with nutrition for considerably longer, by increasing caloric needs and impairing efficient and effective feeding. Children with feeding impairment have a slower convalescence from illness because of their inability to increase their energy consumption.[36]

Concurrent, acute and chronic disorders such as food allergies, malabsorption, GER, delayed gastric emptying, metabolic anomalies or congenital defects of the gastrointestinal tract may add another layer of complexity on assuring nutritional adequacy for those who also have neurologic impairment. These medical problems may cause eating to be painful, either directly (as in the case of GER) or indirectly (when illness causes general malaise or nausea, which becomes associated with eating). Again, the association of the presentation of food with pain may produce aversions to food. Temperature of food and texture sensitivity can play a big role in acceptance of food.

It appears that nausea, in particular, plays an important role in the development of aversions to food.[37] When nausea is paired with eating, aversions to tastes may develop after only one or a few trials, and may generalize to many foods. In addition, studies on conditioned food aversions show that when these aversions develop they can be long-lasting. Children with a complex medical history also miss early critical experiences with feeding. These early opportunities to feed are important for the development of appropriate oral motor skills such as tongue lateralization and elevation.

Studies on hospitalized children indicate that recurrent or chronic hospitalization may have a negative impact on behavior.[38] For example, medically unstable children exhibit distressed behaviors during both invasive and non-invasive caregiving activities.[39] The results of Gorski et al.[39] suggest that *negative behaviors* such as crying are likely to carry over into the feeding situation in children with a history of hospitalization. In addition, infants with a complex medical history also are subjected to numerous invasive diagnostic tests and procedures, which may involve manipulation of the face and mouth (e.g. laryngoscope, NG tube). These invasive procedures are associated with increases in problem behaviors.[10] From the child's perspective, a spoon may not appear to be substantially different from a laryngoscope or other devices that are used during invasive tests and procedures. Therefore, the child may associate the presentation of objects to the face and mouth (e.g. a spoon) with these early negative experiences and exhibit behaviors such as crying, batting and head turning when objects are presented to the face and mouth. Parents of hospitalized and medically fragile children often report 'oral aversions' that affect feeding and other behaviors associated with the face and mouth (e.g. tooth brushing, face washing).

Although these food aversions and biobehavioral resistances to feeding may result from underlying medical problems, their presence can evolve into a dominant issue. In a study of 103 children referred to an interdisciplinary feeding team, 85% had a behavioral component to their feeding dysfunction irrespective of the underlying medical disorder, with only 12% having an isolated behavioral issue.[6]

The parents' or *caregiver's involvement* is important throughout the entire range of events surrounding feeding. This obvious statement extends beyond a parent's normal expectation of parenthood. Unless ultrasonography or amniocentesis indicates a problem with the fetus prenatally, parents are often ill prepared to raise a child who may not be completely healthy. Feeding often becomes the quintessential embodiment of their parenting and nurturing. In addition to learning the basics of infant feeding, they need to recognize problems quickly and carry out a plan to solve or ameliorate any problems. The caretakers' active involvement and competence is absolutely necessary, but may require considerable support and education.

Problems for the teenager with a developmental disability emanate from the increased quantity of nutrients and calories needed because of increased body size. The same may be true for adults, depending on their feeding skills and access to repletional fluids and calories. Decreased feeding efficiency occurs in individuals with cerebral palsy: chewing and swallowing that takes 12 to 15 times longer than in normal controls translates into extended mealtimes. Even then, longer feeding times may not be sufficient to compensate for caloric and nutritional needs,[40] with caregivers often overestimating the individual's caloric intake and the time spent feeding their child with a developmental disability.[41] For those who are not self-feeders, feeding can be further compromised by an oral aversion that develops because of the times that the caregiver must approach the mouth with distasteful medications and foods that are difficult for the child to handle because of delayed oral motor skills.

The combined issues of nutriture become complex because most individuals with developmental disabilities have somewhat *different nutritional requirements*. Body composition is leaner, with eventual height shorter.[19,42] Those who also have oral motor dysfunction have lower Z scores for weight, height and weight-for-height.[43] Physical activity, intake and often energy needs are less.[44,45] Additionally a decreased ability to communicate can make it difficult for the caregiver to appreciate hunger or satiety. When oral feedings are supplemented or replaced by nasogastric or gastrostomy feedings, the issues of oral resistance, interpretation of hunger signals, and feeding time are largely obviated, with rapid[46] and sustained[14–16] weight gain and small increments of height growth achieved. (Please refer to the sections on Physical assessment and Enteral feedings for a more detailed discussion.)

Proper nutriture assumes that nutritious foods are available and provided, and that nutrient needs are adequately met. However, with our still limited knowledge of specific nutrient needs for the individual with neurological impairment, and with costs high and insurance reimbursement low for medically necessary nutrition, nutrient sufficiency cannot be assumed for any given individual. Indeed, individual metabolic variation and physical activity may be different from one individual to another, and even at different points in time (with increased seizure activity or change in neurologic status with an intercurrent or concurrent illness). Feeding time may also need to change for a particular child or adult based on oral consumption or the schedule for enteral feedings.

Each of the etiologic factors in Figure 78.1 can be seen with its own dynamic continuum impacting and interrelating to the other factors. For example, a child's oral aversion may at times be greater than at others, perhaps affected by, and then further affecting, the parent or caregiver's efforts and abilities (in a bidirectional biofeedback loop). Underlying this could be the degree to which the child's GER is active, which might be exacerbated by a meal containing acidic foods or spicy food such as tomato sauce, or the position in which the child was fed. Thus, an understanding of the nutritional consequences of feeding for the child or adult with developmental disabilities requires a broad understanding of the numerous factors that inform each other and continue to change.

PRESENTATION AND EVALUATION

The complex etiology of feeding problems necessitates an interdisciplinary approach to assessment and treatment. The purpose of a thorough medical and nutritional evaluation is:

- To recognize the patient with, or at risk for, chronic malnutrition and/or specific nutrient deficiencies
- To assess the extent of those problems or potential issues
- To identify underlying, contributory or resultant conditions and behaviors
- To determine the sufficiency of current intake.

This information will allow the medical and therapeutic team to recommend continuation or modifications in the nutritional approach (including the food to be offered, the mechanics of delivery, and any therapies or behavioral changes that may improve of both these), with a plan for ongoing reassessment.

Thus, the medical evaluation (Table 78.2) should document the full context and evolving *history of the underlying illness*, its resulting impairments and associated conditions. The child's medications should be noted in detail, because as many as 25% of non-ambulatory patients who receive anticonvulsants may have rickets.[47–49] Impairment or associated conditions should be noted as these conditions may require specific medical, nutritional or other types of intervention (e.g. a child with VACTERL may have a ventriculoseptal defect requiring fluid limitations or additional

Comprehensive evaluation
History Illness, level of function
Development and acquisition of oral motor skills
Medications, associated conditions
Bowel habits
Dietary/feeding history
- Appetite, intake, schedule
- Allergies, intolerances, preferences
- Nutritional, vitamin and mineral supplements
- Changes in activity, weight, appetite, function
- Dysfunction with feeding, swallowing, reflux
Physical (in addition to routine)
Height, weight, triceps skinfold thickness, vital signs
Observation and general impression
Abdomen for constipation
Spine for kyphoscoliosis, sacral anomalies
Neurologic for tone and level of function
Oral for gag, swallow, seal, drooling, mucosal problems
Signs of deficiency state or chronic illness (clubbing or ridging of nails, skin turgor and texture, bruises, decubitus)
Laboratory (when indicated)
Complete blood count – hemoglobin, red blood cell indices, lymphocyte population
Electrolytes with urea nitrogen
Proteins – albumin, prealbumin, transferrin
Calcium, phosphorus, alkaline phosphatase
Vitamin, mineral levels (rarely needed)
Anticonvulsant levels
Thyroid function
Radiography
- Radiography of hand for osteomalacia, bone age
- Ultrasonography or scan of head for hydrocephalus
- Technetium-99 milk scan
- Upper gastrointestinal series
- Oropharyngeal motility study (modified barium swallow)
Videofluoroscopy
pH esophagraphy

Table 78.2 Medical evaluation for nutritional abnormalities

calories, or they may have had anorectal surgery necessitating nutritional attention to bowel habits and delayed oropharyngeal skills and tracheo-esophageal fistulae that would dictate the amount, texture and delivery of foods needed). Furthermore, the presence of feeding problems may be significant diagnostically, as indicated above.[2]

Specific focus on the *development of oral motor skills* will help to recognize those with malnutrition[50] or feeding dysfunction. The acquisition of feedings skills seems to parallel speech abilities as concurrent oral motor activities, with delayed or anomalous speech patterns often indicative of pervasive oral dysfunction.[51] Refusal to eat contributes further to the child's failure to develop appropriate oral motor skills and failure to gain weight. The *individual's level of function* and oral motor skill should be assessed carefully. The parent should be queried about the time required to feed the child, their own desire and ability to continue, and the quality of the interaction. If there are other caretakers at home or school, the success of those feedings should be discussed as well. The less skilled the child is in terms of oral competency, the more likely the child is to refuse food and fail to gain weight. In children with cerebral palsy, failure to thrive is contributory to poor feeding skills as undernourished children have lower feeding competency than children who are adequately nourished.[50] A circle then develops in which the child refuses food, fails to learn that eating is no longer painful, misses opportunities to practise and develop oral motor skills and fails to gain weight, which then reduces the child's motivation to eat even further.[50]

Dietary history, including a 3-day food record, should document the child's actual food and fluid intake and schedule, any food intolerances, preferences and supplements. Past and current medications should be noted in detail, because as many as 25% of non-ambulatory patients who receive anticonvulsants may have osteomalacia or rickets. The patient or parents also should be asked about any herbal, nutraceutical or other formulations they are administering, and whether these have been recommended or self-prescribed. They may be reluctant initially to admit to alternative therapies, but use of these may alert the physician to the degree of the parent's frustration with their child's medical progress and to possible interactions of these substances with other foods or medications. Any changes in appetite, intake, oral function, weight or activity should be addressed as part of an expanded systems review. The patient's bowel habits and urine output may have an important relation to the feedings and should be noted.

This family-centered history should include:

- Degree of self-feeding and tube feedings, as well as the timing and duration of each – occasionally the timing of tube feedings or the parents' efforts to get their child 'to eat anything' may be counterproductive and interfere with the child developing hunger; the duration may be overly long and fatigue a child's efforts; dependent feeders have a higher risk of aspiration.[52]
- Textures, types and amounts of foods offered and consumed – children with a developmental disability often do not consume nearly the volume that is offered. Taste, temperature and texture may change the acceptance of a given food.
- Presentation of food, the setting and circumstances – distraction by ambient television may lessen or increase the food consumed. Children with oral defensiveness may suck a bottle better when first falling asleep or may feed better as they imitate others
- The individual's position – ached extensor tone, common in individuals with cerebral palsy, can increase the risk for aspiration.[53] Additionally, adults with developmental disability who are tube-fed in a horizontal position have a lower life expectancy.[54]
- Troublesome aspects of the feedings (e.g. choking, gagging, change in respiration, regurgitation, feeding refusal) and the stage at which these occur – problems later in the feedings often appear to have a greater correlation with medical issues such as cardiopulmonary problems, dysphagia or GER, whereas problems at the onset may relate to positioning, parent–child interaction or oral defensiveness.[53]
- Interaction with the different caregivers, and the amounts consumed with each – different feeding patterns and techniques are often seen with specific caregivers. Those forcing feedings may find an inability to achieve optimal feeding.

Anthropometrics will corroborate and amplify the physician's general clinical impression about the individual's nutritional status. Height and weight should be measured when possible. Specific growth charts are available for patients with Down's syndrome[55] and cerebral palsy.[56] The latter uses single leg lengths to achieve better approximation of expected growth, as children and adults with developmental disabilities often have contractures or severe spasticity, countering any attempts at obtaining an accurate measurement of height or length. However, an estimate to use for standard growth charts can be calculated by multiplying the tibial length (measured from the medial popliteal line to the bottom of the medial malleolus) by a constant of 3.26 and adding 30.8 cm:

$$\text{Stature} = 3.26 \times \text{tibial length} + 30.8\text{cm}$$

Similarly, upper arm measures can be utilized in patients with myelomeningocele to assess their growth on normalized curves.[57]

We must rely on measures that evaluate growth and malnutrition in terms of calculations based on bodyweight and height for other neurodevelopmental conditions. Height and weight measurements in former premature infants must be adjusted for the months of prematurity in the first 3 years of life, with the expectation that those with 32-week gestations will catch up by 2 years of age and those with gestations of shorter duration may take 3 years to achieve their genetic growth potential. Body mass index (BMI) establishes a ratio between weight and height with comparative percentiles for the general population. Although easily calculated, this measure has not been tested adequately in those at different ages and levels of developmental disability. A single study in adults evaluated 44 men and 33 women with cerebral palsy. At a mean age of 27 years they had a mean±SD BMI of 22.6 ± 3.6 and 23.6 ± 7.2 respectively, with the percentage of body fat at 13.5 ± 6.0% and 23.2 ± 7.4%.[21]

A weight for height should be obtained by first finding the patient's height age (the age at which the patient's current length would be at the 50th percentile on the appropriate National Center for Health Statistics (NCHS) growth chart). The ideal weight is traditionally the 50th percentile weight at that height. However, this may overestimate the ideal weight for those with neurodevelopmental impairment. The 25th percentile, or lower perhaps, is more appropriate. The patient's actual weight as a percentage of the ideal weight for height then can be used to assess the stage of wasting from malnutrition according to Waterlow criteria[58] (Table 78.3).

The limitations of this calculation, resulting from an individual's genetic and ethnic background, must be recognized. Discrepancies within the height age that may not have been reflected by the previous NCHS editions should now be corrected by the more heterogeneous populations that were used to standardize the current version. However, attempts to use height measures as a valid measure of stunting are fraught with difficulty in patients with developmental disabilities because of contractures and scoliosis.

More sophisticated measurements, using mid arm circumference and triceps or subscapular skinfold thickness, may be worthwhile as a measure of muscle mass and energy stores, especially if they are used to monitor a patient's progress. A study of 69 children with cerebral palsy demonstrated that body fat (derived from skinfold thickness) and percentage weight compared to height age (calculated from upper arm length) differentiated children with malnutrition from those with seemingly sufficient energy stores and better growth.[59]

Physical examination is useful in detecting dehydration, malnutrition or specific nutritional deficiencies. Thus, as part of a comprehensive evaluation, the examiner should document the individual's skin turgor, subcutaneous tissue and muscle mass carefully, noting any bruising, clubbing, edema or rashes (these may be the result of specific nutrient deficiency states). If a feeding tube is in place, the site should be examined for erythema, edema, granulation tissue, herniation or the satellite lesions of a cutaneous yeast infection.

The physical examination also should focus on the sufficiency of oral motor skills as well as posture, tone and neurodevelopmental function. Arching, spasticity and neck position should be noted. Respiratory signs including stridor or wheezing are important indicators of the potential for aspiration. The characteristic of an infant's cry may allude to intrinsic laryngeal abnormalities or those that are secondary to GER. Specific anomalies may cause disordered swallowing, which may preclude safe oral feeding. Particular attention to swallowing dysfunction is necessary in muscular dystrophy and similar myopathic disorders. Drooling, mouth closure and pocketing of food in the mouth during meals are all factors that require careful consideration as feeding therapy is planned, because these may be indicators of oral motor dysfunction. Any evidence of regurgitation, choking or possible aspiration should be evaluated. Well trained members of the team may observe the individual eating for a better understanding of his or her oral motor competencies.

If the individual's ability to swallow is questioned, or if he or she appears to aspirate, an oropharyngeal motility study (known in some institutions as a modified barium swallow) fluoroscopically evaluates oral/laryngeal mechanisms and protection of the airway. While the patient is normally seated, different textures (at specific temperatures) are offered to the individual while fluoroscopic images are viewed, allowing visualization of chewing and swallowing mechanics (Fig. 78.2).

Infants, children and adolescents with the primary diagnosis of severe spastic cerebral palsy who were slow, inefficient eaters demonstrated severe dysphagia on videofluorographic swallow studies, and a significant number (68.2%) had significant silent aspiration during videofluorographic swallow study.[13] Decreased or poorly coordinated pharyngeal motility was predictive of silent aspiration, whereas moderately to severely impaired oral–motor coordination was indicative of severity of feeding complications. Furthermore, the data on the 22 individuals evaluated suggested that early diagnostic workup, including baseline and comparative videofluoroscopic

	% ideal weight
Mild malnutrition	<90
Moderate	<80
Severe	<70

Actual weight as a percentage of ideal weight for height.

Table 78.3 Stages of wasting from malnutrition

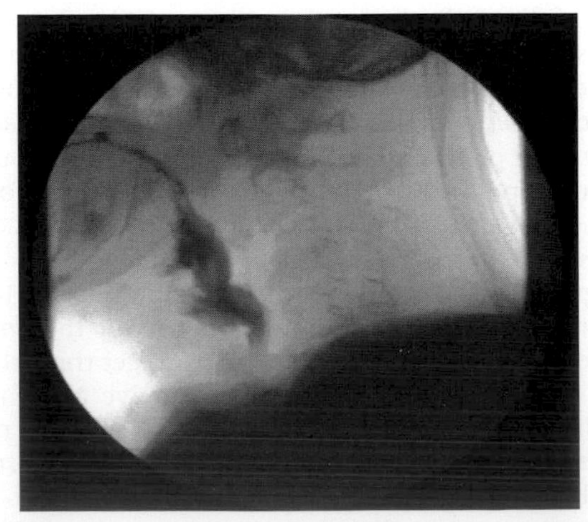

Figure 78.2: Laryngeal penetration demonstrated on oral pharyngeal motility study.

swallow studies, could be helpful in managing the feeding difficulties in these children and preventing chronic aspiration, malnutrition and unpleasant lengthy mealtimes.[13]

Biochemical studies, such as determination of serum zinc or vitamin B_{12} levels, have limited use for nutritional evaluation in these individuals, unless they have concomitant problems with malabsorption. Blood tests primarily measure the quality of the diet, whereas they are insensitive to quantitative insufficiencies, which are more frequent problems for these individuals.[36] Protein status is usually normal, when reflected by albumin, transferrin or prealbumin levels (their half-lives reflecting protein status in the last month, 2 weeks and week respectively). Hemoglobin can screen for iron deficiency anemia, which is common. A hand or limb radiograph may indicate the presence of osteopenia or osteomalacia, particularly in the non-weight-bearing individual, as a more sensitive measure than chemical analysis for calcium, phosphorus or alkaline phosphatase levels. Radiography also can approximate a child's bone age. Anticonvulsant levels and liver/renal function tests may be obtained when indicated.

Currently, bone densitometry may not be cost-effective, as many non-weight-bearing patients can be presumed to develop osteopenia eventually. Bone mineral content and density are reduced in nutritionally adequate children with spastic cerebral palsy, with an even greater reduction in non-independent ambulators.[18] Hair and nail analyses have not proven useful clinically in most cases, although they remain available, but expensive.

GER may be assessed with a 24-h pH esophagraphy. A technetium-99m milk scan may quantify reflux in a child unable to complete 24-h esophagraphy, and may differentially diagnose pulmonary aspiration from the feeding itself or from GER if an image taken 2–4 h later is stained over the lungs. An upper gastrointestinal barium study may be used to assess the suspicion of an anatomic abnormality (but does not diagnose or denote the presence of GER). Gastroesophageal reflux disease may not become obvious until children who have not been fed for prolonged periods actually commence oral food intake during the treatment process.

INTERVENTION

A regimen for feeding the child or adult with a developmental disability must provide adequate nutritional substrates and sufficient energy intake to maintain the individual's metabolic and fluid requirements, with additional energy and micronutrient stores to withstand stressful events, such as infection. Malnutrition and nutrient deficiencies should be corrected and prevented. Each child with a developmental disability, at whatever level should be able to optimize his or her growth. The question is: how much growth is optimal? In the context of achievable height, children with neurologic impairment historically have been smaller.[10,18,60] Short-term studies with aggressive nutritional regimens have been able to increase weight, but not height.[8,11,15,16] Additionally, optimal size for a bed-bound, bedridden child or adult who is severely impaired and requires assistance to move from bed to wheelchair to toilet is perhaps more of an ethical or pragmatic concern. The ease and practicality of providing care for that child or adult may determine the quality of his or her care and the length of time the caregiver can continue to manage that individual's needs in the home setting. Normal weight for height is at the 50th percentile for those with normal activity, the 25th percentile for those able to perform independent transfers, and the 10th percentile for those who are bedridden, with the exception that those under 3 years of age who should be maintained at the 25th to 50th percentile to assure sufficient growth.[61]

Thus, the goals for nutritional management and rehabilitation (Table 78.4) must be considered, with attention to physiologic function as well as the ethics and practical factors in the delivery of care. Importantly, an individual must be medically monitored to adjust for changes in his or her physical condition and for the caregiver's status as well.[8,10,11,15,16]

As nutrient requirements generally parallel energy needs, focus is usually directed towards caloric requirements. Because of the disproportion between weight and height, calculations are usually conceived in terms of body surface area or height. These can be modified for activity level (or lack thereof) and weight repletion. Normally growing children with spastic quadriplegic cerebral palsy have an energy intake of 60 ± 15% of the recommended daily allowance (RDA) for sex and age, and 103 ± 32% of that for weight, when exclusively gastrostomy fed.[45] Patients who are non-ambulatory require an average of 75% of the calories needed by ambulatory patients of comparable height.[45]

Total energy expenditure is reduced relative to resting metabolic rate because both fat-free mass and activity are decreased, even in patients with spastic, quadriplegic cerebral palsy.[42] Resting energy expenditure (REE) correlates poorly with body cell mass in patients with spastic quadriplegia. Accretion of fat-free mass is significantly reduced in these patients. Moreover, the range of REE in adults extends from 16 to 39 kcal per kg per day when measured, and is significantly less than would be predicted by Harris–Benedict and World Health Organization (WHO) equations.[22] Total energy needs for children with spastic quadriplegic cerebral palsy (1.1 × measured REE)[46] are considerably less than the 1.5–1.6 × calculated REE suggested by WHO standards.[32] Should REE be used to calculate

Physiologic maintenance
Rehabilitation of malnutrition
Prevention or correction of nutritional deficiencies
Assist ease of care
Support caregivers in their efforts
When possible:
• Tailor weight/growth to home care need
• Treat feeding problems and behaviors
• Assist development of self-feeding skills
• Regulate bowel habits

Table 78.4 Goals of intervention

Condition	kcal/cm height
Cerebral palsy (5–11 years)	13.9 if mild–moderate activity 11.1 if severely restricted
Down's syndrome (1–3 years)	16.1 males 14.3 females
Myelomeningocele (over 8 years)	7 to achieve weight loss 50% of normal RDA for age/sex for maintenance
Prader–Willi syndrome	10–11 for maintenance 8.5 for weight loss

Table 78.5 Caloric requirements for specific disabilities[56]

patient needs, it must be modified by factors that address muscle tone (increasing 10% for hypertonicity; decreasing 10% for hypotonicity), activity (increasing 15% for those bedridden, and 30% for those ambulating) and growth.[62]

Even though measurement of each individual's REE by indirect calorimetry or bioelectrical impedance might be optimal, repeated measurements may be impractical or at least difficult. Initially, at least, the primary physician or practitioner can calculate caloric needs based on height in centimeters[62] (Table 78.5) and add 5 kcal per gram of weight repletion needed (5000 kcal per kg) divided by the time of acceptable accretion (e.g. 30–90 days). Another technique[63] employs a calculation based on height with modifications: 11.1 kcal/cm for non-ambulatory children with motor dysfunction, 13.9 kcal/cm in those who are ambulatory without motor dysfunction, and 14.7 kcal/cm for children without motor dysfunction. Estimations can also encompass basal metabolic rate and growth, with variations applied for muscle tone and activity.[56]

ORAL FEEDING

The technique of feeding and the food provided are interrelated. Standard, grocery-shelved foodstuffs are the cheapest and simplest means of providing oral feedings. Moreover, the social and emotional pleasures and the expectations of mealtimes often are important for the caregiver, even if only a portion of the individual's nutrient needs can be delivered by mouth. Taste and texture can be varied if the child or adult is identified as a safe oral feeder. Children and adults who can swallow safely but cannot chew effectively may be able to receive the same foods blenderized into a puree or acceptable consistency. Those who can tolerate solids but not liquids can have commercial thickeners added to their fluids. It is important in these children and adults that optimal feeding posture and appropriate food temperature be maintained, as these subtle nuances can make a real difference in feeding tolerance and the prevention of aspiration.

For infants, breast-feeding should be encouraged for its various benefits. Human Milk Fortifier® or proprietary formulas, when used, can be concentrated an additional 10–50% by decreasing free water for children whose nutritional status is compromised (Table 78.6). This allows feedings to lessen critical feeding rates and volumes, with some infants and children unable to sustain growth on standard 20-kcal/oz products because of their volume sensitivity. Small quantities of carbohydrate polymers, cereal or lipids (as long- or medium-chain triglycerides) may be added progressively to either breast milk or formula (Table 78.7), titrating to increase caloric density to 30 kcal or more,[64] while carefully monitoring the child for tolerance to assure adequate urination and to avoid diarrhea, vomiting and/or feeding refusal.

Numerous proprietary products are now available as liquids or puddings to supplement calories, protein and various nutrients. A particular product can be chosen based on the patient's need for fiber in regulating bowel movements and the patient's tolerance of the product's components and taste. Other methods of calorie loading include modification of the foods added to a milk or soy base, which can be adapted for calories, fluid and fiber content, vitamin and mineral requirements, and allergy restrictions according to the child's needs. Potentially, these modular feedings or 'homebrews' (the technique is provided in Table 78.8) are less expensive and offer the caregiver the perception of providing their child 'real food' and 'hands-on care'.

The modular feedings are easily adapted to enteral needs, where taste fatigue will not become an issue. Milk, soymilk or formula can be used as the base ingredient for 'homebrew' feeding. Various calorie-strength recipes can be prepared according to a child's nutritional needs (see Table 78.6). For those children who are volume sensitive, nutrient-dense formulations may be appropriate. Others with relative gastroparesis may need to meet their fluid and nutritional requirements from less dense, lower-fat formulations.

A variety of foods can be blended finely together to make the homebrew nutritionally balanced to meet the child's individual needs (Tables 78.7, 78.8 & 78.9). Mixing the foods in a blender and/or straining results in a smooth, thin consistency that will avoid clogging a gastrostomy or NG tube. Vitamin and mineral supplement may be needed to ensure adequate nutritional status. The feeding tube

	20 kcal/oz	22 kcal/oz[a]	24 kcal/oz	26 kcal/oz
Powder[b]	4 scoops	4½ scoops	4¾ scoops	5¼ scoops
Water to make	8 oz	8 oz	8 oz	8 oz
Powder[b]	1 cup	1 cup	1 cup	1 cup
Add	29 oz	26 oz	24 oz	21.5 oz
Concentrate	13 oz	13 oz	13 oz	13 oz
Water	13 oz	10½ oz	8½ oz	7 oz

[a] Concentrations are approximate, and useful for parental instruction.
[b] Scoops (equivalent to 1 tablespoon) and cups should be level, not pressed or packed.

Table 78.6 Increased calorie concentrations of standard 20-kcal/oz infant formulas

	kcal/g	kcal/tbs	Nutrient source
Human Milk Fortifier®		3.5 per packet	Whey, sodium caseinate, corn syrup solids, lactose
Promod (protein)	4.7	18	Whey
Casec	3.8	17	Calcium caseinate, soy, lecithin
Formula powder[a]		40	Variable
Non-fat dry milk	8.7	27	Milk
MCT oil	8.2	115	Medium-chain triglycerides
Vegetable oil	8.9	124	Variable
Polycose	3.8	23	Glucose polymer
Moducal	3.7	30	Glucose polymer
Duocal	4.9	42	Hydrolyzed corn starch, refined vegetable oils, fractionated coconut oil
Additions	5.2	43	Sodium caseinate, whey protein
Benecalorie (liquid)	1 kcal/ml	110	High oleic sunflower oil, calcium caseinates, sodium ascorbate, polysorbate, zinc, etc.
Rice cereal	4.2	15	Rice flour, soy oil, barley malt

[a]20 cal/oz infant formula.
tbs, tablespoon.

Table 78.7 Modular high-calorie additions

should be flushed with tap water before and after delivering feedings and medication.

As homebrew feedings may be thicker than commercial formulas, a large-size feeding tube may be necessary. Bolus feedings may work better for homebrew tube feedings than a continuous drip because of the thicker consistency and increased risk of bacterial contamination without refrigeration. As always, aseptic techniques, proper handling of utensils and handwashing should be used to

1 Measure all ingredients carefully, using measuring cups
2 Pour ingredients into a large mixing bowl and stir contents to combine
3 Mix well, using blender or mixer method
Blender method: Blend at medium speed for 3 min or until mixed thoroughly
Mixer method: Mix at medium speed for 5 min or until mixed thoroughly
4 There should be no lumps in the formula
5 If the mixture is thick, thin it with water as recommended by dietitian
6 Pour formula into a clean container or individual jars. Cover and refrigerate immediately
7 The refrigerated formula may be safely used within 24–36 h
8 Before each feeding, the amount of formula needed should be measured into a separate container, covered and warmed slightly before use
9 To warm formula: place the container with one feeding into a pan of hot water for 15–20 min, or use a microwave oven on a low setting for approximately 1 min
10 Do not overheat the formula
11 Shake the formula or stir it to avoid hotspots
12 Do not use formula that has been heated or removed from the refrigerator for more than 2 h. Discard immediately
13 Flush tube with 15–30 ml water, or as recommended
14 If any problems are noted (intolerance to formula, diarrhea, thickness of formula), please review with registered dietitian

Note: Once you know your child is tolerating this recipe, it maybe helpful to 'stock up' on all of the ingredients, because each one is *important*. The simple omission of one ingredient could have a serious impact, so call your dietitian if you have any questions or concerns about this recipe before changing it.
Courtesy of Aruna Navathe, Children's Healthcare of Atlanta.

Table 78.8 Directions for preparation of home tube-feeding

For: .... Date: ....

Home Tube-Feeding Recipe
'Home Brew'

The feeding formula should be prepared fresh daily. To prepare this formula safely, you must always:
1 Wash your hands
2 Use clean mixing bowls, equipment and utensils
3 Sanitize the blender or mixer bowl by filling with boiling water. Allow to stand for 3 minutes and then discard water

Recipe:
In a large clean mixing bowl or blender combine the following ingredients:

___ ounces or ___ cups of milk or formula
___ teaspoon(s) vegetable oil
tablespoon(s) cereal (¼ cup)
packet Carnation Instant Breakfast
table salt

Strained baby food:
___ jar(s) fruit (4 oz)
___ jar(s) vegetable (4 oz)
___ jar(s) meat (2.5 oz)

Note: You may vary the selection of strained baby foods daily.

Volume: oz
Calories: cal/recipe Per ounce: cal/oz
Protein: g/recipe Per ounce: g/oz
Fat: g/recipe
Carbohydrate: g/recipe
kcal distribution: % protein, % fat, % carbohydrate
Rate: ml/h
Flushes: 20–30 ml water
Vitamins/minerals: This will meet RDA for all nutrients.

Courtesy of Aruna Navathe, Children's Healthcare of Atlanta.

78.9 Modular formula instructions for parents

prepare formula to avoid cross-contamination and assure food safety.

Assessment of nutritional status and determination of an optimal nutritional plan to meet the child's needs should be done initially, with reassessments of formulation and nutritional needs at 1-, 3-, 6- and 12-month intervals as needed.

If a currently available proprietary formula is used, the physician must recognize that these have fixed nutrient/energy ratios, so that reducing the prescribed calories proportionate to the debilitated patient's needs based on height also may reduce that individual's intake of all other nutrients significantly below the RDA for age. The potential reduction in calcium, phosphorus and vitamin D poses risks of bone disease in these individuals, with other vitamin and mineral deficiencies possible as well, although many vitamin and mineral needs do parallel caloric requirements. In a study of children with cerebral palsy, most nutrient levels exceeded two-thirds of the RDA, but the serum level for calcium was decreased below normal levels.[65] Another study demonstrated increased alkaline phosphatase levels in institutionalized children and adolescents on anticonvulsants.[66] Thus, intervention with maintenance doses of vitamin D and calcium may be prudent as the individual ages, if he or she is not at particular risk for nephrolithiasis.

ORAL FEEDING PROBLEMS

Oral feeding is an option when the child or adult is identified as a safe oral feeder. A primary consideration in treatment of children with feeding problems is that the child with food refusal has a different history or experience of food than the typically eating child, with the problems often persisting and worsening over time.[67] Therefore, the techniques or recommendations that are used for typically eating children may not apply to children with food refusal.

As indicated above, the first step is a comprehensive evaluation. Specificity of diagnosis allows targeted therapy. GER, renal disorders and brain tumors may create a loss of intake, vomiting or weight loss. Moreover, Zangen et al.[29] have demonstrated that 43% of the medically fragile toddlers (most of whom had cerebral palsy) responded to medication, using nifedipine and dicyclomine for diffuse esophageal spasm; dicyclomine for continuous duodenal contractions; imipramine or amitripyline and/or gabapentin and/or ondansetron for raising the gastric pain threshold; octreotide or erythromycin for inducing phase three migrating motor complexes; and cyproheptadine for increasing appetite. Additionally, attention should focus on the amount of enteral feeding, as large volumes may satiate the child, and the protein predominance of the formula. Whey-based formulas markedly reduce gastric emptying time and decrease the frequency of emesis in gastrostomy-fed children with spastic quadriplegia.[68]

Effective, empirically supported, interventions in the treatment of complex feeding problems are those contingency management treatments that include positive reinforcement of appropriate feeding responses and ignoring or guiding inappropriate responses.[69]

Oral competency and painful feedings greatly impact on nutritional status in a cyclical devolution, unless the cycle can be interrupted. Poor oral motor feeding skills result in an inability to eat, subsequent inadequate weight gain and failure to thrive. This leads to lessened motivation and ability to learn these skills (J. Fagan and A. Navathe, unpublished observations).

Thus the main goals of oral feeding are:

- To increase oral intake
- To meet the child's nutritional needs
- To decreasing G-tube dependence
- To increase the texture
- To increase the vasriety of foods
- To decrease bottle dependence
- To increase self-feeding
- To decrease inappropriate behaviors
- To support parental nurturance of the child
- To maintaining family stability.

Initially, treatment for children with total food refusal and inappropriate mealtime behavior (e.g. crying, head turning, batting at the spoon, refusal to open the mouth) should focus on reducing these inappropriate behaviors and increasing more appropriate eating-related behaviors (e.g. opening the mouth) to establish that eating is no longer painful.[70,71] Meals should be time limited and focus on a specific end-goal (e.g. having the child taste one bite of food[72].) It is also important to understand what additional gains the child may achieve by avoiding food or engaging in inappropriate mealtime behavior. For example, if refusal of a non-preferred food (e.g. peas) results in the presentation of a more preferred food (e.g. peanut butter and jelly sandwich), these 'secondary' gains should be eliminated.[37] Strategies used by the caregivers to get their children to eat (i.e. distraction, coaxing, allowing breaks from eating, or providing toys or preferred food) actually worsened behavior in 10 of the 15 participants in one study.[73] From a parental perspective, strategies such as terminating the meal or coaxing may produce the immediate effect of temporarily stopping the undesirable child behavior. However, problem behavior and food refusal appear to produce a favorable outcome from the child's perspective (e.g. avoidance of eating, increased parental attention, preferred foods or toys), and these refusal behaviors are likely to be repeated during subsequent meals. Interestingly, 89% of the children studied had earlier medical conditions (e.g. GER) that probably caused eating to be painful. Even though these medical conditions were resolved at the time of the study, the children had continued feeding refusal.

Often it is necessary to reduce the texture of presented food[74] when the child has limited experiences with oral intake because the child's oral motor skills are not sufficiently well developed to consume age-appropriate textures successfully (i.e. without choking, gagging or fatiguing). Some less complex textures should be presented to prevent fatigue and frustration. Small amounts of greater textures should continue to be presented to enable the child to maintain and advance his or her oral motor skills.

If the child consumes some foods, albeit a limited variety, these preferences can be used to increase the variety of foods consumed by allowing the child to (a) consume a preferred food following consumption of a non-preferred food,[75] (b) avoid consumption of a non-preferred food by consuming a more preferred food[76] or (c) consume preferred and non-preferred foods simultaneously by blending them together.[77]

Because the etiology of the feeding problem is multidetermined, treatment should focus on all of the components (physiologic, oral motor and psychologic) that contribute to feeding problems. A multidisciplinary approach, combining the services of a psychologist, occupational therapist, speech therapist, dietitian and pediatric gastroenterologist, is the most effective means for successful treatment, particularly for difficult feeding problems. Often the programs provide a continuum of services (evaluation, outpatient therapy, day treatment and hospitalization, based on the patient's individual needs.[12,78,79] Rapid (2–3 weeks) success has been described with inpatient care, specifically selected candidates and a consistent approach to overcoming the child's resistence.[80]

Successful treatment of feeding problems should include measurable goals for each child's feeding behaviors that are developed by the interdisciplinary team and caregivers. Feeding behaviors (e.g. amounts consumed, acceptance of bites of food) should be measured objectively and treatment decisions should be data based. Outcomes should be assessed regularly throughout the duration of treatment. A primary goal should be to establish feeding patterns that can be maintained by the caregivers in the home and in other environments. Thus, caregiver training should be an essential component to the success of the program.

Goals are individualized based on the child's problem. For example, children with failure to thrive or G-tube dependence have a goal of increasing oral intake and decreasing G-tube dependence. Other goals include, but are not limited to, increasing the texture and variety of foods consumed, decreasing bottle dependence, decreasing inappropriate mealtime behavior, and increasing self-feeding or self-drinking skills. Goals also are set for training parents to implement treatment procedures both in the clinic and in home and community settings (i.e. generalization).

Preliminary analysis of the outcome measures for one program with approximately 50 children, half of whom had been diagnosed with a developmental disability,[80] indicated that over 87% of the goals for treatment were met by the time of discharge. All of the children met their goals for increasing texture, decreasing bottle dependence, increasing self-feeding skills and increasing variety of foods consumed. When increases in oral calories were the goal of treatment, 70% of the children reached their goal for caloric intake. When increases in liquid intake (for children who did not consume liquids by mouth) were the goal of treatment, 80% of the children reached their goal for oral liquid intake. All others increased solid or liquid intake over baseline levels, but did not reach their final goal during the day treatment admission. Even though not all of the children reached their goal for oral intake, the mean percentage of the p.o. goal met was 82%, suggesting that even when children did not reach 100% of their oral intake goal, their levels of oral intake were increased substantially and within 20% of the goal. Progress towards increasing oral intake continued during outpatient follow-up.[80]

Levels of enteral feedings were decreased for all children who entered the program receiving nutritional supplementation via tube, and 70% of children met their goals for decreases in enteral feedings. Children who entered the program with a NG tube either left the program without the tube (75%) or the tube was removed shortly after discharge (100%). Thus, surgical placement of a gastric (G) tube was avoided for 100% of children who entered the program as candidates for G tubes as a result of the presence of failure to thrive and a NG tube at admission. The goals for decreasing inappropriate mealtime behaviors were met for 97% of the children. Some 88% of caregivers were trained to implement the treatment protocols with greater than 90% accuracy, and the treatment was transferred successfully to the home and community in 100% of cases.

Preliminary analysis of follow-up data indicates that the majority of children (87%) continue to be followed after discharge from the day treatment program. Of those who are currently followed, 85% have continued to make progress toward age-typical feeding, which included further volume increases, further G-tube decreases and G-tube removal, increases in the variety of foods consumed, texture advances, initiation of cup drinking, and initiation of self-feeding.

Additionally, structured diagnosis-specific treatment has resulted in increased tissue stores and decreased hospitalization.[12] When combined with pharmacotherapy to treat esophageal spasm and duodenal dysmotility, to reduce gastric pain threshold and/or to increase appetite, 80% had improved emotional health, with 43% able to eat orally.[29]

ENTERAL DELIVERY

When necessary, proprietary and homemade supplemental formulas can be delivered via non-oral means. A NG tube may be used in the infant needing a brief (less than 2 months) infusion to allow acquisition of feeding skills. Similarly, a child needing perioperative intervention to prevent negative nitrogen balance may benefit from a short-term infusion by NG tube. Any enteral therapy that is expected to extend for a longer duration (greater than 2–3 months) should employ a tube placed directly into the stomach or intestine. In most situations, a G tube will function well for the delivery of nutrition and medication. The tube can be converted to a 'button' device with internal bolsters to decrease traction and any interference with the child's activity and therapies. Gastrostomy placement has been shown to reduce feeding time, food-related choking episodes, frequency of chest infections and family stress, and to improve weight gain and nutritional status significantly in children with severe neurologic impairment.[11,16]

However, percutaneous gastrostomy (PEG) is not without complications or concerns. In a review of a 10-year experience with 220 children, Gauderer[81] reported four minor catheter infections and 13 more significant complications. This included two deaths with underlying cardiac disease. In another series, perforation occurred with 15% of the tubes.[11] Population-based data compiled from the roles of the California Department of Developmental Services[54,82,83] and elsewhere[84] reveal that feeding tubes in severely disabled children with a tracheostomy reduce the risk of mortality, but significantly shorten survival in adults and increase mortality risk by 2.1 in children without a tracheostomy.

Use of the feeding tube is not necessarily causal, as factors such as immobility, malnutrition, oral motor dysfunction and recurrent aspiration that require the use of an alternative nutritional method may contribute to the patient's morbidity. However, the protection offered by a tracheostomy does suggest that the potential for aspiration in patients with gastrostomy devices is considerable; even though quality of life may be improved with the use of enteral feedings through a gastrostomy, the length of survival may be lessened.

Therefore, the anatomy and function of the stomach should be evaluated prior to the placement of the feeding tube. The coexistence of GER may require a simultaneous fundoplication, and delayed gastric emptying must necessitate pyloroplasty or duodenal placement of the distal portion of the tube. Of importance, symptomatic GER may be recognized only after gastrostomy placement, even though it is not demonstrated initially.[85–87] In children with recurrent aspiration, fundoplication and gastrostomy are not able to lower the rate of postoperative aspiration.[88,89] Moreover, recurrent GER can occur after fundoplication and may be increased in children with profound neurologic disability.[90–93] Attempts to identify the risk factors that increase morbidity and mortality include stratifying the disabled population by degree of impairment[94,95] and using serum albumin[96] to predict at least early survival after PEG placement.

Physiologically designed formulas of increased caloric and protein density can be used for gastric and nasogastric infusion, as palatability is no longer an issue. Modifications must be made for osmolality and speed of delivery with a feeding tube in the duodenum or jejunum. Lower osmotic or predigested formulas are needed for duodenal or jejunal infusions and must be delivered by a slow drip to avoid dumping or discomfort. Bolus or cyclic drip feedings may be chosen for the patient with a G or NG tube. The choice between bolus and drip may depend on esphagogastric function, the volume to be delivered, or the home care needs of the child and his or her caregivers. Often nocturnal drip feedings can provide 30–50% of the child's nutrient needs, so that daytime meals can be offered orally without the pressure and large blocks of time that have to be devoted when all requirements need to be met by three or four daily meals.

Gastric emptying has been shown to be delayed in children with cerebral palsy and contributes to GER, which in itself contributes to recurrent vomiting, with the most common manometric abnormality being a reduction in lower esophageal pressure.[97] Whey-based formulas do lessen that impact, however, by decreasing gastric emptying time and reducing the frequency of emesis in gastrostomy-fed children with spastic quadriplegia.[68] The choice of formula may be less of an issue than the volume delivered children and adults with developmental disabilities with these assistive feedings. The amount ingested is no longer defined by appetite, but determined by caregivers and medical providers. Long-term overnutrition presents as much risk as undernutrition. Hypertension and obesity can increase cardiovascular concerns in these patients, especially those with neuromuscular disorders. Moreover, overweight and obese children or adults with developmental disabilities present increased problems for caretakers, who have to risk their own health in lifting or assisting movement. Therefore, calculations must approximate a patient's need for calories and nutrients.

As these prescriptions for volume may overestimate or underestimate actual requirements, and because growing children increase their nutritional needs as they age and grow, re-evaluation at appropriate intervals for serial examination and measurement with the calculations revisited is perhaps more important than any individual prescription.

When safety of oral feeding is not an issue, these enteral techniques can merely supplement the child's own nutrition, with the caregivers continuing to feed the child actively. This dual feeding method often provides great satisfaction to parents and caregivers, because the mealtime interaction is improved when there is no longer any need for force-feeding of medication or nourishment. However, the risk of satiation (i.e. that the patient will not be motivated to feed orally) must be considered in conjunction with the schedule of feedings. Even overnight tube feedings may produce satiation and unwillingness of the child to orally feed concomitant with NG- or G-tube feedings.

Many parents are apprehensive about feeding and assuring adequate nutrition for their children. Understandably, caregivers for children with a developmental disability may be even more anxious. Based on the method of delivery, the caregivers should be trained carefully in the preparation and delivery of the feeding. Parents should be reassured and provided with information about medical, nutritional and home-care agencies that can serve as resources. They should be informed that success may be most dependent on appropriate follow-up visits to assess the patient's progress and adjust the feeding regimens. Moreover, social service agencies and/or medical care facilities should be encouraged to facilitate these efforts. In one study,[98] a hospital providing high-calorie, ready-to-feed nutritional supplementation at cost improved compliance with dietary recommendations. Such a policy has the potential to increase the effectiveness of nutrition intervention.

SUMMARY

Children with chronic illnesses often are debilitated further as a result of secondary nutritional problems that require the attention of their primary care physicians and subspecialists. Recent advancements in understanding and meeting the nutritional needs of children and adults with developmental disabilities have resulted in an improved quality and length of life. Small studies have demonstrated improved weight for height, muscle mass, subcutaneous energy stores, peripheral circulation, healing of decubitus ulcers and general well-being with enteral feedings, with decreased irritability and spasticity.

However, these children do not follow the same patterns for linear growth as other children. The goals for weight accretion must be considered when determining the actual caloric needs for each child. Alternative methods using height or, preferably, single limb length to calculate caloric needs are recommended.

The delivery of nutrient and energy sources should be based on the child's neurologic function, oral motor skills, the presence of GER or other superimposed conditions. The use of proprietary formulas with fixed nutrient/energy ratios may provide sufficient calories, but also have the potential for specific nutrient deficiencies; most notably calcium, phosphorus and vitamin D. In addition, the placement of a gastrostomy device is not without controversy, as there is an increased mortality rate in adults with developmenta; disability without a tracheostomy tube, and this may be related to the underlying condition of these patients or their increased risk of aspiration.

The complex etiology of feeding problems requires a multidisciplinary approach for successful treatment. Goals for treatment should be specified in measurable terms, and outcomes should be tracked during treatment and over time. An intensive, data-based, multidisciplinary approach is successful in more than 85% of children. The highest levels of success (95% or better) are achieved in avoiding G-tube placement in patients with failure to thrive and NG tubes, and for patients with some preliminary oral intake (such as those with food selectivity, texture inadequacies, skill deficits or bottle dependence).

Even though the outcomes for G-tube dependence are *slightly* lower over the short term, progress continues during follow-up with caregiver cooperation, with most individuals continuing to make significant progress toward their goals. Caregiver training and generalization to the home and community environments can also be achieved with high levels of success (over 90%) and is critical to long-term maintenance of program gains. Two of the most important long-term aspects of the feeding program are to assure that once the ethical and technical issues are addressed: (1) the caregivers are adequately instructed, trained and reassured; and (2) appropriate follow-up is arranged to assess the patient's progress and adjust the regimen to achieve an optimal outcome. However, clinical research trials and critical analysis are needed in many areas in order to determine and then disseminate best practices and optimal nutrition.

References

1. Dahl M, Thommessen M, Rasmussen M, Selberg T. Feeding and nutritional characteristics in children with moderate or severe cerebral palsy. Acta Paediatr1996; 6:697–701.
2. Reilly S, Skuse D, Poblete, X. Prevalence of feeding problems and oral motor dysfunction in children with cerebral palsy: a community survey. J Pediatr 1996; 129:877–882.
3. Griggs CA, Jones PM, Lee RE. Videofluoroscopic investigation of feeding disorders of children with multiple handicaps. Dev Med Child Neurol 1989; 31:303–308.
4. Reilly S, Skuse D. Characteristics and management of feeding problems of young children with cerebral palsy. Dev Med Child Neurol 1992; 34:379–388.
5. Babbitt RL, Hoch TA, Coe DA, et al. Behavioral assessment and treatment of pediatric feeding disorders. J Dev Behav Pediatr 1994; 15:278–291.
6. Burklow KA, Phelps AN, Schultz JR, et al. Classifying complex pediatric feeding disorders. J Pediatr Gastroenterol Nutr 1998; 27:143–147.
7. Crist W, Napier-Phillips A. Mealtime behaviors of young children: a comparison of normative and clinical data. J Dev Behav Pediatr 2001; 22:279–286.
8. Patrick J, Boland M, Stoski D, Murray GE. Rapid correction of wasting in children with cerebral palsy. Dev Med Child Neurol 1986; 28:734–739.
9. Rogers B, Stratton P, Msall M, et al. Long-term morbidity and management strategies of tracheal aspiration in adults with severe developmental disabilities. Am J Ment Retard 1994; 98:490–498.
10. Stallings VA, Cronk CE, Zemel BS, Charney EB. Body composition in children with spastic quadriplegic cerebral palsy. J Pediatr 1995; 126:833–839.
11. Brant CQ, Stanich P, Ferrari AP Jr. Improvement in children's nutritional status after enteral feeding by PEG: an interim report. Gastrointest Endosc 1990; 50:183–188.
12. Schwartz SM, Corredor J, Fisher-Medina J, Cohen J, Rabinowitz S. Diagnosis and treatment of feeding disorders in children with developmental disabilities. Pediatrics 2001; 108:671–676.
13. Mirrett PL, Riski JE, Glascott J, Johnson V. Videofluoroscopic assessment of dysphagia in children with severe spastic cerebral palsy. Dysphagia 1994; 9:174–179.
14. Shapiro BK, Green P, Krick J, Allen D, Capute AJ. Growth of severely impaired children: neurological versus nutritional factors. Dev Med Child Neurol 1986; 28:729–733.
15. Rempel GR, Colwell S, Nelson RP. Growth in children with cerebral palsy fed via gastrostomy. Pediatrics 1988; 82:857–862.
16. Sanders KD, Cox K, Cannon R, et al. Growth response to enteral feeding by children with cerebral palsy. JPEN J Parenter Enteral Nutr 1990; 14:23–26.
17. Pryor HB, Thelander HE. Growth deviations in handicapped children. An anthropometric study. Clin Pediatr 1967; 6:501–512.
18. Chad KE, McKay HA, Zello GA, Bailey DA, Failkener RA, Snyder RE. Body composition in nutritionally adequate ambulatory and nonambulatory children with cerebral palsy and a healthy reference group. Dev Med Child Neurol 2000; 42:334–339.
19. Krick J, Murphy-Miller P, Zeger S, Wright E. Pattern of growth in children with cerebral palsy. J Am Diet Assoc 1996; 96:680–685.
20. Rapp CE, Torres MM. The adult with cerebral palsy. Arch Fam Med 2000; 9:466–472.
21. Ferrano TM, Johnson RK, Ferrara MS. Dietary and anthropometric assessment of adults with cerebral palsy. J Am Diet Assoc 1992; 92:1083–1086.
22. Dickerson RN, Brown RO, Gervasio JG, Hak EB, Hak LJ. Measured energy expenditure of tube-fed patients with severe neurodevelopmental disabilities. J Am Coll Nutr 1999; 18:61–68.

23. Cohen SA, Navathe AS. Feeding the developmentally delayed child. J Med Assoc Ga 1999; 88:71–76.
24. Beautrais AL, Fergusson DM, Shannon FT. Family life events and behavioral problems in preschool-aged children. Pediatrics 1982; 70:774–779.
25. Iwata BA, Riordan MM, Wohl MG, Finney JW. Pediatric feeding disorders. Behavioral analysis and treatment. In: Accardo PJ, ed. Failure to Thrive in Infants and Early Childhood: A Multidisciplinary Team Approach. Baltimore, MD: University Park Press; 1982:297–325.
26. Forsyth BW, Leventhal JM, McCarthy PJ. Mothers' perception of feeding and crying behaviors. Am J Dis Child 1985; 139:269–272.
27. Dietz, WH. Body composition and nutritional assessment of the undernourished child. In: Cohen SA, ed. The Underweight Infant, Child, and Adolescent. Norwalk, CT: Appleton, Century, Crofts; 1986:1–14.
28. Dellert SF, Hyams JS, Treem WR, Geertsma MA. Feeding resistance and gastroesophageal reflux in infancy. J Pediatr Gastrointest Nutr 1993; 17:66–71.
29. Zangen T, Ciarla C, Zangen S, et al. Gastrointestinal motility and sensory abnormalities may contribute to food refusal in medically fragile toddlers. J Pediatr Gastroenerol Nutr 2003; 37:287–293.
30. Rudolph CD, Link DT. Feeding disorders in infants and children. Pediatr Clin North Am 2002; 49:79–112.
31. Kleinman R (ed.). Nutritional support for children who are nutritionally impaired. In: Pediatric Nutrition Handbook. Elk Grove Village, IL: American Academy of Pediatrics; 2004:629–642.
32. Hammond MI, Lewis MN, Johnson EW. A nutritional study of cerebral palsied children. J Am Diet Assoc 1996; 49:196–201.
33. Palmer MM, Heyman MB. Assessment and treatment of sensory-versus motor-based feeding problems in very young children. Infants Young Child 1993; 6:67–73.
34. Rudolph CD. Feeding disorders in infants and children. J Pediatr 1994; 125:S116–S124.
35. Kleinman R (ed.) Pediatric feeding and swallowing disorders. In: Pediatric Nutrition Handbook. Elk Grove Village, IL: American Academy of Pediatrics; 2004:425–442.
36. Patrick J, Gisel E. Nutrition for the feeding impaired child. J Neurol Rehab 1990; 4:115–119.
37. Schafe GE, Bernstein IL. Taste aversion learning. In: Capaldi ED, ed. Why We Eat What We Eat: The Psychology of Eating. Washington, DC: American Psychological Association; 1997:31–51.
38. Cataldo MF, Bessman CA, Parker LH, Pearson JE, Rogers MC. Behavioral assessment for pediatric intensive care units. J Appl Behav Anal 1979; 12:83–97.
39. Gorski PA, Hole WT, Leonard CH, Martin JA. Direct computer recording of premature infants and nursery care: distress following two interventions. Pediatrics 1983; 72:198–202.
40. Gisel EG, Patrick J. Identification of children with cerebral palsy unable to maintain a normal nutritional state. Lancet. 1988; i:283–286.
41. Stallings VA, Zemel BS, Davies JC, Cronk CE, Charney EB. Energy expenditure of children and adolescents with severe disabilities: a cerebral palsy model. Am J Clin Nutr 1996; 64:627–634.
42. Stevenson RD. Measurement of growth in children with developmental disabilities. Dev Med Child Neurol 1996; 38:855–860.
43. Krick J, Van Duyn MA. The relationship between oral–motor involvement and growth: a pilot study in a pediatric population with cerebral palsy. J Am Diet Assoc 1984; 84:555–559.
44. Fried MD, Pencharz PB. Energy and nutrient intakes of children with spastic quadriplegia. J Pediatr 1991; 119:947–949.
45. Azcue MP, Zello GA, Levy LD, Pencharz PB. Energy expenditure and body copmposition in children with spastic quadriplegic cerebral palsy. J Pediatr 1996; 129:870–876.
46. Patrick J, Boland M, Stoski D, Murry GE. Rapid correction of wasting in children with cerebral palsy. Dev Med Child Neurol 1994; 36:135–142.
47. Tolman KG, Jubiz W, Sannella JJ. Osteomalacia associated with anticonvulsant drug therapy in mentally retarded children. Pediatrics 1975; 56:45–50.
48. Lifshitz F, Maclaren NK. Vitamin D dependent rickets in institutionalized, mentally retarded children receiving long term anticonvulsant therapy: a survey of 288 patients. J Pediatr 1973; 83:612–620.
49. Crosley CJ, Chee C, Berman PH. Rickets associated with long term anticonvulsant therapy in a pediatric outpatient population. Pediatrics 1975; 56:52–57.
50. Troughton KE, Hill AE. Relation between objectively measured feeding competence and nutrition in children with cerebral palsy. Dev Med Child Neurol 2001; 43:187–190.
51. Croft, RD. What consistency of food is best for children with cerebral palsy who cannot chew? Arch Dis Child 1992; 67:269–271.
52. Arvedson J, Roders B, Buck G, Smart P, Msall M. Silent aspiration in children with dysphagia. Int J Pediatr Otorhinolaryngol 1994; 28:173–181.
53. Arvedson JC, Rogers BT. Pediatric swallowing and feeding disorders. J Med Speech-Lang Pathol 1993; 1:203–221.
54. Eyman RK, Grossman HJ, Chaney RH, Call TL. The life expectancy of profoundly handicapped people with mental retardation. N Engl J Med 1995; 323:584–589.
55. Cronk C, Crocker AC, Pueschel SM, et al. Growth charts for children with Down syndrome: 1 month to 18 years of age. Pediatrics 1988; 81:102–110.
56. Spender QW, Cronk CE, Charney EB, Stallings VA. Assessment of linear growth of children with cerebral palsy: use of alternative measures to height or length. Dev Med Child Neurol 1989; 31:206–214.
57. Belt B, Ekvall S, Cook C, Oppenheimer S, Wessel J. Linear growth measurements: a comparison of single arm lengths and arm span. Dev Med Child Neurol 1986; 28:319.
58. Waterlow JC. Classification and definition of protein-calorie malnutrition. BMJ 1972; 3:566–569.
59. Davies JC, Antonucci DL, Charney EB, Stallings VA. Use of upper-arm length and per cent body fat for nutritional assessment of children with cerebral palsy. Dev Med Child Neurol 1989; 31(Suppl 59):39–40.
60. Stevenson RD, Hayes RP, Carter LV, Blackman JA. Clinical correlates of linear growth in children with cerebral palsy. Dev Med Child Neurol 1994; 34:135–142.
61. Krick J, Murphy PE, Markham JF, Shapiro BK. A proposed formula for calculating energy needs of children with cerebral palsy. Dev Med Child Neurol 1992; 6:481–487.
62. Bandini LG, Schoeller DA, Fukagawa NK, Wykes LJ, Dietz WH. Body composition and energy expenditure in adolescents with cerebral palsy or myelodysplasia. Pediatr Res 1991; 29:70–77.
63. Culley WJ, Middleton TO. Caloric requirements of mentally retarded children with and without motor dysfunction. J Pediatr 1969; 75:380–384.
64. Davis A, Baker S. The use of modular nutrients in pediatrics. J Pediatr Gastroentoral Nutr 1996; 20:228–237.
65. Hammond MI, Lewis MN, Johnson EW. A nutritional study of cerebral palsied children. J Am Diet Assoc 1966; 49:196–201.

66. Pesce KA, Wodarski LA, Wang M. Nutritional status of institutionalized children and adolescents with developmental disabilities. Res Dev Disabil 1989; 10:33–52.

67. Lindberg L, Bohlin G, Hagekull B. Early feeding problems in a normal population. Int J Feeding Disord 1991; 10:395–405.

68. Fried MD, Khoshoo V, Seckler DJ, et al. Decrease in gastric emptying time and episodes of regurgitation in children with spastic quadriplegia fed a whey-based formula. J Pediatr 1992; 120:569–572.

69. Kerwin ME. Empirically supported treatments in pediatric psychology: severe feeding problems. J Pediatr Psychol 1999; 24:193–214.

70. Patel MR, Piazza CC, Martinez CJ, Volkert VM, Santana CM. An evaluation of two differential reinforcement procedures with escape extinction to treat food refusal. J Appl Behav Anal 2000; 35:363–374.

71. Piazza CC, Patel MR, Gulotta CS, Sevin BS, Layer SA. On the relative contribution of positive reinforcement and escape extinction in the treatment of food refusal. J Appl Behav Anal 2003; 36:309–324.

72. Freeman KA, Piazza CC. Combining stimulus fading, reinforcement, and extinction to treat food refusal. J Appl Behav Anal 1998; 31:691–694.

73. Piazza CC, Fisher WW, Brown KA, et al. Functional analysis of inappropriate mealtime behaviors. J Appl Behav Anal 2003; 36:187–204.

74. Patel MR, Piazza CC, Santana CM, Volkert VM. An evaluation of food type and texture in the treatment of a feeding problem. J Appl Behav Anal 2002; 35:183–186.

75. Kelley ME, Piazza CC, Fisher WW, Oberdorff AJ. Acquisition of cup drinking using previously refused foods as positive and negative reinforcement. J Appl Behav Anal 2003; 36:89–93.

76. Piazza CC, Patel MR, Santana CM, Goh H, Delia MD, Lancaster BM. An evaluation of simultaneous and sequential presentation of preferred and nonpreferred food to treat food selectivity. J Appl Behav Anal 2002; 35:259–270.

77. Patel MR, Piazza CC, Kelly ML, Ochsner CA, Santana CM. Using a fading procedure to increase fluid consumption in a child with feeding problems. J Appl Behav Anal 2001; 34:357–360.

78. Byars KC, Burklow KA, Ferguson K, O'Flaherty T, Santoro K, Kaul A. A multicomponent behavioral program for oral aversion in children dependent on gastrostomy feedings. J Pediatr Gastroenterol Nutr 2003; 37:473–480.

79. Piazza CC. Marcus Institute Pediatric Feeding Disorders Program (unreported data).

80. Blackman JA, Nelson CLA. Rapid introduction of oral feedings to tube-fed patients. Dev Behav Pediatr 1987; 8:63–66.

81. Gauderer MW. Percutaneous endoscopic gastrostomy: a 10-year experience with 220 children. J Pediatr Surg 1991; 26:288–292.

82. Eyman RK, Grossman HJ, Chaney RH, Call TL. Survival of profoundly disabled people with severe mental retardation. Am J Dis Child 1993; 147:329–336.

83. Ashwal S, Eyman RK, Call TL. Life expectancy of children in a persistent vegetative state. Pediatr Neurol 1994; 10:27–33.

84. Strauss D, Kastner T, Ashwal S, White J. Tubefeeding and mortality in children with severe disabilities and mental retardation. Pediatrics 1997; 99:358–362.

85. Wesley JR, Coran AG, Sarahan TM, Klein MD, Whilte SJ. The need for evaluation of gastroesophageal reflux in brain-damaged children referred for feeding gastrostomy. J Pediatr Surg 1981; 16:866–871.

86. Mollitt DL, Golladay S, Seibert JJ. Symptomatic gastro-esophageal reflux following gastrostomy in neurologically impaired patients. Pediatrics 1985; 75:1124–1126.

87. Langer JC, Wesson DE, Ein SH, et al. Feeding gastrostomy in neurologically impaired children: is an antireflux procedure necessary? J Pediatr Gastroenterol Nutr 1988; 7:837–841.

88. Bui HD, Dang CV, Chaney RH, Vergara LM. Does gastrostomy and fundoplication prevent aspiration pneumonia in mentally retarded persons? Am J Mental Retard 1989; 94:16–20.

89. Kastner TA. Association between gastrostomy and death: cause or effect? Am J Mental Retard 1992; 97:327–328.

90. Fonkalsrud EW, Ellis DG, Shaw A, et al. A combined hospital experience with fundoplication and gastric emptying procedure for gastroesophageal reflux in children. J Am Coll Surg 1995; 180:449–455.

91. Parikh D, Yam PKH. Results of fundoplication in a UK paediatric centre. Br J Surg 1991; 78:346–348.

92. Caniano DA, Ginn-Pease ME, King DR. The failed antireflux procedure: analysis of risk factors and morbidity. J Pediatr Surg 1990; 25:1022–1026.

93. Wheatley MJ, Wesley JR, Tkach DM, Coran AG. Long-term follow-up of brain damaged children requiring feeding gastrostomy: should an antioreflux procedure always be performed? J Pediatr Surg 1991; 26:301–305.

94. Martinez DA, Ginn-Pease ME, Caniano DA. Recogntion of recurrent gastroesophageal reflux following antireflux surgery in the neurologically disabled child: high index of suspicion and definitive evaluation. J Pediatr Surg 1992; 27:983–990.

95. Smith CD, Othersen HB Jr, Gogan NJ, Walker JD. Nissen fundoplication in children with profound neurologic disability: high risks and unmet goals. Ann Surg 1992; 215:654–659.

96. Friedenberg F, Jensen G, Gujral N, Braitman LE, Levine GM. Serum albumin is predictive of 30 day survival after percutaneous endoscopic gastrostomy. J Parenter Enteral Nutr 1997; 21:72–74.

97. SondheimerJM, Morris BA. Gastroesophageal reflux among severely retarded children. J Pediatr 1979; 94:710–714.

98. Johnson RK, Maeda M. Establishing outpatient nutrition services for children with cerebral palsy. J Am Diet Assoc 1989; 89:1504–1506.

99. Cohen SA The Underweight Infant, Child, and Adolescent. Norwalk, CT: Appleton, Century, Crofts; 1986.

Chapter 79
Gastrointestinal pathology

Robert E. Petras and Terry L. Gramlich

INTRODUCTION

Histopathologic interpretation of endoscopic gastrointestinal biopsies requires adequate clinical information as well as sufficient tissue. The clinical history should include appropriate medication history and any known illnesses that may have associated gastrointestinal findings. The clinical history can alert the pathologist to perform appropriate special studies in addition to the standard hematoxylin and eosin staining. Precise identification of the biopsy site enables the pathologist to provide the most accurate and definitive diagnosis. This is most evident in the diagnosis of inflammatory bowel disease (IBD).

In the absence of granulomas, the distinction between ulcerative colitis and Crohn's disease is based on the distribution of the colitis. Specifically, the presence or absence of rectal involvement as well as documentation of diffuse disease (ulcerative colitis) *vs* skip lesions (Crohn's disease) requires the gastroenterologist to submit separate, labelled containers with biopsies from each region of the colon. The endoscopist should attempt to obtain the largest possible piece of tissue. Multiple biopsies for each site often provide the best information. If special studies such as culture for micro-organisms, electron microscopy or flow cytometry are required, communication with the laboratory prior to biopsy is recommended. Standard histopathologic evaluation is best performed on tissue immediately placed in fixative. The resulting 'final diagnosis' may require review if additional clinical findings are obtained.

ESOPHAGEAL BIOPSY

Gastroesophageal reflux

Gastroesophageal reflux disease (GERD) describes a symptomatic clinical condition related to reflux of gastric and/or duodenal contents into the esophagus that usually presents with pyrosis (heartburn), acid regurgitation and dysphagia. The term reflux esophagitis refers to a subset of patients, usually with symptoms of GERD, who show endoscopic and/or histologic manifestations of inflammation within squamous and/or gastric cardia type mucosa.[1] Many consider esophagogastroduodenoscopy with biopsy the prudent initial evaluation of patients with symptoms of GERD.[1] It quickly excludes other conditions in the clinical differential such as infective esophagitis and 'pill esophagitis'.

The endoscopic changes described with GERD are seen more often in severe cases and include erosions, ulcers and stricture. Biopsy specimens are generally obtained to confirm reflux, to rule out infection or to establish a diagnosis of Barrett's esophagus. Erosive lesions are often sampled to rule out *Candida* species and herpes virus infection. Approximately one-third of patients with reflux have endoscopically normal or only slightly hyperemic esophageal mucosa; however, endoscopic biopsy specimens show characteristic histologic changes (see below).[2] Though debated, some investigators consider histologic evaluation of biopsy specimens the 'gold standard' in the diagnosis of GERD and reflux esophagitis.[3]

Histologic changes – squamous mucosa

Well oriented normal esophageal squamous mucosa demonstrates a basal cell layer that is usually one to three cells thick. These basal cells can be discerned by their smaller size and their more basophilic cytoplasm compared with normal surface squamous cells. The cytoplasmic appearance of basal cells and their relative lack of glycogen can be highlighted with a periodic acid–Schiff (PAS) stain. Lamina propria papillae are present, but make up only one-half of the total epithelial thickness.[4,5]

Biopsy specimens from endoscopically demonstrable lesions in GERD (erosions, ulcers) show acute inflammation of the mucosa and submucosa. Exudates containing neutrophils and eosinophils often overlie an erosion or an ulcer with an inflamed granulation tissue base. Acute inflammation is fairly specific but insensitive for reflux esophagitis.[5,6] Many patients with clinical symptoms and the acid abnormalities of GERD, as measured by intraesophageal pH probes, have an endoscopically normal-appearing esophagus or show only minimal esophageal changes such as hyperemia. Although acute inflammation may be lacking, many patients show characteristic squamous mucosal changes of reflux consisting of hyperplasia (lamina propria papilla greater than 67% of the thickness of the squamous mucosa) and an increase in the basal cell layer (more than 15% of the squamous mucosal thickness).[5–7] These abnormalities are often accompanied by increased numbers of intraepithelial eosinophils and lymphocytes[5,6,8–11] (Fig. 79.1). The squamous mucosa adjacent to ulcers and erosions can show striking regenerative features, with basal cells occupying the full thickness of the squamous mucosa and papillomatosis that may mimic squamous carcinoma or dysplasia.

Histologic changes – glandular mucosa

Several investigators have suggested that the presence of gastric cardia-type mucosa in the esophagus at or near the squamocolumnar junction may be metaplastic, and that

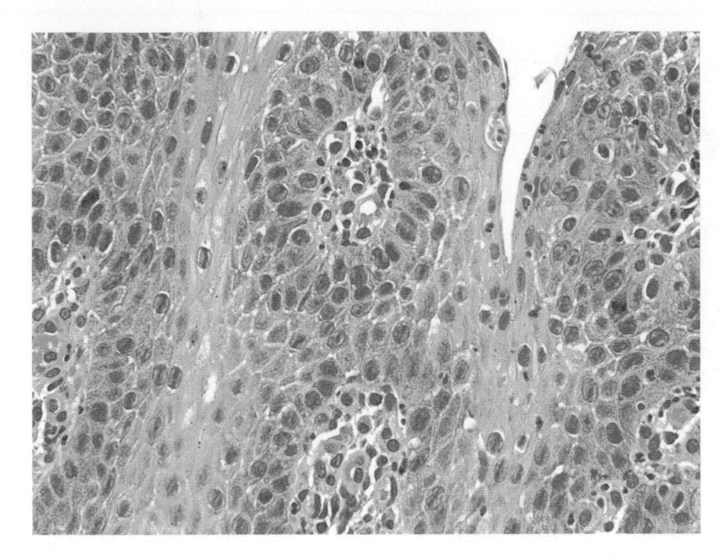

Figure 79.1: Esophageal squamous epithelial changes of reflux. In addition to papillomatosis, an increase in the squamous basal cell layer and increased intraepithelial lymphocytes and eosinophils, surface neutrophils are also present. (*See plate section for color.*)

inflammation of this metaplastic gastric cardia-type mucosa (so-called 'carditis') correlates strongly with GERD.[12,13] In contrast, other investigators have concluded that this 'carditis' is a manifestation of gastric *Helicobacter pylori* infection.[14,15]

The present authors believe that these apparent disparate viewpoints can be reconciled based on methodologic differences and inherent biases within these studies, and that, depending on the patient population and biopsy location, both schools of thought may be correct. Biopsy specimens from the stomach, even millimeters below the squamocolumnar junction, reflect disease processes of the stomach. Therefore, inflammation and intestinal metaplasia in that area correlate with *Helicobacter pylori* infection. However, 'carditis' at the esophagogastric junction or above is characteristic of patients with gastroesophageal reflux as demonstrated by symptoms, manometric and pH probe abnormalities, and probably comprises more than 90% of the gastric carditis seen in practice.

Differential diagnosis

Infectious esophagitis

Herpetic esophagitis typically occurs in immunosuppressed patients, for example those with acquired immune deficiency syndrome, those receiving chemotherapy and following bone marrow transplantation.[16] Endoscopically, ulcers occur that are typically described as shallow and 'punched out' with adjacent normal-appearing squamous mucosa. Biopsy specimens demonstrate an ulcer base that is relatively bland in terms of acute inflammation but may have prominent aggregates of larger mononuclear cells.[16] The diagnostic epithelial changes are found in the adjacent squamous mucosa with giant cell formation, ground-glass nuclei and eosinophilic intranuclear (Cowdry type A) inclusions.[17,18] Occasional multinucleated squamous epithelial giant cells without viral inclusion may occur as part of reflux esophagitis and should not be confused with herpetic infection.[19]

Inclusions of cytomegalovirus (CMV) can be seen in the base of some esophageal ulcers. The role played by CMV as a primary etiologic agent may be difficult to prove. CMV inclusions typically affect mesenchymal cells such as fibroblasts, smooth muscle and endothelial cells, and usually spare the epithelium[20,21] (Fig. 79.2).

Esophagitis due to *Candida* species usually presents endoscopically as brownish-white plaques with exudate that has been described as 'cheesy'. *Candida* esophagitis often occurs in patients with other debilitating illnesses such as immunosuppression, diabetes mellitus and long-term antibiotic therapy. The diagnosis of *Candida* esophagitis requires the identification of budding yeast and pseudohyphae, usually within the inflammatory exudate. Their identification is certainly enhanced by using special stains for fungi. The authors recommend the routine use of the Alcian blue–PAS combination stain for all esophageal biopsy specimens because it is a useful fungal stain, it highlights the basal cell layer, it vividly decorates signet ring cell adenocarcinoma, making it easier to identify, and can be used to verify the specialized columnar epithelium of Barrett's esophagus.

Allergic (eosinophilic) esophagitis

Symptomatic and histologic reflux esophagitis occurs in children.[22] One should, however, be wary of diagnosing reflux esophagitis in the presence of large numbers of eosinophils because many of these cases represent so-called 'allergic (eosinophilic) esophagitis', a condition related to eosinophilic gastroenteritis.[23–25] Children with allergic esophagitis usually present with dysphagia or 'food-catch-

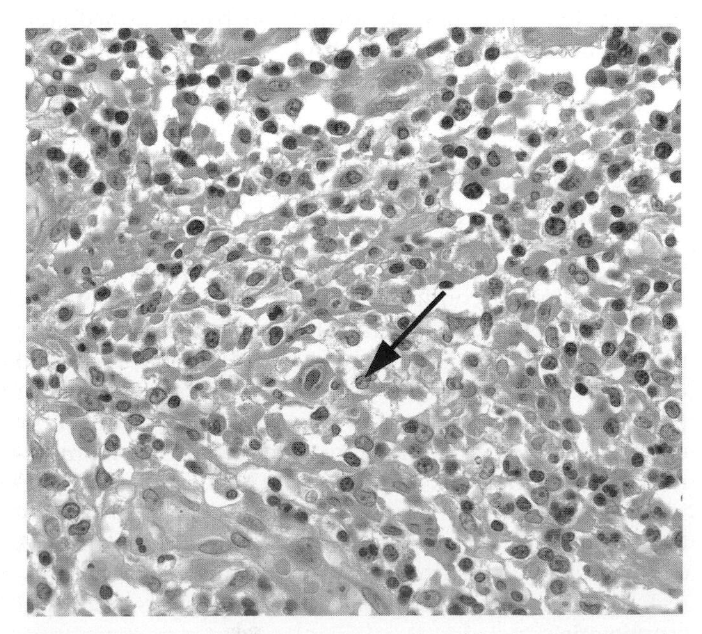

Figure 79.2: Cytomegalovirus inclusion found in ulcer base (center). The infected mesenchymal cell shows cellular enlargement. The nucleus contains a large basophilic inclusion body with surrounding halo and preservation of the nucleolus. (*See plate section for color.*)

ing' and often have an 'allergic history'. Endoscopic erosions or ulcers are seldom seen, but many patients exhibit longitudinal esophageal furrows, rings, stenosis, or small white vesicles or plaques.[26] Esophageal pH probe studies show normal or borderline acid levels in these children, and the symptoms of allergic esophagitis do not respond to acid suppression therapy. Walsh et al.[23] have found that the most useful histologic criteria to differentiate allergic esophagitis from reflux esophagitis are: large numbers of intraepithelial eosinophils (more than 15 per high-magnification field), intramucosal eosinophilic aggregates and superficial eosinophils (Fig. 79.3). Patients with allergic esophagitis may respond to drugs that stabilize mast cells, and may require corticosteroids.

'Pill esophagitis'

Esophageal injury can occur with prolonged direct mucosal contact with medicinal tablets or capsules, even in therapeutic doses.[27,28] Symptomatic 'pill esophagitis' has been associated with odynophagia (pain on swallowing) or the feeling of a 'lump in the throat'. Patients frequently take pills with little or no water. Endoscopic erosions and ulcers are found in more proximal locations of the esophagus (*vs* GERD), often in areas of external esophageal compression such as near the arch of the aorta or near the left atrial appendage, especially in patients with cardiomegaly. The histology of 'pill esophagitis' is non-specific.

Barrett's esophagus

Barrett's esophagus, the eponym given to columnar epithelium-lined esophagus, is acquired through chronic gastroesophageal reflux and occurs rarely in children. The American College of Gastroenterology (ACG) defines Barrett's esophagus as an endoscopic change in esophageal epithelium of any length proved by biopsy to contain intestinal metaplasia.[29]

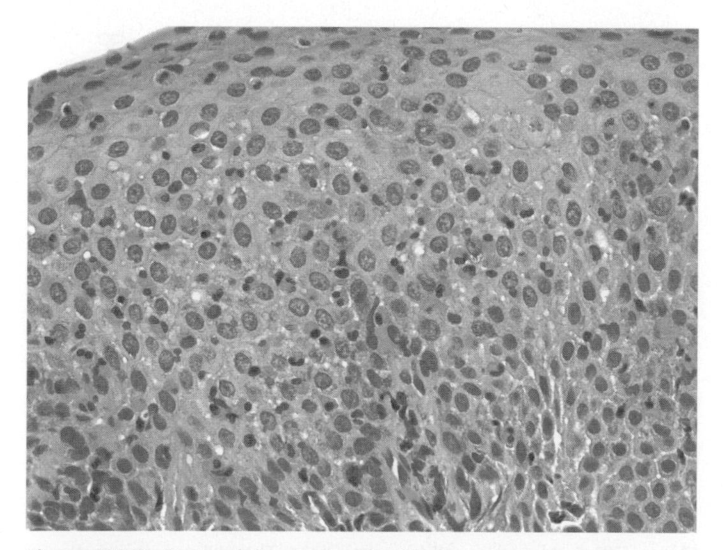

Figure 79.3: Eosinophilic esophagitis. Sections show squamous papillomatosis, a marked increase in the squamous epithelial basal cell layer and numerous intraepithelial eosinophils leukocytes. (*See plate section for color.*)

Endoscopy has become the mainstay in the diagnosis of Barrett's esophagus.[30] In general, the color (orange-red) and appearance (velvety) of Barrett's epithelium as seen through the endoscope is similar to that of normal gastric mucosa. Barrett's epithelium can appear as circumferential or tongue-like extensions of orange-red mucosa into the tubular esophagus. Occasionally, Barrett's epithelium can present as an island of orange-red mucosa entirely surrounded by the more pale pink to gray-white squamous epithelium of normal esophagus. As other conditions can sometimes mimic Barrett's esophagus endoscopically, the endoscopist's impression must be confirmed histologically.[29,30]

Specialized columnar epithelium (incomplete intestinal metaplasia) is the distinctive epithelial type considered diagnostic for Barrett's esophagus.[29] Specialized columnar epithelium can occur in a flat or villous configuration, and consists of goblet cells and columnar cells. The goblet cells contain mucin that stains positively with both PAS and alcian blue at pH 2.5. The columnar cells between goblet cells most often resemble gastric foveolar epithelium, or rarely intestinal absorptive cells.

Barrett's esophagus is encountered only rarely in children undergoing upper endoscopy, with an estimated prevelance of 0.02–0.5%. These patients often have comorbidities that predispose to severe reflux, such as neurologic impairment, chronic lung disease, repaired esophageal atresia or treated intrathoracic malignancy.[31] Dysplasia or carcinoma complicating Barrett's esophagus in children is even rarer. Guidelines have been proposed for surveillance endoscopy with biopsy in children with Barrett's esophagus.[31]

STOMACH BIOPSY

Endoscopy and biopsy in children is used to establish a diagnosis of gastritis and to look specifically for *Helicobacter* infection, eosinophilic gastroenteritis (see below) or Crohn's disease.

H. pylori is responsible for up to 70% of cases of chronic gastritis and can be found in the stomachs of more than 90% of children who have a duodenal ulcer.[32] *H. pylori* infection is easily diagnosed in endoscopic biopsy specimens. Typical patterns of inflammation include chronic inflammation of antral mucosa (chronic antral gastritis) and lymphoplasmacytic infiltration of the lamina propria adjacent to gastric pits (chronic superficial gastritis) (Fig. 79.4); either pattern can be associated with acute inflammation. The organisms can be seen on routine hemotoxylin and eosin-stained sections, but identification is enhanced by use of special stains such as Giemsa (Fig. 79.5), Steiner or immunoperoxidase. The comma-shaped bacilli are typically encountered in the mucous layer overlying gastric foveolar epithelium. The principal differential diagnostic consideration is acute erosive gastritis/reactive gastropathy, often referred to as chemical-type gastritis because of its association with bile reflux, steroid use and non-steroidal anti-inflammatory drugs (NSAIDs). The gastric mucosa may be erythematous with areas of erosion or ulcer. Histologically,

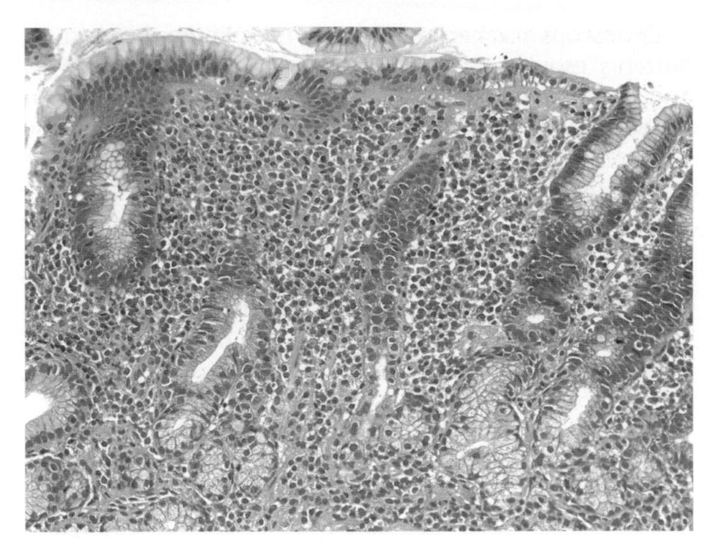

Figure 79.4: *Helicobacter pylori*-associated gastritis. Sections show a dense chronic inflammatory cell infiltrate of the lamina propria associated with some acute inflammation. (*See plate section for color.*)

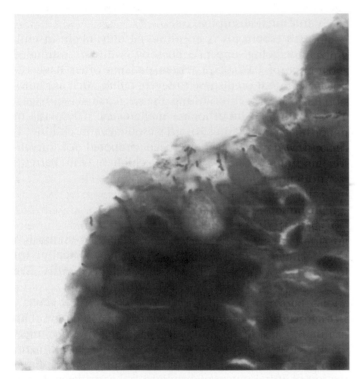

Figure 79.5: *Helicobacter pylori*-associated gastritis, Giemsa stain. Note the curved bacilli within the mucous layer. (*See plate section for color.*)

erosions or fibromuscular change are seen in the lamina propria, associated with loss of mucin in the foveolar epithelium and foveolar hyperplasia.

Gastric inflammatory lesions of Crohn's disease usually occur in association with Crohn's disease lesions elsewhere in the gastrointestinal tract. Granulomatous inflammation can be seen; however, focally enhanced chronic active gastritis seen in the absence of *H. pylori* is a pattern more often seen in patients with Crohn's disease.[33]

Ménétrièr's-type gastritis with foveolar hyperplasia and protein loss has been described in children in whom it is usually associated with CMV infection. Unlike Ménétrièr's disease of adults, the pediatric lesion is usually self-limiting.[34]

SMALL INTESTINAL BIOPSY

Specimen procurement and processing

Small bowel biopsy remains one of the most important steps in evaluating malabsorption. Most specimens are obtained via a gastroscope.[35] Proper evaluation of the specimen requires examination of optimally oriented intestinal villi obtained from the central region of the biopsy specimen. The authors suggest that the small bowel biopsy procedure consist of obtaining multiple endoscopic biopsy specimens. These tissue samples are fixed in 4% formaldehyde solution and processed routinely. Three to four step-section slides are obtained, with one stained with alcian blue–PAS, and the rest stained routinely.

Normal small intestinal histology

The ratio of villus : crypt length approximates 3 : 1 to 5 : 1.[36] Inflammatory cells, including plasma cells, are normally present in the lamina propria. Intraepithelial lymphocytes are present in a ratio of approximately one lymphocyte per five enterocytes. A brush border is often discernible on the enterocyte. The enterocyte nuclei should be basilar in location and evenly aligned. In general, identification of four normal villi in a row indicates that the villous architecture of the whole biopsy specimen is probably normal[36,37] (Fig. 79.6). This does not mean that biopsy specimens with fewer than four aligned normal villi should be considered inadequate for evaluation, because even one normal villus in a proximal small bowel biopsy

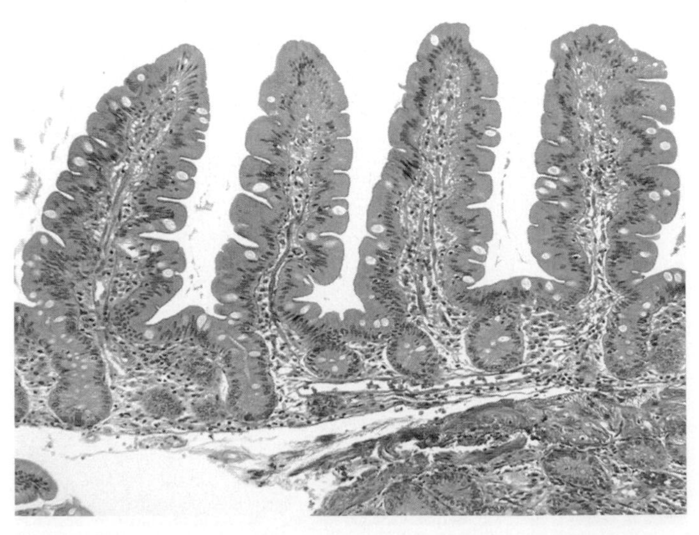

Figure 79.6: Normal small-bowel mucosa. The villi are long and slender. The ratio of villus : crypt length is approximately 4 : 1. Enterocyte nuclei are basilar in location and evenly aligned. Occasional intraepithelial lymphocytes are present. (*See plate section for color.*)

specimen rules out celiac sprue. Conversely, finding four normal villi in a row does not necessarily rule out focal lesions, although it almost always does.

Patterns of abnormal small bowel architecture

The small bowel mucosal responses to injury are limited, and recognition of a response pattern can be useful in differential diagnosis (Table 79.1). In this chapter, the term *severe villus abnormality* describes a flat intestinal mucosa in which no villi are seen or the villi are markedly shortened (villus : crypt length approximately 1 : 1). Usually, this change is diffuse, accompanied by epithelial lymphocytosis (more than 40 intraepithelial lymphocytes per 100 enterocytes) and associated with crypt hyperplasia, evidenced by numerous mitotic figures. The term *variable villus abnormality* describes specimens in which the villi are either only focally flat or are less than flat (mild or moderate villus shortening). Many specimens in this category also show increased intraepithelial lymphocytes. These changes may be associated with features that suggest a specific diagnosis (e.g. numerous eosinophils, granulomas, parasites) or may be non-specific.

Pattern	Conditions
Entities usually associated with a diffuse severe villus abnormality and crypt hyperplasia	Celiac sprue Refractory or unclassified sprue Other protein allergies Lymphocytic enterocolitis
Entities usually associated with a variable villus abnormality and crypt hypoplasia	Kwashiorkor, malnutrition Megaloblastic anemiavariable Radiation and chemotherapeutic effect Microvillus inclusion disease End-stage refractory or unclassified sprue
Entities usually associated with a non-specific variable villus abnormality, usually not flat	Changes associated with dermatitis herpetiformis Partially treated or clinically latent celiac sprue Infection Stasis Tropical sprue Mastocytosis Non-specific duodenitis Autoimmune enteropathy
Entities associated with variable villus abnormalities illustrating specific diagnostic changes	Collagenous sprue Common variable immunodeficiency Whipple's disease *Mycobacterium avium-intracellulare* complex infection Eosinophilic gastroenteritis Parasitic infestation Lymphangiectasia Abetalipoproteinemia Tufting enteropathy

Table 79.1 Patterns of abnormal small bowel architecture

Entities associated with a diffuse severe villus abnormality and crypt hyperplasia

Celiac sprue Celiac sprue, also known as *gluten-induced enteropathy, gluten-sensitive enteropathy* and *non-tropical sprue,* is a major cause of malabsorption.[38] The pathogenesis of celiac sprue involves immunologic injury to the enterocyte associated with the ingestion of the protein gluten, which is found in cereal grains such as wheat, rye and barley. Celiac sprue is clearly an HLA-associated condition, primarily associated with the major histocompatibility complex class II alleles DQA1*0501 and DQB1*0201. This HLA-DQ2 allelic combination is found in 98% of patients with celiac sprue.[38] Patients with celiac sprue usually show a quick and dramatic clinical and histologic improvement following removal of gluten from the diet, and quickly relapse after its reintroduction.[39]

The severe villus abnormality of celiac sprue is associated with increased lymphocytes and plasma cells in the lamina propria and increased intraepithelial lymphocytes (Fig. 79.7). The enterocyte nuclei lose their basilar alignment and become stratified. The histologic abnormality is most severe in the proximal intestinal mucosa and gradually lessens distally. With gluten withdrawal, the abnormalities recede from distal to cephalad in the small intestinal mucosa. Thus, proximal small bowel biopsy specimens may remain abnormal for quite some time, even in patients showing marked clinical improvement. A pathologist does not make the diagnosis of celiac sprue. All that can be said is that the specimens contain a severe villus abnormality that is consistent with celiac sprue. Definitive diagnosis depends on demonstration of a suitable clinical presentation; compatible serologic tests (e.g. IgA-antiendomesial antibodies, anti-tissue transglutaminase antibodies) and small bowel histology; clinical and, ideally, histologic response to a gluten-free diet; and relapse following gluten challenge if performed, although rechallenge is falling out of favor.[38–41]

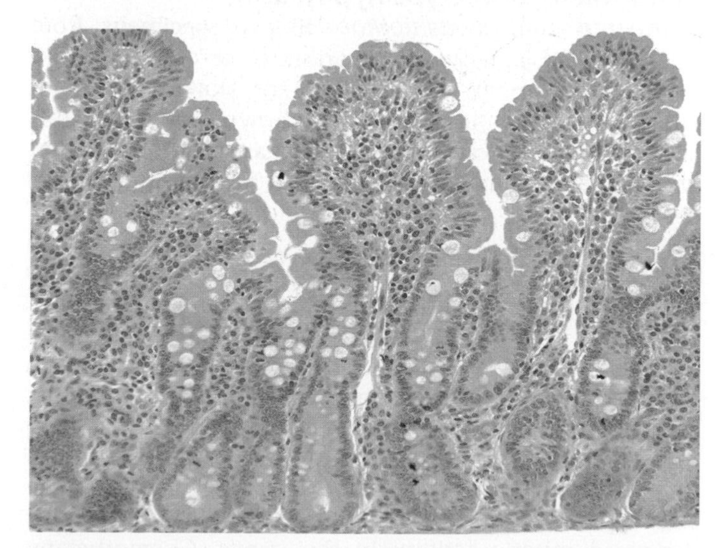

Figure 79.7: Severe villous abnormality typical of celiac sprue. The villus:crypt length is less than 1:1. Inflammatory cells are increased within the lamina propria. Numerous intraepithelial lymphocytes are also present. (*See plate section for color.*)

The histologic differential diagnosis includes all entities that may cause at least a focal severe villus abnormality: immunodeficiency syndromes, protein allergies other than gluten, some cases of infectious gastroenteritis,[42] tropical sprue,[43] stasis,[44] IBD including Crohn's disease,[45] and non-specific duodenitis. Clinicopathologic correlation is essential for proper diagnosis. All biopsy specimens should be evaluated carefully for plasma cells, because their absence in common variable immunodeficiency syndrome (CVID) is easy to overlook. Numerous neutrophils, cryptitis and crypt abscess formation are usually not part of celiac sprue, and entities such as infectious gastroenteritis, Crohn's disease, non-specific duodenitis and stasis syndromes should therefore be considered.

The most common cause of unresponsiveness after implementing a gluten-free diet is that the diet is not really gluten free.[37] If dietary indiscretions are ruled out, patients may have refractory or unclassified sprue,[38] which may respond to the administration of corticosteroids. Refractory sprue can also be associated with cavitation of mesenteric lymph nodes and hyposplenism.[46] Persistent symptoms despite gluten withdrawl with small-bowel histologic improvement should be a clue to search for co-morbidities that may cause persistent diarrhea, such as pancreatic insufficiency, secondary lactase defınciency, bacterial overgrowth or coexisting IBD.[47]

Other protein allergies Patients with allergic reactions to chicken, soy protein, milk, eggs and tuna fish have been reported to show a flat small-bowel mucosa similar to that seen in celiac sprue.[47–51] Definitive diagnosis depends on identifying the offending protein, showing a response to its withdrawal from the diet, and demonstrating recrudescence of symptoms and pathology with its reintroduction.

Entities associated with a variable villus abnormality and crypt hypoplasia

Marasmus and kwashiorkor Biopsy specimens from malnourished patients with marasmus (severe calorie and protein deficiency) and kwashiorkor (low protein but adequate caloric intake) have shown variable villus abnormality associated with increased intraepithelial lymphocyte lesions indistinguishable from those of celiac sprue.[52–54]

Megaloblastic anemia – radiation and chemotherapy effect Nutritional deficiency of folate and vitamin B_{12} may result in impaired epithelial cell replacement because of decreased DNA synthesis. Consequently, a variable villus abnormality with or without megaloblastic epithelial changes can be seen.[55,56] Because radiation therapy and chemotherapeutic agents inhibit DNA synthesis, the intestinal mucosal changes are similar to those in folate and vitamin B_{12} deficiency, and are associated with decreased mitotic activity in the crypts. Chemotherapy and irradiation may also cause focal necrosis of epithelial cells (apoptosis) and increased numbers of chronic inflammatory cells within the mucosa and submucosa.[57,58]

Microvillus inclusion disease Microvillus inclusion disease, which also includes cases classified as microvillus dystrophy, is an inherited autosomal recessive condition causing intractable diarrhea with steatorrhea in infants. It was first reported under the designation *familial enteropathy*.[59] Diarrhea persists despite total parenteral nutrition, and patients rarely survive beyond the age of 2 years. The entity should be recognized so that genetic counseling can be offered.[60] Small-bowel biopsy specimens show a severe villus abnormality with crypt hypoplasia. In general, the mucosal specimen may resemble celiac sprue, but intraepithelial lymphocyte levels are usually not increased. Transmission electron microscopy establishes the diagnosis by identifying abnormal microvillus structures at the luminal border of the enterocyte and apical intracytoplasmic inclusions lined by microvilli in the same cells.[61] The intracytoplasmic vacuoles can also be detected with PAS stain or with carcinoembryonic antigen (CEA) immunostaining.[62] Prominent surface enterocyte CD10 immunoreactivity is also described in microvillus inclusion disease.[63]

Entities associated with a non-specific variable villus abnormality

Many diseases are associated with non-specific variable villus abnormalities that are usually not flat. Although most biopsy specimens showing this change are from patients with clinically latent or partially treated celiac sprue,[38,64] other conditions entering the differential diagnosis include dermatitis herpetiformis, tropical sprue, infectious gastroenteritis, stasis of small intestinal contents, Zollinger–Ellison syndrome, mastocytosis, duodenitis and peptic ulcer disease, and autoimmune enteropathy.[65]

The term *autoimmune enteropathy* has been applied to an intractable watery diarrhea syndrome occurring in infants that has been associated with circulating autoantibodies against intestinal epithelial cells.[66,67] The patients often have variable immunodeficiency and autoimmune phenomena such as juvenile-onset diabetes mellitus, rheumatoid arthritis and hemolytic anemia.[68,69] The small bowel mucosa shows a variable villus abnormality that is often severe and resembles that of celiac sprue. Surface and crypt epithelial degenerative and regenerative changes occur, but many illustrated cases show few intraepithelial lymphocytes, a feature that may distinguish autoimmune enteropathy from celiac sprue. Some patients with autoimmune enteropathy have also had colitis. In some cases the associated colitis resembles lymphocytic colitis, whereas in others the endoscopic and histologic picture is similar to that of ulcerative colitis.[70] Autoimmune enteropathy is usually severe and intractable, often requiring total parenteral nutrition. There have been scattered reports of favorable responses to cyclosporin,[71] tacrolimus[70] and infliximab.[72]

Entities associated with variable villus abnormalities illustrating specific diagnostic changes

Collagenous sprue The term *collagenous sprue* describes the excessive subepithelial deposition of collagen associated with a severe villus abnormality noted in small-bowel biopsy specimens from some patients with malabsorption unresponsive to gluten-free diet.[73] Although some patients with this finding have ultimately responded to a gluten-free diet,[74] many have followed a fulminant and generally fatal course.

Immunodeficiency syndromes (excluding acquired immune deficiency syndrome) Normal small-bowel morphology seen on routine light microscopy is the rule in selective IgA deficiency, although nodular lymphoid hyperplasia may be present.[75] Decreased numbers of IgA-containing plasma cells can be demonstrated by immunocytochemical techniques.

Patients with CVID may have chronic diarrhea, malabsorption and recurrent gastrointestinal giardiasis.[76,77] The morphology of small intestinal biopsy specimens may vary from normal to a severe abnormality mimicking celiac sprue.[76–80] In contrast to celiac sprue, plasma cells in CVID are decreased and IgA-containing plasma cells are absent. Occasionally in CVID, the mucosa demonstrates nodular lymphoid hyperplasia associated with absent or markedly reduced numbers of plasma cells. Giardiasis is commonly found with either histology. Nodular lymphoid hyperplasia without plasma cell changes may also be seen in asymptomatic patients without an immunodeficiency syndrome, especially in children, in whom it may be considered a normal finding. An injury pattern resembling acute graft-*vs*-host disease, with numerous apoptotic bodies deep in crypts, can also be seen in CVID.[80]

Whipple's disease Whipple's disease, a chronic systemic illness with numerous gastrointestinal features such as diarrhea and malabsorption, is caused by *Tropheryma whipplei*, a rod-shaped micro-organism.[81,82] The diagnosis of Whipple's disease is usually based on the identification of PAS-positive, diastase-resistant bacilli in small intestinal biopsy specimens.

Eosinophilic gastroenteritis The term *eosinophilic gastroenteritis* has been used to describe a collection of clinical syndromes that are usually seen in children or young adults and that have in common infiltration of the gastrointestinal tract by large numbers of eosinophilic leukocytes.[83,84] Infiltration primarily in the mucosa of the esophagus is associated with dysphagia and mucosal furrows or rings endoscopically (see above). Mucosal involvement of the stomach and small intestine is associated with diarrhea and malabsorption, whereas eosinophils predominantly in the submucosa and muscularis propria are associated with intestinal obstruction. Ascites is a major manifestation when the eosinophils infiltrate the subserosa.[83–87]

The histologic diagnosis of eosinophilic gastroenteritis may be difficult. Infiltration of the submucosa, muscularis propria and subserosal connective tissue by eosinophils is always abnormal and, when corroborated clinically, is diagnostic of eosinophilic gastroenteritis; however, this type of evaluation does, in general, require a resection specimen. The diagnosis of the mucosal pattern of eosinophilic gastroenteritis in biopsy specimens can be particularly challenging to the pathologist. Scattered intramucosal eosinophils are normal in the gastrointestinal tract, and their mere presence should not prompt a diagnosis of eosinophilic gastroenteritis. However, collections of eosinophils not associated with other inflammatory cells, groups of eosinophils associated with focal mucosal architectural distortion or injury (cryptitis, crypt abscesses), and infiltration of the muscularis mucosae by eosinophils are all abnormal and, in a corroborative clinical setting, are diagnostic of eosinophilic gastroenteritis (Fig. 79.8). The mucosal involvement in eosinophilic gastroenteritis is notoriously patchy; therefore, if the clinical suspicion is great, multiple or additional biopsy specimens should be obtained.

Parasitic infestations A large number of parasites may infect the gastrointestinal tract including *Giardia* (Fig. 79.9), *Strongyloides*, *Capillaria*, *Cryptosporidium* species, *Microsporidia* species and *Isospora* species.[65] Enteric parasites are discussed in greater detail in Chapter 37.

Intestinal lymphangiectasia Intestinal lymphangiectasia is characterized by focal or diffuse dilation of the mucosal, submucosal and subserosal lymphatics that may be

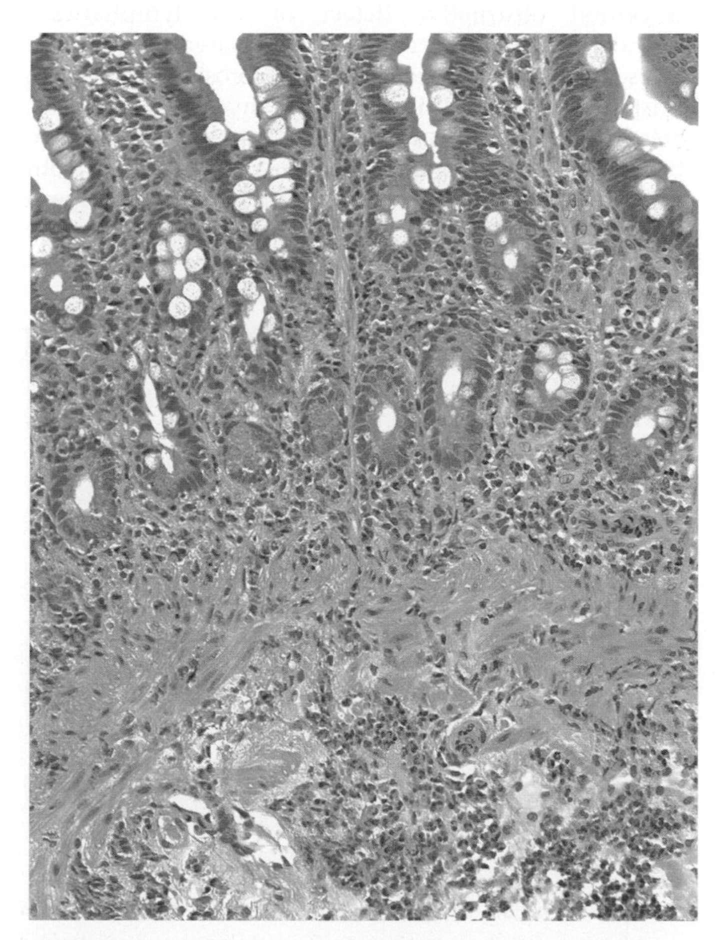

Figure 79.8: Small bowel with eosinophilic gastroenteritis. Note the large collection of eosinophils within the submucosa with lesser numbers infiltrating the muscularis mucosae and lamina propria. (*See plate section for color.*)

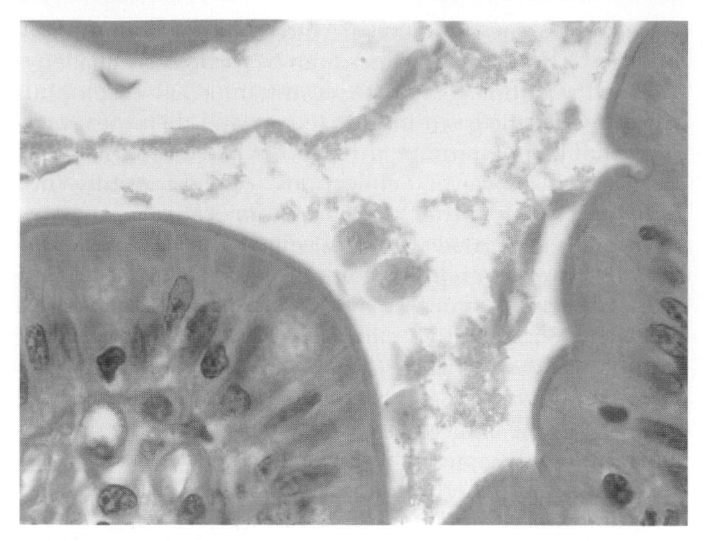

Figure 79.9: Giardiasis. In this small bowel specimen, the diagnosis rests on demonstration of the trophozoite in tissue section. Seen *en face*, *Giardia lamblia* is pear-shaped and demonstrates prominent paired nuclei. (*See plate section for color.*)

associated with protein-losing enteropathy, hypoalbuminemia, hypoproteinemic edema and lymphocytopenia.[88,89] It can occur in a primary or secondary form. The primary form has a predilection for children and is caused by a congenital obstructive defect of the lymphatics.[89] Secondary lymphangiectasia is associated with many diseases, including retroperitoneal fibrosis, pancreatitis, constrictive pericarditis, primary myocardial disease, intestinal Behçet's disease, intestinal malignancy, Waldenström's macroglobulinemia and sarcoidosis.[89,90] In both forms, the histologic appearance of mucosal biopsy specimens is identical: dilated lymphatics located in otherwise normal tissue (Fig. 79.10). Therapy includes treatment of

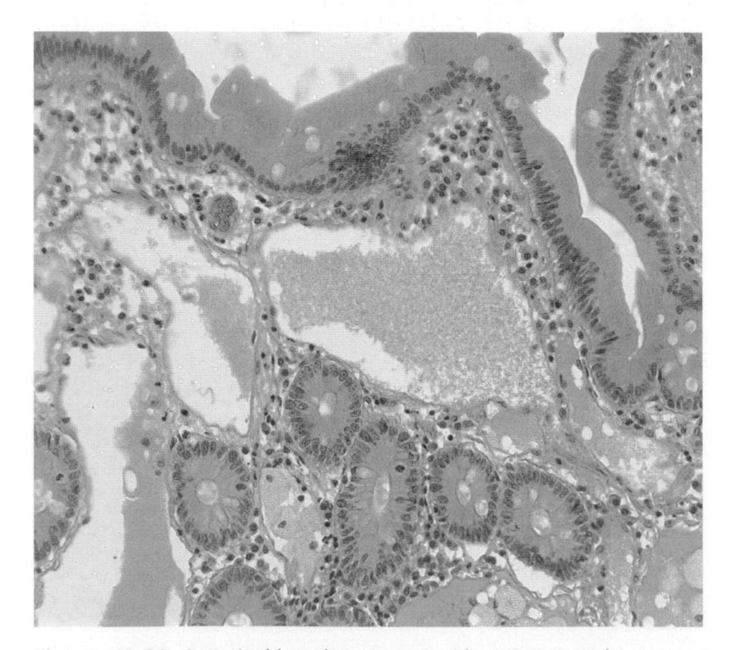

Figure 79.10: Intestinal lymphangiectasia. The primary and secondary forms appear identical in histologic sections, demonstrating dilated lymphatic located in otherwise normal mucosa. (*See plate section for color.*)

underlying conditions, dietary manipulation and, in some localized forms of lymphangiectasia, resection.[88]

Abetalipoproteinemia In abetalipoproteinemia, a condition inherited as an autosomal recessive trait,[91] patients are unable to synthesize apoprotein B. Therefore, fatty acids within intestinal absorptive cells can be re-esterified to triglyceride but cannot be changed into chylomicrons for transport. As a result, fat accumulates in the absorptive cells. Biopsy specimens have a normal villus architecture. Enterocytes, however, have cytoplasm packed with droplets of lipid that appear optically clear or foamy. The changes are most prominent at the tips of the villi. This enterocyte vacuolization, although characteristic, is not pathognomonic, because similar vacuolar change has been described in megaloblastic anemia, celiac sprue and tropical sprue.[92] The present authors have occasionally observed it in patients with no apparent disease process.

Tufting enteropathy The term *tufting enteropathy* has been applied to a sometimes familial intractable diarrhea syndrome in children.[93–96] Symptoms usually begin in the neonatal period with the patient requiring total parenteral nutrition. Small-bowel biopsy specimens have demonstrated a variable villus abnormality that is usually not associated with epithelial lymphocytosis, as well as a distinctive surface epithelial change consisting of epithelial crowding, disorganization and focal tufting. Abnormalities of basement membrane structure have been described.

INTERPRETATION OF COLONIC MUCOSAL BIOPSY SPECIMENS IN THE EVALUATION OF SUSPECTED INFLAMMATORY BOWEL DISEASE

The pathologist plays an increasingly important role in the diagnosis and management of patients with colitis. Patterns of inflammation (chronic colitis, diffuse active colitis, focal active colitis, ischemic-type colitis, trauma change and apoptotic colopathy) can be identified and may be helpful in assessing patients by creating differential diagnostics possibilities.

Chronic colitis – differential diagnosis

Chronic colitis, the pattern of abnormality in chronic ulcerative colitis in remission (quiescent), includes mucosal atrophy and mucosal architectural distortion.[65,97,98] The luminal border is irregular. The number of crypts is decreased; in addition, the remaining crypts appear short (i.e. they do not touch the muscularis mucosae) and lose their parallel arrangement, becoming branched and budded. The goblet cell population is usually preserved. Numbers of chronic inflammatory cells are only mildly increased in the lamina propria. Paneth cells may be present. Although almost all patients with this pattern of injury have ulcerative colitis, it can also be seen in healing Crohn's disease, ischemia, irradiation, chemotherapy and chronic infections (e.g. tuberculosis, schistosomiasis)

Active colitis – differential diagnosis

The term *active colitis* is used to describe an inflammatory condition in which neutrophils are present in the lamina propria, within epithelial cells (cryptitis) or within crypt lumens (crypt abscesses). Included under this heading are:[99,100]

- Ulcerative colitis in an active phase
- Most examples of Crohn's colitis
- Infectious colitis/acute self-limiting colitis.

Recognition of an inflammatory pattern coupled with clinical and endoscopic correlation allows a fairly specific diagnosis to be made in many cases.

Diffuse active colitis

Untreated ulcerative colitis in an active phase represents the prototypic diffuse active colitis. Biopsy specimens demonstrate a diffuse abnormality, meaning that changes are of approximately the same intensity in all areas of the tissue (Fig. 79.11). The luminal border of the mucosa is irregular.[98,101,102] Increased numbers of chronic inflammatory cells are present in the lamina propria. Cryptitis and crypt abscess formation are often prominent. It is surprising that, even in ulcerative colitis of extremely short overt clinical duration, some atrophy, branching and budding of crypts are already apparent in many specimens. This crypt distortion, coupled with basal plasmacytosis (increased numbers of plasma cells in the lower fifth of the mucosa), has been proposed as the most useful criterion to differentiate ulcerative colitis from infectious colitis/acute self-limiting colitis.[98–100] The most a pathologist can conclude from a biopsy specimen showing this pattern is that the changes are consistent with ulcerative colitis in an active phase because the diffuse active colitis pattern can also be seen in some examples of Crohn's colitis and in some cases of documented infectious colitis.

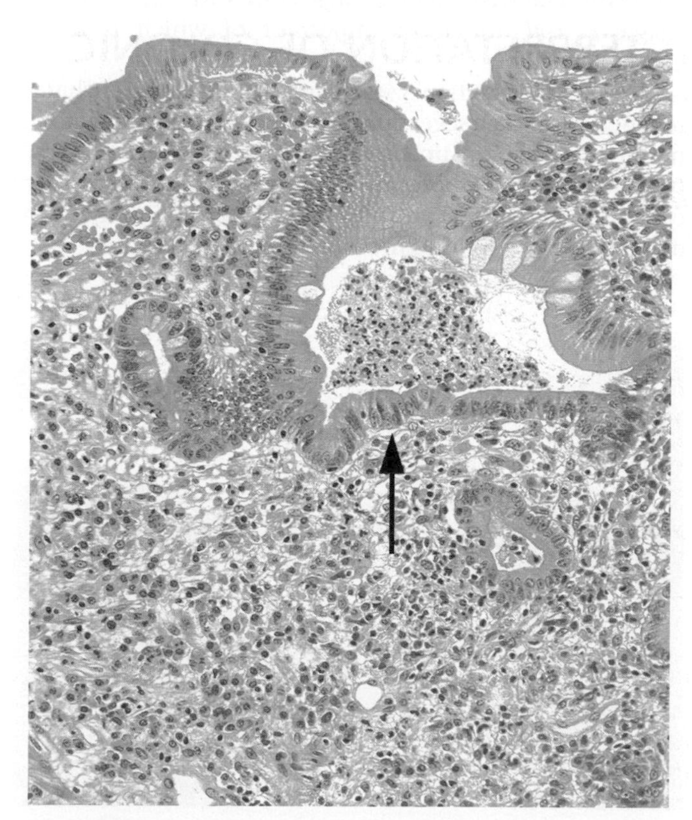

Figure 79.11: Ulcerative colitis in an active phase. Sections show diffuse architectural change, prominent lamina proprial plasmacytosis and crypt abscess formation (arrow). (*See plate section for color.*)

Focal active colitis

Focal active colitis refers to the patchy distribution of inflammation with or without architectural change in a mucosal biopsy specimen.[65] Characteristically, some areas of the biopsy specimen maintain an essentially normal appearance. The focal active colitis pattern is usually not seen with ulcerative colitis and, when present, suggests Crohn's colitis[103] or infectious colitis/acute self-limiting colitis[98–100,104] (Fig. 79.12). However, the active colitis pattern can be seen in resolving ulcerative colitis under medical treatment,[102,105] and areas of previously inflamed colon and rectum in ulcerative colitis can return, with therapy, to an almost normal histologic appearance. The focal active colitis pattern has been described in some patients with ischemia, and has been linked to NSAIDs and to bowel preparation itself.[103,104,106]

The definitive classification of IBD rests on clinicopathologic correlation. The pathologist should convey the histologic pattern of injury to the clinician, who then collates that information with the clinical history and data obtained from endoscopic and radiologic examination. Through consideration of all this information, an accurate diagnosis can be rendered.

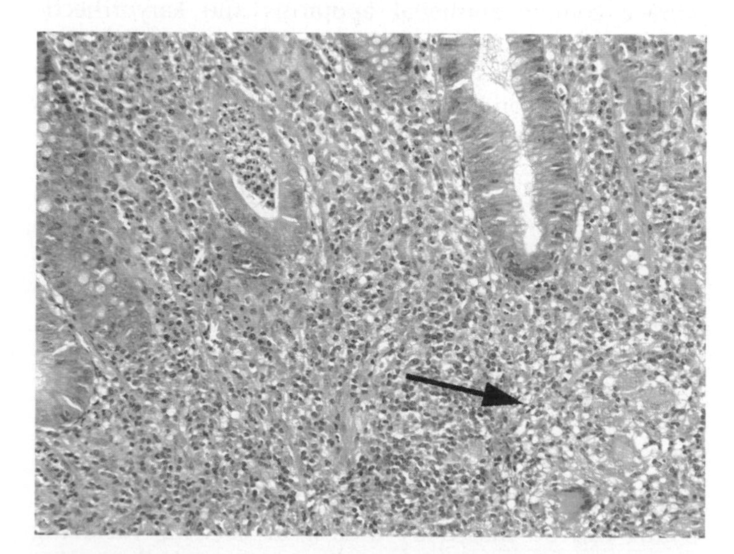

Figure 79.12: Colonic Crohn's disease showing focal active colitis with an intramucosal non-necrotizing granuloma (arrow). (*See plate section for color.*)

Acute ischemic-type change

The characteristic pattern of acute ischemic-type injury consists of hemorrhage into the lamina propria associated with superficial epithelial coagulative necrosis, with sparing of the deep portions of the crypts.[93] These changes may occasionally be associated with more extensive necrosis of superficial epithelium with inflammatory pseudomembrane formation. Surprisingly, acute and chronic inflammatory cells (e.g. plasma cells) are typically few in number in ischemic-type damage and this feature can be helpful in differentiating ischemic-type damage from primary IBD.

The differential diagnosis of acute ischemic-type damage is very wide and includes all causes of true ischemia such as inadequate perfusion, narrowing of blood vessels for any reason, obstructing lesions of the bowel and bowel distention. Ischemic-type change is also associated with a wide variety of drugs including vasopressors, NSAIDs and gluteraldehyde (used to clean endoscopes).[107–109] Some infectious agents, such as CMV, *Clostridium difficile*, *Clostridium septicum* and the enterohemorrhagic *Escherichia coli*, typically cause ischemic-type damage.

Trauma-type change

Trauma-type histologic changes frequently coexist clinically with mucosal ulcers. The characteristic trauma-type histopathology is found in the mucosa adjacent to ulcers or in polypoid areas, and consists of fibromuscular obliteration of the lamina propria associated with mucosal architectural distortion and capillary ectasia. The trauma-type histology can be seen in the solitary rectal ulcer syndrome, localized colitis cystica profunda and inflammatory cloacogenic polyp, and are a frequent finding in the vicinity of the ileocecal valve.[65]

Apoptotic colopathies

Surface colonic epithelial apoptosis and karyorrhectic debris in the superficial lamina propria are commonly seen in mucosal biopsy specimens and are widely attributed to bowel preparation.[65] Apoptotic bodies in the deep crypts are rarely seen (fewer than 1 per 20 crypts) outside pathologic conditions. Increased deep apoptotic bodies are characteristic in ischemic-type damage, CMV infection and chemotherapy/radiation. Although seen in association with a variety of injurious agents, apoptosis is the characteristic form of cell death in cell-mediated immune cytotoxicity as demonstrated in grade I graft-*vs*-host disease, other immune deficiency syndromes and patients with thymoma.[80]

Specific infectious colitides

Common bacterial agents

Colitis can be caused by a host of bacteria, including *Campylobacter* species, *Salmonella* species, *Shigella* species, *Staphylococcus aureus*, *Neisseria gonorrheae*, *E. coli*, *Treponema pallidum*, *Yersinia* species and *Mycobacterium* species. Although the colonic mucosal biopsy appearance in these infections can vary greatly (from essentially normal to lesions like those of idiopathic ulcerative colitis), a large number of specimens demonstrate the focal active pattern of injury outlined above, that strongly suggests infectious colitis/acute self-limiting colitis.[69,107,108] The definitive diagnosis of infectious colitis requires recovery of the offending organism or demonstration of a fourfold increase in specific antibody titer. In general, invasive organisms cause greater changes in morphology than those that produce their effect by toxins.

Histologic evaluation, although helpful in suggesting an infectious etiology, can only rarely suggest a specific agent. True granulomas can be seen in tuberculosis, syphilis, *Chlamydia* species infection, and *Yersinia pseudotuberculosis* infection. Microgranulomas are described in infection with *Salmonella* species, *Campylobacter* species and *Yersinia enterocolitica*. Isolated mucosal giant cells, although non-specific, have been described in *Chlamydia trachomatis* infection.[99,110] Identification of adherent organisms is characteristics of enteroadherent *E. coli* and spirochetosis[65] (Fig. 79.13).

Hemorrhagic colitis syndrome

The clinical syndrome of hemorrhagic colitis is characterized by abdominal cramping, bloody diarrhea, and no or low-grade fever.[111] Patients typically demonstrate right-sided colonic edema, erosions and hemorrhage. Investigations of epidemic outbreaks have confirmed the association between hemorrhagic colitis and enterohemorrhagic *E. coli*, the most important of which is *E. coli* O157:H7.[111,112]

Symptoms in patients with hemorrhagic colitis characteristically present several days after ingestion of contaminated food – usually undercooked hamburger. In almost all patients the disease resolves spontaneously, but severe cases can be complicated by the hemolytic uremic syndrome and thrombotic thrombocytopenic purpura.[112,113]

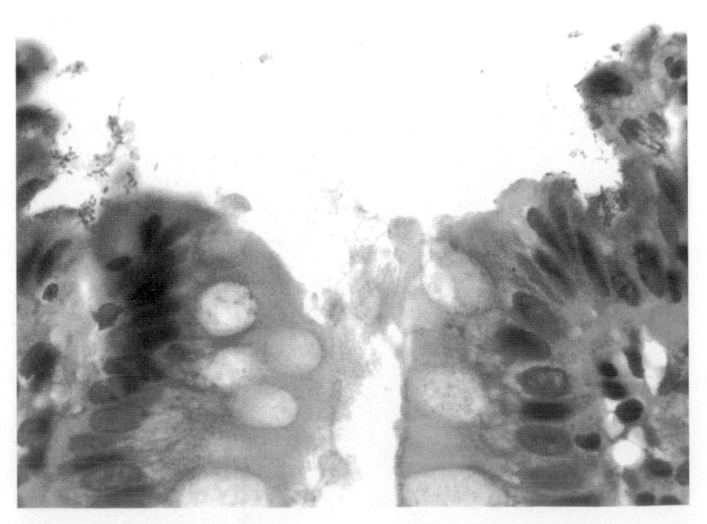

Figure 79.13: Enteroadherent *Escherichia coli.* Note the surface epithelial changes with adherent rod-shaped bacteria. (*See plate section for color.*)

Most patients demonstrate focal necrosis of the superficial mucosa, associated with hemorrhage and acute inflammation, and preservation of the deep portion of the colonic crypts, an appearance similar to the pattern of injury described with acute ischemic colitis.[111] Some specimens have shown the focal active colitis pattern of injury (see Focal active colitis) (Fig. 79.14). Because routine stool culture media do not distinguish *E. coli* O157:H7 from other strains of *E. coli* normally present in the stool, physicians suspecting hemorrhagic colitis caused by enterohemorrhagic *E. coli* should specifically request that stools be screened for these organisms.

Antibiotic-associated colitis and pseudomembranous colitis

Toxin-producing *C. difficile* may cause some antibiotic-associated diarrheas but is more strongly associated with pseudomembranous colitis. Administration of any antibiotic that favors the growth of *C. difficile* can lead to pseudomembranous colitis.[114] Characteristic lesions occur only early in the disease. Endoscopically, the surface of the mucosa contains focal plaque-like cream to yellow pseudomembranes;[115] some early lesions resemble aphthoid ulcers of Crohn's disease. Histologically, there is patchy necrosis of the superficial portions of the colonic crypts, not unlike that seen in ischemia, although true ischemia tends to show more extensive hyalinization of the lamina propria[116] (Fig. 79.15). The affected crypts become dilated, and an inflammatory pseudomembrane exudes from the superficial aspects of the degenerating crypt in an eruptive or mushroom-like configuration. This pseudomembrane extends laterally to overlie adjacent virtually normal colonic mucosa. The karyorrhectic debris and neutrophils within the pseudomembrane often align in a curious linear configuration within the mucin. Very early lesions (as well as the mucosa between diagnostic lesions) can, on occasion, show the focal active colitis pattern of inflammation associated with infectious colitis/acute self-limiting colitis. With progression of disease, the plaques become confluent and the crypt necrosis becomes complete. At this point, pseudomembranous colitis becomes indistinguishable from ischemic colitis. Toxic megacolon and perforation can occur.

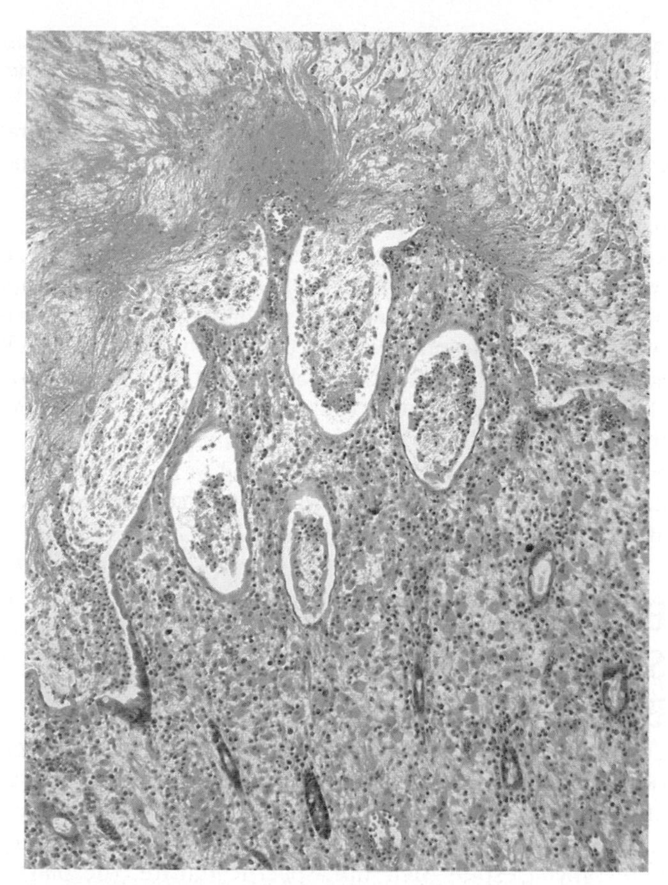

Figure 79.15: *Clostridium difficile*-associated pseudomembranous colitis. An inflammatory pseudomembrane exudes from dilated degenerating crypts in an erosive fashion. The karyorrhectic debris and neutrophils within the pseudomembrane tend to align in a linear configuration within the mucus. (*See plate section for color.*)

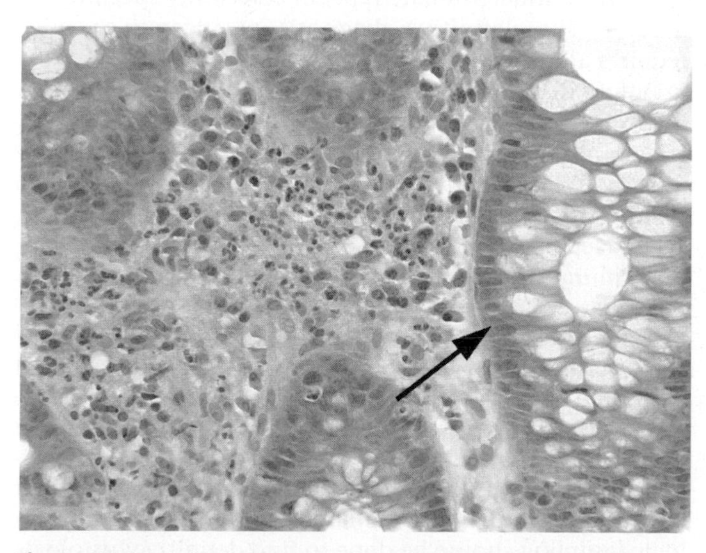

Figure 79.14: Infectious-type focal active colitis pattern of injury from a patient with culture-proved *E. coli* O157:H7 infection. Sections show a collection of lamina proprial neutrophils adjacent to a relatively normal colonic crypt (arrow). (*See plate section for color.*)

Viral agents

Norwalk agent and rotavirus, common causes of viral gastroenteritis, are not known to cause morphologic changes in the colon. CMV and herpes simplex virus (HSV) may cause proctitis and colitis.

Specific forms of colitis

Eosinophilic colitis/proctitis

Infiltration of the large intestine by large numbers of eosinophils correlates with a variety of clinical syndromes. One variant is probably an extension of the eosinophilic gastroenteritis discussed above. Peripheral eosinophilia is marked, and a history of atopy is common[117–120] A second type, primarily in adolescents and adults, previously termed *allergic proctitis*, is, in the authors' opinion, a form of ulcerattive colitis.[121] Whenever large numbers of eosinophils are encountered in colonic biopsy specimens, this should prompt a thorough search for parasites, especially *Strongyloides* species.

The most common type of primary colorectal eosinophilic infiltrate is confined to the mucosa and occurs in infants and young children as a result of dietary-related (protein) allergy (allergic proctitis/colitis).[122,123] These children typically have rectal bleeding with or without diarrhea, and many show peripheral blood eosinophilia. Colonic biopsy specimens may show increased numbers of eosinophils within the lamina propria, often accompanied by a mild focal active colitis. Precise biopsy classification may be difficult. In general, however, more than 60 eosinophils per 10 high-magnification fields and eosinophils in the muscularis mucosae or as the predominant cell in crypt abscesses are features suggestive of an allergic etiology.[123]

Feature	Crohn's enteritis	Crohn's colitis	Ulcerative colitis
Serositis	Yes	Yes	No, except in fulminant colitis
Thick bowel wall	Yes	Yes	No, except when complicated by carcinoma
Stricture	Often	Sometimes	No, except when complicated by carcinoma
Mucosal edema	Yes	Yes	Usually no
Discrete mucosal ulcers	Yes	Yes	Usually no, except in fulminant colitis
Fat wrapping	Often present	Often present	Usually no
Fistula	Common	Sometimes	No
Distribution	Focal	Usually focal	Diffuse
Rectal involvement	No	Sometimes	Yes

Table 79.2 Distinguishing gross features of Crohn's disease and ulcerative colitis

EVALUATION OF RESECTION SPECIMENS IN INFLAMMATORY BOWEL DISEASE

Once specific causes of enteritis and colitis have been ruled out, what is left is a group of diseases referred to as *idiopathic IBD*. IBD describes at least three entities: Crohn's disease, ulcerative colitis and colitis of indeterminate type. Despite their non-specific nature, the pathologic features of Crohn's disease and ulcerative colitis are sufficiently distinctive that they can usually be distinguished from each other and from other kinds of bowel inflammation.

Crohn's disease and ulcerative colitis

The distributional features, gross appearance and histologic characteristics of typical cases of Crohn's disease and ulcerative colitis have been well described;[124–127] the distinguishing features are summarized in Tables 79.2 and 79.3. In the colon, rectal sparing, skip areas of involvement and preferential right-sided localization are gross features favoring Crohn's disease over ulcerative colitis. Discriminating microscopic features of Crohn's disease include non-necrotizing granulomas, fissuring ulcers and transmural inflammation. The granulomas, noted in 50–70% of patients, are generally poorly formed, few in number and seen more often in Crohn's enteritis. The fissuring ulcers are lined by granulation tissue rather than neutrophils, and extend into the deep submucosa, muscularis propria or beyond. Transmural inflammation is usually in the form of lymphoid aggregates with a propensity to localize around lymphatic vessels and small blood vessels.

Colitis-type indeterminate

The term *colitis-type indeterminate* describes approximately 5–10% of operative specimens, almost always from patients with acute or severe clinical disease requiring urgent or emergent colectomy (fulminant colitis), in which pathologic features are ambiguous and do not permit precise separation of Crohn's disease from ulcerative colitis.[126,127] In fulminant colitis, fissuring ulcers and transmural inflammation (normally major criteria of Crohn's disease) may be seen in otherwise typical cases of ulcerative colitis. Although fulminant colitis with toxic megacolon is strongly associated with ulcerative colitis, many of such patients do, in fact, follow a clinical course indicative of Crohn's disease. A three-tiered classification system for primary IBD (ulcerative colitis, Crohn's disease or colitis of indeterminate type) in colectomy specimens is used.[127] The definitive diagnosis of ulcerative colitis requires all of the following features:

- Diffuse disease limited to the large intestine
- Involvement of the rectum
- More proximal colonic disease occurring in continuity with an involved rectum (i.e. no gross or histologic skip lesions)
- No deep fissural ulcers
- No mural sinus tracts
- No transmural lymphoid aggregates or granulomas.

The definitive diagnosis of Crohn's disease requires histologic verification, with the demonstration of transmural lymphoid aggregates in areas not deeply ulcerated or the presence of non-necrotizing granulomas. In patients win whom the gross and clinical features suggest Crohn's disease (e.g. skip lesions, linear ulcers, cobblestoning, fat wrapping, terminal ileal inflammation), extensive histologic sampling should be done to find definitive histologic features of Crohn's disease.

Several studies have apparently concluded that indeterminate colitis clinically acts like ulcerative colitis.

Feature	Crohn's enteritis	Crohn's colitis	Ulcerative colitis
Granulomas	Common	Sometimes	No
Fissuring ulcer	Common	Common	No, except in fulminant colitis
Transmural inflammation	Yes	Yes	No, except in fulminant colitis
Submucosal edema	Yes	Yes	Usually no
Submucosal inflammation	Yes	Yes	Usually no
Neuronal hyperplasia	Yes	Sometimes	Usually no
Thickening of muscularis mucosae	Yes, patchy	Yes, patchy	Yes, diffuse (in chronic mucosal ulcerative colitis)
Pyloric gland metaplasia	Common	Rare	Rare
Mucosal inflammation and architectural distortion	Focal	Usually focal	Diffuse
Paneth cell metaplasia	No	Yes	Yes

Table 79.3 Distinguishing histologic features of Crohn's disease and ulcerative colitis

However, recent reports outline a pouch failure rate in indeterminate colitis (19%) that is intermediate between that seen with overt Crohn's disease (34%) and ulcerative colitis (8%).[127–131]

Lesions associated with surgical procedures

Diversion colitis/defunctionalized bowel

A rectum surgically placed out of circuit acquires histologic changes associated with defunctioning alone, regardless of the original reason for diversion.[132,133] The changes probably reflect a physiologic response to stasis and the loss of trophic factors in the feces, most notably short-chain fatty acids. The mucosa of the diverted segment appears erythematous, granular and friable. Histologic changes include marked lymphoid hyperplasia with germinal center formation, usually accompanied by mild colitis with crypt abscess formation. The changes may be indistinguishable from follicular proctitis (ulcerative proctitis or localized ulcerative colitis). The mucosal lymphoid hyperplasia may be accompanied by lymphoid aggregates scattered in the deep submucosa, muscular wall and perirectal adipose tissue. Because these changes may occur in diverted segments in patients without IBD, care must be taken not to base a diagnosis of primary IBD, especially Crohn's disease, solely on the histologic changes seen in such specimens. In many patients, the rectum is placed out of circuit during an operation for IBD. In these instances, the rectum can show changes of both primary IBD and diversion colitis. The histologic changes in defunctioned rectums do not, in general, correlate with the original diagnosis or clinical outcome.[133]

Ileal reservoirs (pouches) and pouchitis

For patients requiring total colectomy, several surgical operations have been developed that either create continence in an ileostomy (Kock's ileostomy) or preserve anal sphincter function and restore the continuity to the bowel (ileal pouch–anal anastomosis). These operations have in common the creation of a reservoir (pouch), which is formed by interconnecting loops of terminal ileum. These pouch procedures are contraindicated in patients with Crohn's disease because of increased morbidity (e.g. fistula and abscess).

Pouch complications include fistula, obstruction, incontinence and anastomotic leaks.[134] Although many complications result from surgical and mechanical difficulties, and others relate to the development of primary inflammation in the pouch ('pouchitis'), some of these complicated cases likely represent pouch recurrence of initially undiagnosed Crohn's disease. These cases illustrate the pathologists' inability reliably to differentiate ulcerative colitis from Crohn's disease in severe colitis, even after examination of the colectomy specimen (see Colitis-type indeterminate). Virtually all reports of surgical experiences with ileal pouch–anal anastomosis for presumed ulcerative colitis contain approximately 2–7% of patients in whom the actual diagnosis proved to be Crohn's disease.[127–129,135]

A late complication of pouch construction is the development of primary inflammation in the pouch with its associated clinical syndrome, termed *pouchitis*,[136] which affects almost one-half of patients. Nausea, vomiting, malaise, fever and abdominal cramping develop. There is increased effluent and stool from the pouch that may be watery, foul smelling or grossly bloody; patients often become incontinent. Pouch bacterial ecology is often altered, and patients usually respond to antibiotics, suggesting a bacterial etiology. However, some patients require sulfasalazine, corticosteroids, immunomodulator therapy or even pouch excision for management of pouchitis.

Pouch biopsy may be performed to confirm the presence of inflammation or to evaluate the possibility of Crohn's disease.[137] Biopsy specimens obtained from nondysfunctional pouches may show mild villus shortening and increased chronic inflammation with increased crypt mitoses, but, in the authors' experience, most specimens appear similar to the normal terminal ileum. A few neutrophils in the surface epithelium and lamina propria are commonly seen. In contrast, pouches with pouchitis often have decreased epithelial cell mucin and decreased or absent lymphoid follicles. The most consistent findings in pouchitis have been ulcers with granulation tissue and patchy accumulations of neutrophils in the lamina propria, with cryptitis and crypt abscess formation.[137,138]

Many investigators report an inconsistent relationship between endoscopic and histologic changes in the pouch and patient symptoms. Therefore, many clinicians diagnose pouchitis solely on clinical grounds and reserve endoscopic examination with biopsy for those patients with refractory pouchitis or possible Crohn's disease. There are no reliable endoscopic or histologic criteria to differentiate most examples of pouchitis from new onset or recurrence of Crohn's disease in the pouch.

Although debated,[127,139] missed Crohn's disease is more likely to present as a late pouch fistula than as refractory pouchitis. However, refractory pouchitis has been seen in which pouch biopsy specimens contained granulomas or in which the excised pouch has shown major histologic criteria for Crohn's disease.[137] Invariably, the original pathology of the colectomy specimen was either missed Crohn's colitis or indeterminate colitis. Ulcers in the afferent limb of a pelvic pouch correlate with a diagnosis of Crohn's disease or with the use of NSAIDs in patients without Crohn's disease.[140]

Some investigators have identified histologic patterns of mucosal adaption in pouches.[141–144] Approximately 60% of patients exhibit what has been called type A mucosa with normal small-bowel biopsy histologic appearance or only mild mucosal atrophy with no or minimal inflammation. The so-called type B mucosa, characterized by transient atrophy with temporary moderate to severe inflammation followed by normalization of the intestinal mucosa, is seen in 40% of patients. The type C mucosa with permanent persistent atrophy and severe inflammation occurs in approximately 10% of pouches. Colonic-type features have been reported at least focally in pouches of all types by routine morphology, mucin histochemistry, immunohistochemistry, lectin binding or electron microscopy. This colonic-type metaplasia is most well developed in the type C mucosa, but is never complete. All pouches seem to retain mostly small-bowel properties regardless of mucosal type or the duration of the pouch.

DISORDERS OF INTESTINAL MOTILITY

Intestinal pseudo-obstruction

Intestinal pseudo-obstruction is the term used to describe patients with signs and symptoms of intestinal obstruction in whom no mechanical obstructive lesion can be demonstrated.[145] Intestinal pseudo-obstruction may be caused by a heterogeneous group of lesions. In some cases, the condition is associated with a familiar disease or drug. The bowel obstruction is considered a local manifestation of the more generalized disease process or drug effect and, in general, the intestinal pathology is either unknown or non-specific. In other cases, pseudo-obstruction is associated with a familiar disease in which pathologic changes can be seen in the intestine (e.g. scleroderma). Finally, there are several intestinal motility disorders in which the primary pathologic changes and clinical manifestations are gastrointestinal.

Visceral myopathies

There are multiple variants of familial visceral myopathy that demonstrate differences in the mode of inheritance (autosomal dominant *vs* recessive), sites of involvement in the gut, clinical symptoms and extraintestinal manifestations. Visceral myopathies also occur in a sporadic form.[146]

The intestinal pathologic changes in familial and sporadic hollow visceral myopathies are identical and consist of muscle cell degeneration, muscle cell loss and fibrosis of the muscularis propria. The degenerative fibers appear swollen and rarefied. Collagen may encircle the residual muscle fibers in areas of muscle fiber dropout and impart a vacuolated appearance.[146–148] These changes are limited to, or more severe in, the external layer of the muscularis propria. The small intestinal mucosa may show changes associated with stasis; these include a variable villus abnormality with increased chronic inflammatory cells, occasionally mixed with acute inflammatory cells.

Visceral neuropathies

The visceral neuropathies form a complex group of unusual entities that vary in their pattern of inheritance (familial *vs* sporadic), the extent of intestinal and extraintestinal involvement, and the nature of the histopathologic changes in the intramural neural plexi of the gut. Many of the neuronal and axonal changes are subtle; with the exception of inflammatory neuropathies or, perhaps, familial neuropathies associated with intranuclear inclusions, they cannot be recognized in routine sections and special silver-staining techniques are needed to demonstre them.[149] Difficult and unusual cases should probably be referred for consultation to pathology departments with particular expertise in evaluating visceral neuropathies. Some sporadic cases demonstrate mononuclear inflammation in the myenteric plexus, and these can be identified by routine light microscopy alone.[150]

An increasing role for the interstitial cells of Cajal as gut pacemakers and mediators of neurotransmission has been proposed. Interstitial cells of Cajal stain specifically with the tyrosine kinase receptor, c-kit. Immunohistochemistry for c-kit (CD117) and CD34 (which reacts with many c-kit receptors) represents a relatively easy way to study severe constipation and intestinal pseudo-obstruction. Streutker et al.[151] have described completely absent or markedly reduced numbers of interstitial cells of Cajal in intestinal pseudo-obstruction. Although these observations could be an epiphenomenon, they might form the basis of an alternate classification system for pseudo-obstruction.

Ceroidosis: the 'brown bowel syndrome'

Severe intestinal malabsorption, for whatever reason, can be associated with dark brown or orange-brown discoloration of the bowel wall,[152,153] owing to deposition of a granular material that has the characteristics of lipofuscin in the smooth muscle of the muscularis propria and, to a lesser degree, the muscularis mucosae. This excessive accumulation of lipofuscin is termed *ceroidosis,* or the 'brown bowel syndrome'. Whether this pigment deposition adversely affects muscle function is debated.

Melanosis coli

Melanosis coli is a condition in which macrophages filled with lipofuscin-like pigment are found within the lamina propria or deeper in the wall of the colon. They may be of such numbers as to impart a brown or black color to the colon. Melanosis coli has been associated with increased apoptosis, which is often linked to ingestion of purgatives of the anthracene group (cascera, sagrada, aloe, rhubarb, senna, frangula)[154,155] and is often seen in severely constipated patients.

Hirschsprung's disease and allied conditions

Hirschsprung's disease

Hirschsprung's disease (aganglionic megacolon) demonstrates a predilection for male patients. Approximately 90% of patients are first seen in infancy, usually with constipation, abdominal distention, vomiting and delay of meconium stool; diarrhea may occur[156,157] and some patients may even be affected by life-threatening enterocolitis. Hirschsprung's disease has been linked to inactivating mutations of the *RET* proto-oncogene.[158] Several cases of familial Hirschsprung's disease have been associated to mutations of the endothelin receptor B gene.[159] In the typical clinical picture, the anus is normal; the anal canal and rectum are usually small and devoid of stool. In classic cases, these physical findings are confirmed by barium enema: The contrast material flows into an unexpanded distal segment, then passes through a cone-shaped area, and finally into the dilated proximal bowel. The pathologic change is aganglionosis. The narrowed distal segment shows complete absence of ganglion cells from both the submucosal and myenteric plexi, usually accompanied by hypertrophy of the muscularis mucosae and increased numbers and size of nerves in the submucosa and between the muscle layers of the muscularis propria[160] (Fig. 79.16). In the tapered or cone-shaped region, the number of ganglion cells may be decreased.

Historically, histologic diagnosis was made on full-thickness rectal biopsy specimens. However, this procedure requires general anesthesia and risks the development of stricture and perforation. Because the submucosal and myenteric plexi stop at about the same level in Hirschsprung's disease,[161] suction biopsy sampling the mucosa and submucosa is considered the method of choice for the diagnosis. All rectal biopsy specimens for suspected Hirschsprung's disease should be serially sectioned throughout the block, and each section examined. If no ganglion cells are found, then some comment should be made concerning the adequacy of the specimen. Biopsy specimens devoid of ganglion cells, but in which the amount of submucosa is less than the thickness of the mucosa, should be considered as insufficient to diagnose Hirschsprung's disease.[160] If biopsy specimens contain epithelium of the anal canal, this specimen should be considered inadequate, because the anal canal and distal 2 cm of rectum typically are relatively hypoganglionated or aganglionated.

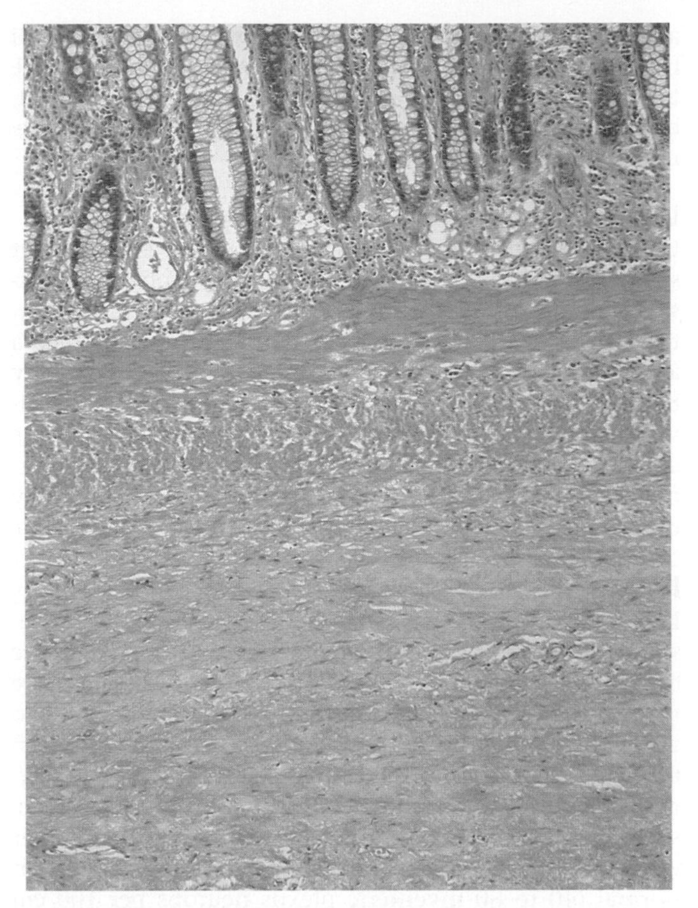

Figure 79.16: Biopsy specimen from patient with Hirschsprung's disease illustrating an absence of ganglion cells associated with marked hypertrophy of the muscularis mucosae. (*See plate section for color.*)

Many pathologists prefer to examine a frozen-section slide stained for acetylcholinesterase in addition to standard hematoxylin and eosin-stained sections.[162] In Hirschsprung's disease, the acetylcholinesterase stain demonstrates a marked increase in acetylcholinesterase-positive nerve fibers in the lamina propria and muscularis mucosae. The utility of this technique as an adjunct to diagnosis is debated. False-positive and false-negative reactions have been reported, and its use is a matter of personal preference.[160,163–165]

Occasionally, ganglion cells may be difficult to identify using light microscopy alone, especially in the neonate.[160] In such cases, a positive immunocytochemical reaction for neuron-specific enolase can be helpful in documenting ganglion cells.[166] Other immunostains such as cathepsin D and protein gene product (PGP) 9.5 can also decorate ganglion cells.[167] Frozen-section evaluation is often used as an adjunct to visual inspection to select the site for colostomy. However, use of frozen section to establish a primary diagnosis of Hirschsprung's disease is best avoided because of the high rate of interpretative errors.[168]

Long-segment Hirschsprung's disease

In 90% of patients with Hirschsprung's disease, the aganglionosis involves segments of colon less than 40 cm in length. The remaining cases demonstrate a longer aganglionic segment that may even extend into the small intestine.[146] Microscopically, the hypertrophied nerve trunks of short-segment Hirschsprung's disease are absent, but the increased number of acetylcholinesterase-positive mucosal nerve fibers can be seen.[162]

Ultrashort-segment Hirschsprung's disease

Ultrashort-segment Hirschsprung's disease (segment smaller than 2 cm) reportedly exists but is probably impossible for a pathologist to document by routine hematoxylin and eosin staining of rectal mucosa and submucosa alone, because this segment of rectum is relatively hypoganglionated or aganglionated, even in normal individuals. Rectal manometry plays a premier role in the diagnosis of this lesion. Acetylcholinesterase nerve abnormalities similar to those of Hirschsprung's disease may complement that study.

Hypoganglionosis

Hypoganglionosis is regularly observed in the cone-shaped transition zone between normal and aganglionic bowel in Hirschsprung's disease.[146] Some authors believe that diffuse hypoganglionosis of the colon may give rise to megacolon similar to that observed in Hirschsprung's disease.[162,169] There is no accepted definition of hypoganglionosis; however, guidelines are offered by Meier-Ruge, suggesting that a decrease by a factor of 10 in the number of ganglion cells per centimeter of bowel compared with normal (40 to 80 myenteric plexus neurons per 100 cm bowel) is diagnostic of hypoganglionosis.[162] In general, the condition has not been well characterized, and many reports lack quantitation.[146] Diverse abnormalities have been described by special silver stains in cases that would have been called hypoganglionosis by routine microscopy,[170] and some cases of hypoganglionosis may be similar to those reported as severe idiopathic constipation or cathartic colon.

Intestinal neuronal dysplasia (hyperganglionosis)

Intestinal neuronal dysplasia is characterized by hyperplasia of myenteric plexi, increased acetylcholinesterase activity in nerves of the lamina propria and submucosa, and increased numbers of ganglion cells with formation of giant ganglions.[171,172] These giant ganglions typically contain more than seven to ten neurons (normal three to five), make up only 3–5% of all ganglions in a given case, and are usually not seen in the distal rectum. Occasionally, ganglion cells may be found within the lamina propria.[169] The condition may give rise to signs and symptoms similar to those of Hirschsprung's disease. It may occur in a localized or disseminated form. Similar lesions, sometimes referred to as ganglioneuromatosis, may be observed in patients with von Recklinghausen's disease or the multiple endocrine neoplasia (MEN) syndrome type IIB.[146,172] Although some investigators diagnose intestinal neuronal dysplasia based on abnormal acetylcholinesterase staining in specimens containing ganglion cells, others believe that acetylcholinesterase staining alone cannot be relied upon for the diagnosis.[173,174] Diagnostic criteria for intestinal neuronal dysplasia and even its existence are challenged[174] because 95% of infants so diagnosed experience normalization of gut motility within 1 year. Therefore, many of the observed abnormalities could be within normal range and, in general, the diagnosis should be reserved for florid pathologic cases.[175]

Other related conditions

In zonal aganglionosis or 'skip-segment' Hirschsprung's disease, ganglion cells are found distal to one or more aganglionic segments.[175–177] The problem here is that a rectal biopsy specimen may yield ganglion cells despite an authentic, more proximal, Hirschsprung's-like aganglionic lesion. Immaturity of ganglion cells[146,162] and hypogenesis of the myenteric plexus[162] have also been reported to cause signs and symptoms similar to those of Hirschsprung's disease.

GASTROINTESTINAL POLYPS AND POLYPOSIS SYNDROMES

Familial adenomatous polyposis

Familial adenomatous polyposis (FAP) is inherited as an autosomal dominant trait. Bussey[178] recognized that 100 or more colonic adenomas (recognized grossly) phenotypically identified patients with FAP and distinguished them from patients with multiple adenomas in whom inheritance was not seen (Fig. 79.17). In typical FAP, hundreds to thousands of adenomas develop within the colon (Fig. 79.18). The adenomas begin to appear in the second decade of life and are surprisingly asymptomatic considering their usually large numbers. Symptomatic patients present with signs and symptoms of increased bowel motility and the passage of blood and/or mucus, which often heralds the onset of carcinoma. Two-thirds of these so-called propositus cases present with carcinoma and nearly

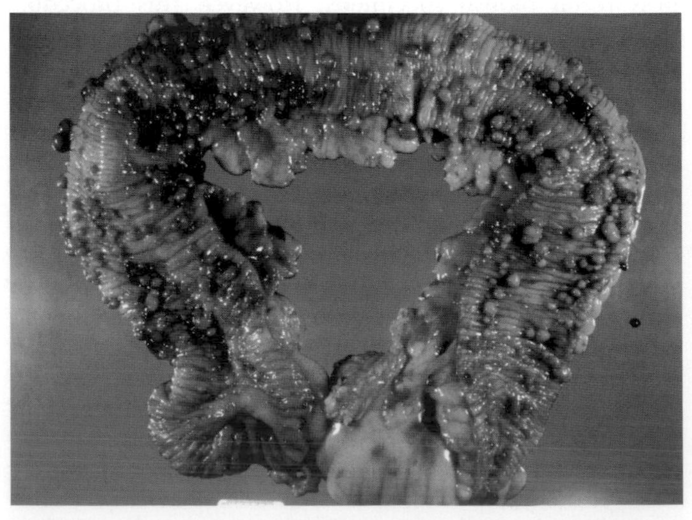

Figure 79.17: Resected colonic resection specimen from familial adenomatous polyposis. (*See plate section for color.*)

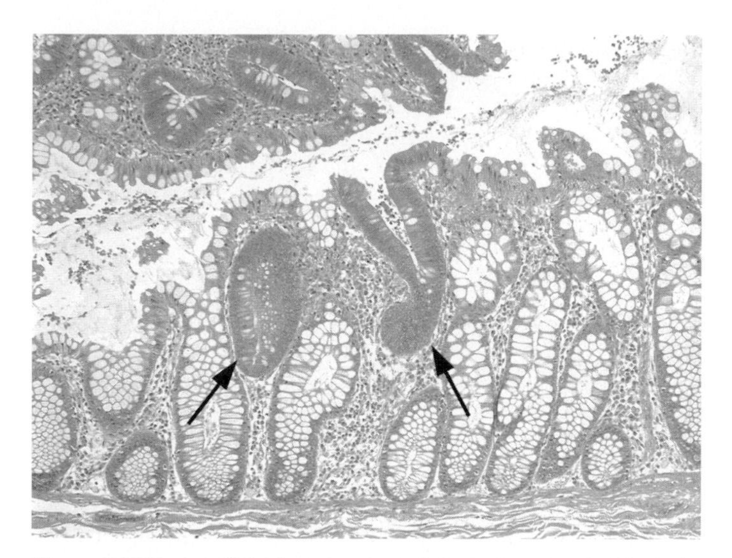

Figure 79.18: Familial adenomatous polyposis. Sections show tubular adenomas including one gland adenomas (arrow) typical for the syndrome. (*See plate section for color.*)

one-half of them will have more than one carcinoma in the colon. This high risk of invasive cancer in symptomatic patients forms the basis for polyposis registries and the extensive screening of asymptomatic kindred at risk for FAP.

Screening recommendations have evolved with increased genetic information. Screening of primary relatives of affected individuals should begin at the age of 10 years, usually with the truncated protein assay protein truncation test (PTT).[179] In the absence of genetic testing, endoscopic screening is still useful to detect FAP. All affected patients have adenomas within the range of the sigmoidoscope. It is therefore recommended that screening sigmoidoscopy begin at age 10–12 years, with re-examination every 2 years. The diagnosis of FAP must be confirmed with biopsy because lymphoid polyposis and hyperplastic polyposis can mimic FAP grossly and endoscopically. Once a diagnosis of FAP has been established, prophylactic proctocolectomy is recommended. Most investigators recommend sigmoidoscopy for mutation negative kindred at the age of 12 years, just in case the genetic test is erroneous. Thyroid examination and serum α-fetoprotein determination to screen for hepatoblastoma are recommended.

Regular upper endoscopy should be done. Gastric and duodenal polyps develop in 30–90% of patients with FAP.[180,181] The gastric lesions are usually fundic gland polyposis, whereas the duodenal polyps are usually adenomas. The incidence of duodenal adenomas and FAP increases with increasing age. There is a propensity for these to develop in the periampullary region. Adenomas everywhere are prone to the dysplasia–carcinoma sequence. The relative risk of duodenal/periampullary carcinoma is approximately 125–350 times that seen in the general population, and duodenal/periampullary carcinoma has become a major cause of morbidity and mortality in patients with FAP in the post-prophylactic colectomy era.[182]

Genetics of familial adenomatous polyposis and related syndromes

The gene responsible for familial adenomatous polyposis (*APC* gene) has been localized to the long arm of chromosome 5 (5q21-q22) and has been cloned.[183,184] Mutation in most patients with FAP and its variants creates a stop codon resulting in a truncated protein product.

Most patients are now diagnosed using an assay (PTT) to detect the truncated APC protein. The conversion variant of this test, in which each strand of the DNA is examined separately, may be able to detect more than 96% of mutations.[179] Direct mutational analysis of the *APC* gene can be performed.[185]

Localization of mutations within the *APC* gene locus correlates with phenotype. For example, germline mutations between codons 1250 and 1464 are associated with very large numbers of colonic adenomas, whereas mutations elsewhere, especially near the 5′ or 3′ end of *APC*, yield lesser numbers of colonic adenomas (see Attenuated familial adenomatous polyposis below).[179,186]

Gardner's and some Turcot's syndromes are variants of FAP. In Gardner's variant, in addition to colonic adenomas and upper gastrointestinal polyps, patients can exhibit a number of extraintestinal manifestation such as osteomas, epidermal inclusion cysts, other benign skin tumors, desmoid tumors of the abdomen/abdominal wall, fibrosis of mesentery, dental abnormalities, carcinoma of the periampullary region/duodenum and carcinoma of the thyroid. Turcot's syndrome describes the association of colonic adenomas with tumors of the central nervous system. In many investigators' zeal to publish, the phenotypic spectrum had been unduly broad, with colonic manifestations ranging from a single adenoma to a virtual carpeting of the colonic mucosa with polyps. Furthermore, the brain tumors have comprised almost every conceivable histologic type. Molecular studies have clarified the situation.[187] Turcot's syndrome families with germline mutations of the *APC* gene tend to develop a typical FAP colonic phenotype and often develop medulloblastomas. Other patients reported as having Turcot's syndrome have mutations in DNA mismatch repair genes that are characteristic of those in families with hereditary non-polyposis colonic cancer syndrome. The brain tumors in this group are usually gliobastoma multiform.

Mutations of the *APC* gene near the 5′ and 3′ ends may have fewer adenomas (fewer than 100), a tendency for the adenomas to be macroscopically flat, and a propensity for these adenomas to cluster in the right colon. Originally reported as hereditary flat adenoma syndrome, this form is now more accurately referred to as attenuated familial adenomatous polyposis.[179,186] Like typical FAP, these patients can develop fundic gland polyposis, duodenal adenomas and periampullary carcinoma. The risk of colorectal carcinoma is increased in these patients, albeit to a lesser degree than in other forms of FAP, and the cancers tend to occur later in life.

Recently, inherited variants of the base excision repair gene mutY homolog (*MYH*) have been associated with colorectal polyposis with an autosomal recessive mode of inheritance.[188,189] Cases phenotypically resemble FAP or attenuated FAP, and are referred to as 'MYH polyposis'.[190]

Juvenile polyps and juvenile polyposis syndromes

Juvenile polyps can occur in a sporadic form or be part of juvenile polyposis as a syndrome. In the sporadic form, juvenile polyps have their peak prevalence in children aged between 1 and 7 years. There is some evidence that juvenile polyps can regress, but they are certainly seen in adults. Sporadic juvenile polyps typically occur singly, although patients may have up to five, usually in the rectum. Juvenile polyps typically range in size from millimeters to 2 cm in size (Fig. 79.19). As they are often attached only by a small pedicle, these polyps are particularly prone to auto-amputation. Histologically, typical juvenile polyps consists of a hamartomatous overgrowth of the lamina propria accompanied by elongation and cystic dilation of crypts lined by non-dysplastic colonic epithelium[191] (Fig. 79.20). The inflammatory component of juvenile polyps can be quite prominent, with neutrophils and lymphoid follicles in the lamina propria. Frequently, the distinction between juvenile polyps and inflammatory polyps of primary IBD cannot be made by histologic examination alone, and requires clinical correlation. Solitary juvenile polyps appear to have no malignant potential.[192]

Juvenile polyposis syndromes can be familial or non-familial, and usually becomes clinically apparent within the first decade of life with painless rectal bleeding, prolapse and iron deficiency anemia, or by passing an auto-amputated polyp. The following diagnostic criteria have been applied. A patient is considered to have juvenile polyposis syndrome if they have six or more juvenile polyps in the colon and rectum, have juvenile polyps throughout the gastrointestinal tract, or have any number of juvenile polyps in association with a positive family history.[193,194] In the non-familial form of juvenile polyposis syndrome (approximately 30% of the total), patients frequently have associated abnormalities, such as cardiac defects, hydrocephalus, malrotation, undescended testes and skull abnormalities. The familial form usually lacks these extra-intestinal manifestations. Inheritance has varied, although almost all are autosomal dominant with variable penetrance. Familial forms of juvenile polyposis syndrome appear to be associated with an increased risk of colorectal carcinoma;[194] prophylactic colectomy may be prudent in juvenile polyposis syndrome.

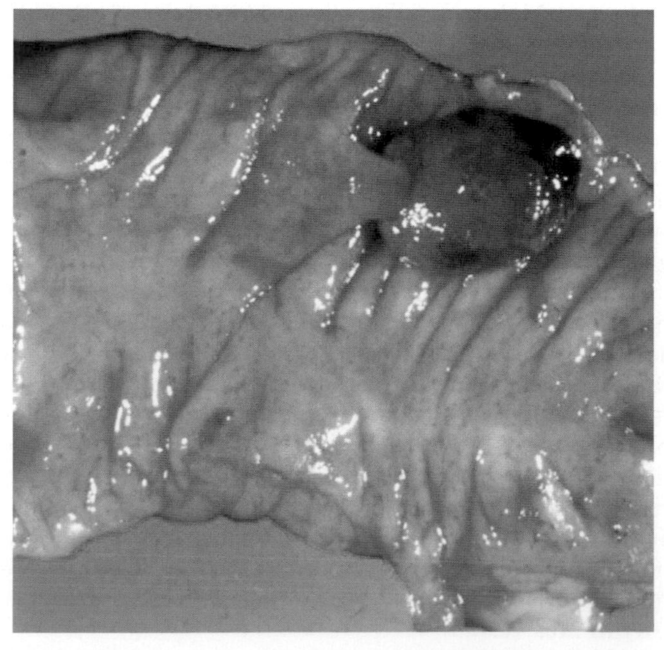

Figure 79.19: Resected colonic juvenile polyp. Note the spherical red polyp attached by an elongate pedicle. (*See plate section for color.*)

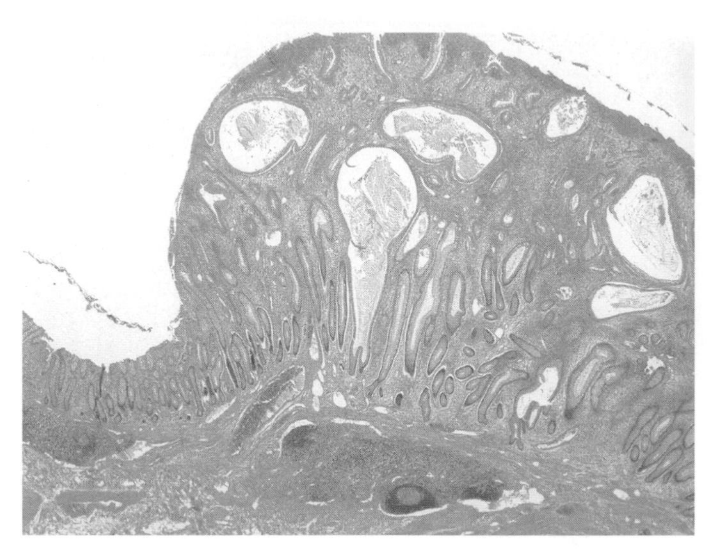

Figure 79.20: Juvenile polyp demonstrating edematous and inflammatory expansion of the lamina propria with colonic mucosal epithelial microcyst formation. (*See plate section for color.*)

The number of polyps in juvenile polyposis syndrome typically ranges from a few dozen to several hundred. Phenotypically, juvenile polyposis syndrome appears to occur in three varieties: (1) polyps limited to the colon; (2) polyps limited to the stomach; and (3) polyps throughout the entire gastrointestinal tract.[195–197] The mucosal polyps found in the context of juvenile polyposis syndromes are often unusual histologically. In addition to typical juvenile polyps (described above), one can find juvenile polyps with unusual features in which there is much more mucosa than lamina propria. In addition, mixture polyps (juvenile polyps with areas of adenoma/dysplasia) are quite frequent.[194] A family showing an autosomal dominant inheritance of atypical juvenile polyps, adenomas, hyperplastic polyps and polyps showing a mixture of all three types (hereditary mixed polyposis syndrome)[198] may be a variant of juvenile polyposis.[199]

Two genes are linked to familial juvenile polyposis syndrome, *SMAD-4* (18q21.1) and *BMPR1A* (10q22.3).[191,200,201] Juvenile polyps can be found in patients with other hamartomatous syndromes of the colon, such as intestinal ganglioneuromatosis/ganglioneurofibromatosis (see below).[202,203]

Patients can sometimes be managed with endoscopy and polypectomy (every 1–3 years); however, colectomy must be considered for patients with large numbers of polyps, polyps with dysplasia, or complications (e.g. bleeding).[191] Upper endoscopy is also recommended in patients with juvenile polyposis syndrome.

Ruvalcabas–Myhe–Smith syndrome (Bannayan–Riley–Ruvalcabas syndrome)

The Ruvalcabas–Myhe–Smith syndrome consists of macrocephaly, intelletual impairment, unusual craniofacial appearance, pigmented macules on the penis and hamartomatous polyps in the gastrointestinal tract. The syndrome may be passed on in an autosomal dominant pattern, although there are too few cases to be sure.[204] The gastrointestinal polyps have been indistinguishable from juvenile polyps and, in rare instances, intestinal ganglioneuromatosis has also been described. The syndrome has been linked to mutations in the *PTEN* gene (10q23.3).[205]

Peutz–Jeghers syndrome

Peutz–Jeghers polyps can be found throughout the gastrointestinal tract and are most commonly seen as part of the Peutz–Jeghers syndrome.[206] The polyp itself is characterized by fairly normal epithelium and lamina propria lining an abnormal arborizing network of smooth muscle that represents hamartomatous overgrowth of the muscularis mucosae[206,207] (Fig. 79.21). Peutz–Jeghers syndrome, usually inherited as an autosomal dominant trait, is the combination of skin hyperpigmentation and Peutz–Jeghers polyps in the gastrointestinal tract. The pigmentation consists of clusters of black-brown freckles about lips of buccal mucosa, perianal and genital area. Pigmented areas can occasionally be seen on the fingers and toes. The spots appear in the first year of life and tend to fade toward middle age. The polyps usually number only in the dozens and are found throughout the gastrointestinal tract. However, there is a propensity for these polyps to form in the small intestine, where they often cause intussusception. There are rare kindred in which Peutz–Jeghers polyps have been limited to the large bowel. Cases of complicating gastrointestinal carcinoma have been reported.[208] Approximately 5% of females with Peutz–Jeghers syndrome have a peculiar ovarian tumor, namely sex cord tumor with annular tubules.[209] Males with Peutz–Jeghers syndrome occasionally have unilateral or bilateral Sertoli cell tumors of the testes.[210] The gene for Peutz–Jeghers syndrome has been linked to the *SKT11* gene on chromosome 19.[211]

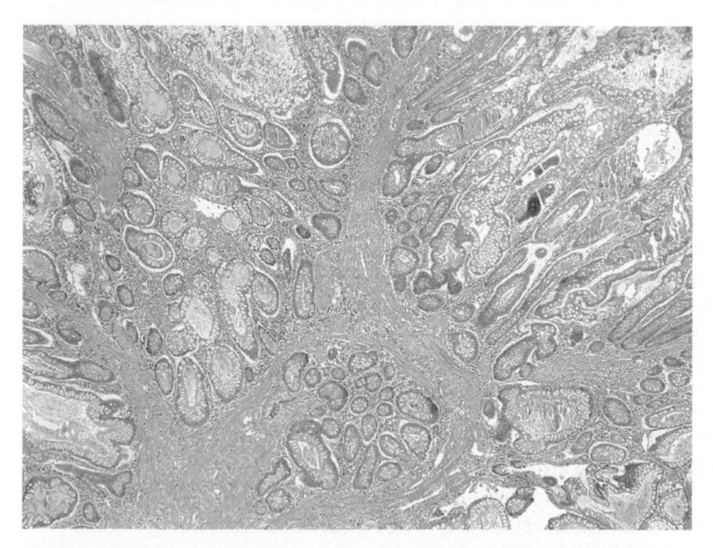

Figure 79.21: Peutz–Jeghers polyp composed of fairly normal epithelium and lamina propria lining an abnormal arborizing overgrowth of the smooth muscle of the muscularis mucosae. (*See plate section for color.*)

Esophagogastroduodenoscopy, colonoscopy, upper gastrointestinal series with small bowel follow-through are recommended in patients with Peutz–Jeghers syndrome, starting at the age of 10 years and every 2 years thereafter, although in some cases follow-up radiologic and endoscopic examination are based on clinical course and symptoms. Testicular examination starting at age 10 years, pelvic examination by age 20 years, mammographic exam by age 25 years and endoscopic ultrasonography of the pancreas by age 30 years have also been recommended.[212]

Intestinal ganglioneuromatosis

Intestinal ganglioneuromatosis is defined as proliferation of ganglion cells, neurites and supporting cells that can affect any layer of the gastrointestinal wall.[204] These proliferations often present as mucosal polyps. Although these lesions can occur as an isolated phenomenon, the importance of intestinal polypoid ganglioneuromatosis is in recognizing the other settings in which it occurs, such as von Recklinghausen's disease (*NF-1* mutation), MEN type IIB (*RET* gene mutation), Cowden's syndrome (*PTEN* mutation) and tuberous sclerosis (*TSC1* [9q34] or *TSC2* [16p13] mutation).[213–216] Intestinal ganglioneuromatosis can coexist with juvenile polyps.

Cowden's syndrome

Cowden's syndrome describes a multiple hamartoma syndrome in which patients have multiple orocutaneous hamartomas (e.g. facial trichilemmomas, mucosal papillomas), fibrocystic disease of the breast, an increased risk of breast carcinoma, thyroid abnormalities and hamartomatous polyps in the stomach, small intestine and colon. Polyps of the gastrointestinal tract, when described, have often demonstrated an abnormal proliferation of the smooth muscle lamina propria and have generally resembled the polypoid variant of solitary rectal ulcer syndrome. Intestinal ganglioneuromatosis has also been described.[216] The gene (*PTEN*) for Cowden's disease has been mapped to chromosome 10 (10q22-23).[217,218]

ACKNOWLEDGMENTS

The authors acknowledge and thank Deanna Hanson for secretarial assistance in preparing this manuscript.

References

1. Kahrilas PJ. Gastroesphageal reflux disease and its complications. In: Feldman M, Scharschmidt BF, Sleisenger MH, eds. Sleisenger and Fordtran, Gastrointestinal and Liver Disease, 6th edn. Philadelphia, PA: WB Saunders; 1998:498–517.
2. Knuff TE, Benjamin SB, Worsham GF, Hancock JE, Castell DO. Histologic evaluation of chronic gastroesophageal reflux: an evaluation of biopsy methods and diagnostic criteria. Dig Dis Sci 1984; 29:194–201.
3. Schindlbeck NE, Wiebeike B, Klauser AG, et al. Diagnostic value of histology in non-erosive gastro-esophageal reflux disease. Gut 1996; 39:151–154.
4. DeNardi FG, Riddell RH. Esophagus. In: Sternberg SS, ed. Histology for Pathologists, 2nd edn. Philadelphia, PA: Lippincott-Raven; 1997:461–493.
5. Frierson HF Jr. Histological criteria for the diagnosis of reflux esophagitis. Pathol Annu 1992; 27:87–104.
6. Collins BJ, Elliott H, Sloan JM, McFarland RJ, Love AHG. Oesophageal histology in reflux esophagitis. J Clin Pathol 1985; 38:1265–1272.
7. Ismail-Beigi F, Horton PF, Pope CE II. Histologic consequences of gastroesophageal reflux in man. Gastroenterology 1970; 58:163–174.
8. Behar J, Sheahan DC. Histologic abnormalities in reflux esophagitis. Arch Pathol 1975; 99:387–391.
9. Johnson LF, DeMeester TR, Haggitt RC. Esophageal epithelial response to gastroesophageal reflux: a quantitative study. Am J Dig Dis 1978; 23:498–509.
10. Tummala V, Barwick KW, Sontag SJ, Vlahcevic RZ, McCallum RW. The significance of intraepithelial eosinophils in the histologic diagnosis of gastroesophageal reflux. Am J Clin Pathol 1987; 87:43–48.
11. Brown LF, Goldman H, Antonioli DA. Intraepithelial eosinophils in endoscopic biopsies of adults with reflux esophagitis. Am J Surg Pathol 1984; 8:899–905.
12. Oberg S, Peters JH, DeMeester TR, et al. Inflammation and specialized intestinal metaplasia of cardiac mucosa is a manifestation of gastroesophageal reflux disease. Ann Surg 1997; 226:522–532.
13. Nandurkar S, Talley NJ, Martin CJ, et al. Short segment Barrett's esophagus: prevalence, diagnosis and associations. Gut 1997; 40:710–715.
14. Goldblum JR, Vicari JJ, Falk GW, et al. Inflammation and intestinal metaplasia of the gastric cardia: the role of gastroesophageal reflux and *H. pylori* infection. Gastroenterology 1998; 114:633–639.
15. Genta RM, Huberman RM, Graham DY. The gastric cardia in *Helicobacter pylori* infection. Hum Pathol 1994; 25:915–919.
16. Greenson JK, Beschorner WE, Boitnott JK, Yardley JH. Prominent mononuclear cell infiltrate is characteristic of herpes esophagitis. Hum Pathol 1994; 22:541–549.
17. Nash C, Ross JS. Herpetic esophagitis: a common cause of esophageal ulceration. Hum Pathol 1974; 5:339–345.
18. McKay JS, Day DW. Herpes simplex oesophagitis. Histopathology 1983; 7:409–420.
19. Singh SP, Odze RD. Multinucleated epithelial giant cell changes in esophagitis. Am J Surg Pathol 1998; 22:93–99.
20. Henson D. Cytomegalovirus inclusion bodies in the gastrointestinal tract. Arch Pathol 1972; 93:477–482.
21. Wilcox CM, Diehl DL, Cello JP, Margaretten W, Jacobson MA. Cytomegalovirus esophagitis in patients with AIDS. A clinical, endoscopic and pathologic correlation. Ann Intern Med 1990; 13:589–593.
22. Black DD, Haggitt RC, Orenstein SR, Whitington PF. Esophagitis in infants. Morphometric histological diagnosis and correlation with measures of gastroesophageal reflux. Gastroenterology 1990; 98:1408–1414.
23. Walsh SV, Antonioli DA, Goldman H, et al. Allergic esophagitis in children: a clinicopathological entity. Am J Surg Pathol 1999; 23:390–396.
24. Mahajau L, Wyllie R, Petras R, Steffan R, Kay M. Idiopathic eosinophilic esophagitis with stricture formation in a patient with longstanding eosinophilic gastroenteritis. Gastrointest Endosc 1997; 46:557–560.
25. Lee RG. Marked eosinophilia in esophageal mucosal biopsies. Am J Surg Pathol 1985; 9:475–479.
26. Orenstein SR, Shalaby TM, DiLorenzo C, Putnam PE, Sigurdson L, Kocoshis SA. The spectrum of pediatric eosinophilic esophagitis beyond infancy: a clinical series of 30 children. Am J Gastroenterol 2000; 95:1422–1430.
27. Bott S, Prakash C, McCallum RW. Medication-induced esophageal injury: survey of the literature. Am J Gastroenterol 1987; 82:758–763.
28. Kikendall JW, Friedman AC, Oyewole MA, et al. Pill induced injury. Case report and review of the medical literature. Dig Dis Sci 1983; 28:174–182.
29. Sampliner RE and the Practice Parameters Committee of the American College of Gastroenterology. Updated practice guidelines on the diagnosis, surveillance and therapy of Barrett's esophagus. Am J Gastroenterol 2002; 97: 1888–1895.
30. Petras RE, Sivak MV Jr, Rice T. Barrett's esophagus: a review of the pathologist's role in diagnosis and management. Pathol Annu 1991; 26:1–32.
31. Hassall E. Columnar-lined esophagus in children. Gastroenterol Clin North Am 1997; 26:533–548.
32. Drumm B, Sherman P, Cutz E, et al. Association of *Camyilobacter pylori* on the gastric mucosa with antral gastritis in children. N Engl J Med 1987; 316:1557–1561.
33. Shapiro JL, Goldblum, JR, Petras RE. A clinicopathologic study of 42 cases of granulomatous gastritis: is there really an isolated granulomatous gastritis? Am J Surg Pathol 1996; 20:462–470.
34. Qualman SJ, Hamoudi AB. Pediatric hypertrophic gastropathy (Ménétrièr's disease). Pediatr Pathol 1992; 12:263–268.
35. Dandalides WM, Carey WD, Petras RE, Achkar E. Endoscopic small bowel mucosal biopsy: a controlled trial evaluating forcep size and biopsy location in the diagnosis of normal and abnormal mucosal architecture. Gastrointest Endosc 1989; 35:197–200.
36. Segal GH, Petras RE. The small intestine. In: Sternberg SS, ed. Histology for Pathologists, 2nd edn. Philadelphia, PA: Lippincott-Raven; 1997:495–518.
37. Perera DR, Weinstein WM, Rubin CE. Small intestinal biopsy. Hum Pathol 1975; 6:157–217.
38. Ciclitira PJ, DeMaertelaer V, LeMoine O, Deviere J. AGA technical review on celiac sprue. Gastroenterology 2001; 120:1526–1540.
39. Walker-Smith JA, Guardlini S, Schmitz J, Shmerling PH, Visakorpi JK. Revised criteria for diagnosis of coeliac disease. Arch Dis Child 1990; 65:909–911.

40. Fasano A, Catassi C. Current approaches to diagnosis and treatment of celiac disease: an evolving spectrum. Gastroenterology 2001; 120:636–651.

41. Vogelsang H, Genser O, Wyatt J, et al. Screening for celiac disease: a prospective study on the value of noninvasive tests. Am J Gastroenterol 1995; 90:394–398.

42. Barnes GL, Townley RRW. Duodenal mucosal damage in 31 infants with gastroenteritis. Arch Dis Child 1973; 48:343–349.

43. Swanson VL, Thomasson RW. Pathology the jejunal mucosa in tropical sprue. Am J Pathol 1965; 46:511–551.

44. Ament ME, Shimoda SS, Saunders DR, Rubin CE. Pathogenesis of steatorrhea in three cases of small intestinal stasis syndrome. Gastroenterology 1972; 63:728–747.

45. Valdez R, Appelman HD, Bronner MP, Greenson JK. Diffuse duodenitis associated with ulcerative colitis. Am J Surg Pathol 2000; 24:1407–1413.

46. Matucharski C, Colin R, Hemet J, et al. Cavitation of mesenteric lymph nodes, splenic atrophy, and a flat small intestinal mucosa. Gastroenterology 1984; 87:606–614.

47. Ryan BM, Kelleher D. Refractory celiac disease. Gastroenterology 2000; 119:243–251.

48. Baker AL, Rosenberg IH. Refractory sprue: recovery after removal of nongluten dietary proteins. Ann Intern Med 1978; 89:505–508.

49. Kuitenen P, Visakorpi JK, Savilahti E, et al. Malabsorption syndromes with cow's milk intolerance. Arch Dis Child 1975; 50:351–356.

50. Ament ME, Rubin CE. Soy protein – another cause of the flat intestinal lesion. Gastroenterology 1972; 62:227–234.

51. Nagata S, Yamashiro Y, Ohtsuka Y, et al. Quantitative analysis and immunohistochemical studies on small intestinal mucosa of food-sensitive enteropathy. J Pediatr Gastroenterol Nutr 1995; 20:44–48.

52. Romer H, Urbach R, Gomez MA, Lopez A, Perozo-Ruggeri G, Vegas ME. Moderate and severe protein energy malnutrition in childhood: effects on jejunal mucosal morphology and disaccharidase activities. J Pediatr Gastroenterol Nutr 1983; 3:459–464.

53. Brunser O, Reid A, Monckeberg F, Maccioni A, Contreres I. Jejunal biopsies in infant malnutrition: with special reference to mitotic index. Pediatrics 1966; 38:605–611.

54. Barbezat GO, Bowie MD, Kaschula ROC, Hansen JDL. Studies on the small intestinal mucosa of children with protein-calorie malnutrition. S Afr Med J 1967; 41:1031–1036.

55. Arvanitakis C. Functional and morphological abnormalities of the small intestinal mucosa in pernicious anemia – a prospective study. Acta Hepatogastroenterol 1978; 25:313–318.

56. Foroozan P, Trier JS. Mucosa of the small intestine in pernicious anemia. N Engl J Med 1967; 277:553–559.

57. Smith FP, Kisner DL, Widerlite L, Schein PS. Chemotherapeutic alteration of small intestinal morphology and function: a progress report. Clin Gastroenterol 1979; 1:203–207.

58. Houtman PM, Hofstra SS, Spoelstra P. Non-celiac sprue possibly related to methotrexate in a rheumatoid arthritis patient. Neth J Med 1995; 47:113–116.

59. Davidson GP, Cutz E, Hamilton JR, et al. Familial enteropathy: a syndrome of protracted diarrhea from birth, failure to thrive, and hypoplastic villus atrophy. Gastroenterology 1978; 75:783–790.

60. Bell SW, Kerner JA Jr, Sibley RK. Microvillus inclusion disease. The importance of electron microscopy for diagnosis. Am J Surg Pathol 1991; 15:1157–1164.

61. Cutz E, Rhoades JM, Drumm B, Sherman PN, Durie PR, Forstner GG. Microvillus inclusion disease; an inherited defect of brush-border assembly and differentiation. N Engl J Med 1989; 320:646–651.

62. Groisman GM, Ben-Izhak O, Schwersenz A, Berant M, Fyfe B. The value of polyclonal carcinoembryonic antigen immunostaining in the diagnosis of microvillus inclusion disease. Hum Pathol 1993; 24: 1232–1237.

63. Groisman GM, Amar M, Livne E. CD10: a valuable tool for the light microscopic diagnosis of microvillous inclusion disease (familial microvillous atrophy). Am J Surg Pathol 2002; 26:902–907.

64. Goldstein NS, Underhill J. Morphologic features suggestive of gluten sensitivity in architecturally normal duodenal biopsy specimens. Am J Clin Pathol 2001; 116:63–71.

65. Petras R. Non-neoplastic intestinal diseases. In: Mills SE, ed. Sternberg's Diagnostic Surgical Pathology, 4th edn. Philadelphia, PA: Lippincott, Williams & Wilkins; 2004:1475–1541.

66. Unsworth J, Hutchins P, Mitchell J, et al. Flat small intestinal mucosa and auto-antibodies against the gut epithelium. J Pediatr Gastroenterol Nutr 1982; 1:503–513.

67. Mirakian R, Richardson A, Milla PJ, et al. Protracted diarrhoea of infancy: evidence in support of an autoimmune variant. BMJ 1986; 293:1132–1136.

68. Pearson RD, Swebsib I, Schaenk EA, Klish WJ, Brown MR. Fatal multisystem disease with immune enteropathy heralded by juvenile rheumatoid arthritis. J Pediatr Gastroenterol Nutr 1989; 8:259–265.

69. Catassi C, Mirakian R, Natalini G, et al. Unresponsive enteropathy associated with circulating enterocyte autoantibodies in a boy with common variable hypogammaglobulinemia and type I diabetes. J Pediatr Gastroenterol Nutr 1988; 7:608–613.

70. Steffen R, Wyllie R, Kay M, Kyllonen K, Gramlich T, Petras R. Autoimmune enteropathy in a pediatric patient: partial response to tacrolimus therapy. Clin Pediatr 1997; 36:295–299.

71. Sanderson IR, Phillips AD, Spencer J, Walker-Smith JA. Response of autoimmune enteropathy to cyclosporin A therapy. Gut 1991; 32:1421–1425.

72. Vanderhoof JA, Young RJ. Autoimmune enteropathy in a child: response to infliximab therapy. J Pediatr Gastroenterol Nutr 2002; 34:312–316.

73. Weinstein WM, Saunders DR, Tytgat GN, Rubin CE. Collagenous sprue – an unrecognized type of malabsorption. N Engl J Med 1970; 283:1297–1301.

74. Robert ME, Ament ME, Weinstein WM. The histological spectrum and clinical outcome of refractory and unclassified sprue. Am J Surg Pathol 2000; 24:676–687.

75. Hammarstrom L, Vorechovsky I, Webster D. Selective IgA deficiency (SIgAD) and common variable immunodeficiency (CVID). Clin Exp Immunol 2000; 120:225–231.

76. Cunningham-Rundles C, Bodian C. Common variable immunodeficiency: clinical and immunological features of 248 patients. Clin Immunol 1999; 92:34–48.

77. Eidelman S. Intestinal lesions in immune deficiency. Hum Pathol 1976; 7:427–434.

78. Teahon K, Webster AD, Price AB, Weston J, Bjarnason I. Studies on the enteropathy associated with primary hypogammaglobulinaemia. Gut 1994; 35:1244–1249.

79. Eidelman S, Davis SD, Rubin CE. Immunologic studies in 'hypogammaglobulinemic sprue'. Clin Res 1968; 16:117.

80. Washington K, Stenzel TT, Buckley RH, Gottfried MR. Gastrointestinal pathology in patients with common variable

immunodeficiency and X-linked agammaglobulinemia. Am J Surg Pathol 1996; 20:1240–1252.

81. Raoult D, Birg ML, La Scola B, et al. Cultivation of the bacillus of Whipple's disease. N Engl J Med 2000; 342:620–625.

82. Raoult D, La Scola B, Lecocq P, et al. Culture and immunologic detection of *Tropheryma whippelii* from the duodenum of a patient with Whipple disease. JAMA 2001; 285:1039–1043.

83. Johnstone JM, Morson BC. Eosinophilic gastroenteritis. Histopathology 1978; 2:335–348.

84. Steffen RM, Wyllie R, Petras RE, et al. The spectrum of eosinophilic gastroenteritis: report of six pediatric cases and review of the literature. Clin Pediatr 1991; 30:404–411.

85. Goldman H, Proujanksy R. Allergic proctitis and gastroenteritis in children. Am J Surg Pathol 1986; 10:75–86.

86. McNabb PC, Fleming CR, Higgins JA, Davis GL. Transmural eosinophilic gastroenteritis with ascites. Mayo Clin Proc 1979; 54: 119–122.

87. Lee M, Hodges WG, Huggins TL. Eosinophilic gastroenteritis. South Med J 1996; 89:189–194.

88. Vardy PA, Lebenthal E, Shwachman H. Intestinal lymphangiectasia: a reappraisal. Pediatrics 1975; 55:842–851.

89. Waldmann TA. Protein-losing enteropathy. Gastroenterology 1966; 50:422–443.

90. Popovic OS, Brkic S, Bojic P, et al. Sarcoidosis and protein-losing enteropathy. Gastroenterology 1980; 78:119–125.

91. Greenwood N. The jejunal mucosa in two cases of A-beta-lipoproteinemia. Am J Gastroenterol 1976; 65:160–162.

92. Joshi M, Hyams J, Treem W, Ricci AJ. Cytoplasmic vacuolization of enterocytes: an unusual histopathologic finding in juvenile nutritional megaloblastic anemia. Mod Pathol 1991; 4:62–65.

93. Reifen RM, Cutz E, Griffiths AM, Ngan BY, Sherman PM. Tufting enteropathy: a newly recognized clinicopathological entity associated with refractory diarrhea in infants. J Pediatr Gastroenterol Nutr 1994; 18:379–385.

94. Goulet O, Kedinger M, Brousse N, et al. Intractable diarrhea of infancy with epithelial and basement membrane abnormalities. J Pediatr 1995; 127:212–219.

95. Goulet OJ, Brousse N, Canioni D, et al. Syndrome of intractable diarrhea with persistent villous atrophy in early childhood: a clinicopathological survey of 47 cases. J Pediatr Gastroenterol Nutr 1998; 26:151–161.

96. Cutz E, Sherman PM, Davidson GP. Enteropathies associated with protracted diarrhea of infancy: clinicopathological features, cellular and molecular mechanisms. Ped Pathol Lab Med 1997; 17:335–367.

97. Goldman H, Antonioli DA. Mucosal biopsy of the rectum, colon, and distal ileum. Hum Pathol 1982; 13:981–1012.

98. Seldenrijk CA, Morson BC, Meuwissen SGM, Schipper NW, Lindermand J, Meijer CJLM. Histopathological evaluation of colonic mucosal biopsy specimens in chronic inflammatory bowel disease: diagnostic implications. Gut 1991; 32:1514–1520.

99. Surawicz CM, Belic L. Rectal biopsy helps to distinguish acute self-limited colitis from idiopathic inflammatory bowel disease. Gastroenterology 1984; 86:104–113.

100. Norstrant TT, Kumar NB, Appelman HD. Histopathology differentiates acute self-limited colitis from ulcerative colitis. Gastroenterology 1987; 92:318–328.

101. LeBerre N, Heresback O, Kerbaol M, et al. Histological discrimination of idiopathic inflammatory bowel disease from other types of colitis. J Clin Pathol 1995; 48:749–753.

102. Surawicz CM. Mucosal biopsy diagnosis of colitis. Semin Colon Rectal Surg 1992; 3:154–159.

103. Volk EE, Shapiro BD, Easley KA, Goldblum JR. The clinical significance of a biopsy-based diagnosis of focal active colitis: a clinicopathologic study of 31 cases. Mod Pathol 1998; 11:789–794.

104. Xin W, Brown PI, Greenson JK. The clinical significance of focal active colitis in pediatric patients. Am J Surg Pathol 2003; 27:1134–1138.

105. Odze R, Antonioli D, Peppercorn M, Goldman H. Effect of topical 5-aminosalicylic acid (5-ASA) therapy on rectal mucosal biopsy morphology in chronic ulcerative colitis. Am J Surg Pathol 1993; 17:869–875.

106. Goldstein NS, Cinenza AN. The histopathology of nonsteroidal anti-inflammatory drug-associated colitis. Am J Clin Pathol 1998; 110:622–628.

107. Deana DG, Dean PJ. Reversible ischemic colitis in young women: association with oral contraceptive use. Am J Surg Pathol 1995; 19:454–462.

108. West AB, Kuan S, Bennick M, Lagarde S. Glutaraldehyde colitis following endoscopy: clinical and pathological features and investigation of an outbreak. Gastroenterology 1005; 108:1250–1255.

109. Bjarnason I, Hayllar J, Macpherson AJ, Russell AS. Side effects of nonsteroidal anti-inflammatory drugs on the small and large intestines in humans. Gastroenterology 1993; 104:1832–1847.

110. Surawicz CM, Goodell SE, Quinn TC, et al. Spectrum of rectal biopsy abnormalities in homosexual men with intestinal symptoms. Gastroenterology 1986; 91:651–659.

111. Griffin PM, Olmstead LC, Petras RE. *Escherichia coli* O157:H7-associated colitis: a clinical and histologic study of 11 cases. Gastroenterology 1990; 99:142–149.

112. Griffin PM, Tauxe RV. The epidemiology of infections caused by *Escherichia coli* O157:H7, other enterohemorrhagic *E. coli* and the associated hemolytic uremic syndrome. Epidemiol Rev 1991; 13:60–68.

113. Griffin PM, Ostroff SM, Tauxe RV, et al. Illness associated with *Escherichia coli* O157:H7 infections: a broad clinical spectrum. Ann Intern Med 1988; 109:705–712.

114. Bartlett JG. Antibiotic associated diarrhea. N Engl J Med 2002; 346:334–339.

115. Price AB, Davies DR. Pseudomembranous colitis. J Clin Pathol 1977; 30:1–12.

116. Dignan CR, Greenson JK. Can ischemic colitis be differentiated from *C. difficile* colitis in biopsy specimens? Am J Surg Pathol 1998; 22:773–774.

117. Schulze K, Mitros FA. Eosinophilic gastroenteritis involving the ileocecal area. Dis Colon Rectum 1979; 22:47–50.

118. Tedesco FJ, Huckaby CB, Hamby-Allen M, Ewing GC. Eosinophilic ileocolitis: expanding spectrum of eosinophilic gastroenteritis. Dig Dis Sci 1981; 26:943–948.

119. Haberkern CM, Christie DL, Haas JE. Eosinophilic gastroenteritis presenting as ileocolitis. Gastroenterology 1978; 74:896–899.

120. Partyka EK, Sanowski RA, Kozarek RA. Colonoscopic features of eosinophilic gastroenteritis. Dis Colon Rectum 1980; 23:353–356.

121. Rosekrans PCM, Meijer CJLM, Van Der Wal AM, Lindeman J. Allergic proctitis, a clinical and immunopathologic entity. Gut 1980; 21:1017–1023.

122. Jenkins HR, Pincott JR, Soothill JF, Milla PJ, Harries JT. Food allergy: the major cause of infantile colitis. Arch Dis Child 1984; 59:326–329.

123. Winter HS, Antonioli DA, Fukaguwa N, Marcial M, Goldman H. Allergy-related proctocolitis in infants: diagnostic usefulness of rectal biopsy. Mod Pathol 1990; 3:5–10.

124. Warren S, Sommers SC. Pathology of regional ileitis and ulcerative colitis. JAMA 1954; 154:189–193.

125. Farmer RG, Hawk WA, Turnbull RB Jr. Regional enteritis of the colon: a clinical and pathologic comparison with ulcerative colitis. Am J Dig Dis 1968; 13:501–514.

126. Farmer M, Petras RE, Hunt LE, Janosky JE, Galandiuk S. The importance of diagnostic accuracy in colonic inflammatory bowel disease. Am J Gastroenterol 2000; 95:3184–3188.

127. Rudolph WG, Uthoff SMS, McAuliffe TL, Goode ET, Petras RE, Galandiuk S. Indeterminate colitis: the real story. Dis Colon Rectum 2002; 45:1528–1534.

128. Pezim ME, Pemberton JH, Beart RW Jr, et al. Outcome of 'indeterminant' colitis following ileal pouch–anal anastomosis. Dis Colon Rectum 1989; 32:653–658.

129. McIntyre PB, Pemberton JH, Wolff BG, Dozois RR, Beart RG Jr. Indeterminate colitis: long-term outcome in patients after ileal pouch–anal anastomosis. Dis Colon Rectum 1995; 38:51–54.

130. Wells AD, McMillian I, Price AB, et al. Natural history of indeterminate colitis. Br J Surg 1991; 78:179–181.

131. Phillips RKS. Ileal pouch–anal anastomosis for Crohn's disease. Gut 1998; 43:303–308.

132. Warren BF, Shepherd NA, Bartolo DC, Bradfield JW. Pathology of the defunctioned rectum in ulcerative colitis. Gut 1993; 34:514–516.

133. Asplund S, Gramlich T, Fazio V, Petras R. Histologic changes in defunctioned rectums in patients with inflammatory bowel disease: a clinicopathologic study of 82 patients with long follow-up. Dis Colon Rectum 2002; 45:1206–1213.

134. Cranley B. The Kock reservoir ileostomy: a review of its development, problems and role in modern surgical practice. Br J Surg 1983; 70:94–99.

135. Koltun WA, Schoetz DJ Jr, Roberts PK, et al. Indeterminate colitis predisposes to perineal complications after ileal pouch–anal anastomosis. Dis Colon Rectum 1991; 34:857–860.

136. Sandborn WJ. Pouchitis following ileal pouch–anal anastomosis: definition, pathogenesis, and treatment. Gastroenterology 1994; 107: 1856–1860.

137. Petras R. Role of the pathologist in evaluating chronic pouches. In: Hanauer SB, Bayless TM, eds. Advanced Therapy of Inflammatory Bowel Disease, 2nd edn. Hamilton, ON: BC Decker; 2001:229–232.

138. Shepherd NA, Jass JR, Duval I, et al. Restorative proctocolectomy with ileal reservoir: pathologic and histochemical study of mucosal biopsy specimens. J Clin Pathol 1987; 40:601–607.

139. Goldstein NS, Sandford WW, Bodzin JH. Crohn's-like complications in patients with ulcerative colitis after total proctocolectomy and ileal pouch–anal anastomosis. Am J Surg Pathol 1997; 21:1343–1353.

140. Wolf JM, Achkar JP, Lashner B, et al. Afferent limb ulcers predict Crohn's disease in patients with ileal pouch–anal anastomosis. Gastroenterology 2004; 126:1686–1691.

141. Setti Carraro P, Talbot JC, Nicholls RJ. Longterm appraisal of the histological appearances of the ileal reservoir mucosa after restorative proctocolectomy for ulcerative colitis. Gut 1994; 35:1721–1727.

142. Veress B, Reinholt FP, Lindquist K, et al. Long-term histomorphological surveillance of the pelvic ileal pouch: dysplasia develops in a subgroup of patients. Gastroenterology 1995; 109:1090–1097.

143. Gullberg K, Stahlberg D, Liljeqvist L, et al. Neoplastic transformation of the pelvic pouch mucosa in patients with ulcerative colitis. Gastroenterology 1997; 112:1487–1492.

144. Sarigol S, Wyllie R, Gramlich T, et al. Incidence of dysplasia in pelvic pouches in pediatric patients after ileal pouch–anal anastomosis for ulcerative colitis. J Pediatr Gastroenterol Nutr 1999; 28:429–434.

145. Faulk DL, Anuras S, Christensen J. Chronic intestinal pseudoobstruction. Gastroenterology 1978; 74:922–932.

146. Krishnamurthy S, Schuffler MD. Pathology of neuromuscular disorders of the small intestine and colon. Gastroenterology 1987; 93:610–639.

147. Schuffler MD, Beegle RG. Progressive systemic sclerosis of the gastrointestinal tract and hereditary visceral myopathy: two distinguishable disorders of intestinal smooth muscle. Gastroenterology 1979; 77:664–671.

148. Mitros FA, Schuffler MD, Teja K, Anuras S. Pathologic features of familial visceral myopathy. Hum Pathol 1982; 13:825–833.

149. Schuffler MD, Jonak Z. Chronic idiopathic intestinal pseudo-obstruction caused by a degenerative disorder of the myenteric plexus: the use of Smith's method to define neuropathology. Gastroenterology 1982; 82:476–486.

150. Schuffler MD, Baird HW, Fleming CR, et al. Intestinal pseudo-obstruction as the presenting manifestations of small-cell carcinoma of the lung: a paraneoplastic neuropathy of the gastrointestinal tract. Ann Intern Med 1983; 98:129–134.

151. Streutker CJ, Huizinga JD, Campbell F, Ho J, Riddell RH. Loss of CD117 (c-kit) and CD34-positive ICC and associated CD34-positive fibroblasts defines a subpopulation of chronic intestinal pseudo-obstruction. Am J Surg Pathol 2003; 27:228–235.

152. Gallager RL. Intestinal ceroid deposition – 'brown bowel syndrome': a light and electron microscopic study. Virchows Arch [A] Pathol Anat Histopathol 1980; 389:143–151.

153. Hitzman JL, Weiland LH, Oftedahl GL, Lie JT. Ceroidosis in the 'brown bowel syndrome'. Mayo Clin Proc 1979; 54:251–257.

154. Byers RJ, Marsh P, Parkinson D, Haboubi NY. Melanosis coli is associated with an increase in colonic epithelial apoptosis and not with laxative use. Histopathology 1997; 30:160–164.

155. Walke NI, Bennett RE, Axelsen RA. Melanosis coli: a consequence of anthraquinone-induced apoptosis of colonic epithelial cells. Am J Pathol 1988; 131:465–476.

156. Nixon HH. Hirschsprung's disease in the newborn. In: Holschneider AM, ed. Hirschsprung's disease. New York: Thieme-Stratton, 1982:103–113.

157. Molenaar JC. Pathogenetic aspects of Hirschsprung's disease. Br J Surg 1995; 82:145–147.

158. Eng C. The *RET* proto-oncogene in multiple endocrine neoplasia type 2 and Hirschsprung's disease. N Engl J Med 1996; 335:943–951.

159. Robertson K, Mason I, Hall S. Hirschsprung's disease: genetic mutation in mice and men. Gut 1997; 41:436–441.

160. Yunis EJJ, Dibbins AW, Sherman FE. Rectal suction biopsy in the diagnosis of Hirschsprung's disease in infants. Arch Pathol Lab Med 1976; 100:329–333.

161. Aldrige RT, Campbell PE. Ganglion cell distribution in the normal rectum and anal canal: a basis for the diagnosis of Hirschsprung's disease by anorectal biopsy. J Pediatr Surg 1968; 3:475–490.

162. Meier-Ruge W. Morphological diagnosis of Hirschsprung's disease. In: Holschneider AM, ed. Hirschsprung's disease. New York: Thieme-Stratton; 1982:62–71.

163. Hamoudi AB, Reiner CB, Boles ET Jr, McClung HJ, Kerzner B. Acetylthiocholinesterase staining activity of rectal mucosa. Its

use in the diagnosis of Hirschsprung's disease. Arch Pathol Lab Med 1982; 106:670–672.

164. Ariel I, Vinograd I, Lernav OZ, Nissan S, Rosenmann E. Rectal mucosal biopsy in aganglionosis and allied conditions. Hum Pathol 1983; 14:991–995.

165. Doody DP, Kim SH. Pathology of Hirschsprung's disease and related neuroenteric disorders. Semin Colon Rectal Surg 1992; 3:207–212.

166. Vinores SA, May E. Neuron-specific enolase as an immunohistochemical tool for the diagnosis of Hirschsprung's disease. Am J Surg Pathol 1985; 9:281–285.

167. Abu-Alfa AK, Kuan S, West AB, Reyes-Mugica M. Cathespin D in intestinal ganglion cells: a potential aid to diagnosis in suspected Hirschsprung's disease. Am J Surg Pathol 1997; 21:201–205.

168. Maia DM. The reliability of frozen-section diagnosis in the pathologic evaluation of Hirschsprung's disease. Am J Surg Pathol 2000; 24:1675–1677.

169. Munakata K, Okabe I, Morita K. Histologic studies of rectocolic aganglionosis and allied disease. J Pediatr Surg 1978; 13:67–75.

170. Krishnamurthy S, Heng Y, Schuffler MD. Chronic intestinal pseudo-obstruction in infants and children caused by diverse abnormalities of the myenteric plexus. Gastroenterology 1993; 104:1398–1408.

171. Scharli AF, Meier-Ruge W. Localized and disseminated forms of neuronal intestinal dysplasia mimicking Hirschsprung's disease. J Pediatr Surg 1981; 16:164–170.

172. Reiffersheid P, Flach A. Particular forms of Hirschsprung's disease. In: Holschneider AM, ed. Hirschsprung's disease. New York: Thieme-Stratton; 1982:133–142.

173. Meier-Ruge WA, Bronnimann PB, Gambazzi F, Schmid PC, Schmidt CP, Stoss F. Histopathological criteria for intestinal neuronal dysplasia of the submucosal plexus (type B). Virchows Arch 1995; 426:549–556.

174. Lake BD. Intestinal neuronal dysplasia: why does it only occur in parts of Europe? Virchows Arch 1995; 426:537–539.

175. Qualman SJ, Murray R. Aganglionosis and related disorders. Hum Pathol 1994; 25:1141–1149.

176. Yunis E, Sieber WK, Ackers DR. Does zonal aganglionosis really exist? Report of a rare variety of Hirschsprung's disease and review of the literature. Pediatr Pathol 1983; 1:33–49.

177. Seldenrijk CA, van der Harten HJ, Kluck P, Tibboel D, Moorman-Voestermans K, Meijer CJLM. Zonal aganglionosis: an enzyme and immunohistochemical study of two cases. Virchows Arch [A] Pathol Anat Histopathol 1986; 410:75–81.

178. Bussey HJR. Familial polyposis coli. Baltimore, MD: Johns Hopkins University Press; 1975.

179. Giardiello FM, Brensinger JD, Peterson GM. AGA technical review on hereditary colorectal cancer and genetic testing. Gastroenterology 2001; 121:198–231.

180. Burt RW. Hereditary polyposis syndromes and inheritance of adenomatous polyps. Semin Gastrointest Dis 1992; 3:13–21.

181. Sarre R, Frost A, Jagelman D, Petras R, Sivak M, McGannon E. Gastric and duodenal polyps in familial adenomatous polyposis: a prospective study of the nature and prevalence of upper gastrointestinal polyps. Gut 1987; 28:306–314.

182. Offerhaus GJA, Giardiello FM, Krush AJ, et al. The risk of upper gastrointestinal cancer in familial adenomatous polyposis. Gastroenterology 1992; 102:1980–1982.

183. Kinzler KW, Nilbert MC, Su LK, et al. Identification of FAP locus genes from chromosome 5q21. Science 1991; 253:661–665.

184. Burt RW, Groden J. The genetic and molecular diagnosis of adenomatous polyposis coli. Gastroenterology 1993; 104:1211–1214.

185. Powell SM, Petersen GM, Krush AJ, et al. Molecular diagnosis of familial adenomatous polyposis. N Engl J Med 1993; 329:1982–1987.

186. Lynch HT, Smyrk T, McGinn T, et al. Attenuated familial adenomatous polyposis (AFAP). A phenotypically and genotypically distinctive variant of FAP. Cancer 1995; 76:2427–2433.

187. Hamilton SR, Liu B, Parsons RE, et al. The molecular basis of Turcot's syndrome. N Engl J Med 1995; 332:839–847.

188. Sieber OM, Lipton L, Crabtree M, et al. Multiple colorectal adenomas, classic adenomatous polyposis, and germ-line mutations in *MYH*. N Engl J Med 2003; 348:791–799.

189. Wang L, Baudhuin LM, Boardman LA, et al. *MYH* mutations in patients with attenuated and classic polyposis and with young-onset colorectal cancer without polyps. Gastroenterology 2004; 127:9–16.

190. Boland CR. Understanding familial colorectal cancer – finding the corner pieces and filling the center of the puzzle. Gastroenterology 2004; 127:334–343.

191. Wirtzfeld DA, Petrelli NJ, Rodriquez-Bigas MA. Hamartomatous polyposis syndromes: molecular genetics neoplastic risk, and surveillance recommendations. Ann Surg Oncol 2001; 8:319–327.

192. Nugent KP, Talbot IC, Hodgson SV, Phillips RKS. Solitary juvenile polyps: not a marker for subsequent malignancy. Gastroenterology 1993; 105:698–700.

193. Aaltonen LA, Jass JR, Howe JR. Juvenile polyposis. In: Hamilton SR, Aaltonen LA, eds. World Health Organization Classification of Tumours: Pathology and Genetics of Tumours of the Digestive System. Lyons: International Agency for Research on Cancer; 2000:130–133.

194. Jass JR, Williams CB, Bussey HJR, Morson BC. Juvenile polyposis – a precancerous condition. Histopathology 1998; 13:619–630.

195. Grotsky HW, Rickert RR, Smith WD, Newsome JF. Familial juvenile polyposis coli. A clinical and pathologic study of a large kindred. Gastroenterology 1992; 82:494–501.

196. Sachatello CR, Pickren JW, Grace JT. Generalized juvenile gastrointestinal polyposis. A hereditary syndrome. Gastroenterology 1970; 58:699.

197. Watanabe A, Nagashima H, Motoi M, Ogawa K. Familial juvenile polyposis of the stomach. Gastroenterology 1979; 77:148–151.

198. Whitelaw SC, Murday VA, Tomlinson IPM, et al. Clinical and molecular features of the hereditary mixed polyposis syndrome. Gastroenterology 1997; 112:327–334.

199. Giardello FM, Hamilton SR. Hereditary mixed polyposis syndrome: a zebra or a horse dressed in pinstripes. Gastroenterology 1997; 112:643–659.

200. Howe JR, Roth S, Ringold JC, et al. Mutations in the *SMAD4/DPC4* gene in juvenile polyposis. Science 1998; 280:1086–1088.

201. Zhou XP, Woodford-Richens K, Lehtonen R, et al. Germline mutations in *BMPR1A/ALK3* cause a subset of cases of juvenile polyposis syndrome and of Cowden and Bannayan–Riley–Ruvalcaba syndromes. Am J Hum Genet 2001; 69:704–711.

202. Weidner N, Flanders DJ, Mitros FA. Mucosal ganglioneuromatosis associated with multiple colonic polyps. Am J Surg Pathol 1984; 8:779–786.

203. Pham BN, Villanueva RP. Ganglioneuromatosis proliferation associated with juvenile polyposis coli. Arch Pathol Lab Med 1989; 113:91–94

204. Haggitt RC, Reid BJ. Hereditary gastrointestinal polyposis syndromes. Am J Surg Pathol 1986; 10:871–887.

205. Zigman AF, Lavin JE, Jones MC, Boland CR, Carethers JM. Localization of the Bannayan–Riley–Ruvalcaba syndrome gene to chromosome 10q23. Gastroenterology 1997; 113:1433–1437.

206. Spigelman AD, Arese P, Phillips RKS. Polyposis: the Peutz–Jeghers syndrome. Br J Surg 1995; 82:1311–1314.

207. Estrada R, Spjut HJ. Hamartomatous polyps in Peutz–Jeghers syndrome. A light, histochemical and electron-microscopic study. Am J Surg Pathol 1983; 7:747–754.

208. Giardiello FM, Welsh SB, Hamilton SR, et al. Increased risk of cancer in the Peutz–Jeghers syndrome. N Engl J Med 1987; 316:1511–1514.

209. Scully RE. Sex cord tumor with annular tubules – a distinctive ovarian tumor of the Peutz–Jeghers syndrome. Cancer 1970; 25:1107–1121.

210. Wilson DM, Pitts WC, Hintz RL, Rosenfeld RG. Testicular tumors with Peutz–Jeghers syndrome. Cancer 1986; 57:2238–2240.

211. Trojan J, Brieger A, Raedle J, Roth WK, Zeuzem S. Peutz–Jeghers syndrome: Molecular analysis of a three-generation kindred with a novel defect in the serine threonine kinase gene *STK11*. Am J Gastroenterol 1999; 94:257–261.

212. McGarrity TJ, Kulin HE, Zaino RJ. Peutz–Jeghers syndrome. Am J Gastroenterol 2000; 95:596–604.

213. Devroede G, Lemieux B, Masse S, LaMarche J, Herman PS. Colonic hamartomas in tuberous sclerosis. Gastroenterology 1988; 94:182–188.

214. Shekitka KM, Sobin LH. Ganglioneuromas of the gastrointestinal tract. Relation to VonRecklinghausen disease and other multiple tumor syndromes. Am J Surg Pathol 1994; 18:250–257.

215. d'Amore ESG, Manivel C, Pettinato G, Neihans GA, Snover DC. Intestinal ganglioneuromatosis: mucosal and transmural types. A clinicopathologic and immunohistochemical study of six cases. Hum Pathol 1991; 22:276–286.

216. Lashner BA, Riddell RH, Winans CS. Ganglioneuromatosis of the colon and extensive glycogenic acanthosis in Cowden's disease. Dig Dis Sci 1986; 31:213–216.

217. Marsh DJ, Dahia PL, Coulon V, et al. Allelic imbalance, including deletion of *PTEN/MMACI*, at the Cowden disease locus on 10q22-23, in hamartomas from patients with Cowden syndrome and germline *PTEN* mutation. Genes Chromosomes Cancer 1998; 21:61–69.

218. Tsou HC, Pink XL, Xie XX, et al. The genetic basis of Cowden's syndrome: three novel mutations in *PTEN/MMAC1/TEP1*. Human Genetics 1998; 102:467–473.

Chapter 80
Endoscopic retrograde cholangiopancreatography

Lisa Feinberg and Moises B. Guelrud

INTRODUCTION

Endoscopic retrograde cholangiopancreatography (ERCP) is a technique used to acquire diagnostic information and to perform therapy for disorders of the biliary tree and pancreas in patients of all ages. The procedure requires an endoscopist skilled in the placement of a specialized side-viewing duodenoscope and provides direct radiographs of the biliary tree and pancreatic duct. Extensive experience with ERCP in the adult literature accrued in the 1970s, and the first reports of ERCP in infants and children were chiefly from adult gastroenterologists experienced with the technique. The use of this technique in children is limited, in part due to the lack of pediatric gastroenterologists trained in ERCP, and also due to the relatively low incidence of disease requiring this type of evaluation in the pediatric population. As a result, adult gastroenterologists in collaboration with their colleagues in pediatric gastroenterology are often called upon to perform this highly useful procedure.

Soon after the gastroscope was introduced and the papilla of Vater was visualized in the duodenum, placement of a catheter through the endoscope to cannulate the major papilla with subsequent injection of contrast material to fill the common bile duct and pancreatic ducts became possible. McCune et al.[1] described the first endoscopic cannulation of the ampulla of Vater in 1968. A lateral-viewing duodenoscope became available outside of Japan in 1970, and the literature that followed described new aspects of diseases such as sclerosing cholangitis and sophisticated therapeutic applications. In 1976, Waye[2] reported the first ERCP in a pediatric patient by performing the procedure on a 6.0-kg 14-week-old jaundiced infant with the standard adult cannulating instrument. One of the authors (M.G.) has performed the procedure successfully in infants weighing as little as 2.5 kg with a smaller instrument designed for pediatric patients.[3]

ERCP is safe in infants and children, and can be performed with intravenous medication for conscious sedation or under general anesthesia for very young infants, children or adolescents unable to cooperate under sedation alone. Success rates of cannulating the relevant duct(s) in pediatric patients are as high as 95–96%.[4,5] Several series have been reported evaluating the diagnostic yield, therapeutic uses and complications of ERCP examinations in pediatric patients.[3–19]

ALTERNATE METHODS FOR IMAGING THE LIVER AND PANCREAS

Several imaging modalities are available for the diagnosis of pancreaticobiliary disease. Ultrasonography is the screening method of choice for gallstones at any age and for pancreaticobiliary ductal dilation, and is frequently used by pediatric gastroenterologists because it is non-invasive, readily available and does not expose the patient to radiation. Ultrasonography is helpful in detecting and estimating the degree of biliary and pancreatic ductal dilation or in detecting pseudocysts, but may fail to provide accurate information about the distal common bile duct and mid to distal pancreas due to overlying bowel gas. Computed tomography (CT) is useful for evaluating hepatic parenchymal lesions, and has application for defining liver and pancreatic abnormalities. However, it provides only limited information about ductal anatomy, although advances in CT technique have improved ductal visualization. CT and ultrasonography may fail to detect stones or lesions in the distal common bile duct.[20]

Appropriate selection of the imaging technique depends on the pathologic process.[21] Barium contrast examination may show displacement of the duodenal C-loop or stomach secondary to mass effect from pancreatic or biliary lesions, but otherwise has a minor role in the diagnosis of pancreaticobiliary lesions. Radionuclide scanning is discussed in detail below in the section on biliary atresia.

Percutaneous transhepatic cholangiography (PTC) is another method used to image the biliary tree. This invasive procedure requires adequately sized or dilated bile ducts in order to inject contrast material, may not image the distal common bile duct, cannot image the pancreatic duct (unless anomalous connection is present) and adds risk owing to hepatic puncture.[22] A randomized trial of 60 consecutive patients comparing ERCP with PTC found comparable success rates and complications bewteen the procedures. Both procedures may need to be followed by surgical intervention in patients with obstruction diagnosed at the time of the procedure in order to avoid septic compications.[23] If required, bilary drains may be placed at the time of PTC. PTC should be considered when prior surgery or malrotations of the small bowel prevent duodenal intubation with the endoscope. Hemorrhage and bile peritonitis may complicate PTC, and a laparotomy may be needed for management of these complications.[23] The availability of these tests and local resources may influence the choice of studies for initial evaluation.

Magnetic resonance cholangiopancreatography (MRCP) is a useful tool for imaging the bile ducts and pancreatic ducts. It is non-invasive and can provide information about the patient's anatomy and the presence of obstruction, stricture, neoplasm or injury following trauma.[24,25] Disadvantages of MRCP include the need for sedation in younger or uncooperative patients. MRCP is also operator dependent and requires a radiologist experienced in its performance and interpretation. ERCP remains the most useful study when therapy is required.

TECHNIQUE OF ERCP

A well equipped endoscopy suite, including equipment for monitoring vital signs and oxygen saturation, and medications for resuscitation, is required for patients of all ages. Occasionally ERCP is done in the operating room, and fluoroscopic equipment is required. Pediatric endoscopy assistants and specially trained nurses can help reduce pre-procedure anxiety, monitor the clinical status of the patient, and assist in holding and reassuring the child,[26,27] medication administration, handling of biopsy forceps and injection of contrast material.

Preparation for ERCP is the same as for upper gastrointestinal endoscopy except for requirements for antibiotic prophylaxis and the potential need for pre-procedure laboratory work.[26] A period of fasting precedes sedation and intubation with the endoscope, and this is age dependent. An intravenous line is placed for sedation and administration of glucagon or other medications to reduce duodenal peristalsis.

Premedication can be administered to sedate the child, minimize discomfort and induce amnesia. General anesthesia may be necessary for very young infants and children or selected older patients. A combination of meperidine (1–2 mg/kg, to a maximum of 100 mg) and midazolam (0.05–0.15 mg/kg, usually to a maximum of 5 mg) is administered slowly.[27] Occasionally atropine or glucagon is given when the duodenum is intubated to reduce peristalsis to allow for cannulation of the ampulla. Somatostatin is being used in clinical trials during ERCP because of its effect on decreasing gastrointestinal secretions[28] and producing transient small-bowel atony.

Antibiotic prophylaxis for prevention of infective endocarditis is given according to the current guidelines of the American Heart Association for children with congenital and rheumatic heart disease.[29,30] For patients with suspected obstructive jaundice or an obstructed biliary tree, and those with a pancreatic pseudocyst, antibiotics are also administered to prevent septic complications from cholangitis or pancreatic abscess formation from injection of contrast material into an inadequately drained space. Antibiotics are also recommended when a stricture, stone or space-occupying lesion is seen on ERCP.[31] Current guidelines should be followed for children with a valvular prosthesis, vascular graft material and indwelling catheters, or status following organ transplant and in immunosuppressed patients. These are discussed in Chapter 81 and elsewhere.[29,30]

The standard adult side-viewing duodenoscope and therapeutic adult-sized duodenoscopes have been used in infants younger than 1 year of age.[2,14] Specialized smaller-caliber pediatric side-viewing instruments are now available (Olympus Corporation, Lake Success, NY, USA). The initial pediatric side-viewing duodenoscope was manufactured without a cannula elevator mechanism and was used successfully in very young infants.[3,32] The commercial model includes an elevator and has an insertion tube with an outer diameter of 7.5 mm, an 80° field of view, and deflection capability of 120° upwards and 90° to the right, left and down. A 2-mm channel is designed to exit the side of the endoscope. The arrival of videoendoscopy using a charge-couple device with a television system has added several new dimensions of maneuverability and a lighter weight to the instrument, as well as the ability to store and retrieve the endoscopic images.[33] A different pediatric ERCP scope has an insertion tube outer diameter of 8.0 mm, a cannula with an elevator, a 100° field of view and a 2-mm instrument channel, and has been used recently in a series of pediatric patients reported by Kato et al.,[34] with a 90% success rate and no reported complications.

Operator experience correlates with the degree of technical success in ERCP.[35] Care is taken to disinfect the equipment before and after each use, but the procedure is not sterile as the insertion tube passes through the oropharynx. Use of pharyngeal sprays to anesthetize the pharynx is not required, but can be used at the operator's discretion. After adequate intravenous sedation, a plastic bite-block is inserted between the teeth, and intubation of the esophagus is done 'blindly'. After the endoscope is guided into the descending duodenum, the papilla is brought into close position so the desired target duct may be cannulated from an *en face* position. The patient is lying in the left lateral decubitus position on a padded table, and is later adjusted to the prone position for more favorable angle of access to the papilla. A Teflon catheter is manipulated into the papilla, and the gastrointestinal assistant injects contrast material through the primed tubing into the pancreatic and bile ducts. Care must be taken to remove any air in the syringe containing contrast material because the introduction of air bubbles into the liver and pancreas will appear as rounded filling defects, simulating stones. Tilting the patient on the table will cause air to rise and heavier filling defects to settle downward. Diluted contrast material is preferred for optimal visualization if filling defects are anticipated in the ducts. Special tapered-tip cannulae should be available for pediatric patients and for negotiating the accessory papilla if necessary. Most endoscopists use a sphincterotome instead of a cannula as a primary cannulation device. The sphincterotome has the ability to flex the tip, increasing the likelihood of cannulating the desired duct. Selected fluoroscopic images are recorded, and therapeutic maneuvers may be performed.

After removal of the endoscope, placing the patient in the supine position and reverse Trendelenburg facilitates filling

Congenital anomalies
Biliary atresia *vs* neontal hepatitis
Alagille's syndrome and paucity syndrome
Congenital hepatic fibrosis
Caroli's disease and Caroli's syndrome
Biliary strictures due to cystic fibrosis
Choledochal cyst
Benign biliary strictures
Acquired diseases
Bile plug syndrome
Primary sclerosing cholangitis
Biliary obstruction due to parasitic infestation
Choledocholithiasis
Benign biliary strictures
Common bile duct complications after liver transplantation

Table 80.1 Biliary conditions identified at ERCP in neonates and children

of the upper hepatic ducts by gravity.[2] Spot films may be taken fluoroscopically without the endoscope in the field. Photo-documentation of the ampullary region is possible.

Small 'daughter' or 'baby' cholangioscopes have been designed to pass through the 'mother' duodenoscope and into the biliary and pancreatic ducts for choledochoscopy, cholangioscopy and pancreatoscopy. This technical advancement has limited application in children and, to date, has been reported only in older patients.

INDICATIONS

The only indication for ERCP in neonates and young infants is cholestasis. Biliary indications for ERCP in children older than 1 year and in adolescents include obstructive jaundice, known or suspected choledocholithiasis, abnormal liver enzymes in children with inflammatory bowel disease, evaluation of biliary ductal leaks after cholecystectomy or liver transplantation, evaluation of abnormal scans (ultrasonography, CT or MRCP) and therapeutic ERCP.

Pancreatic indications for ERCP in children include non-resolving acute pancreatitis, idiopathic recurrent pancreatitis, chronic pancreatitis, evaluation of persistently increased levels of pancreatic enzymes, evaluation of abnormal scans (ultrasonography, CT or MRCP), evaluation of pancreatic pseudocysts and pancreatic ascites, evaluation of pancreatic ductal leaks from blunt abdominal trauma, and therapeutic ERCP. In patients whose liver is transplanted, the integrity of the anastomosis can be studied, and dilated if necessary; bile leaks may also be found.[36]

Biliary disorders

Diagnosis of biliary atresia and neonatal hepatitis

The neonatal liver is susceptible to a wide variety of injuries, but the histologic reaction is often stereotypic. Liver biopsy may demonstrate cholestasis, giant cell transformation, inflammation, hepatocellular necrosis, extramedullary hematopoiesis, fibrosis and bile duct proliferation. The findings on biopsy of several cholestatic diseases of the liver may overlap in early infancy.[37] The differential diagnosis of idiopathic neonatal obstructive cholangiopathies is critical in the first weeks of life because early performance of a hepatoportoenterostomy in patients with biliary atresia is known to reduce morbidity and mortality.[38–43]

Exclusion of infectious, metabolic and other causes of prolonged cholestasis in the newborn will leave 70–80% of patients with a conjugated hyperbilirubinemia; the key differentiation in these patients is between extrahepatic biliary atresia and neonatal hepatitis.[44] Without treatment, patients with biliary atresia will ultimately develop cirrhosis, and rapid identification of this condition is necessary because the success rate of establishing bile flow declines after 2 months of age.[45] None of the available tests or combinations of them have been 100% reliable in diagnosing biliary atresia.[46,47] Although various methods of collecting duodenal fluid for the presence of bile have been promising,[48] diagnosis of biliary atresia has been described in an infant who produced green duodenal fluid at 2 weeks of age.[49]

Cox et al.,[45] in a prospective study of 33 neonates with conjugated hyperbilirubinemia, compared the results of serum liver enzymes, ultrasonography and liver biopsy with technetium-99m-disofenin scanning. When excretion of radioisotope was seen, biliary atresia was excluded, but scanning required a week and was less specific than ultrasonography and liver biopsy. Liver biopsy was 100% sensitive and 87% specific for biliary atresia, and technetium-99m-disofenin scanning was 100% sensitive and only 67% specific. Ultrasonography was 78% sensitive and 75% specific. Measurement of liver enzymes in that study[45] and their rate of increase in another study[50] lacked sensitivity and specificity for biliary atresia. The authors concluded that radionuclide liver scanning was no more reliable than the other available tests and consumed valuable time in the preoperative period. Administration of 5 mg per kg per day of phenobarbital for 5 days before radionuclide scanning is known to enhance and accelerate biliary excretion of the technetium tracer, thereby increasing the accuracy of the test. In one study,[51] phenobarbital pretreatment identified six infants with neonatal hepatitis whose previous scans showed no excretion by the liver in one study. When delayed or absent excretion of tracer is encountered, the scan can be carried out over 1–2 days. This may add up to a week for the evaluation, and decrease the chance of a favorable response to a Kasai procedure.[52] Severe neonatal hepatitis can also show lack of excretion of radionuclide label and cause a false-positive reading of biliary atresia. Absent gallbladder activity is characteristic of biliary atresia on scanning. Some 20% of patients with biliary atresia will have a gallbladder seen on ultrasonography.[51] Apparent gut excretion of tracer on technetium-99m-DISIDA (di-isopropyl-acetanilido-imino-diacetic acid; disofenin) scanning can lead to false-negative results for biliary atresia that has been diagnosed by liver biopsy.[52]

Laparotomy with intraoperative cholangiography and wedge hepatic biopsy has been considered the best available method to establish the presence or absence of biliary atresia. If biliary atresia is identified, the surgeon can proceed with a Kasai procedure. The chief disadvantage of this approach is that many infants with neonatal hepatitis will undergo surgery to exclude biliary stresia, and some infants with other diseases causing cholestasis, such as arteriohepatic dysplasia (Alagille's syndrome),[53] will have a hepatoportoenterostomy but remain cholestatic. Although failure of contrast material to flow retrogradely into the liver despite clamping of the distal common bile duct is accepted as diagnostic of biliary atresia, this cholangiographic appearance may also be seen with Alagille's syndrome. Proliferation of bile ducts on liver biopsy is typical for biliary atresia, but percutaneous liver biopsy may result in insufficient tissue for diagnosis, and early biopsy may not be diagnostic. Another approach taken by some authors is laparoscopy by 4 weeks of age with liver biopsy and simultaneous cholangiography by transhepatic puncture of the gallbladder. Hirsig and Rickham[43] have suggested then proceeding to the Kasai operation, utilizing the same general anesthesia.

In 1979, Lebwohl and Waye[54] published the first report of ERCP in a 4-month-old infant with biliary atresia, using the adult side-viewing instrument. There were no complications and the authors believed the study would be of value in identifying infants who required surgery that could be done expediently in the first 1–2 months of life, when biliary drainage had a higher chance of being successful. Many examinations have subsequently been accomplished using standard lateral-viewing duodenoscopes in infants for this indication.[14] Reported post-procedure problems include duodenal erosions, abdominal distention and retching from air insufflation, but these conditions may be seen to occur after any upper endoscopic procedure and are not thought to be clinically significant.

In a series of 23 jaundiced infants ranging in age from 19 to 150 days, Guelrud et al.[3] used a miniaturized prototype pediatric duodenoscope to perform ERCP. The insertion tube was 8.5 mm in diameter and had a field view of 80°. Four-way tip deflection to 120° upwards and 90° in the other planes was possible. The instrument has a forceps channel of 2 mm in diameter. Cannulation of the papilla was successful in 22 infants, and in 13 of 14 patients with neontal hepatitis, opacification of the common bile duct was thought to exclude biliary atresia. In six of seven infants with biliary atresia, only a pancreatogram was obtained, and biliary atresia was suspected; unnecessary surgery was avoided in most of these infants with neonatal jaundice. In very young infants, little or no sedation was needed. These infants ranged in size from 2.4 to 7.3 kg. Examinations were performed quickly, within a mean of 8 (range 2–18) min, and no complications were reported. Bile was seen in the duodenum in 12 patients, a finding believed to exclude biliary atresia; however, some infants with biliary atresia may have partial or segmental drainage.

In their larger published series of 32 cholestatic infants in whom ERCP was performed with the Olympus PJF prototype duodenoscope, Guelrud et al.[7] distinguished three types of biliary atresia (Fig. 80.1). In type 1, there is no visualization of the biliary tree. Type 2 describes visualization of the distal common bile duct and gallbladder, with no visualization of the main hepatic or intrahepatic ducts. In type 3, there is visualization of the distal common bile duct, gallbladder and segment of the main hepatic duct, with biliary lakes at the porta hepatis.[7] In some infants with biliary atresia with type 2 ERCP findings, there can be normal ultrasonographic emptying of the gallbladder despite the absence of the main hepatic duct. In addition, in one series three of six infants with type 3 ERCP findings had bile in the duodenum.[7] Neonatal hepatitis (Fig. 80.2) and biliary atresia (Figs 80.3–80.5) are illustrated radiographically.

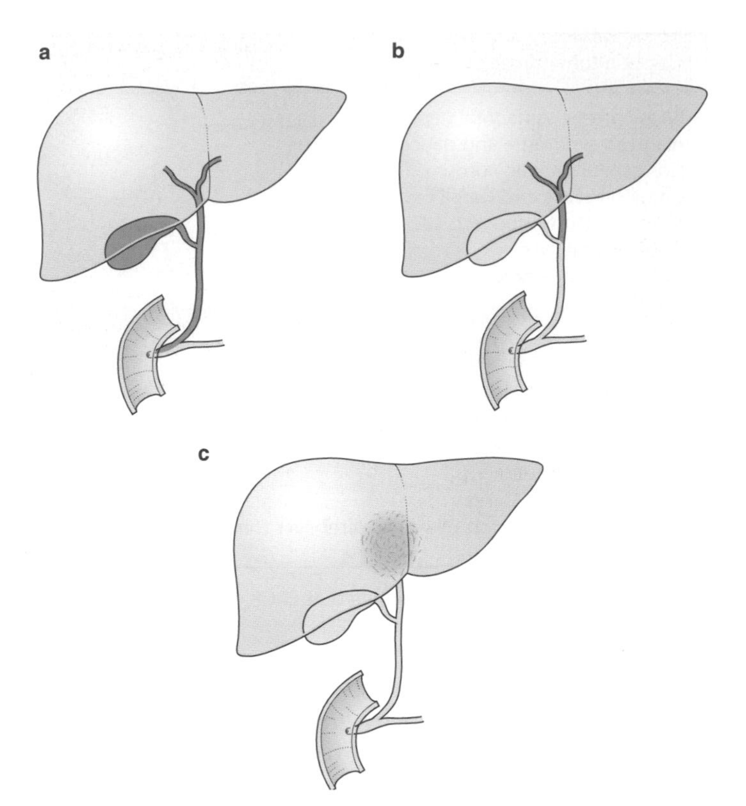

Figure 80.1: Schematic representation of the radiologic findings at ERCP in biliary atresia. In type 1 (**a**) there is no visualization of biliary tree. Type 2 (**b**) involves opacification of the distal common duct and gallbladder without visualization of the main hepatic duct. Type 3 (**c**) is divided in two subtypes: in Type 3a there is visualization of the distal common duct, the gallbladder and a segment of the main hepatic duct with biliary lakes at the porta hepatis; and in Type 3b both hepatic ducts are seen with biliary lakes.

Matsuo et al.[55] used two modified fiberscopes with an outside diameter of 5 mm for assessment of the porta hepatis in a group of nine Japanese children with biliary atresia to evaluate of biliary drainage after surgery and to determine the success of the hepatic portoenterostomy. They reported removal of bile clots from the tiny ducts and endoscopic washing or brushing to treat postoperative complications such as cholangitis.

Ohnuma et al.[17] performed a total of 75 ERCPs in 73 infants with an age range of 8–300 (mean 71) days; 52 patients were found to have biliary atresia, 10 had infantile hepatitis, 5 had congenital biliary dilation, 3 had bile duct

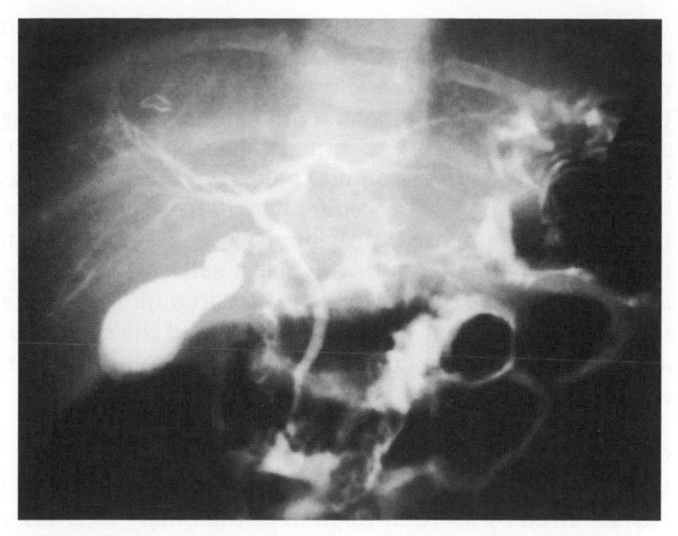

Figure 80.2: Neonatal hepatitis in a 41-day-old infant. A normal biliary tree is observed.

paucity, 2 had duodenal atresia and 1 had postoperative jaundice after surgery for hepatoblastoma. The ampulla of Vater was identified and cannulated successfully in 88% of patients. These authors reported four patterns on ERCP, classified according to the degree of filling of portions of the biliary and pancreatic ducts. In pattern 1, the pancreatic duct alone, or the pancreatic duct and a choledochal cyst, was visualized. Pattern 2 consisted of visualization of the pancreatic duct and a short, dilated common bile duct. Pattern 3 demonstrated the pancreatic duct and the entire length of the common bile duct, but no filling of the common hepatic duct or gallbladder. In pattern 4 the pancreatic duct, common bile duct and gallbladder were visualized, but the common hepatic duct was not seen. During the study, patients' urinary and serum amylase levels were monitored and they were observed for evidence of

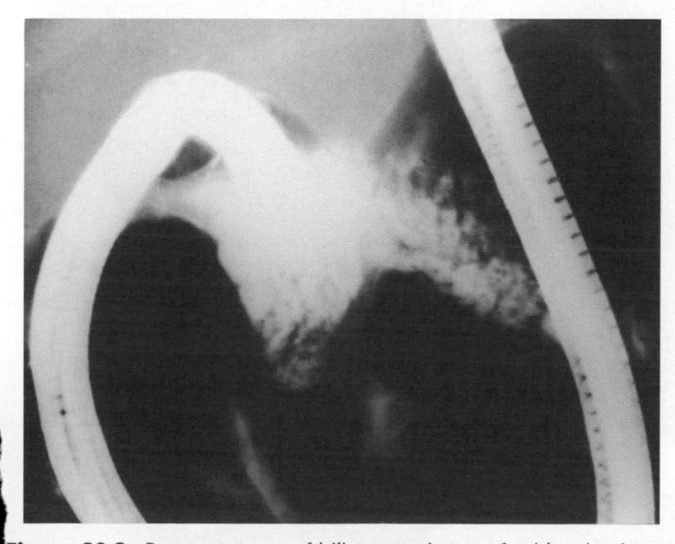

Figure 80.3: Pancreatogram of biliary atresia type 1 with acinarization. No opacification of the biliary tree is seen despite several maneuvers to opacify the common duct.

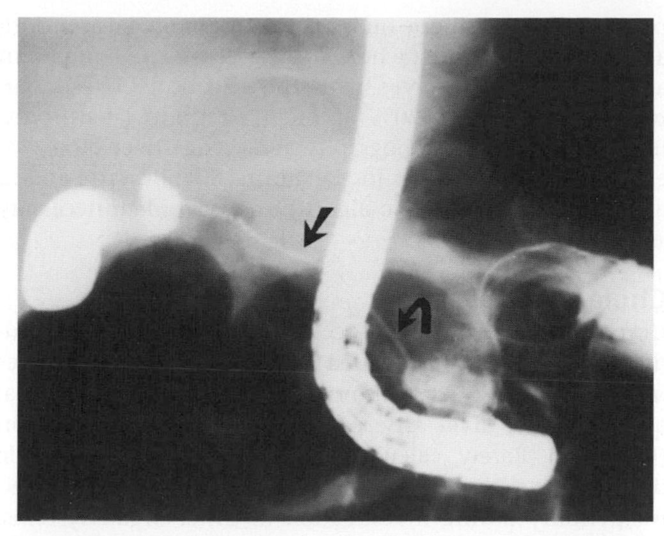

Figure 80.4: Biliary atresia type 2. A distal, narrowed and irregular common bile duct is seen (curved arrow). The cystic duct is wider than the common duct (straight arrow). The gallbladder is normal. No opacification of the main hepatic ducts or the intrahepatic ducts is seen.

infection, pain and vomiting. There were no complications caused by ERCP or anesthesia.[17]

ERCP is the most direct method of establishing a diagnosis of biliary atresia in the hands of endoscopists able to

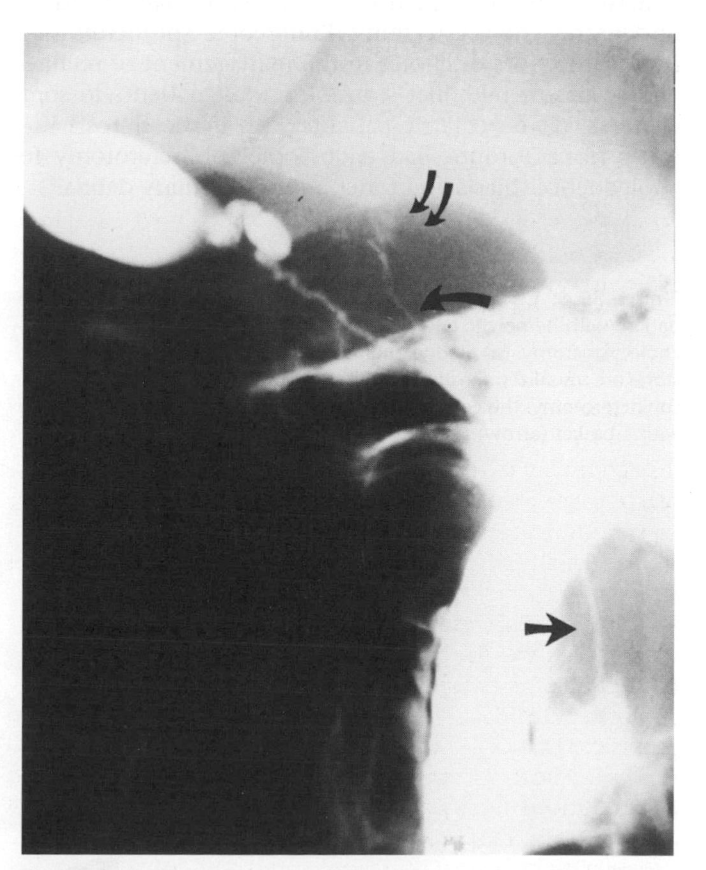

Figure 80.5: Biliary atresia type 3 in a 31-day-old neonate. A distal narrow common bile duct (straight arrow) and a main narrowed hepatic duct (single curved arrow) are visualized. Multiple biliary lakes are seen at the porta hepatis (double curved arrows). The gallbladder is normal.

perform this technique on neonates, and may be appropriate as the first-line test when such expertise and equipment are available.[56] However, with the selection of tests currently available, 10–20% of infants require laparotomy, intraoperative cholangiography and wedge liver biopsy to establish the diagnosis. In the future, ERCP may be used earlier in the diagnostic algorithm to avoid unnecessary surgical interventions.

Choledocholithiasis

Common bile duct calculi occur rarely in infants and children.[57] Conditions associated with the presence of stones include biliary tract malformations such as choledochal cyst, chronic liver disease,[58] hemolysis and infection (Fig. 80.6). Rarely, calculi are noted in the common bile duct without any known etiology. These may be found incidentally during investigation of other organ systems, and may pass spontaneously. Larger stones, however, may have impact at the distal common bile duct and result in clinical and biochemical obstructive jaundice, even in infants. Ultrasonography and MRCP are useful as diagnostic modalities, but interventions require ERCP. Endoscopic sphincterotomy with clearing of the duct by dragging out debris using a Fogarty catheter has been reported in a 3-year-old child.[59] Guelrud et al.[60] have used endoscopic sphincterotomy to remove common bile duct stones in six jaundiced children (aged 6–12 years) who had previously undergone cholecystectomy. Endoscopic sphincterotomy is the procedure of choice in the management of retained and recurrent bile duct stones for adult patients in some centers.[61] Five pediatric patients with cystic fibrosis in a series from Toronto had endoscopic sphincterotomy for choledocholithiasis and for clearance of biliary debris.[4]

Manometric studies of the sphincter of Oddi have been combined with ERCP in the investigation of biliary dyskinesia, by sliding a water-perfused catheter with a pressure transducer into the papilla and recording pressures during a pull-through maneuver. Normal values have been established in adults,[62] and endoscopic sphincterotomy has been done during the procedure when increased pressures have been documented, providing relief of symptoms in the majority of patients in this select subset.[63, 64] Opiates are not used for sedation with this procedure because of their known effect on the smooth muscle of the sphincter, and therefore higher doses of benzodiazepines are often administered.

Choledochal cyst

Choledochal cyst is a malformation of the biliary tract characterized by saccular dilation of the biliary tree. They were classified into three types by Alonso-Lej et al. in 1959.[65] It is speculated that anomalous connection of the pancreatic and bile ducts is a factor in the development of a choledochal cyst, and that the cyst itself may be acquired. A long common channel[66] distal to the anomalous junction of the pancreatic and biliary ducts is present, with or without stenosis at the papilla.[67] Okada et al.[68] reported a series of six patients. All were very young children with common channel syndrome characterized by jaundice, abdominal pain, vomiting and fever. The diagnosis was confirmed by ERCP. Only 20–40% of patients present with the triad of jaundice, right upper quadrant mass and pain, and signs may be intermittent. Recurrent pancreatitis may also occur secondary to a choledochal cyst or anomaly of the distal shared pancreaticobiliary duct.[69,70]

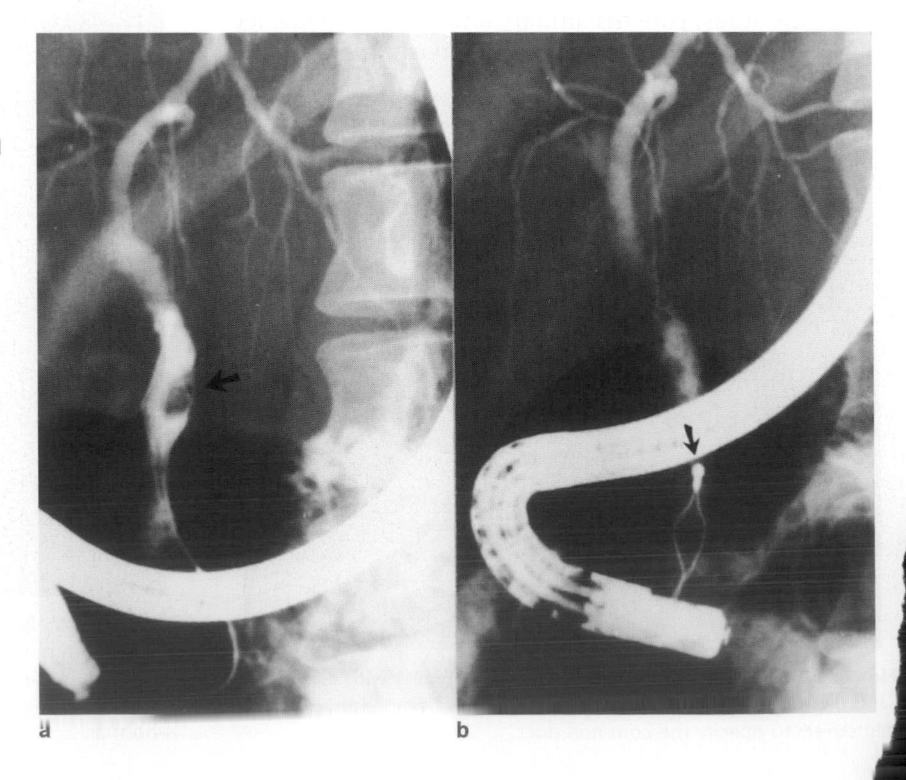

Figure 80.6: Choledocholithiasis in a 12-year-old patient with hemolytic anemia after cholecystectomy. (**a**) Sludge and a common bile stone are visualized (arrow). (**b**) After endoscopic sphincterotomy, the common duct stone is retrieved with a basket (arrow).

The first and most common type of choledochal cyst is congenital cystic dilation of the common bile duct, in which the terminal common bile duct is frequently narrowed as it enters the duodenum (Figs 80.7–80.9). The size of type I cysts is variable, their form is cylindrical or fusiform, and they account for 90% of all choledochal cysts.[71] Type II is a rare congenital diverticulum of the common bile duct; this lesion is not accompanied by jaundice. The term choledochocele is applied to a type III cyst that is limited to the small intraduodenal segment of the common bile duct that herniates into the duodenal lumen. There is no mass, but nausea and vomiting are usually present. Todani et al.[72] expanded the classification in 1977 to include Caroli's disease as type IV-A biliary cystic dilation with multiple intrahepatic and extrahepatic cysts; type IV-B are cysts in the extrahepatic duct system only. Solitray liver cysts are a type V lesion.[73–76] Congenital hepatic fibrosis in the infant will demonstrate a normal common bile duct and irregular intrahepatic ducts with multiple small cysts in the liver (Fig. 80.10).

ERCP is of value in outlining these cysts and their relationship to both ductal systems, providing a roadmap for the surgical approach.[77,87] Ultrasonography,[79] CT and radionuclide scans do not provide the same quality of anatomic detail as the ERCP, but these methods can provide data regarding size, contour, position and the presence of stones.[80] MRCP has been shown to be equivalent to ERCP in defining the morphology of these cysts and in detecting anomalous union of the duct.[25] Cystolithiasis and cholangiocarcinoma[81] are associated phenomena, presumably owing to biliary stasis, reflux of pancreatic secretions and recurrent infections. Retrograde injection of contrast material into the ampulla of Vater or the minor (accessory) papilla in cases of the anomalous pancreaticobiliary junction may simultaneously opacify both ductal systems.

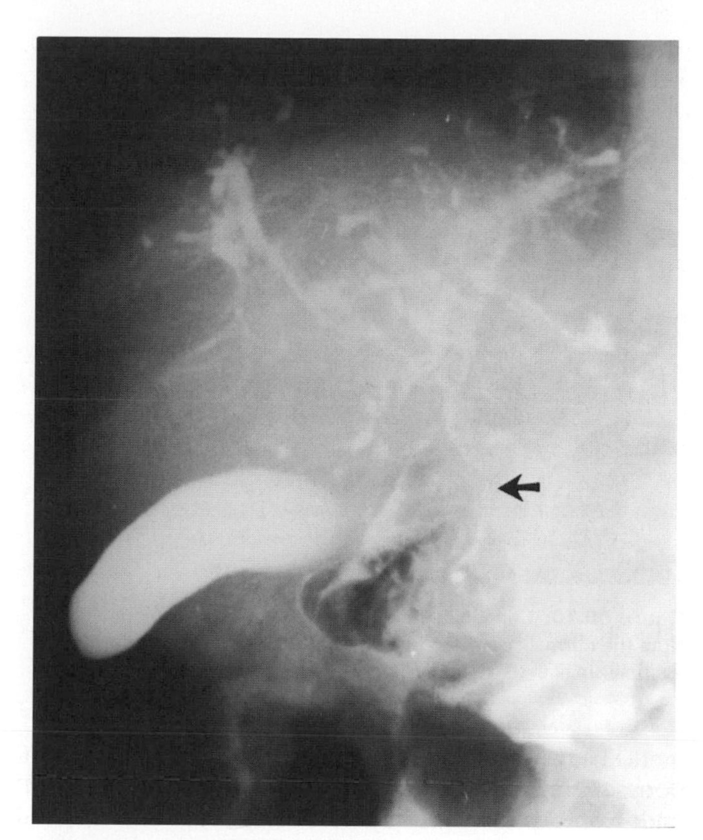

Figure 80.8: Choledochal cyst type IV in a 12-year-old girl. Note the multiple cystolithiasis (arrow) with a stricture of the distal common duct.

There are a few reported series describing therapeutic endoscopic sphincterotomy for type III cysts,[82] with a the-

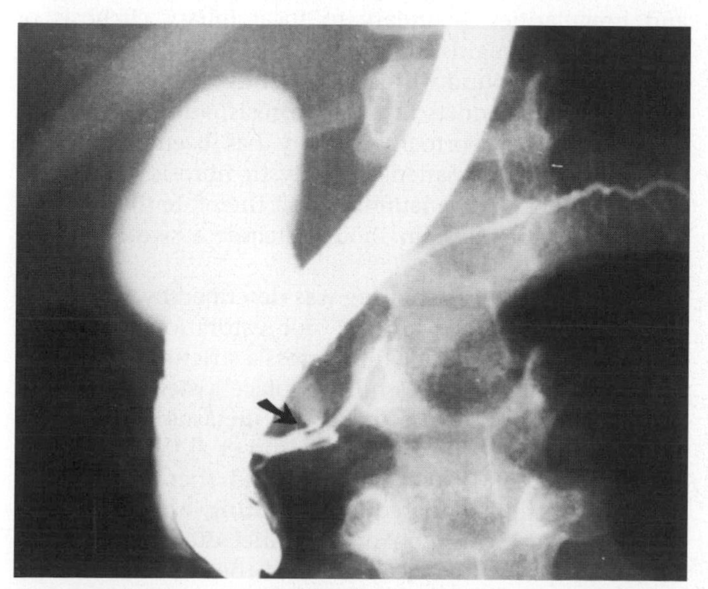

Figure 80.7: Choledochal cyst type I in a 3-year-old boy. Note the segmental choledochal dilation with a stricture of the distal common duct (arrow).

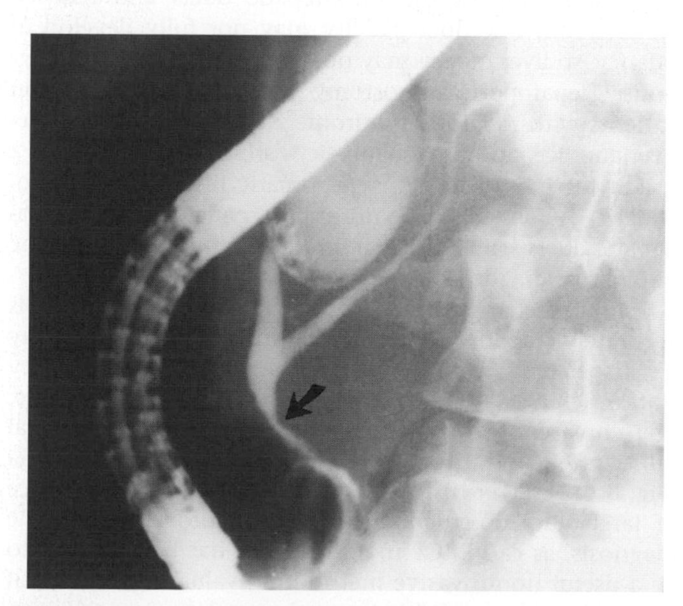

Figure 80.9: Choledochal cyst in an 11-year-old girl. Note an abnormal pancreaticobiliary duct junction with a long common channel (arrow) in a type I cyst.

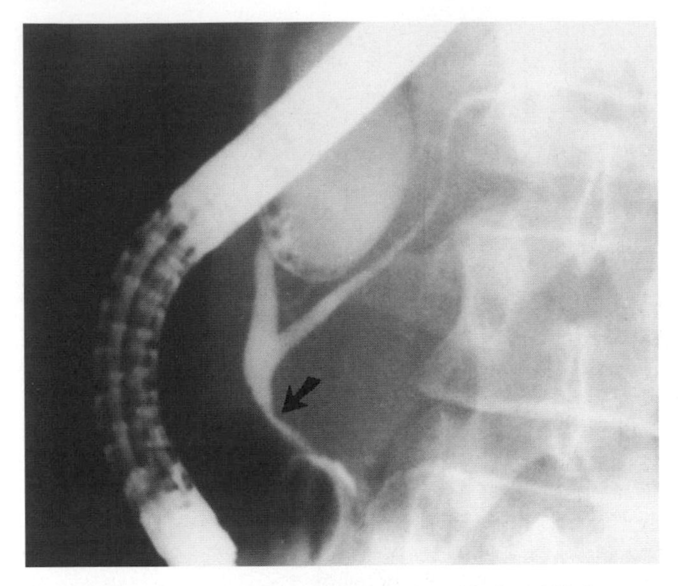

Figure 80.10: Congenital hepatic fibrosis in a 38-day-old infant. Note the normal common duct and irregular intrahepatic ducts with multiple small cysts in the liver.

oretical advantage of avoiding the postoperative complications of stagnation referred to as the sump syndrome.[83] Endoscopic sphincterotomy has been performed with good results in six symptomatic patients with a common channel and distal stenosis.[84] However, some authors consider anomalous drainage into a common channel a contraindication to endoscopic sphincterotomy.[77,85]

Other biliary disorders

Other biliary disorders have been studied with ERCP, and their characteristic anatomic patterns give a precise diagnosis. ERCP in Alagille's syndrome[86,87] shows a marked and diffuse narrowing of the extrahepatic biliary ducts with uniform narrowing of the intrahepatic ducts and reduced arborization. Bile duct paucity may not fully develop in infancy, so liver biopsy may not provide a conclusive diagnosis. Hepatoportoenterostomy has been performed on patients with Alagille's syndrome[88] for prolonged obstructive jaundice, and the diagnostic work-up should include a search for the associated syndromatic findings of arteriohepatic dysplasia. Non-syndromatic paucity of the intrahepatic ducts (Fig. 80.11) should also be considered in the differential diagnosis.

Primary sclerosing cholangitis (PSC)[89,90] in children is accurately diagnosed with ERCP as in adult patients. It may be associated with histiocytosis X, immune deficiency states, sickle cell disease and inflammatory bowel disease. The cholangiogram will show pruning of the peripheral biliary tree and irregular areas of stenosis and ectasia (Fig. 80.12). Liver histology can only suggest the presence of large duct obstruction but cannot provide a specific diagnosis, as can ERCP in PSC. MRCP has been shown to be a useful non-invasive method of evaluating the ductal system for stricture. With more advanced disease, palliative relief of jaundice can be accomplished by therapeutic dilation of a dominant stricture in a major duct with hydro-

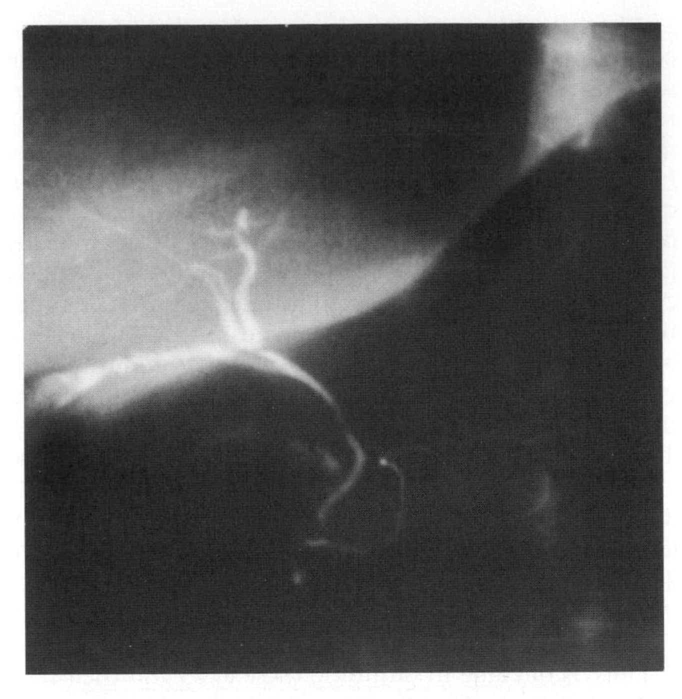

Figure 80.11: Non-syndromic paucity of the bile ducts. A normal extrahepatic biliary ducts is seen. Uniform narrowing of the intrahepatic ducts and reduced arborization are visualized.

static balloon bougienage.[85] A subset of patients with PSC have a dominant extrahepatic biliary stricture that is potentially amenable to endoscopic therapy. One report included 63 adult patients treated with repeated balloon dilation of a dominant biliary stricture. The observed 5-year survival rate was significantly higher than predicted from the Mayo risk score (83% *vs* 65%). These data suggest that repeated endoscopic attempts to maintain biliary patency may improve the survival of patients with PSC and dominant strictures.[91]

The biliary tree may be characterized by cystic dilation and irregularities secondary to focal biliary cirrhosis or recurrent cholangitis in patients with cystic fibrosis.[92] Stones may be found within the liver as well as within the extrahepatic bile ducts in cystic fibrosis, and may be seen on ERCP. Hepatoportoenterostomy has been inappropriately performed on patients with cystic fibrosis[88] who have prolonged obstructive jaundice, and therefore the preoperative diagnostic work-up should include a sweat chloride test.

Endoscopic biliary stenting was described by Soehendra and Reynders-Frederix in 1980[93] for restoration of bile flow via placement of a plastic tube across a stricture. Bickerstaff et al.[94] used ERCP successfully to place a stent, providing palliation of jaundice secondary to metastatic neuroblastoma in a 2-year-old patient. Guelrud et al.[95] reported the usefulness of ERCP for diagnosis and therapy in a 21-month-old child who required stenting of a malignant stricture in the common hepatic duct due to neuroblastoma. A papillotomy was done, and the stent was moved into position over a guidewire. Repeat ERCP 7 months later showed disappearance of the compression, and the biliary endoprosthesis was removed (Fig. 80.13).

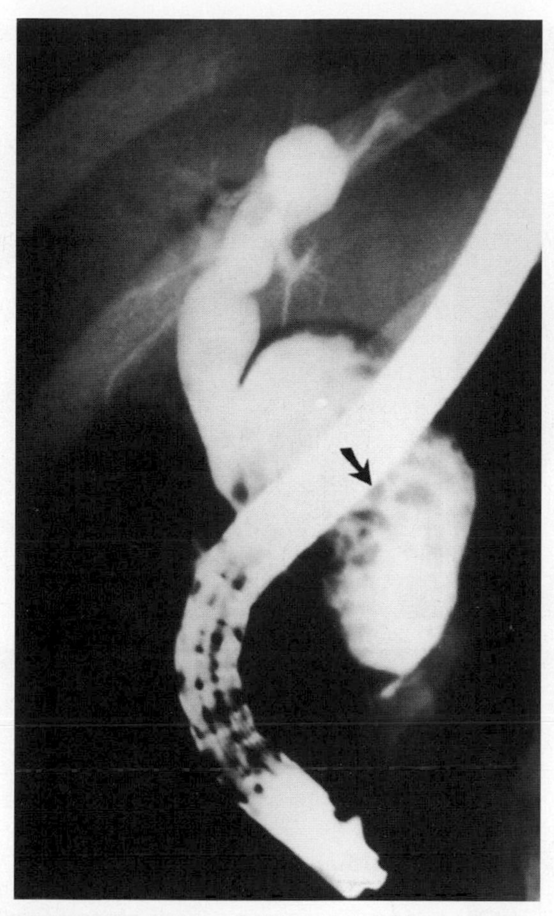

Figure 80.12: Primary sclerosing cholangitis in a 12-year-old girl without an associated underlying condition. Note the narrow and irregular common bile duct (arrow) with pruning of the peripheral biliary tree and irregular areas of stenosis and ectasia.

Diagnostic specimens evaluating for cholangiocarcinoma may be obtained by biopsy forceps or brush cytology through the therapeutic channel on the duodenoscope.[96,97] In older patients a 'daughter' cholangioscope can be introduced through the 'mother' duodenoscope for detailed cholangioscopy. ERCP can help differentiate extrinsic *vs* intrinsic compression by masses. Collection of uncontaminated bile and pancreatic juice, with or without cholecystokinin or secretin stimulation, is possible with directed duct cannulation.[98]

Pancreatic disorders

Congenital malformations

Variants of the pancreatic duct system have been studied in autopsy series. The most common variant is pancreas divisum, occurring at a frequency of 3–10%.[99] The normal relationship of the main pancreatic duct is derived from union of the dorsal and ventral buds of pancreatic tissue in the embryo. When these buds do not fuse, a separate drainage system forms in which the accessory duct of Santorini becomes the main drainage for the gland, and the small ventral duct drains the head and uncinate process via the duct of Wirsung in the main papilla or through the ampulla of Vater. Some studies suggest that this anomaly occurs in equal frequency in patients with and without pancreatitis.[100] There is controversy in the literature about pancreas divisum as a cause of pancreatitis. Reports of divisum and pancreatitis in children[101–106] began to appear with the advent of ERCP. Cotton[105] found an incidence of pancreas divisum of 3.6% in 169 patients with primary biliary tract disease, but in 78 patients with recurrent pancreatitis the incidence was 25.6%. In the author's experience with 272 consecutive cases of successful ERCP performed in children, pancreas divisum was found in 9 (3.4%) children.[103] Recurrent pancreatitis has been reported in pediatric patients with pancreas divisum,[104] and stones may be present in the pancreatic ducts.[106] ERCP is the best way to diagnose pancreas divisum, and cannulation of the minor papilla is necessary to demonstrate the complete pancreatic ductal system. Cannulation of the major papilla shows a short duct of Wirsung (ventral pancreas) that quickly tapers and undergoes arborization (Fig. 80.14). To confirm the diagnosis, it is most important to cannulate the minor papilla to demonstrate the dorsal pancreas. Endoscopic sphincterotomy of the minor papilla is indicated in patients with disabling symptoms. It has led to improvement in approximately 75% of children.[107,108] Overall, these results indicate that, in certain children with recurrent pain or pancreatitis and pancreas divisum,

Recurrent pancreatitis due to conditions indicated below
Congenital disorders
Biliary anomalies
Choledochal cyst Anomalous pancreaticobiliary union
Pancreatic anomalies
Pancreas divisum Annular pancreas Short pancreas Cystic dilation of the pancreatic duct (pancreatocele)
Duodenal anomalies
Duodenal or gastric duplication cysts Duodenal diverticulum
Acquired disorders
Parastic infestation: *Ascaris* Sphincter of Oddi dysfunction Pancreatic trauma Acquired immune deficiency syndrome
Chronic pancreatitis Pseudocysts

Table 80.2 Pancreatic disorders for which ERCP may be indicated

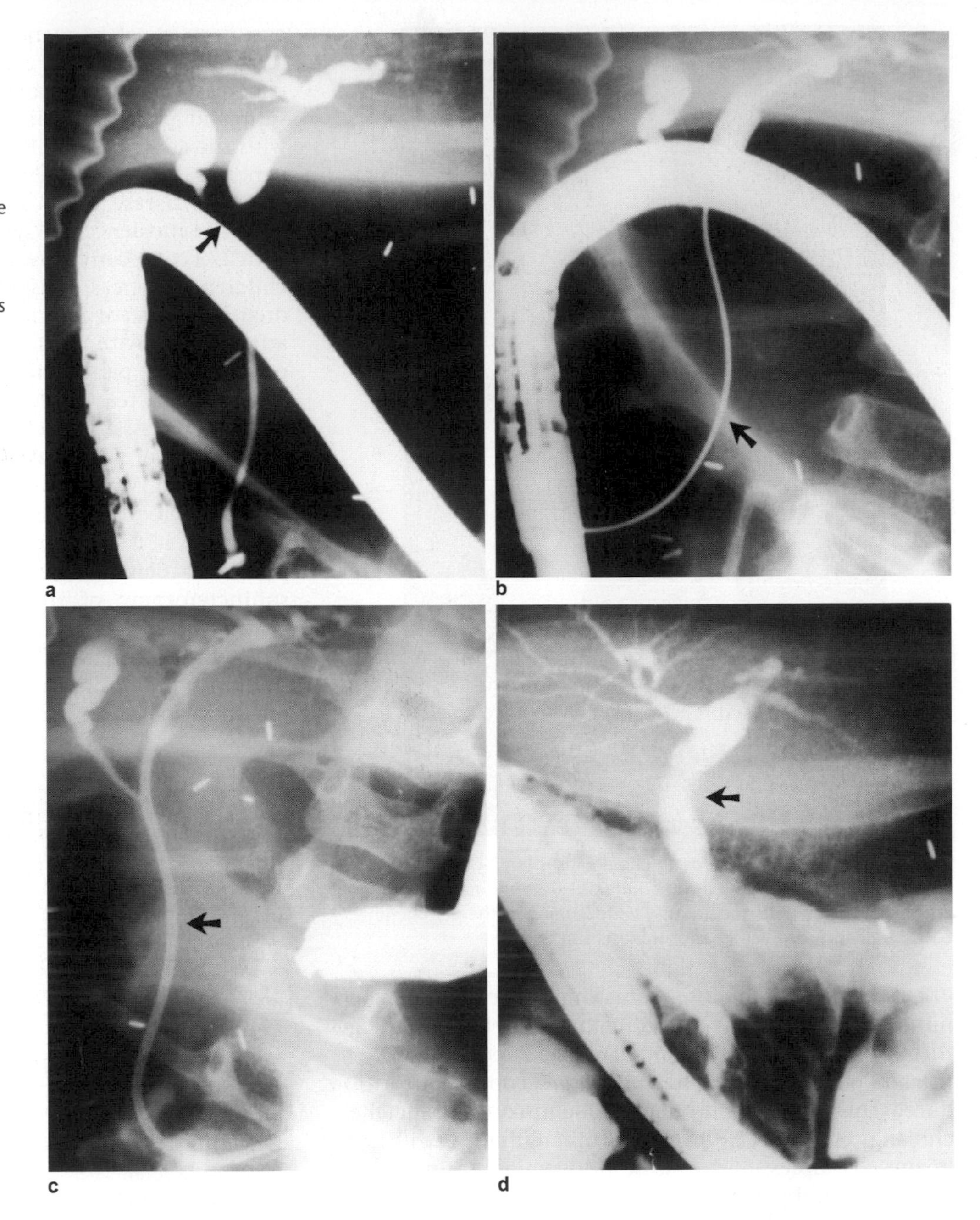

Figure 80.13: Malignant stricture at the common hepatic duct in a 21-month-old child with jaundice secondary to metastatic neuroblastoma. (**a**) Note stricture at the main hepatic duct (arrow) with dilation of intrahepatic ducts. The gallbladder and common bile duct are normal. (**b**) After sphincterotomy, a guidewire (arrow) is introduced into the left hepatic duct. (**c**) A double-pigtail biliary stent, 7 Fr in diameter, is placed (arrow). (**d**) After 4 months of chemotherapy, the biliary stent is removed and the common hepatic duct is free of stricture (arrow).

endoscopic therapy can offer relief or improvement in symptoms.

Annular pancreas is a term denoting a ring of pancreatic tissue surrounding the duodenum that may cause symptoms and can present from the newborn period to advanced age. The ERCP appearance of this congenital anomaly has been reported in a series of four patients from Japan.[109] Annular pancreas may be seen coexistent with pancreas divisum, which may explain the occurrence of pancreatitis in some of these patients.[110]

Acquired disorders

Hydatid disease Hydatid disease, a parasitic infection with *Echinococcus granulosus*, involves the liver and has been confirmed by cholangiography and treated with endoscopic sphincterotomy in 10 patients with good decompression and no complications.[111] Prior to the availability of endoscopic sphincterotomy, stenosis of the papilla had to be treated surgically, but ERCP now has a place in the preoperative and postoperative management in these patients. The presence of *Ascaris* worms is also a cause of obstructive jaundice, and these worms may be removed from the biliary tree with a tripod snare and other special instruments.[12]

Sphincter of Oddi dysfunction Sphincter of Oddi dysfunction is also thought to be a potential cause of recurrent pancreatitis. Guelrud et al.[70] evaluated sphincter of Oddi function in children with anomalous pancreaticobiliary union and recurrent pancreatitis. In a retrospective review of 128 ERCP studies in children older than 1 year, nine patients underwent sphincter of Oddi

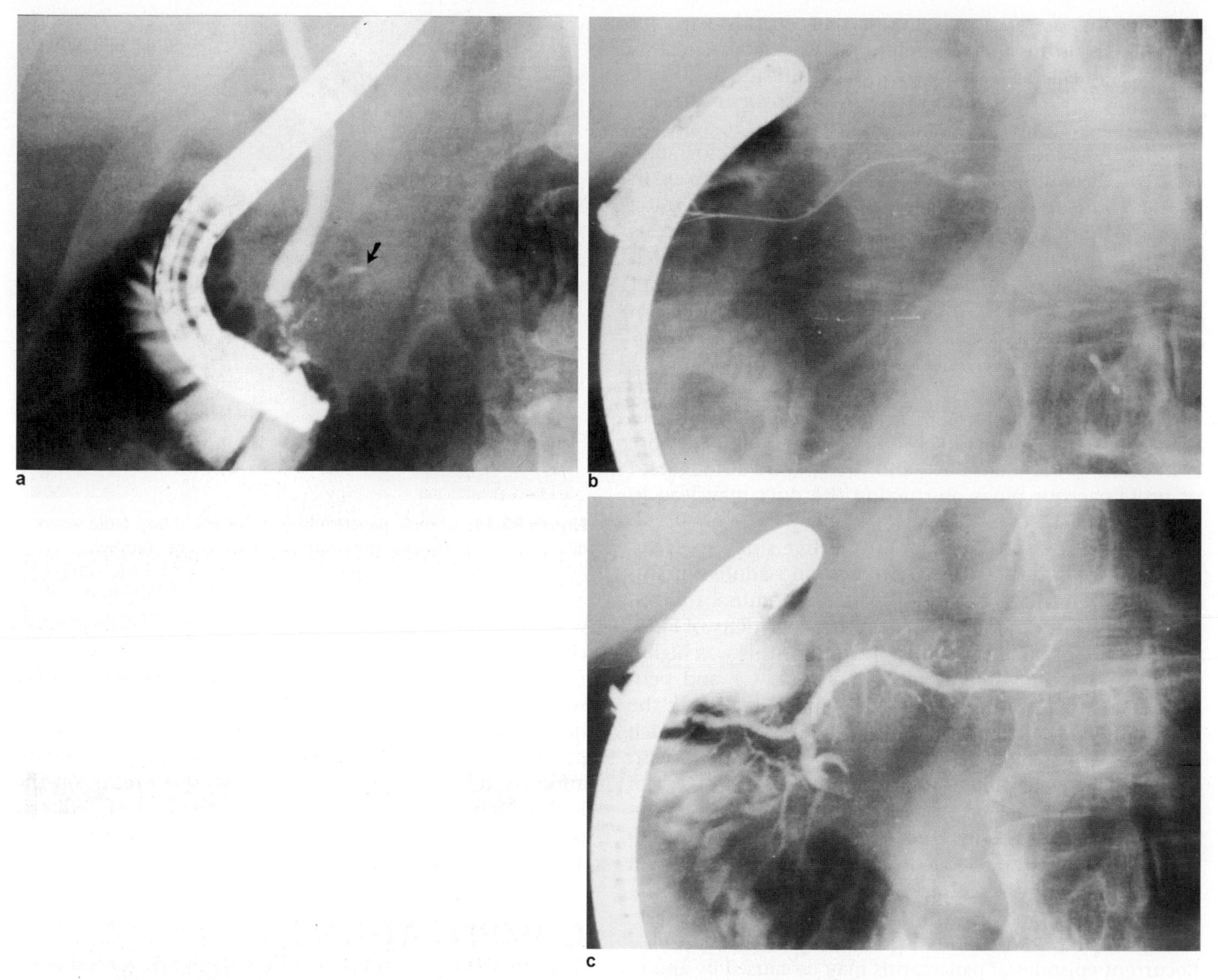

Figure 80.14: Pancreas divisum in a 17-year-old boy. (**a**) Cannulation of the papilla of Vater shows a normal common duct with a small duct of the ventral pancreas (arrow). (**b**) A thin guidewire is introduced into the duct of the dorsal pancreas. A tapered cannula is introduced into the secondary papilla and the guidewire is then withdrawn. (**c**) Contrast medium is injected and a dilated, irregular, dorsal pancreatic duct is visualized.

manometry. Correlation was found between patients with anomalous pancreaticobiliary union, recurrent pancreatitis and abnormal sphincter function.[70] In another series ERCP was performed 34 times in a series of 22 patients. Nine of these included sphincter manometry with abnormal results, leading to sphincterotomy in four. There was a significant reduction in the frequency and severity of pain after intervention.[108] In a third series, Guelrud et al.[107] performed ERCP in 51 patients, 6% of whom had findings suggestive of sphincter of Oddi dysfunction.

Dual endoscopic sphincterotomy of the pancreatic and common duct sphincters may be necessary to improve outcome. However, safety and efficacy of sphincter of Oddi manometry and sphincterotomy in the pediatric population requires further study.

Abdominal trauma Injury by motor vehicle accidents and other causes of blunt or penetrating trauma may cause pancreatic ductal disruption in children and adults. Delayed recognition is not uncommon, especially as injuries to the body and tail of the pancreas may be indolent in their presentation.[112] The pancreas is positioned over the spine; its location makes the organ vulnerable to injury by blunt abdominal trauma, which may fracture or sever the ducts. The retroperitoneal location of the pancreas has made it relatively inaccessible to physical examination and difficult to image with older techniques prior to surgical exploration. ERCP is diagnostic for pancreatic duct laceration, showing extravasation of contrast material at the point of disruption.[113] Hall et al.[114] reported four cases of pancreatic trauma in children aged 2–13 years and recommend early cholangiography to identify the presence and location of duct leakage for patients requiring urgent surgery. Traumatic pancreatitis and its sequelae are associated with significant morbidity and mortality.[112,115] Diagnosis with subsequent therapy should be accomplished as soon as possible to improve outcome.[116] Patients with normal findings on ductography are treated conservatively. ERCP has been reported to aid in the diagnosis and management of an internal pancreatic fistula with ascites in a 5-year-old patient.[117] There is potential for infection caused by injecting a fistula, which may communicate with a semi-closed pseudocyst. Prompt surgery is recommended by several authors. In patients with a large pseudocyst, ERCP is probably unnecessary because the cyst may be imaged by other modalities.[118] Spontaneous resolution of even very large pseudocysts is known to occur. Salinas et al.[119] suggest a role for ERCP in identifying pseudocysts likely to resolve because they are connected to the main duct, and therapeutic dislodgment of proteinaceous plugs obstructing the duct may lead to resolution of the cyst.

Barkin et al.[120] conducted a prospective study to evaluate the use of ERCP in both children and adults for suspected pancreatic ductal rupture after abdominal trauma. They found both the sensitivity and the specificity of ERCP to be 100% for pancreatic duct disruption; this was higher than any combination of serum amylase, CT and peritoneal lavage for establishing the diagnosis. Neither the presence of hyperamylasemia nor the peak level separated patients with a fractured pancreatic duct from those with intact ducts. Determination of the location and extent of the ductal tear directed surgical intervention in the pancreas, where contusion with edema, hematoma, surrounding injuries and the retroperitoneal location of the organ may obscure injury.[121–123]

Chronic pancreatitis and pseudocyst

Recurrent episodes of pancreatitis may be caused by anomalies and abnormalities of the pancreatic and biliary ducts,[69,124,125] which can now be defined precisely by ERCP, lessening the number of patients thought to have 'idiopathic' pancreatitis.[126] Blustein et al.[127] recommend ERCP as the procedure of choice in children with relapsing pancreatitis because of the high yield of surgically correctable lesions. Another series of 10 children with chronic pancreatitis studied with ERCP emphasized that fibrosing pancreatitis needs to be considered in the differential diagnosis of obstructive jaundice.[128] A pancreatic or biliary ductal abnormality was found in 16 of 35 patients with recurrent pancreatitis in a series of children and adults who underwent ERCP.[129,130] The subsequent surgical approach was based on the ERCP findings of potentially correctable lesions in these patients. A dilated, irregular main pancreatic duct with or without strictures and stones may be seen (Fig. 80.15). Therapeutic maneuvers such as placement of a nasobiliary drain[131] and nasopancreatic drain, placement of a pancreatic duct endoprosthesis and pancreatic stone extraction, as reported in a series of 32 patients aged 12–68 years,[132] are viable endoscopic alternatives to surgery. A longer follow-up period will be necessary to determine whether endoscopic success produces long-standing clinical improvement.

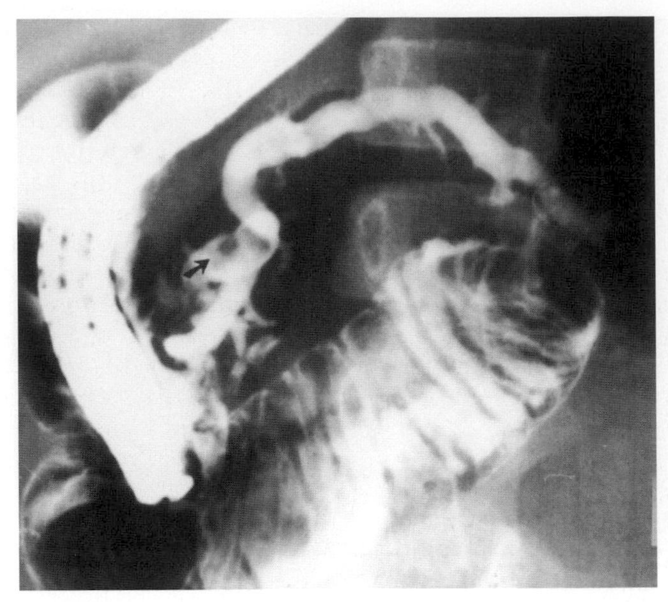

Figure 80.15: Chronic pancreatitis in a 9-year-old boy. Note severe dilation of the pancreatic duct with pancreatic stones (arrow).

Correlation between the degree of structural changes seen on ERCP and functional impairment of the pancreas has been noted in pediatric and adult patients.[133] When pseudocysts complicate pancreatitis, the appropriate operation is determined by location and duration of the lesion,[134] and improvements in management of pediatric patients with acute and chronic pancreatitis have been attributed to ERCP.[135,136]

COMPLICATIONS

Reactions to medications used for sedation or general anesthesia may occur as with upper endoscopy; however, these are usually mild and infrequent. Endoscopic complications are discussed in greater detail in Chapter 81. The most common complication following ERCP in adults is pancreatitis,[137] and the reported incidence varies from 1 to 8%; however, clinical pancreatitis is rare. When measured, serum pancreatic enzyme levels are raised, as expected following cannulation and injection of the pancreatic duct even in totally asymptomatic patients, and this is rarely of clinical significance.[138–140] Correlation has been noted between the force of injection of the pancreatic ducts with contrast material, degree of acinarization seen on fluoroscopy, urographic visualization,[141] and subsequent development of pancreatitis. Attempts to monitor the pressure of injection with manometers have been reported;[142] however, this has not proved to be practical or necessary. Care is taken to fill the ducts with minimal pressure, to stop the procedure if repeated injection of the pancreatic duct occurs when attempting to cannulate the bile duct,[143] and to establish the anatomy of the main pancreatic duct with as little filling of the secondary and tertiary pancreatic radicles as possible.

Bilbao et al.[144] retrospectively surveyed 10 435 ERCP examinations in a multicenter study and noted that experienced endoscopists had a 3% reported incidence of complications in adults, whereas inexperienced workers had four times the failure rate in cannulating the desired duct(s) and twice the complications (7%). Fluoroscopic time also decreases with growing experience of the endoscopist.[145] Data obtained on 3884 examinations in the study of Nebel et al.[146] revealed a complication rate of 2.16%, with pancreatitis, cholangitis, cardiopulmonary problems, perforation and bleeding being the chief complications in decreasing order of frequency. The incidence of complications in pediatric patients is unknown because there are only a few large series, in one of which[4] oversedation and transient tracheal compression were reported in 10% of the infants. Mild pancreatitis occurred in two of 42 children undergoing ERCP, and endoscopic papillotomy was successful in five patients in this series.[4] In a series of 42 ERCP examinations in 37 children and one young adult, mild pancreatitis ensued in three patients (8%), all of whom had a history of pancreatitis.[14] Abnormalities were detected in 22 of 38 (58%) of patients in this series, 11 of whom required surgery.

In patients with pseudocyst formation, injection of the pancreatic duct with contrast material from an endoscope that has been passed through the unsterile oropharynx may potentially seed the cyst with bacteria and cause pancreatic abscess. There is controversy in the literature about performing ERCP in patients with pancreatic pseudocysts, but most authors favor waiting until the patient has recovered from the acute illness. One pediatric death caused by infection of a pancreatic pseudocyst after ERCP has been reported.[8] When ERCP is done to plan the operative approach, the interval to surgery should not exceed 24 h.[118] When ductal obstruction is found, prompt surgical intervention is recommended because of the risk of sepsis.[146]

Acute ascending cholangitis may complicate ERCP[147] and is potentially fatal; however, this risk was described in adults with malignant and other forms of stenotic obstruction of the biliary tree. Antibiotic prophylaxis is recommended in the setting of biliary obstruction because 90% of cases of cholangitis occur with biliary obstruction.[144] In adults, septic complications and perforation have accounted for a mortality rate of 0.1–0.2%. Occasionally intramural injection of contrast material or extravasation of contrast material occurs, but in the pediatric ERCP literature this has not been noted as a complication.

Infections with *Pseudomonas aeruginosa* have been linked to contamination of endoscopes and closed water reservoirs,[148–150] and this has prompted changes and new guidelines for disinfection of the instruments and endoscopy suite. Another prospective evaluation of 51 consecutive patients to determine the frequency of bacteremia with ERCP showed only one patient (2%) with multiple strictures of the main pancreatic duct who had transient bacteremia, but no septic illness ensued.[31] Patients found to have a stricture should be given antibiotics following the procedure. Bleeding may occur with ERCP and is more likely when therapeutic procdeures such as sphincterotomy are performed.

CONTRAINDICATIONS

Contraindications include inability of the patient to cooperate, perforation of a hollow viscus, shock, cervical spine injury, intestinal obstruction and other cardiopulmonary conditions that would not permit safe use of sedation. Fever is a contraindication to ERCP in biliary obstruction, unless followed by immediate ductal drainage.[147] Relative contraindications are coagulopathy, coma, and the presence of pancreatitis or cholangitis, unless therapeutic ERCP could treat the underlying cause of the infection. Certain structural abnormalities may preclude ERCP, such as esophageal stricture, postoperative changes in anatomy, and large paraesophageal hernia.[151]

SUMMARY

The approach to diagnostic studies of the pancreaticobiliary system depends on knowledge of available techniques and resources. ERCP has not commonly been used with pediatric patients, but advances in technology of prototype duodenoscopes and catheters used to cannulate the papilla in the past two decades have established its role in obstructive jaundice and recurrent pancreatitis. Because it is an invasive procedure, its place in the definition of pancreaticobiliary anatomy is being replaced by MRCP. As an interventional tool it has proved safe and effective for certain conditions. The diagnostic yield for ERCP in otherwise unexplained abdominal pain is low, and it is not indicated for this. Special advanced training and continuing experience in ERCP are needed beyond general endoscopic competence.[152] The procedure is of value in assessing surgically correctable lesions of the pancreas and biliary tree, and has defined the cause of neonatal cholestasis in many infants, avoiding the need for surgery and intraoperative cholangiography. Careful patient selection and knowledge of available local skills and alternative methods will influence utilization and referral for ERCP in pediatric patients.

References

1. McCune WS, Shorb PE, Moscovitz H. Endoscopic cannulation of the ampulla of Vater. Ann Surg 1968; 167:752–756.
2. Waye JD. Endoscopic retrograde cholangiopancreatography in the infant. Am J Gastroenterol 1976; 65:461–463.
3. Guelrud M, Jaen D, Torres P, et al. Endoscopic cholangiopancreatography in the infant: evaluation of a new prototype pediatric duodenoscope. Gastrointest Endosc 1987; 33:4–8.
4. Buckley A, Connon JJ. The role of ERCP in children and adolescents. Gastrointest Endosc 1990; 36:360–372.
5. Cotton PB, Laage NJ. Endoscopic retrograde cholangiopancreatography in children. Arch Dis Child 1982; 57:131–136.
6. Guelrud M. Endoscopic retrograde cholangiopancreatography. Gastrointest Endosc Clin North Am 2001; 11:585–601.
7. Guelrud M, Jaen D, Mendoza S, et al. ERCP in the diagnosis of extrahepatic biliary atresia. Gastrointest Endosc 1991; 37:522–526.

8. Wilkinson ML, Mieli-Vergani G, Ball C, et al. Endoscopic retrograde cholangiopancreatography in infantile cholestasis. Arch Dis Child 1991; 66:121–123.
9. Fox VL, Werlin SL, Heyman HB. Endoscopic retrograde cholangiopancreatography in children. Subcommittee on Endoscopy and Procedures of the Patient Care Committee of the North American Society for Pediatric Gastroenterology and Nutrition. J Pediatr Gastroenterol Nutr 2000; 30:335–342.
10. Riemann JF, Koch H. Endoscopy of the biliary tract and pancreas in children. Endoscopy 1978; 10:166–172.
11. Heyman MB, Shapiro HA, Thaler MM. Endoscopic retrograde cholangiography in the diagnosis of biliary malformations in infants. Gastrointest Endosc 1988; 34:449–453.
12. van der Spuy S. Endoscopic retrograde cholangiopancreatography (ERCP) in children. Endoscopy 1978; 10:173–175.
13. Urakami Y, Seki H, Kishi S. Endoscopic retrograde cholangiopancreatography (ERCP) performed in children. Endoscopy 1977; 9:86–91.
14. Putnam PE, Kocoshis SA, Orenstein SR, Schade RR. Pediatric endoscopic retrograde cholangiopancreatography. Am J Gastroenterol 1991; 86:824–830.
15. Allendorph M, Werlin SL, Geenan JE, et al. Endoscopic retrograde cholangiopancreatography in children. J Pediatr 1986; 110:206–211.
16. Derkx HH, Hiubregtse K, Taminiau JA. The role of endoscopic retrograde cholangiopancreatography in infants with cholestasis. Endoscopy 1994; 26:724.
17. Ohnuma N, Takahashi T, Tanabe M, et al. The role of ERCP in biliary atresia. Gastrointest Endosc 1997; 45:365–370.
18. Dite P, Vacek E, Stefan H, Koudelka J. Pozler O, Kralova M. Endoscopic retrograde cholangiopancreatography in childhood. Hepatogastroenterology 1992; 39:291–293.
19. Pfau PR, Chelimsky GG, Kinnard MF, et al. Endoscopic retrograde cholangiopancreatography in children and adolescents. J Pediatr Gastroenterol Nutr 2002; 35: 619–623.
20. Scharschmidt BF, Goldberg HI, Schmid R. Approach to the patient with cholestatic jaundice. N Engl J Med 1983; 308:1515–1519.
21. Riddlesberger MM. Diagnostic imaging of the hepatobiliary system in infants and children. J Pediatr Gastroenterol Nutr 1984; 3:653–664.
22. Schiff ER. Diagnostic percutaneous transhepatic cholangiography. Sem Liver Dis 1982; 2:49–56.
23. Elias E, Hamlyn AN, Jain S, et al. A randomized trial of percutaneous transhepatic cholangiography with the Chiba needle versus endoscopic retrograde cholangiography for bile duct visualization in jaundice. Gastroenterology 1976; 71:439–443.
24. Katon RM, Lee TG, Parent JA, et al. Endoscopic retrograde cholangiopancreatography (ERCP): experience with 100 cases. Am J Dig Dis 1974; 19:295–306.
25. Fulcher AS, Turner MA. MR cholangiopancreatography. Radiol Clin North Am 2002; 40:1363–1376.
26. Caulfield M, Wyllie R, Sivak MV, et al. Upper gastrointestinal tract endoscopy in the pediatric patient. J Pediatr 1989; 115:339–345.
27. Steffen RM, Wyllie R, Sivak MV, et al. Colonoscopy in the pediatric patient. J Pediatr 1989; 115:507–514.
28. Guelrud M, Mendoza S, Viera L, Gelrud D. Somatostatin prevents acute pancreatitis after pancreatic duct sphincter hydrostatic balloon dilation in patients with idiopathic recurrent pancreatitis. Gastrointest Endosc 1991; 37:44–47.
29. Hirota WK, Petersen K, Baron TH, et al. Standards of Practice Committee of the American Society for Gastrointestinal Endoscopy. Guidelines for antibiotic prophylaxis for GI endoscopy. Gastrointest Endosc 2003; 58:475–482.
30. Dajani AS, Taubert KA, Wilson W, et al. Prevention of bacterial endocarditis. Recommendations by the American Heart Association. JAMA 1997; 277:1794–1801.
31. Dutta SK, Cox M, Williams RB, et al. Prospective evaluation of the risk of bacteremia and the role of antibiotics in ERCP. J Clin Gastroenterol 1983; 5:325–329.
32. Mauer K, Waye JD. A new pediatric duodenoscope: successful cannulation without a cannula elevator. Gastrointest Endosc 1989; 35:437–439.
33. Sivak MV. Video endoscopy. Clin Gastroenterol 1986; 15:205–234.
34. Kato S, Kamagata S, Asakura T, et al. A newly developed small caliber videoduodenoscope for endoscopic retrograde cholangiopancreatography in children. J Clin Gastroenterol 2003; 37:173–176.
35. Classen M, Phillip J. Newer endoscopic techniques for image diagnosis and management of hepatobiliary disease. Sem Liver Dis 1982; 2:67–74.
36. Dominguez R, Young LW, Ledesma-Medina J, et al. Pediatric liver transplantation. Part II: Diagnostic imaging in postoperative management. Radiology 1985; 157:339–344.
37. Freese D. Intracellular cholestatic syndromes of infancy. Sem Liver Dis 1982; 2:255–270.
38. Alagille D. Cholestasis in the first three months of life. Prog Liver Dis 1979; 6:471–485.
39. Ferry GD, Selby MJ, Udall J, et al. Guide to early diagnosis of biliary obstruction in infancy. Clin Pediatr 1985; 24:305–311.
40. Mowat AP: Biliary disorders in childhood. Sem Liver Dis 1982; 2:271–281.
41. Odievre M, Hadchouel M, Landrieu P, et al. Long-term prognosis for infants with intrahepatic cholestasis and patent extrahepatic biliary tract. Arch Dis Child 1981; 56:373–376.
42. Mowat AP, Psacharopoulos HT, Williams R. Extrahepatic biliary atresia versus neonatal hepatitis. Review of 137 prospectively investigated infants. Arch Dis Child 1976; 51:763–770.
43. Hirsig J, Rickham PP. Early differential diagnosis between neonatal hepatitis and biliary atresia. J Pediatr Surg 1980; 15:13–15.
44. Balistreri WF. Neonatal cholestasis. J Pediatr 1985; 106:171–184.
45. Cox KL, Stadalnik RC, McGahan JP, et al. Hepatobiliary scintigraphy with technetium-99m disofenin in the evaluation of neonatal cholestasis. J Pediatr Gastroenterol Nutr 1987; 6:885–891.
46. Manolaki AG, Larcher VF, Mowat AP, et al. The prelaparotomy diagnosis of extrahepatic biliary atresia. Arch Dis Child 1983; 58:591–594.
47. Kirks DR, Coleman RE, Filston HC, et al. An imaging approach to persistent neonatal jaundice. AJR Am J Roentgenol 1984; 142:461–465.
48. Greene HL, Helinek GL, Moran R, O'Neill J. A diagnostic approach to prolonged obstructive jaundice by 24-hour collection of duodenal fluid. J Pediatr 1979; 95:412–414.
49. Dorney SFA, Kamath KR, Middleton AW, Kan A. Diagnosis of biliary atresia. N Engl J Med 1983; 308:968.
50. Fung KP, Lau SP. Gamma-glutamyl transpeptidase activity and its serial measurement in differentiation between extrahepatic biliary atresia and neonatal hepatitis. J Pediatr Gastroenterol Nutr 1985; 4:208–213.

51. Majd M, Reba RC, Altman RP. Effect of phenobarbital on ^{99m}Tc-IDA scintigraphy in the evaluation of neonatal jaundice. Semin Nucl Med 1981; 11:194–204.
52. Kasai M, Suzuki H, Ohashi E. Technique and results of operative management of biliary atresia. World J Surg 1978; 2:571–580.
53. Markowitz J, Daum F, Kahn EI, et al. Arteriohepatic dysplasia I: Pitfalls in diagnosis and management. Hepatology 1983; 3:64–66.
54. Lebwohl O, Waye JD. Endoscopic retrograde cholangiopancreatography in the diagnosis of extrahepatic biliary atresia. Am J Dis Child 1979; 133:647–648.
55. Matsuo S, Yoshiie K, Ikeda K. Endoscopic evaluation of the porta hepatis in patients with biliary atresia. Endoscopy 1985; 17:54–59.
56. Ament M. Is endoscopic cholangiopancreatography needed for the jaundiced infant? Gastrointest Endosc 1987; 33:49–52.
57. Shaw PJ, Spitz L, Watson JG. Extrahepatic biliary obstruction due to stone. Arch Dis Child 1984; 59:896–897.
58. Lilly JR. Common bile duct calculi in infants and children. J Pediatr Surg 1980; 15:577–580.
59. Man DWK, Spitz L. Choledocholithiasis in infancy. J Pediatr Surg 1985; 20:65–68.
60. Guelrud M, Mendoza S, Jaen D, et al. ERCP and endoscopic sphincterotomy in infants and children with jaundice due to common bile duct stones. Gastrointest Endosc 1992; 38:450–453.
61. Broughan TA, Sivak MV, Hermann RE. The management of retained and recurrent bile duct stones. Surgery 1985; 98:746–751.
62. Guelrud M, Mendoza S, Rossiter G, Villegas MI. Sphincter of Oddi manometry in healthy volunteers. Dig Dis Sci 1990; 35:38–46.
63. Guelrud M. Papillary stenosis. Endoscopy 1988; 20:193–202.
64. Geenan JE, Hogan WJ, Dodds WJ, et al. The efficacy of endoscopic sphincterotomy after cholecystectomy in patients with sphincter-of-Oddi dysfunction. N Engl J Med 1989; 320:82–87.
65. Alonso-Lej F, Rever WB, Pessagno DJ. Congenital choledochal cyst, with a report of 2, and an analysis of 94 cases. Int Abstr Surg 1959; 108:1–30.
66. Wiedmeyer DA, Stewart ET, Dodds WJ, et al. Choledochal cyst: findings on cholangiopancreatography with emphasis on ectasia of the common channel. AJR Am J Roentgenol 1989; 153:969–972.
67. Wood WJ, Trump DS. Pancreaticobiliary common channel associated with common duct stricture. J Pediatr Surg 1986; 21:738–740.
68. Okada A, Oguchi Y, Kamata S, et al. Common channel syndrome – diagnosis with endoscopic retrograde cholangiopancreatography and surgical management. Surgery 1983; 93:634–642.
69. Karp MP, Jewett TC, Cooney DR. Chronic relapsing pancreatitis in childhood caused by pancreaticobiliary ductal anomaly. J Pediatr Gastroenterol Nutr 1983; 2:324–328.
70. Guelrud M, Morera C, Rodriguez M, Jaen D, Pierre R. Sphincter of Oddi dysfunction in children with recurrent pancreatitis and anomalous pancreaticobiliary union: an etiologic concept. Gastrointest Endosc 1999; 50: 189–193.
71. Little KH, Loeb PM. Choledochal cyst. South Med J 1989; 82:255–258.
72. Todani T, Watanabe Y, Narusue MEA. Congenital bile duct cysts: classification, operative procedures, and review of 37 cases including cancer arising from choledochal cyst. Am J Surg 1977; 134:263–269.
73. Perisic V. Role of PTC and ERCP in diagnostic imaging of the hepatobiliary tree: Caroli's disease in two siblings. J Pediatr Gastroenterol Nutr 1987; 6:647–648.
74. Perisic V. Role of percutaneous transhepatic cholangiography and endoscopic cholangiopancreatography in the diagnostic imaging of hepatobiliary system in infants and children. J Pediatr Gastroenterol Nutr 1985; 4:846–847.
75. Misavage AE, Sugawa C. Caroli's disease: role of endoscopic retrograde cholangiopancreatography. Am J Gastroenterol 1983; 78:815–817.
76. Hermansen MC, Starshak RJ, Werlin SL. Caroli disease: the diagnostic approach. J Pediatr 1979; 94:879–882.
77. Thatcher BS, Sivak MV, Hermann RE, Esselstyn CB. ERCP in evaluation and diagnosis of choledochal cyst: report of five cases. Gastrointest Endosc 1986; 32:27–31.
78. Guelrud M, Jaen D, Mendoza S, Torres P. Usefulness of endoscopic retrograde cholangiopancreatography in diagnosis of choledochal cysts in children. G E N 1989; 43:9–12.
79. Chang M, Wang T, Chen C, Hung W. Congenital bile duct dilatation in children. J Pediatr Surg 1986; 21:112–117.
80. Sherman P, Kilster E, Davies C, et al. Choledochal cysts: heterogeneity of clinical presentation. J Pediatr Gastroenterol Nutr 1986; 5:867–872.
81. Bloustein PA. Association of carcinoma with congenital cystic conditions of the liver and bile ducts. Am J Gastroenterol 1977; 67:40–46.
82. Venu RP, Geenan JE, Hogan WJ, et al. Role of endoscopic retrograde cholangiopancreatography in the diagnosis and treatment of choledochocele. Gastroenterology 1984; 87:1144–1149.
83. Siegel JH, Harding GT, Chateau F. Endoscopic incision of choledochal cysts (choledochocele). Endoscopy 1981; 13:200–202.
84. Ng WD, Liu K, Wong MK, et al. Endoscopic sphincterotomy in young patients with choledochal dilatation and long common channel: a preliminary report. Br J Surg 1992; 79:550–552.
85. Siegel JH, Guelrud M. Endoscopic cholangiopancreatoplasty: hydrostatic balloon dilation in the bile duct and pancreas. Gastrointest Endosc 1983; 29:99–103.
86. Morelli A, Pelli MA, Vedovelli A, et al. Endoscopic retrograde cholangiopancreatography study in Alagille's syndrome: first report. Am J Gastroenterol 1983; 78:241–244.
87. Gorelick FS, Dobbins JW, Burrell M, Riely CA. Biliary tract abnormalities in patients with arteriohepatic dysplasia. Dig Dis Sci 1982; 25:815–820.
88. Perkins WG, Klein GL, Beckerman RC. Cystic fibrosis mistaken for idiopathic biliary atresia. Clin Pediatr 1985; 24:107–109.
89. Classen M, Gotze H, Richter HJ, Bender S. Primary sclerosing cholangitis in children. J Pediatr Gastroenterol Nutr 1987; 6:197–202.
90. Johnson DA, Cattau EL, Hancock JE. Pediatric primary sclerosing cholangitis. Dig Dis Sci 1986; 31:773–777.
91. Baluyut AR, Sherman S, Lehman GA, Hoen H, Chalasani N. Impact of endoscopic therapy on the survival of patients with primary sclerosing cholangitis. Gastroentest Endosc 2001; 53: 308–312.
92. Bass S, Connon JJ, Ho CS. Biliary tree in cystic fibrosis: biliary tract abnormalities in cystic fibrosis demonstrated by endoscopic retrograde cholangiography. Gastroenterology 1983; 84:1592–1596.

93. Soehendra N, Reynders-Frederix V. Palliative bile duct drainage – a new endoscopic method of introducing a transpapillary drain. Endoscopy 1980; 12:8–11.
94. Bickerstaff KI, Britton BJ, Gough MH. Endoscopic palliation of malignant biliary obstruction in a child. Br J Surg 1989; 76:1092–1093.
95. Guelrud M, Mendoza S, Zager A, Noguera C. Biliary stenting in an infant with malignant obstructive jaundice. Gastrointest Endosc 1989; 35:259–261.
96. Rustgi AK, Kelsey PB, Guelrud M, et al. Malignant tumors of the bile ducts; diagnosis by biopsy during endoscopic cannulation. Gastrointest Endosc 1989; 35:248–251.
97. Soehendra N, Grimm H, Berger B, Nam VC. Malignant jaundice: results of diagnostic and therapeutic endoscopy. World J Surg 1989; 13:171–177.
98. Cotton PB. Progress report; ERCP. Gut 1977; 18:316–341.
99. Sigfusson BF, Wehlin L, Lindstrom CG. Variants of pancreatic duct system of importance in endoscopic retrograde cholangiopancreatography. Observations on autopsy specimens. Acta Radiol Diagn Stockh 1983; 24:113–128.
100. Mitchell CJ, Lintott DJ, Ruddell WS, et al. Clinical relevance of an infused pancreatic duct system. Gut 1979; 20:1066–1071.
101. Wagner CW, Golladay ES. Pancreas divisum and pancreatitis in children. Am Surg 1988; 54:22–26.
102. Yaffe MR, Gutenberger JE. Chronic pancreatitis and pancreas divisum in an infant: diagnosed by endoscopic retrograde cholangiopancreatography and treated with somatostatin analog. J Pediatr Gastroenterol Nutr 1989; 9:108–111.
103. Guelrud M. The incidence of pancreas divisum in children (letter). Gastrointest Endosc 1996; 43:83–84.
104. Yedlin ST, Dubois RS, Philippart AI. Pancreas divisum: a cause of pancreatitis in childhood. J Pediatr Surg 1984; 19:793–794.
105. Cotton PB. Congenital anomaly of pancreas divisum as cause of obstructive pain and pancreatitis. Gut 1980; 21:105–114.
106. Yvergneaux JP, Van den Boer H, De Keyser R, Brys R. Pancreas divisum: a teenager with calculi in the duct of Santorini. Report of a case treated by double drainage procedure. Acta Chir Belg 1985; 85:67–70.
107. Guelrud M, Mujica C, Jaen D, et al. The role of ERCP in the diagnosis and treatment of idiopathic recurrent pancreatitis in children and adolescents. Gastrointest Endosc 1994; 40:428–436.
108. Hsu RK, Draganov P, Leung JW, et al. Therapeutic ERCP in the management of pancreatitis in children. Gastrointest Endosc 2000; 51:396–400.
109. Yogi Y, Shibue T, Hashimoto S. Annular pancreas detected in adults, diagnosed by endoscopic retrograde cholangiopancreatography: report of four cases. Gastroenterol Jpn 1987; 22:92–99.
110. Lehman GA, O'Connor KW. Coexistence of annular pancreas and pancreas divisum–ERCP diagnosis. Gastrointest Endosc 1985; 25–28.
111. Vignote ML, Mino G, de la Mata M, et al. Endoscopic sphincterotomy in hepatic hydatid disease open to the biliary tree. Br J Surg 1990; 77:30–31.
112. Taxier M, Sivak MV, Cooperman AM, Sullivan BH. Endoscopic retrograde pancreatography in the evaluation of trauma to the pancreas. Surg Gynecol Obstet 1980; 150:65–68.
113. Rawlings W, Bynum TE, Pasternak G. Pancreatic ascites: diagnosis of leakage site by endoscopic pancreatography. Surgery 1977; 81:363–365.
114. Hall RI, Lavelle MI, Venables CW. Use of ERCP to identify the site of traumatic injuries of the main pancreatic duct in children. Br J Surg 1986; 73:411–412.
115. Vane DW, Grosfeld JL, West KW, Rescorla FJ. Pancreatic disorders in infancy and childhood: experience with 92 cases. J Pediatr Surg 1989; 24:771–776.
116. Whittwell AE, Gomez GA, Byers P, et al. Blunt pancreatic trauma: prospective evaluation of early endoscopic retrograde pancreatography. South Med J 1989; 82:586–591.
117. Filston HC, McLeod RM, Jones RS: Improved management of pancreatic lesions in children aided by ERCP. J Pediatr Surg 1980; 15:121–128.
118. Wind GG, Rubin P, Waye JD, Bauer JJ. Pancreatic pseudocyst: is endoscopic retrograde cholangiopancreatography contraindicated? Mt Sinai J Med 1976; 43:558–564.
119. Salinas A, Rodriguez J, Guelrud M, et al. Resolution of pancreatic pseudocysts: when should we wait? Mt Sinai J Med 1986; 53:470–477.
120. Barkin JS, Ferstenberg RM, Panullo W, et al. Endoscopic retrograde cholangiopancreatography in pancreatic trauma. Gastrointest Endosc 1988; 34:102–165.
121. Belohlavek D, Merkle P, Probst M. Identification of traumatic rupture of the pancreatic duct by endoscopic retrograde pancreatography. Gastrointest Endosc 1978; 24:255–256.
122. Bozymski EM, Orlando RC, Holt JW. Traumatic disruption of the pancreatic duct demonstrated by endoscopic retrograde pancreatography. J Trauma 1981: 21:244–245.
123. Tim LO, Thompson PM, Segal I, Lawson HH. Endoscopic retrograde cholangiopancreatography in the management of traumatic pancreatic pseudocysts. South Am Med J 1979; 5:767–770.
124. Perisic VN, Mihailovic T, Filipovic D. Congenital hepatic fibrosis, bile duct abnormality, long pancreaticobiliary common channel, and pancreatitis. J Pediatr Gastroenterol Nutr 1988; 7:790–791.
125. Crombleholme TM, deLorimer AA, Way LW, et al. The modified Puestow procedure for chronic relapsing pancreatitis in children. J Pediatr Surg 1990; 25:749–754.
126. Rosch W. ERCP in acute and chronic pancreatitis. In: Sivak MV, ed. Gastroenterologic Endoscopy. Philadelphia, PA: WB Saunders; 1987:780–793.
127. Blustein PK, Gaskin K, Filler R, et al. Endoscopic retrograde cholangiopancreatography in pancreatitis in children and adolescents. Pediatrics 1981; 68:387–393.
128. Ghishan FK, Greene HL, Avant G, et al. Chronic relapsing pancreatitis in childhood. J Pediatr 1983; 102:514–518.
129. Cooperman M, Ferrara JJ, Carey LC, et al. Idiopathic acute pancreatitis: the value of endoscopic retrograde cholangiopancreatography. Surgery 1981; 90:666–670.
130. Cooperman AM, Sivak MV, Sullivan BH, Hermann RE. Endoscopic pancreatography: its value in preoperative and postoperative assessment of pancreatic disease. Am J Surg 1975; 129:38–43.
131. Wurbs D, Phillip J, Classen M. Experiences with the long standing nasobiliary tube in biliary diseases. Endoscopy 1980; 12:219–223.
132. Huibregtse K, Schneider B, Vrij AA, Tytgat GNJ. Endoscopic pancreatic drainage in chronic pancreatitis. Gastrointest Endosc 1988; 34:9–15.
133. Girdwood AH, Hatfield ARW, Bornman PC, et al. Structure and function in noncalcific pancreatitis. Dig Dis Sci 1984; 29:721–726.
134. Cooney DR, Grosfeld JL. Operative management of pancreatic pseudocysts in infants and children: a review of 75 cases. Ann Surg 1975; 182:590–596.
135. Tam PKH, Saing H, Irving IM, Lister J. Acute pancreatitis in children. J Pediatr Surg 1985; 20:58–60.
136. O'Neill JA, Greene H, Grishan FK. Surgical implications of chronic pancreatitis. J Pediatr Surg 1982; 17:920–926.

137. LaFerla G, Gordon S, Archibald M, Murray WR. Hyperamylasaemia and acute pancreatitis following endoscopic retrograde cholangiopancreatography. Pancreas 1986; 1:160–163.

138. Okuno M, Himeno S, Kurokawa M, et al. Changes in serum levels of pancreatic isoamylase, lipase, trypsin, and elastase 1 after endoscopic retrograde pancreatography. Hepatogastroenterology 1985; 32:87–90.

139. Weaver HA, Sugawa C, Bouwman DL, Altshuler J. Isoamylase determinations in patients undergoing endoscopic retrograde cholangiopancreatography. Surg Gastroenterol 1984; 3:59–62.

140. Brandes JW, Scheffer B, Lorenz–Meyer H, et al. Complications and prophylaxis, a controlled study. Endoscopy 1981; 13:27–30.

141. Roszler MH, Campbell WL. Post-ERCP pancreatitis: association with urographic visualization during ERCP. Radiology 1985; 157:595–598.

142. Kasugai T, Kuno N, Kizu M. Manometric endoscopic retrograde pancreatocholangiography. Am J Dig Dis 1974; 19:485–502.

143. Hamilton I, Lintott DJ, Rothwell J, Axon AT. Acute pancreatitis following endoscopic retrograde cholangiopancreatography. Clin Radiol 1983; 34:543–546.

144. Bilbao MK, Dotter CT, Lee TG, Katon RM. Complications of endoscopic retrograde cholangiopancreatography (ERCP). Gastroenterology 1976; 70:314–320.

145. van Husen N, Hogemann B, Egen V, Mehnert C. Radiation exposure in endoscopic retrograde cholangiopancreatography. Endoscopy 1984; 16:112–114.

146. Nebel OT, Silvis SE, Rogers G, et al. Complications associated with endoscopic retrograde cholangiopancreatography. Gastrointest Endosc 1975; 22:34–39

147. Lai ECS, Lo C, Choi T, et al. Urgent biliary decompression after endoscopic retrograde cholangiopancreatography. Am J Surg 1989; 157:121–125.

148. Classen DC, Jacobson JA, Burke JP, et al. Serious *Pseudomonas* infections associated with endoscopic retrograde cholangiopancreatography. Am J Med 1988; 84:590–596.

149. Doherty DE, Falko JM, Lefkovitz N, et al. *Pseudomonas aeruginosa* sepsis following retrograde cholangiopancreatography (ERCP). Dig Dis Sci 1982; 27:169–170.

150. Elson CO, Hattori K, Blackstone MO. Polymicrobial sepsis following endoscopic retrograde cholangiopancreatography. Gastroenterology 1975; 69:507–510.

151. Ferguson DR, Sivak MV. Indications, contraindications and complications of ERCP. In: Sivak MV, ed. Gastroenterologic Endoscopy. Philadelphia, PA: WB Saunders; 1987:581–598.

152. Wigton RS, Vennes JA. Clinical competence in diagnostic endoscopic retrograde cholangiopancreatography. Ann Intern Med 1988; 108:142–144.

Chapter 81
Esophagogastroduodenoscopy, colonoscopy and related techniques

Marsha Kay and Robert Wyllie

INTRODUCTION

The earliest gastrointestinal endoscopies were performed in the late 1880s using rigid instruments, looking initially at the esophagus and rectum. The semi-flexible gastroscope was developed in the early 1930s by Schindler and Wolf utilizing a series of short focal-length lenses and a semi-flexible tube.[1] Fiberoptic endoscopes representing a significant advance in endoscopy were popularized in the late 1960s and early 1970s, based on the principle of total internal reflection of light along cylindrical glass rods coated with a material of low refractive index. As light enters one end and strikes the interface between the highly refractive glass and the low refractive index of the glass coating, it is advanced by a series of internal reflections and emitted at the opposite end of the rod. Its position is maintained by maintaining the same relative position of each rod at both ends of the endoscope. With the advent of fiberoptic endoscopes came the availability of both tip control and biopsy capability. The first small-diameter instrument used for esophagogastroduodenoscopy (EGD) in a child was a fiberoptic bronchoscope.[2]

The development of the colonoscope followed that of upper pan-endoscopes. Rigid proctoscopes were developed in the late 1800s, and fiberoptic techniques were adapted to visualize the sigmoid and descending colon in the 1960s. In the 1970s the colonoscope was lengthened with four-way tip deflection, allowing for modern-day colonoscopic techniques.

Gastrocameras were used for still photographs in the late 1940s, but video endoscopy has been developed over the last three decades, with the first mass-produced video instruments introduced in the 1980s. Currently, video endoscopes have all but replaced fiberoptic endoscopes for EGD, endoscopic retrograde cholangiopancreatography (ERCP) and colonoscopy. Present-day trainees are unlikely to have used or even seen a fiberoptic endoscope, with the exception of some endoscopes still utilized for endoscopic ultrasonography (EUS). Dedicated pediatric video endoscopes with a narrow instrument diameter and preserved optic clarity are now widespread in their availability. with instrument outer diameters in the range of 6 mm. These small-caliber endoscopes have found widespread application for both children and adults, and are now being used with increased frequency in adults undergoing unsedated endoscopic procedures.

Pediatric gastrointestinal endoscopists are able to perform almost all of the endoscopic techniques of their adult counterparts. At the same time, they are developing unique applications of these techniques for pediatric patients. The advantage of pediatric gastrointestinal endoscopists is familiarity not only with age-related physiology but also with the spectrum of disease in pediatric patients. The referring physician and endoscopist should be familiar with the risks and benefits of endoscopy and those clinical situations in infants and children in which it is most likely to be useful.

PERSONNEL

Specially trained pediatric endoscopy assistants are an important component of the endoscopy team. Procedure anxiety can be diminished by an assistant who has previously met the child and parent(s), explained the procedure, and greeted them in the endoscopy suite. The same person can then hold and reassure the child throughout the procedure. A second assistant is typically needed to help obtain and process tissue during the procedure and assist with other equipment. Specially trained child life personnel can also be utilized to reduce procedure-related anxiety. Psychologic preparation prior to endoscopy has been shown to reduce procedure-related anxiety, improve patient cooperation, decrease autonomic nervous system stimulation during the procedure and reduce the amount of medication required.[3]

Physicians performing endoscopy on infants and children should have completed a pediatric gastroenterology fellowship or have experience with pediatric gastrointestinal diseases and adequate training in pediatric endoscopy. Guidelines for the minimal number of procedures to establish competency have been established by the North American Society for Pediatric Gastroenterology, Hepatology and Nutrition and the American Society for Gastrointestinal Endoscopy.[4,5] Intravenous sedation should be used only by physicians competent in the administration of drugs and resuscitation in children. Levels of sedation must be carefully and continuously assessed. There is a continuum from conscious sedation to deep sedation to general anesthesia. Physicians administering sedation should be familiar with the definitions of these three levels of sedation and appropriately credentialed for sedation administration, with appropriate equipment available for monitoring and resuscitation.[6]

FACILITIES

Routine endoscopy in infants and children is typically performed in an outpatient setting using parenteral sedation. Large series have reported on the efficacy and safety of this type of sedation with combined minor and major complication rates of less than 0.5% for both EGD and colonoscopy.[7] Occasionally it is necessary to perform endoscopy at the hospital bedside or in an operating room. In many institutions anesthesiologists are utilized to administer sedation for more invasive or therapeutic procedures such as foreign body removal (see Ch. 17), placement of percutaneous tubes (gastrostomy or cecostomy), dilation of strictures and pneumatic dilation, variceal band ligation and therapeutic endoscopy for gastrointestinal bleeding. Some endoscopists may also prefer the assistance of an anesthesiologist for younger patients or those in whom cooperation may be impaired.

The endoscopy suite should be equipped with instruments to monitor blood pressure, pulse rate and oxygen saturation. Pediatric resuscitation equipment including emergency medications and reversal agents, intravenous fluids, appropriately sized endotracheal tubes and laryngoscopes, oxygen and resuscitation bags should be available. Newer methods of non-invasive monitoring such as capnography are being evaluated primarily in the operating room setting and, if found to be helpful, may be adapted for use with procedures being performed utilizing conscious sedation.

EQUIPMENT

There are two main types of upper endoscopes: video endoscopes and fiberoptic endoscopes. Almost all endoscopes currently utilized are video endoscopes, although some EUS scopes are fiberoptic. Upper gastrointestinal endoscopes may also be divided on the basis of their angle of viewing: either forward or side viewing. Currently, side-viewing endoscopes are used only for ERCP and will be discussed in that context.

The video endoscope, an adaption of the fiberoptic instrument, is composed of a control handle that is attached to an insertion tube with a charge coupled device (CCD) located at its distal tip behind the objective lens.[8] The objective lens focuses a miniature picture on the surface of the CCD. The pattern of light falling on the CCD is converted to an array of electrical charges, transforming the optical image into an electronic representation. The charges developed in the CCD are 'read' and processed to reproduce the image ultimately being transmitted to a video processor for display on a television monitor.[8] Images are 'colorized' by different color imaging systems such as RGB (red, green, blue) sequential imaging system or color chip imaging technology. Each of the systems has advantages, descriptions of which are beyond the scope of this text. Differential color imaging systems are currently being studied in adults as a component of chromoendoscopy, used, for example, to distinguish dysplastic from non-dysplastic epithelium, and may some day find similar application in pediatric patients.

The control section of the endoscope is attached via a universal cord to a light, water, suction and electrical source. On the control handle, dials control the up–down and right–left angulation of the instrument tip. Lateral to each dial is a locking mechanism that increases the resistance to turning the dial. On the proximal shaft of the endoscope there are two valves. The more proximal valve is for suction, and the distal one controls air and water. Air is insufflated through the endoscope by lightly occluding the distal button. Firmly pushing down on the button provides a stream of water for irrigation through the endoscope. The control handle contains additional buttons to freeze or alter the image on the video screen. Parts or all of the procedure can be recorded for later review, and digital video recorders are now available for image storage and later retrieval.

Further down the endoscope is a channel with a biopsy valve, through which can be passed various instruments including biopsy forceps, cytology brushes, needles for sclerotherapy or injection, guidewires, coagulation probes, heater probes, polypectomy snares and other instruments. The endoscopic field can be irrigated manually by using a blunt-ended needle attached to a syringe and manually flushing the channel. The rate of irrigation that can be achieved by this method is greater than the rate achieved by occluding the button on the endoscope. If the air button does not function properly during endoscopy, air can also be injected with a syringe via this channel to avoid switching endoscopes in mid-procedure. At the endoscope tip are various openings: an air–water outlet (for lens cleaning), the objective lens, a light guide, and an instrument channel for suction and biopsy forceps. Large-diameter therapeutic instruments may contain an auxiliary water channel or a second suction/instrument channel, or both. The tip of the endoscope has a certain degree of angulation possible in an up or down, right or left direction. The flexible portion of the endoscope is the 'working length' of the instrument. Equipment such as a friction fit adaptor or hood has been developed to attach to the endoscope tip. The friction fit adaptor is used primarily to deploy bands for esophageal variceal ligation but can also be used in the treatment of esophageal meat impactions. The endoscopic hood is used primarily to assist with endoscopic mucosal resection (EMR), a new technique that has been developed primarily in adult patients for resection of large mucosal lesions including dysplastic epithelium or carcinomas.

There are two main types of small bowel enteroscopes. The first is the push-type enteroscope, which represents a modification of the pediatric colonoscope with an increased working length. The second type of small bowel endoscope is the passive enteroscope, also known as the Sonde-type small intestinal fiberscope. It is of much smaller diameter than the push-type enteroscope and is a forward-viewing instrument with a balloon cuff located at the scope tip to facilitate advancement of the scope by peristalsis into the small intestine. Most small bowel enteroscopies are currently performed using the push-type endoscope. Various adaptations of the push-type endoscopes are being developed to allow for examination and treatment of lesions identified in the more distal small bowel. The advantage of push-type endoscopes is that they have a working channel to perform therapeutic procedures such as polypectomy, biopsy, injection or coagulation. The endoscopes being developed have various balloon or stiffening devices to allow for more distal examination; some have recently become available for commercial use and may eventually be utilized for pediatric patients. Video capsule endoscopy (discussed below) will likely compete with small bowel enteroscopy as a method to examine the small bowel distal to the ligament of Treitz. Although capsules are not currently able to be read in real time and do not allow for tissue sampling or endoscopic therapy, future modifications of this technology may allow for these types of advancement, increasing the utility of this technology.

Colonoscopes are similar in construction to the upper endoscopes, with different diameters, instrument lengths, range of tip bending and fields of view. Colonoscopes of variable stiffness have been developed to decrease loop formation and assist with loop reduction. Although they are available for use in pediatric patients, variable stiffening of the endoscope should not be used to replace good endoscopic technique with the emphasis on minimal loop formation and rapid loop reduction.

The most important issues related to pediatric endoscopy equipment are the diameter and length of the insertion tube, the degree of tip angulation and the depth of field. In term infants, the esophagus measures only 4–6 mm in diameter and 9–10 cm in length.[9] Some of the earliest EGDs were performed using small-diameter bronchoscopes with an insertion tube diameter of 5 mm. However, the tubes were too short to allow adequate visualization of the small bowel. Despite theoretical concerns of trauma, perforation or airway compression, early pediatric endoscopists found that they could safely and effectively examine a neonate's digestive tract with an instrument of 7 mm in diameter without complication, due to distensibility of the esophagus. Newer gastrointestinal endoscopes have a 5–6 mm outer diameter with a 2-mm instrument channel and side viewing endoscopes have an outer diameter in the range of 7–8 mm. Standard upper endoscopes have an external diameter in the range of 8.0–9.8 mm with a 2.4–2.8-mm channel. Therapeutic channel scopes have an outer diameter in the range of 9.8–13.2 mm with an instrument channel of 3.2– 3.7 mm, and in the larger scopes dual channels up to 3.8 mm in diameter.

Colonoscopy in infants is usually performed with instruments designed for upper endoscopy because of their smaller diameter. Polypectomy snares can be passed via an upper endoscope with a 2.8-mm channel. Colonoscopy in normally developed children over 2 years of age can usually be performed with a colonoscope designed specifically for pediatric patients. Pediatric colonoscopes, including those with variable stiffness capabilities, have a distal end with an outer diameter in the range of 11.3–11.6 mm with a 3.2–3.8-mm channel, compared with an outer diameter of 12.8 mm for adult colonoscopes. (Endoscope information courtesy of Olympus America Inc., Melville, NY, and Pentax Precision Instrument Corporation, Orangeburg, NY)

INDICATIONS

The indications for gastrointestinal endoscopy vary with the age of the patient. The need for endoscopy in neonates and infants is usually suggested by physical signs reported by parents or other observers, and include vomiting, hematemesis, hematochezia, melena, hypotension, respiratory distress, abnormal posturing or anemia. With toddlers and older children the history is of greater importance in identifying gastrointestinal disorders. The sensitivity of gastrointestinal endoscopy in establishing a diagnosis varies with the indication for the procedure (Table 81.1).

Esophagogastroduodenoscopy

The yield of upper endoscopic examination in pediatric patients differs with the age of the child and the indication for the procedure. Younger patients with specific complaints such as failure to thrive and weight loss appear to have an increased incidence of pathology on endoscopic examination compared with older children with non-specific abdominal pain. In addition, endoscopies performed for gastrointestinal bleeding are more likely to identify a cause than procedures for non-specific complaints. Endoscopy can be performed for diagnosis (gastroe-

Esophagogastroduodenoscopy

Acid peptic disease
Suspicion of mucosal inflammation (including infection); biopsy, brushing and cytology examination
Acute epigastric or right upper quadrant pain
Hematemesis or melena
Dysphagia or odynophagia
Caustic ingestion or foreign-body ingestion
Recurrent vomiting
Therapeutic intervention
- Injection, coagulation or ligation of a bleeding lesion
- Stricture dilation or dilation of gastric outlet obstruction
- Pneumatic dilation
- PEG
- Catheter placement

Colonoscopy

Gastrointestinal hemorrhage
Chronic diarrhea
Suspected inflammatory bowel disease
Cancer surveillance
- Inflammatory bowel disease
- Polyposis syndromes

Therapeutic intervention
- Polyp removal
- Foreign-body removal
- Decompression of toxic megacolon
- Dilation of stricture
- Cautery or injection/ablation of bleeding lesion
- Percutaneous cecostomy
- Stricture dilation

Table 81.1 Indications for esophagogastroduodenoscopy and colonoscopy

sophageal reflux (GER), eosinophilic esophagitis and gastroenteritis, celiac disease, small bowel enteropathy, evaluation of graft-*vs*-host disease and surveillance for Barrett's esophagus, polyposis syndromes or following transplantation), therapy (stricture dilation, foreign body removal, percutaneous endoscopic gastrostomy (PEG) insertion, pyloric dilation, pneumatic dilation, catheter placement) or a combination of diagnosis and therapy (evaluation and treatment of gastrointestinal bleeding including that from acid peptic disease and variceal sources, evaluation of injury following a caustic ingestion).[10–12] Current guidelines and standards of practice should be followed in terms of the yield of endoscopy.[10,13] New endoscopic techniques continue to be developed, will be applied increasingly to pediatric patients, and are discussed at the end of this chapter.

Colonoscopy

The major indications for colonoscopy in infants and children include rectal bleeding, unexplained diarrhea, and abdominal pain with abnormal growth, weight loss or other constitutional symptoms. Colonoscopy is also performed to investigate abnormalities suspected on barium enema, small-bowel follow-through or computed tomography. Colonoscopy is typically the first line of investigation for patients with suspected mucosal disease, and barium enema is infrequently performed for this indication. If inflammatory bowel disease is suspected, endoscopy can provide visual evidence of the nature and extent of disease, and biopsies obtained at the time of the procedure may define the nature of the underlying inflammation. Infectious colitis may be difficult to distinguish visually from inflammatory bowel disease of recent onset, both visually and histologically, especially in patients less than 10 years of age.[14,15] Crohn's disease involving only the colon may also present with a focal active colitis pattern of injury similar to that seen with infection. Some patients may require follow-up endoscopic examination with biopsy to look for evidence of chronicity prior to establishing a firm diagnosis of inflammatory bowel disease. Visualization and biopsy of the terminal ileum may be helpful in the diagnosis of infectious ileitis. In some infections, such as ileocecal tuberculosis, colonic schistosomiasis and amebiasis, stool cultures are usually negative but the organisms can be identified on biopsy specimens or cytologic brushing.

Lymphonodular hyperplasia of the colon, although not an indication for colonoscopy, may be a cause of painless rectal bleeding identified at endoscopy. Thinning of the surface epithelium over the protruding lymphatic tissue with subsequent trauma from the passage of fecal material is thought to lead to ulceration and hematochezia. Prominent lymphatic nodules can be found throughout the large and small bowel. They appear as smooth, round, 2–4-mm nodules with normal overlying mucosa. Occasionally larger nodules may have central umbilication or overlying erosion. This nodular lymph node tissue is thought to represent a self-limiting response to antigenic stimulation and does not require any additional evaluation or therapy.

In children with suspected polyps, colonoscopy is both diagnostic and therapeutic. In diseases associated with an increased rate of malignancy, such as ulcerative colitis, Crohn's disease or familial polyposis, colonoscopic surveillance for dysplastic changes is usually performed at regular intervals. Colonoscopy has been reported for the diagnosis and evaluation of smooth muscle tumors in children with acquired immune deficiency syndrome. These lesions may appear as a submucosal nodule with central umbilication.[16] Colonoscopy is usually not indicated in children complaining of chronic abdominal pain or constipation with unremarkable physical examinations and laboratory studies. However, changes of mucosal prolapse in patients with chronic constipation may on occasion be noted at endoscopy (Fig. 81.1).

Indications for therapeutic colonoscopy include polypectomy, vascular ablation, retrieval of a foreign body, placement of a percutaneous cecostomy and colonic decompression in toxic megacolon. Colonoscopy with therapeutic intervention for vascular lesions can eliminate the need for surgery in many cases. The types of lesion encountered include cavernous hemangiomas and small telangiectasias. Syndromes associated with vascular lesions in the gastrointestinal tract, include Osler–Weber–Rendu, CREST syndrome (calcinosis cutis, Raynaud phenomenon, sclerodactyly and telangiectasis), dyschondroplasia (Maffucci's syndrome), blue rubber bleb nevus syndrome, diffuse neonatal hemangiomatosis, Turner's syndrome and pseudoxanthoma elasticum.

Colonic strictures can also be dilated through the endoscope using through the channel controlled external diameter balloon dilators. Intussusception has been identified and reduced during colonoscopy, but air–contrast reduction remains the procedure of choice. Recently colonoscopy has been employed as an alternative to surgery to direct colonic Gastrografin administration in patients with

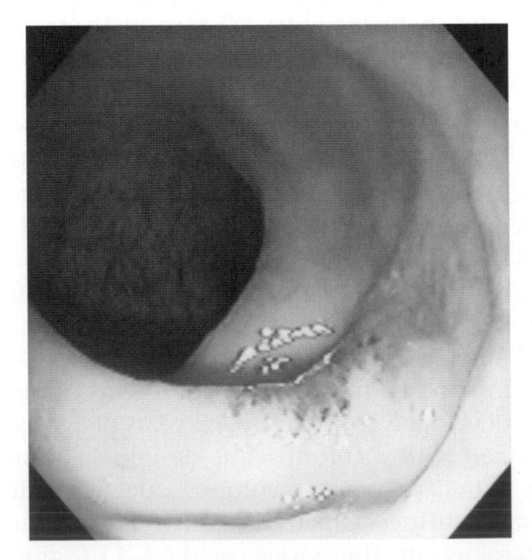

Figure 81.1: Endoscopic appearance of the rectum in a patient with mucosal prolapse. Note localized friability due to repetitive prolapse with an otherwise normal mucosal appearance. (*See plate section for color.*)

cystic fibrosis and distal intestinal obstruction syndrome refractory to medical therapy.[17] Only practitioners with adequate experience should undertake technically advanced therapeutic endoscopic procedures.

CONTRAINDICATIONS

Absolute contraindications to gastrointestinal endoscopy include suspected perforation of the intestine and peritonitis in a toxic patient. There are several relative contraindications, including patients who are severely neutropenic or have bleeding disorders and children with a recent history of bowel surgery. In addition, patients with connective tissue disease, especially Ehlers–Danlos and Marfan's syndromes, are at increased risk of perforation during endoscopy.[18] Toxic dilation of the bowel carries an increased risk of perforation during colonoscopy, although the procedure may relieve the distention. Other relative contraindications include partial or complete bowel obstruction and aneurysm of the abdominal and iliac aorta. In all endoscopic procedures the clinician and endoscopist must determine whether the potential information or therapeutic intervention outweighs the risk of the procedure (Table 81.2).

ANTIBIOTIC PROPHYLAXIS

The incidence of bacteremia after gastrointestinal endoscopy varies according to the patient's underlying medical problem and the procedure performed: EGD 0–8% (mean 4.4%), colonoscopy 0–25% (mean 4.4%), sclerotherapy 31%, endoscopic variceal ligation 1–25% (mean 8.8%) and esophageal dilation 12–22%.[19] Certain bacteria are more likely to be the cause of bacteremia after a procedure. These include *Escherichia coli*, *Bacteroides*, *Pseudomonas*, *Veillonella* and *Peptostreptococcus*, especially after a lower gastrointestinal procedure.[20] However, other bacteria may be more virulent and more likely to cause endocarditis, especially *Streptococcus viridans* and enterococcus.[21] Prophylaxis is directed by the frequency and virulence of the anticipated organisms that may be encountered during the procedure.

Absolute contraindications
Suspected bowel perforation Acute peritonitis
Relative contraindications
Bleeding disorders and/or impaired platelet function Neutropenia Patients with increased risk of bowel perforation, including: • Connective tissue disorders (Ehlers–Danlos and Marfan syndromes) • Toxic dilation of the bowel • Partial or complete intestinal obstruction • Recent bowel surgery

Table 81.2 Contraindications to endoscopy in infants and children

The actual incidence of bacterial endocarditis following gastrointestinal procedures is quite low, with fewer than 20 cases reported. Antibiotic recommendations are based on a combination of procedure-related risk of bacteremia and patient risk, and should be reassessed periodically as new data and guidelines become available.[19,22]

Patients at high risk for infective endocarditis are those with prosthetic heart valves, including bioprosthetic and homograft valves, a previous history of bacterial endocarditis, a surgically constructed systemic pulmonary shunt or conduit, and complex cyanotic congenital cardiac malformations including single ventricle states, transposition of the great arteries and tetralogy of Fallot. Prophylaxis is usually given prior to the procedure, but is no longer repeated 6–8 h after the procedure except in the case of PEGs or other special procedures.

Intermediate-risk patients include most other congenital cardiac malformations, acquired valvular dysfunction (e.g. rheumatic heart disease), hypertrophic cardiomyopathy, mitral valve prolapse with valvular regurgitation and/or thickened leaflets.

Prophylaxis is not required in patients considered not to be at increased risk, including those with physiologic functional or 'innocent' murmurs, and following surgery for coronary artery bypass graft, cardiac pacemakers or implanted defibrillators. Patients with a history of Kawasaki disease without valvular dysfunction, mitral valve prolapse, or rheumatic heart disease without valvular dysfunction do not routinely require prophylaxis. Patients who are status post repair of atrial septal defects, ventricular septal defects or patent ductus arteriosus without residual dysfunction, or those who have secundum atrial septal defects, also are not routinely given antibiotics prior to endoscopic procedures. The current antibiotic recommendations for prophylaxis are outlined in Table 81.3.

For most endoscopic procedures, including EGD, sigmoidoscopy, colonoscopy with or without biopsy, polypectomy and non-variceal hemostasis, antibiotic prophylaxis is not indicated for patients at intermediate risk or no increased risk. Decisions regarding high-risk patients should be made on a case-by-case basis. For endoscopy procedures associated with an increased risk of transient bacteremia including dilation of an esophageal stricture, varix sclerotherapy and ERCP, prophylaxis is recommended for high-risk patients; decisions regarding intermediate-risk patients should be made on a case-by-case basis, and no prophylaxis is recommended for patients at no increased risk.

Antibiotic prophylaxis is recommended for all patients prior to PEG placement and for all patients undergoing ERCP for known or suspected biliary obstruction or known pancreatic pseudocyst, including those who are undergoing pseudocyst drainage or aspiration. In the case of ERCP, antibiotics should be directed against biliary flora including enteric Gram-negative organisms, enterococci and possibly *Pseudomonas* species. Prior to PEG placement,

1 Amoxicillin 2.0 g by mouth (adult) or 50 mg/kg by mouth (child) 60 min before procedure. Alternative for those unable to take by mouth: ampicillin 2.0 g IV or IM (adult) or 50 mg/kg IV or IM (child) within 30 min before procedure
2 *For patients who are penicillin allergic*: Clindamycin 600 mg by mouth (adult) or 20 mg/kg by mouth (child) 1 h before procedure. Alternatives: cephalexin or cefadroxil 2.0 g by mouth (adult) or 50 mg/kg (child) 1 h before procedure; azithromycin or clarithromycin 500 mg by mouth (adult) or 15 mg/kg by mouth (child) 1 h before procedure
3 *For patients who are penicillin allergic and unable to take by mouth*: Clindamycin 600 mg IV (adult) or 20 mg/kg IV (child) within 30 min before procedure. Alternatives: cefazolin 1.0 g IV or IM (adult) or 25 mg/kg IV or IM (child) within 30 min before procedure; vancomycin 1.0 g IV (adult) or 10–20 mg/kg (child)
4 *PEG prophylaxis*: Parenteral cefazolin (or an antibiotic with equivalent coverage) 30 min before the procedure; additional doses following the procedure may be indicated

From Hirota et al., 2003.[19]

Table 81.3 Regimen for endocarditis prophylaxis

parenteral coverage with cefazolin or an equivalent antibiotic is indicated.[19]

Other special patient populations include those with a prosthetic joint or orthopedic prosthesis, in whom antibiotics are generally not recommended; patients with gastrointestinal hemorrhage, in whom antibiotics are generally recommended; patients with cirrhosis, especially those with ascites; patients following transplantation; or other immunocompromised patients undergoing high-risk procedures where prophylaxis should be considered on a case by case basis.[19]

PREPARATION

Esophagogastroduodenoscopy

Preparation for upper gastrointestinal endoscopic procedures involves a period of fasting except in emergency situations. Infants less than 6 months of age are not fed for 2–4 h prior to endoscopy, and children over 2 years of age fast for 6–8 h. Recent studies have suggested that a shorter period of pre-endoscopy fasting may be possible.[23] Although fasting for milk and solids for 4–8 h, depending on patient age, prior to endoscopy is still required, it may be possible to decrease the pre-endoscopy fasting interval for clear liquids to 2–3 h.[24]

Colonoscopy

In addition to a period of fasting, lower pan-endoscopy can be accomplished successfully only if the colon is free of fecal debris. Large amounts of stool compromise the ability to negotiate the curves of the large bowel and prohibit complete visualization of the mucosa. Stool adherent to the lens often requires additional maneuvering and added air–water insufflation to clear the field of vision. Liquid stool can be aspirated through the suction channel but increases the examination time.

Many bowel preparations have been utilized successfully to cleanse the colon. The method depends on the age and cooperation of the child and the individual experience of the examiner. In infants who are totally breast- or bottle-fed, adequate preparation can usually be obtained with the use of small-volume enemas and substituting clear liquids for breast- or bottle-feeding for 12–24 h. In older children and adolescents, the best preparation is usually obtained with the use of colonic lavage solutions that contain a non-absorbable solution of polyethylene glycol and electrolytes (PEG-ELS), which causes an osmotic diarrhea.[25] The risk of dehydration is minimal because of the limited transmural flux of sodium and water. To be effective, a large volume of solution must be ingested over a relatively short period of time. In adolescents of adult size, the usual regimen is 240 ml every 10 min until the fecal effluent is clear. This often requires 3 or 4 l of solution. Smaller volumes are recommended for younger children (Table 81.4). Occasionally, nasogastric administration may be necessary. The rate of nasogastric administration is 20–30 ml/min, or 1.2–1.8 l/h in an older child or adolescent. Appropriate volume reductions can be made for infants and smaller children.

Oral cleansing solutions are effective in over 95% of the patients who drink adequate amounts of the fluid. An occasional patient may experience presumed allergic reactions manifested as dermatitis, urticaria and rhinorrhea.[26] Recently, combination regimens have been evaluated in adults using bisacodyl in addition to PEG-ELS. Addition of bisacodyl may allow for a reduction in the volume of PEG-ELS required, or allow for the use of split-dose regimens.[27] Recently, non-absorbable polyethylene glycol without electrolytes has been reported as an effective bowel-cleansing regimen in children.[28] Minor electrolyte changes may be noted with this regimen.

If the child cannot comply with a large-volume lavage preparation, most endoscopists use an alternative regimen of clear liquids for 48–72 h, accompanied by magnesium citrate the night before the procedure and saline enemas

Weight of child (kg)	Volume (ml) each 10 min until passage of clear fecal effluent	Maximum volume (ml)
<10	80	1100
10–20	100	1600
20–30	140	2200
30–40	180	2900
40–50	200	3200
>50	240	4000

Adapted from Bines and Winter, 1991, with permission.[140]

Table 81.4 Bowel preparation using PEG-ELS oral solutions

administered the night before and the morning of the procedure to clear any residual stool (Table 81.5).

Oral sodium phosphate is an alternative regimen, available in both liquid and tablet form. The cathartic action of oral sodium phosphate is due to its osmotic properties. Oral sodium phosphate solutions are generally safe and effective in patients without significant co-morbid conditions.[29] However, there are a number of case reports of serious adverse effects, related primarily to inappropriate dosing or non-compliance with the prescribed regimen of medication dilution or administration of additional fluids.[30,31] The cathartic effects of oral sodium phosphate may result in significant hypovolemia.[32] Extra caution must be used in patients vulnerable to minor shifts in intravascular volume or transient increases in serum phosphate levels.[31,32] Aphthous ulceration of the colon has been observed following sodium phosphate bowel preparation.

SEDATION AND MONITORING

Sedation is used in most pediatric patients not only to minimize discomfort but also to provide amnesia for the procedure. This helps to prevent the child from becoming fearful of contact with the physician, which is especially important in pediatric patients with chronic conditions that may require repeated procedures. Most pediatric endoscopists have replaced general anesthesia with intravenous sedation for routine upper and lower endoscopy. General anesthesia may be required for therapeutic procedures such as foreign body removal, dilation or PEG placement, or in

Product	Dose	Duration	Maximum	Additional comments	Side-effects (non-inclusive)	References
PEG (Miralax)	1.5 g/kg daily divided bid or tid	4 days	102 g/day (adult)	± Normal saline enema. Clears day before. Mixing beverage: patient choice	Nausea, abdominal pain, vomiting, mild electrolyte changes (K, CO_2, BUN)	28
Oral sodium phosphate	*Adults*: 45 ml/dose 1–2 doses 5–12 h apart, *must be diluted* and *followed by* 64 oz *liquid* per manufacturer's instruction *Pediatric*: Single dose Age 5–9 years: 5–10 ml ×1 Age 10–12 years: 10–20 ml ×1 diluted in 4 oz and follow with >8 oz liquid, as above	Day before colonoscopy	*Adults*: 90 ml total or 40 tablets of Visicol	Follow manufacturer's precautions. May be contraindicated in congenital megacolon, bowel obstruction, renal or cardiac disease, electrolyte imbalance, patient at risk for increased phosphate absorption, and dehydrated patient	Nausea, abdominal pain, vomiting, hyperphosphatemia, hypocalcemia, hypomagnesemia, seizure or fatality secondary to above, volume contraction, colonic mucosal changes (aphthous ulceration)	29, 30,32, 141
Magnesium citrate	1 oz per year of age	Evening prior to procedure	10 oz	± Saline enema		
Magnesium citrate with X-prep	Age 2–5 years: 4 oz magnesium citrate and 2.5 oz X-prep Age >5 years: 6 oz magnesium citrate and 2.5 oz X-prep	1 dose on day prior to colonoscopy				25
Bisacodyl (Dulcolax)	Age 2–5 years: 5 mg Age 5–12 years: 10 mg ≥12 years: 15 mg	Each day for 2 days prior to colonoscopy		Fleets enema on morning of colonoscopy. May be associated with inadequate mucosal visualization		25

*Clear liquids for 24–48 h required in association with the above preparations. BUN, blood urea nitrogen.

Table 81.5 Alternate bowel preparation regimens (non-PEG–electrolyte)*

patients in whom cooperation is not anticipated. A variety of regimens have been tried in pediatric patients, although there are few comparative trials. Most pediatric endoscopists use a combination of a benzodiazepine and a narcotic such as midazolam and meperidine for conscious sedation. A variety of other agents, such as fentanyl, ketamine–midazolam and, more recently, propofol administered by an anesthesiologist and considered a sedative anesthetic, have also been used in pediatric patients.[33–37] Oral midazolam premedication prior to conscious sedation with a combination of a benzodiazepine and a narcotic has also been reported.[34] In selected highly motivated pediatric patients, unsedated endoscopy has been successful.[38]

When used together, meperidine 1–2 mg/kg bodyweight to a maximum of 100 mg is administered by slow infusion followed by midazolam 0.1–0.2 mg/kg bodyweight. The dose of midazolam is titrated according to the patient's level of consciousness, but rarely exceeds 5 mg as a total dose. Meperidine is usually given first to decrease the discomfort at the site of injection associated with intravenous midazolam. Younger children may require more midazolam per kilogram of bodyweight. Occasionally, it may be necessary to administer additional amounts of these medications during the procedure.

Transient reactions at the site of medication administration are not unusual and include cutaneous erythema distal to the site of injection not associated with clinically significant thrombophlebitis. Other reactions include coughing and a characteristic taste with meperidine infusion. In a prospective evaluation of this method of sedation in 100 pediatric endoscopic procedures at the Cleveland Clinic, approximately 50% of the patients had generalized cutaneous flushing, and urticaria without audible wheezing developed in 12 children. Rechallenge with the same sedative in two patients did not result in a more severe reaction.[39] Endoscopy in neonates may be performed with or without sedation, depending on the indication for the procedure. Sedation is helpful if the procedure will last more than a few minutes or interventional endoscopy is anticipated.

General anesthesia is necessary when a patient is uncooperative, requires a lengthy or complicated procedure, or has extenuating medical problems.

During the endoscopic procedure, arterial oxygen saturation and electrocardiographic tracings are routinely monitored. Patients aged less than 1 year, compared with patients more than 1 year of age and those with underlying cardiopulmonary disease, have a greater tendency for decreased mean oxygen saturation with endoscopy.

Oxygen desaturation during sedation may occur without clinically apparent signs and symptoms. For this reason, pulse oximetry should be monitored during endoscopy. Neurologically impaired patients often have gastrointestinal problems that require endoscopy. Sedation in these patients can be unpredictable, and respiratory depression is more common. The dosage of meperidine is therefore reduced to 0.5–1.0 mg/kg bodyweight, and the dosage of midazolam, if this drug is used, is titrated very slowly. Careful and attentive monitoring of the cardiopulmonary status is essential. Medication dosages are also reduced in patients who have undergone a recent weight loss where the volume of distribution may be altered. These include patients with inflammatory bowel disease, malignancy and anorexia nervosa. A number of other adverse effects, including respiratory depression, pulmonary edema, allergic reactions, arrhythmias, hypotension, paradoxical reactions and hallucinations, have been reported following a variety of sedation regimens.[36,40] Endoscopists should counsel patients and their families based on the specific known risks associated with their preferred sedation regimen.

Naloxone is indicated only for narcotic-induced respiratory depression, because its use is usually associated with marked irritability in infants and young children. Flumazenil (Mazicon) is a intravenous benzodiazepine antagonist that competitively blocks the effects of benzodiazepines on γ-aminobutyric acid pathway-mediated inhibition in the central nervous system.[41] Experience is limited with this agent; side-effects with administration include facial erythema, dizziness, hyperexcitability, seizures and serious cardiac arrhythmias. Because its half-life is shorter than that of benzodiazepines, re-sedation after reversal of benzodiazepine sedation may occur, and patients should be monitored accordingly. Routine administration after endoscopy appears to be of questionable benefit in pediatric patients.[42] Recommended doses for intravenous sedation medications and reversal agents are indicated in Table 81.6.

ANATOMY

Esophagogastroduodenoscopy

The esophagus is located posterior to the trachea in the neck. It ranges in diameter from 4 to 6 mm and in length from 9 to 10 cm in the term infant, to a length of approximately 25 cm in the adult.[2] It begins distal to the cricoid cartilage and ends at the cardiac orifice of the stomach.

The esophagus opens with swallowing, unlike the trachea, which is always open except with vocal cord movement. The esophageal opening appears lateral and posterior to each side of the trachea with swallowing. The trachea is easily distinguished from the esophagus by the presence of bilateral vocal cords on its anterolateral aspects and, if intubated, by the circular tracheal rings along its length.

The esophagus is narrowed at four locations: (1) at the level of the cricopharyngeus, (2) where the esophagus is crossed by the aortic arch, (3) where it is crossed by the left mainstream bronchus and (4) at the lower esophageal sphincter. Of these, the regions just below the cricopharyngeus and just above the lower esophageal sphincter are often the sites where foreign bodies lodge after ingestion. The lower esophageal sphincter plays an important role in certain diseases, such as achalasia and GER.

The stomach is usually located beneath the diaphragm and, in an adult, is approximately 10 cm distal to the incisors. The right aspect of the esophagus is in continuity

Medication	Dose	Maximum total dose	Onset (min)	Duration of action
Benzodiazepines				
Midazolam	0.05–0.4 mg/kg	≤5 years: 6 mg >5 years: 10 mg	1–5	1–5 h IM 20–30 min IV
Diazepam	0.1–0.3 mg/kg	10 mg	5–30	30–60 h
Narcotics				
Meperidine	1–2 mg/kg	100 mg/dose	5–15	3–5 h IM 2–3 h IV
Fentanyl	1–5 µg/kg	100 µg	1–5	0.5–1 h
Antagonists				
Flumazenil	0.01 mg/kg	0.2 mg/dose or 1.0 mg total	1–2	20–60 min
Naloxone	0.1 mg/kg	2 mg/dose or 10 mg total	2–5	20–60 min

From Nowicki and Vaughn, 2002, with permission.[36]

Table 81.6 Recommended doses for intravenous sedation medications and reversal agents

with the lesser curvature of the stomach, whereas the left margin of the esophagus joins the greater curvature (Fig. 81.2). The gastric rugae are most prominent along the greater curvature. The area of the stomach where the esophagus enters is known as the gastric cardia. The portion of the stomach above the junction of the esophagus and stomach is known as the fundus; it is also the most posterior aspect of the stomach. The majority of the stomach is known as the body of the stomach. On occasion, the esophagogastric junction is located above the diaphragm, representing a hiatal hernia. Along the lesser curvature of the stomach is the incisura. This notch divides the body of the stomach from the gastric antrum. The pylorus is the muscular junction between the stomach and the small intestine. The pyloric canal is 2–3 cm in length in the adult. The diameter of the pyloric opening may vary according to patient age and size, and may be affected or altered in certain disease states.

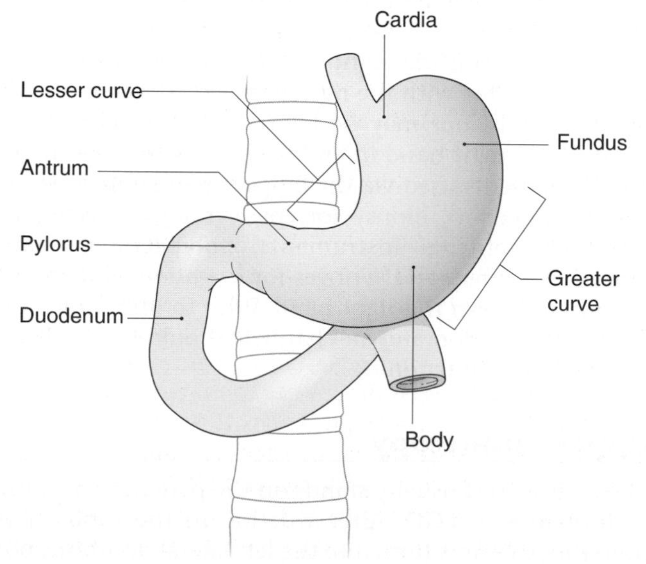

Figure 81.2: Endoscopic anatomy of the stomach and duodenum.

The most proximal portion of the small intestine is the duodenum. The average duodenal length in a full-term infant is 5 cm.[43] The duodenal bulb is an expanded region immediately distal to the pylorus. The duodenum then forms a C-shaped loop and, from the endoscopist's point of view, turns posteriorly and to the right for 2.5 cm in the older child and adult, then inferiorly for 7.5–10 cm (descending portion), then anteriorly and to the left for approximately 2.5 cm, finally connecting to the jejunum at the level of the ligament of Treitz. When it joins the jejunum, it turns abruptly forward.

The common bile duct and pancreatic duct enter the duodenal wall obliquely and join together in the ampulla of Vater, which opens into the descending portion of the duodenum via the duodenal papilla. The papilla is usually located approximately 8–10 cm distal to the pylorus in adults. The pancreatic duct may also empty via an accessory pancreatic duct, which is usually located proximal to the major duodenal papilla. The duodenum, unlike the jejunum or ileum, does not have a mesentery.

The jejunum and ileum form a series of loops attached to the posterior abdominal wall via a mesentery. In a newborn, the average small intestinal length is 266 ± 56 cm.[44] In adults, the jejunum represents the proximal 2 m and the ileum represents the distal 3 m of the small bowel. Although the point of transition is often unclear, the jejunum is initially located in the left upper and left lower quadrants. Intraluminally, the jejunum is characterized by large thick folds, large villi and a luminal diameter of approximately 4 cm. The ileum is thinner walled than the jejunum, with an inner diameter of 3.5 cm, smaller villi and an increased amount of lymphoid tissue compared with the jejunum.

Colonoscopy

The small intestine and transverse and sigmoid colons are attached to mesentery and shift positions freely (Fig. 81.3). Their excursion during a procedure is limited by the length of bowel and length of their attachment. Disease processes, masses or adhesions may influence their configuration or limit their mobility. The ascending colon and descending colon are relatively fixed in the retroperitoneum. The rectum is also relatively fixed as it passes through the pelvic connective tissue, with only a short segment free within the peritoneal cavity.

From the endoscopist's point of view, the anus is first intubated, then the rectum courses posteriorly to the coccyx and follows the gentle angle of the sacrum to the peritoneal reflection. Three 'valves of Houston', two on the right and the middle one on the left, are encountered. These are crescentic, or semilunar, folds and are due to tension by the longitudinal muscle fibers of the teniae coli. These folds assume a more circular pattern in the sigmoid and descending colon, and a characteristic triangular pattern in the transverse colon.

The sigmoid colon is attached to a mesentery and is relatively mobile. The descending colon is usually straight and ends at the splenic flexure, which forms an acute angulation with the transverse colon, turning abruptly to the right and anteriorly. The hepatic flexure forms the distal margin of the transverse colon and forms another abrupt, but inferior and posterior, angle with the descending colon. The transverse colon has a variable configuration and is suspended on a mesentery between the two fixed flexures. The ascending colon is fixed in the retroperitoneum and is relatively straight, ending in the mobile cecum. At the pole of the cecum the tenia fuse to cause a marked cecal haustration, often forming a 'crow's foot' or 'Mercedes Benz' sign. The appendiceal orifice is usually a crescentic opening slightly to the left of the midline (Fig. 81.4). Occasionally it may appear as a tubular diverticulum. The post-appendectomy opening appears identical unless the appendiceal stump has been inverted.

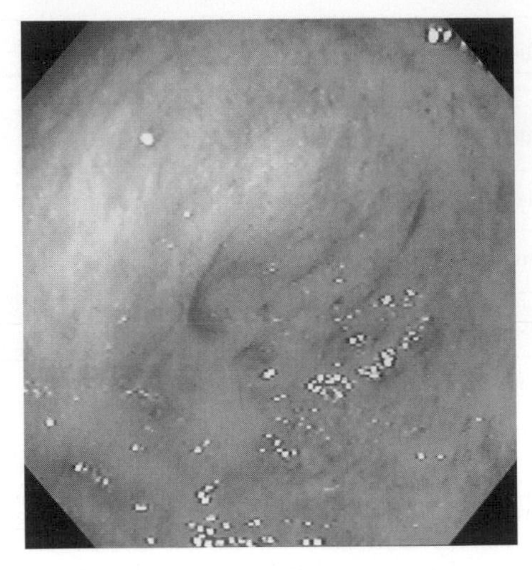

Figure 81.4: Typical appearance of the appendiceal orifice at colonoscopy. (*See plate section for color.*)

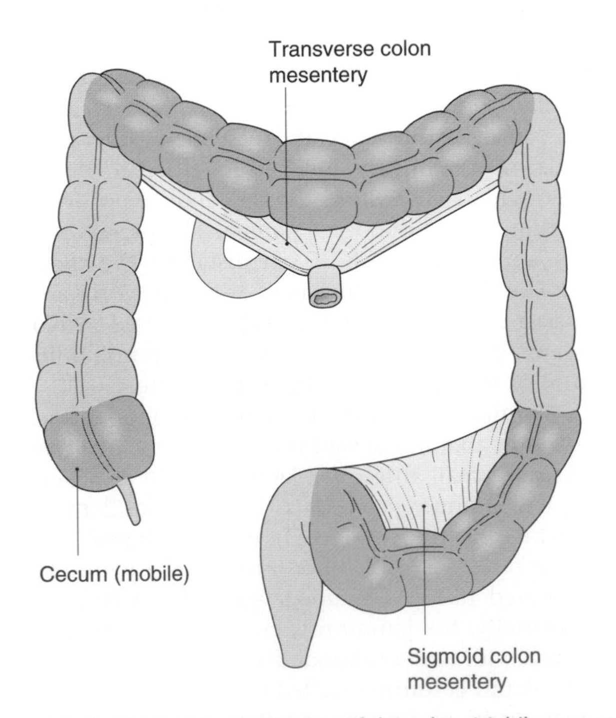

Figure 81.3: Mesenteric attachments of the colon. Mobile areas are darkened.

The ileocecal valve lies proximal to the cecal pole on the prominent ileocecal fold. It usually cannot be directly visualized but is recognizable by a slight irregularity of the fold, with the ileum passing obliquely downward from its cecal opening. The ileum is characterized by the circumferential valvular conniventes and a predominance of lymphoid tissue, especially in younger children (Fig. 81.5).

TECHNIQUE

The endoscope is held in the left hand. The thumb is used to turn the large dial; the index finger and sometimes the middle finger are used to control the suction, air and water valves; and the remaining fingers hold the control handle. The insertion tube is held in the right hand. The lateral wheel, which controls right and left tip deflection, is usually manipulated with the right hand by endoscopists with smaller hands, but may be controlled by either the left hand or the right hand in endoscopists with larger hands. The instruments used via the biopsy channel include needles for injection, biopsy forceps, cytology brushes, foreign-body retrieval instruments, polypectomy snares, probes for cautery and syringes for irrigation, and are usually inserted with the right hand. Prior to initiating a procedure, the suction and air channels should be checked to ensure proper functioning.

Upper endoscopy

The endoscopist usually stands on the patient's left during performance of EGD. After sedation in the supine position, the patient is turned to the left lateral decubitus position with the neck flexed downward in preparation for the

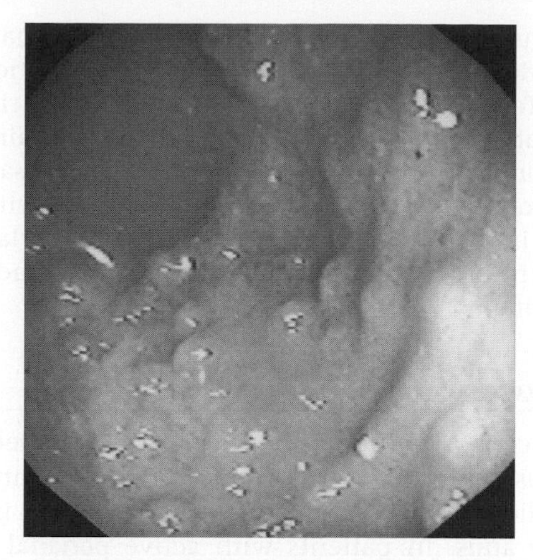

Figure 81.5: Lymphonodular hyperplasia of the terminal ileum. Note glistening mucosa and nodularity without erosions, which is characteristic. (*See plate section for color.*)

procedure. Patients undergoing endoscopy under general anesthesia are usually left in the supine position rather than being placed in the lateral decubitus position for ease of airway management. Prior to insertion of the endoscope into the oral cavity, a bite block is placed in the mouth of the non-intubated patient. The endoscope dials are placed in a neutral position. Some operators prefer to lock the right–left dial during esophageal intubation. The endoscope is guided through the bite block over the tongue to the back of the oropharynx by directing the endoscope tip posteriorly and somewhat laterally to the trachea; lateral motion is obtained by right and left torque on the shaft rather than by turning the dial. Some individuals use their forefinger to direct the tip and blindly advance the instrument. As the patient swallows, the cricopharyngeus relaxes and the esophagus, located posteriorly to the trachea and between the pyriform sinuses, can be intubated under direction vision. If the patient is unwilling or unable to swallow after the tip of the instrument is positioned at the esophageal inlet, gentle pressure will usually ease the tip through the cricopharyngeus into the proximal esophagus. The position of the endoscope during this procedure usually makes the patient gag, and if the instrument cannot be passed expeditiously it should be withdrawn.

After intubating the esophagus, the instrument is advanced down the esophageal lumen while simultaneously examining the mucosa for any lesions. The mucosa is examined as the instrument is inserted to avoid misinterpreting mucosal changes caused by passage of the endoscope. The esophagus is examined for evidence of inflammation, ulcerations, varices, hernias and strictures. The location of the lower esophageal sphincter should be noted. The transition between squamous esophageal and gastric columnar mucosa is called the ‘Z line’. At this point, the mucosa changes from a pale pink to a deep red. The diaphragmatic constriction of the lumen should be noted within 2 cm of the squamocolumnar junction unless a hiatal hernia or Barrett’s esophagus is present.

When the stomach is entered, suction is utilized to remove any residual gastric secretions. After the gastric secretions are removed, air is insufflated to separate the gastric rugae. The endoscope is then advanced while torquing to the right. This can be accomplished by applying pressure to the shaft or by the endoscopist twisting to the right; with video instruments, torque can also be achieved by dropping the handle to the right or left, depending on the desired direction of torque. The endoscope is advanced along the lesser curve toward the pylorus, but it is usually necessary to fill the greater curvature with the endoscope prior to cannulating the pyloric canal (Fig. 81.6).

The pylorus appears as a small opening with radiating folds around it. Periodic antral waves may pass to the pylorus, changing its location and the size of the canal opening. The pylorus is entered by nudging the tip of the endoscope up to the opening and then directly cannulating the pyloric canal.

The duodenal bulb should be examined upon endoscope insertion rather than during withdrawal because of possible mucosal changes caused by passage of the instrument. After examination of all four quadrants, the scope is advanced to the posterior aspect of the bulb where the duodenum takes a sharp right and downward turn. The instrument is advanced using the dials and shaft torque, usually down and to the right followed by an upward spin of the dial, bringing the tip into the descending duodenum. Once the lumen of the descending duodenum is seen, a straightening maneuver is performed. This consists of pulling the endoscope slowly backward while maintaining the lumen in view. This reduces the loop along the greater curvature of the stomach and usually, paradoxically, advances the endoscope into the distal duodenum (Fig. 81.7). The duodenal mucosa, including

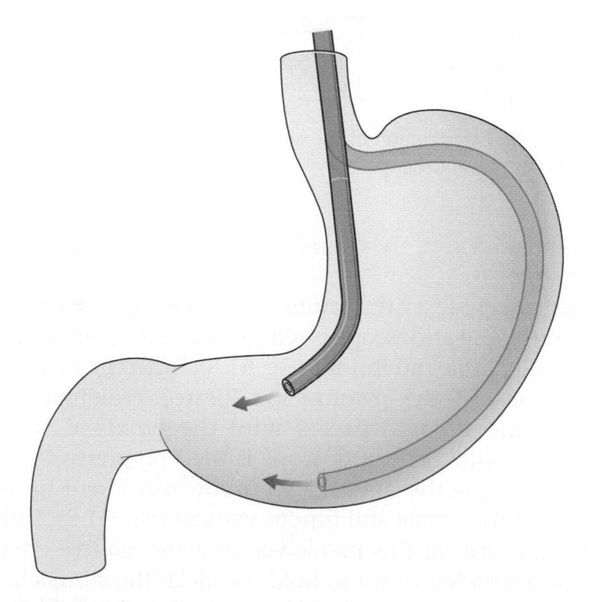

Figure 81.6: Advancement of the endoscope to the duodenum by filling the loop of the greater curvature.

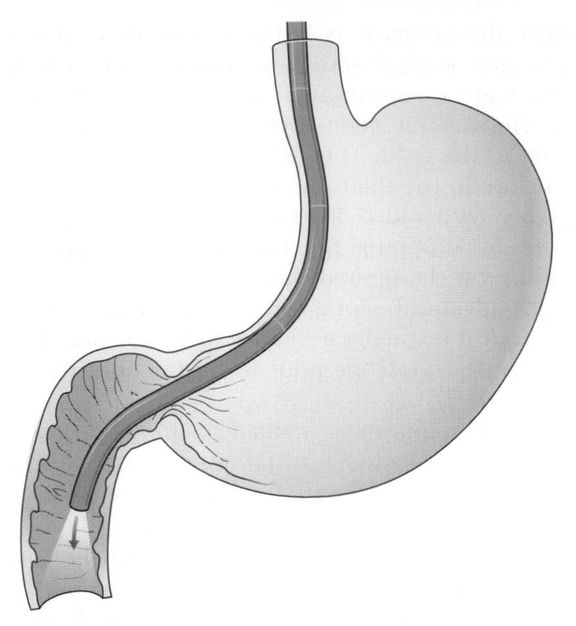

Figure 81.7: Duodenal straightening maneuver that paradoxically advances the endoscope into the distal duodenum by scope withdrawal.

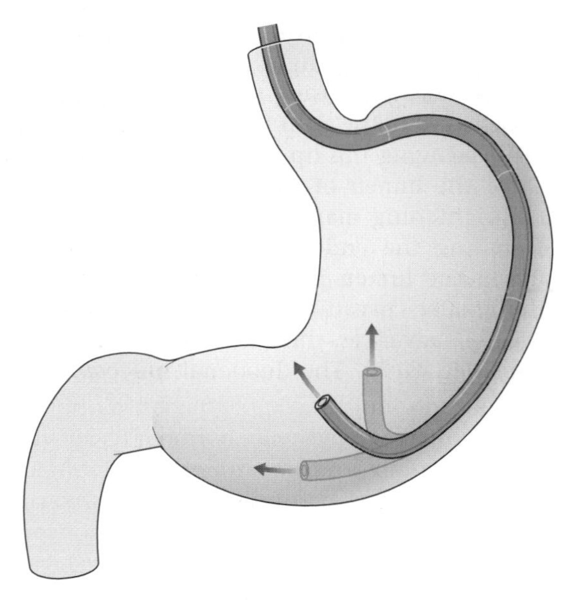

Figure 81.8: Examination of the antrum and incisura by upward deflection of the endoscope tip.

ampulla of Vater, is examined while withdrawing the endoscope.

After adequate examination of the antrum, pylorus and duodenum, the endoscope is retroflexed to look for lesions in the gastric cardia and fundus (Fig. 81.8). With the instrument looking toward the pylorus and located proximal to the incisura, the tip is deflected until the proximal stomach comes into view. The endoscope is then progressively withdrawn, bringing the cardia closer to the instrument tip while distending the cardia and fundus with air (Fig. 81.9). Patients often burp during this maneuver, and cooperative children may be instructed to try to hold the air in the stomach. The endoscope is then rotated 180° in each direction by torquing the insertion tube in a clockwise or counterclockwise manner.

The instrument is then straightened, the remainder of the gastric mucosa is examined and biopsies, if necessary, are performed. The endoscope is then withdrawn. Immediately prior to its leaving the stomach, air is aspirated from the stomach. The esophageal mucosa is once again examined. The endoscope is usually withdrawn rapidly in children when the level of the larynx is reached in order to increase patient comfort and diminish gagging.

Colonoscopy

Colonoscopy is traditionally performed in the left lateral decubitus position with the knees bent. A lubricant is usually applied to the tip of the instrument prior to insertion into the anus. In patients with active perianal disease, lubrication with viscous lidocaine may relieve some discomfort. It is usually necessary to reapply lubricant during the procedure, as the lubricant tends to dry as the endoscope is serially advanced and withdrawn. The endoscopist may mistake the increased resistance secondary to poor lubrication as coming from the more proximal colon.

The anus is inspected visually, examining for fissures, fistulae or skin tags, and the instrument is inserted into the anus and advanced into the rectum. The anal canal is 2–3 cm long (in the older child and adolescent) and is angled toward the umbilicus. The instrument is inserted until there is an abrupt decrease in resistance, indicating that the tip has passed from the anal canal into the rectal ampulla. Following insertion, the scope tip usually comes to rest near the anterior wall of the rectum, because the junction of the rectum and anal canal forms an angle of approximately 90°. If the lumen is not in view, a small puff of air or withdrawing the endoscope a few centimeters will usually locate the lumen. Negotiating the colon is similar

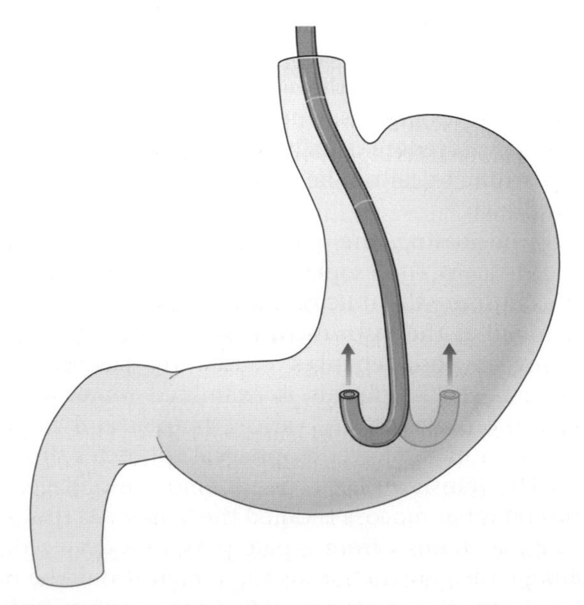

Figure 81.9: Examination of the gastric cardia and fundus by retroflexion, scope withdrawal and rotation.

to the examination of the duodenum. Rather than simply 'pushing', the instrument should be subtly advanced using the dials for tip deflection, and the techniques of air insufflation and suction, rotation or torquing of the insertion tube, external pressure applied to the abdomen, and changing the position of the patient. The elastic nature of the colon allows it to become long and tortuous when it is stretched by the colonoscope. Alternatively, it can be telescoped onto the instrument with little stretching by experienced endoscopists. The fundamentals of colonoscopy are:[45]

- To advance the endoscope under direct observation
- To use as little air as possible while maintaining adequate visualization
- To avoid forming loops, but when loops are formed to reduce them as quickly as possible
- To pull back and telescope the bowel onto the colonoscope whenever possible.

The most prominent landmarks in the rectum are the fixed '"valves of Houston'. These folds are accentuated haustral markings, and the lumen will veer toward the side of the fold. The endoscope is advanced with a series of short movements, jiggling motions or torquing technique, depending on the skill and preference of the examiner. The junction of the rectum and sigmoid usually presents the first major problem and opportunity to form a loop. If the endoscopist simply advances the instrument, the force of the colonoscope is transmitted to the wall of the colon, with progressive distention of the bowel and its mesentery; the patient usually experiences pain and the examiner feels increasing resistance to forward motion. This is often accompanied by the failure of the tip to advance despite insertion of the colonoscope. Paradoxical movement may occur when the tip recedes as the instrument is advanced and a larger loop is formed.

Early colonoscopes with limited tip deflection and fields of view required a 'slide by' technique, as the lumen could not always be kept in view. The instrument was advanced while the endoscopist had only a red field of view as the mucosa moved past the tip of the instrument. Advancement was halted when the mucosa was no longer slipping past the instrument tip or the mucosa took on a whitish hue, suggesting that compression of the bowel wall by the colonoscope was decreasing perfusion to the mucosa.

The instruments currently available reduce some of the technical difficulties, and the instrument should be advanced under direct visualization and not by the 'slide by' technique. The skillful negotiation of the rectosigmoid junction is the key to successful colonoscopy. The experienced endoscopist will anticipate many of the potential problems. Several loops may be formed in the sigmoid colon. Names have been given to various configurations as they were seen under the fluoroscope with the patient positioned in the anterior posterior position (Fig. 81.10). The alpha loop resembles the Greek letter α and may occur in either a normal or reversed configuration. The most common loop is the 'N' loop, which is shaped like the letter N. Each of these loops has a similar appearance when viewed from the lateral position. The sigmoid colon is usually directed upward and then forms a caudad-directed convex loop in the anterior–posterior plane and a second cephalad convex loop with an oblique orientation to the anterior–posterior plane (Fig. 81.11). Less common loops such as the double alpha loop can occur in a forward or backward orientation (Fig. 81.12). Regardless of the anatomy in the individual patient, the endoscopist is unaware of the anatomy unless fluoroscopy or another form of scope position tracking is used during the procedure. As it is rarely needed to complete the procedure and exposes the patient, physician and equipment to radiation, the experienced endoscopist will anticipate the potential problems rather than utilizing fluoroscopy. New equipment utilizing non-fluoroscopic external monitoring devices is being developed that helps the endoscopist to be aware of the position of the endoscope within the patient and detects the presence of loops; however, this is not yet available for widespread commercial application.

Advancing the endoscope through the sigmoid colon should be a smooth and coordinated procedure. This often involves torquing the instrument along its shaft with the right hand and using the left hand to control the tip deflection. Repeated backward and forward motions are usually needed to telescope the colon onto the instrument. As the tip of the instrument reaches a bend, the dials or a combination of dials and torque are used to rotate the tip around the bend into the lumen.

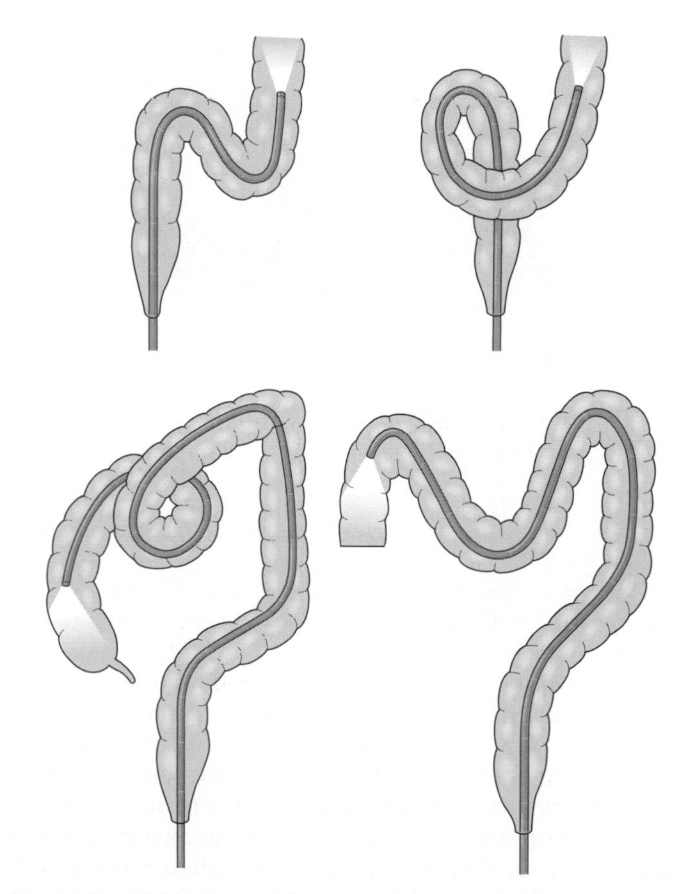

Figure 81.10: Common loops: 'N' loop, alpha loop, gamma loop and 'U' loop.

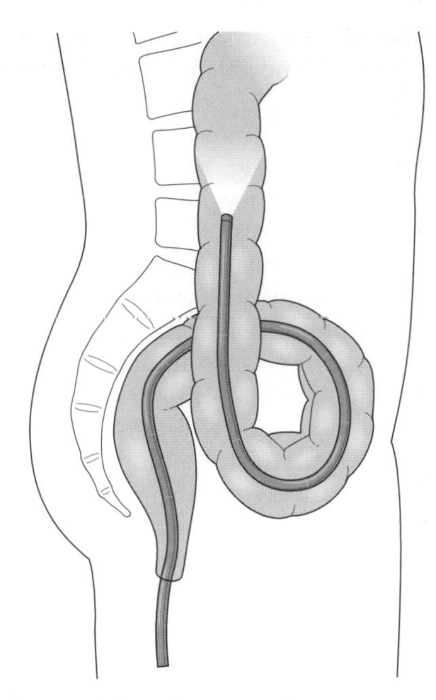

Figure 81.11: Lateral view of common loops.

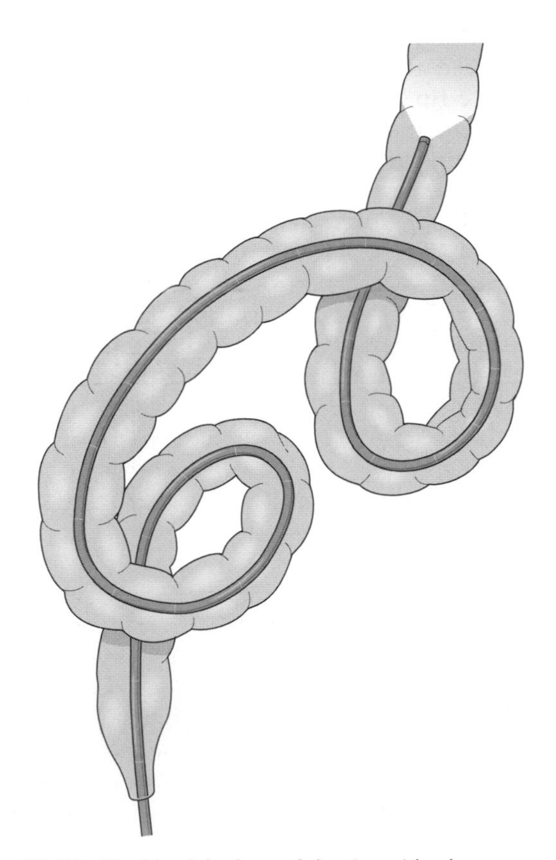

Figure 81.12: Double-alpha loop of the sigmoid colon.

Withdrawing the instrument will often straighten the loop and allow advancement to the next bend. To reduce an alpha loop, the scope is withdrawn so the tip lies just distal to the rectosigmoid junction and then rotated 180° (Fig. 81.13). Failure of 'one to one' movement, increasing patient discomfort and increased resistance to insertion of the endoscope are usually signs of loop formation. Repeated attempts at loop removal are often necessary to traverse the sigmoid colon. In an occasional patient it may be necessary to push through the loop and then reduce it after the instrument reaches the more proximal colon. Hand pressure by an assistant on the anterior abdominal wall may be beneficial during this maneuver (Fig. 81.14). This should be done with caution only by an experienced endoscopist.

Alpha sigmoid loops, with the endoscope advanced into the distal descending colon, can be reduced by rotation (usually clockwise) and withdrawal. N loops can usually be removed with simple withdrawal. Occasionally an N loop has to be converted to an alpha loop for reduction to be successful. This can be done by withdrawal and counter-clockwise rotation. The conversion usually allows the endoscope to be advanced to the level of the descending colon, as most of the forward force on the N loop is directed at the apex of the loop and the forces in the alpha loop are more radially distributed. This permits advancement of the instrument despite the presence of the alpha loop. When the instrument reaches the descending colon, the loop can be reduced. Attempted examination of the proximal colon is usually limited if there is a residual sigmoid loop.

There is no anatomic demarcation between the sigmoid and descending colon, but there is a tendency for the descending colon to be slightly smaller in diameter and to contain residual fecal debris because of its dependent position. Often a long tunnel view may be obtained, and if the sigmoid loops have been reduced the endoscope can usually be advanced to the level of the splenic flexure without difficulty. A straight sigmoid colon is essential for successful maneuvering around the splenic flexure. Paradoxical motion is often noted as the endoscope is advanced into the transverse colon. The configuration and forces resemble those of the N loop in the sigmoid colon. To reduce this tendency, the patient is often rotated from the left lateral to the supine position. Clockwise rotation of the endoscope may also be helpful. The relationship of the transverse colon and splenic flexure also varies with respiration. Deep sustained inspiration in the cooperative child may decrease the acute angle of the splenic flexure and allow easier passage of the endoscope. If the endoscopist is unsuccessful, the instrument should be withdrawn to ensure reduction of a sigmoid loop that may not have been reduced or one that may have reformed during maneuvers to negotiate the flexure (Fig. 81.15). Multiple attempts by trial and error may be necessary to advance the instrument into the transverse colon.

The transverse colon is characterized by triangular-shaped haustral folds (Fig. 81.16). The endoscope can usually be advanced without difficulty to the hepatic flexure, which is easily identified by the bluish discoloration of the outer wall caused by its close approximation to the liver. Occasionally a U-shaped loop is formed; this requires reduction prior to attempted negotiation of the hepatic flexure (see Fig. 81.10). If the transverse colon is redundant, a gamma loop may form. Reduction of this loop is

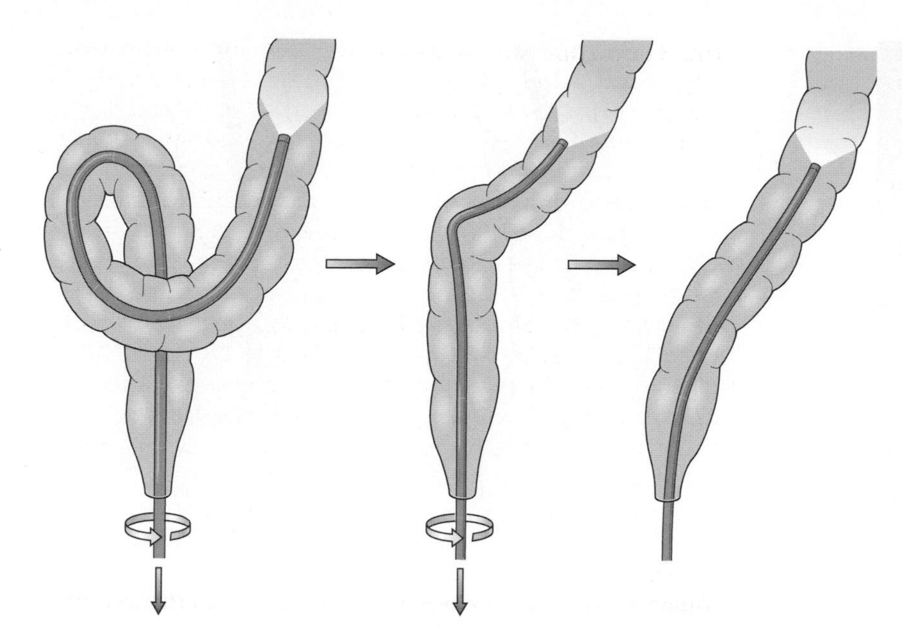

Figure 81.13: Alpha loop. Note initial posterior, then anterior, configuration of the sigmoid colon. Clockwise torque and scope withdrawal allows reduction of the loop and straightening of the sigmoid colon.

difficult because rotational forces are poorly transmitted and the loop is usually large. Reduction is less difficult if the instrument can be advanced into the ascending colon and then withdrawn to reduce the loop.

The fixed position of the splenic flexure acts as a fulcrum while trying to negotiate the hepatic flexure. Suctioning in the region of the hepatic flexure usually draws the mucosa to the tip of the endoscope, and subsequently the tip can be maneuvered around the flexure into the ascending colon. If the flexure cannot be negotiated, withdrawal, manual rotation of the insertion tube, suctioning, manual compression of the abdominal wall and/or sustained deep inspiration may be attempted to facilitate passage. If these measures fail, it may still be possible to advance the endoscope, but the patient usually experiences some discomfort. Rotation of the patient from

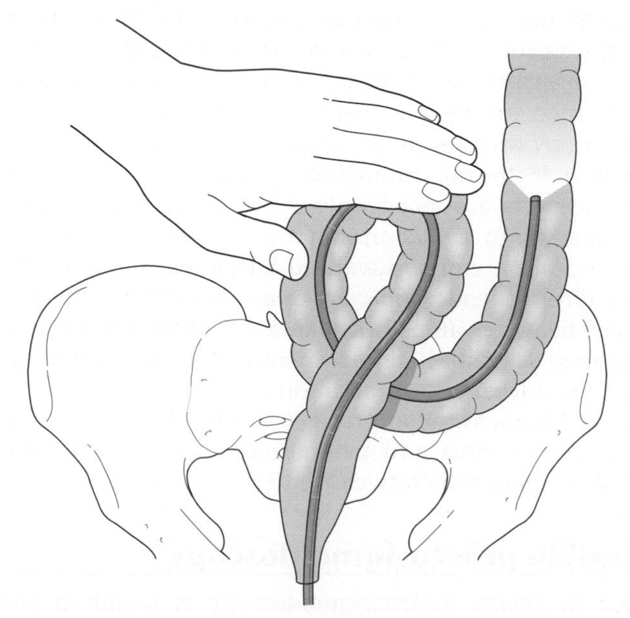

Figure 81.14: Anterior abdominal pressure may facilitate scope advancement by increasing resistance to loop formation.

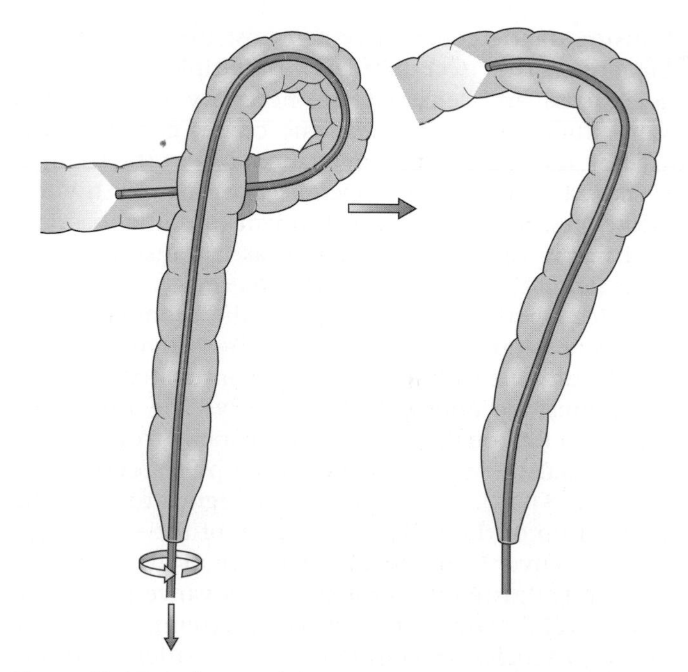

Figure 81.15: Reduction of the splenic flexure loop after intubation of the transverse colon. Without straightening, further advancement of the endoscope is difficult and uncomfortable.

the left lateral position to a supine or right lateral decubitus position may also facilitate scope advancement from the hepatic flexure in to the ascending colon. Reduction of sigmoid looping is key to successful negotiation of the hepatic flexure.

To advance the endoscope into the ascending colon, the tip of the instrument is usually turned into the lumen with the dials. Additional procedures such as withdrawal and rotation may be necessary if paradoxical movement is encountered. Deep inspiration may be effective in 'pushing' the instrument into the ascending colon. After the tip is aligned with the lumen, suctioning will also collapse the cecum toward the tip of the instrument. If there have been any difficulties with the

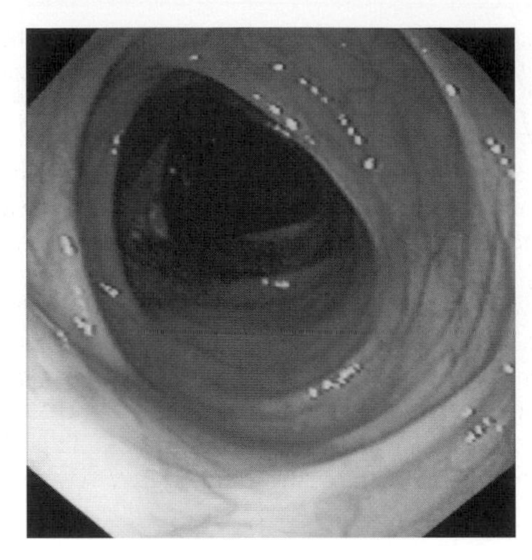

Figure 81.16: Normal colonic mucosal appearance of the transverse colon. Triangular shape of the folds is typical of this area. (*See plate section for color.*)

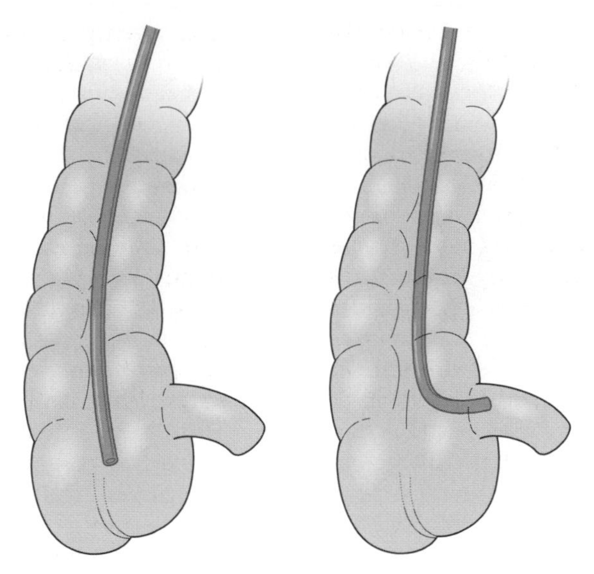

Figure 81.17: The ileocecal valve is intubated by tip deflection rather than *en face.*

cleansing of the colon, they are most likely to become apparent in the ascending colon. Multiple washings of the mucosa and lens may be necessary to allow full examination of the mucosa. The cecum can be recognized by the typical anatomic landmarks of the triangular-shaped folds and the appendiceal orifice. With video endoscopes, the tip of the instrument can often be identified in the right lower quadrant as it transilluminates the anterior abdominal wall. The ileocecal valve can be identified on the lateral surface of the prominent ileal fold as a slight irregularity of the valve contour. Occasionally the valve can be directly intubated, but usually it must be approached indirectly. The tip of the endoscope is brought to a position parallel to the valve, and the dials are used to deflect the tip 90° towards the valve (Fig. 81.17). The maneuver is designed to catch the proximal lip of the valve with the tip of the endoscope. If the maneuver is successful, the lumen of the ileum will open, and adjustment of the tip will advance the instrument several centimeters. Several attempts may be needed to achieve success. Rotating the patient and suctioning the air from the cecum to draw the valve opening closer to the endoscope may be helpful. The mucosa of the ileum is easily identified by the presence of valvula conniventes and lymphoid aggregates, which appear as submucosal 2–4-mm mounds of tissue with normal overlying mucosa. The presence of lymphoid aggregates in adults has been associated with immunoglobulin A deficiency, but is normal in children and even adolescents; the amount tends to decrease with advancing age. If the valve cannot be cannulated and pathologic evaluation is needed, the forceps can sometimes be gently advanced through the valve and biopsy material obtained.

Examination of the mucosa and therapeutic procedures such as polypectomy are conducted principally as the instrument is withdrawn. All areas must be routinely examined, paying special attention to the areas behind folds. Observation of areas around flexures may not be adequate if the scope slips back rapidly, and the instrument may have to be advanced back through areas not well visualized. Observation of the distal rectum requires a retroflexed maneuver for complete examination. This is done by turning the dials to their maximum deflection in the mid-rectum. The endoscope is then slowly rotated to obtain an unobstructed view. The scope must be straightened before removal from the anus.

Colostomies and ileostomies can usually be examined as long as the openings are large enough to admit the tip of the instrument. Regular surveillance ileoscopy is being utilized increasingly in pediatric patients who have undergone a small intestinal transplantation. Depending on the size, an appropriate scope should be chosen after a finger has been inserted into the opening. The length of bowel that can be examined is usually dependent on whether adhesions have formed. Advancement of the instrument around flexures in the bowel again involves repeated advancement, withdrawal and torque of the insertion tube. Ileoscopy of the allograft after transplantation is typically performed using an instrument designed for upper endoscopy with antibiotic prophylaxis but usually without sedation.[46] In the immediate postoperative period the endoscope is advanced only 5–10 cm with minimal air insufflation to avoid anastomotic trauma. Subsequently the endoscope can be advanced further with both random and directed endoscopic biopsies. Indications for small bowel ileoscopy after transplantation include routine surveillance, fever, bacteremia, increased stoma output, diarrhea and bleeding.[46] In addition to detection of rejection, this technique is helpful for detection of infection such as Epstein–Barr virus and cytomegalovirus, and post-transplant lymphoproliferative disorder.[46]

Flexible proctosigmoidoscopy

Routine flexible proctosigmoidoscopy is useful in some pediatric patients. In compliant, usually older, children with a chronic illness such as ulcerative colitis, routine office examination to assess the extent and severity of disease when the history is in doubt or prior to initiating topical therapy for localized disease is useful. Examinations can be performed routinely with the same instruments that are used for full colonoscopy. Examination using either short (35 cm) or long (60 cm) flexible instruments in adults has produced similar pathologic yields. No comparable information is available for the pediatric population, but, when it is necessary to sedate pediatric patients for their comfort, it is usually appropriate to be prepared to perform a full colonoscopic examination. If pathology is encountered that is compatible with the patient's symptoms and therapeutic options do not rest on establishing the extent of the disease, the procedure can be terminated without attempting to examine the entire colon. Flexible sigmoidoscopy with biopsy is frequently performed in the infant with rectal bleeding with suspected cow's milk or soy protein allergy. Use of a small-diameter upper endoscope in the range of 6 mm and the brief nature of the examination often allow the procedure to be performed without sedation.

Anoscopy and rigid proctosigmoidoscopy

Anoscopy and rigid proctosigmoidoscopy are infrequently used procedures in the pediatric patient. Most pediatric gastroenterologists prefer flexible instruments when examination is required. The anoscope, however, remains a useful office instrument for better visualization of the anal canal and identification of sources of bleeding.

BIOPSY TECHNIQUE

Histopathologic evaluation of the gastrointestinal tract is helpful in differentiating infectious, inflammatory and malignant processes. Tissue biopsy is routinely obtained from suspicious lesions during endoscopic examination, but when the gross endoscopic appearance reveals a specific diagnosis, tissue analysis is unnecessary if the result will not alter therapy. However, recent advances in our understanding of the pathogenesis of disease, such as the relationship of *Helicobacter pylori* and peptic ulcer disease, indicate that tissue biopsy may be indicated even when the source of gastrointestinal bleeding, for example, is apparent. Numerous techniques and devices have been designed to obtain tissue samples. A variety of pinch biopsy forceps are available that are coordinated in size with endoscopic channel diameter. Standard-size biopsy forceps are fenestrated with a needle so that two sequential biopsies may be performed without removing the forceps from the endoscope. 'Spiked' forceps that fit through a 2.0-mm channel are not yet available. Fine-needle biopsy may have an advantage when biopsy material from submucosal lesions is sought. Suction biopsy, which has been adapted to the endoscope, is designed to obtain deeper samples, and jumbo biopsy forceps are also available. Larger-sized biopsy specimens may also be obtained with a turn and suction technique. Multiple biopsy specimens improve the diagnostic yield, but the size and location of the biopsies are probably more important. Brush cytology or other combinations of techniques can increase diagnostic yield. Snare excision is usually reserved for large polyps. For a more detailed discussion, see Chapter 79.

The technique of biopsy varies according to the lesion to be biopsied. To perform a routine biopsy, the closed pinch biopsy forceps are advanced through the biopsy channel to a point just past the tip of the endoscope; they are then opened immediately adjacent and perpendicular to the lesion if possible. This angulation may be difficult to achieve in the esophagus, small bowel and terminal ileum. The open forceps are then advanced and closed, and the tissue removed through the endoscope. The depth of biopsy is determined by the lesion being sought and the application force of the forceps.

Esophagus

Reflux esophagitis is traditionally diagnosed by clinical criteria. Endoscopy and biopsy is indicated in patients refractory to therapy. Biopsy increases the diagnostic yield compared with visual examination alone. There is a high rate of interobserver variability in the diagnosis of milder forms of esophagitis when 'erythema and edema' are the only diagnostic findings. There is a greater uniformity of diagnosis when esophageal erosions are present. Prolonged pH probe monitoring appears to be the current 'gold standard' for the diagnosis of GER, which is discussed in further detail in Chapter 20.[47] Numerous eosinophils found in the esophagus can be due to reflux esophagitis or due to eosinophilic esophagitis (Fig. 81.18). The two conditions are distinguished by histologic findings, clinical course and response to therapy.[48–51] The finding of the highly specialized columnar epithelium of Barrett's esophagus necessitates multiple biopsies to screen for dysplasia or adenocarcinoma. Fungal and viral (cytomegalovirus, herpes simplex virus) esophagitis occur in both immunocompromised and immunocompetent hosts. Biopsy, cytology and cultures aid in the diagnosis.[52] Malignant tumors of the esophagus are diagnosed by biopsy in the majority of cases. The addition of brush cytology increases the diagnostic yield in cancerous lesions, and EUS is frequently

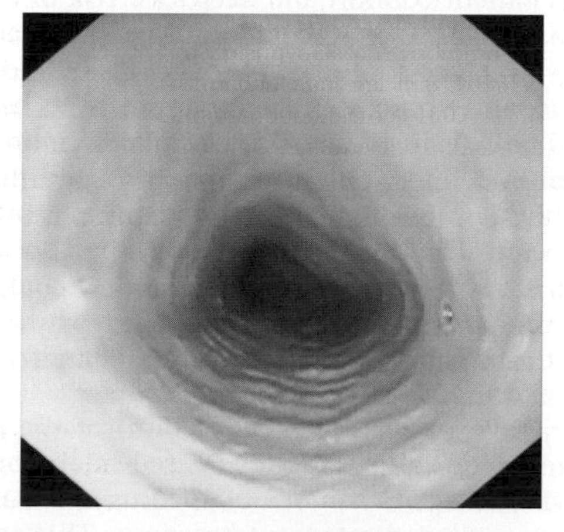

Figure 81.18: Rings of the proximal and mid-esophagus in a patient with eosinophilic esophagitis. (*See plate section for color.*)

used to stage lesions. Although exceedingly uncommon, adenocarcinoma of the esophagus has been reported in adolescent patients.

Stomach

The base of gastric ulcers is not routinely biopsied because ulcerating gastric malignancies are rare in pediatric patients. Biopsies should be obtained from the edge rather than the base of the lesion to look for *H. pylori*, but biopsies may be relatively contraindicated if a visible vessel is present. Complications include perforation and bleeding.

Gastritis secondary to drug administration does not usually require biopsy. Gastritis and duodenitis due to nonsteroidal inflammatory drug use may be significant even in otherwise healthy patients, and can be associated with the presence of gastric or duodenal erosions.[53] Generalized gastritis especially in the setting of a nodular appearing mucosa may suggest the diagnosis of *H. pylori* infection, confirmed by Giemsa staining or urease testing of antral biopsies.[54] Gastric biopsy may also aid in the diagnosis of idiopathic granulomatous gastritis, Crohn's disease, eosinophilic gastroenteritis, sarcoidosis and Ménétrièr's disease.

Gastric neoplasia, although uncommon in pediatrics, may appear as an ulcerative, polypoid or submucosal deformity, or as thickened gastric folds. Pinch biopsy is the preferred technique for ulcerative or small polypoid lesions. Adenomas or hyperplastic polyps of 1.0 cm or more in size should be removed if feasible. Submucosal deformities may be evaluated by deep biopsies from a single site, with or without fine-needle aspiration. EUS examination may assist with evaluation of the submucosal extent of disease in worrisome lesions.

Small intestine

Endoscopic pinch biopsy of the small bowel is helpful in the diagnosis of celiac disease, intestinal lymphangiectasia and Crohn's disease. Multiple directed specimens obtained from the descending duodenum or the more distal bowel have replaced capsule biopsy, with comparable accuracy, increased patient comfort and decreased risk of complications. Characteristic endoscopic findings of celiac disease in children include scalloping of folds, loss of folds, visible vasculature and a mucosal mosaic pattern, especially in the duodenal bulb. This mosaic pattern may be more evident when chromoendoscopy is utilized.[55,56] Intestinal lymphangiectasia in the duodenum and jejunum is often characterized endoscopically by a change in the appearance of the mucosa to white. Specific findings include diffuse whitish mucosa, scattered white spots, white nodules 3–8 mm in size with sharply demarcated margins and submucosal elevations.[57]

Jumbo forceps (open diameter 9 mm) or the turn and suction technique allows for larger-sized small bowel specimens. Distal biopsies can be obtained using small-caliber colonoscopes or dedicated enteroscopes. This technique may be especially useful for lesions that characteristically have a patchy distribution. Biopsy of macroscopically normal tissue may occasionally establish the diagnosis and allows for determination of disaccharidase levels if appropriate.

Small bowel parasitic infection may be identified by direct observation or pathologic identification of removed worms. Aspiration of duodenal contents and histologic examination can identify parasites such as *Giardia lamblia* or *Strongyloides*, which may not produce visible mucosal changes.[58] Duodenal tumors are rare and can be biopsied utilizing either the forward- or side-viewing endoscopes.

Ileum and colon

The colonoscope can be used to obtain biopsy material and collect specimens for culture from the distal small bowel and colon. Histopathologic examination is useful in the differentiation of infectious, inflammatory and malignant processes. Guidelines have outlined the general indications for colonoscopy and biopsy in patients with colonic polyps and inflammatory bowel disease.[59,60] Visual evidence of a suspicious lesion warrants histopathologic evaluation and most pediatric gastroenterologists routinely biopsy normal tissue including the terminal ileum if inflammatory bowel disease is suspected. Methods for obtaining tissue include snare excision, forceps biopsy, hot biopsy forceps, needle biopsy and brushings for cytology. Needle biopsy and brush cytology are utilized mainly in the adult population to enhance the yield in patients with suspected colorectal malignancy. Additional screening tests for colorectal malignancy including fecal DNA testing are being studied in adults.[59] Flow cytometry of colonoscopically obtained tissue has recently been employed as part of a dysplasia screening protocol in adolescent patients with long-standing ulcerative colitis or Crohn's disease.[61] Needle biopsy has the theoretical advantage in ulcerated lesions of providing histologic material not only from the surface but also from areas deeper within the lesion. Needle biopsy may be useful in submucosal lesions that are difficult to access by biopsy forceps, and may be performed using EUS. In most diseases involving pediatric patients, the forceps for pediatric-size instruments or standard forceps provide adequate tissue for mucosal evaluation.

Endoscopy and biopsy can be useful in the diagnosis of infection and in the diagnosis and management of inflammatory bowel disease (Fig. 81.19). Biopsy specimens (one or two using routine forceps) obtained during the acute phase of a bloody diarrheal illness may differentiate acute self-limiting colitis from an initial or recurrent attack of chronic ulcerative colitis. During the resolving phase of acute self-limiting colitis, histologic changes may mimic those of Crohn's disease. Bacterial cultures may be obtained during the procedure by the attachment of a 'trap' to the suction equipment that gathers fecal effluent. Colonic biopsy has also been shown to be helpful in human immunodeficiency virus-infected

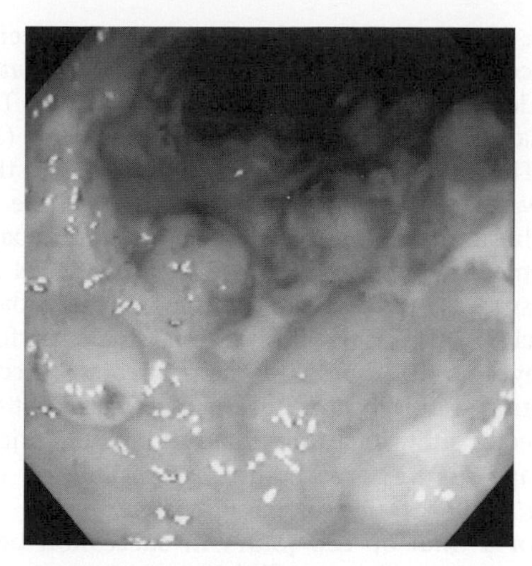

Figure 81.19: Endoscopic appearance of Crohn's colitis involving the transverse colon. Note marked nodularity, mucosal erosions and overlying exudate in contrast to the appearance in Figure 81.16. (*See plate section for color.*)

patients with chronic unexplained diarrhea, and appears to be superior to flexible sigmoidoscopy in this patient population.[62]

Terminal ileal examination may be useful in the diagnosis of Crohn's disease and in the differentiation of Crohn's disease from lymphonodular hyperplasia. Ileal visualization and biopsy may occasionally be useful in patients with infectious ileitis.

Ulcerative colitis and Crohn's disease are predisposing risk factors for the development of colorectal cancer.[63] Routine colonoscopy is usually initiated after 7–8 years in patients with colitis due to ulcerative colitis or Crohn's disease.[61] Biopsies should be taken from any suspicious areas, and serial biopsies should be taken from representative areas of the bowel for detection of dysplasia. Typically a total of 36 to 40 specimens is taken from 10 sites throughout the colon for dysplasia screening.

Biopsies from macroscopically normal mucosa may be useful in the diagnosis of disease. Collagenous colitis or lymphocytic colitis, both with associated chronic diarrhea, may present with macroscopically normal mucosa but characteristic histologic abnormalities.[64] Other diseases, such as amyloidosis, inflammatory bowel disease, 'microscopic colitis in children' and chronic schistosomiasis, have been diagnosed by biopsy of the colon when the mucosa has been macroscopically normal. Complications after biopsy may include perforation and bleeding. For a more detailed discussion, see the section on complications.

THERAPEUTIC ENDOSCOPY

During the early years of gastrointestinal endoscopy, endoscopic examination was primarily a diagnostic tool. As technology advanced and procedural skills developed, the endoscope became a therapeutic instrument. Endoscopes have been used in children to remove foreign bodies and polyps, insert tubes into various organs and stop bleeding lesions. For detailed discussions, the reader is also referred to Chapters 17, 25, 64 and 79.

Acute gastrointestinal hemorrhage is an indication for therapeutic endoscopic intervention, but emergent gastrointestinal endoscopy is associated with an increased risk of complications.[65] This includes a risk of aspiration of gastric contents and a higher risk associated with sedating an actively bleeding patient or a patient with decompensated cardiopulmonary or hepatic function.[65] Upper gastrointestinal lesions that may be amenable to endoscopic therapy include ulcers with evidence of active bleeding, oozing from beneath a clot overlying an ulcer (sentinel clot), or an ulcer with a visible vessel at its base that is not actively bleeding but appears as a red, blue or white plug.[66] These same lesions have a high rate of rebleeding, approximately 50%, compared with an incidence of 10% or less of rebleeding with other lesions, including those with an overlying clot without oozing or flat spots.

Bleeding from esophageal varices can also be treated by endoscopic sclerotherapy, band ligation or a combination of the techniques.[67–71] Therefore, ongoing therapy to ablate distal esophageal varices is usually undertaken after the initial bleeding episode has resolved (see Ch. 64).

Diffuse mucosal bleeding from duodenitis or gastritis is usually not responsive to endoscopic interventions. Colonic lesions treatable with endoscopic therapy include bleeding ulcers, angiomata, polyps and bleeding polyp stalks, an adherent clot in a single diverticulum, or an ulcerative lesion that is resistant to washing, with fresh blood nearby and no other visible lesion in the colon. As in upper gastrointestinal tract disease, diffusely bleeding colonic lesions cannot be controlled successfully by endoscopic intervention.

There are five well established types of therapeutic intervention for acute gastrointestinal bleeding: injection, coagulation or thermal therapy including the recently developed argon plasma coagulator (APC), laser therapy, endoscopic hemostatic devices and ligation therapy. The specific techniques employed depend on equipment availability and experience of the endoscopist. The techniques appear to have roughly equivalent efficacy but some lesions are more amenable to a particular type of therapy.

Therapeutic endoscopy is most easily accomplished using a two-channeled therapeutic scope so that therapy (injection, coagulation, etc.) may be accomplished via one channel and simultaneous suction or irrigation may be performed using the second channel to keep the field in view. Unfortunately, therapeutic endoscopes are of a large diameter compared with standard pediatric endoscopes and often cannot be used in the pediatric patient. Therapeutic endoscopy may still be performed using a single-channel scope, but depending on the modality employed may be technically more difficult.

INJECTION

Injection therapy is used for both variceal and non-variceal bleeding. The technique of esophageal sclerotherapy for varices is discussed elsewhere (see Ch. 64). Non-variceal injection therapy is usually performed by injecting a sclerosing agent at three to four sites around an exposed bleeding vessel (Fig. 81.20). Maximal volumes of sclerosant have been established in adults to minimize the risk of ulcer extension or perforation. Maximal volumes of sclerosants in pediatric patients have not been studied; however, maximal adult volumes should not be exceeded. Complications including perforation may occur with volumes of injection even less than the recommended maximum volumes. Table 81.7 lists the most commonly used solutions, their concentrations and estimated maximal volumes. Several general principles should be noted. First, except under unusual circumstances, injection therapy should be confined to a single solution (single agent or a combination agent) during a given injection episode. Utilizing two sequential solutions may increase the risk of complication with smaller volumes of sclerosant than would be required by using a single agent alone. Second, the injection site (into vessel *vs* surrounding vessel *vs* submucosal) is specific for certain agents. Without appropriate clinical trials, changing the site of injection is probably hazardous. Third, the risks with injection therapy include increased bleeding, rebleeding, bowel ischemia and perforation. Fourth, precise volumes of injection are required. Those that involve smaller volumes may be more technically difficult. Fifth, although submucosal injection has been employed to assist in resection of colonic polyps, optimal volumes of injection of a number of agents have not been established for the large bowel.

THERMOCOAGULATION

A second method of establishing hemostasis is thermocoagulation, utilizing the heater probe, monopolar or bipolar (multipolar) coagulators (Table 81.8). The heater probe is composed of Teflon-coated hollow aluminum cylinders with an inner heater coil and a maximum internal temperature. The probe is water perfused to prevent tissue adherence, an advantage over monopolar coagulation, and heat is delivered via conduction to the tissue. There are small-diamter (2.4 mm) and large-diameter (3.2 mm) probes. The patient should be positioned so that the blood flows away from the ulcer base if possible. The probe is passed through the therapeutic channel, and coagulation is performed by tamponading the bleeding vessel by direct firm pressure using the heater probe and then coagulating the vessel (Fig. 81.21). Coagulation is usually performed in adults by two to four 30-joule pulses in succession.[72] Coagulation should be around the bleeding point first, and then directly on it. In studies of adult patients, the greatest success appears to be with firm tamponade on the ulcer bleeding point or non-bleeding visible vessel, and four pulses for a total of 120 joules in succession before the probe position is changed.[72,73] This technique, however, may increase the risk of complications when applied to other types of lesion, specifically Mallory–Weiss tears or angiomata, that occur in areas with a thinner gut wall.[72] The heater probe may also be used in cases of colonic bleeding. The number of joules per pulse should be reduced, especially in right-sided colonic lesions.

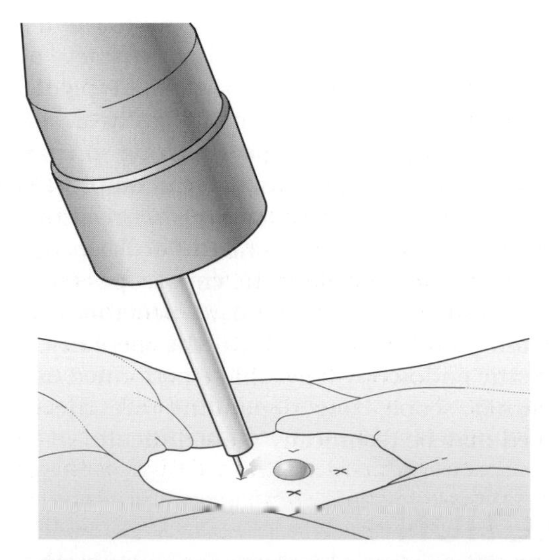

Figure 81.20: Injection circumferentially around a visible vessel in an ulcer base. Injection is performed at three to four sites around the exposed vessel.

ELECTROCOAGULATION

There are two main types of electrocoagulation probes, monopolar and bipolar. In monopolar coagulation, a continuous or intermittent current is passed via the tip or side of the probe. The current is conducted to the patient's ground plate. The current is converted to high-temperature heat at the tissue contact point, which coagulates the tissue, causing collagen contraction and vessel shrinkage. For vessels less than 1 mm in diameter, the electrode is placed directly on the vessel and pressure is applied directly on the vessel to coapt it. With larger vessels, the coagulating current is placed circumferentially around the vessel until bleeding stops. Usually a midrange setting is used for 1–2 s per pulse at a distance of 2–3 mm from the vessel. This is because an artery in an ulcer base may bleed from either side if it is not an end artery; therefore, a ring of tissue must be treated around the bleeding point to ensure adequate hemostasis. The aim is to achieve hemostasis of the underlying artery and not the overlying clot. There are two main problems with monopolar coagulation. The first is that the depth of the burn is very difficult to regulate, and perforation is possible. This is especially true in the colon, where deep necrosis, perforation and delayed massive bleeding have been reported with monopolar electrocoagulation. The second problem is that there is a moderate amount of electrode adherence to the underlying tissue at the treated site and therefore poor visibility, especially in non-irrigated systems. A third technical problem is the need to clean the tip of the probe as the coagulum accumulates during electrocoagulation.

Currently bipolar or multipolar coagulation is the most popular method with endoscopists. Unlike monopolar coagulation, a grounding plate is not required. Current is transmitted from one electrode on the probe to another,

Solution	Concentration	Volume/no. of injections/location	Maximum volume	Comments
Hypertonic saline–epinephrine combination	3.6% saline + 1:20 000 epinephrine or 7.2% saline + 1:20 000 epinephrine[a]	3 ml/3–4 injections at base of bleeding vessel 1 ml/3–4 injections	9–12 ml	Repeat prophylactic injections if visible vessel present 24–48 h after first hemostasis for lesions with extensive fibrosis[a]
Epinephrine with normal saline	1 ml 1:1000 epinephrine + 9 ml normal saline	0.5–2.0 ml injected in multiple sites around bleeding vessel and into bleeding point itself	10 ml	Range 1.5–10 ml, mean 4.1 ml; larger volumes in range for spurting vessels
Epinephrine followed by polidocanol	5–10 ml 1:10 000 epinephrine 5 ml 1% polidocanol	Inject epinephrine into the submucosa directly around blood vessel to achieve hemostasis by compression/vasoconstriction, then obliterate vessel with polidocanol	Epinephrine 5–10 ml Polidocanol 5 ml	May substitute bipolar coagulation or Nd:YAG laser for polidocanol
Thrombin in normal saline	100 IU thrombin in 3 ml normal saline	Inject into bleeding vessel, 10–15 ml total volume	10–15 ml	
Absolute ethanol	98% dehydrated ethanol	0.1–0.2 ml/injection at 3–4 sites surrounding bleeding vessel and 1–2 mm away from vessel	0.6–1.22 ml total	Inject via tuberculin syringe *slowly* (0.2 ml/3 s); extesion/perforation significant risk if maximum volume exceeded; may be technically more difficult to control volume
Epinephrine with normal saline for polypectomy[b]	1 ml 1:1000 epinephrine + 9 ml normal saline	1.0–2.0 ml per injection injected in multiple sites (3–4) around the polyp to be raised up	30 ml	Goal is lack of vascular markings within injection site

[a] 3.6%/0.005% epinephrine prepared by combining 1 part of solution A (20 ml 15% NaCl solution and 1 ml 0.1% epinephrine) to 3 parts of solution B (20 ml distilled water, with 1 ml 0.1% epinephrine). 7.2%/0.005% prepared by combining equal parts (1 : 1) of solutions A and B. Adapted from Sugawa, 1989, with permission.[65]
[b] From Waye, 2001.[104]

Table 81.7 Sclerosants for non-variceal bleeding

and energy is delivered when any pair of electrodes is in contact with the bleeding target. The BICAP (multipolar) probe has six points through which current can be passed; contact between any two is sufficient. This has the advantage of allowing for tangential contact.[74] The maximal temperature achieved with this method is significantly less than that of monopolar coagulation or the Nd:YAG laser, causing less tissue injury and having greater efficacy for vessels less than 2 mm in diameter. Two sizes of probe are available: 2.3 and 3.2 mm. Like the heater probe, the correct technique is to compress the bleeding vessel first, then to coagulate. Forceful application of the larger-size probe appears to increase hemostatic bond strength and the area and depth of coagulation.[75] The greatest depth of coagulation is usually achieved with a low to midrange setting (15–25 watts). Pulses should be applied as short, multiple pulses (2 s in duration) or a single long pulse of up to 14 s in duration.[75] The longer, lower-voltage pulse is thought to work by increasing the depth of coagulation by decreasing tissue desiccation. In adults, a total of up to 40 s of electrocoagulation is required.[75] Increased bleeding after bipolar coagulation has been reported in cases with a visible vessel; usually this bleeding is controllable with further bipolar coagulation, but on occasion surgery has been required.

Bipolar electrocoagulation appears to be equally effective to the heater probe in terms of hemostasis, incidence of rebleeding, transfusion requirement and need for emergency surgery. Several studies report a hemostasis rate in the 90% range for both modalities.[75] Bipolar electrocoagulation also appears to be as efficacious as the laser at a marked reduction in cost. The angulation of the probe, or use of a bipolar electrode compared with a laser, does not appear to affect the rebleeding rate. However, poor angulation along the lesser curvature of the stomach or in a deformed duodenum may make pressure application more difficult.

Method	Site	Setting	Application time	No. of applications	Technique	Notes
Heater probe	Upper GI tract	30 joules		2–4	Firm tamponade, then coagulate around bleeding point, then on it	Decreased setting/time of application in colon or thinner gut wall
Monopolar	Upper GI tract	Mid-range	1–2 s/pulse		Directly on vessel <1 mm in diameter; circumferentially around vessel >1 mm in diameter	Perforation likely in colon
Bipolar/ multipolar	Upper GI tract	15–25 W	2 s/pulse or Up to 14-s pulse	Multiple Single	Firm tamponade, then coagulate	Difficult angulation in lesser curve or deformed duodenum
	Colon	5 W	2 s/pulse	Multiple		
Argon plasma coagulator	Upper GI tract	40–50 W 0.8 l/min	0.5–2 s	Multiple	Operative distance 2–8 mm	Paint confluent or near-confluent areas; avoid tissue contact with probe tip; surface should be free of liquid
Hot biopsy forceps	Cecum and ascending colon	10–15 W	1–2 s		Tent mucosa away	Polyps ≤5 mm in size; contraindicated in upper GI tract
	Left colon	15–20 W	2 s			

Table 81.8 Thermocoagulation

Angiodysplasia, predominantly of the colon, has been treated successfully by endoscopic electrocoagulation. Hemorrhagic proctocolitis with recurrent bleeding after radiation therapy has also been successfully treated with a bipolar probe at a power setting of 5 W with short 2-s pulses by coagulating at multiple bleeding sites. Late rebleeding has been reported, and was treated successfully by repeat electrocoagulation. In some cases, surgery is still required.

A further coagulation technique used primarily in the colon is the hot biopsy forceps. This technique combines the principles of endoscopic biopsy and monopolar electrocoagulation. The lesion to be biopsied is grasped in the jaw of insulated biopsy forceps, including polyps of up to 5 mm in size. The forceps are used to tent the mucosa upward away from the colonic muscular layer (Fig. 81.22). A brief electrocoagulating current passes through the forceps to the mucosa and sometimes the submucosa, producing coagulation at its base, while preserving the histologic integrity of the specimen. The unit is set on coagulation, at a setting of 10–15 W for 1–2 s in the cecum and ascending colon, and up to 15–20 W for 2 s in the left colon. Higher settings or longer application times have been associated with an increased risk of perforation, especially in the right colon.[76]

Perforation has been reported at an increased rate with application of the technique to the upper gastrointestinal tract, both in the stomach (secondary to increased gastric thickness, limiting tenting of the mucosa) and in the duodenum and ileum (secondary to thinness of the bowel wall and variable depth of penetration).[76] In the colon, the risk of perforation appears to be intermediate at 0.05%, less than that associated with snare polypectomy but greater than that of routine colonoscopy. However, for lesions greater than 5 mm, snare polypectomy is the preferred technique.

Another complication of the hot biopsy forceps is major hemorrhage, which may occur in 0.41% of cases.[76] This is especially likely if the forceps are not held perpendicular to the mucosa. Short-circuiting of the current has been reported between the forceps tip and the non-insulated portion of the forceps with massive hemorrhage, if the forceps are held at an angle of 15° or less to the bowel wall.[77] Hemorrhage may be immediate or delayed for up to 1 week after biopsy, and may not respond to conservative therapy.

Results of comparative trials of injection, coagulation and heater probe therapy vary according to the method used; however, in many studies the different techniques are of comparable efficacy given established volumes of injection, thermocoagulation settings, appropriate indica-

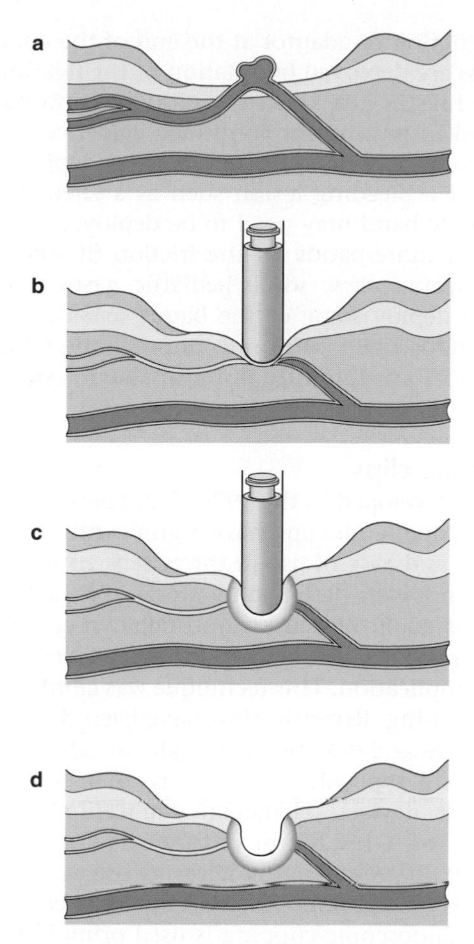

Figure 81.21: Coaptive coagulation utilizing the heater probe. (**a**) Visible vessel in an ulcer base. Note vessel is not an end artery. (**b**) Tamponade with probe initially. (**c**) Coagulation after tamponade. (**d**) 'White footprint' at coagulation site.

tions and times of application.[74] Injection therapy in the setting of peptic ulcer disease has been shown to decrease the rate of rebleeding, the transfusion requirement, the need for emergency surgery and the length of hospital stay. Similar results have been noted in trials comparing multipolar electrocoagulation, heater probe and Nd:Yag laser therapy, with higher costs noted for laser therapy.[74]

In some circumstances, one method of achieving hemostasis may be technically easier than other techniques. With BICAP probes, the depth of coagulation is limited to 2 mm, which limits its use with larger vessels. However, it has the advantage of a built-in wash system, aiding visibility in cases of brisk bleeding compared with injection therapy. The choice of therapeutic endoscopic technique depends to a significant extent on the training of the endoscopist and equipment availability. If the technique is properly performed, the results are similar using injection or thermal coagulation. Certain lesions, based on their anatomic location or briskness of bleeding, may be more amenable to one method than another. Equipment portability may also be an issue, with injection therapy and coagulation techniques such as the heater probe or multipolar probe, or even the argon plasma coagulator, being significantly more portable than laser techniques.

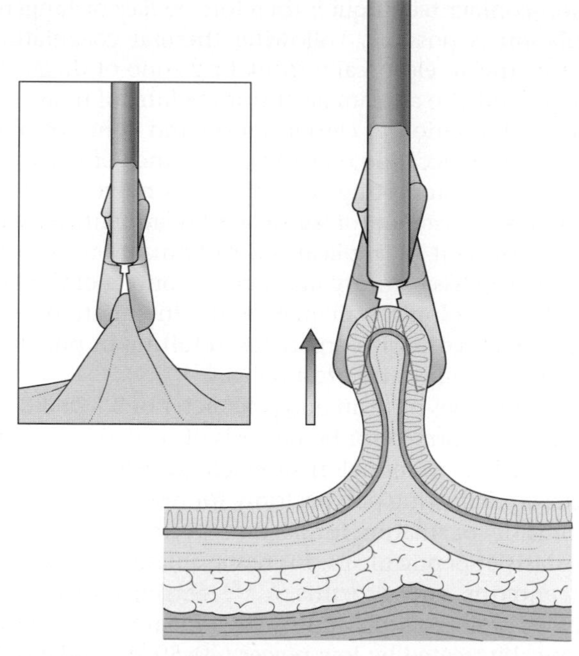

Figure 81.22: Insulated hot biopsy forceps. The mucosa is tented away from the colonic wall prior to electrocoagulation. (From Wadas and Sanowski, Complications of the hot biopsy forceps technique. 1988; 34(1) : 32–37, with permission.[76] copyright of the American Society for Gastrointestinal Endoscopy.)

Complication rates may vary among the techniques, with perforations and rebleeding being reported after monopolar, multipolar coagulation, laser therapy and APC application.[74] Injection therapy is rarely associated with perforation unless non-standard volumes of injection are employed.[74] Similarly hemostatic clips (discussed below), when properly applied, are rarely associated with the development of complications.

Argon plasma coagulation (APC)

The APC was initially used for surgery, both open and laparoscopic, with endoscopic applications after 1991. It is a non-contact method delivered via the accessory channel of the endoscope. The major benefit of this technique is that it is a quick method of therapy deliverable over a large treatment area. The principle of APC is that high-frequency monopolar current is conducted to target tissues *through* ionized argon gas (argon plasma). Argon gas passes through the coagulation probe with an electrode at its tip. The foot switch activates the electrode. Electrons flow through the channel of electrically activated ionized argon gas from the probe to the tissue.[78] The arrival of the current density at the tissue surface results in coagulation. The grounding pad completes the circuit. If electrical energy is not discharged by arcing to nearby tissues, there is no ignition and therefore activation of the foot switch causes insufflation of inert argon gas only. The depth of coagulation using this technique is dependent on the generator power setting, flow rate of argon gas, duration of application, and distance between the probe tip and target tissue. The arc contacts the tissue closest to the electrode (keeping in mind that this is a non-contact technique); therefore *en face* or tangential coagulation is possible. Following thermal coagulation a thin, superficial, electrically insulating zone of desiccation develops, and also a steam layer from boiling of tissue. Both result in a limitation of carbonization and depth of coagulation. After desiccation, electrical resistance of the treated area increases, prompting the current to move to another area of lower resistance for subsequent treatment. With prolonged treatment or application, carbonization, vaporization and deep tissue injury may occur. Contact of the probe tip with the colonic wall may result in inflation of the colonic submucosa with argon gas, resulting in pneumatosis and potentially extraintestinal gas.[74]

Current probes have an outer diameter of 2.3 or 3.2 mm. Therapy is performed for hemostasis of superficial vascular ectasias such as watermelon stomach (gastric antral vascular ectasia), following polypectomy for resection of residual adenoma or coagulation for postpolypectomy bleeding, for hemostasis of peptic ulcers, for tissue ablation and for radiation enteritis and proctitis.[73,78–81] Settings vary significantly by indication. In adults, superficial vascular lesions are typically treated by low power (40–50 W) and gas flow rates (0.8 l/min) with an operative distance between the tissue and the probe of 2–8 mm.[78] Closer contact is used with lower power settings to allow for contact between the plasma and the targeted tissue. Application times are in the range of 0.5–2.0 s. Similar settings have been reported in a pediatric series.[82] The technique is to paint confluent or near-confluent surface areas. Use of a two-channel endoscope, if possible, allows for aspiration of argon gas. If the probe tip contacts the bowel wall, it becomes similar to a grounded monopolar probe (discussed above) and may result in deep tissue injury. The surface to be treated needs to be clear of liquid and blood; if not, coagulated film develops and the tissue beneath may not be adequately treated, limiting the usefulness of this technology in patients with active bleeding.

Endoscopic hemostatic devices including bands and clips

Band ligation

Band ligation was initially utilized for the management of esophageal variceal hemorrhage starting in the late 1980s. This technique has subsequently been used for the management of bleeding gastric, intestinal and colonic varices, Dieulafoy lesions, bleeding hemorrhoids, Mallory–Weiss tears, angiectasias, polypectomy sites and duodenal ulcers.[74] Band ligation is most effective for bleeding lesions in non-fibrotic tissue. Typically, after a diagnostic endoscopy to identify the source of bleeding, the endoscope is withdrawn. The ligating device composed of a control handle and attached adaptor is loaded via the biopsy channel and a friction fit adaptor with the ligating bands is placed at the end of the endoscope (usually a standard-size adult upper endoscope). Ligation kits contain a variable number of bands, but typically multi-band ligators are utilized. After passage of the endoscope to the desired location, suction is applied to draw the lesion to be ligated into the friction fit adaptor at the end of the endoscope.[70] The bands are deployed by rotation of the ligating control handle while in the locked position. Positional adjustments and inspection for continued evidence of bleeding can be made between subsequent band deployments. In the case of a bleeding lesion such as a Dieulafoy lesion, only a single band may need to be deployed. Because the presence of more bands on the friction fit adaptor limits the endoscopic view, some pediatric gastroenterologists choose to deploy some of the bands outside the patient prior to endoscope insertion to improve the field of view. Band ligators are currently not available for smaller pediatric-size endoscopes.

Hemostatic clips

Originally developed in the 1970s for deployment through the endoscope, endoclips have significantly increased in popularity and ease of use in the past 5–10 years.[83] Originally the clips were designed to be placed on a deployment device that could be reused, and deployment of the clip resulted in the need to remove and reload the device after each clip application. This technique was cumbersome and time consuming. Recently clips have been developed that are preloaded and designed for single use, although single-use clips are typically more costly than the multi-use deployment devices. Hemoclip application requires an endoscope with a 2.8-mm channel. Preloaded clips are available in different lengths, allowing use with both upper endoscopes and colonoscopes. Rotatable clips are also available. Endoscopic clipping is used primarily for endoscopic hemostasis, but has also been applied for binding tubes or catheters to the gastrointestinal wall (stent, feeding tube, manometry catheter), closure of fistulae, leaks and perforations, and marking anatomic landmarks for subsequent therapy or surgery.[83,84] Lesions amenable to clip application for hemostasis include gastric and duodenal ulcers with high-risk stigmata, Mallory–Weiss tears and Dieulafoy's lesion. Endoclip application for ulcer bleeding is associated with a high primary hemostatic rate (85–100%), depending on the series, and a low recurrent bleeding rate (2–20%).[83] Ulcers most amenable to endoclip therapy include those with small arteries and those not located on the difficult areas for endoscopic therapy: the proximal posterior wall of the stomach, high on the lesser curvature of the stomach and the posterior duodenal wall. Clips have also been used for lower gastrointestinal bleeding, including hemorrhoids, solitary rectal ulcer syndrome, following biopsy and, most commonly, for bleeding polypectomy stalks.[74]

Endoclips are deployed by the following technique. After passage through the endoscope channel, the stopper on the clip is removed and the cylinder is pulled back, exposing the clip. The slider is slowly pulled back, opening the clip to its maximum width. The clip is pressed against the lesion, a small amount of suction is applied prior to deployment allowing the lumen to collapse, and the slider is quickly pulled back; this closes the clip and deploys it. Typically more than one clip is deployed in a single endoscopic session. The first clip is placed on the bleeding point and subsequent clips may be placed around the bleeding point to occlude the submucosal vessel (opposite to the technique of heater probe application).[83] The clips dislodge spontaneously after application and have not been associated with long-term sequelae.

Endoloops

Endoloops are utilized primarily for the management of potential or actual postpolypectomy hemorrhage. Detachable loops have also been used in the management of gastric varices.[74] Loops, deployed through the biopsy channel, are placed either prior to placement of the standard polypectomy snare or following polypectomy to the transected stalk to reduce the rate of postpolypectomy hemorrhage. Detachable loops work mechanically as a ligating device but are not capable of electrocautery.

When placed prior to polypectomy, if placed too tightly they may result in inadvertent transection of the polyp stalk with resultant bleeding (due to the lack of cautery); if placed too loosely, bleeding can occur following polypectomy. Correct placement is indicated by change in the color of the polyp head without transection. Loop placement prior to snare polypectomy can also be associated with entanglement of the loop within the polypectomy snare.

Loop placement on a polyp stalk after polypectomy may be complicated by difficult placement due to retraction of the stalk. One method to overcome this technique is the lift and ligate technique using a two-channel scope, where the stalk is lifted by forceps from one channel and ligated using a detachable snare from the second channel.[85] When using this technique, the loop is placed first around the stalk but not tightened; the forceps are then placed to lift the stalk and the endoloop is tightened.

Laser photocoagulation

Laser photocoagulation is another modality occasionally used to achieve endoscopic hemostasis. There are two main types of laser: the argon and the Nd:YAG laser. The argon laser's usefulness is limited because of light absorption by surrounding red blood. Therefore, to use the argon laser, overlying blood must be eliminated with a coaxial air jet. Clinically, the argon laser is used primarily for right-sided colonic lesions. When compared with the Nd:YAG laser, it has a lower power and depth of tissue penetration.

The Nd:YAG laser is the most popular laser used in endoscopy. The laser admits a continuous wave of infrared light of wavelength 1064 nm with a power up to 100 W. This light is transmitted via a 600-μm glass fiber in a 2.5-mm Teflon catheter passed down the endoscope biopsy channel. Carbon dioxide is passed coaxially along the catheter to clear blood from the bleeding site and to keep the fiber tip cool and free from debris. A filter is attached to the eyepiece to prevent reflected laser light from entering the endoscopist's eye. The intense laser light is directed to coagulate tissue circumferentially around the bleeding site. Contact and non-contact applications are possible.[74] The current recommendation for adults is to deliver 0.5-s pulses, at 80 W of energy, from a distance of 1 cm, and at least 2–3 mm away from visible arterial segments for upper gastrointestinal lesions.[86]

Lasers in colonoscopy and small bowel enteroscopy have been used for congenital vascular lesions (hereditary hemorrhagic telangiectasia, blue rubber bleb nevi syndrome) as well as superficial vascular lesions, including angiodysplasia, telangiectasia and arteriovenous malformation. Asymptomatic, non-bleeding angiodysplasias are usually not treated. One problem after laser photocoagulation of a lesion is that the histologic diagnosis is difficult to confirm.

Like the heater probe, laser therapy can also provoke bleeding, which can usually be stopped with further laser coagulation.[86] In addition, there is an increased chance of full-thickness perforation of the gut wall. Application of the laser in the colon requires modification of both technique and power settings. The thermal effects of a laser beam on tissue vary according to the power density (the amount of energy converted to heat at the point where the laser beam strikes tissue) and the size of the contact area. Although the power setting and exposure time can be preset, movement, especially in the right colon, and varying wall thickness, especially the thin ascending colon, can change the exposure time required to produce perforation. Instead of coagulating tissue, vaporization of tissue can occur.

There is a long learning curve associated with use of the laser, and this modality should be used only by experienced operators. Currently the laser seems to offer little advantage over the heater probe, multipolar probe or APC, and because of its increased cost and decreased portability the other modalities are likely to predominate in the foreseeable future.

STRICTURE DILATION

Esophageal dilation can be performed with a variety of instruments, but only endoscopic dilation is discussed in this section. The advantage of endoscopic dilation is the ability to visualize the stenotic area, estimate its size, select an appropriately sized dilator and, if necessary, pass a guidewire beyond the stenotic area. Dilation techniques can be divided into those performed using the endoscope itself, those performed over a wire (OTW) and those using through the endoscope dilators (TTS).

Savary–Gillard dilators are among the most frequently used types of dilator. They are hollow bougies of plastic-coated polyvinyl ranging in size from 5 to 15 mm (15–45 Fr). The tip is tapered and flexible, and the shaft is more rigid. Endoscopy is initially performed to the level of the stenosis, or beyond the stenosis if possible. A flexible-tip guidewire is then advanced via the biopsy through the stricture under direct observation. When it passes the stricture, the endoscope is removed while the wire is kept in place by advancing it as the endoscope is withdrawn. Typically a wire with a spring coiled tip is utilized. The wire is advanced into the gastric antrum, for example, in patients with esophageal stricture. The coil at the tip of the wire helps to reduce the incidence of perforation due to the wire. The lubricated bougie is then threaded over the guidewire, which is held taut. Serial dilations are performed by progressively increasing the bougie size according to the amount of resistance encountered. The dilators should be checked for blood after each dilation. Strictures typically need to be dilated over several sessions rather than on a single occasion. The guidewire must be held in place in between application of serial bougies in order to avoid slippage.

In a large French–American series, larger-diameter dilations could be performed using the Savary system than with the Eder–Puestow dilating system. There was no statistically significant difference in the incidence of complications between the two methods.[87] The occurrence of esophageal perforation may relate more to the reason for dilation (e.g. caustic ingestion or malignancy *vs* peptic stenosis) than the dilating method used. Also, the success of dilation may relate to the indication. Dilating congenital stenosis is usually more effective than dilating achalasia or postsurgical stenosis.

Endoscopic balloon dilation may also be performed utilizing TTS balloon dilators. After visualizing the stricture, these types of balloon can be passed through an endoscope with a 2.8-mm channel under direct vision. These single-use dilators have an inflatable balloon at their tip. The balloon is inflatable to a preset maximum diameter and pressure. If the pressure is exceeded, the balloon ruptures, reducing the risk of esophageal perforation. Inflation exerts only radially directed forces as opposed to the shearing longitudinal forces that occur with conventional bougienage. The dilator is positioned through the endoscope with or without the use of a guidewire. The balloon is inflated with water or, occasionally, Gastrografin, and held in inflation for 30–90 s, then deflated.[88] Usually two or three inflations are performed per endoscopic session, with repositioning of the balloon in between inflations. Sessions are repeated over several weeks or months with progressively larger-diameter balloons. This technique has been utilized for esophageal atresia with postoperative strictures and is especially useful for strictures of recent onset. Endoscopically directed hydrostatic balloon dilation has also been reported in obstructive gastroduodenal Crohn's disease. Cicatricial anastomotic strictures of the colon have also been dilated with air-and-water-filled balloons or with a mechanical dilator (e.g. Savary dilator) placed over an endoscopically directed guidewire. Recently successful endoscopic guided OTW balloon dilation of esophageal strictures has been reported in recessive dystrophic epidermolysis bullosa, a condition associated with proximal esophageal strictures and an increased vulnerability of the esophageal mucosa to minor injury.[89,90]

During the past 5 years, balloons that can be inflated to three distinct diameters have been developed and are now widely available. These balloons exert a high degree of radial vector force at each of the different standardized pressures, but are still designed to rupture if preset pressures are exceeded. They represent a potential cost saving to the patient if progressive serial diameter dilations are performed on the same day, and may decrease the time of the endoscopic procedure because of decreased need to exchange balloons during the procedure.

Intralesional steroid injection of peptic and caustic esophageal strictures has been reported as an adjuvant to endoscopic dilation. Small volumes (0.25–1.0 ml per injection) of triamcinolone acetonide (Kenalog 10 mg/ml; Bristol Meyers Squibb Princeton, NJ, USA) are injected in four quadrants of the narrowest stricture segment. The efficacy of triamcinolone appears to be based on its interference with collagen synthesis and subsequent scar formation.[88] This technique has been associated with increased efficacy of dilation and longer symptom-free intervals between endoscopic dilations.[91]

Esophageal dilation can also be performed by passage of progressively larger-sized endoscopes. This is usually performed for esophageal strictures with an outer diameter in the range of 6–8 mm. Typically a gastroscope with an outer diameter of 6 mm is passed initially across the stricture. Subsequently gastroscopes with an outer diameter of 8–9 mm can be passed under direct endoscopic vision using careful steady pressure. Perforation is a potential complication of this technique and the endoscopist must use judgment as to appropriate dilating diameter and the amount of pressure to be exerted, as with any endoscopic technique. The advantage of serial endoscopic dilation compared with OTW dilation is that the length of the stricture can be carefully visualized and assessed, irregularities of the stricture such as shelves can be identified, the direction of the dilating force can be more directly controlled, and bleeding or excessive trauma is identified immediately.

Eosinophilic esophagitis has been identified as a cause of esophageal strictures and ringed esophagus. This condition and its management are discussed elsewhere in the text. This condition can be associated with short or long esophageal strictures and/or diffuse narrowing of the esophagus. Dilation of strictures associated with this condition may require special precautions. The esophagus in this condition appears to be especially susceptible to shear injury, and longitudinal tears of the esophagus have been reported following endoscopy without dilation and after small-diameter dilations.[92,93] Strictures in this condition may occur throughout the length of the esophagus, and there is a higher incidence of proximal strictures compared with reflux-related strictures, which are more typically distal. TTS balloon dilation under direct endoscopic vision may be one method to manage these proximal esophageal strictures effectively.

SMALL BOWEL ENTEROSCOPY

There are two primary techniques of small bowel enteroscopy currently applicable to pediatric patients. In children, this technique is used primarily for the evaluation of gastrointestinal bleeding of unknown origin. It may occasionally be indicated for small bowel biopsy, although this can usually be accomplished utilizing the standard upper endoscopes.

In addition, this technique is utilized for jejunal polypectomy and can be used in conjunction with open or laparoscopic surgical procedures as a method of evaluating the distal small bowel. Additional indications include evaluation of extent of inflammatory bowel disease or polyposis syndromes, including surveillance, evaluation of lymphoma or lymphangiectasia, graft assessment after small bowel transplant, dilation of strictures and directed tube placement such as percutaneous jejunostomy (PEJ) placement (discussed below) and nasojejunal tube placement.[94]

The most popular type of small bowel endoscopic examination is push enteroscopy. The limitation of this technique is that the angulation of the duodenum dissipates the propelling force transmitted to the shaft of the endoscope and subsequently creates a large loop in the stomach and duodenum. Gastroduodenal loops can occasionally be reduced by use of a straightening tube, but are more often reduced by endoscopic techniques of withdrawal and torque similar to those utilized in colonoscopy. This type of enteroscopy is performed with either a sterilized pediatric colonoscope or a special push-type enteroscope. Both of these endoscopes have a larger diameter than standard pediatric gastroscopes, limiting their usefulness in infants and small children. These endoscopes do, however, have a biopsy channel, and angulation of the tip is possible. Therefore, therapeutic interventions such as biopsy, injection, coagulation and polypectomy are possible. The exact extent of evaluation is variable, based on patient size and anatomy, but distances of 120–180 cm beyond the ligament of Treitz have been visualized with this technique, and full examination to the terminal ileum may be possible using a combined enteroscopic–operative advancement technique.[94] After the scope is fully inserted, glucagon may be administered to decrease intestinal peristalsis. The lumen is visualized primarily upon scope withdrawal, combining air insufflation and slow withdrawal of the scope. This technique is useful to detect a diffuse lesion and the causes of small bowel bleeding, especially arteriovenous malformations.

The second type of small bowel endoscopy is passive, using a Sonde-type enteroscope passed intranasally. These instruments have a balloon at their tip and, when it is inflated, bowel peristalsis acts to pull the endoscope through the small bowel. This procedure may take 12–24 h. Compared with the push-type enteroscopes, the Sonde scope has a much narrower diameter for greater patient comfort. It has no tip control for angulation, however, and no biopsy channel. The Lewis–Way modification involved transnasal passage of the passive enteroscope with a suture at its tip. The pediatric colonoscope is then passed orally and the suture is grabbed using the biopsy forceps through the pediatric colonoscope channel. The pediatric colonoscope guides the passive enteroscope into the duodenum and is then carefully withdrawn. The balloon is inflated and its passage is monitored fluoroscopically. Metoclopramide and neostigmine may be given to facilitate scope movement. As with the push-type enteroscope, the lumen is visualized using glucagon paralysis upon scope withdrawal. Sonde small bowel enteroscopy has decreased significantly in popularity compared with push enteroscopy, and with the development of video capsule endoscopy (discussed below) will likely become obsolete.

In July 2004 a double-balloon small bowel enteroscope was released for clinical use in the USA. This scope employs a combination of balloon inflation and deflation, and a small bowel overtube for visualization of the distal small bowel. The scope can also be passed via the rectum for evaluation of the proximal ileum. The scope is 2 m in length, has an 8.5-mm outer diameter (10.5-mm outer diameter with overtube) and a 2.2-mm working channel through which biopsies and other procedures can be performed. A 1.5-mm APC probe is also currently under development, designed to be compatible with this endoscope. (Information courtesy of Fujinon Inc., Wayne, NJ, USA.) Although not yet used in pediatric patients, this endoscope may offer therapeutic advantages compared with wire capsule endoscopy, discussed below.

WIRELESS CAPSULE ENDOSCOPY

Wireless capsule endoscopy has largely replaced passive small bowel enteroscopy as a method to evaluate the distal small bowel between the ligament of Treitz and the distal ileum.

The currently available disposable capsule is 26.4 mm in length and 11 mm in diameter.[95] It is composed of a battery-powered flashing light source, a chip camera sensor and a micro-transmitter. The lens of the capsule is of high resolution (0.1 mm), allowing for high-quality evaluation of mucosal detail. The capsule transmits images at a rate of 2 per second via digital radiofrequency to a data recorder worn on a belt outside the body.[95] The batteries allow an average recording time of 8 h and potentially more than 50 000 images. After completion of the study, data are transferred from the recorder to a computer workstation for evaluation and ultimately storage. Capsule images can roughly be correlated to the location of identified small bowel lesions.

Patients take nothing by mouth for at least 8 h prior to capsule endoscopy. Bowel preparation or a clear liquid diet the day before the study may improve the diagnostic yield. Clear liquids can be taken 1–2 h after the test has begun, and a light meal can generally be taken 2 h or more into the study.[95]

In patients who are unable to swallow the capsule, those with pyloric narrowing or delayed gastric emptying, the capsule can be deployed into the duodenum endoscopically. This is done by preloading the capsule on the upper endoscope, holding the capsule in place using a snare or a Roth retrieval net. Band ligators have been placed around the capsule to help prevent slippage from a polypectomy snare.[95] Release of the capsule from the net may be difficult, especially in small patients.[95] A 'through the endoscope channel' capsule delivery device has recently been introduced, designed specifically to allow capsule deployment to the small intestine. This device may increase the likelihood of small intestinal visualization in patients with impaired or delayed gastric emptying. (Information courtesy of US Endoscopy, Mentor, OH, USA.)

Potential indications for wireless capsule endoscopy are similar to those discussed above for small bowel enteroscopy, and include evaluation of gastrointestinal bleeding of unknown origin, evaluation of extent of inflammatory bowel disease or polyposis syndromes, evaluation of medication-induced mucosal injury (including non-steroidal anti-inflammatory drugs), evaluation of suspected lymphoma or lymphangiectasia, and graft assessment after small bowel transplant or suspected graft-*vs*-host disease. Current limitations of the technique include capsule size, particularly in small patients, failure of capsule passage at several potential locations including the pylorus, areas of anatomic narrowing such as strictures and the ileocecal valve, failure of the capsule completely to image the small bowel within the available battery life in patients with impaired motility, time delay between imaging and image evaluation, time required to evaluate the images, lack of ability to perform therapy or obtain biopsies of abnormalities detected, and lack of ability to direct the capsule to desired areas of image acquisition.

The presence of strictures or other obstructions in the intestinal tract is currently a contraindication to the use of capsule endoscopy. Capsules have become impacted at the site of strictures, and have required endoscopic or surgical removal. A lactose-based patency capsule without recording capabilities but with radiologic markings is currently undergoing evaluation. The capsule can be administered to patients with suspected anatomic narrowing to determine whether the standard capsule device is likely to become lodged. Capsules that are unable to pass are designed to dissolve, but still may require removal from areas of significant anatomic narrowing. Capsule endoscopy has been employed in children as young as 6 years of age, and future technological innovations may allow for applications in even younger patients.

PERCUTANEOUS ENDOSCOPIC GASTROSTOMY AND PERCUTANEOUS ENDOSCOPIC JEJUNOSTOMY

The first report of successful PEG tube placement was in a 1980 by Gauderer, Ponsky and Izant.[96] PEG tube insertion is one of the unique endoscopic procedures that originated in pediatric patients, was subsequently popularized in adults and was later reintroduced in children by pediatric gastroenterologists. Although initially developed by surgeons, it is now performed at an equal or greater frequency by adult and pediatric gastroenterologists. Despite many similarities in the indications and some technical aspects of the procedure between children and adults, there are also significant differences in the indications, limitations and technical aspects of the procedure.

Indications

PEG tubes are appropriate in any pediatric patient who requires a gastrostomy tube (G tube) and does not require an open surgical procedure at the same time as the gastrostomy tube placement. Patients undergoing a simultaneous fundoplication, pyloroplasty or pyloromyotomy would in all likelihood not derive additional benefit from placement of a PEG tube *vs* a surgical gastrostomy at the time of surgery. PEG tube placement does not interfere with subsequent fundoplication, pyloroplasty or pyloromyotomy in patients who may have reflux or gastric emptying issues unresponsive to medical or endoscopic therapy. Benefits of PEG tube insertion *vs* surgical gastrostomy include: reduced procedure time with reduced cost, smaller incision, shorter length of hospital stay, potentially decreased incidence of severe GER in the postoperative period, decreased incidence of postoperative complications including wound infection, dehiscence at operative site, bowel obstruction, pain, atelectasis and impaired mobility. Contraindications are limited. Placement of a PEG tube should not be attempted if there are patient factors that would interfere with successful transillumination of the gastric wall and identification of the indentation performed during the procedure, or if there is a suspicion that the anterior gastric wall is not opposed to the abdominal wall, as in the case of an intervening colon or other abdominal organ. As with any endoscopic procedure, the patient should be medically stable to undergo the procedure; airway protection and management is imperative and the endoscopist should be willing to abort the procedure if it is not progressing as anticipated. This may be due, for example, to positioning of the colon between the stomach and the anterior abdominal wall. This problem may often not be identified before surgery, and may necessitate conversion to an open procedure. PEG tubes may be more difficult to place, should be placed with increased caution, and may require additional pre-procedure evaluation in patients with the following conditions: ascites or peritoneal dialysis, scoliosis or spine abnormalities, small size, ventriculoperitoneal shunt, prior abdominal surgery, congenital abnormalities such as situs inversus, hepatomegaly or splenomegaly or other abdominal masses, patients with small laryngeal or tracheal size, or compromise or ventilatory issues.

PEGs can be placed for medication administration, feeding administration, gastric decompression or a combination of these reasons. The pre-procedure evaluation may vary based on the indication. For example, in a well nourished, neurologically impaired child who is having the PEG tube placed for medication administration only, a preoperative evaluation for reflux may not be indicated. In the same child who has severe vomiting and failure to thrive, additional testing including 24-h pH probe testing may be indicated before surgery to determine whether he or she is a candidate for a simultaneous anti-reflux procedure. Open gastrostomy does not reduce the incidence of severe postoperative GER in neurologically impaired children compared with PEG placement, and is associated with a higher likelihood of severe reflux requiring a fundoplication (odds ratio 6–7 : 1).[97] Potential contributing factors include alteration of the angle of His and reduced lower esophageal sphincter pressure by an open gastrostomy. In many centers, evaluation prior to PEG includes upper gastrointestinal radiography to exclude malrotation and, if possible, to identify whether a portion of the stomach is located below the rib cage. In patients who are having PEGs placed for feeding, a trial of nasogastric feedings (usually outpatient) for approximately 10 days prior to placement of the PEG tube may offer a functional preoperative evaluation of GER. Patients who are intolerant of nasogastric feeds can undergo additional evaluation for an anti-reflux procedure. Patients who tolerate the feedings generally gain weight and improve their nutritional status prior to the anesthetic and operative procedure.

Technique

In most pediatric centers, two physicians perform PEGs; one physician performs the endoscopic portion of the procedure and the other performs the abdominal portion. The physicians may be two pediatric gastroenterologists, a pediatric gastroenterologist and a pediatric surgeon or an interventional radiologist. Insertion of a PEG tube should be considered an advanced endoscopic procedure with a higher rate of associated complications than standard endoscopy. Patients should be nil per os prior to the procedure. Administration of preoperative antibiotics with good coverage for skin flora and two additional peri/postoperative doses has been shown to decrease the incidence of postoperative wound infection.[19,22,98] The abdomen should be prepped and draped in a sterile fashion. Frequently the procedure is performed utilizing a general anesthetic or sedation provided by a pediatric intensivist. Deep sedation has been employed successfully for this procedure. The endoscopist will pass the appropriately sized endoscope and fill the greater curvature of the stomach without intubating the pylorus. Initially, excessive air insufflation should be avoided as this may distend the small bowel loops and interfere with the gastric impression. The other physician, who is 'sterile' throughout the procedure, then performs finger indentation to identify an impression along the anterior gastric wall, preferably away from the gastric cardia and located near the junction of the gastric body and antrum (Fig. 81.23) The optimal indentation is perpendicular to the anterior gastric wall to avoid entering the stomach inferiorly, as this may increase the risk of entering the colon or its mesentery. The indentation should allow enough space for tube insertion away from the costal margin, as tubes too close to the ribs can be associated with significant pain. After identification of a good impression, the sterile physician will inset a 25- or 21-G needle attached to a syringe, usually filled with 1% lidocaine solution to test the tract identified by the gastric indentation. This needle should pass into the stomach under the direct vision of the endoscopist in the same length as the anticipated internal length of the PEG tube. Failure to see passage of the needle into the stomach when it is inserted to its hub suggests that repositioning of the PEG site is necessary or that there is an intervening organ such as colon or bowel mesentery. Lidocaine for local anesthesia is usually injected with needle withdrawal. Some

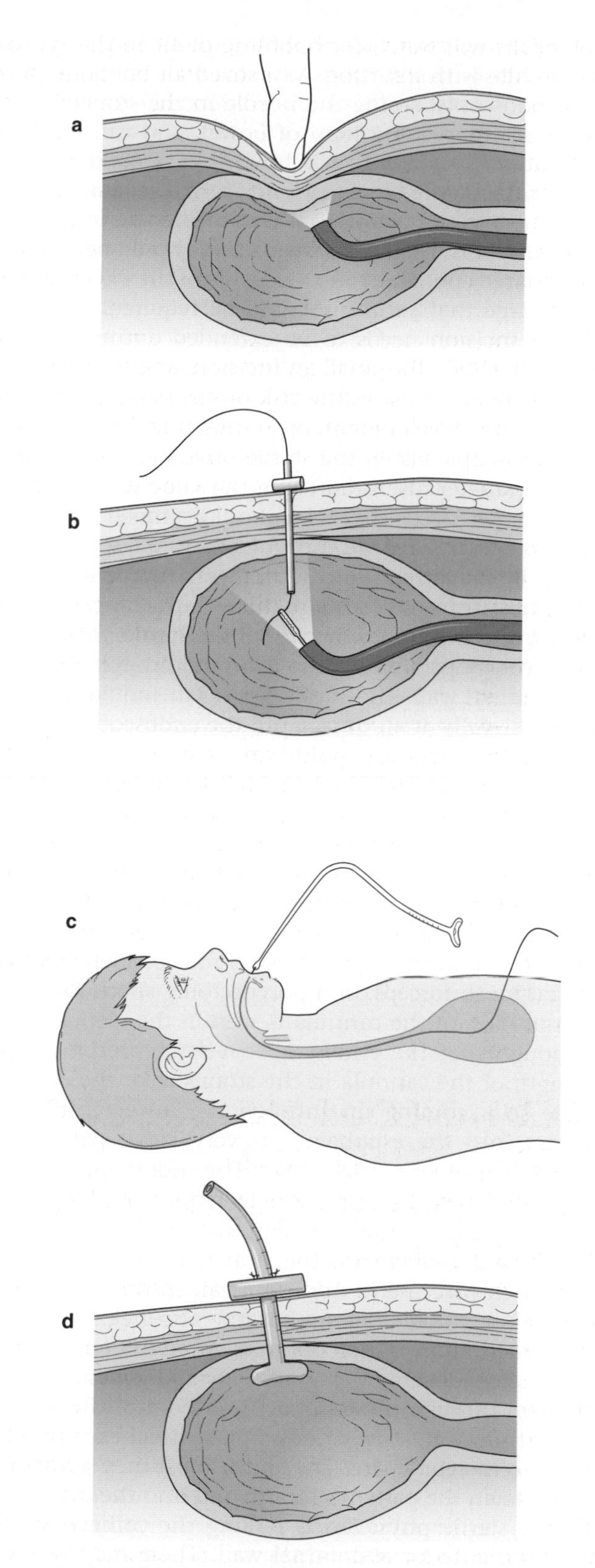

Figure 81.23: PEG placement. (**a**) Finger indentation is performed to identify the optimal position. (**b**) After trochar introduction through the anterior abdominal wall, a suture or guidewire is passed through the trochar and grasped with a snare or forceps. (**c**) The PEG is positioned by pulling the tube through the stomach and into position. (**d**) The PEG catheter may be secured to the anterior abdominal wall with an external bolster. (From George and Dokler, 2002, with permssion.)[139]

endoscopists will watch for bubbling of air in the syringe of the needle with insertion. Visualized air bubbling prior to the endoscopist seeing the needle in the stomach may indicate an intervening loop of bowel, and can result in complications as described below. After a good site has been identified, the sterile physician makes a small incision in the anterior abdominal wall at the site of catheter insertion. This is usually transverse and should be through the skin, large enough to allow passage of the PEG tube but not too large that suturing would be required. On occasion, this incision needs to be extended during the pull aspect of the PEG. Too small an incision, and therefore too tight a catheter, increases the risk of postoperative wound infection and development of granulation tissue. Under direct endoscopic vision the sterile physician then repeats the angiocatheter insertion, using the same technique but with a larger sized (14 G) cannula/catheter that will accommodate passage of the guidewire. As soon as the catheter is visualized in the stomach, the endoscopist passes biopsy forceps or a snare through the biopsy port in order to grasp the guidewire, which the sterile physician is simultaneously passing via the cannula through the anterior abdominal wall. The sterile physician should hold the catheter carefully at all times until the endoscopist secures the guidewire. Once the guidewire is secured, the procedure can almost always be completed safely, but accidental dislodgment of the cannula prior to guidewire insertion can result in a free perforation or other complication. For smaller endoscopes with a 2.0-mm channel, guidewires are grasped utilizing small forceps. For standard endoscopes with a 2.8-mm channel, the guidewire can be grasped using standard forceps, foreign-body forceps such as alligator or rat tooth forceps, or a polypectomy snare. On occasion, a portion of the cannula is seen in the stomach, but not enough that the endoscopist feels comfortable with the length of the cannula in the stomach, or the cannula may be seen coming up through the lower esophageal sphincter into the esophagus in very small patients or across to the posterior gastric wall. The endoscopist can use very gentle endoscopic traction to reduce tenting of the gastric wall on the cannula, which will allow advancement of the cannula safely into the stomach without through and through placement. Additional air insufflation *immediately* before catheter puncture may also help when the gastric indentation is not optimal. After the endoscopist grasps the guidewire, the guidewire and endoscope are withdrawn through the esophagus and out of the mouth. After withdrawal, the endoscopist attaches the PEG catheter to the guidewire. The endoscopist then guides the catheter down the patient's mouth and into the esophagus while the sterile physician is pulling the catheter gently though the anterior abdominal wall. There may be some resistance when the guidewire catheter knot reaches the abdominal wall. In this case, slightly extending the incision may help pull the catheter through the wall, and circular rotation of the guidewire with steady traction by the sterile physician will facilitate this maneuver. In the off-chance that the guidewire breaks as it is coming through the abdominal wall, hemostats can be used to bring the guidewire and catheter though the abdominal wall. Care should be taken to avoid pulling too hard as the catheter is coming though the abdominal wall, especially in small, malnourished or immunocompromised patients, as there have been reports of pulling the catheter entirely through the abdominal wall. The endoscopist will verify the position of the PEG tube and the length to the skin. An excess length to the skin (i.e. 5–6 cm) should raise the possibility that something may be trapped between the stomach and the anterior abdominal wall. An external bumper secures the PEG, leaving room for swelling in the immediate perioperative period. The incision is dressed with antibiotic ointment, and additional intravenous antibiotics are administered in the postoperative period, usually for two further doses. The tubes can generally be used within 6–24 h.

Indications of a potential problem and when to abort include:

- Failure to identify a good gastric impression
- Excess angiocatheter length without seeing the tip in the stomach, or air bubbling in the needle syringe without seeing the needle tip in the stomach
- Gastric varices or significant ulceration
- Identification of stool at any point during the procedure.

Catheters are not changed until 6 weeks after the PEG procedure, and preferably after 2 months to allow the tract to mature.[99] Percutaneous replacement of PEG tubes following accidental dislodgment has been reported within a couple of weeks of placement. Catheters can be changed by traction removal or endoscopically, where the catheter is cut and retrieved like a foreign body. Cut and await passage technique has resulted in intestinal obstruction, impaction and perforation. Endoscopic visualization of placement of the new gastrostomy button at the time of initial conversion from a PEG tube is helpful. If the button is placed in the tract but is not visualized in the stomach, there may be a false tract, a portion of the colon or small bowel may have been trapped between the PEG tube and the abdominal wall, and the button may be located in the colon, small bowel or mesentery. Surgical consultation is appropriate at this point.

Multiple complications have been reported in the literature after PEG placement. Rates in the literature vary, but are generally in the range of 5–30%. Some are preventable with appropriate antibiotic prophylaxis, good endoscopic/percutaneous technique, and recognition by the physicians performing the procedure that things are not going well with a decision to abort the procedure and proceed with open gastrostomy. Some complications may be unavoidable due to patient anatomy or underlying disease. Reported minor complications include cellulitis, uncomplicated pneumoperitoneum, tube defects/disconnection, GER, granulation tissue or pain at the insertion site. Major complications include gastrocolic fistula, gastroileal fistula, gastro (colo/ileal) cutaneous fistulae, placement of catheter through the liver, duodenal hematoma, complicated pneumoperitoneum, aspiration, peritonitis and catheter complications, including migration, buried bumper syndrome, partial gastric separation, catheter/

bumper impaction if not retrieved, ventriculoperitoneal shunt infection, gastric perforation or death.[99] Late complications include gastrocolic fistula, gastroileal fistula, catheter migration/buried bumper syndrome/partial gastric separation, gastric ulceration, cellulitis, fasciitis, gastric perforation, catheter migration or other catheter-related complications, bronchoesophageal fistula (following removal) and aortic perforation (following cut and pass catheter removal).[99]

PERCUTANEOUS ENDOSCOPIC JEJUNOSTOMY

Direct PEJ has also been reported and is indicated in patients prone to aspiration, with complete or partial gastric or duodenal obstruction, or gastric motility disorders. Because of the smaller jejunal size and its variable position, the technique is technically more difficult than PEG. The procedure is performed utilizing a push enteroscope, which is advanced into the jejunum up to 24 inches distal to the ligament of Treitz in adult-size patients. The endoscope tip is used to transilluminate the abdominal wall in a 2–3-cm area. The second physician uses direct fingertip pressure to identify a discrete intrajejunal indentation to the endoscopist. Placement is similar to the PEG technique described above. Catheter size is limited because of the narrower jejunal lumen, and feeding schedules are modified accordingly. In some instances a PEJ tube may not be able to be placed because of inability to appose and transilluminate a jejunal segment adjacent to the abdominal wall. Theoretical problems with PEJ insertion include increased technical difficulty, including maintenance of correct jejunal position and risk of needle entry into the abdomen either directly or through the posterior jejunal wall secondary to diminished luminal size. This technique may prove to be especially difficult in pediatric patients because of the reduced diameter of the intestinal lumen. As with PEG procedures, prophylactic antibiotics are administered routinely.

PERCUTANEOUS CECOSTOMY (PEC)

Recently, percutaneous cecostomy and percutaneous colostomy of the left colon have been reported.[100,101] These techniques were developed to assist in the management of intractable constipation in children. After placement, the PEC tube is used to administer antegrade continence enemas, and represents a modification of the surgical approach to this problem introduced by Malone et al. in 1990.[101] After bowel preparation, prophylactic antibiotic administration (metronidazole and gentamycin, or cefotaxime and metronidazole) and a sterile skin preparation, colonoscopy is performed to the cecum. The bowel is transilluminated, a small incision is made and a trocar is passed into the cecum under direct vision, using a technique similar to PEG placement described above. For left-sided tube placement, tubes have been placed at the junction of the descending and sigmoid colon.[101] The guidewire is passed, grasped via a snare passed via the colonoscope, and pulled out through the anus. A 12–20-Fr pull-type PEG tube is attached to the wire, and subsequently the PEG tube is pulled in a retrograde fashion through the colon and out through the anterior abdominal wall. The position of the PEC tube in the cecum or alternate location is verified endoscopically.[100] PEC tubes are flushed in the postoperative period, usually starting 24 h after surgery, and subsequently can be used for antegrade enema administration of standard concentration solutions. Prophylactic antibiotics are typically administered for 24 h. After development of a mature tract, tubes can be changed to a low-profile device. Complications of this procedure include granulation tissue formation, local or generalized infection, dislodgment of the tube, misplacement of the tube, pain, pressure necrosis and abdominal distention.[100,101]

POLYPECTOMY

The rationale for colonoscopy for suspected polyps in adults is based on the assumption that cancers arise from pre-existing adenomas or neoplastic polyps. Screening has been suggested for patients as they enter higher-risk age groups, for those with a family or personal history of colonic cancer, and for those who have an underlying disease process that would make them more susceptible to the development of carcinoma. Most polyps in the pediatric population are simple juvenile polyps and have no premalignant potential. Recently, however, a greater frequency of adenomas has been identified in pediatric patients. In addition, an increasing percentage of pediatric patients are recognized to have more than one polyp at the time of colonoscopy.[102] Juvenile polyps or adenomas, when multiple, recurrent or associated with extraintestinal abnormalities in pediatric patients, may occur as part of a polyposis syndrome. With advances in genetic testing, these syndromes have been further characterized and are discussed in more detail elsewhere in the text. Up to one-third of patients with simple juvenile polyps develop an iron deficiency anemia and require polypectomy to prevent ongoing blood loss.

Prior to polypectomy the patient must be cleansed of fecal debris. A poorly prepared colon limits visualization and increases the technical difficulty of the procedure. Excessive fecal debris or the use of certain gavage solutions such as mannitol places the patient at risk for explosion during attempted polypectomy.[103] The patient's risk of bleeding should be assessed by history, and studies such as a complete blood count, coagulation profile and blood typing may be indicated.

Diminutive polyps of 5 mm or less in diameter are typically removed with biopsy forceps. Use of hot biopsy monopolar forceps or routine forceps biopsy followed by coagulation, if necessary, allows for histologic evaluation. If lesions are too numerous for removal, representative samples should be obtained. Cold snare technique should be avoided in pediatric patients.

Large polyps (more than 5 mm in diameter) are usually removed with snare electrocautery. The minimal channel diameter for current polypectomy snares is 2.8 mm; therefore, the minimum endoscope outer diameter for polypectomy is 9.0 mm. The snare is inserted into the endoscope with the wire loop retracted. The endoscope tip should be stabilized prior to advancing the polypectomy snare. The polyp, and therefore the snare, is optimally positioned in the 5–7 o'clock position.[104] Only the amount of snare necessary fully to encompass the polyp should be extended. The polyp is then lassoed and the sheath maneuvered to the stalk (Fig. 81.24). The endoscopist should ensure that the snare encompasses only the polyp head and stalk, and that normal bowel is not within in the snare.

Most polyps in the pediatric population are pedunculated with a moderate to long stalk. The snare should be positioned to perform electrocautery closer to the polyp head than to the bowel wall or base of the polyp stalk. This allows for grasping of the stalk and coagulation if post-polypectomy bleeding occurs. This is in distinction to adenomas in the adult patient, where carcinoma *in situ* may be suspected and the endoscopist is trying to achieve as complete a resection as possible. The head of the polyp should be lifted off the mucosa prior to electrocautery; contact between the polyp head and opposing mucosa should be avoided to prevent a mucosal burn on the opposite colonic wall. The shaft of the snare should be approximated to the polyp head as the endoscopist closes the polypectomy snare, bringing the distal aspect of the snare towards the polyp head. To remove large polyps of 2 cm or more in size, piecemeal resection may be necessary. After the head is reduced in size, it is usually possible to snare the stalk and safely remove the remainder of the polyp.

After the polyp has been snared, a current is passed through the snare, which is slowly closed by the assistant. Rapid closure results in bleeding from vessels in the stalk that have been amputated but not coagulated. Most endoscopists use a combination of coagulation and cutting settings for snare polypectomy. Use of cutting current alone, particularly with vascular juvenile polyps, is likely to result in significant postpolypectomy bleeding. Coagulation current alone without cutting may also be effective due to the cutting properties of the snare. Lower settings are typically used in the right side of the colon compared with the left. As the polyp coagulates, there is a whitish discoloration of the polyp (Fig. 81.25).

Large or broad-based polyps must be removed with care (Fig. 81.26). Transection of the polyp close to the bowel wall risks perforation. The colonic wall is thin, in the range of 1.7–2.2 mm, especially on the right side.[104] Submucosal injection of saline (saline-assisted polypectomy) can be employed to elevate the polyp onto a submucosal saline cushion, allowing for safer resection[104,105] (Fig. 81.27). Sterile normal saline or hypertonic saline with epinephrine is typically injected to raise a sessile polyp prior to cautery, increasing the distance between the base of the polyp and the serosa. If the polyp is large, injection should initially be performed behind the polyp (proximally). This technique may require three to four injections of 1 ml or more per injection. Signs of a good submucosal injection include raising of the polyp and lack of vascular markings within the injection site.[105] If there is no submucosal bleb, the injection needle may have penetrated the serosa, and may require repositioning. Care should be taken to avoid snaring submucosal tissue. In the case of large sessile polyps, the endoscopist must assess the risk of polypectomy and the nature of the information to be gained before deciding whether the polyp should be removed endoscopically or surgically. Often segmental resection or multiple biopsies of sessile or broad-based polyps remove adequate tissue for pathologic differentiation. Occasionally large polyps may need to be reduced in multiple sessions for complete obliteration.

When multiple polyps are encountered, the most proximal should be removed first so that subsequent passage of the endoscope will not precipitate hemorrhage over the base of an already amputated polyp. In the patient with large numbers of polyps, representative polyps should be removed or biopsied for pathologic analysis. In patients with familial

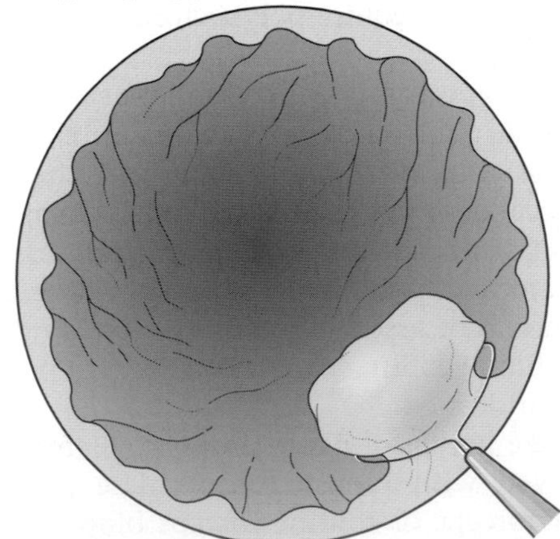

Figure 81.24: Snare polypectomy of a pedunculated polyp. After ensnarement, the loop is advanced to the polyp neck prior to closure, in order to allow sufficient length to resnare a bleeding polyp stalk and avoid thermal injury to the bowel wall.

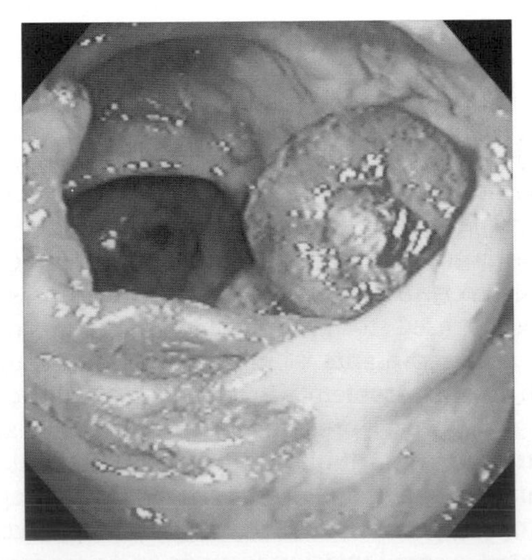

Figure 81.25: Head of a resected and coagulated juvenile polyp. Note the whitish area in the center of the polyp representing the area of coagulation. (See *plate section for color*)

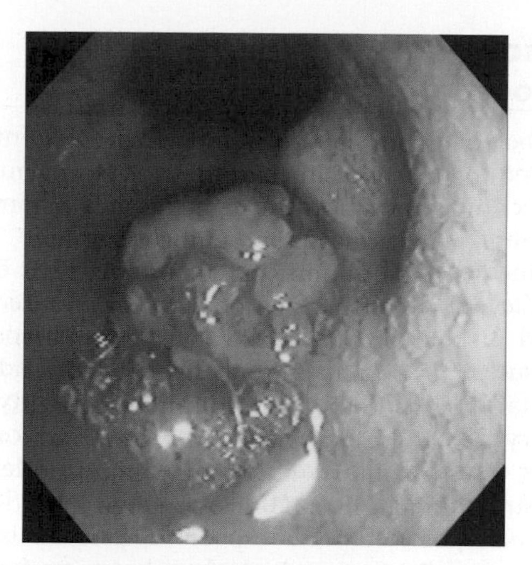

Figure 81.26: Large right-sided sessile polyp in a patient with long-standing Crohn's disease. (*See plate section for color.*)

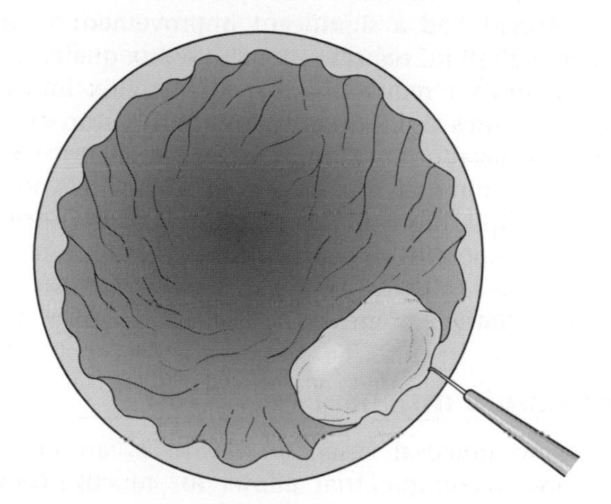

Figure 81.27: Saline-assisted polypectomy of a large sessile polyp. Saline is injection submucosally to elevate the polyp prior to application of electrical current.

adenomatous polyposis, there are too many polyps typically present to biopsy or remove all of them. Larger polyps should be biopsied or removed for histologic analysis. Dysplasia screening in this condition is discussed elsewhere.

After amputation, polyps should be retrieved. Small polyps can be suctioned through the endoscope and the polyp retrieved in a trap. Large polyps can usually be retrieved with the snare, standard or foreign-body forceps such as the Pentapod forceps, or by using the Roth retrieval net.[106] If the endoscopist is unable to retrieve the polyp, the patient can be given an enema or the parents can be asked to strain the stool and submit the tissue for later analysis.

Ancillary equipment should be available prior to starting polypectomy, including needles for injection of saline or epinephrine. In addition to epinephrine injection, detachable polypectomy loops and hemostatic clips are useful for postpolypectomy bleeding. Detachable polypectomy loops should be used with caution due to the possibility of inadvertent transection or inadequate hemostasis.[107] Sterile India ink can be injected for tattooing if the polyp site needs to be marked for future surgical or endoscopic procedures. This tattooing is permanent and should be used for limited indications.[108,109]

Polyps may be encountered elsewhere in the gastrointestinal tract, including the stomach and small bowel. Small bowel polyps are generally amenable to snare removal. Small bowel enteroscopy, either alone or intraoperatively, can be employed for resection of larger small-bowel polyps in patients with Peutz–Jeghers syndrome or other conditions presenting with polyps of the small intestine.[110] Hot biopsy forceps should generally not be used in the stomach or at any location where adequate tenting of the mucosa is not possible. Patient grounding is always required with any form of monopolar coagulation. Gastric polyps may be more amenable to snare removal with or without a submucosal injection technique.

SPECIAL ENDOSCOPIC TECHNIQUES

Pyloric balloon dilation

With advances in endoscopic equipment and accessories such as the development of controlled radial expansion (CRE) through the scope (TTS) balloons have come new applications of older endoscopic techniques. Endoscopic pyloric balloon dilation (PBD) represents a modification of techniques employed for esophageal stricture dilation. Initially reported in 2001 in pediatric patients, this technique has been successfully employed by other centers.[111,112] The primary indication for this procedure is delayed gastric emptying. PBD is performed by passage of a CRE TTS balloon through the endoscopic channel. The balloon is positioned across the pylorus and under direct endoscopic vision is inflated to a controlled pressure for a period of time, usually 60–90 s. Inflation pressures vary based on balloon size. Several inflations are typically employed in a single endoscopic session, often of progressively larger balloons. Patients may need to undergo more than one session depending on their response to therapy.[112] Outer diameters of balloons used are typically in the range of 10–16 mm in adult-sized pediatric patients, but therapy should be individualized for the patient and smaller balloons are employed in younger patients. Depending on the etiology of delayed gastric emptying or the procedure indication, symptom resolution may be seen in 27–68% and symptomatic improvement may be seen in 26–57% of patients.[111,112] Response to PBD can also be used to assess likelihood of response to surgical pyloroplasty.

Endoscopic therapy for achalasia

Pneumatic dilation has long been considered the 'gold standard' for non-operative management of achalasia. Dilators were positioned fluoroscopically and dilation was performed until obliteration of the 'waist' was identified. Patients often required several dilation procedures, resulting in a cumulative radiation exposure for the patient and for physicians performing the procedure. Balloon dilation using Rigiflex dilators (dilators that maintain a similar pressure and diameter along the entire length of the balloon) can be performed under direct endoscopic vision or with fluoroscopic guidance.[88] When performed endoscopically, the dilator is advanced across the lower esophageal sphincter over an endoscopically placed guidewire, which is usually positioned in the antrum. Positioning of the dilator can be monitored by simultaneous endoscopy with the scope positioned adjacent and proximal to the balloon during dilation.[88] This allows for direct visualization of obliteration of the 'waist' and early recognition of mucosal or deeper injury during the dilation procedure. Serial inflations of 60–90 s in duration are usually performed. Dilation is usually initiated with 30-mm outer-diameter balloons and advanced over subsequent sessions to balloons of 40-mm outer diameter, based on patient size and response.[88]

Placement of motility catheters

There have been significant recent advances in the area of gastrointestinal motility. Antroduodenal and colonic motility procedures to evaluate patients with conditions such as chronic intestinal pseudo-obstruction are becoming increasingly common in pediatric centers with a special interest in gastrointestinal motility, and are discussed in Chapters 27 and 42. Unlike rectal motility, in which catheter placement is straightforward, antroduodenal and colonic motility procedures require the monitoring catheter to be placed in the small intestine or cecum respectively. Many centers use endoscopy for initial catheter placement. For antroduodenal motility, a standard EGD is performed. The catheter can be advanced adjacent to the endoscope under direct endoscopic vision or with the aid of forceps across the pylorus and into the small intestine. A loop of suture can also be attached to the end of the catheter. The loop is the grabbed with endoscopic forceps and the catheter can then be guided to its position in the small intestine. Care must be taken not to pull back the catheter when the endoscope is removed. Colonic motility catheters are usually placed after a standard colonoscopy. Once the colonoscope is in the cecum, a guidewire is advanced via the endoscope channel to the cecum. The colonoscope is withdrawn, taking care to advance the guidewire in equal increments with scope withdrawal so that the guidewire stays in the cecum; over-advancement of the guidewire should be avoided because of the risk of perforation. After the endoscope has been removed, the motility catheter is advanced over the guidewire to the cecum. The wire is withdrawn, the catheter secured in place, and monitoring can be initiated once the effects of anesthesia have worn off. Colonic motility catheter placement is facilitated by performing a relatively 'loopless' colonoscopy, allowing for 'one to one' movement of the catheter over the wire. Abdominal radiography is performed prior to the either motility procedure to verify catheter placement.

Endoscopic therapy for gastroesophageal reflux

A number of endoscopic techniques have recently been developed in adults to assist with the management of GER. These techniques are in various stages of development and are currently being evaluated in comparative trials to determine the optimal long-term therapy with a high rate of efficacy and low risk of complications. Techniques reported in adults include full-thickness plication, endoscopic suturing/endoluminal gastroplication (Endocinch), implantation of Plexiglas microspheres (polymethylmethacrylate; PMMA) or a non-resorbable biocompatible polymer (Enteryx) and radiofrequency energy delivery to the gastroesophageal junction (Stretta).[113–118] The only technique reported to date in pediatric patients is endoluminal gastroplication, which has been performed in patients with symptoms of GER dependent on or refractory to proton pump inhibitor therapy. Patients undergoing this treatment had a significant improvement in heartburn, regurgitation, nausea score and reflux quality of life, and a significant reduction in median reflux index and DeMeester scores and a decrease in proton pump inhibitor use.[119] Complications of the procedure in pediatric patients included bleeding necessitating transfusion.[119] A number of other complications of the various anti-GER procedures have been reported in adults and further evaluation is likely required prior to recommendation of these procedures in pediatric patients.

Endoscopic mucosal resection

Endoscopic mucosal resection (EMR) is an emerging endoscopic technique that allows for mucosectomy or mucosal resection without surgery. Resection levels are typically into the middle or deeper layers of the submucosa when performed. Four types of EMR are performed: inject and cut; inject, lift and cut; cap-assisted EMR; and EMR with ligation.[120] Injection is used in a similar fashion to saline-assisted polypectomy (discussed above) to increase the safety of the procedure while allowing for a complete mucosal injection. EMR is often performed using the adjunctive technique of chromoscopy to allow for identification of lesion margins. Indications for this type of procedure are primarily cancer related in adults (esophageal, gastric or colonic carcinoma). Additional potential indications include resection of Barrett's esophagus with high-grade dysplasia, diagnosis and resection of submucosal tumors with low potential for metastases, and resection of small carcinoid tumors found incidentally.[120] Unique pediatric indications for this procedure have not yet been established. Reported complications include pain, bleeding, perforation and stricture formation. Endoscopic clipping may be used at the time of EMR because of the potential perforation risk with this technique.

Several other new techniques have been reported. Okamatsu et al.[121] performed a successful endoscopic membranectomy on a 60-day-old infant with trisomy 21 syndrome and a congenital duodenal membrane. Endoscopic obliteration of a recurrent tracheo-esophageal fistula and obliteration of an esophagobronchial fistula have been reported using Histoacryl or fibrin glue.[122,123]

COMPLICATIONS

Esophagogastroduodenoscopy

As with any procedure, the benefits of the endoscopic procedure and the diagnostic information obtained should outweigh the relative risk to the patient. Endoscopic complications can be classified into four types: sedation related, procedure related, those associated with therapeutic interventions, and those related to the patient's underlying disease or reason for endoscopy. In some cases, the cause of the complication may be multifactorial or remain indeterminate. When reviewing risks of various endoscopic procedures it is important to identify patient- and procedure-related factors that may increase the risk of the procedure (i.e. increased risk of sedation in child with cyanotic congenital heart disease or cystic fibrosis). Limited studies are available that have assessed the risk of complications of endoscopy, especially in pediatric patients. In a large retrospective series of 2711 upper and lower endoscopies in pediatric patients primarily utilizing conscious sedation, minor complications occurred in 0.3 % of patients, including oxygen desaturation that responded to narcotic reversal and medication-related urticaria.[7] In the same series, one patient had a major complication (1 of 1653, rate of 0.06%), which was a guidewire-related perforation. In a 30-day telephone follow-up survey of 393 children undergoing EGD under general anesthesia, 42% reported a complication or adverse event, although only 6% sought medical advice regarding their symptoms.[124] In that series the vast majority of adverse events were minor, such as sore throat or hoarseness, fatigue, cough or headache, and were thought to be related to anesthesia rather than the procedure; no major complications were reported.[124] The American Society for Gastrointestinal Endoscopy (ASGE) reviewed 21 011 gastrointestinal endoscopies to determine the relative rate of drug-related complications.[125] In a group consisting primarily of adult patients, the overall medication complication rate was 13.5 per 1000 procedures; of these, 5.4 per 1000 represented serious cardiac or respiratory complications, with a fatality rate of 0.3 per 1000 procedures. Patients at highest risk for medication-related complications were those who received narcotics, were undergoing an emergent or urgent procedure, or were undergoing colonoscopy. The medication dosage did not correlate with the complication rate.[125] In a recent very large prospective series from Germany, most of the adverse effects associated with diagnostic endoscopy were attributable to medication use.[126] In that series of more than 190 000 endoscopies, the overall complication rates were low for EGD, colonoscopy and polypectomy (0.009%, 0.02% and 0.36% respectively). The overall complication rate for procedures performed by gastroenterologists in that series was 1 per 5155 procedures (0.019%).[126]

A number of mechanical complications have been reported after upper gastrointestinal endoscopy. In the 1974 ASGE survey, the major complication rate was 1.32 per 1000 upper endoscopies, including infection, perforation, bleeding, cardiopulmonary complications and death.[127] In the same series, esophageal dilation was associated with a much higher complication rate, ranging from 4.25 per 1000 cases using mercury bougies, to 6.1 per 1000 using metal olives, and up to 18.1 per 1000 when pneumatic or mechanical dilation was performed. Recent series have reported lower complication rates with wire-guided polyvinyl dilators or balloon dilators.[128] Strictures following caustic ingestion are associated with a higher rate of perforation at the time of dilation compared with other benign strictures. Despite the age of the 1974 series, large series prospectively reporting complication rates of diagnostic endoscopies are infrequent.[128]

Intramural duodenal hematoma resulting in complete bowel obstruction and necessitating blood transfusion has been reported after duodenal biopsies in children. Contributing factors include the fixed third portion of the duodenum, the rich submucosal vascular plexus, lack of a well developed serosal layer in the retroperitoneum and variations of biopsy technique.[129,130] Spontaneous bowel perforation has been reported in patients with Ehlers–Danlos syndrome type 4.[18] These patients may theoretically be at higher risk for perforation during or after gastrointestinal endoscopy.

Serious complications have also been reported after therapeutic injection for bleeding. Full-thickness gastric necrosis has been reported after injection of 12 ml 5% ethanolamine oleate (a sclerosant) into and around a benign actively bleeding ulcer,[131] and following injection of a combination of 4 ml 1% polidocanol and 8 ml 1:10 000 epinephrine solution in a small posterior gastric ulcer.[132] Complications have also been reported after endoscopic laser therapy with a Nd:YAG laser with coaxial carbon dioxide, including free perforation, pneumoperitoneum (thought to occur because of dissection of high-pressure carbon dioxide gas through a laser-induced mucosal erosion and subsequent rupture of the gas-filled bleb) and delayed massive hemorrhage following laser coagulation of angiodysplasia.

There have been two cases of fatal air embolism reported in pediatric patients who had undergone a Kasai procedure for biliary atresia and who were undergoing upper gastrointestinal endoscopy under general anesthesia. The first occurred in a 4-month-old baby undergoing endoscopy to determine the etiology of a diminished stomal bile output. Air apparently was infused into the bed of the porta hepatis, and the authors proposed that, under pressure, this air dissected across diseased liver tissue into a large hepatic vein.[133]

A second similar case was reported in a 10-year-old girl who, also after a Kasai procedure, developed a stricture at the anastomotic site with a stone above it. Under general anesthesia she underwent an endoscopic procedure to remove the stone and dilate the stricture through a percutaneous jejunal loop. The patient developed circulatory collapse and died from a massive air embolus.[134] Because the mechanism of death in these two cases is not entirely clear, extra caution is required in endoscopic procedures involving an exteriorized loop in a patient who has undergone a Kasai procedure. PEG-related complications were discussed above, and complications related to foreign bodies, caustic ingestions and therapy for varices are discussed in other chapters.

Colonoscopy

Sedation complications during colonoscopy are similar to those reported during upper gastrointestinal tract examination. Several series have demonstrated a correlation between the frequency of technical complications during colonoscopy and the experience of the endoscopist. Gastroenterologists treating adults have their highest complication rates during the first 50 to 100 colonoscopic procedures.[135]

Bleeding after colonoscopy is usually minimal but may follow mucosal biopsy or polypectomy. Bleeding following a diagnostic procedure has been reported in 0.008–0.17% of procedures in adults and is likely as rare in children. Bleeding following polypectomy is also uncommon, but may occur in 0.26–2.5% of patients depending on the series.[126,136] Techniques to reduce the risk of postpolypectomy bleeding were discussed above.[126] Perforation is the most serious complication of colonoscopy in children. It is usually related to polypectomy and successfully managed with surgical intervention. The risk of perforation, based primarily on series of adult patients, is increased in patients with severe active colitis, strictures, diverticula, large polyps and adhesions due to prior surgery. The risk ranges from 0.06% to 0.3%.[126,137] Some centers attempt to manage small perforations of the rectum and distal sigmoid colon conservatively.[126,138] Clinically silent diastatic tears have been reported in children, but are thought to be unusual. Advanced endoscopic procedures such as percutaneous cecostomy are likely to be associated with a higher complication rate, and further studies are indicated.

References

1. Gordon ME, Kirsner JB. Rudolf Schindler, pioneer endoscopist. Glimpses of the man and his work. Gastroenterology 1979; 77:354–361.
2. Freeman NV. Clinical evaluation of the fiberoptic bronchoscope (Olympus BF 5B) for pediatric endoscopy. J Pediatr Surg 1973; 8:213–220.
3. Mahajan L, Wyllie R, Steffen R, et al. The effects of a psychological preparation program on anxiety in children and adolescents undergoing gastrointestinal endoscopy. J Pediatr Gastroenterol Nutr 1998; 27:161–165.
4. Position statement. Maintaining competency in endoscopic skills. American Society for Gastrointestinal Endoscopy. Gastrointest Endosc 1995; 42:620–621.
5. Hassall E. Requirements for training to ensure competence of endoscopists performing invasive procedures in children. Training and Education Committee of the North American Society for Pediatric Gastroenterology and Nutrition (NASPGN), the Ad Hoc Pediatric Committee of American Society for Gastrointestinal Endoscopy (ASGE), and the Executive Council of NASPGN. J Pediatr Gastroenterol Nutr 1997; 24:345–347.
6. American Academy of Pediatrics Committee on Drugs. Guidelines for monitoring and management of pediatric patients during and after sedation for diagnostic and therapeutic procedures. Pediatrics 1992; 89:1110–1115.
7. Balsells F, Wyllie R, Steffen R, Kay M. Use of conscious sedation for esophagogastroduodenoscopy in children, adolescents and young adults. A 12 year review. Gastrointest Endosc 1995; 41:375–380.
8. Barlow DE. Flexible endoscope technology: the video image endoscope. In: Sivak MV Jr, ed. Gastroenterologic Endoscopy. Philadelphia, PA: WB Saunders; 2000:29–49.
9. Freeman NV. Clinical evaluation of the fiberoptic bronchoscope (Olympus BF 5B) for pediatric endoscopy. J Pediatr Surg 1973; 8:213–220.
10. Squires RH Jr, Colletti RB. Indications for pediatric gastrointestinal endoscopy: a medical position statement of the North American Society for Pediatric Gastroenterology and Nutrition. J Pediatr Gastroenterol Nutr 1996; 23: 107–110.
11. Wakui M, Okamoto S, Ishida A, et al. Prospective evaluation for upper gastrointestinal tract acute graft-versus-host disease after hematopoietic stem cell transplantation. Bone Marrow Transpl 1999; 23:573–578.
12. Murch SH. Unusual enteropathies. Gastrointest Endosc Clin North Am 2001; 11:741–766.
13. Modifications in endoscopic practice for pediatric patients. Gastrointest Endosc 2000; 52:838–842.
14. Robert ME, Tang L, Hao LM, Reyes-Mugica M. Patterns of inflammation in mucosal biopsies of ulcerative colitis: perceived differences in pediatric populations are limited to children younger than 10 years. Am J Surg Pathol 2004; 28:183–189.
15. Glickman JN, Bousvaros A, Farraye FA, et al. Pediatric patients with untreated ulcerative colitis may present initially with unusual morphologic findings. Am J Surg Pathol 2004; 28:190–197.
16. Molle ZL, Moallem H, Desai N, Anderson V, Rabinowitz SS. Endoscopic features of smooth muscle tumors in children with AIDS. Gastrointest Endosc 2000; 52:91–94.
17. Shidrawi RG, Murugan N, Westaby D, Gyi K, Hodson ME. Emergency colonoscopy for distal intestinal obstruction syndrome in cystic fibrosis patients. Gut 2002; 51:285–286.
18. Stillman AE, Painter R, Hollister DW. Ehlers–Danlos syndrome type IV: diagnosis and therapy of associated bowel perforation. Am J Gastroenterol 1991; 86:360–362.
19. Hirota WK, Petersen K, Baron TH, et al. Guidelines for antibiotic prophylaxis for GI endoscopy. Gastrointest Endosc 2003; 58:475–482.
20. Low DE, Shoenut JP, Kennedy JK, et al. Prospective assessment of risk of bacteremia with colonoscopy and polypectomy. Dig Dis Sci 1987; 32:1239–1243.
21. Neu HC, Fleischer D. Controversies, dilemmas, and dialogues. Recommendations for antibiotic prophylaxis before endoscopy. Am J Gastroenterol 1989; 84:1488–1491.
22. Snyder J, Bratton B. Antimicrobial prophylaxis for gastrointestinal procedures: current practices in North American academic pediatric programs. J Pediatr Gastroenterol Nutr 2002; 35:564–569.
23. Crawford M, Lerman J, Christensen S, Farrow-Gillespie A. Effects of duration of fasting on gastric fluid pH and volume in healthy children. Anesth Analg 1990; 71:400–403.

24. Ingebo KR, Rayhorn NJ, Hecht RM, Shelton MT, Silber GH, Shub MD. Sedation in children: adequacy of two-hour fasting. J Pediatr 1997; 131:155–158.

25. Dahshan A, Lin CH, Peters J, Thomas R, Tolia V. A randomized, prospective study to evaluate the efficacy and acceptance of three bowel preparations for colonoscopy in children. Am J Gastroenterol 1999; 94:3497–3501.

26. Michael KA, DiPiro JT, Bowden TA, Tedesco FJ. Whole-bowel irrigation for mechanical colon cleansing. Clin Pharm 1985; 4:414–424.

27. El S, Kanafani ZA, Mourad FH, et al. A randomized single-blind trial of whole versus split-dose polyethylene glycol-electrolyte solution for colonoscopy preparation. Gastrointest Endosc 2003; 58:36–40.

28. Pashankar DS, Uc A, Bishop WP. Polyethylene glycol 3350 without electrolytes: a new safe, effective, and palatable bowel preparation for colonoscopy in children. J Pediatr 2004; 144:358–362.

29. da Silva MM, Briars GL, Patrick MK, Cleghorn GJ, Shepherd RW. Colonoscopy preparation in children: safety, efficacy, and tolerance of high-versus low-volume cleansing methods. J Pediatr Gastroenterol Nutr 1997; 24:33–37.

30. Shaoul R, Wolff R, Seligmann H, Tal Y, Jaffe M. Symptoms of hyperphosphatemia, hypocalcemia, and hypomagnesemia in an adolescent after the oral administration of sodium phosphate in preparation for a colonoscopy. Gastrointest Endosc 2001; 53:650–652.

31. Nelson DB, Barkun AN, Block KP, et al. Technology status evaluation report. Colonoscopy preparations. May 2001. Gastrointest Endosc 2001; 54:829–832.

32. Hookey LC, Depew WT, Vanner S. The safety profile of oral sodium phosphate for colonic cleansing before colonoscopy in adults. Gastrointest Endosc 2002; 56:895–902.

33. Gilger MA, Spearman RS, Dietrich CL, Spearman G, Wilsey MJ Jr, Zayat MN. Safety and effectiveness of ketamine as a sedative agent for pediatric GI endoscopy. Gastrointest Endosc 2004; 59:659–663.

34. Liacouras CA, Mascarenhas M, Poon C, Wenner WJ. Placebo-controlled trial assessing the use of oral midazolam as a premedication to conscious sedation for pediatric endoscopy. Gastrointest Endosc 1998; 47:455–460.

35. Kaddu R, Bhattacharya D, Metriyakool K, Thomas R, Tolia V. Propofol compared with general anesthesia for pediatric GI endoscopy: is propofol better? Gastrointest Endosc 2002; 55:27–32.

36. Nowicki MJ, Vaughn CA. Sedation and anesthesia in children for endoscopy. Tech Gastrointest Endosc 2002; 4:225–230.

37. Elitsur Y, Blankenship P, Lawrence Z. Propofol sedation for endoscopic procedures in children. Endoscopy 2000; 32:788–791.

38. Bishop PR, Nowicki MJ, May WL, Elkin D, Parker PH. Unsedated upper endoscopy in children. Gastrointest Endosc 2002; 55:624–630.

39. Wyllie R. Esophagogastroduodenoscopy in the pediatric patient. In: Sivak MV Jr, ed. Gastroenterologic Endoscopy. Philadelphia, PA: WB Saunders; 1987:307–320.

40. Tai YT, Yao CT, Yang YJ. Acute pulmonary edema after intravenous propofol sedation for endoscopy in a child. J Pediatr Gastroenterol Nutr 2003; 37:320–322.

41. Gemlo BT, Wong WD, Rothenberger DA, Goldberg SM. Ileal pouch–anal anastomosis. Patterns of failure. Arch Surg 1992; 127:784–786.

42. Peters JM, Tolia V, Simpson P, Aravind MK, Kauffman RE. Flumazenil in children after esophagogastroduodenoscopy. Am J Gastroenterol 1999; 94:1857–1861.

43. Benson CD. Resection and primary anastomosis of the jejunum and ileum in the newborn. Ann Surg 1955; 142:478–485.

44. Reiquam CW, Allen RP, Akers DR. Normal and abnormal small bowel lengths. Am J Dis Child 1965; 109:447–451.

45. Cotton PB, Williams CB. Practical Gastrointestinal Endoscopy. Oxford: Blackwell; 1980.

46. Sigurdsson L, Reyes J, Putnam PE, et al. Endoscopies in pediatric small intestinal transplant recipients: five years experience. Am J Gastroenterol 1998; 93:207–211.

47. Mahajan L, Wyllie R, Oliva L, Balsells F, Steffen R, Kay M. Reproducibility of 24-hour intraesophageal pH monitoring in pediatric patients. Pediatrics 1998; 101:260–263.

48. Gupta SK, Fitzgerald JF, Chong SK, Croffie JM, Collins MH. Vertical lines in distal esophageal mucosa (VLEM): a true endoscopic manifestation of esophagitis in children? Gastrointest Endosc 1997; 45:485–489.

49. Cheung KM, Oliver MR, Cameron DJ, Catto-Smith AG, Chow CW. Esophageal eosinophilia in children with dysphagia. J Pediatr Gastroenterol Nutr 2003; 37:498–503.

50. Teitelbaum JE, Fox VL, Twarog FJ, et al. Eosinophilic esophagitis in children: immunopathological analysis and response to fluticasone propionate. Gastroenterology 2002; 122:1216–1225.

51. Liacouras CA, Markowitz JE. Eosinophilic esophagitis: a subset of eosinophilic gastroenteritis. Curr Gastroenterol Rep 1999; 1:253–258.

52. Miller TL, McQuinn LB, Orav EJ. Endoscopy of the upper gastrointestinal tract as a diagnostic tool for children with human immunodeficiency virus infection. J Pediatr 1997; 130:766–773.

53. Lanza FL, Codispoti JR, Nelson EB. An endoscopic comparison of gastroduodenal injury with over-the-counter doses of ketoprofen and acetaminophen. Am J Gastroenterol 1998; 93:1051–1054.

54. Bahu M, da S, Maguilnick I, Ulbrich-Kulczynski J. Endoscopic nodular gastritis: an endoscopic indicator of high-grade bacterial colonization and severe gastritis in children with *Helicobacter pylori*. J Pediatr Gastroenterol Nutr 2003; 36:217–222.

55. Olds G, McLoughlin R, O'Morian C, Sivak MVJ. Celiac disease for the endoscopist. Gastrointest Endosc 2002; 56:407–415.

56. Ravelli AM, Tobanelli P, Minelli L, Villanacci V, Cestari R. Endoscopic features of celiac disease in children. Gastrointest Endosc 2001; 54:736–742.

57. Aoyagi K, Iida M, Yao T, et al. Characteristic endoscopic features of intestinal lymphangiectasia: correlation with histological findings. Hepatogastroenterology 1997; 44:133–138.

58. Monroe LS. The endoscopic encounter with parasites. Gastrointest Endosc 1984; 30:113–114.

59. Winawer S, Fletcher R, Rex D, et al. Colorectal cancer screening and surveillance: clinical guidelines and rationale – update based on new evidence. Gastroenterology 2003; 124:544–560.

60. Bond JH. Polyp guideline: diagnosis, treatment, and surveillance for patients with colorectal polyps. Practice Parameters Committee of the American College of Gastroenterology. Am J Gastroenterol 2000; 95:3053–3063.

61. Markowitz J, McKinley M, Kahn E, et al. Endoscopic screening for dysplasia and mucosal aneuploidy in adolescents and young adults with childhood onset colitis. Am J Gastroenterol 1997; 92:2001–2006.

62. Bini EJ, Weinshel EH. Endoscopic evaluation of chronic human immunodeficiency virus-related diarrhea: is

colonoscopy superior to flexible sigmoidoscopy? Am J Gastroenterol 1998; 93:56–60.

63. Kay M, Wyllie R, Steffen R. Carcinoma of the colon in pediatric Crohn's disease. J Pediatr Gastroenterol Nutr 1995; 21:341 (Abstract).
64. Salt WB, Llaneza PP. Collagenous colitis: a cause of chronic diarrhea diagnosed only by biopsy of normal appearing colonic mucosa. Gastrointest Endosc 1986; 32:421–423.
65. Sugawa C. Endoscopic diagnosis and treatment of upper gastrointestinal bleeding. Surg Clin North Am 1989; 69:1167–1183.
66. Wyllie R, Kay MH. Therapeutic intervention for nonvariceal gastrointestinal hemorrhage. J Pediatr Gastroenterol Nutr 1996; 22:123–133.
67. Zargar SA, Yattoo GN, Javid G, et al. Fifteen-year follow up of endoscopic injection sclerotherapy in children with extrahepatic portal venous obstruction. J Gastroenterol Hepatol 2004; 19:139–145.
68. Zargar SA, Javid G, Khan BA, et al. Endoscopic ligation compared with sclerotherapy for bleeding esophageal varices in children with extrahepatic portal venous obstruction. Hepatology 2002; 36:666–672.
69. Molleston JP. Variceal bleeding in children. J Pediatr Gastroenterol Nutr 2003; 37:538–545.
70. Fox VL, Carr-Locke DL, Connors PJ, Leichtner AM. Endoscopic ligation of esophageal varices in children. J Pediatr Gastroenterol Nutr 1995; 20:202–208.
71. Goncalves ME, Cardoso SR, Maksoud JG. Prophylactic sclerotherapy in children with esophageal varices: long-term results of a controlled prospective randomized trial. J Pediatr Surg 2000; 35:401–405.
72. Jensen DM. Heat probe for hemostasis of bleeding peptic ulcers: technique and results of randomized controlled trials. Gastrointest Endosc 1990; 36(Suppl):S42–S49.
73. Cipolletta L, Bianco MA, Rotondano G, Piscopo R, Prisco A, Garofano ML. Prospective comparison of argon plasma coagulator and heater probe in the endoscopic treatment of major peptic ulcer bleeding. Gastrointest Endosc 1998; 48:191–195.
74. Nelson DB, Barkun AN, Block KP, et al. Technology status evaluation report. Endoscopic hemostatic devices. Gastrointest Endosc 2001; 54:833–840.
75. Laine L. Therapeutic endoscopy and bleeding ulcers. Bipolar/multipolar electrocoagulation. Gastrointest Endosc 1990; 36(Suppl):S38–S41.
76. Wadas DD, Sanowski RA. Complications of the hot biopsy forceps technique. Gastrointest Endosc 1988; 34:32–37.
77. Quigley EM, Donovan JP, Linder J, Thompson JS, Straub PF, Paustian FF. Delayed, massive hemorrhage following electrocoagulating biopsy ('hot biopsy') of a diminutive colonic polyp. Gastrointest Endosc 1989; 35:559–563.
78. Ginsberg GG, Barkun AN, Bosco JJ, et al. The argon plasma coagulator. Gastrointest Endosc 2002; 55:807–810.
79. Zlatanic J, Waye JD, Kim PS, Baiocco PJ, Gleim GW. Large sessile colonic adenomas: use of argon plasma coagulator to supplement piecemeal snare polypectomy. Gastrointest Endosc 1999; 49:731–735.
80. Canard JM, Vedrenne B. Clinical application of argon plasma coagulation in gastrointestinal endoscopy: has the time come to replace the laser? Endoscopy 2001; 33:353–357.
81. Vargo JJ. Clinical applications of the argon plasma coagulator. Gastrointest Endosc 2004; 59:81–88.
82. Khan K, Schwarzenberg SJ, Sharp H, Weisdorf-Schindele S. Argon plasma coagulation: clinical experience in pediatric patients. Gastrointest Endosc 2003; 57:110–112.
83. Raju GS, Gajula L. Endoclips for GI endoscopy. Gastrointest Endosc 2004; 59:267–279.
84. Tsunada S, Ogata S, Ohyama T, et al. Endoscopic closure of perforations caused by EMR in the stomach by application of metallic clips. Gastrointest Endosc 2003; 57:948–951.
85. Soetikno RM, Friedland S, Lewit V, Woodford S. Lift and ligate: a new technique to treat a bleeding polypectomy stump. Gastrointest Endosc 2000; 52:681–683.
86. Matthewson K, Swain CP, Bland M, Kirkham JS, Bown SG, Northfield TC. Randomized comparison of Nd YAG laser, heater probe, and no endoscopic therapy for bleeding peptic ulcers. Gastroenterology 1990; 98:1239–1244.
87. Dumon JF, Meric B, Sivak MVJ, Fleischer D. A new method of esophageal dilation using Savary–Gilliard bougies. Gastrointest Endosc 1985; 31:379–382.
88. Wyllie R, Kay M. Pediatric therapeutic endoscopy: strictures of the upper gastrointestinal tract and achalasia. Pract Gastroenterol 1997; 21:9–21.
89. Castillo RO, Davies YK, Lin YC, Garcia M, Young H. Management of esophageal strictures in children with recessive dystrophic epidermolysis bullosa. J Pediatr Gastroenterol Nutr 2002; 34:535–541.
90. Kay M, Wyllie R. Endoscopic dilatation of esophageal strictures in recessive dystrophic epidermolysis bullosa: new equipment, new techniques. J Pediatr Gastroenterol Nutr 2002; 34:515–518.
91. Berenson GA, Wyllie R, Caulfield M, Steffen R. Intralesional steroids in the treatment of refractory esophageal strictures. J Pediatr Gastroenterol Nutr 1994; 18:250–252.
92. Straumann A, Rossi L, Simon HU, Heer P, Spichtin HP, Beglinger C. Fragility of the esophageal mucosa: a pathognomonic endoscopic sign of primary eosinophilic esophagitis? Gastrointest Endosc 2003; 57:407–412.
93. Fox VL, Nurko S, Furuta GT. Eosinophilic esophagitis: it's not just kid's stuff. Gastrointest Endosc 2002; 56:260–270.
94. Thomson M. Colonoscopy and enteroscopy. Gastrointest Endosc Clin North Am 2001; 11:603–639.
95. Seidman EG, Sant'Anna AM, Dirks MH. Potential applications of wireless capsule endoscopy in the pediatric age group. Gastrointest Endosc Clin North Am 2004; 14:207–217.
96. Gauderer MW, Ponsky JL, Izant RJJ. Gastrostomy without laparotomy: a percutaneous endoscopic technique. J Pediatr Surg 1980; 15:872–875.
97. Cameron BH, Blair GK, Murphy JJ, Fraser GC. Morbidity in neurologically impaired children after percutaneous endoscopic versus Stamm gastrostomy. Gastrointest Endosc 1995; 42:41–44.
98. Panigrahi H, Shreeve DR, Tan WC, Prudham R, Kaufman R. Role of antibiotic prophylaxis for wound infection in percutaneous endoscopic gastrostomy (PEG): result of a prospective double-blind randomized trial. J Hosp Infect 2002; 50:312–315.
99. Wyllie R. Changing the tube: a pediatrician's guide. Curr Opin Pediatr 2004; 16:542–544.
100. Rivera MT, Kugathasan S, Berger W, Werlin SL. Percutaneous colonoscopic cecostomy for management of chronic constipation in children. Gastrointest Endosc 2001; 53:225–228.
101. Rawat DJ, Haddad M, Geoghegan N, Clarke S, Fell JM. Percutaneous endoscopic colostomy of the left colon: a new technique for management of intractable constipation in children. Gastrointest Endosc 2004; 60:39–43.
102. Gupta SK, Fitzgerald JF, Croffie JM, et al. Experience with juvenile polyps in North American children: the need for pancolonoscopy. Am J Gastroenterol 2001; 96:1695–1697.

103. Bigard MA, Gaucher P, Lassalle C. Fatal colonic explosion during colonoscopic polypectomy. Gastroenterology 1979; 77:1307–1310.
104. Waye JD. Endoscopic mucosal resection of colon polyps. Gastrointest Endosc Clin North Am 2001; 11:537–548.
105. Zuccaro GJ. The difficult colon polyp. Am J Gastroenterol 2004; 99:11–12.
106. Miller K, Waye JD. Polyp retrieval after colonoscopic polypectomy: use of the Roth retrieval net. Gastrointest Endosc 2001; 54:505–507.
107. Matsushita M, Hajiro K, Takakuwa H, et al. Ineffective use of a detachable snare for colonoscopic polypectomy of large polyps. Gastrointest Endosc 1998; 47:496–499.
108. Askin MP, Waye JD, Fiedler L, Harpaz N. Tattoo of colonic neoplasms in 113 patients with a new sterile carbon compound. Gastrointest Endosc 2002; 56:339–342.
109. Ginsberg GG, Barkun AN, Bosco JJ, et al. Endoscopic tattooing. Gastrointest Endosc 2002; 55:811–814.
110. Seenath MM, Scott MJ, Morris AI, Ellis A, Hershman MJ. Combined surgical and endoscopic clearance of small-bowel polyps in Peutz–Jeghers syndrome. J R Soc Med 2003; 96:505–506.
111. Israel DM, Mahdi G, Hassall E. Pyloric balloon dilation for delayed gastric emptying in children. Can J Gastroenterol 2001; 15:723–727.
112. Ogunmola N, Kay M, Wyllie R, Hupertz V. Endoscopic pyloric balloon dilatation in pediatric patients with delayed gastric emptying. J Pediatr Gastroenterol Nutr 2002; 35:447 (Abstract).
113. Chuttani R, Sud R, Sachdev G, et al. A novel endoscopic full-thickness plicator for the treatment of GERD: a pilot study. Gastrointest Endosc 2003; 58:770–776.
114. Filipi CJ, Lehman GA, Rothstein RI, et al. Transoral, flexible endoscopic suturing for treatment of GERD: a multicenter trial. Gastrointest Endosc 2001; 53:416–422.
115. Feretis C, Benakis P, Dimopoulos C, et al. Endoscopic implantation of Plexiglas (PMMA) microspheres for the treatment of GERD. Gastrointest Endosc 2001; 53: 423–426.
116. Triadafilopoulos G, Dibaise JK, Nostrant TT, et al. Radiofrequency energy delivery to the gastroesophageal junction for the treatment of GERD. Gastrointest Endosc 2001; 53:407–415.
117. Johnson DA, Ganz R, Aisenberg J, et al. Endoscopic implantation of enteryx for treatment of GERD: 12-month results of a prospective, multicenter trial. Am J Gastroenterol 2003; 98:1921–1930.
118. Triadafilopoulos G. Stretta: an effective, minimally invasive treatment for gastroesophageal reflux disease. Am J Med 2003; 115(Suppl 3A):192S–200S.
119. Thomson M, Fritscher-Ravens A, Hall S, et al. Endoluminal gastroplication in children with significant gastro-oesophageal reflux disease. Gut 2004; 53:1745–1750.
120. Soetikno RM, Gotoda T, Nakanishi Y, Soehendra N. Endoscopic mucosal resection. Gastrointest Endosc 2003; 57:567–579.
121. Okamatsu T, Arai K, Yatsuzuka M, et al. Endoscopic membranectomy for congenital duodenal stenosis in an infant. J Pediatr Surg 1989; 24:367–368.
122. Al Samarrai AY, Jessen K, Haque K. Endoscopic obliteration of a recurrent tracheoesophageal fistula. J Pediatr Surg 1987; 22:993.
123. Ogunmola N, Wyllie R, McDowell K, Kay M, Mahajan L. Endoscopic closure of esophagobronchial fistula with fibrin glue. J Pediatr Gastroenterol Nutr 2004; 38:539–541.
124. Samer Ammar M, Pfefferkorn MD, Croffie JM, Gupta SK, Corkins MR, Fitzgerald JF. Complications after outpatient upper GI endoscopy in children: 30-day follow-up. Am J Gastroenterol 2003; 98:1508–1511.
125. Arrowsmith JB, Gerstman BB, Fleischer DE, Benjamin SB. Results from the American Society for Gastrointestinal Endoscopy/US Food and Drug Administration collaborative study on complication rates and drug use during gastrointestinal endoscopy. Gastrointest Endosc 1991; 37:421–427.
126. Sieg A, Hachmoeller-Eisenbach U, Eisenbach T. Prospective evaluation of complications in outpatient GI endoscopy: a survey among German gastroenterologists. Gastrointest Endosc 2001; 53:620–627.
127. Mandelstam P, Sugawa C, Silvis SE, Nebel OT, Rogers BH. Complications associated with esophagogastroduodenoscopy and with esophageal dilation. Gastrointest Endosc 1976; 23:16–19.
128. Eisen GM, Baron TH, Dominitz JA, et al. Complications of upper GI endoscopy. Gastrointest Endosc 2002; 55:784–793.
129. Ramakrishna J, Treem WR. Duodenal hematoma as a complication of endoscopic biopsy in pediatric bone marrow transplant recipients. J Pediatr Gastroenterol Nutr 1997; 25:426–429.
130. Guzman C, Bousvaros A, Buonomo C, Nurko S. Intraduodenal hematoma complicating intestinal biopsy: case reports and review of the literature. Am J Gastroenterol 1998; 93:2547–2550.
131. Chester JF, Hurley PR. Gastric necrosis: a complication of endoscopic sclerosis for bleeding peptic ulcer. Endoscopy 1990; 22:287.
132. Loperfido S, Patelli G, La T. Extensive necrosis of gastric mucosa following injection therapy of bleeding peptic ulcer. Endoscopy 1990; 22:285–286.
133. Lowdon JD, Tidmore TLJ. Fatal air embolism after gastro-intestinal endoscopy. Anesthesiology 1988; 69:622–623.
134. Desmond PV, MacMahon RA. Fatal air embolism following endoscopy of a hepatic portoenterostomy. Endoscopy 1990; 22:236.
135. Rankin GB. Indications, contraindications and complications of endoscopy. In: Sivak MV Jr, ed. Gastroenterologic Endoscopy. Philadelphia, PA: WB Saunders; 1987:868–880.
136. Nelson DB, McQuaid KR, Bond JH, Lieberman DA, Weiss DG, Johnston TK. Procedural success and complications of large-scale screening colonoscopy. Gastrointest Endosc 2002; 55:307–314.
137. Korman LY, Overholt BF, Box T, Winker CK. Perforation during colonoscopy in endoscopic ambulatory surgical centers. Gastrointest Endosc 2003; 58:554–557.
138. Orsoni P, Berdah S, Verrier C, et al. Colonic perforation due to colonoscopy: a retrospective study of 48 cases. Endoscopy 1997; 29:160–164.
139. George DE, Dokler M. Percutaneous endoscopic gastrostomy in children. Techn Gastrointest Endosc 2002; 4:201–206.
140. Bines JE, Winter HS. Lower endoscopy. In: Walker WA, Durie PR, Hamilton JR, Walker-Smith JA, Watkins JB, eds. Pediatric Gastrointestinal Disease: Pathophysiology, Diagnosis, Management. Philadelphia, PA: BC Decker; 1991:1257–1271.
141. Anonymous. Sodium phosphate: drug information. Lexi-Comp Online, editor. Online. Available: http://www.uptodate.com.

Index

Page numbers in *italics* represent figures, those in **bold** represent tables

D

E

O

P